GUIDELINES
FOR PERIOPERATIVE PRACTICE
2018 EDITION

Association of periOperative Registered Nurses

Editor-in-Chief
Ramona Conner, MSN, RN, CNOR, FAAN

Contributing Authors
Byron Burlingame, MS, RN, CNOR
Jan Davidson, MSN, RN, CNOR, CASC
Bonnie Denholm, DNP, RN, CNOR
Mary C. Fearon, MSN, RN, CNOR
Sharon Giarrizzo-Wilson, MS, RN-BC, CNOR
Esther M. Johnstone, DNP, RN, CNOR
Terri Link, MPH, BSN, CNOR, CIC
Mary J. Ogg, MSN, RN, CNOR
Lisa Spruce, DNP, RN, CNS-CP, ACNS, ACNP, CNOR, FAAN
Cynthia Spry, MA, MS, RN, CNOR, CBSPDT
Sharon A. Van Wicklin, MSN, RN, CNOR, CRNFA(E), CPSN-R, PLNC, FAAN
Amber Wood, MSN, RN, CNOR, CIC, FAPIC

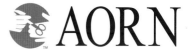

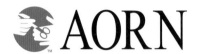

2170 South Parker Road
Suite 400
Denver, CO 80231-5711
(800) 755-2676
(303) 755-6300

Guidelines for Perioperative Practice, 2018 Edition
Copyright © 2018 AORN, Inc

CEO/Executive Director: Linda Groah, MSN, RN, CNOR, NEA-BC, FAAN
Director of Publications & Product Strategy: Richard L. Wohl, MFA, MBA
Senior Managing Editor: Liz Cowperthwaite
Clinical Research Librarian: Kristyn Beaty, MLS, BSN, RN, CNOR
Graphic Designer/Illustrator: Kurt Jones
Senior Creative Services Manager: Colleen Ladny

ISBN 978-0-939583-04-1

Printed

TABLE OF CONTENTS

Guidelines for Perioperative Practice

Aseptic Practice

Equipment and Product Safety

Patient and Worker Safety

Documents appearing in print for the first time in 2018 and new/revised items published electronically in 2017.

Amb *Indicates that an Ambulatory Supplement is available for the preceding topic.*

TABLE OF CONTENTS

* Documents appearing in print for the first time in 2018 and new/revised items published electronically in 2017.

INTRODUCTION TO THE AORN
GUIDELINES FOR PERIOPERATIVE PRACTICE

AORN is committed to promoting excellence in perioperative nursing practice, advancing the profession, and supporting the professional perioperative registered nurse (RN). AORN promotes safe care for patients undergoing operative and other invasive procedures by creating this collection of evidence-based and evidence-rated perioperative guidelines. The descriptive and comprehensive documents in this publication reflect the perioperative RN's scope of professional responsibility. The guidelines are intended to be achievable and represent what is believed to be an optimal level of patient care and workplace safety. Each guideline contains recommendations that are broad statements to be used to guide the development of policies, procedures, and criteria for measuring individual competency in a variety of practice settings. These guidelines represent AORN's official position on questions regarding perioperative practice, and they have been approved by the AORN Guidelines Advisory Board.

Evidence-based practice is essential to improving patient care by promoting decisions based on evidence rather than on the opinion of an individual health care provider. The Institute of Medicine defines clinical practice guidelines as "systematically developed statements to assist practitioner and patient decisions about appropriate health care for specific clinical circumstances."[1(p38)] AORN's guidelines meet this definition. The AORN guidelines are based on a comprehensive, systematic review of research and non-research evidence; the individual references are appraised and scored, and the recommendations are rated according to the strength and quality of the evidence supporting each recommendation.

The guidelines are authored by perioperative practice specialists in the AORN Nursing Department with assistance from members of the AORN Guidelines Advisory Board and in collaboration with liaisons representing the American Association of Nurse Anesthetists, the American College of Surgeons, the American Society of Anesthesiologists, the Association for Professionals in Infection Control and Epidemiology, the International Association of Healthcare Central Service Materiel Management, and the Society for Healthcare Epidemiology of America.

Each guideline is reviewed and updated on a -year cycle. This approach enables AORN to meet the submission criteria for acceptance by the National Guideline Clearinghouse as nationally recognized guidelines for perioperative practice. When adhering to the AORN *Guidelines for Perioperative Practice,* perioperative clinicians can be confident that they are following trustworthy guidelines developed in accordance with the principles set forth by the Institute of Medicine.

Because only a portion of the guidelines are updated for publication in any given year, differences in format, content organization, and design may occur. The titles of previously released recommended practices documents have been changed to "Guideline." However, the name "Recommended Practices" will continue to appear within the text and references of some of the documents until these documents are fully reviewed and revised.

As used within the context of the guidelines, the word "should" indicates that a certain course of action is recommended. "Must" is used only to describe requirements mandated by government regulation. Use of "may" indicates that a course of action is permissible within the limits of the guideline, and "can" indicates possibility and capability.

Evidence Review

Evidence-based guidelines provide a sound foundation that perioperative RNs can use to provide the highest quality patient care possible. Perioperative practices based on science and the professional literature instead of tradition or personal preference are of the utmost importance for protecting patients and health care personnel from harm.

AORN began writing the guidelines using a systematic review of the evidence in 2012. The *Johns Hopkins Nursing Evidence-Based Practice Model and Guidelines*[2] and the *Oncology Nursing Society Putting Evidence Into Practice* (ONS PEP®)[3] schema initially served as the foundation for the evidence review process. After gaining experience in the evidence review process, AORN created the Evidence Appraisal tools and AORN Evidence Rating Model in 2013 to better meet the unique needs of the perioperative practice guidelines. The AORN Model was further refined in 2015 (See Appendix A).

Evidence Rating

Each guideline focuses on a specific question or topic. A clinical research librarian employed by AORN conducts a systematic literature search using the MEDLINE®, CINAHL®, and Scopus® databases and the Cochrane Database of Systematic Reviews to identify meta-analyses, randomized and nonrandomized trials and studies, systematic and nonsystematic reviews, and opinion documents and letters related to the topic. The hierarchy of evidence (Figure 1) is a visual depiction of the types of evidence used in the AORN Guidelines and demonstrates the weakest to the strongest types of evidence.

FIGURE 1. HIERARCHY OF EVIDENCE

AORN Hierarchy of Evidence

RESEARCH

I
SYSTEMATIC REVIEW – All studies RCTs
RANDOMIZED CONTROLLED TRIAL (RCT)

II
SYSTEMATIC REVIEW – All studies Quasi-Experimental or a combination of RCTs and Quasi-Experimental
QUASI-EXPERIMENTAL

III
SYSTEMATIC REVIEW – All studies Non-Experimental or a combination of RCTs, Quasi-Experimental, and Non-Experimental
Any or all studies Qualitative
NON-EXPERIMENTAL
QUALITATIVE

NON-RESEARCH

IV
CLINICAL PRACTICE GUIDELINE
CONSENSUS or POSITION STATEMENT

V
LITERATURE REVIEW
CASE REPORT
EXPERT OPINION
ORGANIZATIONAL EXPERIENCE

As relevant research and other evidence is located, it is independently evaluated and critically appraised according to the strength and quality of the evidence using the AORN Evidence Appraisal Tools (See Appendices B, C, and D). The reviewers participate in conference calls to discuss their individual appraisal scores and to establish consensus. Each article or study is assigned an appraisal score as agreed upon by the reviewers. Each appraisal score includes a Roman numeral (ie, I, II, III, IV, or V) and an alphabetical character (ie, A, B, or C). The Roman numeral represents the level of strength, and the alphabetical character represents the level of quality. The appraisal scores of individual references are noted in brackets after each citation in the references section of the guideline as applicable.

After the evidence is individually appraised, the collective evidence supporting each intervention within a specific recommendation is rated using the AORN Evidence Rating Model. Factors considered when applying the evidence-rating model to the collective body of evidence are the quality of research, the quantity of similar studies on a given topic, and the consistency of results supporting a recommendation. The recommendations in each guideline are given one of the following ratings:

- 1: Strong Evidence
- 1: Regulatory Requirement
- 2: High Evidence
- 3: Moderate Evidence
- 4: Limited Evidence
- 5: Benefits Balanced with Harms

The evidence ratings are noted in brackets after each recommended intervention and activity statement within the guideline (See Appendix E).

Document Structure

Each evidence-rated guideline is composed of eight elements.

1. Introduction: a general introductory statement.
2. Purpose: a description of the intent and scope of the document.

3. Evidence Review: a description of the systematic literature search and review of the evidence and the processes used to evaluate and rate the evidence.

4. Recommendations: broad recommendations for optimal practice. The recommendation statements are in a bold font and identified by a Roman numeral (eg, I). Each recommendation statement is followed by a rationale.

5. Interventions: specific recommendations for treatment or action. Interventions are identified by an alphabetic character after the recommendation Roman numeral (eg, I.a.). The intervention statement is followed by a rationale detailing the evidence that supports the recommendation. The level of each intervention is rated using the AORN Evidence Rating Model. The evidence rating is noted in brackets after the intervention statement (eg, *[1: Strong Evidence]*).

6. Activities: statements that describe the actions necessary to implement the intervention. Activities are noted by a number following the recommendation Roman numeral and the intervention alphabetic character (eg, I.a.1.). The level of each activity may be rated using the AORN Evidence Rating Model. If so, the evidence rating is noted in brackets after the activity statement (eg, *[1: Strong Evidence]*).

7. Glossary: a list of definitions for terms used in the document with which the reader may be unfamiliar.

8. References: a list of all references used within the document and the assigned appraisal scores. The appraisal score is noted in brackets after each citation (eg, [IA], [IVA]).

Ambulatory Supplements

Each document is reviewed and vetted for applicability to ambulatory surgery centers, and supplemental information is provided related to recommendations that may have additional considerations for these perioperative practice settings. The Ambulatory Supplements are intended to be used as additional information for the perioperative RN practicing in a freestanding ambulatory surgery center or a physician office-based surgery center.

The Amb symbol in the text of a guideline indicates that there is additional information in the Ambulatory Supplement following the document. Relevant text from the guideline is repeated in the Supplement for easy reference and to give context to the ambulatory considerations. New text is denoted with the Amb symbol in the Supplement (See Appendix F). Where applicable, the Ambulatory Supplements include text from the Centers for Medicare & Medicaid Services *State Operation Manual Appendix L—Guidance for Surveyors: Ambulatory Surgical Centers*.

The Ambulatory Supplement is an adjunct to the guideline on which it is based and is not intended to be a replacement for that document. Perioperative personnel who are developing and updating organizational policies and procedures should review and cite the full guideline.

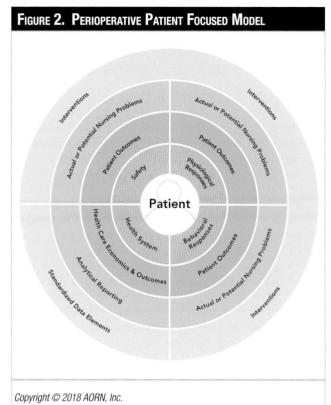

FIGURE 2. PERIOPERATIVE PATIENT FOCUSED MODEL

Copyright © 2018 AORN, Inc.

AORN Guidelines and the PNDS

The Perioperative Nursing Data Set (PNDS) is the standardized nursing language developed and refined by AORN and recognized by the American Nurses Association to describe the nursing care, from preadmission to discharge, of patients undergoing operative or other invasive procedures.[4] The PNDS enables nursing care to be documented in a standardized manner and allows the collection of reliable and valid comparable clinical data to evaluate the effectiveness of nurse-sensitive interventions and the relationship between these interventions and patient outcomes.

The *Guidelines for Perioperative Practice* is the foundation of clinical knowledge from which the PNDS is derived. This standardized language consists of a collection of unique concepts that reflect the nursing process as described in the *Guidelines for Perioperative Practice*. The perioperative patient and his or her family members are at the core of the Perioperative Patient Focused Model (Figure 2), the conceptual framework for the PNDS. The model depicts perioperative nursing in four domains and illustrates the relationship among the patient, his or her family members, and the care provided by the professional perioperative RN. Within the PNDS, the Safety, Physiological Responses, and Behavioral Responses domains contain actual or potential nursing problems, interventions, and patient outcomes representing patient care concerns. The Health System domain focuses on standardized data elements that describe the environment in which care is provided. Each uniquely identified concept in the PNDS is clearly defined, is common to all procedures, relates to the delivery of care, and is appropriate for use in any surgical setting.

The *Guidelines for Perioperative Practice* and the PNDS concepts are mapped to the clinical content within the AORN Syntegrity® perioperative documentation solution for the electronic health record. The AORN Syntegrity solution provides standardized content for electronic perioperative nursing documentation. The PNDS is distributed only through an AORN Syntegrity license. To learn more about the AORN Syntegrity solution and implementation of the PNDS within the electronic health record, contact the AORN Syntegrity team via e-mail at syntegrity@aorn.org or visit http://www.aorn.org/syntegrity.

Implementation in Practice

Individual commitment, professional conscience, and the setting in which perioperative nursing is practiced should guide the RN in implementing these guidelines. Implementation of the guidelines in perioperative settings requires close examination of existing policies and procedures. This review may indicate that new or revised policies and procedures are needed. Although the guidelines are considered to represent the optimal level of practice, variations in practice settings and clinical situations may limit the degree to which each guideline can be implemented. AORN has created a comprehensive set of implementation tools to help health care organizations implement the guidelines. For more information, visit http://www.aorn.org.

New in this Edition

The 2018 edition of this book includes six new evidence-rated guidelines:
- Manual Chemical High-Level Disinfection
- Medical Device and Product Evaluation
- Medication Safety
- Positioning the Patient
- Prevention of Venous Thromboembolism
- Team Communication

Editor's note: ONS PEP is a registered trademark of the Oncology Nursing Society, Pittsburgh, PA. MEDLINE is a registered trademark of the US National Library of Medicine's Medical Literature Analysis and Retrieval System, Bethesda, MD. CINAHL, Cumulative Index to Nursing and Allied Health Literature is a registered trademark of EBSCO Industries, Birmingham, AL. Scopus is a registered trademark of Elsevier B.V., Amsterdam, Netherlands. Syntegrity is a registered trademark of AORN, Inc, Denver, CO.

REFERENCES

1. Institute of Medicine. Field MJ, Lohr KN, eds. *Clinical Practice Guidelines: Directions for a New Program.* Washington, DC: National Academy Press; 1990:38.

2. Newhouse RP, Dearholt SL, Poe SS, Pugh LC, White KM. *Johns Hopkins Nursing Evidence-Based Practice Model and Guidelines.* Indianapolis, IN: Sigma Theta Tau International; 2007.

3. ONS-PEP®—Putting Evidence into Practice. Oncology Nursing Society. https://www.ons.org/practice-resources/pep. Accessed October 5, 2017.

4. Petersen C, ed. *Perioperative Nursing Data Set.* 3rd ed. Denver, CO: AORN, Inc; 2011.

AORN gratefully acknowledges the work of the 2017-2018 Guidelines Advisory Board

Chair
Judith L. Goldberg, DBA, MSN, RN, CNOR, CSSM, CHL, CRCST
Director Perioperative and Procedural Services
Yale New Haven Health
Lawrence + Memorial Hospital
New London, Connecticut
Chair 2007-2009, AORN Board Liaison 2013-2014,
Member 2004-2007, 2009-2010, 2011-2012, 2015-2016,
Chair 2016-2018)

Members
Marie A. Bashaw, DNP, RN, NEA-BC
Assistant Professor
Wright State University
Dayton, Ohio
2016-2018)

Jennifer L. Butterfield, MBA, RN, CNOR, CASC
Administrator/CEO
Surgery Partners – Lakes Surgery Center
West Bloomfield, Michigan
2016-2018)

Jocelyn M. Chalquist, BSN, RN, CNOR
Surgical Services Educator
Aurora Medical Center – Kenosha
Kenosha, Wisconsin
2015-2018)

Gerald McDonnell, PhD, BSc
Senior Director
Johnson & Johnson Family of Companies
Raritan, New Jersey
2017-2018)

Barbara L. Nalley, MSN, CRNP, CNOR
Surgical Assist RNFA Nurse Practitioner
Anne Arundel Medical Group &
Chesapeake Women's Care
Crofton, Maryland
2014-2018)

Donna A. Pritchard, MA, BSN, RN, NE-BC, CNOR
Director of Perioperative Services
Interfaith Medical Center
Brooklyn, New York
2017-2018)

Diana L. Wadlund, MSN, ACNP-BC, FNP-C, CRNFA
Nurse Practitioner
Paoli Hospital
West Chester, Pennsylvania
(2015-2018)

Advisory Board Liaisons
Bernard Camins, MD, MSc
Society for Healthcare Epidemiology of America
(2016-2018)

Leslie Ann Jeter, MSNA, RN, CRNA
American Association of Nurse Anesthetists
(2013-2018)

Sue G. Klacik, BS, CRCST, ACE, CHL, FCS
International Association of Healthcare Central Service
Materiel Management
(2017-2018)

Susan Ruwe, MSN, RN, CPHQ, CIC
Association for Professionals in Infection Control and
Epidemiology
(2017-2018)

David R. Urbach, MD, MSc
American College of Surgeons
(2016-2018)

Mentor
Joanne M. Epstein, BSN, RN, CNOR
Educator/Staff Development/CTOR Coordinator
St Francis Hospital
Wilmington, Delaware
(Member 2014-2017, Mentor 2017-2018)

AORN Board Liaison
Dawn Myers Yost, MSN, RN, CNOR, CSSM
Manager, Training & Development Surgical Services/
Business Manager for Perioperative Services
West Virginia University Hospitals/WVU Medicine
Morgantown, West Virginia
(2016-2018)

AORN and Perioperative Nursing

AORN is a nonprofit membership association that represents the professional interests of more than 160,000 perioperative nurses by providing nursing education, standards, and clinical practice resources to enable optimal outcomes for patients undergoing operative and other invasive procedures. AORN's 41,000 registered nurse members manage, teach, and practice perioperative nursing, are enrolled in nursing education, or are engaged in perioperative research.

AORN Mission, Vision, and Values

Mission
AORN's mission is to promote safety and optimal outcomes for patients undergoing operative and other invasive procedures by providing practice support and professional development opportunities to perioperative nurses. AORN will collaborate with professional and regulatory organizations, industry leaders, and other health care partners who support the mission.

Vision
AORN will be the indispensable resource for evidence-based practice and education that establishes the standards of excellence in the delivery of perioperative nursing care.

Values
AORN's core values reflect what is important to the association:
- Communication—open, honest, respectful
- Innovation—creative, risk taking, leading edge
- Quality—reliable, timely, accountable
- Collaboration—teamwork, inclusion, diversity

ASEPTIC
PRACTICE

GUIDELINE FOR ENVIRONMENTAL CLEANING

The Guideline for Environmental Cleaning was approved by the AORN Recommended Practices Advisory Board. It was presented as proposed recommendations for comments by members and others. The guideline is effective November 15, 2013. The recommendations in the guideline are intended to be achievable and represent what is believed to be an optimal level of practice. Policies and procedures will reflect variations in practice settings and/or clinical situations that determine the degree to which the guideline can be implemented. AORN recognizes the many diverse settings in which perioperative nurses practice; therefore, this guideline is adaptable to all areas where operative and other invasive procedures may be performed.

Purpose

Historically, perioperative registered nurses (RNs) have played a critical role in providing a clean environment for patients undergoing operative or other invasive procedures. In recent years, researchers have developed an increasing awareness of the role of the environment in the development of health care-associated infections and transmission of multidrug-resistant organisms (MDROs).[1-4]

The literature describes a high risk of pathogen transmission in the perioperative setting due to multiple contacts among patients, perioperative team members, and environmental surfaces.[1] Thus, thorough cleaning and disinfection of perioperative areas is essential to preventing the spread of potentially pathogenic microorganisms.[1] Because surfaces that health care providers touch frequently may present a high risk for pathogen transmission to patients,[2] routine cleaning of high-touch objects is an effective approach to limiting transmission of pathogens[5] when implemented as part of a comprehensive environmental cleaning and disinfection program.

Researchers have shown that cleaning practices in the operating room (OR) have not been adequately thorough or consistent with the policies of the health care organization.[1,6,7] Jefferson et al observed a mean cleaning rate of 25% for objects monitored in the OR setting in six acute care hospitals.[7] These findings demonstrate that some ORs may not be as clean as previously thought,[1] although the literature has not defined the concept of cleanliness. All perioperative team members have a responsibility to provide a clean environment for patients. Perioperative and environmental services leaders can cultivate an environment where perioperative and environmental services personnel work collaboratively to accomplish adequately thorough cleanliness in a culture of safety and mutual support.

This document provides guidance for environmental cleaning and disinfection in the perioperative practice setting and are based on the highest quality evidence available. The quality of the research investigating environmental cleaning has not yet achieved a level of rigor to thoroughly define and evaluate best practices for environmental cleaning in health care, including the perioperative setting.[3] According to Carling, published studies have not separated cleaning thoroughness from the cleaning chemicals being evaluated, and there is a need for outcome studies to determine the impact of environmental cleaning on the transmission of disease.[3]

Donskey found that although much of the evidence for environmental disinfection as a control strategy for reducing health care-associated infections is suboptimal, the practice of environmental cleaning is supported by several high-quality investigations.[8] Conscientious application of these recommendations should result in a clean environment for perioperative patients and minimize the exposure risk of health care personnel and patients to potentially infectious microorganisms. Any patient could be infected with bloodborne or other pathogens, so all surgical procedures should be considered potentially infectious. This document provides specific guidance for cleaning procedures; selection of appropriate cleaning chemicals, materials, tools, and equipment; ongoing education and competency verification; policies and procedures; and quality assurance and performance improvement processes.

Although these recommendations include references to cleaning a wide variety of surfaces, the focus of this document is specific to the environmental cleaning of perioperative areas. These recommendations may be applicable to sterile processing areas. Laundering of textiles is outside the scope of these recommendations. Environmental cleaning includes considerations for a safe environment of care, prevention of transmissible infections, and hand hygiene. These topics are addressed in other AORN guidelines, and although they are mentioned briefly where applicable (eg, standard precautions), broader discussions are outside the scope of this document.[9-11]

Evidence Review

A medical librarian conducted systematic searches of the databases MEDLINE, CINAHL, and the Cochrane Database of Systematic Reviews for meta-analyses, systematic reviews, randomized controlled and nonrandomized trials and studies, opinion documents, case reports, letters, reviews, and guidelines. Scopus was also consulted, although not searched systematically.

ENVIRONMENTAL CLEANING

Search terms included *operating room, operating theater, operating suite, surgical suite, recovery room, post-anesthesia, post-anaesthesia, perioperative nursing, ambulatory care facilities, surgicenters, ambulatory surgery, outpatient surgery, healthcare facilities, terminal cleaning, terminal disinfecting, terminal decontamination, cleaning schedule, cleaning program, cleaning regimen, prior patient, prior room occupant, previous patient, cleaning standard, cleaning policies, cleaning guideline, cleaning protocol, routine cleaning, hospital housekeeping, housekeeping department, environmental services, cross infection, infection control, decontamination, room decontamination, disinfection, disinfectants, adenosine triphosphate, detergents, solvents, phenols, disinfectants, hydrogen peroxide, ultraviolet rays, fluorescent light, quaternary ammonium disinfectant, sodium hypochlorite, ozone, silver, copper, gram-negative bacteria, gram-positive bacteria, viruses, Staphylococcus aureus, methicillin resistance, vancomycin, multi-drug resistant organism, clostridium, chickenpox, measles, varicella, rubeola, tuberculosis, prion diseases, prions, Creutzfeldt-Jakob, disease reservoir, dust, surgical wound infection, blood, body fluids, tissues, blood spill, semen, cerebrospinal fluid, synovial fluid, vaginal secretions, pericardial fluid, peritoneal fluid, saliva, amniotic fluid, air microbiology, air pollution, bacterial load, microbial colony count, environmental microbiology, environmental cleaning, green cleaning, mop, mopping, bucket, wringer, brush, buffers, floor machine, sweepers, microfiber, microfibre, paper towel, cloths, wiping, vacuum, environmental surface, contact surface, fomites, floors and floor coverings, interior design and furnishings, mites, lice, fleas, cockroaches, vermin, flies, ants, insects, pest control, textiles, bedding and linens, beds and mattresses, curtains, laundry, laundry service, cellular phone, cellphones, cell phones, telephones, wireless communications, mobile devices, iPad, tablets, laptops, computer systems, computers, keyboards, mouse, tables, beds, operating tables, mattress, stretcher, examination tables, patient transfer board, trolleys, carts, scrub sink, durable medical equipment, disposable equipment, equipment reuse, storage areas, hospitals, eye wash, operating room waste, clinical waste, medical waste, medical waste disposal, biohazardous waste, hazardous materials, formaldehyde, formalin, methyl methacrylate, storage, disposal, transport, handling, safety management, occupational health, occupational-related injuries, occupational exposure, contact precautions, standard precautions, droplet precautions, universal precautions, eye protective devices, masks, respiratory protective devices, protective clothing, gloves, goggles, gowns, environmental monitoring, luminescent measurements, checklists, visual inspection, fluorescent light, audit, tacky mat, sticky mat, hospital design and construction, demolition, construction materials, aspergillus, aspergillosis, central service department, sterile processing, sterile supply, central supply, central processing, task performance and analysis, job performance, competency-based education, continuing education,* and *human factors.*

The search was originally limited to literature published in English between 2008 and 2013. The lead author and the medical librarian identified relevant guidelines from government agencies and standards-setting bodies, and the lead author requested additional articles that either did not fit the original search criteria or were discovered during the evidence appraisal process. The medical librarian also established continuing alerts on the environmental cleaning topics and provided relevant results to the lead author.

Articles identified by the search were provided to the project team for evaluation. The team consisted of the lead author, three members of the Recommended Practices Advisory Board, and two doctorally prepared evidence appraisers. The lead author divided the search results into topics and assigned members of the team to review and critically appraise each article using the Johns Hopkins Evidence-Based Practice Model and the Research or Non-Research Evidence Appraisal Tools as appropriate. The literature was independently evaluated and appraised according to the strength and quality of the evidence. Each article was then assigned an appraisal score. The appraisal score is noted in brackets after each reference, as applicable.

The collective evidence supporting each intervention within a specific recommendation was summarized and used to rate the strength of the evidence using the AORN Evidence Rating Model. Factors considered in review of the collective evidence were the quality of research, quantity of similar studies on a given topic, and consistency of results supporting a recommendation. The evidence rating is noted in brackets after each intervention.

Editor's note: *MEDLINE is a registered trademark of the US National Library of Medicine's Medical Literature Analysis and Retrieval System, Bethesda, MD. CINAHL, Cumulative Index to Nursing and Allied Health Literature, is a registered trademark of EBSCO Industries, Birmingham, AL. Scopus is a registered trademark of Elsevier B.V., Amsterdam, Netherlands.*

Recommendation I

A multidisciplinary team should establish cleaning procedures and frequencies in the perioperative practice setting.

Involvement of a multidisciplinary team (eg, perioperative nursing, sterile processing, environmental services, infection prevention) allows input from personnel who perform environmental cleaning in perioperative areas and from personnel with expertise beyond clinical end-users (eg, infection prevention personnel). As part of a bundled approach to implementing best practices for environmental cleaning, Havill recommended developing cleaning procedures as part of a multidisciplinary team.[12]

Operational guidelines for frequency of cleaning in the perioperative setting were identified as a gap in the literature based on the evidence review.

I.a. A multidisciplinary team should select cleaning chemicals for use in the perioperative setting. *[2: High Evidence]*

A standardized product selection process assists in the selection of functional and reliable products that are safe, cost-effective, and environmentally friendly and promote quality care, as well as decreases duplication or rapid obsolescence.[13]

I.a.1. A multidisciplinary team should evaluate the following factors during selection of a cleaning detergent or disinfectant chemical:
- Environmental Protection Agency (EPA) registration and rating as hospital grade[14,15]; *[1: Strong Evidence]*
- targeted microorganisms[14]; *[1: Strong Evidence]*
- dwell times (ie, contact times)[14]; *[1: Strong Evidence]*
- chemical manufacturers' instructions for use[14,15]; *[1: Strong Evidence]*
- compatibility with surfaces, cleaning materials, and equipment[15]; *[4: Limited Evidence]*
- patient population (eg, neonatal)[14,15]; *[1: Strong Evidence]*
- cost[15]; *[4: Limited Evidence]*
- safety[15-17]; *[3: Moderate Evidence]* and
- effect on the environment.[15] *[4: Limited Evidence]*

I.a.2. High-level disinfectants or liquid chemical sterilants should not be used to clean and disinfect environmental surfaces or noncritical devices.[14] *[1: Strong Evidence]*

These chemicals are not intended for use on environmental surfaces and are not labeled for use as low-level disinfectants.[14]

I.a.3. Alcohol should not be used to disinfect large environmental surfaces.[14] *[1: Strong Evidence]*

Alcohol is not an EPA-registered disinfectant. Alcohol is an antiseptic and not a detergent. Alcohol does not remove soil or debris.

I.a.4. An EPA-registered disinfectant in the concentration indicated in the manufacturer's instructions for nurseries and neonatal patient care areas should be used when the perioperative patient population includes neonates and infants.[14,15] *[1: Strong Evidence]*

Hyperbilirubinemia in newborns has been linked to poor ventilation and cleaning of incubators and other nursery surfaces with inadequately diluted phenolic solutions.[14]

I.b. A multidisciplinary team should select cleaning materials, tools, and equipment for use in the perioperative practice setting.[13,15] *[3: Moderate Evidence]*

A standardized product selection process assists in the selection of functional and reliable products that are safe, cost-effective, and environmentally friendly and promote quality care, as well as decreases duplication or rapid obsolescence.[13,15]

I.b.1. A multidisciplinary team should evaluate the following factors during selection of cleaning materials, tools, and equipment:
- manufacturers' instructions for use on surfaces to be cleaned[15];
- manufacturers' instructions for use for cleaning materials and equipment[15];
- compatibility with detergents and disinfectants[15];
- effect on environmental conditions in the OR (eg, temperature, humidity);
- cost[15];
- personnel ergonomics and safety[15]; and
- effect on the environment.[15]

I.b.2. Reusable or single-use disposable cleaning materials (eg, mop heads, cloths) may be used.[14]

I.b.3. Mops that dispense cleaning solutions may be used.

Using mops that dispense cleaning solutions may decrease the risk of contaminating multi-use containers of cleaning solution and reduce the risk of chemical splashes.

I.b.4. Microfiber or low-linting cotton cleaning materials (eg, mop heads, cloths) may be used.[15,18,19]

In a comparative study, Rutala et al reported that microfiber mopping systems were more effective than cotton string mops at microbial removal, 95% and 68% respectively, and that microbial removal with microfiber was equally effective with and without use of a disinfectant.[18] Diab-Elschahawi et al found in another comparative study that although microfiber cloths were best for decontamination, cotton was most effective after multiple launderings.[19] However, the laundering methods used to process the microfiber cloths in this study were at a higher temperature than that recommended by the Centers for Disease Control and Prevention (CDC), which may have altered their effectiveness.

Additional research is needed to determine the most effective material for cleaning and disinfecting environmental surfaces in perioperative areas.

I.c. A multidisciplinary team should establish cleaning frequencies for high-touch objects and surfaces.[2,14,20,21] *[1: Strong Evidence]*

In a literature review, Dancer found that contamination of environmental surfaces that are touched frequently provides an opportunity for hands to acquire pathogens, which could be transmitted to patients.[2,20] Stiefel et al demonstrated in an observational study that touching environmental surfaces in the inpatient room of a patient colonized with methicillin-resistant *Staphylococcus aureus* (MRSA) was just as likely to contaminate the gloved hands of health care personnel as was touching the patient's skin.[21] The results of this study showed that environmental surfaces may be a reservoir for pathogens that can contaminate the hands of health care personnel.[21]

I.d.   A multidisciplinary team and the infection prevention committee should determine when enhanced environmental cleaning procedures should be implemented to prevent the spread of infections or outbreaks.[22-26] (See Recommendation VII.) *[1: Strong Evidence]*

I.e.   A multidisciplinary team should designate personnel responsible for cleaning perioperative areas and equipment.[15,20] *[3: Moderate Evidence]*

Designating cleaning responsibilities is an important component of defining cleaning procedures. In a literature review, researchers identified the importance of assigning cleaning responsibilities to reduce the number of items that personnel forget to clean.[20]

I.f.   A multidisciplinary team should develop cleaning and disinfection procedures for construction, renovation, repair, demolition, or disaster remediation.[14] (See Recommendation VII.) *[1: Strong Evidence]*

Development of cleaning procedures during construction is a critical component of an infection control risk assessment that should be completed before the start of any construction project.[14]

I.g.   A multidisciplinary team should develop cleaning and disinfection procedures for managing environmental contamination (eg, condensation, air contamination).[14] (See Recommendation VII.) *[1: Strong Evidence]*

Defining cleaning procedures before contamination occurs will guide personnel in selecting appropriate actions to decrease the risk of transmitting pathogens in the event of environmental contamination.[14]

Recommendation II

The patient should be provided with a clean, safe environment.

In a literature review by Ibrahimi et al, the authors stated that the amount of bacteria present in the operative site is one of the most important factors associated with surgical site infection (SSI) development, although the minimum number of bacteria that causes an infection varies depending on the qualities of the organism, the host, and the procedure being performed. The authors also found that fomites near the surgical field may harbor bacteria. These fomites may serve as a reservoir for wound contamination and SSI development through either fomite-to-skin contact with the patient or personnel contact with fomites and subsequent skin-to-skin contact with the patient.[27]

In another literature review, Dancer found that unless a pathogen is removed from fomite surfaces by some cleaning process, the microorganism may persist in the environment for weeks, depending on the qualities of the organism, and may contaminate the hands of perioperative personnel or be deposited on or near a patient if the organism is uplifted by air currents.[20]

II.a.   The perioperative RN should assess the perioperative environment frequently for cleanliness and take action to implement cleaning and disinfection procedures. *[4: Limited Evidence]*

Environmental cleaning and disinfection is a team effort involving perioperative personnel and environmental services personnel. The responsibility for verifying a clean surgical environment before the start of an operative or invasive procedure rests with perioperative nurses.[28]

II.a.1.   The perioperative RN should visually inspect the OR for cleanliness before case carts, supplies, and equipment are brought into the room.

II.b.   All horizontal surfaces in the OR (eg, furniture, surgical lights, booms, equipment) should be damp dusted before the first scheduled surgical or other invasive procedure of the day.[14,20,29] *[1: Strong Evidence]*

Dust is known to contain human skin and hair, fabric fibers, pollens, mold, fungi, insect parts, glove powder, and paper fibers, among other components.[10,14] Airborne particles range from 0.001 micrometers to several hundred micrometers. In settings with dry conditions, gram-positive cocci (eg, coagulase negative *Staphylococcus* species) found in dust may persist; in settings with surfaces that are moist and soiled, the growth of gram-negative bacilli may persist.[14]

II.b.1.   Damp dusting of the OR should be completed before case carts, supplies, and equipment are brought into the room.

II.b.2.   A clean, low-linting cloth moistened with an EPA-registered hospital-grade disinfectant should be used to damp dust.[15]

The purpose of damp dusting is to remove dust, not to perform surface disinfection, which is completed after each procedure and at terminal cleaning. Therefore, achieving disinfectant dwell times for surface disinfection is not necessary when using disinfectants for damp dusting purposes.

II.b.3.   Damp dusting should be performed methodically, from top to bottom.[15]

II.c. Environmental protection agency-registered hospital-grade disinfectants should be used to disinfect surfaces in the perioperative practice setting. *[1: Strong Evidence]*

The CDC recommends that EPA-registered disinfectants be used in health care settings.[14,30]

II.c.1. Environmental surfaces should be cleaned with a detergent prior to disinfection, according to the manufacturer's instructions for use, in either a one-step (ie, combined detergent and disinfectant product) or two-step (ie, two separate detergent and disinfectant products) process.[15]

The presence of visible soil, dirt, and organic material inhibits the process of disinfection by preventing the disinfectant from interacting with the surface.[15]

II.c.2. Safety data sheets must be available and reviewed for each cleaning chemical used in the perioperative setting.[10]

II.c.3. Cleaning chemicals must be prepared, handled, stored, and disposed of according to manufacturers' instructions for use and local, state, and federal regulations.[10,14,30]

Microbial contamination of disinfectants has been reported with improper dilution of the disinfectant.[30]

II.c.4. If the cleaning chemical is removed from the original container, the secondary container should be labeled with the chemical name, concentration, and expiration date.

II.c.5. Disinfectants should be applied and reapplied as needed, per manufacturers' instructions, for the dwell time required to kill the targeted microorganism (eg, *Clostridium difficile*).[30]

II.c.6. Spray and misting methods (eg, a spray bottle) should not be used to apply cleaning chemicals in the perioperative practice setting.[14]

Cleaning chemicals that are sprayed produce more aerosols than solutions that are poured or ready to use.[14] If the cleaning solution is contaminated, the spray mechanism may provide a route for airborne transmission of disease.[14] Aerosols generated may contaminate the surgical wound, sterile supplies, or the sterile field, or may cause respiratory symptoms (acute or chronic) in personnel and patients.

II.d. Floors should be mopped with damp or wet mops. Dry methods of environmental cleaning (ie, dusting, sweeping) should not be used in semi-restricted and restricted areas.[14,31] *[1: Strong Evidence]*

In an observational study, Andersen et al found that wet and moist mopping was most effective in reducing organic soil on floors.[31] Although all methods of mopping in the study increased bacterial counts in the air just after mopping, wet methods of mopping produced fewer aerosols than dry methods.[31]

II.e. Floors in the perioperative practice setting should be considered contaminated at all times.[1,31] *[3: Moderate Evidence]*

Munoz-Price et al found that the OR floor was a potential reservoir for microorganisms due to inadvertent contamination of items during routine patient care.[1] When patient care items (eg, intravenous tubing, safety straps) inadvertently touched the floor, the items were potentially contaminated by the floor and could transmit pathogens to the patient if they were not disinfected before contact with the patient.[1] Andersen et al investigated the reduction of bacterial contamination of the floor using various cleaning methods, and found that even with the best results, the floor was contaminated with more than 25 colony-forming units and the air was contaminated after use of each method.[31] Even in the best scenario, the floor is essentially contaminated as soon as it is cleaned due to air contaminants settling on the floor after mopping and new contaminants being introduced by air currents or traffic.

II.e.1. Items that contact the floor for any amount of time should be considered contaminated. Noncritical items (eg, safety straps, positioning devices) should be disinfected after contact with the floor per manufacturers' instructions before patient use.[14,30]

II.e.2. Reusable cleaning materials should be changed after each use.[14] Disposable cleaning materials should be discarded after each use.

Using a dirty mop or cloth on a clean area or to clean for multiple patients may increase the possibility of cross-contamination.

I.e.3. Used cleaning materials (eg, mop heads, cloths) should not be returned to the cleaning solution container.[14,15]

Used cleaning materials are considered contaminated and returning them to the cleaning solution container contaminates the solution.[15]

II.e.4. Tacky mats should not be used to decrease floor contamination in the OR.[14]

Tacky mats have not been shown to reduce the number of organisms on shoes or equipment wheels, nor do they reduce the risk of SSI.[14]

II.f. A protective barrier covering should be used to protect noncritical equipment surfaces if the surface cannot withstand disinfection or is difficult to clean (eg, computer keyboards, foot pedals).[14] *[1: Strong Evidence]*

Protecting surfaces that cannot withstand disinfection, in accordance with the equipment manufacturer's instructions for cleaning, provides a mechanism to prevent surfaces from becoming a reservoir for microorganisms. Equipment that is difficult to clean may harbor pathogens in crevices that are not amenable to disinfection. Using a barrier covering may prevent contamination of these areas and other areas that are difficult to reach.[14]

II.f.1. Noncritical items in the perioperative setting that cannot be covered and cannot withstand disinfection (eg, monitor screens, telephones, other electronic devices) should be cleaned in accordance with the equipment manufacturers' cleaning recommendations.[14]

Computers and other sensitive electronic devices are likely to become contaminated and may be difficult to clean. Sensitive computer components, such as monitors, may be damaged by cleaning disinfectants.

II.f.2. If a protective barrier covering is used, the cover should be removed or cleaned and disinfected per the manufacturer's instructions after each patient use.

II.g. Equipment should be cleaned and disinfected before being brought into the semi-restricted area. *[5: Benefits Balanced with Harms]*

Equipment may harbor dust and microorganisms that can contaminate the OR environment.

II.h. Mattresses and padded positioning device surfaces (eg, OR beds, arm boards, patient transport carts) should be moisture-resistant and intact.[14] *[1: Strong Evidence]*

Absorbent or nonintact surfaces may become reservoirs for microorganisms and may harbor pathogens.

II.h.1. Damaged or worn coverings should be replaced.[14]

II.h.2. Penetration of the mattress cover by needles and other sharp items should be avoided.[14]

II.i. Cleaning equipment should be disassembled according to manufacturers' instructions for use, cleaned, disinfected with an EPA-registered disinfectant, and dried before storage and reuse.[14] *[1: Strong Evidence]*

Cleaning the equipment prevents the growth of microorganisms during storage and prevents subsequent contamination of the perioperative area.[14]

II.j. Measures should be taken to prevent vermin infestation of the perioperative environment.[14] These measures should include removing food sources or environmental factors that attract pests and keeping windows and doors closed. *[1: Strong Evidence]*

Vermin may cause disease and microorganism transmission by serving as a vector.[14,32-38]

Insects in health care settings have been shown to carry more pathogens than insects in residential settings. Pathogens isolated from insects in health care settings also have been shown to have antibiotic resistance.[14]

II.j.1. If preventive measures fail, a credentialed pest control specialist should be contracted to eliminate the cause of the infestation.

II.j.2. After an infestation is resolved, the area should be terminally cleaned. (See Recommendation V.)

Recommendation III

A clean environment should be reestablished after the patient is transferred from the area.[14,15,39,40]

Reestablishing a clean environment after the patient leaves the area decreases the risk of cross-contamination and disease transmission. Environmental cleaning has been associated with a decreased risk of the patient acquiring MRSA or vancomycin-resistant enterococci (VRE) when the previous room occupant was infected or colonized with one of these MDROs.[23] In an observational study, Morgan et al demonstrated that contamination of health care workers' clothing, gloves, and gowns with MDROs was mainly attributed to contact with contaminated environmental surfaces.[25]

III.a. Reusable noncritical, nonporous surfaces such as mattress covers, pneumatic tourniquet cuffs, blood pressure cuffs, and other patient equipment should be cleaned and disinfected according to manufacturers' instructions after each patient use.[14] *[1: Strong Evidence]*

The CDC recommends low-level disinfection of noncritical patient care items.[14]

III.a.1. Single-use items should be discarded after each patient use.

III.b. Cleaning of high-touch objects after each patient use should include cleaning of any soiled surface of the item and any frequently touched areas of the item (eg, control panel, switches, knobs, work area, handles).[14] *[1: Strong Evidence]*

Contamination of environmental surfaces that are touched frequently provides a risk for hands to acquire pathogens, which could be transmitted to patients.[2,20]

III.c. Operating and procedure rooms must be cleaned after each patient.[14,39,40] (Figure 1) *[1: Regulatory Requirement]*

III.c.1. Environmental cleaning, including trash and contaminated laundry removal, should not begin until the patient has left the area.

III.c.2. Trash and used linen should be removed from the room.[15] (See Recommendation VI.)

FIGURE 1. EXAMPLE OF CLEANING FREQUENCIES: OPERATING AND PROCEDURE ROOMS

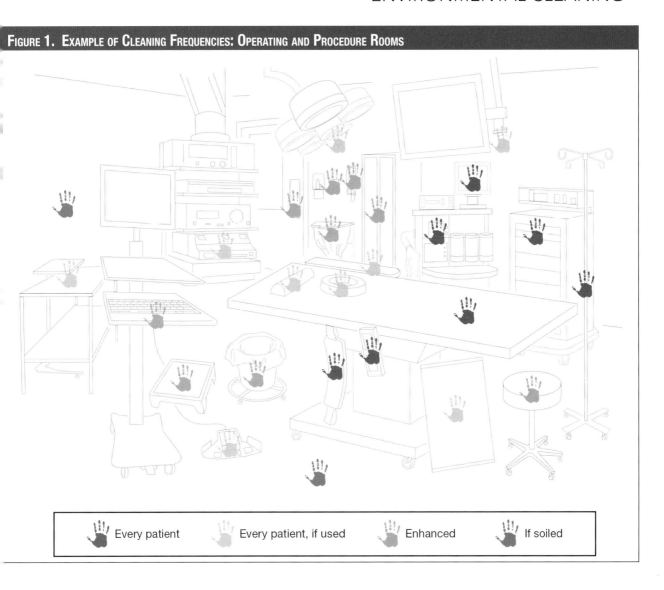

Every patient	Every patient, if used	Enhanced	If soiled

III.c.3. Items that are used during patient care should be cleaned and disinfected after each patient use, including
- anesthesia carts and equipment (eg, IV poles, IV pumps)[1,15];
- anesthesia machines[1,7,41];
- patient monitors[42];
- OR beds[1,14,15]; and
- reusable table straps.[5,15]

III.c.4. Items that are used during a surgical or invasive procedure should be cleaned and disinfected, including
- OR bed attachments (eg, arm boards, stirrups, head rests)[1,15];
- positioning devices (eg, viscoelastic polymer rolls, vacuum pack positioning devices);
- patient transfer devices (eg, roll boards)[43];
- overhead procedure lights[1,5,7,15];
- tables and Mayo stands[1,15]; and
- mobile and fixed equipment (eg, suction regulators, medical gas regulators, imaging viewers, viewing monitors, radiology equipment, electrosurgical units, microscopes, robots, lasers).[7,15]

III.c.5. The floors and walls of operating and procedure rooms should be cleaned and disinfected after each surgical or invasive procedure if soiled or potentially soiled (eg, by splash, splatter, or spray).[1,14,15,18,31]

III.d. Preoperative and postoperative patient care areas must be cleaned after each patient has left the area.[14,15,39,40] (Figure 2) *[1: Regulatory Requirement]*

III.d.1. Items that are used during patient care should be cleaned and disinfected after every patient use, including
- patient monitors,[42]
- patient beds,[2,42,44-48]
- over-bed tables,[2,6,42,45-52]
- television remote controls,[45-48,52] and
- call lights.[2,6,44,49,50]

III.d.2. Mobile and fixed equipment (eg, suction regulators, medical gas regulators, imaging

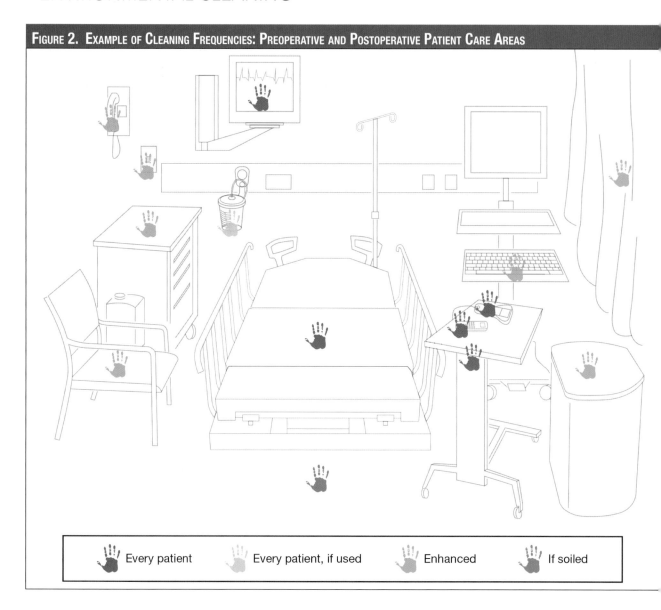

FIGURE 2. EXAMPLE OF CLEANING FREQUENCIES: PREOPERATIVE AND POSTOPERATIVE PATIENT CARE AREAS

Every patient   Every patient, if used   Enhanced   If soiled

viewers, radiology equipment, warming equipment) that is used during patient care should be cleaned and disinfected after each patient use.[7,15]

III.d.3. Preoperative and postoperative patient care area floors and walls should be cleaned after each patient has left the area, if soiled or potentially soiled (eg, by splash, splatter, or spray) during patient care.[1,14,15,18,31,42]

III.e. Patient transport vehicles including the straps, handles, side rails, and attachments should be cleaned and disinfected after each patient use.[14] *[1: Strong Evidence]*

The CDC recommends that noncritical surfaces be cleaned and disinfected after each use.[14,30]

III.e.1. Single-use straps should be discarded after one use according to the manufacturer's instructions.

Recommendation IV

Perioperative areas should be terminally cleaned.

Terminal cleaning and disinfection of the perioperative environment decreases the number of pathogens and the amount of dust and debris.[29] The CDC recommends that floors in the OR be wet vacuumed or mopped after the last procedure of the day or night.[14,29] The Centers for Medicare & Medicaid Services (CMS) states that surveyors should inspect inpatient and outpatient operative rooms and suites at participating hospitals and ambulatory surgery centers to observe that "appropriate terminal cleaning [is] applied," although the procedures and frequencies of appropriate terminal cleaning are not defined.[53,54]

IV.a. Terminal cleaning and disinfection of perioperative areas, including sterile processing areas should be performed daily when the areas are being used.[14,29,55] *[1: Strong Evidence]*

The Association for the Advancement of Medical Instrumentation recommends that floors and horizontal work surfaces in sterile processing areas be cleaned daily.[55] However, neither the CMS nor the CDC provides guidance for the time frame required for terminal cleaning frequencies in perioperative areas. The literature search did not reveal any studies related to the optimal frequency of terminal cleaning.

IV.a.1. For terminal cleaning in semi-restricted and restricted areas (eg, operating or procedure rooms, sterile processing areas, corridors, storage areas), a multidisciplinary team should determine the frequency and extent of cleaning required when areas are not occupied (eg, unused rooms, weekends).

- If the area is closed with no personnel present, the team may determine that terminal cleaning is unnecessary.
- If perioperative team members are present in the area briefly, the team may determine that the area may only need damp dusting on horizontal surfaces.
- If perioperative team members are present in the area for an extended period or are performing patient care activities, the team may determine that thorough terminal cleaning of the area is necessary.

The presence of personnel generates dust from shedding skin squames, which can harbor bacteria.[14,20,56] However, further evidence is needed to determine ideal terminal cleaning frequencies and the extent of cleaning required in perioperative areas.

V.b. All floors in the perioperative and sterile processing areas should be disinfected.[14,15] *[1: Strong Evidence]*

Floor cleaning procedures and frequencies were identified as a gap in the literature during the evidence review, although guidance is provided by the CDC Healthcare Infection Control Practices Advisory Committee and the Association for the Healthcare Environment.[14,15] Additional research is needed in perioperative areas to define the role of the floor in disease transmission and recommendations for cleaning procedures and frequencies.

IV.b.1. Floors may be terminally cleaned with either a wet vacuum or a single-use mop and a disinfectant.[14,15] The floor should be wet with the disinfectant for the dwell time indicated on the manufacturer's instructions for use.[15]

IV.b.2. Cleaning should progress from the cleanest to dirtiest areas of the floor.

IV.b.3. Floor surfaces at the perimeter of the room should be disinfected before floor surfaces in the center of the room.

The center of the room, where the majority of patient care occurs, is most likely to be have higher levels of contamination.

IV.b.4. The entire floor surface should be disinfected, including areas under the OR bed and mobile equipment.

IV.c. Terminal cleaning of operating and procedure rooms should include cleaning and disinfecting of all exposed surfaces, including wheels and casters, of all items, including

- anesthesia carts and equipment (eg, IV poles, IV pumps)[1,15];
- anesthesia machines[1,7,41];
- patient monitors[42];
- OR beds[1,14,15];
- reusable table straps[5,15];
- OR bed attachments (eg, arm boards, stirrups, head rests)[1,15];
- positioning devices (eg, viscoelastic polymer rolls, vacuum pack positioning devices);
- patient transfer devices (eg, roll boards)[43];
- overhead procedure lights[1,5,7,15];
- tables and Mayo stands[1,15];
- mobile and fixed equipment (eg, suction regulators, medical gas regulators, imaging viewers, viewing monitors, radiology equipment, electrosurgical units, microscopes, robots, lasers)[7,15];
- storage cabinets, supply carts, and furniture[7,15];
- light switches[5,7,15];
- door handles and push plates[5,7,15,57];
- telephones and mobile communication devices[5,15,58];
- computer accessories (eg, keyboard, mouse, touch screen)[1,51,59];
- chairs, stools, and step stools[15]; and
- trash and linen receptacles.[7,14,15,29] *[1: Strong Evidence]*

IV.d. Terminal cleaning of preoperative and postoperative patient care areas should include cleaning and disinfecting all exposed surfaces, including wheels and casters, of all items, including

- patient monitors[42];
- patient beds[2,42,44-48];
- over-bed table[2,6,42,45-52];
- television remote controls[45-48,52];
- call lights[2,6,44,49,50];
- mobile and fixed equipment (eg, suction regulators, medical gas regulators, imaging viewers, radiology equipment, warming equipment)[7,15];
- storage cabinets, supply carts, and furniture[7,15];
- light switches[5,7,15];
- door handles and push plates[5,7,15,57];
- telephones and mobile communication devices[5,15,58];
- computer accessories (eg, keyboard, mouse, touch screen)[1,51,59];
- chairs and stools[15]; and
- trash and linen receptacles.[14,15,60,61] *[1: Strong Evidence]*

IV.e. Sterile processing areas should be terminally cleaned.[55] *[4: Limited Evidence]*

Sterile processing personnel conduct critical processes, such as decontaminating, assembling, and sterilizing surgical instrumentation, in support of operating and invasive procedure rooms. As such, the recommendations for terminal cleaning apply in sterile processing areas as in areas where surgical and other invasive procedures are performed. Furthermore, sterile processing areas where decontamination occurs have some of the highest risks for environmental contamination of all perioperative areas. Environmental cleaning in sterile processing areas is critical for reducing the risk of disease transmission from reservoirs of bloodborne pathogens and microorganisms in the decontamination environment.

IV.e.1. During cleaning of sterile processing areas, the clean work areas, such as the packaging area and sterile storage area, should be cleaned before the dirty work areas, such as the decontamination area, to reduce the possibility of contaminating the clean areas.[55]

IV.e.2. All horizontal surfaces (eg, sterilizers, countertops, furniture, shelving) should be damp dusted daily with an EPA-registered disinfectant and a clean, low-linting cloth.[55]

IV.e.3. All work surfaces and high-touch objects should be cleaned with an EPA-registered disinfectant and a clean, low-linting cloth.[55]

IV.e.4. Trash should be removed from receptacles in sterile processing areas when they are full, but at least daily.[55]

IV.e.5. Terminal cleaning should not commence when personnel are actively decontaminating instruments.

IV.f. A multidisciplinary team may choose to evaluate emerging technologies for room decontamination (eg, ozone, peroxide vapor,[62-67] ultraviolet light,[42,48,68-70] saturated steam[71]) as adjuncts to terminal cleaning procedures.[20] (See Recommendation I.) *[3: Moderate Evidence]*

Barbut et al demonstrated in a randomized controlled trial that a hydrogen peroxide mist system was significantly more effective than 0.5% sodium hypochlorite solution at eradicating *C difficile* spores in patient rooms at two French hospitals.[62] Bartels et al used a dry-mist hydrogen peroxide and silver ion vapor to decrease environmental contamination in intensive care unit (ICU) settings as an adjunct to terminal cleaning procedures, but did not find sustained lowering of contamination in ICUs with a MRSA epidemic.[63] Boyce et al found that a hydrogen peroxide vapor effectively eradicated *C difficile* spores from contaminated surfaces in patient rooms.[64] Chan et al used hydrogen per-

oxide vapor to effectively decontaminate ward rooms in an Australian hospital.[65] Manian et al reported that hydrogen peroxide vapor, in addition to a round of cleaning and disinfection, effectively reduced the number of persistently contaminated room sites in hospital rooms contaminated with MRSA.[66] Passaretti et al found a reduction of patient acquisition of MDROs when a hydrogen peroxide vapor system was used as part of room cleaning procedures.[67]

In a prospective cohort study by Anderson et al, the researchers found a significant decrease in environmental contamination of VRE, *C difficile*, and *Acinetobacter* spp in patient rooms after exposure to an automated ultraviolet (UV)-C emitter.[68] Boyce et al found that use of a mobile UV-C light in conjunction with routine terminal cleaning procedures significantly reduced colony counts and *C difficile* spores on five high-touch surfaces in patient rooms.[4] Nerandzic et al reported that a novel automated UV-C emitting device significantly reduced hospital surface contamination of *C difficile*, MRSA, and VRE.[69] Rutala et al determined that a UV-C emitting device effectively eliminated vegetative bacteria from contaminated surfaces within approximately 15 minutes and eliminated *C difficile* spores within 50 minutes.[4] Umezawa et al reported that a portable pulsed UV device was practical for daily disinfection of housekeeping surfaces and decreased the labor burden.[70]

Sexton et al showed that a portable steam vapor system effectively reduced microbial contamination of high-touch objects in patient rooms.[71]

Use of emerging technologies may enhance environmental cleanliness, although additional clinical studies are needed to determine their applicability in the perioperative setting.[72]

Recommendation V

All areas and equipment that are not terminally cleaned should be cleaned according to an established schedule.

A clean environment will reduce the number of microorganisms present.

V.a. A multidisciplinary team should establish a cleaning schedule for perioperative areas and equipment that should be cleaned on a regular (eg, weekly, monthly) basis.[14,15] (See Recommendation I.) *[1: Strong Evidence]*

Areas and equipment that are not cleaned according to a schedule may be missed during routine cleaning procedures and become environmental reservoirs for dust, debris, and microorganisms.

V.a.1. Areas and items that should be cleaned on a schedule include
- clean and soiled storage areas;
- sterile storage areas;

- shelving and storage bins;
- corridors, including stairwells and elevators;
- walls and ceilings;
- privacy curtains;
- pneumatic tubes and carriers;
- sterilizers and loading carts;
- sterilizer service access rooms;
- unrestricted areas (eg, lounges, waiting rooms, offices); and
- environmental services closets.

V.b. Ventilation ducts, including air vents and grilles, should be cleaned and have their filters changed on a routine basis according to manufacturers' instructions for use.[14] *[1: Strong Evidence]*

Clean ventilation ducts and filters support optimal performance of the ventilation system.

V.c. Linen chutes in the perioperative environment should be cleaned and disinfected on a routine basis.[14] *[1: Strong Evidence]*

Linen chutes become contaminated by dirt and debris with use.

V.d. All refrigerators and ice machines in perioperative patient care areas should be cleaned and disinfected on a routine basis according to manufacturers' instructions for use.[14] *[1: Strong Evidence]*

Refrigerators and ice machines become contaminated with use.

V.e. Sinks and wash basins, including eye wash stations, should be cleaned and disinfected on a routine basis.[14] *[1: Strong Evidence]*

V.e.1. Aerators on faucets should be cleaned and disinfected.

Recommendation VI

All personnel should take precautionary measures to limit transmission of microorganisms when performing environmental cleaning and handling waste materials.

The Occupational Safety and Health Administration (OSHA) regulates the implementation of the bloodborne pathogens standard to protect health care workers from exposure to bloodborne pathogens.[73] Because of the increased risk for exposure to bloodborne pathogens during cleaning procedures in the perioperative practice setting, personnel must comply with the bloodborne pathogens standard to protect themselves, their colleagues, and patients from exposure to blood, body fluids, and other potentially infectious materials.

VI.a. Health care personnel who are cleaning must follow standard precautions to prevent contact with blood, body fluids, or other potentially infectious materials.[11,73] *[1: Regulatory Requirement]*

All body fluids except sweat (eg, semen, vaginal secretions, cerebrospinal fluid, synovial fluid, pleural fluid, pericardial fluid, peritoneal fluid, amniotic fluid, saliva) are potentially infectious.[73]

VI.a.1. Health care personnel handling contaminated items or cleaning contaminated surfaces must wear personal protective equipment (PPE) to reduce the risk of exposure to blood, body fluids, and other potentially infectious materials.[14,73]

VI.a.2. Personnel must wear gloves when it is reasonably anticipated that they may have contact with blood, body fluids, or other potentially infectious materials while handling or touching contaminated items or surfaces.[73]

VI.a.3. Personnel must wear masks, eye protection, and face shields whenever contact with splashes, spray, splatter, or droplets of blood, body fluids, or other potentially infectious materials is anticipated.[73]

VI.a.4. If cleaning procedures are expected to generate infectious aerosols, personnel should wear proper respiratory protection (ie, an N95 respirator, a powered air-purifying respirator).[14]

VI.a.5. Hand hygiene should be performed when PPE is removed and as soon as possible after hands are soiled.[9]

VI.b. Cleaning and disinfection activities should be performed in a methodical pattern that limits the transmission of microorganisms.[15,74] *[4: Limited Evidence]*

Cleaning an area in a methodical pattern establishes a routine for cleaning so that items are not missed during the cleaning process.[15] The method for cleaning may limit the transmission of microorganisms to reduce the risk of cross contamination of environmental surfaces.[74]

In an observational study, Bergen et al evaluated the spread of bacteria on surfaces when cleaning with microfiber cloths in a 16-side method and found that although bacterial counts (*Enterococcus faecalis, Bacillus cereus*) were decreased after cleaning, the bacteria from contaminated surfaces were spread to clean surfaces.[74] Additional research is needed to determine optimal cleaning methods for the perioperative setting and to evaluate the risk for microbial transmission across environmental surfaces during cleaning and disinfection activities.

VI.b.1. Cleaning should progress from clean to dirty areas.[15,74]

VI.b.2. Cleaning should progress from top to bottom areas.[15]

During cleaning of top areas, dust, debris, and contaminated cleaning solutions may contaminate bottom areas. If bottom areas are cleaned first, these areas could

ENVIRONMENTAL CLEANING

potentially be recontaminated with debris from the top areas.[15]

VI.b.3. Clockwise or counter-clockwise cleaning may be performed when used in conjunction with clean-to-dirty and top-to-bottom methods.[15]

VI.c. When visible soiling by blood, body fluids, or other potentially infectious materials appears on surfaces or equipment, the area must be cleaned and disinfected as soon as possible.[14,73] The responsibility for verifying disinfection of a contaminated surface rests with the perioperative team member who is aware of the contamination. *[1: Regulatory Requirement]*

Soil on environmental surfaces increases the risk of cross-contamination and is more difficult to remove the longer it remains on the surface.

VI.c.1. If perioperative team members are performing critical patient care activities when the contamination occurs, the contaminated surface should be cleaned as soon as a perioperative team member is available.

VI.c.2. Spills that contain blood, body fluids, or other potentially infectious materials must be removed with an absorbent material as soon as possible, and then the area must be cleaned and disinfected.[14,73] *[1: Regulatory Requirement]*

VI.c.3. If the spill involves a large amount of blood, a 1:10 dilution of sodium hypochlorite solution (5,000 ppm to 6,150 ppm available chlorine), preferably an EPA-registered product, should be applied to the spill before cleaning when feasible.[14]

VI.d. Items that are contaminated with blood or tissue and that would release blood, body fluids, or other potentially infectious materials in a liquid or semi-liquid state if compressed, and items that are caked with dried blood, body fluids, or other potentially infectious materials must be placed in closable, leak-proof containers or bags that are color coded, labeled, or tagged for easy identification as biohazardous waste.[73] *[1: Regulatory Requirement]*

Leak-proof containers prevent exposure of personnel to blood, body fluids, and other potentially infectious materials and prevent contamination of the environment. Color coding and/or labeling alert personnel and others to the presence of items potentially contaminated with infectious microorganisms, prevent exposure of personnel to infectious waste, and prevent contamination of the environment.[73]

VI.d.1. Single-use items that do not release blood, body fluids, or other potentially infectious materials in a liquid or semi-liquid state if compressed and that are not caked with dried blood, body fluids, or other potentially infectious materials are considered

noninfectious and should be placed in a separate receptacle designated for noninfectious waste.[73]

VI.d.2. Waste generated during care of patients on isolation precautions should be managed with the same methods as waste in other patient care areas.[14,75]

VI.e. Contaminated sharps (eg, needles, blades, sharp disposable instruments) must be discarded immediately in a closeable, puncture-resistant container that is leakproof on its sides and bottom and is labeled or color coded.[14,73] *[1: Regulatory Requirement]*

VI.e.1. Sharps containers should be replaced routinely and not overfilled.[73]

VI.e.2. Broken glassware must not be handled with unprotected hands.[73]

VI.f. Contaminated liquid waste must be disposed of according to state and federal regulations (eg, by adding a solidifying powder to the liquid, using a medical liquid waste disposal system, pouring the liquid down a sanitary sewer).[14] *[1: Regulatory Requirement]*

VI.g. Laundry contaminated with blood, body fluids or other potentially infectious materials must be handled as little as possible.[14,73] *[1: Regulatory Requirement]*

Handling contaminated laundry with a minimum of agitation avoids contamination of air, surfaces, and personnel.[14]

VI.g.1. Contaminated laundry must be placed in labeled or color coded containers or bags at the location where it was used.[14,73]

VI.g.2. Contaminated laundry that is wet and may soak or leak through the container or bag must be placed and transported in containers or bags that prevent soak-through or leakage of fluids to the exterior.[14,73]

VI.h. Regulated waste must be stored in a ventilated area that is inaccessible to pests until transported for treatment and disposal according to state and federal regulations.[14] *[1: Regulatory Requirement]*

VI.i. Containers or bags containing regulated medical waste must be transported in closed, impervious containers, according to state and federal regulations.[14] *[1: Regulatory Requirement]*

Recommendation VII

Procedures for environmental cleaning and disinfection should be established for circumstances that may require special cleaning procedures (ie, multidrug-resistant organisms, C difficile, prion diseases, construction, environmental contamination).

Some situations require a deviation from routine cleaning procedures. Having cleaning procedures in place

ASEPTIC PRACTICE

18

or special cleaning situations guides personnel in cleaning the perioperative environment in an efficient and consistent manner in accordance with the health care organization's policies and procedures.

VII.a. Enhanced environmental cleaning procedures, which are intended to decrease environmental contaminates on high-touch surfaces, should be implemented for cleaning following the care of patients who are infected or colonized with MDROs, including

- MRSA,
- VRE,
- Vancomycin-intermediate *Enterococcus* spp,
- Vancomycin-resistant *Staphylococcus aureus*,
- Vancomycin-intermediate *Staphylococcus aureus*,
- Carbapenem-resistant enterobacteriacae,
- Multidrug-resistant *Acinetobacter* spp,
- Extended spectrum beta-lactamase-producing organisms, and
- *Klebsiella pneumoniae* carbapenemase-producing organisms.[22-26,75] (See Recommendation I.) [1: Strong Evidence]

Decreasing environmental contaminates on high-touch surfaces may decrease the risk of MDRO transmission. In a randomized controlled trial, Hess et al evaluated enhanced cleaning procedures in the ICU setting and found that intense cleaning of patient rooms contaminated with identified MRSA or multi-drug-resistant *Acinetobacter baumanii* did not significantly decrease contamination of health care workers' gowns and gloves.[26] However, an observational study by Morgan et al found that environmental contamination was the main determinant of transmission of MDROs to health care workers' clothing, gloves, and gowns.[25]

In a quasi-experimental study, Datta et al found that enhanced cleaning may reduce MRSA and VRE contamination and decrease the risk of transmission from the room's previous occupant.[23]

VII.a.1. All high-touch objects, in addition to objects cleaned as part of routine cleaning, should be cleaned and disinfected as part of enhanced environmental cleaning procedures after the patient leaves the room or area (ie, bay), including

- storage cabinets, supply carts, and furniture[7,15];
- light switches[5,7,15];
- door handles and push plates[5,7,15,57];
- telephones and mobile communication devices[5,15,58];
- computer accessories (eg, keyboard, mouse, touch screen)[1,51,59];
- chairs, stools, and step stools[15];
- trash and linen receptacles[15]; and

- privacy curtains in the perioperative patient care areas.[60,61]

VII.a.2. In addition to standard precautions, perioperative personnel should wear gowns and gloves when performing enhanced environmental cleaning procedures.[11,14]

VII.b. An EPA-registered disinfectant that is effective against *C difficile* spores should be used during cleaning following the care of patients diagnosed with or suspected of infection with *C difficile*.[11,14,30] [1: Strong Evidence]

C difficile presents unique challenges for environmental cleaning. In its spore form, *C difficile* can survive for prolonged periods of time, up to five months, on environmental surfaces. *C difficile* spores also are resistant to several cleaning chemicals (eg, alcohols, phenols, quaternary ammonium compounds).[51] Selection of a cleaning chemical that is effective against *C difficile* spores and removal of the spores from environmental surfaces are crucial when disinfecting a surface contaminated with *C difficile*. Thorough cleaning of environmental surfaces using a chemical that effectively kills *C difficile* spores remains a foundational requirement for preventing the transmission of *C difficile* infection and colonization.[2,51,62,64,76-79]

VII.c. Room access should be restricted following the care of patients diagnosed with or suspected of infection with an airborne transmissible disease (eg, tuberculosis) and following aerosolization activities (eg, intubation, extubation, cough-generating activities) of a droplet transmissible disease (eg, influenza) until adequate time has passed for air exchanges per hour to clean 99% of airborne particles from the air (eg, 15 air exchanges per hour for 28 minutes to remove 99.9% of airborne contaminants).[11,14,80] [1: Strong Evidence]

Patients and personnel entering a room that has transmissible disease particles in the air are at risk for contracting the disease.[11]

VII.c.1. Personnel entering the room before a complete air exchange occurs must wear respiratory protection (eg, an N95 respirator).[11]

VII.c.2. After the air has exchanged by 99%, personnel may proceed with environmental cleaning without respiratory protection.

VII.d. Special cleaning procedures should be used if environmental contamination with high-risk tissue (ie, brain, spinal cord, eye tissue) from a patient who is diagnosed with or suspected of having Creutzfeldt-Jakob disease (CJD) occurs. If the environment is not contaminated with high-risk tissue, routine cleaning procedures should be used.[14,30,81] [1: Strong Evidence]

Currently, no EPA-registered disinfectants claim to inactivate prions on environmental surfaces.[81] When the environment is contaminated with tissue that is high risk for containing prions, the causative infectious agent in CJD, extraordinary cleaning procedures are necessary in accordance with recommendations from the CDC and the Society for Healthcare Epidemiology of America.[14,30,81]

VII.d.1. Before the operative or invasive procedure begins, personnel should cover work surfaces with a disposable, impervious material that can be removed and decontaminated after the procedure if contaminated with high risk tissue.[14,81]

Covering environmental surfaces minimizes contamination of the environment.

VII.d.2. If not contaminated with high-risk tissue, linens may be laundered in accordance with routine laundering processes when the patient is suspected of having CJD.[81]

VII.d.3. Noncritical environmental surfaces contaminated with high-risk tissues should be cleaned with a detergent and then decontaminated with a solution of either sodium hypochlorite (1:5 to 1:10 dilution with 10,000 ppm to 20,000 ppm available chlorine) or sodium hydroxide (1N NaOH), depending on surface compatibility.[14,81]

No transmissions of prion diseases from environmental surfaces have been reported; however, it remains prudent to eliminate highly infectious material from OR surfaces that will be contacted during subsequent surgeries.[14,30,81]

VII.d.4. Cleaning and disinfection of surfaces contaminated with high-risk tissues should be performed in the following order:
1. Remove the gross tissue from the surface.
2. Clean the area with a detergent solution.[81]
3. Apply the disinfectant solution for a contact time of 30 minutes to one hour.[14]
4. Use an absorbent material to soak up the solution.
5. Discard the cleaning material in an appropriate waste container.
6. Rinse the treated surface thoroughly with water.

VII.d.5. Standard cleaning procedures should be used to disinfect surfaces that are not contaminated with high-risk tissue.[81]

VII.d.6. Regulated medical waste generated during patient care, including waste contaminated by high-risk tissue that is decontaminated, should be managed in accordance with standard waste management procedures per local, state, and federal regulations.[14]

No epidemiological evidence has linked CJD transmission to waste disposal practices.[14]

VII.e. Cleaning and disinfection procedures should be implemented for construction, renovation, repair,

demolition, and disaster remediation.[14] *[1: Strong Evidence]*

According to the CDC, cleaning and disinfection measures during internal and external construction projects reduce contamination of environmental air and surfaces with dust and potential pathogens, such as *Aspergillus* and *Bacillus*, and are key elements of an infection prevention program.[14] Several reports have linked environmental air and surface contamination from construction projects to outbreaks of infection in the health care setting.[82-85]

VII.e.1. Cleaning and disinfection of environmental surfaces should be performed to remove dust and debris caused by construction, renovation, remediation, repair, or demolition.[14,85] If dust is contaminating areas outside of the construction barriers, the barrier should be assessed to determine their effectiveness and reestablished.

While investigating an outbreak of deep bacterial eye infections, Gibb et al reported that fine dust from a construction project was found on horizontal surfaces in the OR. After the ORs were cleaned of dust and reopened, no additional eye infections were reported during the surveillance period.[85]

VII.e.2. Terminal cleaning should be performed before equipment and supplies are placed in the area where the construction, renovation, repair, demolition, or disaster remediation has been completed.[14] (See Recommendation IV.)

VII.e.3. A cleaning and disinfection process should be implemented when environmental contamination occurs.[14]

VII.e.4. If flooding or a water-related emergency occurs, including sewage intrusion, terminal cleaning of the affected areas should be performed after the water is removed; the area is inspected for water damage according to local, state, and federal regulations; and remediation for identified water damage is completed.[14] (See Recommendation IV.)
- When hard surfaces remain in good repair, these areas should be allowed to dry for 72 hours prior to cleaning.[14]
- If items cannot be thoroughly cleaned and dried within 72 hours, the surface should be replaced with new material after the facility engineer determines that the underlying structure is dry.[14]

VII.e.5. When condensation is observed on surfaces in the semi-restricted and restricted areas, terminal cleaning of the affected area should be performed. (See Recommendation IV.) *[5: Benefits Balanced with Harms]*

VII.e.6. When contamination of the air occurs, terminal cleaning of the affected areas, including ventilation ducts, air vent, and grilles, should be performed and air filters should be changed after the source of the contamination is identified and contained.[82] [3: Moderate Evidence]

Recommendation VIII

Perioperative and environmental services personnel should receive initial and ongoing education and competency verification on their understanding of the principles and the performance of the processes for environmental cleaning in perioperative areas.[86]

Health care organizations are responsible for providing initial and ongoing education and evaluating the competency of perioperative and environmental services personnel on the principles of and the performance of environmental cleaning.

Initial and ongoing education of perioperative and environmental services personnel on the principles of and the performance of environmental cleaning facilitates the development of knowledge, skills, and attitudes that affect safe patient care. Ongoing development of knowledge and skills and documentation of personnel participation is a regulatory and accreditation requirement for both hospitals and ambulatory settings.[53,54,87-90]

Periodic education programs provide the opportunity to reinforce the principles and processes of environmental cleaning and to introduce relevant new equipment or practices.

Competency assessment measures individual performance, provides a mechanism for documentation, and verifies that perioperative personnel have an understanding of facility policies and potential environmental hazards to patients and personnel. Every nurse is personally accountable for maintaining competency.[28,91]

There are no universally accepted or mandated ways to perform or verify competency, and strategies to accomplish this differ among states. The goal of competency verification is to reassure the public that nurses have the knowledge, skills, and judgment to provide safe and effective care.[92]

VIII.a. Perioperative and environmental services personnel must receive education and complete competency verification activities that address specialized knowledge and skills related to the principles and processes of environmental cleaning.[39,40] [1: Regulatory Requirement]

Hota et al found that surface contamination with VRE was related to a failure to clean rather than failure of a product or cleaning procedure; cleaning thoroughness and site contamination improved significantly after implementation of an education program for housekeeping personnel.[93]

In a literature review, Dancer found that cleaning processes were often no more than a "perfunctory introduction to the cleaning process" and that a lack of understanding of the basic microbiologic principles underlying cleaning processes can allow potential reservoirs of pathogens in the environment to go unrecognized.[20] Dancer further described the consequences of limited training in environmental cleaning, such as improper maintenance of cleaning equipment, inappropriate use of cleaning chemicals, and exposure of the patient to contaminated surfaces.[20]

VIII.a.1. Education and competency verification should include topics related to the principles and processes of environmental cleaning, including
- basic principles of microbiology[20];
- explanation of signs and labels and/or color coding required for contaminated items;
- an explanation of the modes of transmission of bloodborne pathogens and an explanation of the employer's exposure control plan[73];
- an explanation of the use and limitation of methods for reducing the exposure (eg, engineering controls, work practices, PPE)[73];
- information on the hepatitis B vaccine, its efficacy and safety, the method of administration, and the benefits of vaccination[73];
- location and use of eye wash stations[10];
- information on the types, proper selection, proper use, location, removal, handling, decontamination, and disposal of PPE[11,73];
- location of safety data sheets[10];
- hazardous and medical waste disposal[10];
- handling of hazardous chemicals[10];
- review of the organization's policies and procedures;
- selection of cleaning chemicals, materials, and equipment based on the intended use; and
- access to manufacturers' instructions for cleaning and disinfection.[14]

VIII.a.2. Educational materials should be appropriate in content, vocabulary level, literacy, and language for the target personnel.[73]

VIII.a.3. Continuing education should be provided when new equipment or processes are introduced.

VIII.b. Personnel who are occupationally exposed to blood, body fluids, or other potentially infectious materials must receive training before assignments to tasks where occupational exposure may occur, at least annually, and when changes to procedures or tasks effect occupational exposure.[73] [1: Regulatory Requirement]

Employers are required by OSHA to provide training on the bloodborne pathogens standard during working hours at no cost to employees.[73]

VIII.c. Perioperative and environmental services personnel should receive education that addresses human factors related to the principles and processes of environmental cleaning.[94,95] *[3: Moderate Evidence]*

Human factors include the interpersonal and social aspects of the perioperative environment (eg, coordination of activities, teamwork, collaboration, communication). Effectively implementing the principles and processes of environmental cleaning requires that perioperative and environmental services personnel demonstrate not only procedural knowledge and technical proficiency but also the ability to anticipate needs, coordinate multiple activities, work collaboratively with other team members, and communicate effectively.

Matlow et al conducted focus groups and administered questionnaires to evaluate ICU environmental service workers' attitudes and beliefs and intent about their jobs and found that the environmental services workers' attitudes and beliefs may affect intent and effectiveness of their cleaning practices.[95]

Recommendation IX

Policies and procedures for environmental cleaning processes and practices should be developed, reviewed periodically, revised as necessary, and readily available in the practice setting.

Policies and procedures assist in the development of patient and workplace safety, quality assessment, and performance improvement activities. Policies and procedures establish authority, responsibility, and accountability within the facility. Policies and procedures also serve as operational guidelines that are used to minimize patient and health care worker risks, standardize practice, and direct perioperative personnel.

IX.a. Policies and procedures for the implementation of environmental cleaning must be developed. *[1: Regulatory Requirement]*

Policies and procedures that guide and support patient care, treatment, and services are regulatory and accreditation requirements for both hospitals and ambulatory settings.[39,40,89,96-98]

IX.a.1. Policies and procedures regarding the principles and processes of environmental cleaning should include
- standard cleaning and disinfection procedures[14,30];
- frequency of cleaning and disinfection[99];
- identification of responsible personnel[20,100,101];
- cleaning chemicals, materials, and equipment approved for use[14,30];
- preparation, handling, storage, and disposal of cleaning chemicals;
- required PPE[11,14,30,73];
- enhanced cleaning procedures; and
- special cleaning and disinfection procedures for MDROs, *C difficile*, prion diseases, construction, and environmental contamination.[11,14,30]

IX.b. Policies and procedures designed to minimize or eliminate exposure of health care personnel to blood, body fluids, and other potentially infectious materials must be developed and implemented.[73] *[1: Regulatory Requirement]*

A written bloodborne pathogens exposure plan consistent with federal, state, and local rules and regulations that is readily available in the practice setting promotes safety.[73]

IX.c. Policies and procedures must include processes for initial education, training, ongoing competency verification, and annual review for issues related to environmental cleaning. *[1: Regulatory Requirement]*

Policies and procedures assist in the development of activities that support patient safety, quality assessment, and the establishment of guidelines for continuous performance improvement.[39,40,89,96-98]

Recommendation X

Perioperative personnel should participate in a variety of quality assurance and performance improvement activities that are consistent with the health care organization's plan to improve understanding of and compliance with the principles and processes of environmental cleaning.

Quality assurance and performance improvement programs assist in evaluating worker safety and formulating plans for corrective actions. These programs provide data that may be used to determine whether an individual organization is within benchmark goals and, if not, identify areas that may require corrective actions. These programs also may provide ongoing feedback regarding whether problems are improving, stabilizing, or worsening.

X.a. Process monitoring must be a part of every perioperative setting as part of an overall environmental cleaning program.[39,40,89,96-98] Process monitoring should include
- compliance with regulatory standards[39,40];
- a review of products and manufacturers instructions for use[14];
- cleaning procedures;
- monitoring cleaning and disinfection practices; and
- reporting and investigation of adverse events (eg, outbreaks, product issues, corrective actions, evaluation). *[1: Regulatory Requirement]*

X.b. Performance improvement should focus on thoroughness of cleaning.[1] *[2: High Evidence]*

In a prospective study conducted at a large teaching hospital affiliated with the University of Miami, Munoz et al used UV markers and cultures of environmental surfaces to evaluate cleaning thoroughness in the OR. The researchers found that improvement in thoroughness of cleaning practices in the OR significantly decreased surface contamination with organisms that are potentially pathogenic.[1]

X.c.   Cleaning practices should be measured with qualitative measures[6,7,46,49,50,102] (eg, visual observation of cleaning process, visual inspection of cleanliness, fluorescent marking) and quantitative measures[5,45,100,101,103-105] (eg, culture, adenosine triphosphate [ATP] monitoring).[106-108] Multiple measures should be used as part of a comprehensive assessment of environmental cleaning practices.[6,46,103] *[3: Moderate Evidence]*

Carling and Bartley reported that environmental monitoring programs allow health care organizations to provide measurable, objective data to support proof of a clean environment.[106] The CDC tool kit *Options for Evaluating Environmental Cleaning* describes a multidisciplinary approach to implementing a comprehensive environmental monitoring program that is specific to the level of monitoring desired by the health care organization.[108]

Malik et al found in an observational study that visual inspection of cleanliness was less effective than use of an audit tool for inspecting cleanliness.[102] Jefferson et al used a novel fluorescent technique and found improved thoroughness of daily terminal cleaning in the OR.[7] Boyce et al determined that fluorescent marking is useful for determining the frequency of high-touch surface cleaning during terminal cleaning.[46] Carling et al evaluated environmental hygiene in 27 ICUs and found that an objective fluorescent targeting method and feedback to environmental services personnel led to significant improvements in room cleaning.[49] In 23 acute care hospitals, Carling et al found that use of a novel fluorescent targeting method provided significant opportunity to improve cleaning of high-touch objects in the patient's immediate environment.[50]

Aiken determined in a laboratory study that although there is no ideal method for detecting bacteria on hospital surfaces, the viable count culture technique was the most suitable for detecting *Staphylococcus aureus*.[104] Vande Leest et al used ATP and culture methods to evaluate the effectiveness of cleaning five high-touch locations in ORs at an ambulatory surgery center. These researchers determined that their cleaning practices were effective, and they gained insight into the practical applications of cleaning procedures in the perioperative setting.[5] Boyce et al reported that use of an ATP assay showed suboptimal cleaning practices and improved cleaning of high-touch objects

when implemented with an education and feedback program.[45] Sherlock et al found in an observational study that ATP may be useful to assess cleaning efficacy because ATP trends can identify surfaces that need additional cleaning or need to be cleaned more frequently.[105] Dumigan et al used an ATP monitoring system to quantitatively measure cleanliness after delegating cleaning responsibilities and found that the program improved cleanliness across the nursing service.[100] Havill et al also used an ATP monitoring system in combination with aerobic cultures to assess cleaning practices among nurses; the results suggested that periodic education of nurses and monitoring of cleaning practices was warranted.[101]

In a study of 36 acute care hospitals, Carling et al found that cleaning can be significantly improved with a combined approach of a highly objective targeting method, repeat performance feedback to environmental services personnel, and administrative interventions.[6] Al-Hamad and Maxwell reported that combined methods for assessing hospital cleanliness may be useful.[103] Boyce et al found that although fluorescent marking was useful for determining cleaning frequency, this method was not as reliable for detecting surface contamination levels as were quantitative measures.[46]

Data generated by measurement of cleaning practices provides complementary information that can be used to drive process improvement activities, encourage compliance with established cleaning protocols, educate personnel, and verify personnel competency.

X.c.1.   Immediate feedback of assessment findings should be provided to perioperative and environmental services personnel when possible.[45,49]

Boyce et al reported in a prospective intervention study conducted at a university-affiliated community teaching hospital that use of an ATP assay showed suboptimal cleaning practices and implementation of an education and feedback program improved cleanliness of high-touch objects in patient rooms. The researchers found that the instant results of the ATP assay were useful in improving cleaning practice.[45]

Carling et al found that repeated performance feedback to environmental services personnel as part of an objective fluorescent targeting method led to significant improvements in ICU room cleaning.[49]

X.d.   Completion of terminal and scheduled cleaning procedures should be documented on a checklist or log sheet.[109] *[3: Moderate Evidence]*

Checklists that outline the health care organization's cleaning procedures guide cleaning personnel in performing terminal and scheduled cleaning procedures so that items are not missed due to human factors. A checklist or log sheet also facilitates communication between perioperative team members and environmental services personnel that the environment is safe and clean for patients.

Glossary

Clean: The absence of visible dust, soil, debris, blood, or other potentially infectious material.

Disinfection: A process that kills most forms of microorganisms on inanimate surfaces. Disinfection destroys pathogenic organisms (excluding bacterial spores) or their toxins or vectors by direct exposure to chemical or physical means.

Dwell time: The amount of time required for contact of a chemical agent with a surface.

Enhanced environmental cleaning: Environmental cleaning practices implemented to prevent the spread of infections or outbreaks; enhanced cleaning practices promote consistent and standardized cleaning procedures that extend beyond routine cleaning.

Fomite: An inanimate object which, when contaminated with a viable pathogen (eg, bacterium, virus), can transfer the pathogen to a host.

High touch: Frequently touched object or surface.

Low-level disinfection: A process by which most bacteria, some viruses, and some fungi are killed.

Noncritical item: An item or instrument that comes in contact with intact skin, but not with mucous membranes, sterile tissue, or the vascular system.

Noninfectious waste: Materials with no inherent hazards or infectious potential (eg, packaging materials, paper).

Personal protective equipment (PPE): Specialized equipment or clothing for eyes, face, head, body, and extremities; protective clothing; respiratory devices; and protective shields and barriers designed to protect the worker from injury or exposure to a patient's blood, tissue, or body fluids. Used by health care workers and others whenever necessary to protect themselves from the hazards of processes or environments, chemical hazards, or mechanical irritants encountered in a manner capable of causing injury or impairment in the function of any part of the body through absorption, inhalation, or physical contact.

Regulated medical waste: Liquid or semi-liquid blood or other potentially infectious materials, contaminated items that would release blood or other potentially infectious materials in a liquid or semi-liquid state if compressed, items that are caked with dried blood or other potentially infectious materials and are capable of releasing these materials during handling, contaminated sharps, and pathological and microbiological wastes containing blood or other potentially infectious materials.

Standard precautions: The primary strategy for successful infection control and reduction of worker exposure. Precautions used for care of all patients regardless of their diagnosis or presumed infectious status.

Terminal cleaning: Thorough environmental cleaning that is performed at the end of each day when the area is being used.

REFERENCES

1. Munoz-Price LS, Birnbach DJ, Lubarsky DA, et al. Decreasing operating room environmental pathogen contamination through improved cleaning practice. *Infec Control Hosp Epidemiol.* 2012;33(9):897-904. [IIIA]

2. Dancer SJ. The role of environmental cleaning in the control of hospital-acquired infection. *J Hosp Infect* 2009;73(4):378-385. [VB]

3. Carling PC, Huang SS. Improving healthcare environmental cleaning and disinfection: current and evolving issues. *Infect Control Hosp Epidemiol.* 2013;34(5):507-513. [VA]

4. Otter JA, Yezli S, French GL. The role played by contaminated surfaces in the transmission of nosocomial pathogens. *Infect Control Hosp Epidemiol.* 2011;32(7):687-699. [VA]

5. Vande Leest L, Kawczynski R, Esser Lipp F, Barrientos R. Identifying potential areas of infectivity on high touch locations in the OR. *AORN J.* 2012;96(5):507-512 [IIIC]

6. Carling PC, Parry MM, Rupp ME, et al. Improving cleaning of the environment surrounding patients in 36 acute care hospitals. *Infect Control Hosp Epidemiol.* 2008;29(11):1035-1041. [IIIA]

7. Jefferson J, Whelan R, Dick B, Carling P. A novel technique for identifying opportunities to improve environmental hygiene in the operating room. *AORN J.* 2011;93(3):358-364. [IIIB]

8. Donskey CJ. Does improving surface cleaning and disinfection reduce health care-associated infections? *Am J Infect Control.* 2013;41(5 Suppl):S12-S19. [VB]

9. Guideline for hand hygiene. In: *Guidelines for Perioperative Practice.* Denver, CO: AORN, Inc; 2015:31-42 [IVB]

10. Guideline for a safe environment of care, part 1. In *Guidelines for Perioperative Practice.* Denver, CO: AORN Inc; 2015:239-263. [IVA]

11. Guideline for prevention of transmissible infections In: *Guidelines for Perioperative Practice.* Denver, CO: AORN, Inc; 2015:419-451. [IVA]

12. Havill NL. Best practices in disinfection of noncritical surfaces in the health care setting: creating a bundle for success. *Am J Infect Control.* 2013;41(5 Suppl):S26-S30. [VB]

13. Guideline for product selection. In: *Guidelines for Perioperative Practice.* Denver, CO: AORN, Inc; 2015:179-186. [IVB]

14. Sehulster L, Chinn RY; CDC, HICPAC. Guidelines for environmental infection control in health-care facilities Recommendations of CDC and the Healthcare Infection Control Practices Advisory Committee (HICPAC). *MMWR Recomm Rep.* 2003;52(RR-10):1-42. [IVA]

15. *Practice Guidance for Healthcare Environmental Cleaning.* 2nd ed. Chicago, IL: Association for the Healthcare Environment; 2012. [IVC]

16. Arif AA, Delclos GL. Association between cleaning related chemicals and work-related asthma and asthma symptoms among healthcare professionals. *Occup Environ Med.* 2012;69(1):35-40. [IIIB]

17. Bello A, Quinn MM, Perry MJ, Milton DK. Characterization of occupational exposures to cleaning products used for common cleaning tasks—a pilot study of hospital cleaners. *Environ Health.* 2009;8:11. [IIIB]

18. Rutala WA, Gergen MF, Weber DJ. Microbiologic evaluation of microfiber mops for surface disinfection. *Am J Infect Control.* 2007;35(9):569-573. [IIIB]

19. Diab-Elschahawi M, Assadian O, Blacky A, et al. Evaluation of the decontamination efficacy of new and reprocessed microfiber cleaning cloth compared with other commonly used cleaning cloths in the hospital. *Am J Infect Control.* 2010;38(4):289-292. [IIIB]

20. Dancer SJ. Hospital cleaning in the 21st century. *Eur J Clin Microbiol Infect Dis.* 2011;30(12):1473-1481. [VA]

21. Stiefel U, Cadnum JL, Eckstein BC, Guerrero DM, Tima MA, Donskey CJ. Contamination of hands with methicillin-resistant *Staphylococcus aureus* after contact with environmental surfaces and after contact with the skin of colonized patients. *Infect Control Hosp Epidemiol.* 2011;32(2):185-187. [IIIC]

22. Siegel JD, Rhinehart E, Jackson M, Chiarello L; Healthcare Infection Control Practices Advisory Committee. *Management of Multidrug-Resistant Organisms in Healthcare Settings.* Atlanta, GA: Centers for Disease Control and Prevention; 2006. [IVA]

23. Datta R, Platt R, Yokoe DS, Huang SS. Environmental cleaning intervention and risk of acquiring multidrug-resistant organisms from prior room occupants. *Arch Intern Med.* 2011;171(6):491-494. [IIB]

24. Landman D, Babu E, Shah N, et al. Transmission of carbapenem-resistant pathogens in New York City hospitals: progress and frustration. *J Antimicrob Chemother.* 2012;67(6):1427-1431. [IIIA]

25. Morgan DJ, Rogawski E, Thom KA, et al. Transfer of multidrug-resistant bacteria to healthcare workers' gloves and gowns after patient contact increases with environmental contamination. *Crit Care Med.* 2012;40(4):1045-1051. [IIIA]

26. Hess AS, Shardell M, Johnson JK, et al. A randomized controlled trial of enhanced cleaning to reduce contamination of healthcare worker gowns and gloves with multidrug-resistant bacteria. *Infect Control Hosp Epidemiol.* 2013;34(5):487-493. [IA]

27. Ibrahimi OA, Sharon V, Eisen DB. Surgical-site infections and routes of bacterial transfer: which ones are most plausible? *Dermatol Surg.* 2011;37(12):1709-1720. [VB]

28. Standards of perioperative nursing. In: *Perioperative Standards and Recommended Practices.* Denver, CO: AORN, Inc; 2012:3-20. [IVC]

29. Mangram AJ, Horan TC, Pearson ML, Silver LC, Jarvis WR. Guideline for prevention of surgical site infection, 1999. Centers for Disease Control and Prevention (CDC) Hospital Infection Control Practices Advisory Committee. *Am J Infect Control.* 1999;27(2):97-132. [IVA]

30. Rutala WA, Weber DJ; Healthcare Infection Control Practices Advisory Committee. *Guideline for Disinfection and Sterilization in Healthcare Facilities, 2008.* Atlanta, GA: Centers for Disease Control and Prevention; 2008. [IVA]

31. Andersen BM, Rasch M, Kvist J, et al. Floor cleaning: effect on bacteria and organic materials in hospital rooms. *J Hosp Infect.* 2009;71(1):57-65. [IIIB]

32. Cotton MF, Wasserman E, Pieper CH, et al. Invasive disease due to extended spectrum beta-lactamase-producing *Klebsiella pneumoniae* in a neonatal unit: the possible role of cockroaches. *J Hosp Infect.* 2000;44(1):13-17. [IIIB]

33. Faulde M, Spiesberger M. Role of the moth fly *Clogmia albipunctata* (Diptera: Psychodinae) as a mechanical vector of bacterial pathogens in German hospitals. *J Hosp Infect.* 2013;83(1):51-60. [IIIB]

34. Fotedar R, Nayar E, Samantray JC, et al. Cockroaches as vectors of pathogenic bacteria. *J Commun Dis.* 1989;21(4):318-322. [IIIA]

35. Lemos AA, Lemos JA, Prado MA, et al. Cockroaches as carriers of fungi of medical importance. *Mycoses.* 2006;49(1):23-25. [IIIC]

36. Munoz-Price LS, Safdar N, Beier JC, Doggett SL. Bed bugs in healthcare settings. *Infect Control Hosp Epidemiol.* 2012;33(11):1137-1142. [VB]

37. Pai HH, Chen WC, Peng CF. Cockroaches as potential vectors of nosocomial infections. *Infect Control Hosp Epidemiol.* 2004;25(11):979-984. [IIIC]

38. Saitou K, Furuhata K, Kawakami Y, Fukuyama M. Biofilm formation abilities and disinfectant-resistance of Pseudomonas aeruginosa isolated from cockroaches captured in hospitals. *Biocontrol Sci.* 2009;14(2):65-68. [IIIB]

39. *42 CFR 416: Ambulatory Surgical Services.* 2011. US Government Printing Office. http://www.gpo.gov/fdsys/granule/CFR-2011-title42-vol3/CFR-2011-title42-vol3-part416/content-detail.html. Accessed September 30, 2013.

40. *42 CFR 482: Conditions of Participation for Hospitals.* US Government Printing Office. http://www.gpo.gov/fdsys/granule/CFR-2011-title42-vol5/CFR-2011-title42-vol5-part482/content-detail.html. Accessed September 30, 2013.

41. Loftus RW, Brown JR, Koff MD, et al. Multiple reservoirs contribute to intraoperative bacterial transmission. *Anesth Analg.* 2012;114(6):1236-1248. [IIA]

42. Rutala WA, Gergen MF, Weber DJ. Room decontamination with UV radiation. *Infect Control Hosp Epidemiol.* 2010;31(10):1025-1029. [IIIB]

43. van 't Veen A, van der Zee A, Nelson J, Speelberg B, Kluytmans JA, Buiting AG. Outbreak of infection with a multiresistant *Klebsiella pneumoniae* strain associated with contaminated roll boards in operating rooms. *J Clin Microbiol.* 2005;43(10):4961-4967. [VB]

44. Blue J, O'Neill C, Speziale P, Revill J, Ramage L, Ballantyne L. Use of a fluorescent chemical as a quality indicator for a hospital cleaning program. *Can J Infect Control.* 2008;23(4):216-219. [IIIC]

45. Boyce JM, Havill NL, Dumigan DG, Golebiewski M, Balogun O, Rizvani R. Monitoring the effectiveness of hospital cleaning practices by use of an adenosine triphosphate bioluminescence assay. *Infect Control Hosp Epidemiol.* 2009;30(7):678-684. [IIB]

46. Boyce JM, Havill NL, Havill HL, Mangione E, Dumigan DG, Moore BA. Comparison of fluorescent marker systems with 2 quantitative methods of assessing terminal cleaning practices. *Infect Control Hosp Epidemiol.* 2011;32(12):1187-1193. [IIIA]

47. Boyce JM, Havill NL, Lipka A, Havill H, Rizvani R. Variations in hospital daily cleaning practices. *Infect Control Hosp Epidemiol.* 2010;31(1):99-101. [IIIC]

48. Boyce JM, Havill NL, Moore BA. Terminal decontamination of patient rooms using an automated mobile UV light unit. *Infect Control Hosp Epidemiol.* 2011;32(8):737-742. [IIIB]

49. Carling PC, Parry MF, Bruno-Murtha LA, Dick B. Improving environmental hygiene in 27 intensive care units to decrease multidrug-resistant bacterial transmission. *Crit Care Med.* 2010;38(4):1054-1059. [IIA]

50. Carling PC, Parry MF, Von Beheren SM; Healthcare Environmental Hygiene Study Group. Identifying opportunities to enhance environmental cleaning in 23 acute care hospitals. *Infect Control Hosp Epidemiol.* 2008;29(1):1-7. [IIIB]

51. Weber DJ, Rutala WA, Miller MB, Huslage K, Sickbert-Bennett E. Role of hospital surfaces in the

ENVIRONMENTAL CLEANING

ASEPTIC PRACTICE

transmission of emerging health care-associated pathogens: norovirus, *Clostridium difficile*, and Acinetobacter species. *Am J Infect Control.* 2010;38(5 Suppl 1):S25-S33. [VA]

52. Friedman ND, Walton AL, Boyd S, et al. The effectiveness of a single-stage versus traditional three-staged protocol of hospital disinfection at eradicating vancomycin-resistant Enterococci from frequently touched surfaces. *Am J Infect Control.* 2013;41(3):227-231. [IIIB]

53. Centers for Medicare & Medicaid Services. *State Operations Manual Appendix A: Survey Protocol, Regulations and Interpretive Guidelines for Hospitals.* Rev 78; 2011.

54. Centers for Medicare & Medicaid Services. *State Operations Manual Appendix L: Guidance for Surveyors: Ambulatory Surgical Centers.* Rev 76; 2011.

55. *ANSI/AAMI ST79:2010 & A1:2010, & A2:2011, & A3:2012: Comprehensive Guide to Steam Sterilization and Sterility Assurance in Health Care Facilities.* Arlington, VA: Association for the Advancement of Medical Instrumentation; 2012. [IVC]

56. Carlesso AM, Artuso GL, Caumo K, Rott MB. Potentially pathogenic acanthamoeba isolated from a hospital in Brazil. *Curr Microbiol.* 2010;60(3):185-190. [IIIB]

57. Wojgani H, Kehsa C, Cloutman-Green E, Gray C, Gant V, Klein N. Hospital door handle design and their contamination with bacteria: a real life observational study. Are we pulling against closed doors? *PLoS ONE.* 2012;7(10):e40171. [IIIC]

58. Brady RR, Verran J, Damani NN, Gibb AP. Review of mobile communication devices as potential reservoirs of nosocomial pathogens. *J Hosp Infect.* 2009;71(4):295-300. [VA]

59. Wilson AP, Ostro P, Magnussen M, Cooper B; Keyboard Study Group. Laboratory and in-use assessment of methicillin-resistant *Staphylococcus aureus* contamination of ergonomic computer keyboards for ward use. *Am J Infect Control.* 2008;36(10):e19-e25. [IIIB]

60. Trillis F 3rd, Eckstein EC, Budavich R, Pultz MJ, Donskey CJ. Contamination of hospital curtains with healthcare-associated pathogens. *Infect Control Hosp Epidemiol.* 2008;29(11):1074-1076. [IIIC]

61. Ohl M, Schweizer M, Graham M, Heilmann K, Boyken L, Diekema D. Hospital privacy curtains are frequently and rapidly contaminated with potentially pathogenic bacteria. *Am J Infect Control.* 2012;40(10):904-906. [IIIB]

62. Barbut F, Menuet D, Verachten M, Girou E. Comparison of the efficacy of a hydrogen peroxide dry-mist disinfection system and sodium hypochlorite solution for eradication of *Clostridium difficile* spores. *Infect Control Hosp Epidemiol.* 2009;30(6):507-514. [IB]

63. Bartels MD, Kristoffersen K, Slotsbjerg T, Rohde SM, Lundgren B, Westh H. Environmental methicillin-resistant *Staphylococcus aureus* (MRSA) disinfection using dry-mist-generated hydrogen peroxide. *J Hosp Infect.* 2008;70(1):35-41. [IIIB]

64. Boyce JM, Havill NL, Otter JA, et al. Impact of hydrogen peroxide vapor room decontamination on *Clostridium difficile* environmental contamination and transmission in a healthcare setting. *Infect Control Hosp Epidemiol.* 2008;29(8):723-729. [IIIB]

65. Chan HT, White P, Sheorey H, Cocks J, Waters MJ. Evaluation of the biological efficacy of hydrogen peroxide vapour decontamination in wards of an Australian hospital. *J Hosp Infect.* 2011;79(2):125-128. [IIB]

66. Manian FA, Griesenauer S, Senkel D, et al. Isolation of *Acinetobacter baumannii* complex and methicillin-resistant *Staphylococcus aureus* from hospital rooms

following terminal cleaning and disinfection: can we do better? *Infect Control Hosp Epidemiol.* 2011;32(7):667-672. [IIIB]

67. Passaretti CL, Otter JA, Reich NG, et al. An evaluation of environmental decontamination with hydrogen peroxide vapor for reducing the risk of patient acquisition of multidrug-resistant organisms. *Clin Infect Dis.* 2013;56(1):27-35. [IIA]

68. Anderson DJ, Gergen MF, Smathers E, et al. Decontamination of targeted pathogens from patient rooms using an automated ultraviolet-C-emitting device. *Infect Control Hosp Epidemiol.* 2013;34(5):466-471. [IIIB]

69. Nerandzic MM, Cadnum JL, Pultz MJ, Donskey CJ. Evaluation of an automated ultraviolet radiation device for decontamination of *Clostridium difficile* and other healthcare-associated pathogens in hospital rooms. *BMC Infect Dis.* 2010;10:197. [IIB]

70. Umezawa K, Asai S, Inokuchi S, Miyachi H. A comparative study of the bactericidal activity and daily disinfection housekeeping surfaces by a new portable pulsed UV radiation device. *Curr Microbiol.* 2012;64(6):581-587. [IIA]

71. Sexton JD, Tanner BD, Maxwell SL, Gerba CP. Reduction in the microbial load on high-touch surfaces in hospital rooms by treatment with a portable saturated steam vapor disinfection system. *Am J Infect Control.* 2011;39(8):655-662. [IIIB]

72. Otter JA, Yezli S, Perl TM, Barbut F, French GL. The role of "no-touch" automated room disinfection systems in infection prevention and control. *J Hosp Infect.* 2013;83(1):1-13. [VB]

73. *29 CFR 1910.1030. Occupational Exposure. Blood-borne Pathogens.* 2012. Occupational Safety & Health Administration. https://www.osha.gov/pls/oshaweb/owadisp.show_document?p_table=standards&p_id=10051. Accessed September 30, 2013.

74. Bergen LK, Meyer M, Hog M, Rubenhagen B, Andersen LP. Spread of bacteria on surfaces when cleaning with microfibre cloths. *J Hosp Infect.* 2009;71(2):132-137. [IIIB]

75. Siegel JD, Rhinehart E, Jackson M, Chiarello L; Health Care Infection Control Practices Advisory Committee. 2007 Guideline for isolation precautions: preventing transmission of infectious agents in health care settings. *Am J Infect Control.* 2007;35(10 Suppl 2):S65-S164. [IVA]

76. Abbett SK, Yokoe DS, Lipsitz SR, et al. Proposed checklist of hospital interventions to decrease the incidence of healthcare-associated *Clostridium difficile* infection. *Infect Control Hosp Epidemiol.* 2009;30(11):1062-1069. [IIB]

77. Carter Y, Barry D. Tackling *C difficile* with environmental cleaning. *Nurs Times.* 2011;107(36):22-25. [IIIB]

78. Doan L, Forrest H, Fakis A, Craig J, Claxton L, Khare M. Clinical and cost effectiveness of eight disinfection methods for terminal disinfection of hospital isolation rooms contaminated with *Clostridium difficile* 027. *J Hosp Infect.* 2012;82(2):114-121. [IA]

79. Dubberke E. Strategies for prevention of *Clostridium difficile* infection. *J Hosp Med.* 2012;7(Suppl 3): S14-S17. [IVA]

80. Jensen PA, Lambert LA, Iademarco MF, Ridzon R; CDC. Guidelines for preventing the transmission of *Mycobacterium tuberculosis* in health-care settings, 2005. *MMWR Recomm Rep.* 2005;54(RR-17):1-141. [IVA]

81. Rutala WA, Weber DJ, Society for Healthcare Epidemiology of America. Guideline for disinfection and sterilization of prion-contaminated medical instruments. *Infect Control Hosp Epidemiol.* 2010;31(2):107-117. [IVA]

82. Balm MN, Jureen R, Teo C, et al. Hot and steamy: outbreak of *Bacillus cereus* in Singapore associated with

construction work and laundry practices. *J Hosp Infect.* 2012;81(4):224-230. [VA]

83. Campbell JR, Hulten K, Baker CJ. Cluster of Bacillus species bacteremia cases in neonates during a hospital construction project. *Infect Control Hosp Epidemiol.* 2011;32(10):1035-1038. [VA]

84. Fournel I, Sautour M, Lafon I, et al. Airborne Aspergillus contamination during hospital construction works: efficacy of protective measures. *Am J Infect Control.* 2010;38(3):189-194. [IIIB]

85. Gibb AP, Fleck BW, Kempton-Smith L. A cluster of deep bacterial infections following eye surgery associated with construction dust. *J Hosp Infect.* 2006;63(2):197-200. [VB]

86. Kak N, Burkhalter B, Cooper M-A. *Measuring the Competence of Healthcare Providers.* Operations Research Issue Paper 2(1). Bethesda, MD: Quality Assurance Project for the US Agency for International Development; 2001. http://www.hciproject.org/sites/default/files/Measuring%20the%20Competence%20of%20HC%20Providers_QAP_2001.pdf. Accessed September 30, 2013. [VA]

87. HR.01.05.03: Staff participate in ongoing education and training. In: *Comprehensive Accreditation Manual: CAMH for Hospitals.* Oakbrook Terrace, IL: Joint Commission Accreditation; 2012.

88. Quality management and improvement. In: *2012 Accreditation Handbook for Ambulatory Health Care.* Skokie, IL: Accreditation Association for Ambulatory Health Care; 2012:34-39.

89. Personnel: personnel records. In: *Procedural Standards and Checklist for Accreditation of Ambulatory Surgery Facilities.* Version 3 ed. Gurnee, IL: American Association for Accreditation of Ambulatory Surgery Facilities; 2011:77-79.

90. Quality assessment /quality improvement: quality improvement. In: *Procedural Standards and Checklist for Accreditation of Ambulatory Surgery Facilities.* Version 3 ed. Gurnee, IL: American Association for Accreditation of Ambulatory Surgery Facilities; 2011:67.

91. Sportsman S. Competency education and validation in the United States: what should nurses know? *Nurs Forum.* 2010;45(3):140-149. [VA]

92. Jordan C, Thomas MB, Evans ML, Green A. Public policy on competency: how will nursing address this complex issue? *J Contin Educ Nurs.* 2008;39(2):86-91. [VA]

93. Hota B, Blom DW, Lyle EA, Weinstein RA, Hayden MK. Interventional evaluation of environmental contamination by vancomycin-resistant enterococci: failure of personnel, product, or procedure? *J Hosp Infect.* 2009;71(2):123-131. [IIIA]

94. Gillespie BM, Hamlin L. A synthesis of the literature on "competence" as it applies to perioperative nursing. *AORN J.* 2009;90(2):245-258. [VA]

95. Matlow AG, Wray R, Richardson SE. Attitudes and beliefs, not just knowledge, influence the effectiveness of environmental cleaning by environmental service workers. *Am J Infect Control.* 2012;40(3):260-262. [IIIC]

96. Governance. In: *2012 Accreditation Handbook for Ambulatory Health Care.* Skokie, IL: Accreditation Association for Ambulatory Health Care; 2012:20-27.

97. LD.04.01.07: The hospital has policies and procedures that guide and support patient care, treatment, and services. In: *Hospital Accreditation Standards 2012.* 2012 ed. Oakbrook Terrace, IL: Joint Commission Resources; 2012.

98. LD.04.01.07: The organization has policies and procedures that guide and support patient care, treatment, or services. In: *Standards for Ambulatory Care 2012:*

Standards, Elements of Performance Scoring Accreditation Polices. Oakbrook Terrace, IL: The Joint Commission; 2012.

99. Rutala WA, Weber DJ. Sterilization, high-level disinfection, and environmental cleaning. *Infect Dis Clin North Am.* 2011;25(1):45-76. [VA]

100. Dumigan DG, Boyce JM, Havill NL, Golebiewski M, Balogun O, Rizvani R. Who is really caring for your environment of care? Developing standardized cleaning procedures and effective monitoring techniques. *Am J Infect Control.* 2010;38(5):387-392. [VB]

101. Havill NL, Havill HL, Mangione E, Dumigan DG, Boyce JM. Cleanliness of portable medical equipment disinfected by nursing staff. *Am J Infect Control.* 2011;39(7):602-604. [IIIB]

102. Malik RE, Cooper RA, Griffith CJ. Use of audit tools to evaluate the efficacy of cleaning systems in hospitals. *Am J Infect Control.* 2003;31(3):181-187. [IIIC]

103. Al-Hamad A, Maxwell S. How clean is clean? Proposed methods for hospital cleaning assessment. *J Hosp Infect.* 2008;70(4):328-334. [IIIC]

104. Aiken ZA, Wilson M, Pratten J. Evaluation of ATP bioluminescence assays for potential use in a hospital setting. *Infect Control Hosp Epidemiol.* 2011;32(5):507-509. [IIIB]

105. Sherlock O, O'Connell N, Creamer E, Humphreys H. Is it really clean? An evaluation of the efficacy of four methods for determining hospital cleanliness. *J Hosp Infect.* 2009;72(2):140-146. [IIIA]

106. Carling PC, Bartley JM. Evaluating hygienic cleaning in health care settings: what you do not know can harm your patients. *Am J Infect Control.* 2010;38(5 Suppl 1):S41-S50. [IIB]

107. Carling P. Methods for assessing the adequacy of practice and improving room disinfection. *Am J Infect Control.* 2013;41:S20-25. [VA]

108. Guh A, Carling P; Environmental Evaluation Workgroup. CDC toolkit: options for evaluating environmental cleaning. 2010. Centers for Disease Control and Prevention. http://www.cdc.gov/HAI/toolkits/Evaluating-Environmental-Cleaning.html. Accessed September 30, 2012. [VC]

109. Gawande A. *The Checklist Manifesto: How to Get Things Right.* New York, NY: Metropolitan Books; 2010. [VA]

Acknowledgements

LEAD AUTHOR
Amber Wood, MSN, RN, CNOR, CIC, CPN
Perioperative Nursing Specialist
AORN Nursing Department
Denver, Colorado

CONTRIBUTING AUTHOR
Ramona Conner, MSN, RN, CNOR
Manager Standards and Guidelines
AORN Nursing Department
Denver, Colorado

The authors and AORN thank Philip Carling, MD, Department of Clinical Medicine, Boston University School of Medicine, Department of Infectious Diseases, Carney Hospital, Boston, Massachusetts; George Allen, PhD, MS, RN, CNOR, CIC, Director Infection Control, Downstate Medical Center and

ENVIRONMENTAL CLEANING

Clinical Assistant Professor, SUNY College of Health Related Professions, Brooklyn, New York; Marcia R. Patrick, MSN, RN, CIC, Association for Professionals in Infection Control and Epidemiology liaison to the AORN Recommended Practices Advisory Board and Independent Consultant, Tacoma, Washington; Deborah F. Mulloy, PhD, RN, CNOR, Associate Chief Nurse, Quality & Center for Nursing Excellence, Brigham and Women's Hospital, Boston, Massachusetts; Lisa Spruce, DNP, RN, ACNS, ACNP, ANP, CNOR, Director of Evidence-based Perioperative Practice, AORN, Inc, Denver, Colorado; Elayne Kornblatt Phillips, PhD-BSN, MPH, RN, International Healthcare Worker Safety Center, University of Virginia, Charlottesville; and Janice A. Neil, PhD, RN, Associate Professor and Chair, Department of Undergraduate Nursing Science, College of Nursing, East Carolina University, Greenville, North Carolina, for their assistance in developing this guideline.

PUBLICATION HISTORY

Originally published June 1975, *AORN Journal*, as "Recommended practices for sanitation in the surgical practice setting."

Format revised March 1978; March 1982; July 1982 Revised April 1984; November 1988; December 1992.

Revised June 1996; published October 1996, *AORN Journal*. Reformatted July 2000.

Revised; published December 2002, *AORN Journal*.

Revised 2007; published in *Perioperative Standards and Recommended Practices*, 2008 edition.

Minor editing revisions made to omit PNDS codes reformatted September 2012 for publication in *Perioperative Standards and Recommended Practices*, 2013 edition.

Revised September 2013 for online publication in *Perioperative Standards and Recommended Practices*.

Minor editing revisions made in November 2014 for publication in *Guidelines for Perioperative Practice*, 2015 edition.

Evidence ratings revised in *Guidelines for Perioperative Practice*, 2018 edition, to conform to the current AORN Evidence Rating Model.

ASEPTIC PRACTICE

GUIDELINE FOR HAND HYGIENE

ASEPTIC PRACTICE

The Guideline for Hand Hygiene has been approved by the AORN Guidelines Advisory Board. It was presented as a proposed guideline for comments by members and others. The guideline is effective September 1, 2016. The recommendations in the guideline are intended to be achievable and represent what is believed to be an optimal level of practice. Policies and procedures will reflect variations in practice settings and/or clinical situations that determine the degree to which the guideline can be implemented. AORN recognizes the many diverse settings in which perioperative nurses practice; therefore, this guideline is adaptable to all areas where operative or other invasive procedures may be performed.

Purpose

This document provides guidance for hand hygiene and surgical hand antisepsis in the perioperative setting. Hand hygiene is widely recognized as a primary method to prevent health care-associated infections and the transmission of pathogens in the health care setting.[1] Health care-associated infections can result in untoward patient outcomes, such as morbidity and mortality, pain and suffering, longer lengths of hospital stay, delayed wound healing, increased use of antibiotics, and higher costs of care.[2] Thus, prevention of health care-associated infections is a priority for all health care personnel. Hand hygiene and surgical hand antisepsis are effective and cost-efficient ways to prevent and control infections in the perioperative setting.

Normal skin flora on the hands include transient and resident microorganisms. Transient flora are microorganisms that colonize the superficial layers of the skin. Perioperative team members acquire these microorganisms while caring for patients and when coming into contact with contaminated environmental surfaces. Transient microorganisms are easier to remove by hand hygiene than are resident microorganisms, which are seated in the deeper layers of the skin. Skin and nail condition and the presence of jewelry contribute to the number of transient microorganisms on the hands.

The goal of surgical hand antisepsis is to remove soil and transient microorganisms from the hands of perioperative team members and suppress the growth of resident microorganisms for the duration of the surgical procedure to reduce the risk that the patient will develop a surgical site infection (SSI).[3] Safe and effective surgical hand antiseptics rapidly and persistently remove transient microorganisms and suppress the growth of resident microorganisms with minimal skin and tissue irritation.[2]

The perioperative registered nurse (RN) plays a crucial role in developing and implementing protocols for hand hygiene and surgical hand antisepsis in the perioperative setting, including involvement in the selection of surgical hand antiseptics and hand hygiene products. This guideline provides perioperative RNs and other perioperative team members with evidence-based practice guidance for hand hygiene and surgical hand antisepsis to promote patient and personnel safety and reduce the risk for health care-associated infections, especially SSIs.

Hand hygiene in health care settings other than the perioperative setting is outside the scope of this document.

Evidence Review

A medical librarian conducted a systematic search of the databases Ovid MEDLINE®, EBSCO CINAHL®, Scopus®, and the Cochrane Database of Systematic Reviews. The search was limited to literature published in English from January 2010 through September 2015. Between September 2015 and February 2016, the results of alerts established at the time of the initial search were assessed, and the lead author requested additional articles that either did not fit the original search criteria or were discovered during the evidence appraisal process. Finally, the lead author and the medical librarian identified relevant guidelines from government agencies, professional organizations, and standards-setting bodies.

The search was limited to the concept of hand hygiene to the perioperative setting. Hand hygiene search terms included the subject headings *handwashing* and *hand disinfection*, supplemented by the keywords *hand washing, handwashing, hand hygiene, hand antisepsis, hand contamination*, and *hand decontamination*. Search terms related to the perioperative setting included the subject headings *operating rooms, surgicenters, anesthesia, perioperative care, perioperative period, perioperative nursing*, and *operating room personnel* and keywords such as *operating theater, surgical suite, operating suite*, and *perioperative setting*. To retrieve additional relevant articles, the keywords *surgical, preoperative, preoperative, presurgical*, and *pre-surgical* were combined with the keywords *hand antisepsis, wash, scrub, rub*, and *hand preparation*. Subject headings and keywords for cross-contamination and infection, fingernails and jewelry, skin irritation and inflammation, and specific antiseptic agents and products also were included.

Inclusion criteria were research and non-research literature in English, complete publications, and publication dates within the time restriction unless none were available. Excluded were non-peer-reviewed publications and literature on hand hygiene in patient care settings other than the perioperative setting. Editorials, news, and brief items were excluded.

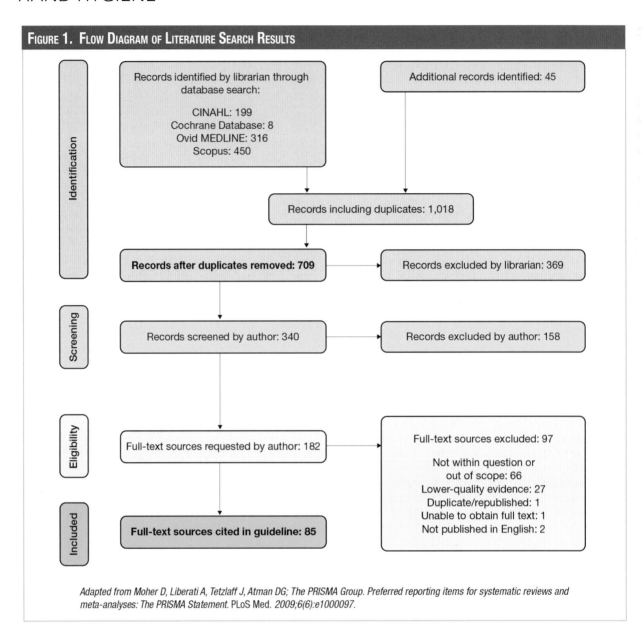

FIGURE 1. FLOW DIAGRAM OF LITERATURE SEARCH RESULTS

Identification

Records identified by librarian through database search:

CINAHL: 199
Cochrane Database: 8
Ovid MEDLINE: 316
Scopus: 450

Additional records identified: 45

Records including duplicates: 1,018

Records after duplicates removed: 709

Records excluded by librarian: 369

Screening

Records screened by author: 340

Records excluded by author: 158

Eligibility

Full-text sources requested by author: 182

Full-text sources excluded: 97

Not within question or out of scope: 66
Lower-quality evidence: 27
Duplicate/republished: 1
Unable to obtain full text: 1
Not published in English: 2

Included

Full-text sources cited in guideline: 85

Adapted from Moher D, Liberati A, Tetzlaff J, Atman DG; The PRISMA Group. Preferred reporting items for systematic reviews and meta-analyses: The PRISMA Statement. PLoS Med. 2009;6(6):e1000097.

Low-quality evidence was excluded when higher-quality evidence was available, and literature outside the time restriction was excluded when literature within the time restriction was available (Figure 1).

Articles identified in the search were provided to the project team for evaluation. The team consisted of the lead author and two evidence appraisers. The lead author divided the search results into topics and assigned members of the team to review and critically appraise each article using the AORN Research or Non-Research Evidence Appraisal Tools as appropriate. The literature was independently evaluated and appraised according to the strength and quality of the evidence. Each article was then assigned an appraisal score. The appraisal score is noted in brackets after each reference as applicable.

The collective evidence supporting each intervention within a specific recommendation was summarized, and the AORN Evidence Rating Model was used to rate the strength of the evidence. Factors considered in the review of the collective evidence were the quality of the evidence, the quantity of similar evidence on a given topic, and the consistency of evidence supporting a recommendation. The evidence rating is noted in brackets after each intervention.

Note: The evidence summary table is available at http://www.aorn.org/evidencetables/.

Editor's note: MEDLINE is a registered trademark of the US National Library of Medicine's Medical Literature Analysis and Retrieval System, Bethesda, MD. CINAHL, Cumulative Index to Nursing and Allied Health Literature, is a registered trademark of EBSCO Industries, Birmingham, AL. Scopus is a registered trademark of Elsevier B.V., Amsterdam, The Netherlands.

Recommendation I

All perioperative team members should maintain healthy fingernail and hand skin condition.

The collective evidence and guidance from professional organizations[1,3-5] indicate that having unhealthy skin or fingernails may impede the removal of microorganisms from the hands during hand hygiene.

Hand hygiene is critical for preventing the transmission of microorganisms from the hands of perioperative team members to the patient and the environment. Transmission to the patient of microorganisms that are harbored in unhealthy skin or fingernails may result in the patient developing a health care-associated infection.

I.a. Perioperative team members should maintain short, natural fingernails. Fingernail tips should be no longer than 2 mm (0.08 inch).[6,7] *[3: Moderate Evidence]*

The collective evidence and guidance from professional organizations support that health care personnel should maintain their fingernails at a short length.[1,3,4,6-10] The most recent research found in the evidence review supports maintaining fingernails at a length no longer than 2 mm (Figure 2).[6,7] Benefits of maintaining short nails include reducing the risk of harboring potential pathogens under fingernails. In addition, the harms of having long nails may include puncturing gloves,[1,3,9] limiting the effectiveness of hand hygiene,[3,8] or injuring patients during patient handling.

Historical studies cited by the Centers for Disease Control and Prevention (CDC)[4] and the World Health Organization (WHO)[3] have found that the areas under the fingernails can harbor high concentrations of bacteria (eg, coagulase-negative staphylococci, gram-negative rods *[Pseudomonas]*, Corynebacteria) and yeasts, which can remain present even after careful hand hygiene or surgical hand antisepsis. Based on this evidence, in 2002, the CDC[4] recommended keeping natural nail length shorter than 0.25 inches. In 2009, the WHO[3] also recommended that health care personnel who have direct contact with patients keep natural nails short, with tips shorter than 0.25 inches or 0.5 cm. Rather than providing a specific recommendation on fingernail length, the Association of Surgical Technologists (AST)[9] recommended in 2008 that fingernail length not extend beyond the fingertips due to the risk for glove puncture.

More recent research has indicated that the 6 mm (0.25 inch) recommendation for length of the fingernail is too long. In 2008, Rupp et al[7] conducted a prospective controlled cross-over trial to introduce alcohol-based hand rubs in two medical-surgical intensive care units at a tertiary care teaching hospital. This study was designed to investigate whether the introduction of an alcohol-based hand rub improved

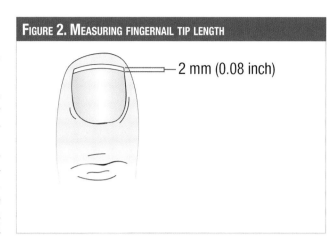

FIGURE 2. MEASURING FINGERNAIL TIP LENGTH

2 mm (0.08 inch)

hand hygiene compliance, affected patient outcomes, or altered the microbial flora on the hands of health care personnel. The researchers used a modified glove juice method to culture the hands of personnel (N = 174) and found that fingernail length longer than 2 mm (0.08 inches) was significantly associated with a higher number of microorganisms compared with fingernail lengths shorter than 2 mm.

Fagernes and Lingaas[6] evaluated the microflora on the hands of 465 Norwegian health care personnel by using the glove juice method in a 2011 observational study. The researchers found that fingernails longer than 2 mm were significantly associated with the prevalence of *Staphylococcus aureus*. Thus, they recommended that the fingernails of health care personnel be no longer than 2 mm.

In a prospective observational study with an educational intervention, Hautemaniere et al[8] evaluated factors associated with hand hygiene effectiveness for 3,067 hospital personnel in France. The researchers evaluated hand hygiene before and after an educational intervention, which consisted of a 30-minute session to teach best practices for use of alcohol-based hand rub. Evaluation of hand hygiene effectiveness was determined using a validated technique of observation of rubbing time (limit 30 seconds), adherence to the application method protocol, and evaluation by visual criteria. The evaluation of visual criteria was assessed by applying fluorescent alcohol-based hand rub and using ultraviolet light to evaluate the percentage of hand coverage. In this study, having long nails was associated with ineffective hand rub use by the evaluation criteria. However, the researchers did not describe the nail length that was used to classify nails as long in this study.

I.b. Artificial fingernails or extenders should not be worn in the perioperative setting.[1,3-5,9] *[1: Strong Evidence]*

Artificial nails have been associated with hand contamination and epidemiologically implicated in outbreaks caused by gram-negative bacteria and yeasts.[1,3,4] Based on this historical evidence, professional organizations recommend that personnel who have direct contact with patients not wear artificial nails or extenders.[1,3-5,9]

Clinical trials of artificial nails may expose patients to harm and, thus, may not be ethical. Further research is needed to determine whether the length of the fingernail or the artificial nail itself poses a risk for the transmission of microorganisms.[3,4]

I.c. A multidisciplinary team that includes perioperative RNs, physicians, and infection preventionists should determine whether fingernail polish may be worn in the perioperative setting.[3] *[1: Strong Evidence]*

The collective evidence is inconclusive regarding the effect of fingernail polish on hand hygiene. Professional organizations provide differing opinions on the wearing of nail polish based on the inconclusive evidence. For example, the WHO[3] recommends that health care facilities develop policies on the wearing of nail polish by health care personnel. The CDC does not make any recommendation on the wearing of nail polish, although the CDC guideline for hand hygiene discusses the evidence on nail polish.[4] The National Institute for Health and Care Excellence (NICE)[5] guidelines in the United Kingdom recommend that the operating team remove nail polish before surgeries because of the lack of evidence on the effect of nail polish on hand contamination. The AST[9] recommends that nail polish be freshly applied and free of chips if the health care facility allows nail polish to be worn.

Arrowsmith and Taylor[11] conducted a systematic review with meta-analysis of one small randomized controlled trial (RCT) published in 1994. The RCT compared the bacterial counts measured in colony-forming units (CFU) on the hands of perioperative nurses (N = 102) with and without nail polish before and after surgical hand antisepsis. In the study, the participants had either unpolished nails (n = 34), freshly applied nail polish that was less than two days old (n = 34), or old nail polish that was either obviously chipped or more than four days old (n = 34). The researchers found a significantly higher median number of CFU after surgical hand antisepsis in the group wearing old or chipped nail polish compared with the groups with unpolished nails or freshly-applied nail polish. However, in the meta-analysis of this RCT, Arrowsmith and Taylor[11] did not find significant differences in the mean CFU between any of the study groups.

A limitation of the RCT is that the data were skewed because of a contaminated sample in the freshly applied nail polish group before surgical hand antisepsis. Thus, the researchers used the median CFU values rather than the mean CFU values to test for statistical significance. Although the median values showed a statistically significant difference in CFU in the old or chipped nail polish group after surgical hand antisepsis, the mean values did not show any difference. Arrowsmith and Taylor[11] describe as a limitation of this RCT that it was underpowered to detect clinically important differences in colonization. Limitations of Arrowsmith and Taylor's systematic review are that the review and meta-analysis was limited to one RCT and the median CFU values were not included in the analysis.

In their observational study, Fagernes and Lingaas[6] cultured the hands of 465 Norwegian health care personnel. They recorded the presence of nail polish for each study participant as either no polish present (n = 377), intact polish (n = 35), or chipped polish (n = 51), or nail polish status was not registered (n = 2). Previous studies of nail polish sampled only the fingernails for culturing, whereas this study cultured the whole hand using the glove juice method. The researchers found no effect of nail polish status on the bacterial count for the whole hand. A limitation of this study is that there was no power analysis to determine whether the sample size was sufficient to determine an effect of nail polish on hand colonization.

A limitation of the evidence on nail polish is that the quality of the research is low. Further research is needed to determine whether wearing nail polish affects hand contamination or patient outcomes, including the rate of SSI.

Although evidence is lacking to determine any harms of wearing nail polish, the potential harms could include nail polish hindering the effectiveness of hand hygiene, transmission to a patient of pathogens harbored in chipped or old nail polish, or chipped polish becoming deposited in the sterile field or wound.

I.c.1. A multidisciplinary team that includes perioperative RNs, physicians, and infection preventionists should determine whether ultraviolet (UV)-cured nail polish (eg, gel, Shellac®) may be worn in the perioperative setting.[1] *[1: Strong Evidence]*

The evidence review found no research to support or refute wearing UV-cured nail polish. The Society for Healthcare Epidemiology of America (SHEA)/Infectious Diseases Society of America (IDSA) hand hygiene practice recommendations[1] also cite a lack of evidence-based guidance on wearing UV-cured nails and nail enhancements in the patient care setting. A conservative approach recommended by SHEA/IDSA[1] is for the health care organization to consider UV-cured nails as artificial and to not allow health care personnel to wear this type of polish in high-risk areas, such as the operating room (OR). Research is needed to determine whether UV-cured nail polish affects the performance of hand hygiene and the microflora on the hands of health care personnel.

Whether UV-cured nail polish carries the same risk of harboring pathogens or transmission of infection to patients as artificial nails is unknown. The harms of wearing UV-cured nail polish may include damage to the natural fingernail and harboring of pathogens in the gaps created as the nail and cuticle grow.

.d. Perioperative team members should take measures to prevent hand dermatitis.[3] *[1: Strong Evidence]*

The collective evidence indicates that hand dermatitis may have a negative effect on hand hygiene.[3,12] According to the WHO,[3] damage to the skin may change skin flora and has been associated with more frequent colonization by staphylococci and gram-negative bacilli.

Personnel with hand dermatitis and eczema are less likely to perform hand hygiene.[12] In an RCT conducted by van der Meer et al,[12] personnel in 48 departments of a hospital in the Netherlands were randomly assigned by department to either a control group or a group that participated in an educational intervention to prevent hand eczema. Participants (N = 1,649) self-reported hand eczema and preventive behavior. The researchers found that 12 months after the baseline report, the intervention group was significantly more likely to report hand eczema, less hand washing, more frequent moisturizer use, and more use of cotton undergloves. The researchers suggested that increased awareness of hand eczema symptoms may have led to the increased reporting of hand eczema in the intervention group.

The limitations of the evidence are that research has not confirmed the effect of dermatitis on hand hygiene or the effect of prevention strategies on the development of hand dermatitis.

Having hand dermatitis may result in hand colonization with pathogens, less hand washing, and increased risk for infection of both patients and perioperative team members. The benefits of preventing hand dermatitis outweigh the harms. Benefits of using hand dermatitis preventative measures may include preventing skin damage and promoting optimal hand hygiene.

I.d.1. Perioperative team members should use moisturizing skin care products approved by the health care organization.[1,3,4,13] *[1: Strong Evidence]*

The collective evidence and guidance from professional organizations support the use of moisturizing skin care products to maintain healthy skin condition.[1,3,4,13] Further research is needed to determine the

effect of hand lotion use on bacterial colonization (See Recommendation V.d. for guidance on selection of skin care products).

The WHO[3] recommends that health care personnel use moisturizing skin care products after hand cleansing to minimize irritant contact dermatitis caused by hand hygiene. The CDC[4] and the SHEA/IDSA[1] also encourage the use of lotion by health care personnel as a strategy to prevent and manage hand hygiene-related irritant contact dermatitis.

Harnoss et al[13] conducted a survey of 16,000 German surgeons and received 1,433 responses (response rate 11%). Although 50% of the respondents reported having experienced skin irritation or discomfort, only 5% reported that they used skin protection or skin care products at the beginning of their shifts. Ten percent of the surgeons refused to use skin care products because of concern that the product would reduce the antimicrobial efficacy of the surgical hand rub. A limitation of this survey is the risk of participation bias by respondents who may have had a personal interest in hand hygiene or skin disorders.

Following the survey, Harnoss et al[13] conducted an experimental crossover study (N = 26) using European Norm standards for testing to determine the effect of skin protection and skin care products on surgical hand antisepsis and glove microperforations after 3 hours of glove wear at rest. After using the skin care products three times daily for 8 days, the participants in the intervention group (n = 13) had significantly higher skin moisture with no significant changes in surgical hand rub effectiveness or glove microperforations than the group that did not use any skin care products (n = 13). Although the study did not find a statistically significant rate of glove microperforations, the group with no skin care product use had a higher perforation rate (23.1%) than the group that used skin care products (7.7%), which may indicate that having dry hands increases the microperforation rate. However, this study was not designed to examine the correlation of dry skin to glove microperforation, so further research is needed to evaluate this relationship. In the interpretation of this study, Harnoss et al[13] cautioned readers to assess the compatibility of skin care products with hand hygiene products during the product selection process.

In an observational study, Fagernes and Lingaas[6] cultured the hands of 465 Norwegian health care personnel using the glove juice method. For each study participant, the minutes between application of hand lotion and hand culturing were recorded. The researchers found that 10 health care personnel used hand lotion within 5 minutes before sampling, and this was significantly associated with the presence of *Staphylococcus aureus*. The researchers postulated that use of hand lotion may increase the efficiency of the skin to acquire staphylococci or may cause better recovery in culturing methods during sampling due to surface-active ingredients or that the findings might be a result of statistical chance. However, the researchers cited a historical report of increased hand bacterial counts after hand lotion use, which supported their findings. A limitation of this study is that there was no power analysis to determine whether the sample size was sufficient to determine the effect of hand lotion on hand colonization.

I.d.2. Hands should be completely dry before gloves are donned.[3] *[1: Strong Evidence]*

The WHO[3] recommends that health care personnel allow hands to dry completely before donning gloves after either hand washing or use of an alcohol-based hand rub because of an increased risk for skin irritation from wearing gloves on wet hands.

I.d.3. Water temperature for hand hygiene should be controlled between 70° F and 80° F (21.1° C and 26.7° C).[14] *[4: Limited Evidence]*

The Facility Guidelines Institute (FGI)[14] recommends controlling water temperature at hand washing stations between 70° F and 80° F (21.1° C and 26.7° C). Water temperatures higher than 80° F (26.7° C) are conducive to the growth of Legionella bacteria.[14]

The WHO,[3] the CDC,[4] and the SHEA/IDSA[1] recommend avoiding hand washing in hot water because repeated exposure to hot water can irritate the skin and may lead to dermatitis or bacterial colonization. As an alternative, the SHEA/IDSA[1] recommends using either warm or cold water for hand washing due to a lack of evidence that either water temperature is superior. Notably, these professional organizations do not define temperature ranges for hot, warm, and cold water. Further research is needed to determine the effect of water temperature on hand dermatitis and bacterial colonization.

I.d.4. In the absence of visible soil, hands should be disinfected with an alcohol-based hand rub rather than washed with soap and water.[1,3] *[1: Strong Evidence]*

The WHO[3] and the SHEA/IDSA[1] recommend promoting the use of alcohol-based hand rub for routine hand hygiene over hand washing with soap and water because

alcohol-based hand rubs are well tolerated and associated with less irritant contact dermatitis.

I.d.5. Cotton glove liners may be worn under nonsterile gloves. Sterile cotton glove liners may be worn under sterile gloves.[1] *[1: Strong Evidence]*

The SHEA/IDSA[1] recommends use of cotton glove liners for individuals with irritant contact dermatitis to maintain healthy skin condition when extended use of gloves is anticipated.

I.d.6. Single-use cotton glove liners should be discarded after each use. Reusable cotton glove liners should be reprocessed in accordance with the manufacturer's instructions for use. *[5: Benefits Balanced with Harms]*

I.d.7. The health care organization should provide education to perioperative team members on the recognition and prevention of hand dermatitis.[1,3,12] *[1: Strong Evidence]*

The WHO[3] and the SHEA/IDSA[1] recommend educating health care personnel on hand care practices to prevent irritant contact dermatitis and other skin damage from hand hygiene practices.

van der Meer et al[12] studied use of an educational intervention to prevent hand eczema in the Netherlands. The multifaceted intervention included education, participatory work groups, and role models. The study found that the educational intervention was effective in influencing personnel to implement evidence-based hand eczema preventative measures, including more frequent moisturizer use and more use of cotton undergloves in the intervention group. Further research is needed to determine the effect of education on the prevalence of hand eczema in health care personnel.

I.e. The activities of health care personnel with dermatitis, infections, exudative lesions, and nonintact skin should be restricted when these activities pose a risk for transmission of infection to patients and other health care providers.[15] State, federal, and professional guidelines and strategies should be followed to determine the need for work restrictions for health care personnel with bloodborne infections.[16,17] *[1: Strong Evidence]*

Perioperative team members with breaks in skin integrity or infections of the nails, hands, or arms may be at risk for acquiring infection or transmitting infection to patients (See the AORN Guideline for Prevention of Transmissible Infections[15] for additional guidance).

ASEPTIC PRACTICE

Recommendation II

Perioperative team members should not wear jewelry (eg, rings, watches, bracelets) on the hands or wrists.

The collective evidence and guidance from professional organizations indicate that wearing jewelry may impede the removal of microorganisms from the hands during hand hygiene.[1,3-5]

Transmission to the patient of microorganisms that are harbored on jewelry worn by perioperative team members may result in the patient developing a health care-associated infection.

II.a.   Perioperative team members should not wear jewelry on the hands or wrists in patient care areas.[3,5,6,8,9,18] *[1: Strong Evidence]*

The collective evidence and guidance from professional organizations support perioperative team members removing rings, watches, and bracelets before caring for patients in the perioperative setting.[3,5,6,8,9] Wearing jewelry on the hands and wrists has been associated with increased bacterial counts on the hands[6] and ineffective use of alcohol-based hand rubs.[8]

Several professional organizations have provided guidance on the wearing of jewelry in the health care setting. The WHO[3] strongly discourages the wearing of rings or other jewelry in the health care setting and recommends that all rings or jewelry be removed in the OR. The WHO[3] recognizes that religious and cultural attitudes may strongly condition health care workers' attitudes toward removing their wedding rings. Thus, the WHO[3] advises that for these individuals, wearing a simple wedding band may be acceptable except in a high-risk setting such as the OR. The NICE[5] guidelines recommend that the operating team remove hand jewelry before surgeries as a measure to decrease the risk for SSI. The AST[9] recommends that all jewelry including rings, bracelets, and watches be removed before surgical hand antisepsis is performed. The AORN Guideline for Surgical Attire[18] recommends that jewelry that cannot be contained within the surgical attire not be worn in the semi-restricted or restricted areas. The CDC[4] makes no recommendation for the wearing of rings in health care settings, designating the issue as unresolved due to the lack of evidence to determine whether wearing rings results in increased transmission of pathogens.

Although a systematic review by Arrowsmith and Taylor[11] did not find any RCTs to evaluate the effect of wearing rings on the effectiveness of surgical hand antisepsis or SSI rates, other types of evidence were found in the evidence review for this guideline.

Fagernes and Lingaas[6] evaluated the microflora on the hands of 465 Norwegian health care personnel by using the glove juice method and found that wearing a wristwatch (n = 79) was significantly associated with a higher total bacteria count on hands than not wearing a watch (n = 121). Wristwatch status was not recorded for 265 study participants. The study also found that wearing one ring (n = 192) increased the rate of colonization with Enterobacteriaceae. However, there was insufficient statistical power to detect a significant difference between wearing of a single decorative ring (n = 50) or wearing of multiple rings (n = 10).

Fagernes and Lingaas[6] also found that wearing rings was associated with a higher total number of bacteria on hands. However, they found that study participants wearing rings were more likely to also wear watches. Because of this confounding factor, the researchers did not use these data in statistical analysis. Based on their findings, they recommended that health care personnel not wear finger rings or watches.

The study conducted by Hautemaniere et al,[8] as described in Recommendation I.a., also evaluated the wearing of jewelry on hand hygiene effectiveness. This study found that wearing a watch, bracelet, and rings other than a wedding ring was significantly associated with ineffective hand rub use by the evaluation criteria. Wearing a wedding ring was not independently associated with hand hygiene ineffectiveness in this study. Notably, the researchers did not describe characteristics of a wedding ring, such as the band type or stone setting. However, they discussed that even though wedding rings had a strong symbolic and sentimental value to the health care personnel, some personnel became aware of the importance of removing their rings because the alcohol solution did not penetrate under the ring, and thus the ring could harbor microorganisms.

A limitation of the evidence is that research has not confirmed the risk of direct transmission of microorganisms to the patient from health care personnel wearing jewelry or watches on the hands or wrists. Further research is needed to determine the effectiveness of hand hygiene in the presence of jewelry on the hands and wrists of health care personnel.

Recommendation III

Perioperative team members should perform hand hygiene.[1,3,4]

The collective evidence and guidance from professional organizations support that hand hygiene reduces the incidence of health care-associated infections.[1,3,4]

Observational research studies have demonstrated that IV stopcocks become contaminated with bacteria in the perioperative setting.[19,20] Loftus et al[21] found that IV stopcock contamination is significantly associated with patient mortality and 30-day postoperative infections. Although the source remains unclear, potential sources of IV stopcock contamination include the patient, the environment, and the hands of anesthesia professionals.

A limitation of the evidence is that current hand hygiene guidelines have not taken into account the rapid pace and task density associated with the administration of anesthesia in the perioperative setting.[22-26] Further research is needed to establish hand hygiene protocols that are feasible for anesthesia professionals and do not compromise patient safety.

Another limitation of the evidence is that research has not established the clinical benefit of performing hand hygiene prior to donning gloves for patient contact that is not associated with a clean or sterile task.[1] Some evidence suggests that glove boxes may be contaminated by the hands of health care personnel retrieving gloves, which may be an indication for performing hand hygiene before donning gloves or for the need for a solution to reduce box contamination during glove dispensing.[1] Further research is also needed to determine the benefits of performing hand hygiene before donning gloves for patient contact.[1]

The benefits of performing hand hygiene outweigh the harms. Benefits include removal of soil and transient microorganisms from the hands of perioperative team members, possibly reducing occupational exposure and the risk for the patient to develop a health care-associated infection.

III.a. Personnel should perform hand hygiene
- before and after patient contact,[1,3,4,19,22,23,27-29]
- before performing a clean or sterile task,[3]
- after risk for blood or body fluid exposure,[1,3,4]
- after contact with patient surroundings,[1,3,4]
- when hands are visibly soiled[1,3,4]
- before and after eating,[4] and
- after using the restroom.[3,4]

[1: Strong Evidence]

The WHO[3] and the CDC[4] recommend performing hand hygiene before and after patient contact, before performing a clean or sterile task, after risk for blood or body fluid exposure, after contact with patient surroundings, and any time hands are visibly dirty or soiled. Table 1 provides examples of hand hygiene indications in the perioperative setting.

III.a.1. Hand hygiene should be performed before and after patient contact, including
- performing a physical exam,[27,29,30]
- marking the site,[27]
- transferring or positioning the patient,[27,30]
- assessing an invasive device (eg, vascular catheter [peripheral, arterial, central], urinary catheter),[27] and
- assessing wound dressing.[27]

[3: Moderate Evidence]

III.a.2. Hand hygiene should be performed before a clean or sterile task, including
- inserting an invasive device (eg, vascular catheter[31] [peripheral,[29,30,32-34] arterial,[30] central[22,23,32]], urinary catheter[35])[1,3,4,10,27,36]; [1: Strong Evidence]
- accessing a vascular device (eg, port,[10] stopcock,[19-21] IV tubing[23,27,33,36])[31]; [1: Strong Evidence]

- moving from a contaminated body site (eg, perineum) to a clean body site (eg, face) on the same patient[1,3,4]; [1: Strong Evidence]
- administering or preparing medication including delivery of medications to the sterile field and preparation of IV fluids[1,3,27,30,33,36]; [1: Strong Evidence]
- performing neuraxial procedures (eg, epidural, spinal, lumbar puncture, spinal tap, epidural blood patch, epidural lysis of adhesions, intrathecal chemotherapy, lumbar or spinal drainage catheters, spinal cord simulation trials)[10,23,27,32,37,38]; [2: High Evidence]
- administering regional anesthesia[30,32,38]; [3: Moderate Evidence]
- performing phlebotomy[30]; [3: Moderate Evidence]
- opening sterile supplies[27,30,33,36]; [3: Moderate Evidence] and
- performing patient skin antisepsis.[27] [3: Moderate Evidence]

III.a.3. Hand hygiene should be performed after risk for blood or body fluid exposure, including
- removing personal protective equipment (eg, gloves, mask)[1,3,4,10,22,23]; [1: Strong Evidence]
- having contact with blood, body fluids, excretions, mucous membranes, non-intact skin, or wound dressings[1,3,4]; [1: Strong Evidence]
- inserting or assessing an invasive device (ie, vascular catheter [peripheral, arterial, central], urinary catheter)[27,30,32]; [3: Moderate Evidence]
- performing airway manipulation (ie, intubation, suctioning)[27,29,30,32,33,36] as patient safety allows[10,23,25]; [3: Moderate Evidence]
- handling used sponges[27,33]; [3: Moderate Evidence]
- handling specimens[27]; [3: Moderate Evidence]
- draining urinary catheter bags, colostomy bags, or other drains[27,33]; [3: Moderate Evidence] and
- removing surgical drapes.[27,33] [3: Moderate Evidence]

III.a.4. Hand hygiene should be performed after contact with patient surroundings, including
- inanimate surfaces and objects, including medical equipment, in the immediate vicinity of the patient[1,3,4]; [1: Strong Evidence]
- OR bed controls[29]; [2: High Evidence]
- patient bed and linens[34]; [3: Moderate Evidence] and

TABLE 1. EXAMPLES OF HAND HYGIENE INDICATIONS IN THE PERIOPERATIVE SETTING

Hand Hygiene Indications	Perioperative Examples
Before and after patient contact[1,3,4,19,22,23,27-29]	• Performing a physical exam[27,29,30] • Marking the site[27] • Transferring or positioning the patient[27,30] • Assessing an invasive device (eg, vascular catheter [peripheral, arterial, central], urinary catheter)[27] • Assessing wound dressing[27]
Before performing a clean or sterile task[3]	• Inserting an invasive device (eg, vascular catheter [peripheral, arterial, central], urinary catheter)[1,3,4,10,22,23,27,29-36] • Accessing a vascular device (eg, port, stopcock, IV tubing)[10,19-21,23,27,31,33,36] • Moving from a contaminated body site (eg, perineum) to a clean body site (eg, face) on the same patient[1,3,4] • Administering or preparing medication, including delivery of medications to the sterile field and preparation of IV fluids[1,3,27,30,33,36] • Performing neuraxial procedures (eg, epidural, spinal, lumbar puncture, spinal tap, epidural blood patch, epidural lysis of adhesions, intrathecal chemotherapy, lumbar or spinal drainage catheters, spinal cord simulation trials)[10,23,27,32,37,38] • Administering regional anesthesia[30,32,38] • Performing phlebotomy[30] • Opening sterile supplies[27,30,33,36] • Performing patient skin antisepsis[27]
After risk for blood or body fluid exposure[1,3,4]	• Removing personal protective equipment (eg, gloves, mask)[1,3,4,10,22,23] • Having contact with blood, body fluids, excretions, mucous membranes, non-intact skin, or wound dressings[1,3,4] • Inserting or accessing an invasive device (ie, vascular catheter [peripheral, arterial, central], urinary catheter)[27,30,32] • Performing airway manipulation (ie, intubation, suctioning) as patient safety allows[10,23,25,27,29,30,32,33,36] • Counting used sponges[27,33] • Handling specimens[27] • Draining urinary catheter bags, colostomy bags, or other drains[27,33] • Removing surgical drapes[27,33]
After contact with patient surroundings[1,3,4]	• Inanimate surfaces and objects, including medical equipment, in the immediate vicinity of the patient[1,3,4] • OR bed controls[29] • Patient bed and linens[34] • The floor or items that have come in contact with the floor[23,30,39]
Other	• Before and after assembling items for sterilization • When hands are visibly dirty or soiled[1,3,4] • Before and after eating[4] • After using the restroom[3,4]

Note: The reference numbers in this table correspond to the numbers in the reference list at the end of the guideline.

• the floor or items that have come in contact with the floor.[23,30,39] *[1: Strong Evidence]*

III.a.5. When gloves are worn and hand hygiene is indicated, the gloves should be removed to perform hand hygiene.[3,4] *[1: Strong Evidence]*

The use of gloves does not replace the need for hand hygiene.[3,4]

III.a.6. Performing a single act of hand hygiene may fulfill multiple indications (eg, opening multiple sterile items sequentially).[3] *[1: Strong Evidence]*

Multiple indications for hand hygiene may arise simultaneously that create a single opportunity to perform hand hygiene.[3]

III.b. In the event that performing hand hygiene would put the patient's safety at risk, the perioperative team member should weigh the risks and benefits of delaying hand hygiene. *[5: Benefits Balanced with Harms]*

The benefits of performing hand hygiene may not outweigh the harms, depending on the clinical situation. Benefits include reducing the risk for the patient developing a health care-associated infection. The harms may include patient injury or delaying necessary, possibly life-saving interventions, such as ventilation.

III.b.1. The anesthesia professional may wear two pairs of gloves (ie, double glove), remove the contaminated outer gloves after airway manipulation, and continue patient care until the patient's status allows for removal of the inner gloves and performance of hand hygiene.[10,40,41] *[2: High Evidence]*

The American Association of Nurse Anesthetists (AANA)[10] recommends that anesthesia professionals double glove during airway manipulation. The AANA[10] recommends maintaining patient oxygenation by ventilating immediately after airway manipulation, auscultating breath sounds, and confirming end-tidal carbon dioxide. Removing gloves to perform hand hygiene immediately after airway management may jeopardize patient safety. As an alternative, the AANA[10] recommends that anesthesia professionals don two pairs of gloves before airway manipulation, remove the outer gloves after the airway device is inserted, and perform hand hygiene when the patient is stable.

Birnbach et al[40] conducted an RCT to assess contamination of the OR surfaces during simulated laryngoscopy and intubation by anesthesiology residents (N = 22). The intervention group members (n = 11) wore two pairs of gloves and removed the outer pair of gloves after intubation, whereas the control group members (n = 11) each wore a single pair of gloves. The study found that the group wearing two pairs of gloves during intubation and removing the outer gloves immediately after intubation contaminated significantly fewer surfaces, as measured by fluorescent marking gel.

In a similar RCT with anesthesiology residents in simulations (N = 45), Birnbach et al[41] compared the level of OR surface contamination after single gloving (n = 15), double gloving with the outer gloves removed (n = 15), and double gloving with the outer gloves used to cover the laryngoscope (n = 15). The study found that both double-gloving techniques were associated with significantly less contamination than single gloving. Use of the outer pair as a sheath for the laryngoscope immediately after intubation was associated with the least contamination of the IV hub, patient, and intraoperative environment.

III.c.   Perioperative personnel should perform hand washing with soap and water
- after being exposed to blood or body fluids,[3,4]
- after using the restroom,[3,4]
- when hands are visibly soiled,[1,3,4] and
- when caring for patients with spore-forming organisms (eg, *Clostridium difficile, Bacillus anthracis*) or norovirus.[1,3,4]

[1: Strong Evidence]

Performing hand hygiene with an alcohol-based hand rub may not be effective when hands are visibly or potentially soiled with organic matter, such as blood and body fluids. Also, spores may be removed from the hands more effectively with soap and water than with an alcohol-based hand rub.[1,3,4]

III.c.1.   A standardized hand washing protocol using soap and water should be performed in the following order:
1. Remove jewelry from hands and wrists (eg, rings, watches, bracelets).[3,4]
2. Adjust water for a comfortable temperature, avoiding hot water.[3]
3. Wet hands thoroughly with water.[3,4]
4. Apply the amount of soap needed to cover all surfaces of the hands.[3,4]
5. Rub hands together vigorously covering all surfaces of the hands and fingers for at least 15 seconds.[4]
6. Rinse with water to remove all soap.[3,4]
7. Dry hands thoroughly with a disposable paper towel.[3,4]
8. When hand-free controls are not available on the sink, use a clean paper towel to turn off the water.[4]

[1: Strong Evidence]

III.d.   When hands are not visibly soiled or dirty, hand hygiene should be performed using an alcohol-based hand rub according to the manufacturer's instructions for use.[3,4] *[1: Strong Evidence]*

The WHO[3] and the CDC[4] recommend performing hand hygiene with an alcohol-based hand rub when hands are not visibly soiled or dirty.

III.d.1.   A standardized hand hygiene protocol using an alcohol-based hand rub should be performed in the following order:
1. Remove jewelry from hands and wrists (eg, rings, watches, bracelets).[3,4]
2. Apply the amount of alcohol-based hand rub recommended by the manufacturer to cover all surfaces of the hands.[3,4]
3. Rub hands together, covering all surfaces of the hands and fingers until dry.[3,4]

[1: Strong Evidence]

III.e.   Hand washing stations should be placed in convenient locations as determined in an infection control risk assessment and in accordance with federal, state, and local regulatory requirements and applicable construction guidelines. *[4: Limited Evidence]*

The FGI[14] has established the minimum number and locations for hand washing stations. The FGI recommends conducting an infection control risk assessment to evaluate the convenience of hand washing station locations for clinical use and to further identify locations that will enhance accessibility to hand hygiene products.

III.e.1.   For areas with multiple patient care stations, at least one hand washing station should be provided for every four patient care stations. The hand washing station should be positioned to be approximately an equal distance between the furthest stations.[14] *[4: Limited Evidence]*

III.e.2. Sinks designated for hand hygiene should only be used for hand hygiene. *[5: Benefits Balanced with Harms]*

Performing activities other than hand washing or surgical hand antisepsis could contaminate the sink, faucet, or hands of personnel subsequently using the sink.

III.f. Hand washing station sinks should have controls that can be operated without using hands, including single-lever or wrist blade devices and electronic sensor controls. When the operation of the scrub sink is dependent on the building electrical service, the controls should be connected to the essential electrical system.[14] *[4: Limited Evidence]*

Hands-free sinks reduce the risk of cross-contamination after hand hygiene is performed.

III.g. Paper towel dispensers should be provided at hand washing stations. The dispenser should dispense paper towels without the need to touch the dispenser.[14] *[4: Limited Evidence]*

III.h. Alcohol-based hand rub product dispensers (eg, wall-mounted, table-top) should be placed in convenient locations as determined by the infection control risk assessment and in accordance with federal, state, and local regulatory requirements.[1,3,4] *[1: Strong Evidence]*

The infection control risk assessment identifies locations that will enhance accessibility to hand hygiene products and evaluates the convenience of locations for clinical use.

Professional organizations support placement of alcohol-based hand rub products at the point of use.[1,3,4] The WHO[3] recommends that hand hygiene product dispensers be as close as possible, ideally within arm's reach, to where patient contact is taking place, to avoid personnel having to leave the care or treatment zone. The CDC[4] and the SHEA/IDSA[1] recommend having alcohol-based hand rub products available at the patient's bedside and in other convenient locations to promote hand hygiene adherence by personnel who perform a high volume of patient care.

III.h.1. Dispenser placement and storage of flammable alcohol-based hand hygiene products must be in compliance with local, state, and federal regulations.[42-44] *[1: Regulatory Requirement]*

The Centers for Medicare & Medicaid Services[42,45] states in §482.41(c)(2) that "facilities, supplies, and equipment must be maintained to ensure an acceptable level of safety and quality," including storage in compliance with fire codes. The National Fire Protection Association[44] makes recommendations for storage of flammable solutions.

III.h.2. Alcohol-based hand hygiene product dispensers should
- be at least 4 ft apart;
- hold a maximum of 1.2 L in rooms, corridors, and areas open to corridors;
- not be placed above an ignition source (eg, electrical outlet, switch) or within 1 inch of the ignition source; and
- not total more than 10 gallons (37.8 L) outside of a storage cabinet in a single smoke compartment.[44]

[4: Limited Evidence]

III.i. Health care organizations may permit use of personal dispensers of alcohol-based hand hygiene products.[3,4] *[1: Strong Evidence]*

The collective evidence and guidance from professional organizations support use of personal dispensers of alcohol-based hand hygiene product in the perioperative setting.[3,4,23,46-48]

The CDC[4] recommends having alcohol-based hand rub available at the patient's bedside and in other convenient locations, including in individual containers carried by health care workers, to promote hand hygiene adherence by personnel who perform a high volume of patient care.

The WHO[3] supports use of personal hand hygiene product containers when combined with wall-mounted dispensing systems to increase access to hand hygiene products at the point of care. However, the WHO[3] discusses the limitations of using personal hand hygiene products in the clinical setting:
- Many of the personal dispensers are not transparent and may be found to be empty when needed.
- The amount of hand rub may be so small (10 mL to 20 mL) that several containers per person are needed each day.
- The personal dispensers may not be cost effective, and maintaining the dispenser supply may be challenging if dependent on a single manufacturer.
- Using disposable dispensers may have a negative impact on the environment.
- The external surface of the bottle may become contaminated, although this may be considered to be negligible because of the excess spillage of the disinfectant and the overall short time until replacement.

Several experts support the use of personal hand hygiene dispensers in the perioperative setting, especially to increase access to hand hygiene products for anesthesia professionals.[23,46,47] In an RCT conducted at a tertiary care and Level 1 trauma center, Koff et al[48] examined the effect of personal hand hygiene product dispenser use by anesthesia professionals (N = 111) on hourly hand decontamination events, contamination of the anesthesia work area and IV tubing, and health care-associated infection rates. As a reminder to the anesthesia professional, the personal dispenser sounded an audible alarm every 6 minutes if no product had been dispensed. Wall-mounted and table-top dispensers were also available in the clinical setting. Use of the personal dispenser was associated with significantly more hourly hand decontamination events, less IV tubing contamination, and lower health care-associated infection rates. A limitation of this study was that a standardized system was not used for health care-associated infection surveillance.

III.j. Hand hygiene product dispenser function should be verified in accordance with the manufacturer's instructions each time a new refill is installed.[44] *[4: Limited Evidence]*

III.k. Hand washing stations and products should be accessible to patients and visitors in unrestricted areas (eg, waiting room, preoperative area, postoperative area) unless contraindicated for a specific patient population or individual patient. *[5: Benefits Balanced with Harms]*

Providing opportunities to perform hand hygiene engages the patient and visitors in the mission of the perioperative team to prevent the patient from developing a health care-associated infection and may reduce the contamination of the patient's environment.

The SHEA/IDSA[1] recommends conducting a point-of-care risk assessment to guide placement of dispensers. Based on the risk assessment, the health care organization may decide to provide patients and visitors with nontoxic hand hygiene products because cognitively impaired, behavioral health, or substance abuse patients may be injured by ingestion of alcohol-based hand rub.

The WHO[3] also recommends careful consideration for placement of dispensers in areas with patients who are likely to ingest the product, such as disoriented elderly patients, psychiatric patients, young children, or patients with alcohol dependence.

III.l. Perioperative team members should receive education and complete competency verification activities that address performance of hand hygiene in accordance with the product manufacturer's instructions and the health care organization's policies and procedures.[1,3,4] *[1: Strong Evidence]*

Lack of knowledge, experience, and education are factors associated with low hand hygiene compliance.[3] The collective evidence and guidance from professional organizations support educating health care personnel on hand hygiene indications and performance as part of a multifaceted hand hygiene program (eg, education, training, observation, feedback).[1,3,4,8,28,29,33,34,36,49-54]

Gould et al[49] conducted a systematic review to evaluate the success of strategies to improve hand hygiene compliance. The researchers found that using multiple strategies for educa-

tion and training, such as engaging personnel in planning and social marketing strategies, may be helpful for improving hand hygiene compliance. However, the quality of the evidence was insufficient to allow for drawing a firm conclusion, and further research is needed to evaluate the effectiveness of educational interventions in increasing hand hygiene compliance.

Several studies have found low compliance with hand hygiene protocols in the perioperative setting[28,32-34,50,54] and knowledge deficits among perioperative team members.[29,36,51,52] In an organizational experience report from Brazil, Santos et al[50] found a significant improvement in hand hygiene rates in an endoscopy unit after a hand hygiene education intervention that included task-oriented training and live demonstrations.

In an organizational report from Australia, Bellaard-Smith and Gillespie[33] found a significant improvement in hand hygiene compliance after they implemented multiple hand hygiene strategies in the operating suite, including education about the WHO five moments of hand hygiene specific to the perioperative setting, appropriate glove use, correct hand hygiene technique, and hand care.

Jericho et al[54] investigated two interventions to improve hand hygiene compliance in the perioperative setting: use of educational posters and including hand hygiene in the time-out process. The researchers found that compliance with using an alcohol-based hand foam was significantly improved after educational posters were placed in strategic locations and hand hygiene was included in the time-out process.

Elkaradawy et al[51] studied the effect of a hand hygiene educational intervention for anesthesia professionals and found a significant reduction in bacterial contamination of the anesthesia machine and the hands of personnel after the intervention.

Some researchers have suggested that use of a fluorescent indicator is an effective hand hygiene education intervention to enhance active participation.[8,53] Pan et al[53] assessed the thoroughness of health care personnel hand hygiene by using a fluorescent substance to simulate hand contamination. The personnel (N = 388) then performed hand hygiene with soap and water, and the researchers used an ultraviolet light detector to identify missed areas where the fluorescent substance remained after the hand wash. The researchers found that the most missed areas of the hand were the nails. The researchers recommended using fluorescent products as part of a "seeing is believing" hand hygiene campaign to encourage active participation.

Hautemaniere et al[8] used a fluorescent alcohol-based hand rub solution to assess thoroughness of hand coverage by using an ultraviolet light to identify any missed areas of the hand that were not covered by the solution. The study found that health care personnel (N = 3,067) significantly improved compliance with a hand hygiene protocol after an educational intervention.

The limitations of the evidence are that the quality of evidence for educational interventions is low, and research has not confirmed the most effective and sustainable education methods to improve hand hygiene compliance. Further research is needed to determine the most effective method to educate health care personnel regarding activities that can result in hand contamination during patient care.[3]

III.l.1. Education and competency verification should be performed when new hand hygiene products or processes are introduced. [5: Benefits Balanced with Harms]

Recommendation IV

Perioperative team members should perform surgical hand antisepsis before donning sterile gowns and gloves for operative and other invasive procedures.[1,3,4,9,55]

Surgical hand antisepsis is the primary line of defense to protect the patient from pathogens on the hands of perioperative team members, whereas sterile surgical gloves are the secondary line of defense.[55] Due to the risk for glove failure,[56] the performance of surgical hand antisepsis is critical for the prevention of SSIs.[3,4,55]

The limitation of the evidence is that due to low quality, the available research has not confirmed the effect of surgical hand antisepsis on the development of SSIs.[2] Although research has demonstrated that surgical hand antisepsis reduces the number of bacteria on the hands of health care personnel, a systematic review by Tanner et al[2] found that the evidence is unclear about how the number of bacteria correlates to the likelihood of a patient developing an SSI. However, further research to confirm this correlation is not ethical to conduct in clinical trials because it may expose patients to harm.[3]

There is indirect historical evidence that supports the correlation of bacteria on the hands of health care personnel with patient infection. For example, historical evidence has shown that bacteria on the hands of surgeons can cause wound infections if introduced to the sterile field during surgery.[4] Older studies have also shown that bacteria multiply rapidly under surgical gloves when hands are washed with non-antimicrobial soap[4] and that switching to the use of a non-antimicrobial surgical scrub was implicated in an outbreak of SSIs.[3]

The benefits of surgical hand antisepsis outweigh the harms. Benefits include reduction of transient and resident microorganisms on the hands of perioperative team members, which may lower the risk of the patient developing an SSI.[2]

IV.a. Surgical hand antisepsis using a surgical hand rub should be performed according to the manufacturer's instructions for use. [5: Benefits Balanced with Harms]

The evidence review found no literature related to application technique. Antiseptic manufacturers' instructions for use convey important safety and efficacy instructions to the user. Failure to adhere to the manufacturer's instructions for use may result in harm or ineffectiveness of the surgical hand antiseptic.

IV.a.1. A standardized surgical hand antisepsis protocol using a surgical hand rub should be performed in the following order:
1. Remove jewelry from hands and wrists (eg, rings, watches, bracelets).[3,4]
2. Don a surgical mask.[3,56]
3. If hands are visibly soiled, wash hands with soap and water.[3,4]
4. Remove debris from underneath fingernails using a disposable nail cleaner under running water.[3,4]
5. Dry hands and arms thoroughly[3,4] with a disposable paper towel.
6. Apply the surgical hand rub product to the hands and arms according to the manufacturer's instructions for use (eg, amount, method, time).[3,4]
7. Allow hands and arms to dry completely[3,4] before using sterile technique to don a surgical gown and gloves.[56]
[1: Strong Evidence]

IV.b. Surgical hand antisepsis using a surgical hand scrub should be performed according to the manufacturer's instructions for use. [5: Benefits Balanced with Harms]

The evidence review found no literature related to application technique, including sequence of scrubbing, alternating between arms, and the need to scrub above the elbow. Antiseptic manufacturers' instructions for use convey important safety and efficacy instructions to the user. Failure to adhere to the manufacturer's instructions for use may result in harm or ineffectiveness of the surgical hand antiseptic.

IV.b.1. A standardized surgical hand antisepsis protocol using a surgical hand scrub should be performed in the following order:
1. Remove jewelry from hands and wrists (eg, rings, watches, bracelets).[3,4]
2. Don a surgical mask.[3,56]
3. If hands are visibly soiled, wash hands with soap and water.[3,4]
4. Remove debris from underneath fingernails using a disposable nail cleaner under running water.[3,4]
5. Apply the amount of surgical hand scrub product recommended by the manufacturer to the hands and forearms using a soft, nonabrasive sponge.
6. Visualize each finger, hand, and arm as having four sides. Wash all four sides

effectively, keeping the hands elevated.[3]

7. Scrub for length of time recommended by the manufacturer.[4] The scrub should be timed to allow adequate product contact with skin.[3]

8. For water conservation, turn off water when it is not in use, if possible.

9. Avoid splashing surgical attire.[3]

10. Discard sponges, if used.

11. Rinse hands and arms under running water in one direction from fingertips to elbows.[3]

12. Hold hands higher than elbows and away from surgical attire.

13. In the OR or procedure room, dry hands and arms with a sterile towel using sterile technique before donning a surgical gown and gloves.[3,56]

[1: Strong Evidence]

IV.b.2. The surgical hand scrub should not be performed using a brush.[3,4,57-59] *[1: Strong Evidence]*

Scrubbing with a brush may damage skin and increase the amount of bacteria shedding from the hands.[4] Several studies have shown that use of a brush is not necessary to reduce the number of bacteria on the hands.[3,4,57-59]

IV.c. A hand scrub sink should be located in the semi-restricted area near the entrance to the OR or procedure room.[14] One hand scrub sink with two scrub positions may serve two operating or procedure rooms if located next to the entrance to each room.[14] *[4: Limited Evidence]*

The FGI[14] recommends that hand scrub facilities be located near the entrance of each cesarean delivery, trauma, operating, interventional imaging procedure, and procedure room in hospitals, outpatient facilities, and office-based surgery settings.

IV.d. Hand scrub sinks should have foot, knee, or electronic sensor controls.[14] When the operation of the scrub sink is dependent on the building electrical service, the controls should be connected to the essential electrical system.[14] *[4: Limited Evidence]*

Operating the scrub sink with hands-free controls allows perioperative team members to maintain sterile technique during surgical hand antisepsis. The FGI[14] recommends that hand scrub sinks have foot, knee, or electronic sensor controls.

IV.e. Perioperative team members should receive education and complete competency verification activities that address performance of surgical hand antisepsis in accordance with the product manufacturer's instructions for use. *[5: Benefits Balanced with Harms]*

Two studies found that misuse of a surgical hand rub product may have contributed to an increase in SSI rates and that peer education in a skills lab may increase compliance with a surgical hand antisepsis protocol.[60,61]

Haessler et al[60] described an investigation of an SSI cluster at an academic, Level 1 trauma, tertiary care medical center. As part of the investigation, direct observations of surgical hand antisepsis, including scrub and alcohol rub products, were performed. Observers noted inadequate pre-washing when required (eg, for soiled hands), lack of use of a nail pick, and incorrect application of the alcohol surgical hand rub product. Interviews revealed that the surgeons lacked understanding about correct alcohol rub product usage. After the product being misused was removed and the surgeons received education on proper surgical hand antisepsis technique, the SSI rate returned to a level at or below the medical center's historical rates.

In a pilot study, Fichtner et al[61] studied the effect of a skills lab on the surgical hand scrubbing compliance of fourth year medical students (N = 161) in Germany. Students randomly assigned to the intervention group underwent a 45-minute standardized peer training session of practical competencies on surgical hand scrubbing according to the European standard EN1500. Compliance was measured by hand coverage with a fluorescent surgical hand scrub antiseptic. The researchers found that the intervention group (n = 80) had significantly better hand coverage than the control group (n = 81), which received training after the test.

IV.e.1. Education and competency verification should be performed when new surgical hand antiseptic products or processes are introduced. *[5: Benefits Balanced with Harms]*

Recommendation V

A multidisciplinary team should select hand hygiene products to be used in the perioperative setting following an analysis of product effectiveness, user acceptance, and cost.[3]

The WHO[3] recommends that a multidisciplinary team evaluate the antimicrobial efficacy, user acceptance, and cost during the selection of hand hygiene products.

V.a. The multidisciplinary team should include the infection prevention committee or designated authority with specialized knowledge in infection prevention. Committee representatives should include perioperative RNs and other perioperative team members. *[5: Benefits Balanced with Harms]*

Members of the infection prevention committee have specialized knowledge in the selection of hand hygiene products.

V.b. The multidisciplinary team should develop a mechanism for product evaluation and selection of hand hygiene products.[62] *[2: High Evidence]*

Developing a mechanism for hand hygiene product selection provides a structured process for product evaluation by the health care organization.

V.c. The multidisciplinary team should evaluate the safety and efficacy of hand hygiene products.[3,4] *[1: Strong Evidence]*

The WHO[3] and the CDC[4] recommend evaluating the safety and efficacy of hand hygiene products during the product selection process.

In a systematic review, Tanner et al[2] found that no one surgical hand antiseptic was more effective than another for preventing surgical site infection. The evidence involving surgical hand antiseptic efficacy conflicts. Some research indicates that alcohol-based antiseptics may be more effective for reducing bacterial counts on hands than aqueous-based solutions.[2,63-67] However, some studies have found that aqueous-based solutions are as effective as alcohol-based antiseptics for reducing bacterial counts.[68,69] Some of these studies indicated a preference for alcohol-based antiseptics because of efficiency and user acceptance.[70,71]

The evidence on the effectiveness of chlorhexidine gluconate (CHG) in surgical hand antiseptics also conflicts. Research indicates that aqueous CHG scrubs may reduce bacterial counts on hands more effectively than aqueous povidone iodine.[2,72] With regard to alcohol-based CHG products, some research indicates that alcohol combined with CHG is superior to other alcohol-based surgical hand antiseptics.[67,73] However, some researchers found that other alcohol-based antiseptics were equally or more effective than the alcohol-and-CHG combination surgical hand antiseptics.[74,75]

Tanner et al[2] found the available evidence on surgical hand antisepsis to be of low quality. Another limitation of some evidence, as described in a laboratory study by Kampf et al,[76] is that studies assessing the efficacy of CHG without using neutralizing agents in the culture sampling fluid may be flawed by overestimating efficacy.

With a gap in the evidence to guide practice, decisions about which surgical hand antiseptic to select for use in the practice setting are complex. This is an unresolved issue that warrants additional research. A variety of products may be necessary to meet the needs of various perioperative team members with skin sensitivities and allergies. Input from a multidisciplinary team with diverse experience and knowledge of hand antiseptics is helpful during review of research, clinical guidelines, and literature from the product manufacturers.

V.c.1. The multidisciplinary team should select products for hand hygiene and surgical hand antisepsis that meet US Food and Drug Administration (FDA) requirements.[77] *[5: Benefits Balanced with Harms]*

The FDA approval process includes evaluation of product efficacy and safety. For efficacy, the FDA requires surgical hand antiseptic products to be fast acting (ie, within 1 minute), broad spectrum, and persistent (ie, no return to baseline flora count at 6 hours post application).[77,78] Health care hand wash or rub products must reduce the bacteria on the hands within 5 minutes.[77,78] The FDA approval process also includes evaluating the safety of hand hygiene and surgical hand antiseptics by reviewing human safety studies (eg, maximal use trials), nonclinical safety studies (eg, developmental and reproductive toxicity studies, carcinogenicity studies), data to characterize hormonal effects, and data to evaluate the development of antimicrobial resistance.[77,78]

The FDA currently categorizes active ingredients in the 1994 Tentative Final Monograph (TFM) for hand antiseptic products as either Category I, II, or III.[77]

- Category I means that the product is generally recognized as safe and effective;
- Category II means that the product is not generally recognized as safe and effective; and
- Category III means that available data is insufficient to classify the product as safe and effective, and additional testing is required.

Due to the availability of advanced understanding in safety and efficacy testing methods, however, in a 2015 proposed rule to finalize the TFM by 2018, the FDA requested additional scientific evidence from manufacturers to evaluate whether the ingredients in certain antiseptic products are safe and effective.[78] Thus, the proposed rule categorizes all the antiseptics as IIISE, until the FDA has received all requested safety and efficacy data for each antiseptic. While the FDA gathers scientific evidence from the manufacturers, they recommend that health care personnel continue to use health care antiseptics to maintain a standard of care to prevent patient infection.[79]

The proposed rule also recommended changes to the FDA clinical simulation testing efficacy requirements for health care personnel hand wash or rub and surgical hand scrub or rub.[78] Table 2 provides a summary of the TFM and proposed rule clinical simulation testing protocols and efficacy requirements.

HAND HYGIENE

Product	Testing Method	1994 Tentative Final Monograph	Proposed Rule
Hand wash or rub	ASTM E-1174 • Artificial contamination with *Serratia marcescens* and *Escherichia coli* • Test solution applied to hands and lower 1/3 of forearms for 30 seconds and rinsed with water • Sterile loose fitting gloves donned and secured at wrist, 75 mL of eluent added and kneaded for 1 minute, and eluate cultured for bacteria	1st wash • 2 $\log_{10}$ reduction, each hand, within 5 minutes 10th wash • 3 $\log_{10}$ reduction, each hand, within 5 minutes	Single wash or rub • 2.5 $\log_{10}$ reduction, each hand, within 5 minutes
Surgical hand scrub or rub	ASTM E-1115 • No artificial contamination, resident skin flora • Volunteer cleans under fingernails with nail stick, clips fingernails, and removes all jewelry from the hands and arms • Hands and lower 2/3 of forearms rinsed with water for 30 seconds, washed with non-antimicrobial soap for 30 seconds, and rinsed with water for 30 seconds • Test solution is applied per manufacturer's instructions • Sterile loose fitting gloves donned and secured at wrist, 75 mL of eluent added and kneaded for 1 minute, and eluate cultured for bacteria	1st wash, Day 1 • 1 $\log_{10}$ reduction, each hand, within 1 minute • Does not exceed baseline at 6 hours Day 2 • 2 $\log_{10}$ reduction, each hand, within 1 minute Last wash, Day 5 • 3 $\log_{10}$ reduction, each hand, within 1 minute	Single wash or rub • 2 $\log_{10}$ reduction, each hand, within 1 minute • Does not exceed baseline at 6 hours

TABLE 2. US FOOD AND DRUG ADMINISTRATION CLINICAL SIMULATION TESTING PROTOCOL[1,2]

REFERENCES

1. *US Food and Drug Administration. Tentative final monograph for healthcare antiseptic drug products proposed rule. Fed Regist. 1994;59(116):31402-31452.*
2. *CFR part 310 safety and effectiveness of health care antiseptics; topical antimicrobial drug products for over-the-counter human use; proposed amendment of the tentative final monograph; reopening of administrative record; proposed rule. Fed Regist. 2015;80(84):25166-25205.*

A limitation of using FDA testing requirements as a tool for evaluating product safety and efficacy is that the FDA testing protocols are based on simulation with volunteers in the laboratory setting. The laboratory protocols may not accurately reflect actual use of hand wash and surgical hand scrub or rub products in the clinical setting.[3,4] Further research is needed to determine the generalizability of these studies and protocols to the clinical setting.

V.c.2. Non-antimicrobial and antimicrobial soaps may be selected for evaluation. *[1: Strong Evidence]*

The CDC[4] and the SHEA/IDSA[1] recommend using either non-antimicrobial or antimicrobial soaps in the health care setting.

V.c.3. Soaps containing triclosan should not be selected for evaluation.[1] *[1: Strong Evidence]*

The SHEA/IDSA[1] recommends avoiding use of soaps containing the antiseptic triclosan in the health care setting due to an assessment of benefits and harms. Evidence is lacking to establish clinical benefit from use of triclosan compared to other antiseptics. The harms of triclosan may include environmental contamination and the potential for development of bacterial resistance.[1] Further research is needed to assess the benefits and harms of triclosan use in the perioperative setting.

V.d. The multidisciplinary team should evaluate the compatibility of hand hygiene products with skin care products (eg, lotions, moisturizers) and types of gloves used at the facility.[3, *[1: Strong Evidence]*

The WHO[3] and the CDC[4] recommend reviewing information from the manufacturer regarding any known interactions between products used to clean hands, skin care products, and gloves. Oil-containing lotions have been associated with altered integrity of latex rubber gloves, reduced persistent effects of hand antiseptics, and bacterial contamination of the lotion.[3,4]

V.e. Cost of hand hygiene products should be evaluated, but cost should not be the primary factor for selection.[3,4] *[1: Strong Evidence]*

The WHO[3] and the CDC[4] recommend evaluating cost during the selection of hand hygiene products. However, both organizations emphasize the importance of product effectiveness and user acceptance over cost.

ASEPTIC PRACTICE

V.f. End-user evaluations should be conducted to determine acceptability of the hand hygiene and skin care products to perioperative team members.[1,3,4] *[1: Strong Evidence]*

Acceptability of hand hygiene products is a key factor that influences health care personnel compliance with hand hygiene.[1,3,4] The WHO,[3] the CDC,[4] and the SHEA/IDSA[1] recommend involving health care personnel in the choice of hand hygiene and skin care products.

V.f.1. The multidisciplinary team should determine the time frame and season for end-user evaluation of hand hygiene products. When more than one product is evaluated, the multidisciplinary team should establish a mechanism for a time period between product evaluations.[3] *[1: Strong Evidence]*

The WHO[3] recommends end-user evaluation for at least 2 to 3 weeks, although a fast-track method has also been validated. When more than one product is being evaluated, the WHO[3] recommends either a period of routine product use or a 2-day period between product evaluations when feasible.

The WHO[3] recommends avoiding the testing of new hand hygiene products during seasons of low humidity because health care personnel may have more skin reactions in this weather and the results of the end-user evaluation could be affected by this seasonal variation. In a European field study, Girard et al[80] investigated factors that influenced the testing of alcohol-based hand rubs and found that test periods during colder seasons were significantly associated with skin reactions.

V.f.2. End-user evaluations should include
- skin tolerance,
- skin reactions,
- ease of use (eg, volume, dry time),
- feel (eg, consistency, texture),
- color, and
- fragrance.[3,4]

[1: Strong Evidence]

As part of the end-user evaluations, the WHO[3] and the CDC[4] recommend that skin tolerance, skin reactions, ease of use, and the aesthetic preferences (ie, fragrance, color, texture) of health care personnel be considered in the selection of hand hygiene products.

V.f.3. Patients should be included in end-user evaluations of hand hygiene products.[3] *[1: Strong Evidence]*

The WHO[3] recommends that the patient's aesthetic preferences (ie, fragrance, color, texture, ease of use) be considered in the selection of hand hygiene products. Patients may be especially sensitive to the fragrance of hand hygiene products.[3]

V.f.4. End-user evaluations should be written and reviewed by the multidisciplinary team. *[5: Benefits Balanced with Harms]*

Written questionnaires or evaluations provide the multidisciplinary team with data to assess acceptability to end-users.

V.g. Hand hygiene product dispensers (eg, wall-mounted, table-top, personal) should be evaluated for adequate, reliable function and delivery of the recommended product volume.[3,4] *[1: Strong Evidence]*

The WHO[3] and the CDC[4] recommend evaluating hand hygiene product dispensers for adequate and reliable function in the delivery of hand hygiene products.

V.g.1. The multidisciplinary team may evaluate automated wall-mounted dispensers.[3] *[5: Benefits Balanced with Harms]*

The evidence is inconclusive regarding the benefits of automated wall-mounted dispensers. The theoretical benefit of automated wall-mounted dispensers is that they can be used without being touched and potentially contaminating the hands of the perioperative team member.[3] The German and Austrian Society for Hospital Hygiene[81] requires that hand hygiene dispensers be triggered without using hands, operated either by a sensor or an elbow.

In an observational study, Assadian et al[82] cultured 17 hand sanitizer dispensers in a 12-bed intensive care unit at an urban teaching hospital. The dispensers were disinfected on a daily basis. This study found that all dispensers were contaminated with bacteria, both from common skin flora and gram-negative bacteria, and that contamination was greatest on the lever. The results of this study implicate hand sanitizer dispensers as potential reservoirs for bacteria in the health care environment. The researchers recommended cleaning the dispensers to reduce contamination and suggested that automated or pedal-operated dispensers may reduce the risk of dispenser contamination. A limitation of this study is that it was not designed to evaluate the effect of disinfection on contamination. Another limitation is that the small sample size may limit the generalizability of the study findings.

The WHO[3] discusses that the downside to automated wall-mounted dispensers is that they have a higher chance for malfunction and are more expensive to maintain than non-automated dispensers.

Further research is needed to determine the effect of contaminated dispensers on hand hygiene effectiveness, the best method for preventing contamination of hand hygiene product dispensers, and the optimal method for dispensing hand hygiene products.

V.g.2. Dispensers of alcohol-based hand hygiene products should
- not release products except when the dispenser is activated,
- only activate when an object is placed within 4 inches of the sensor,
- only activate once when an object is left in place in the activation zone,
- not dispense more product than the amount recommended by the manufacturer for hand hygiene, and
- be designed to prevent accidental or malicious activation of the dispenser.[44]

[4: Limited Evidence]

Recommendation VI

Perioperative personnel should participate in a variety of quality assurance and performance improvement activities that are consistent with the facility or health care organization plan to improve understanding and compliance with the principles and processes of hand hygiene.

Quality assurance and performance improvement programs assist in evaluating and improving the quality of patient care and formulating plans for corrective action. These programs provide data that may be used to determine whether an individual organization is within benchmark goals and, if not, to identify areas that may require corrective action.

VI.a. Barriers for performing hand hygiene in the perioperative setting should be identified and addressed through interventions to improve hand hygiene compliance.[1] [1: Strong Evidence]

Identifying barriers to hand hygiene allows the health care organization to develop relevant interventions to improve hand hygiene compliance.[1] The SHEA/IDSA[1] recommends identifying unit-specific barriers and creating interventions specific to the unit's needs.

VI.b. The health care organization should monitor adherence to policies and procedures for hand hygiene as part of quality assurance and process improvement initiatives.[1,3,4] [1: Strong Evidence]

Professional organizations recommend monitoring health care personnel adherence to recommended hand hygiene practices.[1,3,4] According to the WHO,[3] monitoring hand hygiene adherence as a performance indicator serves several functions including system monitoring, incentive for performance improvement, outbreak investigation, and infrastructure design.

VI.b.1. Hand hygiene in the perioperative setting should be measured by direct observation.[1,3,4,83] [1: Strong Evidence]

The SHEA/IDSA[83] recommends performing direct observation audits of hand hygiene in the perioperative setting as a strategy to prevent SSIs. The authors of several studies and organizational experience reports monitored hand hygiene compliance in the perioperative setting using direct observation.[24,25,28,30,32-34,36,50,52,54,84] Limitations of direct observation are the risk for selection and observer bias[3] and that the method is subject to the Hawthorne effect. Direct observation audits are performed by a human observer, either in person or by video recording, which can be labor intensive. Video observations may be beneficial in the perioperative setting due to the high number of hand hygiene indications and numerous perioperative team members. However, video observations may also compromise patient privacy.[1]

Rowlands et al[26] used video observations of anesthesia professionals to evaluate hand hygiene compliance with WHO criteria. Three perioperative team members (ie, an anesthesiologist, an anesthesiology resident, and a perioperative RN) reviewed the videos independently. The researchers found that hand hygiene compliance in the anesthesia work area was low and that compliance with current hand hygiene guidelines was not feasible. A limitation of the study was that the perioperative team being observed was aware of the recording, which could have biased the observations by creating a Hawthorne effect.

VI.b.2. Other measures to evaluate hand hygiene practices may include product usage or automated monitoring.[1,3,4] [1: Strong Evidence]

Measuring product usage, such as of alcohol-based hand rub products, provides an indicator of overall hand hygiene activity.[3] However, this method does not reliably measure hand hygiene based on opportunities,[1,3] and the CDC-recommended measurement of product volume usage per 1,000 patient-days[4] is not a perioperative indicator of patient volume. This evidence review found no literature to support or refute the use of product usage measurement as a hand hygiene indicator in the perioperative setting.

Automated hand hygiene monitoring is an emerging technology that may detect hand hygiene opportunities within the patient encounter.[1,3] The evidence review found no literature to support or refute the use of automated hand hygiene monitoring systems in the perioperative setting.

VI.b.3. Feedback on hand hygiene performance should be provided to perioperative team members.[1,3,4] [1: Strong Evidence]

Professional organizations[1,3,4] recommend providing health care personnel with performance feedback when monitoring adherence to hand hygiene practices.

VI.c. Patients and visitors should be encouraged to remind perioperative team members to perform hand hygiene before care.[1,3,4,85] *[1: Strong Evidence]*

The collective evidence and guidance from professional organizations support encouraging patients and their family members to remind health care personnel to clean their hands before care episodes.[1,3,4,85] The WHO[3] recommends a structured approach to incorporating patient engagement into the hand hygiene promotion strategy, including developing ownership and shared responsibility for the program at the health care organization, reviewing existing empowerment programs, and developing the program based on organization-specific factors such as culture, program implementation, and evaluation.

The WHO[3] conducted a global survey of patient experiences with hand hygiene (N = 459) and found that 29% of respondents had asked health care personnel to wash their hands, and 25% reported receiving a negative response to the request. The survey found that patients were more likely to feel comfortable reminding health care personnel to wash their hands when encouraged by health care personnel. Patients with direct experience of a health care-associated infection were more likely to question the health care personnel.

In another patient survey, Ottum et al[85] surveyed 200 patient respondents (response rate 94.78%) about their comfort in reminding health care personnel to perform hand hygiene. The study found that 99.5% of patients surveyed believed that personnel were supposed to wash their hands before and after care and that 90.5% believed in reminding health care personnel to wash their hands only if they forgot. However, only 14% of patients reported having asked personnel to wash their hands, with 64% comfortable reminding nurses and 54% comfortable reminding physicians. Patients who had worked in health care were significantly more likely to be comfortable asking personnel to wash their hands than patients who had not worked in health care. The implications of these findings are that the baseline beliefs of the patients about the importance of hand hygiene were universally high, which suggests that more education would be unlikely to empower their participation further. Thus, the researchers recommended focusing interventions on making patients more comfortable with asking health care personnel to wash their hands.

Editor's note: *Shellac is a registered trademark of Creative Nail Design, Inc, San Diego, CA.*

Glossary

Alcohol-based hand rub: An alcohol-containing preparation (eg, liquid, gel, foam) designed for application to the hands to inactivate microorganisms and temporarily suppress their growth.

Antimicrobial soap: Soap containing an antiseptic at a concentration sufficient to inactivate microorganisms and temporarily suppress their growth.

Artificial nails: Substances or devices applied or added to the natural nails to augment or enhance the wearer's own nails. They include, but are not limited to, bonding, extensions, tips, wraps, gel and acrylic overlays, and tapes.

Eluent: A solvent used for separating material from a surface.

Glove juice method: A method for culturing the hands that involves donning a sterile glove, instilling an eluent solution into the glove, securing the glove at the wrist, kneading the gloved hand in a standardized manner for 60 seconds, and extracting the eluent fluid (glove juice) for culture.

Hand hygiene: Any activities related to hand condition and cleansing.

Hand washing station: An area that includes a sink, a hands-free faucet, cleansing solutions, and a means for drying the hands.

Invasive procedure: The surgical entry into tissues, cavities, or organs or the repair of major trauma injuries.

Surgical hand antisepsis: Hand wash or hand rub using a surgical hand antiseptic, performed preoperatively by the surgical team to remove transient flora and reduce resident skin flora.

Surgical hand antiseptic: A product that is a broad-spectrum, fast-acting, and nonirritating preparation containing an antimicrobial ingredient designed to significantly reduce the number of microorganisms on intact skin. Surgical hand antiseptic agents demonstrate both persistent and cumulative activity.

Ultraviolet-cured nail polish: Nail polish created by polymerization of a methacrylate or acrylate that hardens when exposed to ultraviolet (UVA) light.

REFERENCES

1. Ellingson K, Haas JP, Aiello AE, et al. Strategies to prevent healthcare-associated infections through hand hygiene. *Infect Control Hosp Epidemiol.* 2014;35(8):937-960. [IVA]

2. Tanner J, Dumville JC, Norman G, Fortnam M. Surgical hand antisepsis to reduce surgical site infection. *Cochrane Database Syst Rev.* 2016;1:CD004288. [IB]

3. *WHO Guidelines on Hand Hygiene in Health Care.* Geneva, Switzerland: World Health Organization; 2009. [IVA]

4. Boyce JM, Pittet D; Healthcare Infection Control Practices Advisory Committee. Society for Healthcare Epidemiology of America. Association for Professionals in Infection Control. Infectious Diseases Society of America. Hand Hygiene Task Force. Guideline for Hand Hygiene in Health-Care Settings: recommendations of the Healthcare Infection Control Practices Advisory Committee and the HICPAC/SHEA/APIC/IDSA Hand Hygiene Task Force.

Infect Control Hosp Epidemiol. 2002;23(12 Suppl):S3-S40. [IVA]

5. *Surgical Site Infection: Evidence Update June 2013* [Evidence Update 43]. Manchester, United Kingdom: National Institute for Health and Care Excellence; 2013. [IVA]

6. Fagernes M, Lingaas E. Factors interfering with the microflora on hands: a regression analysis of samples from 465 healthcare workers. *J Adv Nurs.* 2011;67(2):297-307. [IIIB]

7. Rupp ME, Fitzgerald T, Puumala S, et al. Prospective, controlled, cross-over trial of alcohol-based hand gel in critical care units. *Infect Control Hosp Epidemiol.* 2008;29(1):8-15. [IIB]

8. Hautemaniere A, Cunat L, Diguio N, et al. Factors determining poor practice in alcoholic gel hand rub technique in hospital workers. *J Infect Public Health.* 2010;3(1):25-34. [IIB]

9. *AST Standards of Practice for Surgical Attire, Surgical Scrub, Hand Hygiene and Hand Washing.* April 13, 2008. Association of Surgical Technologists. http://www.ast.org/uploadedFiles/Main_Site/Content/About_Us/Standard_Surgical_Attire_Surgical_Scrub.pdf. Accessed June 27, 2016. [IVC]

10. *Infection Prevention and Control Guidelines for Anesthesia Care.* 2015. American Association of Nurse Anesthetists. http://www.aana.com/resources2/professionalpractice/Pages/Infection-Prevention-and-Control-Guidelines-for-Anesthesia-Care.aspx. Accessed June 27, 2016. [IVB]

11. Arrowsmith VA, Taylor R. Removal of nail polish and finger rings to prevent surgical infection. *Cochrane Database Syst Rev.* 2014;8:CD003325. [IC]

12. Van Der Meer EWC, Boot CRL, Van Der Gulden JWJ, et al. Hands4U: The effects of a multifaceted implementation strategy on hand eczema prevalence in a healthcare setting. Results of a randomized controlled trial. *Contact Derm.* 2015;72(5):312-324. [IB]

13. Harnoss JC, Brune L, Ansorg J, Heidecke C-D, Assadian O, Kramer A. Practice of skin protection and skin care among German surgeons and influence on the efficacy of surgical hand disinfection and surgical glove perforation. *BMC Infect Dis.* 2014;14:315. [IB]

14. Facility Guidelines Institute, US Department of Health and Human Services, American Society for Healthcare Engineering. *Guidelines for Design and Construction of Hospitals and Outpatient Facilities.* Chicago, IL: American Society for Healthcare Engineering of the American Hospital Association; 2014. [IVC]

15. Guideline for prevention of transmissible infections. In: *Guidelines for Perioperative Practice.* Denver, CO: AORN, Inc; 2016:471-506. [IVA]

16. Bolyard EA, Tablan OC, Williams WW, Pearson ML, Shapiro CN, Deitchmann SD. Guideline for infection control in healthcare personnel, 1998. Hospital Infection Control Practices Advisory Committee. *Infect Control Hosp Epidemiol.* 1998;19(6):407-463. [IVA]

17. Henderson DK, Dembry L, Fishman NO, et al. SHEA guideline for management of healthcare workers who are infected with hepatitis B virus, hepatitis C virus, and/or human immunodeficiency virus. *Infect Control Hosp Epidemiol.* 2010;31(3):203-232. [IVA]

18. Guideline for surgical attire. In: *Guidelines for Perioperative Practice.* Denver, CO: AORN, Inc; 2016:95-118. [IVA]

19. Loftus RW, Muffly MK, Brown JR, et al. Hand contamination of anesthesia providers is an important risk factor for intraoperative bacterial transmission. *Anesth Analg.* 2011;112(1):98-105. [IIIA]

20. Mermel LA, Bert A, Chapin KC, LeBlanc L. Intraoperative stopcock and manifold colonization of newly inserted peripheral intravenous catheters. *Infect Control Hosp Epidemiol.* 2014;35(9):1187-1189. [IIIB]

21. Loftus RW, Brown JR, Koff MD, et al. Multiple reservoirs contribute to intraoperative bacterial transmission. *Anesth Analg.* 2012;114(6):1236-1248. [IIIA]

22. Cosgrove MS. Infection control in the operating room. *Crit Care Nurs Clin North Am.* 2015;27(1):79-87. [VB]

23. Munoz-Price LS, Birnbach DJ. Hand hygiene and anesthesiology. *Int Anesthesiol Clin.* 2013;51(1):79-92. [VA]

24. Munoz-Price LS, Lubarsky DA, Arheart KL, et al. Interactions between anesthesiologists and the environment while providing anesthesia care in the operating room. *Am J Infect Control.* 2013;41(10):922-924. [VA]

25. Munoz-Price LS, Riley B, Banks S, et al. Frequency of interactions and hand disinfections among anesthesiologists while providing anesthesia care in the operating room: induction versus maintenance. *Infect Control Hosp Epidemiol.* 2014;35(8):1056-1059. [IIIB]

26. Rowlands J, Yeager MP, Beach M, Patel HM, Huysman BC, Loftus RW. Video observation to map hand contact and bacterial transmission in operating rooms. *Am J Infect Control.* 2014;42(7):698-701. [IIIA]

27. Allen G. Hand hygiene and the surgical team. *Perioper Nurs Clin.* 2010;5(4):411-418. [VA]

28. Krediet AC, Kalkman CJ, Bonten MJ, Gigengack ACM, Barach P. Hand-hygiene practices in the operating theatre: an observational study. *Br J Anaesth.* 2011;107(4):553-558. [IIIB]

29. Fernandez PG, Loftus RW, Dodds TM, et al. Hand hygiene knowledge and perceptions among anesthesia providers. *Anesth Analg.* 2015;120(4):837-843. [IIIA]

30. Biddle C, Shah J. Quantification of anesthesia providers' hand hygiene in a busy metropolitan operating room: what would Semmelweis think? *Am J Infect Control.* 2012;40(8):756-759. [IIIB]

31. O'Grady NP, Alexander M, Burns LA, et al. Guidelines for the prevention of intravascular catheter-related infections. *Am J Infect Control.* 2011;39(4 Suppl 1):S1-S34. [IVA]

32. Sahni N, Biswal M, Gandhi K, Yaddanapudi S. Quantification of hand hygiene compliance in anesthesia providers at a tertiary care center in northern India. *Am J Infect Control.* 2015;43(10):1134-1136. [VB]

33. Bellaard-Smith ER, Gillespie EE. Implementing hand hygiene strategies in the operating suite. *Health Infect.* 2012;17(1):33-37. [VA]

34. Megeus V, Nilsson K, Karlsson J, Eriksson BI, Andersson AE. Hand hygiene and aseptic techniques during routine anesthetic care—observations in the operating room. *Antimicrob Resist Infect Control.* 2015;4(1):5. [IIIB]

35. Gould CV, Umscheid CA, Agarwal RK, Kuntz G, Pegues DA; Healthcare Infection Control Practices Advisory Committee. Guideline for prevention of catheter-associated urinary tract infections 2009. *Infect Control Hosp Epidemiol.* 2010;31(4):319-326. [IVA]

36. Andersson AE, Bergh I, Karlsson J, Eriksson BI, Nilsson K. The application of evidence-based measures to reduce surgical site infections during orthopedic surgery—report of a single-center experience in Sweden. *Patient Saf Surg.* 2012;6(1):11. [IIIB]

37. American Society of Anesthesiologists Task Force on Infectious Complications Associated with Neuraxial Techniques. Practice advisory for the prevention, diagnosis, and management of infectious complications associated with neuraxial techniques: a report by the American

Society of Anesthesiologists Task Force on Infectious Complications Associated with Neuraxial Techniques. *Anesthesiology.* 2010;112(3):530-545. [IVB]

38. Jochum D, Iohom G, Bouaziz H. Asepsis in regional anesthesia. *Int Anesthesiol Clin.* 2010;48(4):35-44. [VB]

39. Guideline for environmental cleaning. In: *Guidelines for Perioperative Practice.* Denver, CO: AORN, Inc; 2016:7-28. [IVA]

40. Birnbach DJ, Rosen LF, Fitzpatrick M, Carling P, Arheart KL, Munoz-Price LS. Double gloves: a randomized trial to evaluate a simple strategy to reduce contamination in the operating room. *Anesth Analg.* 2015;120(4):848-852. [IB]

41. Birnbach DJ, Rosen LF, Fitzpatrick M, Carling P, Arheart KL, Munoz-Price LS. A new approach to pathogen containment in the operating room: sheathing the laryngoscope after intubation. *Anesth Analg.* 2015;121(5):1209-1214. [IB]

42. *State Operations Manual Appendix A—Survey Protocol, Regulations and Interpretive Guidelines for Hospitals.* Rev 151; 2015. Centers for Medicare & Medicaid Services. https://www.cms.gov/Regulations-and-Guidance/Guidance/Manuals/downloads/som107ap_a_hospitals.pdf. Accessed June 27, 2016.

43. Guideline for a safe environment of care, part 1. In: *Guidelines for Perioperative Practice.* Denver, CO: AORN, Inc; 2016:237-262. [IVA]

44. *NFPA 101: Life Safety Code.* Quincy, MA: National Fire Protection Association; 2015.[IVC]

45. *State Operations Manual Appendix L—Guidance for Surveyors: Ambulatory Surgical Centers.* Rev 137; 2015. Centers for Medicare & Medicaid Services. https://www.cms.gov/Regulations-and-Guidance/Guidance/Manuals/downloads/som107ap_l_ambulatory.pdf. Accessed June 27, 2016.

46. Petty WC. Closing the hand hygiene gap in the postanesthesia care unit: a body-worn alcohol-based dispenser. *J Perianesth Nurs.* 2013;28(2):87-97. [VB]

47. Loftus RW, Koff MD, Birnbach DJ. The dynamics and implications of bacterial transmission events arising from the anesthesia work area. *Anesth Analg.* 2015;120(4):853-860. [VA]

48. Koff MD, Loftus RW, Burchman CC, et al. Reduction in intraoperative bacterial contamination of peripheral intravenous tubing through the use of a novel device. *Anesthesiology.* 2009;110(5):978-985. [IB]

49. Gould DJ, Moralejo D, Drey N, Chudleigh JH. Interventions to improve hand hygiene compliance in patient care. *Cochrane Database Syst Rev.* 2010;9:CD005186. [IIC]

50. Santos LX, Souza Dias MB, Borrasca VL, et al. Improving hand hygiene adherence in an endoscopy unit. *Endoscopy.* 2013;45(6):421-425. [VA]

51. Elkaradawy SA, Helaly GF, Abdel Wahab MM. Effect of an infection control educational programme on anaesthetists' attitude and anaesthetic field bacterial contamination. *Egypt J Anaesth.* 2012;28(2):149-156. [IIA]

52. Swenne CL, Alexandrén K. Surgical team members' compliance with and knowledge of basic hand hygiene guidelines and intraoperative hygiene. *J Infect Prev.* 2012;13(4):114-119. [IIIB]

53. Pan S-C, Chen E, Tien K-L, et al. Assessing the thoroughness of hand hygiene: "Seeing is believing." *Am J Infect Control.* 2014;42(7):799-801. [IIA]

54. Jericho BG, Kalin AM, Schwartz DE. Improving hand hygiene compliance by incorporating it into the verification process in the operating room. *Internet J Anesthesiol.* 2013;32(3):2. [VA]

55. Adams AB. Surgical hand antisepsis: where we have been and where we are today. *Perioper Nurs Clin.* 2010;5(4):443-448. [VB]

56. Guideline for sterile technique. In: *Guidelines for Perioperative Practice.* Denver, CO: AORN, Inc; 2016:65-94. [IVA]

57. Abdelatiff DA, El-Haiyk KS, Ghobashi NH, El-Qudaa RF, El-Sabouni RS. Comparing of using sterile brush during surgical scrubbing versus brushless for surgical team in operating room. *Life Sci J.* 2014;11(1):387-393. [IC]

58. da Cunha ÉR, Matos FGOA, da Silva AM, de Araújo EAC, Ferreira KASL, Graziano KU. The efficacy of three hand asepsis techniques using chlorhexidine gluconate (CHG 2%). *Rev Esc Enferm USP.* 2011;45(6):1440-1445. [IIB]

59. Okgün Alcan A, Demir Korkmaz F. Comparison of the efficiency of nail pick and brush used for nail cleaning during surgical scrub on reducing bacterial counts. *Am J Infect Control.* 2012;40(9):826-829. [IB]

60. Haessler S, Connelly NR, Kanter G, et al. A surgical site infection cluster: the process and outcome of an investigation—the impact of an alcohol-based surgical antisepsis product and human behavior. *Anesth Analg.* 2010;110(4):1044-1048. [VB]

61. Fichtner A, Haupt E, Karwath T, Wullenk K, Pöhlmann C, Jatzwauk L. A single standardized practical training for surgical scrubbing according to EN1500: effect quantification, value of the standardized method and comparison with clinical reference groups. *GMS Z Med Ausbild.* 2013;30(2):Doc24. [IC]

62. Guideline for product selection. In: *Guidelines for Perioperative Practice.* Denver, CO: AORN, Inc; 2016:177-184. [IVB]

63. Barbadoro P, Martini E, Savini S, et al. Invivo comparative efficacy of three surgical hand preparation agents in reducing bacterial count. *J Hosp Infect.* 2014;86(1):64-67. [IIC]

64. Shen N-J, Pan S-C, Sheng W-H, et al. Comparative antimicrobial efficacy of alcohol-based hand rub and conventional surgical scrub in a medical center. *J Microbiol Immunol Infect.* 2015;48(3):322-328. [IIIB]

65. Lai KW, Foo TL, Low W, Naidu G. Surgical hand antisepsis—a pilot study comparing povidone iodine hand scrub and alcohol-based chlorhexidine gluconate hand rub. *Ann Acad Med Singapore.* 2012;41(1):12-16. [IIC]

66. Chen S-H, Chou C-Y, Huang J-C, Tang Y-F, Kuo Y-R, Chien L-Y. Antibacterial effects on dry-fast and traditional water-based surgical scrubbing methods: a two-time points experimental study. *Nurs Health Sci.* 2014;16(2):179-185. [IIB]

67. Hamed Mahmoud M, Morad Asaad A, Ansar Qureshi M. Hand rubbing and scrubbing in relation to microbial count among surgical team members in a Saudi hospital. *Life Sci J.* 2013;10(3):198-205. [IIB]

68. Ghorbani A, Shahrokhi A, Soltani Z, Molapour A, Shafikhani M. Comparison of surgical hand scrub and alcohol surgical hand rub on reducing hand microbial burden. *J Perioper Pract.* 2012;22(2):67-70. [IC]

69. Howard JD, Jowett C, Faoagali J, McKenzie B. New method for assessing hand disinfection shows that preoperative alcohol/chlorhexidine rub is as effective as a traditional surgical scrub. *J Hosp Infect.* 2014;88(2):78-83. [IIB]

70. Chen C-F, Han C-L, Kan C-P, Chen S-G, Hung PW. Effect of surgical site infections with waterless and traditional hand scrubbing protocols on bacterial growth. *Am J Infect Control.* 2012;40(4):e15-e17. [IIC]

ASEPTIC PRACTICE

71. Weight CJ, Lee MC, Palmer JS. Avagard hand anti-sepsis vs. traditional scrub in 3600 pediatric urologic procedures. *Urology*. 2010;76(1):15-17. [IIC]

72. Jarral OA, McCormack DJ, Ibrahim S, Shipolini AR. Should surgeons scrub with chlorhexidine or iodine prior to surgery? *Interact Cardiovasc Thorac Surg*. 2011;12(6):1017-1021. [IIIB]

73. Olson LKM, Morse DJ, Duley C, Savell BK. Prospective, randomized in vivo comparison of a dual-active waterless antiseptic versus two alcohol-only waterless antiseptics for surgical hand antisepsis. *Am J Infect Control*. 2012;40(2):155-159. [IIA]

74. Macinga DR, Edmonds SL, Campbell E, McCormack RR. Comparative efficacy of alcohol-based surgical scrubs: the importance of formulation. *AORN J*. 2014;100(6):641-650. [IB]

75. Cargill DI, Roche ED, Van Der Kar CA, et al. Development of a health care personnel handwash with 6-hour persistence. *Am J Infect Control*. 2011;39(3):226-234. [IIA]

76. Kampf G, Reichel M, Hollingsworth A, Bashir M. Efficacy of surgical hand scrub products based on chlorhexidine is largely overestimated without neutralizing agents in the sampling fluid. *Am J Infect Control*. 2013;41(1):e1-e5. [IIB]

77. US Food and Drug Administration. Tentative final monograph for healthcare antiseptic drug products proposed rule. *Fed Regist*. 1994;59(116):31402-31452.

78. 21 CFR Part 310. Safety and effectiveness of health care antiseptics; topical antimicrobial drug products for over-the-counter human use; proposed amendment of the tentative final monograph; reopening of administrative record; proposed rule. *Fed Regist*. 2015;80(84):25166-25205.

79. Q&A for consumers: health care antiseptics. US Food and Drug Administration. http://www.fda.gov/Drugs/DrugSafety/InformationbyDrugClass/ucm445063.htm. Accessed June 27, 2016.

80. Girard R, Carre E, Mermet V, et al. Factors influencing field testing of alcohol-based hand rubs. *Infect Control Hosp Epidemiol*. 2015;36(3):302-310. [IIIB]

81. Eiref SD, Leitman IM, Riley W. Hand sanitizer dispensers and associated hospital-acquired infections: friend or fomite? *Surg Infect*. 2012;13(3):137-140. [IIIB]

82. Assadian O, Kramer A, Christiansen B, et al. Recommendations and requirements for soap and hand rub dispensers in healthcare facilities. *GMS Krankenhhyg interdiszip*. 2012;7(1):Doc03. [IVC]

83. Anderson DJ, Podgorny K, Berrios-Torres SI, et al. Strategies to prevent surgical site infections in acute care hospitals: 2014 update. *Infect Control Hosp Epidemiol*. 2014;35(6):605-627. [IVA]

84. Homa K, Kirkland KB. Determining next steps in a hand hygiene improvement initiative by examining variation in hand hygiene compliance rates. *Qual Manage Health Care*. 2011;20(2):116-121. [VB]

85. Ottum A, Sethi AK, Jacobs EA, Zerbel S, Gaines ME, Safdar N. Do patients feel comfortable asking healthcare workers to wash their hands? *Infect Control Hosp Epidemiol*. 2012;33(12):1283-1284. [IIIB]

Acknowledgements

LEAD AUTHOR
Amber Wood, MSN, RN, CNOR, CIC
Senior Perioperative Practice Specialist
AORN Nursing Department
Denver, Colorado

CONTRIBUTING AUTHOR
Ramona L. Conner, MSN, RN, CNOR
Editor-in-Chief, Guidelines for Perioperative Practice
AORN Nursing Department
Denver, Colorado

The authors and AORN thank Rodney W. Hicks, PhD, RN, FNP-BC, FAANP, Professor, Western University of Health Sciences, Pomona, California; Bernard C. Camins, MD, MSc, Associate Professor of Medicine Division of Infectious Diseases, University of Alabama at Birmingham Healthcare Epidemiologist, UAB Health System, Medical Director, UAB Hospital Employee Health and UA HSF Employee Health, Birmingham; Barbara L Nalley, MSN, CRNP, CNOR, Manager, Anne Arundel Medical Group, Annapolis, Maryland; Heather A Hohenberger, BSN, RN, CIC, CNOR, CPHQ, Quality Improvement Consultant, Perioperative Services, Indiana University Health, Indianapolis; Jocelyn M. Chalquist, BSN, RN, CNOR, Surgical Services Educator, Aurora Medical Center-Kenosha, Wisconsin; Lisa Spruce, DNP, RN, CNS-CP, ACNS, ACNP, CNOR, FAAN, Director of Evidence-based Perioperative Practice, AORN Nursing Department, Denver, Colorado; Mary C. Fearon, MSN, RN, CNOR, Perioperative Practice Specialist, AORN Nursing Department, Denver, Colorado; Jay Bowers, BSN, RN, CNOR, TNCC, Clinical Educator, WVU Health Care, Morgantown, West Virginia; Missi Merlino, MHA, RN-BC, CNOR, Staff Nurse II, Baylor Scott & White Health, Temple, Texas; Nathalie Walker, MBA, RN, CNOR, Member of the Louisiana Nursing Supply and Demand Commission, a subcommittee of the Health Works Commission of Louisiana, Metairie; and Sandy Albright, MSHM, BSN, RN, CNOR, Clinical Consultant, Cardinal Health, Dublin, Ohio, for their assistance in developing this guideline.

PUBLICATION HISTORY
Originally published May 1976, *AORN Journal*, as "Recommended practices for surgical hand scrubs."

Revised March 1978, July 1982, May 1984, October 1990. Published as proposed recommended practice August 1994.

Revised November 1998; published April 1999, *AORN Journal*. Reformatted July 2000.

Revised November 2003; published in *Standards, Recommended Practices, and Guidelines*, 2004 edition. Reprinted February 2004, *AORN Journal*.

Revised March 2009 for online publication in *Perioperative Standards and Recommended Practices*. Revised July 2009 for online publication in *Perioperative Standards and Recommended Practices*.

Minor editing revisions made in October 2009 for publication in *Perioperative Standards and Recommended Practices*, 2010 edition.

Reformatted September 2012 for publication in *Perioperative Standards and Recommended Practices*, 2013 edition.

Minor editing revisions made in November 2014 for publication in *Guidelines for Perioperative Practice*, 2015 edition, as Guideline for Hand Hygiene.

Revised September 2016 for publication in *Guidelines for Perioperative Practice* online.

GUIDELINE FOR PREOPERATIVE PATIENT SKIN ANTISEPSIS

The Guideline for Preoperative Patient Skin Antisepsis has been approved by the AORN Guidelines Advisory Board. It was presented as a proposed guideline for comments by members and others. The guideline is effective August 15, 2014. The recommendations in the guideline are intended to be achievable and represent what is believed to be an optimal level of practice. Policies and procedures will reflect variations in practice settings and/or clinical situations that determine the degree to which the guideline can be implemented. AORN recognizes the many diverse settings in which perioperative nurses practice; therefore, this guideline is adaptable to all areas where operative and other invasive procedures may be performed.

Purpose

This document provides guidance for preoperative patient skin preparation, including preoperative patient bathing; preoperative hair removal; selection of skin antiseptics; application of antiseptics; and safe handling, storage, and disposal of antiseptics.

The goal of preoperative patient skin antisepsis is to reduce the risk of the patient developing a surgical site infection (SSI) by removing soil and transient microorganisms at the surgical site.[1] Reducing the amount of bacteria on the skin near the surgical incision lowers the risk of contaminating the surgical incision site.[1] As part of preparing the skin for antisepsis, preoperative bathing and hair management at the surgical site contribute to a reduction of microorganisms on the skin.[2-4] Effective skin antiseptics rapidly and persistently remove transient microorganisms and reduce resident microorganisms to subpathogenic levels with minimal skin and tissue irritation.[1]

Perioperative registered nurses (RNs) play a critical role in developing protocols for preoperative bathing, selecting and applying preoperative patient skin antiseptics, and facilitating appropriate hair removal when necessary. The guideline provides the perioperative RN and other perioperative team members with evidence-based practice guidance for preoperative patient skin antisepsis to promote patient safety and reduce the risk of SSI.

The following topics are outside the scope of this document: patient skin antisepsis after incision; antiseptic irrigation; preoperative patient skin antisepsis with no incision; patient skin antisepsis for postoperative wound care, including suture removal; preoperative patient bathing not intended for surgical preparation; preoperative patient bathing for decolonization of *Staphylococcus aureus*; mechanical and oral antimicrobial bowel preparation; adhesive incise drapes; microbial sealants; and antimicrobial prophylaxis to reduce the microbial load on skin.

Evidence Review

A medical librarian conducted a systematic literature search of the databases MEDLINE®, CINAHL®, and the Cochrane Database of Systematic Reviews for meta-analyses, systematic reviews, randomized controlled and nonrandomized trials and studies, case reports, letters, reviews, and guidelines. Search terms included *surgical skin preparation, skin preparation, skin prep, skin antisepsis, skin antiseptic, sterile preparation, disinfectants, local anti-infective agents, antiseptic solution, preoperative care, perioperative nursing, preoperative, surgical procedures, surgical wound infection, skin, skin care, paint, scrub, antiseptic shower, antiseptic cloth, chlorhexidine wipe, preoperative shower, preoperative wash, preoperative bathing, bathing and baths, hair removal, shaving, depilation, depilatory, nonshaved, razor, clipping, clipper, povidone-iodine, chlorhexidine, iodine, iodophors, iodine compounds, 2-propanol, alcohols, baby shampoo, isopropyl alcohol, alcohol-based, parachoroxylenol, chloroxylenol, PCMX, DuraPrep, pHisoHex, Prevantics, Hibiclens, Techni-Care, ChloraPrep, Betadine, Betasept, PVP-I Prep, ExCel AP, Castile, iodophor, cyanoacrylates, tissue adhesives, chemical burns, skin diseases, dermatitis, skin sensitivity, surgical fires, fires, flammability, flammable, penis, vagina, mucous membrane, stoma, fingernails, nail polish, artificial nails, jewelry, body piercing, body jewelry,* and *subdermal implant.*

The initial search, conducted on December 5, 2013, was limited to literature published in English between January 2006 and December 2013; however, the time restriction was not considered in subsequent searches. At the time of the search, the librarian also established weekly alerts on the topics included in the search and until February 2014, presented relevant alert results to the lead author.

Before the systematic search, the medical librarian had provided the lead author with a list of the citations from the 2008 revision of the AORN Recommended Practices for Preoperative Patient Skin Antisepsis for consideration for the 2014 revision. During the development of the guideline, the lead author requested additional articles that either did not fit the original search criteria or were discovered during the evidence appraisal process. Finally, the lead author and medical librarian identified relevant guidelines

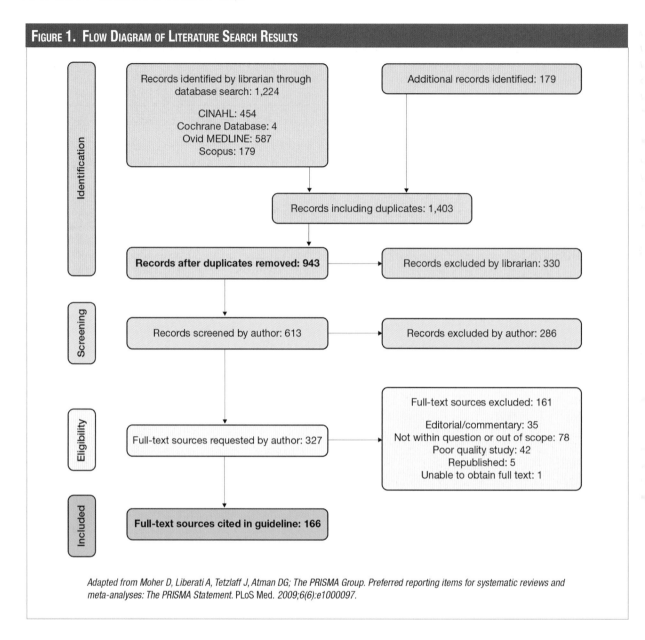

FIGURE 1. FLOW DIAGRAM OF LITERATURE SEARCH RESULTS

Identification

Records identified by librarian through database search: 1,224

CINAHL: 454
Cochrane Database: 4
Ovid MEDLINE: 587
Scopus: 179

Additional records identified: 179

Records including duplicates: 1,403

Records after duplicates removed: 943

Records excluded by librarian: 330

Screening

Records screened by author: 613

Records excluded by author: 286

Eligibility

Full-text sources requested by author: 327

Full-text sources excluded: 161

Editorial/commentary: 35
Not within question or out of scope: 78
Poor quality study: 42
Republished: 5
Unable to obtain full text: 1

Included

Full-text sources cited in guideline: 166

Adapted from Moher D, Liberati A, Tetzlaff J, Atman DG; The PRISMA Group. Preferred reporting items for systematic reviews and meta-analyses: The PRISMA Statement. PLoS Med. 2009;6(6):e1000097.

from government agencies and standards-setting bodies.

Excluded were non-peer–reviewed publications, studies that evaluated skin antisepsis as part of a bundle to prevent SSI, and low-quality evidence when higher-quality evidence was available (Figure 1).

Articles identified in the search were provided to the project team for evaluation. The team consisted of the lead author and three evidence appraisers. The lead author divided the search results into topics and assigned members of the team to review and critically appraise each article using the AORN Research or Non-Research Evidence Appraisal Tools as appropriate. The literature was independently evaluated and appraised according to the strength and quality of the evidence. Each article was then assigned an appraisal score. The appraisal score is noted in brackets after each reference, as applicable.

The collective evidence supporting each interven tion within a specific recommendation was summa rized, and the AORN Evidence-Rating Model was used to rate the strength of the evidence. Factors considered in the review of the collective evidence were the qual ity of evidence, the quantity of similar evidence on a given topic, and the consistency of evidence support ing a recommendation. The evidence rating is noted in brackets after each intervention.

Note: The evidence summary table is available a http://www.aorn.org/evidencetables/.

Editor's note: *MEDLINE is a registered trademark of the US National Library of Medicine's Medical Litera ture Analysis and Retrieval System, Bethesda, MD CINAHL, Cumulative Index to Nursing and Allied Health Literature, is a registered trademark of EBSCC*

Industries, Birmingham, AL. DuraPrep is a registered trademark of 3M, St Paul, MN. pHisoHex is a registered trademark of Aspen Pharmacare Australia Pty Ltd, New South Wales, Australia. Prevantics is a registered trademark of Professional Disposables International, Inc, Parippany, NJ. Hibiclens is a registered trademark of Mölnlycke Health Care AB, Gothenburg, Sweden. Techni-Care is a registered trademark of Care-Tech Laboratories, Inc, St Louis, MO. ChloraPrep is a registered trademark of CareFusion, San Diego, CA. Betadine and Betasept are registered trademarks of The Purdue Frederick Company, South Norwalk, CT. ExCel AP is a registered trademark of Aplicare, Meriden, CT.

Recommendation I

Patients should bathe or shower before surgery with either soap or an antiseptic.

The collective evidence supports that preoperative patient bathing may reduce the microbial flora on the patient's skin before surgery.

The limitations of the evidence are that research has not confirmed the effect of preoperative bathing on SSI development. Additional research is needed to define optimal preoperative bathing procedures, including whether antiseptics are more effective than soaps (eg, plain, antimicrobial), whether bathing the whole body or only the surgical site is more effective, the optimal timing of bathing before surgery, and the optimal number of baths or showers before surgery.

The benefits of preoperative patient bathing outweigh the harms. Benefits include reduction of transient and resident microorganisms on the skin that may lower the risk of the patient developing an SSI.[2] The harms of preoperative patient bathing with an antiseptic may include skin irritation, allergic reaction, or unnecessary treatment with antiseptics.[2]

I.a. The patient should be instructed to bathe or shower before surgery with either soap or a skin antiseptic on at least the night before or the day of surgery.[2,4-14] *[1: Strong Evidence]*

Preoperative patient bathing before surgery may reduce microbial skin contamination. Additional research is needed to determine the optimal soap or antiseptic product, interval between bathing and surgery, and number of baths or showers.

In 1973, findings of a nonexperimental study of 23,649 surgical wounds suggested that preoperative bathing was effective by showing a 2.3% infection rate for patients who did not bathe, 2.1% for patients who bathed with soap, and 1.3% for patients who bathed with an antiseptic before surgery.[5] No similar study has since been published that compares bathing with antiseptics or soaps to not bathing.

Three clinical practice guidelines make recommendations for preoperative bathing. National Institute for Health and Care Excellence (NICE) guidelines advise that the patient should shower or bathe with soap the day of or the day before surgery.[4] The NICE guidelines state that the evidence on the use of antiseptics is inconclusive.[4] The Society for Healthcare Epidemiology of America (SHEA) guidelines note gaps in evidence related to preoperative bathing, such as the effect of bathing on SSI development and the effectiveness of chlorhexidine gluconate (CHG).[6] Guidelines from the National Association of Orthopaedic Nurses (NAON) support the nursing practice of providing the patient with instructions for preoperative bathing protocols and advise providing written instructions.[7]

In a Cochrane systematic review of seven randomized controlled trials (RCTs), Webster and Osborne[2] concluded that there is not a soap or antiseptic product that is clearly the best to use for preoperative bathing for reducing the incidence of SSI. One of the RCTs included in the Cochrane review was a classic European study by Rotter et al[8] that compared a whole-body, two-bath protocol of CHG (n = 1,413) with placebo (n = 1,400) in 2,813 patients. This study found that preoperative bathing had no effect on SSI rates.[8] Another RCT in this Cochrane review, conducted by Veiga et al[9] in Brazil, compared 150 patients undergoing clean plastic surgery: one group took 4% CHG showers two hours before surgery (n = 50), one group showered with a placebo (n = 50), and one group received no instructions for showering (n = 50). The researchers found that the CHG showers effectively reduced skin contamination with coagulase-negative *Staphylococcus* but found no differences in postoperative infection rates.[9]

Randomized controlled trials with conflicting results were examined in the evidence review. A trial by Veiga et al[10] examined preoperative showers with 10% povidone-iodine two hours before surgery (n = 57) compared with no showering instruction (n = 57) for 114 patients. This study found that the povidone-iodine showers effectively reduced *Staphylococcus* colonization of the skin for clean plastic surgery procedures on the thorax and abdomen.[10] In an RCT studying healthy volunteers (n = 60) in the United Kingdom, Tanner et al[14] found that CHG preoperative body washes were more effective than soap for reducing microbial growth immediately and at six hours after the intervention, and that CHG had superior antibacterial activity in the groin area.

Evidence from two systematic reviews is inconclusive. A systematic review with meta-analysis of eight RCTs and eight quasi-RCTs found that routine preoperative whole-body bathing with CHG was not effective in preventing SSI.[13] Although the authors suggested that additional research in this area is needed, they also suggested that the low risk and low cost of preoperative bathing may be worth the marginal benefits of reducing SSI risk.[13] The second systematic review of 20 studies including RCTs, quasi-experimental studies, and nonexperimental studies found that antiseptic showers may reduce skin colonization and may prevent SSI, but data were inconclusive about which antiseptic was most effective.[12]

The number of preoperative baths or showers was the subject of another systematic review of 10 RCTs. Jakobsson et al[11] concluded that there was insufficient evidence to recommend a number of baths or showers to prevent SSI. The authors reverted to a previous recommendation of three to five showers until more evidence becomes available.[11]

There is a growing body of evidence supporting the use of 2% CHG-impregnated cloth products for preoperative bathing. Based on the collective evidence, this practice remains an unresolved issue and warrants additional generalizable, high-quality research to confirm the benefit of CHG-impregnated cloths. The results of studies involving the use of 2% CHG cloths for preoperative bathing conflict. Three RCTs,[15-17] six quasi-experimental studies,[18-23] and two organizational experiences[24,25] support the use of 2% CHG cloths for preoperative bathing. The limitations of two of the RCTs were that the studies were conducted in healthy volunteers and may not be generalizable to select patient populations.[16,17] Eight of these studies were conducted in patients undergoing orthopedic procedures and may also be limited in generalizability.[15,18,20-25]

A systematic review[26] and a literature review[27] also supported the practice of preoperative bathing with 2% CHG cloths, although the systematic review authors recommended additional studies to confirm their findings because of the observational nature of the studies and variations in the quality of data collection and analysis. One quasi-experimental study[28] refuted the use of 2% CHG cloths for preoperative bathing by finding no reduction in SSI with use of the cloths before total joint arthroplasty. Although many studies support the use of 2% CHG cloths for preoperative bathing, additional research is needed before a practice recommendation can be made.

I.a.1.   The patient should be instructed to follow the product manufacturer's instructions for use. [5: Benefits Balanced with Harms]

I.a.2.   After the preoperative bath or shower, the patient should be instructed not to apply
• alcohol-based hair or skin products,
• lotions,
• emollients, or
• cosmetics.
Patients should not apply deodorant for procedures involving the axilla. [5: Benefits Balanced with Harms]

The collective evidence does not suppor or refute this recommendation. Alcohol based products in the hair or on the skin a the surgical site may pose a fire hazar when an ignition source is used near th site. Lotions, emollients, cosmetics, an deodorants used at the surgical site ma reduce the effectiveness of preoperativ patient skin antiseptics or reduce the abilit of patient monitors, adhesive surgica drapes, and adhesive dressings to adhere t the patient's skin.

I.a.3.   For surgery on the hand or foot, the patien should be instructed that the nails on th operative extremity should be clean an natural, without artificial nail surfaces (eg extensions, overlays, acrylic, silk wraps enhancements).[29-31] [3: Moderate Evidence]

The evidence review found no cases o patient incision-site contamination relate to the wearing of artificial nails or nail pol ish on the operative hand or foot. This is a unresolved issue that warrants additiona research.

Two quasi-experimental studies evalu ated the effect of health care personnel wearing of artificial nails on surgical han antisepsis. In these studies, researcher showed that the variety and amount o potentially pathogenic bacteria culture from the fingertips of health care personne wearing artificial nails was greater than fo those with natural nails, both before an after hand washing.[30,31] With regard to nai polish, authors of a Cochrane systemati review found insufficient evidence to deter mine whether the fresh or chipped nail pol ish of health care personnel increased th risk of the patient developing an SSI.[29]

Although these studies showed nail con tamination in health care personnel, thes data may be extrapolated to the patient Patients' wearing of artificial nails or nai polish at the surgical site may harbor micro organisms, which could contaminate th surgical site or reduce the effectiveness o preoperative patient skin antisepsis Removal of artificial nails and nail polis that is near the surgical site may reduc contaminants on and under the nail.

I.a.4.   The patient undergoing head or neck sur gery should be instructed to shampoo his o her hair before surgery.[32] [2: High Evidence]

The results from one RCT showed tha shampooing with either 4% CHG or 7.5% povidone-iodine was effective in reducin resident flora on the scalp. No studies hav compared other types of shampoo with anti septics. The optimal preoperative shampo product is an unresolved issue that war rants additional research.

Leclair et al[32] conducted an RCT of preoperative shampooing with a skin antiseptic by comparing scalp cultures, wound cultures, and SSI rates for 151 patients in four groups:

- preoperative shampoo and preoperative skin antisepsis with 4% CHG,
- no preoperative shampoo and preoperative skin antisepsis with 4% CHG,
- preoperative shampoo and preoperative skin antisepsis with 7.5% povidone-iodine, and
- no preoperative shampoo and preoperative skin antisepsis with 7.5% povidone-iodine.[32]

Patients randomly assigned to a shampoo group in the study were instructed to perform two preoperative shampoos with either CHG or povidone-iodine at least one hour apart during the two- to 24-hour period before surgery. All study patients had their hair clipped, scalp wetted with the assigned antiseptic, hair shaved with a razor, scalp scrubbed with the assigned antiseptic for a minimum of five minutes and blotted dry with a sterile towel, and an adherent plastic drape applied over the incision site. The researchers concluded that preoperative shampooing suppressed the emergence of resident flora on the scalp during neurosurgery and that CHG appeared to be superior to iodophors because of its residual antimicrobial activity.[32]

Prescribing 4% CHG shampoo is a medical decision. This practice contradicts the 4% CHG manufacturer's instructions for use, which state not to use the product on the head. The decision of the prescribing physician to order 4% CHG for preoperative shampooing constitutes off-label use. The benefits of a 4% CHG shampoo may not outweigh the potential harms of CHG causing injury by contact with the eyes, ears, or mouth.

b.   A multidisciplinary team that includes perioperative RNs, physicians, and infection preventionists should develop a mechanism for evaluating and selecting products for preoperative patient bathing.[33] [2: High Evidence]

Involvement of a multidisciplinary team allows input from personnel with clinical expertise.[33]

Recommendation II

Hair removal at the surgical site should be performed only in select clinical situations.

The collective evidence supports that hair at the surgical site should be left in place. When hair removal is necessary, clipping the hair may be associated with a lower risk of SSI development than hair removal with a razor.

The limitations of the evidence include that some studies had an inadequate sample size (ie, were underpowered) to determine the effect of hair removal on the development of SSI, the studies did not use a standardized definition of SSI, and the majority of the studies included in the systematic reviews are approximately 20 years old.

The benefits of leaving hair in place at the surgical site include preventing potential skin trauma from hair removal and potentially reducing the risk for SSI.[3] The harms of leaving the hair in place at the surgical site may include risk of fire.[34] The risk of fire may be minimized by confining the hair with a water-soluble gel and non-metallic ties or with braids for longer hair. No studies evaluated the use of alternative hair management techniques or products to reduce the risk of fire. The AORN Guideline for a Safe Environment of Care, Part 1 recommends coating facial hair with water-soluble gel for surgical procedures that involve the head and neck to minimize the risk of combustion.[34]

II.a.   Hair at the surgical site should be left in place.[3-6,35,36] [1: Strong Evidence]

Removing hair at the surgical site has long been believed to be associated with an increased rate of SSI. In a landmark nonexperimental study of 23,649 surgical wounds, Cruse[5] found a 2.3% infection rate for surgical sites shaved with a razor, 1.7% for sites that were clipped, and 0.9% when no hair removal was performed. The researcher concluded that shaving should be kept to a minimum but did not suggest that hair should be left in place.[5]

Clinical practice guidelines from SHEA[6] and NICE[4] support the practice of leaving hair at the surgical site, unless the hair will interfere with the procedure. Conflicting evidence was examined in a Cochrane systematic review of 14 studies, including RCTs and quasi-RCTs, of a variety of procedure types. Tanner et al[3] concluded that the evidence sample sizes were too small and the studies were methodologically flawed, which prevented them from drawing strong conclusions that routine hair removal at the surgical site reduces the incidence of SSI.

A systematic review of 21 studies, including RCTs, quasi-experimental studies, and nonexperimental studies, found no evidence to suggest that hair should be routinely removed for neurosurgery procedures.[35] Another systematic review evaluated 18 studies and also determined that cranial surgeries should be performed without shaving.[36]

II.a.1.   The patient should be instructed to leave hair in place at the surgical site before surgery.[37] [3: Moderate Evidence]

One nonexperimental study investigated patient compliance with not removing hair at the surgical site for cesarean deliveries. Ng et al[37] used an educational intervention campaign targeted toward prenatal patients to discourage pre-hospital hair removal after 36 weeks gestation. The researchers concluded that the patient education improved patient compliance with non-removal of hair at the surgical site from 41% to 27% in a three-year period.

Although the researchers noted that other evidence-based practices for reduction of SSI, including switching to an alcohol-based skin antiseptic, were implemented during the time of this investigation, they also saw a reduction in SSI rates for cesarean procedures and considered this educational campaign to be an important part of their multimodal approach to reducing SSI.[37] Additional research is needed to determine whether hair removal by the patient has an effect on risk for SSI.[37]

II.b. When necessary, hair at the surgical site should be removed by clipping or depilatory methods in a manner that minimizes injury to the skin.[3,4,6,7,35,38-40] *[1: Strong Evidence]*

When hair removal is necessary, hair removal by clippers may be associated with lower risk of SSI than when hair is removed by razors. No studies were found comparing clipping to depilatory methods. Additional research is needed to determine the most effective method of hair removal, the effect of hair removal on SSI development, and the optimal amount of time between hair removal at the surgical site and the surgical incision.

In a Cochrane systematic review, Tanner et al[3] concluded that although the patient sample size from the collective studies was too small to draw strong conclusions, use of clippers has been associated with lower SSI rates than use of razors. One of the RCTs included in this Cochrane review was a study of 789 spine procedures.[39] In this study, Celik and Kara[39] compared hair removal at the surgical site with a razor (n = 371) to no hair removal (n = 418) and found that shaving with a razor just before skin preparation increased the SSI rate. This study was limited by incomplete data because the researchers were not able to collect follow-up data on 47 shaved patients. In another systematic review of hair removal for neurosurgical procedures, Broekman et al[35] did not find any evidence that shaving decreased the incidence of SSIs, with a possibility that, conversely, shaving increased infections in neurosurgical patients. The authors recommended additional research in this area. A literature review also concluded that clipping and depilatory methods caused fewer SSIs than shaving with a razor.[38]

Studies involving removal of hair in the male genital area are limited and may conflict with recommendations to clip hair rather than shave hair with a razor, although additional research is needed. In an RCT of 217 procedures involving male genitalia, Grober et al[40] compared hair removal on the scrotum with clippers (n = 107) and razors (n = 108), with outcomes of quality of hair removal, skin trauma, and SSI events. The researchers concluded that hair removal by a razor on the scrotum prevented skin trauma and achieved better quality hair removal than clippers, with no apparent increase in infection rate.[40] The study did not describe whether wet or dry methods were used for either clipping or shaving and was limited by not being statistically powered to determine the effect on SSI.

There is consensus among professional associations to recommend hair removal with clipping or depilatory methods rather than shaving with a razor. The SHEA guidelines recommend removing hair by clipping or depilatory methods and specifically recommend not using a razor.[6] Guidelines from NICE advise removing hair with single-use clippers and also advise against using razors.[4] The NAON guidelines recommend using clippers for hair removal but do not address depilatory or shaving methods. With regard to the timing of hair removal, the NAON guidelines recommend removing hair as close to the incision time as possible.[7]

II.b.1. The patient's hair should be removed in location outside the operating or procedure room. *[5: Benefits Balanced with Harms]*

II.b.2. When removing hair outside the operating or procedure room is contraindicated (eg, by emergency, because of patient anxiety), the patient's hair should be removed in a manner that prevents dispersal of hair into the air of the operating or procedure room. Prevention of hair dispersal may be achieved by wet clipping, use of suction, or other methods. *[5: Benefits Balanced with Harms]*

II.b.3. Single-use clipper heads should be used and disposed of after each patient use. The reusable clipper handle should be disinfected after each use, in accordance with the manufacturer's instructions for use.[4] *[1: Strong Evidence]*

Guidelines from NICE recommend using single-use clipper heads to reduce the risk of cross-contamination of bloodborne pathogens between patients.[4]

II.b.4. When using depilatories for hair removal, the perioperative team member should follow the manufacturer's instructions for use, including testing skin for skin allergy and irritation reactions in an area away from the surgical site.[3] *[1: Strong Evidence]*

In a Cochrane systematic review, the authors discussed that depilatories may cause skin irritation and allergic reactions and recommended patch testing at least 24 hours before the cream is applied.[3]

II.b.5. The perioperative RN should document in the patient's health care record the hair removal method, time of removal, and area of hair removal. [5: Benefits Balanced with Harms]

Recommendation III

A multidisciplinary team including perioperative RNs, physicians, and infection preventionists should select safe and effective antiseptic products for preoperative patient skin antisepsis.

The collective evidence indicates that there is no one antiseptic that is more effective than another for preventing SSI.

The limitations of the evidence review include that the literature has not determined which antiseptic is most effective for preoperative skin antisepsis because existing studies had inadequate sample sizes (ie, were underpowered) to determine the effect on SSI and are limited in quality. The evidence suggests that selection of a safe and effective preoperative skin antiseptic should be based on individual patient need.

III.a. The multidisciplinary team should develop a mechanism for product evaluation and selection of preoperative skin antiseptics.[33] [2: High Evidence]

Involvement of a multidisciplinary team allows input from all departments in which the product will be used and from personnel with clinical expertise.[33]

III.a.1. The multidisciplinary team should select antiseptic skin preparation products based on a review of the current research literature. [5: Benefits Balanced with Harms]

No one antiseptic has been found to be better than another for preventing SSI, although alcohol-based antiseptics may be more effective than aqueous-based povidone-iodine when not contraindicated. This is an unresolved issue that warrants additional research. With a gap in the evidence to guide practice, decisions about which preoperative skin antiseptic to use in the practice setting are complex. A variety of products may be necessary to meet the needs of various patient populations. Input from a multidisciplinary team with diverse experience and knowledge of skin antiseptics is helpful during review of research, clinical guidelines, and literature from the manufacturers.

The evidence involving preoperative skin antiseptic selection conflicts. The NICE guidelines have no recommendation for skin antiseptic selection, citing a lack of evidence, although the document mentions that CHG and povidone-iodine are most suitable for preoperative skin antisepsis.[4] The NAON guidelines recommend using povidone-iodine, iodine-based alcohol, or CHG for preoperative skin antisepsis.[7] In a Cochrane systematic review of 13 RCTs, Dumville et al[1] concluded that the evidence for skin antisepsis was lacking in quality, and no determination could be made regarding the most effective skin antiseptic for clean surgery. One literature review recommended aqueous povidone-iodine for use on mucous membranes (eg, gynecological, genitourinary) and alcohol-based antiseptics for longer, open procedures.[41]

A nonexperimental study determined that iodine-based alcohol was an effective antiseptic for preoperative patient skin antisepsis.[42] In another paper describing the efficacy of skin antiseptics, a literature review supported the efficacy of CHG for reducing the risk of SSI.[43]

The evidence review also evaluated several studies that compared various skin antiseptic products, including aqueous povidone-iodine, CHG-alcohol, and iodine-based alcohol.

Some research studies support CHG-alcohol as more effective than aqueous povidone-iodine antiseptics.[44-47] A systematic review[48] and two literature reviews[49,50] found that CHG-alcohol was more effective than aqueous povidone-iodine.

Other evidence has indicated that CHG was more effective than povidone-iodine without accounting for the role of alcohol.[51,52] In a systematic review and meta-analysis, Maiwald and Chan[53] concluded that the role of alcohol has been overlooked in the literature and that studies showing a perceived efficacy of CHG actually demonstrate the effectiveness of CHG-alcohol.

Conversely, researchers who conducted an RCT involving 556 patients undergoing clean hernia surgeries compared aqueous 10% povidone-iodine (n = 285) to CHG-alcohol (n = 271) and concluded that there was no difference in reduction of bacterial counts.[54] A quasi-experimental cohort study also found that there was no difference in the rate of SSIs when either aqueous povidone-iodine (n = 29) or CHG-alcohol (n = 25) was used for cesarean delivery surgical site antisepsis.[55]

In an RCT involving 866 patients undergoing clean procedures, Berry et al[56] found there was no gold standard antiseptic for clean procedures and concluded that neither CHG-alcohol (n = 453) nor alcoholic povidone-iodine (n = 413) antiseptic was

TABLE 1. US FOOD AND DRUG ADMINISTRATION CATEGORIES OF PATIENT PREOPERATIVE SKIN PREPARATIONS[1]

Active ingredient	Category
Benzalkonium chloride	IIIE
Chlorhexidine gluconate	"New drug"
Chloroxylenol	IIIE
Hexachlorophene	II
Iodine tincture USP	I
Iodine topical solution USP	I
Povidone-iodine 5% to 10%	I
Triclosan	IIIE
Iodine Povacrylex/Isopropyl Alcohol[2]	New drug[2]

E = Effectiveness

REFERENCES

1. *US Food and Drug Administration. Tentative Final Monograph for Healthcare Antiseptic Drug Products proposed rule. Fed Regist. 1994;59(116):31402-31452.*
2. *US Food and Drug Administration. New Drug Application (NDA) #21-586.*

superior for reducing the risk of SSI. One RCT of 100 patients undergoing lumbar spine surgery also concluded that CHG-alcohol and iodine-based alcohol were equally effective for removing common pathogens at the surgical site.[57]

A systematic review of eight studies, including RCTs and quasi-RCTs, that compared foot and ankle surgery skin preparation techniques found that CHG-alcohol was more effective than iodine-based alcohol in reducing bacteria in the hallux nail fold area and that the antiseptics were equally effective at reducing bacterial counts in toe web spaces.[58] An RCT of 150 patients undergoing shoulder surgery found that CHG-alcohol was more effective than iodine-based alcohol and povidone-iodine for removing bacteria at the surgical site.[46] A conflicting quasi-experimental comparison of alcoholic iodine and CHG-alcohol products demonstrated that iodine-based alcohol antiseptics were more effective than CHG-alcohol antiseptics.[59]

Two RCTs compared preoperative skin antisepsis with aqueous two-step povidone-iodine products to skin antisepsis with one-step iodine-based alcohol products in cardiovascular procedures. These studies concluded that the iodine-based alcohol products were more effective than aqueous povidone-iodine solutions.[60,61]

III.a.2. The multidisciplinary team should select products for preoperative skin antisepsis that either meet US Food and Drug Administration (FDA) requirements as Category I in the Tentative Final Monograph (TFM) for Over-the-Counter (OTC) Healthcare Anti-

septic Drug Products or are FDA-approve by the "New Drug Approval" (NDA) an "Abbreviated New Drug Approval" (ANDA processes.[62] *[5: Benefits Balanced wit Harms]*

The TFM approval process require patient preoperative skin preparation dru products to be fast acting (ie, a 2-log reduc tion on the abdomen and 3-log reduction o the groin within 10 minutes), broad spec trum, and persistent (ie, no return to baselin flora count at six hours post application and to significantly reduce the number o microorganisms on intact skin.[62] The FD categorizes active ingredients in the TFM fo patient preoperative skin preparation dru products as either Category I, II, or III. Cate gory I means that the ingredient meets mono graph conditions, and Category II or I means that the ingredient does not mee monograph conditions. In previous regula tory documents, Category I meant the prod uct was generally recognized as safe, effec tive, and not misbranded; Category II mean that the product was not generally recog nized as safe and effective or could be mis branded; and Category III meant that avail able data were insufficient to classify th product as safe and effective, and additiona testing was required. Although the languag in the TFM refers to monograph condition the document retains the previous concep of the categories relating to safety and effi cacy. Table 1 provides a summary of FD categories for active ingredients in patien preoperative skin preparations. Table 2 pro vides a summary of the characteristics o commonly used skin antiseptics.

Table 2. Activity and Considerations for Preoperative Patient Skin Antiseptics

	Aqueous iodine/ iodophors (10%)[1]	Chlorhexidine gluconate (CHG) (4%)[2]	*Alcohol (70%-91.3%)[3]	Alcoholic iodine/ iodophors[3]	CHG-alcohol[3]
Mechanism of action[1-3]	Oxidation/substitution with free iodine	Disrupts cell membrane	Denatures cell wall proteins, concentration determines effectiveness	See Aqueous Iodine/ Iodophors and Alcohol	See CHG and Alcohol
Effectiveness against microorganisms[1-3]	Gram + and gram - bacteria, tubercle bacillus, fungi, and viruses	Gram + and gram - bacteria, yeasts, and some viruses	Gram + and gram - bacteria, mycobacteria, fungi, and viruses	See Aqueous Iodine/ Iodophors and Alcohol	See CHG and Alcohol
Rapidity of action[1-3]	Moderate	Moderate	Most rapid	Rapid	Rapid
Residual activity[1-3]	Moderate	Excellent	None	Moderate	Excellent
Use on eyes, ears, or mouth[1,2,4]	Yes, ears and mouth. For eyes, use 5% ophthalmic solution.	No, eyes and ears. Can cause corneal damage or deafness if contacts middle ear. For mouth, use 0.12% CHG oral rinse.	Yes, ears. No, eyes and mouth. Can cause corneal damage or nerve damage.	No. Can cause corneal damage or nerve damage.	No. Can cause corneal damage. Can cause deafness if contacts middle ear.
Use in genital area[1,2,4]	Yes. Use with caution in patients susceptible to iodism.[5]	No[4]	No	No	No
Use internally[1,2,4]	No, external use only.	No, external use only. Do not use on wounds that involve more than superficial layers of skin.	No, external use only.	No, external use only. Do not use on open wounds.	No, external use only. Do not use on open wounds.
Contraindications[1,2,4]	Sensitivity or allergy to drug or any ingredients.	Sensitivity or allergy to drug or any ingredients. Do not use for lumbar puncture or in contact with meninges.	Sensitivity or allergy to drug or any ingredients.	Sensitivity or allergy to drug or any ingredients.	Sensitivity or allergy to drug or any ingredients. Do not use for lumbar puncture or in contact with meninges.
Cautions[1,2,4]	Use with caution in patients susceptible to iodism (eg, patients with burns, patients with thyroid disorders, neonates, pregnant women, lactating mothers). Prolonged exposure may cause irritation. Inactivated by blood.	Use with caution in premature infants or in infants younger than 2 months old, may cause chemical burns.	Flammable.	Flammable. Do not use in infants younger than 2 months old. Use with caution in nursing mothers. Use caution when removing adhesive drapes to avoid skin injury.	Flammable. Use with caution in premature infants or infants younger than 2 months old, may cause chemical burns.

*Isopropyl alcohol (70%-91.3%) is a classified as Category I for patient preoperative skin preparation for the limited indication of "for the preparation of the skin prior to an injection."[6(p31434)]

References

1. Zamora JL. Chemical and microbiologic characteristics and toxicity of povidone-iodine solutions. Am J Surg. 1986;151(3):400-406.
2. Lim K-S, Kam PCA. Chlorhexidine—pharmacology and clinical applications. Anaesth Intensive Care. 2008;36(4):502-512.
3. Reichman DE, Greenberg JA. Reducing surgical site infections: a review. Rev Obstet Gynecol. 2009;2(4):212-221.
4. DailyMed. US National Library of Medicine. http://dailymed.nlm.nih.gov/. Accessed July 14, 2014.
5. American College of Obstetricians and Gynecologists Women's Health Care Physicians, Committee on Gynecologic Practice. Committee Opinion No. 571: Solutions for surgical preparation of the vagina. Obstet Gynecol. 2013;122(3):718-720.
6. US Food and Drug Administration. Tentative Final Monograph for Healthcare Antiseptic Drug Products proposed rule. Fed Regist. 1994;59(116):31402-31452.

III.a.3. Selected products should be purchased in single-use containers.[63] [1: Regulatory Requirement]

In November 2013, the FDA issued a Drug Safety Communication requesting that manufacturers package antiseptics indicated for preoperative skin preparation in single-use containers to reduce the risk of infection from improper antiseptic use and contamination of products during use.[63]

III.a.4. Unless contraindicated (eg, antisepsis of split-thickness skin graft donor sites), the multidisciplinary team should select products for preoperative patient skin antisepsis that are colored or tinted (ie, not clear).[64] *[3: Moderate Evidence]*

Use of colored antiseptics was supported in a quasi-experimental study of skin preparation in upper-limb surgery.[64] This study showed that use of clear antiseptics resulted in more missed spots, mostly in finger areas, than did colored antiseptics.[64] Flammable clear antiseptics may also pose a fire or chemical burn hazard if unseen solution is allowed to drip or pool on or near the patient, although no evidence was found in the evidence review to evaluate the effect of visibility on reducing fire or chemical hazards.

III.b. The perioperative RN, in collaboration with the surgeon and anesthesia professional, should select a safe, effective, health care organization-approved preoperative antiseptic for the individual patient based on the patient assessment, the procedure type, and a review of the manufacturer's instructions for use and contraindications.[65,66] *[3: Moderate Evidence]*

Selection of a preoperative skin antiseptic based on individual patient assessment may reduce the risk for patient complications. One literature review discussed the various preoperative skin antiseptics and concluded that perioperative RNs should evaluate and select the most appropriate antiseptic for each patient.[65] Another literature review concluded that the patient assessment was critical to selection of the correct preoperative skin antiseptic.[66]

III.b.1. The perioperative RN should assess the patient for allergies and sensitivities to preoperative skin antiseptics.[67-78] *[3: Moderate Evidence]*

In an in vitro study, Quatresooz et al[67] found that the skin reacts differently to the action of chemicals in various anatomic sites of the body. These researchers found that, in the laboratory setting, povidone-iodine (100 mg/mL) produced less irritation in the stratum corneum than two other antiseptics (ie, povidone-iodine 70 mg/mL, chlorhexidine digluconate 50 mg/mL), but in in vivo settings the severity of skin irritation depends on individual susceptibility and the site of exposure.[67]

In a case report, Sanders and Hawken[68] described three cases of chemical skin reactions to CHG that provide an example of how anatomic location may cause the skin

to react differently to chemicals. In this report, three patients undergoing shoulder arthroscopy developed partial thickness chemical burns on the shoulder from a CHG-alcohol preoperative skin antiseptic.[6] The authors determined that the occurrences of chemical skin injury were related to alteration of the skin at the shoulder from traction and to local swelling from the procedure.[68]

A 2004 position statement from the American Academy of Allergy Asthma and Immunology (AAAAI) asserted that fish or seafood allergies do not indicate allergy to iodine. According to the position statement, contact dermatitis related to topically applied iodine antiseptics does not indicate an iodine allergy; rather, this is a reaction to chemicals in the product. Anaphylaxis to topical iodine antiseptic solutions is exceedingly rare and not proven to be related to iodine.[69] The AAAAI posts this position statement for reference only, and it does not reflect the current position of the academy. Limited evidence was found describing the relationship between seafood and iodine allergies. One nonexperimental survey study[71] and one literature review[7] support the assertion in the AAAAI position statement that seafood allergy is not related to iodine allergy.

Two case reports describe patients who developed anaphylactic reactions to povidone-iodine solution: one is a report of a pediatric patient with broken skin[7] and one is a report of vaginal application of povidone-iodine to a hypersensitized patient.[73]

In a case report, Sivathasan and Goodfellow[74] discussed the potential dangers of chlorhexidine and recommended caution when using CHG as an antiseptic in patients with a history of contact dermatitis. They recommended that clinicians consider CHG allergy in the event of an allergic reaction.[2] Case reports of anaphylaxis from CHG have been reported in the literature.[75-77]

Although isopropyl alcohol is a rare allergen, there are reports of allergic reactions in the literature.[78] In a case report of delayed hypersensitivity to isopropyl alcohol, Vujevich and Zirwas[78] recommended that clinicians consider alcohol as an allergen when contact dermatitis is suspected after a surgical procedure. The authors hypothesized that the combination of isopropyl alcohol application and alteration of the skin from a needle injection may have allowed isopropyl alcohol to penetrate the stratum corneum and cause an allergic reaction.[78]

III.b.2. The perioperative RN should assess the skin integrity at the surgical site before selecting a preoperative patient skin antiseptic. *[5: Benefits Balanced with Harms]*

III.b.3. The preoperative antiseptic product should be selected based on the procedure type. *[5: Benefits Balanced with Harms]*

Several studies evaluated the efficacy of preoperative patient skin antisepsis based on procedure type. The evidence involving the various procedure-specific preoperative skin antisepsis selection is limited, and this subject warrants additional research.

Several studies support preoperative eye antisepsis with 5% povidone-iodine ophthalmic solution irrigation to reduce rates of conjunctival bacterial load and risk of endophthalmitis from intraocular surgery.[79-83] Although researchers who conducted an RCT of 271 cataract surgeries concluded that 10% povidone-iodine was more effective than 1% or 5% povidone-iodine solutions for reducing bacterial load of the eye,[84] an international laboratory study in Taiwan warned of risk for corneal cell death by cytotoxicity from fixation during exposure to high concentrations of povidone-iodine (ie, 5% to 10%).[85] Researchers in Germany also discussed safety concerns regarding povidone-iodine and recommended use of 1.25% povidone-iodine for ocular antisepsis, citing concern for exacerbating untreated hyperthyroidism and that additional research is needed to evaluate the effect of ophthalmic povidone-iodine on thyroid function.[86,87]

The collective evidence indicates that povidone-iodine is commonly used for vaginal antisepsis in gynecological procedures. There are currently no FDA-approved antiseptic alternatives on the market for use in the vaginal vault when povidone-iodine is contraindicated (eg, by patient allergy). Two alternatives to vaginal povidone-iodine, sterile saline[88] and baby shampoo,[89] were discussed in the literature. Both studies suggested that these alternatives were as effective as povidone-iodine for preoperative vaginal antisepsis.

In a position statement from the American Congress of Obstetricians and Gynecologists (ACOG), the committee recommends off-label use of 4% CHG with low alcohol content (eg, 4%) as a safe and effective alternative for vaginal preparation when povidone-iodine is contraindicated or CHG is preferred by the surgeon.[90]

In an RCT of 1,570 abdominal hysterectomy procedures, Eason et al[91] compared preoperative vaginal antisepsis with a povidone-iodine gel (n = 780) to no gel (n = 790). The researchers found that the povidone-iodine gel group had a lower risk of developing abscesses, but there was no significant difference in infection rates.[91]

Performing preoperative antisepsis of the vagina for cesarean deliveries is supported in a Cochrane systematic review, although the reviewers concluded that evidence on the type of solution and method is lacking.[92] For cesarean procedures, two RCTs[93,94] and one quasi-experimental study[95] found that a vaginal preparation with povidone-iodine was effective for prevention of endometritis and SSI. One nonexperimental study suggested that abdomen preparation with CHG-alcohol was more effective than povidone-iodine.[47] A quasi-experimental study found that povidone-iodine and CHG-alcohol were equally effective in reducing SSI as preoperative abdominal skin antisepsis in cesarean procedures.[55] Authors of a Cochrane systematic review concluded that more research is needed to determine an ideal skin antiseptic for cesarean delivery incisions.[96]

Authors of a systematic review with meta-analysis[58] of eight RCTs and quasi-RCTs of foot and ankle surgery concluded that alcohol antiseptic solutions performed more effectively than aqueous iodine[97] for reducing bacterial load of the foot, and CHG-alcohol was more effective than iodine-based alcohol[98] for reducing foot flora. Researchers who conducted two small RCTs came to conclusions that conflict with this systematic review, including that alcohol gives no added benefit to antiseptic solutions[99] and that iodine-based alcohol is more effective at reducing bacterial load of the foot.[100]

Saltzman et al[46] conducted an RCT of 150 shoulder surgeries by comparing reduction of bacteria at the surgical site after skin antisepsis with three antiseptics: CHG-alcohol, iodine-based alcohol, and povidone-iodine. The researchers concluded that CHG-alcohol was most effective for reducing overall bacteria in the shoulder area and that povidone-iodine was the least effective for removing coagulase-negative *Staphylococcus* from the shoulder.[46]

In an RCT of 100 lumbar spine procedures, Savage et al[57] compared preoperative skin antisepsis with CHG-alcohol (n = 50) and iodine-based alcohol (n = 50). They concluded that the antiseptics were equally effective in removing bacterial pathogens at the surgical site. They also discussed that the skin flora of the lumbar spine differs from other locations of the body and that more research is needed to determine effective antiseptics for lumbar spine procedures.[57]

III.b.4. The perioperative RN should assess the surgical site for the presence of hair.[101] When an alcohol-based skin antiseptic is used for a procedure involving an ignition source, hair at the surgical site should be clipped before application of the antiseptic. *[5: Benefits Balanced with Harms]*

The presence of hair may contraindicate the use of flammable antiseptics according to manufacturers' instructions for use. A flammable antiseptic for preoperative skin antisepsis is contraindicated when the procedure involves an ignition source (eg, electrosurgical unit [ESU], laser) and the solution is unable to dry completely in hair. According to the Centers for Medicare & Medicaid Services (CMS), alcohol-based skin antiseptics that wick into the patient's hair result in prolonged drying times.[102,103] No evidence was found that describes the length or amount of hair that constitutes a fire risk during use of alcohol-based skin antiseptics.

In a case report, a patient described as having copious body hair was burned on the neck and shoulders while undergoing a tracheostomy.[101] After the patient's neck was prepared with an alcohol-based skin antiseptic, the surgical team allowed the solution to dry for three minutes before draping. Activation of electrocautery ignited the fire, which was fueled by the skin antiseptic and the patient's body hair and oxidized in an oxygen-enriched environment. The authors of the case report recommended that the alcohol-based skin antiseptic product not be used for a hirsute patient because the hair can impede drying of the solution.[101]

III.b.5. The perioperative RN should consult the physician when selecting iodine and iodophor-based preoperative patient skin antiseptics for patients susceptible to iodism (eg, patients with burns, patients with thyroid disorders, neonates, pregnant women, lactating mothers).[104] *[3: Moderate Evidence]*

Some patients are susceptible to iodism from preoperative skin antisepsis with iodine and iodophor-based antiseptics.

Three reports in the literature demonstrated that repeated application of povidone-iodine to the skin of burn patients may cause iodine absorption,[105] induced hyperthyroidism,[106] and metabolic acidosis.[107] A review explained that the amount of iodine absorption from polyvinylpyrrolidone-iodine in burn patients depends on the concentration applied, frequency of application, type and total surface area of the burn, and the patient's renal function.[104]

The author of a literature review concluded that most patients can tolerate excess quantities of iodine without negative effects, although iodine-induced hyperthyroidism may occur in patients with underlying hyperthyroidism or goiter.[104] In an RCT (n = 68), Tomoda et al[108] compared preoperative patient skin antisepsis with povidone-iodine (n = 47) to CHG (n = 21) in patients with thyroid carcinoma who were on an iodine-restricted diet and undergoing total thyroidectomy. The researchers demonstrated that iodism resulted from a single application of povidone-iodine for skin antisepsis. In this study, the patients' postoperative iodine levels in the urine were nearly seven times the preoperative levels. The researchers theorized that cutaneously absorbed iodine could potentially interfere with iodine therapy or cause thyroid dysfunction in susceptible patients.[108]

Researchers in Germany cautioned that ophthalmic application of povidone-iodine may cause thyroid disturbances, specifically exacerbation of untreated hyperthyroidism.[86,87] These researchers recommended additional research to evaluate the effect on the thyroid of administering ophthalmic povidone-iodine.

Several case reports and studies have demonstrated iodism in neonates[109] and advise cautious use of iodine-based antiseptics in neonates because of the risk for transient hypothyroidism[104,110,111] or iodine-induced hyperthyroidism.[112] A literature review recommended minimizing neonatal iodine exposure because of the risk of significant iodine overload and severe transient hypothyroidism, especially in premature neonates with increased skin permeability and immature thyroid glands.[113] The authors of the review recommended monitoring thyroid-stimulating hormone levels in neonates exposed to iodine skin antiseptics.[113] Two nonexperimental studies also recommended that iodine-based antiseptics be used with caution, including thyroid function monitoring, in premature infants who require repeated antiseptic applications because transient thyroid alterations may be detrimental to neurologic development in this vulnerable population.[110,111]

A literature review recommended using iodine-based antiseptics with caution in pregnant mothers because iodine crosses the placental barrier.[104] In a Cochrane systematic review, Hadiati et al[96] discussed an abstract of one French RCT (n = 22) that compared CHG 0.5% with 70% alcohol to use of an antiseptic-impregnated adhesive incise drape and found a higher concentration of iodine in the cord blood of newborns in the antiseptic-impregnated adhesive incise drape group, but no significant difference in iodine of 48-hour urine or thyroid-stimulating hormone blood levels on the fifth day. The authors of the systematic review did not make a recommendation based on this abstract.

In a Cochrane systematic review that recommended the use of vaginal povidone-iodine immediately before cesarean deliveries, Haas et al[92] did not discuss any risk of iodism in either the mother or the newborn. In a nonexperimental study of nonpregnant women (n = 12), Vorherr et al[114] demonstrated iodism after a two-minute vaginal antisepsis with povidone-iodine. The researchers advised against treating vaginitis in pregnant women with repeated applications of povidone-iodine because of the risk for development of iodine-induced goiter and hypothyroidism in the fetus and newborn. They explained that this risk is especially high with repeated use of povidone-iodine.[114]

Manufacturer's instructions for use of one iodine-based alcohol skin antiseptic recommend caution when using the product for women who are lactating (ie, breastfeeding) because of potential transient hypothyroidism in the nursing newborn.[115] The evidence review found no research evidence on iodine application in lactating mothers.

III.b.6. The perioperative RN should consult with the physician when selecting CHG and alcohol-based preoperative patient skin antiseptics for neonates.[113,116-118] *[3: Moderate Evidence]*

Neonates, especially extremely premature neonates, are at an increased risk for skin irritation and chemical burns of the skin from both CHG and alcohol-based skin antiseptics. In a literature review, Afsar[113] recommended that alcohol antisepsis be avoided in neonates because alcohol can cause hemorrhagic necrosis and skin burns, especially in extremely low-birth-weight infants and suggested that CHG alone may be a safer alternative for antisepsis.

In one case report of an extremely premature infant with aqueous 2% CHG chemical burns, Lashkari et al[116] found that the chemical exposure could have been limited by immediately wiping excess CHG with normal saline to avoid burns. Another case report of two extremely premature neonates with severe chemical burns as a result of 70% isopropyl alcohol applications for skin antisepsis found that pressure and decreased perfusion also played a role in the skin injury.[117] The authors of this case report advised exercising extreme caution

with use of alcohol for skin antisepsis in severely premature infants.[117]

In another case report, Harpin and Rutter[118] described cutaneous alcohol absorption and hemorrhagic skin necrosis in a 27-week gestation twin pre-term infant from skin antisepsis with methylated spirits (95% ethanol and 5% wood naphtha, which is 60% methanol). In this case, the extremely premature neonate died. Although the role of alcohol intoxication in the neonate's death was unknown because blood alcohol levels were not drawn until 18 hours after the alcohol application, the authors suspected that the maximum alcohol level from cutaneous alcohol absorption was in the potentially fatal range.[118]

III.b.7. When FDA-approved (ie, Category I, NDA, ANDA) antiseptic products are contraindicated, the perioperative team members should collaboratively evaluate the risks and benefits of using Class II or Class III FDA-approved antiseptics or other alternative solutions (eg, soaps, saline). *[5: Benefits Balanced with Harms]*

The evidence review found no literature regarding the efficacy of alternative antiseptic products. When a patient has an allergy or a condition such as a large open wound, all available Class I FDA-approved products for antisepsis might be contraindicated. In this situation, the perioperative team is challenged to select a safe, effective alternative for the individual patient. (See Recommendation III.a.)

Recommendation IV

Perioperative team members should apply the preoperative patient skin antiseptic in a safe and effective manner.

The collective evidence suggests that following the antiseptic manufacturer's instructions for use and applying preoperative patient skin antiseptics in a safe and effective manner may prevent patient harm (eg, inadequate skin antisepsis, fire, chemical injury).

The limitations of the evidence include the limited quality of existing studies and a lack of procedure-specific clinical research evaluating the effectiveness of various skin preparation and antisepsis techniques.

IV.a. Perioperative team members should confirm the surgical site before performing preoperative patient skin antisepsis.[119] *[2: High Evidence]*

The evidence review found no research evidence to support or refute this recommendation. Performing preoperative skin antisepsis at the wrong surgical site may result in a cascade of events leading to wrong site surgery. Confirmation of the location of the surgical site before the time-out process increases communication and consistent documentation and may reduce the likelihood of error. The AORN Guideline for Transfer of Patient Care Information recommends verifying the surgical site as part of the time-out process.[119]

IV.a.1. The surgical site mark should remain visible after preoperative patient skin antisepsis.[120-124] *[3: Moderate Evidence]*

Marking the surgical site with a nonsterile permanent marker is a safe practice for identifying the surgical site. Two quasi-experimental studies, each of 20 healthy volunteers, evaluated the effect of site marking on the sterility of skin antisepsis.[120,121] The researchers concluded that skin marking with a nonsterile permanent marker did not effect the sterility of skin antisepsis with povidone-iodine, as evidenced by no culture growth at the treated areas.[120,121]

Researchers in a nonexperimental study investigated the potential for the surgical site marker to serve as reservoir for transmissible infections.[122] In this study, Wilson and Tate[122] compared two types of markers, water-based and alcohol-based, and determined that transmission of methicillin-resistant *Staphylococcus aureus* (MRSA) is feasible with water-based skin markers. They recommended against using water-based skin markers for multiple patients because of the theoretical risk of transmitting MRSA.[122]

The evidence review also evalutated studies that examined the erasure of the surgical site marking during preoperative patient skin antisepsis. In these experimental studies, each of which involved permanent, alcohol-based markers and had a sample size of 20, the researchers found that a CHG-alcohol antiseptic product erased more site markings than did an iodine-based alcohol antiseptic product.[123,124]

IV.b. The perioperative RN should assess the condition of the patient's skin at the surgical site[125] and prepare the skin for antisepsis. *[4: Limited Evidence]*

The evidence review found no literature to support or refute this recommendation. Patient assessment before an intervention is a standard of perioperative nursing practice.[125]

IV.b.1. The skin at the surgical site should be free of soil, debris, emollients, cosmetics, and alcohol-based products. *[5: Benefits Balanced with Harms]*

The evidence review found no literature to support or refute this recommendation. Removal of superficial soil, debris, emollients, and cosmetics is generally accepted as a practice that may improve the effectiveness of preoperative patient skin antisepsis by decreasing the organic debris on the skin at the surgical site. Alcohol-based products

on the skin or hair at the surgical site may pose a fire hazard if an ignition source will be used during the procedure.

IV.b.2. The patient's jewelry (eg, rings, piercings) at the surgical site should be removed before preoperative skin antisepsis.[29,126] *[5: Benefits Balanced with Harms]*

No literature was found regarding patients' wearing of jewelry and its effect on preoperative patient skin antisepsis. Jewelry at the surgical site may harbor microorganisms and trap these organisms on adjacent skin, which may contaminate the surgical site or reduce the effectiveness of preoperative patient skin antisepsis.

Two studies evaluated health care workers' wearing of jewelry on the effectiveness of surgical hand antisepsis. A Cochrane systematic review of health care workers wearing finger rings during surgical hand antisepsis found that no studies evaluated the effect of this practice on SSI, although there was a common theoretical concern that rings could harbor bacteria and reduce the effectiveness of surgical hand antisepsis.[2] In a quasi-experimental study of health care worker hand contamination, Trick et al[12] found that ring wearing increased the frequency of hand contamination with pathogens, although the levels of contamination were significantly reduced when alcohol-based hand rubs were used.

Although these studies showed hand contamination in health care personnel wearing rings, these data may be extrapolated to the patient. Patients' jewelry at the surgical site may harbor microorganisms, which could contaminate the surgical site or reduce the effectiveness of preoperative patient skin antisepsis. Removal of jewelry near the surgical site may reduce contaminants on the skin.

IV.b.3. If the patient did not bathe or shower preoperatively, the perioperative team member may wash the skin at the surgical site with soap or an antiseptic before performing preoperative skin antisepsis.[127] *[2: High Evidence]*

Preoperative washing is supported by one prospective case-control study.[127] This quasi-experimental study demonstrated that patients undergoing emergency hip arthroplasty who had not followed preoperative bathing protocols were more likely to have more-abundant and different microbial flora at the surgical site before preoperative patient skin antisepsis.[127]

The presence of transient microorganisms has not been proven to be related to the development of SSI. There is a theoretical hypothesis that reducing the microbial load at the surgical site before antisepsis may lower the risk of a transient microorganism contaminating the surgical site. Preoperative washing also may remove gross soil, spores, and oils that may limit the effectiveness of the antiseptic. This is an unresolved issue that warrants additional research.

IV.b.4. Areas of greater contamination (ie, umbilicus, foreskin, under nails, intestinal or urinary stoma) in the surgical field should be cleansed before preoperative patient skin antisepsis is performed. *[5: Benefits Balanced with Harms]*

The evidence review found no literature to support or refute this recommendation. Some anatomic areas may contain more debris than other sites. Cleaning these areas before preoperative patient skin antisepsis may prevent contamination of the surgical site and allow the antiseptic to achieve its intended level of effectiveness.

Organic and inorganic material in the umbilicus (eg, detritus) may reduce the effectiveness of the skin antiseptic and contaminate the surgical site for abdominal procedures. Areas under nails (ie, subungual areas) also may harbor organic and inorganic material, including microorganisms, that could limit the effectiveness of antisepsis for procedures involving the hand or foot. Similarly, surgical sites including the penis may harbor microorganisms that accumulate in the area under the foreskin (ie, prepuce), if present, including organic material (ie, smegma). Intestinal or urinary stomas are also highly likely to contain organic material, such as mucin, that could render some antiseptics ineffective.

IV.b.5. Highly contaminated areas (eg, anus, colostomy) near the surgical site should be isolated with a sterile barrier drape. *[5: Benefits Balanced with Harms]*

V.c. A nonscrubbed perioperative team member should apply the skin antiseptic using sterile technique. *[5: Benefits Balanced with Harms]*

The evidence review found no research evidence to support or refute this recommendation. The risk of contamination of a scrubbed perioperative team member's sterile gown and gloves may be high during preoperative patient skin antisepsis activities.

IV.c.1. The perioperative team member should perform hand hygiene before applying the preoperative patient skin antiseptic.[128] *[2: High Evidence]*

IV.c.2. The perioperative team member should wear sterile gloves when performing preoperative patient skin antisepsis. Nonsterile gloves may be worn if the antiseptic applicator is of sufficient length to prevent contact of the gloved hand with the antiseptic solution and the patient's skin. *[5: Benefits Balanced with Harms]*

The evidence review found no literature to support or refute this recommendation. This is an unresolved issue that warrants additional research.

IV.c.3. The perioperative team member should wear surgical attire that covers his or her arms while performing preoperative patient skin antisepsis.[129] *[2: High Evidence]*

IV.c.4. The perioperative team members should use sterile supplies to apply preoperative patient skin antiseptics. *[5: Benefits Balanced with Harms]*

One RCT compared povidone-iodine skin antisepsis using both clean and sterile kits and found no difference in microbial counts on patients' skin.[130] This study has not been replicated, and no similar studies were found in the evidence review. This is an unresolved issue that warrants additional research.

IV.c.5. Items that touch the patient's skin after preoperative skin antisepsis should be sterile to prevent introduction of microorganisms at the surgical site.[131] *[1: Strong Evidence]*

IV.d. Skin antiseptics should be applied using aseptic technique and according to the manufacturer's instructions for use. *[5: Benefits Balanced with Harms]*

The evidence review found no literature related to application technique. The benefit of using aseptic technique for applying preoperative skin antiseptics outweighs the harm of contaminating the surgical site.

Antiseptic manufacturers' instructions for use convey important safety and efficacy instructions to the user. Failure to adhere to manufacturers' instructions for use may result in patient harm or ineffectiveness of the preoperative patient skin antisepsis.

IV.d.1. The perioperative team member should apply the skin antiseptic to an area large enough to accommodate potential shifting of the surgical drapes, extension of the incision (eg, during conversion of a minimally invasive procedure to an open procedure), potential additional incisions, and all potential drain sites. *[5: Benefits Balanced with Harms]*

IV.d.2. The skin antiseptic should be applied starting at the incision site and moving away toward the periphery of the surgical site. The applicator should be discarded after contact with a peripheral or contaminated area. Another sterile applicator should be used for additional applications. *[5: Benefits Balanced with Harms]*

IV.d.3. When the incision site is more highly contaminated than the surrounding skin (eg, anus, perineum, stoma, open wound, catheter, drain, axilla), the area with a lower bacterial count should be prepped first, followed by the area of higher contamination, as opposed to working from the incision toward the periphery. *[5: Benefits Balanced with Harms]*

The evidence review found no studies related to the sequence of skin antisepsis involving highly contaminated areas. This is an unresolved issue that warrants additional research.

IV.d.4. When using a pre-filled antiseptic applicator, the perioperative team member should follow the manufacturer's instructions for use (eg, maximum and minimum surface area per applicator) to apply the skin antiseptic with uniform distribution. *[5: Benefits Balanced with Harms]*

IV.d.5. The antiseptic should be applied with care (eg, gentle friction) on fragile tissue, burns, open wounds, or malignant areas.[66] *[3: Moderate Evidence]*

Fragile skin or tissue, burns, and open wounds are at a high risk for skin injury during preoperative patient skin antisepsis. Vigorous skin antisepsis in areas of malignancy may potentially spread cancer cells. The practice of using gentle friction when performing antisepsis in an area of malignancy is supported in one literature review.[66]

IV.d.6. For preoperative patient skin antisepsis with aqueous povidone-iodine, either scrub (ie, 7.5% povidone-iodine) and paint (ie, 10% povidone-iodine) or paint alone may be used.[132-136] *[2: High Evidence]*

Literature related to the comparison of scrub versus paint application techniques for preoperative patient skin antisepsis conflicts. Some RCTs support[132-135] and one quasi-experimental study refutes[136] the benefits of scrubbing the patient's skin with 7.5% povidone-iodine before painting with 10% povidone-iodine. This issue is unresolved and warrants additional research.

IV.d.7. When performing preoperative skin antisepsis of the hand or foot, care should be taken to apply the antiseptic to all surfaces between fingers or toes.[58,137-140] *[3: Moderate Evidence]*

Antisepsis may be difficult in the areas between fingers and toes because of difficulty reaching all surfaces of the skin. The collective evidence did not reveal the most effective preparation techniques for the hands and feet, and this warrants additional research.

A systematic review of eight studies, including RCTs and quasi-RCTs, comparing skin preparation techniques for foot and ankle surgery found that although some studies did not clearly describe scrubbing techniques, the use of vigorous foot scrubbing may reduce fungal contamination of the foot.[58] In one RCT of 50 patients undergoing foot surgery, Brooks et al[137] compared the standard foot antisepsis technique of placing antiseptic solution between the toes (n = 24) to a method with additional cleansing of the toe clefts with an antiseptic-soaked gauze (n = 26). The researchers reported a significant reduction in bacterial recolonization of the foot for the method involving additional cleaning of the toe clefts (ie, 7.7% versus 20.8%).[137]

International studies from England, Australia, and New Zealand describe a preoperative patient skin antisepsis technique in which a sterile bag is used to apply 10% povidone-iodine solution to either the foot or hand.[138-140] Researchers have found the bag technique to be equally effective as painting techniques in reducing bacterial counts and more efficient (ie, 24 seconds versus 85 seconds).[138-140] One quasi-experimental study of the sterile bag application technique for antisepsis also discussed a potential benefit of reducing musculoskeletal injury for perioperative personnel who use the bag technique.[138]

IV.d.8. When performing preoperative patient skin antisepsis of the mouth, care should be taken to prevent patient aspiration of the antiseptic solution.[141] *[3: Moderate Evidence]*

In one case report, a patient developed povidone-iodine aspiration pneumonitis after treatment of the oral and nasal cavity with irrigation of a diluted povidone-iodine solution, even though a throat pack was in place. To prevent aspiration, the authors of this report advised against irrigating the oral cavity with povidone-iodine.[141]

IV.e. The antiseptic should be allowed to dry for the full time recommended in the manufacturer's instructions for use before sterile drapes are applied.[34,66,102,103,142-151] *[3: Moderate Evidence]*

Allowing the skin antiseptic to dry completely according to the manufacturer's instructions for use improves the safety and efficacy of preoperative patient skin antisepsis.

Several case reports of patients chemically injured by wet antiseptics dripping or pooling beneath them recommend allowing the skin antiseptic to dry fully before surgical draping to prevent these types of injury.[143-149]

Flammable skin antiseptics pose a risk for fire when dry times are not achieved. The CMS guidelines[102,103] and several clinical practice guidelines[34,150,151] advise allowing flammable skin antiseptics to dry completely in accordance with the manufacturer's instructions for use. (See Recommendation IV.g.)

In a nonexperimental study, Stinner et al[142] determined that application of 4% CHG for preoperative patient skin antisepsis required a two-minute dry time to achieve effectiveness, which was in accordance with the manufacturer's instructions for use. The manufacturer's instructions for use are the result of rigorous testing under specific conditions and contact times.[62] Compliance with contact times and allowing the skin antiseptic to dry facilitates effectiveness of the antiseptic.

IV.f.   Protective measures should be taken to prevent prolonged contact with skin antiseptics.[143-149,152] *[3: Moderate Evidence]*

There are several case reports of patients experiencing chemical skin injury caused by prolonged contact with skin antiseptics.[143-149,152]

IV.f.1.   Sheets, padding, positioning equipment, and adhesive tape should be protected from the dripping or pooling of skin antiseptics beneath and around the patient.[66,143,144] *[3: Moderate Evidence]*

Three case reports found that the dripping of antiseptic solution onto fabric and positioning equipment prevented the solution from drying, which prolonged patient skin contact with the wet solution and caused patient skin injury.[66,143,144]

IV.f.2.   Electrodes (eg, electrocardiogram [ECG], ESU dispersive electrode) and tourniquets should be protected from contact with skin antiseptics.[143,145,149,152] *[3: Moderate Evidence]*

There have been several case reports of injury caused by contact of electrodes and tourniquets with skin antiseptics. One review of multiple cases described patient injuries, including chemical and thermal burns, from skin antiseptic contact with electrodes and tourniquets.[143] Other case reports have described patient injury from skin antiseptic contact with an ESU dispersive electrode[145] and tourniquets.[149,152] Antiseptic contact between the skin and electrode increases impedance and the risk of skin injury or equipment malfunction. When tourniquets cuffs are in contact with antiseptics, compression and occlusion of the wet material against the patient's skin increases the likelihood of a chemical burn.

IV.f.3.   A fluid-resistant pad should be placed under the patient's buttocks during preoperative patient skin antisepsis for patients in the lithotomy position.[146-148] The pad should

be removed after the antiseptic is dry and before sterile drapes are applied. *[3: Moderate Evidence]*

There have been several case reports of patients sustaining chemical burn injury by prolonged contact with antiseptic solution that pooled beneath them while they were in the lithotomy position.[146-148] When a patient is in the lithotomy position, antiseptic solution dripping down the gluteal cleft may not be visible to perioperative team members.

IV.f.4.   Any material near the patient that is in contact with the skin antiseptic solution, including electrodes (eg, ECG, ESU) and tourniquet materials (ie, cuff, padding), should be removed and replaced as necessary. *[5: Benefits Balanced with Harms]*

IV.g.   Protective measures should be taken to minimize the risk of fire when flammable preoperative patient skin antiseptics are used.[34,102,103,150,151] *[1: Regulatory Requirement]*

Flammable skin antiseptics are a fuel source and pose a fire hazard. The prevention of pooling of flammable skin antiseptics and allowing for the complete drying of the antiseptic to minimize the fire hazard is supported by the CMS[102,103] and several clinical practice guidelines, including guidance from the National Fire Protection Association (NFPA),[151] the American Society of Anesthesiologists (ASA),[150] and the AORN Guideline for a Safe Environment of Care, Part 1.[34]

IV.g.1.   Flammable skin antiseptics should be prevented from pooling or soaking into linens or the patient's hair by
- use of reusable or disposable sterile towels to absorb drips and excess solution during application,
- removal of materials that are saturated with the skin antiseptic before the patient is draped, and
- wicking of excess solution with a sterile towel to help dry the surgical prep area completely.[153-155]

[3: Moderate Evidence]

The practice of preventing pooling or soaking into linens or the patient's hair is supported by NFPA guidance[155] and the ECRI Institute.[153,154]

IV.g.2.   Adequate time should be allowed for the flammable skin antiseptic to dry completely and for any fumes to dissipate before surgical drapes are applied or a potential ignition source is used.[150,153-156] *[1: Strong Evidence]*

The practice of allowing flammable skin antiseptics to dry completely and allowing any fumes to dissipate before applying surgical drapes is supported by guidelines from the ASA,[150] ECRI,[153,154] and the NFPA[155] and by a literature review.[156] Allowing adequate time for skin antiseptics to dry before applying drapes helps prevent the accumulation of volatile fumes beneath the drapes.[156] The volatile fumes are flammable and may ignite without a connection between the ignition source and the actual antiseptic solution.[153,154]

IV.g.3. Perioperative team members should communicate use of flammable skin antiseptics as part of the fire risk assessment involving the entire perioperative team before beginning a surgical procedure.[34,150,155] *[1: Strong Evidence]*

The NFPA,[155] the ASA,[150] and the AORN Guideline for a Safe Environment of Care, Part 1[34] support the importance of completing a fire risk assessment. Active communication regarding the use of flammable skin antiseptics alerts all perioperative team members to the inherent risks and allows appropriate precautions to be taken.

IV.g.4. Flammable skin antiseptics should not be heated. *[5: Benefits Balanced with Harms]*

The evidence review found no literature to support or refute this recommendation. Heating flammable antiseptics may pose a serious risk of fire. When the temperature of flammable chemicals increases, they become more unstable and may ignite easily.

IV.h. When lifting and holding the patient's extremity or head during preoperative patient skin antisepsis, the perioperative team member should minimize his or her muscle fatigue by using two hands for holding the extremity or head, obtaining assistance from another team member, using an assistive device, or using a combination of these methods.[157] *[2: High Evidence]*

The evidence review found no literature to support or refute this recommendation. The AORN Guidance Statement: Safe Patient Handling and Movement in the Perioperative Setting supports this practice as part of an ergonomic tool that includes a chart outlining recommended holding techniques based on the patient's weight to help prevent muscle fatigue and musculoskeletal disorders.[157]

IV.i. At the end of the surgical procedure, the skin antiseptic should be removed from the patient's skin before application of an occlusive dressing or tape, unless otherwise indicated by the manufacturer's instructions for use.[66,144] *[3: Moderate Evidence]*

The removal of skin antiseptics from the skin at the end of the surgical procedure is supported by one literature review[66] and one case report of a chemical burn from povidone-iodine.[144] Residual skin antiseptics may cause skin irritation and contact dermatitis in sensitive individuals. Removing the solution as soon as possible after completion of the procedure minimizes the risk on ongoing irritation.

IV.j. The perioperative RN should assess the patient's skin for injury after surgery.[125] A thorough evaluation of the patient's skin may be postponed until the patient is transferred to the postoperative area, depending on the patient's condition. *[4: Limited Evidence]*

No research evidence was found to support or refute this recommendation. Evaluating the patient's progress toward attaining outcomes after an intervention is a standard of perioperative nursing practice.[125] Reassessing the patient's skin after the procedure is an important method for evaluating the patient for injury.

IV.k. Preoperative patient skin antisepsis should be documented in the patient's record. Documentation should include the
   ○ removal and disposition of any jewelry;
   ○ condition of the skin at the surgical site (eg, presence of rashes, skin eruptions, abrasions, redness, irritation, burns);
   ○ antiseptic used;
   ○ person performing preoperative patient skin antisepsis;
   ○ area prepped; and
   ○ postoperative skin condition, including any skin irritation, hypersensitivity, or allergic response to preparation solutions.
[5: Benefits Balanced with Harms]

Recommendation V

Perioperative team members should review and follow the skin antiseptic manufacturer's instructions for use and safety data sheets (SDSs) for handling, storing, and disposing of skin antiseptics.

The collective evidence found that following the antiseptic manufacturer's instructions for use and the SDS is the safest method for handling, storing, and disposing of skin antiseptics.

The evidence review identified a lack of research in the clinical setting for safe handling, storing, and disposing of skin antiseptics.

V.a. Skin antiseptics must be stored in the original single-use container.[63,158-163] *[1: Regulatory Requirement]*

In November 2013, the FDA issued a drug safety communication requesting label changes and single-use packaging of over-the-counter topical antiseptic products to decrease risk of infection.[63] Topical antiseptics are not required by the FDA to be manufactured as sterile although most are manufactured with a sterile process. Nonsterile antiseptics may be contaminated with bacteria during or after manufacturing.[63] As a result of reported outbreaks involving contaminated antiseptic products, the FDA requested that manufacturers package antiseptics for preoperative skin preparation in single-use containers, to be used only one time for one patient.

In several case reports and nonexperimental studies, antiseptics have been linked to patient infections from both intrinsic[159,160,162,163] and extrinsic[161] contamination. In a laboratory study, Anderson et al[158] found that *Pseudomonas cepacia* survived up to 29 weeks in the laboratory setting, which confirmed the plausibility of a case of *P cepacia* surviving in povidone-iodine for 68 weeks after contamination during manufacturing.

V.a.1.   Skin antiseptics in single-use containers must be discarded after use and not refilled.[63] *[1: Regulatory Requirement]*

V.b.   Skin antiseptics must not be diluted after opening.[63] *[1: Regulatory Requirement]*

In a drug safety communication, the FDA states that health care professionals should not dilute antiseptic products after opening them to reduce the possibility of these products becoming contaminated.[63]

V.c.   Heating of nonflammable skin antiseptics should only be performed in accordance with the manufacturers' instructions for use.[164] *[3: Moderate Evidence]*

Heating may alter the chemical composition of the skin antiseptic and may alter the effectiveness of the antiseptic. In a 1985 expert opinion paper, Gottardi[164] described that the heating of povidone-iodine alters the equilibrium of the iodine content. No other evidence was found describing the effect of heating on antiseptics.

Heating antiseptics may also cause thermal or chemical burns. No case reports of injury were found in the evidence review.

V.c.1.   Skin antiseptics should not be warmed in a microwave oven or autoclave. *[5: Benefits Balanced with Harms]*

The evidence review found no literature to support or refute this recommendation. The temperature of the skin antiseptic is uncontrolled when heated in a microwave or autoclave, and temperature extremes may result in a patient injury.

V.d.   Safety data sheets for all skin antiseptics used must be readily available in the practice area.[165] *[1: Regulatory Requirement]*

The SDS provides information about the flammability of the antiseptic and the maximum safe storage temperature. The Occupational Safety and Health Administration requires that SDSs be available for all chemicals used in the practice setting.[165] These documents outline the hazards related to the chemicals and appropriate action to take in the event of a chemical exposure (eg, splash to the eyes).

V.e.   Storage of flammable skin antiseptics must be in compliance with local, state, and federal regulations.[34,102,103,151,155] *[1: Regulatory Requirement]*

The NFPA has recommendations for storage of flammable solutions.[151,155] The CMS states in §482.41(c)(2) that "facilities, supplies, and equipment must be maintained to ensure an acceptable level of safety and quality," including storage in compliance with fire codes.[102,103] The AORN Guideline for a Safe Environment of Care, Part 1 also recommends following local and state fire regulations for storage of flammable liquids, such as alcohol-based skin antiseptic solutions.[34]

V.f.   Disposal of unused flammable skin antiseptics must be handled in a manner to decrease the risk of fire and in accordance with local, state, and federal regulations.[102,103,166] *[1: Regulatory Requirement]*

Disposal of residual flammable antiseptics is regulated by the Environmental Protection Agency (EPA).[166] The CMS regulations state that trash must be stored and disposed of in accordance with federal, state, and local laws and regulations, including those from the EPA.[102,103] No reports of improper disposal of antiseptics were found. There is a risk that fires can occur when flammable antiseptics are discarded in nonhazardous trash, and incineration or autoclaving of biohazardous waste can rapidly ignite flammable antiseptics.

Glossary

Antiseptic: A product with antimicrobial activity applied to the skin to reduce the number of microbial flora.

Iodism: Poisoning by iodine, a condition marked by severe rhinitis, frontal headache, emaciation, weakness, and skin eruptions. Caused by the administration of iodine or one of the iodides.

Log reduction: The logarithmic death progression of microorganisms after exposure to a sterilant or antiseptic agent. The reduction difference between average surviving microbes for control and test carriers used as an efficacy parameter.

References

1. Dumville JC, McFarlane E, Edwards P, Lipp A, Holmes A. Preoperative skin antiseptics for preventing surgical wound infections after clean surgery. *Cochrane Database Syst Rev*. 2013;3:CD003949. [IA]

2. Webster J, Osborne S. Preoperative bathing or showering with skin antiseptics to prevent surgical site infection. *Cochrane Database Syst Rev*. 2012;9:CD004985. [IA]

3. Tanner J, Norrie P, Melen K. Preoperative hair removal to reduce surgical site infection. *Cochrane Database Syst Rev*. 2011;11:CD004122. [IA]

4. Surgical site infection. National Institute for Health and Care Excellence. https://www.nice.org.uk/Guidance/QS49. Accessed July 14, 2014. [IVA]

5. Cruse PJ. A five-year prospective study of 23,649 surgical wounds. *Arch Surg.* 1973;107(2):206-210. [IIIA]

6. Anderson DJ, Kaye KS, Classen D, et al. Strategies to prevent surgical site infections in acute care hospitals. *Infect Control Hosp Epidemiol.* 2008;2(9 Suppl 1):51-61. [IVA]

7. Smith MA, Dahlen NR. Clinical practice guideline surgical site infection prevention. *Orthop Nurs.* 2013;32(5):242-248. [IVB]

8. Rotter ML, Larsen SO, Cooke EM, et al. A comparison of the effects of preoperative whole-body bathing with detergent alone and with detergent containing chlorhexidine gluconate on the frequency of wound infections after clean surgery. The European Working Party on Control of Hospital Infections. *J Hosp Infect.* 1988;11(4):310-320. [IA]

9. Veiga DF, Damasceno CA, Veiga-Filho J, et al. Randomized controlled trial of the effectiveness of chlorhexidine showers before elective plastic surgical procedures. *Infect Control Hospital Epidemiol.* 2009;30(1):77-79. [IB]

10. Veiga DF, Damasceno CA, Veiga Filho J, et al. Influence of povidone-iodine preoperative showers on skin colonization in elective plastic surgery procedures. *Plast Reconstr Surg.* 2008;121(1):115-118. [IA]

11. Jakobsson J, Perlkvist A, Wann-Hansson C. Searching for evidence regarding using preoperative disinfection showers to prevent surgical site infections: a systematic review. *Worldviews Evid Based Nurs.* 2011;8(3):143-152. [IIA]

12. Kamel C, McGahan L, Polisena J, Mierzwinski-Urban M, Embil JM. Preoperative skin antiseptic preparations for preventing surgical site infections: a systematic review. *Infect Control Hosp Epidemiol.* 2012;33(6):608-617. [IIA]

13. Chlebicki MP, Safdar N, O'Horo JC, Maki DG. Preoperative chlorhexidine shower or bath for prevention of surgical site infection: a meta-analysis. *Am J Infect Control.* 2013;41(2):167-173. [IIA]

14. Tanner J, Gould D, Jenkins P, Hilliam R, Mistry N, Walsh S. A fresh look at preoperative body washing. *J Infect Prev.* 2012;13(1):11-15. [IB]

15. Murray MR, Saltzman MD, Gryzlo SM, Terry MA, Woodward CC, Nuber GW. Efficacy of preoperative home use of 2% chlorhexidine gluconate cloth before shoulder surgery. *J Shoulder Elbow Surg.* 2011;20(6):928-933. [IA]

16. Edmiston Jr CE, Krepel CJ, Seabrook GR, Lewis BD, Brown KR, Towne JB. Preoperative shower revisited: can high topical antiseptic levels be achieved on the skin surface before surgical admission? *J Am Coll Surg.* 2008;207(2):233-239. [IB]

17. Edmiston CE Jr, Seabrook GR, Johnson CP, Paulson DS, Beausoleil CM. Comparative of a new and innovative 2% chlorhexidine gluconate-impregnated cloth with 4% chlorhexidine gluconate as topical antiseptic for preparation of the skin prior to surgery. *Am J Infect Control.* 2007;35(2):89-96. [IB]

18. Kapadia BH, Issa K, McElroy MJ, Pivec R, Daley JA, Mont MA. Advance pre-operative chlorhexidine preparation reduces periprosthetic infections following total joint arthroplasty. *Semin Arthroplasty.* 2013;24(2):83-86. [IIA]

19. Graling PR, Vasaly FW. Effectiveness of 2% CHG cloth bathing for reducing surgical site infections. *AORN J.* 2013;97(5):547-551. [IIB]

20. Johnson AJ, Kapadia BH, Daley JA, Molina CB, Mont MA. Chlorhexidine reduces infections in knee arthroplasty. *J Knee Surg.* 2013;26(3):213-218. [IIB]

21. Zywiel MG, Daley JA, Delanois RE, Naziri Q, Johnson AJ, Mont MA. Advance pre-operative chlorhexidine reduces the incidence of surgical site infections in knee arthroplasty. *Int Orthop.* 2011;35(7):1001-1006. [IIB]

22. Johnson AJ, Daley JA, Zywiel MG, Delanois RE, Mont MA. Preoperative chlorhexidine preparation and the incidence of surgical site infections after hip arthroplasty. *J Arthroplasty.* 2010;25(6 Suppl):98-102. [IIB]

23. Kapadia BH, Johnson AJ, Daley JA, Issa K, Mont MA. Pre-admission cutaneous chlorhexidine preparation reduces surgical site infections in total hip arthroplasty. *J Arthroplasty.* 2013;28(3):490-493. [IIB]

24. Kapadia BH, Johnson AJ, Issa K, Mont MA. Economic evaluation of chlorhexidine cloths on healthcare costs due to surgical site infections following total knee arthroplasty. *J Arthroplasty.* 2013;28(7):1061-1065. [VA]

25. Eiselt D. Presurgical skin preparation with a novel 2% chlorhexidine gluconate cloth reduces rates of surgical site infection in orthopaedic surgical patients. *Orthop Nurs.* 2009;28(3):141-145. [VA]

26. Karki S, Cheng AC. Impact of non-rinse skin cleansing with chlorhexidine gluconate on prevention of healthcare-associated infections and colonization with multi-resistant organisms: a systematic review. *J Hosp Infect.* 2012;82(2):71-84. [IIIA]

27. Edmiston CE Jr, Okoli O, Graham MB, Sinski S, Seabrook GR. Evidence for using chlorhexidine gluconate preoperative cleansing to reduce the risk of surgical site infection. *AORN J.* 2010;92(5):509-518. [VB]

28. Farber NJ, Chen AF, Bartsch SM, Feigel JL, Klatt BA. No infection reduction using chlorhexidine wipes in total joint arthroplasty. *Clin Orthop Relat Res.* 2013;471(10):3120-3125. [IIA]

29. Arrowsmith VA, Maunder JA, Sargent RJ, Taylor R. Removal of nail polish and finger rings to prevent surgical infection. *Cochrane Database Syst Rev.* 2001;4:CD003325. [IA]

30. Hedderwick SA, McNeil SA, Lyons MJ, Kauffman CA. Pathogenic organisms associated with artificial fingernails worn by healthcare workers. *Infect Control Hosp Epidemiol.* 2000;21(8):505-509. [IIB]

31. McNeil SA, Foster CL, Hedderwick SA, Kauffman CA. Effect of hand cleansing with antimicrobial soap or alcohol-based gel on microbial colonization of artificial fingernails worn by health care workers. *Clin Infect Dis.* 2001;32(3):367-372. [IIA]

32. Leclair JM, Winston KR, Sullivan BF, O'Connell JM, Harrington SM, Goldmann DA. Effect of preoperative shampoos on resident scalp flora. *Todays OR Nurse.* 1988;10(3):15-21. [IB]

33. Guideline for product selection. In: *Guidelines for Perioperative Practice.* Denver, CO: AORN, Inc; 2015:179-186. [IVB]

34. Guideline for a safe environment of care, part 1. In: *Guidelines for Perioperative Practice.* Denver, CO: AORN Inc; 2015:239-263. [IVA]

35. Broekman ML, van Beijnum J, Peul WC, Regli L. Neurosurgery and shaving: what's the evidence? *J Neurosurg.* 2011;115(4):670-678. [IIIA]

36. Sebastian S. Does preoperative scalp shaving result in fewer postoperative wound infections when compared with no scalp shaving? A systematic review. *J Neurosci Nurs.* 2012;44(3):149-156. [IIIA]

37. Ng W, Alexander D, Kerr B, Ho MF, Amato M, Katz K. A hairy tale: successful patient education strategies to reduce prehospital hair removal by patients undergoing elective caesarean section. *J Hosp Infect.* 2013;83(1):64-67. [IIIB]

38. Jose B, Dignon A. Is there a relationship between preoperative shaving (hair removal) and surgical site infection? *J Perioper Pract.* 2013;23(1-2):22-25. [VB]

39. Celik SE, Kara A. Does shaving the incision site increase the infection rate after spinal surgery? *Spine.* 2007;32(15):1575-1577. [IA]

40. Grober ED, Domes T, Fanipour M, Copp JE. Preoperative hair removal on the male genitalia: clippers vs razors. *J Sex Med.* 2013;10(2):589-594. [IB]

41. Hemani ML, Lepor H. Skin preparation for the prevention of surgical site infection: which agent is best? *Rev Urol.* 2009;11(4):190-195. [VB]

42. Tschudin-Sutter S, Frei R, Egli-Gany D, et al. No risk of surgical site infections from residual bacteria after disinfection with povidone-iodine-alcohol in 1014 cases: A prospective observational study. *Ann Surg.* 2012;255(3):565-569. [IIIA]

43. Edmiston CE Jr, Bruden B, Rucinski MC, Henen C, Graham MB, Lewis BL. Reducing the risk of surgical site infections: does chlorhexidine gluconate provide a risk reduction benefit? *Am J Infect Control.* 2013;41(5 Suppl):S49-S55. [VB]

44. Darouiche RO, Wall MJ Jr, Itani KM, et al. Chlorhexidine-alcohol versus povidone-iodine for surgical-site antisepsis. *N Engl J Med.* 2010;362(1):18-26. [IA]

45. Nishihara Y, Kajiura T, Yokota K, Kobayashi H, Okubo T. Evaluation with a focus on both the antimicrobial efficacy and cumulative skin irritation potential of chlorhexidine gluconate alcohol-containing preoperative skin preparations. *Am J Infect Control.* 2012;40(10):973-978. [IB]

46. Saltzman MD, Nuber GW, Gryzlo SM, Marecek GS, Koh JL. Efficacy of surgical preparation solutions in shoulder surgery. *J Bone Joint Surg Am.* 2009;91(8):1949-1953. [IA]

47. Amer-Alshiek J, Alshiek T, Almog B, et al. Can we reduce the surgical site infection rate in cesarean sections using a chlorhexidine-based antisepsis protocol? *J Matern Fetal Neonatal Med.* 2013;26(17):1749-1752. [IIIB]

48. Lee I, Agarwal RK, Lee BY, Fishman NO, Umscheid CA. Systematic review and cost analysis comparing use of chlorhexidine with use of iodine for preoperative skin antisepsis to prevent surgical site infection. *Infect Control Hosp Epidemiol.* 2010;31(12):1219-1229. [IA]

49. Al Maqbali MA. Preoperative antiseptic skin preparations and reducing SSI. *Br J Nurs.* 2013;22(21):1227-1233. [VA]

50. Lim K-S, Kam PCA. Chlorhexidine—pharmacology and clinical applications. *Anaesth Intensive Care.* 2008;36(4):502-512. [VA]

51. Noorani A, Rabey N, Walsh SR, Davies RJ. Systematic review and meta-analysis of preoperative antisepsis with chlorhexidine versus povidone-iodine in clean-contaminated surgery. *Br J Surg.* 2010;97(11):1614-1620. [IIB]

52. Paocharoen V, Mingmalairak C, Apisarnthanarak A. Comparison of surgical wound infection after preoperative skin preparation with 4% chlorhexidine [correction of chlohexidine] and povidone iodine: a prospective randomized trial. *J Med Assoc Thai.* 2009;92(7):898-902. [IB]

53. Maiwald M, Chan ES-Y. The forgotten role of alcohol: a systematic review and meta-analysis of the clinical efficacy and perceived role of chlorhexidine in skin antisepsis. *PLoS One.* 2012;7(9):e44277. [IIA]

54. Sistla SC, Prabhu G, Sistla S, Sadasivan J. Minimizing wound contamination in a "clean" surgery: comparison of chlorhexidine-ethanol and povidone-iodine. *Chemotherapy.* 2010;56(4):261-267. [IA]

55. Menderes G, Athar Ali N, Aagaard K, Sangi-Haghpeykar H. Chlorhexidine-alcohol compared with povidone-iodine for surgical-site antisepsis in cesarean deliveries. *Obstet Gynecol.* 2012;120(5):1037-1044. [IIA]

56. Berry AR, Watt B, Goldacre MJ, Thomson JW, McNair TJ. A comparison of the use of povidone-iodine and chlorhexidine in the prophylaxis of postoperative wound infection. *J Hosp Infect.* 1982;3(1):55-63. [IB]

57. Savage JW, Weatherford BM, Sugrue PA, et al. Efficacy of surgical preparation solutions in lumbar spine surgery. *J Bone Joint Surg Am.* 2012;94(6):490-494. [IA]

58. Yammine K, Harvey A. Efficacy of preparation solutions and cleansing techniques on contamination of the skin in foot and ankle surgery: a systematic review and meta-analysis. *Bone Joint J.* 2013;95(4):498-503. [IB]

59. Swenson BR, Hedrick TL, Metzger R, Bonatti H, Pruett TL, Sawyer RG. Effects of preoperative skin preparation on postoperative wound infection rates: a prospective study of 3 skin preparation protocols. *Infect Control Hosp Epidemiol.* 2009;30(10):964-971. [IIB]

60. Segal CG, Anderson JJ. Preoperative skin preparation of cardiac patients. AORN J. 2002;76(5):821-828. [IA]

61. Roberts A, Wilcox K, Devineni R, Osevala M. Skin preparation in CABG surgery: a randomized control trial. *Comp Surg.* 1995;14(6):724, 741-744, 747. [IB]

62. US Food and Drug Administration. Tentative final monograph for healthcare antiseptic drug products proposed rule. *Fed Regist.* 1994;59(116):31402-31452.

63. Over-the-counter topical antiseptic products: drug safety communication—FDA requests label changes and single-use packaging to decrease risk of infection. http://www.fda.gov/safety/medwatch/safetyinformation/safetyalertsforhumanmedicalproducts/ucm374892.htm Accessed July 14, 2014.

64. Sullivan PJ, Healy CE, Hirpara KM, Hussey AJ, Potter SM, Kelly JL. An assessment of skin preparation in upper limb surgery. *J Hand Surg Eur* Vol. 2008;33(4):513-514. [IIB]

65. Digison MB. A review of anti-septic agents for pre-operative skin preparation. *Plast Surg Nurs.* 2007;27(4):185-189. [VB]

66. Murkin CE. Pre-operative antiseptic skin preparation. *Br J Nurs.* 2009;18(11):665-669. [VA]

67. Quatresooz P, Xhauflaire-Uhoda E, Pierard-Franchimont C, Pierard GE. Regional variability in stratum corneum reactivity to antiseptic formulations. *Contact Derm.* 2007;56(5):271-273. [IIIB]

68. Sanders TH, Hawken SM. Chlorhexidine burns after shoulder arthroscopy. *Am J Orthop* (Belle Mead NJ). 2012;41(4):172-174. [VB]

69. *Academy Position Statement: The Risk of Severe Allergic Reactions from the Use of Potassium Iodide for Radiation Emergencies.* February 2004. American Academy of Allergy Asthma and Immunology. https://www.aaaai.org/Aaaai/media/MediaLibrary/PDF%20Documents/Practice%20and%20Parameters/Potassium-iodide-in-radiation-emergencies-2004.pdf. Accessed July 14, 2014. [IVB]

70. Schabelman E, Witting M. The relationship of radiocontrast, iodine, and seafood allergies: a medical myth exposed. *J Emerg Med.* 2010;39(5):701-707. [VA]

71. Huang SW. Seafood and iodine: an analysis of a medical myth. *Allergy Asthma Proc.* 2005;26(6):468-469. [IIIC]

72. Yoshida K, Sakurai Y, Kawahara S, et al. Anaphylaxis to polyvinylpyrrolidone in povidone-iodine for impetigo contagiosum in a boy with atopic dermatitis. *Int Arch Allergy Immunol.* 2008;146(2):169-173. [VB]

73. Adachi A, Fukunaga A, Hayashi K, Kunisada M, Horikawa T. Anaphylaxis to polyvinylpyrrolidone after vaginal application of povidone-iodine. *Contact Dermatitis.* 2003;48(3):133-136. [VA]

74. Sivathasan N, Goodfellow PB. Skin cleansers: the risks of chlorhexidine. *J Clin Pharmacol.* 2011;51(5):785-786. [VA]

75. Garvey LH, Roed-Petersen J, Husum B. Anaphylactic reactions in anaesthetised patients - four cases of chlorhexidine allergy. *Acta Anaesthesiol Scand.* 2001;45(10):1290-1294. [VA]

76. Toomey M. Preoperative chlorhexidine anaphylaxis in a patient scheduled for coronary artery bypass graft: a case report. *AANA J.* 2013;81(3):209-214. [VA]

77. Khan RA, Kazi T, O'Donohoe B. Near fatal intraoperative anaphylaxis to chlorhexidine—is it time to change practice? *BMJ Case Rep.* 2011;2011. [VA]

78. Vujevich J, Zirwas M. Delayed hypersensitivity to isopropyl alcohol. *Contact Dermatitis.* 2007;56(5):287. [VC]

79. Baillif S, Roure-Sobas C, Le-Duff F, Kodjikian L. Aqueous humor contamination during phacoemulsification in a university teaching hospital. *J Fr Opthalmol.* 2012;35(3):153-156. [IIIB]

80. Quiroga LP, Lansingh V, Laspina F, et al. A prospective study demonstrating the effect of 5% povidone-iodine application for anterior segment intraocular surgery in Paraguay. *Arq Bras Oftalmol.* 2010;73(2):125-128. [IIA]

81. Ou JI, Ta CN. Endophthalmitis prophylaxis. *Ophthalmol Clin North Am.* 2006;19(4):449-456. [VA]

82. Wu PC, Li M, Chang SJ, et al. Risk of endophthalmitis after cataract surgery using different protocols for povidone-iodine preoperative disinfection. *J Ocul Pharmacol Ther.* 2006;22(1):54-61. [IIA]

83. Trinavarat A, Atchaneeyasakul LO, Nopmaneejumruslers C, Inson K. Reduction of endophthalmitis rate after cataract surgery with preoperative 5% povidone-iodine. *Dermatology.* 2006;212(Suppl 1):35-40. [IB]

84. Li B, Nentwich MM, Hoffmann LE, et al. Comparison of the efficacy of povidone-iodine 1.0%, 5.0%, and 10.0% irrigation combined with topical levofloxacin 0.3% as preoperative prophylaxis in cataract surgery. *J Cataract Refract Surg.* 2013;39(7):994-1001. [IA]

85. Chou SF, Lin CH, Chang SW. Povidone-iodine application induces corneal cell death through fixation. *Br J Ophthalmol.* 2011;95(2):277-283. [IIIB]

86. Below H, Behrens-Baumann W, Bernhardt C, Volzke H, Kramer A, Rudolph P. Systemic iodine absorption after preoperative antisepsis using povidone-iodine in cataract surgery—an open controlled study. *Dermatology.* 2006;212(Suppl 1):41-46. [IIB]

87. Razavi B, Zollinger R, Kramer A, et al. Systemic iodine absorption associated with the use of preoperative ophthalmic antiseptics containing iodine. *Cutan Ocul Toxicol.* 2013;32(4):279-282. [IIB]

88. Amstey MS, Jones AP. Preparation of the vagina for surgery. A comparison of povidone-iodine and saline solution. *JAMA.* 1981;245(8):839-841. [IIIB]

89. Lewis LA, Lathi RB, Crochet P, Nezhat C. Preoperative vaginal preparation with baby shampoo compared with povidone-iodine before gynecologic procedures. *J Minim Invasive Gynecol.* 2007;14(6):736-739. [IIA]

90. American College of Obstetricians and Gynecologists Women's Health Care Physicians, Committee on Gynecologic Practice. Committee Opinion No. 571: Solutions for surgical preparation of the vagina. *Obstet Gynecol.* 2013;122(3):718-720. [IVB]

91. Eason E, Wells G, Garber G, et al. Antisepsis for abdominal hysterectomy: a randomised controlled trial of povidone-iodine gel. *BJOG.* 2004;111(7):695-699. [IA]

92. Haas DM, Morgan S, Contreras K. Vaginal preparation with antiseptic solution before cesarean section for preventing postoperative infections. *Cochrane Database Systematic Rev.* 2013;1:CD007892. [IB]

93. Guzman Melissa A, Prien Samuel D, Blann David W. Post-cesarean related infection and vaginal preparation with povidone-iodine revisited. *Prim Care Update Ob Gyns.* 2002;9(6):206-209. [IB]

94. Haas DM, Pazouki F, Smith RR, et al. Vaginal cleansing before cesarean delivery to reduce postoperative infectious morbidity: a randomized, controlled trial. *Am J Obstet Gynecol.* 2010;202(3):310.e1-310.e6. [IB]

95. Asghania M, Mirblouk F, Shakiba M, Faraji R. Preoperative vaginal preparation with povidone-iodine on post-caesarean infectious morbidity. *J Obstet Gynaecol.* 2011;31(5):400-403. [IIA]

96. Hadiati DR, Hakimi M, Nurdiati DS. Skin preparation for preventing infection following caesarean section. *Cochrane Database Syst Rev.* 2012;9:CD007462. [IA]

97. Bibbo C, Patel DV, Gehrmann RM, Lin SS. Chlorhexidine provides superior skin decontamination in foot and ankle surgery: a prospective randomized study. *Clin Orthop Relat Res.* 2005;438:204-208. [IB]

98. Ostrander RV, Botte MJ, Brage ME. Efficacy of surgical preparation solutions in foot and ankle surgery. *J Bone Joint Surg Am.* 2005;87(5):980-985. [IA]

99. Hort KR, DeOrio JK. Residual bacterial contamination after surgical preparation of the foot or ankle with or without alcohol. *Foot Ankle Int.* 2002;23(10):946-948. [IB]

100. Becerro de Bengoa Vallejo R, Losa Iglesias ME, Alou Cervera L, Sevillano Fernandez D, Prieto Prieto J. Preoperative skin and nail preparation of the foot: comparison of the efficacy of 4 different methods in reducing bacterial load. *J Am Acad Dermatol.* 2009;61(6):986-992. [IB]

101. Weber SM, Hargunani CA, Wax MK. DuraPrep and the risk of fire during tracheostomy. *Head Neck.* 2006;28(7):649-652. [VA]

102. *State Operations Manual Appendix A—Survey Protocol, Regulations and Interpretive Guidelines for Hospitals.* Rev 89; 2013. Centers for Medicare & Medicaid Services. http://www.cms.gov/Regulations-and-Guidance/Guidance/Manuals/downloads/som107ap_a_hospitals.pdf. Accessed July 14, 2014.

103. *State Operations Manual Appendix L—Guidance for Surveyors: Ambulatory Surgical Centers.* Rev. 89; 2013. Centers for Medicare & Medicaid Services. http://www.cms.gov/Regulations-and-Guidance/Guidance/Manuals/downloads/som107ap_l_ambulatory.pdf. Accessed July 14, 2014.

104. Zamora JL. Chemical and microbiologic characteristics and toxicity of povidone-iodine solutions. *Am J Surg.* 1986;151(3):400-406. [VA]

105. Lavelle KJ, Doedens DJ, Kleit SA, Forney RB. Iodine absorption in burn patients treated topically with povidone-iodine. *Clin Pharmacol Ther.* 1975;17(3):355-362. [VB]

106. Rath T, Meissl G. Induction of hyperthyroidism in burn patients treated topically with povidone-iodine. *Burns Incl Therm Inj.* 1988;14(4):320-322. [VA]

107. Pietsch J, Meakins JL. Complications of povidone-iodine absorption in topically treated burn patients. *Lancet.* 1976;1(7954):280-282. [VA]

108. Tomoda C, Kitano H, Uruno T, et al. Transcutaneous iodine absorption in adult patients with thyroid cancer disinfected with povidone-iodine at operation. *Thyroid.* 2005;15(6):600-603. [IB]

109. Pyati SP, Ramamurthy RS, Krauss MT, Pildes RS. Absorption of iodine in the neonate following topical use of povidone iodine. *J Pediatr.* 1977;91(5):825-828. [IIB]

110. Linder N, Davidovitch N, Reichman B, et al. Topical iodine-containing antiseptics and subclinical hypothyroidism in preterm infants. *J Pediatr*. 1997;131(3):434-439. [IIIA]

111. Smerdely P, Lim A, Boyages SC, et al. Topical iodine-containing antiseptics and neonatal hypothyroidism in very-low-birthweight infants. *Lancet*. 1989;2(8664):661-664. [IIIB]

112. Bryant WP, Zimmerman D. Iodine-induced hyperthyroidism in a newborn. *Pediatrics*. 1995;95(3):434-436. [VB]

113. Afsar FS. Skin care for preterm and term neonates. *Clin Exp Derm*. 2009;34(8):855-858. [VA]

114. Vorherr H, Vorherr UF, Mehta P, Ulrich JA, Messer RH. Vaginal absorption of povidone-iodine. *JAMA*. 1980;244(23):2628-2629. [IIIC]

115. DailyMed. US National Library of Medicine. http://dailymed.nlm.nih.gov. Accessed July 14, 2014.

116. Lashkari HP, Chow P, Godambe S. Aqueous 2% chlorhexidine-induced chemical burns in an extremely premature infant. *Arch Dis Child Fetal Neonatal Ed*. 2012;97(1):F64. [VB]

117. Schick JB, Milstein JM. Burn hazard of isopropyl alcohol in the neonate. *Pediatrics*. 1981;68(4):587-588. [VB]

118. Harpin V, Rutter N. Percutaneous alcohol absorption and skin necrosis in a preterm infant. *Arch Dis Child*. 1982;57(6):477-479. [VA]

119. Guideline for transfer of patient care information. In: *Guidelines for Perioperative Practice*. Denver, CO: AORN, Inc; 2015: 583-588. [IVB]

120. Cronen G, Ringus V, Sigle G, Ryu J. Sterility of surgical site marking. *J Bone Joint Surg Am*. 2005;87(10):2193-2195. [IIB]

121. Rooney J, Khoo OKS, Higgs AR, Small TJ, Bell S. Surgical site marking does not affect sterility. *ANZ J Surg*. 2008;78(8):688-689. [IIB]

122. Wilson J, Tate D. Can pre-operative skin marking transfer methicillin-resistant Staphylococcus aureus between patients? A laboratory experiment. *J Bone Joint Surg Br*. 2006;88(4):541-542. [IIIA]

123. Mears SC, Dinah AF, Knight TA, Frassica FJ, Belkoff SM. Visibility of surgical site marking after preoperative skin preparation. *Eplasty* [Electronic Resource]. 2008;8:e35. [IIB]

124. Thakkar SC, Mears SC. Visibility of surgical site marking: a prospective randomized trial of two skin preparation solutions. *J Bone Joint Surg Am*. 2012;94(2):97-102. [IB]

125. Standards of perioperative nursing. In: *Perioperative Standards and Recommended Practices*. Denver, CO: AORN, Inc; 2014:3-18. [IVC]

126. Trick WE, Vernon MO, Hayes RA, et al. Impact of ring wearing on hand contamination and comparison of hand hygiene agents in a hospital. *Clin Infect Dis*. 2003;36(11):1383-1390. [IIA]

127. Bonnevialle N, Geiss L, Cavalie L, Ibnoulkhatib A, Verdeil X, Bonnevialle P. Skin preparation before hip replacement in emergency setting versus elective scheduled arthroplasty: bacteriological comparative analysis. *Orthop Traumatol Surg Res*. 2013;99(6):659-665. [IIA]

128. Guideline for hand hygiene. In: *Guidelines for Perioperative Practice*. Denver, CO: AORN, Inc; 2015:31-42. [IVB]

129. Guideline for surgical attire. In: *Guidelines for Perioperative Practice*. Denver, CO: AORN, Inc; 2015:97-120. [IVB]

130. Pearce BA, Miller LH, Martin MA, Roush DL. Efficacy of clean v sterile surgical prep kits. *AORN J*. 1997;66(3):464-470. [IB]

131. Guideline for sterile technique. In: *Guidelines for Perioperative Practice*. Denver, CO: AORN, Inc; 2015:67-96. [IVA]

132. Cheng K, Robertson H, St Mart JP, Leanord A, McLeod I. Quantitative analysis of bacteria in forefoot surgery: a comparison of skin preparation techniques. *Foot Ankle Int*. 2009;30(10):992-997. [IB]

133. Ellenhorn JD, Smith DD, Schwarz RE, et al. Paint-only is equivalent to scrub-and-paint in preoperative preparation of abdominal surgery sites. *J Am Coll Surg*. 2005;201(5):737-741. [IC]

134. Gilliam DL, Nelson CL. Comparison of a one-step iodophor skin preparation versus traditional preparation in total joint surgery. *Clin Orthop Relat Res*. 1990;250:258-260. [IB]

135. Vagholkar Ketan, Julka Karan. Preoperative skin preparation: which is the best method? *Internet J Surg*. 2012;28(4):1-1. [IA]

136. Weed S, Bastek JA, Sammel MD, Beshara M, Hoffman S, Srinivas SK. Comparing postcesarean infectious complication rates using two different skin preparations. *Obstet Gynecol*. 2011;117(5):1123-1129. [IIA]

137. Brooks RA, Hollinghurst D, Ribbans WJ, Severn M. Bacterial recolonization during foot surgery: a prospective randomized study of toe preparation techniques. *Foot Ankle Int*. 2001;22(4):347-350. [IB]

138. Naderi N, Maw K, Thomas M, Boyce DE, Shokrollahi K. A quick and effective method of limb preparation with health, safety and efficiency benefits. *Ann R Coll Surg Engl*. 2012;94(2):83-86. [IIB]

139. Incoll IW, Saravanja D, Thorvaldson KT, Small T. Comparison of the effectiveness of painting onto the hand and immersing the hand in a bag, in pre-operative skin preparation of the hand. *J Hand Surg Eur Vol*. 2009;34(3):371-373. [IIB]

140. Chou J, Choudhary A, Dhillon RS. Comparing sterile bag rubbing and paint on technique in skin preparation of the hands. *ANZ J Surg*. 2011;81(9):629-632. [IIC]

141. Chepla KJ, Gosain AK. Interstitial pneumonitis after betadine aspiration. *J Craniofac Surg*. 2012;23(6):1787-1789. [VA]

142. Stinner DJ, Krueger CA, Masini BD, Wenke JC. Time-dependent effect of chlorhexidine surgical prep. *J Hosp Infect*. 2011;79(4):313-316. [IIIB]

143. Borrego L. Acute skin lesions after surgical procedures: a clinical approach. *Actas Dermo-Sifiliogr*. 2013;104(9):776-781. [VA]

144. Rees A, Sherrod Q, Young L. Chemical burn from povidone-iodine: case and review. *J Drugs Dermatol*. 2011;10(4):414-417. [VB]

145. Demir E, O'Dey DM, Pallua N. Accidental burns during surgery. *J Burn Care Res*. 2006;27(6):895-900. [IIIB]

146. Hodgkinson DJ, Irons GB, Williams TJ. Chemical burns and skin preparation solutions. *Surg Gynecol Obstet*. 1978;147(4):534-536. [IIIB]

147. Lowe DO, Knowles SR, Weber EA, Railton CJ, Shear NH. Povidone-iodine-induced burn: case report and review of the literature. *Pharmacotherapy*. 2006;26(11):1641-1645. [VA]

148. Murthy MB, Krishnamurthy B. Severe irritant contact dermatitis induced by povidone iodine solution. *Indian J Pharmacol*. 2009;41(4):199-200. [VB]

149. Chiang YC, Lin TS, Yeh MC. Povidone-iodine-related burn under the tourniquet of a child—a case report and literature review. *J Plast Reconstr Aesthet Surg*. 2011;64(3):412-415. [VA]

150. Apfelbaum JL, Caplan RA, Barker SJ, et al. Practice advisory for the prevention and management of operating room fires: an updated report by the American Society of Anesthesiologists Task Force on Operating Room Fires. *Anesthesiology.* 2013;118(2):271-290. [IVA]

151. *NFPA 101: Life Safety Code.* 2012 ed. Quincy, MA: National Fire Protection Association; 2012. [IVB]

152. Palmanovich E, Brin YS, Laver L, Nyska M, Kish B. Third-degree chemical burns from chlorhexidine local antisepsis. *Isr Med Assoc J.* 2013;15(6):323-324. [VA]

153. ECRI. New clinical guide to surgical fire prevention. Patients can catch fire—here's how to keep them safer. *Health Devices.* 2009;38(10):314-332. [VA]

154. ECRI. Fighting airway fires. *Healthc Risk Control.* 2010;4 (Surgery and Anesthesia):1-11. [IVC]

155. *Health Care Facilities Code Handbook.* 9th ed. Quincy, MA: National Fire Protection Association; 2012. [IVB]

156. Rinder CS. Fire safety in the operating room. *Curr Opin Anaesthesiol.* 2008;21(6):790-795. [VC]

157. AORN guidance statement: Safe patient handling and movement in the perioperative setting. In: *Perioperative Standards and Recommended Practices.* Denver, CO: AORN, Inc; 2014:615-634. [IVB]

158. Anderson RL, Vess RW, Panlilio AL, Favero MS. Prolonged survival of Pseudomonas cepacia in commercially manufactured povidone-iodine. *Appl Environ Microbiol.* 1990;56(11):3598-3600. [IIIB]

159. Berkelman RL, Lewin S, Allen JR, et al. Pseudobacteremia attributed to contamination of povidone-iodine with *Pseudomonas cepacia. Ann Intern Med.* 1981;95(1):32-36. [IIIB]

160. Craven DE, Moody B, Connolly MG, Kollisch NR, Stottmeier KD, McCabe WR. Pseudobacteremia caused by povidone-iodine solution contaminated with *Pseudomonas cepacia. N Engl J Med.* 1981;305(11):621-623. [IIIA]

161. O'Rourke E, Runyan D, O'Leary J, Stern J. Contaminated iodophor in the operating room. *Am J Infect Control.* 2003;31(4):255-256. [VA]

162. Panlilio AL, Beck-Sague CM, Siegel JD, et al. Infections and pseudoinfections due to povidone-iodine solution contaminated with *Pseudomonas cepacia. Clin Infect Dis.* 1992;14(5):1078-1083. [IIIA]

163. Parrott PL, Terry PM, Whitworth EN, et al. Pseudomonas aeruginosa peritonitis associated with contaminated poloxamer-iodine solution. *Lancet.* 1982;320(8300): 683-685. [VA]

164. Gottardi W. The influence of the chemical behaviour of iodine on the germicidal action of disinfectant solutions containing iodine. *J Hosp Infect.* 1985;6(Suppl A):1-11. [VA]

165. 29 CFR 1910.1200: Occupational safety and health standards. Toxic and hazardous substances. Hazard communication. July 2013. Occupational Safety and Health Administration. https://www.osha.gov/pls/oshaweb/owa-disp.show_document?p_table=standards&p_id=10099. Accessed July 14, 2014.

166. RCRA Online. US Environmental Protection Agency. http://www.epa.gov/epawaste/inforesources/online/index.htm. Accessed July 14, 2014.

Acknowledgements

LEAD AUTHOR
Amber Wood, MSN, RN, CNOR, CIC, CPN
Perioperative Nursing Specialist
AORN Nursing Department
Denver, Colorado

CONTRIBUTING AUTHOR
Ramona Conner, MSN, RN, CNOR
Manager Standards and Guidelines
AORN Nursing Department
Denver, Colorado

The authors and AORN thank Deborah S. Hickman, MS, RN, CNOR, CRNFA, Renue Plastic Surgery, Brunswick, Georgia; Melanie L. Braswell, DNP, RN, CNS, CNOR, Indiana University Health Arnett, Lafayette, Indiana; Judith R. Garcia, MHSS, MS, BSN, RN, CNOR, Perioperative Department, Ohio State University Wexner Medical Center James Cancer Hospital and Solove Research Institute, Columbus, Ohio; J. Hudson Garrett Jr, PhD, MSN, MPH, FNP-BC, Director, Clinical Affairs, PDI Healthcare, Atlanta, Georgia; and Lisa Spruce, DNP, RN, ACNS, ACNP, ANP, CNOR, Director of Evidence-based Perioperative Practice, AORN, Inc, Denver, Colorado, for their assistance in developing this guideline.

PUBLICATION HISTORY
Originally published May 1976, *AORN Journal,* as "Standards for preoperative skin preparation of patients." Format revision March 1978, July 1982.

Revised February 1983, November 1988, November 1992, June 1996. Published November 1996, *AORN Journal;* reformatted July 2000.

Revised November 2001; published January 2002, *AORN Journal.*

Revised 2007; published as "Recommended practices for preoperative patient skin antisepsis" in *Perioperative Standards and Recommended Practices,* 2008 edition.

Minor editing revisions made to omit PNDS codes; reformatted September 2012 for publication in *Perioperative Standards and Recommended Practices,* 2013 edition.

Revised July 2014 for online publication in *Perioperative Standards and Recommended Practices.*

Minor editing revisions made in November 2014 for publication in *Guidelines for Perioperative Practice,* 2015 edition.

Evidence ratings revised in *Guidelines for Perioperative Practice,* 2018 edition, to conform to the current AORN Evidence Rating Model.

ASEPTIC PRACTICE

GUIDELINE FOR STERILE TECHNIQUE

The Guideline for Sterile Technique was approved by the AORN Recommended Practices Advisory Board. It was presented as proposed recommendations for comments by members and others. The guideline is effective December 15, 2012. The recommendations in this guideline are intended to be achievable and represent what is believed to be an optimal level of practice. Policies and procedures will reflect variations in practice settings and/or clinical situations that determine the degree to which the guideline can be implemented. AORN recognizes the various settings in which perioperative nurses practice; therefore, this guideline is adaptable to various practice settings. These practice settings include traditional operating rooms (ORs), ambulatory surgery centers, physicians' offices, cardiac catheterization laboratories, endoscopy suites, radiology departments, and all other areas where surgery and other invasive procedures may be performed.

Purpose

This document provides guidance for establishing and maintaining a sterile field by following the principles and implementing the processes of sterile technique. Sterile technique involves the use of specific actions and activities to prevent contamination and maintain sterility of identified areas during operative and other invasive procedures. Implementing sterile technique when preparing, performing, or assisting with surgical and other invasive procedures is the cornerstone of maintaining sterility and preventing microbial contamination.

The creation and maintenance of a sterile field can directly influence patient outcomes.[1] All individuals who are involved in operative or other invasive procedures have a responsibility to provide a safe environment for patients. Perioperative team members must be vigilant in safeguarding the sterility of the field and ensuring that the principles and processes of sterile technique are followed and implemented. Perioperative leaders can promote a culture of safety by creating an environment where perioperative personnel are encouraged to identify, question, or stop practices believed to be unsafe without fear of repercussion.

The perioperative registered nurse (RN) uses ethical principles to make clinical decisions and act on them.[2] Adhering to the principles of and implementing the processes for sterile technique is a matter of individual conscience and an ethical obligation that applies to all members of the perioperative team. Perioperative team members should understand the professional responsibility to ensure that contamination of the sterile field is remedied immediately, and to make certain that any item for which sterility is in question is not used. Adhering to the principles of and implementing the processes for sterile technique and taking immediate action to protect the patient when breaks in sterile technique occur meets the maxim, "first, do no harm." The perioperative team serves as the protective intermediary between patients and personnel whose practices do not meet the highest standards of sterile technique. Perioperative nurses have a long-standing reputation of advocating for patients and working together with members of the health care team to provide a safe perioperative environment for patients undergoing operative or other invasive procedures.

Although these recommendations include several references to surgical attire (including surgical masks) and hand hygiene, the focus of this document is on sterile technique. Surgical attire and hand hygiene are outside the scope of these recommendations. The reader should refer to the AORN Guideline for Surgical Attire[3] and Guideline for Hand Hygiene[4] for additional guidance.

Evidence Review

A medical librarian conducted a systematic review of MEDLINE®, CINAHL®, Scopus®, and the Cochrane Database of Systematic Reviews for meta-analyses, randomized and nonrandomized trials and studies, systematic and nonsystematic reviews, and opinion documents and letters. Search terms included *sterile field, sterile technique, aseptic technique, aseptic practices, surgical drapes, double-gloving, assisted gloving, closed gloving, time-related sterilization, event-related sterilization, surgical attire, protective clothing, sterile supplies, sterile barriers, barrier precautions, body-exhaust suits, space suits, laminar air flow, bowel technique, (glove expansion and fluids), (glove perforation and electrosurgery), strikethrough, Spaulding's criteria, product packaging,* and *equipment contamination.*

The lead author and medical librarian identified and obtained relevant guidelines from government agencies, other professional organizations, and standards-setting bodies. The lead author assessed additional professional literature, including some that initially appeared in other articles provided to the author.

The initial search was confined to 2006 to 2011, but the time restriction was not considered in subsequent searches. The librarian also established continuing alerts on the topics included in this guideline and provided relevant results to the lead author.

Articles identified by the search were provided to the project team for evaluation. The team consisted of the lead author, two members of the Recommended Practices Advisory Board, and a member of the Research Committee. The lead author divided the search results into topics and assigned members of the team to review and critically appraise each article using the Johns Hopkins Evidence-Based Practice Model and the Research or Non-Research Evidence Appraisal Tools as appropriate. The literature was independently evaluated and appraised according to the strength and quality of the evidence. Each article was then assigned an appraisal score as agreed upon by consensus of the team. The appraisal score is noted in brackets after each reference, as applicable.

The collective evidence supporting each intervention within a specific recommendation was summarized and used to rate the strength of the evidence using the AORN Evidence Rating Model. Factors considered in review of the collective evidence were the quality of research, quantity of similar studies on a given topic, and consistency of results supporting a recommendation. The evidence rating is noted in brackets after each intervention.

Editor's note: MEDLINE is a registered trademark of the US National Library of Medicine's Medical Literature Analysis and Retrieval System, Bethesda, MD. CINAHL, Cumulative Index to Nursing and Allied Health Literature, is a registered trademark of EBSCO Industries, Birmingham, AL. Scopus is a registered trademark of Elsevier B.V., Amsterdam, Netherlands.

Recommendation I

Perioperative personnel should implement practices that reduce the spread of transmissible infections when preparing or working in the OR or invasive procedure room and when performing or assisting with operative or other invasive procedures.

Protecting patients and safeguarding health care providers from potentially infectious agent transmission is a key focus of perioperative nurses.[5] Hand hygiene has been recognized as a primary method of decreasing health care-associated infections.[4,6] Surgical attire and personal protective equipment (PPE) are worn to support cleanliness and hygiene, promote patient and health care provider safety, and aid in preserving the integrity of the sterile field within the perioperative environment.[3,5]

I.a. Perioperative personnel entering the OR or invasive procedure room for any reason (eg, stocking supplies, bringing procedural supplies and equipment into clean rooms) should wear clean

- scrub attire,[1] including a freshly laundered or single-use, long-sleeved jacket snapped closed with the cuffs down to the wrists, and
- surgical head covers or hoods that cover all hair and scalp skin, including facial hair, sideburns, and the hair at the nape of the neck.[1]

[1: Strong Evidence]

Surgical attire helps contain bacterial shedding and promotes environmental cleanliness.[1,3]

Head coverings and hoods minimize microbial dispersal by containing hair and scalp skin.[1,3]

I.b. Perioperative personnel should perform hand hygiene before entering the OR or invasive procedure room and areas where sterile supplies have been opened. *[1: Strong Evidence]*

Following regular hand hygiene practices helps prevent transmission of infection and reduces health care-associated infections for patients and health care personnel.[4,6]

Prevention of health care-associated infections is a priority of all health care providers. Health care-associated infections can result in untoward outcomes such as increased morbidity and mortality, longer length of stay, increased pain and suffering, and escalating cost of care. Hand hygiene, hand washing, and surgical hand scrubs are the most effective way to prevent and control infections and represent the least expensive means of achieving both.[4]

I.c. Perioperative personnel should wear a clean surgical mask that covers the mouth and nose and is secured in a manner to prevent venting when open sterile supplies are present[1] and when preparing, performing, or assisting with surgery and other invasive procedures including

- central venous catheter (CVC) insertion, peripherally inserted central catheters (PICCs), and guidewire exchange[8-10];
- regional anesthesia procedures[11]; or
- high-risk spinal canal procedures (eg, myelogram, lumbar puncture, spinal anesthesia).[10,12-20]

[1: Strong Evidence]

A clean surgical mask helps protect the patient and procedure site from microbial contamination by organisms carried in the provider's mouth or nose.[1,3,10,21]

Researchers studied the effectiveness of surgical masks in reducing the dispersal of bacterial contamination from the upper airways of 25 volunteers. The volunteers were asked to speak directly at an agar plate for five minutes. A surgical mask was applied and the volunteers were instructed to speak at the agar plate for three additional periods of five minutes each. The results showed a marked reduction in the bacterial contamination of the agar plates while the volunteers were wearing surgical masks.[21]

In a study investigating the possibility that surgical masks increase vertical shedding of bacteria from the face during facial movement, volunteers were asked to speak for 20 minutes while moving their heads from side to side without a surgical mask for the first five minutes and then with a surgical mask for three additional five-minute periods. A blood agar plate was positioned 30 cm below the volunteers' faces. The results showed a statistically significant reduction in the number of colony-forming units on the agar plate when the volunteers were wearing surgical masks. The researchers recommended wearing a surgical mask, particularly when the perioperative team member's face is in close proximity to the procedural site and when the need for speaking during the procedure is anticipated.[22]

In a prospective, randomized, controlled trial of 221 patients, researchers assessed the need for surgical masks during cataract surgery. Patients were randomly assigned to group A, in which the surgeon wore a clean surgical mask, or group B, in which the surgeon did not wear a surgical mask. A settle plate was secured adjacent to the patient's head on the operative side within the sterile field during all procedures. The results showed a significant reduction of bacterial organisms falling on the operative side when the surgeon wore a surgical mask.[23]

In a study exploring the relationship between the use and position of a surgical mask during 30 cardiac catheterization procedures, researchers obtained bacterial samples within the draped, operative site adjacent to the femoral artery. Surgical masks were either not worn by perioperative team members, or worn in positions above and below the nose. The number of bacterial colonies recovered when no mask was worn was significantly greater than when a surgical mask was worn. Mask placement below the nose also was associated with a higher colony count than when the mask was worn above the nose. The researchers voluntarily discontinued the study after 30 patients in the interest of patient safety because of the high bacterial count associated with not wearing surgical masks.[24]

Surgical masks are effective in limiting the dispersal of oropharyngeal droplets[21,25] and are recommended by the Centers for Disease Control and Prevention (CDC) for the placement of CVCs, PICCs, and guidewire exchange.[8-10]

The American Society of Regional Anesthesia and Pain Medicine recommends the use of surgical masks during regional anesthesia as a method to reduce the likelihood of site contamination from microorganisms that may be present in the upper airway of providers.[11]

Oropharyngeal flora was found to be the source of contamination in a number of reported cases of bacterial meningitis after lumbar puncture, spinal and epidural anesthesia, and intrathecal chemotherapy.[12-19]

In 2004, the CDC investigated eight instances in which patients contracted meningitis after procedures that involved placing a catheter or injecting material into the spinal canal or epidural space. The cases involved blood or cerebrospinal fluid contaminated with streptococcal species or other pathogens consistent with oropharyngeal fluid. None of the clinicians wore surgical masks during the procedures. Equipment and products used during these procedures were excluded as sources of contamination.[10] In June 2007, the Healthcare Infection Control Practices Advisory Committee reviewed the cases and determined there was sufficient evidence to warrant the wearing of a surgical mask by the individual placing a catheter or injecting material into the spinal or epidural space.[10]

In September 2008, three cases of bacterial meningitis in postpartum women were reported to the New York State Department of Health. Two additional cases of meningitis were reported to the Ohio Department of Health in May 2009. All of the patients had received intrapartum spinal anesthesia. The investigators concluded that the New York incidents were associated with a single anesthesiologist. The anesthesiologist reported wearing a surgical mask; however, personnel reported that the presence of unmasked visitors in the procedure area was common. The Ohio incidents were found to be associated with a second anesthesiologist who did not wear a surgical mask. The findings underscore the need for adhering to aseptic practices and wearing surgical masks during spinal procedures.[20]

Recommendation II

Surgical gowns, gloves, and drape products for use in the perioperative setting should be evaluated and selected for safety, efficacy, and cost before purchase or use.

The safety and efficacy of surgical gowns, gloves, and drape products depends on the design of the item and the materials from which they are made.[26]

Quality, patient and worker safety, and cost containment are primary concerns for perioperative RNs when they participate in evaluating and selecting medical devices and products for use in practice settings.[27]

II.a. Surgical gowns, gloves, and drape products should be evaluated and selected for use in the perioperative setting according to
- product-specific requirements[27,28];
- procedure-related requirements[27];
- end-user requirements and preferences[27,28];
- patient-related requirements[27];
- environmental considerations[29];
- compliance with federal, state, and local regulatory agencies[5,30,31]; and
- compliance with standards-setting bodies.[32]
[3: Moderate Evidence]

Product-specific requirements include contractual agreements, compatibility with existing products, and implementation of new products of differing material or construction.[27,28]

Procedure-related requirements define what is necessary for the procedure where the surgical gowns, gloves, and drape products will be used, such as resistance to penetration by blood

STERILE TECHNIQUE

and other body fluids, or the presence of adhesive apertures.[27]

End-user requirements, such as the degree of protection from blood, body fluids, and other potentially infectious materials, and preferences, such as comfort, vary depending on how the surgical gowns, gloves, and drape products are used.[27]

Patient-related requirements define the ability of the product to meet the needs of the individual patient, such as being appropriately sized or able to conform to patient contours.[27]

Environmental considerations, such as the potential for recycling or reprocessing, may reduce waste, conserve resources, and decrease costs without compromising quality of care.[29]

Mandatory Occupational Safety and Health Administration regulations require that personal protective equipment such as surgical gowns and gloves do not permit blood or other potentially infectious material to "pass through to or reach the employee's work clothes, street clothes, undergarments, skin, eyes, mouth, or other mucous membranes under normal conditions of use and for the duration of time which the protective equipment will be used."[30(1910.1030(d)(3)(i)]

Surgical gowns and drape products are surgical devices, and as such are regulated by the US Food and Drug Administration (FDA).[31] Failure of these devices is subject to medical device reporting requirements according to the Safe Medical Devices Act of 1990 as amended in March 2000[33] and MedWatch: The FDA Safety Information and Adverse Event Reporting Program.[34]

The American National Standards Institute and Association for the Advancement of Medical Instrumentation standard PB70:2012, "Liquid barrier performance and classification of protective apparel and drapes intended for use in health care facilities," establishes a common system of classification and specifies labeling requirements for manufacturers of protective apparel and drapes used in health care facilities.[32] The classification system is based on standardized test methods for determining liquid barrier performance and compliance. The implementation of consistent classification and labeling requirements by the manufacturer aids in evaluation and selection of the most appropriate protective products for the health care organization.[32]

II.a.1. Surgical gowns, gloves, and drape products used during operative and other invasive procedures must provide a barrier[1,30,32] and should be resistant to tears, punctures, and abrasions.[28]

Tears, punctures, and abrasions may allow for the passage of microorganisms, particulates, and fluids between sterile and unsterile areas and expose patients and perioperative personnel to microbial contamination and bloodborne pathogens.

Abrasions may adversely affect barrier properties by weakening the material and causing it to tear or generate lint.[26]

In a study evaluating bacterial penetration of disposable, non-woven drapes used during total hip arthroplasty, six brands of drapes were tested after 30 and 90 minutes. The results showed that bacterial penetration was time dependent. Most of the drapes remained impenetrable or allowed passage of fewer than 100 colony forming units at 90 minutes; however, none of the drapes tested were completely impenetrable, and certain brands were more resistant to bacterial penetration than others.[35]

In another study considering the effects of moisture and physical stress on surgical draping materials, researchers found that materials differ dramatically in the ability to resist bacterial penetration.[36]

II.a.2. Seams and points of attachment of surgical gowns should minimize liquid penetration and passage of potential contaminants.[1,32]

Wicking or pressure on a seam or point of attachment may cause liquid transfer between sterile and unsterile surfaces, and one or both sides of the gown may become contaminated.

II.a.3. Surgical gowns, gloves, and drape products used during operative or other invasive procedures should be non-abrasive and non-toxic.[28]

Products that are abrasive and contain chemicals and other toxic materials may irritate tissue, damage the skin, and injure patients and perioperative personnel.[26]

II.a.4. Barrier materials used for surgical gowns and drape products should be as lint free as possible.[28]

Lint particles are disseminated into the environment where bacteria attach to them.[37] Bacteria-carrying lint may settle in surgical sites and wounds and may increase postoperative patient complications.

II.a.5. Surgical gowns and drape products should be functional and flexible.[28]

Gowns and drape products that do not adequately perform and are unable to conform to and closely cover the user's body or equipment may be difficult to use and may not provide protection from contamination by blood, body fluids, and other potentially infectious materials.[26]

II.b. Perioperative personnel should select surgical gowns, gloves, and drape products for the procedure according to the barrier performance class of the product as stated on the label and the anticipated degree of exposure to blood,

ASEPTIC PRACTICE

78

body fluids, and other potentially infectious materials.[30,32] *[1: Regulatory Requirement]*

Surgical gowns and drapes are labeled by the manufacturer with the level of performance determined by the barrier properties of the area of the gown or drape where direct contact with blood, body fluids, and other potentially infectious materials is most likely to occur.[32]

Surgical gowns, gloves, and drape products are used to establish a barrier that minimizes the passage of microorganisms, body fluids, and particulate matter between sterile and unsterile areas.[1,30,32,38,39]

Surgical gloves are worn to protect patients and perioperative team members from transmission of pathogens. The process of surgery subjects gloves to mechanical stresses (eg, twisting, pulling, stretching) and exposure to fluids, fats, and chemical substances (eg, methyl methacrylate) that may affect the integrity of the glove barrier. The barrier properties of surgical gloves may be affected by the strength of the glove material and also may be compromised by hand and finger movements and other tasks (eg, holding retractors) that are required during invasive procedures.

In a study evaluating and comparing the barrier performance characteristics of latex, vinyl, and nitrile gloves under simulated use conditions, researchers tested a total of 2,000 gloves (800 latex, 800 vinyl, 400 nitrile) from seven different manufacturers. The gloves were purchased specifically for the study, taken directly from the packages, and immediately tested. A comparative baseline was established by leak-testing 100 gloves of each brand and type. The study gloves were consistently manipulated in a manner simulating patient care activities for a period of 20 minutes. The results showed that the barrier performance of latex and nitrile gloves is comparable, and both materials are much less susceptible to material breakdown and leakage than vinyl.[40]

To compare the frequency of glove defects in latex and nonlatex surgical gloves during routine surgery, researchers collected gloves at the end of 2,318 surgical procedures. They tested a total of 6,386 gloves used by 101 surgeons and residents representing 15 surgical services. Six brands of nonlatex and two brands of latex gloves were tested. The results showed that both latex and nonlatex gloves performed adequately during routine surgical use; however, nonlatex surgical gloves had a higher rate of defects than latex gloves. The data also indicated that nonlatex gloves were nearly twice as likely to fail when used in certain high-risk surgical specialties (eg, oral, dental, cardiac) that require fine motor movement, increased hand dexterity, or contact with hard surfaces and sharp bone.[41]

II.b.1.   Factors that should be considered when selecting surgical gowns, gloves, and drape products for surgical or other invasive procedures include the

- anticipated blood loss;
- volume of irrigation fluid;
- potential for splash, spray, pooling, or soaking;
- duration of the procedure;
- potential for leaning or pressure;
- type of procedure (eg, minimally invasive versus open, superficial incision versus deep body cavity); and
- team member's role.[26]

II.c.   Perioperative personnel should select surgical gowns of appropriate size and sleeve length. *[5: Benefits Balanced with Harms]*

When a gown is of insufficient size or sleeve length to cover the perioperative team member's body, it may restrict movement, increase the potential for the scrubbed team member's unsterile skin or clothing to contact the sterile field, or fail to provide adequate coverage to prevent the scrubbed team member from exposure to blood, body fluids, or other potentially infectious materials.

When a gown is of excessive size or sleeve length, the extra gown material may brush against unsterile objects and surfaces.

II.c.1.   Surgical gowns should be large enough to adequately wrap around the perioperative team member's body and completely cover the back.

In one study evaluating various combinations of surgical attire, the addition of a wrap-around gown reduced environmental microbial contamination by 51% when compared with scrub attire worn without a gown.[42]

II.c.2.   Surgical gowns should be selected so the lower sleeves and gown cuffs

- conform to the shape of the wearer's arms,[32]
- are short enough to allow gloves to fully cover the cuffs and mate properly with the lower sleeves,[32] and
- are of sufficient length to prevent the gown cuffs from pulling out of the gloves when the wearer's arms are extended.[32]

Recommendation III

Perioperative personnel should use sterile technique when donning and wearing sterile gowns and gloves.

Implementing sterile technique when donning and wearing sterile gowns and gloves reduces the risk of wound contamination and surgical site infections that may result from direct contact of surgical team members' skin or clothing with the sterile field.[1]

III.a. Perioperative team members should perform a surgical hand scrub before donning sterile gowns and gloves. *[1: Strong Evidence]*

Surgical hand antisepsis decreases transient and resident microorganisms on the skin, which may reduce health care-associated infections.[4,6] Prevention of health care-associated infections is a priority of all health care providers. Health care-associated infections can result in untoward outcomes, such as increased morbidity and mortality, greater pain and suffering, longer length of stay, and escalated cost of care.[7] Hand hygiene, hand washing, and surgical hand scrubs are the most effective way to prevent and control infections and represent the least expensive means of achieving both.[4]

III.b. Scrubbed team members should don sterile gowns and gloves in a sterile area away from the main instrument table and in a manner to prevent contamination of surgical attire. *[4: Limited Evidence]*

Donning gowns and gloves in a separate area may help prevent contamination of the main instrument table by droplets of water or skin antiseptic solution from the scrubbed team member's wet hands. Donning gowns and gloves in a separate area also may reduce the risk of contamination of the main instrument table from potential contact with the unprotected skin and clothing of the scrubbed team member as they don sterile gown and gloves.

In a non-experimental, two-part study with a small sample size, researchers cultured water droplets from 15 surgeons' arms after a five-minute standardized surgical hand scrub with 10% povidone-iodine followed by thorough rinsing with tap water. The water droplets from each of the surgeons' arms were collected and cultured. Pathogenic and environmental bacteria were recovered from the water droplets from the surgeons' scrubbed arms. In the second part of the study, the wrapping paper from two different brands of gloves was investigated for permeability and bacterial penetration. The paper packaging was found to be permeable. The researchers concluded that pathogenic bacteria could be transferred from the surgeons' arms to the gloves by water dropped on the glove packaging during the gowning and gloving process, and this represented a theoretical source of wound contamination.[43]

III.b.1. Sterile gloves should not be opened directly on top of the sterile gown that has been opened for donning by the scrubbed team member.

When the gown is retrieved, droplets of water or skin antiseptic solution from the scrubbed team member's wet hands may drip onto the glove wrapper and contaminate the sterile gloves.[43]

III.b.2. The scrubbed team member's hands and arms should be completely dry before donning a sterile gown.

Droplets of water or skin antiseptic solution from the scrubbed team member's wet hands and arms may drip onto the gown or gown wrapper and contaminate the sterile gown.[43]

III.b.3. Only the inside of the sterile gown should be touched when it is picked up for donning by the scrubbed team member.

Touching only the inside of the gown when picking it up prevents the scrubbed team member's hands from contaminating the front of the gown.

III.b.4. The sterile glove wrapper or gloves should not be touched until the sterile gown has been donned.

After donning the sterile gown, the scrubbed team member's hands are covered by the impervious gown sleeves, which prevents the scrubbed team member's unprotected hands from contaminating the glove wrapper and gloves.[43]

III.c. The front of a sterile gown should be considered sterile from the chest to the level of the sterile field. *[4: Limited Evidence]*

In a study evaluating the most sterile areas of surgical gowns, researchers obtained samples from 50 surgical gowns at the end of 29 spinal procedures. The samples were taken at six-inch increments beginning at the neck of the gown and ending at the bottom of the gown. An additional 50 gowns were swabbed immediately after donning and before entering the sterile field to serve as negative controls. When compared with the negative controls, the contamination rates of the gowns worn during the procedures were lowest in the section between the chest and the operative field. Bacterial growth was highest in the areas above the chest and below the OR table. The researchers theorized that the increased levels of bacterial growth in the areas above the chest were likely related to microbial shedding from the scrubbed team member's head or mask, whereas the portion of the gown below the operating table was likely contaminated by direct contact with unsterile objects below the level of the operative field. The researchers concluded the front of the gown between the chest and the sterile field to be the area of greatest sterility.[44]

III.c.1. The neckline, shoulders, and axillary regions of the surgical gown should be considered contaminated.

The neckline, shoulders, and axillary regions are areas of friction and may not provide effective microbial barriers.

III.c.2. The surgical gown back should be considered unsterile.

The back of the gown cannot be constantly monitored.

II.d. Gown sleeves should be considered sterile from two inches above the elbow to the cuff, circumferentially. *[4: Limited Evidence]*

From two inches above the elbow to the cuff, gown sleeves are adjacent to the area of the gown that is considered sterile (ie, the front of the gown from the chest to the level of the sterile field[44]). Circumferential sterility of the gown sleeves is necessary because the scrubbed team member's arms move across the sterile field.

III.d.1. Sleeve cuffs of the surgical gown should be considered contaminated when the scrubbed team member's hands pass through and beyond the cuff.

Sleeve cuffs are not impervious and could allow for microbial transfer from the scrubbed team member's hand.[36]

III.d.2. Sleeve cuffs should be completely covered by sterile gloves and should not be exposed.

Permeable sleeve cuffs that are not completely covered by sterile gloves may allow for microbial transfer and contact from the scrubbed team member's arms to the patient, and for contact with blood and body fluids from the patient to the scrubbed team member.

II.e. The closed assisted gloving method should be used to glove team members during initial gowning and gloving for operative or other invasive procedures (Figure 1). *[3: Moderate Evidence]*

The risk for glove cuff contamination increases when open assisted gloving is used. In a blinded, randomized study comparing contamination of the inside of the glove cuff during open and closed assisted gloving, two surgeons were gloved 20 times after covering their fingers and hands with a fluorescent powder. One surgeon was gloved by the closed assisted method and the other by the open assisted method. The results showed that open assisted gloving led to significantly greater glove cuff contamination than the closed assisted gloving method.[45]

III.e.1. During closed assisted gloving, the gown cuff of the team member being gloved should remain at or beyond the fingertips. The glove to be donned should be held open by a scrubbed team member, and the team member being gloved should insert his or her hand into the glove with the gown cuff touching only the inside of the glove.

III.e.2. Open assisted gloving, where the team member's gown sleeve is pulled up so that the gown cuff is at wrist level, leaving the

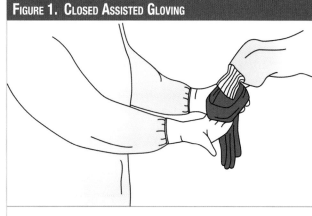

FIGURE 1. CLOSED ASSISTED GLOVING

During closed assisted gloving, the gown cuff should remain at or beyond the fingertips.
Illustration by Colleen Ladny.

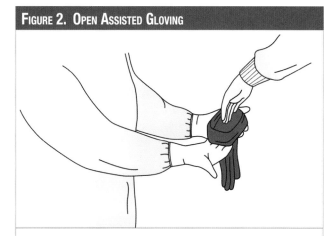

FIGURE 2. OPEN ASSISTED GLOVING

During open assisted gloving, the gown cuff is at wrist level, leaving the fingers and hand exposed.
Illustration by Colleen Ladny.

fingers and hand exposed, should be used when closed assisted gloving is not possible or practical (Figure 2).

III.f. Scrubbed team members should wear two pairs of surgical gloves, one over the other, during surgical and other invasive procedures with the potential for exposure to blood, body fluids, or other potentially infectious materials.[1,5] *[1: Strong Evidence]*

To provide an effective sterile barrier and prevent microbial transfer from surgical team members' hands to the patient, and to protect surgical team members from blood, body fluids, and other potentially infectious materials from the patient, surgical gloves must be intact and without perforations. Wearing two pairs of gloves helps to reduce glove perforations to the inner glove.

A systematic review of 31 randomized controlled trials measuring glove perforations showed that the addition of a second pair of surgical gloves significantly reduced perforations to the inner glove. Triple gloving, knitted outer gloves, and glove liners also significantly reduced perforations to the inner glove. More inner glove perforations were detected during surgery when perforation indicator systems were used.[46]

The CDC, the American College of Surgeons, and the American Academy of Orthopedic Surgeons support double gloving during invasive surgical procedures.[1,47,48]

III.f.1.   When double gloves are worn, perforation indicator systems should be used.

A perforation indicator system is a double gloving system comprising a colored pair of surgical gloves worn beneath a standard pair of surgical gloves. When glove perforation occurs, moisture from the surgical field seeps through the perforation between the layers of gloves, allowing the site of perforation to be seen more easily (Figure 3).

A meta-analysis of five randomized, controlled trials with a combined sample size

---

FIGURE 3. PERFORATION INDICATOR SYSTEMS

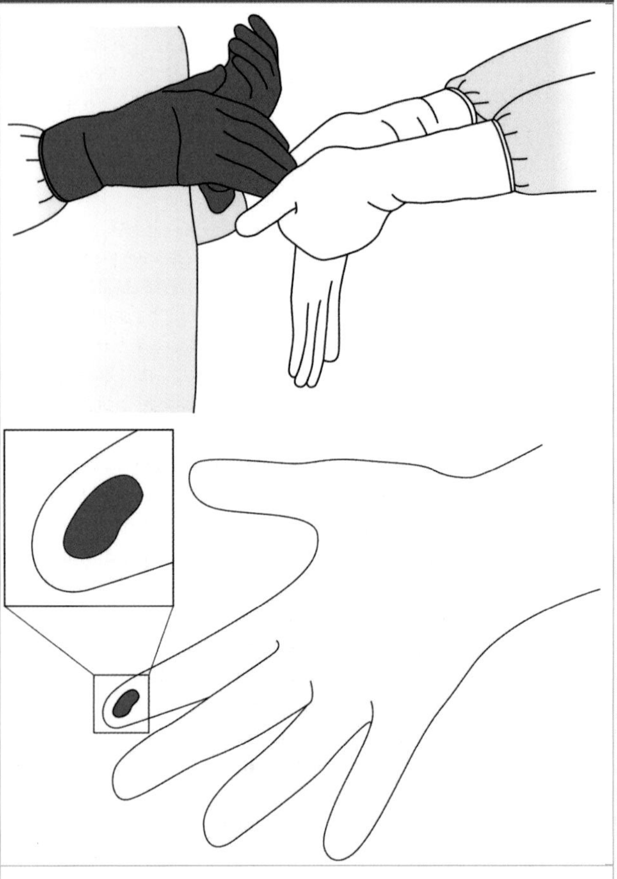

The use of perforation indicator systems may increase safety and reduce the potential for exposure to blood, body fluids, or other potentially infectious materials. When glove perforation occurs, the site of perforation can be more easily seen because of the colored gloves worn beneath the standard gloves.

Illustration by Colleen Ladny.

---

of 582 gloves showed significantly fewer perforations detected by scrubbed team members wearing standard double gloves compared with scrubbed team members using perforation indicator systems. When wearing standard double gloves, 21% of perforations were detected by the scrubbed team member. When wearing perforation indicator systems, 77% of perforations were detected.[46]

III.g.   Scrubbed team members should inspect gloves for integrity after donning, before contact with the sterile field, and throughout use. *[3: Moderate Evidence]*

Careful inspection of glove integrity after donning and before contact with the sterile field may reveal holes and defects in the unused product that may have occurred during the manufacturing or donning process and could allow for the passage of microorganisms, particulates, and fluids between sterile and unsterile areas.

Careful inspection of glove integrity throughout the procedure may prevent unnoticed glove perforation. Unnoticed glove perforation during operative or other invasive procedures may present an increased risk for bloodborne pathogen transmission to perioperative team members related to prolonged exposure to blood, body fluids, or other potentially infectious materials, and also may increase the patient's risk for wound infection related to transfer of microorganisms from the hands of surgical team members.[1]

To investigate the frequency of undetected glove perforation, researchers studied glove perforations from 24 thoracoscopic and 23 open thoracotomy procedures and found that unnoticed glove perforation occurred in 25% of the gloves worn by the primary surgeon and in 12% of all gloves worn during the procedures.[49]

III.h.   Surgical gloves worn during invasive surgical procedures should be changed
  ○ after each patient procedure[6]; *[1: Strong Evidence]*
  ○ when suspected or actual contamination occurs; *[5: Benefits Balanced with Harms]*
  ○ after touching surgical helmet system hoods and visors[50,51]; *[4: Limited Evidence]*
  ○ after adjusting optic eyepieces on the operative microscope[52]; *[3: Moderate Evidence]*
  ○ immediately after direct contact with methyl methacrylate[53-55]; *[1: Strong Evidence]*
  ○ when gloves begin to swell, expand, and become loose on the hands as a result of the material's absorption of fluids and fats[56]; *[3: Moderate Evidence]*
  ○ when a visible defect or perforation is noted or when a suspected or actual perforation from a needle, suture, bone, or other object occurs[1,57]; *[1: Strong Evidence]* and

o every 90 to 150 minutes.[47,57-59] *[1: Strong Evidence]*

Failure to change gloves after each patient procedure may lead to transmission of microorganisms from one patient to another.[6]

Sterile gloves that have contacted unsterile items may transfer microorganisms or other unsterile particulates to the sterile field.

Surgical helmet systems consist of an unsterile reusable helmet with a built-in ventilation fan covered with a single-use disposable sterile visor mask hood. The unsterile helmet is donned before the surgical hand scrub is performed. The sterile visor mask hood that covers the unsterile helmet is applied during the gowning and gloving process (Figure 4).

In a study to evaluate the sterility of a surgical helmet system during six hip arthroplasty and 14 knee arthroplasty procedures, researchers sampled hoods at 30-minute intervals during, as well as at the end, of procedures. Although the small sample size was a limitation of the study, the results showed that 80% of the hoods were contaminated intraoperatively. The hoods were contaminated within 30 minutes of use and showed heavy growth of coagulase-negative *Staphylococcus aureus*. The researchers recommended avoiding direct contact with the surgical helmet hood system during surgical procedures or changing gloves if contact does occur.[50]

In another study evaluating microbial contamination of a surgical helmet system, researchers tested hoods used in 61 hip arthroplasty and 41 knee arthroplasty procedures. Samples were collected immediately after the hood was placed over the helmet and at the conclusion of the procedure. The contamination rate was 47%. The organisms found included coagulase-negative staphylococci, *Micrococcus,* methicillin-susceptible *S aureus*, and methicillin-resistant *S aureus*. The researchers recommended changing gloves if the hood or visor is touched or adjusted during the procedure.[51]

Researchers conducted a study to assess the contamination rates of sterile microscope drapes used during spine surgery. The study included 25 surgical spine procedures requiring the use of the operative microscope. The microscope drapes were swabbed immediately after application as negative controls. Postoperatively, the microscope drapes were sampled in seven different places. When compared with the negative controls, all of the sampled areas were found to be contaminated with bacteria. Four of the seven areas, including the shafts of the optic eyepieces, were found to have significant contamination rates. The regions above the eyepieces and the overhead portion of the drape also were contaminated. The researchers recommended avoiding contact with the upper portion of the drape and changing gloves after adjusting the optic eyepieces.[52]

Studies have demonstrated that surgical gloves are permeable to methyl methacrylate.[53,54] The amount of permeation depends on the type of glove and the duration it is worn.[53,54] A full discussion of methyl methacrylate is outside the scope of this document. The reader should refer to the AORN Guideline for a Safe Environment of Care, Part 1[55] for additional guidance.

Researchers studied the effectiveness of the barrier provided by latex surgical gloves and found that latex is subject to hydration (ie, the absorption of fluid molecules). Hydration rates are highly variable and depend on the properties of the individual glove product, the amount of perspiration from the scrubbed team member's hand, and the amount of body fluid exposure during the procedure. Hydrated gloves showed increased permeability and porosity and a significant reduction of electrical and mechanical resistance. The researchers concluded that latex is an effective barrier; however, the combined effects of the mechanical and biological stress to which the glove is subjected require careful monitoring by the user and changing gloves before the integrity of the glove is lost.[56]

Surgical gloves that are intact and without defects or perforations provide an effective sterile barrier and may prevent microbial transfer from perioperative team members' hands to the patient, and also protect the perioperative team members from transfer of blood, body fluids, and other potentially infectious materials from the patient.[1,57]

In a study measuring the concentration of bacteria passing through glove punctures under

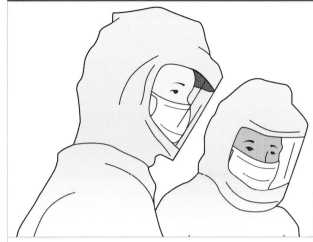

FIGURE 4. SURGICAL HELMET SYSTEMS

Surgical helmet systems consist of an unsterile reusable helmet covered with a single-use disposable sterile visor hood.

Illustration by Colleen Ladny and Kurt Jones.

surgical conditions, 128 outer and 122 inner gloves used by surgical team members during 20 septic laparotomy procedures were tested. The rate of outer glove perforation averaged 15%; however, nearly 82% of the perforations went undetected. The frequency of perforation was directly correlated with the length of time the gloves were worn for both inner and outer gloves. Direct bacterial passage from the patient through a glove puncture occurred in almost 5% of all gloves worn. The researchers recommended a strict policy of changing gloves every 90 minutes.[57]

In a study measuring bacterial translocation through puncture holes in surgical gloves, 98 outer and 96 inner gloves worn by surgical team members during 20 consecutive surgical laparotomy procedures were examined. Ten outer gloves and one inner glove were perforated; however, seven of the perforations were detected because of the indicator glove system worn by surgical team members. Bacterial migration was demonstrated in five of the outer gloves and one of the inner gloves. The frequency of perforation increased with the length of time the gloves were worn. The researchers recommended double gloving and a change of gloves at least every 90 minutes.[58]

In another prospective study, researchers from one facility collected 898 consecutive pairs of surgical gloves used during all general surgery procedures during a nine-month period. There was a positive correlation between the rate of perforation and the duration of time the gloves were worn. Gloves worn for 90 minutes or less showed a perforation rate of 15%. Gloves worn for 91 to 150 minutes showed a perforation rate of 18%, while gloves worn longer than 150 minutes showed a perforation rate of 24%. There was no significant difference in the perforation rates of gloves worn by surgeons, first assistants, or scrub persons. Previously undetected perforations were found in 19% of the gloves worn by all team members. The researchers recommended that surgeons, first assistants, and scrub persons directly assisting at the operative field change gloves after 90 minutes of surgery.[59]

The American Academy of Orthopedic Surgeons recommends changing the outer pair of gloves at least every two hours to prevent skin exposure from perforations that may occur in the gloves with use over time.[47]

III.h.1.   Perioperative team members should develop and implement strategies for changing gloves during operative and other invasive procedures and for identifying appropriate precautions to prevent microbial contamination and transmission of bloodborne pathogens.

The unique and critical factors associated with the immediate situation require thoughtful assessment and the application of informed clinical judgment.

Published literature does not provide conclusive evidence as to whether the outer gloves only or both the inner and outer gloves should be changed, or whether a surgical hand scrub should be performed each time gloves are changed. If the outer glove is contaminated by contact with an unsterile item (eg, surgical helmet hood), it may be sufficient to change only the outer gloves; however, if an outer glove has been perforated, the potential exists that the inner glove also may be perforated. In this case, the safest practice for both patient and surgical team member may be to remove gown and gloves, perform a surgical hand scrub, and don a clean gown and gloves.

III.i.   Perioperative team members who must change their sterile gloves during operative or other invasive procedures should use the assisted gloving method. *[4: Limited Evidence]*

When using the assisted gloving method, one scrubbed team member touches only the outside of the new sterile glove when applying the glove to another scrubbed team member's hand.

Researchers evaluated glove donning techniques for microbial contamination by comparing open, closed, and assisted gloving techniques. After applying an ultraviolet luminescent cream to the tips of each of the fingers on both hands, 13 individuals were observed donning surgical gowns and gloves 20 times each. Contamination of the front and back cuff areas of the gown was noted in all 20 donning procedures using the open gloving method. Contamination of the back cuff areas of the gown was noted in all 20 donning procedures using the closed gloving method. No contamination of any areas of the gown was noted when using the assisted gloving method.[60]

III.i.1.   If possible, the unscrubbed team member should remove the glove to be changed from the sterile team member without altering the position of the gown cuff (ie, pulling the cuff down over the scrubbed team member's hand).

III.i.2.   When assisted gloving is not possible or practical, perioperative team members should change gowns and gloves using the closed gloving technique.

Recommendation IV

Sterile drapes should be used to establish a sterile field.

Sterile drapes provide a barrier that minimizes the passage of microorganisms from unsterile to sterile areas and reduces the risk of health care-associated infections.[1]

V.a. Perioperative team members should place sterile drapes on the patient, furniture, and equipment in the sterile field and should handle them in a manner that prevents contamination.[1] *[1: Strong Evidence]*

In a randomized controlled trial comparing the use of maximal sterile barrier precautions (ie, sterile gown, sterile gloves, surgical cap, full body drape) with the use of only sterile gloves and a small drape during CVC insertion, results showed that maximal sterile barrier precautions led to fewer episodes of catheter colonization and catheter-related bloodstream infections.[61] One program that included using maximal sterile barriers during CVC insertion in 103 intensive care units in Michigan resulted in a 66% decrease in infection rates.[62]

The CDC recommends maximum sterile barrier precautions, including the use of a full body drape, during the placement of CVCs, PICCs, and guidewire exchanges.[8,9]

IV.a.1. Unsterile equipment (eg, Mayo stands) should be covered on the top, bottom, and sides with sterile barrier materials before being introduced to or brought over a sterile field. Sterile barrier material also should be applied to the portion of the equipment that will be positioned immediately adjacent to the sterile field.

IV.a.2. Sterile drapes should be handled as little as possible.

Rapid movement of draping materials creates air currents on which dust, lint, and other particles can migrate.[37]

IV.a.3. Draping materials should be held in a controlled manner that prevents the sterile drape from coming into contact with unsterile surfaces.

IV.a.4. During draping, gloved hands should be shielded by cuffing the drape material over the gloved hands.

Keeping the gloved hands beneath the cuff of the draping material may protect gloves from contact with unsterile items or areas.

Researchers tested 275 outer and inner gloves that were used during 10 total hip replacements for microbial contamination. The results indicated that contamination occurred most frequently on the outside of the gloves that were used exclusively for draping.[63]

IV.a.5. Surgical drapes should be placed in a manner that does not require scrubbed team members to lean across an unsterile area and prevents the front of the surgical gown from contacting an unsterile surface.

IV.a.6. Sterile drapes should be placed from the surgical site to peripheral areas.

IV.a.7. The portion of the surgical drape that establishes the sterile field should not be moved after it has been positioned.

IV.a.8. Only the top surface of a sterile, draped area should be considered sterile. Items that fall below the sterile area should be considered contaminated.

IV.b. Surgical equipment (eg, tubing, cables) should be secured to the sterile drapes with nonperforating devices. *[3: Moderate Evidence]*

Perforation of barrier materials may provide portals of entry and exit for microorganisms, blood, and other potentially infectious materials.[57]

IV.c. The upper portion of the C-arm drape should be considered contaminated. *[3: Moderate Evidence]*

In a prospective study evaluating the sterility of 25 C-arm drapes used during spinal surgery, researchers obtained samples postoperatively from five different locations on a standard fluoroscopic C-arm drape. The researchers also sampled the drapes preoperatively immediately after they were applied to establish a negative control. The results showed that bacterial contamination was present at all sampled locations; however, the samples at the top of the C-arm had the greatest degree of contamination when compared with the negative controls (ie, 56% at the top and 28% at the upper front of the receiver). Lower rates of contamination were observed on the lower front, receiver plate, and mid-portion of the C-arm drape (ie, 12% to 20%), but these were not considered significant. The researchers recommended the top portion of the C-arm drape be considered unsterile, and suggested that avoiding contact with these areas may decrease the risk of postoperative infection[64] (Figure 5).

IV.d. Plastic adhesive incise drapes should not be used for prevention of surgical site infection. *[1: Strong Evidence]*

In a systematic review of seven randomized, controlled studies involving 4,195 patients, researchers concluded there was no evidence to support the use of plastic adhesive incise drapes as a method for reducing infection, and that there was some evidence that infection rates may be increased when adhesive incise drapes are used. A meta-analysis of five studies included in the review, which included 3,082 participants, compared plain plastic adhesive incise drapes with no drape and showed a significantly higher number of patients developed a surgical site infection when the adhesive incise drape was used. There was no effect on surgical site infection rates according to a meta-analysis of two additional studies, including 1,113 participants, which compared iodine-impregnated plastic adhesive incise drapes

FIGURE 5. C-ARM DRAPE CONTAMINATION

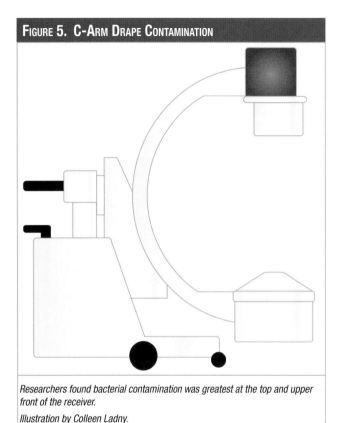

Researchers found bacterial contamination was greatest at the top and upper front of the receiver.

Illustration by Colleen Ladny.

with no drape. The researchers theorized that the patient's skin is not likely to be a primary cause of surgical site infection if it is properly disinfected, and they concluded that attempting to isolate the skin from the surgical wound is of no benefit and may create increased moisture and bacterial growth under adhesive drapes.[65]

Recommendation V

A sterile field should be prepared for patients undergoing surgical or other invasive procedures.

Preparing a sterile field for patients undergoing surgical or other invasive procedures reduces the risk of microbial contamination and is a cornerstone of infection prevention. Failure to adhere to aseptic practices during invasive procedures has been associated with surgical site infections.[1]

V.a. The sterile field should be prepared in the location where it will be used and should not be moved. *[5: Benefits Balanced with Harms]*

Moving the sterile field from one location to another increases the potential for contamination.

V.b. The sterile field should be prepared as close as possible to the time of use. *[1: Strong Evidence]*

The potential for bacterial growth and contamination increases with time because dust and other particles present in the ambient environment settle on horizontal surfaces. Particulate matter can be stirred up by personnel

movement and can settle on opened sterile supplies.[1,37,66-70]

There is no specified amount of time that opened sterile supplies in an unused room can remain sterile. The sterility of an opened sterile field is event-related.[71]

V.c. Sterile supplies should be opened for only one patient at a time in the OR or other procedure room. *[5: Benefits Balanced With Harms]*

Opening sterile supplies for multiple patients in a single OR or other procedure room increases the risk of cross contamination.

V.d. One patient at a time should occupy the OR or other procedure room. *[1: Strong Evidence]*

Concurrent procedures performed on multiple patients in the same OR or other procedure room at the same time may expose patients to a variety of hazards and increase the risk of contamination and infection.

Infectious diseases may be transmitted by airborne, contact, and droplet methods.[10] The risk of cross contamination may be increased when two sterile fields, two surgical teams, and two open surgical wounds are confined to a single OR or other procedure room.

V.e. Perioperative personnel should perform a surgical hand scrub and don a sterile gown and gloves before setting up sterile supplies. *[1: Strong Evidence]*

Surgical hand hygiene decreases transient and resident microorganisms on the skin which may reduce health care-associated infections.[4,6]

Donning a sterile gown and gloves before setting up sterile supplies minimizes the potential for wound contamination and reduces patient risks for surgical site infections that may result from contact with perioperative team members' skin or clothing.[1]

V.f. Only sterile items should come in contact with the sterile field. *[1: Strong Evidence]*

The creation and maintenance of a sterile field may influence patient outcomes.[1]

Using sterile items during invasive procedures minimizes the risk of infection and provides the highest level of assurance that procedural items are free of microorganisms.[72]

V.g. Sterile fields and instrumentation used during procedures that involve both the abdominal and perineal areas should be kept separate and should not be used interchangeably. *[3: Moderate Evidence]*

The perineal area has a higher microbial count than the abdominal area.[73] Placing instruments and other items that have been used in the perineal area into the abdominal area can transfer microorganisms from the perineum to the abdomen and cause an infection. Meticulous sterile technique is required during gynecologic laparoscopic procedures when transurethral instruments and catheters are passed to prevent infections of the urinary tract. These infections are the most common type of health care-associated infection reported to the National Healthcare Safety Network.[74]

The defense system of the peritoneum also may be negatively affected by the pneumoperitoneum used in laparoscopic procedures.[75] The mechanical distension changes the peritoneal microstructure, allowing passage of bacteria[76] to the bloodstream, lungs, and kidneys.[77] This is important because intra-abdominal infections often begin in the peritoneal cavity.[76] Systemic response coupled with the amount of tissue damage and the duration of the procedure may potentially lead to a higher risk for infection.[75]

V.h. Isolation technique should be used during bowel surgery. [2: High Evidence]

Isolation technique, also known as bowel or contamination technique, is implemented to reduce the potential for microorganisms that exist in the bowel to be transferred into the abdominal cavity, tissues of the abdominal wall, and the surgical site. Isolation technique includes

○ no longer using instruments or equipment that have contacted the inside of the bowel or the bowel lumen after the bowel lumen has been closed,

○ using clean instruments to close the wound, and

○ either removing contaminated instruments and equipment from the sterile field or placing them in a separate area that will not be touched by members of the sterile team.

The distal ileum is an area of transition between the small populations of bacteria in the proximal small intestine and the large numbers of bacteria and anaerobic microorganisms in the large bowel.[73,78-80] Only small numbers of bacteria are normally present in the duodenum and proximal jejunum.[73,78-80] Excessive colonization of bacteria in the small bowel is prevented by the destructive action of gastric acid and bile, digestion by proteolytic enzymes, and bacterial clearance by intestinal peristalsis.[73,78-80] Some gastrointestinal disorders that require surgical repair may be associated with an increase in the number of bacteria in the upper gastrointestinal tract (eg, obstruction, diverticula, fistula)[78-80] and may warrant the implementation of isolation technique.

In a study evaluating contamination of surgical instruments that have contacted bowel mucosa and whether isolation technique decreases contamination of the abdominal wall and peritoneal cavity, researchers compared contamination levels of instruments used during procedures involving the large bowel (ie, cecum, ascending, transverse, descending, and sigmoid colon, rectum) with contamination levels of instruments used during procedures involving the small bowel (ie, duodenum, jejunum, ileum). Researchers cultured the needle drivers used to grasp the needles that perforated mucosa when the bowel was anastomosed and the tissue forceps that were used to grasp the edge of the bowel during anastomosis from 20 procedures involving the large bowel. The same two types of instruments from 10 procedures involving the small bowel also were cultured. The study results showed that instruments that come into contact with the bowel lumen during bowel resection surgery become contaminated if they are not isolated, which increases the potential for contamination of the peritoneal cavity and abdominal wall from bowel organisms. The total number of organisms isolated was greater for the large bowel than for the small bowel, and the proportion of anaerobic organisms was greater in the large bowel group.[81]

In a prospective study assessing the risk factors for surgical site infection during gastrointestinal surgery, researchers conducted surveillance of 941 patients in 27 hospitals and found the overall infection rate was 15.5%; the incidence of infection after gastric surgery was 8%; and the incidence of infection after small bowel, colorectal, appendectomy, and stoma surgeries was as high as 20% to 30%. Researchers found that strict adherence to sterile technique and minimal blood loss were associated with a lower incidence of surgical site infection.[82]

V.h.1. The health care organization should develop and implement a standardized procedure for isolation technique.[81,83,84]

A standardized procedure for isolation technique (ie, following the same patterns and processes each time) assists in achieving accuracy, efficiency, and continuity among perioperative team members. Studies of human error have shown that many errors involve a deviation from routine practice.[85]

V.h.2. The use of isolation technique should begin when the gastrointestinal tract is transected and end when the anastomosis is closed.[83]

V.h.3. Isolation technique should be implemented using either a single setup or a dual setup.[83,84]

Single setup:
• Prepare one setup for the procedure, including anastomosis and closure.
• Before transection of the bowel, place clean sterile towels or a wound protector around the surgical site.
• Segregate all contaminated instruments and other items that have contacted the

bowel lumen to a designated area (eg, Mayo stand, basin).
- Refrain from touching the sterile back table while the bowel is open.
- When the anastomosis is complete, remove the contaminated instruments, towel drapes, wound protector, and any other potentially contaminated items (eg, electrosurgical pencil, suction, light handles) from the sterile field, or place them in a separate area that will not be touched by perioperative team members.
- Irrigate the wound and apply moist counted sponges or towels to protect the tissue.
- Initiate team communication announcing the change to clean closure.
- One scrubbed team member should remain at the sterile field while all other team members change into clean gowns and gloves.
- The scrubbed team member who remained at the field should remove the moist counted sponges or towels and then change into a clean gown and gloves.
- Initiate accounting procedures.
- Apply clean light handles.
- Apply clean drapes to cover the existing drapes, which may be soiled with bowel contents.
- Secure a clean electrosurgical pencil and suction to the field.
- Proceed with wound closure using only clean instrumentation and other items.

Dual setup:
- Prepare one setup for the procedure and one for the closure.
- Before transection of the bowel, place clean sterile towels or a wound protector around the surgical site.
- When the anastomosis is complete, remove the contaminated instruments, towel drapes, wound protector, and any other potentially contaminated items (eg, electrosurgical pencil, suction, light handles) from the sterile field or return all contaminated instruments and other items to the procedure setup that will not be touched by perioperative team members.
- Irrigate the wound and apply moist counted sponges or towels to protect the tissue.
- Initiate team communication announcing the change to clean closure.
- One scrubbed team member should remain at the sterile field while all other team members change into clean gowns and gloves.
- The scrubbed team member who remained at the field should remove the

moist counted sponges or towels and then change into a clean gown and gloves.
- Initiate accounting procedures.
- Apply clean light handles.
- Apply clean drapes to cover the existing drapes, which may be soiled with bowel contents.
- Secure a clean electrosurgical pencil and suction to the field.
- Proceed with wound closure using only instrumentation and other items from the closure setup.

V.i. Isolation technique should be used during procedures involving resection of metastatic tumors. [3: Moderate Evidence]

The use of isolation technique is a primary precaution to prevent the potential spread of cancer cells. There have been reports of local and distant implantation of tumor cells associated with the use of instrumentation used for both resection and closure or reconstruction.[86-88]

In one case, a 52-year-old man underwent a subtotal resection of a metastatic gliosarcoma in the right frontal region, a second surgery four months later, and a third surgery with complete resection five months after that. The dural defect that occurred as a result of the total resection was reconstructed using a tensor fascia lata graft from the right leg. Two months later, the patient presented with subcutaneous masses in the frontal and right temporal scalp and in the right upper leg in the area where the donor graft was taken. Pathologic examination of the excised masses verified the presence of cells identical to the primary tumor mass. The patient died two months later with multiple subcutaneous masses in the scalp. Implantation of tumor cells by the use of contaminated surgical instruments used for tumor resection was believed to be the cause of the development of local and distant recurrences.[86]

In another case, a 42-year-old man underwent sublabial transrhinoseptal incomplete resection of a clival chondroid chordoma and postoperative proton beam radiotherapy that resulted in stabilization of the residual tumor remnant. The patient experienced a painless loosening of an upper incisor 31 months later. Computerized tomography revealed a bone defect between the 11th and 12th teeth. Curettage biopsy and pathological examination showed a chondroid clival chordoma resembling the initial chordoma. The patient underwent two additional resections for intracranial recurrences and died at the age of 49 from infectious complications. Seeding during resection is believed to be the cause of the recurrence. The authors recommended removing resection instrumentation before closure and abundantly rinsing the surgical field.[87]

In another case, a 37-year-old woman who was diagnosed at age 10 with a low-grade oligoastrocytoma underwent craniotomy with surgical resection of the tumor at the time of diagnosis. The patient underwent a second craniotomy and surgical resection of the tumor followed by chemoradiation for progression of the tumor. Seven months later, the patient noticed an area of thickening in the scalp incision and underwent resection of the scar for what was believed to be poor wound healing. Pathological examination of the skin from the scalp revealed fibrosis and subcutaneous fat necrosis with chronic inflammation and foreign body giant cell reaction; however, the deep aspect of the subcutaneous tissue showed clusters and infiltrating cords of atypical cells morphologically similar to those of the resected tumor. The development of subcutaneous scalp involvement was believed to be from tumor implantation and seeding during surgical resection.[88]

Recommendation VI

Items introduced to the sterile field should be opened, dispensed, and transferred by methods that maintain the sterility and integrity of the item and the sterile field.

Sterile items that are not opened, dispensed, and transferred by methods that maintain sterility and integrity may contaminate the sterile field.

VI.a. Perioperative team members should inspect sterile items for proper processing, packaging, and package integrity immediately before presentation to the sterile field. *[1: Strong Evidence]*

Inspecting items before presentation to the sterile field helps verify that conditions required for sterility have been met and helps prevent microbial contamination that might occur if the integrity of the container has been breached and the item is placed on the sterile field.

Sterility is event-related and depends on maintenance of the integrity of the package.[71,89,90] The sterility of an item does not change with the passage of time but may be affected by particular events (eg, amount of handling) or environmental conditions (eg, humidity).

In a study of time-related contamination rates of sterilized dental instruments, researchers removed 25 sterilized examination mirrors from their packages and tested them for aerobic and anaerobic microbial contamination immediately after sterilization and at 31, 60, 90, and 124 days. Researchers found no contamination on any of the items at any time.[91]

In another study that evaluated whether storage time has any effect on the susceptibility of sterile packages to contamination under deliberate bacterial exposure, researchers prepared 700 packages containing six porcelain cylinders using four different types of packaging, including one cloth wrap, one paper wrap, and two peel pouches (ie, 175 of each packaging type). As a control group, 100 packages (ie, 25 of each packaging type) were immediately opened and tested for contamination. The outside of the remaining packages were deliberately contaminated with *Serratia marcescens* and opened at intervals of seven, 14, 28, 90, and 180 days. The packages were handled weekly and transferred from one container to another. The results showed no growth in the interior of any of the packages. Researchers concluded that the packages were able to protect the contents for up to six months, even with external contamination.[92]

Researchers tested 7,200 sterile packages to examine the effect of time on internal package sterility. The packages were tested immediately after sterilization and at monthly intervals during a 12-month period after storage in cabinet drawers in 24 different dental procedure rooms. No evidence of increased contamination over time was found for any of the packages. The researchers concluded that a 12-month or longer storage period is acceptable for sterile packages.[93]

To evaluate the sterility of packaged items in a variety of environmental conditions, researchers distributed 152 wrapped and packaged items to five different areas within a single hospital. Every three months over a two-year period, a number of items were removed from their packaging and tested for sterility. All of the tested items were found to be sterile. The results of this study demonstrated that unless the packaging is damaged, properly wrapped or packaged and sterilized items remain sterile. The researchers also concluded that although the study was conducted during a two-year period, there is no reason to suggest that this should be considered as a time limit for sterility.[94]

VI.a.1. If an expiration date is provided, perioperative team members should check the date before the package is opened and the contents are delivered to the sterile field. Items should not be used after the labeled expiration date.

VI.a.2. Perioperative team members should inspect the sterilization chemical indicator in the sterile package to verify the appropriate color change for the sterilization process used.[90]

VI.b. Items should be delivered to the sterile field in a manner that prevents unsterile objects or unscrubbed team members from leaning or reaching over the sterile field. *[1: Strong Evidence]*

Microorganisms are shed from the skin of perioperative personnel.[1,37] Maintaining distance from the sterile field decreases the potential for contamination when items are passed from unsterile to sterile areas.

VI.c. Sterile items should be presented directly to the scrubbed team member or placed securely on the sterile field. *[5: Benefits Balanced with Harms]*

Items tossed onto a sterile field may roll off the edge, create a hole in the sterile drape, or cause other items to be displaced, leading to contamination of the sterile field.

VI.c.1. Heavy items or items that are sharp and may penetrate the sterile barrier should be presented directly to the scrubbed team member or opened on a separate clean, dry surface.

VI.d. Perioperative personnel should open wrapped sterile supplies by opening
1. the farthest wrapper flap,
2. each of the side flaps, and
3. the nearest wrapper flap.
[5: Benefits Balanced with Harms]

Opening the wrapper flap that is farthest away first prevents contamination that might occur from passing an unsterile arm over sterile items.

VI.d.1. Wrapper edges should be secured when supplies are opened and presented to the scrubbed team member or sterile field.[90]

Wrapper edges are considered contaminated. Securing the loose wrapper edges helps prevent them from contaminating sterile areas or items.

VI.d.2. Instrument tray wrappers should be visually inspected for moisture and integrity before the contents are placed on the sterile field.[90]

VI.e. Peel pouches should be presented to the scrubbed team member or opened onto the sterile field by pulling back the flaps without touching the inside of the package or allowing the contents to slide over the unsterile edges of the package. *[5: Benefits Balanced with Harms]*

Touching the inside of the package or allowing the contents to slide over the unsterile edges may contaminate the contents of the package.

VI.f. Rigid sterilization containers should be inspected and opened on a clean, flat, and dry surface.[90] *[4: Limited Evidence]*

Opening rigid sterilization containers on a clean, flat, and dry surface facilitates removing sterile items from their containers without contaminating the items or sterile field.

VI.f.1. Perioperative team members should verify that external locks, latch filters, valves, and tamper-evident devices are intact before opening rigid sterilization containers.[90]

Ensuring container locks, latch filters, valves, and temper-evident devices are intact helps to verify there has not been a breach of the container seal.

VI.f.2. Perioperative team members should verify that the external chemical indicator has changed as appropriate before opening rigid sterilization containers.

Checking for the appropriate chemical indicator change verifies that the container has been through the sterilization process and reduces the potential for opening items that have not been sterilized.

VI.f.3. The rigid sterilization container should be opened according to the manufacturer's written instructions for use. The lid should be lifted up and toward the person opening the container and away from the container.
- The lid should be inspected for the integrity of the filter or valve and the integrity of the filter or valve and the gasket.[90]
- The container contents should be considered contaminated if the filter is damp or dislodged, or has holes, tears, or punctures.

Opening the container according to the manufacturer's written instructions for use facilitates aseptic removal of the contents.[9] Lifting the lid up and away from the container and toward the person removing the lid helps to prevent potential contamination from contact between the unsterile lid and the sterile inner rim, contents, and inside of the container system, and also helps to prevent the unscrubbed person from leaning over the sterile contents of the container.

VI.f.4. The scrubbed team member should avoid contacting the unsterile surfaces of the table or container while lifting the inner basket(s) out and above the container.[90] Before the instruments are placed on the sterile field, the internal chemical indicator should be examined for the appropriate color change and the inside surface of the container inspected for debris, contamination, or damage.[90]

VI.g. Medications and sterile solutions (eg, normal saline) should be transferred to and handled on the sterile field using sterile technique. *[2: High Evidence]*

Transferring and handling medications and solutions on the sterile field poses increased risk for contamination of the medication, solution, sterile field, and surgical site because medications and solutions are removed from their original containers, stored on the sterile field, and passed from a scrubbed team member to a licensed practitioner for administration.[95] Using sterile technique helps prevent microbial contamination of the sterile field or medication.

VI.g.1. Medications and solutions should be visually inspected immediately before transfer to the sterile field and should not be used if the expiration date has passed or if there is any indication that the medication or solution has been compromised (eg, discoloration, particulate formation).[95]

Compromised and outdated medications and solutions may be contaminated or have reduced effectiveness.

VI.g.2. Sterile transfer devices (eg, sterile vial spike, filter straw, plastic catheter) should be used when transferring medications or solutions to the sterile field.[95]

Transfer devices are designed to reduce the potential for contamination of the sterile field by minimizing splashing and spilling and the need to reach over the sterile field.

VI.g.3. When solutions are dispensed to the sterile field, the entire contents of the container should be poured slowly into a solution receptacle that is placed near the sterile table's edge or is held by a scrubbed team member and labeled immediately.

Pouring the entire contents of the container slowly prevents splashing. Splashing may cause strike-through and splash-back from unsterile surfaces to the sterile field.

Placing the solution receptacle near the edge of the sterile table or having the scrubbed team member hold the receptacle reduces the potential for contamination of the sterile table and allows the unscrubbed team member to pour fluids without leaning over the sterile field.

VI.g.4. The edge of the container should be considered contaminated after the contents have been poured.

VI.g.5. The cap should not be replaced on opened medication or solution containers and any remaining fluids should be discarded.

The sterility of the contents of opened medication or solution containers cannot be ensured if the cap is replaced.

Reuse of open containers may contaminate solutions from drops contacting unsterile areas and then running back over container openings.

VI.g.6. Medications and solutions should be dispensed to the sterile field as close as possible to the time they will be used.[95]

VI.g.7. Stoppers should not be removed from vials for the purpose of pouring medications unless specifically designed for removal and pouring by the manufacturer.[95]

VI.g.8. Unused, opened irrigation or IV solutions should be discarded at the end of the procedure.[95]

Irrigation and IV containers and supplies are considered single-use. Using surplus volume from any irrigation or IV solution container or supplies for more than one patient increases the risk of cross-contamination.

Recommendation VII

Sterile fields should be constantly monitored.

The sterile field is subject to unrecognized contamination by personnel, vectors (eg, insects), or breaks in sterile technique if left unobserved.

VII.a. Once created, a sterile field should not be left unattended until the operative or other invasive procedure is completed. *[5: Benefits Balanced with Harms]*

Observation increases the likelihood of detecting a breach in sterility.

VII.a.1. The doors to the OR or other procedure room should not be taped closed or otherwise secured as an alternative to monitoring the sterile field.

VII.b. When there is an unanticipated delay, or during periods of increased activity, a sterile field that has been prepared and will not immediately be used may be covered with a sterile drape. *[2: High Evidence]*

To evaluate the contamination rate of sterile trays that have been opened in a controlled OR environment and the effect of traffic on the contamination rate, researchers opened 45 sterile trays in a positive air-flow OR and randomly assigned them to one of three groups:

○ Trays were opened and left uncovered in a locked OR.
○ Trays were opened and left uncovered in an OR with single-person traffic flowing in and out every 10 minutes from an unsterile corridor.
○ Trays were opened, immediately covered with a sterile surgical towel, and left in a locked OR.

All trays were opened using sterile technique and were exposed for a total of four hours. Cultures of the trays were taken immediately after they were opened and every 30 minutes during the exposure period. The contamination rates for the uncovered trays were 4% at 30 minutes, 15% at 60 minutes, 22% at two hours, and 30% at four hours. There was no difference in the contamination rates between the uncovered trays in the room with traffic and those in the room without traffic. The covered trays had no contamination during the exposure period. The researchers recommended covering sterile trays that are not immediately used to minimize exposure to environmental contaminants.[96]

In a study of 41 total joint replacements (27 hip, 14 knee) that was conducted to evaluate the effectiveness of covering instruments, researchers found that covering the instruments during periods of increased activity (eg, patient transfer to the procedure bed, skin preparation) shortened the overall exposure time and shielded the instruments from bacterial dispersal, resulting in a 28-fold reduction of instrument contamination.[97]

VII.b.1. When sterile fields are covered, they should be covered in a manner that allows the cover to be removed without bringing the part of the cover that falls below the sterile field above the sterile field. When covering the sterile field, two sterile "cuffed" drapes should be used as follows:

- The first drape should be placed horizontally over the table or other area to be covered with the cuff at or just beyond the halfway point. The second drape should be placed from the opposite side of the table and the cuff positioned so that it completely covers the cuff of the first drape (Figure 6).
- The drapes should be removed by placing hands within the cuff of the top drape and lifting the drape up and away from the table and toward the person removing the drape. The second drape should be removed from the opposite side in a similar manner.

FIGURE 6. COVERING A STERILE TABLE

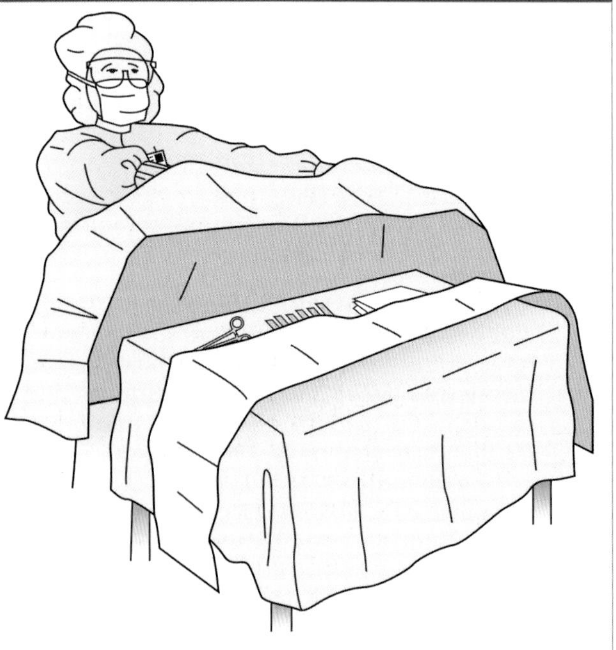

The first drape is placed with the cuff at the halfway point. The second drape is placed from the opposite side and completely covers the cuff of the first drape.
Illustration by Colleen Ladny and Kurt Jones.

Removing the cover from the sterile field may result in a part of the cover that was below the sterile field being drawn above the sterile field, which may allow air currents to draw microorganisms and other contaminants (eg, dust, debris) from an unsterile area (eg, floor) and deposit them in sterile areas.[37]

VII.b.2. The health care organization should develop a standardized procedure in collaboration with infection prevention personnel for covering sterile fields to delineate the specific circumstances when sterile fields may be covered and to specify the method of covering and the length of time a sterile field may be covered.

Standardized procedures (ie, following the same patterns and processes each time) assist in achieving accuracy, efficiency, and continuity among perioperative team members. Studies of human error have shown that many errors involve a deviation from routine practice.[85]

VII.c. Perioperative personnel should observe for, recognize, and immediately correct breaks in sterile technique when preparing, performing, or assisting with operative or other invasive procedures and should implement measures to prevent future occurrences. [1: Strong Evidence]

Breaks in sterile technique may expose the patient to increased microbial contamination. The risk for infection increases with increased amounts of microbial contamination.[1] Preventing, observing for, recognizing, and taking immediate corrective action for breaks in sterile technique may prevent or reduce microbial contamination and help minimize the risk of surgical site infection.

VII.c.1. When a break in sterile technique occurs, corrective action should be taken immediately unless the patient's safety is at risk. When a break in sterile technique cannot be corrected immediately, corrective action should be taken as soon as it is safe for the patient.

The greater the length of time until the break in sterile technique is recognized, the more complex and difficult containment becomes and the more likely it becomes that full containment may not be possible.[98]

VII.d. If organic material (eg, blood, hair, tissue, bone fragments) or other debris (eg, bone cement, grease, mineral deposits) is found on an instrument or item in a sterile set, the entire set should be considered contaminated and perioperative team members should take corrective actions immediately. [1: Strong Evidence]

Organic and inorganic material that remains on a surgical instrument may be transferred to the surgical wound or other areas of the body which increases the risk for surgical site infection or other postoperative complications.

Sterilization or high-level disinfection can only be achieved if all surfaces of an item have contacted the sterilizing agent or disinfectant under the appropriate conditions and for the appropriate amount of time. Organic materials and other debris may act as barriers that interfere with sterilization or high-level disinfection or may combine with and deactivate the sterilant or disinfectant.[71,89,90] If organic material or other debris is found on an instrument that has been through sterilization or high-level disinfection, there is no way to ensure that the sterilant or high-level disinfectant made contact with all surfaces of the item and with other items in the set. Sterility or high-level disinfection may not have been achieved; therefore, the sterility of the entire set is in question.

VII.d.1. Corrective actions should include, at a minimum, removing the entire set and any other items that may have come in contact with the contaminated item from the sterile field and changing the gloves of any team member who may have touched the contaminated item. Additional corrective actions may be required subject to thoughtful assessment and the application of informed clinical judgment based on the specific factors associated with the individual event.

VII.e. If an instrument in a sterile set is found assembled or clamped closed, the entire set should be considered contaminated and perioperative team members should take corrective actions immediately. [1: Strong Evidence]

Sterilization or high-level disinfection can only be achieved if all surfaces of an instrument have contacted the sterilizing or disinfecting agent under the appropriate conditions and for the appropriate amount of time.[71,89,90] If an instrument has not been correctly disassembled or is clamped closed before sterilization or high-level disinfection, there is no way to ensure that the sterilant or high-level disinfectant made contact with all surfaces of the item and with other items in the set. Sterility or high-level disinfection may not have been achieved; therefore, the sterility of the entire set is in question.

VII.e.1. Corrective actions should include, at a minimum, removing the entire set and any other instruments that may have come in contact with the contaminated instrument from the sterile field and changing the gloves of any team member who may have touched the contaminated item. Additional corrective actions may be required subject to thoughtful assessment and the application of informed clinical judgment based on the specific factors associated with the individual event.

Recommendation VIII

All personnel moving within or around a sterile field should do so in a manner that prevents contamination of the sterile field.

Airborne contaminants and microbial levels in the surgical environment are directly proportional to the amount of movement and the number of people in the OR or other procedure room.[37,66-70]

VIII.a. Scrubbed team members should remain close to the sterile field and touch only sterile areas or items. [5: Benefits Balanced with Harms]

Walking outside the periphery of the sterile field or leaving and then returning to the OR or other procedure room in sterile attire increases the potential for contamination.

VIII.a.1. Scrubbed team members should not leave the sterile field to retrieve items from the sterilizer.

VIII.a.2. Scrubbed team members should wear protective devices (eg, lead aprons) that reduce radiological exposure so they are not required to leave the sterile field when x-rays are taken.[99]

VIII.b. Scrubbed team members should keep their hands and arms above waist level at all times. [5: Benefits Balanced with Harms]

Keeping the hands and arms above waist level allows the perioperative team member to see them constantly. Contamination may occur when a perioperative team member moves his or her hands or arms below waist level.

VIII.b.1. Scrubbed team members' arms should not be folded with the hands in the axillary area.

The axillary area has the potential to become contaminated by perspiration, allowing for strike-through of the gown and potential contamination of the gloved hands. The axillary area of the gown is an area of friction and is not considered an effective microbial barrier.

VIII.c. Scrubbed team members should avoid changing levels and should be seated only when the entire procedure will be performed at that level. [4: Limited Evidence]

When scrubbed team members change levels, the unsterile portion of their gowns may come into contact with sterile areas.

To evaluate whether the surgical field could be contaminated by a perioperative team member stepping on and off of a footstool, researchers sprinkled starch powder on the portion of the drape below the level of the sterile field. A surgeon wearing a surgical gown made contact with the drape, and then stepped on and off a 6-inch footstool twice. The contamination level rose 6 inches with each movement. The researchers recommended that scrubbed team members reduce the number of times they step on a footstool.[100]

VIII.d. When changing position with each other, scrubbed team members should turn back to back or face to face while maintaining distance from each other, the sterile field, and unsterile areas. *[5: Benefits Balanced with Harms]*

Contamination of sterile gowns and gloves and the sterile field may be prevented by scrubbed team members maintaining distance from each other and the sterile field when changing position, and by establishing patterns of movement that reduce the risk of contact with unsterile areas.

VIII.e. Unscrubbed personnel should face the sterile field on approach, should not walk between sterile fields or scrubbed persons, and should maintain a distance of at least 12 inches from the sterile field and scrubbed persons at all times. *[5: Benefits Balanced with Harms]*

Contamination of the sterile field or scrubbed team members may be prevented by unscrubbed team members maintaining distance from the sterile field and scrubbed persons and establishing patterns of movement that reduce the risk of contact with sterile areas and scrubbed persons.

VIII.f. Conversations in the presence of a sterile field should be kept to a minimum. *[3: Moderate Evidence]*

Microorganisms are transported on airborne particles including respiratory droplets.[37]

Researchers studied the role of conversation in the OR by using small spherical particles of human albumin ranging in size from 10 to 35 micrometers in diameter to simulate particles that carry bacteria. Approximately 300,000 albumin particles were sprayed on the faces and in the nostrils beneath the surgical masks of the study participants. The participants read aloud continuously for periods of five, 10, 20, 30, 40, 50, and 60 minutes from a position 30 cm above a water bath simulating a surgical wound. The researchers collected particles from the water bath and processed them after each reading session. The results of the study showed that the longer the period of conversation, the greater the number of particles in the simulated wound. The effects of both time and conversation were found to be significant. The researchers concluded that conversation contributes to airborne contamination of surgical wounds.[68]

VIII.g. The number and movement of individuals involved in an operative or other invasive procedure should be kept to a minimum.[1,66,69] *[1: Strong Evidence]*

Bacterial shedding increases with activity. Air currents can pick up contaminated particles shed from patients, personnel, and drapes and distribute them to sterile areas.[37,67,70]

Researchers conducted a prospective, observational study in three pediatric ORs. During a two-week period, surgeons, anesthesia professionals, and perioperative team members were observed during 14 surgical procedures. A medical student observer recorded parameters including the

○ minimum and maximum numbers of personnel in the room during the procedure,

○ number of personnel in the procedure room at each 30-minute interval, and

○ number of personnel changes during the procedure.

There was a positive correlation between the length of the surgery and the number of personnel changes during the procedure, and a statistically significant increase in the number of personnel during spine procedures and procedures that lasted longer than 120 minutes. The researchers also noted a trend toward increased numbers of personnel during the middle of the procedure, especially during longer procedures. It was observed that personnel frequently entered the OR to check on the progress of the procedure, ask questions, or process paperwork. The researchers noted that these factors, in combination with frequent changes in personnel for breaks and shift changes, were a cause of distraction during the procedure, which could potentially lead to errors. Although this study was limited by its small sample size, the results support the need to limit the number of people and distractions in the OR during operative or other invasive procedures.[66]

In a study evaluating whether the behavior and number of OR personnel can predict the density of airborne bacteria at the surgical site, researchers measured the number of airborne particulates and viable bacteria during 22 joint arthroplasty procedures with a range of five to 12 team members in the OR. The results indicated a relationship between the number and activity of team members present in the periphery of the OR and the number of particulates and colony forming units at the surgical site. The researchers recommended minimizing the number of team members who are present during the procedure.[101]

As part of a non-experimental study with two phases, researchers examined the levels of environmental contamination in ORs without personnel and the effect of unscrubbed persons on environmental contamination. The ORs without personnel showed a mean of 13.3 colony forming units per square foot per hour. When five persons wearing scrub suits, shoe covers, hoods, and masks were present, the number of colony forming units increased significantly to 447.6 per square foot per hour. The researchers concluded that people are the major source of environmental contamination in the OR.[67]

In response to an unexplained increase in surgical site infections at one facility, an observational study was conducted to monitor and record behaviors in the OR. Researchers theorized that the number of door openings increased in direct proportion to procedure length, but also had an exponential relationship with the number of team members in the OR. They randomly selected and audited 28 procedures in multiple services (eg, cardiac, orthopedic, neurosurgery, plastic, general). Data collection included the

○ number of people entering and exiting the procedure room,

○ role of the individuals, and

○ reason for entering the room.

Researchers found that the number of door openings in some spinal procedures was as high as one door opening per minute, and there was an average rate of 40 door openings per hour during total joint procedures. With such high numbers of door openings, researchers noted that it was conceivable the door to the OR could remain open for as long as 15 to 20 minutes per hour. The greatest number of door openings occurred during the preincision period, and the most frequent reason for the door opening was requests for information. Personnel entering and exiting the room for breaks accounted for approximately 25% of door openings across every specialty. Retrieving and delivering supplies accounted for approximately 20% of door openings, and the RN circulator was responsible for 37% to 50% of door openings. The cumulative effect of increased door openings is the potential for increased numbers of microorganisms and other contaminants in the air and the surgical site. The researchers also noted that frequent door openings are distracting and have the potential to lead to errors.[102]

In another study of door openings, researchers used an electronic door counter and computer software to calculate and analyze the number of door openings during 46 cardiac procedures. Perioperative team members were blinded to the study. The total number of door openings was 4,273. After adjusting for procedure length and the time required for the door to close, it was found that the door to the OR was open approximately 11% of every hour. A direct correlation was found between the length of the procedure and the frequency of door openings. The data also indicated a trend toward surgical site infections with increased frequency of door openings and patients of advanced age. The researchers hypothesized that increased numbers of personnel and door openings are a distraction to the surgical team and may lead to surgical errors.[103]

Recommendation IX

Perioperative team members should receive initial and ongoing education and competency verification on their understanding of the principles of and performance of the processes for sterile technique.

It is the responsibility of the health care organization to provide initial and ongoing education and to verify the competency of perioperative team members to deliver safe care to patients undergoing operative or other invasive procedures.[2]

Initial and ongoing education of perioperative personnel on the principles and processes of sterile technique facilitates the development of knowledge, skills, and attitudes that affect safe patient care.

Periodic education programs provide the opportunity to reinforce the principles and processes of sterile technique and to introduce relevant new equipment or practices.

Competency verification measures individual performance and provides a mechanism for documentation, and may verify that perioperative personnel have an understanding of the principles and processes of sterile technique.

IX.a.   Perioperative team members should receive education and competency verification that addresses specialized knowledge and skills related to the principles and processes of sterile technique. *[1: Regulatory Requirement]*

    Specialized knowledge includes empirical knowledge (eg, technical understanding), practical knowledge (eg, clinical experience), and aesthetic knowledge (eg, patient advocacy).

    Ongoing development of knowledge and skills and documentation of personnel participation is a regulatory and accreditation requirement for both hospitals and ambulatory settings.[104-114]

IX.a.1.   Education regarding the principles and processes of sterile technique may include a review of the policies and procedures and protocols for

• surgical attire[3];

• surgical hand hygiene[4];

• preparation of ORs or other procedure rooms;

• selection and evaluation of surgical gowns, gloves, and drape products[27];

• assistance with operative or other invasive procedures;

• proper use of sterile gowns and gloves, including double gloving;

• proper use of sterile drape products;

• the use of sterile items during operative or other invasive procedures;

• preparation of a sterile field for patients undergoing operative or other invasive procedures;

• isolation technique;

- how to introduce items to the sterile field, including the transfer of medications[95] and solutions;
- how to maintain a sterile field, including recognition and correction of breaks in sterile technique;
- movement within and around a sterile field;
- the number of people who are permitted in the procedure room; and
- operative or invasive procedure documentation,[115] including reporting of breaks in sterile technique.

IX.b. Perioperative personnel should receive education that addresses human factors related to the principles and processes of sterile technique. *[3: Moderate Evidence]*

Human factors includes the interpersonal and social aspects of the perioperative environment (eg, coordination of activities, teamwork, collaboration, communication). Effectively implementing the principles and processes of sterile technique requires that perioperative personnel demonstrate not only procedural knowledge and technical proficiency, but also demonstrate the ability to anticipate needs, coordinate a multitude of activities, work collaboratively with other team members, and communicate effectively.

In a synthesis of the literature on perioperative nursing competency published between 2000 and 2008, researchers identified two domains of perioperative competency:

- specialized knowledge, described as familiarity with standards and guidelines of perioperative practice, and
- human factors, described as interpersonal and social team interactions.

The researchers recognized teamwork and communication as important aspects of patient safety and indicators of perioperative competency.[116]

In a qualitative, focus group study exploring the perceptions of perioperative nurses on competency, researchers identified three themes:

- technical and procedural knowledge—the knowledge, psychomotor skills, and situational awareness required for competency in the perioperative setting;
- communication skills—the need for communication and team building skills, collegial support, and the ability to decipher and share complex clinical information; and
- managing and coordinating flow—the ability to anticipate needs, organize and prioritize resources, manage conflicts, and grasp the full perspective of the situation.

The findings of the study highlight the importance of human factors as a competency requirement for perioperative nurses.[117]

In a review of the literature exploring the cognitive and social skills used by scrub persons, researchers identified communication, teamwork, and situational awareness as the most valuable and relevant skills.

- Communication is vitally important because of the need to listen and interpret what is being said, to clarify any issues that are unclear, and to convey critical information accurately. The need to communicate using eye contact and nonverbal cues and to speak up when necessary while working at the sterile field was recognized as a required skill for the scrub person.
- Teamwork is an important skill because of the need for scrub persons to share information to aid the team and to establish good working relationships between team members.
- Situational awareness is an important skill that includes the ability of scrub persons to anticipate the actions of the surgeon and to make decisions regarding the need for additional supplies or actions that must be taken and to anticipate future requirements of the procedure.[118]

IX.c. Relative to the principles and processes of sterile technique, the perioperative RN should

- participate in ongoing educational activities[2]
- identify personal learning needs[2];
- seek experiences to acquire, maintain, and augment personal knowledge and skill proficiency[2];
- share knowledge and skills[2];
- communicate pertinent information to perioperative team members[2];
- contribute to a healthy work environment by using appropriate and courteous verbal and nonverbal communication techniques[2]; and
- develop and implement conflict resolution skills to manage difficult behavior, promote positive working relationships, and advocate for patient safety.[2]

[2: High Evidence]

Education, collegiality, and collaboration are standards of perioperative nursing and a primary responsibility of the perioperative RN who practices in the perioperative setting.[2,119]

Recommendation X

Nursing activities related to sterile technique should be documented in a manner consistent with health care organization policies and procedures and regulatory and accrediting agency requirements.

Documentation of nursing activities serves as the legal record of care delivery. Documentation of nursing activities is dictated by health care organization policy and regulatory and accrediting agency requirements and is necessary to inform other health care professionals involved in the patient's care. Highly reliable data collection is not only necessary to chronicle patient responses to nursing interventions, but also to demonstrate the health care organization's progress toward quality care outcomes.[115]

X.a. Significant or major breaks in sterile technique that are not immediately corrected should be documented or reported per organizational policy in consultation with infection prevention personnel. *[1: Regulatory Requirement]*

Perioperative documentation that accurately reflects the patient experience is essential for the continuity of outcome-focused nursing care and for effective comparison of realized versus anticipated patient outcomes.[115]

Effective management and collection of health care information that accurately reflects the patient's care, treatment, and services is a regulatory and accreditation requirement for both hospitals and ambulatory settings.[104,105,120-127]

Recommendation XI

Policies and procedures for the implementation of sterile technique should be developed, reviewed periodically, revised as necessary, and readily available in the practice setting.

Policies and procedures assist in the development of patient safety, quality assessment, and performance improvement activities. Policies and procedures establish authority, responsibility, and accountability within the organization. Policies and procedures also serve as operational guidelines that are used to minimize patient risk for injury or complications, standardize practice, direct perioperative personnel, and establish continuous performance improvement programs.

XI.a. Policies and procedures regarding the implementation of sterile technique should be developed. *[1: Regulatory Requirement]*

Policies and procedures that guide and support patient care, treatment, and services is a regulatory and accreditation requirement for both hospitals and ambulatory settings.[104,105,109,110,128-130]

XI.a.1. Policies and procedures regarding the principles and processes of sterile technique may include
- surgical attire[3];
- surgical hand hygiene[4];
- selection and evaluation of surgical gowns, gloves, and drape products[27];
- proper use of sterile gowns and gloves, including double gloving;
- proper use of sterile drape products;
- isolation technique;
- the numbers of people who are permitted in the OR or other procedure room; and
- reporting of breaks in sterile technique.

Recommendation XII

Perioperative personnel should participate in a variety of quality assurance and performance improvement activities that are consistent with the health care organization's plan to improve understanding of and compliance with the principles and processes of sterile technique.

Quality assurance and performance improvement programs assist in evaluating and improving the quality of patient care and formulating plans for corrective actions. These programs provide data that may be used to determine whether an individual organization is within benchmark goals and, if not, to identify areas that may require corrective actions.

XII.a. Performance improvement activities for sterile technique should include monitoring personnel for understanding of the principles of and compliance with the processes of sterile technique. *[1: Regulatory Requirement]*

Collecting data to monitor and improve patient care, treatment, and services is a regulatory and accreditation requirement for both hospitals and ambulatory settings.[104,105,108,131-135]

XII.a.1. Process monitoring for activities related to sterile technique may include monitoring compliance with policies and procedures for
- surgical attire[3];
- surgical hand hygiene[4];
- preparation of the OR or other procedure room;
- selection and evaluation of surgical gowns, gloves, and drape products[27];
- performance of or assistance with operative or other invasive procedures;
- proper use of sterile gowns and gloves, including double gloving;
- proper use of sterile drape products;
- isolation technique;
- introduction of items to the sterile field, including transfer of medications[95] and solutions;
- recognition and correction of breaks in sterile technique;
- movement within and around a sterile field;
- the number of people permitted in the OR or other procedure room; and
- reporting of breaks in sterile technique.

XII.a.2. The quality assurance and performance improvement program for sterile technique should include
- periodically reviewing and evaluating activities to verify compliance or to identify the need for improvement,
- identifying corrective actions directed toward improvement priorities, and
- taking additional actions when improvement is not achieved or sustained.

Reviewing and evaluating quality assurance and performance improvement activities may identify failure points that contribute to errors in sterile technique and help define actions for improvement and increased competency.

STERILE TECHNIQUE

Taking corrective actions may improve patient safety by enhancing understanding of the principles of and compliance with the processes for sterile technique.

XII.b. Perioperative RNs should participate in ongoing quality assurance and performance improvement activities related to sterile technique by
- identifying processes that are important for quality monitoring (eg, double gloving);
- developing strategies for compliance;
- establishing benchmarks to evaluate quality indicators;
- collecting data related to the levels of performance and quality indicators;
- evaluating practice based on the cumulative data that are collected;
- taking action to improve compliance; and
- assessing the effectiveness of the actions taken.

[2: High Evidence]

Participating in ongoing quality assurance and performance improvement activities is a standard of perioperative nursing and a primary responsibility of the perioperative RN who is engaged in practice in the perioperative setting.[2]

Glossary

Aseptic: The absence of all pathogenic microorganisms. Synonym: sterile.

Aseptic practices: Patterns of behavior and processes that are implemented to prevent microbial contamination.

Assisted gloving: Technique used when changing a contaminated glove. One scrubbed team member assists another to don a new sterile glove by touching only the outside of the new sterile glove when applying the glove to another scrubbed team member's hand.

Barrier material: Material that minimizes or retards the penetration of microorganisms, particulates, and fluids.

Closed assisted gloving: Technique for donning sterile gloves during which the gown cuff of the team member being gloved remains at or beyond the fingertips. The glove to be donned is held open by a scrubbed team member, while the team member being gloved inserts his or her hand into the glove with the gown cuff touching only the inside of the glove.

Closed gloving: Technique used when donning surgical gloves. The scrubbed team member dons the gloves without assistance by keeping his or her hands inside the gown sleeves.

Colony forming unit: A measure of the number of viable bacterial cells in a sample.

Event-related sterility: Concept that the sterility of an item does not change with the passing of time but may be affected by particular events (eg, amount of handling), or environmental conditions (eg, temperature, humidity).

Invasive procedure: The surgical entry into tissues, cavities, or organs, or the repair of major traumatic injuries.

Isolation technique: Instruments and equipment that have contacted the inside of the bowel, or the bowel lumen, are no longer used after the lumen has been closed. Clean instruments are used to close the wound. The contaminated instruments and equipment are either removed from the sterile field or placed in a separate area that will not be touched by members of the sterile team. Synonyms: bowel technique, contamination technique.

Open assisted gloving: Technique for donning sterile gloves during which the gown sleeve of the team member being gloved is pulled up so that the gown cuff is at wrist level, leaving the fingers and hand exposed. The glove to be donned is held open by a scrubbed team member, while the team member being gloved inserts his or her hand into the glove without touching the outside of the glove.

Open gloving: Technique used to don sterile gloves without assistance. The cuff of each glove is everted to allow the team member to don sterile gloves by touching only the inner side of the glove with ungloved fingers and the outer sterile side of the glove with gloved fingers.

Perforation indicator system: A double gloving system comprising a colored pair of surgical gloves worn beneath a standard pair of surgical gloves. When a glove perforation occurs, moisture from the surgical field seeps through the perforation between the layers of gloves, allowing the site of perforation to be more easily seen.

Sterile: The absence of all living microorganisms. Synonym: aseptic.

Sterile field: The area surrounding the site of the incision or perforation into tissue, or the site of introduction of an instrument into a body orifice that has been prepared for an invasive procedure. The area includes all working areas, furniture, and equipment covered with sterile drapes and drape accessories, and all personnel in sterile attire.

Sterile technique: The use of specific actions and activities to prevent contamination and maintain sterility of identified areas during operative or other invasive procedures.

Surgical hand scrub: Antiseptic hand wash or antiseptic hand rub performed preoperatively by perioperative personnel to eliminate transient bacteria and reduce resident hand flora.

Surgical helmet system: An unsterile, reusable helmet with a built-in ventilation fan covered with a single-use, disposable sterile visor mask hood. The unsterile helmet is donned before the surgical hand scrub is performed. The sterile visor mask hood that covers the unsterile helmet is applied during the gowning and gloving process.

REFERENCES

1. Mangram AJ, Horan TC, Pearson ML, Silver LC, Jarvis WR; Centers for Disease Control and Prevention (CDC) Hospital Infection Control Practices Advisory Committee.

ASEPTIC PRACTICE

Guideline for prevention of surgical site infection, 1999. *Am J Infect Control*. 1999;27(2):97-132. [IVA]

2. Standards of perioperative nursing. In: *Perioperative Standards and Recommended Practices*. Denver, CO: AORN, Inc; 2012:3-20. [IVB]

3. Guideline for surgical attire. In: *Guidelines for Perioperative Practice*. Denver, CO: AORN, Inc; 2015:97-120. [IVB]

4. Guideline for hand hygiene. In: *Guidelines for Perioperative Practice*. Denver, CO: AORN, Inc; 2015:31-42. [IVB]

5. Guideline for prevention of transmissible infections. In: *Guidelines for Perioperative Practice*. Denver, CO: AORN, Inc; 2015:419-451. [IVA]

6. Boyce JM, Pittet D; Healthcare Infection Control Practices Advisory Committee; HICPAC/SHEA/APIC/IDSA Hand Hygiene Task Force. Guideline for Hand Hygiene in Health-Care Settings. Recommendations of the Healthcare Infection Control Practices Advisory Committee and the HICPAC/SHEA/APIC/IDSA Hand Hygiene Task Force. Society for Healthcare Epidemiology of America/Association for Professionals in Infection Control/Infectious Diseases Society of America. *MMWR Recomm Rep*. 2002;51(RR-16):1-45. [IVA]

7. Graves PB, Twomey CL. Surgical hand antisepsis: an evidence-based review. *Perioper Nurs Clin*. 2006;1(3): 235-249. doi:10.1016/j.cpen.2006.06.002. [VA]

8. Weber DJ, Rutala WA. Central line-associated bloodstream infections: prevention and management. *Infect Dis Clin North Am*. 2011;25(1):77-102. [IVB]

9. O'Grady NP, Alexander M, Burns LA, et al; Healthcare Infection Control Practices Advisory Committee (HICPAC). *Guidelines for the Prevention of Intravascular Catheter-Related Infections, 2011*. Atlanta, GA: Centers for Disease Control and Prevention; 2011. [IVA]

10. Siegel JD, Rhinehart E, Jackson M, Chiarello L; Healthcare Infection Control Practices Advisory Committee. *2007 Guideline for Isolation Precautions: Preventing Transmission of Infectious Agents in Healthcare Settings*. Atlanta, GA: Centers for Disease Control and Prevention; 2007. http://www.cdc.gov/ncidod/dhqp/pdf/isolation2007.pdf. Accessed October 18, 2012. [IVA]

11. Hebl JR. The importance and implications of aseptic techniques during regional anesthesia. *Reg Anesth Pain Med*. 2006;31(4):311-323. [IVB]

12. Watanakunakorn C, Stahl C. Streptococcus salivarius meningitis following myelography. *Infect Control Hosp Epidemiol*. 1992;13(8):454. [VA]

13. Schlesinger JJ, Salit IE, McCormack G. Streptococcal meningitis after myelography. *Arch Neurol*. 1982;39(9):576-577. [VB]

14. Schlegel L, Merlet C, Laroche JM, Fremaux A, Geslin P. Iatrogenic meningitis due to Abiotrophia defectiva after myelography. *Clin Infect Dis*. 1999;28(1):155-156. doi:10.1086/517189. [VB]

15. Veringa E, van Belkum A, Schellekens H. Iatrogenic meningitis by *Streptococcus salivarius* following lumbar puncture. *J Hosp Infect*. 1995;29(4): 316-318. [VA]

16. Couzigou C, Vuong TK, Botherel AH, Aggoune M, Astagneau P. Iatrogenic *Streptococcus salivarius* meningitis after spinal anaesthesia: need for strict application of standard precautions. *J Hosp Infect*. 2003;53(4):313-314. [VA]

17. Torres E, Alba D, Frank A, Diez-Tejedor E. Iatrogenic meningitis due to Streptococcus salivarius following a spinal tap. *Clin Infect Dis*. 1993;17(3):525-526. [VB]

18. Schneeberger PM, Janssen M, Voss A. Alpha-hemolytic streptococci: a major pathogen of iatrogenic meningitis following lumbar puncture. Case reports and a review of the literature. *Infection*. 1996;24(1):29-33. [VB]

19. Yaniv LG, Potasman I. Iatrogenic meningitis: an increasing role for resistant viridans streptococci? Case report and review of the last 20 years. *Scand J Infect Dis*. 2000;32(6):693-696. [VB]

20. Centers for Disease Control and Prevention (CDC). Bacterial meningitis after intrapartum spinal anesthesia—New York and Ohio, 2008-2009. *MMWR*. 2010;59(3):65-69. [VA]

21. Philips BJ, Fergusson S, Armstrong P, Anderson FM, Wildsmith JA. Surgical face masks are effective in reducing bacterial contamination caused by dispersal from the upper airway. *Br J Anaesth*. 1992;69(4):407-408. [IIC]

22. McLure HA, Talboys CA, Yentis SM, Azadian BS. Surgical face masks and downward dispersal of bacteria. *Anaesthesia*. 1998;53(7):624-626. [IIB]

23. Alwitry A, Jackson E, Chen H, Holden R. The use of surgical facemasks during cataract surgery: is it necessary? *Br J Ophthalmol*. 2002;86(9):975-977. [IB]

24. Berger SA, Kramer M, Nagar H, Finkelstein A, Frimmerman A, Miller HI. Effect of surgical mask position on bacterial contamination of the operative field. *J Hosp Infect*. 1993;23(1):51-54. [IB]

25. Baer ET. Iatrogenic meningitis: the case for face masks. *Clin Infect Dis*. 2000;31(2):519-521. doi:10.1086/313991. [VB]

26. AAMI TI11: Selection and use of protective apparel and surgical drapes in health care facilities. Arlington, VA: Association for the Advancement of Medical Instrumentation; 2005. [IVC]

27. Guideline for product selection. In: *Guidelines for Perioperative Practice*. Denver, CO: AORN, Inc; 2015:179-186. [IVB]

28. Rutala WA, Weber DJ. A review of single-use and reusable gowns and drapes in health care. *Infect Control Hosp Epidemiol*. 2001;22(4):248-257. doi:10.1086/501895. [VA]

29. Position statement on environmental responsibility. AORN, Inc. http://www.aorn.org/WorkArea/DownloadAsset.aspx?id=21920. Accessed October 18, 2012. [IVB]

30. Occupational Safety and Health Standards, Toxic and Hazardous Substances: Bloodborne Pathogens, 29 CFR §1910.1030 (2012). Occupational Safety and Health Administration. http://www.osha.gov/pls/oshaweb/owadisp.show_document?p_table=STANDARDS&p_id=10051. Accessed October 18, 2012.

31. Medical Devices, General and Plastic Surgery Devices, 21 CFR §878 (2008).

32. AAMI PB70: Liquid barrier performance and classification of protective apparel and drapes intended for use in health care facilities. Arlington, VA: Association for the Advancement of Medical Instrumentation; 2012. [IVC]

33. Medical Device Reporting, 21 CFR §803 (2012).

34. MedWatch: the FDA safety information and adverse event reporting program. US Food and Drug Administration. http://www.fda.gov/Safety/MedWatch/default.htm. Accessed October 18, 2012.

35. Blom AW, Barnett A, Ajitsaria P, Noel A, Estela CM. Resistance of disposable drapes to bacterial penetration. *J Orthop Surg*. 2007;15(3):267-269. [IIIC]

36. Laufman H, Eudy WW, Vandernoot AM, Harris CA, Liu D. Strike-through of moist contamination by woven and nonwoven surgical materials. *Ann Surg*. 1975;181(6):857-862. [IIIC]

37. Edmiston CE Jr, Sinski S, Seabrook GR, Simons D, Goheen MP. Airborne particulates in the OR environment. *AORN J*. 1999;69(6):1169-72, 1175-7, 1179 passim. [IIB]

38. Surgical Apparel, 21 CFR §878.4040 (2000).

39. Surgical Drape and Drape Accessories, 21 CFR §878.4370.

40. Rego A, Roley L. In-use barrier integrity of gloves: latex and nitrile superior to vinyl. *Am J Infect Control.* 1999;27(5):405-410. [IB]

41. Korniewicz DM, Garzon L, Seltzer J, Feinleib M. Failure rates in nonlatex surgical gloves. *Am J Infect Control.* 2004;32(5):268-273. doi:10.1016/j.ajic.2003.12.005. [IIB]

42. Ritter MA, Eitzen HE, Hart JB, French ML. The surgeon's garb. *Clin Orthop Relat Res.* 1980;153:204-209. [IIB]

43. Heal JS, Blom AW, Titcomb D, Taylor A, Bowker K, Hardy JR. Bacterial contamination of surgical gloves by water droplets spilt after scrubbing. *J Hosp Infect.* 2003;53(2):136-139. [IIIC]

44. Bible JE, Biswas D, Whang PG, Simpson AK, Grauer JN. Which regions of the operating gown should be considered most sterile? *Clin Orthop Related Res.* 2009;467(3):825-830. [IIC]

45. Jones C, Brooker B, Genon M. Comparison of open and closed staff-assisted glove donning on the nature of surgical glove cuff contamination. *ANZ J Surg.* 2010;80(3):174-177. [IIIB]

46. Tanner J, Parkinson H. Double gloving to reduce surgical cross-infection. *Cochrane Database Syst Rev.* 2009;3:CD003087. doi:10.1002/14651858.CD003087.pub2. [IA]

47. Information statement: preventing the transmission of bloodborne pathogens. American Academy of Orthopedic Surgeons, American Association of Orthopaedic Surgeons. http://www.aaos.org/about/papers/advistmt/1018 .asp. Accessed October 18, 2012. [IVB]

48. ST-58: Statement on sharps safety. American College of Surgeons. http://www.facs.org/fellows_info/statements/ st-58.html. Accessed October 18, 2012. [IVB]

49. Kojima Y, Ohashi M. Unnoticed glove perforation during thoracoscopic and open thoracic surgery. *Ann Thorac Surg.* 2005;80(3):1078-1080. [IIB]

50. Singh VK, Hussain S, Javed S, Singh I, Mulla R, Kalairajah Y. Sterile surgical helmet system in elective total hip and knee arthroplasty. *J Orthop Surg (Hong Kong).* 2011;19(2):234-237. [IIIC]

51. Kearns KA, Witmer D, Makda J, Parvizi J, Jungkind D. Sterility of the personal protection system in total joint arthroplasty. *Clin Orthop Relat Res.* 2011;469(11):3065-3069. doi:10.1007/s11999-011-1883-1. [IIIC]

52. Bible JE, O'Neill KR, Crosby CG, Schoenecker JG, McGirt MJ, Devin CJ. Microscope sterility during spine surgery. *Spine (Phila Pa 1976).* 2012;37(7):623-267. doi:10.1097/BRS.0b013e3182286129. [IIB]

53. Thomas S, Padmanabhan TV. Methyl methacrylate permeability of dental and industrial gloves. *N Y State Dent J.* 2009;75(4):40-42. [IIIB]

54. Waegemaekers TH, Seutter E, den Arend JA, Malten KE. Permeability of surgeons' gloves to methyl methacrylate. *Acta Orthop Scand.* 1983;54(6):790-795. [IIIB]

55. Guideline for a safe environment of care, part 1. In: *Guidelines for Perioperative Practice.* Denver, CO: AORN, Inc; 2015:239-263. [IVA]

56. Hentz RV, Traina GC, Cadossi R, Zucchini P, Muglia MA, Giordani M. The protective efficacy of surgical latex gloves against the risk of skin contamination: how well are the operators protected? *J Mater Sci Mater Med.* 2000;11(12):825-832. [IIB]

57. Harnoss JC, Partecke LI, Heidecke CD, Hubner NO, Kramer A, Assadian O. Concentration of bacteria passing through puncture holes in surgical gloves. *Am J Infect Control.* 2010;38(2):154-158. [IIA]

58. Hubner NO, Goerdt AM, Stanislawski N, et al. Bacterial migration through punctured surgical gloves under real surgical conditions. *BMC Infectious Diseases.* 2010;10:192. [IIIB]

59. Partecke LI, Goerdt AM, Langner I, et al. Incidence of microperforation for surgical gloves depends on duration of wear. *Infect Control Hosp Epidemiol.* 2009;30(5):409-414. [IA]

60. Newman JB, Bullock M, Goyal R. Comparison of glove donning techniques for the likelihood of gown contamination. An infection control study. *Acta Orthop Belg.* 2007;73(6):765-771. [IIIC]

61. Raad II, Hohn DC, Gilbreath BJ, et al. Prevention of central venous catheter-related infections by using maximal sterile barrier precautions during insertion. *Infec Control Hosp Epidemiol.* 1994;15(4 Pt 1):231-238. [IA]

62. Pronovost P, Needham D, Berenholtz S, et al. An intervention to decrease catheter-related bloodstream infections in the ICU. *N Engl J Med.* 2006;355(26):2725-2732. doi:10.1056/NEJMoa061115. [IIIB]

63. McCue SF, Berg EW, Saunders EA. Efficacy of double-gloving as a barrier to microbial contamination during total joint arthroplasty. *J Bone Joint Surg Am* 1981;63(5):811-813. [IIB]

64. Biswas D, Bible JE, Whang PG, Simpson AK, Grauer JN. Sterility of C-arm fluoroscopy during spinal surgery. *Spine (Phila Pa 1976).* 2008;33(17):1913-1917 doi:10.1097/BRS.0b013e31817bb130. [IIB]

65. Webster J, Alghamdi A. Use of plastic adhesive drapes during surgery for preventing surgical site infection. *Cochrane Database Syst Rev.* 2011;1. [IA]

66. Parikh SN, Grice SS, Schnell BM, Salisbury SR. Operating room traffic: is there any role of monitoring it? *J Pediatr Orthop.* 2010;30(6):617-623. doi:10.1097/ BPO.0b013e3181e4f3be. [IIC]

67. Ritter MA, Eitzen H, French ML, Hart JB. The operating room environment as affected by people and the surgical face mask. *Clin Orthop Relat Res.* 1975;111:147-150 [IIIC]

68. Letts RM, Doermer E. Conversation in the operating theater as a cause of airborne bacterial contamination. *J Bone Joint Surg Am.* 1983;65(3):357-362. [IIB]

69. Ritter MA. Operating room environment. *Clin Orthop Relat Res.* 1999;369:103-109. [IIB]

70. Howard JL, Hanssen AD. Principles of a clean operating room environment. *J Arthroplasty.* 2007;22(7 Suppl 3):6-11. doi:10.1016/j.arth.2007.05.013. [VB]

71. Guideline for sterilization. In: *Guidelines for Perioperative Practice.* Denver, CO: AORN, Inc; 2015:665-692 [IVA]

72. Spaulding EH, Cundy KR, Turner FJ, SS Block Chemical disinfection of medical and surgical materials In: SS Block, ed. *Disinfection, Sterilization, and Preservation.* 2nd ed. Philadelphia, PA: Lea & Febiger; 1977:654-684. [VB]

73. Gengelkirk P, Duben-Engelkirk J. Microbial ecology and microbial technology. In: Gengelkirk P, Duben-Engelkirk J, eds. *Burton's Microbiology for the Health Sciences.* 9th ed. 2011:158-170.

74. Healthcare-associated infections (HAIs): Catheter-associated urinary tract infections (CAUTI). Centers for Disease Control and Prevention. http://www.cdc.gov/HAI/ ca_uti/uti.html. Accessed October 18, 2012. [IVA]

75. Ahmad A, Schirmir BD. Summary of intraoperative physiologic alterations associated with laparoscopic surgery. In: *The SAGES Manual of Perioperative Care in Minimally Invasive Surgery.* New York: Springer-Verlag 2006:56-62. [VA]

ASEPTIC PRACTICE

76. Strickland AK, Martindale RG. The increased incidence of intraabdominal infections in laparoscopic procedures: potential causes, postoperative management, and prospective innovations. *Surg Endosc.* 2005;19(7):874-881. doi:10.1007/s00464-004-8211-8. [VA]

77. Ozmen MM, Col C, Aksoy AM, Tekeli FA, Berberoglu M. Effect of CO(2) insufflation on bacteremia and bacterial translocation in an animal model of peritonitis. *Surg Endosc.* 1999;13(8):801-803. [IIB]

78. Hao WL, Lee YK. Microflora of the gastrointestinal tract: a review. *Methods Mol Biol.* 2004;268:491-502. doi:10.1385/1-59259-766-1:491. [VA]

79. Bures J, Cyrany J, Kohoutova D, et al. Small intestinal bacterial overgrowth syndrome. *World J Gastroenterol.* 2010;16(24):2978-2990. [VA]

80. Husebye E. The pathogenesis of gastrointestinal bacterial overgrowth. *Chemotherapy.* 2005;51(Suppl 1):1-22. doi:10.1159/000081988. [VA]

81. Porteous J, Gembey D, Dieter M. Bowel technique in the O.R. Is it really necessary? *Can Oper Room Nurs J.* 1996;14(1):11-14. [IIA]

82. Watanabe A, Kohnoe S, Shimabukuro R, et al. Risk factors associated with surgical site infection in upper and lower gastrointestinal surgery. *Surg Today.* 2008;38(5):404-412. [IIIB]

83. Zach J. A review of the literature on bowel technique. *ACORN.* 2004;17(4):14-19. [VB]

84. Bruen E. Clean/dirty scrub technique. Is it worth the effort? *Br J Perioper Nurs.* 2001;11(12):532-537. [VA]

85. Reason J. Safety in the operating theatre—Part 2: human error and organisational failure. *Qual Saf Health Care.* 2005;14(1):56-60. [VA]

86. Bekar A, Kahveci R, Tolunay S, Kahraman A, Kuytu T. Metastatic gliosarcoma mass extension to a donor fascia lata graft harvest site by tumor cell contamination. *World Neurosurg.* 2010;73(6):719-721. doi:10.1016/j.wneu.2010.03.015. [VA]

87. Zemmoura I, Ben Ismail M, Travers N, Jan M, Francois P. Maxillary surgical seeding of a clival chordoma. *Br J Neurosurg.* 2012;26(1):102-103. doi:10.3109/02688697.2011.595844. [VB]

88. McLemore MS, Bruner JM, Curry JL, Prieto VG, Torres-Cabala CA. Anaplastic oligodendroglioma involving the subcutaneous tissue of the scalp: report of an exceptional case and review of the literature. *Am J Dermatopathol.* 2012;34(2):214-219. doi:10.1097/DAD.0b013e318230655c. [VA]

89. *Guideline for Disinfection and Sterilization in Healthcare Facilities, 2008.* Atlanta, GA: Centers for Disease Control and Prevention; 2008. [IVA]

90. ANSI/AAMI ST79:2010 & A1:2010 & A2:2011 Consolidated Text). Arlington, VA: Association for the Advancement of Medical Instrumentation; 2011. [IVC]

91. Barker CS, Soro V, Dymock D, Fulford M, Sandy JR, Ireland AJ. Time-dependent recontamination rates of sterilised dental instruments. *Br Dent J.* 2011;211(8): E17. doi:10.1038/sj.bdj.2011.869; 10.1038/sj.bdj.2011.869. [IIB]

92. de Araújo Moriya GA, de Souza RQ, Gomes Pinto FM, Graziano KU. Periodic sterility assessment of materials stored for up to 6 months at continuous microbial contamination risk: laboratory study. *Am J Infect Control.* 2012;May 25. Epub ahead of print. doi:10.1016/j.ajic.2012.01.020. [IA]

93. Butt WE, Bradley DV Jr, Mayhew RB, Schwartz RS. Evaluation of the shelf life of sterile instrument packs. *Oral Surg Oral Med Oral Pathol.* 1991;72(6):650-654. [IA]

94. Webster J, Lloyd W, Ho P, Burridge C, George N. Rethinking sterilization practices: evidence for event-related outdating. *Infect Control Hosp Epidemiol.* 2003;24(8):622-624. doi:10.1086/502264. [IIB]

95. Guideline for medication safety. In: *Guidelines for Perioperative Practice.* Denver, CO: AORN, Inc; 2015:291-329. [IVB]

96. Dalstrom DJ, Venkatarayappa I, Manternach AL, Palcic MS, Heyse BA, Prayson MJ. Time-dependent contamination of opened sterile operating-room trays. *J Bone Joint Surg Am.* 2008;90(5):1022-1025. [IC]

97. Chosky SA, Modha D, Taylor GJ. Optimisation of ultraclean air. The role of instrument preparation. *J Bone Joint Surg Br.* 1996;78(5):835-837. [IB]

98. Hopper WR, Moss R. Common breaks in sterile technique: clinical perspectives and perioperative implications. *AORN J.* 2010;91(3):350-364. doi:10.1016/j.aorn.2009.09.027. [VB]

99. Guideline for reducing radiological exposure. In: *Guidelines for Perioperative Practice.* Denver, CO: AORN, Inc; 2015:335-344. [IVB]

100. Saito S, Kato W, Uchiyama M, Usui A, Ueda Y. Frequent stepping on and off the footstool contaminates the operative field. *Am J Infect Control.* 2007;35(1):68-69. doi:10.1016/j.ajic.2006.08.013. [IIIC]

101. Stocks GW, Self SD, Thompson B, Adame XA, O'Connor DP. Predicting bacterial populations based on airborne particulates: a study performed in nonlaminar flow operating rooms during joint arthroplasty surgery. *Am J Infect Control.* 2010;38(3):199-204. doi:10.1016/j.ajic.2009.07.006. [IIB]

102. Lynch RJ, Englesbe MJ, Sturm L, et al. Measurement of foot traffic in the operating room: implications for infection control. *Am J Med Qual.* 2009;24(1):45-52. doi:10.1177/1062860608326419. [IIIB]

103. Young RS, O'Regan DJ. Cardiac surgical theatre traffic: time for traffic calming measures? *Interac Cardiovasc Thorac Surg.* 2010;10(4):526-529. [IIIC]

104. Centers for Medicare & Medicaid Services. *State Operations Manual Appendix A—Survey Protocol, Regulations and Interpretive Guidelines for Hospitals.* Rev. 78; 2011.

105. Centers for Medicare & Medicaid Services. *State Operations Manual Appendix L: Guidance for Surveyors: Ambulatory Surgical Centers.* Rev. 76; 2011.

106. HR.01.05.03: Staff participate in ongoing education and training. In: *Comprehensive Accreditation Manual: CAMH for Hospitals.* Oakbrook Terrace, IL: The Joint Commission; 2012.

107. HR.01.05.03: Staff participate in ongoing education and training. In: *Comprehensive Accreditation Manual for Ambulatory Care.* Oakbrook Terrace, IL: Joint Commission; 2012.

108. Quality management and improvement. In: *2012 Accreditation Handbook for Ambulatory Health Care.* Skokie, IL: Accreditation Association for Ambulatory Health Care; 2012:34-39.

109. Personnel: personnel records. In: *Procedural Standards and Checklist for Accreditation of Ambulatory Surgery Facilities.* Version 3. Gurnee, IL: American Association for Accreditation of Ambulatory Surgery Facilities; 2011:77-79.

110. Personnel: personnel records; resumes. In: *Regular Standards and Checklist for Accreditation of Ambulatory Surgery Facilities.* Version 13. Gurnee, IL: American Association for Accreditation of Ambulatory Surgery Facilities; 2011:77-78.

111. Personnel: knowledge, skill & CME training. In: *Procedural Standards and Checklist for Accreditation of Ambulatory Surgery Facilities.* Version 3. Gurnee, IL:

American Association for Accreditation of Ambulatory Surgery Facilities; 2011:79.

112. Personnel: personnel safety. In: *Procedural Standards and Checklist for Accreditation of Ambulatory Surgery Facilities*. Version 3. Gurnee, IL: American Association for Accreditation of Ambulatory Surgery Facilities; 2011:79-80.

113. Personnel: knowledge, skill & CME training. In: *Regular Standards and Checklist for Accreditation of Ambulatory Surgery Facilities*. Version 13. Gurnee, IL: American Association for Accreditation of Ambulatory Surgery Facilities; 2011:78-79.

114. Personnel: personnel safety. In: *Regular Standards and Checklist for Accreditation of Ambulatory Surgery Facilities*. Version 13. Gurnee, IL: American Association for Accreditation of Ambulatory Surgery Facilities; 2011:80.

115. Guideline for perioperative health care information management. In: *Guidelines for Perioperative Practice*. Denver, CO: AORN, Inc; 2015:491-512. [IVB]

116. Gillespie BM, Hamlin L. A synthesis of the literature on "competence" as it applies to perioperative nursing. *AORN J*. 2009;90(2):245-258. doi:10.1016/j.aorn.2009.07.011. [VA]

117. Gillespie BM, Chaboyer W, Wallis M, Chang HY, Werder H. Operating theatre nurses' perceptions of competence: a focus group study. *J Adv Nurs*. 2009;65(5):1019-1028. [IIIB]

118. Mitchell L, Flin R. Non-technical skills of the operating theatre scrub nurse: literature review. *J Adv Nurs*. 2008;63(1):15-24. doi:10.1111/j.1365-2648.2008.04695.x. [VB]

119. Jordan C, Thomas MB, Evans ML, Green A. Public policy on competency: how will nursing address this complex issue? *J Contin Educ Nurs*. 2008;39(2):86-91. [VA]

120. RC.01.01.01: The hospital maintains complete and accurate medical records for each individual patient. In: *Hospital Accreditation Standards 2012*. Oakbrook Terrace, IL: Joint Commission on Resources; 2012.

121. RC.01.01.01: The organization maintains complete and accurate clinical records. In: *Standards for Ambulatory Care 2012 : Standards, Elements of Performance Scoring Accreditation Polices*. Oakbrook Terrace, IL: The Joint Commission; 2012.

122. Clinical records and health information. In: *2012 Accreditation Handbook for Ambulatory Health Care*. Skokie, IL: Accreditation Association for Ambulatory Health Care; 2012:40-42.

123. Medical records: procedure room records. In: *Procedural Standards and Checklist for Accreditation of Ambulatory Surgery Facilities*. Version 3. Gurnee, IL: American Association for Accreditation of Ambulatory Surgery Facilities; 2011:64-66.

124. Medical records: operating room records. In: *Regular Standards and Checklist for Accreditation of Ambulatory Surgery Facilities*. Version 13. Gurnee, IL: American Association for Accreditation of Ambulatory Surgery Facilities; 2011:64-66.

125. Medical records: general. In: *Procedural Standards and Checklist for Accreditation of Ambulatory Surgery Facilities*. Version 3. Gurnee, IL: American Association for Accreditation of Ambulatory Surgery Facilities; 2011:60-61.

126. Medical records: general. In: *Regular Standards and Checklist for Accreditation of Ambulatory Surgery Facilities*. Version 13. Gurnee, IL: American Association for Accreditation of Ambulatory Surgery Facilities; 2011:61.

127. Medical records: pre-operative medical record. In: *Regular Standards and Checklist for Accreditation of Ambulatory Surgery Facilities*. Version 13. Gurnee, IL: American Association for Accreditation of Ambulatory Surgery Facilities; 2011:62-63.

128. LD.04.01.07: The hospital has policies and procedures that guide and support patient care, treatment, and services. In: *Hospital Accreditation Standards 2012*. Oakbrook Terrace, IL: Joint Commission on Resources; 2012.

129. LD.04.01.07: The organization has policies and procedures that guide and support patient care, treatment or services. In: *Standards for Ambulatory Care 2012 Standards, Elements of Performance Scoring Accreditation Polices*. Oakbrook Terrace, IL: The Joint Commission 2012.

130. Governance. In: *2012 Accreditation Handbook for Ambulatory Health Care*. Skokie, IL: Accreditation Association for Ambulatory Health Care; 2012:20-27.

131. PI.03.01.01: The hospital improves performance on an ongoing basis. In: *Hospital Accreditation Standards 2012*. Oakbrook Terrace, IL: The Joint Commission; 2012.

132. PI.03.01.01: The organization improves performance. In: *Standards for Ambulatory Care 2012: Standards, Elements of Performance Scoring Accreditation Polices*. Oakbrook Terrace, IL: The Joint Commission 2012.

133. Quality improvement/quality assessment: quality improvement. In: *Procedural Standards and Checklist for Accreditation of Ambulatory Surgery Facilities*. Version 3. Gurnee, IL: American Association for Accreditation of Ambulatory Surgery Facilities; 2011:67.

134. Quality assessment/quality improvement: quality improvement. In: *Regular Standards and Checklist for Accreditation of Ambulatory Surgery Facilities*. Version 13. Gurnee, IL: American Association for Accreditation of Ambulatory Surgery Facilities; 2011:67.

135. Quality assessment/quality improvement: unanticipated operative sequelae. In: *Regular Standards and Checklist for Accreditation of Ambulatory Surgery Facilities*. Version 13. Gurnee, IL: American Association for Accreditation of Ambulatory Surgery Facilities 2011:69-71.

Acknowledgments

LEAD AUTHOR
Sharon A. Van Wicklin, MSN, RN, CNOR, CRNFA CPSN, PLNC
Perioperative Nursing Specialist
AORN Nursing Department
Denver, Colorado

CONTRIBUTING AUTHOR
Ramona Conner, MSN, RN, CNOR
Manager, Standards and Guidelines
AORN Nursing Department
Denver, Colorado

The authors and AORN thank Paula J. Morton, MS RN, CNOR, Director Perioperative Services, Sherman Health, Elgin, Illinois; Catherine M. Moses, RN CNOR, CPHQ, QM Coordinator, Medical Arts Surgical Centers/BHSF, Miami, Florida; Christine Anderson PhD, RN, Clinical Assistant Professor, University of Michigan School of Nursing, Ypsilanti, Michigan and Annette Wasielewski, BSN, RN, CNOR, Senior

Consultant, Lodi, New Jersey, and Bariatric Coordinator, Hudson Valley Hospital Center, Cortlandt Manor, New York, for their assistance in developing this guideline.

PUBLICATION HISTORY

Originally published March 1978, *AORN Journal*, as "Recommended practices for aseptic technique." Format revision July 1982. Revised March 1987, October 1991.

Revised June 1996; published November 1996, *AORN Journal*.

Revised and reformatted; published February 2001, *AORN Journal*.

Revised November 2005; published as "Recommended practices for maintaining a sterile field" in *Standards, Recommended Practices, and Guidelines*, 2006 edition. Reprinted February 2006, *AORN Journal*.

Revised and reformatted December 2012 for online publication as "Recommended practices for sterile technique" in *Perioperative Standards and Recommended Practices*.

Evidence ratings revised 2013 to conform to the AORN Evidence Rating Model.

Minor editing revisions made in November 2014 for publication in *Guidelines for Perioperative Practice*, 2015 edition.

Evidence ratings revised in *Guidelines for Perioperative Practice*, 2018 edition, to conform to the current AORN Evidence Rating Model.

GUIDELINE FOR SURGICAL ATTIRE

T he Guideline for Surgical Attire has been approved by the AORN Guidelines Advisory Board. It was presented as a proposed guideline for comments by members and others. The guideline is effective November 15, 2014. The recommendations in the guideline are intended to be achievable and represent what is believed to be an optimal level of practice. Policies and procedures will reflect variations in practice settings and/or clinical situations that determine the degree to which the guideline can be implemented. AORN recognizes the many diverse settings in which perioperative nurses practice; therefore, this guideline is adaptable to all areas where operative and other invasive procedures may be performed.

Purpose

This document provides guidance for surgical attire including scrub attire, shoes, jewelry, head coverings, and masks worn in the semi-restricted and restricted areas of the perioperative practice setting. This document also provides guidance for personal items such as stethoscopes, backpacks, briefcases, cell phones, and tablets.

The human body and inanimate surfaces inherent in the surgical environment are major sources of microbial contamination and transmission.[1] Surgical attire and personal protective equipment (PPE) are worn to provide a high level of cleanliness and hygiene within the perioperative environment and to promote patient and worker safety. Reducing the patient's exposure to microorganisms that are shed from the skin and hair of perioperative personnel may reduce the patient's risk for surgical site infection (SSI). Patient safety is the primary consideration for perioperative personnel.

This document does not address patient clothing or linens used in health care facilities. A complete discussion of the use of PPE and sterile attire worn at the surgical field is outside the scope of this document. The reader should refer to the AORN Guideline for Sterile Technique,[2] Guideline for Prevention of Transmissible Infections,[3] and Guideline for Sharps Safety[4] for additional information. The use of nail polish, artificial nails, or other nail enhancements and the recommended fingernail length for perioperative personnel is outside the scope of this document. The reader should refer to the AORN Guideline for Hand Hygiene[5] for additional information. Ensuring and monitoring personnel compliance with policies and procedures for surgical attire and personal hygiene is a responsibility of the facility or health care organization administrators.

Evidence Review

On June 25 and June 27, 2013, a medical librarian conducted a systematic search of the databases MEDLINE® and CINAHL® and the Cochrane Database of Systematic Reviews for meta-analyses, systematic reviews, randomized controlled and non-randomized trials and studies, case reports, letters, reviews, and guidelines. The librarian also searched the Scopus database, although not systematically. The search was limited to literature published in English from January 2008 through June 2013.

Search terms included *surgical attire, clothing, personal protective equipment, protective gloves, respiratory protective devices, masks, eye protection, goggles, scrubs, surgical gown, jumpsuit, head covering, surgical cap, hoods, coveralls, bunny suit, textiles, bedding and linens, privacy curtain, hospital laundry service, laundering, laundry, washing machine, tie, backpack, fanny pack, fleece, briefcase, purse, stethoscope, lanyard, badge, patient attire, patient clothing, colonization, fomites, tattooing, body piercing, jewelry, ring, wedding band, fingernails, eyelashes, facial hair, beard, groin, armpit, scalp, skin, squames, dandruff, epithelial cells, seborrheic dermatitis, computers, mobile communication device, mobile phone, cell phone, cellular phone, tablet computer, smartphone, iPad, iPhone, text messaging, pollen, dust, fungi, mold, equipment contamination, nosocomial, cross infection, infectious disease transmission, surgical wound infection, bacterial load,* and *infection control.*

At the time of the search, the librarian established weekly alerts on the search topics and until March 2014, presented relevant results to the lead author.

Prior to the search, the medical librarian provided to the lead author the results of literature searches conducted for the 2010 edition of the AORN Recommended Practices for Surgical Attire. These articles had no time restriction. During the development of this edition, the authors also requested supplementary literature searches and additional literature that either did not fit the original search criteria or was discovered during the evidence-appraisal process. The time restriction was not considered in these subsequent searches. Relevant guidelines from government agencies and standards-setting bodies also were identified.

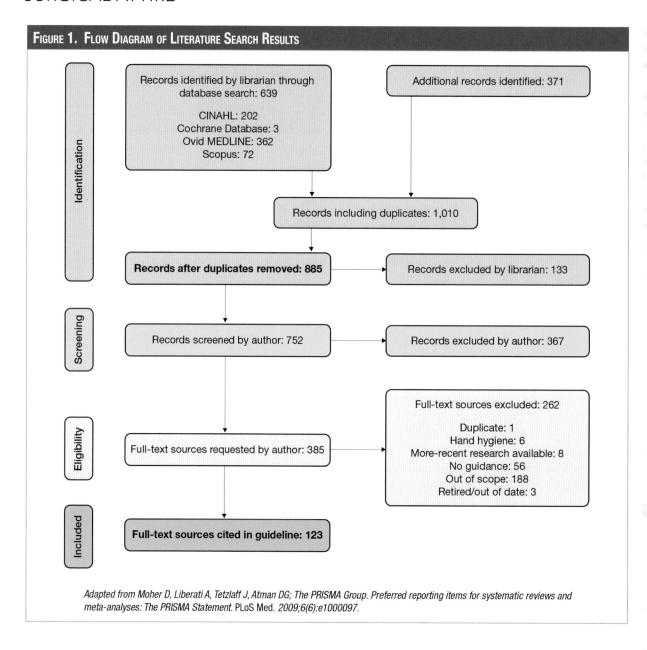

FIGURE 1. FLOW DIAGRAM OF LITERATURE SEARCH RESULTS

Identification

Records identified by librarian through database search: 639

CINAHL: 202
Cochrane Database: 3
Ovid MEDLINE: 362
Scopus: 72

Additional records identified: 371

Records including duplicates: 1,010

Records after duplicates removed: 885

Records excluded by librarian: 133

Screening

Records screened by author: 752

Records excluded by author: 367

Eligibility

Full-text sources requested by author: 385

Full-text sources excluded: 262

Duplicate: 1
Hand hygiene: 6
More-recent research available: 8
No guidance: 56
Out of scope: 188
Retired/out of date: 3

Included

Full-text sources cited in guideline: 123

Adapted from Moher D, Liberati A, Tetzlaff J, Atman DG; The PRISMA Group. Preferred reporting items for systematic reviews and meta-analyses: The PRISMA Statement. PLoS Med. 2009;6(6):e1000097.

Inclusion criteria were research and non-research literature in English, complete publications, relevance to the key questions, and publication dates within the time restriction unless none were available. Excluded were non-peer-reviewed publications; literature that examined the use of sterile gowns, drapes, and masks worn for maintaining sterile technique; low-quality evidence when higher quality evidence was available; and literature outside the time restriction when literature within the time restriction was available. In total, 885 research and non-research sources of evidence were identified for possible inclusion, and of these, 123 were cited in the guidance document (Figure 1).

Articles identified by the search were provided to the project team. The team consisted of the lead author, a co-author, five members of the Guidelines Advisory Board, and two evidence appraisers. The lead author and the evidence appraisers reviewed and

critically appraised each article using the AORN Research or Non-Research Evidence Appraisal Tools as appropriate. The literature was independently evaluated and appraised according to the strength and quality of the evidence. Each article was then assigned an appraisal score. The appraisal score is noted in brackets after each reference, as applicable.

Notably, much of the evidence related to surgical attire is not recent evidence. There are no randomized controlled trials (RCTs) or systematic reviews that show a direct causal relationship between surgical attire and SSI. There are many confounding variables that affect a patient's risk for SSI, and this makes it extraordinarily difficult to identify surgical attire as a singular source of SSIs. It is a well-accepted scientific principle that increased numbers of microorganisms in the perioperative environment will increase the patient's risk for SSI. It is unnecessary, and it may be unethical, for researchers to perform new studies for the sole purpose of demonstrating this recognized concept.

The methodology of the research and non-research evidence used to support this document was critically evaluated by the authors for validity and generalizability to current practice. The collective evidence supporting each intervention within a specific recommendation was summarized by the authors, and the AORN Evidence Rating Model was used to rate the strength of the evidence. Factors considered in the review of the collective evidence were the quality of evidence, the quantity of similar evidence on a given topic, and the consistency of evidence supporting a recommendation. The evidence rating is noted in brackets after each intervention.

Note: *The evidence summary table is available at http://www.aorn.org/evidencetables/.*

Editor's note: *MEDLINE is a registered trademark of the US National Library of Medicine's Medical Literature Analysis and Retrieval System, Bethesda, MD. CINAHL, Cumulative Index to Nursing and Allied Health Literature, is a registered trademark of EBSCO Industries, Birmingham, AL. Scopus is a registered trademark of Elsevier B.V., Amsterdam, The Netherlands. iPad and iPhone and registered trademarks of Apple, Inc, Cupertino, CA.*

Recommendation I

Clean surgical attire should be worn in the semi-restricted and restricted areas of the perioperative setting.

The collective body of evidence supports wearing clean surgical attire in the perioperative setting to reduce the number of microorganisms in the environment and the patient's risk for developing an SSI (Figure 2). Clean scrub attire has been laundered in a health care-accredited laundry facility and has not been previously worn.

The limitations of the evidence are that some research studies were underpowered, did not look at SSIs as an outcome, or did not control for factors contributing to SSIs (eg, antibiotic use, glucose levels). There was no clear definition of "tightly woven fabric."

The benefit of wearing clean surgical attire may include a reduction of microorganisms in the perioperative environment that may in turn lower the patient's risk for developing an SSI and reduce the potential for health care workers to transport microorganisms from the facility or health care organization into the home or community.

I.a. Fabrics used for scrub attire should be tightly woven, low linting, stain resistant, and durable. *[4: Limited Evidence]*

One quasi-experimental[6] and four nonexperimental[7-10] studies compared airborne bacterial

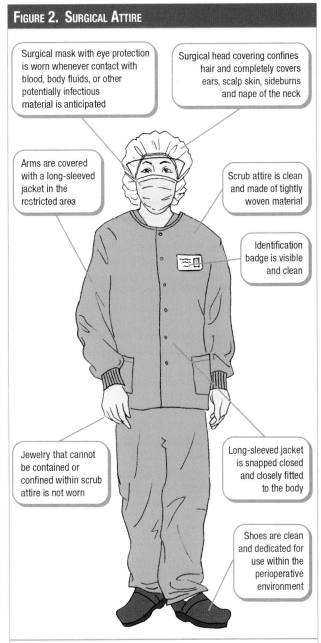

FIGURE 2. SURGICAL ATTIRE

Surgical mask with eye protection is worn whenever contact with blood, body fluids, or other potentially infectious material is anticipated

Surgical head covering confines hair and completely covers ears, scalp skin, sideburns and nape of the neck

Arms are covered with a long-sleeved jacket in the restricted area

Scrub attire is clean and made of tightly woven material

Identification badge is visible and clean

Jewelry that cannot be contained or confined within scrub attire is not worn

Long-sleeved jacket is snapped closed and closely fitted to the body

Shoes are clean and dedicated for use within the perioperative environment

Surgical attire and personal protective equipment are worn to provide a high level of cleanliness and hygiene within the perioperative environment, and to promote patient and worker safety.

Illustration by Kurt Jones.

contamination levels when perioperative team members wore various types of scrub attire. The results of four of the studies indicated that tightly woven scrub attire was superior to other types of scrub attire in decreasing bacterial contamination of the air.[6-9] One study concluded that use of disposable scrub attire was better for achieving improved OR air quality.[10] Tammelin et al[6,8] defined conventional scrub attire as 50% cotton/50% polyester woven with 270 x 230 threads/10 cm and tightly woven scrub attire as 50% cotton/50% polyester woven with 560 x 395 threads/10 cm.

In a nonexperimental study conducted in a day surgery clinic at a university hospital after eight incidents of postoperative endophthalmitis, Andersen and Solheim[7] found there was a significant reduction of more than 50% of the bacterial load in the air when team members (N = 12) wore tightly woven polypropylene scrub attire (100% spunbond polypropylene [50 g/m³]) than when they wore traditional cotton scrub attire. No additional cases of endophthalmitis occurred when team members wore the tightly woven scrub attire. The researchers did not define thread counts for the traditional cotton scrub attire or the tightly woven polypropylene scrub attire.

Tammelin and colleagues conducted four studies of surgical scrub attire.[6,8-10] In the first, quasi-experimental study, conducted in a university hospital in 2000, Tammelin et al[6] examined methicillin-resistant *Staphylococcus epidermidis* (MRSE) shedding into the air to determine whether the amount of shedding could be reduced if team members wore tightly woven scrub attire. The scrubbed and non-scrubbed personnel (N = 40) participated in 33 surgical procedures while dressed in conventional scrub attire (ie, 50% cotton/50% polyester woven with 270 x 230 threads/10 cm) and in 32 surgical procedures while dressed in tightly woven scrub attire (ie, 50% cotton/50% polyester woven with 560 x 395 threads/10 cm). The researchers found that 25% of women and 43% of men dispersed MRSE that was shed into the air in the OR. The median number of colony-forming units (CFUs) dropped significantly from 14.5/m3 to 7.7/m³ when perioperative team members wore the tightly woven scrub attire. The researchers recommended wearing tightly woven scrub attire to decrease the risk of airborne bacterial transmission from shed skin squames.

In a second, nonexperimental study, conducted in a university hospital in 2001, Tammelin et al[8] examined whether team members wearing conventional scrub attire (ie, 50% cotton/50% polyester blend, 270 x 230 threads/10 cm) with shirts untucked (n = 33) or wearing scrub attire with a tighter weave (ie, 50% cotton/50% polyester blend, 560 x 365 threads/10 cm) with shirts tucked (n = 32) could reduce surgical wound contamination in patients undergoing cardiothoracic surgery. The investigators specifically investigated MRSE strains. They found that wearing the tightly woven scrub attire did not reduce the amount of MRSE in air samples compared with wearing conventional scrub attire.

In a third, nonexperimental study, conducted in 2012 in a hospital in which more than 6,000 orthopedic procedures were performed per year, Tammelin et al[9] compared levels of airborne bacterial contamination when 21 team members wore scrub attire made of one of three different types of fabric during orthopedic procedures in four operating rooms (ORs). The three fabrics were

- mixed material (69% cotton/30% polyester/1% carbon fiber, weight 150 g/m²),
- polyester material (99% polyester/1% carbon fiber, weight 100 g/m²), and
- polyester material (99% polyester/1% carbon fiber, weight 120 g/m²).

All team members wore scrub attire made from the same material during each procedure. The mean value of CFUs emitted by each team member was calculated for each of the three garments worn. The researchers found that wearing scrub attire made of either type of polyester material significantly reduced the number of CFUs/m³ emitted compared with wearing scrub attire made from mixed material. The results of this study indicated that airborne bacteria from the emitted skin flora of perioperative team members may reach the surgical site. The researchers emphasized the importance of having perioperative team members wear scrub attire that contains skin squames. The researchers recommended that additional studies be conducted to determine the protective efficacy of these materials.[9]

Tammelin et al[10] conducted a nonexperimental study in a 100-bed acute care hospital in 2013 that compared two types of scrub attire for bacterial dispersal levels:

- reusable scrub attire made of 69% cotton/30% polyester/1% carbon fiber, weight 150 g, washed 50 times (n = 32) and
- single-use scrub attire made of nonwoven, spun-bonded polypropylene, weight 35 g (n = 29).

Dispersal tests were conducted with team members wearing both types of scrub attire in a closed chamber and in an OR during 10 surgical procedures. Air sampling was conducted and CFUs were measured in both settings. The researchers found the number of CFUs was significantly lower when team members wore the single-use scrub attire compared with the reusable scrub attire in both the dispersal chamber and the OR. The researchers concluded that there can be a difference in protective capacity between different types of scrub attire.[10]

In a nonexperimental study, Noble et al[1] examined skin dispersal rates among men and women. The researchers found that the men had higher populations of skin organisms than the women. The researchers concluded that scrub attire made of tightly woven fabric is necessary to contain shed skin squames so they cannot pass through the pores of the fabric.

Lidwell et al[11] conducted a quasi-experimental study to determine the number of bacteria-carrying particles in the air during prosthetic joint surgery procedures in 15 hospitals. The researchers found coagulase-negative *Staphylococcus* in

51% of the air samples and *Staphylococcus aureus* in 39% of the air samples. Pulse-field gel electrophoresis showed the *S aureus* was identical to that carried by the study participants. There was a strong correlation between sepsis rates and the degree of bacterial air contamination. The researchers recommended limiting the number of persons present in the OR, avoiding unnecessary activity, and wearing closely woven fabrics with barrier qualities.

Wearing scrub attire that is lint-free may help prevent lint particles from being disseminated into the environment where bacteria may attach to them and settle in surgical sites and wounds and increase the potential for postoperative patient complications.[12] Scrub attire that is stain-resistant and durable promotes a professional appearance and is better able to withstand the rigorous laundering process necessary to maintain a high level of cleanliness.

I.a.1. Scrub attire may be made of antimicrobial fabric. *[3: Moderate Evidence]*

There is emerging evidence on the use of fabrics with antimicrobials incorporated into yarns during processing or during finishing to prevent bacteria and fungi from adhering to the fabric. Incorporating this technology into the material used for scrub attire and other garments worn by health care personnel may help to protect the patient from the risk of SSIs.[13-19] This issue warrants further research.

In a quasi-experimental study to examine whether antibacterial finishes on fabric could effectively reduce the presence of bacteria on fabric used for health care worker's uniforms, Chen et al[18] found that the antibacterial finishes provided a significant reduction of *Staphylococcus aureus* and *Klebsiella pneumoniae*. The researchers concluded that adding antibacterial finishes to fabric was an effective method of reducing bacterial contamination.

Mariscal et al[17] conducted a quasi-experimental study to evaluate the action of a commercially available antimicrobial textile (80% polyester/20% cotton containing silver [180 parts per million]) on 33 strains of bacteria. They found that the antimicrobial fabric significantly reduced the numbers of four reference microorganisms (ie, *Escherichia coli, Pseudomonas aeruginosa, Morganella morgannii, Staphylococcus aureus*) compared with the numbers of reference microorganisms on the control fabric (80% polyester/20% cotton without silver).

Bearman et al[19] conducted an RCT to determine the effectiveness of antimicrobial fabric for reducing the bacterial burden on the hands of and scrub attire worn by health care workers in an intensive care unit (ICU) setting of an academic medical center. All study participants (N = 30) were randomly assigned to wear either traditional scrub attire or scrub attire made of antimicrobial fabric during a clinical shift during a four-week period. Each health care worker underwent unannounced weekly garment and hand cultures. Cultures taken at the beginning and end of the shifts included garment cultures taken from the abdominal and leg pockets of the scrub attire. The researchers did not specify the length of the clinical shifts.

The researchers found a significant difference (ie, a 4 to 7 mean log reduction) in the number of methicillin-resistant *Staphylococcus aureus* (MRSA) CFUs in both the leg and abdominal area of antimicrobial scrub attire and traditional scrub attire at the beginning and end of shifts. However, the researchers found no differences in the number of CFUs of vancomycin-resistant *Enterococcus* or gram-negative rods, and no difference was observed in the number or percentage of health care workers with positive hand cultures wearing either type of scrub attire.[19]

In a quasi-experimental study to evaluate the bactericidal effects of woven and nonwoven fabrics coated with a hydroxyapatite-binding silver/titanium dioxide ceramic composite, Kasuga et al[16] found that bacterial cell counts of *Staphylococcus aureus* and *Escherichia coli* on both the woven and nonwoven fabrics decreased to below 2-log_{10} CFU/mL within six hours and were undetectable at the end of the 18 hour incubation period. Bacterial cell counts of *Pseudomonas aeruginosa* could not be detected after three to six hours. The researchers found that bacterial counts on the coated woven fabric decreased more rapidly than counts on the coated nonwoven fabric. The bacterial counts on the uncoated woven and nonwoven fabric did not decrease during the 18-hour incubation period.

Sun et al[14] quantitatively and qualitatively evaluated 100% cotton and 35% cotton/65% polyester fabrics treated with antimicrobial chemicals in a nonexperimental study. The researchers found that even after 50 washings, the treated fabrics exhibited antibacterial properties against gram-negative (ie, *Escherichia coli*) and gram-positive (ie, *Staphylococcus aureus*) bacteria and fungi (ie, *Candida albicans*) within a two-minute contact time. Despite the biocidal properties of the antimicrobial fabric, the researchers found it was nontoxic to human skin. They concluded that antimicrobial fabrics were effective and suitable for medical use.

I.b. Personnel should don clean scrub attire daily. *[2: High Evidence]*

The primary source of bacteria dispersed into the air in the OR or procedure room comes from health care providers' skin.[20] Noble[20] reported that humans disseminate more than 10^7 skin particles every day. Approximately 10% of disseminated skin squames carry viable microorganisms that can pose a potential threat of SSI to perioperative patients.[20] Benediksdottir and Hambraeus[21] found that the highest density of bacteria was on the face and upper trunk of the health care worker and the highest yield of dispersed bacteria came from the lower trunk.

Weiner-Well et al[22] investigated the rate of potentially pathogenic organisms on 135 physicians' (n = 60) and nurses' (n = 75) uniforms in a nonexperimental study. The physicians and nurses reported that they changed attire daily, and 77% (n = 104) described their level of personal hygiene as fair to excellent. Sixty-three percent of the attire showed pathogenic organisms on at least one area (n = 85), and 20% (n = 17) of those were antibiotic-resistant organisms. The researchers did not determine whether these bacteria could be transmitted to patients and contribute to health care-associated infections (HAIs).

In an observational study conducted to determine the presence of bacteria in 10 locations on 30 sets of scrub attire worn by three orthopedic residents, Krueger et al[23] found that 41% of scrub attire had at least one bacterial species on it at the beginning of the work day; however, 89% of scrub attire had bacterial species on it at the end of the work day. The researchers did not specify the length of the residents' work day. Most of the organisms found were common skin flora and not multidrug-resistant microorganisms (MDROs). The researchers concluded that personnel should change into clean scrub attire before performing or assisting with surgical procedures, and they noted the need for further research to investigate how contaminated scrub attire contributes to SSIs.

I.b.1. Scrub attire should be donned in a designated dressing area before entry from the outdoors into the semi-restricted and restricted areas. *[5: Benefits Balanced with Harms]*

Changing from street apparel into clean or disposable scrub attire in a designated area assists in maintaining a clean environment and decreases the possibility of transferring microorganisms from street apparel to patients.

I.b.2. When donning scrub attire, perioperative team members should avoid contact of the clean attire with the floor or other potentially contaminated surfaces. *[5: Benefits Balanced with Harms]*

Scrub attire that contacts the floor could become a vehicle for transferring microorganisms from the floor to perioperative patients or surfaces.

I.b.3. When a two-piece scrub suit is worn, the top of the scrub suit should be secured at the waist or tucked into the pants or should fit close to the body. *[3: Moderate Evidence]*

Loose scrub tops may allow skin squames from the axilla and chest to disperse into the environment. A literature review by Ibrahimi et al[24] examined routes of bacterial transfer during surgery and found that one route that could potentially contribute to contamination of the air in the OR was skin cells dispersed through the openings of clothing by the bellows action of clothing that occurs with movement.

I.b.4. Scrub dresses may be worn over scrub pants or leggings that are laundered in a health care-accredited laundry facility after each daily use and when contaminated. *[5: Benefits Balanced with Harms]*

I.b.5. Personal clothing that cannot be contained within the scrub attire either should not be worn or should be laundered in a health care-accredited laundry facility after each daily use and when contaminated. *[5: Benefits Balanced with Harms]*

I.c. When in the restricted areas, all nonscrubbed personnel should completely cover their arms with a long-sleeved scrub top or jacket. *[3: Moderate Evidence]*

The collective body of evidence supports perioperative team members covering their arms to help contain skin squames.

Several studies have shown that human skin squames and bacteria are dispersed into the air.[1,11,21,25] A literature review by Noble[20] found 11 studies demonstrating that the skin is a source of multiple organisms and more than 10 million particles are shed from skin every day. The act of walking releases 1,000 skin scales per minute.[20]

In a nonexperimental study, May et al[25] examined dispersal of skin organisms. The results of this study demonstrated that skin squames were shed at varying rates from the test participants.

Benediktsdottir and Hambraeus[21] examined air dispersal of bacteria in a quasi-experimental study and determined that any organism present on the skin can be dispersed into the air. The dominant anaerobic bacteria dispersed were *Propionibacterium acnes*; however, *Propionibacterium avidum*, *Propionibacterium granulosum*, and gram-positive cocci also were isolated from the dispersal samples. The researchers did not determine the effect, if any, that the dispersed organisms had on the infection rates of patients.

Tammelin et al[6] conducted a quasi-experimental study to examine the dispersal of MRSE by personnel in a cardiothoracic operating suite. They found that dispersal of MRSE occurred in 25% of women and 43% of men. The researchers concluded that MRSE was a possible source of airborne contamination, and personnel should be covered by tightly woven scrub attire to help prevent dispersal of the organisms into the air.

Tammelin et al[9] conducted a nonexperimental study confirming that airborne bacteria from the skin flora of perioperative team members can reach the surgical site. The researchers emphasized the importance of surgical team members wearing scrub attire that contains skin squames.

In a literature review, Ibrahimi et al[24] found that the bacterial transfer of organisms during surgery included respiratory droplets, skin scales carried on air currents, direct contact with the perioperative team member's skin, and contaminated fomites (eg, clothing, identification badges, pens). The authors concluded that actions to decrease the bacterial load at the surgical site were prudent to reduce the risk of SSI. These actions included reducing the patient's exposure to the perioperative team member's skin.

I.c.1. The perioperative team member should wear scrub attire that covers the arms while performing preoperative patient skin antisepsis.[26] *[3: Moderate Evidence]*

Wearing long-sleeved attire helps contain skin squames shed from bare arms.[7] Performing the preoperative skin antisepsis without wearing a long-sleeved jacket may allow skin squames from the perioperative team member's bare arms to drop onto the area that is being prepped and may increase the patient's risk for an SSI.

For more information on preoperative patient skin antisepsis, the reader should refer to the AORN Guideline for Preoperative Patient Skin Antisepsis.[26]

I.c.2. The perioperative or sterile processing team member should wear scrub attire that covers the arms while preparing and packaging items in the clean assembly section of the sterile processing area. *[3: Moderate Evidence]*

Wearing long-sleeved attire helps contain skin squames shed from bare arms.[7] Not wearing a long-sleeved jacket while preparing and packaging items that will be used during operative or other invasive procedures may allow skin squames from the bare arm to drop onto the item that is being prepared or packaged and may increase the patient's risk for SSI. This organic material may be transferred to the surgical wound or

other areas of the body and may increase the patients risk of SSI or other postoperative complications.[2]

I.c.3. Long-sleeved jackets and scrub attire tops should fit closely to the arms and torso to prevent the jacket or top from potentially contaminating the surgical site during preoperative patient skin antisepsis or other activities (eg, application of surgical dressings). *[5: Benefits Balanced with Harms]*

I.c.4. When a long-sleeved jacket is worn, it should be snapped closed or buttoned up the front. *[5: Benefits Balanced with Harms]*

Wearing the jacket snapped or buttoned closed helps prevent the edges of the front of the jacket from contaminating sterile areas.

I.d. Persons entering the semi-restricted or restricted areas of the surgical suite for a brief time (eg, law enforcement officers, parents, biomedical engineers) should don either clean scrub attire; single-use scrub attire; or a single-use jumpsuit (eg, coveralls, bunny suit) designed to completely cover personal apparel. *[5: Benefits Balanced with Harms]*

Donning clean scrub attire, single-use scrub attire, or single-use jumpsuits before entry into the semi-restricted and restricted areas may help to maintain a clean environment and decrease the possibility of transferring microorganisms from external areas and personal attire to perioperative surfaces and patients.

I.e. Health care personnel should change into street clothes whenever they go outside of the building. *[3: Moderate Evidence]*

Surgical attire may become contaminated by contact with the external environment. Changing into clean surgical attire before entering the semi-restricted area(s) decreases the possibility of contamination with microorganisms present in the external environment.

A prospective case control study by Sivanandan et al[27] compared the level and type of contamination of surgical attire worn inside and outside the perioperative suite within the facility. The researchers determined that there was no increased bacterial contamination of surgical attire worn in the facility; however, they did not evaluate contamination levels of surgical attire worn outside the facility. This is an unresolved issue that warrants further research.

A quasi-experimental study by Neeley and Maley,[28] and a nonexperimental study by Neeley and Orloff,[29] found that microorganisms such as enterococci and fungi can survive on fabrics and plastics for at least one day, and many can survive for as long as 90 days. These studies demonstrate that potentially pathogenic organisms can survive on many objects and fabrics. These pathogenic organisms may contaminate

SURGICAL ATTIRE

surgical attire when it is worn outside of the facility. When this contaminated attire is subsequently worn inside the facility, it could potentially increase the risk for SSIs via transfer of microorganisms from the contaminated attire to patients and surfaces within the perioperative environment. In addition, pathogenic microorganisms can be carried on contaminated surgical attire and transferred to a variety of external environments (eg, home, car, community).

I.f. Cover apparel (eg, lab coats) worn over scrub attire should be clean or be for single use. Reusable cover apparel should be laundered in a health care-accredited laundry facility after each daily use and when contaminated (Figure 3). *[3: Moderate Evidence]*

The collective evidence does not support wearing of cover apparel to protect scrub attire from contamination, and there is evidence that lab coats worn as cover apparel can be contaminated with large numbers of pathogenic microorganisms.[30-34] Researchers have found that cover apparel is not always discarded daily after use or laundered on a frequent basis.[30,31]

Kaplan et al[35] enrolled 75 participants in three groups for a quasi-experimental study to determine the effectiveness of cover apparel in preventing contamination of scrub attire.

- Group 1 participants wore a cover garment over their scrub attire,
- Group 2 participants wore scrub attire without a cover garment, and
- Group 3 participants wore scrub attire without a cover garment and also wore their scrub attire outdoors.

The researchers found there was no significant difference between the three groups, and they concluded that wearing cover apparel over scrub attire did not prevent contamination of scrub attire.[35]

A nonexperimental study conducted by Munoz-Price et al[31] examined the association between bacterial contamination of 119 health care workers' hands, lab coats, and scrub attire in five ICUs at a university medical center. Bacterial growth was detected on 104 hands; 13 grew *Staphylococcus aureus*, seven grew *Acinetobacter*, two grew enterococci, and 83 grew normal skin flora. The presence of pathogens on health care workers' hands was associated with an increased likelihood of the presence of pathogens on lab coats.

Loh et al[36] examined lab coats worn by 100 physicians in a nonexperimental study. *Staphylococcus aureus* was isolated from 25 of the lab coats, and the researchers found that the cuffs and pockets of the coats were the most contaminated areas.

In a nonexperimental study of 100 medical students' cover apparel, Banu et al[37] found microorganisms on the cuffs and side pockets of the cover apparel. Contamination was found on the

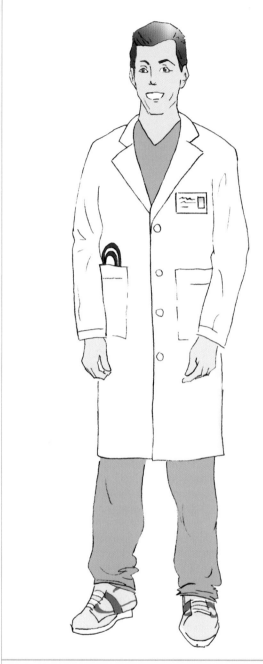

FIGURE 3. COVER APPAREL AND STETHOSCOPES

Reusable cover apparel should be laundered in a health care-accredited laundry facility after each daily use and when contaminated. Stethoscopes should not be worn around the neck and should be cleaned before and after each use with a low-level disinfectant.

Illustration by Kurt Jones.

dominant hand sleeve cuffs and the backs of the cover apparel 10 cm down from the collar. These areas were contaminated with *Staphylococcus* species on all cover apparel, *Acinetobacter* species on seven students' cover apparel, and diphtheroids on 12 students' cover apparel.

In a nonexperimental study, Munoz-Price et al[31] investigated the laundering practices of 160 health care providers related to scrub attire and

ASEPTIC PRACTICE

lab coats. Overall, lab coats were washed every 12.4 days and scrub attire every 1.7 days. Ninety percent of respondents laundered their lab coats only once per month, and four people washed their lab coats only once every 90 days to 12 months. Water temperature used by health care providers to launder their lab coats included cold (11%), warm (21%), and hot (52%); 11% did not know the temperature used; and 6% dry-cleaned their lab coats. A total of 145 health care providers (90%) acknowledged that their lab coats were potentially contaminated with hospital pathogens. The researchers recommended that lab coats be laundered regularly (ie, at least once or twice per week) and whenever dirty or soiled with body fluids. The researchers also recommended that the lab coats be laundered in hot water with bleach to reduce or eliminate potential pathogens.

In a nonexperimental study of contamination levels of health care practitioners' cover apparel, Treakle et al[30] found that cover apparel in inpatient and outpatient areas, ICUs, administrative areas, and the OR was contaminated with *Staphylococcus aureus* that included both susceptible and resistant isolates. Two-thirds of the health care practitioners perceived their cover apparel to be dirty because it had not been washed in more than one week. Notably, health care personnel with contaminated cover apparel were more likely to have home laundered their cover apparel.

I.g. Perioperative personnel should wear clean shoes that are dedicated for use within the perioperative area. *[3: Moderate Evidence]*

In a quasi-experimental study, Amirfeyz et al[38] examined shoes worn outdoors and shoes worn only in the surgical suite (N = 120). The results of the study demonstrated that 98% of the outdoor shoes were contaminated with coagulase-negative staphylococci, coliform, and *Bacillus* species compared with 56% of the shoes worn only in the surgical suite. Bacteria on the perioperative floor may contribute up to 15% of CFUs dispersed into the air by walking. The researchers concluded that shoes worn only in the perioperative area may help to reduce contamination of the perioperative environment.

I.g.1. Shoes worn within the perioperative environment must have closed toes and backs, low heels, and nonskid soles and must meet Occupational Safety and Health Administration (OSHA) and the health care organization's safety requirements.[39] *[1: Regulatory Requirement]*

Shoes that enclose the foot with backs, low heels, and nonskid soles may reduce the risk for injury from slips and falls and from dropped items. The OSHA regulations require the use of protective footwear in areas where there is a danger of foot injuries from falling or rolling objects or objects piercing the sole. The employer is responsible for determining whether foot injury hazards exist and what, if any, protective footwear is required. The OSHA regulations mandate that employers perform a workplace hazard risk assessment and ensure that employees wear protective footwear to provide protection from identified potential hazards (eg, needle sticks, scalpel cuts, splashing from blood or other potentially infectious materials).[39]

Shoes that have holes or perforations may not protect health care workers' feet from exposure to blood, body fluids, or other liquids that may contain potentially infectious agents. Shoes made of cloth, that are open-toed, or that have holes on the top or sides do not offer protection against spilled liquids or sharp items that may be dropped or kicked.

In a quasi-experimental study, Barr and Seigel[40] examined 15 different types of shoes and tested them with an apparatus that measured resistance to penetration by scalpels. The materials of the shoes included leather, suede, rubber, and canvas. Sixty percent of the shoes sustained scalpel penetration through the shoe into a simulated foot. Only six materials prevented complete penetration. These materials included sneaker suede, suede with inner mesh lining, leather with inner canvas lining, non-pliable leather, rubber with inner leather lining, and rubber. Wearing shoes made of these materials could potentially prevent harm to the perioperative team member.

I.g.2. Shoe covers or boots must be worn in instances when gross contamination can reasonably be anticipated (eg, orthopedic surgery).[39] *[1: Regulatory Requirement]*

I.g.3. Single-use shoe covers worn as PPE must be removed immediately after use and discarded, and hand hygiene should be performed.[39] *[1: Regulatory Requirement]*

I.h. Surgical masks in combination with eye protection devices, such as goggles, glasses with solid side shields, or chin-length face shields, must be worn whenever splashes, spray, spatter, or droplets of blood, body fluids, or other potentially infectious materials may be generated and eye, nose, or mouth contamination can be reasonably anticipated.[41] *[1: Regulatory Requirement]*

Wearing surgical masks and face and eye protection is recommended by the Centers for Disease Control and Prevention (CDC)[42] and is a regulatory requirement.[41]

Surgical masks worn in the perioperative setting serve two purposes. First, they help protect the patient and environment from microbial contamination by organisms carried in the provider's mouth or nose. Second, they provide protection for the wearer from exposure to blood, body fluids, or other potentially infectious materials.

The results of an observational, descriptive, nonexperimental study conducted by White et al[43] involving 8,500 surgical procedures showed that 26% of exposures to blood were to the heads and necks of scrubbed personnel, and 17% of blood exposures were to circulating personnel outside the sterile field.

For additional information on surgical masks, the reader should refer to the AORN Guideline for Sterile Technique[2] and Guideline for Prevention of Transmissible Infections.[3]

I.h.1. Reusable eye protection devices worn with surgical masks, such as goggles, or personal glasses supplemented with solid side shields, should be cleaned according to the manufacturer's instructions for use before and after the health care worker performs or assists with each new procedure. *[5: Benefits Balanced with Harms]*

Reducing the number of microorganisms present on eye protection devices and glasses may protect patients from SSIs resulting from the transfer of microorganisms from the devices or hands of health care workers to patients or environmental surfaces.

I.h.2. The surgical mask should cover the mouth and nose and be secured in a manner that prevents venting at the sides of the mask (Figure 4). *[1: Strong Evidence]*

Masks with ear loops may not have been designed and intended for use as surgical masks and may not provide a secure facial fit that prevents venting at the sides of the mask. A mask that conforms to the perioperative team member's face decreases the risk that the health care worker will transmit nasopharyngeal and respiratory microorganisms to the patient or the sterile field.[42]

I.h.3. A fresh surgical mask should be donned before the health care worker performs or assists with each new procedure. The mask should be replaced and discarded whenever it becomes wet or soiled or has been taken down. *[5: Benefits Balanced with Harms]*

The filtering capacity of a surgical mask becomes compromised when it is wet or soiled. In a controlled, quasi-experimental study to determine whether filtration efficiency of surgical masks decreased with the length of time the mask was worn, Barbosa and Graziano[44] evaluated 32 individuals wearing surgical masks and 32 individuals without masks. The surgical masks used during the study had a bacterial filtration

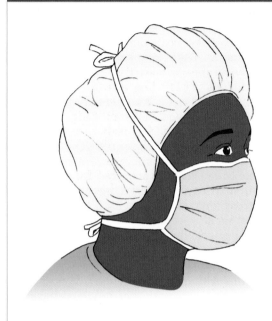

FIGURE 4. SURGICAL MASKS

Surgical masks should cover the mouth and nose and be secured in a manner that prevents venting at the sides of the mask.

Illustration by Kurt Jones.

efficiency of 95%. Researchers took air samples from the surgical field at one, two, four and six hours. The results of the study showed an increase in contamination of the filter portion of the mask after four hours. The researchers concluded that the microbial barrier of surgical masks decreased significantly after four hours.

I.h.4. Surgical masks should not be worn hanging around the neck. *[5: Benefits Balanced with Harms]*

The filter portion of a surgical mask harbors bacteria collected from the nasopharyngeal airway. The contaminated mask may cross-contaminate the scrub attire top or long-sleeved jacket when the mask is worn hanging around the neck.

I.h.5. Surgical masks should be removed and discarded by handling only the mask ties. Hand hygiene should be performed after removal of masks.[42] *[1: Strong Evidence]*

The filter portion of the mask harbors bacteria collected from the nasopharyngeal airway. Removing masks by the ties prevents possible contamination of the hands from the filter portion of the mask.

I.i. Identification badges should be worn secured on the scrub attire top or long-sleeved jacket and should be visible. Lanyards should not be worn. Badges should be cleaned with a low-level disinfectant (eg, 70% isopropyl alcohol) regularly and when the badge becomes soiled. *[2: High Evidence]*

Health care personnel as well as patients should be able to identify caregivers. Visible identification badges support security measures and assist in identifying persons authorized to be in the perioperative setting.

In a cross-sectional, quasi-experimental study, Kotsanas et al[45] examined the pathogenic contamination of identification badges and lanyards and found that the median bacterial load was tenfold greater for lanyards (3.1 CFUs/cm²) than for identification badges (0.3 CFUs/cm²). The microorganisms recovered from lanyards and identification badges were methicillin-sensitive *Staphylococcus aureus*, MRSA, *Enterococcus* species, and *Enterobacteriaceae*. The researchers concluded that identification badges should be clipped on and disinfected regularly and that lanyards should be changed frequently or not be worn.

I.j. Jewelry (eg, earrings, necklaces, bracelets, rings) that cannot be contained or confined within the scrub attire should not be worn in the semi-restricted or restricted areas. *[3: Moderate Evidence]*

Wearing earrings, watches, and rings was found to increase bacterial counts on skin surfaces both when the jewelry is in place and after its removal. The literature search did not find any research or non-research evidence related to bacterial contamination from necklaces. Four quasi-experimental studies[46-49] and three nonexperimental studies[50-52] collectively support the removal of rings, the removal or containment of watches, and the complete covering of ear and nose piercings with a surgical mask or head covering in the surgical setting.

A systematic review conducted by Arrowsmith and Taylor[53] determined there were no RCTs that compared ring wearing with the removal of rings in the prevention of SSIs.

In a quasi-experimental study, Trick et al[54] compared ring wearing to no ring wearing and determined that ring wearing was associated with a tenfold higher median skin organism count on the hands. The researchers recommended that all health care workers remove rings and perform hand hygiene before caring for patients.

Kelsall et al[49] found that finger rings increased skin surface bacterial counts in a quasi-experimental study. Although hand hygiene reduced bacterial skin counts, there were more bacteria under rings than on the adjacent skin or on the opposite hand. Pathogens identified by the researchers in this study included coagulase-negative staphylococci, gram-negative cocci, *Pseudomonas* species, *Staphylococcus aureus*, and other skin flora.

The results of a nonexperimental, retrospective, cohort study by Stein and Pankovich-Wargula[55] that compared SSI rates of a single surgeon over four years (ie, wearing a ring for two years versus not wearing a ring for two years) contradicted the results of other studies. The SSI rates were 19 infections in 987 surgeries in the no ring group (1.9%), and 6 infections in 1,140 surgeries in the ring group (0.53%)

I.k. Stethoscopes should not be worn around the neck and should be cleaned with a low-level disinfectant before and after each use. *[3: Moderate Evidence]*

Stethoscopes are one of the most commonly and frequently used medical devices in a health care facility. Stethoscopes come in direct contact with patients' skin and could provide an opportunity for transmission of microbes from patient to patient, from patient to health care worker, or from health care worker to patient.

The literature search found six quasi-experimental,[56-61] and 10 nonexperimental studies[62-71] of good or high quality that investigated stethoscope contamination. Contaminated stethoscope tubing and diaphragms may transmit pathogens such as MRSA by direct contact (eg, by using a contaminated stethoscope on a patient) or by indirect contact (eg, by wearing the stethoscope around the neck and contaminating the skin and scrub attire and subsequently transferring the microorganisms from the contaminated skin or attire to the patient). The collective evidence showed that hand hygiene and stethoscope cleaning by health care personnel decreased the possibility of transmitting pathogens to patients and environmental surfaces.

A quasi-experimental study by Denholm et al[60] examined the microbial contamination levels of the stethoscopes of 155 physicians and medical students and compared personal stethoscopes with facility-owned stethoscopes. The researchers isolated significantly more organisms from personal stethoscopes than from facility-owned stethoscopes; however, there was no significant relationship between the frequency of stethoscope cleaning and the degree of contamination. The researchers concluded that even regular cleaning of stethoscopes may be insufficient to prevent colonization with pathogenic organisms and that stethoscopes used for patients at high risk for HAIs should be restricted to single-patient use.

In a nonexperimental cross-sectional study, Campos-Murguia et al[68] examined the number of potentially pathogenic organisms present on stethoscopes by analyzing 112 stethoscopes from 12 hospital departments. At least 1 CFU was found on 106 stethoscopes (95%). Forty-eight stethoscopes (43%) had microorganisms that were potentially pathogenic. The results of this study showed that stethoscopes could be significant contributors to MRSA infections and that they should be routinely cleaned and disinfected before and after each patient use.

I.k.1. Fabric stethoscope tubing covers should not be used. *[4: Limited Evidence]*

Fabric covers on stethoscope tubing may become contaminated with pathogenic microorganisms and subsequently act as fomites. In a nonexperimental study, Milam et al[72] isolated gram-positive aerobic bacteria, gram-negative aerobic bacteria, anaerobes, and yeast from 18 of 20 fabric stethoscope covers (90%) that had been used for one to 24 months. The researchers found that the average length of time between stethoscope cover laundering was 3.7 months, and some fabric covers were never laundered.

I.l. Briefcases, backpacks, and other personal items that are taken into the semi-restricted or restricted areas should be cleaned with a low-level disinfectant and should not be placed on the floor. *[3: Moderate Evidence]*

Items brought into the OR, such as briefcases, backpacks, and other personal items, may be difficult to clean and may harbor pathogens, dust, and bacteria. Maintaining a clean perioperative environment helps decrease the patient's risk of SSI.[73] Cleaning these items may help to decrease the transmission of potentially pathogenic microorganisms from external surfaces to perioperative surfaces and from perioperative surfaces to external surfaces.

Floors in the OR or procedure room are considered contaminated.[73] Items placed on the floor could become vehicles for transferring microorganisms from the floor to other perioperative or external surfaces.

The literature search did not find any literature that specifically examined the effect on SSIs associated with bringing backpacks, briefcases, or other personal items from an external environment into a surgical environment. Two quasi-experimental studies,[28,74] five nonexperimental studies,[29,75-78] and one literature review[79] addressed the survivability of microorganisms on fabrics, plastics, and other materials. The evidence did not suggest that these items should be prohibited in the health care setting; however, the collective evidence did support the need for thorough cleaning and disinfecting procedures.

In a quasi-experimental study, Neely and Maley[28] examined the ability of gram-positive bacteria (ie, vancomycin-sensitive and -resistant enterococci and methicillin-sensitive and -resistant staphylococci) to survive on five materials commonly found in health care facilities:

- smooth 100% cotton clothing,
- 100% cotton terry cloth towels,
- 60% cotton/40% polyester blend scrub attire and lab coats,
- 100% polyester privacy curtains, and
- 100% polypropylene plastic splash aprons.

The researchers found that all bacteria survived for at least one day, and some survived for more than 90 days. The researchers recommended meticulous cleaning to limit the spread of these bacteria.

Neely and Orloff[29] examined the ability of fungi to survive on seven materials commonly found in health care facilities:

- smooth 100% cotton clothing;
- 100% cotton terrycloth towels and washcloths;
- 60% cotton/40% polyester blend scrub attire lab coats, and other clothing;
- 100% polyester privacy curtains;
- 25% spandex/75% nylon pressure garments;
- 100% polyethylene plastic splash aprons and
- 100% polyurethane keyboard covers.

The researchers found that fungi associated with HAIs survived for at least one day, and some survived for weeks. The researchers recommended meticulous cleaning to reduce the potential for patient infection.

Four nonexperimental studies[75-78] and one literature review[79] supported the findings of Neeley and Maley[28] and Neely and Orloff.[29] Koca et al[76] conducted a nonexperimental study that demonstrated that bacteria and fungi survived for days to months on commonly used hospital fabrics. The researchers recommended that current national guidelines on disinfection and sterilization of fabrics be followed to minimize cross-infection and help prevent HAIs.

In a nonexperimental case control study to determine whether physician's purses were contaminated with microorganisms more frequently than the purses of women who were not physicians, Feldman et al[74] found that five of the 13 physicians' purses (38.5%) were colonized with bacteria compared with two of the 14 nonphysicians' purses (14%). The researchers concluded that there is a potential for physicians' purses to serve as a vector for disease transmission.

I.m. Cell phones, tablets, and other personal communication or hand-held electronic equipment should be cleaned with a low-level disinfectant according to the manufacturer's instructions for use before and after being brought into the perioperative setting. *[3: Moderate Evidence]*

The collective evidence demonstrates that cell phones, tablets, and other personal hand-held devices are highly contaminated with microorganisms, some potentially pathogenic. One RCT,[80] three quasi-experimental studies,[46,81,82] eight nonexperimental studies,[83-90] and one literature review[91] addressed cell phones and other electronic devices brought into the health care setting. All of the researchers recommended regular cleaning of these devices and implementing hand hygiene before and after use. Reducing the numbers of microorganisms present on the devices may protect patients from the risk of HAIs resulting from the transfer of microorganisms from the devices or hands of health care workers to patients.

Datta et al[80] conducted an RCT to investigate the rate of bacterial contamination of the mobile phones of health care workers employed in a tertiary health care teaching hospital and compared the contamination rate with that of a group of individuals not working in a health care environment. Of the 200 health care workers' mobile phones sampled, 144 (72%) were contaminated with bacteria, and 18% of those bacteria were MRSA. Of the 50 non-health care workers' mobile phones sampled, only five (10%) were contaminated with bacteria (ie, coagulase-negative staphylococci). The researchers concluded that simple measures such as regular cleaning of cell phones and other hand-held electronic devices and improving hand hygiene might help to decrease the risk of HAIs from bacteria carried on personal mobile devices.

Tekerekoglu et al[85] conducted a nonexperimental, cross-sectional study to determine the amount of bacterial colonization on the mobile phones of patients, patients' companions, health care workers, and visitors in a university medical center. Two hundred cell phones were tested, and the results showed a significantly higher rate of pathogenic organisms on the patients', patient companions', and visitors' phones than on those of the health care workers. The researchers concluded that the cleaning of phones brought into the health care setting by patients and others is just as important as cleaning the phones of health care workers.

Kilic et al[81] conducted a quasi-experimental study that tested the bacterial levels of 106 mobile phones carried by health care workers in three hospitals and compared them to bacterial levels of 30 phones carried by people who did not work in hospitals. Bacterial growth was observed in 65 of the 106 samples (61%) of the health care workers' phones; the most common pathogens were *Staphylococcus*, *Corynebacterium*, and *Escherichia coli*. Of the control phones carried by non-health care workers, 16 of the samples (53%) were colonized with *Staphylococcus epidermidis* and *Bacillus*.

During a nine-month period, White et al[89] conducted a nonexperimental study of microbial growth on smartphones used by students in the OR. Devices were sampled for two cohort groups (ie, nine devices on six occasions, and seven devices on three occasions), with a four- to five-hour period of use between sampling activity. No device was found to be free of growth. The devices demonstrated multiple species of microbial growth in all cases except one, which was contaminated solely with coagulase-negative *Staphylococcus* species.

Eighty-six percent of the smartphones had three or more types of bacteria on them; some had as many as seven types. The most common pathogen found was coagulase-negative *Staphylococcus*. Other pathogenic organisms found were MRSA, *Micrococcus* species, *Enterococcus* species, and coliforms. The researchers concluded that mobile phones are contaminated with significant numbers of pathogenic bacteria. They recommended cleaning mobile phones with 70% isopropyl alcohol in combination with frequent hand hygiene and other infection prevention measures to reduce the risk for infection from transmission of microorganisms found on mobile phones.[89]

Recommendation II

All individuals who enter the semi-restricted and restricted areas should wear scrub attire that has been laundered at a health care-accredited laundry facility or disposable scrub attire provided by the facility and intended for use within the perioperative setting.

The evidence regarding home laundering of scrub attire compared with health care-accredited laundering conflicts. Some evidence indicates there is a risk for pathogenic organisms to be carried on scrub attire laundered in the home.[92-95] These organisms can potentially put the patient at risk of infection or contaminate the home or community of the perioperative team member.

Limitations of the evidence are that some studies examined in-vitro conditions that may not be applicable to real-life conditions, and some evidence is not specific to the perioperative setting and therefore may not be generalizable to the perioperative environment. Except for one case report by Wright et al,[95] none of the authors considered SSI as an outcome.

The benefits of health care-accredited laundering compared with home laundering are that health care-accredited laundering may protect the patient from potential exposure to microorganisms that could contribute to an SSI and may protect the perioperative team member from contaminating the home or community with pathogenic organisms from the workplace. Health care-accredited laundering provides control of the laundering process and helps ensure that effective laundering standards have been met.

II.a.   Scrub attire should be laundered in a health care-accredited laundry facility after each daily use and when contaminated. *[3: Moderate Evidence]*

   The evidence regarding home laundering compared with health care-accredited laundering of surgical attire conflicts. Fijan and Turk[96] conducted a literature review of laundering practices of hospital textiles. The authors concluded that the available evidence is diverse and contradictory. Effective laundering of scrub attire is dependent on several factors including the duration, type of detergent and disinfectants, ratio of chemicals to water, and type of fabric being laundered.

Eight articles support health care-accredited laundering. In a quasi-experimental study to determine whether enteric and respiratory viruses could survive the wash, rinse, and drying cycles commonly used for home laundering, Gerba et al[92] concluded that common household laundering practices did not eliminate enteric and respiratory viruses from clothing.

In a literature review of laundering practices of nurses' uniforms, Halliwell[97] found a disparity between home and hospital laundering practices, inconsistency between laundering guidelines, and a lack of evidence that uniforms can act as a secondary source of HAIs. The results of the literature review revealed three important concepts:

○ Nurses' uniforms become highly contaminated with microorganisms while they are worn.
○ Contamination is higher on the areas of frequent hand contact, such as pockets, buttocks, and cuffs.
○ Hands that touch the uniform also become contaminated.

The author concluded that nurses' uniforms could be considered "biological hazards" and suggested that legislation be implemented that requires employers to provide and launder uniforms for health care workers.

Lis et al[93] conducted a nonexperimental study to evaluate airborne *Staphylococcus aureus* in the homes of people who had contact with the hospital environment. The researchers found a significant difference in airborne multidrug-resistant *S aureus* strains in the homes of people who had contact with a hospital environment. The researchers suggested that the bacteria may have been transmitted to the home via clothing.

Nguyen et al[98] reported an outbreak of 22 sternal SSIs in a hospital in which approximately 400 open heart surgeries were performed per year. Of the 22 SSIs, four cases were *Gordonia* species. The authors found that antimicrobial dosing was often inadequate, cleaning practices were inadequate, personnel employed poor hand hygiene, there were inadequate environmental controls in place, and home laundered scrub attire was worn.

In a quasi-experimental study to determine whether hospital laundry facilities could adequately decontaminate enterococci from hospital linens, Orr et al[99] found that the organism was successfully decontaminated with a water temperature of 150° F (66° C) for 10 minutes and at a temperature of 160° F (71° C) for three minutes.

Sasahara et al[100] reviewed an outbreak of *Bacillus cereus* bacteremia and found that the hospital laundry and washing machines were highly contaminated with *B cereus*. The organism is resistant to heat and alcohol, and eliminating the organisms requires that laundry be washed at 176° F (80° C) for more than 10 minutes.

In a nonexperimental study to assess the bioburden associated with scrub attire, Twomey and Beitz[94] evaluated single-use, reusable, facility-laundered, third-party laundered, and home laundered scrub attire before and after wear. The researchers measured CFUs for each type of scrub attire. They found no differences in the mean microbial populations among the facility, third-party laundered, or single-use scrub attire before wear. Notably, the home laundered attire had a significantly greater microbial population before use. The home laundered scrub attire was as contaminated after laundering and before being worn as the facility-laundered and third-party laundered attire were at the end of a work day. The researchers concluded that home laundering is not as effective as facility- or third-party laundering for decontaminating scrub attire.

Wright et al[95] reported three cases of postoperative *Gordonia bronchialis* sternal infections after coronary artery bypass grafting surgery. *G bronchialis* was isolated from the scrub attire, axilla, hands, and purse of a nurse anesthetist and was implicated as the cause of the SSIs. Cultures taken from her roommate, who was also a nurse, showed the same microorganism. After notification of the culture results, the nurse anesthetist discarded her front-loading washing machine. During the next year, the nurse anesthetist and her roommate's scrub attire, hands, nares, and scalp tested negative for *G bronchialis*. The authors concluded that the home washing machine was the likely bacterial reservoir. Home laundering may not reliably kill all pathogens, and the pathogens may survive in the form of biofilms within the washing machine. Biofilms have been implicated in the malodor of washing machines. The authors recommended that hospital-laundered scrub attire be implemented as a measure to reduce patients' risk of developing an SSI. This report is the first to demonstrate a causal relationship between home laundering and human disease.

Nine articles support home laundering. Al Benna[101] conducted a literature review to explore home laundering of scrub attire and found there was little scientific evidence that facility laundering was better than home laundering; however, the author recommended the following guidelines for home laundering:

○ Uniforms should be washed as the last laundry load of the day.
○ Bleach should be used.
○ Laundry should be totally submerged.
○ Laundry personnel should wash their hands after handling laundry.

- The lid or door of the washer should be disinfected before clean laundry is removed to avoid contamination.
- Laundry should be dried at the highest temperature possible immediately after washing.
- Laundry should be transported in a manner that maintains cleanliness.

Belkin[102] noted the lack of evidence linking home laundering with SSI or HAIs in an expert opinion article and recommended the addition of a disinfecting agent, such as chlorine bleach to each load of laundry. In a second expert opinion article, Belkin[103] again noted the lack of evidence supporting facility laundering over home laundering and stated that no facilities have reported an increase in SSIs related to home laundering.

In a nonexperimental study to determine whether domestic laundry procedures were effective in eliminating viruses on clothing, Heinzel et al[104] used commercial powdered laundry detergent to test their virucidal performance. The researchers concluded that powdered detergents are able to decontaminate viruses from textiles in a common household laundering process.

Lakdawala et al[105] conducted a nonexperimental investigation of the effect of low-temperature washing cycles (140° F [60° C]) by assessing the amount of bioburden on health care workers uniforms before and after laundering. The researchers concluded that a washing cycle of 140° F (60° C) for 10 minutes was sufficient to decontaminate hospital uniforms and reduce the bacterial load by at least a 7-log reduction. The uniforms could become recontaminated after laundering, but the organisms could be easily removed by ironing.

In a nonexperimental study of OR surgical attire conducted as the result of an increase of MDROs and HAIs, Nordstrom et al[106] took swatches from unwashed, hospital-laundered, new cloth, and disposable scrub attire, and tested them for the presence of microorganisms. The researchers found that the home laundered scrub attire had a significantly higher total bacterial count than the facility laundered attire, and they found no significant difference in bacterial counts between hospital-laundered, unused, or disposable scrub attire. The researchers concluded that although it is not known how contaminated scrub attire contributes to the spread of HAIs, hospital administrators and infection preventionists should consider the potential for transmission of infection versus cost savings by the facility if home laundering is allowed. The researchers advised that health care workers should be made aware of the risks of home laundering and being provided with instructions for best methods for home laundering in order to reduce the risk of infection.

Patel et al[107] conducted a quasi-experimental study to determine the effectiveness of home laundering in removing *Staphylococcus aureus* from scrub attire. The researchers cut hospital laundered scrub attire into squares, inoculated them with *S aureus,* and washed them at a typical household laundry temperature of 104° F (40° C) and a higher temperature of 140° F (60° C). The researchers concluded that the lower 104° F (40° C) temperature did not remove *S aureus*; however, adding sequential tumble drying or ironing reduced the number of bacteria to an undetectable level. Washing at 140° F (60° C) produced a greater reduction in total viable organisms compared with the 104° F (40° C) temperature. The researchers concluded that scrub attire can be safely washed at 104° F (40° C) if tumble dried for 30 minutes or ironed.

Wilson et al[108] reviewed the literature related to health care workers uniforms as a vehicle for microbial transmission and to determine the efficacy of different laundry practices. The authors found limited evidence directly related to decontamination of health care workers' uniforms. They concluded that there was no strong evidence that home laundering of uniforms was inferior to industrial laundry practices; however, the authors recommended that if home laundering is performed, overloading of the machine should be avoided to ensure that a sufficient amount of water is present for adequate agitation and rinsing during the washing process.

In a nonexperimental study to determine the level of contamination of health care workers uniforms before and at the end of a work shift, Perry et al[109] found that the uniforms became progressively more contaminated the longer they were worn. The researchers questioned the ability of home laundering processes to adequately clean the uniforms. The researchers emphasized the importance of daily laundering, and also recommended that if home laundering is practiced, specific guidelines provided by the facility are necessary for standardized laundering, including the need for laundering uniforms separately from other household garments and at a water temperature sufficient to eliminate pathogenic organisms.

Using health care-accredited laundry facilities is recommended because they meet industry standards[110] including the following:

- Textile quality control procedures are defined and implemented.
- The inventory system is adequate to ensure supply.
- Soiled and contaminated textile areas are separated.
- The ventilation is controlled
  - with negative pressure in the soiled area,

- with positive pressure from the clean textile area through the soiled textile area,
- at 6 to 10 air exchanges per hour, and
- with air vented to the outside.

○ Clean textiles are stored at temperatures of 68° F to 78° F (20° C to 25.6° C) in an area free of vermin, dust, and lint.

○ Storage shelves are 1 to 2 inches from the wall, the bottom shelf is 6 to 8 inches from the floor, and the top shelf is 12 to 18 inches below the ceiling.

○ Hand washing facilities are located in all areas with soiled textiles; hand washing or antiseptic dispensers are in the clean textile area; and employees perform hand washing after glove removal and restroom use, before eating, and when hands are contaminated with blood, body fluids, or other potentially infectious materials.

○ Work surfaces are clean and are disinfected if they become contaminated with blood, body fluids, or other potentially infectious materials.

○ The OSHA Exposure Control Plan is in place and PPE is supplied, available, and worn.

○ Quality control monitoring processes are in place.

○ Personnel education and training is provided and documented.

○ Safety data sheets are available for each chemical used.

○ water quality is tested on a regular basis for hardness, alkalinity, iron content, and pH;

○ Soiled health care textiles are handled, collected, and transported according to local, state, and federal regulations.

○ Each laundry cycle is monitored and applicable data for each cycle are recorded, including pre-wash, wash, rinse, and final rinse times, water levels and usage, temperatures, and chemical usage.

○ Water extraction and drying are performed using methods that preserve the integrity of the textiles and minimize bacterial growth.

○ Cleaned textiles are packaged and stored in fluid-resistant bundles or fluid-resistant carts or hampers and are handled as little as possible.

○ Carts used for transport or storage are kept clean and are well maintained.

○ Clean textiles are stored and transported separately from soiled textiles.

○ Vehicles used to transport textiles provide separation of clean and soiled textiles, and the vehicle interiors are cleaned on a regular basis.

The Healthcare Laundry Accreditation Council offers voluntary accreditation for those laundry facilities that process reusable health care textiles and that incorporate OSHA and CDC guidelines and professional association recommended practices.[110]

The benefit of health care-accredited laundering of surgical attire is that it may protect the patient from exposure to pathogenic organisms remaining on the health care worker's attire after home laundering and may prevent the health care worker from transmitting pathogenic organisms from the attire worn in the health care facility into the home or community. Health care-accredited laundering may reduce the potential for allergies to laundry detergents or other chemical additives because the rinsing process leaves little to no soap residue in the fabric.

The potential harm associated with home laundering is that it may not protect patients, health care workers, their family members, or the community from exposure to bloodborne pathogens or other infectious materials during handling and decontamination of scrub attire. To address health hazards posed by pathogens transported from the workplace to the home, the National Institute for Occupational Safety and Health published *Protecting Workers' Families: A Research Agenda*.[111] The authors emphasized that exposure to blood, body fluids, and potentially pathogenic organisms are possible threats for disease transmission that can be carried to the homes of workers on clothing and other objects that have been used in the workplace. To mitigate this risk, the authors recommended that employers institute engineering, administrative, and worker protection techniques, and that health care workers not bring objects used in the work setting into the home.

Home laundering is not monitored for quality, consistency, or safety. Home washing machines may not have the adjustable parameters or controls required to achieve the necessary thermal measures (eg, water temperature); mechanical measures (eg, agitation); or chemical measures (eg, capacity for additives to neutralize the alkalinity of the water, soap, or detergent) to reduce microbial levels in soiled scrub attire.

Scrub attire that is home laundered may not be protected from contaminants in the environment during transport to the practice setting.

II.a.1. Laundered scrub attire should be protected during transport to the practice setting.[112] *[4: Limited Evidence]*

Protecting clean scrub attire from contamination during transport from the laundry facility to the practice setting helps prevent physical damage and minimizes potential contamination from the external environment.[112]

II.a.2. Laundered scrub attire should be transported in enclosed carts or containers and in vehicles that are cleaned and disinfected regularly.[112] *[4: Limited Evidence]*

Carts, containers, and vehicles can be a source of contamination.

II.a.3. Laundered scrub attire should be stored in enclosed carts or cabinets that are cleaned and disinfected regularly.[112] *[4: Limited Evidence]*

Storing laundered surgical attire in clean enclosed carts or cabinets helps prevent contamination. Storing clean attire in a facility locker with personal items from outside of the facility may contaminate the clean scrub attire.

II.a.4. Laundered scrub attire may be stored in dispensing machines. Dispensing machines should be regularly cleaned and disinfected according to the manufacturer's instructions for use. *[5: Benefits Balanced with Harms]*

Scrub attire-dispensing machines may promote cost containment, help to facilitate an adequate supply of scrub attire, provide clean storage for scrub attire, and increase individual accountability.

I.b. Reusable scrub attire should be left at the health care facility for laundering. *[3: Moderate Evidence]*

Callaghan[113] conducted a nonexperimental study to evaluate the amount of bacterial contamination of nurses' uniforms during an eight-hour shift and found that at the end of the shift, the uniforms were highly contaminated with potentially pathogenic microorganisms.

II.b.1. Scrub attire that has been penetrated by blood, body fluids, or other potentially infectious materials must be removed immediately or as soon as possible and replaced with clean attire. When extensive contamination of the body occurs, the health care worker should take a shower or bath before donning fresh attire.[41,114] *[1: Regulatory Requirement]*

Changing contaminated, soiled, or wet attire may reduce the potential for contamination and protect personnel from exposure to potentially pathogenic microorganisms.

II.b.2. Scrub attire contaminated with visible blood or body fluids must remain at the health care facility for laundering or be sent to a health care-accredited laundry facility contracted by the health care organization.[41,111] *[1: Regulatory Requirement]*

Controlled laundering of attire contaminated by blood or body fluids reduces the risk of transferring pathogenic microorganisms from the health care facility to the home or community. Exposure to blood, body fluids, and potentially pathogenic organisms are potential threats to health care workers and their home environments.[111]

II.b.3. Wet or contaminated scrub attire must not be rinsed or sorted in the location of use.[41] *[1: Regulatory Requirement]*

Rinsing or sorting contaminated reusable attire may expose the health care worker to blood, body fluids, or other potentially infectious materials.

II.b.4. Reusable scrub attire that has been worn should not be stored in personal lockers for later use. *[3: Moderate Evidence]*

Scrub attire that has been worn may have bacterial colony counts that are even higher after the attire is removed, stored in a locker, and used again. Microbes have been shown to survive for long periods of time on fabrics.[28,29]

II.b.5. Reusable or single-use contaminated scrub attire should be placed in designated containers after use. *[5: Benefits Balanced with Harms]*

Recommendation III

Personnel entering the semi-restricted and restricted areas should cover the head, hair, ears, and facial hair.

Hair and skin can harbor bacteria that can be dispersed into the environment. The collective body of evidence supports covering the hair and ears while in the semi-restricted or restricted areas.

The limitations of the evidence are that some research studies had small sample sizes, were of low quality, or were conducted in laboratory settings that may not be generalizable to other settings.

The benefit of covering the head, ears, and hair is the reduction of the patient's exposure to potentially pathogenic microorganisms from the perioperative team member's head, hair, ears, and facial hair.

III.a. A clean surgical head cover or hood that confines all hair and completely covers the ears, scalp skin, sideburns, and nape of the neck should be worn. *[3: Moderate Evidence]*

There are several studies that show that hair can be a source of bacterial organisms.[1,115-117] The results of a nonexperimental study conducted by Noble et al[1] found that 10% of individuals had *Staphylococcus aureus* present in their hair. In a quasi-experimental study conducted by Summers et al,[115] the researchers cultured the hair of hospital personnel, inpatients, and outpatients, and found bacteria in the hair of all test participants. *S aureus* was the most common pathogen isolated. The researchers concluded that the exposed hair of health care workers is a potential source of patient infection. They recommended that health care workers cover all hair during even minor surgical procedures.

Dineen and Drusin[116] investigated two outbreaks of postoperative wound infections and found that the infections were directly related to personnel carrying *Staphylococcus aureus* in their hair. Mastro et al[117] investigated a prolonged outbreak of 20 postoperative SSIs caused by group A *Streptococcus*. Two case control studies and a review of records conducted by the researchers failed to identify the carrier. The researchers used bacterial settling plates to sample the air in the OR and identified the source of the outbreak as a surgical technologist who carried the identical type of group A *Streptococcus* on the scalp.

A literature review by McHugh et al[118] identified several conflicting studies related to the need for a surgical head covering. The authors concluded there was little evidence to suggest that covering the hair reduces SSI rates; however, they acknowledged that surgical team members wearing head coverings decreased bacterial contamination of the surgical field.

The results of a literature review conducted by Eisen[119] showed that hair is a potential vehicle for bacterial dispersal and that hair has been shown to carry *Staphylococcus aureus*. The author concluded that there is conflicting evidence about the effect of hair coverings on SSI rates.

Ibrahimi et al[24] conducted a literature review to examine SSIs and routes of bacterial transfer. The authors concluded that there was no convincing evidence that head coverings reduce SSI rates.

Mase et al[120] conducted a quasi-experimental study to determine whether staphylococci that were present on the hair could be removed by shampooing. The results of the study showed that staphylococci become firmly attached to the human hair surface and the edge of hair cuticles. Extensive treatment with neutral detergents did not remove the organism, suggesting that conventional shampooing has little effect on removing staphylococci from hair. Moreover, these neutral detergents had little bactericidal activity on staphylococci. These results suggest that hair could be a source of multidrug-resistant staphylococci in patient infections. The researchers concluded that hair could be a source of MRSA in HAIs.

A nonexperimental study conducted by McClure et al[121] examined dispersal of bacteria by men with and without beards and by women. The results of the study showed that there was significantly more bacterial shedding by bearded men than by clean-shaven men or by women, even when a mask was worn. The researchers suggested that beards may act as a reservoir for bacteria and dead organic material that can be dislodged when a face mask is removed. The researchers recommended that perioperative team members not wear beards.

Owers et al[122] conducted a nonexperimental study in which 20 OR team members had their

foreheads, eyebrows, and ears cultured. The researchers found there was significantly more bacteria isolated from the ears than from the foreheads and eyebrows of the surgical team members. The researchers concluded that the ears should be covered by surgical head covers during surgery.

III.a.1. Personnel wearing scrub attire should not remove the surgical head covering when leaving the perioperative area. *[5: Benefits Balanced with Harms]*

The purpose of the head covering is to contain hair and minimize microbial dispersal. When the head covering is removed, hair and microbes may be shed onto scrub attire.

Head coverings commonly used in the perioperative setting (eg, bouffant caps) are worn for hair and skin containment and are not considered PPE. The Occupational Safety and Health Administration requires that PPE not permit blood, body fluids, or other potentially infectious materials to pass through or reach the employee's clothing, skin, eyes, or other mucous membranes under normal conditions of use.[123]

III.a.2. Personnel should remove surgical head coverings whenever they change into street clothes and go outside of the building. *[5: Benefits Balanced with Harms]*

Removing surgical head coverings when exiting the building decreases the possibility of contamination with microorganisms present in the external environment.

III.a.3. Used single-use head coverings should be removed at the end of the shift or when contaminated and should be discarded in a designated receptacle. *[5: Benefits Balanced with Harms]*

III.a.4. Reusable head coverings should be laundered in a health care-accredited laundry facility after each daily use and when contaminated (see Recommendation II.b). *[3: Moderate Evidence]*

Head coverings are part of the scrub attire.

Glossary

Fomite: An inanimate object which, when contaminated with a viable pathogen (eg, bacterium, virus), can transfer the pathogen to a host.

Health care-accredited laundry facility: An organization that processes health care linens and has successfully passed an inspection of its facility, policies and procedures, training programs, and relationships with customers.

SURGICAL ATTIRE

Low-level disinfectant: An agent that destroys all vegetative bacteria, some fungi, and some viruses but not all bacterial spores.

Scrub attire: Nonsterile apparel designed for the perioperative practice setting that includes two-piece pantsuits, scrub dresses, long-sleeved cover jackets, and head coverings.

Squames: Flat, keratinized, dead cells shed from the outermost layer of stratified squamous epithelium.

Surgical attire: Nonsterile apparel designated for the perioperative practice setting that includes two-piece pantsuits, scrub dresses, cover jackets, head coverings, shoes, masks, and protective eyewear.

Surgical mask: A device worn over the mouth and nose by perioperative team members during surgical procedures to protect both the patient and perioperative team member from transfer of blood, body fluids, and other potentially infectious materials. Surgical masks prevent the transmission of large droplets (ie, greater than 5 microns). Surgical masks are evaluated for fluid resistance, bacterial filtration efficiency, differential pressure, and flammability.

REFERENCES

1. Noble WC, Habbema JD, van Furth R, Smith I, de Raay C. Quantitative studies on the dispersal of skin bacteria into the air. *J Med Microbiol.* 1976;9(1):53-61. [IIIB]

2. Guideline for sterile technique. In: *Guidelines for Perioperative Practice.* Denver, CO: AORN, Inc; 2015:67-76. [IVA]

3. Guideline for prevention of transmissible infections. In: *Guidelines for Perioperative Practice.* Denver, CO: AORN, Inc; 2015:419-451. [IVA]

4. Guideline for sharps safety. In: *Guidelines for Perioperative Practice.* Denver, CO: AORN, Inc; 2015:365-388. [IVA]

5. Guideline for hand hygiene. In: *Guidelines for Perioperative Practice.* Denver, CO: AORN, Inc; 2015:31-42. [VB]

6. Tammelin A, Domicel P, Hambraeus A, Stahle E. Dispersal of methicillin-resistant *Staphylococcus epidermidis* by staff in an operating suite for thoracic and cardiovascular surgery: relation to skin carriage and clothing. *J Hosp Infect.* 2000;44(2):119-126. [IIC]

7. Andersen BM, Solheim N. Occlusive scrub suits in operating theaters during cataract surgery: effect on airborne contamination. *Infect Control Hosp Epidemiol.* 2002;23(4):218-220. [IIIC]

8. Tammelin A, Hambraeus A, Stahle E. Source and route of methicillin-resistant *Staphylococcus epidermidis* transmitted to the surgical wound during cardiothoracic surgery. Possibility of preventing wound contamination by use of special scrub suits. *J Hosp Infect.* 2001;47(4):266-276. [IIIC]

9. Tammelin A, Ljungqvist B, Reinmüller B. Comparison of three distinct surgical clothing systems for protection from air-borne bacteria: a prospective observational study. *Patient Saf Surg.* 2012;6(1):23. [IIIC]

10. Tammelin A, Ljungqvist B, Reinmuller B. Single-use surgical clothing system for reduction of airborne bacteria in the operating room. *J Hosp Infect.* 2013;84(3):245-247. [IIC]

11. Lidwell OM, Lowbury EJL, Whyte W, Blowers R, Stanley SJ, Lowe D. Airborne contamination of wounds in joint replacement operations: the relationship to sepsis rates. *J Hosp Infect.* 1983;4(2):111-131. [IIA]

12. Edmiston CE Jr, Sinski S, Seabrook GR, Simons D, Goheen MP. Airborne particulates in the OR environment. *AORN J.* 1999;69(6):1169-1179. [IIB]

13. Bauer J, Kowal K, Tofail SAM, Podbielska H. MRSA-resistant textiles. In: Tofail SAM, ed. *Biological Interactions with Surface Charge in Biomaterials.* Cambridge, England: RSC Publishing;2012:193-207. [VB]

14. Sun G, Qian L, Xu X. Antimicrobial and medical-use textiles. *Textile Asia.* 2001;32(9):33-35. [IIIB]

15. Rajendran R, Radhai R, Kotresh TM, Csiszar E. Development of antimicrobial cotton fabrics using herb loaded nanoparticles. *Carbohydr Polym.* 2013;91(2):613-617. [IIIA]

16. Kasuga E, Kawakami Y, Matsumoto T, et al. Bactericidal activities of woven cotton and nonwoven polypropylene fabrics coated with hydroxyapatite-binding silver/titanium dioxide ceramic nanocomposite "Earth-plus." *Int J Nanomed.* 2011;6:1937-1943. [IIB]

17. Mariscal A, Lopez-Gigosos RM, Carnero-Varo M, Fernandez-Crehuet J. Antimicrobial effect of medical textiles containing bioactive fibres. *Eur J Clin Microbiol Infect Dis.* 2011;30(2):227-232. [IIB]

18. Chen-Yu JH, Eberhardt DM, Kincade DH. Antibacterial and laundering properties of AMS and PHMB as finishing agents on fabric for health care workers' uniforms. *Clothing Text Res J.* 2007;25(3):258-272. [IIA]

19. Bearman GM, Rosato A, Elam K, et al. A crossover trial of antimicrobial scrubs to reduce methicillin-resistant *Staphylococcus aureus* burden on healthcare worker apparel. *Infect Control Hosp Epidemiol.* 2012;33(3):268-275. [IA]

20. Noble WC. Dispersal of skin microorganisms. *Br J Dermatol.* 1975;93(4):477-485. [VA]

21. Benediktsdottir E, Hambraeus A. Dispersal of non-sporeforming anaerobic bacteria from the skin. *J Hyg (Lond).* 1982;88(3):487-500. [IIA]

22. Wiener-Well Y, Galuty M, Rudensky B, Schlesinger Y, Attias D, Yinnon AM. Nursing and physician attire as possible source of nosocomial infections. *Am J Infect Control.* 2011;39(7):555-559. [IIIA]

23. Krueger CA, Murray CK, Mende K, Guymon CH, Gerlinger TL. The bacterial contamination of surgical scrubs. *Am J Orthoped.* 2012;41(5):e69-e73. [IIIA]

24. Ibrahimi OA, Sharon V, Eisen DB. Surgical-site infections and routes of bacterial transfer: Which ones are most plausible? *Dermatol Surg.* 2011;37(12):1709-1720. [VA]

25. May RK, Pomeroy NP, Hers JFP, Winkler KC. Bacterial dispersion from the body surface. In: Hers JFP, Winkler KC, eds. *Airborne Transmission and Airborne Infection.* Utrecht, The Netherlands: Oosthoek Publishing Company; 1973:426-432. [IIIB]

26. Guideline for preoperative patient skin antisepsis. In: *Guidelines for Perioperative Practice.* Denver, CO: AORN, Inc; 2015:43-66. [IVA]

27. Sivanandan I, Bowker KE, Bannister GC, Soar J. Reducing the risk of surgical site infection: a case controlled study of contamination of theatre clothing. *J Periop Pract.* 2011;21(2):69-72. [IIIB]

28. Neely AN, Maley MP. Survival of enterococci and staphylococci on hospital fabrics and plastic. *J Clin Microbiol.* 2000;38(2):724-726. [IIB]

29. Neely AN, Orloff MM. Survival of some medically important fungi on hospital fabrics and plastics. *J Clin Microbiol.* 2001;39(9):3360-3361. [IIIB]

30. Treakle AM, Thom KA, Furuno JP, Strauss SM, Harris AD, Perencevich EN. Bacterial contamination of

health care workers' white coats. *Am J Infect Control.* 2009;37(2):101-105. [IIIB]

31. Munoz-Price LS, Arheart KL, Lubarsky DA, Birnbach DJ. Differential laundering practices of white coats and scrubs among health care professionals. *Am J Infect Control.* 2013;41(6):565-567. [IIIA]

32. Munoz-Price LS, Arheart KL, Mills JP, et al. Associations between bacterial contamination of health care workers' hands and contamination of white coats and scrubs. *Am J Infect Control.* 2012;40(9):e245-e248. [IIIA]

33. Butler DL, Major Y, Bearman G, Edmond MB. Transmission of nosocomial pathogens by white coats: an invitro model. *J Hosp Infect.* 2010;75(2):137-138. [IIIC]

34. Henderson J. The endangered white coat. *Clin Infect Dis.* 2010;50(7):1073-1074. [VB]

35. Kaplan C, Mendiola R, Ndjatou V, Chapnick E, Minkoff H. The role of covering gowns in reducing rates of bacterial contamination of scrub suits. *Am J Obstet Gynecol.* 2003;188(5):1154-1155. [IIC]

36. Loh W, Ng VV, Holton J. Bacterial flora on the white coats of medical students. *J Hosp Infect.* 2000;45(1):65-68. [IIB]

37. Banu A, Anand M, Nagi N. White coats as a vehicle for bacterial dissemination. *J Clin Diag Res.* 2012;6(8):1381-1384. [IIIA]

38. Amirfeyz R, Tasker A, Ali S, Bowker K, Blom A. Theatre shoes—a link in the common pathway of postoperative wound infection? *Ann R Coll Surg Engl.* 2007;89(6):605-608. [IIB]

39. 29 CFR §1910.136: Personal protective equipment: Occupational foot protection. Occupational Safety and Health Administration. https://www.osha.gov/pls/oshaweb/owadisp.show_document?p_table=standards&p_id=9786. Accessed September 19, 2014.

40. Barr J, Siegel D. Dangers of dermatologic surgery: protect your feet. *Dermatol Surg.* 2004;30(12 Pt 1):1495-1497. [IIB]

41. Occupational Safety and Health Administration. Toxic and Hazardous Substances: Bloodborne Pathogens, 29 CFR §1910.1030 (2012). Occupational Safety and Health Administration. http://www.osha.gov/pls/oshawewb/owadisp.show_document?p_table=STANDARDS&p_id=10051. Accessed September 19, 2014.

42. Siegel JD, Rhinehart E, Jackson M, Chiarello L; the Healthcare Infection Control Practices Advisory Committee. 2007 Guideline for Isolation Precautions: Preventing Transmission of Infectious Agents in Healthcare Settings. 2007. http://www.cdc.gov/ncidod/dhqp/pdf/isolation2007.pdf. Accessed September 19, 2014. [IVA]

43. White MC, Lynch P. Blood contact and exposures among operating room personnel: a multicenter study. *Am J Infect Control.* 1993;21(5):243-248. [IIIA]

44. Barbosa MH, Graziano KU. Influence of wearing time on efficacy of disposable surgical masks as microbial barrier. *Braz J Microbiol.* 2006;37(3):216-217. [IIB]

45. Kotsanas D, Scott C, Gillespie EE, Korman TM, Stuart RL. What's hanging around your neck? Pathogenic bacteria on identity badges and lanyards. *Med J Aust.* 2008;188(1):5-8. [IIA]

46. Saxena S, Singh T, Agarwal H, Mehta G, Dutta R. Bacterial colonization of rings and cell phones carried by health-care providers: are these mobile bacterial zoos in the hospital? *Trop Doct.* 2011;41(2):116-118. [IIB]

47. Bartlett GE, Pollard TC, Bowker KE, Bannister GC. Effect of jewelry on surface bacterial counts of operating theatres. *J Hosp Infect.* 2002;52(1):68-70. [IIB]

48. Field EA, McGowan P, Pearce PK, Martin MV. Rings and watches: should they be removed prior to operative dental procedures? *J Dent.* 1996;24(1-2):65-69. [IIB]

49. Kelsall NKR, Griggs RKL, Bowker KE, Bannister GC. Should finger rings be removed prior to scrubbing for theatre? *J Hosp Infect.* 2006;62(4):450-452. [IIB]

50. Jeans AR, Moore J, Nicol C, Bates C, Read RC. Wristwatch use and hospital-acquired infection. *J Hosp Infect.* 2010;74(1):16-21. [IIIA]

51. Salisbury DM, Hutfilz P, Treen LM, Bollin GE, Gautam S. The effect of rings on microbial load of health care workers' hands. *Am J Infect Control.* 1997;25(1):24-27. [IIIB]

52. Khodavaisy S, Nabili M, Davari B, Vahedi M. Evaluation of bacterial and fungal contamination in the health care workers' hands and rings in the intensive care unit. *Prev Med Hyg.* 2011;52(4):215-218. [IIIB]

53. Arrowsmith VA, Taylor R. Removal of nail polish and finger rings to prevent surgical infection. *Cochrane Database Syst Rev.* 2012;5:003325. [IA]

54. Trick WE, Vernon MO, Hayes RA, et al. Impact of ring wearing on hand contamination and comparison of hand hygiene agents in a hospital. *Clin Infect Dis.* 2003;36(11):1383-1390. [IIA]

55. Stein DT, Pankovich-Wargula AL. The dilemma of the wedding band. *Orthopedics.* 2009;32(2):86. [IIIC]

56. Wood MW, Lund RC, Stevenson KB. Bacterial contamination of stethoscopes with antimicrobial diaphragm covers. *Am J Infect Control.* 2007;35(4):263-266. [IIB]

57. Bernard L, Kereveur A, Durand D, et al. Bacterial contamination of hospital physicians' stethoscopes. *Infect Control Hosp Epidemiol.* 1999;20(9):626-628. [IIB]

58. Russell A, Secrest J, Schreeder C. Stethoscopes as a source of hospital-acquired methicillin-resistant Staphylococcus aureus. *J PeriAnesth Nurs.* 2012;27(2):82-87. [IIA]

59. Mehta AK, Halvosa JS, Gould CV, Steinberg JP. Efficacy of alcohol-based hand rubs in the disinfection of stethoscopes. *Infect Control Hosp Epidemiol.* 2010;31(8):870-872. [IIB]

60. Denholm JT, Levine A, Kerridge IH, Ashhurst-Smith C, Ferguson J, D'Este C. A microbiological survey of stethoscopes in Australian teaching hospitals: potential for nosocomial infection? *Aust Infect Control.* 2005;10(3):79. [IIA]

61. Waghorn DJ, Wan WY, Greaves C, Whittome N, Bosley HC, Cantrill S. Stethoscopes: a study of contamination and the effectiveness of disinfection procedures. *Br J Infect Control.* 2005;6(1):15-17. [IIB]

62. Gopinath KG, Stanley S, Mathai E, Chandy GM. Pagers and stethoscopes as vehicles of potential nosocomial pathogens in a tertiary care hospital in a developing country. *Trop Doct.* 2011;41(1):43-45. [IIIB]

63. Muniz J, Sethi RK, Zaghi J, Ziniel SI, Sandora TJ. Predictors of stethoscope disinfection among pediatric health care providers. *Am J Infect Control.* 2012;40(10):922-925. [IIIA]

64. Hyder O. Cross-sectional study of frequency and factors associated with stethoscope cleaning among medical practitioners in Pakistan. *East Mediterr Health J.* 2012;18(7):707-711. [IIIA]

65. Uneke CJ, Ogbonna A, Oyibo PG, Onu CM. Bacterial contamination of stethoscopes used by health workers: public health implications. *J Infect Develop Countries.* 2010;4(7):436-441. [IIIA]

66. Uneke CJ, Ogbonna A, Oyibo PG, Ekuma U. Bacteriological assessment of stethoscopes used by medical students in Nigeria: implications for nosocomial infection control. *World Health Popul.* 2008;10(4):53-61. [IIIB]

67. Bhatta DR, Gokhale S, Ansari MT, et al. Stethoscopes: a possible mode for transmission of nosocomial pathogens. *J Clin Diag Res.* 2012;5(6):1173-1176. [IIIB]

68. Campos-Murguia A, Leon-Lara X, Munoz JM, Macias AE, Alvarez JA. Stethoscopes as potential intrahospital carriers of pathogenic microorganisms. *Am J Infect Control.* 2013;42(1):82-83. [IIIB]

69. Worster AP, Srigley JA, Main CL. Examination of staphylococcal stethoscope contamination in the emergency department (pilot) study (EXSSCITED pilot study). *Can J Emerg Med.* 2011;13(4):239-244. [IIIB]

70. Williams C, Davis DL. Methicillin-resistant Staphylococcus aureus fomite survival. *Clin Lab Sci.* 2009;22(1):34-38. [IIIB]

71. Mitchell A, Dealwis N, Collins J, et al. Stethoscope or "staphoscope"? Infection by auscultation. *J Hosp Infect.* 2010;76(3):278-279. [IIIB]

72. Milam MW, Hall M, Pringle T, Buchanan K. Bacterial contamination of fabric stethoscope covers: the velveteen rabbit of health care? *Infect Control Hosp Epidemiol.* 2001;22(10):653-655. [IIIC]

73. Guideline for environmental cleaning. In: *Guidelines for Perioperative Practice.* Denver, CO: AORN, Inc; 2015:9-30. [IVA]

74. Feldman J, Feldman J, Feldman M. Women doctors' purses as an unrecognized fomite. *Del Med J.* 2012;84(9):277-280. [IIA]

75. Lankford MG, Collins S, Youngberg L, Rooney DM, Warren JR, Noskin GA. Assessment of materials commonly utilized in health care: implications for bacterial survival and transmission. *Am J Infect Control.* 2006;34(5):258-263. [IIIB]

76. Koca O, Altoparlak U, Ayyildiz A, Kaynar H. Persistence of nosocomial pathogens on various fabrics. *Eurasian J Med.* 2012;44(1):28-31. [IIIA]

77. Huang R, Mehta S, Weed D, Price CS. Methicillin-resistant Staphylococcus aureus survival on hospital fomites. *Infect Control Hosp Epidemiol.* 2006;27(11):1267-1269. [IIIC]

78. Malik YS, Allwood PB, Hedberg CW, Goyal SM. Disinfection of fabrics and carpets artificially contaminated with calicivirus: relevance in institutional and healthcare centres. *J Hosp Infect.* 2006;63(2):205-210. [IIIB]

79. McNeil E. Dissemination of microorganisms by fabrics and leather. *Dev Ind Microbiol.* 1964;5:30-35. [VB]

80. Datta P, Rani H, Chander J, Gupta V. Bacterial contamination of mobile phones of health care workers. *Indian J Med Microbiol.* 2009;27(3):279-281. [IB]

81. Kilic IH, Ozaslan M, Karagoz ID, Zer Y, Davutoglu V. The microbial colonisation of mobile phone used by healthcare staffs. *Pak J Biol Sci.* 2009;12(11):882-884. [IIA]

82. Albrecht UV, von Jan U, Sedlacek L, Groos S, Suerbaum S, Vonberg RP. Standardized, app-based disinfection of iPads in a clinical and nonclinical setting: comparative analysis. *J Med Internet Res.* 2013;15(8):e176. [IIA]

83. Al-Abdalall AH. Isolation and identification of microbes associated with mobile phones in Dammam in eastern Saudi Arabia. *J Family Community Med.* 2010;17(1):11-14. [IIIA]

84. Brady RR, Chitnis S, Stewart RW, Graham C, Yalamarthi S, Morris K. NHS connecting for health: healthcare professionals, mobile technology, and infection control. *Telemed J E-Health.* 2012;18(4):289-291. [IIIB]

85. Tekerekoglu MS, Duman Y, Serindag A, et al. Do mobile phones of patients, companions and visitors carry multidrug-resistant hospital pathogens? *Am J Infect Control.* 2011;39(5):379-381. [IIIA]

86. Sadat-Ali M, Al-Omran AK, Azam Q, et al. Bacterial flora on cell phones of health care providers in a teaching institution. *Am J Infect Control.* 2010;38(5):404-405. [IIIA]

87. Akinyemi KO, Atapu AD, Adetona OO, Coker AO. The potential role of mobile phones in the spread of bacterial infections. *J Infect Dev Countries.* 2009;3(8):628-632. [IIIB]

88. Basol R, Beckel J, Gilsdorf-Gracie J, et al. You missed a spot! Disinfecting shared mobile phones. *Nurs Manage.* 2013;44(7):16-18. [IIIC]

89. White S, Topping A, Humphreys P, Rout S, Williamson H. The cross-contamination potential of mobile telephones. *J Res Nurs.* 2012;17(6):582-595. [IIIB]

90. Ustun C, Cihangiroglu M. Health care workers' mobile phones: a potential cause of microbial cross-contamination between hospitals and community. *J Occup Environ Hyg.* 2012;9(9):538-542. [IIIB]

91. Singh A, Purohit B. Mobile phones in hospital settings: a serious threat to infection. *Occup Health Saf.* 2012;81(3):42-44. [VA]

92. Gerba CP, Kennedy D. Enteric virus survival during household laundering and impact of disinfection with sodium hypochlorite. *Appl Environ Microbiol.* 2007;73(14):4425-4428. [IIA]

93. Lis DO, Pacha JZ, Idzik D. Methicillin resistance of airborne coagulase-negative staphylococci in homes of persons having contact with a hospital environment. *Am J Infect Control.* 2009;37(3):177-182. [IIIB]

94. Twomey CL, Beitz H Johnson BJ. Bacterial contamination of surgical scrubs and laundering mechanisms: infection control implications. *Infection Control Today.* http://www.arta1.com/cms/uploads/Bacterial%20Contamination%20of%20Surgical%20Scrubs%20and%20Laundering%20Mechanisms_%20Infection%20Control%20Implications.pdf. Posted October 19, 2009. Accessed on September 23, 2014. [IIIB]

95. Wright SN, Gerry JS, Busowski MT, et al. Gordonia bronchialis sternal wound infection in 3 patients following open heart surgery: intraoperative transmission from a healthcare worker. *Infect Control Hosp Epidemiol.* 2012;33(12):1238-1241. [VA]

96. Fijan S, Turk SS. Hospital textiles, are they a possible vehicle for healthcare-associated infections? *Int J Environ Res Public Health.* 2012;9(9):3330-3343. [VA]

97. Halliwell C. Nurses' uniforms: off the radar. A review of guidelines and laundering practices. *Healthc Infect.* 2012;17(1):18-24. [VA]

98. Nguyen DB, Gupta N, Abou-Daoud A, et al. A polymicrobial outbreak of surgical site infections following cardiac surgery at a community hospital in Florida, 2011-2012. *Am J Infect Control.* 2014;42(4):432-435. [VB]

99. Orr KE, Holliday MG, Jones AL, Robson I, Perry JD. Survival of enterococci during hospital laundry processing. *J Hosp Infect.* 2002;50(2):133-139. [IIA]

100. Sasahara T, Hayashi S, Morisawa Y, Sakihama T, Yoshimura A, Hirai Y. Bacillus cereus bacteremia outbreak due to contaminated hospital linens. *Eur J Clin Microbiol Infect Dis.* 2011;30(2):219-226. [VB]

101. Al-Benna S. Laundering of theatre scrubs at home. *J Periop Pract.* 2010;20(11):392-396. [VA]

102. Belkin NL. Masks, barriers, laundering, and gloving: where is the evidence? *AORN J.* 2006;84(4):655-657. [VB]

103. Belkin NL. Laundry day: processing linens, textiles and uniforms. *Health Facil Manage.* 2010;23(3):36-38. [VC]

104. Heinzel M, Kyas A, Weide M, Breves R, Bockmühl DP. Evaluation of the virucidal performance of domestic laundry procedures. *Int J Hyg Environ Health.* 2010;213(5):334-337. [IIIB]

105. Lakdawala N, Pham J, Shah M, Holton J. Effectiveness of low-temperature domestic laundry on the decontamination of healthcare workers' uniforms. *Infect Control Hosp Epidemiol.* 2011;32(11):1103-1108. [IIIA]

106. Nordstrom JM, Reynolds KA, Gerba CP. Comparison of bacteria on new, disposable, laundered, and unlaundered hospital scrubs. *Am J Infect Control.* 2012;40(6):539-543. [IIIA]

107. Patel SN, Murray-Leonard J, Wilson AP. Laundering of hospital staff uniforms at home. *J Hosp Infect.* 2006;62(1):89-93. [IIA]

108. Wilson JA, Loveday HP, Hoffman PN, Pratt RJ. Uniform: an evidence review of the microbiological significance of uniforms and uniform policy in the prevention and control of healthcare-associated infections. Report to the Department of Health (England). *J Hosp Infect.* 2007;66(4):301-307. [VA]

109. Perry C, Marshall R, Jones E. Bacterial contamination of uniforms. *J Hosp Infect.* 2001;48(3):238-241. [IIIB]

110. *Accreditation Standards for Processing Reusable Textiles for Use in Healthcare Facilities.* 2011 ed. Frankfort, IL: Healthcare Laundry Accreditation Council; 2011.

111. Protecting Workers' Families—DHHS(NIOSH) Pub No. 2002-113. National Institutes for Occupational Safety and Health. http://www.cdc.gov/niosh/docs/2002-113/2002-113.html. Accessed September 19, 2014. [VB]

112. *ANSI/AAMI. ST65 2008/(R) 2013: Processing of Reusable Surgical textiles for Use in Health Care Facilities.* 2013. Arlington, VA: Association for the Advancement of Medical Instrumentation; 2013. [IVC]

113. Callaghan I. Bacterial contamination of nurses' uniforms: a study. *Nurs Stand.* 1998;13(1):37-42. [IIIB]

114. 29 CFR §1910.132: General requirements. Occupational Safety and Health Administration. https://www.osha.gov/pls/oshaweb/owadisp.show_document?p_id=9777&p_table=STANDARDS. Accessed September 19, 2014.

115. Summers MM, Lynch PF, Black T. Hair as a reservoir of staphylococci. *J Clin Path.* 1965;18(13):13-15. [IIB]

116. Dineen P, Drusin L. Epidemics of postoperative wound infections associated with hair carriers. *Lancet.* 1973;2(7839):1157-1159. [VA]

117. Mastro TD, Farley TA, Elliott JA, et al. An outbreak of surgical-wound infections due to group A streptococcus carried on the scalp. *N Engl J Med.* 1990;323(14):968-972. [IIIB]

118. McHugh SM, Corrigan MA, Hill AD, Humphreys H. Surgical attire, practices and their perception in the prevention of surgical site infection. *Surgeon.* 2014;12(1):47-52. [VA]

119. Eisen DB. Surgeon's garb and infection control: what's the evidence? *J Am Acad Dermatol.* 2011;64(5):960.e1-960.e20. [VA]

120. Mase K, Hasegawa T, Horii T, et al. Firm adherence of Staphylococcus aureus and Staphylococcus epidermidis to human hair and effect of detergent treatment. *Microbiol Immunol.* 2000;44(8):653-656. [IIB]

121. McLure HA, Mannam M, Talboys CA, Azadian BS, Yentis SM. The effect of facial hair and sex on the dispersal of bacteria below a masked subject. *Anaesthesia.* 2000;55(2):173-176. [IIIC]

122. Owers KL, James E, Bannister GC. Source of bacterial shedding in laminar flow theatres. *J Hosp Infect.* 2004;58(3):230-232. [IIIC]

123. Occupational exposure to bloodborne pathogens. OSHA Final rule. *Fed Regist.* 1991;56(235):64004-64182.

Acknowledgements

LEAD AUTHOR
Lisa Spruce, DNP, RN, ACNS, ACNP, ANP, CNOR
Director of Evidence-based Perioperative Practice
AORN Nursing Department
Denver, Colorado

CO-AUTHOR
Sharon A. Van Wicklin, MSN, RN, CNOR, CRNFA, CPSN, PLNC
Perioperative Nursing Specialist
AORN Nursing Department
Denver, Colorado

CONTRIBUTING AUTHOR
Ramona L. Conner, MSN, RN, CNOR
Manager, Standards and Guidelines
AORN Nursing Department
Denver, Colorado

The authors and AORN thank Paula Berrett, BS CRCST, Utah Valley Regional Medical Center, Provo Utah, International Association of Healthcare Centra Service Material Management liaison to the AORN Guidelines Advisory Board; Angela Hewett, MD, MS University of Nebraska Medical Center, Omaha Nebraska, Society for Healthcare Epidemiology o America liaison to the AORN Guidelines Advisory Board; Antonia B. Hughes, MA, BSN, RN, CNOR, Peri operative Education Specialist, Baltimore Washington Medical Center, Glen Burnie, Maryland; Deborah Mulloy, PhD, RN, CNOR, Brigham & Womens Hospi tal, Newtonville, Massachusetts; Janice A. Neil, RN PhD, American Association of Colleges of Nursing Leadership Fellow, Associate Professor and Chair Department of Undergraduate Nursing Science, Eas Carolina University College of Nursing, Greenville North Carolina; and Marcia R. Patrick, MSN, RN, CIC Association for Professionals in Infection Control and Epidemiology liaison to the AORN Guidelines Advi sory Board and Independent Consultant, Tacoma Washington, for their assistance in developing thi guideline.

PUBLICATION HISTORY
Originally published March 1975, *AORN Journal,* a AORN "Standards for proper OR wearing apparel. Format revision March 1978, July 1982.

Revised March 1984, March 1990. Published as pro posed recommended practices, August 1994.

Revised November 1998; published December 1998 Reformatted July 2000.

Revised November 2004; published in *Standard: Recommended Practices, and Guidelines,* 2005 edi tion. Reprinted February 2005, *AORN Journal.*

Revised October 2010 for online publication in *Perioperative Standards and Recommended Practices*.

Reformatted September 2012 for publication in *Perioperative Standards and Recommended Practices*, 2013 edition.

Revised September 2014 for online publication in *Perioperative Standards and Recommended Practices*.

Minor editing revisions made in November 2014 for publication in *Guidelines for Perioperative Practice*, 2015 edition.

Evidence ratings revised in *Guidelines for Perioperative Practice*, 2018 edition, to conform to the current AORN Evidence Rating Model.

ASEPTIC PRACTICE

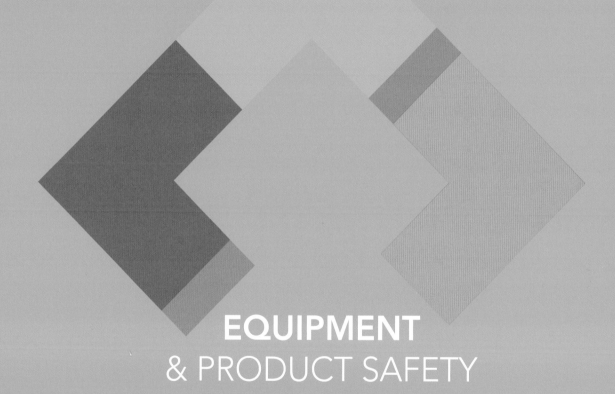

EQUIPMENT
& PRODUCT SAFETY

GUIDELINE FOR SAFE USE OF ENERGY-GENERATING DEVICES

The Guideline for Safe Use of Energy-Generating Devices has been approved by the AORN Guidelines Advisory Board. It was presented as a proposed guideline for comments by members and others. The guideline is effective September 1, 2016. The recommendations in the guideline are intended to be achievable and represent what is believed to be an optimal level of practice. Policies and procedures will reflect variations in practice settings and/or clinical situations that determine the degree to which the guideline can be implemented. AORN recognizes the many diverse settings in which perioperative nurses practice; therefore, this guideline is adaptable to all areas where operative or other invasive procedures may be performed.

Purpose

This document provides guidance to the perioperative team for the safe use and maintenance of energy-generating devices. The types of energy addressed in this document include electricity delivered as radio-frequency waves, ultrasound, and laser.[1,2] The devices that generate the energy include electrosurgical units (ESUs), electrocauteries, ultrasonic instruments, and lasers. The energy produced is transferred to the patient by various methods, including monopolar, bipolar, advanced bipolar (eg, vessel-sealing),[3] and tripolar (eg, plasma knife) devices[4]; class 3 and class 4 lasers; and ultrasound (eg, ultrasonic tissue ablation system, phacoemulsification) and argon-enhanced coagulation (AEC) modalities.

Electrosurgery, which uses high-frequency (ie, radio-frequency) electrical current, is routinely used to cut, coagulate, dissect, ablate, and shrink tissue. Ultrasonic dissectors fragment tissue by vibration. Vessel-sealing or bipolar ligating-cutting devices use a combination of pressure and heat to permanently fuse vessels and tissue.[5] In the literature, the terms *electrosurgery, electrocautery*, and *diathermy* are often used interchangeably. This guideline addresses precautions to be taken during the use of each of these technologies and does not endorse any specific products. Proper care and handling of all energy-generating devices is essential to patient and personnel safety.

This document provides guidance for some elements of surgical fires and electrical safety related to energy-generating devices. For additional guidance on these two topics, the reader should refer to the AORN Guideline for a Safe Environment of Care, Part 1.[6]

The following subjects are outside the scope of this guideline:
- surgical smoke safety,
- endoscopic distention fluid (See the AORN Guideline for Minimally Invasive Surgery),[7]
- procedure-related decisions (eg, the amount of time the tissue is exposed to the energy-generating device active electrode),
- therapeutic diathermy,
- use of electrical dental equipment (eg, battery-operated curing lights, ultrasonic baths, ultrasonic scalers, electric pulp testers, electric toothbrushes), and
- selection of electrosurgical devices.

Evidence Review

A medical librarian conducted a systematic search of the databases MEDLINE®, CINAHL®, and Scopus® and the Cochrane Database of Systematic Reviews in October 2015. Results were limited to literature published in English from January 2009 through October 2015. The medical librarian also established alerts at the time of the initial search. During the development of the guideline, the lead author requested supplementary searches and additional articles that either did not fit the original search criteria or were discovered during the evidence appraisal process. The results of alerts were considered until February 2016.

The search terms included subject headings and keywords that address precautions and injuries related to the use of electrosurgical and laser devices. Terms for procedures included *electrosurgery, ultrasonic therapy, ultrasonic surgical procedures, diathermy, argon plasma coagulation, electrocoagulation, high-intensity focused ultrasound ablation, endometrial ablation techniques*, and *laser therapy*. Subject headings and keywords related to precautions included *adverse effects, accident prevention, patient safety, equipment contamination, equipment safety, equipment failure*, and *risk management*. Special attention was paid to terms that would retrieve literature addressing the potential causes and effects of equipment failure and injuries. Such terms included *burns, fires, implantable electronic devices* (eg, *artificial pacemaker, implanted electrodes, electromagnetic fields*), and *power sources and settings* (eg, *electric power supplies, grounding, capacitive coupling, electric wiring*). Subject headings and keywords for types of personal protective equipment and occupational hazards also were included.

Excluded were non-peer-reviewed publications, evidence from other disciplines when evidence from the perioperative setting was available, and case reports that did not provide recommendations for preventing injuries related to the use of electrosurgical devices. Editorials, news items, and other brief items were excluded. Lower-level or lower-quality

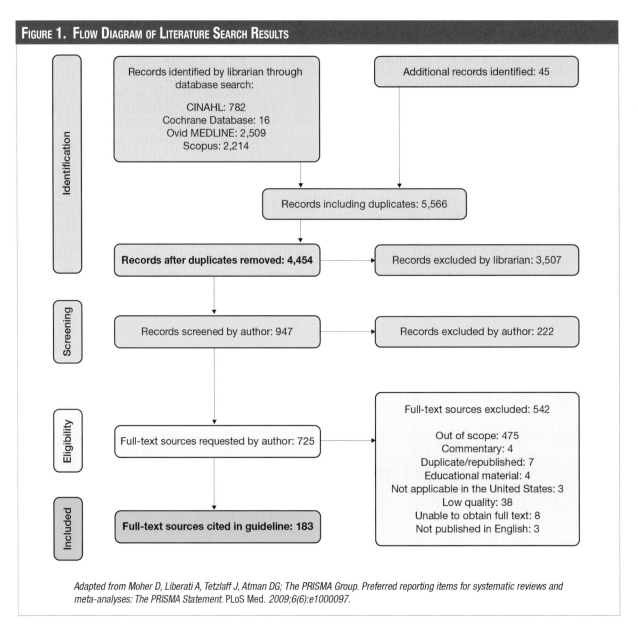

FIGURE 1. FLOW DIAGRAM OF LITERATURE SEARCH RESULTS

Records identified by librarian through database search:

CINAHL: 782
Cochrane Database: 16
Ovid MEDLINE: 2,509
Scopus: 2,214

Additional records identified: 45

Records including duplicates: 5,566

Records after duplicates removed: 4,454

Records excluded by librarian: 3,507

Records screened by author: 947

Records excluded by author: 222

Full-text sources requested by author: 725

Full-text sources excluded: 542

Out of scope: 475
Commentary: 4
Duplicate/republished: 7
Educational material: 4
Not applicable in the United States: 3
Low quality: 38
Unable to obtain full text: 8
Not published in English: 3

Full-text sources cited in guideline: 183

Identification / Screening / Eligibility / Included

Adapted from Moher D, Liberati A, Tetzlaff J, Atman DG; The PRISMA Group. Preferred reporting items for systematic reviews and meta-analyses: The PRISMA Statement. PLoS Med. 2009;6(6):e1000097.

evidence was excluded when higher-level or higher-quality evidence was available (Figure 1).

Articles identified by the search were provided to the project team for evaluation. The team consisted of the lead author and three evidence appraisers. The lead author divided the search results into topics and assigned members of the team to review and critically appraise each article using the AORN Research or Non-Research Evidence Appraisal Tools as appropriate. The literature was independently evaluated and appraised according to the strength and quality of the evidence. Each article was then assigned an appraisal score. The appraisal score is noted in brackets after each reference, as applicable.

The collective evidence supporting each intervention within a specific recommendation was summarized and the AORN Evidence Rating Model was used to rate the strength of the evidence. Factors considered in the review of the collective evidence

were the quality of the evidence, the quantity of similar evidence on a given topic, and the consistency of evidence supporting a recommendation. The evidence rating is noted in brackets after each intervention.

Note: *The evidence summary table is available at http://www.aorn.org/evidencetables/.*

Editor's note: *MEDLINE is a registered trademark of the US National Library of Medicine's Medical Literature Analysis and Retrieval System, Bethesda, MD. CINAHL, Cumulative Index to Nursing and Allied Health Literature, is a registered trademark of EBSCO Industries, Birmingham, AL. Scopus is a registered trademark of Elsevier B.V., Amsterdam, The Netherlands.*

Recommendation I

Precautions should be taken to mitigate the risk for injury to patients and personnel during the use of energy-generating devices.

The collective evidence contains reports of incidents in which patients undergoing various procedures were injured by the use of energy-generating devices.[8-23]

In a descriptive study, Overbey et al[15] reviewed reports to the Manufacturer and User Facility Device Experience (MAUDE) database from January 1, 1994, to December 31, 2013, and found 3,553 injuries and 178 deaths related to energy-generating devices. The energy-generating devices were classified as monopolar "Bovie" instruments (n = 1,670; 44.8%), radio-frequency/microwave ablation devices (n = 728, 19.5%), advanced bipolar devices (n = 538, 14.4%), ultrasonic devices (n = 350, 9.3%), bipolar instruments (n = 270, 7.2%), plasma beam monopolar devices (n = 163, 4.4%), and other (n = 12, 0.3%). The incidents involved thermal burns (n = 2,353, 63.1%), hemorrhage (n = 642, 17.2%), mechanical failure (n = 442, 11.8%), and fire (n = 294, 7.9%). The authors concluded that the risk for injury from surgical energy-generating devices is significant and warrants further research and education.

A review of the MAUDE database by Tremaine and Avram[17] identified 1,212 adverse events resulting from the use of various energy-generating devices in a dermatological setting. The reported injuries to patients included blistering, burns, scarring, changes in skin color, fat loss, and nerve palsy. The devices listed included lasers and electrosurgical devices.

I.a.　Fire safety precautions should be followed during the use of energy-generating devices (See the AORN Guideline for a Safe Environment of Care, Part 1).[6] *[3: Moderate Evidence]*

The collective evidence identifies energy-creating devices as an ignition source.[8,10-14,16,18,19,23-27] In an analysis of 5,297 surgical malpractice claims from 1985 to 2009 in the American Society of Anesthesiologists Closed Claims Database, Mehta et al[9] found 103 claims related to surgical fires. Electrosurgical devices were found to be the ignition source in 93 of the claims. The remaining sources of ignition included lasers (n = 9) and a defibrillator (n = 1).

Smith and Roy[24] surveyed 8,523 members of the American Academy of Otolaryngology—Head and Neck Surgery to obtain information regarding the characteristics and the frequency of OR fires in otolaryngology. Eighty-eight of the 349 surgeons who responded to the survey reported having witnessed at least one OR fire during their careers. For the total of 106 fires reported, the ignition source was an electrosurgical unit (59%), a laser (32%), or a light cord (7%). The researchers concluded that OR fires occur during many procedures and that electro-surgical devices are the most frequent sources of ignition.

I.a.1.　Fire safety precautions to take with all energy-generating devices include
- using technologies other than monopolar or laser devices (eg, bipolar, coblation technology, non-energy applying instruments) in situations determined to be high risk during the fire risk assessment[16,28-31]; *[3: Moderate Evidence]*
- using water-soluble lubricants (eg, eye lubricant) near the surgical site[29,30]; *[3: Moderate Evidence]*
- using moist sponges near the ignition source[11-13,16,26,27,29,30,32,33]; *[2: High Evidence]*
- prohibiting the use of alcohol-soaked sponges on the surgical field[14]; *[4: Limited Evidence]* and
- stopping delivery of oxygen or decreasing the percentage to the lowest tolerable level before activating an energy-generating device near the head, face, or neck.[26,29,32] *[1: Strong Evidence]*

Matt and Cottee[28] conducted a descriptive laboratory study in which they placed a bipolar radio-frequency ablation device in direct contact with flammable materials found in the OR (ie, alcohol, four individual salt packets dissolved in alcohol, two pumps of ethanol-based foam hand sanitizer, saline-dampened gauze, plastic packaging filled with 5 mL of saline, a 4.0 endotracheal tube with 100% oxygen flowing through the tube). The researchers found that the device did not ignite the various materials even when set at the highest settings (ie, 9 ablation, 5 coagulation). The authors concluded that the tested bipolar radio-frequency ablation device did not produce an adequate amount of heat to serve as an ignition source at the surgical site, therefore decreasing the potential for fire.

In a laboratory study, Roy and Smith[31] compared the time to ignition of a chicken (as a human tissue surrogate) when using a standard monopolar device at 15 watts (W) coagulate mode versus a bipolar radio-frequency ablation wand set at 9, 7, and 3 in the ablate mode. An endotracheal tube was inserted into the gut of the chicken, with 100% oxygen flowing through the tube. Contact between the chicken and the device was made near the end of the endotracheal tube. Ignition occurred after 25 to 80 seconds during use of the monopolar device, and no ignition occurred during use of the bipolar device. The researchers concluded that use of a bipolar radio-frequency ablation device eliminates the risk for fire during open cavity surgery.

131

Dhar et al[27] conducted a descriptive laboratory study to determine the difference in time to ignition of dry and moistened neurosurgical patties. At 5 W of laser fire and 50% oxygen, the dry patties ignited in an average of 2.3 seconds and the moist patties ignited in an average of 63.9 seconds. The researchers recommended that only moist patties be used near the laser target area.

I.a.2. Precautions should be taken to mitigate the risk for fire or injury associated with the use of electrocautery devices (eg, battery-powered, hand held devices), including
- applying the protective cap when the cautery is not in use and
- removing the wire loop before discarding the device.[34]

[3: Moderate Evidence]

Unintentional activation of a battery-powered, hand-held cautery unit after disposal has been reported to cause a fire.[34] Axelrod et al[35] described four cases in which the electrocautery device was identified as the ignition source of a fire.

I.b. Precautions for electrical safety should be followed during the use of energy-generating devices (See the AORN Guideline for a Safe Environment of Care, Part 1).[6] *[3: Moderate Evidence]*

I.b.1. Containers of liquids should not be placed on energy-generating devices. *[5: Benefits Balanced with Harms]*

Liquids entering the energy-generating device may cause unintentional activation, device failure, or an electrical hazard.

I.b.2. Foot pedal accessories should be encased in a fluid-resistant cover when there is potential for fluid spills. *[5: Benefits Balanced with Harms]*

I.b.3. Safety and warning alarms and activation indicators should be operational, audible, and visible at all times. *[3: Moderate Evidence]*

Safety and warning alarms alert the operator to potential equipment failure. The indicators and alarms immediately alert the perioperative team when the energy-generating device is activated.[36]

I.c. The device manufacturer's instructions for use (IFU) should be readily available to users. *[5: Benefits Balanced with Harms]*

I.d. The energy-generating device inspection, preventative maintenance, and repair should be performed by a qualified individual in accordance with the manufacturer's IFU and documented according and health care organization policy.[36-40] *[3: Moderate Evidence]*

Periodic preventive maintenance helps support continued safe operation of energy-generating devices.

I.e. The lowest power setting that achieves the desired result should be selected. *[3: Moderate Evidence]*

The collective evidence[11,12,21,25,36,41-71] supports use of the lowest power setting needed to achieve the desired effect. However, the authors of one descriptive study stated that high power settings used during radio-frequency ablation are safe and increase efficacy.[72]

In a randomized controlled trial, Maurins et al[41] compared the amount of analgesic medication required after an endovenous laser ablation using 15 W to the amount required after laser ablation using 25 W. Forty patients undergoing an endovenous laser ablation for an incompetent greater saphenous vein were randomly and equally divided into two groups. The control group was treated using a laser set at 15 W and the study group was treated with a laser set at 25 W. On postoperative days two through 10, the mean number of analgesic tablets taken by the control group was 2.6 and the mean number taken by the study group was 4.6. The researchers concluded that the patients had less pain when a power setting of 15 W was used.

Jones et al[43] found that damage from antenna coupling is decreased with the use of low power settings. In a laboratory study, the researchers measured the tissue temperature in a bovine liver. An L-hook device was used as the active electrode, and an unlit 10-mm laparoscope was used as the instrument receiving the coupled energy. The researchers used a generator set at 15 W or 30 W. The tissue temperature increase was 24.7° C (76.5° F) less at the end of the laparoscope when the lower power setting was used. The researchers recommended using the lowest power setting possible during laparoscopic procedures to decrease the risk of antenna coupling.

Using an ultrasonic scalpel at low power settings is supported in a descriptive study by Druzijanic et al.[55] The researchers measured tissue lateral thermal damage after use of an ultrasonic scalpel (output power of 3 and 5) on 100 patients who underwent peritoneal surgery. Secondary results of the study reported only in the results section of the article and not included in the conclusion or discussion section showed there was significantly less thermal damage with the ultrasonic scalpel at an output power of 3 than at an output power of 5. The thermal damage at an output power of 3 was 90.42 µm and at an output power of 5 was 127.48 µm.

Mantke et al found[73] similar results in a descriptive study. The researchers sealed porcine carotid vessels using an ultrasonic shear set at an output power of 1 (n = 108), power of 3 (n = 114), or power of 5 (n = 125). After the sealing was complete, they tested the failure rate of the seal. In the discussion of the results, the researchers noted that vessels sealed at the power setting of 1 had an initial seal rate failure of 2.44% and vessels sealed at the power setting of 5 had a 10% failure rate. The researchers recommended that a power setting of 1 to 3 be used to seal vessels between 2 mm to 5 mm in diameter.

Munro[56] conducted a laboratory comparative study to identify mechanisms of thermal injury to the lower genital tract during radio-frequency resectoscopic surgery. He used a tissue model to represent the uterus and created defects in the electrode insulation. He found that injuries with a higher severity score resulted from coupling with higher power settings (ie, cut setting at 300 W and coagulation setting at 120 W) than coupling with lower power settings (ie, cut setting at 120 W and coagulation setting at 60 W). Munro concluded that injuries with a higher severity score resulted when a higher power setting was used.

Mitchell et al[57] conducted a laboratory descriptive study to determine the amount of undesirable tissue effect (ie, depth of tissue debridement plus depth of chondrocyte death in underlying cartilage) on bovine patella, using a radio-frequency energy generator set at power settings of 50 W or 110 W during a simulated thermal chondroplasty. The higher power setting resulted in a greater undesirable tissue effect (249 µm to 607 µm) than the lower power setting (121 µm to 364 µm). The researchers concluded that the lowest power setting should be used to reduce undesired tissue injury.

Lowe et al[58] performed a prospective cohort study involving 8,465 patients undergoing tonsillectomy with cold steel dissection and bipolar radio-frequency power for hemostasis. The researchers found the rate of hemorrhage in patients was 1.8% with use of the lowest power settings (6 W to 8 W) and 3.7% when the power settings were above 18 W. The researchers concluded that the risk for postoperative hemorrhage is greater when the bipolar power is increased in patients undergoing tonsillectomy with cold steel dissection and bipolar radio-frequency power for hemostasis.

Kaspar et al[59] conducted an experimental ex vivo study using surgically removed saphenous trunks. The researchers used the number of perforations as the indicator for complications. A higher rate of perforations was found in the vessels that were treated with a laser set at 15 W of power compared to the vessels treated with 8 W to 12 W of power. A limitation of this study was that the results were only presented in a graph and no statistical values were provided. The researchers suggested that low or medium power settings (8 W to 12 W) with slower pull-back speed of the laser fiber (0.2 mm/second to 2 mm/second) will achieve vein shrinkage and adequate obliteration of veins and result in fewer perforations.

Itoi et al[60] measured the effects of radio-frequency ablation with various power settings and exposure times on ex vivo pig livers. The researchers measured the size of the ablation area at 5 W, 10 W, 15 W, and 20 W with each setting applied for 60, 90, and 120 seconds. The researchers found that higher power settings and longer exposure times both resulted in an increased ablation area. The researchers recommended that the time of exposure and the power settings be based on the size of the masses, using this study's results as a basis for the decision.

Huang et al[61] conducted a descriptive study to determine the effects (ie, amount and depth of cell death) of various of bipolar radio-frequency power settings (ie, 2, 4 and 6) and times of application (ie, 2, 5, and 10 seconds) on explanted human articular cartilage. The researchers found that chondrocyte mortality during the treatment time of 2 seconds at a power setting of level 2 was significantly lower compared with the longer durations or when a higher level of power was used. The researchers recommended that a power setting of 2 for 2 seconds be used during arthroscopy procedures.

Goulet et al[62] conducted a blinded quasi-experimental study to determine the relationship between the depth and area of injury and the power setting and duration of energy application. The researchers performed colposcopies on swine and cauterized the colon using an argon plasma coagulator set at 10 W, 20 W, 40 W, and 60 W. Each setting was administered for 1, 3, and 5 seconds. After euthanizing the swine, the researchers examined the amount of deep tissue damage in the colon. They found the depth and the surface of the injury was significantly correlated to the amount of energy delivered. Based on this information, the researchers recommended that the lowest power setting and the lowest duration of energy application be used.

In a laboratory study using fresh bovine muscle fascia, Hefermehl et al[74] measured the thermal spread of two monopolar instruments at power settings of 30 W, 60 W, and 90 W for a 1-second application time. The researchers found the thermal spread of the monopolar devices were

- 16.8 mm and 8.8 mm, respectively, at 30 W;
- 3.5 mm and 2.5 mm at 60 W; and
- 16.8 mm and 8.8 mm at 90 W.

The researchers found a similar increase in the thermal spread using an ultrasonic instrument. The ultrasonic instrument was tested at 1, 3, and 5 power settings for a 1-second duration with spreads of 1.1 mm, 1.3 mm, and 1.8 mm,

ENERGY-GENERATING DEVICES

respectively. They concluded that procedures should be started at the lowest settings. Sutton et al[63] obtained similar results for thermal spread using monopolar and ultrasonic instruments in porcine tissue. They reached the same conclusions as Hefermehl et al.[74]

Govekar et al[65] conducted a laboratory study to determine whether monopolar power settings affected the functionality of a pacemaker in the heart of a pig. The researchers measured the number of missed beats when the active electrode was activated at 30 W or 60 W for 5 seconds at a distance of 7.5 cm from the generator. The researchers found a mean of 2.3 beats were dropped when the power setting was 60 W versus 1.6 beats at 30 W. The researchers concluded that the lowest power setting possible should be used. A limitation of this study is that only one pacemaker was studied, and the results may not be generalizable to all pacemaker types or models.

Martinek et al[44] performed a quasi-experimental study that examined the connection between the development of esophageal ulcerations and generator power settings during radio-frequency ablation. The researchers assigned the patients to one of three groups: a control group that received 25 W of power with long duration (n = 70), a group that received 25 W with short duration (n = 35), and a group that received 15 W with long duration (n = 35). One patient in both the control group and the 25 W/short duration group experienced ulceration compared with no patients in the 15 W group. The researchers concluded that lower energy settings may provide an increase in safety without loss of efficacy.

In a laboratory study, Robinson et al[45] examined the effect of monopolar electrosurgical devices on cardiac implanted electronic devices (CIEDs) in pigs. The researchers measured the amount of electromagnetic interference (EMI) present after they changed the power from 60 W to 30 W. They found significantly less EMI when the power was at 30 W. The researchers concluded that a low power setting should be used in the presence of CIEDs.

An expert opinion recommended that low ESU power settings be used for both cutting and coagulation to reduce the likelihood of insulation failure and capacitive coupling injuries. Low power settings minimize tissue damage from direct coupling when the active electrode is activated in close proximity to another metal device inserted into an adjacent trocar port.[49]

The findings of a study by Metzner et al[72] conflicted with the studies presented above. The researchers assigned 30 patients undergoing endoscopic pulmonary vein isolation using an endoscopic ablation system equally to one of three groups:

- in Group 1, ablation was performed at power settings of 5.5 W and 7.0 W;
- in Group 2, ablation was performed at power settings of 7.0 W and 8.5 W; and
- in Group 3, ablation was performed at power settings of 8.5 W and 10.0 W.

Pulmonary vein isolation was successfully performed in each of the groups (69% in Group 1, 73% in Group 2, 90% in Group 3). One patient in each of Groups 2 and 3 developed esophageal thermal lesions but none were reported in Group 1. The researchers concluded that higher energy settings increase efficacy and are safe to use. They also stated that the study was small and further research should be conducted before final conclusions can be drawn.

I.e.1. The RN circulator should confirm the power settings with the operator before the energy-generating device is activated.[69] *[4: Limited Evidence]*

I.f. The energy-generating device foot pedal activation switch should only be activated by the person in control of the energy-delivering hand piece (eg, ESU active electrode, laser hand piece, ultrasonic wand).[36,69] *[3: Moderate Evidence]*

Activation by the operator of the active electrode prevents unintentional discharge of the device, which minimizes the potential for patient and personnel injury.

I.g. Energy-generating devices should be turned off at the end of the procedure. *[Benefits Balanced with Harms]*

Turning off energy-generating devices may help to prevent an error in power settings for the next procedure and may help to conserve energy and the life of the machine.

I.h. Energy-generating device cords should be secured to the sterile drapes
- with a plastic or other non-conductive device,[36]
- with a non-piercing device, and
- in a manner which does not crush or damage the cord.

[3: Moderate Evidence]

Plastic devices do not conduct electricity if there is leakage. Use of a non-piercing device decreases the potential of contaminating the sterile field by making holes in the drapes. Crushing or damaging the cords may create a place at which the current can escape from the cord, creating a fire on the drapes or causing the device to malfunction.

I.i. Energy-generating device accessories should be inspected for damage (eg, insulation breakage) before and after use and, if reusable, during decontamination and package assembly.[69] *[3: Moderate Evidence]*

Breaks in electrosurgical active electrode internal wires have been reported to cause procedure delays (eg, while replacement equipment is obtained), injury to staff members or patients, and ignition of surgical drapes or clinicians' gowns.[38,75-77]

I.i.1. The number of sterilization cycles should be confirmed for reusable accessory cords before sterilization, and if the maximum number of cycles has been reached, the cord should be handled per the manufacturer's IFU. *[5: Benefits Balanced with Harms]*

Manufacturers' IFU contain instructions on the maximum number of sterilization cycles at which integrity testing has been performed.

I.i.2. Energy-generating device accessories that are not working properly or are damaged should be removed from service immediately and reported to the individual responsible for equipment maintenance (eg, a bioengineering services representative).[69] *[4: Limited Evidence]*

I.j. Energy-generating devices should be inspected before initial use within the facility and should undergo periodic preventive maintenance, per the manufacturer's IFU, by a designated and trained individual (eg, a biomedical engineering services representative).[54,69,78-80] *[3: Moderate Evidence]*

I.j.1. Energy-generating devices that are not working properly or are damaged should be removed from service immediately and reported to the individual responsible for equipment maintenance (eg, a bioengineering services representative).[69] *[4: Limited Evidence]*

I.k. When patient or personnel injuries or equipment failures occur during the use of energy-generating devices,
   ○ the energy-generating device should be removed from service;
   ○ all accessories and packaging should be retained if possible; and
   ○ the adverse event details, including device identification and maintenance and service information, should be reported according to the health care organization's policy and procedures.
   [5: Benefits Balanced with Harms]

Retaining the generator, accessories, and packaging facilitates a complete incident investigation.

I.l. The health care organization should establish policies and procedures for use of all energy-generating devices. These should address
   ○ preoperative, intraoperative, and postoperative patient assessments[81];
   ○ safety precautions to be taken during use[54,81];
   ○ equipment checks before initial use[54,80];
   ○ reporting and impounding of malfunctioning equipment[54,81,82];
   ○ reporting of injuries[54];
   ○ equipment maintenance programs[54]; and
   ○ documentation.[54]
   [2: High Evidence]

The collective evidence supports the creation of policies and procedures.[40,80,81,83]

Recommendation II

Precautions should be taken to mitigate the risk for injury associated with the use of electrosurgical units and electrosurgical accessories.

Electrosurgical devices, including the active and dispersive electrodes, have been implicated as the cause of injuries.[20,51,84,85]

II.a. The ESU should be securely mounted to a tip-resistant cart or shelf.[69] *[2: High Evidence]*

Mounting the ESU on a tip-resistant cart or shelf will help prevent the unit from falling to the floor and possibly causing injury to the patient or personnel.

II.a.1. The ESU should not be used as a shelf or table.[69] *[4: Limited Evidence]*

A case report describes a situation in which a peripheral nerve stimulator generator was placed on top of an ESU during a procedure. The stimulator was turned on and required use of a toggle switch for activation. However, the stimulator was activated simultaneously with the activation of the ESU without use of the toggle switch. The unintentional activation was caused by electromagnetic coupling between the peripheral nerve stimulator's circuitry and the ESU generator. The unintentional activation ceased after the stimulator generator was removed from the top of the ESU.[86]

II.b. The patient's skin condition should be assessed preoperatively, intraoperatively, and postoperatively when there is a potential for or planned use of an ESU. *[5: Benefits Balanced with Harms]*

Preoperative and postoperative assessments are necessary to evaluate the patient's skin condition for injuries at the dispersive electrode site and other locations.

II.c. Precautions should be taken to avoid alternate site injuries. *[3: Moderate Evidence]*

Alternate site injuries are reported to potentially occur because of insulation failure, capacitive coupling, or current leakage. Current leakage occurs when the electricity finds a route to ground that is shorter than the route that includes the dispersive electrode.

In a case report, Sabzi et al[87] described two cases of alternate site burns. In the first case, the burn resulted from a decreased dispersive electrode pad area related to a partially removed dispersive electrode. In the second case, the electrical current found a pathway through the patient's sacrum to ground that was shorter than the distance to the dispersive electrode on the thigh. The risk for alternate site burns related to the phenomenon of stray current leakage has almost been eliminated by technological improvements in ESUs.[88,89]

II.c.1. The ESU active electrode should not be activated until it is in close proximity to or in contact with the target tissue based on the desired effect.[53] *[4: Limited Evidence]*

Makedonov and Lee[90] used a computer-generated model to determine the potential for an alternate site burn. They found that for an alternate site burn to occur, the following conditions needed to be present:
- 20 seconds of continuous ESU activation,
- activation of the ESU without contact between the active electrode and the patient,
- a small alternate return site contact area of 1 cm², and
- the use of a high-power (ie, 200-W) cut mode.

The researchers concluded that to prevent alternate site burns, the active electrode should not be activated prior to contact with the patient.

II.c.2. A patient's metal jewelry that is between the active and dispersive electrode should be removed, or if jewelry is in the pathway, alternate technologies should be used. *[3: Moderate Evidence]*

Metallic jewelry, including body piercings, subdermal implants, and transdermal or microdermal implants, presents a potential risk for burns from directed current (ie, active electrode contact); heat from the active electrode conducted before the electrode cools; capacitive coupling; and rarely, leakage current.[21,71,88-90]

II.c.3. During the use of monopolar devices, contact between the patient and metal objects should be prevented. *[4: Limited Evidence]*

Metal (eg, OR beds, stirrups, positioning devices, safety strap buckles) could offer a potential alternate return path for the electrical current.[69,71,90]

II.d. Precautions should be taken to decrease the risk of antenna coupling, including
○ placing the cord joining the monopolar active electrode to the generator as far as possible from or at 90 degrees to other cords (eg, cardiac and neuromuscular monitoring cords,[46] light cords,[91] second electrosurgery cords)[50,66,68] and
○ placing patient monitoring electrodes (eg, electrocardiogram, oximetry, fetal) as far as possible from the surgical site.[46]
[3: Moderate Evidence]

The collective evidence supports placing the cords as far as possible from or at 90 degrees to other cords to decrease the potential for antenna coupling, which may cause burns in areas remote from the surgical site (eg, under cardiac monitors, at the site of neuromuscular electrodes).[43,46,66,91]

Robinson et al[91] conducted a randomized controlled trial involving 84 patients undergoing laparoscopic cholecystectomy. The amount of thermal injury was measured in patients who were assigned to the control group, for whom the active electrodes and camera cords were oriented parallel and located in close proximity, and the experimental group, for whom the cords were separated. The researchers found that thermal injury, assessed by histological examination of tissue at the camera insertion site, was significantly less in the experimental group than in the control group (31% versus 57%). The researchers concluded that cords should be separated and not oriented parallel or located in close proximity. Robinson et al[66] found similar results and drew the same conclusion in a descriptive laboratory study using bovine muscle tissue.

Jones et al[43] illustrated antenna coupling in a laboratory study. The researchers measured the tissue temperature in a bovine liver using an L-hook device as the active electrode and an unlit 10-mm laparoscope as the instrument receiving the coupled energy. The researchers compared the temperature at the end of the scope when the cords were parallel and bundled to the temperature at the end of the scope and the grasper when the cords were completely separated. The temperature at the end of the laparoscope increased even though there was no contact between the active electrode and the instruments. The increase was greater when the cords were bundled together compared with when the cords were separated (38.2° C [100.8° F] versus 15.7° C [60.3° F]). The researchers recommended separation of the camera/light cord and the wires leading from the generator to the active electrode.

Townsend et al[46] found similar results in a study using a porcine model. The researchers examined the temperature of the surface of the porcine tissue where a neuromuscular and an electrocardiogram lead were attached. The items were tested with an ESU power setting at 30 W and 15 W and cords placed close to or 15 cm away from the electrodes. The researchers noted a significant decrease in the temperature when the lower power setting was used and when the cords were not in close proximity. Based on these findings, they recommended using as low a power as possible and placing the wires as far away from the electrodes as possible.

Hammwohner et al[92] described the effects of antenna coupling in a case report of a patient who developed ventricular tachycardia during radio-frequency ablation. It was determined that the pacemaker leads were acting as antennae and channeling the energy from the radio-frequency ablation catheter into the ventricle, causing the ventricular tachycardia. The authors recommended using bipolar energy to prevent this from occurring because when the generator was switched to 100% bipolar energy, the ventricular tachycardia no longer occurred.

II.d.1. Alternate technologies (eg, bipolar, ultrasonic) should be used instead of monopolar electrosurgery when neuromonitoring electrodes (eg, somatosensory evoked potentials [SSEP]) are present. *[3: Moderate Evidence]*

A laboratory study by Townsend et al[46] supported the use of alternate technologies. This study examined the temperature of the surface of the porcine tissue model onto which a neuromuscular and an electrocardiogram lead were attached. The instruments used included monopolar electrosurgery, an argon beam generator, an advanced bipolar device, and an ultrasonic device. The researchers found an insignificant increase in the temperature with the use of the advanced bipolar and ultrasonic devices compared to the temperature increase with the use of the monopolar electrosurgical unit or the argon beam generator. Based on these findings, the researchers recommended using alternative technologies when neuromonitoring electrodes are required.

II.e. Precautions should be taken when the patient has any implanted electronic device (IED) (eg, gastric or cardiac pacemaker; implantable cardioverter defibrillator; cochlear implant; deep brain, vagal nerve, sacral nerve, phrenic nerve, spinal cord, or bone stimulator). *[3: Moderate Evidence]*

The evidence review found reports of EMI caused by energy-generating devices leading to complications, including ventricular tachycardia[93] and ventricular fibrillation,[94,95] and reports of inappropriate defibrillation caused by EMI from an electrosurgical active electrode being sensed as ventricular fibrillation by an implantable cardioverter defibrillator.[96-99] Electromagnetic interference may cause a pacemaker to oversense, reset, or inhibit pacing or may damage a lead or the pulse generator.[100]

In a bench study, Maheshwari et al[101] tested the amount of EMI created by devices used during dental procedures (ie, heat carrier, electronic apex locator, electric pulp tester, unipolar electrosurgery unit, electric motor, curing light, and three gutta-percha guns) and the interaction of the EMI on a CIED. The researchers found that the monopolar electrosurgery device was the only device that created enough EMI to

affect the CIED. The researchers suggested that the ESU produced enough EMI to interfere with the operation of a CIED.

II.e.1. The perioperative team should consult with the team managing the implanted device before surgery and as needed. Team members for specific devices may include the following:
- Pacemaker—cardiologist, electrophysiology team, manufacturer's representative
- Cochlear implant—implanting surgeon, manufacturer's representative
- Neurostimulator device—implanting surgeon, neurologist
- Implanted infusion pump—implanting surgeon, physician responsible for managing care

[3: Moderate Evidence]

Models of the same type of implant manufactured by the same or different manufacturers may exhibit different responses to the EMI created by the energy-generating device. The team managing the device should have the specific information on the functionality of the device and be able to advise on precautions to take.[21,52,68,69,95,97-100,102-111]

II.e.2. Before the consultation, the following information should be provided to the team managing the patient with an IED:
- the procedure scheduled, including the site[100];
- intraoperative patient positioning[100];
- the potential for EMI based on the type of electrosurgical device to be used (eg, radio-frequency ablation, monopolar, bipolar)[70,100,102,111];
- the procedure room location (eg, OR, interventional radiology)[100]; and
- the post-procedure patient disposition (eg, outpatient, inpatient).[100,112]

[4: Limited Evidence]

This information will help the team managing the patient with an IED to make a determination regarding the interventions to be performed during the perioperative time frame. This information will also assist with scheduling members of the team (eg, a representative who can perform reprogramming) to be present for the procedure.[100]

II.e.3. Interventions to be performed when caring for the patient with an existing IED should be based on the following information that may be obtained from patient assessment, patient caregivers, the identification (ID) card carried by the patient, and the medical record[100,103,104,111]:
- type of implanted device,[70,88,97,100,103-106,110,111,113]
- patient's level of dependence,[70,100,102,103,110,111,113,114]

- location of the device and leads (eg, within or outside the path between the active and dispersive electrode),[50,68,88,95,97,103,104,106,110,115-118]
- device manufacturer and model,[100,103]
- clinical indication for the device,[100,103]
- battery life,[97,100,104,111]
- device settings,[97,100,114] and
- lead placement.[104]

For cardiac devices, the following information is also needed:

- date of the last device interrogation or monitoring,[70,100,102-104,106,110,116,117]
- lead polarity (eg, unipolar or bipolar),[88,97,103,104,106,110]
- need for device programming,[100,102,103,111]
- response of the device to a magnet,[100,104,111,113]
- presence of an alert status on the generator or on the lead,[100] and
- the last pacing threshold.[100]

[3: Moderate Evidence]

Various types of implants and various brands of the same implant may exhibit different responses to the EMI created by the energy-generating device.[68,95,97,98,100,103,111,112]

Use of a magnet is not always indicated because not all pacemakers respond in the same way; for example, use of a magnet on a pacemaker with a low battery may lead to device failure because the power of the battery may become rapidly exhausted.[104]

II.e.4. Interventions that should be performed for a patient with an existing CIED include

- reprogramming the device by a magnet or having equipment reprogrammed by a qualified person, if so advised by the team managing the CIED[52,70,92,100,111]; *[4: Limited Evidence]*
- placing the dispersive electrode as close as possible to the surgical site, verifying the IED is not in the current pathway between the active and dispersive electrode[21,36,45,52,65,68,70,88,97,102,103,106,109,114,117-119]; *[3: Moderate Evidence]*
- using electrocautery,[117] bipolar forceps,[21,36,50,68,88,92,102,103,106,109,114,116-118,120] or other alternative technology (eg, ultrasonic technology, ferromagnetic surgical system)[50,70,97,120-122]; *[3: Moderate Evidence]*
- placing the active electrode cord away from the pulse generator[45]; *[3: Moderate Evidence]*
- using a five-lead ECG system[97]; *[3: Moderate Evidence]*
- using a beat-to-beat indicator (eg arterial line, pulse oximeter)[52,70,97,100,102-104,113]; *[3: Moderate Evidence]*
- having temporary pacing equipment and an external defibrillator readily available[36,70,93,100,104,111]; *[3: Moderate Evidence]*

- keeping a magnet immediately available if the pacemaker will respond to a magnet and one is not used for reprogramming[100]; *[4: Limited Evidence]* and
- employing continuous cardiac monitoring whenever the pacemaker is deactivated.[100] *[4: Limited Evidence]*

The collective evidence[22,52,88,95,98,106,107,109,114,121-123] supports taking precautions in the patient with a CIED.

Pacemakers may incorrectly interpret the electrical signals from an electrosurgical device, leading to a misfiring or not firing that can result in arrhythmia, such as ventricular fibrillation or ventricular tachycardia.[88,106,123] Use of a magnet is not always indicated because not all pacemakers respond in the same way; for example, use of a magnet on a pacemaker with a low battery may lead to device failure because the power of the battery may become rapidly exhausted.[104] Pacemaker leads may act as an antenna, leading to antenna coupling as described in a case report by Hammwohner (See Recommendation II.d).[92]

Bipolar electrosurgery does not produce EMI unless the forceps come into direct contact with the CIED.[100] The tolerance of EMI is different for different types of pacemakers (unipolar, bipolar) and different models and manufacturers of pacemakers.[97]

Use of a five-lead electrocardiogram configuration provides multiple leads to view in case one lead is obscured or difficult to interpret because of electrical interference. Use of a beat-to-beat indicator provides a signal for the pulse in case the electrocardiogram is obscured or difficult to interpret because of EMI.[97,102]

Wiess and Manwaring[122] performed a laboratory study in which they implanted a synthetic surrogate model with a pacemaker and a cardiac defibrillator generator and then cut the model using a ferromagnetic device. The researchers found no disturbance to electrocardiographic monitoring with the use of the ferromagnetic device. They concluded that the ferromagnetic device was safe to use in the patient with a pacemaker and CIED generator.

Paniccia et al[120] measured the average maximum EMI occurring on a cardiac device implanted in a pig during activations of various surgical energy-based devices. The researchers found the EMI transferred to the implanted cardiac device varied for each device:

- 0.01 mV for a traditional bipolar device at 30 W,
- 0.004 mV for an advanced bipolar device,
- 0.01 mV for ultrasonic shears,

- 0.5 mV for a monopolar device at 30 W coagulation,
- 0.92 mV for a monopolar device at 30 W blend,
- 0.21 mV for a monopolar device without a dispersive electrode,
- 3.48 mV for a plasma energy-generating device, and
- 2.58 mV for an argon beam coagulator.

The researchers concluded that bipolar and ultrasonic devices are useful for decreasing the EMI on implanted cardiac defibrillators.

Govekar et al[65] conducted a laboratory study to determine whether the location of the dispersive electrode affected the functionality of a pacemaker in the heart of a pig. The dispersive electrode was placed on the right gluteus, left gluteus, right shoulder, and left shoulder. The ESU was set at a power of 30 W in the coagulation mode. The active electrode was activated for 5 seconds at a distance of 7.5 cm from the pacemaker generator. The researchers found more beats were dropped (1.5 versus 0.2) when the current vector traveled from the active electrode to the dispersive electrode through the pacemaker or through the leads. The researchers concluded that the dispersive electrode should be located such that the current vector does not pass through the pacemaker or the leads.

In a laboratory study, Robinson et al[45] examined the effect of monopolar electrosurgery devices on CIEDs implanted in pigs. The researchers measured the amount of EMI present after changing the orientation of the active electrode cord from across the chest wall to coming from the feet and changing the current vector from flowing across the CIED. The researchers found significantly less EMI when the orientation of the active electrode was from the feet and the current vector avoided the CIED. They concluded that the active electrode cord should be placed at the greatest distance possible from the CIED generator, and the CIED generator should not be in the pathway of the current from the active electrode to the dispersive electrode.

II.e.5. Interventions that should be taken for a patient with an existing non-cardiac IED include
- using alternative technology (eg, electrocautery, bipolar forceps, ultrasonic technology, ferromagnetic surgical system) instead of monopolar electrosurgery when possible,[21,103,111,113] [3: Moderate Evidence]
- activating the ESU for the shortest amount of time possible,[21,103,111] [3: Moderate Evidence]

- placing the grounding pad as far as possible from the device's generator and leads,[103,111] [2: High Evidence]
- verifying that the implanted device and leads are not between the active electrode and the dispersive electrode,[21] [3: Moderate Evidence] and
- turning off the IED if it is safe to do so.[103,111,113,124] [3: Moderate Evidence]

Turning these devices off may mitigate any malfunctioning caused by EMI.[103]

In a case report, Radolec et al[124] described a patient with an implanted vagus nerve stimulator who underwent radio-frequency ablation to treat supraventricular tachycardia. The stimulator was turned off before the procedure. During the procedure, no interaction was noted between the stimulator and energy from the radio-frequency ablation catheter, and postoperatively, there were no noted effects to the stimulator.

A cadaveric study by Jeyakumar et al[125] assessed whether changes to an implanted cochlear device occurred during electrocautery or after failure analysis and if there were changes in the intracochlear temperature. The researchers found no changes in the device, and the temperature of the cochlear device did not increase after 30 minutes of electrosurgical energy delivered at 30 W into the oral cavity. The researchers concluded that no damage or temperature increase occurred, but that further study was required before changing the current practice.

II.e.6. Interventions that should be taken for a patient with an existing cochlear implant include
- not using electrosurgical devices within 2 cm to 3 cm of the implant package and electrodes,[21,117,126] and
- removing all external components,[117,126]
[3: Moderate Evidence]

II.e.7. Precautions that should be taken for patients who have deep brain stimulators, sacral nerve stimulators, spinal cord stimulators, vagal nerve stimulators, or gastric pacemakers include turning off the device if so advised by the implant management team and if it is safe to do so.[103,111] [2: High Evidence]

II.e.8. Patients and their caregivers should receive education on the effects of electrosurgery on IEDs (eg, non-cardiac IEDs, CIEDs, cochlear implants, deep brain stimulators). [3: Moderate Evidence]

Frampton and Mitchell[127] conducted a survey of 50 adults with cochlear implants and the parents of 50 children with cochlear implants to determine their knowledge of the risks for complications when a cochlear implant is present and electrosurgery is used during head and neck procedures. The researchers found that 86% of the adult patients possessed an implant ID card, and 71% carried it with them. Seventy-seven percent stated that if surgery were required, they would show their implant ID card and discuss the issue of electrosurgery with the physician. Eighty-four percent of the parents reported that the child possessed an ID card; 8% of parents ensured the child carried the card at all times, and 12% reported that they carried the card for the child. Seventy-six percent of the parents believed that surgeons would be unaware of the diathermy restrictions, but none of the 12% of parents whose children had undergone surgery had brought the issue to the surgeon's attention. The researchers concluded that cochlear implant recipients and non-cochlear implant surgeons should receive education about the risks of complications that could occur when electrosurgery is used for patients with cochlear implants.

II.f. All components of the circuit (eg, generator, dispersive electrode, active electrode, active electrode tip) should be compatible as defined by the manufacturer.[128] *[3: Moderate Evidence]*

II.g. The active electrode should
- be visually inspected before use for any apparent damage to the cord or hand piece (eg, impaired insulation)[36,53,69,71,99]; *[4: Limited Evidence]*
- have a firm seating of the tip into the hand piece with no gaps between tip insulation and hand piece[53]; *[4: Limited Evidence]*
- be connected directly into a designated receptacle on the ESU; *[5: Benefits Balanced with Harms]* and
- be placed in a clean, dry, nonconductive safety holster when not in use.[25,29,33,36,51,129]

[3: Moderate Evidence]

The use of a holster is supported in case studies and articles expressing expert opinion.[25,29,33,36,51,129] Use of a nonconductive safety holster prevents the active electrode from falling off the sterile field and from unintentional activation.[129]

II.g.1. When needed, only adaptors approved by the manufacturers of both the ESU and the accessory should be used. *[5: Benefits Balanced with Harms]*

II.h. Active electrode tips should
- be used according to the manufacturer's instructions; *[5: Benefits Balanced with Harms]*
- be securely seated into the hand piece[53]; *[4: Limited Evidence]*
- be cleaned

- whenever there is visible eschar present,
- away from the incision,
- with a moistened sponge or instrument wipe for nonstick coated electrosurgical tips, and
- with an abrasive electrode cleaning pad for noncoated electrodes[36];

[3: Moderate Evidence]
- be inspected for insulation failure, if insulation is present[130-132]; *[3: Moderate Evidence]* and
- not be altered (eg, bent) unless this is allowed by manufacturer's IFU. *[5: Benefits Balanced with Harms]*

Eschar buildup on the active electrode tip has been reported to impede the desired current flow, causing the unit to function less effectively.[49]

Burns at the skin surface have been reported to be caused by a break in the insulation during radio-frequency ablation procedures.[130-132]

II.i. A single-use dispersive electrode should
- be used according to the manufacturer's instructions for use[69,88,99,133]; *[3: Moderate Evidence]*
- be placed on the patient after final positioning; *[5: Benefits Balanced with Harms]*
- be placed
  - close to the surgical site,[21,88,98,99,105]
  - on clean, dry skin,[36,48,99]
  - over a large, well-perfused muscle mass,[21,36,48,99]
  - on the surgical side when indicated (eg, left or right shoulder, hip, kidney),[36] and
  - to avoid any metal or monitoring leads between the dispersive and active electrodes[90,105,134];

[3: Moderate Evidence]
- be applied and in uniform contact with the patient's skin[48,88,99,135]; *[3: Moderate Evidence]*
- be of an appropriate size for the patient (eg, neonate, infant, pediatric, adult) based on the patient's weight, as described in the manufacturer's IFU[21,130]; *[3: Moderate Evidence]*
- be checked for flaws, damage, discoloration, adhesiveness, and dryness before application[36,48,69,71,99,133]; *[3: Moderate Evidence]*
- be placed away from a warming device;[105] *[3: Moderate Evidence]*
- be checked for uniform contact if the patient has been moved or repositioned or if any tension has been applied to the dispersive electrode cord[87,88,135]; *[3: Moderate Evidence]*
- not be repositioned or reapplied[36,48]; *[3: Moderate Evidence]*
- not be altered (eg, cut, folded)[36,99]; *[3: Moderate Evidence]* and
- not be placed
  - over bony prominences and potential pressure points,[21,36,48,87] *[3: Moderate Evidence]*
  - over scar tissue,[21,48] *[3: Moderate Evidence]*

- over an implant containing metal components,[21,36,48,90,99,133] *[3: Moderate Evidence]*
- over skin folds,[48] *[3: Moderate Evidence]*
- on areas with dense hair,[36,48,87,99] *[3: Moderate Evidence]* or
- on areas distal to tourniquets.[36,98] *[3: Moderate Evidence]*

Patient skin injuries at the dispersive electrode site have been reported.[48,51,135-138] Specific injuries related to inadequate adhesion of the dispersive electrode have been reported.[85,87,132] A reused single-use dispersive electrode may not adhere uniformly and reuse may be against the manufacturer's IFU. Moving the patient after the application of the dispersive electrode may disrupt the contact to the patient's skin, causing tenting, gapping, or moisture collection under the electrode. Liquids may prevent the electrode from uniformly adhering to the skin. Replacing the dispersive electrode provides an opportunity to examine the amount of contact between the patient's skin and the electrode and to examine the patient's skin for burns or elements that do not allow good contact.

Tissue types differ in respect to electrical resistance. Adipose tissue and bone have high resistance and are poor conductors; in contrast, muscle and skin are better conductors.[21,51] Fatty tissue, tissue over bone, scar tissue, and hair can impede electrosurgical return current flow. High impedance leads to heating of the tissue, arcing to the tissue under the dispersive electrode, and subsequent burns.[21] Adequate tissue perfusion cannot be assured if the dispersive electrode is placed distal to tourniquets or over scar tissue.

Using the appropriately sized dispersive electrode reduces the concentration of current and minimizes the potential for electrosurgical injuries.[51,85]

Placing a dispersive electrode in a location that results in metal being between the dispersive and active electrodes (eg, over the site of a metal implant or prosthesis, metal wires, metal clips, jewelry) may result in super heating of the metal, potentially causing a burn.[90] Nguyen et al[134] conducted a bench study to examine the effect of monopolar radio-frequency energy on the temperature of bovine myocardium tissue surrounding implanted metal objects. The researchers found the temperature was elevated in the tissue surrounding the objects by a mean of 5.8° C to 8.9° C (10.4° F to 16° F) when the objects were between the active and dispersive electrodes and at a distance of 1 mm from the site of the active electrode. The researchers concluded that the dispersive electrode should be placed in a location with no metal objects between it and the active electrode.

Placing the dispersive electrode under a warming blanket may cause synergistic heating of the tissue, which may cause a thermal injury.[105]

II.i.1. When reusable dispersive electrode cables are used,
- the cable and pad should be securely connected,
- the attachment clip should cover the gel-free connecting lugs or tabs, and
- cables should be replaced when worn.[88]

[3: Moderate Evidence]

II.i.2. Dispersive electrode packaging should
- not be opened until needed and
- be checked to confirm the manufacturer's expiration date has not passed.[69]

[3: Moderate Evidence]

The longer the package is opened, the greater the potential for drying of the dispersive electrode's adhesive and the conductive gel.[88,133]

II.i.3. Corrective measures should be performed if inadequate contact between the single-use dispersive electrode and the patient occurs, including
- removing oil, lotion, moisture, or prep solution;
- removing excessive hair;
- changing sites; and
- applying a new pad.

[3: Moderate Evidence]

Injuries have been associated with inadequate adhesion of the dispersive electrode.[85,87,136]

II.j. Reusable, capacitive coupled dispersive electrode pads should
- be used according to manufacturers' IFU in conjunction with a compatible ESU,[133]
- be an appropriate size for the patient (ie, adult, pediatric),
- be used without or with minimal material between the pad and patient,
- be used with an isolated electrosurgical unit,
- be cleaned with a health care facility-approved and Environmental Protection Agency-registered agent between uses in accordance with the manufacturer's IFU,
- be checked for tears or breaks in the surface material before and after use,
- be repaired or replaced if damage is present, and
- be replaced on their labeled expiration dates.

[5: Benefits Balanced with Harms]

II.j.1. Reusable, capacitive coupled dispersive electrode pad cables should be checked for integrity before use and be replaced if damaged. *[5: Benefits Balanced with Harms]*

II.k. Additional precautions should be taken when two ESUs are used simultaneously. *[5: Benefits Balanced with Harms]*

EQUIPMENT AND PRODUCT SAFETY

II.k.1.   When multiple ESUs are used simultaneously, the compatibility of the equipment and proper functioning of corresponding electrode monitoring systems should be verified with the manufacturer. *[5: Benefits Balanced with Harms]*

II.k.2.   The accessories used with each ESU should be labeled to correspond with the ESU to which they are attached. *[3: Moderate Evidence]*

Labeling each individual unit and the accessories was supported in an article describing an organizational experience. Labeling individual ESUs assists in identifying which ESU requires adjustment or, during a move by the operator from one side of the table to the other, which operator is using which unit.[139]

II.k.3.   A single-use dispersive electrode should be used for each ESU;
- the dispersive electrodes should be placed as close as possible to the surgical site,
- the dispersive electrodes should not overlap, and
- the dispersive electrodes should be placed equidistant from the surgical site when it is a single site.[85]

[3: Moderate Evidence]

Equidistant placement is recommended because of the asymmetric distribution of the electrical current.[85]

II.k.4.   When a capacitive coupled dispersive electrode is used with two ESUs, the electrode and ESU manufacturers' IFUs should be followed. *[5: Benefits Balanced with Harms]*

II.l.   When high current is used for a prolonged period of time and there are no specific manufacturer's directions, a second single-use dispersive electrode with an adaptor or a return electrode with a larger conductive surface may be used. *[4: Limited Evidence]*

Dispersive electrode site burns have been reported when high-current, long-activation-time procedures have been performed. Increasing the dispersive area decreases the potential for a burn.[136,137]

II.m.   When a single-use dispersive electrode is used, a generator with return-electrode contact quality monitoring should be used.[140] *[3: Moderate Evidence]*

Return-electrode contact quality monitoring inhibits the output of the ESU if the return electrode is not in contact with the patient and connected to the ESU. Return-electrode contact quality monitoring confirms that there is adequate contact between the return electrode and the patient. An audible alarm and visual indicator signals the user of a misconnection.[21,99,140]

II.n.   If the operator repeatedly requests an increase in power, personnel should confirm the integrity of the entire ESU and accessories circuit including the dispersive electrode and cord connections.[36] *[3: Moderate Evidence]*

Poor contact between the dispersive electrode and the patient may cause ineffective coagulation and cutting, resulting in a request by the user for an increase in the power.[48,87]

II.o.   The health care organization should provide education and verify competency regarding precautions to be taken during use of an ESU, as applicable to the person's job responsibilities.[36,71,133,141] *[3: Moderate Evidence]*

Brown and Blank[142] conducted a review of the MAUDE database that supported the need for education and competency. The authors reviewed reports of serious complications after endometrial ablation and noted that 8% of the 829 reported serious adverse events that occurred during endometrial ablation were related to device use outside of the manufacturers' labeled instructions. The authors concluded that additional education is needed on the correct techniques for use of the devices, which are described in the manufacturers' labeled instructions.

Feldman et al[143] conducted a pretest-posttest study of 48 surgeons and 27 residents to determine the participants' knowledge on use of electrosurgical devices. On the pretest, the median percent of correct answers in the surgeon group was 59% and in the resident group was 55%. After the groups received the education, a median of 90% correct was achieved on the posttest. The researchers concluded that there was a knowledge gap and education was required.

Frampton et al[126] sent a survey to 36 head and neck surgeons and received 35 responses. The survey assessed the surgeons' knowledge of safety considerations when using electrosurgery in the presence of a cochlear implant. Seventy-seven percent of the respondents did not know about the published guidelines covering the use of electrosurgery in the patient with a cochlear implant, and 11% thought it was safe to use monopolar electrosurgery in this group of patients. The researchers concluded that surgeons need education on the safety guidelines regarding the use of electrosurgery when the patient has a cochlear implant.

Ahrens et al[115] conducted a survey of 12 shoulder surgeons and eight residents in the United Kingdom to determine the physicians' knowledge of possible locations for pacemaker lead placement and knowledge of the type of electrosurgery to use in the presence of a pacemaker lead. The researchers found that 65% of the surgeons and 70% of the residents knew that the cephalic vein may be used for the route of the pacemaker electrode. When asked what type of electrosurgery to use on the cephalic vein in the presence of a pacemaker, four surgeons but no residents reported they would use monopolar electrosurgery, 12 surgeons and six residents reported they would use bipolar electrosurgery, and one surgeon and two residents reported they would not use electrosurgery in the presence of a pacemaker. The researchers concluded that education was needed on the proper use of electrosurgery and techniques used in other medical specialities (eg, the path used by the cardiologist to run the pacemaker leads).

No study of other perioperative team member education was found in the literature search; therefore, further research is needed.

II.o.1.   Education and competency verification should include
- principles of electrosurgery including direct, capacitive, and antenna coupling and alternate current pathways;
- risks to patients and personnel[48,144];
- measures to minimize the risks[48,144];
- corrective actions to employ in the event of a fire or injury;
- precautions that must be taken when caring for patients with IEDs[115,126];
- steps for operation, care, and handling of the energy-generating device and accessories before, during, and after use that are in alignment with the manufacturer's IFU[142,144];
- the potential for electrosurgical-induced artefactual changes in patient monitoring devices (eg, cardiac, electroencephalogram, capnograhy, bispectral index)[145]; and
- equipment manufacturers' instructions for use and warnings.
[3: Moderate Evidence]

I.p.   Documentation related to the use of the ESU should be recorded in the patient's medical record in a manner consistent with the health care organization's policies and procedures and should include
- energy-generating device identification (eg, serial or biomedical number),
- location of dispersive electrode placement, and
- the patient's skin condition before application and after removal of the dispersive electrode.[146]
[4: Limited Evidence]

Recommendation III

Precautions should be taken to mitigate the risk for injury associated with the use of electrosurgery during minimally invasive surgery.

Electrosurgery used during minimally invasive surgical procedures has been reported to cause burns from direct and capacitive coupling of current and insulation failure of the active electrode.[1,51,141,147-150]

In a laboratory descriptive study, Abu-Rafea et al[147] used sheep liver, pig bowel, and dog bowel to illustrate burns resulting from direct and capacitive coupling during simulated single-port laparoscopic surgery using monopolar electrosurgery. The researchers used a monopolar surgery generator set at power outputs of 40 W to 60 W and both coagulation and cut waveforms and commercially available single-port devices. The researchers recommended that when monopolar electrosurgery is used during single-port laparoscopic surgery, extreme caution should be used to minimize or avoid the risk for visceral burns.

III.a.   Conductive trocar systems should be used.[51,71,133] *[3: Moderate Evidence]*
Conductive trocar cannulas provide a means for the electrosurgical current to flow safely between the cannula and the abdominal wall. This reduces high-density current concentration and heating of non-target tissue.[49,141]

III.b.   Electrosurgical unit-activated instrumentation (ie, active electrodes) should be examined for intact insulation before use.[36] *[3: Moderate Evidence]*
The collective evidence establishes that electrode insulation failure provides an alternate pathway for the electrical current to exit from the active electrode. There are multiple reports of insulation failure resulting in injuries.[36,49,51,56,141,150,151]

Munro[56] conducted a laboratory comparative study to identify mechanisms of thermal injury to the lower genital tract during radio-frequency resectoscopic surgery. The researcher used a tissue model to represent the uterus and created defects in the insulation on the electrode. He found injuries resulting from capacitive coupling occurred when the insulation had been damaged and concluded that injuries may occur when damage to the insulation is present.

Montero et al[151] examined 165 reusable laparoscopic instruments for breaks in insulation. They found 19% of the instruments had insulation failure. They recommended that surgeons be made aware of the many insulation failures that can occur and adopt practices to decrease the potential for complications related to insulation failure.

III.b.1.   An active electrode monitoring and shielding device should be used at the point of electrosurgery use.[51,140,141,152] *[3: Moderate Evidence]*
Active electrode shielding continuously monitors the endoscopic instruments to minimize the risks for insulation failure or capacitive coupling injuries.[140,141,152]

Mendez-Probst et al[152] conducted a descriptive laboratory study to identify the amount of current leakage in robotic instruments. The researchers measured the amount of current leakage in 37 robotic instruments with visually intact insulation. Stray currents were found in 100% of the instruments with a mean leakage of 4.1 W. The researchers recommended adoption of an active electrode monitoring technology program.

III.b.2. After the instrument is decontaminated, an active electrode insulation integrity tester should be used to examine the instrument for intact insulation. *[3: Moderate Evidence]*

In a descriptive study, Espada et al[153] tested 78 robotic and 298 laparoscopic instruments at 20 W and 2.64 kV in phase A and tested 60 robotic and 308 laparoscopic instruments at 20 W/1 kV and 20 W/4.2 kV in phase B. In phase A, the researchers found insulation failures in 80% of the robotic instruments and in 36% of the laparoscopic instruments. In phase B, they detected failures in 81.7% of the robotic instruments and 19.5% of the laparoscopic instruments. The researchers recommended routine testing of laparoscopic and robotic instruments for insulation failure.

Recommendation IV

A laser safety program should be established for all owned, leased, or borrowed laser equipment in any location where lasers are used.[54,82,154]

A laser safety program establishes requirements for the safe operation of lasers in all locations.

IV.a. A laser safety program should
- delegate authority and responsibility for supervising laser safety to a laser safety officer (LSO)[54,80,82,154];
- establish a multidisciplinary laser safety committee, which may be same as a facility-wide safety committee[54,82,154];
- establish usage criteria and authorized procedures for all health care personnel working in laser nominal hazard zones[54,80,82];
- identify laser hazards (eg, beam and non-beam) and provide requirements for monitoring compliance with applicable administrative, engineering, and procedural control measures[54,82,154];
- identify the type and frequency of medical examinations for personnel[154];
- identify education requirements (eg, competency verification, certification, participating personnel qualifications)[54,80-82,154]; and
- define quality processes, including audits.[82,154]
[3: Moderate Evidence]

A laser safety program manages patient and personnel safety by providing guidance to minimize laser hazards.

IV.a.1. The multidisciplinary laser safety committee, which may include the same members as the facility-wide safety committee, should include the following individuals or departmental representatives:
- administrators,[154]
- the LSO,[154]
- a biomedical engineer and/or clinical biomedical engineer,[154]
- a physician representative from each specialty group that uses lasers,[154]
- anesthesia professionals,
- perioperative services administrators,
- a perioperative educator,[154]
- medical staff education/credentialing personnel,[154]
- quality department personnel, and
- the laser safety specialist (eg, nurse, technician).[154]

One individual may represent more than one area based on the organizational staffing plan. *[4: Limited Evidence]*

The collective evidence supports creating a laser safety committee with a multidisciplinary membership.[54,82,155]

IV.a.2. The responsibilities of the laser safety committee should include
- strategic planning for and acquisition of laser-related technology (eg, technology assessment, cost analysis, product evaluation, review of marketing information from laser vendors)[54];
- establishing requirements for credentialing[54];
- verifying that any physician who operates a laser has completed the health care organization's required education on the operation and safety precautions and coursework in basic laser physics, laser tissue interaction, and clinical applications for the specific laser for which privileges are sought[54,154];
- establishing requirements for hazard assessment[154];
- overseeing the laser safety program;
- developing and enforcing laser-related policy and procedures[54,154];
- overseeing laser-related education and competency verification[54,154];
- setting staffing requirements[54];
- establishing a quality assurance and improvement program[54]; and
- overseeing third-party laser services.
[3: Moderate Evidence]

IV.b. An LSO should be appointed by the laser safety committee and given the authority and responsibility to monitor and oversee the laser safety program.[37,54,79,81-83,154,156-158] *[3: Moderate Evidence]*

IV.b.1. The responsibilities of the LSO should include

- performing a laser hazard evaluation before initial use in the facility[37,83,154];
- overseeing the implementation of the laser manufacturers' IFU[54,154,159];
- administering policies and procedures for control of laser hazards, maintenance, service, and use of lasers[54,81,154,157];
- verifying that protective equipment is available, used correctly, and maintained in working order[54,83,154];
- verifying that American National Standards Institute (ANSI)-compliant warning signs are posted in locations where lasers are in use[83,154];
- approving equipment installation according to the manufacturer's safety recommendations[54,79,81,154];
- coordinating laser safety education programs[54,79,81,83,154];
- confirming that all operators are properly credentialed according to the health care organization's policy;
- maintaining records on the laser's maintenance and service[79];
- verifying that the type of fire extinguisher needed for each specific laser based on manufacturers' IFU is available and located as defined by the health care organization's policy and procedure[6,79];
- performing periodic safety audits[83,154];
- determining the nominal hazard zone for each laser used; and
- performing adverse event investigation.[83]

[3: Moderate Evidence]

IV.b.2. The LSO may fulfill multiple roles (eg, laser operator, laser safety specialist) within the health care organization, depending on the scope of services provided.[82,154] *[4: Limited Evidence]*

IV.b.3. The LSO should have the requisite education and training applicable to the type of lasers used in the facility.[37,154,160] The education topics should include

- laser terminology,
- laser-specific information (eg, wave lengths, pulse shapes, modes, power/energy, classification, controlled areas),[81]
- radiometric units and measurement devices,
- steps and requirements for performing a laser hazard evaluation,
- fundamentals of lasers and optics,
- beam and non-beam hazard control measures,
- regulatory requirements and standards of practice,
- laser safety program administration, and
- maximum permissible exposure values.[154,160]

[3: Moderate Evidence]

Education provides the LSO with a foundation to assist in providing a safe environment for patients and health care personnel.[160]

IV.c. An laser safety specialist (LSS) should be designated and approved by the LSO to oversee laser use for each area when lasers are being used in multiple sites in a health care organization.[82] *[4: Limited Evidence]*

IV.c.1. The LSS may not be needed when the laser is used only in one location and the LSO is available.[82] *[4: Limited Evidence]*

IV.c.2. The responsibilities of the LSS may include
- supervising laser usage in a specific area (eg, ambulatory surgery unit, eye clinic),
- troubleshooting equipment malfunctions,
- monitoring compliance with laser policies and procedures,
- reviewing laser-related documentation (eg, logs, laser manufacturers' IFU),
- acting as a resource to personnel,
- assessing needs for continuing education and training, and
- assisting with data gathering and quality monitoring for the facility (eg, education, credentialing, licensure).[82]

[4: Limited Evidence]

IV.c.3. The LSS should have the requisite education and training applicable to the type of lasers used in the facility and based on job responsibilities. *[5: Benefits Balanced with Harms]*

IV.d. A laser operator who has no competing responsibilities that would require leaving the laser unattended during active use should be assigned for every procedure, except when the laser console is controlled by the laser user.[82,154] *[4: Limited Evidence]*

IV.d.1. The laser operator should have the requisite education and training applicable to the type of lasers used in the facility, including
- laser operation principles;
- clinical applications;
- potential risks to the patient and health care personnel;
- safety procedures;
- care of the laser, safety equipment, and accessories; and
- hands-on use of the laser (eg, setup, testing, control panel use).[82]

[4: Limited Evidence]

IV.e. The health care organization should provide education and verify competency related to use of the laser, as applicable to the person's job responsibilities, periodically and when new laser equipment, accessories, or safety equipment is brought into the practice environment. *[3: Moderate Evidence]*

EQUIPMENT AND PRODUCT SAFETY

The collective evidence supports the need for education on laser use and precautions.[37,38,40,54,78,79,81,83,161]

IV.e.1. Education and competency verification should be specific to the laser used and procedures performed.[38,54,82] The education must include safety precautions for each type of laser used (eg, personal protective equipment required, window coverings, warning signs and alarms, electrical safety, fire safety)[54,81,162] *[1: Regulatory Requirement]* and should include information on
- the laser safety program, *[5: Benefits Balanced with Harms]*
- hazards associated with lasers,[54,79-81,163] *[3: Moderate Evidence]*
- reporting of adverse events,[38,54] *[3: Moderate Evidence]* and
- emergency laser shut off.[81] *[2: High Evidence]*

IV.f. Documentation in the patient's medical record should be recorded in a manner consistent with the health care organization's policies and procedures and include the
- type of laser used (eg, wavelength),[54,81]
- safety measures implemented during laser use,[81]
- laser activation and de-activation times,[54]
- energy-generating device identification (eg, serial or biomedical number),[146] and
- patient protection (eg, type of eyewear, eye shield).[54,81]

[3: Moderate Evidence]

IV.g. Laser safety audits should be completed at least annually or more frequently as determined by the LSO[54,82,83] and should include
- examining all laser-related equipment and safety devices (eg, eyewear, warning signs, inspection tracking indicators),
- verifying competency in laser safety, and
- observing laser practices for compliance with the health care organization's written policies and procedures.

[3: Moderate Evidence]

A laser safety audit helps verify that safety measures are in place and that safe practices are being followed.

IV.g.1. The results of the laser safety audit, including a proposed correction plan for any identified deficits, should be reported to the laser safety committee. *[5: Benefits Balanced with Harms]*

IV.h. An occupational health program should incorporate precautions for personnel participating in laser use. *[3: Moderate Evidence]*

A occupational health program defines the requirements for medical surveillance testing before use of a laser and after an exposure.[54,82,164]

IV.h.1. A physician should perform an examination of the affected body part as soon as possible after a suspected or confirmed laser-induced injury.[82,154] *[3: Moderate Evidence]*

Recommendation V

Precautions should be taken to mitigate the risk for injury associated with the use of a laser.[40,78]

The collective evidence includes reports of injury to health care personnel and patients by unintentional laser beam exposure to the eyes, skin, and respiratory system.[78,165,166]

V.a. Laser warning signs must be placed conspicuously to alert bystanders to potential hazards (eg, at all entrances to laser treatment areas when lasers are in use). *[1: Regulatory Requirement]*

The Occupational Safety and Health Administration requires placement of warning signs.[167]

V.a.1. Warning signs should be specific to the type of laser being used and should meet the ANSI criteria.[54,82] *[3: Moderate Evidence]*

V.b. All persons in the nominal hazard zone must use eye protection selected and approved by the LSO for the specific wavelength and optical density of the laser in use. *[1: Regulatory Requirement]*

The use of eye protection is supported by the collective evidence.[37,38,40,54,82,83,156,157,159,162,164,166,168,169] Eye injury can occur because the beam operates in a millisecond range of pulse duration but the eyelid takes 0.10 seconds to close. The area of the eye that is at risk for injury depends on the wavelength of the laser.[39,78,158,169]

V.b.1. Safety eyewear must be labeled with the appropriate optical density and wavelength for the laser in use.[38,80,82,168,169] *[1: Regulatory Requirement]*

V.b.2. The selection of eye protection should be based on the
- laser manufacturer's protective eyewear specifications,[54]
- wavelength of laser emission,[39,54,158,169]
- optical density of the eyewear,[54,80,169]
- radiant exposure limits,
- need for corrective lenses,
- restriction of peripheral vision, and
- comfort and fit.[37,83]

[3: Moderate Evidence]

V.b.3. Protective eyewear must be available (eg, at the entrance to a room where a laser is in use)[54,80,168] *[1: Regulatory Requirement]* and
- should be inspected for damage and scratches before use,[54,82] *[3: Moderate Evidence]*
- should be removed from use if damaged,[80] *[3: Moderate Evidence]* and

- may be labeled to match a label on the corresponding laser.[54] *[3: Moderate Evidence]*

  Defects in eyewear may allow the beam to enter the eye.[54,83]

V.b.4. Precautions to protect the patient's eyes and eyelids from injury should be performed[82]:

- Patients who remain awake during laser procedures should wear goggles or glasses designated for the type of laser being used. *[3: Moderate Evidence]*
- Patients who undergo general anesthesia should be provided with protection including wet eye pads, laser-specific eye shields, or other devices approved by the LSO. *[3: Moderate Evidence]*
- Patients undergoing laser treatments on or around the eyelids should have their eyes protected by metal corneal eye shields that are approved by the US Food and Drug Administration for use during laser procedures. *[3: Moderate Evidence]*

  The collective evidence supports the use of protective measures for patients' eyes.[37,39,40,54,80,82,83,156]

V.b.5. Laser shutters or filters with the appropriate optical density should be used on microscopes and microscope accessory oculars. *[3: Moderate Evidence]*

  Shutters and laser filters protect the laser user from laser exposure.[54,82]

V.c. Doors in the nominal hazard zone should remain closed and windows, including door windows, should be covered with a barrier that blocks transmission of the beam as applicable to the laser being used.[37-40,54,80,82] *[3: Moderate Evidence]*

  Laser energy, except energy from carbon dioxide (CO_2) wavelength lasers, has the potential to pass through windows.[54,82,83]

V.d. Procedures should be implemented to prevent accidental activation or misdirection of laser beams, including the following:

- Access to laser keys should be restricted to authorized personnel who are skilled in laser operation.[54,80,82,83] *[3: Moderate Evidence]*
- The laser should be calibrated before each use following the manufacturer's IFU.[54,79,80,82,83,159,170,171] *[3: Moderate Evidence]*
- Lasers should be placed in standby mode when not in active use.[33,37,40,54,83] *[3: Moderate Evidence]*
- The laser foot switch should be placed in a position convenient to the user and in a position where it will not be confused with other foot pedals.[54,82,83] *[3: Moderate Evidence]*
- The laser user should be the only one to activate the device.[54,82] *[3: Moderate Evidence]*

  Accidental activation or misdirection of the laser beam may cause eye and skin injury to the patient and health care personnel.[156]

  Attention to placement of the foot switch and use of the standby setting can prevent unintended activation of the laser beam and reduce the potential for injury to the patient or health care personnel.

  Control of activation by the laser user prevents unintentional discharge of laser energy and minimizes the potential for patient or health care personnel injury.

V.e. Use of reflective surfaces should be minimized during laser surgery. *[3: Moderate Evidence]*

  The laser beam may reflect off surfaces onto non-target tissues, potentially causing skin or eye injury.[37,40,54,80,82]

  In a laboratory descriptive study, Hammons et al[172] used a CO_2 laser to determine the results of reflection off of various surfaces on surgical field materials. The researchers found that the reflection off of sandblasted and polished surfaces created a hole in a glove and a flame on a surgical gown. The researchers concluded that there is a risk of damage to surgical field materials from reflected laser beams.

V.e.1. Anodized-, dull-, non-reflective-, or matte-finished instruments should be used near the laser site.[38] *[3: Moderate Evidence]*

  Anodized, dull, non-reflective, or matte finishes decrease the reflectivity of laser beams.[39,54,82,83,157,172]

V.e.2. Instruments that have been coated (ie, ebonized) should be inspected for damage to the integrity of the coating before use, after use, and before packaging and sterilization. If damaged, the instrument should be removed from service and repaired or replaced. *[5: Benefits Balanced with Harms]*

  Damage or scratches to the coating may allow the laser beam to reflect off the instrument, potentially causing skin or eye injury.

V.e.3. Reflective instruments that cannot be ebonized should be covered with materials that will not reflect and will not ignite when exposed to the laser beam (eg, saline saturated radiopaque towels, radiopaque sponges).[82,83] *[3: Moderate Evidence]*

V.f. Backstops (eg, titanium rods, quartz rods) or guards should be used during CO_2 laser surgery to prevent the laser beam from striking normal tissue. *[4: Limited Evidence]*

  The collective evidence supports the use of shielding devices.[54,156] The CO_2 laser beam continues to move through the tissue after it cuts or coagulates. A backstop or guard will prevent the laser beam from affecting non-targeted tissue.[82]

V.g. Exposed tissues around the surgical site should be protected with saline-saturated materials

EQUIPMENT AND PRODUCT SAFETY

(eg, towels, sponges) when lasers are being used.[37,38,40,54,82,83,157] *[3: Moderate Evidence]*

In a laboratory descriptive study, Hammons et al[172] used a CO_2 laser to determine the results of reflection off of various surfaces on surgical field materials. They found there was no reflection off wet gauze. The researchers recommended using a tongue blade covered with a moistened sponge with a wet gauze attached to prevent reflection of the laser beam.

V.h. Fire safety precautions should be taken during laser use (See the AORN Guideline for a Safe Environment of Care, Part 1).[6] *[3: Moderate Evidence]*

Li et al[173] reviewed the records of 704 patients undergoing surgery with a CO_2 laser and found 127 adverse events related to the use of the laser in this group of patients. The adverse events included the endotracheal tube bursting, sparks, dense smoke, and burn smells. The authors concluded that precautions should be taken, including inflating the endotracheal tube with water instead of air.

V.h.1. Precautions should be taken to avoid breaking a laser fiber, including not
- leaning against a fiber,
- clamping a fiber, or
- stressing or bending a fiber beyond what is specified as acceptable in the manufacturer's IFU.[82]

[4: Limited Evidence]

V.h.2. During perineal surgery, moistened radiopaque sponges should be used for rectal packing or for covering the anus. *[3: Moderate Evidence]*

Moist packing prevents the release of methane gas from the rectum. Methane gas is highly flammable and potentially explosive.[54,82]

V.h.3. A laser-resistant endotracheal tube should be used during laser procedures involving the airway.[29,32,54,82,174] *[2: High Evidence]*

Roy and Smith[174] compared the time to ignition of a reinforced "laser safe" endotracheal tube and a traditional endotracheal tube when a CO_2 laser was aimed directly at the tube with 21% to 60% oxygen flowing through it. The researchers fired the laser until time of ignition or a maximum of 2 minutes, whichever was longer. The traditional tube ignited in 1 second to 8 seconds. The time to ignition was decreased when a higher percentage of oxygen was flowing through the tube. The reinforced "laser safe" endotracheal tube did not ignite when the CO_2 laser was fired directly at the tube but did ignite when the laser was aimed at the non-reinforced tip of the tube. The researchers concluded that a reinforced "laser safe" endotracheal tube should be

used during surgery performed with a CO_2 laser and that fires will ignite faster with higher concentrations of oxygen.

V.h.4. Endotracheal tube cuffs should be inflated with normal saline or methylene blue-tinted saline during procedures involving laser treatment of the patient's airway or aerodigestive tract.[82,157] *[3: Moderate Evidence]*

The cuffs of the laser-resistant endotracheal tube may not be laser resistant, and inflating the cuff with a liquid may help decrease the potential for the tube to ignite. Methylene blue is added to the saline to help identify a tube cuff rupture.[54]

Li et al[173] conducted an in vitro experiment to determine whether an endotracheal tube cuff filled with water was more resistant to bursting than a cuff filled with air when exposed to a laser beam. The researchers pointed the laser beam at endotracheal tube cuffs that were inflated with air or filled with water. They found the water-filled cuff to be more resistant to bursting than the air-filled cuff. They recommended that endotracheal tube cuffs be filled with water when a laser is being used in the presence of the endotracheal tube.

V.h.5. Moistened packs should be placed around the endotracheal tube and kept moist during procedures involving lasers and the patient's airway or aerodigestive tract.[16] *[3: Moderate Evidence]*

Moistened packs help protect the endotracheal tube from the laser beam.[54,175]

V.i. When laser transmission is not required, the laser must be turned off or beam shutters or caps used. The laser must be turned off when the laser is not attended.[82,167] *[1: Regulatory Requirement]*

V.j. Precautions should be taken during endoscopic procedures using a laser[176]:
○ Before and after the procedure, the scrub person should inspect the laser catheter sheaths and laser fibers for damage,[159,177] and if the sheaths or fibers are damaged, remove them from service.
○ Before the procedure, the scrub person should confirm that the catheter sheath meets the manufacturer's labeled length and the laser fiber is of sufficient length to extend beyond the catheter. If the length differs from the manufacturer's stated length, the scrub person should remove it from service.
○ After each removal from the patient, the scrub person should confirm that the catheter sheath and the laser fiber are intact and complete. If not, the scrub person should remove it from service, report the situation to the physician, and implement the organization's policy for retained surgical items.

[3: Moderate Evidence]

Precautions may prevent retention of a laser fiber and make the team aware of the missing fiber before the patient leaves the surgical suite.[176] Breakage of the fiber has been reported in a case report.[178] van den Bos et al[177] described a case in which the laser fiber punctured the insertion catheter.

Recommendation VI

Precautions should be taken to mitigate the risk for injury associated with the use of a phacoemulsifier.

VI.a. Precautions that should be taken during use of a phacoemulsifier include
- inspecting the phacoemulsifier hand piece operating tip before and after use,[179]
- performing pre-use testing according to the manufacturer's instructions for use,[180] and
- maintaining a continuous irrigation solution flow.[181]

[3: Moderate Evidence]

Abulafia et al[181] examined the effects of an occluded irrigation port on 36 porcine eyes during the use of a phacoemulsification system. The researchers measured the tissue temperature of the eyes and assessed the eyes for the presence of burns during the use of a phacoemulsification system with the irrigation solution either flowing or occluded. The researchers found that the temperature of the eye rose rapidly when the irrigation solution was occluded, which resulted in tissue burns. The researchers concluded that a continuous flow of irrigation solutions is required to maintain a low temperature.

The evidence review found one case report in which the phacoemulsification sleeve was fractured, resulting in an injury to the patient's eye. Shum et al[179] recommended that the instrument be carefully inspected before introduction into the eye.

VI.b. The health care organization should provide education and verify competency related to the use, cleaning, and maintenance of the phacoemulsification system, as applicable to the person's job responsibilities. *[5: Benefits Balanced with Harms]*

Recommendation VII

Precautions should be taken to mitigate the risk of injury associated with the use of argon enhanced coagulation (AEC).

The evidence review found one case report in which the patient developed a cerebral gas embolism after use of AEC.[182] The case report provides technique-related precautions for the physician to follow for the prevention of embolisms (eg, use of a non-contact technique, minimizing gas flow rates).

VII.a. All safety precautions for monopolar electrosurgery and those described in the AEC manufacturer's IFU should be followed during use of AEC technology. *[4: Limited Evidence]*

In a case report, Law et al[183] discussed a patient who received a burn at a staple line that was near a second surgical site. The authors postulated that the burn was caused by the current seeking the shortest route to ground through the nearby staple line (ie, direct coupling). The authors suggested not using AEC when there is a staple line in the vicinity of the area to be treated. This report did not describe the location of the dispersive electrode.

VII.b. Personnel should be prepared to recognize signs and symptoms of gas emboli and initiate treatment. *[3: Moderate Evidence]*

There is a risk of gas embolism when AEC is used.[182]

Glossary

Active electrode monitoring: A dynamic process of searching for insulation failures and capacitive coupling during monopolar surgery. If the monitor detects an unsafe level of stray energy, it signals the generator to deactivate.

Advanced bipolar device: A bipolar electrosurgery unit that uses a computer-controlled tissue feedback response system to sense tissue impedance, allowing for the continuous adjustment of the voltage and current generated by the unit. This allows the lowest possible power setting to achieve the desired tissue effect.

Alternate site injury: An injury caused by an electrosurgical device that occurs away from the dispersive electrode site.

Anodized finish: A matte finish applied to metal surgical instruments to decrease reflectivity.

Antenna coupling: Radio-frequency energy emitted by a monopolar active electrode and transferred without direct contact through conductive materials (eg, neuromuscular, cardiac monitoring electrode wires).

Argon-enhanced coagulation: Radio-frequency coagulation from an electrosurgical generator that is capable of delivering monopolar current through a flow of ionized argon gas.

Bipolar electrosurgery: Electrosurgery in which current flows between two tips of a bipolar forceps that are positioned around tissue to create a surgical effect. Current passes from the active electrode of one tip of the forceps through the patient's desired tissue to the other dispersive electrode tip of the forceps, thus completing the circuit without entering another part of the patient's body.

Capacitive coupled dispersive electrode: A large, nonadhesive dispersive electrode placed close to and forming a capacitor with the patient, returning electrical current from the patient back to the electrosurgical unit.

Capacitive coupling: Transfer of electrical current from the active electrode through intact insulation to adjacent conductive items (eg, tissue, trocars).

EQUIPMENT AND PRODUCT SAFETY

Class 3 lasers: Lasers that are potentially hazardous for direct exposure to specular (ie, mirror-like) reflection.

Class 4 lasers: Lasers that present significant skin and fire hazards. Most surgical lasers are class 4 lasers.

Current: A movement of electrons analogous to the flow of a stream of water.

Direct coupling: The contact of an energized active electrode tip with another metal instrument or object within the surgical field.

Dispersive electrode: The accessory that directs electrical current flow from the patient back to the electrosurgical generator. Often called the patient plate, return electrode, inactive electrode, or grounding pad.

Ebonized finish: A black finish applied to metal surgical instruments to decrease reflectivity.

Electrocautery: A surgical device, often battery powered, that is used to cauterize blood vessels. Heat is produced in a closed loop. No electrodes are used. Electricity does not pass through the patient or through the tissue. Cauterization is produced by heat.

Electromagnetic interference: The disruption of operation of an electronic device (eg, pacemaker, cochlear implant) when it is in the vicinity of an electromagnetic field in the radio-frequency spectrum that is caused by another electronic device (eg, electrosurgery unit).

Electrosurgery: The cutting and coagulation of body tissue with a high-frequency (ie, radio-frequency) current. The current is passed through the body or the tissue and between two poles. Heat is generated in the tissue through which the current passes.

Electrosurgical accessories: The active electrode with tip(s), dispersive electrode, adapters, and connectors to attach these devices to the electrosurgery generator.

Electrosurgical unit: The generator that produces a high-frequency current waveform that is delivered to tissues, the foot switch with cord (if applicable), the electrical plug, cord, and connections.

Eschar: Charred tissue residue.

Ferromagnetic device: An electrocautery device in which the electricity travels through a closed loop and produces heat by excitation of the ferromagnetic coating on the loop.

Insulation failure: Damage to the insulation of the active electrode that provides an alternate pathway for the current to leave that electrode as it completes the circuit to the dispersive electrode.

Isolated electrosurgical unit: A system in which electrical current is sent to the patient and selectively returns and is grounded through the generator.

Laser: A device that produces an intense, coherent, directional beam of light by stimulating electronic or molecular transitions to lower energy levels. An acronym for "light amplification by stimulated emission of radiation."

Laser operator: The person who sets up the laser and operates the laser console to control the laser parameters under the supervision of the laser user.

Laser safety officer: The person responsible for effecting the knowledgeable evaluation of laser hazards and authorized and responsible for monitoring and overseeing the control of such laser hazards.

Laser safety specialist: The person designated to oversee safe laser use in each area where a laser is used.

Laser user: The person employing the laser for its intended purpose within the user's scope of practice, education, and experience.

Monopolar electrosurgery: Electrosurgery in which only the active electrode is in the surgical wound and the electrical current is directed through the patient's body, received by the dispersive pad, and transferred back to the generator, completing the monopolar circuit.

Nominal hazard zone: The space in which the level of direct, reflected, or scattered radiation used during normal laser operation exceeds the applicable maximum permissible exposure. Exposure levels beyond the boundary of the nominal hazard zone should be below the appropriate maximum permissible exposure level of the laser. Special eye and skin precautions must be enforced in the nominal hazard zone.

Optical density: The ability to absorb a specific laser wavelength.

Return-electrode contact quality monitoring: A dynamic monitoring circuit measuring impedance of the dispersive return electrode. If the dispersive electrode becomes compromised, the circuit inhibits the electrosurgical unit's output.

Tripolar device: An electrosurgical device using a tripolar tip consisting of a central pole and an outer pole on either side. The current flows from the center pole to the outer poles, creating a corona of energy that makes a blade-like incision. The current alternates with a second current that passes from one of the outer poles to the other, resulting in simultaneous cutting and coagulating.

Vessel-sealing device: A device that uses a combination of mechanical pressure and thermal energy to cut and coagulate tissue using radio-frequency current.

REFERENCES

1. van de Berg NJ, van den Dobbelsteen JJ, Jansen FW, Grimbergen CA, Dankelman J. Energetic soft-tissue treatment technologies: an overview of procedural fundamentals and safety factors. *Surg Endosc.* 2013;27(9):3085-3099. [VA]

2. Sutton C, Abbott J. History of power sources in endoscopic surgery. *J Minim Invasive Gynecol.* 2013;20(3):271-278. [VB]

3. Law KS, Abbott JA, Lyons SD. Energy sources for gynecologic laparoscopic surgery: a review of the literature. *Obstet Gynecol Surv.* 2014;69(12):763-776. [VA]

4. Gillespie MB, Stachiw ND, Way J, et al. Neural outcomes after plasma knife dissection: a pathologic study and clinical correlation. *Head Neck.* 2010;32(10):1321-1327. [IB]

5. Sankaranarayanan G, Resapu RR, Jones DB, Schwaitzberg S, De S. Common uses and cited complications of energy in surgery. *Surg Endosc.* 2013;27(9):3056-3072. [VA]

6. Guideline for a safe environment of care, part 1. In: *Guidelines for Perioperative Practice*. Denver, CO: AORN, Inc; 2016:237-262. [IVB]

7. Guideline for minimally invasive surgery. In: *Guidelines for Perioperative Practice*. Denver, CO: AORN, Inc; 2016:589-616. [IVC]

8. Lee JY, Park CB, Cho EJ, et al. Airway fire injury during rigid bronchoscopy in a patient with a silicon stent—a case report. *Korean J Anesthesiol*. 2012;62(2):184-187. [VC]

9. Mehta SP, Bhananker SM, Posner KL, Domino KB. Operating room fires: a closed claims analysis. *Anesthesiology*. 2013;118(5):1133-1139. [VB]

10. Haith LR Jr, Santavasi W, Shapiro TK, et al. Burn center management of operating room fire injuries. *J Burn Care Res*. 2012;33(5):649-653. [VC]

11. Hudson DW, Guidry OF, Abernathy JH 3rd, Ehrenwerth J. Case 4-2012: intrathoracic fire during coronary artery bypass graft surgery. *J Cardiothorac Vasc Anesth*. 2012;26(3):520-521. [VC]

12. Bansal A, Bhama JK, Varga JM, Toyoda Y. Airway fire during double-lung transplantation. *Interact Cardiovasc Thorac Surg*. 2013;17(6):1059-1060. [VC]

13. Moskowitz M. Fire in the operating room during open heart surgery: a case report. *AANA J*. 2009;77(4):261-264. [VA]

14. Herman MA, Laudanski K, Berger J. Surgical fire during organ procurement. *Internet J Anesthesiol*. 2009;19(1):6. [VC]

15. Overbey DM, Townsend NT, Chapman BC, et al. Surgical energy-based device injuries and fatalities reported to the Food and Drug Administration. *J Am Coll Surg*. 2015;221(1):197-205. [IIIA]

16. Raghavan K, Lagisetty KH, Butler KL, Cahalane MJ, Gupta A, Odom SR. Intraoperative fires during emergent colon surgery. *Am Surg*. 2015;81(2):E82-E83. [VB]

17. Tremaine AM, Avram MM. FDA MAUDE data on complications with lasers, light sources, and energy-based devices. *Lasers Surg Med*. 2015;47(2):133-140. [VA]

18. Chae SB, Kim WK, Yoo CJ, Park CW. Fires and burns occurring in an electrocautery after skin preparation with alcohol during a neurosurgery. *J Korean Neurosurg Soc*. 2014;55(4):230-233. [VC]

19. Chung SH, Lee HH, Kim TH, Kim JS. A patient who was burned in the operative field: a case report. *Ulus Travma Acil Cerrahi Derg*. 2012;18(3):274-276. [VC]

20. Kim MS, Lee JH, Lee DH, Lee YU, Jung TE. Electrocautery-ignited surgical field fire caused by a high oxygen level during tracheostomy. *Korean J Thorac Cardiovasc Surg*. 2014;47(5):491-493. [VC]

21. Messenger D, Carter F, Francis N. Electrosurgery and energized dissection. *Surgery (United Kingdom)*. 2014;32(3):126-130. [VB]

22. Gunaruwan P, Barlow M. Diathermy-induced ventricular fibrillation with Riata high-voltage lead insulation failure. *Europace*. 2013;15(4):473. [VC]

23. Mumith A, Thuraisingham J, Gurunathan-Mani S. Ignition of free gas in the peritoneal cavity: an explosive complication. *Case Rep Surg*. 2013;2013:746430. [VC]

24. Smith LP, Roy S. Operating room fires in otolaryngology: risk factors and prevention. *Am J Otolaryngol*. 2011;32(2):109-114. [IIIB]

25. Vo A, Bengezi O. Third-degree burns caused by ignition of chlorhexidine: a case report and systematic review of the literature. *Plast Surg (Oakv)*. 2014;22(4):264-266. [VA]

26. Partanen E, Koljonen V, Salonen A, Back LJ, Vuola J. A patient with intraoral fire during tonsillectomy. *J Craniofac Surg*. 2014;25(5):1822-1824. [VA]

27. Dhar V, Young K, Nouraei SA, et al. Impact of oxygen concentration and laser power on occurrence of intraluminal fires during shared-airway surgery: an investigation. *J Laryngol Otol*. 2008;122(12):1335-1338. [IIA]

28. Matt BH, Cottee LA. Reducing risk of fire in the operating room using coblation technology. *Otolaryngol Head Neck Surg*. 2010;143(3):454-455. [IIIC]

29. Dennis E. Decreasing airway fires. *OR Nurse*. 2012;6(2):37-40. [VB]

30. González Ma CE, Fernández VO. Case report: airway burn. *Rev Colomb Anestesiol*. 2013;41(3):226-228. [VC]

31. Roy S, Smith LP. Device-related risk of fire in oropharyngeal surgery: a mechanical model. *Am J Otolaryngol*. 2010;31(5):356-359. [IIB]

32. Apfelbaum JL, Caplan RA, Connis RT, et al. Practice advisory for the prevention and management of operating room fires: an updated report by the American Society of Anesthesiologists Task Force on Operating Room Fires. *Anesthesiology*. 2013;118(2):271-290. [IVA]

33. Seifert PC, Peterson E, Graham K. Crisis management of fire in the OR. *AORN J*. 2015;101(2):250-263. [VA]

34. Fire caused by improper disposal of a battery-powered electrocautery pen. *Health Devices*. 2013;42(10):346. [VC]

35. Axelrod EH, Kusnetz AB, Rosenberg MK. Operating room fires initiated by hot wire cautery. *Anesthesiology*. 1993;79(5):1123-1126. [IIIB]

36. Potty AG, Khan W, Tailor HD. Diathermy in perioperative practice. *J Perioper Pract*. 2010;20(11):402-405. [VB]

37. Singh S, Gambhir RS, Kaur A, Singh G, Sharma S, Kakar H. Dental lasers: a review of safety essentials. *J Lasers Med Sci*. 2012;3(3):91-96. [VB]

38. De Felice E. Shedding light: laser physics and mechanism of action. *Phlebology*. 2010;25(1):11-28. [VB]

39. Dudelzak J, Goldberg DJ. Laser safety. *Curr Probl Dermatol*. 2011;42:35-39. [VC]

40. Dhepe N. Minimum standard guidelines of care on requirements for setting up a laser room. *Indian J Dermatol Venereol Leprol*. 2009;75(Suppl 2):S101-S110. [IVB]

41. Maurins U, Rabe E, Pannier F. Does laser power influence the results of endovenous laser ablation (EVLA) of incompetent saphenous veins with the 1 470-nm diode laser? A prospective randomized study comparing 15 and 25 W. *Int Angiol*. 2009;28(1):32-37. [IA]

42. Robinson TN, Pavlovsky KR, Looney H, Stiegmann GV, McGreevy FT. Surgeon-controlled factors that reduce monopolar electrosurgery capacitive coupling during laparoscopy. *Surg Laparosc Endosc Percutan Tech*. 2010;20(5):317-320. [IIA]

43. Jones EL, Robinson TN, McHenry JR, et al. Radiofrequency energy antenna coupling to common laparoscopic instruments: practical implications. *Surg Endosc*. 2012;26(11):3053-3057. [IIIB]

44. Martinek M, Bencsik G, Aichinger J, et al. Esophageal damage during radiofrequency ablation of atrial fibrillation: impact of energy settings, lesion sets, and esophageal visualization. *J Cardiovasc Electrophysiol*. 2009;20(7):726-733. [IIB]

45. Robinson TN, Varosy PD, Guillaume G, et al. Effect of radiofrequency energy emitted from monopolar "Bovie" instruments on cardiac implantable electronic devices. *J Am Coll Surg*. 2014;219(3):399-406. [IIIB]

46. Townsend NT, Jones EL, Paniccia A, Vandervelde J, McHenry JR, Robinson TN. Antenna coupling explains unintended thermal injury caused by common operating room monitoring devices. *Surg Laparosc Endosc Percutan Tech*. 2015;25(2):111-113. [IIB]

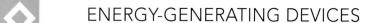

47. Russo V, Rago A, DI Meo F, et al. Ventricular fibrillation induced by coagulating mode bipolar electrocautery during pacemaker implantation in Myotonic Dystrophy type 1 patient. *Acta Myologica.* 2014;33(3):149-151. [VB]

48. Sanders SM, Krowka S, Giacobbe A, Bisson LJ. Third-degree burn from a grounding pad during arthroscopy. *Arthroscopy.* 2009;25(10):1193-1197. [VB]

49. Brill AI. Electrosurgery: principles and practice to reduce risk and maximize efficacy. *Obstet Gynecol Clin North Am.* 2011;38(4):687-702. [VB]

50. Ubee SS, Kasi VS, Bello D, Manikandan R. Implications of pacemakers and implantable cardioverter defibrillators in urological practice. *J Urol.* 2011;186(4):1198-1205. [VA]

51. Alkatout I, Schollmeyer T, Hawaldar NA, Sharma N, Mettler L. Principles and safety measures of electrosurgery in laparoscopy. *JSLS.* 2012;16(1):130-139. [VC]

52. Misiri J, Kusumoto F, Goldschlager N. Electromagnetic interference and implanted cardiac devices: the medical environment (part II). *Clin Cardiol.* 2012;35(6):321-328. [VA]

53. Lowry TR, Workman JR. Avoiding oral burns during electrocautery tonsillectomy. *Ear Nose Throat J.* 2009;88(2):790-792. [VC]

54. ECRI. Laser use and safety. *Operating Room Risk Management.* 2011:IA. [VA]

55. Druzijanic N, Pogorelic Z, Perko Z, Mrklic I, Tomic S. Comparison of lateral thermal damage of the human peritoneum using monopolar diathermy, Harmonic scalpel and LigaSure. *Can J Surg.* 2012;55(5):317-321. [IIA]

56. Munro MG. Mechanisms of thermal injury to the lower genital tract with radiofrequency resectoscopic surgery. *J Minim Invasive Gynecol.* 2006;13(1):36-42. [IIIB]

57. Mitchell ME, Kidd D, Lotto ML, et al. Determination of factors influencing tissue effect of thermal chondroplasty: an ex vivo investigation. *Arthroscopy.* 2006;22(4):351-355. [IIB]

58. Lowe D, Cromwell DA, Lewsey JD, et al. Diathermy power settings as a risk factor for hemorrhage after tonsillectomy. *Otolaryngol Head Neck Surg.* 2009;140(1):23-28. [IIIA]

59. Kaspar S, Siller J, Cervinkova Z, Danek T. Standardisation of parameters during endovenous laser therapy of truncal varicose veins—experimental ex-vivo study. *Eur J Vasc Endovasc Surg.* 2007;34(2):224-228. [IIB]

60. Itoi T, Isayama H, Sofuni A, et al. Evaluation of effects of a novel endoscopically applied radiofrequency ablation biliary catheter using an ex-vivo pig liver. *J Hepatobiliary Pancreat Sci.* 2012;19(5):543-547. [IIB]

61. Huang Y, Zhang Y, Ding X, Liu S, Sun T. Working conditions of bipolar radiofrequency on human articular cartilage repair following thermal injury during arthroscopy. *Chin Med J.* 2014;127(22):3881-3886. [IIB]

62. Goulet CJ, Disario JA, Emerson L, Hilden K, Holubkov R, Fang JC. In vivo evaluation of argon plasma coagulation in a porcine model. *Gastrointest Endosc.* 2007;65(3):457-462. [IIB]

63. Sutton PA, Awad S, Perkins AC, Lobo DN. Comparison of lateral thermal spread using monopolar and bipolar diathermy, the Harmonic Scalpel and the Ligasure. *Br J Surg.* 2010;97(3):428-433. [IIB]

64. Sananes N, Favre R, Koh CJ, et al. Urological fistulas after fetal cystoscopic laser ablation of posterior urethral valves: surgical technical aspects. *Ultrasound Obstet Gynecol.* 2015;45(2):183-189. [IIIB]

65. Govekar HR, Robinson TN, Varosy PD, et al. Effect of monopolar radiofrequency energy on pacemaker function. *Surg Endosc.* 2012;26(10):2784-2788. [IIIC]

66. Robinson TN, Barnes KS, Govekar HR, Stiegmann GV, Dunn CL, McGreevy FT. Antenna coupling—a novel mechanism of radiofrequency electrosurgery complication: practical implications. *Ann Surg.* 2012;256(2):213-218. [IIB]

67. Devassy R, Gopalakrishnan S, De Wilde RL. Surgical efficacy among laparoscopic ultrasonic dissectors: are we advancing safely? A review of literature. *J Obstet Gynecol India.* 2015;65(5):293-300. [VB]

68. Peter NM, Ribes P, Khooshabeh R. Cardiac pacemakers and electrocautery in ophthalmic surgery. *Orbit.* 2012;31(6):408-411. [VC]

69. Rey JF, Beilenhoff U, Neumann CS, Dumonceau JM. European Society of Gastrointestinal Endoscopy (ESGE) guideline: the use of electrosurgical units. *Endoscopy.* 2010;42(9):764-771. [IVC]

70. American Society of Anesthesiologists. Practice advisory for the perioperative management of patients with cardiac implantable electronic devices: pacemakers and implantable cardioverter-defibrillators: an updated report by the American Society of Anesthesiologists Task Force on Perioperative Management of Patients with Cardiac Implantable Electronic Devices. *Anesthesiology.* 2011;114(2):247-261. [IVC]

71. O'Riley M. Electrosurgery in perioperative practice. *J Perioper Pract.* 2010;20(9):329-333. [VC]

72. Metzner A, Wissner E, Schoonderwoerd B, et al. The influence of varying energy settings on efficacy and safety of endoscopic pulmonary vein isolation. *Heart Rhythm.* 2012;9(9):1380-1385. [IIIB]

73. Mantke R, Halangk W, Habermann A, et al. Efficacy and safety of 5-mm-diameter bipolar and ultrasonic shears for cutting carotid arteries of the hybrid pig. *Surg Endosc.* 2011;25(2):577-585. [IIIA]

74. Hefermehl LJ, Largo RA, Hermanns T, Poyet C, Sulser T, Eberli D. Lateral temperature spread of monopolar, bipolar and ultrasonic instruments for robot-assisted laparoscopic surgery. *BJU Int.* 2014;114(2):245-252. [IIIB]

75. Hazard report. Internal wire breakage in reusable electrosurgical active electrode cables may cause sparking and surgical fires. *Health Devices.* 2009;38(7):228-229. [VB]

76. Shah AJ, Janes R, Holliday J, Thakur R. Radiofrequency transseptal catheter electrode fracture. *Pacing Clin Electrophysiol.* 2010;33(6):e57-e58. [VB]

77. El-Damaty A, Love M, Parkash R. Detached tip of a transseptal sheath during left atrial ablation. *Catheter Cardiovasc Interv.* 2012;79(3):444-447. [VC]

78. Hospital eTools. Surgical suite—use of medical lasers. Occupational Safety and Health Administration https://www.osha.gov/SLTC/etools/hospital/surgical.lasers.html. Accessed June 27, 2016. [VC]

79. National Fire Protection Association Technical Committee on Laser Fire Protection. *NFPA 115: Standard for Laser Fire Protection.* Quincy, MA: National Fire Protection Association; 2008. [IVC]

80. Mary S. Laser safety: practical measures and latest legislative requirements. *J Perioper Pract.* 2011;21(9):299-303. [VB]

81. Plauntz L. Guidelines for staff administering laser therapy in an office setting. *Plast Surg Nurs.* 2013;33(1):29-35. [IVB]

82. Z136.3: Safe use of lasers in health care. In: *ANS Z136 Standards.* Orlando, FL: Laser Institute of America; 2011. [IVC]

83. Smalley PJ. Laser safety: risks, hazards, and control measures. *Laser Ther.* 2011;20(2):95-106. [VB]

84. Munro MG. Complications of hysteroscopic and uterine resectoscopic surgery. *Obstet Gynecol Clin North Am.* 2010;37(3):399-425. [VB]

85. Fonseca AZ, Santin S, Gomes LG, Waisberg J, Ribeiro MA Jr. Complications of radiofrequency ablation of hepatic tumors: frequency and risk factors. *World J Hepatol.* 2014;6(3):107-113. [VB]

86. Gil Franco F, Bailard N. Peripheral nerve stimulator response triggered by proximity to electrosurgical unit. *Anesth Analg.* 2012;114(5):1142-1143. [VC]

87. Sabzi F, Niazi M, Ahmadi A. Rare case-series of electrocautery burn following off-pump coronary artery bypass grafting. *J Inj Violence Res.* 2014;6(1):44-49. [VB]

88. Nelson G, Morris ML. Electrosurgery in the gastrointestinal suite: knowledge is power. *Gastroenterol Nurs.* 2015;38(6):430-439. [VA]

89. Vilos GA, Rajakumar C. Electrosurgical generators and monopolar and bipolar electrosurgery. *J Minim Invasive Gynecol.* 2013;20(3):279-287. [VA]

90. Makedonov I, Lee J. An evaluation of potential for alternate return site burns due to capacitive coupling between active electrode and ground while using electrosurgery units. *J Clin Eng.* 2011;36(1):29-31. [IIIC]

91. Robinson TN, Jones EL, Dunn CL, et al. Separating the laparoscopic camera cord from the monopolar "Bovie" cord reduces unintended thermal injury from antenna coupling: a randomized controlled trial. *Ann Surg.* 2015;261(6):1056-1060. [IA]

92. Hammwohner M, Stachowitz J, Willich T, Goette A. Induction of ventricular tachycardia during radiofrequency ablation via pulmonary vein ablation catheter in a patient with an implanted pacemaker. *Europace.* 2012;14(2):298-299. [VC]

93. Goel AK, Korotkin S, Walsh D, Bess M, Frawley S. Monomorphic ventricular tachycardia caused by electrocautery during pacemaker generator change in a patient with normal left ventricular function. *Pacing Clin Electrophysiol.* 2009;32(7):957-958. [VC]

94. Cassagneau R, Hanninen M, Yee R. Electrocautery-induced ventricular fibrillation during routine implantable cardioverter-defibrillator generator replacement. *Europace.* 2014;16(3):319. [VC]

95. Schulman PM, Rozner MA. Use caution when applying magnets to pacemakers or defibrillators for surgery. *Anesth Analg.* 2013;117(2):422-427. [VA]

96. Mohammed I, Ratib K, Creamer J. An unusual intracardiac electrogram showing cause for false electrical discharge from an ICD. *BMJ Case Rep.* 2013;2013. [VC]

97. Castillo JG, Silvay G, Viles-Gonzalez J. Perioperative assessment of patients with cardiac implantable electronic devices. *Mt Sinai J Med.* 2012;79(1):25-33. [VB]

98. King C. Endoscopic electrosurgery—an overview. *Gastrointest Nurs.* 2011;9(4):28-33. [VB]

99. Lomax A. Overview of the principles of electrosurgery and patient safety in the endoscopy room. *J GENCA.* 2009;19(3):14-34. [VC]

100. Crossley GH, Poole JE, Rozner MA, et al. The Heart Rhythm Society (HRS)/American Society of Anesthesiologists (ASA) Expert Consensus Statement on the perioperative management of patients with implantable defibrillators, pacemakers and arrhythmia monitors: facilities and patient management. This document was developed as a joint project with the American Society of Anesthesiologists (ASA), and in collaboration with the American Heart Association (AHA), and the Society of Thoracic Surgeons (STS). *Heart Rhythm.* 2011;8(7):1114-1154. [IVC]

101. Maheshwari KR, Nikdel K, Guillaume G, Letra AM, Silva RM, Dorn SO. Evaluating the effects of different dental devices on implantable cardioverter defibrillators. *J Endod.* 2015;41(5):692-695. [IIIB]

102. Stone ME, Salter B, Fischer A. Perioperative management of patients with cardiac implantable electronic devices. *Br J Anaesth.* 2011;107(Suppl 1):i16-i26. [VA]

103. Petersen BT, Hussain N, Marine JE, et al. Endoscopy in patients with implanted electronic devices. *Gastrointest Endosc.* 2007;65(4):561-568. [VB]

104. Navaratnam M, Dubin A. Pediatric pacemakers and ICDs: how to optimize perioperative care. *Paediatr Anaesth.* 2011;21(5):512-521. [VB]

105. Gallagher K, Dhinsa B, Miles J. Electrosurgery. *Surgery.* 2011;29(2):70-72. [VB]

106. Garcia Bracamonte B, Rodriguez J, Casado R, Vanaclocha F. Electrosurgery in patients with implantable electronic cardiac devices (pacemakers and defibrillators). *Actas Dermosifiliogr.* 2013;104(2):128-132. [VB]

107. Can I, Aribas A, Dereli Y, Tholakanalli V. Inappropriate sensing events revealing electrocautery-induced implantable cardioverter-defibrillator lead failure. *Anatol J Cardiol.* 2015;15(10):E27. [V]

108. Chia PL, Foo D. A practical approach to perioperative management of cardiac implantable electronic devices. *Singapore Med J.* 2015;56(10):538-541. [VB]

109. Santini L, Forleo GB, Santini M. Implantable devices in the electromagnetic environment. *J Arrhythm.* 2013;29(6):325-333. [VB]

110. Stone ME, Apinis A. Current perioperative management of the patient with a cardiac rhythm management device. *Semin Cardiothorac Vasc Anesth.* 2009;13(1):31-43. [VB]

111. Healey JS, Merchant R, Simpson C, et al. Canadian Cardiovascular Society/Canadian Anesthesiologists' Society/Canadian Heart Rhythm Society joint position statement on the perioperative management of patients with implanted pacemakers, defibrillators, and neurostimulating devices. *Can J Anesth.* 2012;59(4):394-407. [IVB]

112. Ogg MJ. Caring for patients with cardiovascular implantable electronic devices [Clinical Issues]. *AORN J.* 2013;98(2):196-197. [VB]

113. Howe N, Cherpelis B. Obtaining rapid and effective hemostasis: part II. electrosurgery in patients with implantable cardiac devices. *J Am Acad Dermatol.* 2013;69(5):677.e1-677.e9. [VC]

114. Rozner MA. Perioperative care of the patient with a cardiac pacemaker or ICD. *Rev Mex Anestesiol.* 2009;32(Suppl 1):S190-S197. [VB]

115. Ahrens PM, Siddiqui NA, Rakhit RD. Pacemaker placement and shoulder surgery: is there a risk? *Ann R Coll Surg Engl.* 2012;94(1):39-42. [IIIC]

116. Pavlovic S, Milasinovic G, Zivkovic M. Approach to patients with implanted pacemaker and scheduled surgical or diagnostic procedure. *Acta Chir Iugosl.* 2011;58(2):25-29. [VC]

117. Voutsalath MA, Bichakjian CK, Pelosi F, Blum D, Johnson TM, Farrehi PM. Electrosurgery and implantable electronic devices: review and implications for office-based procedures. *Dermatol Surg.* 2011;37(7):889-899. [VA]

118. Venkatraghavan L, Chinnapa V, Peng P, Brull R. Non-cardiac implantable electrical devices: brief review and implications for anesthesiologists. *Can J Anaesth.* 2009;56(4):320-326. [VA]

119. Abdelmalak B, Jagannathan N, Arain FD, Cymbor S, McLain R, Tetzlaff JE. Electromagnetic interference in a cardiac pacemaker during cauterization with the coagulating, not cutting mode. *J Anaesth Clin Pharmacol.* 2011;27(4):527-530. [VB]

EQUIPMENT AND PRODUCT SAFETY

120. Paniccia A, Rozner M, Jones EL, et al. Electromagnetic interference caused by common surgical energy-based devices on an implanted cardiac defibrillator. *Am J Surg.* 2014;208(6):932-936. [IIB]

121. Bouyer B, Bachy M, Vermesch AI, Doummar D, Coubes P, Vialle R. The use of Harmonic scalpel in spinal surgery with contraindication to the use of monopolar electrocautery: a case report in a 14-year-old girl with a primary generalized dystonia and a 100° thoracic scoliosis. *Childs Nerv Syst.* 2012;28(8):1251-1255. [VC]

122. Weiss JP, Manwaring P. Freedom from electromagnetic interference between cardiac implantable electronic devices and the FMwand ferromagnetic surgical system. *J Clin Anesth.* 2013;25(8):681-684. [IIC]

123. Asensio EL, Lopez TG, Guerrero MH, et al. Radiofrequency ablation of a hepatic neoplasm in a patient with an abdominal pacemaker. *Cardiol J.* 2009;16(3):264-268. [VB]

124. Radolec MM, Beerman LB, Arora G. Radiofrequency energy ablation in a child with an implanted vagus nerve stimulator. *Cardiol Young.* 2015;25(7):1379-1381. [VB]

125. Jeyakumar A, Wilson M, Sorrel JE, et al. Monopolar cautery and adverse effects on cochlear implants. *JAMA Otolaryngol Head Neck Surg.* 2013;139(7):694-697. [IIIB]

126. Frampton SJ, Ismail-Koch H, Mitchell TE. How safe is diathermy in patients with cochlear implants? *Ann R Coll Surg Engl.* 2012;94(8):585-587. [IIIB]

127. Frampton SJ, Mitchell TE. Surgical safety issues relating to the use of diathermy in patients with cochlear implants: the patient's perspective. *Cochlear Implants Int.* 2014;15(1):48-52. [IIIB]

128. Alternate-site burns from improperly seated or damaged electrosurgical pencil active electrodes. *Health Devices.* 2012;41(10):334. [VB]

129. Flowers J. Fire safety in procedural areas. *J Radiol Nurs.* 2012;31(1):13-19. [VB]

130. Kwon H-J, Kim PN, Byun JH, et al. Various complications of percutaneous radiofrequency ablation for hepatic tumors: radiologic findings and technical tips. *Acta Radiol.* 2014;55(9):1082-1092. [VB]

131. Pompili M, Riccardi L, Garcovich M, Sollazzi L, Seccia A, Rapaccini G. Severe skin burn at needle entry point complicating radiofrequency ablation for hepatocellular carcinoma. *Ultraschall Med.* 2012;33(7):E359-E360. [VB]

132. Ogake K, Yasui C, Aihara T, et al. Analysis of tissue impedance waveform reflecting in a grounding pad burn during radiofrequency ablation. *Acta Hepato Jpn.* 2011;52(6):361-367. [VC]

133. Demircin S, Aslan F, Karagoz YM, Atilgan M. Medicolegal aspects of surgical diathermy burns: a case report and review of the literature. *Rom J Leg Med.* 2013;21(3):173-176. [VB]

134. Nguyen DT, Barham W, Zheng L, Dinegar S, Tzou WS, Sauer WH. Effect of radiofrequency energy delivery in proximity to metallic medical device components. *Heart Rhythm.* 2015;12(10):2162-2169. [IIIB]

135. Saaiq M, Zaib S, Ahmad S. Electrocautery burns: experience with three cases and review of literature. *Ann Burns Fire Disasters.* 2012;25(4):203-206. [VB]

136. Ertugrul I, Karagoz T, Aykan HH. A rare complication of radiofrequency ablation: skin burn. *Cardiol Young.* 2015;25(7):1385-1386. [VC]

137. Dhillon PS, Gonna H, Li A, Wong T, Ward DE. Skin burns associated with radiofrequency catheter ablation of cardiac arrhythmias. *Pacing Clin Electrophysiol.* 2013;36(6):764-767. [VC]

138. Huffman SD, Huffman NP, Lewandowski RJ, Brown DB. Radiofrequency ablation complicated by skin burn. *Semin Intervent Radiol.* 2011;28(2):179-182. [VC]

139. Hachach-Haram N, Saour S, Alamouti R, Constantinides J, Mohanna PN. Labelling of diathermy consoles when multiple systems are used: should this be part of the WHO checklist? *BMJ Qual Saf.* 2013;22(9):775-776. [VB]

140. Odell RC. Surgical complications specific to monopolar electrosurgical energy: engineering changes that have made electrosurgery safer. *J Minim Invasive Gynecol* 2013;20(3):288-298. [VB]

141. Liu Q, Sun XB. Indirect electrical injuries from capacitive coupling: a rarely mentioned electrosurgical complication in monopolar laparoscopy. *Acta Obstet Gynecol Scand.* 2013;92(2):238-241. [VC]

142. Brown J, Blank K. Minimally invasive endometrial ablation device complications and use outside of the manufacturers' instructions. *Obstet Gynecol.* 2012;120(4):865-870. [VC]

143. Feldman LS, Fuchshuber P, Jones DB, Mischna J, Schwaitzberg SD; FUSE (Fundamental Use of Surgical Energy™) Task Force. Surgeons don't know what they don't know about the safe use of energy in surgery. *Surg Endosc.* 2012;26(10):2735-2739. [IIB]

144. AlNomair N, Nazarian R, Marmur E. Complications in lasers, lights, and radiofrequency devices. *Facial Plast Surg.* 2012;28(3):340-346. [VB]

145. Surve R, Madhusudan S, Sriganesh K. Electrocautery interference with intraoperative capnography during neurosurgery. *J Clin Monit Comput.* 2014;28(4):429-430 [VB]

146. Guideline for health care information management. In: *Guidelines for Perioperative Practice.* Denver, CO: AORN, Inc; 2016:577-588. [IVC]

147. Abu-Rafea B, Vilos GA, Al-Obeed O, AlSheikh A, Vilos AG, Al-Mandeel H. Monopolar electrosurgery through single-port laparoscopy: a potential hidden hazard for bowel burns. *J Minim Invasive Gynecol* 2011;18(6):734-740. [IIIB]

148. Cassaro S. Delayed manifestations of laparoscopic bowel injury. *Am Surg.* 2015;81(5):478-482. [VA]

149. Humes DJ, Ahmed I, Lobo DN. The pedicle effect and direct coupling: delayed thermal injuries to the bile duct after laparoscopic cholecystectomy. *Arch Surg* 2010;145(1):96-98. [VC]

150. Cormier B, Nezhat F, Sternchos J, Sonoda Y, Leitao MM Jr. Electrocautery-associated vascular injury during robotic-assisted surgery. *Obstet Gynecol.* 2012;120(2 Pt 2):491-493. [VB]

151. Montero PN, Robinson TN, Weaver JS, Stiegmann GV. Insulation failure in laparoscopic instruments. *Surg Endosc.* 2010;24(2):462-465. [IIIB]

152. Mendez-Probst CE, Vilos G, Fuller A, et al. Stray electrical currents in laparoscopic instruments used in da Vinci robot-assisted surgery: an in vitro study. *J Endourol.* 2011;25(9):1513-1517. [IIIB]

153. Espada M, Munoz R, Noble BN, Magrina JF. Insulation failure in robotic and laparoscopic instrumentation: a prospective evaluation. *Am J Obstet Gynecol.* 2011;205(2):121.e1-121.e5. [IIIB]

154. Z136.1: Safe use of lasers. In: *ANSI Z136 Standards.* Orlando, FL: Laser Institute of America; 2014. [IVC]

155. Dhar P, Malik A. Anesthesia for laser surgery in ENT and the various ventilatory techniques. *Trends Anaesth Crit Care.* 2011;1(2):60-66. [VB]

156. Kyoukai KH. Safety guidelines for the laser removal of dental calculus. *Laser Ther.* 2012;21(2):137-145. [VC]

157. Thomas G, Isaacs R. Basic principles of lasers. *Anaesth Intensive Care Med.* 2011;12(12):574-577. [VC]

158. Kang Y, Rabie AB, Wong RW. A review of laser applications in orthodontics. *Int J Orthod.* 2014;25(1):47-56. [VA]

159. Kaneko S. Safety guidelines for diagnostic and therapeutic laser applications in the neurosurgical field. *Laser Ther.* 2012;21(2):129-136. [IVC]

160. Edwards B, Sams B. Overview of the Board of Laser Safety's professional certification programs for laser safety officers. *Med Laser Appl.* 2010;25(2):70-74. [VB]

161. Osti D, Ferri E, Caggese G, Rinaldi S, Guberti A, Zoppellari R. Probable case of vascular air embolism during endonasal CO2 laser surgery. *Minerva Anestesiol.* 2009;75(5):275-279. [VC]

162. 29 CFR 1910. Subpart I—personal protective equipment. Occupational Safety and Health Administration. https://www.osha.gov/pls/oshaweb/owastand.display_standard_group?p_toc_level=1&p_part_number=1910. Accessed June 27, 2016.

163. Wöllmer W, Schade G, Kessler G. Endotracheal tube fires still happen—a short overview. *Med Laser Appl.* 2010;25(2):118-125. [VA]

164. Russi M, Buchta WG, Swift M, et al. Guidance for occupational health services in medical centers. *J Occup Environ Med.* 2009;51(11):1e-18e. [VC]

165. Pierce JS, Lacey SE, Lippert JF, Lopez R, Franke JE, Colvard MD. An assessment of the occupational hazards related to medical lasers. *J Occup Environ Med.* 2011;53(11):1302-1309. [IIIB]

166. Althunayan AM, Elkoushy MA, Elhilali MM, Andonian S. Adverse events resulting from lasers used in urology. *J Endourol.* 2014;28(2):256-260. [VC]

167. 29 CFR 1926. Safety and health regulations for construction. Occupational Safety and Health Administration. https://www.osha.gov/pls/oshaweb/owastand.display_standard_group?p_toc_level=1&p_part_number=1926. Accessed June 27, 2016.

168. Public Law 91-596. Occupational Safety and Health Act of 1970. December 29, 1970, as amended through January 1, 2004. Occupational Safety and Health Administration. http://www.osha.gov/pls/oshaweb/owadisp.show_document?p_table=OSHACT&p_id=2743. Accessed June 27, 2016.

169. Paulausky C. Laser safety: the eyes have it! *Occup Health Saf.* 2014;83(8):10-12. [VC]

170. Ohshiro T, Ohshiro T, Sasaki K, et al. Correct calibration procedure for the Q-switched ruby laser and checking the treatment irradiation pattern. *Laser Ther.* 2013;22(3):171-180. [VB]

171. Crossley B. New equipment, new challenges: managing a laser safety program. *Biomed Instrum Technol.* 2009;43(4):294. [VC]

172. Hammons MA, Ramey NA, Stinnett S, Woodward JA. Effects of reflected CO2 laser energy on operative field materials: risks to patients and operating room personnel. *Ophthal Plast Reconstr Surg.* 2010;26(5):386-388. [IIIB]

173. Li S, Chen L, Tan F. Laryngeal surgery using a CO2 laser: is a polyvinylchloride endotracheal tube safe? *Am J Otolaryngol.* 2012;33(6):714-717. [IIIA]

174. Roy S, Smith LP. Prevention of airway fires: testing the safety of endotracheal tubes and surgical devices in a mechanical model. *Am J Otolaryngol.* 2015;36(1):63-66. [IIB]

175. Roy S, Smith LP. Surgical fires in laser laryngeal surgery: are we safe enough? *Otolaryngol Head Neck Surg.* 2015;152(1):67-72. [IIB]

176. Lekich C, Hannah P. Retained laser fibre: insights and management. *Phlebology.* 2014;29(5):318-324. [VB]

177. van den Bos RR, Neumann M, Nijsten T. Laser fibre stabs the catheter: a serious complication of endovenous laser ablation. *Phlebology.* 2011;26(3):119-120. [VB]

178. Bozoglan O, Mese B, Inci MF, Eroglu E. A rare complication of endovenous laser ablation: intravascular laser catheter breakage. *BMJ Case Rep.* 2013;2013. [VC]

179. Shum JWH, Chan KSK, Wong D, Li KKW. Intraoperative fracture of phacoemulsification sleeve. *BMC Ophthalmol.* 2010;10:29. [VB]

180. Ogg M. Thermal burns during phacoemulsification [Clinical Issues]. *AORN J.* 2010;92(3):358-359. [VB]

181. Abulafia A, Michaeli A, Belkin A, Assia EI. Temperature profiles of sleeveless and coaxial phacoemulsification. *J Cataract Refract Surg.* 2013;39(11):1742-1748. [IIB]

182. Shaw Y, Yoneda KY, Chan AL. Cerebral gas embolism from bronchoscopic argon plasma coagulation: a case report. *Respiration.* 2012;83(3):267-270. [VA]

183. Law SC, Wong JC, Cheung HY, Chung CC, Li MK. Colonic injury from electric arcing: a significant complication of argon plasma coagulation. *Hong Kong Med J.* 2009;15(3):227-229. [VC]

Acknowledgements

LEAD AUTHOR
Byron L. Burlingame, MS, BSN, RN, CNOR
Senior Perioperative Nursing Specialist
AORN Nursing Department
Denver, Colorado

CONTRIBUTING AUTHOR
Ramona L. Conner, MSN, RN, CNOR
Editor-in-Chief, Guidelines for Perioperative Practice
AORN Nursing Department
Denver, Colorado

The authors and AORN thank Janice Neil, PhD, RN, CNE, Associate Professor, College of Nursing, East Carolina University, Greenville, North Carolina; Mary Lamonte, MPH, MSN, RN, CNOR, Staff Nurse, Stamford Surgical Center, Stamford, Connecticut; Barbara Nalley, MSN, CRNP, CNOR, RN First Assistant, Jackson Surgical Assistant, Crofton, Maryland; Melanie Sandoval, PhD, RN, ACNP, Perioperative Research Nurse Scientist, University of Colorado Hospital, Aurora, Colorado; and Jane Flowers, MSN, RN, CNOR, NEA-BC, Nurse Manager, Shore Health System, Easton, Maryland, for their assistance in developing this guideline.

PUBLICATION HISTORY
Originally published in September 2016 in *Guidelines for Perioperative Practice* online. Supersedes and replaces the Guideline for Electrosurgery and the Guideline for Laser Safety.

GUIDELINE FOR CARE OF PATIENTS UNDERGOING PNEUMATIC TOURNIQUET-ASSISTED PROCEDURES

The following Guideline for Care of Patients Undergoing Pneumatic Tourniquet-Assisted Procedures has been approved by the AORN Recommended Practices Advisory Board. It was presented as proposed recommendations for comments by members and others. The guideline is effective June 15, 2013. The recommendations in this guideline are intended to be achievable and represent what is believed to be an optimal level of practice. Policies and procedures will reflect variations in practice settings and/or clinical situations that determine the degree to which the guideline can be implemented. AORN recognizes the various settings in which perioperative nurses practice; therefore, this guideline is adaptable to various practice settings. These practice settings include traditional operating rooms (ORs), ambulatory surgery centers, physicians' offices, cardiac catheterization laboratories, endoscopy suites, radiology departments, and all other areas where surgery and other invasive procedures may be performed.

Purpose

Pneumatic tourniquets are used to occlude blood flow, obtain a near bloodless field for extremity surgery, and confine a bolus of anesthetic in an extremity for intravenous regional anesthesia. Serious patient injuries related to the use of pneumatic tourniquets are uncommon, but risk is present. The Norwegian Orthopedic Society conducted a survey of 398 surgeons working in 71 health care organizations who performed an estimated 63,484 procedures involving a pneumatic tourniquet. The response rate was 67% (265 surgeons). The researchers determined the incidence of complications was one in 2,442 procedures. Of the 26 complications reported, 15 were nerve injuries; three were blistering or skin necrosis; six were compartment syndrome or deep vein thrombosis (DVT), although these complications may have related more to the injury or surgical procedure than the tourniquet; and two were excluded from the study because of limited specific information. Specific to nerve injuries, the researchers determined the incidence of complications was one in 6,155 procedures involving tourniquets applied to upper limbs and one in 3,752 procedures involving tourniquets applied to lower limbs.[1]

The Arthroscopy Association of North America conducted a national survey and reported 930 complications in 118,590 arthroscopic procedures (0.8%). Sixty-three of the complications were neurological injuries and 80% of those were related to tourniquet use.[2] Researchers from the University of British

Columbia sent an e-mail survey to 1,908 active fellows of the American College of Foot and Ankle Surgeons in the United States and Canada. The response rate was 19% (317 respondents) based on the 1,665 surveys that were successfully delivered. Nerve injury and DVT were listed as the most common concerns of using a tourniquet (ie, cited by 25% of the 73 respondents on tourniquet-related hazards). However, 28 respondents with eight to 31 years of clinical practice commented that complications were rare or had never been encountered (ie, 38% of the 73 respondents on tourniquet-related hazards).[3]

Pain from the tourniquet is one of the most common complications related to pneumatic tourniquet use.[4] Other complications that patients may experience include cardiovascular, respiratory, cerebral circulatory, and hematological effects related to the metabolic changes that result from ischemia caused by the pneumatic tourniquet applied to the extremity during surgery. Temperature changes, prolonged postoperative swelling of the affected limb, and arterial injury are other complications that may occur when a pneumatic tourniquet is used.[4,5]

In reports compiled by the Pennsylvania Patient Safety Authority from December 2004 through December 2009, 140 reported events were associated with pneumatic tourniquet use. The data revealed that 41% of the events were related to limb redness, bruising, or swelling, 19% were related to skin tears or blisters, and more than 40% were related to equipment or safety issues.[6]

This document provides guidance to perioperative team members on the use of pneumatic tourniquets. The guideline provides information about testing, applying, and cleaning pneumatic tourniquet equipment, and the patient care associated with the safe use of this equipment. Pneumatic tourniquet equipment consists of a pressure regulator with display, connective tubing, and an inflatable cuff. The guideline provides general recommendations for developing policies and procedures for safe use of a pneumatic tourniquet in the practice setting. Due to the variety and complexity of pneumatic tourniquet equipment, policies and procedures that reflect considerations for specific pneumatic tourniquet systems are beyond the scope of this guideline. Finger tourniquets and tourniquets used for phlebotomy or traumatic bleeding are outside the scope of this document.

Evidence Review

A medical librarian conducted searches of the databases MEDLINE®, CINAHL®, Scopus®, and the

Cochrane Database of Systematic Reviews for meta-analyses, systematic reviews, randomized controlled and non-randomized trials, guidelines, and case reports. Search terms included *pneumatic tourniquet, tourniquet safety, tourniquet, surgical hemostasis, surgical procedures, nursing care, perioperative care, patient positioning, compartment syndromes, arm injuries, leg injuries, hand injuries, pain measurement, peripheral nervous system, peripheral nervous system diseases, nerve palsy, metabolic phenomena, metabolic changes, metabolic effects, vital signs, respiration, carbon dioxide, intracranial pressure, oxygen consumption, cardiac output, acidosis, hyperemia, venous congestion, blood pressure, lactic acid, hemodynamics, pulse, hypothermia, hyperthermia, systemic inflammatory response, Esmarch bandage, Urias bag, Pomidor roll-cuff, bandage, elastic wrap, intravenous regional anesthesia, Bier block, ankle block, conduction anesthesia, bloodless field, occlusion pressure, ischemia,* and *reperfusion injury.*

The search was limited to articles published in English between January 2006 and February 2012. The search was expanded to include articles published before 2006 when the original search did not identify more recent literature on a particular topic. The librarian established continuing alerts on the pneumatic tourniquet topics. The lead author and librarian identified relevant guidelines from government agencies and standards-setting bodies.

Articles identified in the search were provided to the lead author and a doctorally prepared evidence appraiser for evaluation. Each article was reviewed and critically appraised using the Johns Hopkins Evidence-Based Practice Model and the Research or Non-Research Evidence Appraisal Tools as appropriate. The literature was independently evaluated and appraised according to the strength and quality of the evidence. Each article was then assigned an appraisal score as agreed upon by consensus of the lead author and evidence appraiser. The appraisal score is noted in brackets after each reference, as applicable.

The collective evidence supporting each intervention within a specific recommendation was summarized and used to rate the strength of the evidence using the AORN Evidence Rating Model. Factors considered in review of the collective evidence were the quality of research, quantity of similar studies on a given topic, and consistency of results supporting a recommendation. The evidence rating is noted in brackets after each intervention.

Editor's note: MEDLINE is a registered trademark of the US National Library of Medicine's Medical Literature Analysis and Retrieval System, Bethesda, MD. CINAHL, Cumulative Index to Nursing and Allied Health Literature, is a registered trademark of EBSCO Industries, Birmingham, AL. Scopus is a registered trademark of Elsevier B.V., Amsterdam, Netherlands.

Recommendation I

The perioperative registered nurse (RN) should assess the patient preoperatively for risks and potential contraindications related to the use of a pneumatic tourniquet.

Risks related to the use of a pneumatic tourniquet include nerve injuries,[1-3] skin injuries (eg, blistering, bruising, necrosis),[1,6] compartment syndrome,[1] DVT,[1,3] and pain.[4] When a pneumatic tourniquet is used on a patient's extremity, the patient may experience systemic responses (eg, changes in temperature or blood pressure) related to reperfusion upon cuff deflation.[4,5] Using a pneumatic tourniquet on patients who have preoperative conditions that predispose them to these risks may result in a cumulative effect.

I.a. The perioperative RN should not assume routine use of a pneumatic tourniquet for all extremity procedures. The RN should confirm in the surgeon's or anesthesia professional's plan of care whether a pneumatic tourniquet will be used. *[1: Strong Evidence]*

The surgeon or anesthesia professional determines whether to use a tourniquet based on the risks and benefits to the patient. There is debate in the medical community regarding the use of a pneumatic tourniquet for surgical procedures. Based on the evidence, routine use of a pneumatic tourniquet for limb occlusion can no longer be assumed. Findings from an e-mail survey sent to 1,665 foot and ankle surgeons in North America revealed that 11 respondents (3.4%) rarely or never used a tourniquet.[3]

One researcher used a randomized controlled study to explore tourniquet use in patients undergoing arthroscopic knee surgery. Comparing the outcomes of 56 patients who were assigned either to the control group or the intervention group, the researcher found no significant differences related to operative times, technical difficulties, identification of intra-articular structures, postoperative pain, or postoperative complications when a tourniquet was not used. The researcher suggested the use of a tourniquet may be unnecessary for arthroscopic knee surgery.[7]

Findings from another prospective randomized controlled trial also revealed that knee arthroscopy could be performed successfully without the use of a tourniquet. In this study, tourniquets were applied to all of the 109 patients who participated, with 58 patients assigned to a group that had the tourniquet inflated and the other 51 assigned to a group that did not have the tourniquet inflated. The operative view was rated poor by the surgeon in four procedures (7.8% of procedures performed) in the uninflated tourniquet group, requiring those tourniquets to be inflated for 5% to 60% of the procedure time. The mean procedure time was 27 minutes for the inflated tourniquet group (ie, range 10 minutes to 80 minutes) and 30 minutes for the uninflated tourniquet group (ie, range 10 minutes to 87 minutes). The researchers did not report significant differences between the two groups when measuring the operative view, duration of the procedure, pain scores, analgesic requirements, or complications.[8]

A prospective double-blind randomized clinical trial involved 120 patients who were having routine arthroscopies. Sixty-one patients were randomly assigned to the inflated tourniquet group and 59 patients were assigned to the uninflated tourniquet group. Intraoperatively, for the inflated tourniquet group, surgeons reported they had better ability to see and experienced less technical difficulty; however, the findings revealed that the mean operative time was similar; the average operative time for the inflated tourniquet group was 30.5 minutes compared to an average of 31.1 minutes for the uninflated tourniquet group. The study was designed to be blinded, but the surgeon was able to tell whether the tourniquet cuff was inflated or deflated in all but five of the procedures, thus introducing a potential bias. The researchers discussed the need for further study to determine whether using an infusion pump in combination with intermittent tourniquet inflation would improve the ability to see during procedures on the uninflated tourniquet group. They reported an increase in postoperative pain in the inflated tourniquet group when the tourniquet was inflated for more than 30 minutes.[9]

Researchers conducted a meta-analysis and identified nine studies to compare outcomes of arthroscopic knee procedures in which a tourniquet was used and arthroscopic knee procedures in which a tourniquet was not used. With the exception of the ability to see the operative field, there were no significant differences for all other outcome measures. The researchers reported that there was limited evidence to suggest that a tourniquet assists in arthroscopic knee surgery.[10]

Tourniquet use for total knee replacements was the focus of a study involving 100 patients. Patients were randomly assigned to group A, which involved epinephrine-augmented hypotensive epidural anesthesia, or group B, which involved normotensive epidural anesthesia with use of a tourniquet. The researchers measured perioperative hemoglobin values and transfusion rates postoperatively and for six days after the procedure. They determined that the patients in group A did not experience detrimental effects on their perioperative hemoglobin values or transfusion rates. They also reported that when epinephrine-augmented hypotensive epidural anesthesia was used, it was an effective method to avoid the use of a tourniquet during total knee arthroplasty. The average surgery time for group A was 1.53 hours and for group B was 1.58 hours.[11]

Researchers conducted a meta-analysis and identified 15 studies to compare outcome measures and parameters of 1,040 total knee replacements in 991 patients. The researchers reported a trend for greater complications in the patients who had a tourniquet applied compared to the patients who did not have a tourniquet applied. They also reported that patients who underwent surgeries without a tourniquet had significantly greater intraoperative blood loss compared to patients who underwent tourniquet-assisted surgery; however, they did not identify a significant difference between the two groups for total blood loss or transfusion rate. There was no difference between the groups for any other outcome measure assessed; therefore, the researchers concluded that there was no advantage to using a tourniquet in knee replacement surgery for reduction of transfusion requirements.[12]

In another meta-analysis, researchers explored the correlation between 318 tourniquet-assisted total knee arthroplasties and the risks of complications when compared to 316 non-tourniquet-assisted total knee arthroplasties. They included eight randomized controlled trials and three high-quality prospective studies in the analysis. They reported that the evidence suggests that using a tourniquet in total knee arthroplasty may increase the risk of thromboembolic complications and that use of a tourniquet may save the surgeon time but it may not reduce the patient's blood loss.[13]

Researchers conducted a meta-analysis and identified four studies comparing outcomes of tourniquet-assisted ankle and foot surgery to non-tourniquet-assisted ankle and foot surgery. The analysis concluded that hospital length of stay was significantly shorter and that the postoperative period was less painful, with reduced swelling from the fifth postoperative day in surgeries undertaken without a tourniquet compared to tourniquet-assisted procedures. There may be a greater incidence of wound infection and DVT in tourniquet-assisted foot and ankle procedures. Because of methodological limitations of the reviewed studies, the researchers recommended further study to determine whether a tourniquet should be used during ankle or foot procedures.[14]

Researchers conducted a systematic review and meta-analysis to compare the patient outcomes when a tourniquet was used for orthopedic surgery on upper limbs to the patient outcomes when a tourniquet was not used. In 849 citations, they found only two studies that met their criteria. These two studies involved 55 patients and assessed the surgeon's ability to see, the patient's pain, and the total operative time. From the analysis, the researchers suggested that

EQUIPMENT AND PRODUCT SAFETY

technical difficulties during upper limb surgery may have been reduced when tourniquets were used. However, they were not able to determine whether pain perception or operative time was influenced by the use of a tourniquet. They recommended further studies with stronger methodology.[15]

In another study, researchers followed 138 patients for at least one year after their surgical procedures to repair tibial fractures. The patients were randomly assigned to one of two groups (ie, with or without tourniquet use). The researchers reported that use of a tourniquet did not influence the infection rate or the healing time. They did report that patients' perceptions of pain decreased when a tourniquet was not used. They suggested that a tourniquet may not be necessary when plating tibial fractures because the surgical repair can be a short procedure that does not typically involve severe bleeding.[16]

I.b.   The perioperative RN should assess the patient for considerations related to tourniquet use, including
- planned location of the tourniquet,
- condition of skin under and distal to the planned cuff site,
- size and shape of the extremity, and
- peripheral pulses distal to the cuff.

[3: Moderate Evidence]

Preoperative skin assessment provides a baseline to evaluate skin injuries that may occur at the site of the tourniquet cuff because of pressure necrosis or friction burns. Applying the tourniquet cuff to the proximal portion of the limb in an area of the limb where there is the most soft tissue can help to decrease the risk of injury to underlying nerves and vessels.[5]

Preoperative patient assessment facilitates planning for tourniquet cuff selection. There is a direct correlation between the circumference of the limb at the site of cuff application and the cuff pressure required to suppress circulation. Large limb circumferences indicate a higher tourniquet pressure will be necessary to achieve vessel occlusion.[17] Patients with small limb circumferences (eg, children younger than two years, small adults) will require a tourniquet cuff specifically designed for this patient population.[18,19]

Preoperative assessment of the limb shape also helps to plan for the selection of a properly fitting tourniquet cuff (eg, straight-cylindrical versus wide-contour cuff).[20] The risk of the tourniquet cuff shifting may be increased when the patient is obese or has limb tissue that is loose.[21]

Preoperative assessment of the patient's circulatory system including a baseline measurement of peripheral pulses helps to evaluate the risk of applying a tourniquet to the patient's limb. Indicators of poor circulatory nutrition include brittle, dry nails; shining or scaly skin; and extremity hair loss. Other indicators for circulatory considerations include capillary filling time and the presence of varicose veins.[22]

I.c.   The nursing assessment should include screening for potential contraindications for tourniquet use, including
- venous thromboembolism,[2,3,23-27]
- impaired circulation or peripheral vascular compromise,[17,27-29]
- previous revascularization of the extremity,[22,30]
- extremities with dialysis access (eg, arteriovenous grafts, fistulas),[22]
- acidosis,[31]
- hemoglobinopathy (eg, sickle cell anemia),[17,28,32-34]
- extremity infection,[17]
- tumor distal to the tourniquet,[17]
- medications (eg, antihypertensives)[35,36] and supplements (eg, creatine),[37]
- history of pain[38] or weakness[39] in muscles or bones in extremities,
- open fracture, and
- increased intracranial pressure.[23,28]

[3: Moderate Evidence]

Risk of complications may be higher for certain patient populations. Using a 17-item questionnaire delivered by e-mail, researchers conducted an investigation to determine current practice patterns among members of the American College of Foot and Ankle Surgeons. A total of 317 respondents reported that the most commonly listed contraindications to tourniquet use included vascular disease or previous bypass and DVT.[3]

Researchers conducting a prospective comparison study examined the outcomes of 48 consecutive patients undergoing total knee arthroplasty and reported that the incidence of DVT was high (81.3%) with or without the use of a tourniquet. The first group of 21 patients underwent the surgical procedure without a tourniquet, and the next 27 patients underwent a tourniquet-assisted procedure. The researchers concluded that the use of a tourniquet decreased perioperative blood loss and did not increase the risk of DVT. They identified symptomatic pulmonary embolism in 1.7% of the patients and emphasized the importance of prevention and early detection of DVT to decrease the risk of fatal pulmonary thromboembolism.[24]

Twenty patients participated in a prospective study to determine whether extramedullary guided total knee arthroplasty decreased the severity of embolic showers after tourniquet deflation. The researchers reported that 14 patients experienced large venous emboli and six patients experienced small venous emboli. The researchers concluded that the thrombogenic effect of the tourniquet may be the cause of venous emboli rather than the manipulation of the marrow cavity because they did not find a difference in the incidence of venous emboli with extramedullary guided total knee arthroplasty when compared to the results of previous studies reporting the incidence of venous emboli with intramedullary guided total knee arthroplasty.[25]

Researchers conducted a randomized comparison study to determine the incidence of large venous emboli in 23 patients who underwent total knee arthroplasty procedures (ie, either intramedullary or extramedullary guided) without pneumatic tourniquet inflation. Their findings suggest a 5.33-fold greater risk of experiencing a large emboli for patients who have a knee arthroplasty with a tourniquet inflated, based on comparison with historical controls from a previous investigation.[26]

Patients who have arterial calcification, abnormal clotting times, diabetes, sickle cell trait, tumor, infection, or hypertension may have a higher risk of experiencing negative outcomes when a tourniquet is used.[17] Venous stasis and tissue hypoxia occur with use of a tourniquet, increasing the risk for exaggerated clotting cascade responses and poor wound healing.[23] A case study analysis of a patient with peripheral vascular disease and a femoral artery stent reported the patient developed an asymptomatic thrombosis in the stent between the time the surgeon last saw the patient in the clinic and the day of surgery. The authors recommended that the surgeon obtain a preoperative pedal pulse and perform a vascular examination immediately before marking the surgical site to identify recent changes in vascularity before initiating tourniquet-induced vein occlusion and tissue ischemia.[30]

Using a tourniquet on a limb that has arthrosclerotic vessels increases the risk for poor wound healing and sepsis. When a limb has an arterial prosthesis, there may be insufficient implant elasticity and impaired collateral circulation that cannot accommodate the sudden increased blood flow after tourniquet deflation.[22] One case has been reported in which calcification of an underlying artery may have caused tourniquet failure.[29]

Patients who have cardiopulmonary conditions, renal compromise, or clinically significant acid-base imbalance also have a higher risk of complications with application of a tourniquet.[31] Diabetic patients may already be at a higher risk for poor peripheral circulation, delayed healing, and prolonged infections in distal extremities.

Patients with sickle cell trait are at a higher risk for complications because of the hemostasis, hypoxia, and acidosis that occur beneath the tourniquet cuff and that provide ideal conditions to promote red cell sickling.[28,32] Researchers reviewed four studies that included 96 patients with sickle cell traits or hemoglobinopathies who underwent surgical procedures

with tourniquet inflation. Ten patients who had tourniquet surgery on a lower extremity experienced complications compared to one patient with a complication after tourniquet surgery on an upper extremity. Therefore, the researchers suggested that a stronger correlation may exist between patients with sickle cell trait or hemoglobinopathies who undergo lower extremity tourniquet procedures than those who undergo upper extremity tourniquet procedures.[32] Based on findings from this review and an earlier case study, there is limited evidence to suggest that tourniquets may be safe to use for patients with sickle cell indicators when effective perioperative management is implemented.[32,33] Another case study in which surgeons used a tourniquet safely during a total knee replacement for an 82-year-old woman who was a Jehovah's Witness with sickle cell trait supports this finding.[34]

One case study reported a severe drop in blood pressure followed by myocardial depression at the time of tourniquet deflation. The authors attributed the severe reaction to the patient's preoperative dose of oral clonidine. They recommended using caution when using tourniquets on patients who are taking antihypertensives.[35] After investigating 75 patients who were having elective surgical procedures on their lower limbs, other researchers found that preoperative clonidine was an effective way to prevent systemic arterial pressure increases related to tourniquet use for patients under general anesthesia.[36]

Preoperative assessment is important for young adults as well as older adults. Two case studies have been reported involving younger people undergoing orthopedic procedures. The first case report involved a 21-year-old athlete who experienced rhabdomyolysis and acute renal failure after arthroscopic knee surgery. The authors suggested the patient's risk of tourniquet-related skeletal muscle injury was increased because of the patient's use of creatine supplements.[37]

The second case study did not relate to medications, but highlights the importance of the preoperative interview to reveal a history of pain. A 35-year-old patient undergoing a tourniquet-assisted open reduction-internal fixation of an ankle fracture developed symptoms of anterior compartment syndrome 10 hours after surgery. Preoperatively, the patient stated he had experienced pain in his legs previously while playing football and the pain continued afterward. The authors believed the tourniquet may have contributed to the development of the compartment syndrome. Retrospectively, they also believed that the patient may have had a predisposition to an exercise-induced compartment syndrome and that postoperative pain medications contributed to the delay in diagnosis. They encouraged the

EQUIPMENT AND PRODUCT SAFETY

assessment of pre-injury pain when patients are injured during sporting activities and suggested using tourniquets with caution.[38]

Risks may be higher when a tourniquet is applied to an extremity of a patient who has a condition that causes muscle weakness (eg, myasthenia gravis). Authors of one case study advised caution when using bilateral tourniquets and prolonged tourniquet application in patients who have myasthenia gravis because of the risk of exacerbated symptoms in spite of regional anesthesia and the avoidance of muscle relaxants.[39]

Recommendation II

The perioperative RN should collaborate with the surgeon and anesthesia professional to develop and confirm the plan of care related to the use of a tourniquet.

Variations in patient conditions or the planned procedure influence perioperative plans relating to the use of a tourniquet. Because of these variations, the whole perioperative team should be in alignment. For example, administration of the preoperative antibiotic may be adjusted to coordinate with the timing of tourniquet inflation with the intent of increasing tissue concentrations.[40,41] Anesthesia professionals may plan to implement preconditioning or adjust their anesthetic plan to reduce oxidative stress resulting from tourniquet-induced ischemia-reperfusion.[42-44]

Anesthesia professionals may adjust their anesthesia plan of care (eg, preconditioning, supplementing regional anesthetic with ketamine) to reduce pain or rhabdomyolysis.[45,46] Intravenous regional anesthesia may be planned for upper extremity surgeries, requiring the perioperative nurse to anticipate the need for equipment and medications and be prepared for adverse events including those associated with intravenous regional anesthesia.[47-49]

Findings from the preoperative assessment may provide information that influences the size or shape of the tourniquet cuff to be used to obtain effective vessel occlusion with the lowest possible pressure.[50]

II.a. The timing of preoperative prophylactic antibiotic administration, when ordered, should be based on the health care organization's policy and procedure with a goal of achieving optimal tissue concentration. [3: Moderate Evidence]

Efficacy of prophylactic antibiotics requires tissue perfusion of the surgical site. In studies published in 1994 and 1995, researchers reported that optimal tissue concentrations were found when antibiotics were administered preoperatively, 20 minutes before tourniquet inflation.[51,52]

In a more recent study, researchers conducted a single-center randomized double-blind study of 908 patients who underwent total knee arthroplasty procedures to determine the importance of a "tourniquet-release" dose of antibiotics. One group of patients (n = 442) received the

standard regimen (ie, receiving antibiotics before tourniquet inflation); the other group (n = 466) did not receive antibiotics before inflation but received a "tourniquet release dose" of the same dose of the antibiotic 10 minutes before release of the tourniquet. Both groups received a postoperative dose of the same antibiotic six hours after the procedure. The researchers speculated that the standard regimen (ie, administering antibiotics before tourniquet inflation) may result in a lower serum antibiotic concentration at the end of the surgical procedure and that is when the highest concentrations of antibiotics are needed to prevent growth of microorganisms during the 12 to 24 hours after the surgery. They found the "tourniquet-release" dose was more effective than the standard regimen, but there was not a statistically significant difference. The primary limitation to this study was that more patients were needed to determine statistical significance because the researchers' initial predictions about the difference in infection rate between both groups was higher than what occurred in the study.[41]

In another recent study, researchers measured outcomes for 106 patients, with 54 patients receiving antibiotics before tourniquet inflation and 52 patients receiving antibiotics one minute after tourniquet inflation. More than 70% of the procedures involved open reduction and internal fixation of fractures on lower extremities. The researchers concluded that administering an antibiotic shortly after inflation of the tourniquet did not produce an inferior outcome when compared to administering an antibiotic before exsanguination and inflation of a lower extremity tourniquet.[40]

II.b. The perioperative nurse should collaborate with the surgeon and the anesthesia professional to address DVT risk factors identified during the patient's preoperative assessment.[53] [2: High Evidence]

Researchers in one study hypothesized that systemic thrombin generation begins after tourniquet deflation in total knee arthroplasty procedures. However, they also acknowledged that a tourniquet may damage endothelial vessels and create venous stasis in the extremity, which may increase thrombogenic and fibrinolytic activity. The participating patients were treated preoperatively with thromboprophylaxis. However, the researchers found that the patients' coagulation systems were activated 10 minutes after surgery. They recommended additional studies to explore correlations between preoperative and postoperative thromboprophylaxis and fibrinolytic system activities. Their data indicated that vein occlusion caused by tourniquets may contribute to thrombosis formation during surgery on lower extremities. However, the researchers did not believe the tourniquet inflation alone activated a systemic formation of the thrombosis.[54]

In another study, researchers confirmed that cellular interactions that augment blood coagulability were increased in the perioperative period for patients who underwent total knee arthroplasty. They also concluded that these responses were more prominent during tourniquet-assisted total knee procedures.[55]

II.c. The perioperative nurse should collaborate with the surgeon and anesthesia professional to address considerations related to the plan for anesthesia or ischemic preconditioning.[53] *[2: High Evidence]*

The purpose of ischemic preconditioning is to increase the tolerance of tissue to a longer period of ischemia by initiating brief periods of ischemia[56] or influencing skeletal muscle tolerance with anesthetic regimens.[57] Several studies have investigated the correlation between various anesthesia or preconditioning techniques and oxidative stress related to ischemia and reperfusion that occurs after the release of a tourniquet.[42-44,56-64]

To reduce oxidative stress related to tourniquet inflation, preconditioning techniques may be planned to initiate short intervals of temporary ischemia (eg, three cycles of five minutes, followed by five minutes of reperfusion just before tourniquet inflation).[42,44,59,61] Perioperative nurses may participate in activities related to preconditioning (eg, retrieving medications, setting up equipment, coordinating the timing of skin preparation, documenting intervals of inflation). By collaborating with the surgeon and anesthesia professional, the nurse will be better prepared to assist in preconditioning-related activities.[53]

II.d. Before the patient enters the OR, a pneumatic tourniquet cuff should be selected using the following considerations.
- The width of the tourniquet cuff should be as wide as possible without inhibiting surgical site exposure.[50,65] *[2: High Evidence]*
- Contoured tourniquet cuffs should be used for patient extremities in which there is a tapering of the extremity between the upper and lower edge of the cuff.[23,50,65] *[2: High Evidence]*
- The length of the tourniquet cuff should be sufficient to provide bladder overlap on the limb and full engagement of the hook-and-loop fasteners. *[5: Benefits Balanced with Harms]*

Confirming that a tourniquet with the appropriate cuff size and shape is available before the patient enters the OR decreases the risk of using the wrong cuff size or shape or causing a delay to search for the appropriately sized cuff while the patient is under anesthesia.

Improper tourniquet cuff application may lead to skin injuries (eg, pressure necrosis, friction burns).[5] The risk of injury to tissue and nerves increases when more pressure is required for vessel occlusion. The ratio of the cuff width to the limb circumference has an inverse relationship with limb occlusion pressure (eg, wider cuffs require lower tourniquet pressures, narrower cuffs require higher tourniquet pressures).[20] Choosing the wrong cuff size or shape could lead to unnecessarily higher pressures and increase the risk for injury.

Wider cuffs minimize the risk for injury to underlying tissue by dispersing pressure over a greater surface area. In clinical trials, using a wider cuff has been found consistently to occlude blood flow at a lower pressure in adult patients.[50,65-67] Similar results were found using wider cuffs in children.[18] Contoured tourniquet cuffs have been found in clinical trials to occlude arterial flow at lower pressures than straight tourniquet cuffs of equal width. Contoured tourniquet cuffs minimize the risk of excessive pressure on one edge of the cuff, migration of the cuff, and a shearing injury to underlying tissue.[23,50,65]

II.e. A sterile cuff should be used when the cuff will be very close to the sterile field. A single-use cuff should be used when adequate protection of the cuff from contamination cannot be assured. *[4: Limited Evidence]*

Researchers conducted a study at two hospitals to assess microbial colonization on reusable tourniquet cuffs versus sterile single-use disposable tourniquets. They found that 23 of the 34 reusable tourniquet cuffs were contaminated before surgical application. Although they did not follow the patients to find out the incidence of surgical site infection in the 23 patients who had contaminated cuffs applied, the researchers concluded that sterile single-use tourniquet cuffs are preferred to decrease the bacterial load when the cuff is placed in close proximity to the surgical site.[68]

II.f. Potential risks for patient injuries and complications associated with dual-bladder cuffs used for intravenous regional anesthesia should be identified and safe practices should be established. *[4: Limited Evidence]*

Reports indicate that complications associated with intravenous regional anesthesia include local anesthetic toxicity, seizures, cardiac arrests, compartment syndrome, thrombophlebitis, discoloration, or widespread petechiae.[47] When using intravenous regional anesthesia, there is a risk for local anesthetic toxicity caused by accidental tourniquet failure or leakage around the tourniquet due to high venous pressure.[49,69] Complications can also occur that are related to tubings and misconnections (eg, attaching to distal versus proximal cuffs) when using dual cuffs for intravenous regional anesthesia.[70,71]

II.f.1. Based on the preoperative patient assessment, the perioperative nurse should identify medication allergies, especially sensitivities to local anesthetics, and communicate with the anesthesia professional to clarify the plan for intravenous regional anesthesia before the tourniquet is applied.

II.f.2. The perioperative RN should confirm that
- a dual-bladder tourniquet cuff and extra connective tubing will be used,
- the planned location on the extremity is wide enough to accommodate the additional width of the dual-bladder tourniquet cuff, and
- a higher pressure is planned to compensate for the narrow size of each cuff bladder.[17]

Although intravenous regional anesthesia is more common in upper extremities, dual tourniquet cuffs and injection of local anesthetics have been used for lower extremities.[72] Variation in cuff sizes and the need for dual cuffs versus two separate cuffs will depend on the size of the patient's extremity and the location planned for the regional block.

II.f.3. Members of the perioperative team should clearly communicate with each other about the inflation-deflation sequence when using a dual-bladder cuff and when using two single-bladder cuffs together for intravenous regional anesthesia.

II.f.4. The proximal and distal cuffs and the respective tubing should be clearly identified.

Recommendation III

Patient safety should be the primary consideration when using a pneumatic tourniquet and its accessories.

Patient injury related to pneumatic tourniquet use has been reported. For example, one case report found that if the cuff that is applied to a patient's extremity has a bladder that is bent, folded, or crushed, adequate pressure may be compromised, resulting in bleeding at the surgical site.[73] Excessive pressure from the tourniquet may cause limb redness, bruising, swelling, or nerve injury.[6]

III.a. The tourniquet's tubing and connectors should be incompatible with other tubing (eg, intravenous) or labeled to clearly identify that they are part of the tourniquet system.[70,71] *[4: Limited Evidence]*

Although reports of misconnections involving tourniquet tubing are not common, misconnections of other types of tubing and connectors (eg, blood pressure tubing, Luer connections) have been reported.[70,71]

III.b. Before each use, the perioperative nurse should verify that the entire tourniquet system is complete, clean, and functioning according to the manufacturer's instructions for use.
- The pneumatic tourniquet regulator should be compatible with all associated components, and the connections should be secure.[17]
- The cuff, tubing, connectors, and o-rings should be inspected for cracks, leaks, and other damage.[17]
- The tourniquet should be tested for integrity and function.[17]
- The integrity of the hook-and-loop fasteners and tie ribbons should be inspected.[17]
- A full battery power charge should be confirmed, if applicable.[17]

[4: Limited Evidence]

Ensuring that the tourniquet functions properly before a procedure reduces the risk of pressure loss and patient injury.[17]

Unintentional pressure loss can result from loose tubing connectors, deteriorated tubing, or cuff bladder leaks and may result in patient injury.

III.c. A pneumatic tourniquet that is not working properly or is damaged should be removed from service immediately, along with all its accessories, and reported to the designated individual responsible for equipment maintenance (eg, biomedical engineering personnel).[74] *[3: Moderate Evidence]*

III.d. The perioperative RN should verify the correct surgical site before application of the tourniquet cuff and verify the tourniquet inflation pressure during the time-out process.[75] *[2: High Evidence]*

Placing a tourniquet on the wrong limb may result in a cascade of events leading to wrong site surgery. Confirmation of the location of the tourniquet and its pressure setting during the time-out process increases communication and consistent documentation and reduces the likelihood of error.

III.e. Safety practices should be implemented when applying tourniquet cuffs to the verified operative extremity. *[2: High Evidence]*

When the tourniquet cuff is inflated, nerves and blood vessels are compressed. This poses a potential risk to superficial nerves that are in unprotected areas during cuff placement.[4,23]

Proper application of the cuff decreases the risk for injury or pressure variances.[5,17,76-80] For example, a loose fitting cuff may shift after placement, causing a friction burn on the skin.[5] Higher pressures also may be needed if the cuff is applied too loosely.[17] Patients who are obese or others who have loose skin and adipose tissue at the site of the tourniquet cuff are at risk for the skin folding or puckering beneath the tourniquet cuff. This increases the risk for uneven pressure on vessels and skin injury.[17]

III.e.1. Tourniquet cuffs should be applied snugly to the verified operative extremity[50] and in a position on the extremity that creates a minimal amount of ischemia.[27]

In one quasi-experimental study of 50 patients undergoing surgery for carpal tunnel syndrome under local anesthesia, researchers recommended placement of the tourniquet on the upper arm. They reported that there were not significant differences for patients tolerating tourniquets placed on the upper arm versus the forearm when the tourniquet time was shorter than 20 minutes. In addition, the patient's fingers may curl up and the tourniquet cuff may interfere with the surgical incision when it is placed at the forearm.[81] Researchers have found that patients undergoing foot surgery with local anesthesia have less pain when the cuff is placed at the ankle.[82-84]

III.e.2. When applying the tourniquet cuff to the small limb of a child where space is limited, the perioperative RN should evaluate the size, shape, and fit of the tourniquet to avoid its movement during the procedure. Sterile tourniquets should be considered for use if the tourniquet must be positioned close to the surgical site.[76]

Children's extremities can present unique challenges related to the size of the limb (eg, no space for the tourniquet, acute taper of a young child's thigh). If the tourniquet is not the right shape or is not applied tightly enough, it may slide toward the surgical wound, risking loss of compression or interference at the surgical site.[76]

III.e.3. The cuff should be applied in its final position. If at any time a cuff position change is necessary, the cuff should be removed and reapplied.

Moving a cuff after placement may cause shearing of underlying tissues and subsequent injury.

III.e.4. A low-lint, soft padding (eg, limb protection sleeve, two layers of stockinette) should be placed around the limb according to the cuff manufacturer's instructions for use. The padding should be wrinkle-free and should not pinch the skin.

In two clinical trials, the overall skin complication rate was lower when padding was used.[77,78] However, higher pressures may be needed if a cuff is applied over a thick layer of loose padding.[17]

Avoiding padding materials that may shed fibers (eg, cotton cast padding, sheet padding) will decrease linting. When lint from padding materials becomes embedded in the hook-and-loop fasteners of a tourniquet, it may reduce the effectiveness of the fasteners and potentially lead to an unexpected release of the cuff during a procedure.

III.e.5. The patient's skin under the tourniquet cuff should be protected to prevent fluid accumulation (eg, skin prep solutions, irrigation) under the cuff.

Underpadding and tourniquet cuffs can harbor moisture, resulting in skin breakdown if protective interventions are not taken. Two cases have been reported in which patients had to undergo burn wound excision and skin grafting because of chemical burns caused by pooling of the prep solution under a tourniquet.[80]

III.e.6. Reusable tourniquet cuffs should be protected from contamination by fluid, blood, and other potentially infectious material during surgery. Tourniquet protectors (eg, U-shaped drapes, adhesive drapes, tourniquet covers) should be used to minimize soiling.

Reusable tourniquet cuffs that are not protected from fluid, blood, and other potentially infectious material can be a source of cross contamination.

III.e.7. The cuff tubing should be positioned on or near the lateral aspect of the extremity.

Lateral placement of the cuff tubing may help avoid pressure on nerves of the extremity and prevent kinking of the tubing.

III.f. Procedures involving pneumatic tourniquet control on two extremities should have the tourniquet tubing labeled to clearly identify which tubing belongs to which cuff and which is associated with which components of the tourniquet system(s). The perioperative RN, surgical team members, and anesthesia professionals should confirm the respective placement of the tourniquets and plans for inflation during the time-out process.[75] [3: Moderate Evidence]

The risk for complications and the systemic effects of tourniquet use may increase when ischemia and reperfusion occur in two extremities. However, in one published expert opinion, the authors suggested that the delay between the sequential deflation of the first cuff and inflation of the second cuff allows time for caregivers to assess the systemic response and accommodate for the lactic acid released from the first procedure before the second cuff is inflated. If the patient does not tolerate the reperfusion or if complications occur in the first procedure, the option of aborting the second procedure may be a better choice than performing simultaneous bilateral procedures.[85]

The use of two tourniquet cuffs increases the number of tubings and connections which can increase the opportunity for errors of misconnections or inflation or deflation of the wrong cuff. Labeling the tubing to each cuff minimizes the risk of inflating or deflating the wrong cuff.[70,71]

Recommendation IV

Inflation of the tourniquet cuff should be done under the direction of the surgeon and coordinated with the anesthesia professional.

After limb exsanguination and cuff inflation, there is an increase in blood volume to vital organs and a subsequent increase in systolic blood pressure.[28] Healthy adults may experience only minor hemodynamic changes when a tourniquet is inflated. However, patients who are elderly or have cardiac conditions (eg, cardiac failure, cardiac enlargement) may experience intraoperative hypertension or other complications related to the increased blood volume (eg, 800 mL of blood may be added when exsanguinating a leg).[4,5] Coordination with the anesthesia professional facilitates management of the patient during this rapid physiologic change.

Several cases of fatal complications immediately or within 30 minutes following exsanguination of the operative leg have been reported.[86] Patients who are older than 50 years or who have not been mobile or whose preoperative cardiovascular evaluation suggests higher risk factors for DVT (eg, smoking, obesity, cardiac arrhythmias) are at higher risk for complications during or following exsanguination of the lower limb.[86]

IV.a. The extremity should be exsanguinated before inflation of the tourniquet. *[3: Moderate Evidence]*

When a limb is exsanguinated, an elastic wrap (eg, an Esmarch bandage) compresses superficial blood vessels, forcing blood out of the extremity. Use of an elastic bandage for exsanguination enhances the bloodless field and may minimize the pain associated with tourniquet use.

The surgeon or anesthesia professional determines appropriate use of an elastic wrap, taking into consideration the risks and benefits to the patient. Exsanguination using an elastic wrap may not be appropriate following traumatic injury or if the extremity has been in a cast. In these instances, thrombi in blood vessels may become dislodged, resulting in emboli. Fatal pulmonary emboli have been reported following exsanguination of such extremities.[86]

In a randomized trial, 100 patients were assigned to one of three groups to compare the effectiveness of exsanguination methods (ie, limb elevation, squeezing the limb hand over hand starting distally and moving proximally with the limb elevated, and mechanical exsanguination with a sterile elastic bandage). The researchers concluded that the "squeeze" method and the elastic bandage methods were more effective at providing a bloodless surgical field than the elevation method.[87] However, elevating the extremity may be the preferred method for exsanguination when a patient has an infection or a malignant tumor in the operative extremity and using an elastic wrap for exsanguination is contraindicated.[88,89] Elevation also may be a preferred exsanguination method to reduce the risk for additional tissue damage when the patient has an unstable fracture in the operative extremity or when the patient has a latex allergy and a latex-safe elastic wrap is not available.[89]

IV.a.1. An elastic wrap should be available for exsanguination.

IV.a.2. The extremity should be elevated to allow venous blood to exit the limb.

IV.a.3. If the patient has an infection, malignant tumor, or fractures in the operative extremity, exsanguination should be accomplished by extremity elevation alone.[88,89]

IV.a.4. The anesthesia professional should be alerted before the extremity is wrapped.

Notification of the anesthesia professional facilitates monitoring for potential complications.

IV.b. Tourniquet inflation pressure should be determined by the surgeon[17] or anesthesia professional[4] based on the patient's systolic blood pressure and limb circumference. Inflation should be kept to the minimum effective pressure.[90-94] *[1: Strong Evidence]*

Overpressurization may cause pain at the tourniquet cuff site; muscle weakness; compression injuries to blood vessels, nerves, muscles, or skin; or extremity paralysis. Underpressurization may result in blood in the surgical field, passive congestion of the limb, shock, and hemorrhagic infiltration of a nerve. Sustaining adequate tourniquet pressure decreases the risk for poor visualization at the surgical field and engorgement of the limb or compartment syndrome related to arterial flow entering the limb.[65] Applying lower pressure has been found to result in less postoperative pain.[90,95,96]

Although many surgeons assume that standard tourniquet pressures are appropriate in all cases, researchers have shown that lower pressures than those typically used are effective.[65,94,95,97-100] Standard settings for tourniquet pressures have been identified as 300 mm Hg to 350 mm Hg in lower limbs and 200 mm Hg to 250 mm Hg in upper limbs.[4] In a retrospective study of 3,115 patient records for podiatry procedures, tourniquet pressures for cuffs applied at the ankle averaged 310.52 mm Hg, with 325 mm Hg as the pressure used most often. For tourniquet cuffs applied to the thigh, the average pressure was 398.39 mm Hg, and 400 mm Hg was the most common pressure setting.[27]

A web-based survey was distributed to 350 academic or community-based orthopedic surgeons

EQUIPMENT AND PRODUCT SAFETY

in the United States to identify the tourniquet pressures surgeons routinely used and whether the surgeons based their decision on findings from the literature. There was a response rate of 57% (n = 199), which was further divided into responses for lower extremity (n = 151) or upper extremity (n = 141). For the lower extremity, the mean and the median pressures were 300 mm Hg (range 145 mm Hg to 400 mm Hg). Thirty surgeons (20.5%) reported being able to cite evidence to support the decision. For the upper extremity, the mean tourniquet pressure was 242 mm Hg and the median was 250 mm Hg (range 150 mm Hg to 300 mm Hg). Twenty-five surgeons (17.7%) reported being able to cite evidence to support the decision. The researchers recommended increasing surgeons' awareness through training and daily practice to encourage them to use lower pressures and base their practice on findings in the literature.[93]

In another study of surgeon's practice, 253 surveys were mailed to members of the American Orthopaedic Foot and Ankle Society. The response rate was 55%, with 140 surgeons returning completed surveys. Nine percent of the respondents based their pressure settings on limb occlusion pressure (LOP); however, 73% of the respondents evaluated the patient's blood pressure as a factor to determine the cuff pressure, 65% evaluated the patient's limb size, and 43% evaluated both blood pressure and limb size in their determinations of pressure. Of the responding surgeons, 49% said they applied tourniquet cuffs to the thigh and reported their most common pressures to be 301 mm Hg to 350 mm Hg. For procedures in which a calf or ankle tourniquet cuff was applied, 52% of the surgeons who used calf cuffs and 66% of those who used ankle cuffs reported their most common pressures to be above 201 mm Hg to 250 mm Hg. However, 41% of the surgeons who used calf cuffs and 19% of those who used ankle cuffs reported they often used pressure above 250 mm Hg. The researchers concluded that more surgeons might adopt lower pressures and base their determinations on LOP if there were more explicit recommendations for using LOP.[101]

Research studies have shown that occlusion can be achieved using a lower pressure when an LOP method is used in conjunction with a wide tourniquet cuff in adult patients.[65,67,91,95,98,100] The same was found when studying pediatric patients.[18] Some tourniquet systems are designed to determine LOP automatically and add a safety margin to allow for fluctuations in blood pressure intraoperatively.

When using a wide contoured thigh cuff for patients older than 18 years, the cuff pressure setting researchers have suggested is determined by adding a safety margin to the LOP as follows:
- add 40 mm Hg to 50 mm Hg for LOP less than 130 mm Hg,
- add 60 mm Hg to 75 mm Hg for LOP between 131 mm Hg and 190 mm Hg, and
- add 80 mm Hg to 100 mm Hg for LOP greater than 190 mm Hg.[65,100]

For pediatric patients, the cuff pressure setting should be adjusted by adding 50 mm Hg to the LOP.[19]

IV.b.1. The baseline systolic blood pressure or LOP measurement should be taken when the patient's blood pressure is stabilized to the level expected during surgery and may be taken before or after induction of anesthesia.

IV.b.2. Before inflating the cuff, members of the perioperative team should confirm the setting to be used.

IV.c. Members of the perioperative team should confirm the positioning of the patient's extremity before inflating the tourniquet. *[4: Limited Evidence]*

For a lower extremity, if the invasive procedure is related to the quadriceps muscles, the surgeon may want the knee in a flexed position when inflating the tourniquet to avoid "tethering" of the underlying structures. The surgeon may prefer the knee extended if the invasive procedure involves the hamstring muscles.[102] In a comparative study of 30 patients to determine whether the position of the knee at the time of tourniquet inflation had a correlation with postoperative knee range of motion, researchers found a statistically significant difference in the range of motion between the two groups (ie, knee flexed at the time of inflation, knee extended at the time of inflation) but they did not find the statistical difference to be clinically significant.[102]

IV.d. Pneumatic tourniquets should be inflated under the direction of the surgeon and the anesthesia professional. *[3: Moderate Evidence]*

Inflation of the tourniquet cuff may be associated with hemodynamic changes (eg, hypertension, complications related to increased blood volume after exsanguination).[4,5]

IV.e. Activation indicators and pressure displays should be visible and audible alarms should be sufficiently loud to be heard above other sounds in the OR.[103] *[3: Moderate Evidence]*

Equipment alarms alert personnel to a change in pressure, equipment failure, or lapse of a designated duration of inflation time.

When the pressure gauge or digital display is clearly visible while the tourniquet cuff is inflated, the perioperative team can monitor for excessive fluctuation.

Because nerve damage may result from excessive tourniquet pressure and rhabdomyolysis has been reported with the tourniquet pressure set at an extreme pressure (ie, 520 mm Hg) even though the application time was relatively short (ie, 45 minutes), alarms are necessary to warn about conditions that may cause patient harm.[104,105]

Recommendation V

Tourniquet inflation time and patient condition should be monitored while the tourniquet cuff is inflated.

Tourniquet inflation time has a direct correlation to tourniquet-related complications (ie, increased inflation time increases the risk for injury). The patient's systemic response to ischemia is dependent on both tissue type and tourniquet time.[20] While cardiac muscle has a higher demand for oxygen, skeletal muscle is considered highly susceptible to ischemia.[106,107] This is because of the higher volumes of skeletal muscle mass releasing toxic substances into the circulatory system when reperfusion occurs, which can then lead to a severe inflammatory response.[107,108] Excessive tourniquet inflation time (ie, two to three hours) may result in metabolic changes; muscle damage; impaired pulmonary, hepatic, or renal function; neurological complications; or pain.[108-113]

To determine the efficacy and safety of distally placed pneumatic tourniquets, researchers initiated a retrospective study to review 3,027 procedures during which the surgeons used ankle tourniquets. Following a chart review, the researchers determined that the duration of ankle ischemia was as short as four minutes to as long as 139 minutes. Tourniquet failure was reported in 50 cases. Clinically, five complications were determined (ie, three post-tourniquet syndrome, one sickle cell-related problem, one DVT) and all eventually resolved. Based on the study, the authors concluded that an upper limit of two hours resulted in fewer complications.[27]

In a prospective study of awake patients, researchers investigated tolerance of intraoperative tourniquet pain. The study was designed to include 1,000 patients undergoing elective foot surgery with a local block, but 12 patients were excluded because the surgeon chose not to use a tourniquet. This left a sample size of 988 patients. The researchers found that 31 patients (3.1%) expressed pain during the procedure and eight of those experienced symptoms (eg, breakthrough bleeding from reduced tourniquet pressure, oversedation, excessive restlessness) that required the surgeon to interrupt the procedure. Of those eight patients, the anesthesia professional converted four patients to general anesthesia. The maximum tourniquet inflation time was 90 minutes (ie, range two to 90 minutes, median 18 minutes). The researchers concluded that for foot procedures with local blocks and ankle tourniquets, a tourniquet time of up to 30 minutes is tolerated by patients younger than 70 years of age, but 1% of the patients will report pain for each 11 minutes beyond 30 minutes. They recommended caution when administering local anesthesia to patients older than 70 years, especially if the tourniquet inflation time is expected to be longer than 30 minutes.[84]

In a retrospective review of more than 1,000 patients who had total knee arthroplasties (ie, primary and revision knee replacements), researchers set out to identify risk factors that contribute to neurological complications. All patients had tourniquet times greater than 120 minutes. The researchers reported that 90 patients (7.7%) experienced 129 peroneal and/or tibial nerve palsies. They concluded that extended tourniquet times, the patient's age (ie, postoperative neurological dysfunction was associated with younger age), and the presence of preoperative flexion contractures were contributing factors to neurological complications. The authors also reported that total tourniquet time and a reperfusion interval only modestly decreased the risk of nerve injuries.[111]

Twenty-six patients undergoing arthroscopic anterior cruciate ligament repairs participated in a prospective open randomized study that compared metabolic effects of using wide, curved tourniquet cuffs at a pressure of 250 mm Hg in one group and narrow, straight cuffs at a pressure of 350 mm Hg in the other. The researchers reported a significant correlation between femoral vein lactate levels and tourniquet time. They found the test parameters for measuring muscle injuries and anaerobic metabolism were the same between the two groups for the first hour of tourniquet inflation, but the metabolic changes increased as the tourniquet time increased.[110]

V.a. Pneumatic tourniquet inflation time should be kept to a minimum. *[3: Moderate Evidence]*

Even with relatively short tourniquet inflation times (ie, 26 minutes ± eight minutes), researchers have found significant markers of systemic inflammatory response when they were measured 15 minutes after tourniquet deflation.[106] Inflation times of 60 minutes for an upper extremity and 90 minutes for a lower extremity have been identified as a general guideline for inflation duration.[17] However, some sources indicate that two hours is a safe time limit for tourniquet inflation.[20,31] In pediatric patients, inflation times of less than 75 minutes for lower extremities has been recommended.[114]

Irreversible skeletal muscle damage is thought to begin after three hours of ischemia and is extensive at six hours.[115] Allowing intermittent reperfusion restores oxygenation and releases toxins.[31] Deflating the tourniquet every two hours with at least a 10-minute reperfusion time has been identified as a strategy to consider to decrease the risk for tissue damage.[28] Another approach is to release the tourniquet after 90 minutes for at least 10 to 15 minutes for the first reperfusion period, then 15 to 20 minutes for each subsequent reperfusion period.[17] However, it has also been reported that implementing reperfusion periods after

60 to 90 minutes of ischemia can contribute to muscle injury.[23]

V.a.1. The surgeon should be informed of the tourniquet inflation time at regular, established intervals.[28]

V.a.2. When the duration of tourniquet inflation is longer than two hours, the RN circulator should confer with the surgeon and anesthesia professional about deflating the tourniquet for 10 to 15 minutes to allow tissue reperfusion.[17,28]

V.b. The patient should be monitored for physiological responses to tourniquet cuff inflation. *[3: Moderate Evidence]*

Patients may experience pain or anxiety accompanied by an increase in heart rate and blood pressure when the tourniquet is inflated.[28,116-118] An increase in core body temperature has been reported in both pediatric and adult patients after tourniquet inflation.[119-121]

V.b.1. Care should be exercised to avoid overheating the patient while the tourniquet cuff is inflated, particularly for pediatric patients.[120,122]

V.c. The perioperative nurse should collaborate with the anesthesia professional to prepare for potential patient injuries and complications associated with the inflation rotation sequence used with dual-bladder tourniquet cuffs during intravenous regional anesthesia.[53] *[2: High Evidence]*

Adverse reaction to local anesthetic agents is a potential complication of intravenous regional anesthesia. A bolus of local anesthesia entering the general circulation can occur when there is an unplanned sudden deflation of the tourniquet soon after injection of local anesthetic or when the bolus is released too rapidly at the end of the procedure.[49]

Recommendation VI

The perioperative RN should collaborate with the surgeon and anesthesia professional to implement safe practices when deflating the pneumatic tourniquet.

Physiologic changes resulting from deflation of the tourniquet are dependent on the relative size of the extremity, duration of tourniquet time, and overall physiologic status of the patient. A decrease in blood pressure occurs as blood is shunted back to the extremity.[28] A significant decrease in core body temperature occurs after deflation of a lower extremity cuff.[121,123] Studies measuring emboli released after tourniquet cuff deflation have revealed that the highest number of emboli were released within one minute of deflation.[124,125]

Products of anaerobic metabolism (eg, lactate, hyperkalemia) enter the systemic circulation when the tourniquet cuff is deflated and cause acidosis.[4,28,108]

This can result in severe myocardial depression and possibly cardiac arrest.[35]

Ischemia-reperfusion injury also can cause an increase in intracranial pressure. Three studies have investigated the effect of different anesthetics (eg, isoflurane, sevoflurane, propofol) on the degree of cerebral vasodilation.[126-128] The findings from one study revealed an increase in the velocity of blood flow in the middle cerebral artery for five minutes after tourniquet deflation, with a greater degree of increased flow when isoflurane was used.[126] A study using hyperventilation to decrease the risk of increased cerebral blood flow after tourniquet deflation reported a greater increase in flow with isoflurane when compared to sevoflurane and propofol.[128]

Coordination among members of the perioperative team can facilitate management of the patient's physiologic status during this period of rapid change.

VI.a. Pneumatic tourniquets should be deflated under the direction of the surgeon and anesthesia professional. *[2: High Evidence]*

Hemodynamic changes may occur when the tourniquet is deflated. One prospective, randomized study found that the rate of acute systemic metabolic changes were reduced and there was greater hemodynamic stability when the tourniquet deflation was staggered (ie, deflated for 30 seconds, reinflated, and then repeated twice at three minute intervals).[129]

VI.a.1. The cuff and skin protection (eg, sleeve, padding) should be removed from the extremity after deflation of the tourniquet.

The padding or a deflated cuff may hinder venous return, resulting in congestion and pooling of blood at the surgical site.[17]

VI.b. Timing of the deflation of the pneumatic tourniquet should be coordinated based on the surgical procedure and the anesthesia plan of care. *[1: Strong Evidence]*

A meta-analysis of 11 randomized controlled trials revealed that the tourniquet may be deflated before wound closure (ie, early release) as a strategy to control bleeding during the surgical procedure. There was a significantly higher risk for early postoperative complications when the tourniquet was deflated after wound closure (ie, late release). However, researchers identified a wide diversity in methodologies and clinical strategies and concluded that larger studies are needed to clarify how the timing of tourniquet deflation correlates with the risk of postoperative complications.[130]

In a randomized clinical trial involving 84 patients and 96 total knee arthroplasty procedures, researchers compared blood loss and operative time when no tourniquet was used, when the tourniquet was deflated after implant insertion and cautery was used for hemostasis before closing, and when the tourniquet was deflated after wound closure and application of compression dressings. They did not identify

EQUIPMENT AND PRODUCT SAFETY

any significant differences in blood loss or blood transfusions between the three groups, but they did report a significant increase in operative time when no tourniquet was used (ie, an average of 115 minutes without a tourniquet compared to an average of 82 minutes with intraoperative deflation and an average of 77 minutes with deflation after wound closure).[131] Another study evaluated 939 patients who had total knee replacements. The findings revealed that when the surgeon released the tourniquet after wound closure, there was a significantly higher degree of perioperative blood loss than when the surgeon released the tourniquet intraoperatively.[132]

The anesthesia professional may choose to increase IV fluids immediately before deflating the tourniquet cuff.[35] Hyperventilation before tourniquet cuff deflation also has been recommended to reduce the risk of severe increases in intracranial pressure.[126,128,133]

VI.c. When tourniquets are used on two extremities, the perioperative RN should confirm the sequence and timing of the deflation of each of the tourniquets. *[3: Moderate Evidence]*

The risk of complications and the systemic effects of tourniquet use may be increased when two tourniquets are applied at the same time. Tourniquet inflation causes anaerobic metabolism, which produces lactic acid and other metabolites.[115] Tourniquet deflation returns blood flow into the extremity and also releases the toxins that have built up in the extremity. Systemic responses related to tourniquet deflation on the first limb could occur during the second limb procedure.

A study of 15 healthy children ages six months to 15 years found that systolic blood pressure decreased 8 mm Hg to 10 mm Hg for five to 10 minutes after tourniquet deflation and a greater decrease in pH occurred with simultaneous deflation of bilateral tourniquets.[114]

VI.c.1. The first tourniquet cuff inflated should be completely deflated (and the cuff and limb protection removed, if possible) to assess circulation in the first limb while the procedure on the second limb is being completed.[85]

Sequential deflation lessens the potential for adverse patient reactions from simultaneous release of metabolic by-products from both extremities.[85] Researchers studied 35 patients who underwent bilateral total knee replacements and found the blood pressure changes were more evident after deflation of the tourniquet cuff on the second extremity than after the deflation of the tourniquet cuff on the first extremity.[134]

Respondents from a survey reported one case in which an amputation of the primary limb became necessary because of severe ischemia related to the primary tourniquet cuff remaining inflated unintentionally throughout the secondary procedure.[19]

VI.c.2. The surgeon or anesthesia professional may choose to stagger the tourniquet deflations 30 to 45 minutes apart.[17]

Staggering the tourniquet deflations may reduce the rapid simultaneous release of large amounts of metabolic by-products from both limbs into the vascular system.[17]

VI.d. When dual-bladder tourniquet cuffs are used with intravenous regional anesthesia, the tourniquet should be deflated as determined by the anesthesia professional. *[3: Moderate Evidence]*

As the tourniquet cuff deflates, the anesthetic agent may be released into the circulatory system, causing systemic effects.[135-137] Various techniques for deflation of the tourniquet after intravenous regional anesthesia have been reported.[135,136,138] One case study was reported in which a 21-year-old woman undergoing an open reduction and fixation of a fractured finger with intravenous regional anesthesia experienced temporary bilateral blindness after a member of the perioperative team deflated the tourniquet cuff without consulting the anesthesia professional. The authors of the case study concluded that the bilateral blindness occurred as a result of a toxic overdose of lidocaine. The patient's blindness resolved within 10 minutes postoperatively, and she did not have residual visual symptoms at the one month postoperative examination.[137]

Recommendation VII

The perioperative RN should evaluate the outcome of patient care after the tourniquet has been deflated.

The patient's blood pressure may be low for the first hour after tourniquet cuff deflation because of blood that is shunted to reperfuse the tissue. This is also related to bleeding at the surgical site and reactive vasodilatation and microvascular permeability.[23]

Systemic responses occur in relation to ischemia when a tourniquet is inflated and reperfusion when the tourniquet has been deflated.[139] The amount of time it takes the patient's body to clear the anaerobic metabolites depends on the patient's physiologic status, the extremity involved, and the duration of tourniquet inflation.

During the reperfusion phase, free radicals often are released into the circulatory system resulting in oxidative stress.[107] Several researchers have studied the biochemical mechanisms that contribute to ischemia-reperfusion injury and the appropriate pharmacological interventions to effectively reduce the patient's systemic response to oxidative stress.[42,139-143] In a study of 16 elderly patients undergoing bilateral total knee arthroplasty, researchers evaluated whether the administration of an antioxidant (eg, ascorbic acid, tocopherol, coenzyme Q10) could prevent the decreased vascular compliance and cardiac injury caused by oxidative stress. The researchers found that the administration of a high dose of vitamin C during bilateral total knee arthroplasties could play a part in protecting the myocardium because it prevents the production of oxygen free radicals and lowers arterial oxygen tension and the mean blood pressure caused by ischemia-reperfusion injury.[107] A case report indicated that younger people also can be affected by cardiac ischemia related to tourniquet inflation. A 25-year-old man exhibited respiratory and electrocardiogram changes 20 minutes after the tourniquet had been deflated. His laboratory reports revealed increased serum potassium and metabolic acidosis, which the clinicians believed caused coronary vasospasm. The patient's electrocardiogram and laboratory values reflected resolution of the systematic response to the ischemia-reperfusion injury three hours after surgery.[144]

Other researchers studied cell damage resulting from tourniquet-induced ischemia. Their findings revealed that the highest level of cell damage was measured immediately after reperfusion and that the markers of cell damage remained one hour after tourniquet deflation.[145]

A decrease in core body temperature may occur when a tourniquet cuff that is placed on a lower extremity is deflated.[123] In a randomized single-blind study of 24 older adults undergoing general anesthesia for unilateral total knee arthroplasties, researchers reported that intraoperative forced-air warming prevented hypothermia when the tourniquet was deflated.[146]

VII.a. The perioperative RN should include a report on pressure settings, duration of the pneumatic tourniquet inflation, and patient outcomes when transferring the care of the patient to other caregivers. [2: High Evidence]

Transfer of care reports facilitate continuity in care.[75]

VII.b. The patient should be monitored for systemic responses and blood loss after the pneumatic tourniquet cuff has been deflated. [1: Strong Evidence]

Patients may experience a drop in blood pressure immediately after tourniquet cuff deflation and for an extended time after surgery.[23,121] Systemic responses to anaerobic metabolites and pulmonary emboli may occur after the tourniquet is deflated.[125,139,147]

Postoperative blood loss will vary after tourniquet-assisted procedures. Inflating a pneumatic tourniquet may decrease the blood loss intraoperatively, but researchers in one study found that patients who undergo tourniquet-assisted total knee arthroplasties may have more hidden blood loss and may not be able to participate in rehabilitation exercises as early as those who have the same surgery without a tourniquet.[148] In another study, researchers set out to determine whether post-

operative drainage following knee replacement would be reduced if the release of suction drains was delayed by an hour, thereby allowing tamponade. A total of 100 patients participated in the study and were randomly assigned to either a group in which the drains were released immediately after deflation of the tourniquet or a group in which the drains were clamped until one hour after the tourniquet was deflated. The findings revealed that the group with the clamped drains had a statistically significant reduction in postoperative bleeding and required fewer postoperative transfusions. Furthermore, the researchers reported that one patient in the "immediate release" group experienced a pulmonary embolus, and two in the "clamped" group experienced DVT.[149]

Some researchers have undertaken studies to investigate how medications administered intraoperatively influence postoperative blood loss in total knee arthroplasty procedures. In one study of 84 patients, researchers infused a low dose of norepinephrine (dilution 1:200,000) into the knees of 29 patients before the tourniquets were released. Researchers reported a significant reduction in perioperative blood loss in the group of patients that received the norepinephrine irrigation. They attributed this to the hemostatic effect that norepinephrine had on peak blood flow 20 to 30 minutes after the tourniquet cuff was deflated. The control group patients (n = 55) received a saline wash. The researchers reported that no patients in either group experienced DVT or skin edge necrosis.[150] A different study was designed to explore the effectiveness of tranexamic acid in inhibiting the fibrinolytic system to reduce blood loss without resulting in an increase of DVT. The researchers concluded that there was a significant decrease in the "amount of blood loss in the early postoperative period" when they injected 15 mg/kg of tranexamic acid at the time of cementing the knee implant, before tourniquet deflation. They did not find an increase in thromboembolic complications related to the use of tranexamic acid.[151]

VII.b.1. The postoperative evaluation should include
- vital signs, including oxygen saturation;
- temperature;
- skin condition under the tourniquet (eg, temperature, color, integrity);
- pulses distal to the tourniquet cuff;
- surgical wound site (eg, dressings, drains); and
- blood loss.

VII.c. Complications should be reported to the surgeon and anesthesia professional and discussed during the hand off of care to other caregivers. [2: High Evidence]

PNEUMATIC TOURNIQUET

Pulmonary emboli have been reported to occur after tourniquet cuff deflation.[28,124,152-157] Postoperative neurological complications related to tourniquet use also have been reported.[111,158] Although unusual, compartment syndrome related to tourniquet use has also been reported.[159-161]

Recommendation VIII

The pneumatic tourniquet and accessories should be cleaned after each use according to the manufacturer's written instructions.

Studies have reported microbial growth after culturing of reusable tourniquet cuffs.[162-164] In a limited study, researchers cultured 10 reusable tourniquet cuffs and 10 exsanguinators and compared the findings with microbes found in infected fracture wounds. They found that all 10 of the exsanguinators and eight of the tourniquet cuffs grew pathogens. *Staphylococcus aureus* and *Acinetobacter* were among the pathogens that were isolated, and coagulase-negative staphylococcus was the most commonly cultured pathogen. *Staphylococcus epidermidis* was the coagulase-negative pathogen found in two wound site infections out of 24 ankle fractures. Although the researchers found all of the exsanguinators and the majority of the cuffs they cultured to be contaminated, they could not identify evidence linking exsanguinators and tourniquet cuffs to surgical site infections. Despite this, the researchers recommended autoclaving tourniquet cuffs and using a clean exsanguinator for each procedure.[164]

VIII.a. After use, personnel should turn off the pneumatic tourniquet and clean and inspect it according to the manufacturer's written instructions. *[1: Strong Evidence]*

Cleaning between procedures prevents cross contamination.[165,166] Inspecting equipment after use helps to identify issues that can be handled before the equipment is used again.

VIII.a.1. Single-use cuffs should be discarded in an appropriate receptacle.

VIII.b. Between uses on patients, reusable cuffs and bladders should be cleaned using an Environmental Protection Agency-registered hospital disinfectant and then rinsed and dried.[162-166] *[1: Strong Evidence]*

Rinsing removes residue that may cause skin irritation, increase the chance of allergic reaction, and decrease the life of the cuff and bladder.[17]

VIII.b.1. If a reusable cuff is unable to be cleaned adequately, it should be discarded in an appropriate receptacle.

Recommendation IX

Perioperative team members should receive initial and ongoing education and competency verification on the use of the pneumatic tourniquet and on their understanding of the physiologic responses that influence the care of a patient undergoing pneumatic tourniquet-assisted operative or invasive procedures.

Health care organizations have a responsibility to provide initial and ongoing education and to evaluate the competency of perioperative team members to deliver safe care to patients undergoing pneumatic tourniquet-assisted operative or invasive procedures.[53,167] Every nurse is personally accountable for maintaining competency.[53,168]

Initial and ongoing development of knowledge and skills and documentation of personnel participation is a regulatory and accreditation requirement for both hospitals and ambulatory settings.[169-174]

Two studies evaluating the knowledge of perioperative personnel who used tourniquets identified the need for education on the application of tourniquet cuffs and the use of pneumatic tourniquets to prevent injuries and complications.[164,175] In one study, researchers distributed questionnaires to assistants and orthopedic specialists in the OR from five different hospitals. A total of 54 questionnaires were returned and analyzed. The mean score for the orthopedic specialists was 41.3% (standards deviation 6.85%; range 29.0% to 54.8%). The mean score for the assistants was 46.7% (standard deviation 9.64%; range 23.3% to 62.9%). The researchers concluded that there is a need for standard guidelines on tourniquet use.[175] In another study, researchers distributed a questionnaire to OR personnel who used exsanguinators and pneumatic tourniquets. A total of 74 questionnaires were returned and analyzed. The respondents included eight porters, 12 nurses, 10 senior house officers, 38 registrars, and six consultants. The nursing group had the highest mean score of 38.8%. The other mean scores were reported as 36.1% for the specialist registrars, 33.6% for the consultants, 32.8% for the registrars, 25.5% for the senior house officers, and 11.9% for the porters. The researchers identified the need for providing education to provide the best patient care.[164]

IX.a. Perioperative team members should receive education and competency verification that addresses the care of patients undergoing pneumatic tourniquet-assisted operative or other invasive procedures.[169-174] The education should address
- differentiating indications and contraindications for tourniquet use,
- identifying risks to patients and precautions to minimize these risks,
- selecting appropriate tourniquet cuffs based on patient assessment,
- following specific manufacturers' instructions for use,
- operating the tourniquet regulator according to the manufacturer's recommendations,
- measuring LOP,
- identifying physiologic changes during and after tourniquet use,
- implementing proper care and handling of the tourniquet and its accessories,

EQUIPMENT AND PRODUCT SAFETY

172

- documenting and communicating tourniquet information and its affects during hand offs to facilitate continuity in patient care, and
- employing corrective actions in the event of a patient injury.

[1: Regulatory Requirement]

Tourniquets and accessories have been associated with patient injuries.[106,108,112,113] Education provides a foundation to guide safe patient care and minimize these risks.[111]

Competency verification confirms that personnel have knowledge regarding the use of the pneumatic tourniquet and appropriate corrective action to be taken in the event of a patient injury.[176-179]

IX.b. Perioperative personnel should receive education that addresses human factors related to the management of patient care for patients undergoing pneumatic tourniquet-assisted operative or other invasive procedures. *[3: Moderate Evidence]*

Human factors include the interpersonal and social aspects of the perioperative environment (eg, coordination of activities, teamwork, collaboration, communication).

In a synthesis of the literature on perioperative nursing competency published between 2000 and 2008, researchers identified two domains of perioperative competency:

- specialized knowledge, described as familiarity with standards and guidelines of perioperative practice, and
- human factors, described as interpersonal and social team interactions.

The researchers recognized teamwork and communication as important aspects of patient safety and indicators of perioperative competency.[176]

In a qualitative focus group study exploring the perceptions of perioperative nurses on competency, researchers identified three themes as competency requirements:

- technical and procedural knowledge—the knowledge, psychomotor skills, and situational awareness required for competency in the perioperative setting;
- communication skills—the need for communication and team building skills, collegial support, and the ability to decipher and share complex clinical information; and
- managing and coordinating flow—the ability to anticipate needs, organize and prioritize resources, manage conflicts, and grasp the full perspective of the situation.

The findings of the study highlight the importance of human factors as a competency requirement for perioperative nurses.[180]

Education, collegiality, and collaboration are standards of perioperative nursing and primary responsibilities of the perioperative RN who practices in the perioperative setting.[53,179]

Recommendation X

Documentation should reflect activities related to the care of the patient undergoing pneumatic tourniquet-assisted operative or other invasive procedures.

Documentation is a professional medicolegal standard. Documentation of nursing activities is dictated by the health care organization's policy and regulatory and accrediting agency requirements and is necessary to inform other health care professionals involved in the patient's care. Highly reliable data collection is not only necessary to chronicle patient responses to nursing interventions, but also to demonstrate the health care organization's progress toward quality care outcomes.[181]

X.a. Patient assessments, the plan of care, interventions implemented, and evaluation of care related to use of a pneumatic tourniquet should be documented. *[1: Regulatory Requirement]*

At the patient care level, documentation facilitates continuity of patient care through clear communication and supports collaboration among health care team members.

Perioperative documentation that accurately reflects the patient experience is essential for the continuity of outcome-focused nursing care and for effective comparison of realized versus anticipated patient outcomes.[181]

Effective management and collection of health care information that accurately reflects the patient's care, treatment, and services provided is a regulatory and accreditation requirement for both hospitals and ambulatory settings.[169,170,182-187]

X.a.1. Documentation should include
- pneumatic tourniquet system identification,
- limb occlusion pressure,
- cuff pressure,
- skin protection measures,
- location of the tourniquet cuff,
- skin integrity under the cuff before and after use of the pneumatic tourniquet,
- the person placing the tourniquet cuff,
- time of inflation and deflation,
- assessment and evaluation of the entire extremity including preoperative and postoperative pulses distal to the tourniquet, and
- systemic reactions to ischemia and reperfusion.

X.b. The perioperative RN should include information about pressure settings, the duration of the pneumatic tourniquet inflation, and patient outcomes when transferring the care of the patient to other caregivers. *[2: High Evidence]*

Transfer of care reports facilitate continuity in care.[75]

X.b.1. Complications should be reported to the surgeon and anesthesia professional and included in documentation communicated during the hand off of care to other caregivers.

X.c. The perioperative RN should document all postoperative patient instructions given to the patient and his or her support person(s) related to pneumatic tourniquet-assisted operative or other invasive procedures.[181] *[2: High Evidence]*

Postoperative limb swelling and neurological complications (eg, compression paralysis, cutaneous sensory loss) have been reported to occur in relation to tourniquet use.[158,188,189] Patients and their support person(s) are better prepared to alert the surgeon or surgical facility about unusual symptoms if they have received adequate postoperative and discharge instructions.

X.d. Documentation of tourniquet testing should reflect the biomedical equipment identification number or serial number, date of inspection, preventive maintenance, and status of all equipment.[74] *[3: Moderate Evidence]*

Records of equipment failure and preventative maintenance assist in identifying equipment performance problems or hazards and minimize risk of patient injury and equipment failure.

Recommendation XI

Policies and procedures for use of pneumatic tourniquets should be developed, reviewed periodically, revised as necessary, and readily available in the practice setting.

Policies and procedures assist in the development of patient safety, quality assessment, and performance improvement activities. Policies and procedures establish authority, responsibility, and accountability within the health care organization. Policies and procedures also serve as operational guidelines that are used to minimize patient risk for injury or complications, standardize practice, direct perioperative personnel, and establish continuous performance improvement programs.

XI.a. Policies and procedures for the pneumatic tourniquet should include
- preoperative, intraoperative, and postoperative patient assessments;
- the timing of prophylactic antibiotic administration;
- guidelines for cuff selection (eg, sterile, reusable, width, length, shape) and fit;
- equipment checks before initial use, including cuff compatibility with the regulator and appropriate power or gas source;
- reporting and impounding of malfunctioning equipment[190];
- equipment maintenance programs and intervals for evaluation by designated personnel;
- responsibility for exsanguination;

- responsibility for cuff application;
- precautions during use;
- the interval for reporting tourniquet inflation time to the physician;
- safe parameters for tourniquet inflation times;
- safe parameters for tourniquet inflation pressures;
- parameters for reperfusion following extended inflation times;
- reporting of injuries;
- care and cleaning of the tourniquet and cuffs after use; and
- documentation.

[1: Regulatory Requirement]

Policies and procedures that guide and support patient care, treatment, and services are a regulatory and accreditation requirement for both hospitals and ambulatory settings.[169,170,173,191-193]

XI.b. The pneumatic tourniquet manufacturer's written instructions for cleaning, operation, and maintenance should be reviewed and reflected in policies and procedures. *[5: Benefits Balanced with Harms]*

As new technologies are introduced for use in perioperative practice settings, it is imperative that health care personnel strictly follow manufacturers' written instructions for the operation and maintenance of equipment and be aware of the hazards that the equipment may pose to patients.

XI.b.1. User manuals for pneumatic tourniquets should be readily available and retained for the life of the equipment.

Recommendation XII

Perioperative personnel should participate in quality assurance and performance improvement activities that are consistent with the health care organization's plan to improve understanding of the physiologic responses that influence the care of a patient undergoing pneumatic tourniquet-assisted operative or other invasive procedures and compliance with safe practices when using pneumatic tourniquets.

Quality assurance and performance improvement programs assist in evaluating and improving the quality of patient care and formulating plans for corrective actions. These programs provide data that may be used to determine whether an individual organization is within benchmark goals and, if not, to identify areas that may require corrective actions. Participating in ongoing quality assurance and performance improvement activities is a standard of perioperative nursing and a primary responsibility of the RN who is engaged in practice in the perioperative setting.[53]

Complications related to equipment failure and pneumatic tourniquet use have been reported.[1,2,6]

XII.a. The pneumatic tourniquet system should be evaluated for safe use by designated personnel (eg, biomedical engineering personnel) within the health care organization and at intervals consistent with the manufacturer's written instructions and policies of the health care organization. *[3: Moderate Evidence]*

Periodic preventative maintenance supports continuous safe operation of pneumatic tourniquets.[74]

XII.b. The quality management program should include processes to monitor compliance with patient safety considerations when a pneumatic tourniquet and accessories are used in perioperative settings. Considerations should include
  ○ that tourniquet cuffs are decontaminated after each use,
  ○ that the tourniquet cuff chosen is the right size and shape for the patient's extremity,
  ○ tourniquet inflation times that exceed the health care organization's specified parameters, and
  ○ tourniquet inflation pressures that exceed the health care organization's specified parameters.
  [1: Strong Evidence]

Collecting data to monitor and improve patient care, treatment, and services is a regulatory and accreditation requirement for both hospitals and ambulatory settings.[194-197]

Monitoring cleaning and disinfection practices to ensure adherence can help control transmission of multidrug-resistant organisms and other pathogens that may be residing in the environment.[165,166,198] The information obtained from assessments can be used to develop focused administrative and educational interventions that incorporate ongoing feedback to the environmental services personnel to improve cleaning and disinfection practices in health care institutions.[199] Compliance and adjunct monitoring after terminal cleaning can help prevent cross-contamination of areas that have or have had patients with multidrug-resistant organisms.[198,200]

XII.c. When compliance issues are identified, quality indicators should be developed to measure improvement in compliance with safe practices related to pneumatic tourniquets. *[1: Strong Evidence]*

Quality indicators are measurable and demonstrate that facilities are using specific interventions to provide safe patient care.[201]

According to the Agency for Healthcare Research and Quality, "An adequate quality indicator must have a sound clinical or empirical rationale for its use. It should measure an important aspect of quality that is subject to provider or healthcare system control."[201(p3)] Quality indicators are one response to the need for multidimensional, accessible, quality measures that can be used to gauge performance in health care. The quality indicators are evidence-based and can be used to identify variations in the quality of care provided on both an inpatient and outpatient basis.

XII.d. The health care organization's quality management program should include investigation of adverse events and near misses associated with use of a pneumatic tourniquet.[202,203] *[1: Regulatory Requirement]*

Reporting and investigating adverse events and near misses facilitates identification of trends and patterns and evaluation of the quality of patient care to assist in the formulation of plans for corrective actions.

XII.d.1. If a patient injury or equipment failure occurs, the pneumatic tourniquet system (eg, regulator, tubing, cuff) must be handled in accordance with the Safe Medical Devices Act of 1990, amended in March 2000.[190]

XII.d.2. Device identification, maintenance and service information, and adverse event information should be included in the report from the practice setting. Retaining the regulator, tubing, and cuff allows for a complete systems check to determine the tourniquet system integrity.

Glossary

Compartment syndrome: A pathologic condition caused by the progressive development of arterial compression and consequent reduction of blood supply. Clinical manifestations include swelling, restriction of movement, vascular compromise, and severe pain or lack of sensation.

Contoured tourniquet cuffs: Pneumatic tourniquet cuffs with a distal edge shorter than the proximal edge, creating a funnel-like shape when applied to an extremity.

Exsanguination: The process of forcible expulsion of blood from an extremity before pneumatic tourniquet use.

Limb occlusion pressure (LOP): The pneumatic tourniquet cuff pressure required to occlude arterial flow in the limb.

Preconditioning: Techniques used to reduce oxidative stress and increase skeletal muscle ischemia tolerance related to tourniquet inflation by initiating anesthetic regimens or short intervals of temporary ischemia.

Shearing: A sliding movement of skin and subcutaneous tissue that leaves the underlying muscle stationary.

REFERENCES

1. Odinsson A, Finsen V. Tourniquet use and its complications in Norway. *J Bone Joint Surg Br.* 2006;88(8):1090-1092. [IIIB]

2. Complications of arthroscopy and arthroscopic surgery: results of a national survey. Committee on Complications of Arthroscopy Association of North America. *Arthroscopy.* 1985;1(4):214-220. [IIIC]

3. Kalla TP, Younger A, McEwen JA, Inkpen K. Survey of tourniquet use in podiatric surgery. *J Foot Ankle Surg.* 2003;42(2):68-76. [IIIC]

4. Aziz ES. Tourniquet use in orthopaedic anaesthesia. *Curr Anaesth Crit Care.* 2009;20(2):55-59. [VC]

5. Klenerman L. Effect of a tourniquet on the limb and the systemic circulation. In: *The Tourniquet Manual: Principles and Practice.* London, UK: Springer; 2003:13-38. [VA]

6. Strategies for avoiding problems with the use of pneumatic tourniquets. *Pa Patient Saf Advis.* 2010;7(3):97-101. [VA]

7. Tibrewal SB. The pneumatic tourniquet in arthroscopic surgery of the knee. *Int Orthop.* 2001;24(6):347-349. [IB]

8. Johnson DS, Stewart H, Hirst P, Harper NJ. Is tourniquet use necessary for knee arthroscopy? *Arthroscopy.* 2000;16(6):648-651. [IA]

9. Kirkley A, Rampersaud R, Griffin S, Amendola A, Litchfield R, Fowler P. Tourniquet versus no tourniquet use in routine knee arthroscopy: a prospective, double-blind, randomized clinical trial. *Arthroscopy.* 2000;16(2):121-126. [IA]

10. Smith TO, Hing CB. A meta-analysis of tourniquet assisted arthroscopic knee surgery. *Knee.* 2009;16(5):317-321. [IIB]

11. Kiss H, Raffl M, Neumann D, Hutter J, Dorn U. Epinephrine-augmented hypotensive epidural anesthesia replaces tourniquet use in total knee replacement. *Clin Orthop Relat Res.* 2005;(436):184-189. [IA]

12. Smith TO, Hing CB. Is a tourniquet beneficial in total knee replacement surgery? A meta-analysis and systematic review. *Knee.* 2010;17(2):141-147. [IIB]

13. Tai TW, Lin CJ, Jou IM, Chang CW, Lai KA, Yang CY. Tourniquet use in total knee arthroplasty: a meta-analysis. *Knee Surg Sports Traumatol Arthrosc.* 2011;19(7):1121-1130. [IB]

14. Smith TO, Hing CB. The efficacy of the tourniquet in foot and ankle surgery? A systematic review and meta-analysis. *Foot Ankle Surg.* 2010;16(1):3-8. [IIIB]

15. Smith TO, Hing CB. Should tourniquets be used in upper limb surgery? A systematic review and meta-analysis. *Acta Orthop Belg.* 2009;75(3):289-296. [IIIC]

16. Saied A, Zyaei A. Tourniquet use during plating of acute extra-articular tibial fractures: effects on final results of the operation. *J Trauma.* 2010;69(6):E94-E97. [IA]

17. McEwen JA. Tourniquet use and care. http://www.tourniquets.org/use_care.php. Accessed May 4, 2013. [VC]

18. Lieberman JR, Staheli LT, Dales MC. Tourniquet pressures on pediatric patients: a clinical study. *Orthopedics.* 1997;20(12):1143-1147. [IIB]

19. Tredwell SJ, Wilmink M, Inkpen K, McEwen JA. Pediatric tourniquets: analysis of cuff and limb interface, current practice, and guidelines for use. *J Pediatr Orthop.* 2001;21(5):671-676. [IIIC]

20. Noordin S, McEwen JA, Kragh JF Jr, Eisen A, Masri BA. Surgical tourniquets in orthopaedics. *J Bone Joint Surg Am.* 2009;91(12):2958-2967. [VB]

21. Krackow KA. A maneuver for improved positioning of a tourniquet in the obese patient. *Clin Orthop Relat Res.* 1982;(168):80-82. [VC]

22. Klenerman L. Complications. In: *The Tourniquet Manual: Principles and Practice.* London, UK: Springer; 2003:61-75. [VA]

23. Estebe JP, Davies JM, Richebe P. The pneumatic tourniquet: mechanical, ischaemia-reperfusion and systemic effects. *Eur J Anaesthesiol.* 2011;28(6):404-411. [VB]

24. Fukuda A, Hasegawa M, Kato K, Shi D, Sudo A, Uchida A. Effect of tourniquet application on deep vein thrombosis after total knee arthroplasty. *Arch Orthop Trauma Surg.* 2007;127(8):671-675. [IIIC]

25. Parmet JL, Horrow JC, Pharo G, Collins L, Berman AT, Rosenberg H. The incidence of venous emboli during extramedullary guided total knee arthroplasty. *Anesth Analg.* 1995;81(4):757-762. [IIIB]

26. Parmet JL, Horrow JC, Berman AT, Miller F, Pharo G, Collins L. The incidence of large venous emboli during total knee arthroplasty without pneumatic tourniquet use. *Anesth Analg.* 1998;87(2):439-444. [IIB]

27. Derner R, Buckholz J. Surgical hemostasis by pneumatic ankle tourniquet during 3027 podiatric operations. *J Foot Ankle Surg.* 1995;34(3):236-246. [IIIA]

28. Kam PC, Kavanagh R, Yoong FF. The arterial tourniquet: pathophysiological consequences and anaesthetic implications. *Anaesthesia.* 2001;56(6):534-545. [VB]

29. Barr L, Iyer US, Sardesai A, Chitnavis J. Tourniquet failure during total knee replacement due to arterial calcification: case report and review of the literature. *J Perioper Pract.* 2010;20(2):55-58. [VC]

30. Garabekyan T, Oliashirazi A, Winters K. The value of immediate preoperative vascular examination in an at-risk patient for total knee arthroplasty. *Orthopedics.* 2011;34(1):52. [VB]

31. Wakai A, Winter DC, Street JT, Redmond PH. Pneumatic tourniquets in extremity surgery. *J Am Acad Orthop Surg.* 2001;9(5):345-351. [VB]

32. Fisher B, Roberts CS. Tourniquet use and sickle cell hemoglobinopathy: how should we proceed? *South Med J.* 2010;103(11):1156-1160. [VB]

33. Fanning R, O'Donnell B, Lynch B, Stephens M, O'Donovan F. Anesthesia for sickle cell disease and congenital myopathy in combination. *Paediatr Anaesth.* 2006;16(8):880-883. [VB]

34. Siddiqui FM, Slater RM, Razzaq I, Atkinson M, Ryan K. Tourniquet use during total knee replacement in a Jehovah's Witness with sickle cell trait: a case report. *Eur J Anaesthesiol.* 2010;27(6):581-582. [VC]

35. Gupta K, Aggarwal N, Rao M, Verma UC, Anand R. Re-emphasizing the importance of tourniquet time: severe myocardial depression following tourniquet deflation. *Acta Anaesthesiol Scand.* 2008;52(6):873. [VC]

36. Honarmand A, Safavi MR. Preoperative oral dextromethorphan vs. clonidine to prevent tourniquet-induced cardiovascular responses in orthopaedic patients under general anaesthesia. *Eur J Anaesthesiol.* 2007;24(6):511-515. [IB]

37. Sheth NP, Sennett B, Berns JS. Rhabdomyolysis and acute renal failure following arthroscopic knee surgery in a college football player taking creatine supplements. *Clin Nephrol.* 2006;65(2):134-137. [VB]

38. Seyahi A, Uludag S, Akman S, Demirhan M. Unrecognized anterior compartment syndrome following ankle fracture surgery: a case report. *J Am Podiatr Med Assoc.* 2009;99(5):438-442. [VB]

39. Brodsky MA, Smith JA. Exacerbation of myasthenia gravis after tourniquet release. *J Clin Anesth.* 2007;19(7):543-545. [VC]

40. Akinyoola AL, Adegbehingbe OO, Odunsi A. Timing of antibiotic prophylaxis in tourniquet surgery. *J Foot Ankle Surg.* 2011;50(4):374-376. [IB]

41. Soriano A, Bori G, Garcia-Ramiro S, et al. Timing of antibiotic prophylaxis for primary total knee arthroplasty performed during ischemia. *Clin Infect Dis.* 2008;46(7):1009-1014. [IB]

42. Koca K, Yurttas Y, Cayci T, et al. The role of preconditioning and N-acetylcysteine on oxidative stress resulting from tourniquet-induced ischemia-reperfusion in

arthroscopic knee surgery. *J Trauma*. 2011;70(3):717-723. [IB]

43. Mas E, Barden AE, Corcoran TB, Phillips M, Roberts LJ 2nd, Mori TA. Effects of spinal or general anesthesia on F-isoprostanes and isofurans during ischemia/reperfusion of the leg in patients undergoing knee replacement surgery. *Free Radic Biol Med*. 2011;50(9):1171-1176. [IIIB]

44. Lin LN, Wang LR, Wang WT, et al. Ischemic preconditioning attenuates pulmonary dysfunction after unilateral thigh tourniquet-induced ischemia-reperfusion. *Anesth Analg*. 2010;111(2):539-543. [IC]

45. Viscomi CM, Friend A, Parker C, Murphy T, Yarnell M. Ketamine as an adjuvant in lidocaine intravenous regional anesthesia: a randomized, double-blind, systemic control trial. *Reg Anesth Pain Med*. 2009;34(2):130-133. [IIC]

46. Orban JC, Levraut J, Gindre S, et al. Effects of acetylcysteine and ischaemic preconditioning on muscular function and postoperative pain after orthopaedic surgery using a pneumatic tourniquet. *Eur J Anaesthesiol*. 2006;23(12):1025-1030. [IC]

47. Guay J. Adverse events associated with intravenous regional anesthesia (Bier block): a systematic review of complications. *J Clin Anesth*. 2009;21(8):585-594. [VC]

48. Kol IO, Ozturk H, Kaygusuz K, Gursoy S, Comert B, Mimaroglu C. Addition of dexmedetomidine or lornoxicam to prilocaine in intravenous regional anaesthesia for hand or forearm surgery: a randomized controlled study. *Clin Drug Investig*. 2009;29(2):121-129. [IB]

49. Singh R, Bhagwat A, Bhadoria P, Kohli A. Forearm IVRA, using 0.5% lidocaine in a dose of 1.5 mg/kg with ketorolac 0.15 mg/kg for hand and wrist surgeries. *Minerva Anestesiol*. 2010;76(2):109-114. [IC]

50. Graham B, Breault MJ, McEwen JA, McGraw RW. Occlusion of arterial flow in the extremities at subsystolic pressures through the use of wide tourniquet cuffs. *Clin Orthop Relat Res*. 1993;(286):257-261. [IIIB]

51. Dounis E, Tsourvakas S, Kalivas L, Giamacellou H. Effect of time interval on tissue concentrations of cephalosporins after tourniquet inflation. Highest levels achieved by administration 20 minutes before inflation. *Acta Orthop Scand*. 1995;66(2):158-160. [IIB]

52. Papaioannou N, Kalivas L, Kalavritinos J, Tsourvakas S. Tissue concentrations of third-generation cephalosporins (ceftazidime and ceftriaxone) in lower extremity tissues using a tourniquet. *Arch Orthop Trauma Surg*. 1994;113(3):167-169. [IIIB]

53. Standards of perioperative nursing. In: *Perioperative Standards and Recommended Practices*. Denver, CO: AORN, Inc; 2012:20. [IVB]

54. Reikeras O, Clementsen T. Time course of thrombosis and fibrinolysis in total knee arthroplasty with tourniquet application. Local versus systemic activations. *J Thromb Thrombolysis*. 2009;28(4):425-428. [IIIC]

55. Kageyama K, Nakajima Y, Shibasaki M, Hashimoto S, Mizobe T. Increased platelet, leukocyte, and endothelial cell activity are associated with increased coagulability in patients after total knee arthroplasty. *J Thromb Haemost*. 2007;5(4):738-745. [IB]

56. Van M, Olguner C, Koca U, et al. Ischaemic preconditioning attenuates haemodynamic response and lipid peroxidation in lower-extremity surgery with unilateral pneumatic tourniquet application: a clinical pilot study. *Adv Ther*. 2008;25(4):355-366. [IC]

57. Carles M, Dellamonica J, Roux J, et al. Sevoflurane but not propofol increases interstitial glycolysis metabolites availability during tourniquet-induced ischaemia-reperfusion. *Br J Anaesth*. 2008;100(1):29-35. [IC]

58. Budic I, Pavlovic D, Kocic G, et al. Biomarkers of oxidative stress and endothelial dysfunction after tourniquet release in children. *Physiol Res*. 2011;60(Suppl 1):S137-S145. [IIIC]

59. Murphy T, Walsh PM, Doran PP, Mulhall KJ. Transcriptional responses in the adaptation to ischaemia-reperfusion injury: a study of the effect of ischaemic preconditioning in total knee arthroplasty patients. *J Transl Med*. 2010;8:46. [IC]

60. Erturk E, Cekic B, Geze S, et al. Comparison of the effect of propofol and N-acetyl cysteine in preventing ischaemia-reperfusion injury. *Eur J Anaesthesiol*. 2009;26(4):279-284. [IB]

61. Sullivan PJ, Sweeney KJ, Hirpara KM, Malone CB, Curtin W, Kerin MJ. Cyclical ischaemic preconditioning modulates the adaptive immune response in human limb ischaemia-reperfusion injury. *Br J Surg*. 2009;96(4):381-390. [IB]

62. Yagmurdur H, Ozcan N, Dokumaci F, Kilinc K, Yilmaz F, Basar H. Dexmedetomidine reduces the ischemia-reperfusion injury markers during upper extremity surgery with tourniquet. *J Hand Surg Am*. 2008;33(6):941-947. [IB]

63. Turan R, Yagmurdur H, Kavutcu M, Dikmen B. Propofol and tourniquet induced ischaemia reperfusion injury in lower extremity operations. *Eur J Anaesthesiol*. 2007;24(2):185-189. [IIC]

64. Memtsoudis SG, Valle AG, Jules-Elysse K, et al. Perioperative inflammatory response in total knee arthroplasty patients: impact of limb preconditioning. *Reg Anesth Pain Med*. 2010;35(5):412-416. [IB]

65. Younger AS, McEwen JA, Inkpen K. Wide contoured thigh cuffs and automated limb occlusion measurement allow lower tourniquet pressures. *Clin Orthop Relat Res*. 2004;(428):286-293. [IB]

66. Moore MR, Garfin SR, Hargens AR. Wide tourniquets eliminate blood flow at low inflation pressures. *J Hand Surg Am*. 1987;12(6):1006-1011. [IIIB]

67. Pedowitz RA, Gershuni DH, Botte MJ, Kuiper S, Rydevik BL, Hargens AR. The use of lower tourniquet inflation pressures in extremity surgery facilitated by curved and wide tourniquets and an integrated cuff inflation system. *Clin Orthop Relat Res*. 1993;(287):237-244. [IB]

68. Thompson SM, Middleton M, Farook M, Cameron-Smith A, Bone S, Hassan A. The effect of sterile versus non-sterile tourniquets on microbiological colonisation in lower limb surgery. *Ann R Coll Surg Engl*. 2011;93(8):589-590. [IIC]

69. Guedj MP. Sudden deflation of a tourniquet caused by lowering of the operating table. *Ann Fr Anesth Reanim*. 2007;26(2):174. [VC]

70. Simmons D, Phillips MS, Grissinger M, Becker SC; USP Safe Medication Use Expert Committee. Error-avoidance recommendations for tubing misconnections when using Luer-tip connectors: a statement by the USP Safe Medication Use Expert Committee. *Jt Comm J Qual Patient Saf*. 2008;34(5):293-296, 245. [VC]

71. Paparella S. Inadvertent attachment of a blood pressure device to a needleless IV "Y-site": surprising, fatal connections. *J Emerg Nurs*. 2005;31(2):180-182. [VC]

72. Arslan M, Canturk M, Ornek D, et al. Regional intravenous anesthesia in knee arthroscopy. *Clinics (Sao Paulo)*. 2010;65(9):831-835. [IIC]

73. US Food and Drug Administration. Pneumatic tourniquet cuffs, with the tourniquet systems. *Medical Product Safety News*. 2007;7(1):24. http://www.fda.gov/MedicalDevices/Safety/AlertsandNotices/TipsandArticlesonDeviceSafety/ucm070189.htm. Accessed May 4, 2013. [VB]

74. ECRI. Optimizing an IPM program. *Healthc Risk Control*. 2009;3(Risk Analysis Medical Technology 9). [VB]

75. Guideline for transfer of patient care information. In: *Guidelines for Perioperative Practice*. Denver, CO: AORN, Inc; 2015:583-588. [IVB]

76. Eidelman M, Katzman A, Bialik V. A novel elastic exsanguination tourniquet as an alternative to the pneumatic cuff in pediatric orthopedic limb surgery. *J Pediatr Orthop B*. 2006;15(5):379-384. [IIIC]

77. Olivecrona C, Tidermark J, Hamberg P, Ponzer S, Cederfjall C. Skin protection underneath the pneumatic tourniquet during total knee arthroplasty: a randomized controlled trial of 92 patients. *Acta Orthop*. 2006;77(3):519-523. [IB]

78. Din R, Geddes T. Skin protection beneath the tourniquet. A prospective randomized trial. *ANZ J Surg*. 2004;74(9):721-722. [IC]

79. Guo S. Is Velband still a safe and cost effective skin protection beneath the tourniquet in hand surgery? *Hand Surg*. 2011;16(1):5-8. [IIIB]

80. Hubik DJ, Connors A, Cleland H. Iatrogenic chemical burns associated with tourniquet use and prep solution. *ANZ J Surg*. 2009;79(10):762. [VC]

81. Odinsson A, Finsen V. The position of the tourniquet on the upper limb. *J Bone Joint Surg Br*. 2002;84(2):202-204. [IIC]

82. Finsen V, Kasseth AM. Tourniquets in forefoot surgery: less pain when placed at the ankle. *J Bone Joint Surg Br*. 1997;79(1):99-101. [IIC]

83. Lichtenfeld NS. The pneumatic ankle tourniquet with ankle block anesthesia for foot surgery. *Foot Ankle*. 1992;13(6):344-349. [IIIB]

84. Rudkin AK, Rudkin GE, Dracopoulos GC. Acceptability of ankle tourniquet use in midfoot and forefoot surgery: audit of 1000 cases. *Foot Ankle Int*. 2004;25(11):788-794. [IIIA]

85. Branson JJ, Goldstein WM. Sequential bilateral total knee arthroplasty. *AORN J*. 2001;73(3):610-635; quiz 637-642. [VB]

86. Darmanis S, Papanikolaou A, Pavlakis D. Fatal intraoperative pulmonary embolism following application of an Esmarch bandage. *Injury*. 2002;33(9):761-764. [VB]

87. Blond L, Jensen NV, Soe Nielsen NH. Clinical consequences of different exsanguination methods in hand surgery. a double-blind randomised study. *J Hand Surg Eur Vol*. 2008;33(4):475-477. [IIB]

88. Iyer S, Pabari A, Branford OA. Refinement of a simple technique with new relevance for exsanguination of the upper limb. *Tech Hand Up Extrem Surg*. 2011;15(2):82-83. [VC]

89. Angadi DS, Blanco J, Garde A, West SC. Lower limb elevation: useful and effective technique of exsanguination prior to knee arthroscopy. *Knee Surg Sports Traumatol Arthrosc*. 2010;18(11):1559-1561. [IIIC]

90. Estebe JP, Le Naoures A, Chemaly L, Ecoffey C. Tourniquet pain in a volunteer study: effect of changes in cuff width and pressure. *Anaethesia*. 2000;55(1):21-26. [IIC]

91. McEwen JA, Kelly DL, Jardanowski T, Inkpen K. Tourniquet safety in lower leg applications. *Orthop Nurs*. 2002;21(5):55-62. [IIIB]

92. Tuncali B, Karci A, Tuncali BE, et al. A new method for estimating arterial occlusion pressure in optimizing pneumatic tourniquet inflation pressure. *Anesth Analg*. 2006;102(6):1752-1757. [IIIB]

93. Tejwani NC, Immerman I, Achan P, Egol KA, McLaurin T. Tourniquet cuff pressure: The gulf between science and practice. *J Trauma*. 2006;61(6):1415-1418. [IIIC]

94. Ishii Y, Noguchi H, Matsuda Y, Takeda M, Higashihara T. A new tourniquet system that determines pressures in synchrony with systolic blood pressure in total knee arthroplasty. *J Arthroplasty*. 2008;23(7):1050-1056. [IIB]

95. Newman RJ, Muirhead A. A safe and effective low pressure tourniquet. A prospective evaluation. *J Bone Joint Surg Br*. 1986;68(4):625-628. [IA]

96. Worland RL, Arredondo J, Angles F, Lopez-Jimenez F, Jessup DE. Thigh pain following tourniquet application in simultaneous bilateral total knee replacement arthroplasty. *J Arthroplasty*. 1997;12(8):848-852. [IB]

97. Tuncali B, Karci A, Bacakoglu AK, Tuncali BE, Ekin A. Controlled hypotension and minimal inflation pressure: a new approach for pneumatic tourniquet application in upper limb surgery. *Anesth Analg*. 2003;97(5):1529-1532. [IB]

98. Younger AS, Manzary M, Wing KJ, Stothers K. Automated cuff occlusion pressure effect on quality of operative fields in foot and ankle surgery: a randomized prospective study. *Foot Ankle Int*. 2011;32(3):239-243. [IA]

99. Reilly CW, McEwen JA, Leveille L, Perdios A, Mulpuri K. Minimizing tourniquet pressure in pediatric anterior cruciate ligament reconstructive surgery: a blinded, prospective randomized controlled trial. *J Pediatr Orthop*. 2009;29(3):275-280. [IB]

100. Olivecrona C, Ponzer S, Hamberg P, Blomfeldt R. Lower tourniquet cuff pressure reduces postoperative wound complications after total knee arthroplasty: a randomized controlled study of 164 patients. *J Bone Joint Surg Am*. 2012;94(24):2216-2221. [IA]

101. Younger AS, Kalla TP, McEwen JA, Inkpen K. Survey of tourniquet use in orthopaedic foot and ankle surgery. *Foot Ankle Int*. 2005;26(3):208-217. [IIIB]

102. Zura RD, Adams SB Jr, Mata BA, Pietrobon R, Olson SA. Does knee position at the time of tourniquet inflation affect knee range of motion? *J Surg Orthop Adv*. 2007;16(4):171-173. [IIIC]

103. Guideline for a safe environment of care, part 1. In: *Guidelines for Perioperative Practice*. Denver, CO: AORN, Inc; 2015:239-263. [IVB]

104. Hodgson AJ. A proposed etiology for tourniquet-induced neuropathies. *J Biomech Eng*. 1994;116(2):224-227. [IIIB]

105. Lee YG, Park W, Kim SH, et al. A case of rhabdomyolysis associated with use of a pneumatic tourniquet during arthroscopic knee surgery. *Korean J Intern Med*. 2010;25(1):105-109. [VC]

106. Wakai A, Wang JH, Winter DC, Street JT, O'Sullivan RG, Redmond HP. Tourniquet-induced systemic inflammatory response in extremity surgery. *J Trauma*. 2001;51(5):922-926. [IB]

107. Lee JY, Kim CJ, Chung MY. Effect of high-dose vitamin C on oxygen free radical production and myocardial enzyme after tourniquet ischaemia-reperfusion injury during bilateral total knee replacement. *J Int Med Res*. 2010;38(4):1519-1529. [IC]

108. Gourdin MJ, Bree B, De Kock M. The impact of ischaemia-reperfusion on the blood vessel. *Eur J Anaesthesiol*. 2009;26(7):537-547. [VB]

109. Kim JG, Lee J, Roe J, Tromberg BJ, Brenner M, Walters TJ. Hemodynamic changes in rat leg muscles during tourniquet-induced ischemia-reperfusion injury observed by near-infrared spectroscopy. *Physiol Meas*. 2009;30(7):529-540. [IIB]

110. Kokki H, Vaatainen U, Penttila I. Metabolic effects of a low-pressure tourniquet system compared with a

high-pressure tourniquet system in arthroscopic anterior crucial ligament reconstruction. *Acta Anaesthesiol Scand.* 1998;42(4):418-424. [IIB]

111. Horlocker TT, Hebl JR, Gali B, et al. Anesthetic, patient, and surgical risk factors for neurologic complications after prolonged total tourniquet time during total knee arthroplasty. *Anesth Analg.* 2006;102(3):950-955. [IIIA]

112. Jacobson MD, Pedowitz RA, Oyama BK, Tryon B, Gershuni DH. Muscle functional deficits after tourniquet ischemia. *Am J Sports Med.* 1994;22(3):372-377. [IB]

113. Yassin MM, Harkin DW, Barros D'Sa AA, Halliday MI, Rowlands BJ. Lower limb ischemia-reperfusion injury triggers a systemic inflammatory response and multiple organ dysfunction. *World J Surg.* 2002;26(1):115-121. [IB]

114. Lynn AM, Fischer T, Brandford HG, Pendergrass TW. Systemic responses to tourniquet release in children. *Anesth Analg.* 1986;65(8):865-872. [IIIC]

115. Blaisdell FW. The pathophysiology of skeletal muscle ischemia and the reperfusion syndrome: a review. *Cardiovasc Surg.* 2002;10(6):620-630. [VB]

116. Sunder RA, Toshniwal G. An atypical presentation of tourniquet pain. *Acta Anaesthesiol Scand.* 2006;50(4):525-526. [VC]

117. Burg A, Tytiun Y, Velkes S, Heller S, Haviv B, Dudkiewicz I. Ankle tourniquet pain control in forefoot surgery: a randomized study. *Foot Ankle Int.* 2011;32(6):595-598. [IB]

118. Rastogi S, Brady WJ. Trousseau's sign related to upper arm tourniquet following brachial plexus blockade. *Anaesthesia.* 2011;66(9):846-847. [VB]

119. Goodarzi M, Shier NH, Ogden JA. Physiologic changes during tourniquet use in children. *J Pediatr Orthop.* 1992;12(4):510-513. [IIIB]

120. Bloch EC, Ginsberg B, Binner RA Jr, Sessler DI. Limb tourniquets and central temperature in anesthetized children. *Anesth Analg.* 1992;74(4):486-489. [IIB]

121. Estebe JP, Le Naoures A, Malledant Y, Ecoffey C. Use of a pneumatic tourniquet induces changes in central temperature. *Br J Anaesth.* 1996;77(6):786-788. [IC]

122. Bloch EC. Hyperthermia resulting from tourniquet application in children. *Ann R Coll Surg Engl.* 1986;68(4):193-194. [IIIC]

123. Sanders BJ, D'Alessio JG, Jernigan JR. Intraoperative hypothermia associated with lower extremity tourniquet deflation. *J Clin Anesth.* 1996;8(6):504-507. [IIIC]

124. Hirota K, Hashimoto H, Kabara S, et al. The relationship between pneumatic tourniquet time and the amount of pulmonary emboli in patients undergoing knee arthroscopic surgeries. *Anesth Analg.* 2001;93(3):776-780. [IIIB]

125. Hirota K, Hashimoto H, Tsubo T, Ishihara H, Matsuki A. Quantification and comparison of pulmonary emboli formation after pneumatic tourniquet release in patients undergoing reconstruction of anterior cruciate ligament and total knee arthroplasty. *Anesth Analg.* 2002;94(6):1633-1638. [IIIC]

126. Kadoi Y, Kawauchi CH, Ide M, Saito S, Mizutani A. Differential increases in blood flow velocity in the middle cerebral artery after tourniquet deflation during sevoflurane, isoflurane or propofol anaesthesia. *Anaesth Intensive Care.* 2009;37(4):598-603. [IIC]

127. Hinohara H, Kadoi Y, Takahashi K, Saito S, Kawauchi C, Mizutani A. Time course of changes in cerebral blood flow velocity after tourniquet deflation in patients with diabetes mellitus or previous stroke under sevoflurane anesthesia. *J Anesth.* 2011;25(3):409-414. [IIC]

128. Hinohara H, Kadoi Y, Ide M, Kuroda M, Saito S, Mizutani A. Differential effects of hyperventilation on cerebral blood flow velocity after tourniquet deflation during sevoflurane, isoflurane, or propofol anesthesia. *J Anesth.* 2010;24(4):587-593. [IIB]

129. van der Velde J, Serfontein L, Iohom G. Reducing the potential for tourniquet-associated reperfusion injury. *Eur J Emerg Med.* 2012. [IB]

130. Rama KR, Apsingi S, Poovali S, Jetti A. Timing of tourniquet release in knee arthroplasty. Meta-analysis of randomized, controlled trials. *J Bone Joint Surg Am.* 2007;89(4):699-705. [IA]

131. Yavarikia A, Amjad GG, Davoudpour K. The influence of tourniquet use and timing of its release on blood loss in total knee arthroplasty. *Pak J Biol Sci.* 2010;13(5):249-252. [IA]

132. Bell TH, Berta D, Ralley F, et al. Factors affecting perioperative blood loss and transfusion rates in primary total joint arthroplasty: a prospective analysis of 1642 patients. *Can J Surg.* 2009;52(4):295-301. [IIIB]

133. Conaty KR, Klemm MS. Severe increase of intracranial pressure after deflation of a pneumatic tourniquet. *Anesthesiology.* 1989;71(2):294-295. [VC]

134. Huang CH, Wang MJ, Chen TL, et al. Blood and central venous pressure responses after serial tourniquet deflation during bilateral total knee replacement. *J Formos Med Assoc.* 1996;95(6):496-499. [IIIB]

135. Sukhani R, Garcia CJ, Munhall RJ, Winnie AP, Rodvold KA. Lidocaine disposition following intravenous regional anesthesia with different tourniquet deflation technics. *Anesth Analg.* 1989;68(5):633-637. [IIIB]

136. Rodola F, Vagnoni S, Ingletti S. An update on intravenous regional anaesthesia of the arm. *Eur Rev Med Pharmacol Sci.* 2003;7(5):131-138. [VB]

137. Sawyer RJ, von Schroeder H. Temporary bilateral blindness after acute lidocaine toxicity. *Anesth Analg.* 2002;95(1):224-226. [VB]

138. Barry LA, Balliana SA, Galeppi AC. Intravenous regional anesthesia (Bier block). *Tech Reg Anesth Pain Manag.* 2006;10(3):123-131. [VB]

139. Budic I, Pavlovic D, Cvetkovic T, et al. The effects of different anesthesia techniques on free radical production after tourniquet-induced ischemia-reperfusion injury at children's age. *Vojnosanit Pregl.* 2010;67(8):659-664. [IIIC]

140. Wang L, Wang W, Zhao X, et al. Effect of Shenmai injection, a traditional Chinese medicine, on pulmonary dysfunction after tourniquet-induced limb ischemia-reperfusion. *J Trauma.* 2011;71(4):893-897. [IB]

141. Laisalmi-Kokki M, Pesonen E, Kokki H, et al. Potentially detrimental effects of N-acetylcysteine on renal function in knee arthroplasty. *Free Radic Res.* 2009;43(7):691-696. [IB]

142. Hughes SF, Hendricks BD, Edwards DR, Middleton JF. Tourniquet-applied upper limb orthopaedic surgery results in increased inflammation and changes to leukocyte, coagulation and endothelial markers. *PLoS One.* 2010;5(7):e11846. [IIIC]

143. Lin L, Wang L, Bai Y, et al. Pulmonary gas exchange impairment following tourniquet deflation: a prospective, single-blind clinical trial. *Orthopedics.* 2010;33(6):395. [IIC]

144. Broom MA, Rimmer C, Parris MR. Tourniquet-associated cardiac ischaemia in a healthy patient undergoing trauma hand surgery. *Eur J Anaesthesiol.* 2007;24(8):729-730. [VB]

145. Lialiaris T, Kouskoukis A, Tiaka E, et al. Cytogenetic damage after ischemia and reperfusion. *Genet Test Mol Biomarkers.* 2010;14(4):471-475. [IIIC]

146. Kim YS, Jeon YS, Lee JA, et al. Intra-operative warming with a forced-air warmer in preventing

hypothermia after tourniquet deflation in elderly patients. *J Int Med Res.* 2009;37(5):1457-1464. [IC]

147. Townsend HS, Goodman SB, Schurman DJ, Hackel A, Brock-Utne JG. Tourniquet release: systemic and metabolic effects. *Acta Anaesthesiol Scand.* 1996;40(10):1234-1237. [IIIC]

148. Li B, Wen Y, Wu H, Qian Q, Lin X, Zhao H. The effect of tourniquet use on hidden blood loss in total knee arthroplasty. *Int Orthop.* 2009;33(5):1263-1268. [IA]

149. Roy N, Smith M, Anwar M, Elsworth C. Delayed release of drain in total knee replacement reduces blood loss. A prospective randomised study. *Acta Orthop Belg.* 2006;72(1):34-38. [IA]

150. Gasparini G, Papaleo P, Pola P, Cerciello S, Pola E, Fabbriciani C. Local infusion of norepinephrine reduces blood losses and need of transfusion in total knee arthroplasty. *Int Orthop.* 2006;30(4):253-256. [IIB]

151. Orpen NM, Little C, Walker G, Crawfurd EJ. Tranexamic acid reduces early post-operative blood loss after total knee arthroplasty: a prospective randomised controlled trial of 29 patients. *Knee.* 2006;13(2):106-110. [IB]

152. Asakura Y, Tsuchiya H, Nieda Y, Yano T, Kato T, Takagi H. Deep vein thrombosis: how long will it remain? *J Anesth.* 2010;24(3):490-491. [VC]

153. McGrath BJ, Hsia J, Boyd A, et al. Venous embolization after deflation of lower extremity tourniquets. *Anesth Analg.* 1994;78(2):349-353. [IIIC]

154. Bharti N, Mahajan S. Massive pulmonary embolism leading to cardiac arrest after tourniquet deflation following lower limb surgery. *Anaesth Intensive Care.* 2009;37(5):867-868. [VB]

155. Cohen JD, Keslin JS, Nili M, Yosipovitch Z, Gassner S. Massive pulmonary embolism and tourniquet deflation. *Anesth Analg.* 1994;79(3):583-585. [VB]

156. Watanabe S, Terazawa K, Matoba K, Yamada N. An autopsy case of intraoperative death due to pulmonary fat embolism—possibly caused by release of tourniquet after multiple muscle-release and tenotomy of the bilateral lower limbs. *Forensic Sci Int.* 2007;171(1):73-77. [VB]

157. Sinicina I, Bise K, Hetterich R, Pankratz H. Tourniquet use in childhood: a harmless procedure? *Paediatr Anaesth.* 2007;17(2):167-170. [VC]

158. Maguina P, Jean-Pierre F, Grevious MA, Malk AS. Posterior interosseous branch palsy following pneumatic tourniquet application for hand surgery. *Plast Reconstr Surg.* 2008;122(2):97e-99e. [VC]

159. Kort NP, van Raay JJ, van Horn JR. Compartment syndrome and popliteal vascular injury complicating unicompartmental knee arthroplasty. *J Arthroplasty.* 2007;22(3):472-476. [VB]

160. O'Neil D, Sheppard JE. Transient compartment syndrome of the forearm resulting from venous congestion from a tourniquet. *J Hand Surg Am.* 1989;14(5):894-896. [VC]

161. Kerrary S, Schouman T, Cox A, Bertolus C, Febrer G, Bertrand JC. Acute compartment syndrome following fibula flap harvest for mandibular reconstruction. *J Craniomaxillofac Surg.* 2011;39(3):206-208. [VC]

162. Ahmed SM, Ahmad R, Case R, Spencer RF. A study of microbial colonisation of orthopaedic tourniquets. *Ann R Coll Surg Engl.* 2009;91(2):131-134. [IIIB]

163. Walsh EF, Ben-David D, Ritter M, Mechrefe A, Mermel LA, DiGiovanni C. Microbial colonization of tourniquets used in orthopedic surgery. *Orthopedics.* 2006;29(8):709-713. [IIIB]

164. Daruwalla ZJ, Rowan F, Finnegan M, Fennell J, Neligan M. Exsanguinators and tourniquets: do we need to change our practice? *Surgeon.* 2012;10(3):137-142. [IIIC]

165. Guideline for environmental cleaning. In: *Guidelines for Perioperative Practice.* Denver, CO: AORN, Inc; 2015:9-30. [IVB]

166. Guideline for prevention of transmissible infections. In: *Guidelines for Perioperative Practice.* Denver, CO: AORN, Inc; 2015:419-451. [IVA]

167. Meeting the Ongoing Challenge of Continued Competence. 2005. National Council of State Boards of Nursing. https://www.ncsbn.org/Continued_Comp_Paper_TestingServices.pdf. Accessed May 4, 2013. [VC]

168. Sportsman S. Competency education and validation in the United States: what should nurses know? *Nurs Forum.* 2010;45(3):140-149. [VA]

169. Centers for Medicare & Medicaid Services. State Operations Manual Appendix A: Survey Protocol, Regulations and Interpretive Guidelines for Hospitals. Rev. 78; 2011. http://www.cms.gov/Regulations-and-Guidance/Guidance/Manuals/downloads/som107ap_a_hospitals.pdf. Accessed May 4, 2013.

170. Centers for Medicare & Medicaid Services. State Operations Manual Appendix L: Guidance for Surveyors: Ambulatory Surgical Centers. Rev. 76; 2011. http://www.cms.gov/Regulations-and-Guidance/Guidance/Manuals/downloads/som107ap_l_ambulatory.pdf. Accessed May 4, 2013.

171. The Joint Commission. HR.01.05.03: Staff participate in ongoing education and training. *Comprehensive Accreditation Manual for Ambulatory Care.* Oakbrook Terrace, IL: Joint Commission Accreditation; 2012.

172. The Joint Commission. HR.01.05.03: Staff participate in ongoing education and training. In: *Comprehensive Accreditation Manual: CAMH for Hospitals.* Oakbrook Terrace, IL: Joint Commission Accreditation; 2012.

173. American Association for Accreditation of Ambulatory Surgery Facilities. Personnel: personnel records resumes. In: *Regular Standards and Checklist for Accreditation of Ambulatory Surgery Facilities.* Version 13 ed. Gurnee, IL: American Association for Accreditation of Ambulatory Surgery Facilities; 2011: 77-78.

174. American Association for Accreditation of Ambulatory Surgery Facilities. Personnel: knowledge, skill & CME training. In: *Regular Standards and Checklist for Accreditation of Ambulatory Surgery Facilities.* Version 13 ed. Gurnee, IL: American Association for Accreditation of Ambulatory Surgery Facilities; 2011: 78-79.

175. Sadri A, Braithwaite IJ, Abdul-Jabar HB, Sarraf KM. Understanding of intra-operative tourniquets amongst orthopaedic surgeons and theatre staff—a questionnaire study. *Ann R Coll Surg Engl.* 2010;92(3):243-245. [IIIC]

176. Gillespie BM, Hamlin L. A synthesis of the literature on "competence" as it applies to perioperative nursing. *AORN J.* 2009;90(2):245-258. [VA]

177. Kak N, Burkhalter B, Cooper M-A. Measuring the Competence of Healthcare Providers. Operations Research Issue Paper 2(1). Bethesda, MD: Quality Assurance Project for the US Agency for International Development 2001. http://www.hciproject.org/sites/default/files/Measuring%20the%20Competence%20of%20HC%20Providers_QAP_2001.pdf. Accessed May 4, 2013. [VA]

178. Ringerman E, Flint LJ, Hughes DE. An innovative education program: the peer competency validator model *J Nurses Staff Dev.* 2006;22(3):114-123. [VB]

179. Jordan C, Thomas MB, Evans ML, Green A. Public policy on competency: how will nursing address this complex issue? *J Contin Educ Nurs.* 2008;39(2):86-91. [VA]

180. Gillespie BM, Chaboyer W, Wallis M, Chang HY, Werder H. Operating theatre nurses' perceptions

of competence: a focus group study. *J Adv Nurs.* 2009;65(5):1019-1028. [IIIB]

181. Guideline for perioperative health care information management. In: *Guidelines for Perioperative Practice.* Denver, CO: AORN, Inc; 2015:491-512. [IVB]

182. RC.01.01.01: The hospital maintains complete and accurate medical records for each individual patient. In: *Hospital Accreditation Standards 2012.* Oakbrook Terrace, IL: Joint Commission Resources; 2012.

183. RC.01.01.01: The organization maintains complete and accurate clinical records. In: *Standards for Ambulatory Care 2012: Standards, Elements of Performance Scoring Accreditation Polices.* Oakbrook Terrace, IL: The Joint Commission; 2012.

184. Clinical records and health information. In: *2012 Accreditation Handbook for Ambulatory Health Care.* Skokie, IL: Accreditation Association for Ambulatory Health Care; 2012:40-42.

185. American Association for Accreditation of Ambuatory Surgery Facilities. Medical records: general. In: *Regular Standards and Checklist for Accreditation of Ambulatory Surgery Facilities.* Version 13 ed. Gurnee, IL: American Association for Accreditation of Ambulatory Surgery Facilities; 2011:61.

186. American Association for Accreditation of Ambuatory Surgery Facilities. Medical records: pre-operative medical record. In: *Regular Standards and Checklist for Accreditation of Ambulatory Surgery Facilities.* Version 13 ed. Gurnee, IL: American Association for Accreditation of Ambulatory Surgery Facilities; 2011:62-63.

187. American Association for Accreditation of Ambulatory Surgery Facilities. Medical records: operating room records. In: *Regular Standards and Checklist for Accreditation of Ambulatory Surgery Facilities.* Version 13 ed. Gurnee, IL: American Association for Accreditation of Ambulatory Surgery Facilities; 2011:64-66.

188. Silver R, de la Garza J, Rang M, Koreska J. Limb swelling after release of a tourniquet. *Clin Orthop Relat Res.* 1986;(206):86-89. [IIIC]

189. Subramanian S, Lateef H, Massraf A. Cutaneous sensory loss following primary total knee arthroplasty. A two years follow-up study. *Acta Orthop Belg.* 2009;75(5):649-653. [IIIC]

190. 65 FR 4112. Medical device reporting: manufacturer reporting, importer reporting, user facility reporting, distributor reporting. US Government Printing Office. http://www.gpo.gov/fdsys/granule/FR-2000-01-26/00-1785/content-detail.html. Accessed May 4, 2013.

191. Governance. In: *2012 Accreditation Handbook for Ambulatory Health Care.* Skokie, IL: Accreditation Association for Ambulatory Health Care; 2012:20-27.

192. LD.04.01.07: The hospital has policies and procedures that guide and support patient care, treatment, and services. In: *Hospital Accreditation Standards 2012.* 2012 ed. Oakbrook Terrace, IL: Joint Commission Resources; 2012.

193. LD.04.01.07: The organization has policies and procedures that guide and support patient care, treatment, or services. In: *Standards for Ambulatory Care 2012: Standards, Elements of Performance Scoring Accreditation Polices.* Oakbrook Terrace, IL: The Joint Commission; 2012.

194. PI.03.01.01: The hospital improves performance on an ongoing basis. In: *Hospital Accreditation Standards 2012.* 2012 ed. Oakbrook Terrace, IL: Joint Commission Resources; 2012.

195. American Association for Accreditation of Ambulatory Surgery Facilities. Quality assessment/quality improvement: quality improvement. In: *Regular Standards and Checklist for Accreditation of Ambulatory Surgery Facilities.* Version 13 ed. Gurnee, IL: American Association for Accreditation of Ambulatory Surgery Facilities; 2011:67.

196. American Association for Accreditation of Ambulatory Surgery Facilities. Quality assessment/quality improvement: unanticipated operative sequelae. In: *Regular Standards and Checklist for Accreditation of Ambulatory Surgery Facilities.* Version 13 ed. Gurnee, IL: American Association for Accreditation of Ambulatory Surgery Facilities; 2011:69-71.

197. Quality management and improvement. In: *2012 Accreditation Handbook for Ambulatory Health Care.* Skokie, IL: Accreditation Association for Ambulatory Health Care; 2012:34-39.

198. Carling PC, Bartley JM. Evaluating hygienic cleaning in health care settings: what you do not know can harm your patients. *Am J Infect Control.* 2010;38(5 Suppl 1): S41-S50. [IIB]

199. Carling PC, Parry MF, Von Beheren SM; Healthcare Environmental Hygiene Study Group. Identifying opportunities to enhance environmental cleaning in 23 acute care hospitals. *Infect Control Hosp Epidemiol.* 2008;29(1):1-7. [IIIB]

200. Siegel JD Rhinehart E Jackson M Chiarello L; Healthcare Infection Control Practices Advisory Committee. *2007 Guideline for Isolation Precautions: Preventing Transmission of Infectious Agents in Healthcare Settings.* Atlanta, GA: Centers for Disease Control and Prevention; 2006. [IVA]

201. Farquhar M. AHRQ quality indicators. In: Hughes RG, ed. *Patient Safety and Quality: An Evidence-based Handbook for Nurses.* (Prepared with support from the Robert Wood Johnson Foundation). AHRQ Publication No. 08-0043. Rockville, MD: Agency for Healthcare Research and Quality; 2008. http://www.ahrq.gov/professionals/clinicians-providers/resources/nursing/resources/nurseshdbk/nurseshdbk.pdf. Accessed May 4, 2013. [IA]

202. 42 CFR 416: Ambulatory surgical services. 2011. US Government Printing Office. http://www.gpo.gov/fdsys/granule/CFR-2011-title42-vol3/CFR-2011-title42-vol3-part416/content-detail.html. Accessed May 4, 2013.

203. 42 CFR 482: Conditions of participation for hospitals. US Government Printing Office. http://www.gpo.gov/fdsys/granule/CFR-2011-title42-vol5/CFR-2011-title42-vol5-part482/content-detail.html. Accessed May 4, 2013.

Acknowledgements

LEAD AUTHOR
Bonnie Denholm, MS, BSN, RN, CNOR
Perioperative Nursing Specialist
AORN Nursing Department
Denver, Colorado

CONTRIBUTING AUTHORS
Ramona Conner, MSN, RN, CNOR
Manager, Standards and Guidelines
AORN Nursing Department
Denver, Colorado

Rodney W. Hicks, PhD, RN, FNP-BC, FAANP, FAAN
Professor
Western University of Health Sciences
Pomona, California

The authors and AORN thank Janice A. Neil, PhD, RN, Associate Professor and Chair, Department of Undergraduate Nursing Science, College of Nursing, East Carolina University, Greenville, NC; Jim McEwen, PhD, DSc, PEng, Adjunct Professor, Departments of Orthopaedics & Electrical and Computer Engineering, University of British Columbia, Vancouver, Canada; and Lisa Spruce, DNP, RN, ACNS, ACNP, ANP, CNOR, Director of Evidence-based Perioperative Practice, AORN, Inc, Denver, CO, for their assistance in developing this guideline.

PUBLICATION HISTORY

Originally published April 1984, *AORN Journal.* Revised November 1990.

Published as proposed recommended practices March 1994. Revised November 1998; published December 1998. Reformatted July 2000.

Revised November 2001; published February 2002, *AORN Journal.*

Revised 2006; published in *Standards, Recommended Practices, and Guidelines,* 2007 edition.

Minor editing revisions made to omit PNDS codes; reformatted September 2012 for publication in *Perioperative Standards and Recommended Practices,* 2013 edition.

Revised April 2013 for online publication in *Perioperative Standards and Recommended Practices.*

Evidence ratings revised 2013 to conform to the AORN Evidence Rating Model.

Minor editing revisions made in November 2014 for publication in *Guidelines for Perioperative Practice,* 2015 edition.

Evidence ratings revised in *Guidelines for Perioperative Practice,* 2018 edition, to conform to the current AORN Evidence Rating Model.

EQUIPMENT AND PRODUCT SAFETY

GUIDELINE FOR MEDICAL DEVICE AND PRODUCT EVALUATION

The Guideline for Medical Device and Product Evaluation has been approved by the AORN Guidelines Advisory Board. It was presented as a proposed guideline for comments by members and others. The guideline is effective November 1, 2017. The recommendations in the guideline are intended to be achievable and represent what is believed to be an optimal level of practice. Policies and procedures will reflect variations in practice settings and/or clinical situations that determine the degree to which the guideline can be implemented. AORN recognizes the many diverse settings in which perioperative nurses practice; therefore, this guideline is adaptable to all areas where operative or other invasive procedures may be performed.

Purpose

This document provides guidance to perioperative team members for developing and implementing a process for evaluating US Food and Drug Administration–cleared medical devices and products for use in the perioperative setting. The safety of patients and perioperative team members, optimal patient outcomes, and product quality are the primary concerns of perioperative registered nurses (RNs) as they participate in product review and evaluation.

The evidence regarding best practices for product evaluation in the perioperative setting is limited. The health care system is complex, with many variables that make it difficult to perform research on product selection that is generalizable to all settings. These variables include the size of the organization, financial constraints, group purchasing organization relationships, and contractual agreements.

The following subjects are outside the scope of this guideline: specific processes for cleaning, disinfection, and sterilization; management of products and devices after purchase (eg, equipment maintenance, inventory control); selection of electronic health records (eg, health information technology); processes for product waste disposal; and purchasing processes (eg, supply chain).

Evidence Review

A medical librarian conducted a systematic literature search of the databases Ovid MEDLINE®, EBSCO, CINAHL®, Scopus®, and the Cochrane Database of Systematic Reviews. The search was limited to literature published in English from 2012 through April 2017. At the time of the initial search, weekly alerts were created on the topics included in the search. Results from these alerts were provided to the lead author until July 2017. The lead author requested additional articles that did not fit the original search criteria or were discovered during the appraisal process.

Search terms included *cost control, financial management, materials management, purchasing department, cost savings, value-based purchasing, surgical instruments, operating rooms, costs and cost analysis, decision-making, organizational, cost-benefit analysis, value stream mapping, financial impact analysis, product selection, quality assurance, cost effectiveness, efficiency, perioperative nursing, device approval, surgical equipment, disposable equipment,* and *equipment and supplies.* Key words and phrases included *group purchasing, surgical devices, surgical services, surgical department, consignment, vendor, committee, interdisciplinary communication, cooperative behavior, single-use devices, patient care items, par level,* and *team.*

Included were research and non-research literature in English, complete publications, and publication dates within the time restriction when available. Excluded were non-peer-reviewed publications and older evidence within the time restriction when more recent evidence was available. Editorials, news items, and brief items were excluded. Low-quality evidence was excluded when higher-quality evidence was available, and literature outside the time restriction was excluded when literature within the time restriction was available (Figure 1).

Included articles were independently evaluated and critically appraised according to the strength and quality of the evidence. Articles identified in the search were provided to the project team for evaluation. The team consisted of the lead author and one evidence appraiser. The lead author divided the search results into topics, and both members of the team reviewed and critically appraised each article using the AORN Research or Non-Research Evidence Appraisal Tools as appropriate. The literature was independently evaluated and appraised according to the strength and quality of the evidence. Each article was then assigned an appraisal score. The appraisal score is noted in brackets after each reference, as applicable.

The collective evidence supporting each intervention within a specific recommendation was summarized, and the AORN Evidence Rating Model was used to rate the strength of the evidence. Factors considered in review of the collective evidence were the quality of evidence, the quantity of similar evidence on a given topic, and the consistency of evidence supporting a recommendation. The evidence rating is noted in brackets after each intervention.

Note: The evidence summary table is available at http://www.aorn.org/evidencetables/.

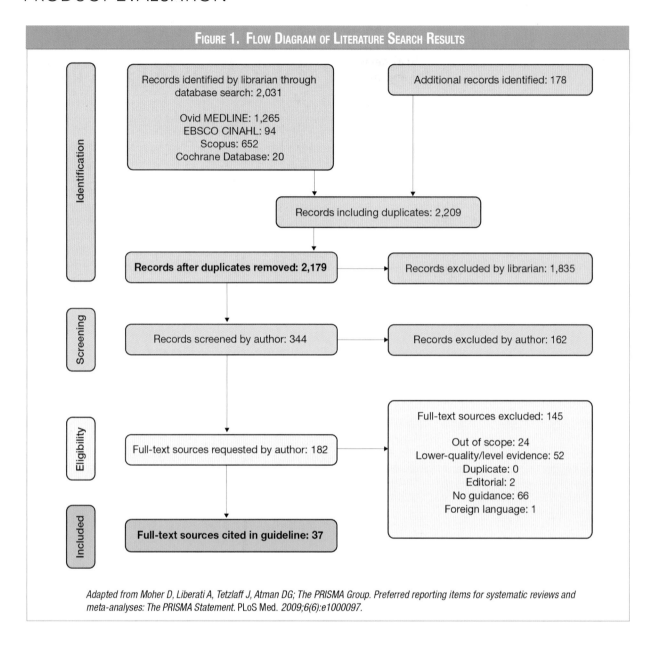

FIGURE 1. FLOW DIAGRAM OF LITERATURE SEARCH RESULTS

Records identified by librarian through database search: 2,031

Ovid MEDLINE: 1,265
EBSCO CINAHL: 94
Scopus: 652
Cochrane Database: 20

Additional records identified: 178

Records including duplicates: 2,209

Records after duplicates removed: 2,179

Records excluded by librarian: 1,835

Records screened by author: 344

Records excluded by author: 162

Full-text sources requested by author: 182

Full-text sources excluded: 145

Out of scope: 24
Lower-quality/level evidence: 52
Duplicate: 0
Editorial: 2
No guidance: 66
Foreign language: 1

Full-text sources cited in guideline: 37

Identification

Screening

Eligibility

Included

Adapted from Moher D, Liberati A, Tetzlaff J, Atman DG; The PRISMA Group. Preferred reporting items for systematic reviews and meta-analyses: The PRISMA Statement. PLoS Med. 2009;6(6):e1000097.

Editor's note: *MEDLINE is a registered trademark of the US National Library of Medicine's Medical Literature Analysis and Retrieval System, Bethesda, MD. CINAHL, Cumulative Index to Nursing and Allied Health Literature, is a registered trademark of EBSCO Industries, Birmingham, AL. Scopus is a registered trademark of Elsevier B.V., Amsterdam, The Netherlands.*

Recommendation I

The health care organization should establish an interdisciplinary team to be responsible for oversight of the medical device and product evaluation process.

Health care organizations use different titles to refer to interdisciplinary teams with responsibility for oversight of medical device and product evaluation; these titles include product selection committee, medical device and product evaluation committee, purchasing committee, and value analysis committee. The collec-

tive evidence supports an interdisciplinary team approach to the medical device and product evaluation process.[1-9]

I.a.   Perioperative RNs should have an active role in the evaluation and selection of perioperative products.[2,3,6,7,10,11] *[3: Moderate Evidence]*

Evidence from qualitative research studies indicates that RNs as stakeholders can provide clinical, safety, and device-user experience that may help to determine the value of a product under evaluation.

In a qualitative study conducted in five hospitals in the United Kingdom, Hinrichs et al[4] identified stakeholders with authority for making purchasing decisions and examined the challenges of promoting patient safety during the purchasing process. The researchers identified the main stakeholders as clinical engineers, clinical end users or device users, health care

EQUIPMENT AND PRODUCT SAFETY

industry representatives, and risk managers. The findings from the study suggest that responsibility for purchasing safe medical devices is shared among clinical end users and financial and technical stakeholders.

Grundy[2] conducted a qualitative research study of purchasing groups at four hospitals in the metropolitan area of a western US city to explore the interactions between nurses and industry representatives in clinical practice. Participants (N = 72) included RNs, supply chain professionals, administrators, and health care industry representatives. The findings indicated that RNs believed it was important for clinicians to be informed on new product developments so they would be prepared when new products were presented for evaluation. The researcher also found that involvement of nurses in hospital value analysis committees could drive quality and cost savings.

Grundy et al[3] conducted another qualitative research study of 72 participants at four acute care hospitals in a western US city to examine in depth the interactions between RNs and health care industry representatives. Data collection processes included observations of nurse-industry interactions in meetings, interviews, and focus groups. Health care industry representatives described RNs as a key audience because RNs have direct contact with patients, prescribers, and purchasers. The researchers found that RNs influenced the distribution of resources that could affect patient care.

.b. The interdisciplinary team should include key stakeholders from within the facility.[1,2,4,8,12] *[3: Moderate Evidence]*

Including key stakeholders in the interdisciplinary team provides the health care organization with relevant knowledge and expertise specific to the organization's structure and patient population.

Vincent and Blandford[13] interviewed 20 purchasing committee participants in four hospitals in the United Kingdom to understand purchasing decisions, with a focus on the usability of infusion devices, purchasing practices, and the factors that shape purchasing decisions. The researchers found that a wide variety of stakeholders, including RNs, were influential in evaluating products and that having an interdisciplinary committee encouraged a holistic approach.

I.b.1. The interdisciplinary team may include
- perioperative RNs,[2,3,7,10,11] *[3: Moderate Evidence]*
- cardiac catheterization lab/electrophysiology lab personnel,[1] *[3: Moderate Evidence]*
- interventional radiology personnel,[1] *[3: Moderate Evidence]*
- laboratory personnel,[1] *[3: Moderate Evidence]*
- materials management/supply chain personnel,[14,15] *[3: Moderate Evidence]*
- surgeons and proceduralists,[7] *[3: Moderate Evidence]*
- surgical technologists,[7] *[3: Moderate Evidence]*
- biomedical engineers,[14,16] *[4: Limited Evidence]*
- sterile processing personnel,[9] *[4: Limited Evidence]*
- perioperative educators, *[5: Benefits Balanced with Harms]*
- anesthesia professionals, *[5: Benefits Balanced with Harms]*
- clinical engineers, *[5: Benefits Balanced with Harms]*
- endoscopy services personnel, *[5: Benefits Balanced with Harms]*
- environmental services personnel, *[5: Benefits Balanced with Harms]*
- infection preventionists, *[5: Benefits Balanced with Harms]*
- pathology personnel, *[5: Benefits Balanced with Harms]*
- pharmacists, *[5: Benefits Balanced with Harms]*
- purchasing personnel, *[5: Benefits Balanced with Harms]*
- quality management personnel, *[5: Benefits Balanced with Harms]*
- risk managers, *[5: Benefits Balanced with Harms]* and
- others as deemed necessary.

Including representatives from affected disciplines in the evaluation process allows input from personnel with expertise beyond clinical end users and may enhance teamwork and end-user compliance with correct use of the product.

I.b.2. The interdisciplinary team composition should be adjusted to include end users for specific medical devices and products under evaluation.[4] *[3: Moderate Evidence]*

Certain medical devices and products do not affect all departments, and input from key end users is needed to provide relevant and specific input.

I.b.3. The health care organization must establish a process for selecting and evaluating sharps safety devices as part of the written bloodborne pathogens exposure control plan.[17,18] *[1: Regulatory Requirement]*

Recommendation II

The interdisciplinary medical device and product evaluation team should establish and implement a process for the pre-purchase evaluation of products.

PRODUCT EVALUATION

A standardized medical device and product evaluation process assists in the selection of functional and reliable products that are safe, cost-effective, and environmentally friendly and that promote quality care. The collective evidence[2,6,12,19] indicates there is a need for health care organizations to be responsible for verifying that medical devices and products used within the organization are effective and safe to use. Regulatory agencies[20,21] require health care organizations to develop and promote a safe health care environment to meet the needs of patients' and personnel.

II.a.   The evaluation process should include use of a decision support framework.[2,6,12,19] *[3: Moderate Evidence]*

A decision support framework provides the team with a standardized tool by which to compare products equally.

Health care organizations have implemented various approaches to product evaluation and purchasing decisions. Grundy[2] developed a framework for value analysis related to medical product decision making. The framework establishes a need for the product, verifies the usability of the product, evaluates the associated costs of the product, and ends with the final decision. The researcher concluded that applying the value analysis framework might assist others in the decision-making process.

Clinical personnel at the University of Pennsylvania used an evidence-based practice center (EPC) as a mechanism for evaluating medical devices and products. The clinical personnel submitted requests to the EPC to conduct an evidence review about a device, equipment, or supply item. The personnel at the EPC reviewed the request, conducted a rapid systematic review of the evidence, translated the evidence, and made recommendations to the purchasing committee. Jayakumar et al[6] found that the EPC process was an effective method for promoting evidence-based purchasing decisions.

Wernz et al[19] conducted a qualitative research study to identify a best practice decision-making process among hospital decision makers. The researchers conducted interviews with key stakeholders from six hospitals in five countries, including the United States. They identified a best practice approach in a US hospital that used a computer-based decision support system. The computer-based support system uses certain criteria (eg, capacity/access, financial reports, infrastructure, implementation, strategic importance, quality) and weighting of organizational goals to assist in decision-making related to the purchase of a medical device. The findings from this study suggest that use of a computer-based decision support tool may be effective for evaluation of medical devices.

Martelli et al[12] developed a criteria-based tool to assist in the analysis and evaluation of medical devices based on results of a literature review and survey that included 25 participants from 18 hospitals in France. The innovative device assessment (IDA) tool is a decision-support tool that combines multi-criteria decision analysis and a mini health technology assessment. The IDA tool consists of five weighted criteria separated into two categories: risk and value. The risk-based criteria included the need for specific expertise and training of users, the number of patients and impact on workflow, cost per patient, additional payments for the device, and the unit cost of the device. The value-based criteria included expected risks or adverse events related to the device, expected clinical benefit for the patient, impact on quality of life, opinion concerning the device, and the quality of the evidence related to the device. The researchers applied the IDA tool at a health care system representing 38 hospitals in Paris for the evaluation of two new drug-eluting beads for transcatheter arterial chemoembolization. The IDA tool revealed that the new drug-eluting beads conferred no additional value relative to drug-eluting beads currently available. The researchers concluded that the use of the IDA tool may promote a more structured approach to health technology assessment and that it is useful as a decision-support tool.

II.b.   A financial impact analysis should be performed on each medical device and product being evaluated. *[3: Moderate Evidence]*

Financial analysis is a key element in product evaluation and selection. The financial analysis assists in determining whether the product fits within the organization's overall fiscal strategy[22] and may provide data that are useful in determining global procedural costs.[2] Understanding the financial impact of a new product or device can also assist with budget development and resource utilization plans.

In some cases a financial analysis may be required for reimbursement.[24] The Centers for Medicare & Medicaid Services[25] Hospital Value Based Purchasing Program is an initiative that connects reimbursement with quality and patient safety. A percentage of a hospital's reimbursement is withheld until the hospital meets required quality measures. The quality measures address patient safety, patient satisfaction, and cost efficiency. The intent is to hold hospitals accountable and to improve the value of health care provided in acute health care settings.[26,27]

II.b.1.   The financial impact analysis should include
- direct costs (eg, cost of the product acquisition, replacement strategy, associated equipment),
- indirect costs (eg, utilities, waste disposal processing, personnel orientation, storage, energy use, depreciation, retrofitting o

existing equipment, renovation or construction),
- reimbursement potential (eg, Centers for Medicare & Medicaid Services Value-Based Purchasing), and
- group purchasing organization contract pricing if applicable.
[5: Benefits Balanced with Harms]

II.c. Elements of the product evaluation should include
- compliance with local, state, and regulatory requirements; [5: Benefits Balanced with Harms]
- clinical usability and cost effectiveness[5,6,13,28]; [3: Moderate Evidence]
- patient and user safety[4,9]; [3: Moderate Evidence]
- improved patient outcomes; [5: Benefits Balanced with Harms]
- product quality[7,29-31]; [3: Moderate Evidence]
- strategic priorities[1,29,32]; [3: Moderate Evidence]
- vendor contractual agreements[7,16]; [3: Moderate Evidence]
- compliance with accrediting organizations; [5: Benefits Balanced with Harms]
- compatibility with existing processing methods; [5: Benefits Balanced with Harms]
- compatibility with existing disposal methods; [5: Benefits Balanced with Harms]
- patient-population needs; [5: Benefits Balanced with Harms] and
- personnel and end-user preferences. [5: Benefits Balanced with Harms]

I.d. The interdisciplinary team should assess the environmental impact of a device or the product. [3: Moderate Evidence]

Perioperative RNs have an ethical obligation and professional responsibility to address environmental exposures and hazards for the health, welfare, and safety of all people. Perioperative RNs can help to mitigate the environmental effects of health care by supporting the selection of environmentally responsible products.[33] Serving as stewards of the environment includes implementing practices that will help preserve natural resources, reduce waste, and minimize exposure to hazardous materials.[34]

In a nonexperimental study, Kaplan et al[35] found that health care organizations are among the country's most energy-intensive facilities, accounting for a significant percentage of US greenhouse gas and carbon dioxide emissions. Health care organizations create 6,600 tons of waste per day and use large amounts of toxic chemicals.[35] Following sustainable practices that include energy-use reduction, recycling, minimization of regulated waste, reduction of landfill waste, reprocessing, reuse of single-use medical devices, and reformulation of OR custom packs may reduce waste.[36,37]

II.d.1. Criteria for determining whether to purchase a single-use or reusable product should include:
- the useful life of the product;
- the intended use of the product;
- the ability to clean the medical device or product;
- the availability of required cleaning, disinfection, and sterilization processes;
- time required for reprocessing;
- if single-use, whether the product can be reprocessed by a US Food and Drug Administration-cleared third party reprocessor;
- if single-use, cost and requirements for disposal;
- inventory required;
- complexity of the manufacturer's instructions for use and the end user's ability to reliably follow instructions;
- competency requirements for personnel who use, maintain, and reprocess instruments, medical devices, and other equipment;
- maintenance, repair, or restoration programs for instruments and equipment; and
- storage requirements.
[5: Benefits Balanced with Harms]

II.e. The interdisciplinary team should obtain and review the manufacturer's technical specifications and clinical use recommendations during the product evaluation process. [5: Benefits Balanced with Harms]

Health care product and device manufacturers provide clinical and technical information related to the product use and safety that is vital for product evaluation.

II.f. The interdisciplinary team should develop and implement a plan to introduce new products and devices into clinical practice, including a plan for education of personnel. [5: Benefits Balanced with Harms]

The development of a comprehensive plan for the introduction of a medical device or product may facilitate smooth implementation.[6]

Recommendation III

The health care organization should establish a quality assurance and performance improvement process for product evaluation.

A quality assurance/performance improvement program provides a mechanism for verifying that new products and devices are meeting expected performance criteria and that the pre-selection evaluation process has met its objectives.

III.a. Personnel should participate in ongoing quality assurance and performance improvement activities. [5: Benefits Balanced with Harms]

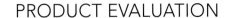

PRODUCT EVALUATION

Participating in ongoing quality assurance and performance improvement activities is a primary responsibility of perioperative personnel engaged in practice.

III.b.   After a product or device has been introduced, a comprehensive plan for post purchase evaluation should be developed and implemented. *[5: Benefits Balanced with Harms]*

Glossary

Financial impact analysis: An estimate of the financial consequences associated with purchasing a new product or medical device.

REFERENCES

1. Atwood D, Larose P, Uttley R. Strategies for success in purchasing medical technology. *Biomed Instrum Technol.* 2015;49(2):93-98. [VB]

2. Grundy Q. "Whether something cool is good enough": the role of evidence, sales representatives and nurses' expertise in hospital purchasing decisions. *Soc Sci Med.* 2016;165:82-91. [IIIB]

3. Grundy Q, Bero LA, Malone RE. Marketing and the most trusted profession: the invisible interactions between registered nurses and industry. *Ann Intern Med.* 2016;164(11):733-739. [IIIB]

4. Hinrichs S, Dickerson T, Clarkson J. Stakeholder challenges in purchasing medical devices for patient safety. *J Patient Saf.* 2013;9(1):36-43. [IIIB]

5. Li CS, Vannabouathong C, Sprague S, Bhandari M. Orthopedic implant value drivers: a qualitative survey study of hospital purchasing administrators. *J Long Term Eff Med Implants.* 2015;25(3):237-244. [IIIC]

6. Jayakumar KL, Lavenberg JA, Mitchell MD, et al. Evidence synthesis activities of a hospital evidence-based practice center and impact on hospital decision making. *J Hosp Med.* 2015;11(3):185-192. [VA]

7. Plonien C, Williams M. Vendor presence in the OR. *AORN J.* 2014;100(1):81-86. [VB]

8. Sohrakoff K, Westlake C, Key E, Barth E, Antognini J, Johnson V. Optimizing the OR: a bottom-up approach. *Hosp Top.* 2014;92(2):21-27. [VB]

9. Vockley M. Choosing wisely: trends and strategies for capital planning and procurement. *Biomed Instrum Technol.* 2016;50(4):230-241. [VC]

10. Lerner DG, Pall H. Setting up the pediatric endoscopy unit. *Gastrointest Endosc Clin N Am.* 2016;26(1):1-12. [IIIB]

11. *NHS Procurement & Commercial Standards.* 2016. https://nhsprocurement.org.uk/files/2016-07/Standards_of_Procurement.pdf. Accessed August 23, 2017. [IVC]

12. Martelli N, Hansen P, van den Brink H, et al. Combining multi-criteria decision analysis and mini-health technology assessment: a funding decision-support tool for medical devices in a university hospital setting. *J Biomed Inform.* 2016;59:201-208. [IIIB]

13. Vincent CJ, Blandford A. How do health service professionals consider human factors when purchasing interactive medical devices? A qualitative interview study. *Appl Ergon.* 2017;59(Pt A):114-122. [IIIA]

14. Lynch PK. Do group purchasing organizations really save money on capital equipment? *Biomed Instrum Technol.* 2017;51(2):170-171. [VC]

15. Walsh SS. Suture cost savings in the OR. *AORN J.* 2012;95(5):631-634. [VB]

16. Kobernick T. How to negotiate with high-pressure vendors. *Biomed Instrum Technol.* 2013;47(1):36-37. [VC]

17. 29 CFR §1910.1030: Bloodborne pathogens. Occupational Safety and Health Administration. https://www.osha.gov/pls/oshaweb/owadisp.show_document?p_id=10051&p_table=STANDARDS. Accessed August 23, 2017.

18. Guideline for sharps safety. In: *Guidelines for Perioperative Practice.* Denver, CO: AORN, Inc; 2017: 423-446. [IVA]

19. Wernz C, Zhang H, Phusavat K. International study of technology investment decisions at hospitals. *Ind Manage Data Syst* [serial online]. 2014;114(4):568-582. [IIIC]

20. 42 CFR 482: Conditions of participation for hospitals. 2011. US Government Publishing Office. https://www.gpo.gov/fdsys/granule/CFR-2011-title42-vol5/CFR-2011-title42-vol5-part482. Accessed August 23, 2017.

21. 42 CFR 416: Ambulatory surgical services. 2011. US Government Publishing Office. https://www.gpo.gov/fdsys/granule/CFR-2011-title42-vol3/CFR-2011-title42-vol3-part416. Accessed August 23, 2017.

22. *ISO 20400:2017. Sustainable Procurement—Guidance.* Geneva, Switzerland: International Organization for Standardization; 2017.

23. Raft J, Millet F, Meistelman C. Example of cost calculations for an operating room and a post-anaesthesia care unit. *Anaesth Crit Care Pain Med.* 2015;34(4):211-215. [IIIA]

24. Sullivan SD, Mauskopf JA, Augustovski F, et al. Budget impact analysis—principles of good practice: report of the ISPOR 2012 Budget Impact Analysis Good Practice II Task Force. *Value Health.* 2014;17(1):5-14. [VA]

25. Hospital value-based purchasing. Centers for Medicare & Medicaid Services. https://www.cms.gov/Medicare/Quality-Initiatives-Patient-Assessment-Instruments/hospital-value-based-purchasing/index.html?redirect=/hospital-value-based-purchasing. Updated February 15, 2017. Accessed August 23, 2017.

26. Stacy KM. Hospital value-based purchasing part 1, overview of the program. *AACN Adv Crit Care* 2016;27(4):362-367. [VA]

27. Stacy KM. Hospital value-based purchasing: part 2 implications. *AACN Adv Crit Care.* 2017;28(1):16-20. [VA]

28. How healthcare executives make buying decisions *Healthc Financ Manage.* 2012;66(6):1-7. [VC]

29. Bosko T, Dubow M, Koenig T. Understanding value based incentive models and using performance as a strategic advantage. *J Healthc Manag.* 2016;61(1):11-14. [VB]

30. Eiferman D, Bhakta A, Khan S. Implementation of a shared-savings program for surgical supplies decreases inventory cost. *Surgery.* 2015;158(4):996-1002. [VB]

31. Farrokhi FR, Gunther M, Williams B, Blackmore CC. Application of lean methodology for improved quality and efficiency in operating room instrument availability. *Healthc Qual.* 2015;37(5):277-286. [VB]

32. Rocchio BJ. Achieving cost reduction through data analytics. *AORN J.* 2016;104(4):320-325. [VB]

33. AORN position statement on environmental responsibility. *AORN J.* 2014;99(1):18-21. [IVB]

34. ANA's Principles of Environmental Health for Nursing Practice with Implementation Strategies. Silver Spring, MD: American Nurses Association; 2007. http://www.nursingworld.org/MainMenuCategories/WorkplaceSafety/Healthy-Nurse/ANAsPrinciplesofEnvironmentalHealthforNursingPractice.pdf. Accessed August 23, 2017 [IVC]

35. Kaplan S, Sadler B, Little K, Franz C, Orris P. Can sustainable hospitals help bend the health care cost curve? *Issue Brief (Commonw Fund).* 2012;29:1-14. [IIIC]

36. Southorn T, Norrish AR, Gardner K, Baxandall R. Reducing the carbon footprint of the operating theatre: a multicentre quality improvement report. *J Perioper Pract.* 2013;23(6):144-146. [VB]

37. Wormer BA, Augenstein VA, Carpenter CL, et al. The green operating room: simple changes to reduce cost and our carbon footprint. *Am Surg.* 2013;79(7):666-671. [VA]

Acknowledgments

LEAD AUTHOR

Esther M. Johnstone, DNP, RN, CNOR
Perioperative Practice Specialist
AORN Nursing Department
Denver, Colorado

CONTRIBUTING AUTHOR

Ramona L. Conner, MSN, RN, CNOR, FAAN
Editor-in-Chief, Guidelines for Perioperative Practice
AORN Nursing Department
Denver, Colorado

The authors and AORN thank Marie Bashaw, DNP, RN, NEA-BC, CNOR, Assistant Professor, Wright State University, Dayton, Ohio; Barbara Nalley, MSN, RN, CRNP, CNOR, Surgical Assist RNFA Nurse Practitioner, Anne Arundel Medical Group & Chesapeake Women's Care, Crofton, Maryland; Susan Klacik, BS, CRCST, ACE, CHL, FCS, Klacik Consulting LLC, Canfield, Ohio; Dawn Yost, MSN, BSDH, RN, RDH, CNOR, CSSM, Manager of Training & Development, Surgical Services, WVU Medicine–Ruby Memorial Hospital, Morgantown, West Virginia; James (Jay) Bowers, BSN, RN, CNOR, Clinical Educator, West Virginia Health- care, Morgantown; Evangeline (Vangie) Dennis, BSN, RN, CNOR, CMLSO, Director of Patient Care Practice, Emory Healthcare and Ambulatory Surgery Centers, Atlanta, Georgia; Sharon Van Wicklin, MSN, RN, CNOR, CRNFA(E), CPSN-R, PLNC, Senior Perioperative Practice Specialist, AORN Nursing Department, Denver, Colorado; and Amber Wood, MSN, RN, CNOR, CIC, FAPIC, Senior Perioperative Practice Specialist, AORN Nursing Department, Denver, Colorado, for their assistance in developing this guideline.

PUBLICATION HISTORY

Originally published April 1989, *AORN Journal*, as "Recommended practices: product evaluation and selection for perioperative patient care."

Revised August 1993.

Revised November 1997; published January 1998, *AORN Journal*, as "Recommended practices for product selection in perioperative practice settings."

Reformatted July 2000.

Revised November 2003; published in *Standards, Recommended Practices, and Guidelines*, 2004 edition. Reprinted March 2004, *AORN Journal*.

Revised January 2010 for online publication in *Perioperative Standards and Recommended Practices*.

Reformatted September 2012 for publication in *Perioperative Standards and Recommended Practices*, 2013 edition.

Minor editing revisions made in November 2014 for publication as "Guideline for product selection" in *Guidelines for Perioperative Practice*, 2015 edition.

Revised November 2017 for publication in *Guidelines for Perioperative Practice* online.

EQUIPMENT AND PRODUCT SAFETY

EQUIPMENT AND PRODUCT SAFETY

PATIENT
& WORKER SAFETY

GUIDELINE FOR AUTOLOGOUS TISSUE MANAGEMENT

The Guideline for Autologous Tissue Management has been approved by the AORN Guideline Advisory Board. It was presented as a proposed guideline for comments by members and others. The guideline is effective November 15, 2014. The recommendations in the guideline are intended to be achievable and represent what is believed to be an optimal level of practice. Policies and procedures will reflect variations in practice settings and/or clinical situations that determine the degree to which the guideline can be implemented. AORN recognizes the many diverse settings in which perioperative nurses practice; therefore, this guideline is adaptable to all areas where operative and other invasive procedures may be performed.

Purpose

This document provides guidance to perioperative personnel for managing autologous tissue in the perioperative setting, including avulsed teeth, cranial bone flaps, parathyroid glands, skin, veins, and dropped autografts. Guidance is provided for transferring tissue from the sterile field, packaging and labeling, transporting and storing, and handling autologous tissue for delayed replantation or autotransplantation within the same facility. Guidance for managing autologous adipose tissue is not provided. Currently, adipose aspirates can only be used for immediate autologous fat grafting at the time of recovery, and there is no reliable method for preserving and storing adipose tissue for delayed autotransplantation.[1,2] Recommendations related to processes for intraoperative storage and cryopreservation of autologous tissue are outside the scope of this document.

A facility that handles autologous tissue for delayed replantation or autotransplantation into the same patient and within the same facility is not required to register with the US Food and Drug Administration (FDA) as a tissue establishment (ie, tissue bank) that manufactures human cells, tissues, and cellular and tissue-based products, nor to follow requirements of 21 CFR Part 1271 (ie, the FDA regulations for these products).[3,4] Facilities or health care organizations that handle autologous tissue are required to recover, process, package, label, store, track, and replant or autotransplant the tissue in a manner that minimizes microbial growth, prevents mix-ups, and reduces the risk for errors.[3] Although the regulation defines manufacturing to include recovery, processing, storage, labeling, packaging, or distribution of any human cell or tissue,[3,5] the FDA considers most procedures related to autologous tissue to be a single procedure encompassed within the element of storage. The reader can refer to section 1271.15(b), in which storage of autologous tissue is exempt if replantation or autotransplantation will occur in the facility where the recovery took place.[4] Similarly, packaging and labeling of autologous tissue can be encompassed within the exception for storage.[4] Freezing autologous tissue as a method of storage does not, in itself, require registration and listing with the FDA as a tissue establishment.[4]

In addition, the FDA has interpreted the "same surgical procedure" language in its final rule to include recovery and storage before replantation or autotransplantation.[3] Retaining autologous tissue to be used in a subsequent application for the same patient is exempt from registration because the two applications are essentially a single, continuous procedure.[4]

The facility is required to register with the FDA if autologous tissue handling includes steps to process the autograft when any step requires specific manufacturing controls to decontaminate the tissue (ie, subjecting the autograft to a steam sterilization process).[4] If autologous tissue-handling functions are expanded to include distribution of the autograft to another facility located at a different address, registration and listing with the FDA using Form FDA 3356 is required.[3]

Whether or not facility registration is required, the federal regulations described in 21 CFR Part 1271 provide good practices for preventing the introduction, transmission, or spread of communicable disease and enhancing patient safety related to autologous tissue management.[3,5]

The reader can also refer to the standards of the American Association of Tissue Banks (AATB), which reflect the collective expertise and efforts of tissue bank professionals to provide a comprehensive foundation to support tissue banking activities, including practices for managing autologous tissue.[6]

Evidence Review

On January 24 and January 27, 2014, a medical librarian conducted a systematic search of the databases MEDLINE®, CINAHL®, and the Cochrane Database of Systematic Reviews for meta-analyses, systematic reviews, randomized controlled and non-randomized trials and studies, case reports, letters, reviews, and guidelines. The librarian also searched Scopus®, although not systematically. Search terms included *autologous transplantation, tissue preservation, organ transplantation, preservation, storage, storage solution, saline solution, isotonic saline, potassium chloride, N-acetylhistidine, ice, cold temperature, bone flap, bone transplantation, skull, bone and bones, surgical flap, saphenous vein, radial artery, renal artery, mammary artery,* and *thoracic artery*. During the development of this document, the lead author also requested supplementary

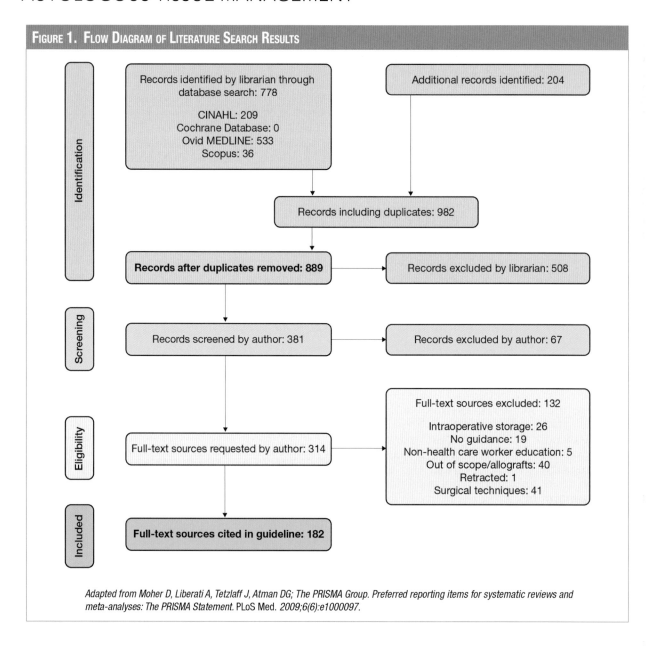

FIGURE 1. FLOW DIAGRAM OF LITERATURE SEARCH RESULTS

Adapted from Moher D, Liberati A, Tetzlaff J, Atman DG; The PRISMA Group. Preferred reporting items for systematic reviews and meta-analyses: The PRISMA Statement. PLoS Med. 2009;6(6):e1000097.

searches on the topics of storage media, preservation of avulsed teeth, and the use of swab cultures.

The initial search was limited to literature published in English since January 2006; however, the time restriction was not considered in subsequent searches. At the time of the initial search, the librarian also established weekly alerts on the topics included in the initial search. The librarian later added terms from subsequent supplementary searches to the alerts and, until May 2014, presented relevant results to the lead author.

The lead author reviewed search results from the medical librarian's literature search for the AORN Guideline for Specimen Management to identify literature specific to management of other tissues and the preservation of avulsed teeth. During the development of the document, the lead author requested additional articles and other literature that either did not fit the original search criteria or was discovered during the evidence appraisal process. Finally, the lead author and the medical librarian identified relevant guidelines from government agencies and standards-setting bodies. In total, 889 research and non-research sources of evidence were identified for possible inclusion, and of these, 182 were cited in the guidance document (Figure 1).

Excluded were non-peer-reviewed or retracted publications; evidence specific to organ transplantations, processes for cryopreservation, and surgical techniques and treatment protocols; and some evidence related to allografts, intraoperative storage of autologous tissue, and educational needs surrounding traumatic dental injuries not specific to health care workers.

Articles identified in the search were provided to the lead author and the assigned evidence reviewer for review and critical appraisal using the AORN Research or Non-Research Evidence Appraisal Tools as appropriate. The literature was independently evaluated and appraised by the lead author and the evidence reviewer according to the strength and quality of the evidence. Each article was then assigned an appraisal score determined by consensus. The appraisal score is noted in brackets after each reference, as applicable. Various articles also were provided to an expert member of the project team for consideration regarding relevance and application of the evidence for determining practice guidelines.

The evidence supporting each intervention and activity statement within a specific recommendation was summarized, and the AORN Evidence-Rating Model was used to rate the strength of the collective evidence. Factors considered in the review of the collective evidence were the quality of the evidence, the quantity of similar evidence on a given topic, the consistency of evidence supporting a recommendation, and the potential benefits and harms. The assigned evidence rating is noted in brackets after each intervention and activity statement.

Note: The evidence summary table is available at http://www.aorn.org/evidencetables/.

Editor's note: MEDLINE is a registered trademark of the US National Library of Medicine's Medical Literature Analysis and Retrieval System, Bethesda, MD. CINAHL, Cumulative Index to Nursing and Allied Health Literature, is a registered trademark of EBSCO Industries, Birmingham, AL. Scopus is a registered trademark of Elsevier B.V., Amsterdam, The Netherlands.

Recommendation I

Avulsed teeth that cannot be immediately replanted in the patient at the time of avulsion should be placed in a storage medium to help maintain periodontal ligament (PDL) cell viability.

Tooth avulsion is characterized by a complete displacement of the tooth from the alveolar socket.[7-14] The avulsion causes a rupture in the PDL tissue as shown in Figure 2. A portion of the PDL tissue remains on the walls of the alveolar socket, and a portion remains attached to the root surface of the avulsed tooth.[15] The PDL cells attached to the alveolar wall maintain viability; however, the PDL cells attached to the root surface are at risk for necrosis[12,16-18] or infection.[9] Neurovascular supply to the tooth is compromised and may result in loss of tooth pulp vitality.[7,8,13,19-22]

The collective evidence indicates that the ability to successfully replant an avulsed tooth often depends on measures taken at the time of the avulsion and immediately afterward.[23-25] Immediate replantation of the tooth at the site of the avulsion injury is the preferred treatment.[8-20,22,25-41] When immediate replantation is not possible, storing the tooth in an effective storage medium can help to maintain the viability of the PDL cells.[7-24,27,32,34-36,38-47] Numerous types of media have been recommended for storage of avulsed teeth. The most effective media to support PDL cell viability are Hank's Balanced Salt Solution (HBSS) or milk. Table 1 provides a list of recommended storage media

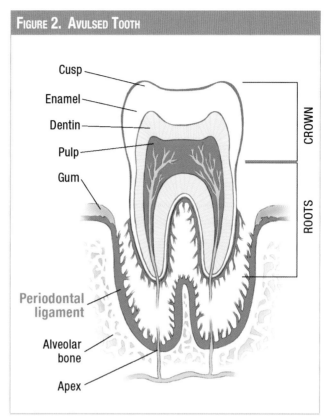

FIGURE 2. AVULSED TOOTH

Cusp

Enamel

Dentin

Pulp

Gum

CROWN

ROOTS

Periodontal ligament

Alveolar bone

Apex

Avulsion causes a rupture in the periodontal ligament (PDL). A portion of the PDL tissue remains on the walls of the alveolar socket, and a portion remains attached to the root surface of the avulsed tooth. Neurovascular supply to the tooth is compromised and may result in loss of tooth pulp vitality.

Illustration by Kurt Jones.

for avulsed teeth, and Table 2 provides information related to the characteristics of various types of storage media.

The limitations of the evidence are that some of the recommended storage media are not likely to be immediately available at the site of the avulsion injury or where treatment of the injury will occur. Some research studies were conducted in laboratory settings, and the results may not be generalizable to settings outside of the laboratory.

The benefit of immediate replantation or storage of avulsed teeth in a medium that will help to maintain PDL cell viability is that it increases the chances for successful replantation of an avulsed tooth. The harms associated with immediate replantation are that the tooth replantation may be performed incorrectly. Replantation of a tooth that is contaminated with debris may increase the patient's risk for infection. There are no harms associated with storing avulsed teeth in a medium that will maintain PDL cell viability.

In a nonexperimental study, Karayilmaz et al[24] reviewed patient records from a university dental health and treatment center during a nine-year period and found that 5.9% of all traumatic dental injuries treated (66 of 1,124) were avulsion injuries. Notably, 64.5% of avulsed teeth (60 of 93) were lost as a result of panic and a lack of knowledge of the individuals at

TABLE 1. RECOMMENDED STORAGE MEDIA FOR AVULSED TEETH

Researchers/authors	CLS	CW	Egg white	Formula	Gatorade®	GTE	HBSS	Milk	Mulberry[a]	NaCl	ORS	Pedialyte®	Probiotic[b]	Propolis	Ricetral	Sage[c]	Saliva	Soymilk	ViaSpan®	Water
Ahangari et al (2013)[47]														+						
Al-Nazhan and Al-Nasser (2006)[30]	+																			
American Association of Endodontists (2013)[53]							+													
Andersson (2012)[25]							+	+		+							+			-
Andreasen et al (1995)[31]										+										+
Ballal and Jothi (2011)[54]	-					+									+					
Brullmann et al (2010)[11]								+		+							+			-
Caglar (2010)[26]							+	+		+			+				+			
Ceallaigh et al (2007)[29]								+												
Chamorro et al (2008)[48]	-				-															
Chen and Huang (2012)[9]						+														
de Sousa et al (2008)[39]			+					+									+			
de Souza et al (2010)[52]							+													-
Doshi (2009)[21]								+												
Eskandarian et al (2013)[34]													+							
Gjertsen et al (2011)[10]															+					
Gopikrishna et al (2008)[13]		+																		
Huang et al (1996)[46]							+	+												
Hwang et al (2011)[37]							+													
Jung et al (2011)[51]						+														
Karayilmaz et al (2013)[24]							+	+												
Khademi et al (2008)[12]			+				+													
Koca et al (2010)[56]																	+			
Krasner (2010)[15]							+													
Lin et al (2007)[22]							+	+		+										
Macway-Gomez and Lallier (2013)[35]		+											+							
Malhotra (2011)[27]							+	+		-				+			-		+	-
Moazami et al (2012)[19]				+			+											+		-
Moradian et al (2013)[16]										+										
Moreira-Neto et al (2009)[38]										+										
Moura et al (2012)[36]																		+		
Mousavi et al (2010)[50]							+						+							-
Ozan et al (2007)[20]															+					
Ozan et al (2008)[41]										+										
Ozan et al (2008)[40]																	+			
Rajendran et al (2011)[44]							+	-							+					
Royal College of Surgeons (2004)[43]								+		+										
Sanghavi et al (2013)[7]			+											+						
Saxena et al (2011)[28]										+				+						
Sigalas et al (2004)[14]	+				+		+	+												-
Silva et al (2013)[33]							+	+									+			
Sonoda et al (2008)[55]																	+			
Souza et al (2010)[32]							+	+												
Souza et al (2011)[18]								+												
Subramaniam et al (2011)[45]													+							
Thomas et al (2008)[8]			+				+													
Udoye et al (2012)[17]								+												

Abbreviations: CLS = contact lens solution; CW = coconut water; GTE = green tea extract; HBSS = Hank's Balanced Salt Solution; NaCl = sodium chloride (saline) solution; ORS = oral rehydration solution.
[a] *Morus rubra (Red Mulberry)*   [b] *Lactobacillus reuteri*   [c] *Salvia officinalis*
+ Recommended   - Not recommended   ▇ Most recommended storage media

Editor's note: *Gatorade is a registered trademark of Stokely-Van Camp, Inc, Chicago, IL. Pedialyte is a registered trademark of Abbott Laboratories, Inc, Abbott Park, IL. ViaSpan is a registered trademark of Barr Laboratories, Inc, Champaign, IL.*

the scene of the accident regarding the need to store the avulsed tooth in an effective storage medium for future replantation.

I.a. Avulsed teeth should be replanted at the time of avulsion. *[2: High Evidence]*

The longer an avulsed tooth is outside of the mouth, the greater the potential for root resorption and reduced pulpal healing.[7,9,10,12-14,17,22,24,28,30,33,35-39,43-45,47,48]

The International Association for Dental Traumatology recommends

TABLE 2. CHARACTERISTICS OF TYPES OF STORAGE MEDIA FOR AVULSED TEETH

Storage medium	Characteristics
Contact lens solution	May be an effective storage medium.[46] The presence of preservatives in contact lens solution may be harmful to periodontal ligament (PDL) cell viability.[17,23,30]
Coconut water	May be effective as a storage medium due to the amino acids, proteins, vitamins and minerals present in coconut water.[7,8,13,23,26] It is an isotonic solution[8,9] that resembles intracellular fluid.[13] Coconut water supports PDL viability and helps to reduce bacterial growth.[35] Coconut water has a pH of 4.1 that may be detrimental for cell metabolism.[17,38]
Egg white	May be an effective storage medium due to osmolality of 251-298 mOsm/Kg that promotes cell growth.[12,23]
Formula	May be as effective as milk as a storage medium, does not require refrigeration, and has a long shelf life.[23]
Gatorade®	Low pH (2.91) may be harmful to PDL cell viability.[17,50] Gatorade is a hypotonic solution that may cause the PDL cells to lose water.[23]
Green tea extract	May be effective as a storage medium due to anti-inflammatory and antioxidant properties that help to preserve tissues and cells.[3,5,9,30] Adding green tea extract to the storage medium may allow for storage periods longer than 14 days.[5]
Hank's Balanced Salt Solution	Contains nutrients and salts that can sustain and reconstitute the cellular components of PDL cells.[4,22] Considered the gold standard of storage mediums.[26,27,32,40] May be effective for an extended time (ie, as long as 48 hours).[26]
Milk	Significantly better than other storage media. Its osmolality, pH, and physiologic properties are compatible with PDL cells.[21,22] Milk also provides nutritional substances, such as amino acids, carbohydrates, and vitamins.[14,22,23,26,27] Chilled milk is preferred over milk at room temperature.[26] The antigens in milk may interfere with the PDL cell reattachment process.[26] The time period during which PDL cell viability is maintained when stored in milk is controversial.[27] Skim milk is not as effective in preserving cell viability as whole milk.[36]
Mulberry (Morus rubra)	May be an effective storage medium due to its antioxidant properties.[41]
Sodium chloride (NaCl)	Osmolality of 280 mOsm/Kg is compatible with PDL cells; however, NaCl lacks essential nutrients (eg, glucose, calcium, magnesium) necessary to maintain the metabolic needs of PDL cells.[17,23,26] May only be effective for a brief period of time (ie, < 2-3 hours).[17,22,26]
Oral rehydration solution	May be an effective storage medium due to its ability to preserve cell viability and its potential regenerative effect.[34]
Pedialyte®	May be an effective storage medium due to its ability to support PDL cell survival and reduce bacterial growth.[35]
Probiotic (Lactobacillus reuteri)	May be as effective as milk, Hank's Balanced Salt Solution (HBBS), or saline as a storage media.[5,23]
Propolis	May be an effective storage medium. Propolis maintains PDL cell viability and is antimicrobial, anti-inflammatory, and antioxidant.[10,17,23,26,28,47,54] Propolis also decreases apoptosis of PDL fibroblasts.[10]
Ricetral	May be effective as a storage medium due to concentrations of glucose and vital salts that are adequate for cell metabolism.[30]
Sage (Salvia officinalis)	May be an effective storage medium due to its antimicrobial properties.[40]
Saliva	Effective for a short period of time (ie, < 60 minutes).[17] Low osmolality of 60-80 mOsm/Kg may increase the harmful effects of bacteria.[8,10,22,23,26,32,39] Saliva is a hypotonic solution that may lead to lysis of the PDL cells.[8,17,26,40]
Soymilk	May be an effective storage medium due to its ability to maintain cell viability at similar levels as milk and HBSS.[19,33,36]
Viaspan	May be an effective long-term storage medium due to pH of 7.4 that is ideal for cell growth.[8,23,26] Viaspan contains a hydrogen ion buffer that may help to maintain pH. Viaspan also contains adenosine which is necessary for cell division and may improve vitality of PDL cells by preventing cell swelling.[32] Requires refrigeration.[17]
Water	One of the least effective storage mediums. It is a hypotonic medium that may lead to rapid lysis of the PDL cells.[5,17,23,26,39,40,43,48] Water has a low osmolality and may contain chlorine.[40]

Editor's note: Gatorade is a registered trademark of Stokely-Van Camp, Inc, Chicago, IL. Pedialyte is a registered trademark of Abbott Laboratories, Inc, Abbott Park, IL. ViaSpan is a registered trademark of Barr Laboratories, Inc, Champaign, IL.

- picking up the tooth by the crown and not touching the root,[15,25,29]
- washing the tooth[29] under cold running water for no longer than 10 seconds,[11,25]
- replanting the tooth if possible and holding it in place,[11,25,29]
- placing the tooth in a glass of milk or other storage medium (eg, HBBS) if immediate replantation is not possible,[25,29] and
- seeking emergency treatment as soon as possible.[25]

The patient's teeth and mouth may be covered in debris that may require removal by gentle washing[29] with a physiologic solution.[15] Lin et al[49] recommended immediate fixation of the tooth by suturing as a method to initiate pulpal and periodontal healing and improve long-term prognosis and stabilization of the tooth.

I.a.1. Members of the health care team should record the events leading to the tooth avulsion in the patient's health record and conduct a thorough patient examination as soon as possible after the event occurs (eg, during intubation) or when the patient arrives at the facility. This should include
- an examination for head injury and facial fracture,[11,22,25,43]
- an examination for signs of external injury (eg, laceration),[22]
- an oral examination[22] that includes accounting for all of the patient's teeth to ensure they have not been inhaled,[29] and
- a review of the patient's tetanus vaccination history.[29]

[2: High Evidence]

I.b. Avulsed teeth that cannot be immediately replanted should be placed in a storage medium. The storage medium should
- maintain viability of the PDL cells,[7,33,38,41,46]
- facilitate repopulation of the denuded root surface and prevent root resorption,[7]
- provide physiological osmolality (230 mOsm/Kg to 400 mOsm/Kg)[8,38] and pH (7.0)[38] to allow optimal cell growth and survival,[7,10,21] and
- be available and readily accessible at the location of the avulsion injury.[7,33-36,38,46]

[2: High Evidence]

Successful replantation of avulsed teeth is directly related to PDL cell viability.[8,13-15,17,20, 21,23,28,30,37,38,41,44,45,48,50,51] Prolonged drying of the tooth reduces the viability of the PDL cells[27,30,44] and leads to dehydration of the tooth pulp.[31,43] Patients with avulsed teeth may have suffered other serious injuries that require immediate treatment. In these cases, it may be necessary to store the avulsed tooth in a medium that will help prevent dehydration and maintain PDL viability until the tooth can be replanted.[7,8,11,13,24,25,33,34,46,49,52,51]

When immediate replantation of the avulsed tooth is not possible, the American Association of Endodontists recommends storing an avulsed tooth in HBBS, milk, normal saline solution, or saliva.[53] The Royal College of Surgeons recommends storing the tooth in cold milk, normal saline solution, or saliva.[43] The International Association for Dental Traumatology recommends placing the tooth in milk, HBSS, or another storage medium.[25]

I.b.1. Avulsed teeth that will not be immediately replanted should be stored in HBSS or milk. *[2: High Evidence]*

Hank's Balanced Salt Solution is an effective medium for maintaining the viability of PDL cells at room temperature[17,27,46] and is considered the gold standard for storage of avulsed teeth.[12,14,18-20,22,24,32,35,40,41,47,49,54] It is often used as a comparison medium for determining the effectiveness of other storage media.[27,40]

Hank's Balanced Salt Solution is available commercially as an emergency tooth preserving system[20,40] that allows the avulsed tooth to be suspended in a basket that helps wash debris off the tooth while preventing damage to the PDL cells.[17,43] The system also allows the tooth to be removed from the basket without being touched by forceps or fingers.[23] The unopened product has a three-year shelf life,[17,27] but it cannot be stored at temperatures above 104° F (40° C).[11] The German Dental Association recommends that all kindergartens, schools, sports centers, dental practices, and medical institutions keep a supply of tooth rescue kits readily available for tooth avulsion injuries.[11]

Milk has been widely accepted as a suitable storage medium for avulsed teeth.[12,14,17,18,20,22,24,26,28-30,32,36,38,42,46,47,54] Milk has a physiological osmolality (230 mOsm/Kg to 270 mOsm/Kg), has a slightly acidic pH (6.5 to 6.8), and contains nutrients and growth factors that support the PDL cells.[22,28,42,47] Moradian et al[16] reported successful replantation of an avulsed maxillary central incisor after 12 hours of storage in milk. The tooth was stable and remained functional and aesthetically acceptable after three years. Storing the avulsed tooth in milk at a cool temperature (32° F to 39° F [0° C to 4° C])[27] may help reduce cell metabolism, limit bacterial growth, and prevent the milk from spoiling.[42]

In a nonexperimental study to assess the viability of PDL cells at room temperature and on ice, Sigalas et al[14] concluded that storage on ice was more beneficial than storage at room temperature. In a quasi-experimental study to investigate apoptosis in PDL cells, Chamorro et al[48] found that storage on ice inhibited cell death.

de Souza et al[42] conducted a quasi-experimental study to determine whether the renewal of milk used as a storage medium with fresh milk every 24 hours for up to 120 hours would improve viability of PDL fibroblasts. They found that, regardless of the temperature, renewal of the milk did not affect the viability of PDL fibroblasts.

In a quasi-experimental study, Moura et al[36] investigated the efficacy of soy milk in maintaining the viability of PDL fibroblasts compared with different cow milks. The researchers found that soy milk was an adequate storage medium for avulsed teeth, but skim milk was not as effective in preserving PDL cell viability.

I.b.2. Avulsed teeth that will not be immediately replanted may be temporarily stored in the patient's saliva if a more effective type of storage medium is not available. *[3: Moderate Evidence]*

The availability of saliva at the moment of avulsion allows for its use as a temporary storage medium until the tooth can be replanted or placed into a more effective medium. Sonoda et al[55] reported the case of a 30-year-old woman with an accidentally avulsed permanent incisor that was kept in her oral cavity from the moment of trauma until its replantation 90 minutes later. Three years later, clinical and radiographic findings showed no root absorption or mobility of the tooth.

Koca et al[56] reported the case of an eight-year-old boy whose avulsed left upper central incisor was kept in his oral cavity in direct contact with saliva for five hours, from the moment of trauma until its replantation. Two years later, clinical and radiographic findings showed no root resorption or mobility of the replanted tooth.

I.b.3. Avulsed teeth that will not be immediately replanted should not be stored in water, unless the only alternative is dry storage. *[2: High Evidence]*

It is not advisable to store an avulsed tooth in water[8,11,17,19,25,27,32,37,39,43,50]; however, dry storage of a tooth is not recommended.[14,23,29,38,43,50] Ize-Iyamu and Saheeb[57] reported two cases of successful replantation of avulsed teeth that occurred after 72 hours of dry storage. In a nonexperimental study that examined pulpal healing of 400 avulsed and replanted teeth, Andreasen et al[31] found an increasing negative effect on pulp healing with increasing periods of dry storage. However, the researchers still recommended replanting teeth that had been kept dry for a long period of time. In a literature review conducted by Goswami et al,[23] the authors concluded that moist storage optimizes PDL cell survival, but no storage medium is ideal, and further research is warranted.

I.c. Education and competency verification activities related to best practices for the management of avulsed teeth should be provided for perioperative or other health care personnel who may be involved in caring for patients who have sustained traumatic tooth avulsion. *[2: High Evidence]*

The collective evidence supports providing education to health care workers and others involved in the care of patients who have sustained traumatic tooth avulsion. The limitations of the evidence are that some studies may not be generalizable outside of the geographic area in which the study was conducted, and some research studies used surveys, so the responses may be subjective and not representative of the broader population.

The benefit of providing education to perioperative or other health care personnel involved in caring for patients who have sustained traumatic tooth avulsion is that it may increase the likelihood of successful replantation of avulsed teeth for patients treated within the facility or health care organization. The benefit will be even greater if parents, school teachers, athletic coaches, and the general public also receive education regarding the protocols for managing traumatic tooth avulsion injuries and if tooth rescue kits are available in schools, sporting facilities, and health care facilities.[21,24,25,27,49] There are no harms associated with providing education and competency verification activities for perioperative and other health care personnel involved in caring for patients who have sustained traumatic tooth avulsion.

In a nonexperimental study conducted to evaluate the knowledge of treatment of tooth avulsion injuries among 50 school nurses in Bialystok, Poland, Baginska and Wilczynska-Borawska[58] found that the nurses had knowledge about the need for an effective storage medium for the avulsed tooth and that they understood the critical need for keeping the time to treatment at a minimum to achieve successful replantation of an avulsed tooth. The researchers found a significant correlation between the level of the nurses' knowledge and the receipt of previous education related to dental trauma.

Ulusoy et al[59] surveyed 69 emergency physicians from one university and 10 public hospitals in Samsun, Turkey, to evaluate their knowledge related to treatment of traumatic tooth avulsion injuries and found that the majority of physicians could not provide correct answers to the survey questions. The researchers concluded there was a need for education of emergency physicians related to treatment of traumatic tooth avulsion injuries.

In a nonexperimental study conducted to investigate dentists' knowledge of procedures for managing traumatic dental injuries in children, Yeng and Parashos[60] surveyed 693 dentists in Victoria, Australia, and found that the respondents demonstrated only a moderate level of knowledge. The researchers concluded that professional education programs on the management of dental trauma in children were needed to improve practice.

Kargul and Welbury[61] conducted a retrospective observational study of the patient records of 75 children with 120 avulsed teeth treated in a dental hospital trauma clinic in Istanbul, Turkey. They found that only 42.5% of avulsed teeth (n = 51) were placed in an effective storage medium before replantation. The researchers determined public education was needed to improve successful tooth replantation in patients treated for avulsion injuries.

To assess the level of dental practitioners' knowledge of recommended guidelines for treatment of tooth avulsion injuries, de Vasconcellos et al[62] surveyed 264 dental practitioners from public and private dental schools in São José dos Campos, Brazil. The results of the study showed that the participants exhibited knowledge of the correct procedures for treatment of traumatic tooth avulsion. However, the results also showed a lack of communication regarding treatment guidelines for avulsion injuries by the dental practitioners to those at risk for avulsion injury (eg, individuals who participate in contact sports).

Zhao and Gong[63] conducted a study to evaluate the knowledge of dentists (N = 258) working in urban and suburban areas of Beijing, China, related to the management and treatment of dental emergencies. The results of the study showed that 87.2% of participants (n = 225) recommended immediate replantation of the avulsed tooth; however, only 15.9% of the participants (n = 41) were able to correctly identify the most effective storage media, and only 55.8% (n = 144) had received any education related to emergency management of avulsed teeth.

Loh et al[64] surveyed 167 dental therapists (formerly known as school dental nurses) in Singapore to gather information on their knowledge related to the management of traumatic dental injuries. The majority of respondents (54.5%; n = 91) were not aware of the most effective storage media for avulsed teeth, and a very high percentage (94.6%; n = 158) indicated there was a need for more education.

In a nonexperimental study, Hugar et al[65] assessed the knowledge of 300 nurses and prospective nurses from a university hospital in Belgaum, India, about emergency management of traumatic dental injuries. The researchers found that only 2.3% (n = 7) were aware of effective storage media for avulsed teeth, and 49.7% (n = 149) had received no education related to the management of traumatic dental injuries. The researchers emphasized the need for education for nurses, as they may be the first health care personnel to provide patient care.

In a survey of Massachusetts emergency department directors (n = 16) and physicians (n = 56), Needleman et al[66] investigated the physicians' knowledge of traumatic dental injury management. The researchers found that none of the emergency departments had a formal, written protocol in place for managing traumatic dental injuries. Most of the physicians who responded to the survey (45 of 56; 80.4%) had received education related to managing traumatic dental injuries during their residency; however, their knowledge of the correct treatment for dental fractures was poor, as indicated by correct responses of only 55.4% or lower to survey questions. The responding physicians scored higher on questions related to management of dislocated or avulsed teeth, with correct responses ranging between 61% and 89%. Physicians who specialized in pediatric emergency medicine were more likely to answer the questions correctly than were emergency medicine physicians. Physicians at hospitals with an academic affiliation scored significantly better than those at nonacademic-affiliated hospitals. The researchers concluded that educational campaigns were needed to improve physicians' knowledge of managing traumatic dental injuries and that education would enhance the long-term outcomes for patients who sustain dental trauma and who present to the emergency department for treatment.

Choi et al[67] conducted a survey of 100 randomly selected public and private school nurses in New York City. The researchers found that 87% of the nurses (n = 87) had not received education in managing traumatic dental injuries in children. Sixty-eight percent of the nurses either thought that the tooth should not be replanted (52%; n = 52), or did not know whether the tooth should be replanted (16%; n = 16). Although school nurses were often the first persons to provide emergency treatment for children with avulsed teeth, they had limited knowledge, resources, and experience to provide the correct treatment. The researchers concluded there was a need to provide educational programs for school nurses to improve the management of traumatic dental injuries in children.

Recommendation II

The patient's autologous cranial bone flap may be preserved and replanted.

The collective evidence indicates that decompressive craniectomy with removal of cranial bone and subsequent replantation with the patient's preserved bone flap or with artificial material is a widely used technique for the management of refractory intracranial hypertension after traumatic brain injury or extensive cerebral infarctions or brain tumors.[68-76] The evidence supports replanting the autologous cranial bone flap compared with using artificial materials for cranial reconstruction.[73,75-82] Autologous bone, such as rib and iliac crest, also may be used for cranial reconstruction; however, it is difficult to shape into the desired configuration, may not be large enough to fill the cranial defect, and may necessitate additional incisions.[81,82] Using autologous bone rather than artificial materials may increase the patient's risk for infection and bone resorption,[68,70,71,79,83] and there may be potential for infection related to the nonviability of the cranial bone flap.[70]

Artificial materials most suitable for use in reconstructive cranioplasty procedures are those that are resistant to infection, radiolucent, protective, thermally nonconductive, non-ionizing, and noncorrosive, and provide aesthetically pleasing results.[79] Artificial materials used for cranioplasty include methyl methacrylate, hydroxyapatite-based ceramics, titanium, and polypropylene polyester.[69,79] Methyl methacrylate is not suited to modeling large areas or reproducing the curved shape of the cranium,[79,84] and using it to reconstruct the cranium may increase the patient's risk for infection compared with using titanium.[83] Hydroxyapatite-based ceramics are expensive, may crack during drilling, and do not allow for the use of screws for fixation.[79] The organic nature and macroporosity of hydroxyapatite allows for osseointegration; however, this process takes several months and does not provide strong protection for the cranium during the early postoperative period.[75] Artificial materials used for cranioplasty may be rejected as foreign bodies even after they have remained in the patient for many years.[81]

The limitations of the evidence are that some research studies had small sample sizes and limited availability of cranial bone; some studies lacked controls; different methods (eg, storage time, storage temperature) may have achieved different results; and the results of the studies may not be generalizable to all settings where autologous cranial bone grafts are replanted.

The benefits of using the patient's autologous bone for cranial reconstruction compared with artificial materials include improved appearance[68,69,71,74,77,79,80,82,85]; increased potential for bone engrafting, remodeling, and growth[68,69,74,82]; reduced potential for immunoreaction or disease transmission[69,71,74,77,79,82]; improved heat conduction[69]; reduced cost[68,69,74,79]; and reduced operating time.[85] The harms associated with the use of autologous bone for reconstructive cranioplasty include the potential for infection from contaminated cranial bone grafts, and bone nonviability and resorption,[68,70,71,79,83] particularly in pediatric patients.[74]

II.a. Cranial bone flaps to be replanted may be frozen or cryopreserved. *[2: High Evidence]*

The collective evidence indicates that freezing and cryopreservation are common methods of preserving excised cranial bone for replantation at a later date[70-72,79,86]; however, the optimal storage temperature has not been determined.[68,72,74] There are gaps in the literature related to best practices for managing frozen or cryopreserved autologous cranial bone flaps. To date, there are no consistent guidelines for preserving cranial bone flaps relative to tempera-

ture settings, length of storage, packaging method, or treatment of the excised flap with antibiotic or antiseptic solutions before storage or replantation.[68,74]

Likewise, the effect of freezing on the biological properties of skull bone and the process of autograft incorporation after replantation of frozen cranial bone warrant further research.[70,72] Understanding the viability of frozen bone cells may have significant ramifications for clinical practice in trauma, orthopedic, plastic and reconstructive, and neurosurgery.[70] Research to determine cell viability after storage of cranial bone flaps under various conditions may help provide insight into the most effective storage methods for improving graft revascularization and incorporation and reducing infection and bone resorption.[70,74]

However, maintaining cell viability in a bone autograft may not be necessary. For replantation success, provision of a suitable bone matrix for partial repopulation by autologous cells may suffice for osteoconduction, osteoinduction, and osseointegration[87] because similar success has been experienced with transplants involving nonviable bone allografts.[88-93] The evidence review did not reveal any evidence that addressed the effect of apoptotic autologous cells on undesirable replantation outcomes, such as resorption. Steps taken to maintain viable cells may also increase the risk that microorganisms will survive if the autograft becomes contaminated because of patient trauma or steps taken in handling or packaging the autologous cranial bone for storage.

The limitations of the evidence are that some research studies had a small sample size, and the results of the studies may not be generalizable to all settings where frozen or cryopreserved autologous cranial bone grafts are used.

The benefits of frozen or cryopreserved storage of autologous cranial bone flaps are that it may preserve the autograft for replantation at a later date and does not require additional surgical time or incisions. The harms associated with frozen or cryopreserved storage of autologous cranial bone flaps are that the autograft may be contaminated during storage or during the recovery or replantation procedure. The process of cryopreservation and long-term storage may lead to mechanical instability (eg, crack formation) of the bone or surface abrasiveness that facilitates bacterial adhesion and colonization.[72] Long-term storage of autologous tissue carries with it the potential for mix-ups if autograft labeling methods are inadequate (eg, smudging of identifiers during cold storage, labels separating from the package), and contamination or cross-contamination if the graft's packaging material is not validated for use at the storage temperature selected.

PATIENT AND WORKER SAFETY

During a seven-month period, Bhaskar et al[74] surveyed 25 neurosurgical centers in public and teaching hospitals in Australia to obtain information related to cranial bone flap preparation after craniectomy, temperature and duration of frozen storage of cranial bone flaps, infection prevention protocols, methods for detecting contamination in the flaps, and procedures for cranial replantation. The results of the study were the following:

○ Neurosurgeons preferred using frozen autologous cranial bone flaps over synthetic materials (96%; n = 24).
○ Cranial bone flaps were prepared for storage by double- or triple-bagging under dry, sterile conditions (88%; n = 22).
○ Cranial bone flaps were irrigated with normal saline solution containing antibiotics or povidone-iodine before cryopreservation (16%; n = 4).
○ Biopsies or cultures were obtained from the cranial bone flaps before cryopreservation to determine contamination levels (68%; n = 17).
○ Cranial bone flaps were cryopreserved at temperatures of -0.4° F to -117.4° F (-18° C to -83° C) for varying time intervals (eg, six months, until the patient died).
○ Cranial bone flaps were stored in facility freezers (52%; n = 13) or in commercial bone banks (48%; n = 12).
○ Some facilities used specific thawing procedures involving immersion of the frozen cranial flap in lactated Ringer's solution, povidone-iodine, or both (24%; n = 6).
○ Biopsies or cultures were obtained from the cranial bone flaps before replantation to determine contamination levels (12%; n = 3).
○ Maximum duration of storage before designation as biohazardous waste and disposal varied between five years (56%; n = 14), two years (8%; n = 2), nine months (4%; n = 1), six months (16%; n = 4), until the patient was deceased (4%; n = 1), and no time limit (12%; n = 3).

The researchers concluded that practices for cryopreservation and storage of autologous cranial bone flaps were highly variable in neurosurgical centers throughout Australia. They also concluded that there was a need for further research to determine the biological and biomechanical effects of frozen storage conditions on cranial bone and to verify best practices for cranial bone flap management.

In a quasi-experimental study to assess whether viable bone cells could be cultured from cranial bone flaps that had been cryopreserved without cryoprotectants for more than six months, Bhaskar et al[70] examined bone cultures from 27 cranial bone flaps harvested from patients who had undergone decompressive craniectomies for intractable intracranial hyperten-

sion at a university medical center. The flaps had been stored at -22° F (-30° C) for 7.6 to 41.8 months. The researchers found that the control samples showed abundant growth of osteoblasts, whereas samples taken from the cryopreserved cranial bone flaps showed no osteoblasts. The researchers concluded that cranial bone flaps cryopreserved without cryoprotectants for longer than six months were not viable.

In a nonexperimental study to evaluate the surface structure of cryopreserved cranial bone flaps, Beez et al[72] used scanning electron microscopy to examine cranial bone flaps removed from five patients during decompressive craniectomy and then stored for six to eight months at -112° F (-80° C) in a university neurosurgical center freezer. During morphological analysis of the bone flaps, the researchers found that two of the flaps had smooth bone surfaces, two had mixed surfaces (ie, smooth and abrasive), and one had an abrasive surface. The researchers found no correlation with any patient variables, such as age, or with the length of the cryopreservation; they determined that the differences in bone surface were reflective of differences in individual human anatomy. The researchers concluded that cryopreservation for as long as eight months did not alter the physiological surface of the skull bone, and they theorized that cryopreservation for longer periods would not harm the surface structure of the bone.

Elwatidy et al[73] conducted a nonexperimental study to evaluate the microbiological and histological characteristics of 14 cranial bone flaps preserved at -0.4° F (-18° C) for two months to five years at a university hospital. The bone flaps were prepared for storage by removal of soft tissue and bone spicules and washing with 1 L normal saline solution containing 80 mg gentamicin followed by 1 L normal saline solution containing 1 g vancomycin. The bone flaps were then dried, wrapped in sterile towels, and placed into two layers of sterile plastic bags. The packages were labeled with the patient's name, identification number, and the date of removal and were stored in the freezer.

On the day of the cranioplasty procedure, the researchers removed the cranial bone flap from its package and obtained swab cultures and histology specimens from the flap. They washed the bone in 1 L normal saline solution containing 80 mg gentamicin followed by 1 L normal saline solution containing 1 g vancomycin and then replanted it. The results of microbiology and histology examination showed no bacterial contamination in any of the cranial bone flaps. All of the flaps were viable except one. The viability of the bone was proportional to the duration of preservation in the freezer. The specimen that showed no viability had been stored in the freezer for five years.[73]

One patient developed a superficial wound infection that resolved after treatment with antibiotics. A second patient experienced partial bone resorption that resolved with spontaneous bone growth a few months later. The researchers concluded that preservation of cranial bone flaps by storage in a freezer at -0.4° F (-18° C) maintained sterility and viability for as long as 12 months. Notably, the swab culture method used by the researchers could not determine graft sterility. The results obtained when using such a method can only be deemed "swab culture negative."

Prolo et al[76] conducted a nonexperimental study in a university medical center to examine and analyze the repair of membranous skull after cranioplasty with frozen preservation of autologous cranial bone flaps. The researchers examined three groups of cranial bone flaps.

For Group 1, fresh cranial bone flaps were obtained from five patients who required a second craniectomy of the same area of the skull where the original craniectomy procedure had been performed 1.25 to 19 years earlier. The researchers examined the flaps visually and microscopically and found that in all patients, the replanted cranial bone flap was grossly thinner than the adjacent skull. They also found variable numbers of osteocytes in the bone flaps. The researchers concluded that segmental portions of skull removed and then replaced during cranioplasty regained viability.

For Group 2, the researchers visually and microscopically examined fragments from 12 excised cranial bone flaps that had been soaked for one to three hours in a bacitracin solution (500 units/mL), frozen in the solution at -4° F (-20° C), and then stored frozen for three to 35 months. They found no bacterial or fungal growth in any of the samples and found variable numbers of osteocytes in the bone flaps. There was no correlation between the length of time the bone flap had been stored and the number of osteocytes present. The researchers concluded that cranial bone removed aseptically during craniectomy and frozen in bacitracin solution for as long as three years was culture negative and not visually or microscopically altered in morphology.

For Group 3, 53 patients who underwent decompressive craniectomy and subsequent cranioplasty with autologous cranial bone flaps soaked in bacitracin (500 units/mL) and stored frozen at either -4° F (-20° C; n = 28) or -94° F (-70° C; n = 25) for a period of three weeks to 19 months were followed postoperatively for one to nine years. The researchers found there was some resorption of the bone in all patients, causing the graft to diminish in size over a period of years. In two children, ages seven months and two years, the amount of bone resorption was considerable; however, in all cases, the graft was functional and retained a cosmetically acceptable appearance. Two grafts were removed because of infection, and two patients died from causes unrelated to the autologous cranioplasty. The researchers concluded that the skull bone was intensely active after replantation and was the ideal material for cranioplasty. The researchers also concluded that freezing cranial bone flaps after decompressive craniectomy was an effective method of preservation for patients from the latter part of the first decade of life through adulthood.

Iwama et al[79] conducted a retrospective study in a university medical center to evaluate the use of frozen autologous cranial bone flaps for delayed cranioplasty in 49 patients during a 12-year period. The cranial bone flaps removed during the initial craniectomy procedure were wiped to remove all blood, sealed in three sterile vinyl bags, and stored at -31° F (-35° C) (n = 37) or -119.2° F (-84° C) (n = 12) for four to 168 days.

On the day of the cranioplasty procedure, the cranial bone flap was removed from the package, thawed at room temperature, and washed in 500 mL normal saline solution supplemented with 60 mg tobramycin. Forty-seven patients (96%) experienced no complications. The clinical and aesthetic results were satisfactory. Bone resorption was observed in one 12-year-old boy, and a 14-year-old boy developed an infection. Both patients underwent a second cranioplasty procedure with ceramic plates. The researchers concluded that delayed cranioplasty using frozen autologous cranial bone flaps achieved satisfactory clinical and aesthetic results.

Grossman et al[71] prospectively reviewed and reported the results of 12 cases of decompressive craniectomy followed by reconstructive cranioplasty performed during a nine-year period at a university medical center. A protocol was developed to prepare the excised cranial bone flaps for replantation. The autologous bone flaps were excised and transferred to the tissue bank within six hours. They were gently rinsed with 1 L to 3 L normal saline solution supplemented with neomycin (926 mg/L), wrapped in two layers of sterile plastic, and preserved at -112° F (-80° C) for 0.25 to 27 months.

On the day of the reconstructive procedure, the cranial bone flap was removed from the freezer and transferred to the OR in an icebox. The flap was allowed to thaw and was then removed from the package and washed with normal saline solution. All of the cranial bone flaps were replanted. The researchers found no bone flap resorption or infection, and the aesthetic results were satisfactory. The researchers concluded that freezing at -112° F (-80° C) was an effective method of preserving autologous cranial bone flaps.

Tahir et al[68] conducted a retrospective review of infection rates in 88 patients who had undergone autologous cranioplasty procedures at a busy neurotrauma center in a university hospital during a 10-year period. The patients' excised cranial bone flaps were wrapped in two layers of sterile, waterproof paper and placed in a close-fitting, sterile, air-tight plastic bag. This package was placed into a second, larger, sterile, air-tight plastic bag. All packages were labeled with the patient's identification and placed into an OR freezer maintained at a constant temperature of -14.8° F (-26° C) for a mean of 78.05 ± 66.7 days.

To minimize exposure time during the replantation procedure, the frozen cranial bone flaps were not removed from the packaging until after the subgaleal pocket was created. The bone flaps were cleaned of bone dust, attached soft tissue, and loose fragments and then immersed in povidone-iodine solution for 10 minutes, followed by irrigation with a solution of equal parts hydrogen peroxide (H_2O_2) and normal saline. The flaps were rinsed with an antibiotic solution immediately before replantation.

Three patients (3.4%) developed infections after the cranioplasty procedure. Two patients developed superficial wound infections, and one patient developed a deep wound infection involving the subgaleal space. The two patients with superficial infections were treated with antibiotics. The patient with the deep wound infection required wound exploration and irrigation and treatment with oral antibiotics. All the postoperative infections resolved completely. The researchers did not provide the formulation for "antibiotic solution" or the strength of the povidone-iodine and H_2O_2 solutions. The researchers concluded that frozen storage of autologous cranial bone flaps at a temperature of -14.8° F (-26° C) was safe, and the risk for infection was low.

To investigate whether cranial bone flaps preserved by freezing could survive and regenerate after autologous replantation, Lu et al[69] followed 16 patients undergoing cranioplasty procedures with replantation of autologous cranial bone flaps in a university hospital during a 16-month period. The bone flaps had been excised and sealed in a double-layer sterile plastic bag under sterile conditions, labeled with the patient's identification, and subsequently frozen at -112° F (-80° C) for 63 to 289 days.

On the day of the reconstructive procedure, the frozen autologous bone graft was thawed for 60 minutes, immersed in 3% povidone-iodine solution for 30 minutes, and then rinsed twice with normal saline solution before replantation. After surgery, the researchers used cranial bone tomography to examine the replanted bone at two-week, three-month, and 12-month periods. The researchers found that the frozen cranial bone was able to survive and regenerate new blood vessels and osteoblasts. They concluded that frozen autologous cranial bone could survive and regenerate after autologous replantation.

II.a.1. Facilities recovering, packaging, labeling, and freezing or cryopreserving autologous cranial bone for storage and replantation within the same facility are not required to register with the FDA as a tissue establishment. *[1: Regulatory Requirement]*

The facility would meet the exception from registration described in section 1271.15(b), in which storage of tissue for autologous use is exempt as long as no other manufacturing controls are performed (ie, subjecting the autograft to the steam sterilization process, distributing the autograft to another facility).[3,4]

II.b. The cranial bone flap to be replanted may be stored in a subcutaneous pocket within the patient in an anatomical location determined by the physician. *[3: Moderate Evidence]*

The collective evidence indicates there are two primary methods for preserving autologous cranial bone flaps: preserving the flap in the patient's body and storing the flap outside of the body.[53,71,86,94] The most commonly used preservation methods are frozen storage or storage in a subcutaneous pocket, most often in the lower abdominal wall, anterolateral thigh, or scalp.

The limitations of the evidence are that some research studies had small sample sizes, and the results of the studies may not be generalizable to all settings where cranial bone grafts are replanted.

The benefits of subcutaneous storage of autologous cranial bone flaps are that it may offer a sterile,[95] physiological storage environment that reduces graft devitalization,[75,78,80] and the autograft cannot be lost when stored within the patient.[95] The benefits of subgaleal storage are that it avoids an abdominal scar and may be less time consuming to perform than subcutaneous abdominal storage.[96]

The harms associated with subcutaneous storage of autologous cranial bone flaps are that the procedure requires additional surgical time and may require an additional surgical incision, and the graft may be contaminated during recovery, during storage, or during the replantation procedure. Patients may experience discomfort from the stored autograft, and osteoclast activity may cause the autograft to diminish in size during subcutaneous storage.[75,78,97]

Zingale and Albanese[86] conducted a meta-analysis of the literature to investigate the best methods for preserving autologous cranial bone flaps for delayed replantation. Statistical analysis showed no significant difference between frozen storage and subcutaneous storage relative to the frequency of postoperative complications (ie, bone resorption, infection). However, the researchers opined that frozen storage was superior to subcutaneous storage because it requires no additional surgical time, and the frozen bone flap may be stronger than the fresh flap. The researchers concluded there was a need for more research in this area.

In a retrospective study to investigate whether differences in the storage method of cranial bone flaps affected the incidence of postoperative surgical site infection (SSI), Inamasu et al[98] compared the incidence of SSI in 70 patients undergoing decompressive craniectomy and subsequent cranioplasty with autologous cranial bone during a nine-year period in a tertiary trauma referral center. Bone flaps for 39 patients were stored subcutaneously in the patient's abdominal wall. Bone flaps for the remaining 31 patients were immersed in 10% povidone-iodine solution immediately after recovery, wrapped in sterile gauze, and stored in the facility freezer at -94° F (-70° C). The frozen bone flaps were thawed at room temperature immediately before cranioplasty. Two patients from the subcutaneous storage group (5.1%), and five patients from the frozen storage group (16.1%) developed an SSI. The difference was not statistically significant. The researchers concluded that subcutaneous storage and frozen storage of cranial bone flaps were equally efficacious storage methods, but subcutaneous storage may be the better method.

Sultan et al[99] conducted a prospective study to compare frozen and subcutaneous storage of cranial bone grafts in rats. The cranial bone grafts (N = 30) were stored in a surgically created subcutaneous pocket in the animals' abdominal walls (n = 15) or wrapped in sterile saline-soaked gauze, placed in a 50 cm³ conical tube, and frozen at -112° F (-80° C) (n = 15). After 10 days of storage, the grafts were either replanted (subcutaneous, n = 3; frozen, n = 3), or analyzed (subcutaneous, n = 12; frozen, n = 12). The researchers found no microbial growth after culturing the frozen bone grafts and found normal skin flora after culturing the subcutaneous grafts. After 12 weeks, the researchers found there was limited bony union and considerable bone resorption in all the replanted grafts. The researchers concluded that neither storage method maintained bone graft viability, but subcutaneous storage might provide a small advantage compared with frozen storage.

In a retrospective study, Shoakazemi et al[77] reviewed the medical records of 100 consecutive patients who underwent decompressive craniectomy, storage of the excised cranial bone flap in a subcutaneous pocket in the abdominal wall, and subsequent replantation at a regional hospital neuroscience unit between 2000 and 2005. The researchers analyzed patient outcomes one year after the replantation procedure. They found eight patients had died before replantation of the stored cranial bone flap, and data were missing for three patients. Of the 89 patients who had their cranial bone flaps replanted, the bone flaps were removed for seven patients (7.8%) because of infection (n = 5; 5.6%) or for cosmetic reasons associated with bone flap resorption (n = 2; 2.2%) and were successfully replanted in 82 patients (92%). The researchers concluded that storage of the excised cranial bone flap in a subcutaneous pouch in the patient's abdominal wall produced a favorable long-term outcome.

Movassaghi et al[78] conducted a retrospective study of 53 of 65 consecutive patients who underwent emergency decompressive craniectomy with autologous cranial bone placement in the abdominal wall for 15 to 388 days. The study was conducted in a medical school general hospital during a six-year period. Clinical outcome after autograft replantation was determined by the ability of the stored cranial bone to achieve a satisfactory cosmetic result, the incidence of infection, and the need for additional surgery.

The researchers found that 49 of the 53 patients (92%) achieved a satisfactory reconstruction. In eight patients (15%), it was necessary to supplement the graft with alloplastic material to achieve the desired contour. One patient (2%) required a secondary procedure to improve the cranial contour. Three patients (6%) developed infections, including one patient whose graft was found to be infected when retrieved from the abdominal pocket.[78]

The researchers also histologically evaluated the bone viability of two autografts after subcutaneous storage and assessed the extent of autograft revascularization using bone scans one year after graft replantation in two patients. They found a mixture of necrotic and newly formed bone during the histological examinations. The bone scans showed that the osteoblast activity of the replanted cranial graft was almost identical to that of the adjacent bone. The researchers concluded that subcutaneous storage preserved the viability of the excised cranial bone graft and that cranioplasty performed with subcutaneously preserved cranial bone graft had low infection and revision rates.[78]

Baldo and Tacconi[75] conducted a prospective pilot study during a one-year period in a university hospital in Trieste, Italy, to assess the effectiveness and safety of reconstructing a cranial bone defect using an autologous cranial bone flap stored subcutaneously in the patient's abdominal wall. The researchers evaluated the infection rate and the need for revision in 12 of 15 consecutive patients who had undergone

203

decompressive craniectomy and subsequent cranioplasty with autologous cranial bone flap stored in the patient's abdominal wall for 15 to 180 days.

To assess the viability of the bone, a bone biopsy was taken at the time the cranial flap was placed into the subcutaneous abdominal pocket and also when the cranial flap was removed for replantation. Cultures were taken from the subcutaneous site where the cranial bone had been stored and also from the site of replantation. A computed tomography (CT) scan was performed a few days after replantation and at six months after surgery to quantify the degree of bone gapping. Technetium bone scans were performed in four patients one year after replantation to assess the extent of graft revascularization. Hospital nurses subjectively assessed cosmetic appearance as good, satisfactory, or poor on postoperative day one, three, five, and seven and at three, six, nine, and 12 months.[75]

Among the 15 consecutive patients, two died and one patient was diagnosed with a malignant brain tumor that prevented replantation of the autologous cranial bone flap. Among the remaining 12 patients, two died from complications not related to the procedure, and one patient was not available for follow up. None of the patients developed an infection, and in all cases, the nurses had rated the patient's overall cosmetic appearance as good. All of the bone samples had a normal histological appearance.[75]

The CT scans showed no significant bone resorption. The technetium bone scans showed an insignificant reduction in perfusion. The researchers concluded that subcutaneous storage of an autologous cranial bone flap was a feasible option that preserved the viability of the autograft, provided good cosmetic results, and resulted in low infection rates.[75]

In 75 cases of cranioplasty with subcutaneously preserved cranial autografts in Kosova during an eight-year period, Morina et al[80] placed the excised cranial bone graft in the patient's left abdomen with the convex part of the autograft on the upper side to prevent interference with potential future appendectomy or cholecystectomy procedures and to prevent skin injury from the bone edges. The duration of subcutaneous abdominal storage ranged from 14 to 232 days. The authors reported that 66 patients (88%) achieved a satisfactory cosmetic result, whereas nine patients (12%) required augmentation of the replanted cranial bone flap with methyl methacrylate to achieve a satisfactory result.

Two patients (2.7%) developed postoperative infections requiring removal of the graft and subsequent replacement with methyl methacrylate after six months. Two patients (2.7%) complained of abdominal pressure. The authors concluded that storage of autologous cranial bone flaps in a subcutaneous pocket of the patient's abdominal wall was a safe and effective method for preserving the cranial bone graft and achieved satisfactory cosmetic results.[80]

Flannery and McConnell[95] described their experience with 20 patients who underwent decompressive craniectomy with subcutaneous placement of the autologous cranial bone graft during an 11-month period at a busy regional trauma center. The autografts were stored subcutaneously in the patient's abdominal wall for a period of six weeks to three months. The authors noted that for patients in whom the autograft was stored for a longer period of time, there was some difficulty in removal as a result of the granulation tissue that had formed around the graft.

The authors reported that all of the cranial bone flaps appeared visually normal after removal from the abdomen. All of the cranioplasty and abdominal wounds healed without any procedure-related complications or evidence of bone resorption, with the exception of one patient who developed a wound infection and one patient who required removal of a loose screw. The authors suggested that preservation of the excised cranial bone flap in a subcutaneous pocket of the patient's abdominal wall provided superior cosmetic results and might represent the best option for the patient.[95]

Krishnan et al[96] described their experience using a technique for preserving excised cranial bone flaps in a subgaleal pocket created over the noninvolved side of the cranium. The authors prospectively analyzed 74 consecutive cases of decompressive craniectomy procedures performed at a national neurosciences center during a two-year period. The cranial bone flap was preserved in a subgaleal pocket in 55 patients (74%), was preserved in a subcutaneous abdominal pocket in nine patients (12%), and was not preserved in 10 patients (14%).

To decrease the potential for abrasion of the overlying skin, the sharp edges of the excised cranial bone were removed before the autograft was placed in the abdominal or subgaleal space. The cranial bone flaps were stored from six weeks to eight months before replantation. After removal from the abdominal or subgaleal pocket, the authors examined the flaps and did not find any macroscopic evidence of bone resorption.[96]

The authors encountered complications in two cases. One patient developed a skin breakdown caused by a sharp bone spicule on the graft, and one patient developed a skin necrosis caused by the storage pocket being too small. The authors suggested that subgaleal preservation of the patient's cranial bone flap provided better physiological and cosmetic results than other methods of storage.[96]

Pasaoglu et al[81] described their experience managing 27 patients undergoing decompressive craniectomy with subgaleal preservation of the autologous cranial bone flap at a university school of medicine during a 30-month period. The cranial bone flaps were stored in a subgaleal pocket for a period of 14 to 98 days before replantation. The macroscopic appearance of the autografts removed from the subgaleal space in preparation for replantation was normal. The authors encountered no bone resorption, infection, or complaints of discomfort during the 26-month follow-up period and found that cosmetic results were excellent.

In a literature review of 18 articles related to subcutaneous storage of excised cranial bone flaps under the scalp (ie, subgaleal) and in the abdominal wall, Joaquim et al[94] concluded that it was not possible to state with certainty that one method was superior to another. They concluded that further research was warranted, and the method of storage should be determined based on factors specific to the patient and situation.

II.c.   Autologous bone should not be subjected to the steam sterilization process unless there is a clinical indication to do so. *[3: Moderate Evidence]*

The collective evidence suggests that subjecting excised cranial bone flaps to the steam sterilization process may denature bone protein and severely damage the bone structure and increase the potential for bone resorption and infection[84]; however, steam sterilization may also destroy and prevent recurrence of tumor cells.[82,85] There are gaps in the literature related to best practices for management of autologous cranial bone flaps removed for treatment of brain tumors and subjected to steam or other sterilization processes. Further research is warranted.

The limitations of the evidence are that some research studies had small sample sizes, and the results of the studies may not be generalizable to all settings in which autologous cranial bone grafts are used.

The benefits of subjecting autologous cranial bone flaps to the steam sterilization process are that it may destroy tumor cells and may allow for reuse of the patient's autologous cranial bone for cranioplasty after tumor removal.[82,85] The harms associated with subjecting autologous cranial bone flaps to the steam sterilization process are that it denatures bone protein and may severely damage the bone structure and increase the potential for bone resorption and infection.[84] The steam sterilization process has not been validated for use with human tissue for transplantation. A significantly high rate of postoperative graft infection was found when cranial bone grafts subjected to the steam sterilization process were used for cranial reconstruction.[83]

Osawa et al[100] described their experience with 27 cases of cranioplasty performed with autologous cranial bone flaps that had been frozen and then subjected to a steam sterilization process before replantation. The excised cranial bone flaps were wrapped in sponges that had been soaked in a solution supplemented with either gentamicin 10 mg or amikacin 200 mg. The researchers did not specify the amount of irrigation solution or how many bone flaps were soaked in each antibiotic. The bone flaps were then sealed in a sterile plastic bag, and stored at -112° F (-80° C) in a facility freezer for 19 to 79 days. The day before the replantation procedure, the bone flaps were thawed and subjected to a steam sterilization process at 270° F (132° C) for 20 minutes. The researchers did not provide information as to the type of cycle that was used (ie, gravity or prevacuum) or whether any dry time was applied.

The authors took samples of the cranial bone flaps and performed histological examination when the cranial bone flap was removed from the patient, after storage at -112° F (-80° C) for seven days, and after the steam sterilization process. The patients were followed for a period of four months to two years. During this time, the authors performed skull radiographs to evaluate the amount of bone resorption. There were no serious complications except in two patients who developed small areas of bone resorption and in one patient who developed an epidural abscess that required removal of the autologous cranial bone flap. The histological examination showed only minimal effects on bone structure from the freezing and steam sterilization process. The authors suggested that subjecting the cranial bone flap to the steam sterilization process did not increase the risk of postoperative complications, such as bone resorption or infection.[100]

In a nonexperimental study to investigate the effects of the steam sterilization process on bone morphology, Vanaclocha et al[82] examined the excised cranial bone flaps of 62 patients undergoing craniectomy procedures for treatment of 64 tumors (meningiomas, n = 35; bone tumors, n = 16; scalp tumors, n = 8; metastasis, n = 5) in a university medical center during a six-year period. The researchers contended that bone flaps infiltrated by tumor cells could not be replanted because of the propensity of the tumor cells to invade and destroy the bone; however, they theorized that although the steam sterilization process destroys living cells and damages bone structure, the remaining bone scaffolding might allow for repopulation of the bone and the creation of new bone through the remodeling process.

The researchers cleaned the excised cranial bone flaps, and subjected them to the steam sterilization process at 273° F (134° C) for 20 minutes. The bone flaps were soaked for 15 minutes in normal saline solution supplemented with rifampicine, rinsed with sterile normal saline solution, and then replanted into the patient. The researchers did not provide information as to the type of cycle that was used (ie, gravity or prevacuum) or whether any dry time was applied, nor did they specify the amount of rifampicine or the amount of normal saline used for the soaking solution.[82]

The researchers followed the patients for 10 to 58 months; in addition to conducting the postoperative clinical examinations, they took radiographs and photographs at each follow-up visit. The thickness of the bone flap was assessed by CT scan as needed. In six patients, bone biopsies of the replanted flaps were taken during a second surgical procedure.[82]

The cosmetic appearance was satisfactory in all patients, there were no postoperative infections, and none of the cranial bone flaps had to be removed because of infection. The histological examination showed complete cellular destruction and preservation of the mineral matrix with severe damage to the protein structure of the bone flap. The radiographs and CT scans showed slow but progressive revitalization of the cranial bone grafts. The researchers observed partial bone resorption in 12 patients (19.4%) and some loss of bone volume manifested as bone thinning in 35 patients (56.5%). A second surgery was required for six patients (9.7%) because of a recurrence of the original tumor. The researchers concluded that

- the steam sterilization process destroyed tumor cells in excised cranial bone flaps and helped to prevent tumor recurrence;
- the steam sterilization process severely damaged the bone structure of cranial bone flaps, but the replanted bone flap was progressively revitalized by the adjacent bone; and
- bone resorption was a common occurrence in cranial bone flaps subjected to the steam sterilization process, but it did not lead to bad cosmetic results.[82]

Wester[85] reported the results of 25 cranioplasty procedures. In six patients, the excised cranial bone graft was macroscopically infiltrated with tumor tissue (meningiomas, n = 5; prostate cancer metastasis, n = 1). The cranial bone flaps were removed, cleaned of all osseous material, subjected to the steam sterilization process at 273° F (134° C) for 20 minutes, and replanted. In nine patients, the excised cranial bone grafts were removed, cleaned of all osseous material, subjected to the steam sterilization process at 273° F (134° C) for 20 minutes, preserved in a freezer for three to six months, subjected to the steam sterilization process at 273° F (134° C) for 20 minutes, washed with normal saline solution supplemented with penicillin, and replanted. The researchers did not specify the temperature of the freezer, the amount of penicillin, or the amount of normal saline solution, nor did they provide information as to the type of cycle that was used for the steam sterilization process (ie, gravity or prevacuum) or whether any dry time was applied.

In 10 patients, the excised cranial bone graft was unavailable for storage and replantation, and a reinforced acrylic prosthesis was used for the cranioplasty. All patients were followed for three months to eight years. The researchers found no tumor recurrence in any of the six patients with tumor-infiltrated cranial bone flaps subjected to the steam sterilization process and replanted. One patient required a second surgery for a recurrence of the intracranial malignant tumor. During the procedure, the researchers found that the bone flap was viable and there was no sign of tumor infiltration. The patient lived for another two years and then died from the intracranial malignant tumor. At the time of the patient's death, there was still no sign of tumor infiltration of the cranial bone flap.[85]

There were no postoperative complications in any of the nine patients replanted with autologous cranial bone grafts. Radiographs and CT scans showed revitalization of all bone flaps without bone resorption. The researchers concluded that cranial bone flaps could be revitalized and safely replanted after being subjected to the steam sterilization process, and that the steam sterilization process effectively killed tumor cells in the bone. The researchers also concluded that there was no difference in infection rates between patients who received autologous cranial bone versus those who received cranial grafts made of artificial material; however, the patient's autologous bone provided a satisfactory cosmetic result with a shorter operative time, and for this reason, the researchers recommended replanting autologous bone whenever possible.[85]

Schultke et al[84] conducted a quasi-experimental study to evaluate different methods for disinfecting cranial bone grafts. In the first part of the experiment, the researchers excised 20 palm-sized cranial flaps immediately after craniectomy. The grafts were cleaned of all adherent tissue, washed in 3% H_2O_2 solution, placed into a sterile double-layer package, placed in a sterile plastic bag, and stored at -5.8° F (-21° C). After storage for various periods of time, the bone flaps were removed, thawed, and boiled in normal saline solution for 30 minutes. The researchers did not provide details regarding the length of time the grafts were stored or the thawing or boiling process that was used. The researchers examined the boiled bone flaps and found a bacterial contamination rate of 20%.

In the second part of the experiment, the researchers compared three methods for disinfecting autologous cranial bone grafts to be replanted. After disinfection as described in the first part of the experiment, eight bone flaps from patients who did not survive their stroke or brain injury were divided into 84 sterile bone pieces. The bone pieces were artificially contaminated with virulent strains of *Serratia marcescens*, *Enterococcus faecium*, or *Staphylococcus aureus*. The pieces from each contamination group were divided, frozen at -5.8° F (-21° C), thawed, and disinfected by boiling in normal saline solution for 15 minutes, boiling in normal saline solution for 30 minutes, immersing in 3% H_2O_2 solution for 60 minutes, or heating at 167° F (75° C) for 20 minutes in a prevacuum steam sterilizer. The researchers did not provide information regarding the length of time the grafts were stored, the thawing or boiling process that was used, or whether any dry time was applied during the sterilization process.[84]

The researchers examined the bone pieces from each group for bacterial contamination and found no bacterial strains in the group treated in the prevacuum steam sterilizer. The researchers concluded that steam disinfection at 167° F (75° C) for 20 minutes in a prevacuum steam sterilizer was an effective method for disinfecting autologous cranial bone grafts before replantation.[84]

To evaluate the effectiveness of using ethylene oxide (ETO) and room temperature storage of excised autologous cranial bone flaps, Jho et al[97] conducted a retrospective review of 103 consecutive patients who underwent decompressive craniectomy and subsequent cranioplasty with autologous cranial bone flap in a university medical center between March 1999 and July 2005. After craniectomy, the excised cranial bone flaps were cleaned of any remaining soft tissue. The flaps were air dried for 72 hours and then placed into two sealed sterilization pouches, one pouch inside of the other. Both pouches were labeled with patient identification information.

The sealed packages were subjected to an ETO sterilization process and aerated for 16 hours to remove residual ETO from the bone flap and packaging. The packaged bone flaps were then stored in a locked cabinet maintained at a temperature of 68° F (20° C) for nine days to 15 months before replantation into the patient. The researchers followed the patients for one to 63 months after the procedure.[97]

Aesthetic and functional results of the cranioplasty procedure were assessed by CT scans and cosmetic appearance. The researchers found that 95 patients (92.2%) had excellent cosmetic and functional results. Eight patients (7.8%) developed postoperative infections requiring removal of the flap and subsequent reconstruction with methyl methacrylate with satisfactory results. A preservation time longer than 10 months was associated with a significantly increased risk of infection. The researchers concluded that subjecting the excised cranial bone flap to the ETO sterilization process and storing at room temperature was simple and effective; however, they suggested that bone flaps preserved beyond 10 months be discarded or reprocessed before use.[97]

II.c.1.   Facilities or health care organizations that subject autologous bone to steam or other sterilization processes that require manufacturing controls must register with the FDA as a tissue establishment that manufactures human cells, tissues, and cellular and tissue-based products and must follow applicable requirements of 21 CFR Part 1271.[3,5] *[1: Regulatory Requirement]*

Subjecting tissue to mechanisms for sterilization, such as the steam sterilization process, for the purpose of inactivating or removing adventitious agents is considered processing under section 1271.3(ff), and under section 1271.220(c), would require manufacturing controls to validate that the correct time, temperature, and pressure has been achieved with each load.[3,5]

Recommendation III

The patient's parathyroid tissue may be cryopreserved and autotransplanted.

The collective evidence suggests there is an indication for autotransplantation of cryopreserved autologous parathyroid tissue in cases of postoperative hypoparathyroidism resulting from the unintentional removal or injury of parathyroid glands during thyroid and parathyroid surgery.[101-103]

A standard protocol for the cryopreservation of parathyroid tissue does not exist.[104] The cryopreservation process may impair cellular function and viability and lead to cell necrosis.[101] Autograft functionality may depend on storage time and may decrease with storage times longer than 22 months.[101] Further research is warranted to determine the optimal process of cryopreservation to enhance cell viability.[105,106]

The limitations of the evidence are that there was an inadequate amount of literature addressing this practice issue. The research studies had small sample sizes, and there was no uniform assessment of cell viability. Although one study included samples that had been cryopreserved for as long as 15 years, there was no controlled method of cryopreservation for the samples included in that study.[105]

The benefits of cryopreservation and autotransplantation of the patient's parathyroid tissue are that it permits storage of parathyroid tissue for later transplantation without compromising cellular integrity or function[107] and also allows the clinician to determine whether any residual parathyroid tissue will recover function or whether a delayed autotransplantation will be required.[101] Autotransplantation of cryopreserved parathyroid tissue can eliminate or minimize the requirements for calcium and vitamin D supplementation required for patients who have lost thyroid function.[105]

The harms associated with cryopreservation and autotransplantation of patients' parathyroid tissue include the need for a secondary surgery, increased cost, and the increased potential for infection from transplanting contaminated or nonviable autologous parathyroid tissue. There is an increased risk of autograft failure with cryopreserved tissue compared with fresh tissue.[106] Parathyroid tissue may be destroyed by the cryopreservation process or degraded to the extent that insufficient parathyroid hormone is released after autotransplantation.[106] Long-term storage of autologous tissue carries with it the potential for mix-ups if autograft labeling methods are inadequate (eg, smudging of identifiers during cold storage, labels separating from the package), and contamination or cross-contamination if the graft's packaging material is not validated for use at the storage temperature selected.

III.a. Parathyroid tissue may be cryopreserved for delayed autotransplantation for as long as 24 months. *[3: Moderate Evidence]*

Agarwal et al[107] described the cryopreservation technique and storage methods used for autologous parathyroid glands in a university medical center since 2002. Within 15 minutes of excision, fragments of parathyroid tissue removed from the patient were minced into 30 to 40 uniform small pieces (ie, 2 mm), suspended in sterile normal saline solution, and drawn into a 1 mL tuberculin syringe. The syringe was capped and labeled, placed into a plastic bag labeled as biohazardous, surrounded by ice, and immediately transported by perioperative personnel to the laboratory where the autologous parathyroid segments were preserved in cryopreservation media and stored in liquid nitrogen.

To prevent storage of cancerous or nonparathyroid tissue, the pathologist histologically confirmed the tissue to be normal parathyroid tissue by frozen section before the cryopreservation process was initiated. Perioperative personnel collected approximately 5 mL to 10 mL of the patient's blood in tubes that contained no additives. The tubes were labeled and transported to the laboratory where the blood was

---

OVERVIEW OF PARATHYROID CRYOPRESERVATION AND AUTOTRANSPLANTATION

Parathyroid cryopreservation is performed to provide a source of viable parathyroid tissue that can be autotransplanted at a later date to treat permanent hypoparathyroidism that may occur after thyroid or parathyroid surgery.[1-3] The risk of hypoparathyroidism is greatest after subtotal or total parathyroidectomy, thyroid resection, nodal dissection for large thyroid cancers, and reoperative neck procedures.[4] Permanent hypoparathyroidism is defined as persistent hypocalcemia requiring calcium and vitamin D supplements six months after surgery.[5] Effective management of hypoparathyroidism requires lifelong medication and frequent laboratory testing and may necessitate frequent hospital admissions.[5] The absence of parathyroid hormone has long-term systemic effects on the body, including the development of osteoporosis, premature cataracts, cardiac dysfunction, and neurologic dysfunction.[5] Hypoparathyroidism that persists longer than six months after parathyroid or thyroid surgery is commonly treated with autotransplantation of cryopreserved autologous parathyroid tissue if it is available.[5]

Intraoperative preparation of parathyroid tissue for cryopreservation most often involves removing the tissue surgically and then dissecting it into small segments approximately 1 mm x 1 mm x 1 mm.[4] The segments are placed into a sterile container, positioned on ice, and transported to the laboratory for cyropreservation.[4] On the day of the autotransplantation procedure, the parathyroid tissue to be transplanted is removed from storage and placed in a warm water bath until thawed.[4] The tissue segments may be rinsed in a serial fashion to remove any cryoprotectant residue or contaminants that may be present on the tissue.[4] Pockets are created in the brachioradialis muscle of the nondominant arm,[4] sternocleidomastoid muscle, thigh muscles, or muscles of the anterior chest or abdominal wall.[5] One to three parathyroid tissue segments are placed into each muscle pocket until a total of 20 to 40 segments has been transplanted.[4] It is important to prevent excess bleeding, because an intramuscular hematoma may compromise graft function.[4]

Success of the autotransplantation is measured by sampling blood from both the grafted and nongrafted arms to determine parathyroid hormone levels at both sites.[4] Transplanted parathyroid segments may require as long as six months to resume adequate function.[5] The autograft is considered to be fully functional when the patient remains asymptomatic and is no longer dependent on calcium and vitamin D supplements.[4] The success of the autotransplantation may depend on the cryopreservation process used, the amount of storage time, and the amount and size of the parathyroid segments transplanted.[5]

REFERENCES

1. Guerrero MA. Cryopreservation of parathyroid glands. Int J Endocrinol. 2010;2010:829540. Epub December 8, 2010.
2. Stotler BA, Reich-Slotky R, Schwartz J, et al. Quality monitoring of microbial contamination of cryopreserved parathyroid tissue. Cell Tissue Bank. 2011;12(2):111-116.
3. Cohen MS, Dilley WG, Wells SA Jr, et al. Long-term functionality of cryopreserved parathyroid autografts: a 13-year prospective analysis. Surgery. 2005;138(6):1033-1040.
4. Agarwal A, Waghray A, Gupta S, Sharma R, Milas M. Cryopreservation of parathyroid tissue: an illustrated technique using the Cleveland Clinic protocol. J Am Coll Surg. 2013;216(1):e1-e9.
5. Guerrero MA, Evans DB, Lee JE, et al. Viability of cryopreserved parathyroid tissue: when is continued storage versus disposal indicated? World J Surg. 2008;32(5):836-839.

used to prepare the cryopreservation media. The cryopreservation process took approximately one to two hours. The tissue was stored for a minimum of two years.[107]

Laboratory personnel were notified the day before the autotransplantation procedure in order to allow sufficient time to thaw the desired quantity of parathyroid tissue. The tissue was gradually thawed and delivered to the operating room (OR) either at room temperature or on ice, based on the surgeon's preference. Perioperative personnel transferred the tissue to a sterile specimen cup and diluted it with sterile normal saline solution.[107]

The surgeon transplanted the parathyroid tissue into several small muscular pockets of the patient's nondominant arm, with one to two fragments transplanted into each pocket. The surgeon determined the amount of parathyroid tissue to be replanted, which was generally an amount equal to two normal-sized parathyroid glands. After surgery, the surgeon closely monitored the patient's serum calcium and parathyroid hormone levels. The authors noted that parathyroid function may take several weeks to manifest as levels detectable with blood samples.[107]

Stotler et al[102] described a university medical center's quality monitoring protocol for detecting the presence of bacterial contamination in parathyroid tissue intended for autotransplantation. Laboratory personnel performed bacterial cultures on all parathyroid tissue immediately before processing of the tissue and at the completion of the cryopreservation process; cultures were also performed on the corresponding cryopreservation medium. If the culture result was positive, they performed a Gram stain and subcultured the samples in cell media. Bacterial identification and antimicrobial susceptibility testing were performed.

Between January 2005 and October 2008, a total of 47 parathyroid tissues were cryopreserved for potential future autotransplantation. The authors found bacterial contamination in 23% of cases (n = 11). Contamination was present before tissue processing in 91% of the contaminated samples (n = 10). In 27% of the contaminated samples (n = 3), contamination was present both before and after processing. In 9% (n = 1), contamination was found only after processing. Of the 11 contaminated samples, 55% (n = 6) grew *Staphylococcus epidermidis*. The authors concluded there is a need to monitor the contamination levels of resected parathyroid tissue that will be cryopreserved and replanted into a patient.[102]

In a study conducted to determine the viability of cryopreserved autologous parathyroid tissue in relation to the length of time in storage and to define the most effective time frame for tissue transplantation and disposal, Guerrero et

al[105] identified all parathyroid autografts cryopreserved at -112° F (-80° C) between 1991 and 2006 at a major medical college. From the 501 cryopreserved parathyroid autografts, four to 12 samples from each year were randomly selected for the study (N = 106).

The researchers assessed cell viability using a hemacytometer to count viable and nonviable cells. Of the 106 autografts, only 11 (10.3%) were found to be viable. The researchers found that one autograft was viable for 120 months, but none of the autografts were viable for longer than 120 months. Of the autografts cryopreserved for 24 months or less, 71.4% (10 of 14) were viable, compared with only 1.1% of autografts (one of 92) stored for more than 24 months. The single autograft with evidence of viability beyond 24 months had only 2% viable cells.[105]

The researchers concluded that the viability of the cryopreserved parathyroid cells was associated with the duration of storage and that parathyroid tissue preserved for longer than 24 months was unlikely to be viable. They recommended limiting the preservation time for parathyroid tissue to 24 months. The researchers noted that knowing the viability of cryopreserved autologous parathyroid tissue could help to minimize ethical concerns and enable more objective decision-making related to establishing time frames for discarding autologous parathyroid tissue.[105]

Alvarez-Hernandez et al[108] conducted a quasi-experimental study to test the viability and functionality of fresh and cryopreserved parathyroid tissue. Small fragments of 18 parathyroid glands removed from 18 patients with secondary hyperparathyroidism were cultured immediately after excision and again after cryopreservation at -112° F (-80° C) for a maximum of 18 months. The researchers found that cell viability at both the beginning and end of the testing period was greater than 85% and concluded there were no differences in viability or functionality between the fresh and cryopreserved parathyroid tissue.

In a prospective study to determine the amount of time that human parathyroid tissue can be stored before cryopreservation, Barreira et al[109] evaluated parathyroid tissue from 11 patients undergoing total parathyroidectomy in a university medical center between April and October 2009. Immediately after surgical resection, the researchers cut the parathyroid tissue intended for pathology examination into 2-mm segments. The resected tissue was equally divided into five groups and examined immediately after resection and after storage at 39.2° F (4° C) in Dulbecco's modified Eagle's medium for two, six, 12, and 24 hours.

The researchers found that 10 (90.9%) of the parathyroid tissue samples maintained structural integrity at the molecular level for up to

12 hours. At 24 hours, all of the samples showed degenerative changes in cell cytoplasm and mitochondria. Two samples (18.2%) showed cellular changes consistent with apoptosis and cell death. The researchers concluded that molecular structural integrity was maintained in the parathyroid tissue segments stored for as long as 12 hours in culture medium at 39.2° F (4° C).[109]

Cohen et al[103] conducted a study of 29 patients who underwent 34 parathyroid autotransplantation procedures in a university medical center between November 1991 and November 2004. After surgical resection, the researchers divided the parathyroid tissue into 30 to 40 segments approximately 1 mm x 1 mm x 3 mm. The fragments were placed in a sterile medicine cup filled with normal saline solution and then placed on ice and submitted to laboratory personnel for cryopreservation. In addition to the parathyroid tissue, perioperative personnel drew 10 mL of the patient's blood and submitted it to the laboratory to prepare autologous serum. The parathyroid tissue was stored in a liquid nitrogen freezer at -274° F (-170° C) for as long as 11 months.

On the day of the procedure, perioperative personnel removed the samples from storage and placed them in a 98.6° F (37° C) water bath. The surgeons placed approximately 20 to 25 pieces of parathyroid tissue (approximately 50 mg to 75 mg) into five to 10 pockets created in the brachioradialis muscle of the patient's forearm. Patients were followed for two months to 11 years, with an average follow-up time of 24 months. Outcomes were determined based on peripheral parathyroid hormone levels. Parathyroid autograft function was defined as

○ completely functional (ie, normal parathyroid hormone and calcium levels with no supplements required),

○ partially functional (ie, normal parathyroid hormone levels and mild hypocalcemia requiring calcium supplementation), or

○ nonfunctional (ie, low parathyroid hormone levels and dependence on calcium and vitamin D supplementation).[103]

Of the 29 patients, prospective data were available for 26 patients undergoing 30 parathyroid autotransplantation procedures. The researchers found that 12 of the 26 patients (46%) had completely functional autografts, six patients (23%) had partially functional autografts, and eight patients (31%) had nonfunctional autografts. The researchers found the duration of cryopreservation was a significant indicator of graft failure.[103]

The 18 functional grafts had an average cryopreservation time of 7.9 months. The eight nonfunctional grafts had an average cryopreservation time of 15.3 months. No autograft was observed to be functional beyond 22 months of cryopreservation, suggesting that shorter cryo-

preservation times may result in an improved functional outcome. None of the patients experienced recurrent hyperparathyroidism. The researchers concluded that delayed replantation of cryopreserved parathyroid tissue is beneficial for patients who have permanent postoperative hypoparathyroidism.[103]

de Menezes Montenegro et al[110] reported successful results with autotransplantation of parathyroid tissue cryopreserved for 21 months. The patient was a 40-year-old woman with renal hyperparathyroidism who underwent total parathyroidectomy with cryopreservation of parathyroid tissue. After 21 months of follow up, she was hypocalcemic and had an undetectable parathyroid hormone level. Approximately 45 cryopreserved parathyroid segments were thawed and transplanted into her forearm. After autotransplantation, the patient's clinical condition improved. Within 18 months, her parathyroid hormone levels were normal, and she did not require any calcium or vitamin D supplements. The authors recommended cryopreservation of excised parathyroid tissue for all cases of hyperparathyroidism should the need to correct postoperative hypoparathyroidism arise.

Saxe et al[106] reported on 12 patients who underwent parathyroid autotransplantation with cryopreserved parathyroid tissue in the forearm between August 1975 and March 1981 in a national cancer institute. The surgeons divided the excised parathyroid tissue into 1 mm x 1 mm x 1 mm segments in the OR in chilled normal saline solution or Roswell Park Memorial Institute 1640 culture medium. Perioperative personnel transported the tissue to the laboratory where it was cryopreserved for two to 18 months.

Two hours before the autotransplantation procedure, perioperative personnel thawed the tissue in a 107.6° F (42° C) water bath. The surgeons placed 20 to 30 segments in an equal number of muscular pockets in the brachioradialis muscle of the nondominant arm. Follow-up ranged from four to 66 months. Because all patients had been dependent on calcium supplements before the autotransplantation procedure, the authors considered freedom from calcium therapy to be the best evidence of autograft function. Six patients (50%) no longer required calcium supplementation and in one patient (8%), the dose was reduced. The researchers concluded that further research was warranted regarding the optimal procedures for cryopreservation of human parathyroid tissue.[106]

To evaluate their experience with parathyroid autotransplantation and analyze the role of cryopreservation and delayed autotransplantation of parathyroid tissue in the treatment of patients with renal hyperparathyroidism, Schneider et al[104] reviewed a university medical center database of 883 patients with renal hyperparathyroidism. They found that 15 patients (1.7%) had undergone delayed parathyroid autotransplantation with parathyroid tissue cryopreserved for one to 86 months between 1976 and 2011. The standardized process used for cryopreservation included first having the pathologist verify parathyroid origin of the excised tissue by histological examination. The surgeons then divided the tissue into 1 mm x 1 mm x 1 mm segments, and perioperative personnel transported the segments to the laboratory in cold normal saline solution.

On the day of the autotransplantation procedure, the pathologist estimated viability of the tissue by histological examination to determine the number of necrotic and viable cells in a sample of the tissue. Laboratory personnel tested the tissue to be autotransplanted for microbial contamination. If the amount of cell necrosis was found to be less than 50% and the sample showed no sign of microbial contamination, laboratory personnel thawed the remaining tissue in a 98.6° F (37° C) water bath, rinsed it, and preserved it on ice during transport to the OR.[104]

During surgery, the surgeons placed approximately 30 segments of parathyroid tissue into muscular pockets in the brachioradialis muscle of the patient's nondominant or non-shunt-bearing arm. The researchers reviewed the histopathology reports and found no necrosis of the tissue in 14 patients (93.3%) and 70% necrosis of the tissue in one patient (6.7%).[104]

The patients' serum calcium and parathyroid hormone levels were closely monitored by the researchers during the follow-up period. The autotransplantation procedure raised serum calcium and parathyroid hormone levels to normal levels in all patients during the 78-month follow-up period. The researchers theorized that the high success rate of the autotransplantation procedure could be explained by the microbiological and histological examinations conducted before autotransplantation because only tissues with low levels of necrosis and no microbial contamination were replanted. They also noted that the time from resection to cryopreservation was always less than one hour. The researchers concluded that the success of the procedure was high; however, because of the low number of patients requiring delayed autotransplantation of parathyroid tissue, the practice of cryopreserving and storing tissue for every patient should be questioned.[104]

III.a.1. Facilities recovering, packaging, labeling, or cryopreserving autologous parathyroid tissue for storage and autotransplantation within the same facility are not required to register with the FDA as a tissue establishment. *[1: Regulatory Requirement]*

The facility would meet the exception from registration described in section 1271.15(b), in which storage of tissue for autologous use is exempt as long as no other manufacturing controls are performed (ie, subjecting the autograft to the steam sterilization process, distributing the autograft to another facility).[3,4]

Recommendation IV

The patient's autologous skin may be preserved and autotransplanted.

The collective evidence indicates that refrigerated storage of split-thickness skin grafts for delayed autotransplantation is a common practice.[111,112] The use of a storage medium may improve and extend the viability of the stored human skin autograft compared with storage in normal saline solution.[113,114] Skin grafts may also be stored at the donor site for delayed autotransplantation.[112] There are gaps in the literature regarding histological changes that occur in stored autologous skin and the optimal storage methods, storage media, storage temperatures, and acceptable length of storage for human skin. Further research is warranted.

Human skin is sometimes meshed before storage. Meshing the skin graft allows the surgeon to stretch the skin graft to cover a larger area and also allows fluid to drain from the underlying wound; however, meshing the skin exposes it to mechanical trauma that may compromise cellular function.[115]

The limitations of the evidence are that only a small amount of literature addressed this practice issue, and the research studies had small sample sizes. One research study did not provide sufficient detail regarding the methods used to prepare human skin autografts for storage, the storage temperatures used, or the time required to thaw frozen autografts.[116]

The benefits of storing autologous skin for delayed autotransplantation include reduced cost and the potential elimination of a secondary donor site. The benefits of storing autologous skin at the donor site for delayed autotransplantation are that it allows the skin graft placement to be performed at the patient's bedside after the initial swelling at the recipient site has gone down.[112] This delayed placement increases the potential for the graft to be accepted by reducing stress on the graft that might occur from its being stretched and pulled over swollen tissue and also helps ensure there is no fluid collection at the recipient site that could collect under the graft, increase tension, and prevent adherence of the graft to the graft site. Storing the patient's skin autograft at the donor site also may prevent the need for an additional surgical procedure.

The harms associated with storing autologous skin for delayed autotransplantation include the increased potential for infection from contaminated or nonviable autologous skin grafts. Long-term storage of autologous tissue carries with it the potential for mix-ups if autograft labeling methods are inadequate (eg, smudging of identifiers during cold storage, labels separating from the package) and for contamination or cross-contamination if the graft's packaging material is not validated for use at the storage temperature selected.

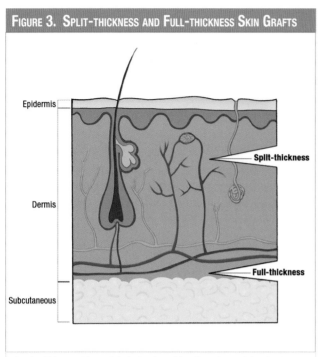

FIGURE 3. SPLIT-THICKNESS AND FULL-THICKNESS SKIN GRAFTS

Epidermis

Dermis

Subcutaneous

Split-thickness

Full-thickness

A split-thickness skin graft includes the epidermis and part of the dermis. A full-thickness skin graft includes the epidermis and all of the dermis.

Illustration by Kurt Jones.

IV.a. Autologous skin for delayed autotransplantation may be refrigerated and stored in normal saline solution or in a storage medium or may be cryopreserved. *[3: Moderate Evidence]*

In a retrospective review conducted between January 1991 and December 1995 in the burn institute of a general hospital and medical school, Sheridan et al[116] found that human skin autografts had been autotransplanted to 42 open wounds in 28 patients. The autografts consisted of remnants of unused skin from the initial split-thickness skin grafting procedure (Figure 3). The remnants of skin had been stored from four to 117 days in one of two ways:

○ If the interval to anticipated autotransplantation was anticipated to be fewer than seven days, the autograft was refrigerated.

○ If the interval to autotransplantation was anticipated to be more than seven days, the skin was treated with 15% glycerol solution; frozen; and stored in a sealed, labeled, plastic envelope.

None of the refrigerated grafts were autotransplanted. The frozen skin was thawed by placing it in room-temperature normal saline solution before replantation. The researchers did not provide information as to the refrigerator or freezer storage temperatures, the method of storage preparation of the refrigerated autografts, the cryopreservation process, or the length of time required to thaw the frozen autografts. Notably, the researchers found documen-

tation of the rate of successful engraftment of the frozen skin in 12 cases. In these cases, the amount of successful engraftment averaged 70%. The researchers recommended autologous skin banking as a method to preserve unused portions of human skin grafts for delayed autotransplantation to minimize the need for obtaining additional tissue from new donor sites.[116]

Sterne et al[115] obtained skin grafts from six patients undergoing abdominoplasty to provide a qualitative description of the histological changes that occurred in split-thickness skin grafts wrapped in saline-soaked gauze and stored at 39.2° F (4° C) during a four-week period. The researchers divided the tissue into two groups of four grafts:

○ unmeshed skin, rolled (ie, folded in half longitudinally with the dermal surfaces contacting each other and rolled);

○ unmeshed skin, flat (ie, folded in half and placed in a sterile plastic cassette and covered with saline-moistened filter paper);

○ meshed skin, rolled; or

○ meshed skin, flat.

The skin grafts were placed on tulle gras, wrapped in saline-soaked gauze, placed into a sterile specimen container, and stored in one of two refrigerators at 39.2° F (4° C). A tissue sample was sent for histological examination at the time of initial storage and after one, seven, 14, 21, and 28 days of refrigeration. The researchers found variability in the size and shape of the cells and cell nuclei beginning at day seven. The meshed skin showed greater swelling and more acute variability in the shape of the cells and cell nuclei. From day 14 through day 21, the structure of the dermal collagen became progressively degraded. From day 21 through day 28, the researchers found extensive separation of the epidermis from its vascular supply. They concluded that the viability of the stored grafts was greatest when the grafts were stored as an unmeshed roll at 39.2° F (4° C) for fewer than seven days.[115]

Titley et al[117] conducted a quantitative and qualitative study of 102 consecutive split-thickness skin grafts to

○ identify the organisms colonizing split-thickness skin grafts at the time of recovery and after three weeks of refrigerated storage,

○ relate the number of organisms on fresh skin to the percentage of successful engraftment, and

○ compare the number of organisms contaminating skin grafts.

The study was conducted in a plastic surgery unit of a regional hospital. The researchers took tissue samples of all skin autografts. The grafts were placed on tulle gras, wrapped in saline-moistened gauze, placed into a sterile specimen container, and stored in the facility refrigerator at 42.8° F to 51.8° F (6° C to 11° C) for as long as three weeks.[117]

When the stored skin was autotransplanted, the researchers took a second sample of the graft. *Staphylococcus aureus* and coagulase-negative staphylococci were the organisms most commonly isolated from the initial skin sample. There was no growth in 56.9% of the grafts (n = 58), but more than one organism was grown from 10.8% of the grafts (n = 11). At three weeks, the remaining stored skin was submitted for microbial examination. The researchers found that coagulase-negative staphylococci were still the predominant organisms on the grafts; however, there was an increase in the number of *Acinetobacter* and *Pseudomonas* species. The researchers also found more organisms on the skin grafts of male patients than of female patients. They theorized that because men have more body hair than women, there may be more preoperative shaving of the male donor sites. The shaving may have caused microscopic wounds that increased bacterial proliferation, particularly if the patient was shaved several hours before the procedure.[117]

During the first dressing change, the researchers recorded the percentage of the graft that had successfully engrafted. They found the percentage of successful engraftment was inversely proportional to the number of microorganisms on the grafts (ie, as the number of microorganisms increased, the percentage of engraftment decreased). Notably, the researchers found a spike in temperature (57° F [13.9° C]) whenever the refrigerator door was opened. The researchers concluded that storage of human skin autografts in refrigerators allowed for significant bacterial proliferation during a three-week storage period. The researchers also concluded there was a need for strict temperature monitoring of refrigerators used for storage of human skin autografts. They suggested that the temperature of the refrigerator be maintained at 39.2° F (4° C) or colder to help prevent bacterial proliferation.[117]

DeBono et al[111] conducted a quasi-experimental study to assess the efficacy of McCoy's 5A medium for human skin storage and to assess whether supplying supplementary oxygen (O_2) to the medium would improve survival of the graft. The researchers stored two 3-mm discs of split-thickness human skin obtained from a single patient in 40 sterile sealable containers in one of four solutions:

- 4.4 mL normal saline solution plus 80 mg gentamicin,
- 4 mL McCoy's 5A medium plus 80 mg gentamicin,
- 4 mL McCoy's 5A medium plus 80 mg gentamicin supplemented with carbon dioxide (CO_2) at 2 L/minute for 30 seconds repeated every seven days, or

- 4 mL McCoy's 5A medium plus 80 mg gentamicin supplemented with O_2 at 2 L/minute for 30 seconds repeated every seven days.

The sealed containers were stored in a temperature-monitored refrigerator at 39.2° F (4° C). A tissue culture of the stored skin was taken every seven days to assess the viability of the stored skin. The researchers found that the skin stored in McCoy's 5A medium supplemented with CO_2 was viable for less than one week. The skin stored in normal saline solution was viable for only one week. The skin stored in McCoy's 5A medium or in McCoy's 5A medium supplemented with O_2 was viable for four weeks. The researchers noted that oxygenating the medium did not improve the viable storage time, and they theorized that the extended skin viability was caused by the nutrients and buffers present in the medium. The researchers concluded that McCoy's 5A medium was an acceptable storage medium that prolonged the viability of the stored skin for as long as four weeks.[111]

IV.a.1. Facilities recovering, packaging, labeling, and refrigerating autologous skin for storage and autotransplantation within the same facility are not required to register with the FDA as a tissue establishment. *[1: Regulatory Requirement]*

The facility would meet the exception from registration described in section 1271.15(b), in which storage of tissue for autologous use is exempt as long as no other manufacturing controls are performed (ie, subjecting the autograft to the steam sterilization process, distributing the autograft to another facility).[3,4]

IV.b. Human skin for delayed autotransplantation may be stored on the patient's donor site. *[3: Moderate Evidence]*

Mardini et al[112] described their experience with 10 patients undergoing voice reconstruction surgery using jejunal and ileocolonic flaps between January and July 2006. Delayed autotransplantation from the thigh to the neck was carried out at the patient's bedside during the third to eighth postoperative day, using skin that had been recovered from and stored at the patients' thighs during the initial reconstructive surgery. Elevation of the stored graft was well tolerated, and there was greater than 95% engraftment in all cases. The authors found all grafts were completely healed during the five- to 12-month follow-up period. They recommended storage of the skin autograft at the donor site for as long as eight days as a reliable technique with diverse clinical applications when traditional skin banking is not feasible.

AUTOLOGOUS TISSUE MANAGEMENT

Recommendation V

The patient's autologous vein may be preserved and autotransplanted.

The collective evidence indicates that storing unused segments of autologous vein grafts after cardiac surgery for delayed autotransplantation in the event of a graft failure is common,[118,119] especially for older patients.[120] The autologous saphenous vein is the most commonly used conduit in cardiac surgery.[118,120] Storing vein grafts in a manner that prevents epithelial injury and maintains vessel function is important for successful autotransplantation.[120] Endothelial injury resulting from storage of autologous veins may promote vessel thrombosis, vessel wall inflammation, and graft failure.[119] Normal saline and lactated Ringer's solutions have commonly been used for storage of autologous vein grafts; however, using culture media may be a better option for maintaining vessel function.[120] Cryopreservation maintains the elastic properties of the vein[118] but destroys the integrity of the endothelial layer of the vessel, and for this reason, it is not considered to be an effective storage mechanism for autologous vein grafts.[118,120]

The limitations of the evidence are that only a small amount of literature addressed this practice issue, and the research studies had small sample sizes.

The benefits of storing the patient's autologous vein for delayed autotransplantation include reduced cost and the potential elimination of a secondary donor site. The harm associated with storing the patient's autologous vein for delayed autotransplantation is the increased potential for infection from contaminated or nonviable autologous vein grafts.

V.a.   Autologous veins for delayed autotransplantation may be refrigerated and stored in normal saline or lactated Ringer's solution or in a storage medium. *[3: Moderate Evidence]*

To identify alterations in the functional, morphologic, and molecular level of blood vessels after cold storage, Ebner et al[119] examined 2-mm segments of mouse aorta placed in TiProtec® solution and stored at 39.2° F (4° C) after two hours and one, two, four, and seven days. The researchers found significant genetic alterations in the vessel segments within the first two hours of storage. They theorized that these molecular alterations could affect graft function. The researchers also found impairment of vessel function after cold storage for two days; however, they did not find any histologic changes in the structure of the vessel segments. The researchers concluded that storage beyond two days impaired vessel function, but further research was warranted to determine whether any comorbidities are associated with the impaired vessel function.

To investigate the effect of storing saphenous vein segments in normal saline solution compared with TiProtec solution, Wilbring et al[120] isolated 19 saphenous vein segments from patients undergoing coronary artery bypass grafting with autologous saphenous veins in a university heart center between October 2008 and March 2010. The veins were extracted without the use of electrocoagulation. Each vein segment was divided into two parts and placed in either normal saline solution or TiProtec. The vein segments were stored at 39.2° F (4° C) for 96 hours and then examined.

The researchers found that the vessel function was significantly reduced after 24 hours of cold storage in normal saline solution. After 96 hours of storage in normal saline solution, there was minimal to no vessel function remaining. Vascular function of the vein segments stored in TiProtec was significantly better preserved. The researchers concluded that cold storage of venous grafts was feasible for as long as 96 hours when the grafts were stored in TiProtec solution; however, storage of venous grafts in normal saline solution was not recommended beyond 24 hours.[120]

Molnar et al[118] conducted a quasi-experimental study to investigate the passive and active biomechanical properties of 72 saphenous vein segments remaining after coronary bypass grafting from 32 patients in a university medical center. The vein segments were divided into eight testing groups:

- fresh, examined immediately after recovery;
- stored in normal Krebs-Ringer solution at 32° F to 39.2° F (0° C to 4° C), examined one week after recovery;
- stored in normal Krebs-Ringer solution at 32° F to 39.2° F (0° C to 4° C), examined two weeks after recovery;
- stored in X-Vivo 10® at 32° F to 39.2° F (0° C to 4° C), examined one week after recovery;
- stored in X-Vivo 10 at 32° F to 39.2° F (0° C to 4° C), examined two weeks after recovery;
- stored in X-Vivo 10 at 32° F to 39.2° F (0° C to 4° C), examined three weeks after recovery;
- stored in X-Vivo 10 at 32° F to 39.2° F (0° C to 4° C), examined four weeks after recovery; or
- cryopreserved at -220° F (-140° C), examined three weeks after recovery.

The cryopreserved samples were thawed by immersion in warm (98.6° F; 37° C) Krebs-Ringer solution. The biomechanical testing showed that the vein segments stored in Krebs-Ringer solution lost their ability to dilate and contract within one week. The segments stored in X-Vivo 10 preserved their contractility after one week, and it only slowly decreased during the four-week study period. There was a slight decrease in vessel wall thickness, but the lumen diameter was not affected. The elastic parameters were almost identical to the fresh segments. The cryopreserved segments narrowed, the vessel wall thickened, and contractility diminished. The

PATIENT AND WORKER SAFETY

214

researchers concluded that storage in X-Vivo 10 helped to preserve the passive and active biomechanical properties of human saphenous vein segments. They also concluded that maintaining these properties could be expected to improve stored autologous vein graft viability.[118]

Baumann et al[121] used light transmission and scanning electron microscopy to investigate the effects of various methods of vein preparation on endothelial and smooth muscle cells in dog cephalic veins. The researchers removed the veins, divided them into 10-cm segments (N = 10), and placed them in one of three solutions (ie, autologous blood [n = 3], Plasma-Lyte® [n = 2], or Plasma-Lyte with 0.6 mg/mL papaverine [n = 5]) containing heparin 10,000 units/L, and then stored them at 50° F (10° C) for either five minutes or one hour.

The researchers found the vein wall was extremely sensitive to dissection, manipulation, or introduction of fixative solutions and reacted to such stimulations with severe contraction that not only diminished the luminal diameter but also resulted in protrusion of endothelial cells into the lumen and the formation of cytoplasmic extensions of medial smooth muscle cells. The veins stored in autologous blood demonstrated the greatest amount of vessel wall contraction and endothelial cell loss. Veins stored in Plasma-Lyte for five minutes showed few contractions; however, after one hour, there were contractions and some endothelial cell loss. Veins stored in Plasma-Lyte supplemented with papaverine had the most relaxed appearance and minimal endothelial cell loss. The researchers recommended mitigating damaging vein graft contractions by

- using gentle surgical dissection to avoid vein spasm;
- instituting and intermittently repeating (ie, every two to three minutes) gentle perfusion with a solution of Plasma-Lyte supplemented with papaverine immediately after exposure of the distal end of the vein and while the rest of the vein is removed;
- avoiding the use of autologous blood for vein immersion, storage, or distention; and
- monitoring the pressure used to check vein grafts for leaks at less than 100 mmHg.[121]

The researchers concluded that attention to the details of vein dissection, preparation, and storage medium could lead to a significant improvement in endothelial preservation and subsequent patency rates after cardiac bypass procedures.[121]

V.a.1. Facilities recovering, packaging, labeling, and refrigerating autologous veins for storage and autotransplantation within the same facility are not required to register with the FDA as a tissue establishment. *[1: Regulatory Requirement]*

The facility would meet the exception from registration described in section 1271.15(b), in which storage of tissue for autologous use is exempt as long as no other manufacturing controls are performed (ie, subjecting the autograft to the steam sterilization process, distributing the autograft to another facility).[3,4]

Recommendation VI

A multidisciplinary team consisting of the surgeon, perioperative RN, and infection preventionist should conduct a risk assessment to consider the benefits and potential harms associated with replantation or autotransplantation of a contaminated autograft compared with other treatment options (eg, discarding the graft and using artificial material).

The collective evidence indicates there are instances in which autologous grafts necessary for replantation or autotransplantation are contaminated or dropped on the OR floor. The collective evidence also indicates that the infection rate associated with replantation or autotransplantation of contaminated grafts is low.[122-124] Various processes for decontaminating the graft have been implemented; however, there is no consistent protocol for managing the event when this occurs.[122-124] Further research is warranted on best practices for decontaminating contaminated autologous tissue, defining the specifications for low-pressure and high-pressure pulsatile lavage, and determining methods to prevent the graft from being dropped or otherwise contaminated.

The limitations of the evidence are that the long-term risk of SSI related to replantation or autotransplantation of contaminated autologous tissue is unknown. The results of surveys related to management of this event may be subjective and may not reflect the true number of incidents in the broader population. One survey had a low response rate (223 of 1,900; 12%) and therefore cannot be construed as representative of all members of the group surveyed.[124] Some research studies had no negative control. Some studies were conducted in controlled laboratory conditions, and the results of these studies may not be generalizable to settings outside of the laboratory.

The benefits of replantation or autotransplantation of contaminated autologous grafts include reduced cost, surgical time, and need for a secondary procedure and may include improved cosmetic appearance. The harm associated with replantation or autotransplantation of contaminated autologous grafts is the increased potential for the patient to develop an SSI.

In a retrospective review of 15,157 craniectomy procedures during a 16-year period in three health care facilities, Jankowitz and Kondziolka[122] assessed when bone grafts were dropped and how these events were managed. They also conducted a survey of 50 neurosurgeons in the United States to determine their experiences and protocols for managing dropped bone grafts.

In their review, the researchers found 14 instances of dropped cranial bone grafts. The cranial bone flaps were dropped

- during elevation of the bone flap from the cranium (n = 4; 28.6%),
- during movement of the bone flap from the surgical field to the back table (n = 4; 28.6%),
- during plating of titanium hardware (n = 4; 28.6%), and
- for unknown reasons (n = 2; 14.3%).[122]

Management of the dropped cranial bone flaps included

- soaking the flap in povidone-iodine or antibiotic solution and replanting (n = 8; 57.1%),
- subjecting the flap to the steam sterilization process and replanting (n = 2; 14.3%),
- discarding the flap and using artificial materials (n = 3; 21.4%), and
- using unknown methods (n = 1; 7.1%).[122]

According to the survey (N = 50), recommendations for managing dropped cranial bone flaps included

- soaking the flap in povidone-iodine solution and replanting (n = 11; 22%),
- soaking the flap in povidone-iodine and antibiotic solution and replanting (n = 16; 32%),
- subjecting the flap to the steam sterilization process and replanting (n = 18; 36%), and
- discarding the flap and using artificial materials to reconstruct the cranium (n = 9; 18%).[122]

After reviewing the records from 2004 and 2005, the researchers found there were 693 and 692 craniectomy procedures, respectively, that involved excising a cranial bone flap with the intention of replanting it. During this time period, a total of five cranial bone flaps were dropped, resulting in an incidence of 3.6 drops per 1,000 craniotomies (0.36%). The results of the survey showed that 66% of the polled neurosurgeons (n = 33) had experienced a dropped cranial bone graft, and 83% (n = 45 of 54) would replant the dropped graft after implementing a method of disinfection (eg, irrigation with antibiotic solution). There was a greater number of responses than polled surgeons because some surgeons reported their treatment of multiple incidents. The patients were followed for two to 176 months. There were no postoperative infections and no long term complications in any of the patients. The researchers concluded that disinfection of a dropped cranial bone graft and replantation is an acceptable option for treatment.[122]

Kang et al[123] conducted a survey of orthopedic surgeons who routinely performed orthopedic trauma surgery to determine how often autologous bone was dropped on the floor during orthopedic trauma surgery and the decontamination protocols that were implemented on these occasions. A total of 104 orthopedic surgeons responded to the survey. Forty surgeons (38%) reported that they had experienced at least one case in which the autologous bone was dropped from the sterile field during surgery. Methods used by the surgeons for decontaminating the dropped autologous bone included

- irrigating the bone with low-pressure pulsatile lavage (n = 36; 90%),
- soaking the bone in bacitracin solution (n = 28; 70%),
- soaking the bone in povidone-iodine solution (n = 26; 65%),
- soaking the bone in H_2O_2 solution (n = 4; 10%),
- subjecting the bone to the steam sterilization process (n = 7; 18%), and
- using other unspecified methods (n = 27; 68%).[123]

The researchers did not provide a definition for "low-pressure" lavage, the formulation for "bacitracin solution," or the strength of the povidone-iodine and H_2O_2 solutions used. None of the surgeons reported that replantation or autotransplantation of the contaminated autograft resulted in an SSI. The results of the survey showed that approximately one in three surgeons had experienced at least one instance in which autologous bone was dropped from the sterile field during surgery and that multiple methods were used for decontamination of the dropped bone, reflecting a lack of consensus on best practices. The researchers concluded that further research was warranted to determine the best procedures for decontamination of autologous bone after exposure to potential contamination and that guidelines reflecting best practices would be helpful for mitigating risk to patients.[123]

Centeno et al[124] conducted an online survey of 1,900 American Society for Aesthetic Plastic Surgery members to determine their practices for managing contaminated autologous grafts and received 223 responses (12%). The survey was designed to obtain information related to frequency of contamination, treatment preferences, clinical outcomes, and patient disclosure. Surgeons were asked whether they had witnessed or experienced a graft contamination. Thirty-three percent of respondents (n = 52 of 156) reported two occurrences and 26% (n = 40 of 156) reported four or more contaminated autologous graft incidents. The researchers allowed multiple responses for many survey questions to capture a fuller range of experience for each question.

Reasons provided by the surgeons for graft contamination (ie, for 312 contamination incidents reported by 160 respondents) included

- the graft falling on the floor (75%),
- the graft being exposed to a nonsterile part of the drape (44.3%),
- the graft being exposed to a nonsterile part of the surgical field (28.7%),
- the graft being discarded in the trash (28.1%),
- the graft being exposed to a nonsterile specimen container (16.9%), and
- unknown reasons (1.9%).[124]

The anatomical areas involved (ie, for 246 contamination incidents reported by 158 respondents) included

- craniofacial (n = 104; 65.8%),
- lower extremity (n = 43; 27.2%),
- breast (n = 40; 25.3%),
- trunk (n = 28; 17.7%),
- upper extremity (n = 27; 17.1%), and
- genitourinary (n = 4; 2.5%).[124]

The types of contaminated autologous grafts (ie, for 284 contamination incidents reported by 158 respondents) included

- skin (n = 97; 61.4%),
- cartilage (n = 62; 39.2%),
- nipple-areolar complex (n = 35; 22.2%),
- bone (n =34; 21.5%),
- composite (n = 20; 12.7%),
- muscle (n = 18; 11.4%),
- fascia (n = 12; 7.6%), and
- fat (n = 6; 3.8%).[124]

Management of the contaminated autologous grafts (ie, based on responses from 160 respondents, with multiple responses allowed) included

- decontaminating and using the graft (n = 151; 94.4%),
- harvesting a graft from another site (n = 11; 6.9%),
- using another reconstructive technique (n = 6; 3.5%),
- using an alloplastic material or implant (n = 3; 1.9%), and
- discarding the graft and ending the surgery (n = 0).[124]

Solutions and methods used for decontaminating the contaminated autologous graft (ie, based on responses from 157 respondents, with multiple responses allowed) included

- povidone-iodine solution (n = 85; 54.1%),
- antibiotic solution (n = 79; 50.3%),
- normal saline solution with a bulb syringe (n = 67; 42.7%),
- normal saline solution with pulsatile lavage (n = 18; 11.5%),
- chlorhexidine gluconate (CHG) solution (n = 1; 0.6%), and
- no decontamination (n = 4; 3.2%).[124]

More than 98% of plastic surgeons responding to the survey (n = 154) who had experienced a contaminated autologous graft and replanted or autotransplanted the graft responded that its use did not lead to an infection. Only three patients with decontaminated grafts (1.9%) were reported to have developed an infection. Notably, 60% of respondents (n = 96 of 160) did not disclose the incident to the patient.[124]

VI.a.   If a decision is made to replant or autotransplant the contaminated autograft, the following steps should be taken:

- ○ Rinse the contaminated graft in sterile normal saline solution to remove surface debris and contaminants.
- ○ Use pulsatile lavage at low-pressure settings (eg, 6 lb to 14 lb per square inch [psi])[125,126] and use sterile normal saline solution for more thorough cleansing of contaminated bone grafts if indicated (eg, adherent debris).
- ○ Use a separate sterile field for decontaminating the dropped graft and exercise care to prevent splashing onto the primary sterile field.
- ○ Implement corrective actions as necessary to maintain the sterility of the primary sterile field (eg, changing gowns and gloves after pulsatile lavage of the contaminated graft).
- ○ Change the wound classification to Class III, Contaminated.[127]
- ○ Document the event in a variance report.
- ○ Conduct a debriefing session and a root cause analysis with members of the surgical team and other individuals who may be helpful in providing a critical analysis and determining the factors that contributed to the event and methods to prevent its recurrence.

[3: Moderate Evidence]

Rinsing the dropped autograft in normal saline solution may be sufficient to remove surface debris and contaminants. In a randomized controlled trial (RCT) conducted to determine the amount of contamination that occurred when a bone graft was dropped on the floor, Presnal and Kimbrough[128] collected bone samples that were to be discarded during 50 orthopedic and neurosurgical procedures. Two bone samples of similar size were collected from each procedure. The first sample was placed directly into a culture tube under sterile conditions. The second sample was dropped on the OR floor near the operating table. The researchers chose this location because it was a high traffic area and also the most likely place that a bone graft would be dropped.

The bone sample was left on the floor for one minute and then retrieved using sterile technique and placed directly into a culture tube. Perioperative personnel then transported both samples to the laboratory for culture studies. No changes were made to the procedures for cleaning the OR floors, and the team members responsible for cleaning the floors were blinded to the study. Samples were obtained from random ORs at various times during the day. The results showed no positive cultures from either study group. The researchers concluded that replanting a dropped bone graft was acceptable without extensive and potentially damaging efforts to disinfect the graft.[128]

Pulsatile lavage may be useful for removing soil or microorganisms that are difficult to kill or remove with rinsing, such as heavy contamination and debris embedded in the tissue (eg, from a traumatic accident). There is no agreement in the literature as to the absolute definition of low-pressure versus high-pressure lavage.[125] Bhandari et al[129] found that high-pressure lavage (ie, 70 psi) may damage the bone and carry surface contaminants deeper into the bone. In another study, Bhandari et al[125] found that low-pressure lavage (ie, 14 psi) was as effective as high-pressure lavage (ie, 70 psi) in removing adherent bacteria from bone and preserved the bony architecture when applied within three hours of contamination. However, the researchers found that after six hours of contamination, low-pressure pulsatile lavage may not effectively remove adherent bacteria from cortical bone.

In a study to investigate the contamination rate of fresh frozen bone allografts after treatment with different decontamination methods, Hirn et al[126] contaminated 103 bone grafts harvested from healthy donors during primary total hip arthroplasty procedures. The researchers contaminated the bone grafts by rubbing them against the OR floor and leaving them on the floor for 60 minutes. The researchers also cultured the OR floor to determine the microorganisms present on the floor. Both coagulase-negative staphylococci and Bacillis species were cultured from the floor. The researchers cultured 23 bone grafts after contamination on the OR floor as a control group and found that 22 (96%) of the grafts were culture positive. The remaining 80 contaminated grafts were divided into groups of 20 grafts:

- Group 1 grafts were rinsed with 3 L normal saline solution.
- Group 2 grafts were rinsed with 3 L normal saline supplemented with 3 g cefuroxime.
- Group 3 grafts were rinsed with 3 L normal saline supplemented with 1.2 g rafampicin solution.
- Group 4 grafts were rinsed with 1 L normal saline using low-pressure lavage (6 psi).

The researchers cultured all grafts after treatment. The results showed that two grafts from Group 1 were culture negative (10%); seven grafts from Group 2 were culture negative (35%); 12 grafts from Group 3 were culture negative (60%); and 14 grafts from Group 4 were culture negative (70%). The researchers concluded that low-pressure lavage with sterile normal saline solution decreased bioburden on the contaminated graft, avoided the potential negative effects on bone that may arise with high-pressure lavage, and was effective when compared with the antibiotic solutions tested.[126]

Using a separate sterile field may help prevent contamination of the primary sterile field by microorganisms on the contaminated autograft and from droplets caused by rinsing or irrigation fluid used to decontaminate the graft. Implementing corrective actions to maintain the sterility of the surgical field may prevent or reduce microbial contamination and help minimize the patient's risk of SSI.

Replantation or autotransplantation of a contaminated autograft constitutes a major break in sterile technique. According to the Centers for Disease Control and Prevention surgical wound classification system, a surgical wound with a major break in sterile technique is classified as Class III, Contaminated.[127]

Variance reports document the steps taken during the event and provide a mechanism for alerting infection preventionists to the need for surveillance. Variance reports can also be useful for quality improvement activities. Implementing a process of debriefing and root cause analysis after the event has occurred may help prevent future incidents by examining underlying factors and system flaws that may have contributed to the event and may be responsive to analysis and correction.[130]

VI.a.1. The following actions may be taken:
- Add antibiotics or antiseptics to the solution used to rinse the autograft.
- Take cultures before and after decontamination of the graft to determine the identity of the contaminating microorganism and the level of contamination.
- Consult with an infection preventionist to assess the benefits versus harms of implementing postoperative broad-spectrum antibiotic prophylaxis therapy.
- Send the autograft to a tissue bank for decontamination and processing.

[3: Moderate Evidence]

Adding antibiotics or antiseptics to the irrigation solution may be unnecessary or potentially harmful. Antibiotics and antiseptics may not have been validated for use in irrigation solutions and may therefore pose a risk to the patient. Tissue proteins may inhibit effectiveness of the antibiotics.[131] Some antibiotics, such as bacitracin,[132] have not been found to be effective for eliminating bone contaminants, whereas others, such as rifamycin,[133] have been found to be effective for decontaminating contaminated bone grafts. Antiseptic solutions are intended for external use and may be ineffective or toxic when used internally. Povidone-iodine solution has been found to provide effective bone decontamination[134] however, the antibacterial activity of 10% povidone-iodine solution is directly related to the level of contamination and the duration of exposure to the contaminated bone.[135]

Lacey[136] found that the antibacterial effect of povidone-iodine solution was inactivated in the presence of blood. Kaysinger et al[13] found that 0.5%, 5%, and 50% povidone iodine solutions and 1.5% and 3% H_2O solutions were cytotoxic to osteoblasts. Bhandari et al[125] found that povidone-iodine solution and bacitracin decreased the number of osteoclasts and impaired osteoblast function. When used to disinfect explanted bone, Schultke et al[84] found that H_2O_2 was ineffective.

Chlorhexidine gluconate has been found to be both effective[134] and ineffective[133] for decontaminating contaminated bone grafts and has also been found to be toxic to bone cells, even at very low concentrations (ie 1%).[132] Using chemical disinfectants (eg glutaraldehyde) on bone may cause tissue damage, or they may be difficult to remove. The steam sterilization process denatures bone protein and may severely damage bone structure and increase the potential for bone resorption and infection.[84]

Bhandari et al[132] conducted a two-part quasi-experimental study to compare the effects of various irrigating solutions on the number and function of osteoblasts and osteoclasts in bone and to examine the effectiveness of these solutions in removing adherent bacteria from bone. In Part 1, the researchers isolated calvarial cells from newborn mice and exposed the cells to equivalent concentrations of

- 1% ethanol,
- 10% ethanol,
- 1% povidone-iodine,
- 10% povidone-iodine,
- 1% soap (10 mL liquid soap/1 L normal saline),
- 10% soap (100 mL liquid soap/1 L normal saline),
- 1% CHG,
- 4% CHG,
- 1% antimicrobial (50 units bacitracin/L normal saline),
- 10% antimicrobial (500 units bacitracin/L normal saline), and
- normal saline solution

for two, 10, and 20 minutes. The researchers found that all of the irrigation solutions decreased the number of viable osteoblasts and osteocytes. The 10% povidone-iodine and 4% CHG solutions caused the most cell destruction. The 1% soap solution provided the least amount of cell destruction and the greatest amount of cell preservation.

In Part 2, the researchers contaminated canine cortical tibias with *Staphylococcus aureus* for six hours, and then subjected them to the same irrigating solutions used in Part 1 of the study with and without low-pressure lavage (ie, 14 psi). The researchers found the fewest number of bacteria on the contaminated tibias after exposure to 1% and 10% povidone-iodine, 1% and 4% CHG, and 1% and 10% soap. Low-pressure pulsatile lavage with 1% soap solution removed the most bacteria from the contaminated tibias. The antimicrobial solutions were the least effective at eliminating bacteria from the tibial samples.[132]

The researchers noted that the optimal technique for bone debridement should maximize the removal of adherent bacteria while preserving the structure and function of bone. They concluded that low-pressure lavage is as effective as high-pressure lavage in removing bacteria from the bone with significantly less macroscopic and microscopic bone damage.[132]

Bruce et al[134] conducted a three-phase quasi-experimental investigation to establish an intraoperative protocol for the management of contaminated autologous bone that will be replanted in the patient.

- Phase 1 of the study was performed to quantify the rate of contamination and the microbial profile of 162 bone fragments dropped on the OR floor. The results showed a contamination rate of 70%, with coagulase-negative staphylococcus being the most commonly cultured organism.
- Phase 2 of the study was performed to assess the feasibility and determine the optimal method of decontaminating 340 bone fragments contaminated with bacteria identified in Phase 1 of the study and decontaminated by methods and with cleansing solutions commonly available in an OR. The researchers tested 10% povidone-iodine, 4% CHG, 70% alcohol/2% CHG, and 0.9% normal saline solutions. The results showed the most effective solutions for decontaminating the bone fragments were 10% povidone-iodine and 4% CHG. Increasing exposure time to the decontaminating solutions from five to 10 minutes did not make a significant difference in contamination levels; however, mechanical scrubbing of the bone provided superior results to irrigating with a bulb syringe.
- Phase 3 of the study was performed to histologically assess the viability of the chondrocyte cells of 101 bone fragments after each decontamination process. The results showed that the bone samples treated with 10% povidone-iodine solution and normal saline solution maintained the greatest number of live cells.

The researchers concluded that five minutes of cleansing with 10% povidone-iodine solution followed by rinsing with normal saline solution provided the optimal balance between effective decontamination and maintaining cellular viability of the bone.[134]

In a systematic review conducted to explore intraoperative anterior cruciate ligament (ACL) graft decontamination, Khan et al[138] analyzed six experimental studies conducted between 1991 and 2012. The experimental groups from the studies included 328 allograft samples composed of fresh-frozen human Achilles tendocalcaneal grafts (n = 15), fresh-frozen human patellar tendon bone grafts (n = 30), excess hamstring graft from ACL reconstructions (n = 90), live human ACLs (n = 150), human cadaveric ACLs (n = 10), and human cadaveric patellar tendons (n = 33).

The allograft samples were contaminated by the researchers using various methods, such as dropping the tissue samples onto the OR floor or directly contaminating the samples with common pathogens (ie, *Staphylococcus aureus*, *Staphylococcus epidermidis*, *Pseudomonas aeruginosa*, *Klebsiella pneumoniae*, diphtheroids, micrococcus species). The researchers decontaminated the allografts using a variety of antiseptic and antibiotic solutions, including 2% and 4% CHG, normal saline solution, antibiotic solutions of polymyxin B and bacitracin or polymyxin B and neomycin, and 10% povidone-iodine. The decontamination protocols included seven to eight minutes of irrigation, mechanical agitation, serial dilution, pulsatile lavage, soaking for a variable duration of time, or a combination of rinsing and soaking. The researchers did not provide a definition for mechanical agitation or serial dilution, nor did they provide information as to the exact composition of the antiseptic and antibiotic solutions used in the studies included in the review.[138]

The researchers found that seven to eight minutes of irrigation with 3 L of 2% CHG and mechanical agitation and serial dilution with a polymyxin B-bacitracin solution provided 100% microbial decontamination (n = 10 of 10 samples). In two studies, they found that soaking the allograft in 4% CHG for 90 seconds provided 98% microbial decontamination (n = 49 of 50 samples) and 97% microbial decontamination (n = 29 of 30 samples), respectively. Soaking the grafts in bacitracin solution provided 97% microbial contamination (n = 29 of 30 samples), and soaking them in a combined solution of neomycin and polymyxin B provided 94% microbial decontamination (n = 47 of 50). Soaking the allografts in normal saline solution provided 70% microbial decontamination (n = 21 of 30). The results from two pooled studies showed that pulsatile lavage with normal saline solution provided 40% microbial decontamination (n = 6 of 15 samples). A combined solution of bacitracin and polymyxin B provided 57% microbial decontamination (n = 17 of 30 samples). Combined data from two studies showed that the least effective microbial decontamination (48%) occurred after soaking the allografts in 10% povidone-iodine (n = 40 of 84 samples).[138]

The researchers concluded the optimal antiseptic for decontaminating a contaminated allograft was CHG. However, they pointed out that the evidence included in the review was laboratory based and might not accurately reflect clinical conditions.

They recommended interpreting the findings of the systematic review with caution.[138]

Tissue cultures may be helpful in determining whether the dropped autograft was contaminated before or after decontamination measures were implemented. The results of the cultures may be useful in guiding treatment after replantation.

Some tissue banks provide services to decontaminate autologous bone skull flaps when contamination is suspected (ie, dropped autograft, head trauma, positive culture result). When sending an autograft to a tissue bank for decontamination and processing, the sending facility is not required to register with the FDA.

VI.a.2. The contaminated graft should not be subjected to the steam sterilization process. *[3: Moderate Evidence]*

The steam sterilization process denatures bone protein and may severely damage the bone structure and increase the potential for bone resorption and infection.[84] The steam sterilization process has not been validated for use with human tissue. A significantly high rate of postoperative graft infection has been found when cranial bone grafts subjected to the steam sterilization process were used for cranial reconstruction.[83]

VI.b. Perioperative team members should develop and implement measures to prevent dropped autografts. *[3: Moderate Evidence]*

In their review of 15,157 craniectomy procedures, Jankowitz and Kondziolka[122] found no consistent association between the dropping of the bone and the type of procedure, location of the surgical site, position of the patient, or activity being performed. To help prevent dropped cranial bone grafts, the researchers recommended that
- surgeons keep one hand on the flap and use the other hand to detach the dura from the bone with an instrument;
- surgeons elevate the bone by positioning themselves on the side exposed to the floor in order to direct the force of the elevation towards the surgical field and allow the excised cranial bone graft to fall onto the sterile drapes rather than the floor;
- surgeons complete the bone plating on a large surface area, such as the back table, while an assistant holds the bone;
- surgical assistants hold the flap with an instrument or position themselves to catch the cranial flap; and
- surgical team members place the bone flap directly onto the Mayo stand or back table rather than handing it to another team member.

Based on a review of the literature, Centeno et al[124] provided the following recommendations for managing contaminated autologous grafts used in plastic surgery:

- Alert all team members during the preoperative briefing or mandatory time out that an autologous graft will be obtained, and ask that all team members be vigilant of the location of the graft at all times during the procedure.
- Place the autologous graft in a labeled container, preferably a lidded container, and keep the labeled container on the largest table in the sterile field (eg, the back table), and away from instruments and the edge of the table.
- Limit handling and exchanging of the autologous graft between personnel as much as possible.
- Include the location of the autograft in the transfer-of-care report when surgical team members are relieved during the procedure.
- Do not discard any tissue without confirmation from the surgeon.
- Include the potential for autograft contamination and replantation or autotransplantation of a decontaminated autologous graft in the informed consent. If the autologous graft is contaminated during the procedure, provide full disclosure to the patient.

Recommendation VII

Autologous tissue that will be stored within the facility or health care organization for delayed replantation or autotransplantation should be transferred from the sterile field in a manner that maintains the sterility and integrity of the tissue and prevents exposure of health care personnel to blood, body fluids, or other potentially infectious materials.

The collective evidence review found gaps in the literature related to best practices for transferring autologous tissue from the sterile field. No research studies were found that compared different methods of transferring autologous tissue from the sterile field. Further research is warranted.

The benefits associated with transferring autologous tissue from the sterile field in a manner that maintains the sterility and integrity of the tissue and prevents exposure of health care personnel to blood, body fluids, or other potentially infectious materials are the reduced potential for compromise and contamination of the tissue that could lead to replantation or autotransplantation failure or infection, and the reduced potential for exposure of health care personnel to blood, body fluids, or other potentially infectious materials. There are no harms associated with transferring autologous tissue from the sterile field in the manner recommended in this document.

VII.a. Autologous tissue that will be stored within the facility or health care organization for delayed replantation or autotransplantation should be passed off the sterile field as soon as possible. *[5: Benefits Balanced with Harms]*

Passing the tissue off the sterile field as soon as possible reduces the potential for the integrity of the tissue to be compromised or for the tissue to be misplaced or lost.

VII.b. Autologous tissue that will be kept on the sterile field before transfer should be sequestered, identified, and monitored.[139] *[5: Benefits Balanced with Harms]*

Isolating, identifying, and monitoring autologous tissue kept on the sterile field reduces the possibility for the tissue to be contaminated, compromised, or lost.[139]

VII.c. Autologous tissue should be kept moist until transfer from the sterile field and should not be placed on dry, absorbent surfaces or materials. *[2: High Evidence]*

Air exposure can lead to desiccation of tissue.[140] Dry, absorbent surfaces or materials may adhere to the tissue.[140] Keeping tissue moist helps prevent drying of the tissue before packaging and storage.[141]

VII.d. Patient and tissue identification should be verified before tissue is transferred from the sterile field. Autologous tissue transferred from the sterile field should be verbally identified by the surgeon and verified by the perioperative RN using a "write down, read back" technique.[142] *[3: Moderate Evidence]*

Verifying patient and tissue identification using a "write down, read back" technique during the transfer process helps prevent misidentification of the patient or tissue and minimizes the potential for labeling errors.[142]

VII.e. Perioperative personnel should use standard precautions when transferring autologous tissue from the sterile field. *[1: Strong Evidence]*

Using standard precautions represents the minimum infection prevention strategy to be applied during all patient care activities (regardless of the suspected or confirmed infection status of the patient) in any setting in which health care is delivered.[143] Implementing standard precautions when autologous tissue is transferred from the sterile field helps prevent exposure of personnel to blood, body fluids, or other potentially infectious materials.[143]

VII.f. Autologous tissue should be transferred from the sterile field by personnel using sterile technique. *[5: Benefits Balanced with Harms]*

Using sterile technique when autologous tissue is transferred from the sterile field helps to prevent microbial contamination of the tissue.[139]

VII.g. The cellular structure of the tissue should be maintained during the transfer process by not crushing, twisting, or otherwise damaging the integrity of the tissue.[139] *[5: Benefits Balanced with Harms]*

Maintaining the cellular structure of the tissue reduces the potential for replantation failure or infection associated with tissue viability and integrity.

Recommendation VIII

Autologous tissue that will be stored within the facility or health care organization for delayed replantation or autotransplantation should be packaged and labeled in a manner that protects and secures the autograft; prevents cross-contamination and mix-ups during storage; facilitates tissue tracking; and prevents exposure of health care personnel to blood, body fluids, or other potentially infectious materials.

The collective evidence review found gaps in the literature related to best practices for packaging and labeling autologous tissue. No research studies were found that compared different packaging materials and methods of packaging and labeling autologous tissue. Further research is warranted.

The benefits associated with packaging and labeling autologous tissue are the reduced potential for mix-ups if autograft labeling methods are inadequate (eg, smudging of identifiers during cold storage, labels separating from the package) and contamination or cross-contamination if the graft's packaging material is not validated for use at the storage temperature selected. Donors of autologous tissue are usually not screened or tested for communicable diseases (eg, HIV, hepatitis B, hepatitis C, syphilis). If the packaging that contains the autograft sufficiently secures the autograft, the potential for cross-contamination of other packages stored with the autograft is reduced. There are no harms associated with packaging and labeling autologous tissue in the manner recommended in this document.

A full discussion of the requirements for packaging systems for sterilization is outside the scope of these recommendations. The reader should refer to the AORN Guideline for Selection and Use of Packaging Systems for Sterilization[144] for additional guidance related to packaging for sterilization.

VIII.a. Autologous tissue intended for delayed replantation or autotransplantation should be contained and labeled immediately after transfer from the sterile field.[139] *[5: Benefits Balanced with Harms]*

Containing and labeling autologous tissue immediately after transfer from the sterile field helps preserve the quality and integrity of the tissue and prevent contamination, damage, or loss of the autograft.[139] Correctly labeling the autologous tissue may also prevent transplantation of the tissue into an unintended recipient.

VIII.b. Packaging materials for autologous tissue must be
- leak proof and punctures resistant[145] and
- designed to prevent the introduction, transmission, or spread of communicable diseases.[3]
[1: Regulatory Requirement]

Using packaging materials and containers that are leak proof, puncture resistant,[145] and designed to prevent the introduction, transmis-

sion, or spread of communicable diseases[3] is a regulatory requirement.

VIII.c. Packaging materials for autologous tissue should be validated to meet the anticipated storage conditions and should
- maintain the integrity and stability of the autograft[139] throughout
  - preparation (eg, exposure to antibiotics or other chemicals),
  - processing (eg, cryopreservation),
  - storage (eg, -148° F [-100° C]), and
  - thawing procedures, if the autograft will be thawed in its package[6];
- not produce toxic residues;
- be large enough and of the correct size to secure the tissue[139]; and
- remain impervious to microorganisms and microscopic particles.
[3: Moderate Evidence]

Using packaging materials that are validated to meet the anticipated storage conditions is an AATB standard.[6] Validated packaging materials help maintain the tissue at the correct temperature.[146]

Verifying that containers are of the correct size to fully secure the tissue may help prevent damage to the autograft. This can also prevent leakage and help protect perioperative personnel or others who handle the container or its contents from unnecessary exposure to blood, body fluids, or other potentially infectious materials.[139]

Using packages or containers that maintain integrity and prevent contamination of the autograft helps prevent compromise of the autograft that could lead to an SSI[139] or the inability to replant or autotransplant the tissue.

VIII.c.1. Packages or containers used for storage of autologous tissue that will be frozen or cryopreserved should be able to withstand temperatures of -4° F (-20° C) or colder.[6,131] *[4: Limited Evidence]*

Frozen storage requires a packaging material that will not become brittle or break when exposed to extremely low temperatures. The minimum acceptable temperature for short-term storage of autologous tissue is -4° F (-20° C) or colder.[6,131] Long-term storage (ie, longer than six months) occurs at temperatures of -40° F (-40° C) or colder.

VIII.d. Autologous bone should not be packaged or stored in solution. *[3: Moderate Evidence]*

Packaging and storing autologous bone while it is still wet or in solution may be harmful to the bone.[131]

During freezing, the graft is biologically inactive. Antibiotic solutions have no effect on bacteria.[126]

VIII.e. When autologous tissue is placed into a storage container, the perioperative RN should confirm and document
- the patient's identity using two unique identifiers (eg, patient name and medical record number) according to the facility or health care organization policy[139];
- the originating source of the tissue including laterality, if applicable;
- the type of tissue;
- the clinical diagnosis; and
- any additional pertinent clinical information.[139]

[4: Limited Evidence]

Maintaining a procedure to verify the accuracy of labels when labeling human tissue is a regulatory requirement for good tissue practice[3] and an AATB standard.[6]

VIII.f. The autograft package must be labeled
- "For Autologous Use Only,"[3,5,6]
- "Not Evaluated for Infectious Substances" (if infectious disease testing has not been performed),[3,5,6,131] and
- "Biohazard" (if infectious disease testing was performed and any results were positive, or if donor screening was performed and risk factors were identified).[3,5,145]

The package should also be labeled with an expiration date.[3,6] *[1: Regulatory Requirement]*

Autologous tissue may not have undergone culturing to detect contaminating microorganisms, and the autologous donor was likely not tested for communicable diseases. Labeling to communicate "For Autologous Use Only" and "Not Evaluated for Infectious Substances" (if infectious disease testing has not been performed),[3] biohazard information,[145] and the expiration date[3,6] are regulatory requirements. Failure to communicate biohazard information could result in exposure or injury to personnel who handle the tissue or to an unintended tissue recipient. Failure to communicate the expiration date could result in expired tissue being replanted into a patient.

VIII.g. The autograft package label should include the
- facility- or health care organization-defined unique patient identifiers (eg, patient name and medical record number)[6,131,139]
- donor classification statement "Autologous Donor"[6];
- procedure, date of recovery, and name of the surgeon[131];
- tissue type and site, including laterality if applicable[131,139];
- identity of the person who packaged and labeled the autograft[131];
- date of tissue recovery[131];
- time the autograft was placed into storage and the identity of the person placing it into storage[131];
- method of preservation, if applicable[6];
- recommended storage temperature and acceptable storage temperature range[6];
- method of decontamination and identification of any potential processing or solution residues (eg, antibiotics) if used[6]; and
- manner in which the tissue was recovered and prepared (eg, under aseptic conditions).[6]

[4: Limited Evidence]

Labeling in the manner described here is an AATB standard.[6,131] Accurate and detailed labeling may help prevent autologous tissue from being transplanted into a recipient other than the original donor.

VIII.h. Dark indelible ink should be used on autograft package labels.[131,139] *[4: Limited Evidence]*

Using dark ink improves visibility on both handwritten and electronic labels.[139] Using indelible ink helps prevent ink from being removed from the label.[139]

VIII.i. A bar-code labeling system should be used and a bar-code label applied to the package or container if the technology is available.[3] *[3: Moderate Evidence]*

Bar-code labeling systems may reduce identification errors by facilitating improved accuracy in matching tissue to the desired recipient[147,148] and may also improve the accuracy of facility or health care organization records. Bar-code labeling also may enhance tissue tracking records.

Implementing a procedure to verify the accuracy of labels for human tissue is a regulatory requirement for good tissue practice.[3]

VIII.j. Identification labels should be securely affixed to the outside of both the inner and outer package or container[131] and should not be secured to a container lid.[148] Labels should adhere to the packaging material under all anticipated storage conditions for the shelf-life of the tissue.[6] *[3: Moderate Evidence]*

Labeling the autograft package in a manner that minimizes the risk for errors is a regulatory requirement for good tissue practice[3] and an AATB standard.[6] Using both an internal and external label is recommended because the outer label may fall off or become unreadable during frozen storage (eg, smudged from condensation).[131] Placing the label on the container instead of the lid may help prevent loss of autograft information after the lid is removed from the container or if the lid becomes detached from the container.[148]

VIII.k. Autograft tissue identification and labeling should be confirmed among surgical team members during the debriefing at the end of the operative or other invasive procedure.[139] Confirmation should include
- visual confirmation that the autograft is in the container and

PATIENT AND WORKER SAFETY

AUTOLOGOUS TISSUE MANAGEMENT

○ verification that the patient and autograft information on the label is correct and legible, including laterality as applicable.[139]

[5: Benefits Balanced with Harms]

Management of autologous tissue is a multidisciplinary process. Postprocedure confirmation of the autograft identification and labeling can improve communication among team members and may help to reduce or eliminate errors[130] in autologous tissue management.

Recommendation IX

Autologous tissue should be transported in a manner that protects and secures the autograft; maintains the integrity of the tissue; prevents exposure of health care personnel to blood, body fluids, or other potentially infectious materials; and ensures the confidentiality of protected patient information.

The collective evidence review found gaps in the literature related to best practices for transporting autologous tissue. No research studies were found that compared different methods of transporting autologous tissue. Further research is warranted.

The benefits associated with transporting autologous tissue in a manner that protects and secures the autograft; maintains the integrity of the tissue; prevents exposure of health care personnel to blood, body fluids, or other potentially infectious materials; and ensures the confidentiality of protected patient information are the reduced potential for compromising and contaminating the tissue that could lead to replantation or autotransplantation failure or infection; the reduced potential for exposing health care personnel to blood, body fluids, or other potentially infectious materials; and the reduced potential for violating the confidentiality of the patient's protected information. There are no harms associated with transporting autologous tissue in the manner recommended in this document.

IX.a. Autologous tissue must be transported in a manner that prevents exposure of health care personnel to blood, body fluids, or other potentially infectious materials.[145] *[1: Regulatory Requirement]*

Transporting tissue in a manner that prevents exposure of health care personnel to blood, body fluids, or other potentially infectious materials is a regulatory requirement.[145]

IX.b. Autologous tissue must be transported in a manner that ensures the confidentiality of protected patient information.[149] *[1: Regulatory Requirement]*

Ensuring the confidentiality of protected health information is a regulatory requirement and a standard of perioperative nursing care.[149-151]

IX.c. Autologous tissue must be transported in a manner that maintains the required temperature and minimizes the risk of degradation or con-

tamination of the autograft.[3,5] *[1: Regulatory Requirement]*

Transporting autologous tissue in a manner that minimizes the risk of degradation or contamination of the autograft is a regulatory requirement for good tissue practice.[3,5]

Maintaining the tissue at the required temperatures during transport reduces the potential for the autograft to become degraded or contaminated. Degradation of the autograft may increase the potential for an adverse reaction and unexpected outcome for the patient.

IX.d. Devices intended for transport of specimens must be labeled with biohazard information.[145] *[1: Regulatory Requirement]*

Labeling to communicate biohazard information is a regulatory requirement.[145] Failure to communicate biohazard information could result in exposure of personnel handling the autograft package to blood, body fluids, or other potentially infectious materials.

Recommendation X

Autologous tissue intended for delayed replantation or autotransplantation should be stored in a manner that protects and secures the autograft, prevents cross-contamination and mixups during storage, and prevents exposure of health care personnel to blood, body fluids, or other potentially infectious materials.

The collective evidence review found gaps in the literature related to best practices for storage of autologous tissue. No research studies were found that compared different storage methods for autologous tissue. Further research is warranted.

The benefits of storing autologous tissue in a manner that protects and secures the autograft, prevents cross-contamination and mix-ups during storage, and prevents exposure of health care personnel to blood, body fluids, or other potentially infectious materials are the reduced potential for compromise and contamination of the tissue that could lead to replantation or autotransplantation failure or infection; the reduced potential for distributing the tissue to an unintended recipient; and the reduced potential for exposing health care personnel to blood, body fluids, or other potentially infectious materials. There are no harms associated with storing autologous tissue in the manner recommended in this document.

X.a. Autologous tissue intended for delayed replantation or autotransplantation must be stored in a manner that prevents exposure of health care personnel to blood, body fluids, or other potentially infectious materials.[145] *[1: Regulatory Requirement]*

Preventing exposure of health care personnel to blood, body fluids, or other potentially infectious materials is a regulatory requirement.[145]

X.b. Autologous tissue that will be stored within the facility or health care organization for delayed

PATIENT AND WORKER SAFETY

224

replantation or autotransplantation must be stored in an area that is controlled to prevent mix-ups, contamination, and cross-contamination of tissue and the potential for tissue to be incorrectly distributed.[3,5,6] *[1: Regulatory Requirement]*

Storing tissue in a controlled area that reduces the potential for tissue contamination or incorrect distribution is a regulatory requirement for good tissue practice[3,5] and an AATB standard.[6]

X.c. Tissue from two or more donors must not be comingled.[3,5,6] *[1: Regulatory Requirement]*

Combining tissue from two or more donors in the same package or container increases the potential for introducing, transmitting, or spreading communicable diseases.

X.d. Autologous tissue should be separated from allografts.[6] *[4: Limited Evidence]*

Tissue from an autologous donor is usually not tested for contaminating microorganisms, and autologous donors are usually not screened or tested for communicable diseases. Separating autologous tissue from allografts minimizes the potential for autologous tissue to be transplanted into a patient who is not the donor.

X.d.1. Autografts and allografts may be stored in the same refrigerator or freezer if
- they are stored separately (eg, allografts stored on the upper shelves and autografts stored on the lower shelves, allografts and autografts placed in separate storage bins),
- they are packaged using validated packaging materials,
- they are prominently labeled, and
- the correct storage conditions exist for all items in the refrigerator or freezer.

[5: Benefits Balanced with Harms]

Using separate storage areas or bins and providing prominent, easy-to-identify labels helps perioperative personal distinguish between the containers and reduces the potential for error.

Using validated packaging materials and ensuring the correct storage conditions exist for all items in the refrigerator or freezer helps ensure the tissue is maintained in optimal condition for replantation or autotransplantation.

X.e. The number of autografts in storage should be inventoried according to an established schedule, and autografts should be removed and discarded by the expiration date. *[5: Benefits Balanced with Harms]*

Inventorying the number of autografts in storage and removing and discarding expired autografts helps ensure autografts are maintained in optimal storage conditions for successful replantation or autotransplantation and helps prevent replantation or autotransplantation of potentially compromised tissue.

X.f. Autologous tissue that may have been compromised should be removed from storage[152,153] and discarded and should not be replanted or autotransplanted. *[5: Benefits Balanced with Harms]*

Removing from storage and discarding autologous tissue that may have been compromised (eg, exposed to incorrect storage temperatures) helps ensure potentially compromised tissue is not replanted or autotransplanted into a patient. Replanting or autotransplanting compromised tissue could lead to serious patient injury.

X.g. Autologous tissue must be stored at temperatures that will prevent contamination or degradation of the tissue.[3,5] Storage temperatures
- must be maintained and periodically reviewed to ensure that temperatures are within acceptable limits[3,5,6] and
- should be established in accordance with federal and state regulations and AATB standards.[6]

[1: Regulatory Requirement]

Maintaining storage temperatures within recommended parameters helps ensure that autografts are maintained in optimal condition for successful replantation or autotransplantation.

X.h. Autologous bone should be stored at -4° F (-20° C) or colder for six months or less.[6] Autologous bone may be stored at -40° F (-40° C) or colder for up to five years; however, this is considered long-term storage and may require registering with the FDA as a tissue establishment.[6,131] *[4: Limited Evidence]*

Storage at -40° F (-40° C) or colder is preferred because tissue enzymes may be active at temperatures warmer than -40° F (-40° C) and may negatively affect tissue if it is stored for an extended time. Temperatures of -94° F (-70° C) or colder may prevent enzymatic destruction of tissue.[131]

Maintaining the storage temperature below -40° F (-40° C) may also be a "buffer" that provides additional time before critical temperatures are reached in the event of a freezer malfunction.[131]

X.i. Autologous skin should be stored between 32° F to 50° F (0° C to 10° C) for no longer than 14 days.[6] Refrigerated skin should be submerged in a storage medium, and the storage medium should be changed every 72 hours.[113] *[3: Moderate Evidence]*

Refrigeration retards autolysis and helps prevent bacterial proliferation.[117] Keeping the skin submerged helps prevent dehydration of the tissue. Changing the storage medium every 72 hours may help to prevent microbial growth and improve skin autograft viability.[113,114]

PATIENT AND WORKER SAFETY

Cram and Domayer[114] stored split-thickness autologous skin grafts from 32 patients in 100 mL Roswell Park Memorial Institute 1640 culture medium supplemented with 25 units/mL penicillin and 25 mcg/mL streptomycin. The skin grafts were stored in a refrigerator at 39.2° F (4° C) for 22 days. The storage medium was changed every three to four days during the storage period. The grafts were rinsed with normal saline solution before autotransplantation. The authors found that 75% of the grafts (n = 24) were successfully engrafted. They concluded that skin autografts could be stored up to 22 days using this technique.

In a quasi-experimental study conducted to evaluate the effects of storage solutions, temperature and the changing of storage media on skin graft anatomy as an indicator of graft viability, Robb et al[113] retrieved split-thickness human skin grafts from cadaveric donors and grafted them to circumferential, full-thickness skin wounds on mice. After three months, samples of the human skin (N = 149) were recovered from the mice and divided into four groups:

○ Group 1: normal saline solution,
○ Group 2: normal saline solution changed every three days,
○ Group 3: Eagle's minimum essential medium, and
○ Group 4: Eagle's minimum essential medium changed every three days.

All sample groups were stored at either room temperature, or in a refrigerator at 39.2° F (4° C) for five, 10, or 21 days. The results showed that skin stored in Eagle's minimum essential medium maintained better histological anatomy than skin stored in normal saline solution. There was also better preservation of skin anatomy after storage at room temperature for 21 days with media changes every three days when compared with changed and unchanged media stored at 39.2° F (4° C). The researchers concluded that storage at room temperature and the increased nutrients in the Eagle's minimum essential medium maintained increased viability of the human skin samples; however, despite replenishment of storage media every three days, the skin samples were no longer viable after 21 days.

X.j. Autologous veins should be stored between 32° F to 50° F (0° C to 10° C) for no longer than 14 days. Refrigerated veins should be submerged in storage medium, and the storage medium should be changed every 72 hours. [3: Moderate Evidence]

Keeping the veins submerged helps prevent dehydration of the tissue. Changing the storage medium every 72 hours may help to prevent microbial growth and improve autograft viability.[114,113]

X.k. Autografts that are to be frozen should be frozen within a few hours of recovery.[131] [4: Limited Evidence]

Warm tissue is a medium for bacterial growth. Freezing the tissue within a few hours of recovery helps decrease the potential for microbial contamination that may lead to an SSI.

X.l. Autologous tissue that will not be immediately transported to the storage area should be temporarily stored in a manner that maintains autograft integrity. Equipment (eg, refrigerators, freezers) or devices used for transport or temporary storage (eg, coolers) should maintain tissue at the AATB recommended temperature.[6] [4: Limited Evidence]

Maintaining optimal integrity of autologous tissue and ensuring the autograft is maintained at the recommended temperature may help prevent degradation of the autograft.

X.m. Documentation should be provided when autologous tissue is placed into the refrigerator or freezer for storage. Documentation should include

○ the facility- or health care organization-defined unique identifiers (eg, patient name and medical record number);
○ the procedure, date of the procedure, and name of the surgeon[131];
○ the date and time of tissue storage and the identity of the person placing it into storage[131];
○ whether the tissue was cultured[131]; and
○ any additional pertinent clinical information (eg, increased potential for autograft contamination because of trauma).[131]

[4: Limited Evidence]

Documentation as described here is recommended by the AATB.[131]

X.n. Equipment and devices used for storage of autologous tissue must be cleaned, sanitized, and maintained according to an established schedule to prevent malfunctions, contamination or cross-contamination, or other events that may result in the introduction, transmission, or spread of communicable diseases.[3,5,6] [1: Regulatory Requirement]

Cleaning, sanitizing, and maintaining equipment and devices used for storage of autologous tissue is a regulatory requirement[3,5] and an AATB standard.[6]

X.n.1. Records of cleaning and sanitation, including cleaning and sanitation methods used, cleaning schedule, and personnel responsible for cleaning and sanitation, must be retained for three years after the record is created.[3,5] [1: Regulatory Requirement]

Retaining cleaning and sanitation records for three years after the record is created is a regulatory requirement.[3,5]

X.o. Refrigerators and freezers used for storage of autologous tissue must have regular calibration checks in accordance with the manufacturer's written instructions for use.[3,5] *[1: Regulatory Requirement]*

Performing regular calibration checks on equipment used for storage of autologous tissue is a regulatory requirement[3,5] and an AATB standard.[6] Performing regular calibration checks helps ensure that tissue is being stored at the correct temperatures.[146]

X.o.1. Maintenance, calibration, and other activities performed on refrigerators and freezers used for storage of autologous tissue must be documented, and the records must be readily available.[3,5] *[1: Regulatory Requirement]*

Documentation and availability of records related to maintenance and calibration of refrigerators and freezers used for storage of autologous tissue is a regulatory requirement.[3,5]

X.p. Freezers and refrigerators used for storage of autologous tissue should provide continuous temperature monitoring[6,131,152,153] and should
○ be monitored regularly with daily temperature checks recorded[152,153];
○ have an alert or alarm system[131,152,153] that notifies personnel when the temperature is not within the acceptable range; and
○ have an emergency power system.
[4: Limited Evidence]

Daily temperature checks of refrigerators and freezers used for storage of autologous tissue is an accreditation standard.[152,153] Maintaining the recommended temperatures for storage of tissue helps ensure tissue integrity. Temperature fluctuations outside of the recommended temperature range may render the tissue unsafe for replantation or autotransplantation.

X.p.1. The alert or alarm system should
• sound in an area where an individual is present at all times to initiate corrective action or
• notify personnel who are available to respond.
[5: Benefits Balanced with Harms]

Temperature fluctuations outside of the recommended temperature range may require rapid corrective action to prevent compromise or degradation of tissue intended for replantation or autotransplantation.

X.q. Processes should be established for
○ maintaining the temperature and integrity of stored autologous tissues in the event of a refrigerator or freezer malfunction (eg, transferring tissue to another storage unit)[6,152,153] and
○ responding to a malfunction of the refrigerator or freezer that occurs when the facility is closed or when the area where the tissue is stored is unoccupied.
[4: Limited Evidence]

Maintaining the recommended temperatures for storage of tissue helps ensure the tissue is not compromised. Temperature fluctuations outside of the recommended temperature range may render the tissue unsafe for replantation or autotransplantation.

X.q.1. Autologous tissue should not be stored on-site if the facility or health care organization does not have the capability of monitoring storage conditions when the facility is closed or when the area where the tissue is stored is unoccupied. *[5: Benefits Balanced with Harms]*

Temperature fluctuations outside of the recommended temperature range may require rapid corrective action to prevent compromise or degradation of tissue intended for replantation or autotransplantation.

Recommendation XI

Autologous tissue intended for replantation or autotransplantation should be handled using sterile technique and in a manner that protects and secures the autograft from damage or contamination.

The collective evidence review found gaps in the literature related to best practices for handling autologous tissue. No research studies were found that compared different protocols for handling autologous tissue. Further research is warranted.

The benefits of handling autologous tissue using sterile technique and in a manner that protects and secures the autograft are that it may help prevent compromise or contamination that may render the autograft unacceptable for replantation or autotransplantation and may decrease the patient's risk for SSI. There are no harms associated with handling autologous tissue in the manner recommended in this document.

XI.a. Autologous tissue management should be assessed and planned among surgical team members during the preoperative briefing before operative or other invasive procedures. *[3: Moderate Evidence]*

Management of autologous tissue is a multidisciplinary process. Collaborative preprocedural assessment and planning may improve efficiency and communication among team members and may help to reduce or eliminate errors[154] in autologous tissue management.

XI.b. Autologous tissue must be released only for replantation or autotransplantation in the donor.[3,6] *[1: Regulatory Requirement]*

Autologous tissue is not tested for infectious organisms or diseases, so release to another recipient could cause serious injury.

XI.b.1. The facility- or health care organization-defined unique identifiers (eg, patient name and medical record number) should be used to verify autologous donor identity for release of autologous tissue. *[5: Benefits Balanced with Harms]*

Using unique identifiers to verify donor identity may help to reduce the potential for errors in donor patient identification.

XI.b.2. Bar-coding technology should be used if available.[3] *[3: Moderate Evidence]*

Bar-code labeling systems may reduce identification errors by facilitating improved accuracy in matching tissue to the desired recipient[147,148] and may also improve the accuracy of facility or health care organization and patient records.

XI.b.3. Removal of the autograft from storage should be documented. Documentation should include the date and time of removal and the identity of the person removing the tissue.[131] *[4: Limited Evidence]*

Documentation as described here is recommended by the AATB.[131]

XI.c. Autologous tissue should not be released for replantation or autotransplantation until all handling criteria (ie, processing, labeling, storage, cultures) have been verified and determined to be satisfactory for release. *[5: Benefits Balanced with Harms]*

Verifying criteria for release helps minimize the potential for errors.

XI.c.1. Autologous tissue that does not meet the release criteria should be considered compromised and should not be used. *[5: Benefits Balanced with Harms]*

Replantation or autotransplantation of compromised tissue could cause serious injury.

XI.d. The perioperative RN should review the culture results for stored autografts before the autograft is replanted or autotransplanted.[131] *[4: Limited Evidence]*

Collecting health data relevant to the patient's situation is necessary to inform other health care professionals involved in the patient's care.[150]

XI.d.1. If the culture result is positive, a multidisciplinary team consisting of the surgeon, perioperative RN, and infection preventionist should determine whether or not the autograft will be replanted or autotransplanted. *[2: High Evidence]*

Chiang et al[155] conducted a prospective cohort study in a university hospital to identify the prevalence of bone flaps with positive cultures and to assess the risk of SSI after replantation of bone flaps with positive cultures. Nursing personnel swabbed all surfaces of the cranial bone flaps of 372 neurosurgery patients undergoing craniectomy procedures between November 1, 2007, and November 30, 2008, and submitted the swab cultures for aerobic and anaerobic testing before soaking the flap in 500 mL normal saline solution supplemented with 50,000 units bacitracin. The bone flaps were then either replanted during the same procedure or wrapped in a sterile towel, labeled with the patient's identifiers, placed into a sterile freezer bag, and cryopreserved at -94° F (-70° C) or colder until the time of replantation. The researchers did not specify how long the bone flaps were soaked before replantation or packaging for cryopreservation and storage.

The researchers found that 50% of the bone flaps were contaminated with microorganisms (n = 186). The microorganisms were primarily skin flora such as *Propionibacterium acnes*, coagulase negative staphylococci, and *Staphylococcus aureus*. Replanting the bone flaps with positive culture results did not increase the patient's risk for infection. The researchers concluded that cranial bone flaps with low numbers of skin flora contaminants could be safely replanted. The researchers did not specify what were considered "low numbers of skin flora." The researchers also found that the risk of SSI increased when the preoperative skin antiseptics were not allowed to dry, and they concluded that operative factors were more important than low numbers of skin flora contaminating the cranial bone flap in the pathogenesis of SSI after craniectomy procedures.[155]

XI.d.2. If a decision is made to replant or autotransplant the tissue, the multidisciplinary team should determine whether any disinfection measures (eg, prophylactic antibiotics, extensive rinsing with or without pulsatile lavage) will be applied to the autograft.[131] *[4: Limited Evidence]*

Autologous tissue management is a multidisciplinary process. Collaborative discussion and decision making may improve patient outcomes.

XI.e. Frozen bone autografts should be removed from the freezer after the surgeon has confirmed the autograft will be replanted or autotransplanted.[131] *[4: Limited Evidence]*

Removing the frozen autograft after the surgeon has confirmed it will be replanted or autotransplanted helps prevent unnecessary thawing and refreezing of autografts.

XI.f. The perioperative RN and a scrubbed team member should verify the contents of the autologous tissue package, patient and tissue identification, expiration date, and other pertinent information before the tissue is transferred to the sterile field. *[5: Benefits Balanced with Harms]*

Verifying identification of the autologous tissue during the transfer process minimizes opportunities for error and helps prevent misidentification of the autograft.

XI.g. Frozen bone autografts should be removed from their packages using sterile technique and placed into

   ○ a sterile basin filled with warm (ie, 98.6° F to 105.8° F [37° C to 41° C]), sterile normal saline or lactated Ringer's solution for 15 to 20 minutes or

   ○ an empty sterile basin and allowed to thaw at room temperature for a minimum of 30 minutes before replantation or autotransplantation.[131]

[4: Limited Evidence]

Using sterile technique to remove autografts from their packages may help to prevent contamination of the autograft. Complete thawing of the frozen autograft reduces bone brittleness.[131] Antibiotics added to the irrigation fluid may not be effective because the autograft contains lipids, red blood cells, and other proteins that may neutralize the intended activity of the antibiotics.[131]

XI.h. Before replantation or autotransplantation, the autograft should be rinsed at least three times with sterile normal saline or lactated Ringer's solution.[131] The volume of fluid used should be at least 10 times the volume of the autograft.[131] *[4: Limited Evidence]*

Rinsing may remove surface contamination. Rinsing as described here is recommended by the AATB.[131]

XI.i. The date and time of replantation or autotransplantation, the procedure used to prepare the autograft, and the names and titles of all individuals involved in preparing the autograft should be documented in the patient's record.[131] *[4: Limited Evidence]*

Documentation as described here is recommended by the AATB.[131]

XI.j. Autologous bone grafts may be refrozen if necessary (eg, an autograft thawed for replantation that is then not replanted).[131] A multidisciplinary team consisting of the surgeon, perioperative RN, and infection preventionist should conduct a risk assessment to consider the benefits and potential harms associated with replanting refrozen bone compared with other treatment options (eg, discarding the graft and using artificial material) and to determine the number of acceptable freeze-thaw cycles. *[4: Limited Evidence]*

Refreezing autologous bone may allow it to be used for cranioplasty; however, additional freeze-thaw cycles may increase the patient's risk for SSI.[131]

XI.j.1. If a decision is made to refreeze the bone graft, cell remnants and nonviable cells within the thawed bone graft should be removed using pulsatile lavage followed by a series of 30-minute soaks in a warm, sterile isotonic solution at a volume 10 times that of the autograft and then rinsing.[131] *[4: Limited Evidence]*

Bone marrow and red blood cell remnants and nonviable cells may be present within the cancellous bone of an autologous bone graft that has been thawed after frozen storage.[131] The cell remnants and nonviable cells may be recognized by the donor's immune system at the time of replantation or autotransplantation and may increase the potential for an inflammatory or immune system response.[131]

XI.k. In the event the autograft is not replanted or autotransplanted and is transferred to another facility or discarded, documentation must be provided so that the autograft can be traced to its final disposition.[3,5,6] *[1: Regulatory Requirement]*

Traceability of the autograft to its final disposition and retention of records related to disposition of autologous tissue are regulatory requirements[3,5] and AATB standards.[6]

XI.l. If it becomes necessary to transfer the autograft to another facility, an AATB-accredited tissue source facility should be contacted for assistance with packaging and shipping.[131] *[4: Limited Evidence]*

Personnel at an AATB-accredited tissue bank can offer expert assistance with packaging and shipping autologous tissue.

XI.l.1. Facilities or health care organizations that distribute autologous tissue to another facility at a different address are required to register with the FDA as a tissue establishment that manufactures human cells, tissues, and cellular and tissue-based products and to follow applicable requirements of 21 CFR Part 1271.[3,5] *[1: Regulatory Requirement]*

Transferring tissue to another facility is considered distribution. The requirement for registration as a tissue establishment exists even if distribution occurs only rarely.[3,5]

XI.m. Autologous human tissue must be treated as biohazardous waste and disposed of in accordance with local and state regulations.[145] *[1: Regulatory Requirement]*

Local and state regulations related to disposal of human tissue vary. Disposal of human tissue as biohazardous waste helps prevent exposure of health care personnel to blood, body fluids, or other potentially infectious materials.

XI.m.1. A multidisciplinary team consisting of surgeons, perioperative RNs, pathology laboratory representatives, infection preventionists,

AUTOLOGOUS TISSUE MANAGEMENT

risk management personnel, and other involved stakeholders should develop a plan for disposal of autologous tissue that addresses the need to contact the patient or patient's legal representative, the patient's cultural preferences, and any requests for release of autologous tissue for burial or cremation before disposal. *[5: Benefits Balanced with Harms]*

Management of autologous tissue is a multidisciplinary process. Collaborative discussion and decision making may improve outcomes.

XI.m.2. Facilities that distribute autologous tissue for burial or cremation are not required to register with the FDA as a tissue establishment. *[1: Regulatory Requirement]*

The facility would meet the exception from registration described in section 1271.15(b), in which storage of tissue for autologous use is exempt as long as no other manufacturing controls are performed (ie, subjecting the autograft to the steam sterilization process, distributing the autograft to another facility).[3,4]

Recommendation XII

Policies and procedures for managing autologous tissue must be developed, reviewed periodically, revised as necessary, and readily available in the practice setting.[3,5,6,152,153,156]

Establishing and maintaining policies and procedures for managing autologous tissue is a regulatory requirement[3,5] and an AATB[6] and accreditation agency standard.[152,153,156]

Policies and procedures assist in the development of patient safety, quality assessment, and performance improvement activities. Policies and procedures establish authority, responsibility, and accountability within the organization. Policies and procedures also serve as operational guidelines used to minimize patient risk for injury or complications, standardize practice, direct perioperative personnel, and establish continuous performance improvement programs.

XII.a. Policies and procedures for autologous tissue management must designate personnel responsible for oversight of autologous tissue and with authority and accountability for all activities performed.[3,5,6,152,153] *[1: Regulatory Requirement]*

Centralized oversight of all aspects of autologous tissue management helps ensure that tissue is
- safe for replantation or autotransplantation;
- managed in compliance with regulatory requirements;
- monitored on an ongoing basis;
- packaged, transported, stored, and handled according to standardized processes; and
- able to be traced to the original source and recalled, if necessary.

Review and approval of all procedures related to autologous tissue management and

designation of the personnel responsible for oversight is a regulatory requirement[3,5] and an AATB[6] and accreditation standard.[152,153]

XII.a.1. A physician or medical advisory committee should be available to provide direction for medical decisions.[6] *[4: Limited Evidence]*

The AATB recommends that a medical director be appointed for oversight.[6]

XII.b. Policies and procedures for managing autologous tissue must be designed to decrease the risk of introducing, transmitting, or spreading communicable diseases (ie, diseases transmitted by viruses, bacteria, fungi, parasites, and transmissible spongiform encephalopathy agents).[3,5] *[1: Regulatory Requirement]*

Developing policies and procedures for tracking, storing, and handling autologous tissue and investigating adverse reactions is a regulatory requirement[3,5] and an AATB[6] and accreditation agency standard.[152,153,156]

XII.c. Policies and procedures for autologous tissue management should be developed by a multidisciplinary team that includes infection preventionists, risk management personnel, pathology laboratory representatives, perioperative RNs, and other stakeholders (eg, surgeons who replant or autotransplant tissue). *[5: Benefits Balanced with Harms]*

Management of autologous tissue is a multidisciplinary process. Collaborative discussion and decision making may improve patient outcomes.

XII.c.1. Policies and procedures related to autologous tissue management may include processes for
- providing care for patients who have sustained traumatic tooth avulsion injuries, including immediate replantation or storage of the tooth in a storage medium;
- providing care for patients who may be undergoing recovery, replantation, or autotransplantation of autologous tissue;
- transferring autologous tissue from the sterile field;
- packaging and labeling autologous tissue;
- transporting autologous tissue;
- preserving and storing autologous tissue;
- determining the maximum storage duration of autologous tissue and ensuring tissue is not replanted or autotransplanted beyond its expiration date;
- cleaning and sanitizing equipment or devices used to transport or store autologous tissue;
- maintaining and monitoring equipment used to store autologous tissue;
- responding to alarms and malfunction of equipment used to store autologous tissue and designating the personnel who are responsible for responding;

- monitoring temperatures of stored autologous tissue;
- maintaining tissue at required temperatures during storage equipment malfunction or a power outage;
- handling autologous tissue using sterile technique;
- culturing autologous tissue;
- thawing frozen autologous tissue;
- determining whether or not contaminated autologous tissue will be replanted or autotransplanted;
- refreezing autologous bone;
- transferring or releasing autologous tissue to another facility or a funeral home[131];
- discarding autologous tissue[131];
- documenting activities related to autologous tissue management;
- responding to and investigating adverse reactions related to autologous tissue[152,153]; and
- determining individual roles and responsibilities.

[5: Benefits Balanced with Harms]

Developing and maintaining policies and procedures that guide and support patient care, treatment, and services is a regulatory requirement[157,158] and an accreditation agency standard[159-162] for both hospitals and ambulatory settings.

Recommendation XIII

Perioperative team members should receive initial and ongoing education and complete competency verification activities on the principles and processes of autologous tissue management.

It is the responsibility of the health care organization to provide initial and ongoing education and to evaluate the competency of perioperative team members to deliver safe care to patients undergoing operative or other invasive procedures.[151]

Initial and ongoing education of perioperative personnel related to autologous tissue management facilitates the development of knowledge, skills, and attitudes that affect safe patient care. Periodic education programs provide the opportunity to reinforce the principles and processes of autologous tissue management and to introduce relevant new equipment or practices. Competency verification measures individual performance, provides a mechanism for documentation, and helps verify that perioperative personnel have an understanding of the principles and processes of autologous tissue management.

XIII.a. Education related to autologous tissue management may include a review of the policies and procedures for
- providing care for patients who have sustained traumatic tooth avulsion injuries, including immediate replantation or storage of the tooth in an effective storage medium;
- providing care for patients who may be undergoing recovery, replantation, or autotransplantation of autologous tissue;
- transferring autologous tissue from the sterile field;
- packaging and labeling autologous tissue;
- transporting autologous tissue;
- preserving and storing autologous tissue;
- determining maximum storage duration of autologous tissue and ensuring tissue is not replanted or autotransplanted beyond its expiration date;
- cleaning and sanitizing equipment or devices used to transport or store autologous tissue;
- maintaining and monitoring equipment used to store autologous tissue;
- responding to alarms and malfunction of equipment used to store autologous tissue;
- monitoring temperatures of stored autologous tissue;
- maintaining tissue at required temperatures during storage equipment malfunction or power outage;
- handling autologous tissue using sterile technique;
- culturing autologous tissue;
- thawing frozen autologous tissue;
- determining whether or not contaminated autologous tissue will be replanted or autotransplanted;
- refreezing autologous bone;
- transferring or releasing autologous tissue to another facility or a funeral home[131];
- discarding autologous tissue[131];
- documenting activities related to autologous tissue management;
- responding to and investigating adverse reactions related to autologous tissue[152,153]; and
- determining individual roles and responsibilities.

[5: Benefits Balanced with Harms]

Ongoing development of knowledge and skills and documentation of personnel participation is a regulatory requirement[157,158] and an accreditation agency standard[163-166] for both hospitals and ambulatory settings.

Recommendation XIV

Nursing activities related to autologous tissue management should be documented in a manner consistent with facility or health care organization policies and procedures, regulatory requirements,[3,5] AORN guidelines,[150] and accreditation agency[152,153,156] and AATB standards.[6]

Documentation of nursing activities serves as the legal record of care delivery. Documentation of nursing activities is dictated by facility or health care organization policy, regulatory requirements, accreditation agency standards, and professional guidelines. Documentation is necessary to inform other health care professionals involved in the patient's care. Perioperative documentation that accurately reflects the patient's experience is essential for the continuity of outcome-focused nursing care and for effective comparison of realized versus anticipated patient outcomes.[150] Highly reliable data collection is not only necessary to chronicle patient responses to nursing interventions, but also to demonstrate the facility or health care organization's progress toward quality care outcomes.[150]

XIV.a. Nursing activities related to autologous tissue management must be documented.[3,5] *[1: Regulatory Requirement]*

Maintaining records related to autologous tissue management is a regulatory requirement[3,5], and an accreditation agency[152,153,156] and AATB standard.[6]

XIV.a.1. Tracking of autologous tissue from its source to its final destination must be included in documentation related to autologous tissue management.[3,5,6,152,153] *[1: Regulatory Requirement]*

Traceability of the autograft to its final disposition and retention of records related to disposition of autologous tissue are regulatory requirements[3,5] and AATB standards.[6]

XIV.a.2. Documentation related to autologous tissue management should include

- a listing of all autologous tissue stored and used[152,153];
- records of informed consent;
- information on
  - recovery,
  - processing,
  - preservation,
  - labeling,
  - storage,
  - tissue culture results, and
  - release or transfer of autologous tissue[152,153];
- dates and times of autologous tissue preparation and the identities of personnel preparing the tissue for preservation;
- dates and times of autologous tissue storage and retrieval and the identities of personnel storing and retrieving tissue;
- quality assurance records; and
- information about transfer or disposal of tissue.

[5: Benefits Balanced with Harms]

Effective management and collection of health care information that accurately reflects the patient's care, treatment, and services is a regulatory requirement[157,158] and an accreditation agency standard[167-170] for both hospitals and ambulatory settings.

XIV.a.3. Records related to autologous tissue must be maintained for a minimum of 10 years after the tissue is dispensed or expired, whichever is longer.[3,5] *[1: Regulatory Requirement]*

Maintaining records related to autologous tissue for 10 years is a regulatory requirement[3,5] and an AATB[6] and accreditation agency standard.[152,153]

Recommendation XV

Perioperative personnel should participate in a variety of quality assurance and performance improvement activities that are consistent with the facility or health care organization plan to improve understanding of and compliance with the principles and processes of autologous tissue management.

Quality assurance and performance improvement programs assist in evaluating and improving the quality of patient care and formulating plans for corrective actions. These programs provide data that may be used to determine whether an individual organization is within benchmark goals and, if not, to identify areas that may require corrective actions.

XV.a. A quality assurance program must be maintained to prevent the introduction, transmission, or spread of communicable disease during every step of the autologous tissue management process.[3] *[1: Regulatory Requirement]*

Maintaining a quality assurance program to prevent the introduction, transmission, or spread of communicable disease during every step of the autologous tissue management process is a regulatory requirement[3] and an AATB[6] and accreditation agency standard.[152,153]

XV.a.1. The quality assurance program should prevent contamination, avoid mix-ups, and promote tissue tracking and investigation and reporting of adverse reactions.[6] *[4: Limited Evidence]*

Maintaining a quality improvement program to prevent contamination, avoid mix-ups, and promote tissue tracking and investigation and reporting of adverse reactions is an AATB standard.[6]

XV.a.2. The quality assurance program for autologous tissue management should

- establish a multidisciplinary committee to perform a baseline assessment of the processes (eg, to verify alignment with federal regulations and AATB and accreditation agency standards)[152,153];
- provide at least annual program reviews to monitor ongoing compliance with regulations and safe autologous tissue management processes[152,153];
- identify quality indicators including
  - tissue-handling protocols,
  - labeling procedures,
  - storage requirements,
  - criteria for release of tissue,
  - verification processes, and
  - record maintenance;
- measure compliance with established policies and procedures; and

- mandate investigation and reporting of adverse reactions and events.

[5: Benefits Balanced with Harms]

Collecting data to monitor and improve patient care, treatment, and services is a regulatory requirement[157,158] and an accreditation agency standard[171-174] for both hospitals and ambulatory settings.

XV.a.3. Performance improvement activities for autologous tissue management should include
- monitoring personnel for compliance with safe practices for autologous tissue management,
- periodically reviewing and evaluating activities to identify the need for improvement,
- identifying corrective actions directed toward improvement priorities, and
- taking additional actions when improvement is not achieved or sustained.

[5: Benefits Balanced with Harms]

Reviewing and evaluating quality assurance and performance improvement activities may identify failure points that contribute to errors in autologous tissue management and help define actions for improvement and increased competency.

Taking corrective actions may improve patient safety by enhancing understanding of and compliance with safe practices for autologous tissue management.

XV.b. Perioperative personnel who may be involved in culturing autologous tissue should participate in quality assurance and performance improvement activities related to effective methods of culturing autologous tissue. *[3: Moderate Evidence]*

The collective evidence indicates that autologous tissue culture results may identify tissue that is not acceptable for replantation or autotransplantation and also provide a baseline for evaluation of processing and storage; however, there is a need to optimize and standardize quality monitoring of autologous tissue and culture methods and protocols.[102] Swab cultures are commonly used to determine the level and identity of microbial growth on a surface. They are convenient and easy to use; however, they may pose potential problems when used for identifying and determining the number of microorganisms on autologous tissue.

Surface swab cultures may have limited sensitivity and specificity even when transferred to culture media for incubation.[175] A negative culture result does not mean the autograft is sterile; likewise, a positive culture does not necessarily indicate that the autograft cannot be replanted.[155] Swab cultures are prone to error as a result of variation in the way the swab is manipulated.[175] It is possible that all of the microorganisms on the surface of the tissue being cultured will not be collected by the swab.[175] In addition, some of the microorganisms that are collected may become trapped in the matrix of the swab itself, not transferred to the culture medium, and not detected.[175]

The ability of the swab to recover microorganisms is dependent on its ability to pick up viable microorganisms from the surface of the item being swabbed and to release those microorganisms from the swab into the culture medium.[176] The swab tip may be relatively small compared with the surface area of an autograft. If the existing amount of bioburden is low, it reduces the potential for the swab to collect all microorganisms on the surface.[177]

Liquid culture methods involving a tissue wash may be more effective. The tissue is submerged in solution, and a portion of the solution is aspirated and incubated in culture medium for a defined period of time.[178] Further research is warranted on best methods for determining microbial presence on autologous tissue and the implications of microorganisms on autologous tissue that will be replanted or autotransplanted into the patient.

The limitations of the evidence are that using different methods of culturing or culturing different tissues may have resulted in different outcomes.

The benefit of culturing tissue to determine the level and identity of microbial growth on autologous tissue surfaces is that it may allow for more effective and directed antibiotic therapy to prevent or treat infection. The harm associated with culturing tissue to determine the level and identity of microbial growth on autologous tissue surfaces is that the patient may receive unnecessary antibiotics or other treatments to prevent infection.

Aggarwal et al[179] prospectively compared the effectiveness of tissue and swab cultures in diagnosing periprosthetic joint infections. The samples were collected during a consecutive series of 156 septic and aseptic arthroplasty revisions from October 2011 through April 2012. Three tissue and three swab cultures were taken in a standardized manner from identical regions of the joint. The tissue samples, approximately 1 cm3 in size, were obtained using sterile instruments and placed directly into sterile specimen containers. The researchers found that
- the tissue cultures were positive in 28 of 30 septic cases (93%),
- the swab cultures were positive in 21 of 30 septic cases (70%),
- the tissue cultures were positive in two of 87 aseptic cases (2%), and
- the swab cultures were positive in 10 of 87 aseptic cases (11%).

The researchers concluded that tissue samples demonstrated higher sensitivity for diagnosing periprosthetic joint infections than swab cultures. The swab cultures had more false-negative and false-positive results than the tissue cultures. The researchers recommended against the use of swab cultures for intraoperative tissue cultures because they posed a higher risk of not identifying or of incorrectly identifying infective organisms.[179]

In a quasi-experimental study, Dennis et al[178] evaluated allograft tissue from 78 musculoskeletal donors by concurrently testing for microorganisms using liquid and swab culture methods. The swab cultures were obtained using a single swab from the surface of the long bones, medullary canal, and joint soft tissue. The liquid cultures were obtained by immersion of the tissue in 4,000 mL of sterile normal saline solution for 10 minutes and then shaking for one minute. A portion of the rinse solution (10 mL) was then injected into a culture medium. The results showed that the swab method detected four of 20 organisms (20%) while the liquid culture method detected 18 of 20 organisms (90%). The researchers concluded that the liquid culture method was superior to the swab method; however, further research was warranted to determine the best method for obtaining optimal culture results when using the liquid culture method.

Ronholdt and Bogdansky[176] conducted an RCT to evaluate the suitability of using swab cultures as a method for determining microbial contamination of allograft tissues. The researchers compared two swab-culturing systems using 168 human allograft tissues sterilized by radiation and then inoculated with low levels of multiple bacterial and fungal microorganisms (ie, *Staphylococcus aureus, Pseudomonas aeruginosa, Bacillus subtillus, Candida albicans, Aspergillus niger, Clostridium sporogenes*). The inoculated allograft tissues were swabbed in a "zigzag" pattern to ensure that the greatest surface area of the allograft was swabbed, and then streaked onto the culture medium three times while the culture plate was turned 120 degrees clockwise each time, for a total of 360 degrees. The swab tip was also rotated 120 degrees each time the plate was turned to ensure the entire surface of the swab contacted the entire surface of the culture medium, thus increasing the likelihood of recovering the challenge microorganisms.

The researchers calculated the average amount of challenge microorganism recovery for each swab system. The results showed that both swab-culturing systems tested exhibited low and variable microorganism recovery from the allograft tissues, and there was not a statistically significant difference between the two systems. No organisms were recovered in 73.8% of cultures (n = 124).

The researchers noted an interesting trend in that the soft tissue allografts (ie, tissues used to repair and reconstruct tendons and ligaments [eg, fascia, Achilles tendon]) (n = 84) had more positive cultures compared with the cut tissue allografts (ie, load-bearing tissues [eg, tricortical wedges, femoral heads]) (n = 84). The researchers theorized that this was because the microorganisms resided on the surface of the soft tissue and were more easily recovered, whereas the porous nature of the cut tissue allowed the microorganisms to be absorbed into the interior of the tissue, making recovery more difficult.

In addition, the researchers noted that a moist swab was more likely to capture and retain microorganisms than was a dry swab. The researchers concluded that swab-culturing methods may not have the sensitivity or reproducibility necessary to be used for final release of allograft tissues. They recommended that alternative, validated microbial detection methods be evaluated and implemented for tissue cultures.

XV.b.1. Microbiologic culture testing should be performed in a laboratory that is either certified under the Clinical Laboratory Improvement Amendments of 1988 (CLIA-88)[180] or is certified or accredited by another laboratory-accrediting organization that has deemed status for CLIA-88.[6] *[4: Limited Evidence]*

Using a certified laboratory for microbiologic culture testing is an AATB standard.[6]

XV.b.2. Cultures obtained for determining the level and identity of microbial growth on autologous tissue should
- be obtained before the tissue is treated with antibiotics or cleansing agents[131] and
- include testing to detect bacteria (ie, aerobic and anaerobic) and fungi.[6]

[4: Limited Evidence]

Using antibiotics or other cleansing agents may inhibit the culture method used to detect viable organisms and may result in a false-negative culture result. Obtaining cultures to detect bacteria and fungi may help to identify tissue that is contaminated and may be unacceptable for replantation.

XV.c. Perioperative personnel must investigate any adverse reaction or event involving a communicable disease related to replanted or autotransplanted autologous tissue.[3,5] An adverse reaction or event involving a communicable disease must be reported if it
○ is life-threatening or fatal;
○ results in permanent impairment of a body function or permanent damage to a body structure; or

necessitates medical or surgical intervention, including hospitalization.[3,5,181]

[1: Regulatory Requirement]

Reporting adverse reactions and events related to replanted or autotransplanted tissue is a regulatory requirement[3,5,181] and an AATB[6] and accreditation agency standard.[152,153]

XV.c.1. Reports should be submitted through Med-Watch: The FDA Safety Information and Adverse Event Reporting Program.[182] [1: Regulatory Requirement]

Editor's note: *TiProtec is a registered trademark of Dr. Franz Köhler Chemie GmbH, Bensheim, Germany. X-Vivo 10 is a registered trademark of BioWhittaker Molecular Applications, Rockland, ME. Plasma-Lyte is a registered trademark of Baxter International, Deerfield, IL.*

Glossary

Adverse reaction: Related to replanted or autotransplanted autologous tissue, a harmful and unintended response to human cells or tissue for which there is a reasonable probability that the human cells or tissue caused the event.

Allograft: A graft taken from a living or nonliving donor for transplantation to a different individual.

American Association of Tissue Banks (AATB): A nonprofit organization that defines the standards for tissue banking.

Apoptosis: A sequence of events leading to cell death by fragmentation of cell particles that are engulfed by other cells.

Autograft: Tissue recovered from an individual for implantation or transplantation exclusively on or in the same individual.

Autologous: Cells or tissues obtained from the same individual.

Autotransplantation: Transplantation of tissue from one site to another in the same individual.

Avulsed tooth: A tooth separated by a traumatic action from the socket in which the roots of the tooth are embedded.

Cancellous bone: Bone with a lattice-like or spongy structure typically found at the ends of long bones, proximal to joints, and within the interior of vertebrae.

Chondrocyte: A cartilage cell.

Computed tomography (CT): A three-dimensional radiograph generated by computer synthesis of multiple cross-sectional images made along an axis.

Craniectomy: Surgical removal of a portion of the skull.

Cranioplasty: Surgical repair of a defect or deformity of the skull.

Cryopreservation: A process for maintaining the viability of resected tissue or organs by storing them at very low temperatures without causing damage from the formation of ice that may occur during freezing.

Cryoprotectant: A chemical substance used to protect biological tissue from damage due to ice formation during the cryopreservation process.

Cytotoxic: A substance that is poisonous to living cells.

Dulbecco's modified Eagle's medium: A modified version of Eagle's minimum essential medium that contains iron, phenol red, four times the amount of vitamins and amino acids, and two to four times as much glucose.

Eagle's minimum essential medium: A cell and culture medium that contains amino acids, salts, glucose, and vitamins.

Engrafting: A process that occurs when a piece of tissue (eg, skin) that has been surgically transplanted begins to function normally.

Fibroblasts: Star-shaped cells capable of forming collagen fibers.

Hank's Balanced Salt Solution: A solution composed of inorganic salts and bicarbonate ions designed to maintain physiological acid-base balance and osmotic pressure necessary for cell growth.

Hemacytometer: A device used to count cells.

Isotonic: Having the same solute concentration as a reference solution.

Krebs-Ringer solution: A balanced salt solution and physiological buffer used to maintain structural integrity of cells in culture.

Lactobacillus reuteri: A Gram-positive, rod-shaped, nonpathogenic bacteria that inhabits the intestinal tract of mammals.

McCoy's 5A medium: A sterile nutrient medium made up of amino acids, vitamins, minerals, antibiotics, and buffers.

Meshed skin: A skin graft with multiple cuts that allow it to be stretched to cover a larger area.

Mitochondria: Structures located in cell cytoplasm that are responsible for energy production.

Morus rubra: A mulberry tree, also known as red mulberry.

Oral rehydration solution: A solution made of water with small amounts of sugar and salt that is used to prevent or correct dehydration.

Osmolality: A measurement of the concentration of chemical particles found in a fluid. The greater the concentration of dissolved particles, the higher the osmolality.

Osseointegration: The structural and functional connection that develops between living bone and the surface of an implant.

Osteoblasts: Large cells responsible for synthesis and mineralization of bone during bone formation and regeneration. Osteoblasts are the major cellular component of bone.

Osteoclasts: Large multinuclear bone cells that resorb bone tissue.

Osteoconduction: Growth of bone tissue into an implant or graft.

Osteocytes: Bone cells located within the bone matrix.

Osteoinduction: Acceleration of new bone formation.

Periodontal ligament: Connective tissue that surrounds the tooth root.

Plasma-Lyte®: An isotonic solution that closely resembles human plasma in its electrolyte content, osmolality, and pH.

Pulsatile lavage: A method of delivering irrigation under pressure with pulsation. Used to remove microorganisms and debris from the surface of a wound.

Replantation: Replacement of an organ or body part (eg, avulsed tooth) into its original site and reestablishing its circulation.

Roswell Park Memorial Institute 1640 culture medium: A cell and culture medium enriched with amino acids and vitamins that contains a bicarbonate buffering system.

Salvia officinalis: An evergreen shrub also known as garden sage or common sage.

Storage medium: A physiologic solution that closely replicates conditions that help to preserve the viability of cells.

Subgaleal: The space between the skin and the skull.

TiProtec®: A sterile, hypothermic solution enriched with potassium chloride and N-acetyl histidine used for long-term protection and storage of tissue.

Tissue bank: A facility that participates in procuring, processing, preserving, or storing human cells and tissue for transplantation.

Tooth pulp: Soft tissue in the center of the tooth that contains blood vessels, connective tissue, and nerves.

Transmissible spongiform encephalopathy agents: Abnormal protein particles known as prions that are believed to be the cause of a group of diseases that affect the brain and nervous system. The development of tiny holes in the brain give it a sponge-like appearance, hence the term *spongiform.*

Tulle gras: A fine-meshed gauze impregnated with vegetable oil or soft paraffin.

X-Vivo 10®: A serum-free, cell media containing human proteins, phenol red, and gentamicin that supports the formation of blood or blood cells.

REFERENCES

1. Pu LL, Cui X, Fink BF, Cibull ML, Gao D. Long-term preservation of adipose aspirates after conventional lipoplasty. *Aesthet Surg J.* 2004;24(6):536-541. [IB]

2. Pu LLQ. Cryopreservation of adipose tissue. *Organogenesis.* 2009;5(3):138-142. [VA]

3. §21 CFR 1271: Human cells, tissues, and cellular and tissue-based products. April;2013. US Food and Drug Administration. http://www.accessdata.fda.gov/scripts/cdrh/cfdocs/cfcfr/CFRSearch.cfm?CFRPart=1271. Accessed September 26, 2014.

4. Human Cells, Tissues, and Cellular and Tissue-Based Products; Establishment Registration and Listing. *Fed Regist.* 2001;66(13):5447-5469. http://www.gpo.gov/fdsys/pkg/FR-2001-01-19/pdf/01-1126.pdf. Accessed September 26, 2014.

5. *Current Good Tissue Practice (CGTP) and Additional Requirements for Manufacturers of Human Cells, Tissues, and Cellular and Tissue-Based Products (HCT/Ps).* Silver Spring, MD: US Food and Drug Administration; 2012.

6. *Standards for Tissue Banking.* McLean, VA: American Association of Tissue Banks; 2012. [IVC]

7. Sanghavi T, Shah N, Parekh V, Singbal K. Evaluation and comparison of efficacy of three different storage media, coconut water, propolis, and oral rehydration solution, in maintaining the viability of periodontal ligament cells. *J Cons Dentistry.* 2013;16(1):71-74. [IIB]

8. Thomas T, Gopikrishna V, Kandaswamy D. Comparative evaluation of maintenance of cell viability of an experimental transport media "coconut water" with Hank's balanced salt solution and milk, for transportation of an avulsed tooth: an in vitro cell culture study. *J Conserv Dentistry.* 2008;11(1):22-29. [IIB]

9. Chen H, Huang B. (-)-Epigallocatechin-3-gallate: a novel storage medium for avulsed teeth. *Dent Traumatol.* 2012;28(2):158-160. [IB]

10. Gjertsen AW, Stothz KA, Neiva KG, Pileggi R. Effect of propolis on proliferation and apoptosis of periodontal ligament fibroblasts. *Oral Surg Oral Med Oral Pathol Oral Radiol Endod.* 2011;112(6):843-848. [IIB]

11. Brullmann D, Schulze RK, d'Hoedt B. The treatment of anterior dental trauma. *Dtsch Arztebl Int.* 2010;108(34-35):565-570. [VB]

12. Khademi AA, Saei S, Mohajeri MR, et al. A new storage medium for an avulsed tooth. *J Contemp Dent Pract.* [Electronic Resource]. 2008;9(6):25-32. [IB]

13. Gopikrishna V, Thomas T, Kandaswamy D. A quantitative analysis of coconut water: a new storage media for avulsed teeth. *Oral Surg Oral Med Oral Pathol Oral Radiol Endod.* 2008;105(2):e61-e65. [IB]

14. Sigalas E, Regan JD, Kramer PR, Witherspoon DE, Opperman LA. Survival of human periodontal ligament cells in media proposed for transport of avulsed teeth. *Dent Traumatol.* 2004;20(1):21-28. [IIIC]

15. Krasner P. Treatment of avulsed teeth by oral and maxillofacial surgeons. *J Oral Maxillofac Surg.* 2010;68(11):2888-2892. [VB]

16. Moradian H, Badakhsh S, Rahimi M, Hekmatfar S. Replantation of an avulsed maxillary incisor after 12 hours: three-year follow-up. *Iranian Endod J.* 2013;8(1):33-36. [VB]

17. Udoye CI, Jafarzadeh H, Abbott PV. Transport media for avulsed teeth: a review. *Austr Endod J.* 2012;38(3):129-136. [VB]

18. Souza BD, Luckemeyer DD, Reyes-Carmona JF, Felippe WT, Simoes CM, Felippe MC. Viability of human periodontal ligament fibroblasts in milk, Hank's balanced salt solution and coconut water as storage media. *Int Endod J.* 2011;44(2):111-115. [IIB]

19. Moazami F, Mirhadi H, Geramizadeh B, Sahebi S. Comparison of soymilk, powdered milk, Hank's balanced salt solution and tap water on periodontal ligament cell survival. *Dent Traumatol.* 2012;28(2):132-135. [IIB]

20. Ozan F, Polat ZA, Er K, Ozan U, Deger O. Effect of propolis on survival of periodontal ligament cells: new storage media for avulsed teeth. *J Endod.* 2007;33(5):570-573. [IIB]

21. Doshi D. Bet 3. Avulsed tooth brought in milk for replantation. *Emerg Med J.* 2009;26(10):736-737. [VB]

22. Lin S, Zuckerman O, Fuss Z, et al. New emphasis in the treatment of dental trauma: avulsion and luxation. *Dent Traumatol.* 2007;23(5):297-303. [VB]

23. Goswami M, Chaitra T, Chaudhary S, Manuja N, Sinha A. Strategies for periodontal ligament cell viability: an overview. *J Conserv Dent.* 2011;14(3):215-220. [VB]

24. Karayilmaz H, Kirzioglu Z, Erken Gungor O. Aetiology, treatment patterns and long-term outcomes of tooth avulsion in children and adolescents. *Pakistan J Med Sci.* 2013;29(2):464-468. [IIIB]

25. Andersson L, Andreasen JO, Day P, et al. International Association of Dental Traumatology guidelines for

PATIENT AND WORKER SAFETY

the management of traumatic dental injuries: 2. Avulsion of permanent teeth. *Dent Traumatol.* 2012;28(2):88-96. [IVB]

26. Caglar E, Sandalli N, Kuscu OO, et al. Viability of fibroblasts in a novel probiotic storage media. *Dent Traumatol.* 2010;26(5):383-387. [IIC]

27. Malhotra N. Current developments in interim transport (storage) media in dentistry: an update. *Br Dent J.* 2011;211(1):29-33. [VB]

28. Saxena P, Pant VA, Wadhwani KK, Kashyap MP, Gupta SK, Pant AB. Potential of the propolis as storage medium to preserve the viability of cultured human periodontal ligament cells: an in vitro study. *Dent Traumatol.* 2011;27(2):102-108. [IIB]

29. Ceallaigh PO, Ekanaykaee K, Beirne CJ, Patton DW. Diagnosis and management of common maxillofacial injuries in the emergency department. Part 5: dentoalveolar injuries. *Emerg Med J.* 2007;24(6):429-430. [VB]

30. Al-Nazhan S, Al-Nasser A. Viability of human periodontal ligament fibroblasts in tissue culture after exposure to different contact lens solutions. *J Contemp Dent Pract.* [Electronic Resource]. 2006;7(4):37-44. [IIC]

31. Andreasen JO, Borum MK, Jacobsen HL, Andreasen FM. Replantation of 400 avulsed permanent incisors. 4. Factors related to periodontal ligament healing. *Endod Dent Traumatol.* 1995;11(2):76-89. [IIIB]

32. Souza BD, Luckemeyer DD, Felippe WT, Simoes CM, Felippe MC. Effect of temperature and storage media on human periodontal ligament fibroblast viability. *Dent Traumatol.* 2010;26(3):271-275. [IIB]

33. Silva EJ, Rollemberg CB, Coutinho-Filho TS, Krebs RL, Zaia AA. Use of soymilk as a storage medium for avulsed teeth. *Acta Odontol Scand.* 2013;71(5):1101-1104. [IIB]

34. Eskandarian T, Badakhsh S, Esmaeilpour T. The effectiveness of oral rehydration solution at various concentrations as a storage media for avulsed teeth. *Iranian Endod J.* 2013;8(1):22-24. [IIB]

35. Macway-Gomez S, Lallier TE. Pedialyte promotes periodontal ligament cell survival and motility. *J Endod.* 2013;39(2):202-207. [IIB]

36. Moura CC, Soares PB, Reis MV, Fernandes Neto AJ, Soares CJ. Soy milk as a storage medium to preserve human fibroblast cell viability: an in vitro study. *Braz Dent J.* 2012;23(5):559-563. [IIB]

37. Hwang JY, Choi SC, Park JH, Kang SW. The use of green tea extract as a storage medium for the avulsed tooth. *J Endod.* 2011;37(7):962-967. [IIB]

38. Moreira-Neto JJ, Gondim JO, Raddi MS, Pansani CA. Viability of human fibroblasts in coconut water as a storage medium. *Int Endod J.* 2009;42(9):827-830. [IIB]

39. de Sousa HA, de Alencar AH, Bruno KF, Batista AC, de Carvalho AC. Microscopic evaluation of the effect of different storage media on the periodontal ligament of surgically extracted human teeth. *Dent Traumatol.* 2008;24(6):628-632. [IIB]

40. Ozan F, Polat ZA, Tepe B, Er K. Influence of storage media containing *Salvia officinalis* on survival of periodontal ligament cells. *J Contemp Dent Pract.* [Electronic Resource]. 2008;9(6):17-24. [IIB]

41. Ozan F, Tepe B, Polat ZA, Er K. Evaluation of in vitro effect of *Morus rubra* (red mulberry) on survival of periodontal ligament cells. *Oral Surg Oral Med Oral Pathol Oral Radiol Endod.* 2008;105(2):e66-e69. [IIB]

42. de Souza BD, Luckemeyer DD, Felippe WT, Alves AM, Simoes CM, Felippe MC. Effect of milk renewal on human periodontal ligament fibroblast viability in vitro. *Dent Traumatol.* 2012;28(3):214-216. [IIB]

43. *Treatment of Avulsed Permanent Teeth in Children.* Rev. 2004. Royal College of Surgeons. http://www.rcseng.ac.uk/fds/publications-clinical-guidelines/clinical_guidelines/documents/avulsed_permanent_treatment.pdf/view. Accessed September 26, 2014. [IVB]

44. Rajendran P, Varghese NO, Varughese JM, Murugaian E. Evaluation, using extracted human teeth, of Ricetral as a storage medium for avulsions—an in vitro study. *Dent Traumatol.* 2011;27(3):217-220. [IC]

45. Subramaniam P, Eswara U, Girish Babu KL, Vardhan B. Oral rehydration salt-liquid as an alternative storage medium—a preliminary study. *J Clin Pediatr Dent.* 2011;35(4):393-395. [IC]

46. Huang SC, Remeikis NA, Daniel JC. Effects of long-term exposure of human periodontal ligament cells to milk and other solutions. *J Endod.* 1996;22(1):30-33. [IIB]

47. Ahangari Z, Alborzi S, Yadegari Z, Dehghani F, Ahangari L, Naseri M. The effect of propolis as a biological storage media on periodontal ligament cell survival in an avulsed tooth: an in vitro study. *Cell J.* 2013;15(3):244-249. [IIB]

48. Chamorro MM, Regan JD, Opperman LA, Kramer PR. Effect of storage media on human periodontal ligament cell apoptosis. *Dent Traumatol.* 2008;24(1):11-16. [IIC]

49. Lin S, Emodi O, Abu El-Naaj I. Splinting of an injured tooth as part of emergency treatment. *Dent Traumatol.* 2008;24(3):370-372. [VB]

50. Mousavi B, Alavi SA, Mohajeri MR, Mirkheshti N, Ghassami F, Mirkheshti N. Standard oral rehydration solution as a new storage medium for avulsed teeth. *Int Dent J.* 2010;60(6):379-382. [IB]

51. Jung IH, Yun JH, Cho AR, Kim CS, Chung WG, Choi SH. Effect of (-)-epigallocatechin-3-gallate on maintaining the periodontal ligament cell viability of avulsed teeth: a preliminary study. *J Periodontal Implant Sci.* 2011;41(1):10-16. [IIB]

52. de Souza BD, Bortoluzzi EA, da Silveira Teixeira C, Felippe WT, Simoes CM, Felippe MC. Effect of HBSS storage time on human periodontal ligament fibroblast viability. *Dent Traumatol.* 2010;26(6):481-483. [IIC]

53. *Recommended Guidelines of the American Association of Endodontists for the Treatment of Traumatic Dental Injuries.* 2013. American Association of Endodontists. http://www.nxtbook.com/nxtbooks/aae/traumaguidelines/. Accessed September 26, 2014. [IVC]

54. Ballal V, V J. Storage media. *Br Dent J.* 2011;211(4):153. [VB]

55. Sonoda CK, Poi WR, Panzarini SR, Sottovia AD, Okamoto T. Tooth replantation after keeping the avulsed tooth in oral environment: case report of a 3-year follow-up. *Am Assoc Endod.* 2008;24(3):373-376. [VB]

56. Koca H, Topaloglu-Ak A, Sutekin E, Koca O, Acar S. Delayed replantation of an avulsed tooth after 5 hours of storage in saliva: a case report. *Dent Traumatol.* 2010;26(4):370-373. [VB]

57. Ize-Iyamu IN, Saheeb B. Reimplantation of avulsed dry permanent teeth after three days: a report of two cases. *Nigerian J Clin Pract.* 2013;16(1):119-122. [VC]

58. Baginska J, Wilczynska-Borawska M. Knowledge of nurses working at schools in Bialystok, Poland, of tooth avulsion and its management. *Dent Traumatol.* 2012;28(4):314-319. [IIIB]

59. Ulusoy AT, Onder H, Cetin B, Kaya S. Knowledge of medical hospital emergency physicians about the first-aid management of traumatic tooth avulsion. *Int J Paed Dent.* 2012;22(3):211-216. [IIIB]

60. Yeng T, Parashos P. An investigation into dentists' management methods of dental trauma to maxillary

permanent incisors in Victoria, Australia. *Dent Traumatol.* 2008;24(4):443-448. [IIIB]

61. Kargul B, Welbury R. An audit of the time to initial treatment in avulsion injuries. *Dent Traumatol.* 2009;25(1):123-125. [IIIB]

62. de Vasconcellos LG, Brentel AS, Vanderlei AD, de Vasconcellos LM, Valera MC, de Araujo MA. Knowledge of general dentists in the current guidelines for emergency treatment of avulsed teeth and dental trauma prevention. *Dent Traumatol.* 2009;25(6):578-583. [IIIB]

63. Zhao Y, Gong Y. Knowledge of emergency management of avulsed teeth: a survey of dentists in Beijing, China. *Dent Traumatol.* 2010;26(3):281-284. [IIIB]

64. Loh T, Sae-Lim V, Yian TB, Liang S. Dental therapists' experience in the immediate management of traumatized teeth. *Dent Traumatol.* 2006;22(2) 66-70. [IIIB]

65. Hugar SM, Suganya M, Kiran K, Vikneshan M, More VP. Knowledge and awareness of dental trauma among Indian nurses. *Int Emerg Nurs.* 2013;21(4):252-256. [IIIB]

66. Needleman HL, Stucenski K, Forbes PW, Chen Q, Stack AM. Massachusetts emergency departments' resources and physicians' knowledge of management of traumatic dental injuries. *Dent Traumatol.* 2013;29(4):272-279. [IIIC]

67. Choi D, Badner VM, Yeroshalmi F, Margulis KS, Dougherty NJ, Kreiner-Litt G. Dental trauma management by New York City school nurses. *J Dent Child.* 2012;79(2):74-78. [IIIB]

68. Tahir MZ, Shamim MS, Sobani ZA, Zafar SN, Qadeer M, Bari ME. Safety of untreated autologous cranioplasty after extracorporeal storage at -26 degree celsius. *Br J Neurosurg.* 2013;27(4):479-482. [IIIB]

69. Lu Y, Hui G, Liu F, Wang Z, Tang Y, Gao S. Survival and regeneration of deep-freeze preserved autologous cranial bones after cranioplasty. *Br J Neurosurg.* 2012;26(2):216-221. [IIIC]

70. Bhaskar IP, Yusheng L, Zheng M, Lee GY. Autogenous skull flaps stored frozen for more than 6 months: do they remain viable? *J Clin Neurosci.* 2011;18(12):1690-1693. [IIB]

71. Grossman N, Shemesh-Jan HS, Merkin V, Gideon M, Cohen A. Deep-freeze preservation of cranial bones for future cranioplasty: nine years of experience in Soroka University Medical Center. *Cell Tissue Bank.* 2007;8(3):243-246. [VB]

72. Beez T, Sabel M, Ahmadi SA, Beseoglu K, Steiger H-J, Sabel M. Scanning electron microscopic surface analysis of cryoconserved skull bone after decompressive craniectomy. *Cell Tissue Bank.* 2013;15(1):85-88. [IIIC]

73. Elwatidy S, Elgamal E, Jamjoom Z, Habib H, Raddaoui E. Assessment of bone flap viability and sterility after long periods of preservation in the freezer. *Pan Arab J Neurosurg.* 2011;15(1):24-28. [IIIC]

74. Bhaskar IP, Zaw NN, Zheng M, Lee GYF. Bone flap storage following craniectomy: A survey of practices in major Australian Neurosurgical centres. *ANZ J Surg.* 2011;81(3):137-141. [IIIC]

75. Baldo S, Tacconi L. Effectiveness and safety of subcutaneous abdominal preservation of autologous bone flap after decompressive craniectomy: a prospective pilot study. *World Neurosurg.* 2010;73(5):552-556. [IIIB]

76. Prolo DJ, Burres KP, McLaughlin WT, Christensen AH. Autogenous skull cranioplasty: fresh and preserved (frozen), with consideration of the cellular response. *Neurosurgery.* 1979;4(1):18-29. [IIIB]

77. Shoakazemi A, Flannery T, McConnell RS. Long-term outcome of subcutaneously preserved autologous cranioplasty. *Neurosurgery.* 2009;65(3):505-510. [IIIB]

78. Movassaghi K, Ver Halen J, Ganchi P, Amin-Hanjani S, Mesa J, Yaremchuk MJ. Cranioplasty with subcutaneously preserved autologous bone grafts. *Plast Reconstr Surg.* 2006;117(1):202-206. [IIIC]

79. Iwama T, Yamada J, Imai S, Shinoda J, Funakoshi T, Sakai N. The use of frozen autogenous bone flaps in delayed cranioplasty revisited. *Neurosurgery.* 2003;52(3):591-596. [IIIB]

80. Morina A, Kelmendi F, Morina Q, et al. Cranioplasty with subcutaneously preserved autologous bone grafts in abdominal wall—experience with 75 cases in a post-war country Kosova. *Surg Neurol Int.* 2011;2:72. [VB]

81. Pasaoglu A, Kurtsoy A, Koc RK, et al. Cranioplasty with bone flaps preserved under the scalp. *Neurosurg Rev.* 1996;19(3):153-156. [IIIC]

82. Vanaclocha V, Saiz-Sapena N, Garcia-Casasola C, De Alava E. Cranioplasty with autogenous autoclaved calvarial bone flap in the cases of tumoural invasion. *Acta Neurochir (Wien).* 1997;139(10):970-976. [IIIC]

83. Matsuno A, Tanaka H, Iwamuro H, et al. Analyses of the factors influencing bone graft infection after delayed cranioplasty. *Acta Neurochir (Wien).* 2006;148(5):535-540. [IIIB]

84. Schultke E, Hampl JA, Jatzwauk L, Krex D, Schackert G. An easy and safe method to store and disinfect explanted skull bone. *Acta Neurochir (Wien).* 1999;141(5):525-528. [IIB]

85. Wester K. Cranioplasty with an autoclaved bone flap, with special reference to tumour infiltration of the flap. *Acta Neurochir (Wien).* 1994;131(3-4):223-225. [VB]

86. Zingale A, Albanese V. Cryopreservation of autogeneous bone flap in cranial surgical practice: what is the future? A grade B and evidence level 4 meta-analytic study. *J Neurosurg Sci.* 2003;47(3):137-139. [IC]

87. Albrektsson T, Johansson C. Osteoinduction, osteoconduction and osseointegration. *Eur Spine J.* 2001;10(Suppl 2):S96-S101. [VA]

88. Gibson S, McLeod I, Wardlaw D, Urbaniak S. Allograft versus autograft in instrumented posterolateral lumbar spinal fusion: a randomized control trial. *Spine (Phila Pa 1976).* 2002;27(15):1599-1603. [IB]

89. Yazici M, Asher MA. Freeze-dried allograft for posterior spinal fusion in patients with neuromuscular spinal deformities. *Spine (Phila Pa 1976).* 1997;22(13):1467-1471. [VB]

90. Bridwell KH, O'Brien MF, Lenke LG, Baldus C, Blanke K. Posterior spinal fusion supplemented with only allograft bone in paralytic scoliosis. Does it work? *Spine (Phila Pa 1976).* 1994;19(23):2658-2666. [IIIC]

91. Gill K, O'Brien JP. Observations of resorption of the posterior lateral bone graft in combined anterior and posterior lumbar fusion. *Spine (Phila Pa 1976).* 1993;18(13):1885-1889. [IIIC]

92. Nasca RJ, Whelchel JD. Use of cryopreserved bone in spinal surgery. *Spine (Phila Pa 1976).* 1987;12(3):222-227. [IIIB]

93. Wimmer C, Krismer M, Gluch H, Ogon M, Stockl B. Autogenic versus allogenic bone grafts in anterior lumbar interbody fusion. *Clin Orthop Relat Res.* 1999;(360)(360):122-126. [IIIB]

94. Joaquim AF, Mattos JP, Neto FC, Lopes A, de Oliveira E. Bone flap management in neurosurgery. *Revi Neuroci.* 2009;17(2):133-137. [VB]

95. Flannery T, McConnell RS. Cranioplasty: why throw the bone flap out? *Br J Neurosurg.* 2001;15(6):518-520. [VB]

96. Krishnan P, Bhattacharyya AK, Sil K, De R. Bone flap preservation after decompressive craniectomy—experience with 55 cases. *Neurol India.* 2006;54(3):291-292. [VC]

PATIENT AND WORKER SAFETY

97. Jho DH, Neckrysh S, Hardman J, Charbel FT, Amin-Hanjani S. Ethylene oxide gas sterilization: a simple technique for storing explanted skull bone. Technical note. *J Neurosurg.* 2007;107(2):440-445. [IIIB]

98. Inamasu J, Kuramae T, Nakatsukasa M. Does difference in the storage method of bone flaps after decompressive craniectomy affect the incidence of surgical site infection after cranioplasty? Comparison between subcutaneous pocket and cryopreservation. *J Trauma-Inj Infect Crit Care.* 2010;68(1):183-187. [IIIB]

99. Sultan SM, Davidson EH, Butala P, et al. Interval cranioplasty: Comparison of current standards. *Plast Reconstr Surg.* 2011;127(5):1855-1864. [IIB]

100. Osawa M, Hara H, Ichinose Y, Koyama T, Kobayashi S, Sugita Y. Cranioplasty with a frozen and autoclaved bone flap. *Acta Neurochir (Wien).* 1990;102(1-2):38-41. [VB]

101. Guerrero MA. Cryopreservation of parathyroid glands. *Int J Endocrinol.* 2010;2010:829540. [VA]

102. Stotler BA, Reich-Slotky R, Schwartz J, et al. Quality monitoring of microbial contamination of cryopreserved parathyroid tissue. *Cell Tissue Bank.* 2011;12(2):111-116. [VB]

103. Cohen MS, Dilley WG, Wells SA Jr, et al. Long-term functionality of cryopreserved parathyroid autografts: a 13-year prospective analysis. *Surgery.* 2005;138(6):1033-1040. [IIIB]

104. Schneider R, Ramaswamy A, Slater EP, Bartsch DK, Schlosser K. Cryopreservation of parathyroid tissue after parathyroid surgery for renal hyperparathyroidism: does it really make sense? *World J Surg.* 2012;36(11):2598-2604. [IIIB]

105. Guerrero MA, Evans DB, Lee JE, et al. Viability of cryopreserved parathyroid tissue: when is continued storage versus disposal indicated? *World J Surg.* 2008;32(5):836-839. [IIIB]

106. Saxe AW, Spiegel AM, Marx SJ, Brennan MF. Deferred parathyroid autografts with cryopreserved tissue after reoperative parathyroid surgery. *Arch Surg.* 1982;117(5):538-543. [IIIC]

107. Agarwal A, Waghray A, Gupta S, Sharma R, Milas M. Cryopreservation of parathyroid tissue: an illustrated technique using the Cleveland Clinic protocol. *J Am Coll Surg.* 2013;216(1):e1-e9. [VA]

108. Alvarez-Hernandez D, Gonzalez-Suarez I, Carrillo-Lopez N, Naves-Diaz M, Anguita-Velasco J, Cannata-Andia JB. Viability and functionality of fresh and cryopreserved human hyperplastic parathyroid tissue tested in vitro. *Am J Nephrol.* 2008;28(1):76-82. [IIC]

109. Barreira CE, Cernea CR, Brandão LG, Custodio MR, Caldini ET, de Menezes Montenegro FL. Effects of time on ultrastructural integrity of parathyroid tissue before cryopreservation. *World J Surg.* 2011;35(11):2440-2444. [IIC]

110. de Menezes Montenegro FL, Custodio MR, Arap SS, et al. Successful implant of long-term cryopreserved parathyroid glands after total parathyroidectomy. *Head Neck.* 2007;29(3):296-300. [VB]

111. DeBono R, Rao GS, Berry RB. The survival of human skin stored by refrigeration at 4 degrees C in McCoy's 5A medium: does oxygenation of the medium improve storage time? *Plast Reconstr Surg.* 1998;102(1):78-83. [IIB]

112. Mardini S, Agullo FJ, Salgado CJ, Rose V, Moran SL, Chen HC. Delayed skin grafting utilizing autologous banked tissue. *Ann Plast Surg.* 2009;63(3):311-313. [VB]

113. Robb EC, Bechmann NRVT, Plessinger RT, Boyce ST, Warden GD, Kagan RJ. Storage media and temperature maintain normal anatomy of cadaveric human skin for transplantation to full-thickness skin wounds. *J Burn Care Rehabil.* 2001;22(6):393-396. [IIB]

114. Cram AE, Domayer MA. Short-term preservation of human autografts. *J Trauma.* 1983;23(10):872-873. [VC]

115. Sterne GD, Titley OG, Christie JL. A qualitative histological assessment of various storage conditions on short term preservation of human split skin grafts. *Br J Plast Surg.* 2000;53(4):331-336. [IIC]

116. Sheridan R, Mahe J, Walters P. Autologous skin banking. *Burns.* 1998;24(1):46-48. [IIIC]

117. Titley OG, Cooper M, Thomas A, Hancock K. Stored skin--stored trouble? *Br J Plast Surg.* 1994;47(1):24-29. [IIIB]

118. Molnar GF, Nemes A, Kekesi V, Monos E, Nadasy GL. Maintained geometry, elasticity and contractility of human saphenous vein segments stored in a complex tissue culture medium. *Eur J Vasc Endovasc Surg.* 2010;40(1):88-93. [IB]

119. Ebner A, Poitz DM, Augstein A, Strasser RH, Deussen A. Functional, morphologic, and molecular characterization of cold storage injury. *J Vasc Surg.* 2012;56(1):189-198.e3. [IIB]

120. Wilbring M, Tugtekin SM, Zatschler B, et al. Preservation of endothelial vascular function of saphenous vein grafts after long-time storage with a recently developed potassium-chloride and N-acetylhistidine enriched storage solution. *Thorac Cardiovasc Surg.* 2013;61(8):656-662. [IIIB]

121. Baumann FG, Catinella FP, Cunningham JN Jr, Spencer FC. Vein contraction and smooth muscle cell extensions as causes of endothelial damage during graft preparation. *Ann Surg.* 1981;194(2):199-211. [IIB]

122. Jankowitz BT, Kondziolka DS. When the bone flap hits the floor. *Neurosurgery.* 2006;59(3):585-589. [IIIB]

123. Kang L, Mermel LA, Trafton PG. What happens when autogenous bone drops out of the sterile field during orthopaedic trauma surgery. *J Orthop Trauma.* 2008;22(6):430-431. [IIIB]

124. Centeno RF, Desai AR, Watson ME. Management of contaminated autologous grafts in plastic surgery. *Eplasty.* April 22, 2008;8:e23. [IIIB]

125. Bhandari M, Schemitsch EH, Adili A, Lachowski RJ, Shaughnessy SG. High and low pressure pulsatile lavage of contaminated tibial fractures: an in vitro study of bacterial adherence and bone damage. *J Orthop Trauma.* 1999;13(8):526-533. [IIB]

126. Hirn M, Laitinen M, Pirkkalainen S, Vuento R. Cefuroxime, rifampicin and pulse lavage in decontamination of allograft bone. *J Hosp Infect.* 2004;56(3):198-201. [IIB]

127. Mangram AJ, Horan TC, Pearson ML, Silver LC, Jarvis WR. Guideline for Prevention of Surgical Site Infection, 1999. Centers for Disease Control and Prevention (CDC) Hospital Infection Control Practices Advisory Committee. *Am J Infect Control.* 1999;27(2):97-132; quiz 133-4; discussion 96. [IVA]

128. Presnal BP, Kimbrough EE. What to do about a dropped bone graft. *Clin Orthop Relat Res.* 1993;Nov;(296):310-311. [IB]

129. Bhandari M, Adili A, Lachowski RJ. High pressure pulsatile lavage of contaminated human tibiae: an in vitro study. *J Orthop Trauma.* 1998;12(7):479-484. [IIB]

130. Makary MA, Holzmueller CG, Sexton JB, et al. Operating room debriefings. *Jt Comm J Qual Patient Saf.* 2006;32(7):407-410, 357. [VB]

131. *Sample Procedure: Handling Autologous Bone Skull Flaps.* Version 14. McLean, VA: American Association of Tissue Banks; 2012. [IVC]

132. Bhandari M, Adili A, Schemitsch EH. The efficacy of low-pressure lavage with different irrigating solutions

to remove adherent bacteria from bone. *J Bone Joint Surg Am.* 2001;83-A(3):412-419. [IIB]

133. Yaman F, Unlu G, Atilgan S, Celik Y, Ozekinci T, Yaldiz M. Microbiologic and histologic assessment of intentional bacterial contamination of bone grafts. *J Oral Maxillofac Surg.* 2007;65(8):1490-1494. [IIB]

134. Bruce B, Sheibani-Rad S, Appleyard D, et al. Are dropped osteoarticular bone fragments safely reimplantable in vivo? *J Bone Joint Surg Am.* 2011;93(5):430-438. [IIB]

135. Soyer J, Rouil M, Castel O. The effect of 10% povidone-iodine solution on contaminated bone allografts. *J Hosp Infect.* 2002;50(3):183-187. [IB]

136. Lacey RW. Antibacterial activity of povidone iodine towards non-sporing bacteria. *J Appl Bacteriol.* 1979;46(3):443-449. [IIB]

137. Kaysinger KK, Nicholson NC, Ramp WK, Kellam JF. Toxic effects of wound irrigation solutions on cultured tibiae and osteoblasts. *J Orthop Trauma.* 1995;9(4):303-311. [IIB]

138. Khan M, Rothrauff BB, Merali F, Musahl V, Peterson D, Ayeni OR. Management of the contaminated anterior cruciate ligament graft. *Arthroscopy.* 2014;30(2):236-244. [IA]

139. Guideline for specimen management. In: *Guidelines for Perioperative Practice.* Denver, CO: AORN, Inc; 2015:389-418. [IVA]

140. Lagios MD. Pathology procedures for evaluation of the specimen with potential or documented ductal carcinoma in situ. *Semin Breast Dis.* 2000;3:42-49. [VB]

141. Wolff AC, Hammond ME, Hicks DG, et al. Recommendations for human epidermal growth factor receptor 2 testing in breast cancer: American Society of Clinical Oncology/College of American Pathologists clinical practice guideline update. *Arch Pathol Lab Med.* 2014;138(2):241-256. [IVB]

142. Greenberg CC, Regenbogen SE, Studdert DM, et al. Patterns of communication breakdowns resulting in injury to surgical patients. *J Am Coll Surg.* 2007;204(4):533-540. [IIIB]

143. Siegel JD, Rhinehart E, Jackson M, Chiarello L, Health Care Infection Control Practices Advisory Committee. 2007 Guideline for Isolation Precautions: Preventing Transmission of Infectious Agents in Health Care Settings. *Am J Infect Control.* 2007;35(10 Suppl 2):S65-S64. [IVA]

144. Guideline for selection and use of packaging systems for sterilization. In: *Guidelines for Perioperative Practice.* Denver, CO: AORN, Inc; 2015:651-664. [IVA]

145. Occupational Safety and Health Administration. Toxic and Hazardous substances: Bloodborne pathogens, 29 CFR §1910.1030 (2012). Occupational Safety and Health Administration. https://www.osha.gov/pls/oshaweb/owadisp.show_document?p_id=10051&p_table=STANDARDS. Accessed September 26, 2014.

146. Benner J. Establish a transparent chain-of-custody to mitigate risk and ensure quality of specialized samples. *Biopreserv Biobank.* 2009;7(3):151-153. [VB]

147. Valenstein PN, Sirota RL. Identification errors in pathology and laboratory medicine. *Clin Lab Med.* 2004;24(4):979-96, vii. [VB]

148. College of American Pathologists. When a rose is not a rose: the problem of mislabeled specimens. *Lab Med DirecTIPs.* http://www.cap.org/apps/portlets/content-Viewer/show.do?printFriendly=true&contentReference=practice_management%2Fdirectips%2Fmislabeled_specimens.html. Updated February 23, 2010. Accessed October 14, 2014. [VB]

149. 45 CFR Parts 160 and 164. Modifications to the HIPAA Privacy, Security, Enforcement, and Breach Notification Rules Under the Health Information Technology for Economic and Clinical Health Act and the Genetic Information Nondiscrimination Act; Other Modifications to the HIPAA Rules; Final Rule. *Fed Regist.* 2013;78(17):5566-5702.

150. Guideline for perioperative health care information management. In: *Guidelines for Perioperative Practice.* Denver, CO: AORN, Inc; 2015:491-512. [IVB]

151. Standards of perioperative nursing practice. In: *Perioperative Standards and Recommended Practices.* Denver, CO: AORN, Inc; 2014:3-42. [IVB]

152. Joint Commission. Transplant safety. In: *Comprehensive Accreditation Manual for Hospitals E-dition.* Washington, DC: The Joint Commission; March 2014.

153. Joint Commission. Transplant safety. In: *Comprehensive Accreditation Manual for Ambulatory Care E-dition.* Washington, DC: The Joint Commission; March 2014.

154. Makary MA, Holzmueller CG, Thompson D, et al. Operating room briefings: working on the same page. Jt Comm *J Qual Patient Saf.* 2006;32(6):351-355. [VB]

155. Chiang HY, Steelman VM, Pottinger JM, et al. Clinical significance of positive cranial bone flap cultures and associated risk of surgical site infection after craniotomies or craniectomies. *J Neurosurg.* 2011;114(6):1746-1754. [IIIA]

156. Surgical and related services. In: *Accreditation Handbook for Ambulatory Health Care.* Skokie, Ill.: Accreditation Association for Ambulatory Health Care; 2014:52-55.

157. Centers for Medicare & Medicaid Services. State Operations Manual Appendix A Survey Protocol, Regulations and Interpretive Guidelines for Hospitals. Rev. 105; 3/21/14. Baltimore, MD: Centers for Medicare & Medicaid; 2014.

158. Centers for Medicare & Medicaid Services. State Operations Manual Appendix L: Guidance for Surveyors: Ambulatory Surgical Centers. Rev. 99; 1/31/14. Baltimore, MD: Centers for Medicare & Medicaid; 2014.

159. LD.04.01.07: The hospital has policies and procedures that guide and support patient care, treatment, and services. In: *Hospital Accreditation Standards 2014.* 2014 ed. Oakbrook Terrace, IL: Joint Commission Resources; 2014.

160. LD.04.01.07: The organization has policies and procedures that guide and support patient care, treatment, or services. In: *Standards for ambulatory care 2014: Standards, Elements of Performance, Scoring, Accreditation Polices.* Oakbrook Terrace, IL: Joint Commission Resources; 2014.

161. Governance. In: *2014 Accreditation Handbook for Ambulatory Health Care.* Skokie, IL: Accreditation Association for Ambulatory Health Care; 2014:19-26.

162. SS.1: Organization. In: *NIAHO Interpretive Guidelines and Surveyor Guidance.* 10.1 ed. Milford, OH: DNV Healthcare Inc; 2012:70-71.

163. HR.01.05.03: Staff participate in ongoing education and training. In: *Comprehensive Accreditation Manual: CAMH for Hospitals. 2014 ed.* Oakbrook Terrace, Ill.: Joint Commission Resources; 2014.

164. HR.01.05.03: Staff participate in ongoing education and training. In: *Comprehensive Accreditation Manual: CAMAC for Ambulatory Care. 2014 ed.* Oakbrook Terrace, Ill.: Joint Commission Resources; 2014.

165. Quality management and improvement. In: *2014 Accreditation Handbook for Ambulatory Health Care.* Skokie, IL: Accreditation Association for Ambulatory Health Care; 2014:32-36.

166. MS.10 Continuing education. In: *NIAHO Interpretive Guidelines and Surveyor Guidance.* 10.1 ed. Milford, OH: DNV Healthcare Inc; 2012:24.

167. RC.01.01.01: The hospital maintains complete and accurate medical records for each individual patient. In: *Hospital Accreditation Standards 2014.* 2014 ed. Oakbrook Terrace, IL: Joint Commission Resources; 2014.

168. RC.01.01.01: The organization maintains complete and accurate clinical records. In: *Standards for ambulatory care 2014: Standards, Elements of Performance Scoring Accreditation Polices.* Oakbrook Terrace, IL: Joint Commission Resources; 2014.

169. Clinical records and health information. In: *2014 Accreditation Handbook for Ambulatory Health Care.* Skokie, IL: Accreditation Association for Ambulatory Health Care; 2014:37-39.

170. MS.16 Medical record maintenance. In: *NIAHO Interpretive Guidelines and Surveyor Guidance. 10.1 ed.* Milford, OH: DNV Healthcare Inc; 2012:29.

171. PI.03.01.01: The hospital improves performance on an ongoing basis. In: *Hospital Accreditation Standards 2014. 2014 ed.* Oakbrook Terrace, IL: Joint Commission Resources; 2014.

172. PI.03.01.01: The organization improves performance. In: *Standards for ambulatory care 2014: Standards, Elements of Performance, Scoring, Accreditation Polices.* Oakbrook Terrace, IL: Joint Commission Resources; 2014.

173. Quality management and improvement. In: *2014 Accreditation Handbook for Ambulatory Health Care.* Skokie, IL: Accreditation Association for Ambulatory Health Care; 2014:32-36.

174. Quality management system. In: *NIAHO Interpretive Guidelines and Surveyor Guidance. 10.1 ed.* Milford, OH: DNV Healthcare Inc; 2012:10-16.

175. International Organization for Standardization. *Sterilization of Medical Devices: Microbiological Methods.* Part 1. Geneva, Switzerland: International Organization for Standardization; 2006. [IVC]

176. Ronholdt CJ, Bogdansky S. The appropriateness of swab cultures for the release of human allograft tissue. *J Industr Microbiol Biotechnol.* 2005;32(8):349-354. [IB]

177. Nguyen H, Morgan DA, Cull S, Benkovich M, Forwood MR. Sponge swabs increase sensitivity of sterility testing of processed bone and tendon allografts. *J Ind Microbiol Biotechnol.* 2011;38(8):1127-1132. [IIB]

178. Dennis JA, Martinez OV, Landy DC, et al. A comparison of two microbial detection methods used in aseptic processing of musculoskeletal allograft tissues. *Cell Tissue Bank.* 2011;12(1):45-50. [IIB]

179. Aggarwal VK, Higuera C, Deirmengian G, Parvizi J, Austin MS. Swab cultures are not as effective as tissue cultures for diagnosis of periprosthetic joint infection. *Clin Orthopaed Rel Res.* 2013;471(10):3196-3203. [IIIB]

180. 42 CFR §493 - Condition of participation: Laboratory Requirements. Washington, DC: Government Printing Office; 2012.

181. Vaccines, Blood and Biologics. Guidance for Industry: MedWatch Form FDA 3500A: Mandatory Reporting of Adverse Reactions Related to Human Cells, Tissues, and Cellular and Tissue-Based Products (HCT/Ps). US Food and Drug Administration. http://www.fda.gov/BiologicsBlood Vaccines/GuidanceComplianceRegulatoryInformation/ Guidances/Tissue/ucm074000.htm. Accessed September 26, 2014.

182. MedWatch: The FDA Safety Information and Adverse Event Reporting Program. US Food and Drug Administration. http://www.fda.gov/Safety/MedWatch/default.htm. Accessed September 26, 2014.

Acknowledgements

LEAD AUTHOR
Sharon A. Van Wicklin, MSN, RN, CNOR, CRNFA, CPSN, PLNC
Perioperative Nursing Specialist
AORN Nursing Department
Denver, CO

CONTRIBUTING AUTHORS
Scott A. Brubaker, CTBS
Chief Policy Officer
American Association of Tissue Banks
McLean, VA

Ramona Conner, MSN, RN, CNOR
Manager, Standards and Guidelines
AORN Nursing Department
Denver, CO

The authors and AORN thank Marie A. Bashaw, DNP, RN, NEA-BC, CNOR, Clinical Assistant Professor, Wright State University College of Nursing and Health, Dayton, OH; Patricia Graybill-D'Ercole, MSN, RN, CNOR, CHL, CRCST, Clinical Specialist, Integra Life Science, York, PA; and Deborah Farina Mulloy, PhD, RN, Associate Chief Nurse, Quality and Center for Nursing Excellence, Brigham and Women's Hospital, Boston, MA, for their assistance in developing this guideline.

PUBLICATION HISTORY
Originally published in November 2014 in *Perioperative Standards and Recommended Practices* online.

Minor editing revisions made in November 2014 for publication in *Guidelines for Perioperative Practice,* 2015 edition.

Evidence ratings revised in *Guidelines for Perioperative Practice,* 2018 edition, to conform to the current AORN Evidence Rating Model.

GUIDELINE FOR A SAFE ENVIRONMENT OF CARE, PART 1

The following Guideline for a Safe Environment of Care, Part 1 has been approved by the AORN Recommended Practices Advisory Board. It was presented as proposed recommendations for comments by members and others. The guideline is effective December 15, 2012. The recommendations in this guideline are intended to be achievable and represent what is believed to be an optimal level of practice. Policies and procedures will reflect variations in practice settings and/or clinical situations that determine the degree to which the guideline can be implemented. AORN recognizes the various settings in which perioperative nurses practice; therefore, this guideline is adaptable to various practice settings. These practice settings include traditional operating rooms (ORs), ambulatory surgery centers, physicians' offices, cardiac catheterization laboratories, endoscopy suites, radiology departments, and all other areas where operative and other invasive procedures may be performed.

Purpose

This document provides guidance for providing a safe environment of care related to patients and perioperative personnel and the equipment used in the perioperative environment. They include information on

- musculoskeletal injury,
- fire safety,
- electrical equipment,
- clinical and alert alarms,
- blanket- and solution-warming cabinets,
- medical gas cylinders,
- waste anesthesia gases,
- latex,
- chemicals including methyl methacrylate bone cement, and
- hazardous waste.

The potential for injuries related to exposure to bloodborne pathogens, radiation, surgical smoke, and chemotherapeutic agents are outside the scope of this document. Patient injuries related to incorrect tubing connections and requirements for heating, ventilation, and air conditioning also are outside the scope of this document. The recommendations for these topics are addressed in other AORN guidelines.

Evidence Review

A medical librarian conducted a systematic literature search of the databases MEDLINE®, CINAHL®, Scopus®, and Cochrane Database of Systematic Reviews for meta-analyses, randomized and non-randomized trials and studies, systematic and non-systematic reviews, and opinion documents and letters. Search terms included *operating room, ambulatory surgery center, perioperative nursing, nursing, nurses, surgical procedures, anesthesia, electrosurgery, diathermy, ventilation, smoke, surgical smoke, security measures, violence, occupational accidents, occupational diseases, musculoskeletal diseases, lifting, transportation of patients, patient positioning, human engineering, ergonomics, latex hypersensitivity, security measures, violence, security risk, fire blanket, fire safety, fires, smoke plume, clinical alarms, anesthetics, gas scavengers, compressed gas, compressed medical gas, methyl methacrylate, occupational exposure, hazardous waste, hazardous substances, waste products, hazardous upon disposal, protective clothing, tubing misconnection, spontaneous abortion, miscarriage,* and *abnormality.*

The search was limited to articles published in English and between the years 2005 and 2011; the librarian also established continuing alerts on the environment of care topics and contacted a federal agency for guidance. The lead author and medical librarian also identified relevant guidelines from government agencies and standards-setting bodies and consulted equipment specifications. In addition, the lead author identified and requested other guidelines and professional literature as deemed appropriate.

Articles identified by the search were provided to the project team for evaluation. The team consisted of the lead author, three members of the Recommended Practices Advisory Board, one member of the Research Committee, and one doctorally prepared evidence appraiser. The lead author divided the search results into topics and assigned members of the team to review and critically appraise each article using the Johns Hopkins Evidence-Based Practice Model and the Research or Non-Research Evidence Appraisal Tools as appropriate. The literature was independently evaluated and appraised according to the strength and quality of the evidence. Each article was then assigned an appraisal score as agreed upon by consensus of the team. The appraisal score is noted in brackets after each reference, as applicable.

The collective evidence supporting each intervention within a specific recommendation was summarized and used to rate the strength of the evidence using the AORN Evidence Rating Model. Factors considered in review of the collective evidence were the quality of research, quantity of similar studies on a given topic, and consistency of results supporting a recommendation. The evidence rating is noted in brackets after each intervention.

Editor's note: *MEDLINE is a registered trademark of the US National Library of Medicine's Medical Literature Analysis and Retrieval System, Bethesda, MD. CINAHL,*

Recommendation I

Precautions should be taken to mitigate the risk of occupational injuries that may result in death, days lost from work, work restrictions, medical treatment beyond first aid, and loss of consciousness.[1]

Occupational injuries include injuries that result in breaking of the skin and musculoskeletal injuries from slips, trips, falls, or ergonomic stressors.[2,3] Musculoskeletal injuries involve the muscles, nerves, tendons, ligaments, joints, cartilage, and spinal discs. Contributing factors, including duration, frequency, and magnitude, determine the effect of each ergonomic stressor. Examples of ergonomic stressors encountered in the perioperative environment include

- forceful tasks (eg, pushing a stretcher and patient up a ramp),
- repetitive motions (eg, passing instruments, opening suture packets, typing),
- awkward postures (eg, holding retractors during a surgical procedure, lifting or holding patient extremities),
- static postures (eg, standing for long periods of time in one position),
- moving or lifting patients and equipment (eg, lifting without assistance),
- carrying heavy instruments and equipment, and
- overexertion (eg, protecting a combative patient emerging from anesthesia).[1,4,5]

Perioperative nurses expressed more complaints regarding neck and shoulder injuries than non-specialized and intensive care nurses in a descriptive study involving 3,169 employees in eight university hospitals in the Netherlands.[6] In another descriptive study of direct patient caregivers (n = 5,991 nurses, n = 1,543 aides), aides had a higher rate of injury than nurses. The back was the most common body part injured that resulted in days away from work. Sharps injury was the most frequent injury that did not require time away from work. The OR had the highest number of injuries that did not require time away from work, and perioperative nurses had the second highest rate of injuries that resulted in days away from work.[1]

A study of musculoskeletal injuries in a tertiary medical center revealed that nurse's aides had a higher rate of injury than nurses, and the stressors for injury were equally distributed between lifting, pushing, and pulling equipment; patient handling; and slips, trips, and falls.[7] A descriptive study of endoscopy nurses showed that about 50% of the sample (N = 38) experienced upper extremity injuries.[8] In a descriptive study, researchers determined that patient transfers, clean-up duties, basic patient care, and bed making all resulted in the nurse assuming a stressful trunk posture, which can lead to back injury.[5]

The advent of laparoscopic surgery has created ergonomic stressors in addition to those usually encountered during open surgery.[9] These stressors are created by the need to view a monitor and the need to maintain a static posture related to holding a camera.[10,11] The instruments may not be configured appropriately for the user or the patient, which can lead to stress on the user's arms and neck.[12]

A 2010 report from the Bureau of Labor Statistics indicated that musculoskeletal disorders accounted for 29% of all workplace injuries that led to time away from work. Back injuries were the most frequent claim overall, and shoulder injuries were the most severe injury for all occupations. Among registered nurses, 55.1% reported back injuries and 13.2% reported shoulder injuries. Although back injuries were the most frequently reported, abdominal injuries and leg injuries resulted in the greatest number of days away from work, at 19 days and 13 days, respectively. The rates for nursing assistants were higher than those for registered nurses.[13]

Perioperative team members are prone to pain and fatigue from the need to maintain static postures during surgical procedures.[4] A cross-sectional study in Greece of 350 nursing personnel revealed that 51% experienced lower back pain and 23% experienced knee pain. Personnel who perceived that their jobs demanded high physical exertion or that they had moderate to bad general health had a higher odds ratio of experiencing low back or knee pain.[14]

A survey of 425 German surgeons indicated that they perceive that OR design, equipment (eg, lights, tables, monitors), cables and tubes, instrument design, and working posture all contribute to ergonomic stressors in the OR.[15]

I.a.   Risk-reduction strategies (ie, administrative, engineering, behavioral controls) for injury prevention should be identified, developed, and implemented. *[3: Moderate Evidence]*

Education on techniques to improve posture and ergonomics has been shown to decrease the incidence of occupational injuries overall.[16] In an endoscopy suite with 120 employees, various strategies that were implemented reduced the number of reported injuries (eg, trips over cords, head traumas, crushing injuries to the hand).[3] In another study of endoscopy suites, strategies such as combining cables into one bundle, covering cables and tubes on the floors, and using electrical plugs anchored in the ceiling were shown to reduce the incidence of team members tripping over exposed wires and tubes.[2]

After changing to a zero-transfer system, one facility reported a 100% decrease in staff member injuries related to patient transfers, which was sustained for two years.[17] The zero-transfer system involved using a chair with wheels that, when in position, became the OR bed. A pre- and post-intervention study of 766 injury cases in six facilities showed that a combination of administrative and engineering controls significantly reduced personnel injuries and disabilities related to patient handling.[18] A qualitative study of 126 patient-caregiver encounters revealed that the complexity of care, patient treatment goals, the amount of time to complete the task, knowledge of patient moving techniques, and equipment issues all influence the nurse's decision on the best way to move a patient.[19] A descriptive, exploratory study in a facility with 950 nurses investigated nurses' satisfaction with the use of mechanical lift equipment, the frequency of use, and the efficacy of employing a hands-on bedside mechanical lift equipment facilitator in increasing the use of lift equipment. The study revealed a decrease in lost work days and in the cost of worker's compensation claims after the interventions were employed.[20]

I.a.1. Administrative controls for an ergonomically healthy perioperative environment should include
- developing a culture of ergonomic safety,
- developing and implementing a policy for manual patient handling,
- using patient care ergonomic assessment protocols,
- educating personnel in the use of patient handling devices and strategies to prevent musculoskeletal injury,[16]
- using ergonomic workstations,
- having adequate personnel present during patient handling and other situations resulting in ergonomic stress, and
- having ergonomic clinical advisors or resources available.[20]

A comparative study involving 16 nurses revealed that education on safe patient handling techniques improves compliance.[21] A report from a 958-bed hospital in Florida showed a 62% reduction in injuries related to patient handling during a six-year period after the creation of a lift team.[22] Similar injury reductions were noted in an Australian study after a no-lift policy was implemented in the entire state of Victoria.[23]

I.a.2. Engineering controls for an ergonomically healthy perioperative environment should include
- having appropriate assistive patient handling equipment available[22,23];
- limiting the weight of instrument trays to 25 lb total weight[24];
- adapting workstations, tools, and equipment for ergonomic safety; and
- providing adequate lighting.[25]

I.a.3. Behavioral controls for an ergonomically healthy perioperative environment include
- wearing nonskid footwear;
- eliminating clutter, including removing wires or tubes from the floor;
- covering equipment cables across the floor;
- keeping cabinet and room doors closed;

- placing monitors straight in front of personnel and slightly lower than eye level[10];
- cleaning up spills or debris as soon as possible;
- using anti-fatigue mats;
- using lift teams and assistive devices to transfer or lift patients; and
- cleaning furniture wheels frequently.

A retrospective study of medical records, employee records, and interviews of personnel who worked in endoscopy rooms showed a decrease in injuries from collisions when spills were cleaned up as soon as possible, booties were not worn over shoes, and monitors were placed at eye level and were replaced with lighter weight models.[3] Another study revealed a reduction in injuries when cords or tubing lying on the floor were removed or were bundled and covered.[2]

I.b. The physical environment should provide
○ hydraulic or electric booms mounted to the ceiling or wall when structurally feasible;
○ adequate room lighting;
○ adequate storage; and
○ floor surfaces that allow for easy movement of patient handling equipment.[26]
[2: High Evidence]
Using hydraulic or electric ceiling-suspended equipment decreases the risk of injuries to perioperative team members.[10,27] Low lighting levels have been shown to increase the risk of tripping.[2,9] A review of accident reports revealed an injury resulting from tripping over an improperly stored wheelchair.[3]

I.c. Perioperative personnel should follow the algorithms outlined in the AORN "Guidance statement: safe patient handling and movement in the perioperative setting"[27] and organizational policies and procedures while completing activities such as
○ performing a lateral patient transfer from a stretcher to the OR bed;
○ positioning or repositioning the patient on the OR bed;
○ lifting and holding the patient's head or extremities for prepping;
○ standing for a prolonged period;
○ retracting tissue;
○ lifting and carrying supplies or equipment; and
○ pushing, pulling, or moving equipment on wheels.[27]
[3: Moderate Evidence]
The AORN guidance statement provides evidence-based directions for decreasing ergonomic stressors that, if they are not recognized, can cause personnel injury.[28-34]

Recommendation II

Potential hazards associated with fire safety in the practice setting should be identified, and safe practices for communication, prevention, suppression, and evacuation should be established and followed.

Fire is a risk to both patients and personnel in the OR because all three elements of the fire triangle (Figure 1) that are necessary for a fire—fuel, oxidizer, ignition source—typically are present.[35,36] Surgical fires are estimated to occur in the United States about 550 to 650 times a year.[36,37] The ECRI Institute states that surgical fires occur most frequently on the patient (70%), and 29% occur in the patient. Forty-four percent of fires occurring on the patient involve the head, neck, and upper chest, and 26% occur elsewhere. Twenty-one percent of fires are located in the airway, and 8% occur at other locations in the body.[36] The majority of fatal fires are airway fires.[37] Fires have been reported to occur during different types of surgical procedures (eg, coronary bypass graft, otolaryngology procedures).[38-40] One explosion was reportedly caused by cutting the wires from the battery pack of a battery-operated lavage system.[41]

II.a.   A written fire prevention and management plan should be developed by a multidisciplinary group composed of key stakeholders within the organization such as
   ○ perioperative RNs,
   ○ perioperative unlicensed assistive personnel,
   ○ anesthesia professionals,
   ○ physicians,
   ○ a local fire department representative,
   ○ risk management personnel,
   ○ the safety officer, and
   ○ facilities/engineering personnel.[35]
   [2: High Evidence]

II.a.1.   The fire prevention and management plan should include
   • perioperative team members' responsibilities, including communication;
   • methods of prevention;
   • processes to safely manage different fire scenarios;
   • alarm activation procedures;
   • methods to extinguish a fire;
   • the preferred routes and levels of evacuation;
   • a description of the facility's fire risk assessment tool (Figure 2); and
   • the required content for and frequency of fire safety education, including frequency of and procedures for fire drills.[35]

II.b.   A fire risk assessment should be completed and communicated to the entire perioperative team before beginning a surgical procedure. *[2: High Evidence]*

   Fire prevention experts and professional associations support the importance of completing the risk assessment.[35,42] In one case report that involved a fire caused by the electrosurgical electrode igniting a sponge during open heart surgery, a lack of communication may have contributed to the fire. In this situation, there was a delay in communicating to the surgeon a decrease in the tidal volumes that was caused by a ruptured bleb. The rupture caused oxygen to leak into the patient's chest cavity and created an oxygen-enriched environment.[39]

II.b.1.   The fire risk assessment should identify
   • fuels that are present,
   • ignition sources that are present,
   • the potential for the presence of an oxygen-enriched environment,
   • the specific type of fire extinguisher that is required based on the fuel and involvement of electrical current, and
   • additional preventive measures that are required as determined by the location of the fire and fuel sources.

II.c.   Ignition sources (eg, active electrosurgical electrodes, lasers, electrocautery devices, fiber-optic light cords) should be used according to manufacturers' instructions for use and AORN guidelines.[9,43,44] *[2: High Evidence]*

   Manufacturers' written instructions for use and labels include fire safety information, such as the laser resistance of the endotracheal tube and methods of disposal for equipment (eg, battery packs).[37,41,45] Electrosurgical units provide the ignition source, especially when they are used in the presence of oxidizers, flammable solutions, or volatile or combustible chemicals or liquids.[36,44] Lasers provide the ignition source

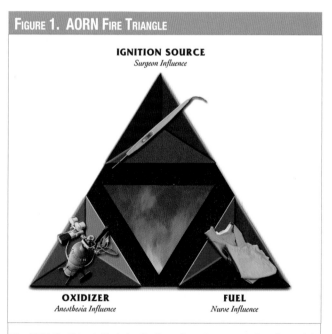

FIGURE 1. AORN FIRE TRIANGLE

IGNITION SOURCE
Surgeon Influence

OXIDIZER
Anesthesia Influence

FUEL
Nurse Influence

The AORN Fire Triangle illustrates the three elements necessary for a fire and the members of the perioperative team who frequently influence the element.

when they are used in the presence of oxidizers, flammable solutions, or volatile or combustible chemicals or liquids.[36,37,43] Fiber-optic light cables may provide an ignition source if they are disconnected from the working element and are allowed to remain in contact with drapes, sponges, or other fuel sources.[9,46]

II.c.1. Saline should be used to cool devices that create heat during use (eg, drills, burrs, saw blades).[36]

II.c.2. Defibrillator paddles and pads should be an appropriate size for the patient and applied using only manufacturer-recommended lubricants.

Using paddles that are the correct size and with manufacturer-recommended lubricants decreases both sparking and the amount of energy required for defibrillation.[36]

II.d. Fuels (eg, alcohol-based skin antiseptic agents, collodion, drapes, gowns, endotracheal tubes) should be managed to prevent contact with ignition sources. [3: Moderate Evidence]

Preventing contact between fuels and ignition sources breaks the fire triangle, thereby preventing fire.[47] Many potential fuels that will not burn in ambient air will burn in an oxygen-enriched environment, which may be present in the OR.[36,37,42]

II.d.1. The flammable or combustible rating of a skin antiseptic agent should be determined by reviewing the applicable material safety data sheet (MSDS) or safety data sheet (SDS).

Prep solutions can be rated as "flammable" or "combustible" on the MSDS or SDS. A combustible solution will burn but requires a higher temperature to cause ignition. A rating of "flammable" indicates a solution that has a flash point of less than 100° F (37.8° C). A solution with a rating of "combustible" has a flash point of greater than 100° F (37.8° C).[48]

II.d.2. Flammable skin antiseptic agents should be prevented from pooling or soaking into linens or the patient's hair by
- using reusable or disposable sterile towels to absorb drips and excess solution during application,
- removing materials that are saturated with the skin antiseptic agent before draping the patient, and
- wicking excess solution with a sterile towel to help dry the surgical prep area completely.[36,37,42]

II.d.3. Adequate time should be provided to allow flammable skin antiseptic agents to dry completely and to allow any fumes to dissipate before applying surgical drapes or using a potential ignition source.[35,42]

FIGURE 2. AORN FIRE RISK ASSESSMENT TOOL

AORN

Fire Risk Assessment Tool

A. Is an alcohol-based skin antiseptic or other flammable solution being used preoperatively?
❏ Yes
❏ No

B. Is the operative or other invasive procedure being performed above the xiphoid process or in the oropharynx?
❏ Yes
❏ No

C. Is open oxygen or nitrous oxide being administered?
❏ Yes
❏ No

D. Is an electrosurgical unit, laser, or fiber-optic light being used?
❏ Yes
❏ No

E. Are there other possible contributors (eg, defibrillators, drills, saws, burrs)?
❏ Yes
❏ No

The AORN Fire Risk Assessment Tool illustrates components that should be included in an assessment tool.

Allowing adequate time for skin antiseptic agents to dry before applying drapes helps prevent the accumulation of volatile fumes beneath the drapes.[47] The volatile fumes are flammable and may ignite without a connection between the ignition source and the actual surgical antiseptic agent.[36,37]

II.d.4. For surgical procedures that involve the head or neck, a water-soluble gel should be used to cover the patient's facial hair, and any eye lubricants that are used should be water based.

The patient's hair is a fuel source, and covering facial hair with water-soluble gel decreases the risk of combustion because it raises the temperature that is required for ignition.[36]

II.d.5. Local and state fire regulations should be followed regarding the storage of flammable liquids (eg, alcohol-based skin antiseptic solutions, hand sanitizer, alcohol, acetone, collodion) and the location of dispensers.[42,49-51]

II.e. Oxidizers (eg, oxygen, nitrous oxide) should be used with caution near any ignition or fuel sources. *[2: High Evidence]*

An oxygen-enriched environment is when the oxygen concentration is greater than 21% by volume.[35] In an oxygen-enriched environment, the temperature and energy required for fuels to ignite is lower than that of ambient or medical air. Nitrous oxide is considered an oxidizer and requires the same precautions that are used with oxygen.[36,37,42,49]

II.e.1. The anesthesia circuit should be free of leaks.

Leaks in the anesthesia circuit can increase the oxygen concentration under the drapes, creating an oxygen-enriched environment that increases the risk of fire.[35,37,52] The anesthesia circuit includes the endotracheal tube, the seal between the tube and the patient's airway, the bag reservoir, and the tubing that leads from the anesthesia machine to the endotracheal tube.

II.e.2. Accumulated anesthetic gas should be evacuated using a metal suction cannula before an ignition source is used in or near an oxygen-enriched environment.

The suction will assist with removing excess oxidizing agents to create an atmosphere that is closer to ambient air.[36,37] A metal suction cannula will not ignite.[37]

II.e.3. The lowest possible concentration of oxygen that provides adequate patient oxygen saturation should be used for a patient who requires supplemental oxygen.[35-37,52,53]

II.e.4. A laryngeal mask airway or an endotracheal tube should be used when the patient requires supplementary oxygen greater than 30% unless using the tube is contraindicated by the procedure (eg, the patient is required to respond verbally during the procedure).

Use of a laryngeal mask airway or an endotracheal tube decreases the risk of fire by decreasing the oxygen concentration under the drapes and in the patient's upper airway.[35-37,54]

II.e.5. Drapes should be placed over the patient's head in a manner that allows the oxygen to flow freely and prevents accumulation under the drapes.[36,37,47,52]

II.e.6. When using a warming blanket with an attached head drape, the following precautions should be used:
- cut a hole in the drape around the endotracheal tube;
- place the drape over the patient's head in a manner that allows the oxygen to flow

freely and prevents accumulation under the drapes;
- lift and reposition the patient's head frequently, if possible; and
- keep the warmer blower on while the drape is in place.

These precautions have been shown to decrease the oxygen concentration under the drapes, which assists in preventing an oxygen-enriched environment.[52]

II.e.7. A second delivery system that administers 5 L/minute to 10 L/minute of medical air should be used when supplemental oxygen is administered under the drapes.

A second delivery system, which consists of a flow meter that is connected to a medical air source and tubing that delivers air beneath the drapes, assists with flushing oxygen from under the drapes. Mixing oxygen with nonflammable gases, such as medical air, reduces the risk of fire by preventing an oxygen-enriched environment.[36,37]

II.e.8. When performing surgical procedures on anatomical structures that present special fire hazards (eg, bowel, trachea), additional precautions should be taken (eg, using a scalpel rather than an electrosurgical active electrode to create the incision).

Hydrogen and methane, which are flammable gases, may be present in the bowel and ignite when they are exposed to an ignition source, such as an active electrosurgical electrode.[36,47,55] An oxygen-enriched environment may be present within the trachea because of the presence of anesthesia gases.[37,55]

II.f. The risk of airway fires should be minimized during surgical procedures involving the airway by placing wet radiopaque sponges in the back of the throat and inflating endotracheal tube cuffs with tinted solutions. *[2: High Evidence]*

Wet radiopaque sponges placed in the back of the throat help decrease or prevent oxygen leaks.[35,40] Inflating endotracheal tube cuffs with tinted solutions improves visibility in the event of a cuff rupture.[35-37]

II.g. Communication, suppression, and evacuation procedures should be followed in the event of a fire. *[3: Moderate Evidence]*

Following established procedures assists in protecting patients and perioperative personnel from injury or may decrease the severity of sustained injuries.[56]

II.g.1. Perioperative team members should be alerted to the presence of a fire by the person who discovers the fire.

Alerting the team allows team members to carry out their responsibilities and decreases the risks of injury to the patient and personnel.[36]

II.g.2. Water or normal saline or a safe method for smothering should be used to extinguish a fire, if it can be accomplished safely.

Extinguishing a fire as soon as possible decreases the risk of injury to the patient and personnel.[36,37]

II.g.3. In the event of an airway fire, the endotracheal tube should be removed and normal saline should be poured into the airway. These steps should occur in collaboration with the anesthesia care professional.

Removing the endotracheal tube removes the source of the fuel, and normal saline cools burned tissue.[35,37,56,57]

II.g.4. In the event of a non-airway fire, the fuel source should be removed from the patient and the fire extinguished. Simultaneously, the anesthesia care professional should discontinue administration of airway gases.[36,56,57]

II.g.5. After the fuel source has been removed from the patient, ventilation should be reestablished, the patient assessed, and the findings reported to the physician.[56,57]

II.g.6. After safely extinguishing the fire, perioperative team members should follow required procedures for reporting and should save all items that were involved in the fire.

Saving all items that are involved in the fire is necessary to provide evidence for an investigation. This investigation may be accomplished by the quality or risk management department personnel but also may involve the local fire department.[36,37]

II.g.7. The OR should be evacuated according to the facility fire plan if perioperative team members are unable to extinguish a fire.

Evacuation protects the patient and perioperative team members from injury from the by-products of fire or the fire itself.[36]

II.h. Equipment that emits unanticipated smoke, whether in use or not, should be disconnected from the electrical current source. The equipment and all of the accessories in use should be moved to a safe area, if this can be done safely. [3: Moderate Evidence]

Smoke suggests the presence of fire, and equipment may be an ignition source for nearby items. Disconnecting the piece of equipment from the electrical current source may remove the ignition source and thereby extinguish the fire. Moving the equipment out of the OR decreases the risk to the patient and perioperative team members in that room.[36] An overheated ventilator circuit has been reported to be the cause of two different fires.[58]

II.h.1. The room should be immediately evacuated if the equipment cannot be removed safely.[36]

II.i. Fire extinguishers should be located within 30 to 75 feet from the center of the OR, or as required by the local authority with jurisdiction, depending on the fuel source and extinguisher.[59] [2: High Evidence]

II.i.1. Fire extinguishers should be selected according to standards established by the National Fire Protection Association (NFPA) and the local authority with jurisdiction. Factors that help determine the appropriate type of fire extinguisher include
- types of fuel that are present,
- potential fire size,
- hazards that are present and may create adverse chemical reactions with the extinguishing agent,
- electrical equipment that is present,
- ease of use,
- physical abilities of potential users, and
- maintenance requirements.[59]

The NFPA recommends either a water mist or carbon dioxide extinguisher be used in the OR. Water mist extinguishers are rated Class 2A:C.[59] Carbon dioxide extinguishers are rated Class B and Class C, but also may be used for Class A fires.[59]

II.i.2. Fire extinguishing equipment and supplies should be regularly inspected, tested, and maintained.[59]

II.i.3. Fire extinguishers should not be used as a first line of defense in a fire.

Extinguishing a fire using noncombustible and nonflammable solutions from the back table or a smothering technique can be faster than obtaining a fire extinguisher.[36]

II.j. All personnel should be able to identify medical gas control valves, including the areas that they control, and have the ability to shut down medical gases in the event of a fire. [3: Moderate Evidence]

Removing the oxidizer by turning off the medical gas supply assists with breaking the fire triangle.[36,42] A medical gas control valve may control more than one OR.

II.k. Equipment (eg, case carts, stretchers, supply carts, patient beds) should not be stored in locations that block access to pull alarms, medical gas control valves, or electrical panels.[49] [2: High Evidence]

II.l. Fire blankets should not be used in an OR.

Fire blankets may trap fire next to or under the patient and cause more harm. Fire blankets are made of wool and can burn in an oxygen-enriched environment.[36,60] During the application of the fire blanket, instruments may be dislodged, causing injury to the patient. Usage can lead to wound contamination or spread the fire.[36,56] [3: Moderate Evidence]

II.m. Evacuation routes should be established for the perioperative environment, be developed in collaboration with local authorities, and be guided by NFPA regulations.[49] *[2: High Evidence]*

II.m.1. Personnel and emergency responders should be educated about how to implement the evacuation plan.[42,49]

II.m.2. Evacuation routes should be clearly displayed in multiple locations throughout the health care facility.[49]

II.m.3. The evacuation destination should be the closest safe location where patient care can be continued.[36]

II.n. All personnel should receive education and competency verification on
- the elements of the fire triangle;
- use of the perioperative fire risk assessment;
- fire extinguisher locations;
- use of fire extinguishers and other fire-fighting equipment;
- evacuation routes for each room;
- medical gas panel locations and operation, including how to turn them off in an emergency;
- the location of shut off controls for ventilation and electrical systems;
- the location of fire alarm pull stations;
- procedures for turning off the ventilation and electrical systems;
- how and when to activate the fire safety and evacuation plan;
- how and when to contact the local fire department; and
- the roles and responsibilities of each team member in various fire scenarios.[36,37,49,56]
[3: Moderate Evidence]

The need for education is identified in a report of a fire simulation in an obstetric OR that revealed personnel did now know the locations of the fire extinguishers or fire safe zones.[61]

II.n.1. Fire drills should occur periodically as required by the local authority with jurisdiction.

The NFPA 101 recommends that fire drills occur at least quarterly on each shift.[49] The NFPA 99 recommends fire drills to include evacuation annually or as determined by the relevant building code.[42] The local authority with jurisdiction may not have adopted the most current NFPA guidelines and therefore may be following the earlier edition.

Recommendation III

Precautions should be taken to mitigate the risk of injury associated with the use of electrical equipment.

Injuries to patients, personnel, or visitors may occur from medical equipment that has frayed cords, from damaged outlets, or from extension cords.[42] In 2011 the Joint Commission received 39 reports of medical equipment–related events, and the ECRI Institute received reports of events related to ceiling-mounted booms that created the potential for or resulted in injuries.[62,63]

III.a. All electrical equipment, including ceiling- and wall-mounted equipment (eg, booms, monitors), and all loaned equipment should be inspected for damage periodically and before each use. Inspection should include checking power cords for fraying and examining strain relief and plugs for damage. *[3: Moderate Evidence]*

Damaged electrical equipment and power cords can cause unsafe conditions. Power cords are frequently subject to damage from daily use.[42] Fires related to improper cleaning or malfunctions of booms and other equipment has been reported.[62,64]

III.b. Equipment, including the electrical cord, that is found to be in disrepair should be removed immediately from service. *[2: High Evidence]*

Using equipment that is in a state of disrepair can create unsafe conditions.[42]

III.c. Device cords should be secured and have the appropriate characteristics for the intended use, including adequate length. *[2: High Evidence]*

Cords that do not lie flat create the risk of tripping or accidental unplugging of the equipment.[2,3] An inappropriate cord may cause damage to the machine if it does not meet the necessary electrical characteristics (eg, grounding resistance, power cord ampacity, correct polarization).[42]

III.c.1. Device cords should not be changed unless the replacement cord meets the electrical characteristics of the original.

Changing the device cord may nullify the device warranty. The cord may cause damage to the equipment if the electrical characteristics do not match the characteristics of the original cord.[42]

III.c.2. Cords should be secured in a safe manner with an "electrically safe device"[42] that is disposable and able to be cleaned.

Safely securing cords helps prevent trips and falls.[2,3] Using an electrically safe device to secure cords decreases the potential for an electrical shock.[42] Using a device that is disposable or that can be cleaned decreases the risk of transmitting an infection to the patient by contact with the contaminated device.[65,66]

III.c.3. An extension cord should be used only if it has the correct electrical characteristics.

Incorrect electrical characteristics can cause damage to the equipment and over heating of the cord.[42]

III.c.4. Multiple outlet connections should be mounted to a movable equipment assembly (eg, cart, table, pedestal, boom), provided that the cord and the connection have the capacity to allow the total number of amps used to pass through the cord without creating unsafe conditions. The total number of amps should be calculated by adding the amps required by each piece of equipment together.

The use of a multiple outlet connection allows for multiple pieces of equipment to be plugged in to one connection. This connection has only one cord on the floor instead of one cord for each piece of equipment.[42]

III.d. All electrical equipment charger adaptor cords should be labeled with the name of the piece of equipment to which they belong. [4: Limited Evidence]

Equipment has been reported to overheat and malfunction when incorrect charger adaptor cords are used.[67]

Recommendation IV

Precautions should be taken to mitigate hazards associated with non-functioning clinical and alert alarms or with personnel failing to hear or failing to act on alarms.

A clinical alarm (eg, cardiac monitor, ventilator, anesthesia machine) is patient specific and used for the purpose of alerting staff members to a patient emergency. An alert alarm (eg, medical gas systems, blood bank refrigerators, fire alarms, code blue alarms, ethylene oxide level alarms, water treatment alarms) is connected to a system and alerts personnel to system failures that would affect multiple patients. Alarms can be auditory, visual, or a combination of both.[68] Patients have experienced injuries and near-misses because of alarms being turned off or being inaudible.[69-71]

IV.a. Clinical and alert alarms should be tested on initial setup.[72] [2: High Evidence]

IV.b. Clinical and alert alarms should be tested according to organizational policy and procedures. [3: Moderate Evidence]

Periodic testing assists with maintaining a working system.[69,71]

IV.c. An inventory of clinical and alert alarms should be conducted periodically as a collaborative effort between clinical engineering and perioperative personnel. [3: Moderate Evidence]

Clinical engineering and perioperative personnel provide a broad spectrum of information for the team.[69,71] Completing an assessment assists with identifying the pieces of equipment that have alarms, maintaining an accurate alarm inventory, and tracking testing. This information also may assist with setting optimal alarm limits.[71]

IV.c.1. The alarm inventory should include all devices with alarms, including
- blood bank refrigerators,
- medication refrigerators,
- security systems,
- electrosurgical units (ESUs),
- pneumatic tourniquets,
- patient monitoring devices (eg, cardiac monitors, oximeters),
- carbon dioxide (CO_2) insufflators,
- anesthesia equipment,
- sequential compression devices, and
- infusion pumps.

IV.d. Clinical and alert alarms should be sufficiently loud to allow them to be heard above competing noise, and competing noise should be reduced so that alarms can be heard. [3: Moderate Evidence]

Competing noise makes it difficult to hear and differentiate between alarms.[69,71] The OR is a very noisy atmosphere with competing noise from alarms on anesthesia monitors and other equipment (eg, tourniquets) and operating alerts, such as the alert on the ESU.[73] A study that evaluated the amount of competing noise in the OR revealed that in 25 consecutive elective cardiac surgery procedures, an anesthesia alarm sounded an average of every 1.2 minutes.[70] AORN recommends that noise-reduction interventions be incorporated into action plans intended to decrease distractions.[74]

IV.e. Changes in alarm default parameters (eg, volume, high or low limits) should be communicated verbally and visually during changes of personnel, including using a clearly distinguishable visual cue, such as posting a sign, to indicate the change in the default. [3: Moderate Evidence]

Communicating changes to alarm settings notifies the oncoming personnel that the default settings have been changed and prepares them to respond appropriately.[75]

Recommendation V

Precautions should be taken to avoid thermal injuries related to warming solutions, blankets, and patient linens in blanket- and solution-warming cabinets.

The danger of burns from heated blankets, solutions, or linens is increased in the perioperative setting because patients are unconscious or sedated and cannot feel an increase in temperature or communicate discomfort. Even when solutions and blankets do not feel warm to the touch, heat continues to build up in these items and can be transferred to the patient.[76] Injuries to the patient can result from irrigation solution being warmed to high temperatures. In one report, a patient experienced full thickness skin burns and joint damage from irrigation solutions that were warmed in a cabinet in which the temperature ranged from 100.4° F (38° C) on the top shelf to 118.4° F (48° C) on the bottom shelf.[77]

V.a. Solutions, blankets, and patient linens should be stored in separate warming cabinets or in cabinets with separate compartments that have independent temperature controls. *[4: Limited Evidence]*

Using separate warming cabinets allows for better temperature control compared to dual compartment or single compartment cabinets. Separate compartments with separate controls allow for each compartment to be set to an individual temperature and for accurate regulation of both cabinets.[76,78] Fluids should not be warmed to the same temperature as blankets because fluids attain a higher temperature and retain that temperature longer, presenting a greater risk of thermal injury.[76]

V.a.1. Warming cabinets should be labeled to identify items that may be placed within the cabinet and the maximum permissible temperature setting. If the cabinet has separate compartments, each compartment should be labeled.[76]

V.b. Warming cabinet temperatures should be set, maintained, monitored, and documented according to organizational policy. *[3: Moderate Evidence]*

Monitoring and documenting the temperature of warming cabinets is necessary to verify that temperature settings are maintained within specified limits.[76] A malfunctioning cabinet can cause temperature variation.[77]

V.b.1. Temperatures should be documented on a temperature log or recorded with an electronic recording system.

V.b.2. A specific team member should be assigned to set, maintain, monitor, and document the temperature of the warming cabinets.[76]

V.b.3. Precautions should be taken when a warming cabinet malfunctions, including
- removing the cabinet from service,
- labeling the cabinet as out of order,
- removing all blankets and solutions from the warmer,
- not using blankets if they are overheated until the temperatures are within the acceptable range,
- following fluid manufacturers' written instructions to determine usability of solutions, and
- reporting the malfunction to the clinical engineering department for maintenance.

V.b.4. Warming cabinet contents should be rotated on a first-in, first-out basis.

V.c. The number of warming cabinets should be sufficient to support the anticipated need for warmed items. *[3: Moderate Evidence]*

Three blankets may be required per patient to decrease the amount of heat loss. Blankets may take eight to 12 hours to reach the set temperature.[76] Perioperative staff members have been reported to use unsafe means to warm blankets, such as in autoclaves or microwaves.[79] When the supply of warm blankets is not sufficient, staff members may increase the temperature of the warmer, which can cause overheating of the blankets and potentially lead to burns. The use of methods such as forced-air warming devices may decrease the number of warming cabinets required.[76,80]

V.d. Warming cabinets should be located close to the point of use. *[3: Moderate Evidence]*

One single-site quality improvement project that measured blanket temperatures showed that if a blanket is warmed to 110° F (43.3° C), its temperature drops to 82° F (27.8° C) within five minutes, and if a blanket is warmed to 150° F (65.6° C), its temperature drops to 83° F (28.3° C) within five minutes.[79]

V.e. Warming cabinet or compartment temperatures used for blankets and other patient linens should not exceed 130° F (54.4° C). *[3: Moderate Evidence]*

In one limited quality improvement project, blankets were warmed to 150° F (65.6° C) without harmful effects to the subjects, who were alert and not under the effects of any anesthetic agents.[79] However, this recommendation is based on stronger evidence that shows temperatures greater than 130° F (54.4° C) increase the potential for burns.[76,78]

V.f. Solution manufacturers' instructions for use should be followed regarding the maximum temperature and length of time solutions should remain in the warming cabinet or compartment and for usability after removal. *[4: Limited Evidence]*

Solution manufacturers' recommendations for maximum temperature setting, time limit that solutions may remain in the warming device, and for solution use after removal vary. Manufacturers' settings may be determined by the stability of the container and the solution.[76]

V.f.1. When solutions are placed in warming cabinets, they should be labeled with the date of insertion or date of removal.

Labeling helps determine when the solution has reached its maximum shelf life and prevents overheating related to being left in the warmer too long.

V.f.2. The temperature of solutions on the sterile field should be remeasured before administration.

Burns have been associated with the administration of overheated solutions.[9,76,77,80]

V.g. Solutions intended for IV administration should only be warmed using technology designed for this purpose. *[4: Limited Evidence]*

Warming IV solutions in warming cabinets can overheat the solution from inconsistencies in temperature within the warming cabinet and variances in the temperature of the cabinet.[76,78]

V.h. Skin antiseptic agents should not be warmed, unless otherwise directed by the manufacturer's instructions for use.[81] *[2: High Evidence]*

Recommendation VI

Precautions should be taken to mitigate risks associated with handling, storage, and use of compressed medical gas cylinders and liquid oxygen containers.

The US Food and Drug Administration (FDA) has received reports of patient deaths and injuries related to hook-up errors in medical gas systems.[82]

VI.a. Storage conditions for medical gases should be determined by the volume stored in a location, the need for immediate use, and regulatory requirements.[42] *[2: High Evidence]*

The NFPA and regulatory agencies have determined and enforce the various medical gas storage condition requirements.[42]

VI.a.1. An adequate emergency supply of oxygen should be stored at the facility to provide an uninterrupted supply for one day.[42] **Amb**

VI.a.2. Medical gases must be stored in a secure area with controlled access and separately from industrial gases.

The FDA considers compressed medical gases to be drugs for dispensing by prescription only.[42,83,84]

VI.a.3. The combined volume of medical gas cylinders not considered to be for immediate patient use should not exceed 3,000 ft³ per smoke compartment.

Cylinders on patient gurneys are considered in use or for immediate patient use. Cylinders and carts directly associated with a specific patient are considered "in use." Cylinders and carts not directly associated with a specific patient for 30 minutes or more are considered not in use or in storage.[42]

VI.a.4. Medical gas cylinders that are not intended for immediate use should be stored indoors and

- in a room with a minimum one-hour fire resistance rating,
- in a room that has negative pressure and eight air exchanges per hour,[26]
- in a holder or storage rack with a chain-like securing device, and
- away from heat sources.

Securing cylinders with a chain-like device or in racks prevents the cylinders from falling over. Cylinders and carts directly associated with a specific patient are considered "in use." Cylinders and carts not directly associated with a specific patient for 30 minutes or more are considered not in use or in storage.[42]

VI.a.5. Medical gas cylinders should not be stored in an egress hallway.[42]

VI.a.6. Empty medical gas cylinders should be marked and segregated from full cylinders.

Segregating empty cylinders from full ones minimizes the risk of connecting to an empty cylinder and delaying administration of vital gases.[42]

VI.b. Medical gas cylinders should be transported and secured in a carrier that is designed to prevent the cylinders from tipping or being dropped or damaged. *[2: High Evidence]*

Transporting a cylinder without using an appropriate carrier increases the potential of damage to the cylinder and causing sudden release of the compressed gas, which can cause propulsion of the cylinder and subsequent injury.[42]

VI.c. Medical gas cylinders used during patient transport should be secured to the transport cart or bed in holders designed for this purpose and not placed on top of the bed or cart next to the patient. *[2: High Evidence]*

Holders minimize the risk of the cylinder falling, which can cause propulsion of the cylinder and subsequent injury. Many transport carts are available with built-in holders.[42]

VI.d. Before use, gas cylinders should be checked for the appropriate label, pin-index safety system connector, and color coding. *[2: High Evidence]*

The color of the cylinder, written labels, and a unique pin-index safety system connector are used to clearly identify the medical gas contained within medical gas cylinders.[42]

The pin-index safety system connector for different medical gases prevents connecting the wrong gas to the delivery system.[85] The Compressed Gas Association has approved standardized colors for identification of different medical gases (eg, green indicates oxygen).[42,86] Serious injuries and deaths have resulted from the use of an incorrectly identified medical gas.[82]

VI.e. Fittings on medical gas cylinders and hoses should not be altered under any circumstances.[42] *[2: High Evidence]*

Serious injuries and deaths have resulted from altering the pin-index safety system, thereby permitting delivery of an incorrect gas into the medical gas administration system.[82,87]

VI.e.1. If the fitting does not easily connect, the label on the gas cylinder or hose should be rechecked to verify that it is correct.[42,87]

VI.e.2.   If the label is correct, the cylinder should be returned to the distributor for examination.[42]

VI.e.3.   If the label is incorrect, the cylinder should be replaced with a correctly labeled gas cylinder.[42]

VI.f.   Only approved regulators or other flow control devices should be used.[42,87] *[2: High Evidence]*

VI.f.1.   The regulator, gasket, and washers should be inspected before use.[87]

VI.f.2.   The regulator should be tightened with a T-handle until it is firmly in place.

VI.g.   Precautions should be followed when using medical gas cylinder valves. *[2: High Evidence]*
    Improper use of medical gas cylinder valves can result in contamination of the gas and leakage of the contents into the environment.[42]

VI.g.1.   When a cylinder valve is opened, a small amount of gas should be released before attaching the regulator.
    Opening the valve removes any dust that may have accumulated.[42,87]

VI.g.2.   The valve should be opened slowly to determine whether there is a leak, and the valve should be closed quickly if a leak is found.

VI.g.3.   Compressed medical gas tank valves should be opened fully during use.[42]

VI.g.4.   The valves on medical gas cylinders should be closed properly to avoid leaking during storage. *Amb*

VI.h.   Liquid oxygen containers must be handled, filled, stored, and transported according to state and federal regulations and manufactures' written instructions and labeling.[42] *[2: High Evidence]*

VI.h.1.   Liquid oxygen containers should be stored
    • in a cool, dry place outside of the building or
    • inside the building, as long as the containers are secured to prevent them from tipping over, they do not interfere with foot traffic, they are not exposed to open flames or high-temperature devices, and they are not subject to damage from falling devices.[42]

Recommendation VII

Precautions should be taken to mitigate hazards related to waste anesthesia gases.

All anesthesia machines have the potential to leak, which increases the level of waste anesthesia gases in the ambient air.[88] A study of 15,317 live births between 1990 and 2000 to 9,433 mothers who were exposed to waste anesthesia gases consisting of halothane, isoflurane, or sevoflurane revealed a potential exposure-response relationship between gas exposure and the development of congenital anomalies in the children, although the study did not establish a causal link. Results suggest the anomalies may correlate with the type of waste anesthesia gas to which the mother was exposed.[89]

A report of two cases from 2008 suggests a potential relationship between personnel exposure to high nitrous oxide concentrations and persistent cognitive deficits.[90] A study in Poland involving 55 female nurses and 29 male anesthesiologists showed a link between the levels of waste nitrous oxide and DNA damage. If the concentration of nitrous oxide exceeded the occupational exposure level of 180 mg/m^3, the genetic injury was aggravated.[91] A British study revealed a link between lower vitamin B12 metabolism and levels of nitrous oxide greater than the occupational exposure level, but no link existed if the level was less than the occupational exposure level.[92]

A correlation between levels of waste anesthesia gases and DNA damage was revealed in a study involving 30 OR personnel compared to 30 non-OR personnel. There also was a correlation between DNA damage and an increased oxidative stress index and total oxidative status.[93] In a study of 50 OR personnel in Croatia, where a scavenging system was in use at the facility, researchers found DNA damage.[94] Similar results were found from a study in India that involved a group of 90 OR personnel.[95] A descriptive study in Turkey revealed that a group of anesthesiologists who were exposed to higher than acceptable levels of waste anesthesia gases experienced higher levels of sister chromatid exchanges (ie, DNA mutation) compared to internists who did not work in the OR, and the levels dropped after a two-month absence from the OR. These ORs did not have scavenging systems or low-leakage anesthesia machines, and no preventative maintenance had been performed.[96]

A literature review revealed that the effects of waste anesthesia gases are controversial and the acceptable occupational levels vary by country.[97] A report by the National Institute for Occupational Safety and Health (NIOSH) showed inconsistencies in the literature regarding the effects of waste anesthesia gases, confirmed the means of exposure, and provided guidance for reducing exposures.[98]

VII.a.   The health care organization should establish a waste anesthesia gas management program to be in compliance with the NIOSH recommendations. *[2: High Evidence]*
    The NIOSH standard for nitrous oxide exposure levels is no more than 25 parts per million (ppm) during an eight-hour period and no more than 2 ppm of any halogenated anesthetic agent in one continuous hour.[99]

VII.a.1.   Anesthesia circuits should be inspected before each use to verify the absence of leaks.[72]
    One study showed various types of leaks were present during anesthesia administration, including within the circuitry and

from inadequate control by the anesthesia professional during administration.[100] Higher levels of waste anesthesia gases related to the use of uncuffed endotracheal tubes and during induction with a mask were reported in a review of the literature.[101] A study comparing four different administration techniques revealed that variance in the level of waste anesthesia gases was related to the administration technique.[102]

VII.a.2. Air sampling for the most frequently used anesthesia gases should be conducted every six months to evaluate occupational exposure and the effectiveness of control measures.[88,99]

VII.b. A scavenging system must be used to remove waste anesthesia gases.[88,99] *[1: Regulatory Requirement]*

A Polish study that involved 35 ORs in 10 hospitals showed that the combination of a scavenging system and air exchanges of more than 12 per hour was required to maintain a level of nitrous oxide below the acceptable occupational exposure limit. Use of ventilation systems with up to 15 air exchanges per hour were not adequate alone to keep the nitrous oxide level below the acceptable occupational exposure limit.[103]

VII.b.1. Scavenging systems should be tested for leaks at installation and daily, and testing compliance documentation should be maintained.[72,99]

VII.b.2. Scavenging systems must be vented to an area where waste anesthesia gases will not be reintroduced into the intake air vents or into the recirculating system.[26,88]

VII.c. Ventilation systems in rooms where anesthesia gases are administered should have an air exchange rate of at least 15 exchanges per hour.[26] *[3: Moderate Evidence]*

A descriptive study revealed less waste anesthesia gases in the ambient air when an air exchange rate of at least 15 exchanges per hour was maintained.[100]

VII.d. Anesthesia delivery systems located throughout the facility must be in proper working order and maintained on a regularly scheduled basis, consistent with the manufacturer's written instructions and organizational policy and procedures.[88,99] *[1: Regulatory Requirement]*

A report summarizing the results of one facility's 24 anesthesia machine testing revealed differing high- and low-level leaks at the time of testing. One group of machines had leaks primarily at the absorbent canister bases. The remainder of the machines had leaks in other locations.[104] It is required by OSHA and recommended by NIOSH that a program for routine inspection and maintenance of all anesthesia machines be in place.[88,99]

Recommendation VIII

A protocol to establish a natural rubber latex–safe environment should be developed and implemented.

In a review of the literature, natural rubber latex was identified as a common cause of anaphylaxis during surgical and interventional procedures.[105-107] An observational study performed at two facilities in Wisconsin determined that health care providers are exposed to latex antigens from airborne sources, and the use of powder-free latex gloves reduces the risk of sensitization.[108]

Health care personnel and patients are at a high risk of developing a latex sensitivity from exposure to latex.[109] There are several routes of exposure to natural rubber latex, including

- direct external contact (eg, gloves, natural rubber latex face masks, blood pressure cuff tubing);
- airborne sources that can affect the mucous membranes of the eyes, nose, trachea, bronchi and bronchioles, and oropharynx;
- particles that are swallowed after entering the nasopharynx or oropharynx;
- direct contact of the mucous membranes with indwelling natural rubber latex devices such as catheters;
- internal patient exposure from health care provider use of natural rubber latex gloves during surgical procedures; and
- internally placed natural rubber latex devices, such as wound drains.[105]

The reactions to latex can include urticaria; blisters; rash; dry, cracked, or irritated skin; bronchospasm; and anaphylactic shock.[105] The quality of life for those allergic to latex is improved by avoiding latex.[110] The symptoms of a reaction may resolve quickly after the source of the latex protein has been removed, but the immunoglobulin E (IgE)—a class of antibody that indicates continued sensitivity—remains in the body for at least five years.[111]

VIII.a. Latex-free products, as determined by their labels, should be purchased, if available. *[4: Limited Evidence]*

In 1997, the FDA required that all medical devices containing latex be labeled as such and carry a warning that latex can cause allergic reactions.[112]

VIII.a.1. A list of supplies for which there are no latex-free alternatives should be maintained.

The American Latex Allergy Association maintains an electronic listing of products that contain latex and alternatives that do not.[113]

VIII.b. All patients should be assessed preoperatively for risk factors for latex sensitivity. *[1: Strong Evidence]*

Early recognition of risk factors for sensitivity can prevent the progression of anaphylaxis. Anaphylaxis to latex usually presents 30 to 60 minutes after induction of anesthesia. Latex sensitization reportedly occurs in as many as 12% of health care workers, in 75% of patients with spina bifida, and in patients with a history of multiple surgical procedures.[109]

VIII.b.1. The preoperative assessment should include risk factors for latex sensitivity, including
- a history of long-term bladder care[114];
- a history of spina bifida and genitourinary abnormalities in children[109,114];
- a history of multiple surgical procedures[109,114];
- occupational exposure to latex, such as work in health care[109];
- food allergies (eg, banana, kiwi, avocado, chestnut, raw potato)[105,114]; and
- a history of symptoms of
  - contact dermatitis (ie, type IV sensitivity), especially of the hands,
  - contact urticaria, or
  - hay fever, rhinitis, or asthma.[114]

In a study of children with latex allergies, the researchers concluded that the greater the total number of risk factors, the greater the seriousness of the allergy.[114] The presence of contact dermatitis may permit greater amounts of latex to penetrate the skin.[105]

VIII.b.2. The perioperative RN should document and communicate patient latex sensitivity or allergy information to the perioperative team.

VIII.c. Latex precautions should be implemented for patients with latex sensitivity or allergy. [3: Moderate Evidence]

A seven-year study involving patients with latex allergies demonstrated the effectiveness of establishing a latex-safe management program, as evidenced by known allergic patients having no allergic reactions.[114]

VIII.c.1. Personnel should remove latex gloves, wash their hands, and don latex-safe gloves before entering the room of a patient with a known or suspected latex sensitivity or allergy.

Natural rubber latex proteins on gloves bind to the glove powder (eg, cornstarch powder) and release allergens into the air when gloves are removed.[108,109]

VIII.c.2. Patients with a sensitivity or allergy to latex should be identified by a wristband or bracelet, as well as a label on the patient's bed and a label or electronic flag on the patient's health record.[105,109]

These interventions provide multiple visual cues for health care team members and promote patient safety.

VIII.c.3. The following steps should be followed during care of a patient with a latex sensitivity who requires surgery or another invasive procedure in a non–latex-safe environment:
- remove all latex-containing products from the room the evening before the procedure, except those that are sealed or contained;
- do not use latex products during terminal cleaning of the room the evening before the procedure;
- schedule an elective surgery as the first procedure of the day;
- restrict traffic and equipment in the OR before and during the procedure; and
- when no latex-safe alternative is available, cover latex-containing equipment that comes into direct contact with the patient with stockinette.

Removing latex-containing products from the room the evening before the procedure and using non-latex products during terminal cleaning is thought to help reduce the release of latex particles.[115] Scheduling elective procedures as the first of the day provides time for room air to be completely exchanged after terminal cleaning. Covering latex-containing equipment with stockinette provides a barrier between the equipment and the skin.[116]

VIII.c.4. Signs indicating "latex allergy" should be posted on all doors leading into the OR where the procedure will be performed before the start of the procedure.[116]

VIII.c.5. Postoperatively, the patient should be transferred to a latex-safe care area.[106]

VIII.c.6. Latex sensitivity should be included in all hand-off communications during the transfer of patient care.[106]

VIII.c.7. Rubber stoppers should not be removed from medication vials when withdrawing the medication. The stopper should only be punctured once.

In a review of the literature, no evidence was found to support the removal of medication vial stoppers. Removing the stopper does not reduce contamination of the contents with latex protein because the medication already may contain latex absorbed from the stopper during transport and storage. Not all stoppers contain latex, and the amount of latex in each stopper varies. Requirements for labeling medication vials regarding the latex content of the stopper have not been established.[107]

Multiple punctures of the stopper increase the opportunity for introducing latex proteins into the contents.[107]

PATIENT AND WORKER SAFETY

VIII.d. Perioperative personnel should wear low-protein, powder-free, natural rubber latex gloves or latex-free gloves. *[1: Strong Evidence]*

Health care personnel are susceptible to developing latex allergies when they are exposed to latex gloves and glove powder.[110] A study that involved 325 health care workers in Kenya showed 16% had an allergy to latex gloves; wearing gloves for more than one hour per day and more years of service increased the risk factors for latex allergy. This study also showed, with statistically marginal significance, that working in an environment where others are wearing latex gloves increases the risk of latex allergy.[117]

Use of low-protein, powder-free natural rubber latex gloves or latex-free gloves can minimize latex exposure and the risk of reactions in both health care workers and patients.[108-110,117,118] A systematic review of the literature showed that using low-protein, powder-free, natural rubber latex gloves or latex-free gloves significantly reduces natural rubber latex aeroallergens in the environment, as well as sensitivity and asthma in health care workers.[118]

Quality-of-life scores improved in health care workers with latex allergies after latex products were removed from the workplace. Participants were asked to complete a questionnaire that addressed quality-of-life scores related to skin, eye, and respiratory symptoms that they experienced as a result of exposure to latex in the workplace.[110]

A study in two hospitals involving 805 health care workers showed that the amount of latex in the air duct systems decreased with the introduction of powder-free gloves. This study also identified a reduction in the latex sensitization of seven of the 28 previously sensitized employees.[108]

Recommendation IX

Precautions must be taken to mitigate the risks associated with the use of chemicals in the perioperative setting (eg, methyl methacrylate, glutaraldehyde, formalin, ethylene oxide).[119,120]

Improper handling of chemicals can result in injury to health care workers and patients. Injuries may result from exposure to any portion of the body, including the integumentary or respiratory systems.[121,122] A study of 12 physicians and eight nurses in 10 states revealed the presence of a variety of chemicals (eg, mercury, tricloscan, perfluorinated compounds [PFCs]) in the participants' blood or urine; however, the levels were consistent with general population studies conducted by the US Centers for Disease Control and Prevention National Report on Biomonitoring.[123]

IX.a. Health care organizations must follow the most stringent federal, state, or local regulations for chemical handling and disposal. *[1: Regulatory Requirement]*

State and local requirements may be more stringent than federal regulations.[119,124,125] The most stringent regulations take precedence over less-restrictive regulations.

IX.b. For every potentially hazardous chemical, MSDSs or SDSs must be readily accessible to employees within the practice setting.[119] *[1: Regulatory Requirement]*

The Occupational Safety and Health Administration (OSHA) has changed the title of the "material safety data sheet" to "safety data sheet" and changed the requirements for what information manufacturers must provide on the sheets. The updated requirements now align with international requirements. The updated SDSs include information on hazard identification, recommendations for precautions or special handling, signs and symptoms of toxic exposure, and first aid treatments for exposure, as well as provide more information, including pictograms and signal words (eg, danger, warning).[119]

IX.c. A chemical hazard risk assessment for all chemicals within the unit or facility must be performed annually using the MSDS or SDS and the manufacturer's instructions for use for each chemical. The assessment should include
- the concentration of each ingredient;
- the means of exposure (eg, respiratory, skin, eye, inhalation);
- handling precautions;
- first aid measures if an exposure occurs;
- spill management procedures;
- storage requirements;
- appropriate disposal methods;
- required personal protective equipment (PPE) for handling and spill management;
- whether a chemical that has less risk of causing and injury can be used[121]; and
- whether a chemical that is present is no longer being used and therefore should be disposed of.

[1: Regulatory Requirement]

The risk assessment helps determine the precautions to take and provides information for developing an action plan in the event of spills or exposures.[119]

IX.d. All chemicals must be handled according to their respective MSDS or SDS and the manufacturer's instructions for use,[119] including
- disinfectants and sterilants (eg, glutaraldehyde, ortho-phthalaldehyde, ethylene oxide, hydrogen peroxide, peracetic acid),[24,126]
- tissue preservatives (ie, formalin),[127] and
- antiseptic agents (eg, hand hygiene products, surgical prep solutions).[42,81,128]

[1: Regulatory Requirement]

IX.e. An emergency spill plan should be developed for all chemicals listed in the chemical hazard risk assessment if required by regulation. *[1: Regulatory Requirement]*

Some chemicals may not require an emergency spill plan, or the requirement may be based on the volume of the chemical spilled (eg, formaldehyde, glutaraldehyde).[125]

IX.f. Chemicals must be stored according to
  ○ MSDS or SDS information;
  ○ manufacturer instructions for use;
  ○ flammability and combustibility;
  ○ patient and perioperative personnel safety requirements; and
  ○ local, state, and federal regulations.[129]
  [1: Regulatory Requirement]

IX.g. Personal protective equipment must be provided, as applicable, for employees who must handle chemicals in the workplace. *[1: Regulatory Requirement]*

Defined as any clothing or other equipment that protects a person from exposure to chemicals, PPE may include gloves, aprons, chemical splash goggles, and impervious clothing.[129] Scrubs and lab coats worn by health care workers are not considered PPE because they are not impervious.

IX.h. A respiratory protection plan applicable to each chemical listed in the chemical hazard risk assessment must be developed. *[1: Regulatory Requirement]*

Respiratory protection includes local exhaust ventilation (eg, hoods) or general ventilation above a designated number of air changes per hour. Respirators are required as a portion of the respiratory protection plan for certain chemicals and if the appropriate ventilation cannot be provided.[130]

IX.i. Eyewash stations, either plumbed or self contained, must be provided where chemicals that are hazardous to the eyes are located.[131] *[1: Regulatory Requirement]*

IX.i.1. Plumbed eyewash stations should deliver warm water (ie, 60° F to 100° F [15.6° C to 37.8° C]) at a rate of 1.5 L/minute.[132]

IX.i.2. Plumbed eyewash stations should be flushed weekly.

Weekly flushing removes stagnant water, which may contain microbial contamination, from the system.[132]

IX.i.3. Eyewash stations should be located so that travel time is no greater than 10 seconds from the location of chemical use or storage, or should be immediately available if the chemical is caustic or is a strong acid.[132]

IX.j. Health care organizations must provide education to employees about the hazardous chemicals in the workplace.[119] *[1: Regulatory Requirement]*

IX.k. Safe practices should be established for the use of methyl methacrylate bone cement. *[1: Regulatory Requirement]*

Bone cement is a combination of methyl methacrylate monomer, which is a liquid, and beads of polymethyl methacrylate or a polymethyl methacrylate-based polymer.[133] The liquid portion of methyl methacrylate can be absorbed through the skin and respiratory tract and by ingestion and may cause irritation to the area exposed.[134,135] The permissible exposure limit that OSHA set for methyl methacrylate is 100 ppm or a time-weighted average of 410 mg/m³.[134,135]

One study revealed that morbidity among orthopedic surgeons was higher than general surgeons related to esophageal and myeloproliferative malignancies, but a direct link to methyl methacrylate was not determined.[122] Methyl methacrylate has not been proven to be carcinogenic.[136]

IX.k.1. Eye protection must be worn when mixing and inserting methyl methacrylate bone cement.[134]

Methyl methacrylate fumes may irritate the eyes.[135,137]

IX.k.2. Mixed cement should not come in contact with gloves until it has reached the dough stage. A second pair of gloves, made of the material recommended in the methyl methacrylate manufacturer's instructions, should be worn and then be discarded after contact with the cement.

Methyl methacrylate can penetrate many plastic and latex compounds and can be absorbed through the skin, leading to contact dermatitis.[135,137]

IX.k.3. A closed mixing system or mixing gun should be used for mixing methyl methacrylate.

Closed mixing systems and mixing guns help reduce chemical handling. Closed mixing systems with or without a vacuum release less methyl methacrylate vapor into the breathing zone of the surgical team compared with open mixing systems.[136]

IX.k.4. Direct contact with methyl methacrylate monomer should be avoided.

The liquid monomer is a mild skin irritant and may induce skin sensitization.[133]

IX.k.5. Discarded bone cement should not be left in contact with the patient's skin.

During the curing process, the cement releases heat and has been shown to cause patient burns during total hip arthroplasty.[138]

IX.k.6. When methyl methacrylate liquid is spilled,
  • the spill area should be ventilated until the odor has dissipated,
  • all sources of ignition should be removed,

- appropriate PPE should be worn during cleanup as required by the MSDS or SDS or the manufacturer's instructions for use,
- the spill area should be isolated,
- the liquid should be covered with an activated charcoal absorbent, and
- the waste product should be disposed of in a hazardous waste container.[134]

IX.k.7. Methyl methacrylate monomer is hazardous waste and must be disposed of according to state, local, and federal requirements.[139]

IX.l. Safe handling practices for glutaraldehyde should be developed as required by federal, state, and local regulation and as described in the AORN "Guideline for high-level disinfection."[124,126] *[3: Moderate Evidence]*

Exposure to glutaraldehyde for greater than one hour continuously has been shown to increase the risk of a spontaneous abortion, according to a study that involved 6,707 live births and 775 spontaneous abortions.[140]

IX.l.1. Alternatives for glutaraldehyde should be considered if any are listed in the manufacturer's instructions for use for the device being high-level disinfected.

Several alternative methods of high-level disinfection or sterilization that are less toxic to humans and the environment than glutaraldehyde are available.[124,126]

IX.m. Safe handling practices must be developed for handling formalin.[127] *[1: Regulatory Requirement]*

Formaldehyde, the active ingredient in formalin, is a known carcinogen and may cause other acute and chronic health conditions, including sensitization leading to asthma and contact dermatitis.[127]

IX.m.1. Locations where formalin is used should
- be free of ignition sources,
- have posted signs warning of formaldehyde use, and
- have ventilation systems with adequate capacity to maintain levels below the permissible exposure limits (ie, eight-hour total weighted average of 0.75 ppm; 15-minute, short-term exposure limit of 2.0 ppm).[127]

Formalin is a combustible liquid. The permissible exposure limits are set by OSHA and individual states.[127,141]

IX.m.2. Formaldehyde should not be stored in the OR unless the ventilation system is adequate to keep the levels within the recommended exposure limits.

IX.m.3. Personnel handling formaldehyde must wear proper PPE based on the potential for exposure, including gloves, impervious clothes, aprons, chemical splash goggles, and respiratory protection.

Latex gloves provide no protection against formaldehyde. Butyl and nitrile gloves provide eight hours of protection, and polyethylene gloves provide four hours of protection. Providing respiratory protection (eg, respirators, ventilation hoods) is required if the levels of formalin in the area are greater than 100 ppm.[141]

IX.m.4. Medical surveillance must be provided if workers are exposed to levels of formaldehyde above the permissible exposure limits.[142]

IX.m.5. Health care organizations must monitor levels of formaldehyde
- when the agent is introduced into the space where it will be stored or used;
- if there is a change in processes or practices involving formaldehyde;
- periodically after introduction,
- after a change in processes or practices unless permission has been granted by the regulatory agency with jurisdiction to stop monitoring after two consecutive measurements that were taken at least seven days apart showed the levels were below the recognized safe limits; and
- when an employee reports symptoms of respiratory or dermal exposure.[127,142]

IX.n. Safe handling precautions for ethylene oxide must be developed as required by federal, state, and local regulations and as described in the AORN "Guideline for sterilization."[24,124,129] *[1: Regulatory Requirement]*

Recommendation X

Precautions should be taken to avoid hazards associated with handling waste.

The types of precautions taken when handling wastes are based on the US Environmental Protection Agency (EPA) classifications (eg, hazardous, non-hazardous). Hazardous waste is further classified by the EPA as listed waste, characteristic waste, universal waste, and mixed waste. Medical waste is considered non-hazardous waste and disposal may or may not be regulated.[143]

X.a. The most stringent of federal, state, or local laws that govern the disposal of hazardous and non-hazardous waste must be followed.[143] *[1: Regulatory Requirement]*

Legal requirements vary by state and local jurisdiction. The most stringent requirement supersedes others.

X.a.1. The appropriate regulatory body should be consulted for the applicable definition of medical waste (ie, regulated, non-regulated), which may include specific requirements (eg, volume of body fluids, type of waste exposed to human body fluids)

to classify the item as a regulated medical waste.[143]

X.b. Waste that is classified as hazardous must be placed in hazardous waste containers at the point of use.[143] *[1: Regulatory Requirement]*

This action alerts handlers to take precautions during disposal.

X.b.1. The waste container must be labeled with the type of waste it contains (eg, red bags indicate regulated medical waste, yellow bags indicate hazardous waste such as waste contaminated by chemotherapy agents).[143]

X.b.2. The waste container must protect the personnel handling the container against exposure to the contents (eg, a container used to dispose of sharps must be puncture-resistant, the container for hazardous liquids must be fracture-resistant, the lid of the waste container must seal).[143]

X.b.3. Batteries that contain cadmium, lead, or silver must be disposed of as hazardous waste.[139]

X.b.4. Any product that contains mercury must be disposed of as a hazardous waste.[139]

X.b.5. Flammable liquids (eg, alcohol, benzoin, collodion, formalin, methyl methacrylate monomer, silver nitrate) are considered characteristic wastes and must be contained and placed into a hazardous waste receptacle for disposal.[143]

These chemicals pose fire and environmental hazards if they are discarded into the regular waste stream.

X.c. Medications should be disposed of in accordance with guidelines from the state or local regulatory body with jurisdiction and the AORN "Guideline for medication safety,"[144] and in consultation with the health care organization's pharmacist. *[1: Regulatory Requirement]*

Regulations that cover medication disposal vary between states and locality. The category of waste, which dictates the method of disposal, may vary based on the volume of waste and other conditions.[143]

Recommendation XI

Perioperative personnel should receive initial and ongoing education and complete competency verification activities for establishing and maintaining a safe environment of care.[50,51]

Initial and ongoing education of perioperative personnel on establishing and maintaining a safe environment of care facilitates the development of knowledge, skills, and attitudes that affect safe patient care.

Periodic educational programs provide the opportunity to reinforce the knowledge of potential environmental hazards to patients and personnel, and to introduce new information on equipment or practice changes.

Competency verification measures individual performance and provides a mechanism for documentation. Competency assessment verifies that perioperative personnel have an understanding of potential environmental hazards to patients and personnel.

XI.a. Perioperative team members should receive education and complete competency verification activities that address specialized knowledge and skills related to providing a safe environment of care. Education and competency verification activities should review topics related to maintaining a safe environment of care, including

- the available ergonomic equipment and safe lifting and moving practices;
- the safe use of medical equipment in the perioperative environment;
- appropriate responses to and the meanings of clinical and alert alarms[69,71];
- the safe use of blanket- and solution-warming cabinets[76];
- fire prevention, suppression, and risk assessment;
- the safe use and handling of medical and anesthetic gases;
- precautions for handling and storage of all chemicals listed in the chemical hazard risk assessment[119];
- latex precautions and procedures for handling latex-related reactions;
- hazardous and medical waste disposal; and
- an introduction to and review of organizational policies and procedures.

[1: Regulatory Requirement]

Specialized knowledge includes empirical knowledge (eg, technical understanding), practical knowledge (eg, clinical experience), and aesthetic knowledge (eg, patient advocacy). Ongoing development of knowledge and skills and documentation of personnel participation is a regulatory and accreditation requirement for both hospitals and ambulatory settings.[145-151]

XI.a.1. Simulation demonstrations, such as fire and other emergency drills, should be used to educate perioperative personnel when applicable.

Simulation has been reported to assist with identifying strengths and weaknesses in systems.[61]

XI.b. Employers must provide education and competency verification for perioperative personnel who work with chemicals and other potentially hazardous agents in the workplace.[119,120] Education should include safe handling practices, a description of potential hazards, exposure prevention practices, and spill management procedures. *[1: Regulatory Requirement]*

Recommendation XII

Documentation reflecting activities related to providing a safe environment of care should be recorded in a manner consistent with the health care organization's policies and procedures.

Documentation demonstrates compliance with regulatory and accrediting agency requirements and identifies trends and quality improvement opportunities. Highly reliable data collection is not only necessary to chronicle patient responses to nursing interventions, but also to demonstrate the health care organization's progress toward quality care outcomes.[152]

XII.a. Documentation related to providing a safe environment of care should include
- the date and the name of the person who performs inspection, testing, and maintenance of equipment and alarms;
- the date and the name of the person who performs inspection, testing, and maintenance of eyewash stations;
- results of blanket- and solution-warming cabinet temperature monitoring[76];
- the date and name of the person who performs testing of anesthesia systems and waste gas scavenging systems[42,139];
- the date and name of the person who performs inspection, testing, and maintenance of fire extinguishing equipment[153];
- employee injuries; and
- patient and visitor injuries.

[1: Regulatory Requirement]

Effective management and collection of health care information that accurately reflects the patient's care and treatment, as well as measures taken to ensure employee, patient, and visitor safety, are regulatory and accreditation requirements for both hospitals and ambulatory settings.[50,51,154-158]

XII.b. Records should be maintained for a time period specified by the health care organization and in compliance with local, state, and federal regulations.[119] *[1: Regulatory Requirement]*

Recommendation XIII

Policies and procedures for the provision of a safe environment of care should be developed, reviewed periodically, revised as necessary, and readily available in the practice setting. Amb

Policies and procedures assist in the development of patient safety, quality assessment, and performance improvement activities. Policies and procedures establish authority, responsibility, and accountability within the organization. Policies and procedures also serve as operational guidelines that are used to minimize patient risk for injury or complications, to standardize practice, to direct perioperative personnel, and to establish continuous performance improvement programs.

XIII.a. Policies and procedures should be consistent across disciplines, be supported by administrative leaders, and reflect the rules and recommendations of regulatory and accreditation bodies.[119,120] Policies and procedures related to maintaining a safe environment of care should describe or define the requirements for
- safe patient handling and movement in the perioperative setting[27];
- processes to effectively manage medical equipment, including selection, purchase, inspection, maintenance, and removal from service in the event of a malfunction;
- the use of extension cords;
- the monitoring and recording of warming cabinet temperatures;
- inspection, testing, and maintenance of fire extinguishing equipment and supplies[42];
- who is responsible for and has the authority to turn off medical gas valves;
- the monitoring of nitrous oxide levels and the levels of other inhalation anesthetics;
- the maintenance of anesthesia delivery systems, including scheduling and testing criteria;
- alert and clinical alarm testing and criteria for setting alarm limits[68,69,75];
- who is permitted to change alarm limits, including default limits[68,69,71,75];
- chemical storage[125]; and
- effective management of patients and health care personnel who are at risk for natural rubber latex sensitivity or allergy.

[1: Regulatory Requirement]

Establishing policies and procedures that guide and support patient care, treatment, and services is a regulatory and accreditation requirement for both hospitals and ambulatory settings.[50,51,159-161]

Recommendation XIV

Perioperative personnel should participate in a variety of quality assurance and performance improvement activities that are consistent with the health care organization's plan to improve understanding of and compliance with the principles and processes of maintaining a safe environment of care.

Quality assurance and performance improvement programs assist in evaluating the quality of patient care, the presence of environmental safety hazards, and the formulation of plans for taking corrective actions. These programs provide data that may be used to determine whether an individual organization is within benchmark goals and meets regulatory requirements, and if not, to identify areas that may require corrective actions.

XIV.a. A quality management plan should be developed by a multidisciplinary team that includes representatives from all disciplines of the perioperative team and should include guidance for

- collecting and analyzing information about adverse outcomes associated with the environment of care (eg, latex allergy) as a part of the organization-wide performance improvement program that addresses adverse events and near misses;
- monitoring actual and potential risks in each care area on a regular basis (eg, at least monthly environment of care rounds) and by a team that includes clinicians, administrators, and support personnel;
- monitoring and reporting incidents of equipment malfunction that lead to patient harm, as outlined in the Safe Medical Devices Act of 1990[162];
- monitoring and reporting incidents of alarm malfunction and events related to the inability of the team members to respond to alarms[68,69,71];
- conducting scheduled "walk around" safety rounds to test clinical and alert alarms and to observe staff member responses to the alarms;
- monitoring compliance with requirements for safe handling of chemicals and hazardous wastes in the workplace;
- developing processes to regularly inspect, test, and maintain fire extinguishing equipment and supplies;
- critiquing fire drill performance by a team that includes representatives from all disciplines of the perioperative department to identify deficiencies and opportunities for improvement; and
- reporting work-related health problems, such as using the E-OSHA 300 log.[163]

[1: Regulatory Requirement]

Collecting data to monitor and improve safety, patient care, treatment, and services is a regulatory and accreditation requirement for both hospitals and ambulatory settings.[50,51,155,164,165]

XIV.a.1. Personnel in the perioperative setting should
- identify safety hazards,
- take appropriate corrective actions, and
- report hazards according to organizational policy.

Glossary

Alert alarm: An alarm connected to a system such as medical gas systems, blood bank refrigerators, and fire alarms.

Characteristic wastes: Wastes that do not meet any of the criteria to be considered a listed waste, but exhibit ignitability, corrosivity, reactivity, or toxicity.

Combustible: A substance that can burn, but requires a flash point that is higher than a flammable substance and is at or above 100° F.

Compressed medical gas: A liquefied or vaporized gas alone, or in combination with other gases, which is defined as a drug by the US Food and Drug Adminis-

tration (eg, oxygen, nitrogen, nitric acid, nitrous oxide, carbon dioxide, helium, medical air).

Flammable: A substance that can burn, but requires a flash point, which is less than a combustable substance, and less than 100° F.

Flash point: The temperature of a liquid at which sufficient vapor is given off forming a mixture with the air that will ignite when exposed to an ignition source.

Industrial gases: Gases that are not filtered to remove oils from the compressor and other contaminants.

References

1. Boden LI, Sembajwe G, Tveito TH, et al. Occupational injuries among nurses and aides in a hospital setting. *Am J Ind Med.* 2012;55(2):117-126. doi:10.1002/ajim.21018; 10.1002/ajim.21018. [IIIA]

2. Cappell MS. Injury to endoscopic personnel from tripping over exposed cords, wires, and tubing in the endoscopy suite: a preventable cause of potentially severe workplace injury. *Dig Dis Sci.* 2010;55(4):947-951. doi:10.1007/s10620-009-0923-0. [VB]

3. Cappell MS. Accidental occupational injuries to endoscopy personnel in a high-volume endoscopy suite during the last decade: mechanisms, workplace hazards, and proposed remediation. *Dig Dis Sci.* 2011;56(2):479-487. doi:10.1007/s10620-010-1498-5. [VB]

4. Esser AC, Koshy JG, Randle HW. Ergonomics in office-based surgery: a survey-guided observational study. *Dermatol Surg.* 2007;33(11):1304-1313. doi:10.1111/j.1524-4725.2007.33281.x. [IIIB]

5. Freitag S, Ellegast R, Dulon M, Nienhaus A. Quantitative measurement of stressful trunk postures in nursing professions. *Ann Occup Hyg.* 2007;51(4):385-395. doi:10.1093/annhyg/mem018. [IIIC]

6. Bos E, Krol B, van der Star L, Groothoff J. Risk factors and musculoskeletal complaints in non-specialized nurses, IC nurses, operation room nurses, and X-ray technologists. *Int Arch Occup Environ Health.* 2007;80(3):198-206. doi:10.1007/s00420-006-0121-8. [IIIC]

7. Pompeii LA, Lipscomb HJ, Dement JM. Surveillance of musculoskeletal injuries and disorders in a diverse cohort of workers at a tertiary care medical center. *Am J Ind Med.* 2008;51(5):344-356. doi:10.1002/ajim.20572. [IVB]

8. Drysdale SA. The incidence of upper extremity injuries in endoscopy nurses. *Gastroenterol Nurs.* 2007;30(3):187-192. [IIIB]

9. Guideline for minimally invasive surgery. *Guidelines for Perioperative Practice.* Denver, CO: AORN, Inc; 2015:525-552. [IVB]

10. van Det MJ, Meijerink WJ, Hoff C, Totte ER, Pierie JP. Optimal ergonomics for laparoscopic surgery in minimally invasive surgery suites: a review and guidelines. *Surg Endosc.* 2009;23(6):1279-1285. doi:10.1007/s00464-008-0148-x. [VB]

11. Lee G, Lee T, Dexter D, et al. Ergonomic risk associated with assisting in minimally invasive surgery. *Surg Endosc.* 2009;23(1):182-188. doi:10.1007/s00464-008-0141-4. [VC]

12. Matern U. Ergonomic deficiencies in the operating room: examples from minimally invasive surgery. *Work.* 2009;33(2):165-168. doi:10.3233/WOR-2009-0862. [VB]

13. Nonfatal occupational injuries and illnesses requiring days away from work, 2010 [news release]. Washington, DC: US Department of Labor Bureau of Labor

Statistics; November 9, 2011. http://www.bls.gov/news.release/pdf/osh2.pdf. Accessed September 27, 2012.

14. Alexopoulos EC, Tanagra D, Detorakis I, et al. Knee and low back complaints in professional hospital nurses: occurrence, chronicity, care seeking and absenteeism. *Work*. 2011;38(4):329-335. doi:10.3233/WOR-2011-1136. [IIIA]

15. Matern U, Koneczny S. Safety, hazards and ergonomics in the operating room. *Surg Endosc.* 2007;21(11):1965-1969. doi:10.1007/s00464-007-9396-4. [IIIB]

16. Reddy PP, Reddy TP, Roig-Francoli J, et al. The impact of the alexander technique on improving posture and surgical ergonomics during minimally invasive surgery: pilot study. *J Urol.* 2011;186(4 Suppl):1658-1662. doi:10.1016/j.juro.2011.04.013. [IC]

17. Timmons L. Creating a no-lift, no-transfer environment in the OR. *AORN J.* 2009;89(4):733-736. doi:10.1016/j.aorn.2008.12.025. [VB]

18. Black TR, Shah SM, Busch AJ, Metcalfe J, Lim HJ. Effect of transfer, lifting, and repositioning (TLR) injury prevention program on musculoskeletal injury among direct care workers. *J Occup Environ Hyg.* 2011;8(4):226-235. doi:10.1080/15459624.2011.564110. [IIIB]

19. de Ruiter HP, Liaschenko J. To lift or not to lift: patient-handling practices. *AAOHN J.* 2011;59(8):337-343. doi:10.3928/08910162-20110718-02; 10.3928/08910162-20110718-02. [IIIB]

20. Meeks-Sjostrom D, Lopuszynski SA, Bairan A. The wisdom of retaining experienced nurses at the bedside: a pilot study examining a minimal lift program and its impact on reducing patient movement related injuries of bedside nurses. *Medsurg Nurs.* 2010;19(4):233-236. [IIC]

21. Resnick ML, Sanchez R. Reducing patient handling injuries through contextual training. *J Emerg Nurs.* 2009;35(6):504-508. doi:10.1016/j.jen.2008.10.017. [IIIC]

22. Kutash M, Short M, Shea J, Martinez M. The lift team's importance to a successful safe patient handling program. *J Nurs Adm.* 2009;39(4):170-175. doi:10.1097/NNA.0b013e31819c9cfd. [VA]

23. Martin PJ, Harvey JT, Culvenor JF, Payne WR. Effect of a nurse back injury prevention intervention on the rate of injury compensation claims. *J Safety Res.* 2009;40(1):13-19. doi:10.1016/j.jsr.2008.10.013. [VC]

24. Guideline for sterilization In: *Guidelines for Perioperative Practice.* Denver, CO: AORN, Inc; 2015:665-692. [IVA]

25. Illuminating Engineering Society of North America. *Lighting for Hospitals and Health Care Facilities.* New York, NY: Illuminating Engineering Society of North America; 2006. [IVC]

26. Facility Guidelines Institute. *Guidelines for Design and Construction of Health Care Facilities.* Washington, DC: American Society for Healthcare Engineering (ASHE) of the American Hospital Association; 2010. [IVC]

27. AORN guidance statement: safe patient handling and movement in the perioperative setting. In: *Perioperative Standards and Recommended Practices.* Denver, CO: AORN, Inc; 2012:689-710. [IVB]

28. Waters T, Lloyd JD, Hernandez E, Nelson A. AORN ergonomic tool 7: pushing, pulling, and moving equipment on wheels. *AORN J.* 2011;94(3):254-260. doi:10.1016/j.aorn.2010.09.035. [VA]

29. Waters T, Baptiste A, Short M, Plante-Mallon L, Nelson A. AORN ergonomic tool 6: lifting and carrying supplies and equipment in the perioperative setting. *AORN J.* 2011;94(2):173-179. doi:10.1016/j.aorn.2010.09.033. [VA]

30. Spera P, Lloyd JD, Hernandez E, et al. AORN ergonomic tool 5: tissue retraction in the perioperative setting. *AORN J.* 2011;94(1):54-58. doi:10.1016/j.aorn.2010.08.031. [VA]

31. Hughes NL, Nelson A, Matz MW, Lloyd J. AORN ergonomic tool 4: solutions for prolonged standing in perioperative settings. *AORN J.* 2011;93(6):767-774. doi:10.1016/j.aorn.2010.08.029. [VA]

32. Waters T, Spera P, Petersen C, Nelson A, Hernandez E, Applegarth S. AORN ergonomic tool 3: lifting and holding the patient's legs, arms, and head while prepping. *AORN J.* 2011;93(5):589-592. doi:10.1016/j.aorn.2010.08.028. [VA]

33. Waters T, Short M, Lloyd J, et al. AORN ergonomic tool 2: positioning and repositioning the supine patient on the OR bed. *AORN J.* 2011;93(4):445-449. doi:10.1016/j.aorn.2010.08.027. [VA]

34. Waters T, Baptiste A, Short M, Plante-Mallon L, Nelson A. AORN ergonomic tool 1: lateral transfer of a patient from a stretcher to an OR bed. *AORN J.* 2011;93(3):334-339. doi:10.1016/j.aorn.2010.08.025. [VA]

35. American Society of Anesthesiologists Task Force on Operating Room Fires; Caplan RA, Barker SJ, Connis RT, et al. Practice advisory for the prevention and management of operating room fires. *Anesthesiology.* 2008;108(5): 786-801. doi:10.1097/01.anes.0000299343.87119.a9. [IVB]

36. ECRI. New clinical guide to surgical fire prevention. *Health Devices.* 2009;38(10):314-332. [IVC]

37. ECRI. Fighting airway fires. *Healthcare Risk Control.* 2010;4(Surgery and Anesthesia 10):1-11. [VC]

38. Friedrich M, Tirilomis T, Schmitto JD, et al. Intrathoracic fire during preparation of the left internal thoracic artery for coronary artery bypass grafting. *J Cardiothorac Surg.* 2010;5:10. doi:10.1186/1749-8090-5-10. [VA]

39. Moskowitz M. Fire in the operating room during open heart surgery: a case report. *AANA J.* 2009;77(4):261-264. [VA]

40. Richter GT, Willging JP. Suction cautery and electrosurgical risks in otolaryngology. *Int J Pediatr Otorhinolaryngol.* 2008;72(7):1013-1021. doi:10.1016/j.ijporl.2008.03.006. [IIIA]

41. Mirsaidi N. Cutting a battery pack cable can start a fire. *Nursing.* 2008;38(8):13-14. doi:10.1097/01.NURSE.0000327465.69676.1c. [IIIA]

42. Bielen RP, Lathrop JK. *Health Care Facilities Code Handbook.* 9th ed. Quincy, MA: National Fire Protection Association; 2012. [IVB]

43. Guideline for laser safety. In: *Guidelines for Perioperative Practice.* Denver, CO: AORN, Inc; 2015:139-152. [IVB]

44. Guideline for electrosurgery. In: *Guidelines for Perioperative Practice.* Denver, CO: AORN, Inc; 2015:121-138. [IVB]

45. Guidleine for product selection. In: *Guidelines for Perioperative Practice.* Denver, CO: AORN, Inc; 2015:179-186. [IVB]

46. ECRI. Reducing the risk of burns from surgical light sources. *Risk Management Reporter.* 2009;28(6):15-17. [VB]

47. Rinder CS. Fire safety in the operating room. *Curr Opin Anaesthesiol.* 2008;21(6):790-795. doi:10.1097/ACO.0b013e328318693a. [VC]

48. NFPA 30: *Flammable and Combustible Liquids Code.* Quincy, MA: National Fire Protection Association; 2012. [IVB]

49. *NFPA 101: Life Safety Code.* Quincy, MA: National Fire Protection Association; 2012. [IVB]

50. Ambulatory Surgical Services, 42 CFR §416 (2011).

51. Conditions of Participation for Hospitals, 42 CFR §482 (2010).

52. Chapp K, Lange L. Warming blanket head drapes and trapped anesthetic gases: understanding the fire risk. *AORN J.* 2011;93(6):749-760. doi:10.1016/j.aorn.2010.08.030. [IIIA]

53. Roy S, Smith LP. What does it take to start an oropharyngeal fire? Oxygen requirements to start fires in the operating room. *Int J Pediatr Otorhinolaryngol.* 2011;75(2):227-230. doi:10.1016/j.ijporl.2010.11.005. [VA]

54. Militana CJ, Ditkoff MK, Mattucci KF. Use of the laryngeal mask airway in preventing airway fires during adenoidectomies in children: a study of 25 patients. *Ear Nose Throat J.* 2007;86(10):621-623. [IIIB]

55. Nishiyama K, Komori M, Kodaka M, Tomizawa Y. Crisis in the operating room: fires, explosions and electrical accidents. *J Artif Organs.* 2010;13(3):129-133. doi:10.1007/s10047-010-0513-0. [VC]

56. Yardley IE, Donaldson LJ. Surgical fires, a clear and present danger. *Surgeon.* 2010;8(2):87-92. doi:10.1016/j.surge.2010.01.005. [VB]

57. Watson DS. Surgical fires: 100% preventable, still a problem. *AORN J.* 2009;90(4):589-593. doi:10.1016/j.aorn.2009.09.012. [VB]

58. Laudanski K, Schwab WK, Bakuzonis CW, Paulus DA. Thermal damage of the humidified ventilator circuit in the operating room: an analysis of plausible causes. *Anesth Analg.* 2010;111(6):1433-1436. doi:10.1213/ANE.0b013e3181ee8092. [VA]

59. National Fire Protection Association Technical Committee on Portable Fire Extinguishers. NFPA 10: Standard for Portable Fire Extinguishers. Quincy, MA: National Fire Protection Association; 2010. [IVB]

60. Water-Jel fire blankets [product sheet]. Carlstadt, NJ: Water-Jel; #FB 1110-0.

61. Berendzen JA, van Nes JB, Howard BC, Zite NB. Fire in labor and delivery: simulation case scenario. *Simul Healthc.* 2011;6(1):55-61. doi:10.1097/SIH.0b013e318201351b. [VA]

62. ECRI. Hazard report: prevent surgical boom fires with routine maintenance. *Health Devices.* 2008;January:24-26. [VC]

63. Sentinel event statistics data—event type by year (1995-2011). The Joint Commission. http://www.jointcommission.org/sentinel_event.aspx. Accessed June 21, 2012. [VB]

64. Kuczkowski KM. Anesthesia machine as a cause of intraoperative "code red" in the labor and delivery suite. *Arch Gynecol Obstet.* 2008;278(5):477-478. doi:10.1007/s00404-008-0610-y. [VC]

65. US Department of Health and Human Services Centers for Disease Control and Prevention. Guidelines for environmental infection control in health-care facilities. http://www.cdc.gov/ncidod/dhqp/pdf/guidelines/Enviro_guide_03.pdf ed. Accessed September 27, 2012. [IVA]

66. Guideline for environmental cleaning. *Guidelines for Perioperative Practice.* Denver, CO: AORN, Inc; 2015:9-30. [IVB]

67. Hargrove M, Aherne T. Possible fire hazard caused by mismatching electrical chargers with the incorrect device within the operating room. *J Extra Corpor Technol.* 2007;39(3):199-200. [VC]

68. Phillips J. Clinical alarms: complexity and common sense. *Crit Care Nurs Clin North Am.* 2006;18(2):145-156. [VB]

69. Clinical Alarms Task Force. Impact of clinical alarms on patient safety: a report from the American College of Clinical Engineering Healthcare Technology Foundation. *J Clin Eng.* 2007;32(1):22-33. [VB]

70. Schmid F, Goepfert MS, Kuhnt D, et al. The wolf is crying in the operating room: patient monitor and anesthesia workstation alarming patterns during cardiac surgery. *Anesth Analg.* 2011;112(1):78-83. doi:10.1213/ANE.0b013e3181fcc504. [IIIB]

71. *A Siren Call to Act: Priority Issues from the Medical Device Alarms Summit.* Arlington, VA: Association for the Advancement of Medical Instrumentation; 2011. [VC]

72. 2008 recommendations for pre-anesthesia checkout procedures. American Society of Anesthesiologists. http://asatest.asahq.org/clinical/fda.htm. Accessed October 9, 2012. [IVB]

73. Hagenouw RR. Should we be alarmed by our alarms? *Curr Opin Anaesthesiol.* 2007;20(6):590-594. doi:10.1097/ACO.0b013e3282f10dff. [VC]

74. Position statement on noise in the perioperative practice setting. AORN, Inc. http://www.aorn.org/WorkArea/DownloadAsset.aspx?id=21925. Accessed September 27, 2012. [IVB]

75. Brown JC, Anglin-Regal P. Patient safety focus. Clinical alarm management: a team effort. *Biomed Instrum Technol.* 2008;42(2):142-144. [VA]

76. Warming cabinets. *Oper Room Risk Manag.* 2010;2(Surgery 7). [VC]

77. Huang S, Gateley D, Moss AL. Accidental burn injury during knee arthroscopy. *Arthroscopy.* 2007;23(12):1363.e1–1363.e3. doi:10.1016/j.arthro.2006.08.015. [VB]

78. Limiting temperature settings on blanket and solution warming cabinets can prevent patient burns. *Health Devices.* 2005;34(5):168-171. [VC]

79. Bujdoso PJ. Blanket warming: comfort and safety. *AORN J.* 2009;89(4):717-722. [VB]

80. Guideline for the prevention of unplanned perioperative hypothermia. In: *Guidelines for Perioperative Practice.* Denver, CO: AORN, Inc; 2015:479-490. [IVB]

81. Guideline for preoperative patient skin antisepsis. In: *Guidelines for Perioperative Practice.* Denver, CO: AORN, Inc; 2015:43-66. [IVB]

82. *Guidance for Hospitals, Nursing Homes, and Other Health Care Facilities.* FDA Public Health Advisory. Rockvill, MD: US Food and Drug Administration Center for Drug Evaluation and Research; 2001. http://www.fda.gov/downloads/Drugs/GuidanceComplianceRegulatoryInformation/Guidances/ucm070285.pdf. Accessed October 9, 2012.

83. US Department of Health and Human Services Food and Drug Administration. Medical gas containers and closures; current good manufacturing practice requirements. *Fed Regist.* 2006;71(68):18039-18053.

84. Compressed Medical Gases Guideline. Revised February 1989. Food and Drug Administration Center for Drug Evaluation and Research. http://www.fda.gov/Drugs/GuidanceComplianceRegulatoryInformation/Guidances/ucm124716.htm. Accessed October 9, 2012.

85. ISO 407:2004. Small medical gas cylinders—Pin-index yoke-type valve connections. ISO. http://www.iso.org/iso/catalogue_detail.htm?csnumber=40148. Accessed October 9, 2012. [IVB]

86. Compressed Gas Association. *Standard Color Marking of Compressed Gas Cylinders Intended for Medical Use.* 4th ed. Chantilly, VA: Compressed Gas Association; 2004. [IVB]

87. ECRI. Compressed gases. *Healthcare Risk Control.* 2007;3(Environmental Issues 17.1). [VB]

88. Anesthetic gases: guidelines for workplace exposures. US Department of Labor Occupational Safety & Health Administration. http://osha.gov/dts/osta/anesthet

icgases/index.html. Published July 20, 1999. Revised May 18, 2000. Accessed October 9, 2012.

89. Teschke K, Abanto Z, Arbour L, et al. Exposure to anesthetic gases and congenital anomalies in offspring of female registered nurses. *Am J Ind Med*. 2011;54(2):118-127. doi:10.1002/ajim.20875; 10.1002/ajim.20875. [IIIB]

90. Dreyfus E, Tramoni E, Lehucher-Michel MP. Persistent cognitive functioning deficits in operating rooms: two cases. *Int Arch Occup Environ Health*. 2008;82(1):125-130. doi:10.1007/s00420-008-0302-8. [VC]

91. Wronska-Nofer T, Palus J, Krajewski W, et al. DNA damage induced by nitrous oxide: study in medical personnel of operating rooms. *Mutat Res*. 2009;666(1-2):39-43. doi:10.1016/j.mrfmmm.2009.03.012. [IIIB]

92. Krajewski W, Kucharska M, Pilacik B, et al. Impaired vitamin B12 metabolic status in healthcare workers occupationally exposed to nitrous oxide. *Br J Anaesth*. 2007;99(6):812-818. doi:10.1093/bja/aem280. [IIIB]

93. Baysal Z, Cengiz M, Ozgonul A, Cakir M, Celik H, Kocyigit A. Oxidative status and DNA damage in operating room personnel. *Clin Biochem*. 2009;42(3):189-193. doi:10.1016/j.clinbiochem.2008.09.103. [IIIB]

94. Rozgaj R, Kasuba V, Brozovic G, Jazbec A. Genotoxic effects of anaesthetics in operating theatre personnel evaluated by the comet assay and micronucleus test. *Int J Hyg Environ Health*. 2009;212(1):11-17. doi:10.1016/j.ijheh.2007.09.001. [IIIB]

95. Chandrasekhar M, Rekhadevi PV, Sailaja N, et al. Evaluation of genetic damage in operating room personnel exposed to anaesthetic gases. *Mutagenesis*. 2006;21(4):249-254. doi:10.1093/mutage/gel029. [IIIB]

96. Eroglu A, Celep F, Erciyes N. A comparison of sister chromatid exchanges in lymphocytes of anesthesiologists to nonanesthesiologists in the same hospital. *Anesth Analg*. 2006;102(5):1573-1577. doi:10.1213/01.ane.0000204298.42159.0e. [IIIB]

97. Oliveira CR. Occupational exposure to anesthetic gases residue. *Rev Bras Anestesiol*. 2009;59(1):110-124. [VC]

98. *Waste Anesthetic Gases: Occupational Hazards in Hospitals* [DHHS (NIOSH) Publication No. 2007-151]. Atlanta, GA: National Institute for Occupational Safety and Health; 2007. [IVB]

99. NIOSH Criteria Documents: Criteria for a Recommended Standard: Occupational Exposure to Waste Anesthetic Gases and Vapors. Atlanta, GA: National Institute for Occupational Safety and Health; 1977:194. http://www.cdc.gov/niosh/docs/1970/77-140.html. Accessed October 9, 2012. [IVB]

100. Sartini M, Ottria G, Dallera M, Spagnolo AM, Cristina ML. Nitrous oxide pollution in operating theatres in relation to the type of leakage and the number of efficacious air exchanges per hour. *J Prev Med Hyg*. 2006;47(4):155-159. [IIIB]

101. Irwin MG, Trinh T, Yao CL. Occupational exposure to anaesthetic gases: a role for TIVA. *Expert Opin Drug Saf*. 2009;8(4):473-483. doi:10.1517/14740330903003778. [VA]

102. Barberio JC, Bolt JD, Austin PN, Craig WJ. Pollution of ambient air by volatile anesthetics: a comparison of 4 anesthetic management techniques. *AANA J*. 2006;74(2):121-125. [IVA]

103. Krajewski W, Kucharska M, Wesolowski W, Stetkiewicz J, Wronska-Nofer T. Occupational exposure to nitrous oxide—the role of scavenging and ventilation systems in reducing the exposure level in operating rooms. *Int J Hyg Environ Health*. 2007;210(2):133-138. doi:10.1016/j.ijheh.2006.07.004. [VB]

104. Smith FD. Management of exposure to waste anesthetic gases. *AORN J*. 2010;91(4):482-494. [VA]

105. Pollart SM, Warniment C, Mori T. Latex allergy. *Am Fam Physician*. 2009;80(12):1413-1418. [VB]

106. Mertes PM, Lambert M, Gueant-Rodriguez RM, et al. Perioperative anaphylaxis. *Immunol Allergy Clin North Am*. 2009;29(3):429-451. doi:10.1016/j.iac.2009.04.004. [VB]

107. Heitz JW, Bader SO. An evidence-based approach to medication preparation for the surgical patient at risk for latex allergy: is it time to stop being stopper poppers? *J Clin Anesth*. 2010;22(6):477-483. doi:10.1016/j.jclinane.2009.12.006. [VC]

108. Kelly KJ, Wang ML, Klancnik M, Petsonk EL. Prevention of IgE sensitization to latex in health vare workers after reduction of antigen exposures. *J Occup Environ Med*. 2011;53(8):934-940. doi:10.1097/JOM.0b013e31822589dc. [IIIC]

109. Lieberman P, Nicklas RA, Oppenheimer J, Kemp SF, Lang DM, eds. The diagnosis and management of anaphylaxis practice parameter: 2010 update [published correction appears in *J Allergy Clin Immunol*. 2010;126(6):1104]. *J Allergy Clin Immunol*. 2010;126(3):477-480.e42. doi:10.1016/j.jaci.2005.01.010. [IVA]

110. Power S, Gallagher J, Meaney S. Quality of life in health care workers with latex allergy. *Occup Med (Lond)*. 2010;60(1):62-65. doi:10.1093/occmed/kqp156. [IIIC]

111. Smith AM, Amin HS, Biagini RE, et al. Percutaneous reactivity to natural rubber latex proteins persists in health-care workers following avoidance of natural rubber latex. *Clin Exp Allergy*. 2007;37(9):1349-1356. doi:10.1111/j.1365-2222.2007.02787.x. [IIIC]

112. Natural rubber-containing medical devices; user labeling. Final rule. *Fed Regist*. 1997;62(189):51021-51030.

113. Online resource manual section 1: latex-free product lists—consumer, dental, hospital. American Latex Allergy Association. http://www.latexallergyresources.org/latex-free-products. Accessed October 9, 2012. [IVC]

114. Gentili A, Lima M, Ricci G, et al. Perioperative treatment of latex-allergic children. *J Patient Saf*. 2007;3(3):166-172. [IIIB]

115. Bernardini R, Catania P, Caffarelli C, et al. Perioperative latex allergy. *Int J Immunopathol Pharmacol*. 2011;24(3 Suppl):S55-S60. [VB]

116. AANA latex protocol. American Latex Allergy Association. http://www.latexallergyresources.org/articles/aana-latex-protocol. Accessed October 9, 2012. [IVC]

117. Amarasekera M, Rathnamalala N, Samaraweera S, Jinadasa M. Prevalence of latex allergy among healthcare workers. *Int J Occup Med Environ Health*. 2010;23(4):391-396. doi:10.2478/v10001-010-0040-5. [IIIB]

118. LaMontagne AD, Radi S, Elder DS, Abramson MJ, Sim M. Primary prevention of latex related sensitisation and occupational asthma: a systematic review. *Occup Environ Med*. 2006;63(5):359-364. doi:10.1136/oem.2005.025221. [IIIB]

119. Hazard Communication: Toxic and Hazardous Substances, 29 CFR §1910.1200 (2012). http://www.osha.gov/pls/oshaweb/owadisp.show_document?p_table=STANDARDS&p_id=10099. Accessed October 9, 2012.

120. Occupational Safety and Health Standards, Toxic and Hazardous Substances, Definition of "Trade Secret" (Mandatory), 29 CFR §1910.1200E (2012). http://www.osha.gov/pls/oshaweb/owadisp.show_document?p_table=STANDARDS&p_id=10104. Accessed October 9, 2012.

121. Gunson TH, Smith HR, Vinciullo C. Assessment and management of chemical exposure in the Mohs laboratory. *Dermatol Surg.* 2011;37(1):1-9. doi:10.1111/j.1524-4725.2010.01807.x; 10.1111/j.1524-4725.2010.01807.x. [VC]

122. Diaz JH. Proportionate cancer mortality in methyl methacrylate-exposed orthopedic surgeons compared to general surgeons. *J Med Toxicol.* 2011;7(2):125-132. doi:10.1007/s13181-011-0134-x. [IIIC]

123. Wilding BC, Curtis K, Welker-Hood K. *Hazardous Chemicals in Health Care: A Snapshot of Chemicals in Doctors and Nurses.* Washington, DC: Physicians for Social Responsibility. http://www.psr.org/assets/pdfs/hazardous-chemicals-in-health-care.pdf. Accessed October 9, 2012. [IIIA]

124. ECRI. Ethylene oxide, formaldehyde, and glutaraldehyde. *Healthcare Risk Control.* 2011;3(Environmental Issues 6). [VC]

125. Occupational Safety and Health Standards, Hazardous Materials, Hazardous Waste Operations and Emergency Response, 29 CFR §1910.120 (2012). http://www.osha.gov/pls/oshaweb/owadisp.show_document?p_table=standards&p_id=9765. Accessed October 9, 2012.

126. Guideline for high-level disinfection. In: *Guidelines for Perioperative Practice.* Denver, CO: AORN, Inc; 2015:601-614. [IVB]

127. Occupational Safety and Health Standards, Toxic and Hazardous Substances, Formaldehyde, 29 CFR §1910.1048 (2012). http://www.osha.gov/pls/oshaweb/owadisp.show_document?p_table=STANDARDS&p_id=10075. Accessed October 9, 2012.

128. Guideline for hand hygiene. In: *Guidelines for Perioperative Practice.* Denver, CO: AORN, Inc; 2015:31-42. [IVB]

129. Occupational Safety and Health Standards, Personal Protective Equipment, General Requirements, 29 CFR §1910.132 (2011). http://www.osha.gov/pls/oshaweb/owadisp.show_document?p_table=STANDARDS&p_id=9777. Accessed October 9, 2012.

130. Occupational Safety and Health Standards, Personal Protective Equipment, Respiratory Protection. 29 CFR §1910.134 (2011). http://www.osha.gov/pls/oshaweb/owadisp.show_document?p_table=STANDARDS&p_id=12716. Accessed October 9, 2012.

131. Occupational Safety and Health Standards, Medical and First Aid, Medical Services and First Aid. 29 CFR §1910.151 (1998). http://www.osha.gov/pls/oshaweb/owadisp.show_document?p_table=STANDARDS&p_id=9806. Accessed October 9, 2012.

132. *ANSI/ISEA Z358.1-2009: American National Standard for Emergency Eyewash and Shower Equipment.* New York, NY: American National Standards Institute; 2009. [IVC]

133. Leggat PA, Smith DR, Kedjarune U. Surgical applications of methyl methacrylate: a review of toxicity. *Arch Environ Occup Health.* 2009;64(3):207-212. doi:10.1080/19338240903241291. [IVC]

134. International Chemical Safety Cards: Methyl methacrylate. International Programme on Chemical Safety. http://www.cdc.gov/niosh/ipcsneng/neng0300.html. Accessed October 9, 2012.

135. Chemical sampling information: methyl methacrylate. Occupational Safety and Health Administration. http://www.osha.gov/dts/chemicalsampling/data/CH_254400.html. Updated April 27, 2007. Accessed October 9, 2012.

136. Ungers LJ, Vendrely TG, Barnes CL. Control of methyl methacrylate during the preparation of orthopedic bone cements. *J Occup Environ Hyg.* 2007;4(4):272-280. doi:10.1080/15459620701223843. [IIIB]

137. Medical devices; reclassification of polymethylmethacrylate (PMMA) bone cement. Final rule. *Fed Regist.* 2002;67(137):46852-46855.

138. Burston B, Yates P, Bannister G. Cement burn of the skin during hip replacement. *Ann R Coll Surg Engl.* 2007;89(2):151-152. doi:10.1308/003588407X168262. [VC]

139. Protection of Environment, Chapter 1: Environmental Protection Agency, Subchapter I: Solid Wastes. 40 CFR §260, 266 (2011).

140. Lawson CC, Rocheleau CM, Whelan EA, et al. Occupational exposures among nurses and risk of spontaneous abortion. *Am J Obstet Gynecol.* 2012;206(4):327.e1–327.e8. doi:10.1016/j.ajog.2011.12.030. [IIIB]

141. Occupational Safety and Health Standards, Toxic and Hazardous Substances, Substance Technical Guidelines for Formalin, 29 CFR §1910.1048A (2006). http://www.osha.gov/pls/oshaweb/owadisp.show_document?p_table=STANDARDS&p_id=10076. Accessed October 9, 2012.

142. Occupational Safety and Health Standards, Toxic and Hazardous Substances, Sampling Strategy and Analytical Methods for Formaldehyde, 29 CFR §1910.1048B. http://www.osha.gov/pls/oshaweb/owadisp.show_document?p_table=STANDARDS&p_id=10077. Accessed October 9, 2012.

143. Wastes. Environmental Protection Agency. http://www.epa.gov/epawaste/index.htm. Accessed October 9, 2012.

144. Guideline for medication safety. In: *Guidelines for Perioperative Practice.* Denver, CO: AORN, Inc; 2015:291-329. [IVB]

145. Centers for Medicare & Medicaid Services. *State Operations Manual Appendix A—Survey Protocol, Regulations and Interpretive Guidelines for Hospitals.* Rev. 78; 2011.

146. Centers for Medicare & Medicaid Services. *State Operations Manual Appendix L: Guidance for Surveyors: Ambulatory Surgical Centers.* Rev. 76; 2011.

147. HR.01.05.03: Staff participate in ongoing education and training. In: *Comprehensive Accreditation Manual: CAMH for Hospitals.* Oakbrook Terrace, IL: The Joint Commission; 2012.

148. HR.01.05.03: Staff participate in ongoing education and training. In: *Comprehensive Accreditation Manual for Ambulatory Care.* Oakbrook Terrace, IL: Joint Commission; 2012.

149. Quality management and improvement. In: 2012 *Accreditation Handbook for Ambulatory Health Care.* Skokie, IL: Accreditation Association for Ambulatory Health Care; 2012:34-39.

150. Personnel. Personnel records. In: *Procedural Standards and Checklist for Accreditation Ambulatory Facilities.* Version 1. Gurnee, IL: American Association for Accreditation of Ambulatory Facilities; 2008:51-52.

151. Knowledge, skill & CME training. In: *Procedural Standards and Checklist for Accreditation Ambulatory Facilities.* Version 1. Gurnee, IL: American Association for Accreditation of Ambulatory Facilities; 2008:53.

152. Guideline for perioperative health care information management. In: *Guidelines for Perioperative Practice.* Denver, CO: AORN, Inc; 2015:491-512. [IVB]

153. *NFPA 99 : Health Care Facilities Code.* 2012 ed. Quincy, MA: National Fire Protection Association; 2011. [IVB]

154. RC.01.01.01: The hospital maintains complete and accurate medical records for each individual patient. In:

Hospital Accreditation Standards 2012. Oakbrook Terrace, IL: Joint Commission on Resources; 2012.

155. PI.03.01.01: The hospital improves performance on an ongoing basis. In: *Hospital Accreditation Standards 2012.* Oakbrook Terrace, IL: Joint Commission on Resources; 2012.

156. Medical records. *Procedure room records.* In: *Procedural Standards and Checklist for Accreditation Ambulatory Facilities.* Version 1. Gurnee, IL: American Association for Accreditation of Ambulatory Facilities; 2008:42-43.

157. Medical records. General. In: *Procedural Standards and Checklist for Accreditation Ambulatory Facilities.* Version 1. Gurnee, IL: American Association for Accreditation of Ambulatory Facilities; 2008:39-40.

158. Clinical records and health information. In: 2012 *Accreditation Handbook for Ambulatory Health Care.* Skokie, IL: Accreditation Association for Ambulatory Health Care; 2012:40-42.

159. LD.04.01.07: The hospital has policies and procedures that guide and support patient care, treatment, and services. In: *Hospital Accreditation Standards 2012.* Oakbrook Terrace, IL: Joint Commission on Resources; 2012.

160. LD.04.01.07: The organization has policies and procedures that guide and support patient care, treatment, or services. In: *Standards for Ambulatory Care 2012: Standards, Elements of Performance Scoring Accreditation Polices.* Oakbrook Terrace, IL: The Joint Commission; 2012.

161. Governance. In: *2012 Accreditation Handbook for Ambulatory Health Care.* Skokie, IL: Accreditation Association for Ambulatory Health Care; 2012:20-27.

162. Safe Medical Devices Act of 1990 and the Medical Device Amendments of 1992. HHS Publication FDA 93-4243. Washington, DC: US Dept. of Health and Human Services, Public Health Service/Food and Drug Administration, Center for Devices and Radiological Health; 1993.

163. Randall SB, Pories WJ, Pearson A, Drake DJ. Expanded occupational safety and health administration 300 log as metric for bariatric patient-handling staff injuries. *Surg Obes Relat Dis.* 2009;5(4):463-468. doi:10.1016/j.soard.2009.01.002. [IIIA]

164. PI.03.01.01: The organization improves performance. In: *Standards for Ambulatory Care 2012: Standards, Elements of Performance Scoring Accreditation Polices.* Oakbrook Terrace, IL: The Joint Commission; 2012.

165. Quality assessment/quality improvement. Quality improvement. In: *Procedural Standards and Checklist for Accreditation Ambulatory Facilities.* Version 1. Gurnee, IL: American Association for Accreditation of Ambulatory Facilities; 2008:44.

Acknowledgments

The authors and AORN thank Antonia B. Hughes, MA, BSN, RN, CNOR, Perioperative Education Specialist, Baltimore Washington Medical Center, Glen Burnie, Maryland; Elizabeth A. P. Vane, MSN, RN, CNOR, Chief, Perioperative Nursing Services, Walter Reed National Military Medical Center, Bethesda, Maryland; Rebecca M. Patton, MSN, RN, CNOR, FAAN, Atkinson Scholar in Perioperative Nursing, Case Western Reserve University, Lakewood, Ohio; and Rev Donna S Nussman, PhD, RN, Surgical Health Care Consultant, and Adjunct Professor, College of Mechanical Engineering/BioEngineering Department, University of North Carolina – Charlotte, for their assistance in developing this guideline.

Publication History

Originally published February 1988, *AORN Journal*, as "Recommended practices for safe care through identification of potential hazards in the surgical environment." Revised March 1992.

Revised November 1995; published March 1996, *AORN Journal*. Reformatted July 2000.

Revised; published March 2003, *AORN Journal*.

Revised 2007; published in *Perioperative Standards and Recommended Practices*, 2008 edition, as "Recommended practices for a safe environment of care."

Revised November 2009 for online publication in *Perioperative Standards and Recommended Practices*.

Minor editing revisions made in November 2010 for publication in *Perioperative Standards and Recommended Practices*, 2011 edition.

Revised and reformatted December 2012 for online publication in *Perioperative Standards and Recommended Practices*.

Evidence ratings revised 2013 to conform to the AORN Evidence Rating Model.

Minor editing revisions made in November 2014 for publication in *Guidelines for Perioperative Practice*, 2015 edition.

Evidence ratings revised in *Guidelines for Perioperative Practice*, 2018 edition, to conform to the current AORN Evidence Rating Model.

LEAD AUTHOR
Byron Burlingame, MS, BSN, RN, CNOR
Perioperative Nursing Specialist
AORN Nursing Department
Denver, Colorado

CONTRIBUTING AUTHOR
Ramona Conner, MSN, RN, CNOR
Manager, Standards and Guidelines
AORN Nursing Department
Denver, Colorado

AMBULATORY SUPPLEMENT: SAFE ENVIRONMENT OF CARE, PART 1

Recommendation VI

Precautions should be taken to mitigate risks associated with handling, storage, and use of compressed medical gas cylinders and liquid oxygen containers.

VI.a.1.   An adequate emergency supply of oxygen should be stored at the facility to provide an uninterrupted supply for one day.[A1]

Amb Oxygen delivery may only be available on certain days, and emergency supplies may be unavailable.

Amb An alarm system should indicate oxygen reserve status and one-day supply.[A2-A4]

Amb Oxygen supply levels should be verified daily when the facility is open for business.[A2,A3]

Amb Surgical procedures should not be started until a sufficient oxygen supply is confirmed.

VI.g.4.   The valves on medical gas cylinders should be closed properly to avoid leaking during storage.

Amb Gas cylinder valves and oxygen delivery unit valves (eg, anesthesia machines, flow meters) should be checked at the close of business to confirm they are in the off position.

A cylinder valve or delivery unit valve left open overnight or over the weekend may deplete the facility's entire oxygen supply.

Recommendation XIII

Policies and procedures for the provision of a safe environment of care should be developed, reviewed periodically, revised as necessary, and readily available in the practice setting.

 Policies and procedures should include
* the minimum oxygen supply level to be maintained,[A4]
* oxygen storage capabilities,[A4]
* the oxygen procurement process,[A4]
* the amount of time needed for routine and emergency oxygen delivery,[A3,A4]
* processes for verifying the daily oxygen supply,[A2,A3] and
* processes for checking gas cylinder valves and oxygen delivery unit valves (eg, anesthesia machines, flow meters) at the close of business to confirm they are in the off position.

REFERENCES

A1. Bielen RP, Lathrop JK. *Health Care Facilities Code Handbook.* 9th ed. Quincy, MA: National Fire Protection Association; 2012. [IVB]

A2. EC.02.05.09: The organization inspects, tests, and maintains medical gas and vacuum systems. In: *Comprehensive Accreditation Manual for Ambulatory Care.* Oakbrook Terrace, IL: Joint Commission; 2013.

A3. Anesthesia services. In: 2013 *Accreditation Handbook for Ambulatory Health Care.* Skokie, IL: Accreditation Association for Ambulatory Health Care; 2013:47.

A4. *NFPA 99: Health Care Facilities Code.* 2012 ed. Quincy, MA: National Fire Protection Association; 2011. [IVB]

GUIDELINE FOR A SAFE ENVIRONMENT OF CARE, PART 2

The Guideline for a Safe Environment of Care, Part 2 has been approved by the AORN Guidelines Advisory Board. It was presented as a proposed guideline for comments by members and others. The guideline is effective May 15, 2014. The recommendations in the guideline are intended to be achievable and represent what is believed to be an optimal level of practice. Policies and procedures will reflect variations in practice settings and/or clinical situations that determine the degree to which the guideline can be implemented. AORN recognizes the many diverse settings in which perioperative nurses practice; therefore, this guideline is adaptable to all areas where operative and other invasive procedures may be performed.

Purpose

The physical design and environment of the perioperative suite should support safe patient care, workplace safety, and security. This document provides guidance for the design of the building structure; movement of patients, personnel, supplies, and equipment through the suite; safety during construction; environmental controls (eg, heating, ventilation, air conditioning [HVAC]); maintenance of structural surfaces; power failure response planning; security; and control of noise and distractions. Disaster response and recovery are outside the scope of this document.

Evidence Review

A medical librarian conducted a systematic review of the MEDLINE®, CINAHL®, and Scopus® databases and the Cochrane Database of Systematic Reviews for meta-analyses, randomized and nonrandomized trials and studies, and systematic and nonsystematic reviews. Search terms included *restricted area, semirestricted area, nonrestricted area, transition zone, traffic patterns, traffic, foot traffic, traffic flow, door swings, hospital design and construction, hospital construction, facility design and construction, Aspergillus, aspergillosis, spores, mycoses, fungi, dust, debris, operating rooms, operating theatres, operating suites, surgicenters, ambulatory surgery centers, hospitals, air microbiology, filtration, indoor air pollution, infection control, surgical site infection, surgical wound infection, Health Insurance Portability and Accountability Act, HIPAA, privacy, confidentiality, controlled environment, heating, ventilation, air conditioning, HVAC, equipment contamination, cardboard, ventilation, heating, laminar flow, laminar airflow, Staphylococcus, enterococcus, enterococci, Staphylococcaceae, microbial colony count, security measures, violence, ultraviolet disinfection, ultraviolet rays, ultraviolet, disinfection, terminal cleaning,* company representatives, industry representatives, sales representatives, equipment manufacturers, humidity, temperature, health personnel, surgical attire, clothing, clothes, textiles, fabric, lighting, illumination, electricity,* and *electric power supplies.*

Articles specific to animals and the topics of refuse disposal, waste management, sanitary engineering, waste products, and the food industry were excluded. In addition, the librarian reviewed the search results related to laminar airflow and removed from them articles that were not relevant to infection or the environment. The lead author and the medical librarian identified and obtained relevant guidelines from government agencies, other professional organizations, and standards-setting bodies.

The initial search was conducted in February 2011; an April 2012 follow-up search included additional topics. In both cases, search results were limited to literature published in the five years prior to the date of the search. The lead author also consulted the results of a 2013 literature search on distractions in the perioperative environment for recent studies on this topic. The librarian established continuing alerts on the topics included in this guideline and provided relevant results to the lead author.

Editor's note: *MEDLINE is a registered trademark of the US National Library of Medicine's Medical Literature Analysis and Retrieval System, Bethesda, MD. CINAHL, Cumulative Index to Nursing and Allied Health Literature, is a registered trademark of EBSCO Industries, Birmingham, AL. Scopus is a registered trademark of Elsevier B.V., Amsterdam, Netherlands.*

Recommendation I

The health care organization should establish a multidisciplinary team that is responsible for the oversight of any surgical suite construction or renovation project.

A multidisciplinary team can provide expertise on functional design, the functional needs of the users, infection prevention, sustainability, and regulatory requirements.[1-3]

I.a.   The multidisciplinary team should consist of
- representatives of the health care organization, including perioperative nurses and an infection preventionist[1,2];
- representatives from all affected disciplines;
- external representatives including the design team (eg, architects, interior designers, engineers); and

○ representatives of equipment manufacturers whose equipment requires provisions for structural support, space, and utilities. *[3: Moderate Evidence]*

Representatives of the health care organization possess the clinical expertise necessary to identify the functional needs of the users and assess the design for possible constraints (eg, infection prevention, functional workflow).[1,3] Representatives of equipment manufacturers can provide critical equipment installation specifications to the design team at the time of planning and design. This information is needed to help avoid costly adjustments to the plan after construction has begun.

I.a.1. A perioperative registered nurse (RN) should provide input into the selection of equipment, proposed flow of people and equipment, and space utilization during the planning stages of the project.

Perioperative RNs possess the clinical expertise to provide input on these topics and to advocate for patient safety.[4]

I.b. The multidisciplinary team should participate in all phases of the project including planning, design, construction, and commissioning.[5-7] *[2: High Evidence]*

Involvement of the multidisciplinary team in the process helps hold all parties responsible for taking the necessary precautions to prevent or decrease the risk to patients.[3]

I.b.1. The multidisciplinary team should create a functional plan to include
- intended use of the space,
- projected volume of procedures,
- utility requirements,
- environmental requirements,
- security requirements,
- communication requirements,
- location of support areas,
- storage requirements, and
- traffic patterns.

The functional plan defines the requirements for the space and provides the framework upon which designers will create the design for the project.[7]

I.b.2. The multidisciplinary team should obtain and be familiar with federal, state, and local regulatory requirements and applicable construction guidelines (eg, Occupational Safety and Health Administration [OSHA], Centers for Medicare & Medicaid Services, National Fire Protection Association [NFPA], Facility Guidelines Institute, American Society for Healthcare Engineering).[6-11]

I.c. The multidisciplinary team should perform an initial and ongoing risk assessment beginning early in the planning phase, continuing throughout the project, and ending at commissioning. *[3: Moderate Evidence]*

The assessment identifies potential risks to patients and personnel that could be caused by the construction and the need for precautions to prevent the spread of infection to patients after the building project is completed.[1-3,12]

I.c.1. The risk assessment should identify factors that support a safe design and create the criteria for the selection of finishes, surfaces, and HVAC systems.

I.c.2. The assessment should identify the risks created during construction that affect patient care and workplace safety, including
- infection prevention,
- air quality,
- utilities,
- noise,
- vibration, and
- security.[3,7]

Recommendation II

The multidisciplinary team should use evidence-based design concepts in the planning and design of the surgical suite.

Evidence-based design can be cost-effective and may positively affect the safety, quality, and efficiency of perioperative patient care. In an analysis of the business case for evidence-based design, Henriksen et al determined that the upfront capital costs related to using evidence-based design would be paid for in two to three years. The hypothetical facility used in this analysis was a 300-bed hospital with an original construction cost of $240 million. The upfront capital costs for the evidence-based design improvements was $12 million. Using the cost data available, the authors determined that the evidence-based design improvements could save the facility $7 million annually by decreasing the cost of operations and increasing revenues.[13]

II.a. During the surgical suite planning and design phase, a simulated room or suite setup should be used. *[3: Moderate Evidence]*

Simulation has been shown to assist in determining factors that affect the performance of tasks in an area.[14] Birnbach et al conducted a quantitative study to determine whether simulation could predict possible errors in design. The indicator measured in this study, which involved 52 physicians and residents, was hand hygiene completion. The variable that was manipulated was the location of the hand hygiene dispenser.[15]

The hand hygiene solution dispenser was placed in the designer's chosen location for group 1 (n = 26). In this group, 11.5% (n = 3) of the participants performed hand hygiene using the dispenser. For group 2 (n = 26), the dispenser was placed in clear view of the physicians as they observed patients. In this group, 53.8% (n = 14) used the dispenser. Based on these data, the researchers concluded that simulation is effective and can be an inexpensive way to quantitatively evaluate proposed design solutions to patient safety hazards.[15]

II.a.1.   The perioperative RN should verify that the components required (eg, surgical table, anesthesia machine, suction canister, back table) in an operating room (OR) are present in the simulated OR.

II.b.   Traffic patterns should be designed to facilitate movement of patients, personnel, equipment, and supplies into, through, and out of defined areas within the surgical suite. *[2: High Evidence]*

The surgical suite design should include three designated areas that are defined by the activities performed in each area (Table 1):

○ **Unrestricted area:** An area of the building that is not defined as semi-restricted or restricted. This area includes a central control point for designated personnel to monitor the entrance of patients, personnel, and materials into the semi-restricted areas. This area may include locker rooms, break rooms, offices, waiting rooms, the preoperative admission area, Phase I and Phase II postanesthesia care units (PACUs), and access to procedure rooms (eg, endoscopy rooms, laser treatment rooms). Street clothes are permitted in this area. Public access to the area may be limited based on the facility's policy and procedures.

○ **Semi-restricted area:** The peripheral support areas of the surgical suite. The area may include storage areas for equipment and clean and sterile supplies; work areas for processing instruments; sterilization processing room(s); scrub sink areas; corridors leading from the unrestricted area to the restricted area of the surgical suite; and the entrances to locker rooms, the preoperative admission area, the PACU, and sterile processing. This area is entered directly from the unrestricted area past a nurses' station or from other areas. Semi-restricted areas have specific HVAC design requirements associated with the intended use of the space (See Recommendation IV).[7] Personnel in the semi-restricted area should wear surgical attire and cover all head and facial hair.[16] Access to the semi-restricted area should be limited to authorized personnel and patients accompanied by authorized personnel.

○ **Restricted area:** A designated space contained within the semi-restricted area and accessible only through a semi-restricted area. The restricted area includes the operating and other rooms in which operative or other invasive procedures are performed. Restricted areas have specific HVAC design requirements associated with the intended use of the space (See Recommendation IV).[7]

Personnel in the restricted area should wear surgical attire and cover head and facial hair. Masks should be worn when the wearer is in the presence of open sterile supplies or of persons who are completing or have completed a surgical hand scrub.[16,17] Only authorized personnel and patients accompanied by authorized personnel should be admitted to this area.

The HVAC, surgical attire, and traffic pattern requirements of the surgical suite are designed to be more stringent as one moves from unrestricted to restricted areas.[2] The progression of restrictions is intended to provide the cleanest environment in the restricted area.

II.b.1.   The designated areas should be separated by

• signage indicating the attire required for entering the area and who may access the area;

• doors separating the restricted area from the semi-restricted area; and

• doors, signage, or a line of demarcation to identify the separation between the unrestricted and semi-restricted areas.

Signs provide a visual cue that alerts persons to the restrictions required for entry into each area. The doors provide a physical barrier to assist in maintaining control of the HVAC.

II.c.   When a hybrid OR is to be included in the construction or renovation project, the hybrid room should

○ be sized to accommodate the equipment to be used based on the manufacturers' specifications;

○ have radiation protection based on the type and amount of protection required for the type of system used;

○ include the size and location of the radiation system control room; and

○ have, at a minimum, the same traffic restrictions and ventilation system requirements as an OR.

[2: High Evidence]

Meeting these recommendations will help provide a safe environment for patients and for personnel working in these areas, help avoid unnecessary construction expenses and late change orders, and help ascertain that the room will accommodate the equipment.[7]

II.d.   Laminar airflow may be used in the restricted area. *[3: Moderate Evidence]*

The results of studies involving laminar airflow conflict; some support and some refute the benefits of laminar airflow in the OR.[18-29] This is an unresolved issue and additional research is needed. The studies define and measure laminar flow differently or do not provide a definition of laminar flow, making comparison and analysis difficult.

TABLE 1: UNIT/AREA DESIGNATION OF RESTRICTION

Unit/area	Level of restriction
Postanesthesia care unit	Unrestricted or semi-restricted
Endoscopy suite	Unrestricted
Pain clinic/procedure room	Unrestricted
Locker room/administrative office/waiting room	Unrestricted
Sterile processing area	Semi-restricted
Equipment and sterile supply storage	Semi-restricted
Sterile processing decontamination area	Semi-restricted
Operating room	Restricted
Invasive procedure room	Restricted
Preoperative/postoperative patient care area	Unrestricted

A review of the literature by Howard and Hanssen concluded that vertical laminar airflow is more effective than horizontal airflow.[22] The authors pointed out that when horizontal laminar airflow is used, persons passing or standing between the unit and the patient can disrupt the airflow. The authors recommended that the patient and all instruments be within the clean air zone during use of a vertical laminar system.[22]

One limited study by Hall suggests that vertical laminar airflow may be affected by the design of the surgical light. In this study, a large dome type light either blocked or altered the airflow.[28]

Researchers conducting an Austrian study of 80 orthopedic surgical procedures that compared no laminar airflow to use of laminar flow systems of 19.83 m² and 4.56 m² found that the 19.83 m² system provided a significant reduction in the number of viable microorganisms on the instrument table and an insignificant reduction on the other locations measured (ie, at the patient's head, the instrument table, the right side of the patient at about waist level, the left side of the patient's head but away from the table).[20]

A retrospective study conducted by Hooper et al in 2011 included 51,485 total hip arthroplasties and 36,826 total knee replacements. The researchers defined laminar flow as 300 air changes per hour (ACH) and conventional airflow rate as 30 ACH. They concluded that the rate of prosthetic revisions for early deep infections was not reduced by using laminar flow and protective suits with hoods and self-contained exhaust systems when compared with procedures performed with a conventional air change rate and without protective suits.[25]

A comparative study conducted in the United Kingdom between the years 2000 and 2004 involved 435 patients who required re-operation after an Austin-Moore hemiarthroplasty. The researchers did not provide a definition of laminar airflow. They determined that the rate of re-operation for all indications in the non-laminar airflow theater group was four times greater than in the laminar airflow group. Based on these findings, they recommended the use of laminar airflow.[24]

In a quasi-experimental study of 140 patients having total hip or total knee replacements (n = 70 in the control group, n = 70 in the experimental group for whom laminar air flow was used), Knobben et al cultured used instruments, unused instruments, and bone removed from each patient. Laminar airflow was defined as an airflow of 8,100 m³/hour; air inflow speed was 20 cm/second, resulting in the total number of air changes in the entire OR of 60 ACH. The standard airflow was 2,700 m³/hour with an air inflow speed of 10 cm/second and 22 ACH. The researchers concluded that use of laminar airflow reduced the occurrence of prolonged wound discharge and superficial surgical site infection (SSI) and, when compared to standard airflow, laminar airflow was shown to decrease intraoperative bacterial contamination.[26]

Friberg and Friberg compared an upward displacement (ie, a thermal convection system) with 17 ACH to a vertical downward flow system with 16 ACH, with bacterial air and surface counts as the measure of performance. Use of the vertical delivery system resulted in lower bacterial counts than use of the thermal convection system. The researchers also found that vertical, horizontal, and exponential laminar airflow systems all performed equally well.[27]

In a quasi-experimental study comparing bacterial contamination of wood (n = 10), plastic (n = 10), and stainless steel (n = 10) tiles placed within and outside the laminar flow area, Da Costa et al found no less contamination of the tiles placed outside the laminar flow than those placed within the laminar flow area. Based on the results of this study, the researchers suggested that placing instruments and implants outside the laminar flow area is a safe practice.[21]

Hirsch et al tested four ventilation systems (ie, window-based ventilation, supported air nozzle canopy, low-turbulence displacement airflow, and low-turbulence displacement airflow with flow stabilizer) for intraoperative contamination using a descriptive study technique. The study included 277 procedures performed in six ORs in five German hospitals. The researchers found that use of the window-based ventilation system resulted in the highest intraoperative contamination and use of the low-turbulence displacement airflow with flow stabilizer system resulted in the lowest intraoperative contamination. The low-turbulence displacement airflow with flow stabilizer system is equivalent to the vertical laminar airflow system used in the United States.[29]

A retrospective study involving 63 surgical departments in 55 German hospitals (N = 99,230 surgical procedures) showed higher SSI rates with use of laminar airflow in the OR when compared with turbulent clean air for hip prosthesis; for knee prosthesis and abdominal surgery (ie, appendectomy, cholecystectomy, colon surgery, herniorrhaphy) no significant differences were found. The researchers performed active SSI surveillance using the methods and definitions of the US National Nosocomial Infection Surveillance system. They suggested that the results may not be generalizable because of factors that were not controlled in the study.[19]

A survey of orthopedic program administrators in 256 hospitals in which 8,288 total knee replacements were performed in 2000 found no significant difference in the rate of deep infection after total knee replacement. The survey asked whether the facility used or did not use laminar airflow or body exhaust suits. The overall 90-day cumulative incidence of deep infection requiring subsequent surgery was used for measurement. Twenty-eight of the 8,288 procedures required subsequent surgery (0.34%) because of the presence of an infection.[23]

II.d.1. If the multidisciplinary team chooses to consider the use of laminar airflow, a risk/benefit/cost analysis should be performed during the planning phase. Analysis should include the direction of the airflow (eg, from ceiling to floor, lateral).

II.e. A ventilation setback strategy may be used for periods when the OR is unoccupied. *[3: Moderate Evidence]*

A ventilation setback strategy provides a cost savings by allowing the amount of air supplied to an OR to be reduced when the room is not in use. The cost savings occurs because the amount of energy used in heating or cooling the air is decreased.[30]

II.e.1. An HVAC system setback that reduces the number of ACH may be used if
- the temperature and humidity settings are maintained within the design parameters as stated in Recommendation IV and
- the positive-pressure relationship of the OR to the adjacent area is maintained.[7,30]

II.e.2. A risk/benefit/cost analysis should be performed during the planning phase to determine whether use of such a system is acceptable. The analysis of ventilation system setback should include
- actual or projected usage;
- the needs, preferences, and perceptions of the system's users;
- local climate;
- facility type (eg, hospital, ambulatory surgery center);
- applicable local building code requirements;
- existing ventilation system design;
- cost of system maintenance;
- energy savings; and
- necessary components of the system (eg, occupancy sensor, manual control, timed control, combined control).[30]

II.f. Ultraviolet (UV) light for air purification may be used in the restricted area. If the multidisciplinary team chooses to consider the use of UV light, a risk/benefit/cost analysis should be performed during the planning phase. *[2: High Evidence]*

There are a number of published studies regarding UV light use for infection prevention. The study designs are varied and not all relate directly to the OR, but the results may be generalizable to the OR.[31-39]

In a study that was performed in a patient room to compare the effects of UV light on methicillin-resistant *Staphylococcus aureus* (MRSA), vancomycin-resistant enterococcus (VRE) and *Clostridium difficile*, Nerandzic and Donskey concluded that UV-C light kills all three of the organisms. A 3-log reduction in *Clostridium difficile* was achieved after an exposure to 20,000-microwatt seconds/cm[2] for 45 minutes. If the *Clostridium difficile* was first exposed to a germination solution, the 3-log reduction occurred in 10 minutes. There was a 3-log reduction in the MRSA and VRE counts with both of the exposure conditions. In this study, the UV light was administered by an automated room decontamination device.[32]

In a single facility comparative study published in 2007, Ritter et al reviewed the records of 5,980 patients undergoing total joint surgery performed by a single surgeon between 1986 and 2005. The study compared the infection

273

rate when laminar flow was used (n = 1,071) to the infection rate when a downward pointing UV light was used (n = 4,909). The infection rate was 1.77% when laminar flow was used and 0.57% when UV light was used. The researchers concluded that when proper safety precautions were taken, use of downward-pointing UV lights appeared to be an effective method of reducing the infection rate in total joint replacement surgeries.[33]

In a report by the National Institute of Occupational Safety and Health (NIOSH), the use of upper room UV lights was found to be beneficial when there were 6 ACH. The air changes in this study were not the same as the recommended changes for the OR (ie, 15 to 25 ACH); therefore, the effect of UV lights in the OR may not match the results in this study.[37] The air exchanges are significant because UV germicidal irradiation is effective at a low air change rate, but its efficacy diminishes as the rate increases. The decrease in efficacy occurs because the kill rate is dependent on the length of exposure of the microbe to the UV light. The high air change rate in an OR decreases the exposure time; therefore, the efficacy is significantly decreased.[35] Similar results were found in other studies and in literature reviews.[35,36,38,39]

A review of the literature published in 2010 concluded that direct down-pointing UV lights should not be used in the OR because of the risk of injury to personnel and the decreased efficacy related to the rate of ACH. This review also suggests that UV light could be used as an adjunct to other infection prevention measures.[35]

II.f.1. The risk/benefit/cost analysis should include
- the design of the light system to be used (eg, within the duct work, upper room, downward pointing, portable),[31]
- the safety measures required (eg, protective clothing, eye wear), and
- room down time and other use restrictions.

Ultraviolet light exposure may cause harmful effects to the eyes and the skin.[34,35] The required safety measures, including wearing protective clothing and keeping the room vacant, are dependent on the type of system used.[35]

II.g. An environmental impact assessment of construction materials and design features should be performed during the planning phase. [3: Moderate Evidence]

If amounts of volatile chemicals are high, "sick building syndrome" may result, which may cause personnel and patients to experience headaches, dizziness, nausea, dry cough, nasal dryness, watery or itchy eyes, skin rashes, and difficulty concentrating.[40]

The literature frequently describes efforts to produce a low environmental impact as *green design*, *green building*, and *sustainable design*, which are synonyms and encompass all aspects of building design.[41] Green design features may include a high-efficiency HVAC system, surfaces and finishes that use low volatile organic compounds, natural lighting, and reclamation or recycling of materials disposed of during construction.[1,42] The financial effects of green design may be short or long term and positive or negative.[41,42]

II.g.1. The environmental impact assessment should include the projected water and energy consumption; the biodegradability and environmental toxicity of the building materials; and the ability to recycle, reuse, or renew building materials.

II.h. The perioperative environment should be planned with electrical safeguards in place as described in *NFPA 70: National Electrical Code*[43]; *Guidelines for Design and Construction of Hospitals and Outpatient Facilities*[7]; and local, state, and national regulations.[10] *[2: High Evidence]*

Electrical hazards in the OR may lead to fires, burns, and electrical shocks. These conditions result from electric current flowing through inappropriate pathways (eg, through the patient's or perioperative team member's body to ground).[44]

II.i. The OR lighting system should be planned and designed to provide
- light for monitoring the patient, illumination of the surgical field, and performance of other patient care tasks;
- dimmable lighting;
- low operating and maintenance cost; and
- surgical field lighting that
  - causes minimal interference with air circulation,
  - has the required ceiling support system,
  - causes minimal interference with other ceiling-mounted equipment,
  - provides the ability to focus and control the spot size,
  - generates minimal heat,
  - requires minimal time and effort for lamp replacement,
  - provides the desired color and temperature,
  - limits the amount of shadow produced,
  - is easy to clean,
  - requires a low amount of energy for movement and focusing, and
  - provides the ability to control settings at the sterile field.

[3: Moderate Evidence]

Lighting in the OR that is comfortable, safe, and provides optimal visibility and color recognition should provide a satisfactory visual environment and meet the requirements of the OR personnel.[45] The shape and size of the surgical lights have been shown to affect the airflow patterns during use of laminar airflow.[28] Surgical lights may produce high amounts of radiant heat that may cause damage to exposed tissues and discomfort to the surgical team.[46] The color of light produced can change the color and appearance of the skin and other tissue.[46,47] Shadows may be produced by equipment that blocks the light.

Lights require frequent cleaning to protect against infections caused by dust.[47] An observational study of 46 hours of surgery revealed that high forces were required to move the lights, and an interruption was caused by adjustment of the lights, which at times required assistance from the RN circulator.[48] In a comparison of different surgical lights, varying levels of inclusion of these criteria (eg, amount of force required to move the lights, amount of interruption caused during adjustment) were found among the different light manufacturers.[49,50]

Incidents of patient burns from surgical lights have been reported. The reported incidents occurred when multiple light heads were aimed at one small area and operating at or near maximum power.[51]

II.j. The building design should provide functionally equivalent space for decontamination and sterilization of surgical instruments in all locations where sterilization processes are performed.[7,52,53] When instrument sterilization is to be performed within the surgical suite, a sterile processing room should have
- separate clean and decontamination spaces, which may be rooms or areas;
- decontamination and clean spaces that are separated by one of three methods:
  - a wall with a door or pass-through,
  - a partial wall or partition that is at least 4-ft high and at least the width of the counter, or
  - a distance of 4 ft between the instrument-washing sink and the area where the instruments are prepared for sterilization;
- provisions for sterilization equipment and storage of related supplies in the clean area;
- separate sinks for washing instruments and washing hands;
- decontaminating equipment (eg, automated washer, ultrasonic cleaner); and
- storage space for personal protective equipment (PPE) and cleaning supplies in the decontamination area.[7]

[2: High Evidence]

The requirements for reprocessing of reusable medical devices do not vary by location. Equivalent procedures, supplies, and equipment are needed in all locations where sterilization is performed.

II.k. All surfaces (eg, floors, walls, ceilings, cabinets) should be durable, smooth, and cleanable. [2: High Evidence]

Surfaces that are durable, smooth, and cleanable allow for ease of cleaning and assist in preventing buildup of dirt and debris in crevices.[2,7,54]

II.k.1. In the semi-restricted and restricted areas,
- surfaces should withstand cleaning chemicals;
- floors should have no seams or have sealed seams and a cove base;
- walls should be smooth with no seams or sealed seams;
- cabinets should have a smooth surface and be made of laminate, stainless steel, or glass; and
- absorbent material, such as exposed wood, should not be used.[2,7]

II.k.2. Ceilings in semi-restricted areas should be smooth and may be either monolithic or drop-in ceiling tiles.

II.k.3. Ceilings in restricted areas should be monolithic. Drop-in ceiling tiles should not be used.[7]

II.l. The surgical suite should have security controls (eg, door security systems, video surveillance, tracking systems, electronic identification access tracking systems, visitor logs).[55,56] [2: High Evidence]

Security controls help limit unauthorized access to the semi-restricted and restricted areas of the surgical suite. Video surveillance assists with monitoring of access at all times. Tracking systems (eg, electronic identification access tracking systems, visitor logs) assist in identifying who is present in the perioperative suite.

II.l.1. Security measures should be selected based on a risk assessment and may include the use of devices (eg, alarm systems, video surveillance, shatter-proof glass, metal detectors, locked doors).

Recommendation III

During renovation and construction in the close vicinity of an occupied health care facility, measures for preventing environmental contamination should be established, maintained, and monitored by perioperative team members and the infection preventionist in accordance with applicable state regulations and the ongoing risk assessment.

Multiple studies have been published that demonstrate contamination of the internal environment by infectious agents present in the external environment during renovation and construction.[57-60]

Pini et al measured *Aspergillus* levels in two units of a facility during construction. The levels were greater in the corridor connected to the construction area in comparison with the restricted access rooms.

The researchers recommended ongoing surveillance of the levels of *Aspergillus* during construction.[57]

III.a.   Infection prevention measures should include
- barriers applicable to the type of construction occurring;
- maintenance of barrier integrity;
- surgical attire for construction workers;
- special construction-related traffic pathways, entrances, and exits;
- negative pressure and use of high-efficiency particulate air (HEPA) filters on the construction side of the barrier;
- regular maintenance of the air-handling system; and
- other infection control prevention and surveillance measures (eg, particulate counts).

[2: High Evidence]

A prospective air and surface sampling study examined the amount of *Aspergillus* in air samples and on surfaces in a facility during construction outside the building. The measurements were completed in three units with high populations of immunocompromised patients. The researchers found no increase in the amount of *Aspergillus* when protective measures, described as use of HEPA filtration systems, wet brooming, and wetting down of the outside construction site, were taken and the importance of environmental cleaning was reinforced.[61]

A limited study conducted during two separate renovation projects requiring exterior demolition at a hospital in Japan compared the effectiveness of adhesive tape with the effectiveness of an adhesive poly film applied to the window frames as a weather stripping for the purpose of creating an additional dust barrier. The amount of dust in the air was measured before construction and during construction. The results revealed that the adhesive tape was more effective than the poly film, but both controlled the amount of dust in the air.[58]

An outbreak of *Bacillus* species in a neonatal care unit was linked to contamination resulting from excavation during construction. After precautions were taken, including replacing air filters, cleaning surfaces in the unit, emphasizing hand hygiene, and relocating the loading dock for linen and supply delivery, the rate of patient infection decreased to zero.[59]

A review of the literature published in 2006 revealed that more than 500 reported cases of surgical infections were caused by airborne *Aspergillus*. This review included patients having surgery in various specialities but did not specify whether the infections occurred during construction. In the majority of the cases, it was presumed that the source of the *Aspergillus* causing the infection was the air in the OR. The authors recommended routine maintenance of the air-handling system.[60]

Infection prevention during construction and renovation is a complex issue dependent on multiple variables specific to the setting.

III.a.1.   High-efficiency particulate air filters should be used to filter the incoming air during construction occurring outside of the building.

III.a.2.   Construction workers should don surgical attire if they are required to enter the semi-restricted area.[16]

III.a.3.   Barriers (eg, solid fiberboard or sheetrock walls, sealed plastic walls) should be placed between the construction site and the perioperative environment and maintained at all times.

III.a.4.   Traffic plans for construction personnel and movement of supplies, equipment, and debris should be developed, communicated, and implemented.

Traffic plans assist surgical team members in moving from place to place without contaminating their surgical attire and in moving supplies and equipment by a route that minimizes contamination from the construction site. The traffic plans also help prevent exposure of construction workers to soiled or potentially infectious materials.

III.a.5.   Perioperative RNs should participate in the construction process by
- verifying the presence and integrity of barriers and infection prevention measures,
- participating in construction meetings,
- monitoring the progress of the project by visual inspection,
- communicating to the perioperative team the progress of the project and information that will affect the daily functions of the surgical suite (eg, presence of new barriers, additional cleaning required, noise and vibration that will be caused by the construction), and
- collaborating with perioperative team members to resolve unanticipated problems as they arise.

Recommendation IV

The health care organization should create and implement a systematic process for monitoring HVAC performance parameters and a mechanism for resolving variances.

Heating, ventilation, and air conditioning systems control room air quality, temperature, humidity, and air pressure of the room in comparison to the surrounding areas. The HVAC system is intended to reduce the amount of environmental contaminates (eg, microbial-laden skin squames, dust, lint) in the surgical suite. The restricted areas are intended to be the cleanest; therefore, the HVAC requirements for the restricted areas are the most stringent. The HVAC system reduces the amount of environmental contamination by carrying airborne contaminates away from the sterile field and removing these contaminants through the return duct vents located at the periphery of the room.[62,63]

IV.a. Designated perioperative team members in collaboration with a multidisciplinary team should perform a risk assessment of the surgical suite if a variance in the parameters of the HVAC system occurs. [5: Benefits Balanced with Harms]

The literature search did not reveal any evidence of clinical significance related to the degree of variance in the HVAC system design parameters. Additional research is needed.

The effect of the HVAC system parameters falling out of range is variable. A small variance for a short period of time may not be of clinical concern, whereas a large variance for a longer period may have clinical significance.

IV.a.1. The multidisciplinary team should include
- a perioperative nurse,
- an infection preventionist,
- a surgeon,
- a facility plant engineer or designated person,
- sterile processing department personnel, and
- facility and perioperative managers.

IV.a.2. Based on the risk assessment, corrective measures may include
- rescheduling or redirecting procedures to areas of the surgical suite where the HVAC system is functioning within parameters,
- delaying elective procedures,
- limiting surgical procedures to emergency procedures only,
- closing the affected OR(s), or
- taking no action.

IV.a.3. Based on the risk assessment, measures that should be taken to restore the surgical suite to full functionality after the HVAC system variance has been corrected may include
- terminal cleaning when there is evidence of contamination on surfaces[54];
- reprocessing or discarding any supplies with packaging that may have been compromised[53]; and
- inventorying discarded, damaged supplies for insurance claim purposes and to obtain replacements.

IV.b. Personnel who identify an unintentional variance in the predetermined HVAC system parameters should report the variance according to the health care organization's policy and procedures. [5: Benefits Balanced with Harms]

Rapid communication between affected and responsible personnel can help facilitate resolution of the variance.

IV.c. The minimum number of ACH including the percentage of outdoor air should be maintained within the HVAC design parameters at the rate that was applicable at the time of design or of the most recent renovation of the HVAC system (Table 2). [3: Moderate Evidence]

Filtered air minimizes the recirculation of indoor contaminants within the perioperative area. In a comparative study conducted in a Turkish hospital OR, researchers compared the number of live airborne microorganisms in the air in one OR in which the HEPA filters were turned on and one OR in which the HEPA filters were turned off during a weekend. The OR in which the HEPA filters were turned off experienced a rise in the air microbial load. The airborne microorganism load in the OR in which the HEPA filter was operating was 222.44 colony-forming units (cfu)/m^3; the airborne microorganism load in the OR in which the HEPA filter was not operating was 536.66 cfu/m^3. The researchers concluded that operational HEPA filtration systems reduce the air microbial load.[64]

Hirsch et al compared four ventilation systems to determine the system with the greatest efficiency at preventing bacterial emission into the sterile field. The study included 277 surgical procedures performed in 60 ORs located in five German hospitals. The ventilation systems tested included window-based, supported air nozzle canopy, low-turbulence displacement airflow, and low-turbulence displacement airflow with flow stabilizer. The low-turbulence displacement airflow with flow stabilizer system was found to be the most efficient in preventing bacterial emission into the sterile field. The low-turbulence displacement airflow with flow stabilizer system described in this document is similar to the system used in the United States.[29]

In a comparative study conducted in Poland, researchers assessed the level of occupational exposure to nitrous oxide using different ventilation and scavenging systems. Thirty-five ORs in 10 hospitals were equipped with different ventilation systems with active or passive scavenging systems. The ventilation systems included natural ventilation with supplementary fresh air provided by a pressure ventilation system at 6 ACH, pressure and exhaust systems equipped with ventilation units supplying fresh air to maintain the ACH rate at about 10 ACH to 15 ACH, and laminar flow air-conditioning systems that maintain the ACH at a rate of 15 or higher. The researchers concluded that at least 12 ACH in addition to use of a scavenging system reduces the levels of waste anesthesia gases below the Polish occupational exposure levels of 180 mg/m^3.[65]

A study conducted in Taiwan compared the air particulate level in two ORs with two different

TABLE 2: HVAC DESIGN PARAMETERS[1-3]

Functional area	Minimum outdoor air changes per hour	Minimum total air changes per hour*	Humidity	Temperature	Settings for airflow patterns (pressure)
Operating room	4	20	20% to 60%	68° F to 75° F (20° C to 24° C)	Positive
Decontamination room	2	6	NR	60° F to 73° F (16° C to 23° C)	Negative
Clean workroom	2	4	Maximum 60%	68° F to 73° F (20° C to 23° C)	Positive
Sterile storage	2	4	Maximum 60%	Maximum 75° F (24° C)	Positive
Restroom/ housekeeping	NR	10	NR	NR	Negative
Postanesthesia care unit	2	6	20% to 60%	70° F to 75° F (21° C to 24° C)	NR
Procedure room	3	15	20% to 60%	70° F to 75° F (21° C to 24° C)	Positive
Endoscopy procedure room	2	6	20% to 60%	68° F to 73° F (20° C to 23° C)	NR
Endoscope processing room	2	10	NR	NR	Negative
Semi-restricted corridor	NR	NR	NR	NR	NR

NR = No recommendation
* Total air changes per hour is the sum of the outdoor air changes plus the recirculated air changes.

REFERENCES
1. Facility Guidelines Institute, US Department of Health and Human Services, American Society for Healthcare Engineering. Guidelines for Design and Construction of Hospitals and Outpatient Facilities. Chicago, IL: American Society for Healthcare Engineering of the American Hospital Association; 2014.
2. Centers for Medicare & Medicaid Services. State Operations Manual Appendix A—Survey Protocol, Regulations and Interpretive Guidelines for Hospitals. Rev. 78; 2011.
3. ANSI/ASHRAE/ASHE Addendum h to ANSI/ASHRAE/ASHE Standard 170-2013: Ventilation of Health Care Facilities. Atlanta, GA: American Society of Heating, Refrigerating and Air-Conditioning Engineers, Inc; 2016. https://www.ashrae.org/File%20Library/docLib/StdsAddenda/170_2013_h_20160523.pdf. Accessed October 3, 2016.

rates of air changes. One OR had an air change rate of 23 ACH and the other OR had a rate of 15 ACH. The comparison revealed that the OR with 23 ACH had lower levels of particulate matter in the air. The researchers concluded that a higher air change rate may reduce microbial contamination in the OR.[66]

Perdelli et al measured airborne microbial concentrations in various environments including ORs in 10 hospitals in Saudi Arabia. They found that the fungal concentration was lower inside the building compared to the outside environment. The fungal concentration levels were the lowest in the ORs that were equipped with HEPA filters (efficiency = 99.97%), had at least 15 ACH, and had positive pressure.[67]

IV.c.1. The ACH in a restricted area should be maintained at 20 total changes per hour, with a minimum of four air changes of outdoor air per hour or at the rate that was applicable at the time of design or of the most recent renovation of the HVAC system.[7]

IV.c.2. The ACH in a semi-restricted area are related to the function performed in that area:
- sterile storage—4 total and 2 outdoor air changes
- decontamination room—6 total and 2 outdoor air changes[7,68]

IV.c.3. The ACH in an unrestricted area are related to the function performed in that area:
- postanesthesia care unit—6 total and 2 outdoor air changes
- procedure room—15 total and 3 outdoor air changes
- endoscopy procedure room—6 total and 2 outdoor air changes[7,68]

IV.d. The incoming air should be sequentially filtered through two filters. The first filter should be rated as 7 MERV (ie, minimum efficiency reporting value) and the second should be rated as 14 MERV.[7] *[2: High Evidence]*

In a comparative study in a French hospital under construction, Fournel et al evaluated the benefits of a filtration system by measuring the amount of *Aspergillus* found inside the facility before and during construction. The study found the levels of *Aspergillus* inside did not increase during construction outside, even though there was a rise in the amount of *Aspergillus* outside. The researchers attributed the results to the use of filtration systems in the building. The filtration systems were either HEPA filters or a mobile air treatment decontamination unit. The decontamination unit used a novel technology based on nonthermal-plasma reactors instead of mechanically filtering the air.[61]

In a study comparing two different hematology departments, one with and one without HEPA filters, Crimi et al found that incoming air filtered with HEPA filters had a lower amount of microbic and *Aspergillus* contamination at the air output grille, in the middle of the room, and at the air intake grille.[69] In another study, researchers found lower airborne particulate counts in the OR when the air was filtered using two filters with efficiency ratings of 30% and 90%.[70]

A study in Taiwan compared two ORs, one with HEPA filtration and 23 ACH and one with no HEPA filtration and 15 ACH. The researchers found the room with HEPA filtration and 23 ACH had significantly reduced levels of particulate matter in the air.[66]

A comparative study measured airborne microbial concentrations in various departments including the OR in 10 hospitals equipped with air conditioning. The researchers found the fungal concentration inside the building was lower than that in the outside environment. The levels were the lowest in the ORs that were equipped with HEPA filters (99.97% efficiency) and had at least 15 ACH and positive pressure. The other areas of the buildings had a lower percentage of filtration and number of air changes. The authors concluded that air-handling systems are effective in reducing fungal concentrations.[67]

The outside air requires filtration continuously because airborne fungi are present at all times, but the level of the fungi can vary with the season. A descriptive study in Egypt investigated the effect of air pollutants and environmental parameters on the survivability of airborne fungi. The researchers found that the amount of airborne fungi and the species of fungi in outdoor air varied among seasons of the year. The two largest predictors of the amount and species of fungus were temperature and relative humidity. The fungi count was the lowest in the summer and highest in the autumn. The researchers concluded that environmental parameters were the most significant indicator of fungal survival.[71]

IV.e.   Relative humidity should be maintained within the HVAC design parameters. *[3: Moderate Evidence]*

The effect of relative humidity on bacterial, fungal, and viral growth is inconclusive. Additional research is required to determine optimal relative humidity levels for control of environmental contamination.

In a descriptive study, Panagopoulou et al examined air and surface fungal levels in four units in a Greek tertiary care hospital during a 12-month period. Two of the units were in building A and two were in building B. In building A, each room had a separate air conditioning unit; building B had a central air conditioning unit. The researchers determined that the fungal levels were higher during the months when the temperature and humidity levels were higher, independent of the method of air conditioning. They also determined that the air conditioning system in building B was more effective.[72]

The authors of a literature review on the effects of humidity on bacterial survival found that various levels of humidity created differing responses in different strains of bacteria. The responses included structural changes and death. The bacterial survival rates are dependent on the species. A generalization of a link between humidity and bacterial survival cannot be made.[73]

In a laboratory setting, Thompson et al found that aerosolized *Staphylococcus epidermidis*, used as a surrogate for *Staphylococcus aureus*, survived at relative humidity levels of < 20%, 40% to 60%, 70% to 80%, and > 90%. The researchers concluded that the *Staphylococcus epidermidis* was not affected by the level of relative humidity.[74]

In a literature review of 120 articles, Memarzadeh found no conclusive evidence to support a maximum or minimum relative humidity level to decrease the survival rate of viruses and the ability of viruses to cause diseases.[75]

IV.e.1.   The relative humidity in a restricted area should be maintained within a range of 20% to 60%.[7]

IV.e.2.   The humidity in a semi-restricted area is related to the function performed in that area:
- sterile storage—maximum 60%
- decontamination room—no recommendations
- semi-restricted corridor—no recommendations[7,68]

IV.e.3. The relative humidity in an unrestricted area is related to the function performed in that area:
- PACU—20% to 60%
- endoscopy procedure room—20% to 60%
- procedure room—20% to 60%[7,68]

IV.f. The temperature should be maintained within the limits recommended for each area (ie, unrestricted, semi-restricted, restricted). The temperature of the room may be intentionally adjusted based on the individual needs of the patient. *[3: Moderate Evidence]*

No research studies linking variations in temperature to SSIs were found in the literature search. However, literature reviews by Tang[73] and Memarzadeh[75] discuss the effect of temperatures on bacterial and viral survival rates. Neither review is directly related to the OR, nor is either review generalizable to the OR because they recommend temperatures that are beyond the OR comfort zone.

The review by Tang details factors affecting the survival of airborne bacteria in hospitals. This review suggests that temperatures above 75° F (24° C) decrease bacterial survival rates by varying amounts for gram-negative, gram-positive, and intracellular bacteria.[73] The review by Memarzadeh, which includes 120 research studies, indicated that temperatures greater than 60° C (140° F) for longer than 60 minutes will inactivate viruses, and the level of inactivation is dependent on the presence of organic materials.[75]

The only literature regarding room temperature ranges for the surgical suite found in the literature search were guidelines developed by the American Society for Healthcare Engineering, which are the accepted professional guidelines for HVAC systems in the United States.[7]

IV.f.1. The temperature range in a restricted area should be 68° F to 75° F (20° C to 24° C) but the range may be intentionally adjusted for a limited time based on the individual needs of the patient.[7]

Individual patients, such as pediatric surgical patients or patients undergoing procedures that require intentional hypothermia, may require that room temperature be adjusted outside of the recommended range.

IV.f.2. The temperature in a semi-restricted area should be dependent on the use of the area:
- sterile storage—maximum 75° F (24° C)
- decontamination room—60° F to 73° F (16° C to 23° C)
- semi-restricted corridor—no recommendations[7,68]

IV.f.3. The temperature of an unrestricted area should be between 70° F and 75° F (21° C and 24° C).[7,68]

IV.f.4. The temperature of an endoscopy procedure room should be between 68° F and 73° F (20° C and 23° C).[7,68]

IV.g. The airflow direction (ie, pressure relationship of one area to adjacent areas) should be maintained within the HVAC design parameters. *[2: High Evidence]*

The direction of the airflow from one room to the adjacent area is designed and engineered to minimize the flow of contaminates from clean to less-clean areas.[76] Disruptions in the airflow patterns within the OR can redirect contaminants onto the sterile field.[62,77]

IV.g.1. The restricted area should have a positive pressure relationship to the adjacent areas.[7]

IV.g.2. The pressure relationship of the semi-restricted area to the adjacent area should be based on the use of the area:
- sterile storage—positive
- decontamination room—negative
- semi-restricted corridor—no recommendations[7,68]

IV.g.3. Equipment and supplies should be located away from return ducts.

An unobstructed airflow out of the room is required to maintain the correct pressure within the area.

IV.h. Free-standing fans, portable HEPA filtering devices, humidifiers, air conditioners, and dehumidifiers should not be used in restricted areas or sterile processing areas. *[3: Moderate Evidence]*

A retrospective study of 180 patients undergoing total knee arthroplasties revealed that 5.6% (n = 10) of the patients developed a superficial infection and 3.9% (n = 7) developed a deep infection. The procedures were performed in an OR with a nonstandard air conditioner installed above a door, which produced a horizontal airflow. An instrument-washing sink was located on the intake side of the air conditioner. After the sink and the air conditioner were removed, a repeat study was completed two years later. In the repeat study, the infection rate fell to 2.2% or one in 45 patients. The investigators concluded that removing the sink and the wall air conditioner resulted in a decrease in SSIs.[78]

Free-standing fans can disrupt airflow patterns, resulting in contamination of the sterile field. A pilot study compared the airflow patterns created by two free-standing HEPA filters and a portable anteroom system with HEPA filtration. The researchers examined a single OR and used smoke plumes to indicate airflow direction. The airflow pattern during use of the free-standing HEPA filter systems moved upward into the breathing zones of the personnel and over the patient. The portable anteroom system maintained the downward airflow pattern. This study also found the noise level was increased with the use of the portable units compared to the portable anteroom system. The authors concluded that use of free-standing HEPA filters in an OR should be avoided and that the portable anteroom system with HEPA filtration was effective in removing airborne infectious agents, which may enhance patient safety.[77]

IV.h.1. For patients who require airborne precautions when no airborne infection isolation room is available, a portable, industrial grade HEPA filter should be used to supplement air cleaning.[79]

IV.i. Preventive maintenance, including regular inspection and changing of filters, should be performed on HVAC systems. *[3: Moderate Evidence]*

A properly functioning HVAC system minimizes the risk of contamination to the sterile field and is an essential component in SSI prevention.[2]

The authors of a study conducted in a Polish hospital concluded that the air filtering system requires regular maintenance, including filter changes, based on the amount of *Aspergillus* in the air samples. The filter should be changed according to the manufacturer's instructions for use because as the air filter ages, its effectiveness decreases.[80]

An investigation of an outbreak of postoperative shoulder arthritis (ie, four cases within one month) caused by *Propionibacterium acnes* infection revealed that the HVAC system was not functioning properly. After repair of the system and increased environmental cleaning, no additional cases were reported.[81]

IV.i.1. Health care personnel in consultation with the HVAC design engineer and plant operations personnel should determine the frequency of filter changes and establish a mechanism for maintaining the system.

IV.j. Doors to the operating or invasive procedure room should be kept closed except during the entry and exit of patients and personnel. *[3: Moderate Evidence]*

Several studies have demonstrated the effects of OR door openings. The studies all support keeping the doors closed during the surgical procedure except when opening is required for a procedure-related reason.[82-87]

A quasi experimental cohort study conducted in a Dutch hospital involved 284 colorectal procedures performed between June 2009 and October 2011. The researchers measured the relationship between personnel compliance with a bundle of interventions and the rate of SSI. The bundle consisted of four interventions including removal of razors previously used for hair removal during preoperative skin preparation, an explicit and uniform protocol for perioperative antibiotic prophylaxis, preoperative application of a warming blanket, and recommendations to reduce the number of OR door openings.

The researchers concluded that a significant relationship existed between the development of an SSI and the higher number of door openings. The primary reasons for door openings were noted to be for non-procedure–related conversation, obtaining equipment required for the procedure, and providing breaks for staff members. A decrease in the number of door openings and a corresponding SSI rate decrease were noted after implementation and enforcement of procedures such as providing breaks at different times and having all necessary equipment in the OR before the beginning of the procedure. The researchers stated that a limitation of the study was not including confounding factors for the door opening, such as complications occurring during surgery.[82]

When the doors are left open, the HVAC system is unable to maintain critical environmental control parameters.[2] Leaving the door open can disrupt pressurization. The ventilation system in the OR is designed to administer air pressure that is greater than the pressure in the semi-restricted area. The ventilation system is also designed to facilitate 20 total room ACH.[7]

In a descriptive study completed in three parallel ORs during 30 orthopedic trauma surgeries, door openings were shown to increase the CFUs present in the air. The characteristics of the ORs in this study included positive pressure in relation to the hallway, one doorway, and an upward air displacement system. The researchers also examined the reasons for the door openings, which included consultation between two experts, obtaining supplies or instruments, relief of personnel, required entrance of personnel while the wound was open, logistic reasons, social visits, and no detectable reason. The researchers concluded that the traffic flow in the OR should be reduced because increased traffic flow has a negative effect on the OR environment.[83]

A descriptive study of the number of door openings during total joint arthroplasties found that the door to the OR was opened 0.69 times per minute. The three most frequent reasons for opening the door were to obtain supplies, to exchange information, and unknown purposes. The door was opened by the RN circulator 26% of the time, by other members of the nursing team 19% of the time, and by the equipment representative 20.3% of the time. The researchers concluded that strategies such as storage of

ENVIRONMENT OF CARE, PART 2

instruments and supplies in the OR will decrease the number of door openings.[84]

In response to an unexplained increase in SSIs, Lynch et al conducted a comprehensive review of infection prevention practices. The review recorded the number of OR door openings, who opened the doors, and the reasons for door openings. The researchers found that during 28 procedures, the door was opened 3,071 times. Door openings varied across specialities and were most often related to requests for information. They also determined that the duration for the OR door to be open was 20 seconds and when multiplied by the number of openings per surgical procedure, the door was open for seven to 20 minutes per hour. The authors suggested that to decrease the number of SSIs, the number of OR door openings should be decreased.[86]

In a descriptive study of 46 consecutive surgical procedures, Young and O'Regan noted an increased potential for the development of an SSI related to the number of door openings during the procedure. There were five infections in 46 procedures; the mean frequency of door openings was 94 times during the procedures that resulted in an infection and 76.4 times during those that did not result in an infection.[85]

A study conducted during 23 surgeries performed in three different ORs evaluated the relationship between biological and dust contamination. Scaltriti et al found that the number of dust particles in the air of the OR decreased as the number of door openings increased, but the presence of bacteria increased as the frequency of door opening increased. The researchers suggested that behaviors such as frequently opening the door may affect the air quality in the OR.[87]

IV.j.1.   The health care organization should have a quality monitoring process to monitor rates of and reasons for OR door openings that occur while sterile supplies are open.

A quality improvement initiative in a pediatric hospital revealed that observation alone did not decrease the number of door openings. This study also revealed that the door was opened frequently for communication, and the number of door openings increased with the length of the procedure and the number of people in the room. The authors recommended that a quality plan include measures that describe the reason for OR door openings.[88]

IV.j.2.   Measures to reduce the number of door openings may include
- preplanning so that turbulence from opening the door is minimized during the procedure or when sterile supplies are opened,[86,88]
- keeping the surgeons' preference cards current,[88]
- confirming that all instruments and supplies are present before the incision is made,
- posting a sign on the door to restrict traffic while a procedure is in progress,[88]
- using means of communication that do not involve opening the door during procedures,[86,88]
- installing locks on OR doors that can be opened from the inside only,
- analyzing the stage of the procedure before relieving for breaks,[86,88]
- analyzing the culture in the perioperative environment, and
- providing education about the effects of opening the doors.[83]

Recommendation V

The integrity of structural surfaces (eg, doors, floors, walls, ceilings, cabinets) should be maintained, and surfaces should be repaired when damaged.

Surfaces can be damaged through use. Damaged surfaces can lead to an inability to clean and could create a fall or other injury hazard.[2,54]

V.a.   Personnel should report damage to floors, walls, ceilings, cabinets, and other structural surfaces according to the health care organization's policy. *[5: Benefits Balanced with Harms]*

Damaged structural surfaces may create a reservoir for the collection of dirt and debris that cannot be removed during cleaning. Damage to floor surfaces may create a trip or fall hazard.

V.a.1.   Repair priorities should be based on a risk assessment.

Recommendation VI

The health care organization emergency preparedness plan should include procedures for power failure.

There have been multiple reports of power failures in ORs.[89-91]

VI.a.   The power failure plan should include procedures for a failure during which the emergency generator works and a failure during which the emergency generator does not work. *[3: Moderate Evidence]*

Advanced preparation will assist in emergency response to an electrical power failure.[90] Generators are designed to operate until there is no fuel; however, generator failure has been reported.[92,93] Reports of organizational experiences and expert opinions recommend various steps to be taken before an electrical outage to assist in preventing negative outcomes.[89-94]

VI.a.1.   The power failure plan should identify which essential equipment should be connected to

PATIENT AND WORKER SAFETY

the outlets powered by the emergency generator.[91]

VI.a.2. The power failure plan should identify alternate power sources, including
- working flashlights in every OR and on every anesthesia machine,
- manual monitoring equipment (eg, blood pressure cuff, stethoscope),
- long extension cords,
- battery-operated communication devices, and
- paper documentation forms/records.

VI.a.3. Personnel should be aware of
- the locations of alternate sources of lighting, power, and supplies for use when the normal power is interrupted and
- which life-sustaining medical equipment has battery backup.[43]

Battery power can assist in keeping the equipment operating in case of a power failure involving the main electrical circuit.[91,92]

VI.a.4. Perioperative personnel should confirm batteries are
- labeled with their expiration date,
- checked monthly for expiration, and
- replaced as needed.[95]

VI.b. The power failure plan should include personnel education, including
○ what equipment can operate on battery power[91,94] and
○ the location and availability of
- charged transport monitors,
- manual monitoring devices (eg, manual blood pressure cuff, stethoscope),
- flashlights,
- the power failure emergency procedures manual,
- back-up resources for documentation and for supplies that are secured in devices that require power to open,
- long extension cords, and
- nonelectrical powered communication devices.[91,92,94]
[2: High Evidence]

VI.c. The power failure plan should include procedures for restoring an OR to service after loss of power, including the required assessment and interventions to perform based on the assessment. *[3: Moderate Evidence]*

The assessment is completed to determine whether there is damage and the extent of damage to equipment, supplies, and the facility.[93]

VI.c.1. Designated perioperative RNs should perform an assessment of the surgical suite in collaboration with a multidisciplinary team that includes
- an infection preventionist,
- a facility plant manager,

- sterile processing personnel, and
- biomedical personnel.

VI.c.2. The assessment should include
- environmental cleanliness (eg, condensation on surfaces including walls and flooring, dirt, debris),
- integrity of sterile supplies (eg, presence of condensation on package surfaces, signs of water damage),
- functionality of the power supply (eg, fully restored, emergency generator in use), and
- availability of water (eg, water pressure, water quality, steam supply).

VI.c.3. Interventions should be completed by the designated perioperative team members to restore the surgical suite to full functionality, based on the results of the assessment (Table 3).

Recommendation VII

The facility-wide security plan should include provisions for security of the surgical suite.

Security measures provide for the safety of patients, personnel, and visitors; prevention of drug diversion and theft; and protection of patient information.[16,96-98] Including the surgical suite in the facility-wide plan takes into consideration the unique security risks created by the presence of high-value equipment, supplies, and pharmaceuticals and the variable hours when the suite may be unoccupied.[99]

Preliminary data released by the US Bureau of Labor Statistics in 2012 shows that in the previous year, there were 11 fatal injuries in which the victim was a nurse.[100]

VII.a. A multidisciplinary team should develop the security plan in consultation with security personnel or law enforcement representatives. *[3: Moderate Evidence]*

Security personnel and law enforcement representatives have expertise in identifying security risks and in prevention and mitigation tactics.[99]

VII.a.1. The security plan should be reviewed and updated based on security breaches that have occurred, potential or actual changes related to construction, and changes in technology.[56,97]

VII.a.2. The security plan should include the prevention of workplace violence and address
- mandatory education,
- tracking and analysis of incidents and potential risk,
- a response plan,
- follow-up care for personnel, and
- the process for event reporting.[55,56]

TABLE 3: ASSESSMENTS AND INTERVENTIONS AFTER A POWER FAILURE[1-3]

Assessment	Intervention
Environmental cleanliness	• Perform terminal cleaning.
Integrity of sterile supplies	• Reprocess or discard any sterile items suspected of damage. • Inventory and record discarded, damaged supplies for insurance claim purposes and to obtain replacements. • Contact manufacturers of sterile supplies to obtain the method of determining package integrity.
Functionality of power supply	• Delay elective procedures until the power supply is restored. • Complete surgeries already in progress. • Redirect procedures to areas of the surgical suite where the power supply is functioning.
Availability of water	• Perform a quality check on steam sterilizers and automated cleaning equipment before returning them to service. • Collaborate with engineering department personnel to determine whether water is safe to use.

REFERENCES

1. *Mangram AJ, Horan TC, Pearson ML, Silver LC, Jarvis WR. Guideline for prevention of surgical site infection, 1999. Hospital Infection Control Practices Advisory Committee.* Infect Control Hosp Epidemiol. *1999;20(4):250-278.*
2. *ANSI/AAMI ST79:2010 & A1:2010 & A2:2011 & A3:2012 (Consolidated Text)* Comprehensive Guide to Steam Sterilization and Sterility Assurance in Health Care Facilities. *Arlington, VA: AAMI; 2012.*
3. *Mitchell L, Anderle D, Nastally K, Sarver T, Hafner-Burton T, Owens S. Lessons learned from Hurricane Ike. AORN J. 2009;89(6):1073-1078.*

Workplace violence is defined by the Federal Bureau of Investigation as violent acts

- directed at anyone within the workplace and committed by criminals not connected to the workplace,
- directed at employees and committed by those who have a direct connection to the workplace (eg, customers, clients, students),
- directed at employees and committed by present or former employees, or
- directed at employees or customers and committed by a person with whom they have had a personal relationship.[55]

Workplace violence is defined by the US Bureau of Labor as "violent acts directed towards a person at work or on duty (eg, physical assaults, threats of assault, harassment, intimidation, or bullying)."[101] In private industry in 2011, 11,760 persons were intentionally injured by another person. None of these injuries resulted in death but the recovery required the injured party to take days off from work.[101]

Incidents of violence against health care workers have been reported including fatal and nonfatal attacks. Between 1997 and 2006, 113 incidents of assault, rape, or homicide were reported to The Joint Commission.[97]

In 2007, 291 nurses in a German hospital participated in a retrospective cross-sectional survey. Seventy-two percent of the nurses reported having experienced verbal violence from a patient or visitor and 42% reported having experienced physical violence from a patient or visitor in the previous 12 months. The violence sometimes resulted in physically injury (23%) and in one or more days of sick leave (14%).[56,102]

A security risk assessment and an analysis of incidents can help identify the actual or potential risk of workplace violence.[55]

VII.a.3. The security plan should include methods for protecting the patient's health information and personal identifiable information, such as during broadcast surgery or use of social media and photography.

The Health Insurance Portability and Accountability Act requires facilities to keep patient's protected health information and personal identifiable information confidential.[94,103] Protected health information includes the information shared during surgery broadcast using any technology.[104]

It has been reported that social media has been used to share confidential information, which may be considered a breach of the confidentiality regulations.[105] One descriptive study on social media involving 88 residents and 127 faculty members at a school of medicine found that 64% and 22% respectively had a Facebook® profile. Fifty percent of the Facebook pages were public; 31% of the public pages were found to have work-related postings, and patient-specific information was shared in 14% of those with work-related postings. The researchers concluded that individuals have personal responsibility for managing their usage of social media. Health care organizations should have guidelines to guard against professional truancy and violation of patient confidentiality.[105]

In a report summarizing malpractice, battery, and invasion-of-privacy cases, Segal and Sacopulos noted that monetary awards have been received by patients whose photographs have been used for purposes other than those intended or whose photograph was taken without the patient's consent. They concluded that the facility should have plans in place and have the necessary forms completed to limit liability when photographs of patients are taken.[106]

A survey of 205 patients undergoing plastic surgery measured patients' perceptions of the correct use of their photographs. Ninety-eight percent of the patients felt their photographs could be used by their treating physicians but other uses had varying lesser percentages of acceptance (eg, by other physicians [74%], for student teaching [82%], for patient education [88%]). The authors concluded that photography is acceptable to most patients and appropriate consents should be obtained to maximize the patient's acceptance of use.[107]

A case involving a breach of confidentiality was reported related to sharing of confidential patient information on the telephone. In this case, the nurse called the patient's home and spoke with a person whom she knew to be the patient's mother and not the patient. The patient had left specific instructions that the home telephone number was not to be used. The jury awarded the patient $365,000. The legal commentary reminds nurses to be aware of the significance of patient confidentiality and their role in it.[108]

VII.b. Identification badges should be worn by all persons entering the perioperative suite. The identification should be worn on the upper body and be visible. *[2: High Evidence]*

Identification badges support security measures and help identify persons authorized to access the surgical suite.[16]

VII.b.1. Individuals with limited or temporary access to the perioperative environment (eg, students, law enforcement agents, parents of pediatric patients, health care industry representatives) should be identified as visitors and should wear temporary identification badges.[109,110]

Recommendation VIII

Noise and distractions that are not related to patient care should be minimized.

Noise and distractions are created by conversation, clinical and alert alarms, HVAC systems, telephones and other communication devices, and tools related to the provision of surgical procedures (eg, instruments, powered instruments, electrosurgical units, smoke evacuators). Some noise is unavoidable in the perioperative environment but certain noises can be controlled.[111-113]

In one investigation, NIOSH measured noise levels in 18 ORs and found that the noise levels were the highest in the orthopedic and neurosurgery rooms. The levels were higher the closer the person was to the source of the sound (eg, higher for the people in the sterile field compared to the RN circulator). The authors concluded that noise protection was not required because the noise levels were below the NIOSH recommended criterion level of 85 decibels A-Scale (dBA). The NIOSH criterion level describes level of noise exposure that can be safely tolerated during an eight-hour shift without ear protection. There were peak levels that exceeded the threshold level of 90 dBA but that lasted for only short periods of time. The researchers also concluded that the levels were high enough to potentially cause interference with understanding of the spoken word.[114]

In a comparative study involving 10 participants performing robotic-assisted suture tying and mesh alignment, Siu et al concluded that music with high rhythmicity (eg, hip-hop, Jamaican music) had a beneficial effect on performance of both tasks, and music played in the surgical environment may improve surgical education and increase the efficiency of the acquisition of surgical skills. The study compared performance when classical, jazz, hip-hop, or Jamaican music was played. The best performance was noted when Jamaican music was played and when the person performing the task liked the music being played. The study did not consider volume as a variable.[115]

In a review of the literature, Joseph and Ulrich found that noise can induce stress and increase work pressure, annoyance, fatigue, emotional exhaustion and burnout, and communication difficulties. The authors found conflicting articles regarding the effect of noise on performance of health care personnel. Based on the studies reviewed, the authors concluded that it took more effort to maintain a high level of performance when loud noise was present. They also conclude that an increased level of noise frequently required raising the volume of the voice to enable accurate comprehension.[116]

In an observational study performed during 10 surgical procedures, Christian et al recorded 11 events that had the potential to compromise patient safety (eg, counting errors, the RN circulator needing to leave the room). They identified communication and information flow problems, work flow, and competing tasks as possible sources of the events.[117]

A total of 9,830 patients were involved in a prospective study assessing underlying errors that contribute to surgical complications. The study was performed during a 12-month period in an academic department of surgery. The tool used was a survey completed by surgeons. Of the 9,830 patients, 322 experienced a complication (eg, prolonged hospitalization, temporary disability, permanent disability, death) related to an error (eg, incomplete understanding of problem, carelessness/inattention to detail, judgment error, error of omission, technique error). The researchers concluded that errors contributed more than 50% to the complications. Two percent of the 322 errors were attributed to communication errors.[118]

In another study, 62 perioperative professionals (ie, physicians, nurses, nurse anesthetists) completed the Disruptions in Surgery Index. The participants perceived that the disruptions had a greater effect on others than on themselves. The number of disruptions was reported to be the highest for the nurses and the least for the surgeons. The issues considered to be disruptions included individuals' personality and skills, the OR environment, communication, coordination/situational awareness, patient-related disruptions, team cohesion, and the organizational culture.[119]

In a 2010 survey of 439 perfusionists, 55.6% of the respondents admitted to using a cell phone while performing cardiopulmonary bypass.[120]

VIII.a. Non-procedure–related conversation and activities should be prohibited during critical phases of the surgical procedure.[121] *[2: High Evidence]*

The effects of interruptions and distractions are well documented in the literature.[122-127] In an observational study, interruptions and distractions diverting the attention of the operator from the task at hand caused 44% of errors in simulated procedures being performed by 18 medical students who had varying amounts of education. The authors concluded that distractions and interruptions in the OR could cause surgical residents to commit operative errors.[122]

In a controlled laboratory study, 12 medical interns performing a task related to laparoscopic surgery experienced a significant decline in performance and an increased level of irritation when distracted by music, conversation, and non-optimal handling of the laparoscope. The researchers concluded that the social and technological sources of irritation should be evaluated with a goal of increasing safety for patients.[123]

In a controlled study involving 96 undergraduate university students, Altmann and Trafton found that after an interruption, it took an average of 3.8 seconds for the students to collect their thoughts and return to the activity. The test group partially completed activity A, which was followed by an interruption, and then the time to return to activity A was measured. The control group completed activity A without interruption and then the time to begin activity B was measured at only 1.9 seconds.[124]

Interruptions were shown to increase error rates in a study involving 300 undergraduate university students performing tasks of various lengths with varying types of interruptions. The researchers found the longer the interruption, the greater the error rate.[125]

An observational study in a hospital setting examined the causes of work interruptions during medication administration. The study involved 59 hours and two minutes of medication administration time. The researchers found the work interruptions were caused primarily by nurse colleagues.[126]

In an observational study that examined distractions and interruptions in anesthesia care, Campbell et al noted 424 distracting events, 22% of which had a negative effect. The study involved 30 surgeries lasting a total of 31 hours and two minutes. The researchers suggested that to decrease the potential for committing errors, the anesthesia professional should ignore inappropriate intrusions or conversations, ask personnel who have entered the OR for non-procedure–related reasons to return later, prepare all supplies well in advance, and not participate in irrelevant conversation.[127]

VIII.b. Noise and distraction created by the following sources should be minimized:
  ○ portable communication devices (eg, beepers, cell phones, personal digital assistants, computers),
  ○ fixed communication devices (eg, overhead pages and announcements, telephones, computers),
  ○ electronic music devices (eg, radios, CD players, digital audio players),
  ○ the environment (eg, HVAC system, pneumatic tube systems),
  ○ medical equipment and devices (eg, radiology equipment, waste management system, smoke evacuator, powered surgical instruments, monitors, clinical and alert alarms, metal instruments),
  ○ electronic activities (eg, e-mail, texting, social media [eg, Facebook, YouTube®, Twitter®, LinkedIn®], Internet, games), and
  ○ behavioral activities (eg, nonessential and extraneous conversations, personnel movement in and out of the room).
[3: Moderate Evidence]

The sources of noise and distractions are well documented in the literature, and minimizing various sources is supported by professional organizations.[112-114,128-142] The American College of Surgeons and the American Association of Nurse Anesthetists both support the creation of a policy that limits the use of mobile communication devices in the OR.[141,142]

In an evaluation of noise pollution in ORs in nine hospitals during 43 surgeries, Tsiou et al found that noise pollution came from many sources including the building, machinery, tools, and people. Based on these findings, they recommended a multidisciplinary approach to solving the noise pollution problem.[132]

In a prospective study including 50 trauma procedures, the average noise level was 85 dB with a range of 40 dB to 130 dB. The researchers also noted an average of 60.8 interruptions and distractions per procedure (range, 5 to 192). The distractions and interruptions were caused by team members entering and leaving the room, equipment alarms, parallel conversations, and telephones or pagers. The main effect of distractions and interruptions was disruption in the continuous flow of surgical activities.[113]

A study involving 15 physicians using simulated OR noise and music showed that when music was added to the noise and a task was being performed, the level of auditory processing was decreased. Auditory processing was measured by the surgeon's ability to understand and repeats words using a revised version of the Speech in Noise Test.[138]

The amount of noise generated by pneumatic power tools during orthopedic procedures includes saws at 95 dBA, drills at 90 dBA, K-wire drivers at 85 dBA, and hammers at 65 dBA.[136] These are short-term exposures, and this level of noise is not consistent for the eight-hour shift required in the NIOSH recommended limits of 85 dBA of noise exposure for an eight-hour shift without ear protection.[114]

The results of a cohort observational study involving 11 nurses showed that higher average sound levels were related to higher self-reported levels of stress and annoyance.[134]

Juang et al studied noise created in the hospital unit and outside the unit at three hospitals in Taiwan. The study, which involved 573 patients and personnel, found noise was created by multiple factors including doors opening and closing, people talking, alarms, and equipment. The effects of the noise on the participants' emotion and physiology varied depending on gender, age, religion, work experience, and other factors.[139]

In a review of the literature on occupational exposure to noise, Oliviera and Arenas concluded that noise pollution in ORs can cause a breakdown in communications.[112] They reported that to enable good communication, the spoken voice needs to be 10 dB higher than the surrounding noise.[112]

In a pilot study involving 35 patients undergoing open abdominal procedures, a connection was found between sound levels and the development of SSIs. The authors speculated this may be caused by decreased concentration or a stressful environment.[133]

Nurses in the ORs in three different facilities identified that speech comprehension difficulties were related to the amount of noise in the OR. This difficulty led to more vocal effort being required to achieve speech comprehension.[140] The procedures performed during this study involved various specialities. Similar results were found in a nine-hospital study in which background noise and average noise were measured during surgical procedures performed in different subspecialties. In this study, Stringer et al found noise levels to be higher than those recommended by the World Health Organization for locations in a hospital where patient care occurs.[140] This study and one by Kracht et al[130] found the orthopedic ORs had the highest levels of noise, and other specialities were less noisy. The comparative specialities varied in these studies.[130,140]

A review of the literature conducted in 2010 revealed that the primary effect of noise on personnel was impaired communication.[129]

Arora et al investigated the frequency of stress being produced by distractions and interruptions and the severity of that stress. The study participants were the personnel involved in 55 elective procedures in the United Kingdom. The participants rated distractions and interruptions as frequent cause of stress but rated these least severe on the severity scale. The example of distractions and interruptions stated in the article was telephone calls that led to conveying and replying to nonurgent messages.[128]

In a study of 78 endo-urological procedures, a distraction occurred every 1.8 minutes. Equipment problems and relevant and irrelevant conversations were rated as the most frequent and most distracting events.[131]

In a study in which 10 participants performed robot-assisted suturing and were simultaneously multitasking, the time to secondary task completion was longer and the speed of the primary task was slower compared with a control group.[135]

One case was reported in which a person texting an order was interrupted by a personal text. The interruption resulted in the order not being completed, and the patient received an overdose of anticoagulation medication.[136]

VIII.b.1. Portable communication devices (eg, pagers, smart phones, cell phones, wireless communication systems, hand held two-way radio transceivers [eg, walkie-talkies]) should be
- placed on vibrate or silent mode,
- off unless directly needed for job performance, or
- left at a common location outside of the OR.

VIII.b.2. Fixed communication devices (eg, overhead paging systems, intercoms, telephones) should be used
- only for essential communications,
- at the lowest volume possible, and

- for essential communication instead of opening the door and entering the OR.

    The use of fixed communication devices is preferred to opening the door because opening the door causes a greater distraction and affects the airflow within the surgical suite.[84]

VIII.b.3. The volume level of electronic music devices (eg, radios, digital audio players, CD players) should be low enough to allow communication among team members.

VIII.b.4. Alarms and verbal communications should be audible above competing environmental noise.

    The level of environmental noise (eg, HVAC system, pneumatic tube systems, radiology equipment, suction, smoke evacuator, drills monitors, alarms) may compete with critical communications.

VIII.b.5. The health care organization should establish a policy and procedure for the use of mobile communication devices that includes
- use of personal devices,
- use of facility-owned devices,
- locations or prohibited locations for use, allowable information that may be conveyed by the mobile device (eg, patient-related information only, photography),
- level of encryption and security controls, and
- device cleaning.

VIII.b.6. The health care organization should establish a policy and procedure for distraction control that includes
- portable communication devices (eg, pagers, cell phones, personal digital assistants, computers),
- fixed communication devices (eg, overhead pages and announcements, telephones, computers),
- electronic music devices (eg, radios, CD players, digital audio players),
- the environment (eg, HVAC system, pneumatic tube systems),
- medical equipment and devices (eg, radiology equipment, waste management system, smoke evacuator, powered surgical instruments, monitors, clinical and alert alarms, metal instruments),
- use of electronic activities (eg, e-mail, texting, social media [eg, Facebook, YouTube, Twitter, LinkedIn], Internet, games), and
- personal conduct (eg, essential and extraneous conversations, personnel movement in and out of the room).

VIII.c. The level of noise generated by a piece of equipment or instrument should be a part of the evaluation criteria for purchasing decisions. *[3: Moderate Evidence]*

A health hazard evaluation report conducted by NIOSH at a large teaching facility demonstrated that different amounts of noise are generated by different type of instruments that perform the same function (eg, a modified design produced less noise than the standard design).[114]

VIII.d. Before use, the user should verify that the mobile communication device is
- approved for sharing patient-related information,
- approved for photography,
- equipped with the required level of encryption and security controls, and
- approved for use within the surgical suite.

[4: Limited Evidence]

    The advantages of mobile communication technology include easy access to clinical data and patient information, ease of bedside documentation, automated reminders, and ease of access to the device. Devices may be easily lost and personal information contained on the device may be stolen.[136,143]

    Cases have been reported in which electromechanical interference was caused by cell phone use (ie, the use of a cell phone changed the operation of a medical device).[143]

Editor's note: Facebook is a registered trademark of Facebook, Inc, Menlo Park, CA. YouTube is registered trademark of Google, Inc, Mountain View, CA. Twitter is a registered trademark of Twitter, Inc, San Francisco, CA. LinkedIn is a registered trademark of LinkedIn Corp, Mountain View, CA.

Glossary

Commissioning: A quality process used to achieve, validate, and document that facilities and component infrastructure systems are planned, constructed, installed, tested, and are capable of being operated and maintained in conformity with the design intent or performance expectations.

Cove base: Molding or trim used to create a curved right-angle transition from the wall to the floor.

Displacement airflow system: An airflow system in which the air entry point is located low on the wall, the air exit point is located near the ceiling, and the filtered air is introduced at a low velocity.

Distraction: An event that causes a diversion of attention during performance of a task or diverts the person's concentration from the task.

Evidence-based design: A process used by architects, interior designers, and facility managers in the planning, design, and construction of health care facilities. Individuals using evidence-based design make decisions based on the best information available from research, project evaluations and evidence gathered from client operations. An evidence-based design should result in improvements to an organization's outcomes, economic performance, productivity, and customer satisfaction.

Interruption: An unplanned or unexpected event causing discontinuation of a task.

Laminar air delivery system: An air delivery system that delivers particle-free air that moves over the sterile field at a uniform velocity of 0.3 to 0.5 micrometers/second. Laminar airflow is recirculated air that is filtered through a HEPA filter. Laminar air flow can be either vertical or horizontal. Synonym: *ultra clean air.*

Monolithic: A surface constructed to be free of fissures, cracks, and crevices.

Noise: Any sound that interferes with normal hearing and is undesired.

Overhead air delivery system: An airflow system in which the air entry point is located in the ceiling, the air exit point is located low on the wall, and the filtered air is introduced at various velocities.

Procedure room: A room designated for the performance of procedures that do not require a restricted environment but may require the use of sterile instruments or supplies.

REFERENCES

1. Bartley JM, Olmsted RN, Haas J. Current views of health care design and construction: practical implications for safer, cleaner environments. *Am J Infect Control.* 2010;38(5 Suppl 1):S1-12. [VB]

2. Allo MD, Tedesco M. Operating room management: operative suite considerations, infection control. *Surg Clin North Am.* 2005;85(6):1291-1297, xii. [VC]

3. Lee L. Clean construction. Infection control during building and renovation projects. *Health Facil Manage.* 2010;23(4):36-38. [VB]

4. Guideline for product selection. In: *Guidelines for Perioperative Practice.* Denver, CO: AORN, Inc; 2015:179-186. [IVA]

5. Chang CC, Athan E, Morrissey CO, Slavin MA. Preventing invasive fungal infection during hospital building works. *Intern Med J.* 2008;38(6b):538-541. [VC]

6. American Society of Heating Refrigerating and Air-Conditioning Engineers. Room design. In: *HVAC Design Manual for Hospitals and Clinics.* 2nd ed. Atlanta, GA: ASHRAE; 2013:151-202. [IVB]

7. Facility Guidelines Institute, US Department of Health and Human Services, American Society for Healthcare Engineering. *Guidelines for Design and Construction of Hospitals and Outpatient Facilities.* Chicago, IL: American Society for Healthcare Engineering of the American Hospital Association; 2014. [IVB]

8. National Fire Protection Association. *NFPA 101: Life Safety Code.* Quincy, MA: National Fire Protection Association; 2012. [IVB]

9. National Fire Protection Association. *NFPA 99: Health Care Facilities Code.* 2012 ed. Quincy, MA: National Fire Protection Association; 2011. [IVB]

10. 42 CFR 482.41—Condition of participation: Physical environment. http://www.gpo.gov/fdsys/granule/CFR-2011-title42-vol5/CFR-2011-title42-vol5-sec482-41/content-detail.html. Accessed April 7, 2014.

11. 42 CFR 416.44—Condition for coverage: Environment. http://www.gpo.gov/fdsys/granule/CFR-2012-title42-vol3/CFR-2012-title42-vol3-sec416-44/content-detail.html. Accessed April 7, 2014.

12. Haiduven D. Nosocomial aspergillosis and building construction. *Med Mycol.* 2009;47(Suppl 1):S210-S216. [VB]

13. Henriksen K, Isaacson S, Sadler BL, Zimring CM. The role of the physical environment in crossing the quality chasm. *Jt Comm J Qual Patient Saf.* 2007;33(11 Suppl):68-80. [VA]

14. Lin F, Lawley M, Spry C, McCarthy K, Coyle-Rogers PG, Yih Y. Using simulation to design a central sterilization department. *AORN J.* 2008;88(4):555-567. [IIIC]

15. Birnbach DJ, Nevo I, Scheinman SR, Fitzpatrick M, Shekhter I, Lombard JL. Patient safety begins with proper planning: a quantitative method to improve hospital design. *Qual Saf Health Care.* 2010;19(5):462-465. [IIB]

16. Guideline for surgical attire. In: *Guidelines for Perioperative Practice.* Denver, CO: AORN; 2015:97-120. [IVB]

17. Guideline for hand hygiene. In: *Guidelines for Perioperative Practice.* Denver, CO: AORN; 2015:31-42. [IVB]

18. Mangram AJ, Horan TC, Pearson ML, Silver LC, Jarvis WR. Guideline for prevention of surgical site infection, 1999. Hospital Infection Control Practices Advisory Committee. *Infect Control Hosp Epidemiol.* 1999;20(4):250-278. [IVA]

19. Brandt C, Hott U, Sohr D, Daschner F, Gastmeier P, Ruden H. Operating room ventilation with laminar airflow shows no protective effect on the surgical site infection rate in orthopedic and abdominal surgery. *Ann Surg.* 2008;248(5):695-700. [IIIA]

20. Diab-Elschahawi M, Berger J, Blacky A, et al. Impact of different-sized laminar air flow versus no laminar air flow on bacterial counts in the operating room during orthopedic surgery. *Am J Infect Control.* 2011;39(7):e25-e29. [IIIB]

21. Da Costa AR, Kothari A, Bannister GC, Blom AW. Investigating bacterial growth in surgical theatres: establishing the effect of laminar airflow on bacterial growth on plastic, metal and wood surfaces. *Ann R Coll Surg Engl.* 2008;90(5):417-419. [IIC]

22. Howard JL, Hanssen AD. Principles of a clean operating room environment. *J Arthroplasty.* 2007;22(7 Suppl 3):6-11. [VC]

23. Miner AL, Losina E, Katz JN, Fossel AH, Platt R. Deep infection after total knee replacement: impact of laminar airflow systems and body exhaust suits in the modern operating room. *Infect Control Hosp Epidemiol.* 2007;28(2):222-226. [IIIB]

24. Kakwani RG, Yohannan D, Wahab KH. The effect of laminar air-flow on the results of Austin-Moore hemiarthroplasty. *Injury.* 2007;38(7):820-823. [IIIB]

25. Hooper GJ, Rothwell AG, Frampton C, Wyatt MC. Does the use of laminar flow and space suits reduce early deep infection after total hip and knee replacement?: the ten-year results of the New Zealand Joint Registry. *J Bone Joint Surg Br.* 2011;93(1):85-90. [IIIA]

26. Knobben BA, van Horn JR, van der Mei HC, Busscher HJ. Evaluation of measures to decrease intra-operative bacterial contamination in orthopaedic implant surgery. *J Hosp Infect.* 2006;62(2):174-180. [IIB]

27. Friberg B, Friberg S. Aerobiology in the operating room and its implications for working standards. *Proc Inst Mech Eng H.* 2005;219(2):153-160. [IIIB]

28. Hall G. Air flow disruption must be minimised. *Health Estate.* 2005;59(3):53-55. [VC]

29. Hirsch T, Hubert H, Fischer S, et al. Bacterial burden in the operating room: impact of airflow systems. *Am J Infect Control.* 2012;40(7):e228-e232. [IIIB]

30. *Operating Room HVAC Setback Strategies.* Chicago, IL: American Society for Healthcare Engineering; 2011. [VB]

31. Chan DWT, Law KC, Kwan CHS, Chiu WY. Application of an air purification system to control airborne bacterial contamination in a University clinic.

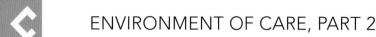

ENVIRONMENT OF CARE, PART 2

Transactions Hong Kong Institution of Engineers. 2005;12(1):17-21. [IIIB]

32. Nerandzic MM, Donskey CJ. Triggering germination represents a novel strategy to enhance killing of *Clostridium difficile* spores. *PLoS One.* 2010;5(8):e12285. [IIB]

33. Ritter MA, Olberding EM, Malinzak RA. Ultraviolet lighting during orthopaedic surgery and the rate of infection. *J Bone Joint Surg Am.* 2007;89(9):1935-1940. [IIIA]

34. ACGIH. *Ultraviolet Radiation: TLV Physical Agents. Documentation.* 7th ed. Cincinnati, OH: American Conference of Industrial Hygienists; 2010. [IVB]

35. Memarzadeh F, Olmsted RN, Bartley JM. Applications of ultraviolet germicidal irradiation disinfection in health care facilities: effective adjunct, but not standalone technology. *Am J Infect Control.* 2010;38(5 Suppl 1):S13-S24. [VA]

36. Escombe AR, Moore DA, Gilman RH, et al. Upperroom ultraviolet light and negative air ionization to prevent tuberculosis transmission. *PLoS Med.* 2009;6(3):e43. [IA]

37. National Institute for Occupational Safety and Health Centers for Disease Control and Prevention. *Environmental Control for Tuberculosis: Basic Upper-Room Ultraviolet Germicidal Irradiation Guidelines for Healthcare Settings.* DHHS (NIOSH) Publication Number 2009-105. Atlanta, GA: National Institute for Occupational Safety and Health. Centers for Disease Control and Prevention; 2009. [IVB]

38. Rutala WA, Gergen MF, Weber DJ. Room decontamination with UV radiation. *Infect Control Hosp Epidemiol.* 2010;31(10):1025-1029. [IIB]

39. McDevitt JJ, Milton DK, Rudnick SN, First MW. Inactivation of poxviruses by upper-room UVC light in a simulated hospital room environment. *PLoS One.* 2008;3(9):e3186. [IIB]

40. Stichler JF. Enhancing safety with facility design. *J Nurs Adm.* 2007;37(7-8):319-323. [VB]

41. Guenther R, Hall AG. Healthy buildings: impact on nurses and nursing practice. *Online J Issues Nurs.* 2007;12(2):2. [VB]

42. Stichler JF. Code green: a new design imperative for healthcare facilities. *J Nurs Adm.* 2009;39(2):51-54. [VC]

43. *NFPA 70: National Electrical Code.* Quincy, MA: National Fire Protection Association; 2011. [IVB]

44. Barker SJ, Doyle DJ. Electrical safety in the operating room: dry versus wet. *Anesth Analg.* 2010;110(6):1517-1518. [VB]

45. Illuminating Engineering Society of North America. *Lighting for Hospitals and Health Care Facilities.* New York, NY: Illuminating Engineering Society of North America; 2006. [IVB]

46. Cockram A. Correct lighting of hospital buildings. 1976. *Health Estate.* 2007;61(4):21-23. [VC]

47. Verrinder J. Use of right lighting levels essential. *Health Estate.* 2007;61(6):31-32. [VC]

48. Knulst AJ, Mooijweer R, Jansen FW, Stassen LP, Dankelman J. Indicating shortcomings in surgical lighting systems. *Minim Invasive Ther Allied Technol.* 2011;20(5):267-275. [VC]

49. Baillie J. Stars of the theatre show true colours. *Health Estate.* 2012;66(1):31-40. [VC]

50. Surgical lights. An illuminating look at the LED marketplace. *Health Devices.* 2010;39(11):390-402. [VB]

51. ECRI Institute. Hazard report. Overlap of surgical lighthead beams may present burn risk. *Health Devices.* 2009;38(10):341-342. [IVC]

52. *ANSI/AAMI ST79:2010 & A1:2010 & A2:2011 & A3:2012 (Consolidated Text) Comprehensive Guide to Steam Sterilization and Sterility Assurance in Health Care Facilities.* Arlington, VA: AAMI; 2012. [IVB]

53. Guideline for sterilization. In: *Guidelines for Perioperative Practice.* Denver, CO: AORN; 2015:665-692. [IVA]

54. Guideline for environmental cleaning. In: *Guidelines for Perioperative Practice.* Denver, CO: AORN; 2015:9-30. [IVA]

55. Warren B. Workplace violence in hospitals: safe havens no more. *J Healthc Prot Manage.* 2011;27(2):9-17. [VC]

56. Guidelines for preventing workplace violence for health care & social service workers. OSHA 3148-01R 2004. Occupational Safety & Health Administration. http://www.osha.gov/Publications/OSHA3148/osha3148. html. Accessed April 7, 2014. [IVA]

57. Pini G, Faggi E, Donato R, Sacco C, Fanci R. Invasive pulmonary aspergillosis in neutropenic patients and the influence of hospital renovation. *Mycoses.* 2008;51(2):117-122. [IIIC]

58. Yahara K, Miura M, Masunaga K, et al. Comparison of two control measures of weatherstripping in reducing blowing dust during hospital renovations. *J Infect Chemother.* 2010;16(6):431-435. [IIIC]

59. Campbell JR, Hulten K, Baker CJ. Cluster of Bacillus species bacteremia cases in neonates during a hospital construction project. *Infect Control Hosp Epidemiol.* 2011;32(10):1035-1038. [IIIC]

60. Pasqualotto AC, Denning DW. Post-operative aspergillosis. *Clin Microbiol Infect.* 2006;12(11):1060-1076. [VA]

61. Fournel I, Sautour M, Lafon I, et al. Airborne Aspergillus contamination during hospital construction works: efficacy of protective measures. *Am J Infect Control.* 2010;38(3):189-194. [IIIB]

62. American Society of Heating Refrigerating and Air-Conditioning Engineers. Infection control. In: *HVAC Design Manual for Hospitals and Clinics.* 2nd ed. Atlanta, GA: ASHRAE; 2013:19-34. [IVB]

63. Eames I, Tang JW, Li Y, Wilson P. Airborne transmission of disease in hospitals. *J R Soc Interface.* 2009;6(Suppl 6):S697-S702. [VB]

64. Aydin Cakir N, Ucar FB, Haliki Uztan A, Corbaci C, Akpinar O. Determination and comparison of microbial loads in atmospheres of two hospitals in Izmir, Turkey. *Ann Agric Environ Med.* 2013;20(1):106-110. [IIIC]

65. Krajewski W, Kucharska M, Wesolowski W, Stetkiewicz J, Wronska-Nofer T. Occupational exposure to nitrous oxide—the role of scavenging and ventilation systems in reducing the exposure level in operating rooms. *Int J Hyg Environ Health.* 2007;210(2):133-138. [IIIB]

66. Wan GH, Chung FF, Tang CS. Long-term surveillance of air quality in medical center operating rooms. *Am J Infect Control.* 2011;39(4):302-308. [IIIB]

67. Perdelli F, Cristina ML, Sartini M, et al. Fungal contamination in hospital environments. *Infect Control Hosp Epidemiol.* 2006;27(1):44-47. [IIA]

68. *ANSI/ASHRAE/ASHE Addendum h to ANSI/ASHRAE/ASHE Standard 170-2013: Ventilation of Health Care Facilities.* Atlanta, GA: American Society of Heating, Refrigerating and Air-Conditioning Engineers, Inc; 2016. https://www.ashrae.org/File%20Library/docLib/StdsAddenda/170_2013_h_20160523.pdf. Accessed October 3, 2016. [IVC]

69. Crimi P, Valgiusti M, Macrina G, et al. Evaluation of microbial contamination of air in two haematology departments equipped with ventilation systems with different filtration devices. *J Prev Med Hyg.* 2009;50(1):33-36. [IIIC]

70. Stocks GW, Self SD, Thompson B, Adame XA, O'Connor DP. Predicting bacterial populations based on airborne particulates: a study performed in nonlaminar flow operating rooms during joint arthroplasty surgery. *Am J Infect Control.* 2010;38(3):199-204. [IIIB]

71. Abdel Hameed AA, Khoder MI, Ibrahim YH, Saeed Y, Osman ME, Ghanem S. Study on some factors affecting survivability of airborne fungi. *Sci Total Environ.* 2012;414:696-700. [IIIC]

72. Panagopoulou P, Filioti J, Farmaki E, Maloukou A, Roilides E. Filamentous fungi in a tertiary care hospital: environmental surveillance and susceptibility to antifungal drugs. *Infect Control Hosp Epidemiol.* 2007;28(1):60-67. [IIIB]

73. Tang JW. The effect of environmental parameters on the survival of airborne infectious agents. *J R Soc Interface.* 2009;6(Suppl 6):S737-S746. [VB]

74. Thompson KA, Bennett AM, Walker JT. Aerosol survival of *Staphylococcus epidermidis. J Hosp Infect.* 2011;78(3):216-220. [IIIB]

75. Memarzadeh F. Literature review of the effect of temperature and humidity on viruses. *ASHRAE Transactions.* 2012;118(1):1046-1060. [VB]

76. American Society of Heating Refrigerating and Air-Conditioning Engineers. Overview of health care HVAC. In: *HVAC Design Manual for Hospitals and Clinics.* Atlanta, GA: American Society of Heating, Refrigerating and Air-Conditioning Engineers, Inc; 2003:33-45. [IVB]

77. Olmsted RN. Pilot study of directional airflow and containment of airborne particles in the size of *Mycobacterium tuberculosis* in an operating room. *Am J Infect Control.* 2008;36(4):260-267. [IIB]

78. Babkin Y, Raveh D, Lifschitz M, et al. Incidence and risk factors for surgical infection after total knee replacement. *Scand J Infect Dis.* 2007;39(10):890-895. [IIIB]

79. Guideline for prevention of transmissible infections. In: *Guidelines for Perioperative Practice.* Denver, CO: AORN, Inc; 2015:419-451. [IVA]

80. Gniadek A, Macura AB. Air-conditioning vs presence of pathogenic fungi in hospital operating theatre environment. *Wiad Parazytol.* 2011;57(2):103-106. [IIIB]

81. Berthelot P, Carricajo A, Aubert G, Akhavan H, Gazielly D, Lucht F. Outbreak of postoperative shoulder arthritis due to *Propionibacterium acnes* infection in nondebilitated patients. *Infect Control Hosp Epidemiol.* 2006;27(9):987-990. [VB]

82. Crolla RM, van der Laan L, Veen EJ, Hendriks Y, van Schendel C, Kluytmans J. Reduction of surgical site infections after implementation of a bundle of care. *PLoS One.* 2012;7(9):e44599. [IIB]

83. Andersson AE, Bergh I, Karlsson J, Eriksson BI, Nilsson K. Traffic flow in the operating room: an explorative and descriptive study on air quality during orthopedic trauma implant surgery. *Am J Infect Control.* 2012;40(8):750-755. [IIIB]

84. Panahi P, Stroh M, Casper DS, Parvizi J, Austin MS. Operating room traffic is a major concern during total joint arthroplasty. *Clin Orthop Relat Res.* 2012;470(10):2690-2694. [VC]

85. Young RS, O'Regan DJ. Cardiac surgical theatre traffic: time for traffic calming measures? *Interact Cardiovasc Thorac Surg.* 2010;10(4):526-529. [IIIC]

86. Lynch RJ, Englesbe MJ, Sturm L, et al. Measurement of foot traffic in the operating room: implications for infection control. *Am J Med Qual.* 2009;24(1):45-52. [VB]

87. Scaltriti S, Cencetti S, Rovesti S, Marchesi I, Bargellini A, Borella P. Risk factors for particulate and microbial contamination of air in operating theatres. *J Hosp Infect.* 2007;66(4):320-326. [IIIB]

88. Parikh SN, Grice SS, Schnell BM, Salisbury SR. Operating room traffic: is there any role of monitoring it? *J Pediatr Orthop.* 2010;30(6):617-623. [VB]

89. Riley RH. Power failure to a tertiary hospital's operating suite. *Anaesth Intensive Care.* 2010;38(4):785. [VB]

90. Yasny J, Soffer R. A case of a power failure in the operating room. *Anesth Prog.* 2005;52(2):65-69. [VB]

91. Carpenter T, Robinson ST. Case reports: response to a partial power failure in the operating room. *Anesth Analg.* 2010;110(6):1644-1646. [VA]

92. Preventing adverse events caused by emergency electrical power system failures. *Sentinel Event Alert.* September 6, 2006;37. The Joint Commission. http://www.jointcommission.org/assets/1/18/SEA_37.PDF. Accessed April 7, 2014.[IVA]

93. Mitchell L, Anderle D, Nastally K, Sarver T, Hafner-Burton T, Owens S. Lessons learned from Hurricane Ike. *AORN J.* 2009;89(6):1073-1078. [VB]

94. Eichhorn JH, Hessel EA 2nd. Electrical power failure in the operating room: a neglected topic in anesthesia safety. *Anesth Analg.* 2010;110(6):1519-1521. [VB]

95. Routine maintenance and operational testing. In: *NFPA 110: Standard for Emergency and Standby Power Systems.* Quincy, MA: National Fire Protection Association; 2013:110-19–110-21. [IVB]

96. 45 CFR Parts 160, 162, 164: General administrative requirements, Administrative requirements, Security and privacy. http://www.gpo.gov/fdsys/search/pagedetails.action?collectionCode=CFR&searchPath=Title+45%2FSubtitle+A%2FSubchapter+C&granuleId=&packageId=CFR-2007-title45-vol1&oldPath=Title+45%2FSubtitle+A%2FSubchapter+A%2FPart+2&fromPageDetails=true&collapse=true&ycord=2372. Accessed April 7, 2014.

97. The Joint Commission. Protecting your health care workers from violence in the workplace. *Joint Commission: The Source.* 2006;4(4):1-2, 10. [VB]

98. Centers for Medicare & Medicaid Services (CMS) DHHS. Medicare and Medicaid programs; hospital conditions of participation: patients' rights. Final rule. *Fed Regist.* 2006;71(236):71378-71428. http://www.cms.gov/CFCsAndCoPs/downloads/finalpatientrightsrule.pdf. Accessed April 7, 2014.

99. Potter AN. Developing a strategic security plan. *J Healthc Prot Manage.* 2011;27(2):59-65. [VC]

100. United States Census of Fatal Occupational Injuries, 2011. Bureau of Labor Statistics. http://www.bls.gov/iif/oshcfoi1.htm. Accessed April 7, 2014. [IIIA]

101. Injuries, illnesses, and fatalities: frequently asked questions (FAQs). US Bureau of Labor Statistics. http://www.bls.gov/iif/oshfaq1.htm#q05. Accessed April 7, 2014. [VA]

102. Hahn S, Muller M, Needham I, Dassen T, Kok G, Halfens RJ. Factors associated with patient and visitor violence experienced by nurses in general hospitals in Switzerland: a cross-sectional survey. *J Clin Nurs.* 2010;19(23-24):3535-3546. [IIIB]

103. Department of Health and Human Services. HIPAA administrative simplification: standard unique health identifier for health care providers; final rule. *Fed Regist.* 2004;69(15):3434-3469. http://frwebgate.access.gpo.gov/cgi-bin/getpage.cgi?dbname=2004_register&position=all&page=3434. Accessed April 7, 2014.

104. Williams JB, Mathews R, D'Amico TA. "Reality surgery"—a research ethics perspective on the live broadcast of surgical procedures. *J Surg Educ.* 2011;68(1):58-61. [VB]

105. Landman MP, Shelton J, Kauffmann RM, Dattilo JB. Guidelines for maintaining a professional compass in the

ENVIRONMENT OF CARE, PART 2

PATIENT AND WORKER SAFETY

era of social networking. *J Surg Educ.* 2010;67(6):381-386. [IIIC]

106. Segal J, Sacopulos MJ. Photography consent and related legal issues. *Facial Plast Surg Clin North Am.* 2010;18(2):237-244. [VA]

107. Lau CK, Schumacher HH, Irwin MS. Patients' perception of medical photography. *J Plast Reconstr Aesthet Surg.* 2010;63(6):e507-e511. [IIIB]

108. How aware of patient confidentiality are you? *Nurs Law Regan Rep.* 2007;48(7):2. [VB]

109. AORN position statement on the role of the health care industry representative in the perioperative/invasive procedure setting. 2006. AORN, Inc. http://www.aorn.org/Clinical_Practice/Position_Statements/Position_Statements.aspx. Accessed April 7, 2014. [VC]

110. Health care industry representatives in the operating room. *Clin Privil White Pap.* 2005;(1010):1-12. [IVB]

111. Healey AN, Sevdalis N, Vincent CA. Measuring intra-operative interference from distraction and interruption observed in the operating theatre. *Ergonomics.* 2006;49(5-6):589-604. [IIIB]

112. Oliveira CR, Arenas GW. Occupational exposure to noise pollution in anesthesiology. *Rev Bras Anestesiol.* 2012;62(2):253-261. [VB]

113. Pereira BM, Pereira AM, Correia Cdos S, Marttos AC Jr, Fiorelli RK, Fraga GP. Interruptions and distractions in the trauma operating room: understanding the threat of human error. *Rev Col Bras Cir.* 2011;38(5):292-298. [IIIB]

114. Chen L, Brueck SE. Health hazard evaluation report: evaluation of potential noise exposures in hospital operating rooms, Morgantown, WV [NIOSH HETA No. 2008-0231-3105]. Cincinnati, OH: US Department of Health and Human Services, Centers for Disease Control and Prevention, National Institute for Occupational Safety and Health; 2010. [IIIB]

115. Siu KC, Suh IH, Mukherjee M, Oleynikov D, Stergiou N. The effect of music on robot-assisted laparoscopic surgical performance. *Surg Innov.* 2010;17(4):306-311. [IIIC]

116. Joseph A, Ulrich R. *Sound Control for Improved Outcomes in Healthcare Settings.* Concord, CA: Center for Health Design; 2007. [VA]

117. Christian CK, Gustafson ML, Roth EM, et al. A prospective study of patient safety in the operating room. *Surgery.* 2006;139(2):159-173. [IIIB]

118. Fabri PJ, Zayas-Castro JL. Human error, not communication and systems, underlies surgical complications. *Surgery.* 2008;144(4):557-563. [IIIC]

119. Sevdalis N, Forrest D, Undre S, Darzi A, Vincent C. Annoyances, disruptions, and interruptions in surgery: the Disruptions in Surgery Index (DiSI). *World J Surg.* 2008;32(8):1643-1650. [IIIB]

120. Smith T, Darling E, Searles B. 2010 Survey on cell phone use while performing cardiopulmonary bypass. *Perfusion.* 2011;26(5):375-380. [IIIB]

121. AORN position statement on noise in the perioperative practice setting. 2009. AORN, Inc. http://www.aorn.org/Clinical_Practice/Position_Statements/Position_Statements.aspx. Accessed April 7, 2014. [VA]

122. Feuerbacher RL, Funk KH, Spight DH, Diggs BS, Hunter JG. Realistic Distractions and interruptions that impair simulated surgical performance by novice surgeons. *Arch Surg.* 2012;147(11):1026-1030. [IIIC]

123. Pluyter JR, Buzink SN, Rutkowski AF, Jakimowicz JJ. Do absorption and realistic distraction influence performance of component task surgical procedure? *Surg Endosc.* 2010;24(4):902-907. [IIB]

124. Altmann EM, Trafton JG. Task interruption: resumption lag and the role of cues. In: *Proceedings of the 26th Annual Conference of the Cognitive Science Society.* Austin, TX: Cognitive Science Society; 2004. [IA]

125. Altmann EM, Trafton JG, Hambrick DZ. Momentary interruptions can derail the train of thought. *J Exp Psychol Gen.* 2014;143(1):215-226. [IIA]

126. Biron AD, Lavoie-Tremblay M, Loiselle CG. Characteristics of work interruptions during medication administration. *J Nurs Scholarsh.* 2009;41(4):330-336. [IIIB]

127. Campbell G, Arfanis K, Smith AF. Distraction and interruption in anaesthetic practice. *Br J Anaesth.* 2012;109(5):707-715. [IIIB]

128. Arora S, Hull L, Sevdalis N, et al. Factors compromising safety in surgery: stressful events in the operating room. *Am J Surg.* 2010;199(1):60-65. [IIIB]

129. Hasfeldt D, Laerkner E, Birkelund R. Noise in the operating room—what do we know? A review of the literature. *J Perianesth Nurs.* 2010;25(6):380-386. [VA]

130. Kracht JM, Busch-Vishniac IJ, West JE. Noise in the operating rooms of Johns Hopkins Hospital. *J Acoust Soc Am.* 2007;121(5 Pt1):2673-2680. [IIIB]

131. Persoon MC, Broos HJ, Witjes JA, Hendrikx AJ, Scherpbier AJ. The effect of distractions in the operating room during endourological procedures. *Surg Endosc.* 2011;25(2):437-443. [IIIB]

132. Tsiou C, Efthymiatos G, Katostaras T. Noise in the operating rooms of Greek hospitals. *J Acoust Soc Am.* 2008;123(2):757-765. [IIIA]

133. Kurmann A, Peter M, Tschan F, Muhlemann K, Candinas D, Beldi G. Adverse effect of noise in the operating theatre on surgical-site infection. *Br J Surg.* 2011;98(7):1021-1025. [IIIC]

134. Morrison WE, Haas EC, Shaffner DH, Garrett ES, Fackler JC. Noise, stress, and annoyance in a pediatric intensive care unit. *Crit Care Med.* 2003;31(1):113-119. [IIIC]

135. Suh IH, Chien JH, Mukherjee M, Park SH, Oleynikov D, Siu KC. The negative effect of distraction on performance of robot-assisted surgical skills in medical students and residents. *Int J Med Robot.* 2010;6(4):377-381. [IIIC]

136. Halamka J. Order interrupted by text: multitasking mishap. *AHRQ Web M&M* [serial online]. http://webmm.ahrq.gov/case.aspx?caseID=257. Published December 2011. Accessed April 7, 2014. [VB]

137. Siverdeen Z, Ali A, Lakdawala AS, McKay C. Exposure to noise in orthopaedic theatres—do we need protection? *Int J Clin Pract.* 2008;62(11):1720-1722. [IIIB]

138. Way TJ, Long A, Weihing J, et al. Effect of noise on auditory processing in the operating room. *J Am Coll Surg.* 2013;216(5):933-938. [IIIC]

139. Juang DF, Lee CH, Yang T, Chang MC. Noise pollution and its effects on medical care workers and patients in hospitals. *Int J Environ Sci Tech.* 2010;7(4):705-716. [IIIB]

140. Stringer B, Haines TA, Oudyk JD. Noisiness in operating theatres: nurses' perceptions and potential difficulty communicating. *J Perioper Pract.* 2008;18(9):384-391. [IIIA]

141. American College of Surgeons Committee on Perioperative Care. Statement on use of cell phones in the operating room. *Bull Am Coll Surg.* 2008;93(9):33-34. [IVB]

142. Position statement number 2.18: mobile device use. *AANA J.* 2013;81(1):12. [IVB]

143. Judgment call. *Health Devices.* 2012;41(10):314-329. [VC]

Acknowledgements

LEAD AUTHOR
Byron Burlingame, MS, BSN, RN, CNOR
Perioperative Nursing Specialist
AORN Nursing Department
Denver, Colorado

CONTRIBUTING AUTHOR
Ramona Conner, MSN, RN, CNOR
Manager, Standards and Guidelines
AORN Nursing Department
Denver, Colorado

The authors and AORN thank Antonia B. Hughes, MA, BSN, RN, CNOR, Perioperative Education Specialist, Baltimore Washington Medical Center, Edgewater, MD; Sandy Albright, MSHM, BSN, RN, CNOR, Nurse Consultant, Synergy Health North America, Tampa, FL; Janice Neil, PhD, RN, Associate Professor and Chair, Department of Undergraduate Nursing Science, College of Nursing, East Carolina University, Greenville, NC; Rodney W. Hicks, PhD, RN, FNP-BC, FAANP, Professor, Western University of Health Sciences, Pomona, CA: Bill Rostenberg, FAIA, FACHA, ACHE, EDAC, Principal and Director of Research, Anshen + Allen Architects, San Francisco, CA, for their assistance in developing this guideline.

PUBLICATION HISTORY
Originally published in May 2014 in *Perioperative Standards and Recommended Practices* online.

Minor editing revisions made in November 2014 for publication in *Guidelines for Perioperative Practice,* 2015 edition.

Minor revisions to functional area terminology and recommendations for facility temperatures made in October 2016 for publication in *Guidelines for Perioperative Practice,* 2017 edition.

Evidence ratings revised in *Guidelines for Perioperative Practice,* 2018 edition, to conform to the current AORN Evidence Rating Model.

PATIENT AND WORKER SAFETY

GUIDELINE FOR MEDICATION SAFETY

The Guideline for Medication Safety has been approved by the AORN Guidelines Advisory Board. It was presented as a proposed guideline for comments by members and others. The guideline is effective September 1, 2017. The recommendations in the guideline are intended to be achievable and represent what is believed to be an optimal level of practice. Policies and procedures will reflect variations in practice settings and/or clinical situations that determine the degree to which the guideline can be implemented. AORN recognizes the many diverse settings in which perioperative nurses practice; therefore, this guideline is adaptable to all areas where operative or other invasive procedures may be performed.

Purpose

This document provides guidance to perioperative team members for developing, implementing, and evaluating safety precautions that may assist with decreasing medication errors throughout the six phases of the medication use process. The medication use process includes procuring medication, prescribing medication, transcribing medication orders, dispensing medication, administering medication, and monitoring patient outcomes. The dispensing of medications from the pharmacy to the caregiver or patient is considered to be outside the role of the perioperative RN and is not covered in this document.

Medication errors can occur at any point in the medication use process and may or may not be detected before administration of the medication. Errors detected before administration are commonly referred to as near miss errors.[1] Reports of medication errors show that errors can be influenced by many factors and may be connected to any person who is involved in the process. Results of medication errors can include substantial threats to patients, increased health care costs, and compromised patient confidence in the health care system.[2]

While the phases of the medication use process are the same in all practice settings where medications are administered, there are unique considerations specific to the perioperative setting, including the following:

- The transcription and documentation phase may be omitted or modified.
- Medication is removed from the original manufacturer's packaging for aseptic delivery to the sterile field.
- An intermediary (eg, scrub person) in sterile attire receives and transfers dispensed medications to the proceduralist or assistant who is in sterile attire.

- Medications dispensed to the sterile field may be handled by multiple individuals before administration.
- Medications may be ordered and administered by multiple health care providers.
- Medications may be labeled one way on the sterile field and a different way off the sterile field.
- Sensory distractions are intrinsic to the environment.[3]

The following topics are outside the scope of this document:

- adverse drug reactions,
- drug-drug interactions,
- dosing recommendations,
- drug diversion prevention,
- medication-specific recommendations for prescribing,
- recommendations for manufacturers (eg, labeling),
- recommendations for specific components of a computerized order entry system,
- interventions that apply to the pharmacy,
- situations involving products contaminated at the manufacturer or compounder,
- regulations and recommendations based on laws that do not apply in the United States,
- antibiotic and anticoagulant stewardship programs,
- situations involving prescription of potentially inappropriate medications,
- dispensing errors,
- management of drug shortages,
- selection and administration of anesthetic agents and medication,
- medication-specific disposal methods,
- the effect of culture on reporting of medication errors,
- off-label use of medications, and
- recommendations for implementation of bar coding.

Evidence Review

A medical librarian conducted a systematic search of the databases Ovid MEDLINE®, EBSCO CINAHL®, Scopus®, and the Cochrane Database of Systematic Reviews. The search was limited to literature published in English from 2011 through 2016. The lead author requested additional articles that either did not fit the original search criteria or were discovered during the evidence appraisal process. The lead author and the medical librarian also identified relevant guidelines from government agencies, professional organizations, and standards-setting bodies.

Search terms included subject headings such as *operating rooms, drug storage, adverse drug event, medication systems, drug labeling, medication errors, medical waste disposal, compounding,* and *drug administration.* Additional keywords and phrases included *drug diversion, name differentiation, verbal*

order, drug storage, medication reconciliation, and *medication cart.*

Included were research and non-research literature in English, complete publications, and publications with dates within the time restriction unless none were available. Excluded were non-peer-reviewed publications and older evidence within the time restriction when more recent evidence was available. Editorials, news, and brief items were excluded. Low-quality evidence was excluded when higher-quality evidence was available, and literature outside the time restriction was excluded when literature within the time restriction was available. Also excluded were articles that presented a bundled approach, articles that described medication errors and corrective situations involving nursing students, and prevalence studies with no interventions for correction. Some international studies were excluded because the results are not generalizable to the United States (Figure 1).

Articles identified in the search were provided to the project team for evaluation. The team consisted of the lead author and three evidence appraisers. The lead author divided the search results into topics and assigned members of the team to review and critically appraise each article using the AORN Research or Non-Research Evidence Appraisal Tools as appropriate. The literature was independently evaluated and appraised according to the strength and quality of the evidence. Each article was then assigned an appraisal score. The appraisal score is noted in brackets after each reference, as applicable.

The collective evidence supporting each intervention within a specific recommendation was summarized and the AORN Evidence Rating Model was used to rate the strength of the evidence. Factors considered in the review of the collective evidence were the quality of the evidence, the quantity of similar evidence on a given topic, and the consistency of evidence supporting a recommendation. The evidence rating is noted in brackets after each intervention.

Note: *The evidence summary table is available at http://www.aorn.org/evidencetables/.*

Editor's note: *MEDLINE is a registered trademark of the US National Library of Medicine's Medical Literature Analysis and Retrieval System, Bethesda, MD. CINAHL, Cumulative Index to Nursing and Allied Health Literature, is a registered trademark of EBSCO Industries, Birmingham, AL. Scopus is a registered trademark of Elsevier B.V., Amsterdam, The Netherlands.*

Recommendation I

The health care organization should establish a multidisciplinary team to be responsible for the oversight of the medication management plan.

The multidisciplinary team may be commonly known as the pharmacy and therapeutics committee or medication safety committee. Including representatives from all disciplines involved in the process strengthens policies and procedures, contributes to interprofessional collaboration, and may enhance teamwork and compliance. The collective evidence supports a multidisciplinary team approach to medication management and error prevention.[4-15]

I.a. The multidisciplinary team should include
  ○ perioperative RNs,
  ○ licensed independent practitioners,
  ○ anesthesia professionals,[16]
  ○ pharmacists,[11,17]
  ○ risk management/quality personnel,
  ○ purchasing personnel,
  ○ infection preventionists, and
  ○ administrators.
  [4: Limited Evidence]

Involving all health care professionals who participate in the medication use process assists with identifying medication error risk factors from a variety of perspectives.

I.a.1. One individual may represent more than one discipline, based on organizational staffing. *[5: Benefits Balanced with Harms]*
Health care organizations may assign multiple roles and responsibilities to a single individual.

I.b. The multidisciplinary team should develop, provide implementation oversight of, and evaluate the perioperative medication management plan. *[5: Benefits Balanced with Harms]*

Developing a medication management plan that incorporates structures, processes, and professional responsibilities into each of the six phases of the medication use process allows for identification of latent and active failures and provides a guideline for performing the steps of the medication use process.

I.b.1. The medication management plan should include a process for
  • procuring, storing, and disposing of all medications[11,18] (See Recommendations II and XI);
  • administering medication (See Recommendation V);
  • performing medication reconciliation (See Recommendation VI);
  • managing hazardous medications, when applicable (See Recommendation X);[19]
  • transcribing medication orders (See Recommendation XIII);
  • monitoring quality assurance and improvement (See Recommendation XV);
  • managing look-alike and sound-alike medications; *[5: Benefits Balanced with Harms]*
  • managing medication shortages, discontinuations, or recalls[14,20,21]; *[3: Moderate Evidence]*
  • managing high-alert medications[22]; *[2: High Evidence]* and
  • creating, maintaining, and reviewing preference cards and standing order forms. *[5: Benefits Balanced with Harms]*

FIGURE 1. FLOW DIAGRAM OF LITERATURE SEARCH RESULTS

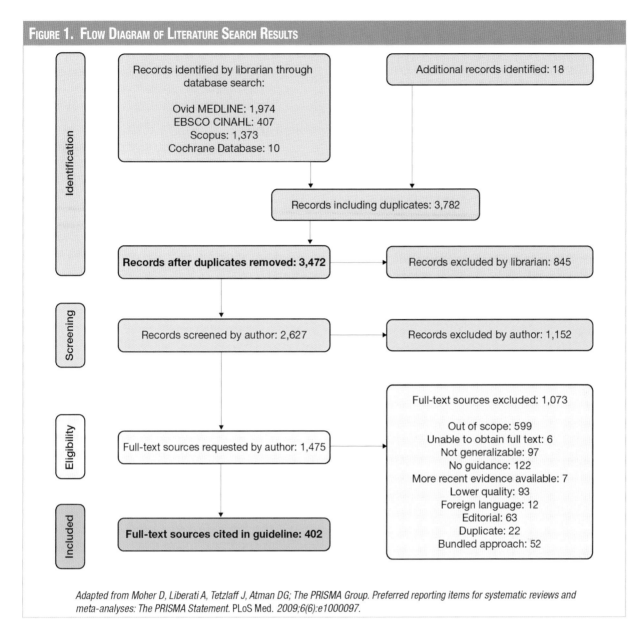

Adapted from Moher D, Liberati A, Tetzlaff J, Atman DG; The PRISMA Group. Preferred reporting items for systematic reviews and meta-analyses: The PRISMA Statement. PLoS Med. 2009;6(6):e1000097.

I.b.2. The perioperative medication plan should align with the facility or health care organization medication plan. *[5: Benefits Balanced with Harms]*

I.b.3. The multidisciplinary team should communicate the medication management plan to all members of the perioperative team. *[4: Limited Evidence]*

Increasing the perioperative team's awareness of the health care organization's medication management plan disseminates a broader picture of medication risk-reduction strategies and can help communicate the interdependence of the team's actions.[14]

I.b.4. The medication management plan should be implemented consistently in all areas where operative and other invasive procedures are performed. *[5: Benefits Balanced with Harms]*

I.c. The multidisciplinary team should

○ establish, monitor, and review the portion of the formulary unique to the perioperative services[11,23]; *[1: Strong Evidence]*

○ establish, monitor, and review medications that are routinely stocked at par level in perioperative medication storage areas; *[5: Benefits Balanced with Harms]*

○ establish the frequency of the review of the formulary and medication stock; *[5: Benefits Balanced with Harms]*

○ establish the type of labels to be used, including preprinted labels for use on the sterile field[24]; *[4: Limited Evidence]*

○ define the scope, role, orientation, and assessment of competency for supplemental personnel (eg, temporary personnel, contracted pharmacist) as related to the medication use process; *[5: Benefits Balanced with Harms]* and

○ standardize medication-related perioperative documents. *[5: Benefits Balanced with Harms]*

The author of an organizational experience report found compliance with labeling of medications improved with the use of preprinted labels.[25]

I.d. The multidisciplinary team should select technological devices (eg, bar-code systems, computerized prescriber order entry system, biometrics, pharmacy automation, radio-frequency identification systems, electronic medication storage and inventory systems, electronic medication administration records, electronic medication reconciliation tools) to be used during all phases of the medication use process based primarily on the safety aspects incorporated into each device. *[2: High Evidence]*

The collective evidence supports the use of technological devices to decrease medication errors[26-47] or the potential for errors.[48-51] In addition, the evidence establishes other benefits for the use of technological devices, including providing nurses with more patient contact time,[52] improving medication order turnaround time,[53-55] and decreasing prescribing time.[55-58]

The use of computerized ordering systems has also been shown to result in fewer illegible and incomplete prescriptions.[59-61] Meisenberg et al[62] conducted a quality study that found preprinted orders contained fewer errors than handwritten orders, and orders entered in a computerized prescriber order entry system contained even fewer errors. Eighty-five (91%) of the 93 physicians who responded to a survey believed that computerized order entry decreased the number of medication errors compared to handwritten prescriptions.[63] In addition, in other nonexperimental studies, use of automated dispensing cabinets has been shown to decrease the number of medication selection and preparation errors[64,65] and increase efficiency.[66]

Conversely, some of the literature documents situations in which medication errors continued to occur or new errors occurred following implementation of computerized medication information systems (eg, selection of the wrong medication from the list on the computer).[47,62,67-84] In addition, in an observational, cross-sectional comparative study, Hinojosa-Amaya et al[85] found that the number of errors decreased but the severity of the errors increased when a computerized prescriber order entry system was instituted. The severity of errors was measured on a 9-point scale ranging from "capacity to cause error" to "contributes to or causes death."

In a review of the literature, Fischer[34] found that the number of errors decreased when computerized order entry was used, but the author could not determine whether there was an association between the errors and patient harm. Another review of the literature identified that some of the medication errors connected with computerized order entry include wrong-patient errors; duplicate orders; and selection of the wrong dose, wrong route, wrong timing, and wrong drug.[86] In a quasi-experimental study, Leung et al[87] found a 45% decrease in the number of preventable adverse drug events with the use of a computerized order entry system with advanced clinical decision support, but the number of potential adverse drug events increased significantly.

In a qualitative study, Hoonakker et al[88] found that computerized prescriber order entry systems disrupted the quality of physician–nurse communication for the short term (ie, 3 months), but the quality of communication returned to pre-implementation levels in the long term (ie, 12 months).

Tschannen et al[89] reviewed the effects of the implementation of a computerized order entry system on nursing workflow and found that the process to confirm orders was lengthened and there was a reduction in communication between medical and nursing personnel. The researchers theorized this could lead to an increase in medication errors.

I.e. The multidisciplinary team should develop and review a list of do-not-use abbreviations and symbols that are inappropriate for inclusion in documentation. *[3: Moderate Evidence]*

Two studies found that even with a "do not use" list, problems persisted because prescribers continued to use other error-prone abbreviations that were not on the list.[90,91]

I.f. The health care organization must provide resources to the perioperative team, such as up-to-date online reference materials and access to drug information centers.[23] *[1: Regulatory Requirement]*

Regulatory and professional guidelines, a review of the literature, and a descriptive study of medication errors in an intensive care unit emphasize the importance of having various resources available to help prevent medication errors.[9,23,92,93]

I.g. Pharmacists should be involved in all phases of medication management. *[3: Moderate Evidence]*

There is general agreement worldwide that benefits are realized when a pharmacist is involved in all phases of the medication use process. These benefits include a decrease in readmissions, decreased medication discrepancies upon discharge, identification of medication errors before administration, and decreased costs.[9,11,94-122] Two studies involving critical access facilities found fewer dispensing errors when the dispensing was done by a pharmacist compared to a telepharmacy service[65] and fewer medication errors when a pharmacist was present at least 40 hours per week.[123]

Conversely, McCoy et al[124] conducted a randomized clinical trial that sought to determine whether pharmacy surveillance of patients with acute kidney injury would detect and prevent medication errors that were not corrected by the electronic clinical support system. The researchers did not find a significant decrease in the number of errors and concluded that pharmacy surveillance did not show an incremental benefit over the clinical decision support systems already in place.

Evidence supports the involvement of a pharmacist in medication reconciliation.[102,125,126] Some of the evidence supports medication reconciliation being performed by a pharmacist instead of nurses,[127,128] a resident/intern,[129] or a pharmacy technician.[128] Aag et al[130] found that the medication reconciliation process was completed in less time by the pharmacist than by a nurse, but there was not a significant difference in the number of discrepancies found. Zemaitis et al[131] found a decrease in readmission rates when a pharmacist performed medication reconciliation.

I.g.1.   The health care organization may contract with a pharmacist to provide consultative services onsite or via telepharmacy.[23,132,133] *[1: Strong Evidence]*

The Centers for Medicare & Medicaid Services (CMS) Conditions of Participation states that "Hospitals must provide pharmaceutical services that meet the needs of their patients."[23] The CMS Conditions of Coverage for ambulatory surgery centers (ASCs) states that a specific licensed health care professional is required to provide direction to the ASC's pharmaceutical service unless the ASC is performing activities that under state law may only be performed by a licensed pharmacist.[132] **Amb**

Recommendation II

Precautions should be taken to mitigate the risks associated with medication and medication-related supply procurement and storage.

The literature, including regulatory requirements, describes several strategies for safe procurement and storage of medication.[14,23,132,134-137]

II.a.   Medications should be procured
- as single-dose units if available,
- in a size as close as possible to the anticipated dose,
- in prefilled syringes if available, and
- in limited concentrations.

[3: Moderate Evidence]

Procurement of single-dose vials in the smallest available size produces less waste,[134-136] and prefilled syringes eliminate the potential for re-labeling errors.[137]

II.b.   All medications and related supplies must be stored securely in areas with limited access, including refrigerated areas, anesthesia carts, and emergency carts.[14,23,138] *[1: Regulatory Requirement]*

The CMS states,

The operating room suite is considered secure when the suite is staffed and staff are actively providing patient care. When the suite is not in use (e.g., weekends, holidays and after hours), it would not be considered secure. A hospital may choose to lock the entire suite, lock non-mobile carts containing drugs and biologicals, place mobile carts in a locked room, or otherwise lock drugs and biologicals in a secure area. If an individual operating room is not in use, the hospital is expected to lock non-mobile carts, and ensure mobile carts are in a locked room. . . . Due to their mobility, mobile nursing medication carts, anesthesia carts, epidural carts and other medication carts containing drugs or biologicals . . . must be locked in a secure area when not in use.[23]

II.c.   Medications should be stored according to the specifications (eg, temperature) stated in the medication manufacturer's instructions for use.[11,14,23] *[2: High Evidence]*

Medications may have sensitive formulations that require storage at specific temperature ranges to maintain stability or avoid inactivation. Failure to control the temperature of medication storage areas may result in decreased therapeutic levels caused by inactivation, a change in pH, a change in concentration, or spoilage. Temperature-sensitive medications have been shown to deteriorate when stored outside of the recommended temperature ranges.[139]

II.c.1.   Medications that require refrigeration must be stored in a segregated area of the refrigerator with restricted access.[132] *[1: Regulatory Requirement]*

II.d.   All Class II, III, IV, and V medications must be stored in a locked location.[23,132] *[1: Regulatory Requirement]* **Amb**

II.e.   Medications in the storage areas including emergency and specialty carts should be organized in a standardized manner using safety considerations, including
- separating medications by generic name and packaging;
- separating high-alert medications;

299

- providing separate bins or dividers for all medications in storage;
- labeling storage bins, using tall man lettering when possible, with both the medication's generic and brand names;
- positioning medication containers so that the labels are visible; and
- avoiding alphabetical storage.

[3: Moderate Evidence]

Placing medications in storage areas using these safety considerations may assist in selection of the correct medication and decrease the potential for medication errors.[140,141]

II.e.1.   Sound-alike and look-alike medications should be separated in storage locations.[10,137,142] *[4: Limited Evidence]*

Incidents of the wrong medication being selected because of look-alike containers and labels have been reported in the literature.[77,137,140,143-149]

Recommendation III

Precautions should be taken to mitigate the risk for medication errors in the prescribing phase of the medication use process.

The collective evidence establishes that medication errors occur during the prescribing phase. The reported errors are related to the use of incorrect abbreviations, illegible handwriting, and incomplete information.[6,70,79,82,150-152]

III.a.   All medications must be prescribed by a licensed independent practitioner in accordance with state and federal regulatory requirements. *[1: Regulatory Requirement]*

Regulatory requirements direct prescriptive authority.[11,14,23,132,153-155]

III.b.   Medication orders
- should not contain trailing zeros;
- should contain leading zeros, if the dose is less than 1 unit of the selected unit of measure; and
- should contain only approved abbreviations.[91,155-157]

[3: Moderate Evidence]

Clinical guidelines provide recommendations for the required elements of medication orders.[9,17,154,158,159] In a nonexperimental study of medication administration, Gimenes et al[82] found that 91.3% of the prescriptions contained abbreviations. The researchers recommended using no abbreviations or acronyms.

III.b.1.   Handwritten medication orders should be legible and include a legible signature of the prescriber initiating the order. *[5: Benefits Balanced with Harms]* Amb

III.c.   Pick lists, preference cards, and protocols that contain orders for medications may be considered preprinted orders if so defined in the facility or health care organization policy and proce-

dure. When considered preprinted orders, these should be placed in the patient's medical record unless the order is recorded by another means. *[5: Benefits Balanced with Harms]*

No evidence defining pick lists, preference cards, or protocols was found in the literature review for this guideline. Use of standing orders is a commonly accepted practice throughout the United States. The literature did not reveal any specific evidence related to medications included in standing orders; however, there are regulatory requirements for documentation of medication orders.[23,132]

III.c.1.   Preprinted orders must be reviewed for accuracy by the prescribing licensed independent practitioner at least annually and after every change.[23,132,159,160] *[1: Regulatory Requirement]*

III.c.2.   A written order to reflect items requiring a prescriber's order must be placed in the patient's medical record.[23] *[1: Regulatory Requirement]*

III.d.   Verbal medication orders, which must only be used when required by clinical necessity, should
- be received and carried out only by persons who are authorized to do so, consistent with federal and state law and the health care organization policy and procedures;
- be confirmed by reading back the order to the prescriber digit by digit and spelling out the medication name if necessary;
- be immediately recorded in the patient's record;
- be reviewed, validated, and signed by the prescriber as close as possible to the time of the medication administration;
- contain a legible signature of the person documenting the order; and
- contain all components of a written order.

[1: Regulatory Requirement]

The CMS regulations and professional practice guidelines identify the necessary elements for safe use of verbal orders.[14,23,132,161,162] Verbal orders can be misinterpreted for a number of reasons, including but not limited to, regional dialects, background noise, muffled voices behind surgical masks, and orders involving sound-alike or commonly confused medication names. Verbal orders have been the source of medication errors.[161]

Recommendation IV

Precautions should be taken to mitigate the risk of medication errors occurring when the medication is obtained and prepared.

Grou Volpe et al[8] conducted a descriptive study of medication errors that involved 484 medication administrations; 293 of the administrations (61%) contained errors that occurred during the preparation phase. Preparation errors were defined as any discrepancy that occurred during the preparation and formulation of the medication. The preparation errors included incorrect dilution, mixing of two incompatible medications, and inadequate packaging. The researchers did not define "inadequate packaging."

IV.a.   Medications should be retrieved from storage bins, automated dispensing storage systems, or a satellite pharmacy for only one patient at a time. *[4: Limited Evidence]*

Retrieving medications for more than one patient at a time may increase the risk for error. Medication administration errors have occurred because a perioperative nurse retrieved the wrong product from an automated dispensing system.[163] If a restocking error has occurred, it is more likely to be detected if the nurse is focused on each medication required for the individual patient at the time the medication is being retrieved.

IV.a.1.   All medications obtained from storage should be verified against the original medication order. *[4: Limited Evidence]*

The original medication order, including preprinted order forms, prescriptions, or preference cards, establishes what medication the prescriber intended the patient to receive. Automated dispensing storage systems have been reported to have up to a 5% misfill rate.[164] As medications are obtained, an additional visual confirmation of the order and product will help establish accuracy in administering the correct medication.

IV.b.   Compounded medications prepared by a compounding pharmacy that meets the standards specified in USP 797 should be used when available.[165] *[2: High Evidence]*

The evidence supports medication compounding in a pharmacy and under sterile conditions to decrease the potential for contamination.[17,165-167]

IV.c.   When medications compounded by a compounding pharmacy that meets the standards specified in USP 797 are not available, medications may be compounded in the perioperative suite for immediate use.[165] *[2: High Evidence]*

IV.c.1.   Perioperative personnel performing compounding in the perioperative suite must
- have completed competency verification;
- combine no more than three medications together;
- perform hand hygiene before compounding;
- disinfect nonsterile surfaces including the medication container;
- use aseptic technique;
- use dispensing equipment or a sterile syringe for removal of medication from the container;
- verify the correct medication, amount, and concentration;
- visually inspect the compounded medication for absence of particulate material; and
- apply a label unless the medication is being immediately administered or verify the label applied by the scrub person if medication is transferred to the sterile field.[23,165]

IV.c.2.   Administration of medications compounded in the perioperative suite must begin within 1 hour of compounding.[23,165] *[1: Regulatory Requirement]*

Medications compounded in the perioperative suite are considered to be at high risk for contamination because they have been compounded in a location where room air quality is less than ISO Class 5.[165]

IV.c.3.   Medications compounded in the perioperative suite must be under continuous observation if not administered immediately. *[1: Regulatory Requirement]*

Continuous observation reduces the potential for contamination or confusion with other compounded preparations.[23,165]

IV.d.   Compounded preparations prepared off the sterile field should be labeled with
- patient identification information,
- the names and amounts of all ingredients,
- the name or initials of the person who prepared the compound,
- the date of preparation, and
- the beyond-use date and time (See Recommendation VII for labeling requirements on the sterile field).[9,23,137,168]

[3: Moderate Evidence]

IV.d.1.   When a medication is compounded off the sterile field and will be either administered immediately or delivered immediately to the sterile field, labeling is not required.

IV.d.2.   When a medication is prepared in multiple concentrations, the labels should be different colors.[166] *[4: Limited Evidence]*

IV.d.3.   The medication label should contain the full medication name; the name should not be abbreviated.[169] *[4: Limited Evidence]*

IV.d.4.   Tall man lettering should be used on labels placed on containers (eg, syringes, sterile medication cups, IV bags) if medications have look-alike or sound-alike names (See Recommendation VII.e.1). *[3: Moderate Evidence]*

The evidence supports the use of tall man lettering to increase name differentiation between look-alike medication names.[9,10,16,17,24,140,142,170-175]

301

Recommendation V

Precautions should be taken to mitigate the risk for errors during medication administration.

The collective evidence describes the causes of medication errors that occur during the administration phase.[8,70,168,176] Causes include dosage miscalculation,[6,177] name mix-ups,[77,143,178-182] omissions errors,[6,8,150,151] wrong time,[6,8,150] and syringe swap.[183]

V.a.   All medications should be administered according to the manufacturer's instructions for use. *[5: Benefits Balanced with Harms]*

Manufacturer's instructions provide specific instructions for dosage and administration.

V.b.   Before administering medication, perioperative personnel who administer medications should verify the
- right patient using at least two patient identifiers,
- right medication,
- right dose,
- right route,
- right time,
- right strength or concentration,
- right medication administration rate, and
- infusion pump settings, if applicable.[3,23,141]
[2: High Evidence]

V.b.1.   Compatibility of medications administered through a single IV line should be verified before concurrent administration. *[2: High Evidence]*

In a descriptive study, Kanji et al[184] reviewed 434 simultaneously administered medication infusions and found that 68% contained medications that were considered to be incompatible but were administered simultaneously through the same IV tubing. The researchers did not report on the outcomes of the patients in the study.

V.b.2.   A dosage calculation tool may be used to calculate maximum dose limits, especially for high-alert medications. *[5: Benefits Balanced with Harms]*

V.c.   Perioperative care providers administering medications should verify that the patient is not allergic to the medication. *[3: Moderate Evidence]*

Adverse events have been reported because allergies were not verified.[185]

V.d.   Perioperative care providers administering medications should verify that the medication dose is correctly adjusted to the patient's weight. *[3: Moderate Evidence]*

Adverse events have been reported because the dosage was not appropriate for the weight of the patient.[9,186]

V.e.   A double-checking system (eg, independent double check) performed by two licensed individuals should be developed and used for predetermined high-alert and high-risk medications (eg, insulin, heparin). *[3: Moderate Evidence]*

The collective evidence supports double checking of high-alert and high-risk medications to decrease medication administration errors.[9,17,137,141,155,168,187-190] However, after conducting a systematic literature review, Alsulami et al[191] concluded that there was insufficient evidence to support or refute the practice of double checking. The review consisted of 16 studies including three qualitative studies and one randomized controlled trial. The researchers recommended that more studies be completed to determine the efficacy of double checking high-alert and high-risk medications.

V.f.   The preoperative RN should confirm that the patient has taken or discontinued medications and herbal supplements on the day of surgery or the designated number of days before surgery as ordered by the licensed independent practitioner. *[5: Benefits Balanced with Harms]*

V.f.1.   The perioperative RN should notify the physician and anesthesia professional if the patient has not taken or has not discontinued medications as ordered. *[5: Benefits Balanced with Harms]*

V.g.   Perioperative personnel who administer medications should not be interrupted or distracted when preparing and administering medications. *[3: Moderate Evidence]*

The collective evidence supports preventing interruptions and distractions during medication administration because interruptions have been shown to be a cause of medication errors.[7,176,192-201]

V.g.1.   A distraction- and interruption-free zone should be used when available.[202] *[3: Moderate Evidence]*

V.g.2.   A do-not-interrupt signal method (eg, a "do not disturb" sign, vest, verbal cue) should be used during medication administration. *[3: Moderate Evidence]*

The use of do-not-interrupt signals to indicate when the person administering or preparing medications should not be disturbed has been shown to contribute to decreasing medication errors.[10,192,193,200-204]

V.g.3.   A standard phrase, such as "I cannot be interrupted now," established by the health care organization's policy and procedure may be used to help prevent interruptions during medication administration.[201,202] *[3: Moderate Evidence]*

V.h.   Single-dose/single-use vials and single-use dispensing devices should be used on only one patient. *[3: Moderate Evidence]*

The collective evidence contains reports of infections being transmitted by the reuse of single-patient vials and single-use dispensing devices (eg, insulin pens) on more than one patient.[134,205-208] The contamination of single-use medication vials has also been demonstrated in laboratory studies.[209] In a nonexperimental study, Baniasadi et al[210] examined opened single and multidose vials that were within their use date and found both types of vials were contaminated after the initial medication withdrawal.

V.h.1.   A sterile needle and a sterile syringe should be used each time a medication is withdrawn from a single-dose/single-use vial. [3: Moderate Evidence]

A Joint Commission *Sentinel Event Alert* and a case study contain reports of bacterial and viral (eg, hepatitis B and C) infections being spread by the reuse of needles and syringes.[134,211]

V.i.   Multidose vials should be used for only one patient when medication is prepared at the point of use. [3: Moderate Evidence]

The collective evidence contains reports of infections being spread by use of a multidose vial for more than one patient.[134,212-214]

V.i.1.   A sterile needle and a sterile syringe should be used each time a medication is withdrawn from a multidose vial. [4: Limited Evidence]

The literature contains reports of infections being spread by the use of a multidose vial for more than one patient and recommends use of a sterile needle and a sterile syringe each time a vial is entered.[134,211,215,216]

V.i.2.   Multidose vials should be labeled at the time of first use with a beyond-use date of 28 days or as specified by the manufacturer.[165] [2: High Evidence]

When a product has been opened or a vial cap has been punctured or removed, the manufacturer's expiration date is no longer valid unless it is within the 28-day limit.[134]

V.i.3.   When a multidose vial is supplied with individual applicator tips, the applicator tip should be changed between uses for different patients. [3: Moderate Evidence]

One nonexperimental study showed no contamination of the solution when a fresh tip was used.[217]

V.j.   Multidose vials should be stored outside the immediate patient treatment area when possible.[134] [3: Moderate Evidence]

V.k.   The rubber septum on all vials should be disinfected with alcohol and allowed to dry before each entry. [3: Moderate Evidence]

The evidence supports disinfecting the rubber septum to remove any contaminant present on the stopper.[134,218]

V.l.   A syringe and needle should be used only once to administer a medication to a single patient, after which the syringe and needle should be discarded. [5: Benefits Balanced with Harms]

V.l.1.   When administering incremental doses to a single patient from the same syringe is an integral part of the procedure, the same syringe and needle may be reused, with strict adherence to aseptic technique. [5: Benefits Balanced with Harms]

V.l.2.   The syringe should never be left unattended and should be discarded immediately at the end of the procedure. [5: Benefits Balanced with Harms]

V.m.   Labels on all containers should be carefully read before contents are removed for preparation or administration. [4: Limited Evidence]

The literature contains reports of medication errors resulting from syringe swaps and clearly labeled syringes not being read carefully by the person administering the medication.[137,168,219] Wearing colored lenses, such as laser goggles, may distort the wearer's ability to determine the color of the label.[220]

V.n.   All medication containers (eg, vials, ampules) for which the sterility has been compromised should be discarded.[134] [3: Moderate Evidence]

V.o.   Unused, opened irrigation or IV solutions should be discarded at the end of the procedure. [5: Benefits Balanced with Harms]

Irrigation and IV containers and supplies are considered to be for single-patient use. Using surplus volume from any irrigation or IV solution containers or supplies for more than one patient increases the risk of cross contamination.

V.p.   Medications that are removed from the original package and found in a secondary container without a label should be discarded. [5: Benefits Balanced with Harms]

Medications that are removed from the original package and not labeled cannot be verified before administration, which may increase the risk for administering the wrong medication.

V.q.   Intravenous solution containers should be punctured (eg, spiked) within 1 hour of the initiation of administration. [2: High Evidence]

The Association for Professionals in Infection Control and Epidemiology supports beginning administration within 1 hour of the medication being spiked.[221]

Haas et al[222] tested lactated Ringer's solution for bacterial contamination at various times (ie, at the time of spiking; 1, 2, 4, and 8 hours after spiking) and found no bacterial growth at any of the time points. The mean number of bags sampled was 16 (range, 15 to 17) at each time point. A limitation of this study is that the test was not conducted on any other solutions used in the clinical setting.

V.r.   Precautions should be taken to mitigate the risk for errors associated with tubing, including
- tracing all tubing to the point of origin and point of insertion,
- labeling all tubing and injection ports with the point of exit (eg, epidural, arterial, venous),
- avoiding the use of y-port extension tubing,
- aligning tubing to avoid tangling and to facilitate easy identification,
- avoiding use of standard Luer-lock syringes for medications intended for oral or enteric administration,
- allowing only individuals who have been deemed competent to manage connections and lines, and
- using only non-Luer-lock connectors on spinal, epidural, and combined spinal/epidural devices.[168]

[4: Limited Evidence]

The literature contains reports of medication errors related to tubing misconnections and tubing mixups that support the use of the precautions listed.[17,146,189,223-230]

V.s.   All used medication vials and delivery devices should be retained in the OR or invasive procedure room until the completion of the procedure.[188] [3: Moderate Evidence]

Recommendation VI

Precautions should be taken to mitigate the risk for errors during the transitions of care between phases of perioperative care.

Evidence from national and international sources supports the use of medication reconciliation as a method for detecting potential medication errors, reducing hospital admissions,[155,231,232] and creating financial savings.[128,231-233] The errors consist of omissions,[234] medications prescribed without indication,[235] incorrect routes, and incorrect dosages.[231,236-259] Conversely, a systematic review of the literature and a quasi-experimental study did not find a benefit to medication reconciliation.[260,261] Medication errors have been reported to occur during all phases of perioperative care.[262,263] This recommendation specifies the role of the perioperative nurse in the reconciliation process and includes the information that should be shared at the time of a transition of care.

VI.a.   The preoperative RN or designated professional should obtain a baseline medication history at admission.[262] [2: Moderate Evidence]

VI.a.1.   The medication history should include
- the patient's allergies and symptoms of reaction and
- all products taken regularly or as needed and administered via all routes, including prescribed and nonprescribed medications and herbal and dietary supplements. [2: High Evidence]

An analysis of medication errors supports including these components in a medication history.[253] This list of medications is the first step in the medication reconciliation process and provides information necessary for reconciling the patient's medications at the time of discharge.[262] Many patients take herbal remedies that may interact with prescribed medications and affect postprocedure patient outcomes.[264]

VI.a.2.   The medication history should include the name, dose, frequency, route, purpose, and date and time of the last dose taken for each item listed. [5: Benefits Balanced with Harms]

VI.a.3.   The medication history should be obtained by interview with the patient or caregivers and, if information is missing, additional sources (eg, the primary physician's office, pharmacy, primary caregivers including home health nurses) may be consulted. [3: Moderate Evidence]

The evidence supports obtaining the list of medications by interview instead of by using only the existing medical record because discrepancies have been found between medical records and patient-stated lists.[265] The evidence also supports use of other sources because inaccuracies have been discovered in medication histories obtained strictly from patients.[266]

VI.b.   The medication history and medications administered during each phase of care should be communicated to the receiving caregiver by a person designated by the health care organization. [5: Benefits Balanced with Harms]

Sharing of information regarding the medication history and medications administered may decrease medication errors.

VI.b.1.   The information provided to the receiving caregiver using the means described in the facility or health care organization policy and procedure should include the following:
- Preoperative to intraoperative phase:
  - medication allergies and reaction,
  - preoperative medication history including the last dose taken,
  - medications administered during the preoperative phase including the dose and time, and
  - effects of medications administered during the preoperative phase.
- Intraoperative change of personnel:
  - medication allergies and reactions,
  - preoperative medication history including the last dose taken,

- medications administered during the preoperative phase including the dose and time,
- effects of medications administered during the preoperative phase,
- medications administered during intraoperative phase including the dose and time,
- IV and irrigation fluids administered intraoperatively,
- anesthesia type and route,
- current or pending laboratory or other test results that relate to medications, and
- medications present on the sterile field.

- Intraoperative to postoperative phase I or phase II:
  - medication allergies and reaction,
  - preoperative medication history including the last dose taken,
  - medications received during the preoperative phase including the dose and time,
  - effects of medications received during the preoperative phase,
  - medications administered during the intraoperative phase including the dose and time,
  - patient responses to medications administered during the intraoperative phase,
  - IV and irrigation fluids administered,
  - anesthesia type and route,
  - current or pending laboratory or other test results that relate to medications,
  - infusion pump settings if applicable, and
  - surgeon's orders for medications if present.

- Postoperative phase I to postoperative phase II or to an inpatient caregiver:
  - medication allergies,
  - preoperative medication history including the last dose taken,
  - medications received during the preoperative phase including the dose and time,
  - effects of medications received during the preoperative phase,
  - medications administered during the intraoperative phase including the dose and time,
  - effects of medications received during the intraoperative phase,
  - IV and irrigation fluids administered,
  - anesthesia type and route,
  - current or pending laboratory or other test results that relate to medications,
  - infusion pump settings if applicable,
  - surgeon's orders for medications if present,

- medications administered during the postoperative phase including the dose and time,
- the patient's responses to medications administered during the postoperative phase, and
- IV fluids administered.
  [5: Benefits Balanced with Harms]

VI.c. The medication reconciliation process should be completed before the patient is discharged. *[3: Moderate Evidence]*

The collective evidence supports performing medication reconciliation during all phases of care to decrease medication errors and unintentional discrepancies.[4,14,216,245,253,262,267-275] The evidence specific to the perioperative setting is limited; however, the evidence derived from other settings is relevant to perioperative care. Some of the literature revealed that medication errors do occur after medication reconciliation[276]; however, the reported errors did not affect patient outcomes.[277]

VI.c.1. The medication reconciliation process should include a comparison of the medication history to the postdischarge medication instructions and verification that medications ordered are indicated and dosages are appropriate. *[5: Benefits Balanced with Harms]*

VI.c.2. The person performing medication reconciliation should consult with or alert the prescriber if discrepancies between the admission history and the discharge medication list are found. *[5: Benefits Balanced with Harms]*

VI.c.3. The person performing medication reconciliation should document the results of the consultation. *[5: Benefits Balanced with Harms]*

VI.d. The medication reconciliation process should
- be standardized for all patients,
- include the use of a standardized medication reconciliation form that may be electronic with a scripted list of questions or prompts,[234] and
- engage patients and their caregivers.[31,278-281]
[2: High Evidence]

Recommendation VII

Precautions should be taken to mitigate the risk for errors during transfer of medications to the sterile field and handling of medications on the sterile field.

The literature contains reports of errors including incorrect medications being drawn up from unlabeled bowls and incorrect medications being administered from unlabeled syringes on the sterile field.[16,24,282]

305

VII.a. Before transferring medication to the sterile field, the RN circulator should check the expiration date and visually inspect the medication for any indication that the medication was compromised during the storage process (eg, particulates, discoloration). If there is any question of compromise, the item should not be transferred to the sterile field and should be discarded according to facility or health care organization policy and procedure. *[5: Benefits Balanced with Harms]*

VII.b. The RN circulator transferring the medication to the sterile field and the person receiving the medication should concurrently verify the medication name, strength, dosage, and expiration date by reading the label aloud.[16,24,140,283] *[3: Moderate Evidence]*

VII.c. Aseptic technique should be used during transfer of medications to the sterile field.[284] *[1: Strong Evidence]*

VII.c.1. Rubber stoppers should not be removed from vials unless they are designed to be removed. *[5: Benefits Balanced with Harms]*

VII.c.2. A commercially available sterile transfer device (eg, sterile vial spike, filter straw, plastic catheter) should be used to deliver medications to the sterile field. *[5: Benefits Balanced with Harms]*

Medication vials are not designed to pour the contents aseptically into a secondary container on the sterile field. Transfer devices are designed to minimize splashing, spilling, and the need to reach over the sterile field, which may cause contamination of the sterile field.

VII.d. Only one medication at a time should be transferred to the sterile field, followed immediately by application of the label before another medication or solution is transferred.[16,24,283] *[4: Limited Evidence]*

VII.e. Containers and syringes on the sterile field that contain medications, solutions, chemicals, and reagents should be labeled immediately after they are received[141] *[3: Moderate Evidence]*

o with the medication name, strength, dilution and diluent if used, date, and time accepted on to the sterile field[141]; *[3: Moderate Evidence]*

o with no abbreviations or only approved abbreviations and dose expressions[175]; *[2: High Evidence]* and

o without unnecessary information.[175] *[2: High Evidence]*

VII.e.1. Tall man lettering should be used on labels placed on containers (eg, syringes, sterile medication cups, IV bags) and shelving and bins containing products with look-alike names. *[3: Moderate Evidence]*

The evidence supports the use of tall man lettering to increase name differentiation between look-alike medication names.[9,10,16,17,24,140,142,170-175] Or and Wang[285] found that tall man lettering increased differentiation accuracy, but other typographic styles were also effective.

VII.f. The RN circulator transferring the medication to the sterile field and the person receiving the medication should concurrently verify the label on the medication container on the sterile field. *[5: Benefits Balanced with Harms]*

VII.g. The label of the medications, solutions, chemicals, and reagents should be verified at the time of relief of the RN circulator or the scrub person.[24,283] *[4: Limited Evidence]*

Hand overs involving multiple personnel increase the risk for miscommunication. Enhancing communication among perioperative team members may help reduce medication errors.

VII.h. Unlabeled solutions on the sterile field should be discarded.[24] *[4: Limited Evidence]*

VII.i. Medications, solutions, chemicals, and reagents should be delivered to the sterile field as close as possible to the time they will be administered.[24,283] *[4: Limited Evidence]*

VII.j. If there is no designated scrub person, the licensed person delivering the medication to the sterile field should confirm the medication visually and verbally with the licensed independent practitioner performing the procedure. *[5: Benefits Balanced with Harms]*

VII.k. Verbal confirmation should be given when a medication is passed to the licensed independent practitioner for subsequent administration, even when only one medication is on the sterile field. *[5: Benefits Balanced with Harms]*

A standardized method of communication may help reduce the risk for error involving medications on the sterile field.

Recommendation VIII

Perioperative team members who are responsible for medication administration must monitor the patient for therapeutic effect or adverse reactions to medications.[23]

Adverse patient outcomes as a result of inadequate monitoring after medication administration are reported in the literature.[6,70,178,286] Assessing the patient's response to medication provides information related to dose effectiveness and the identification of symptoms of a potential medication-related adverse effect (eg, anaphylaxis, toxicity), which facilitates a timely and effective response. Monitoring the patient for effects of medications is consistent with professional standards associated with the medication use process.[287]

VIII.a. Perioperative team members who are responsible for medication administration should monitor and document the patient's physiological and psychological responses. The physiological and psychological responses monitored (eg, heart rate and rhythm, blood pressure, level of consciousness) should be based on the patient's condition and needs and the procedure performed. The frequency should be as described in the facility policy and procedure.[17,23,288,289] *[1: Regulatory Requirement]*

VIII.a.1. Perioperative personnel who are responsible for medication administration should document patient responses as close as possible to the time the medication was administered and the response was observed. *[5: Benefits Balanced with Harms]*

VIII.b. The patient's medication regimen should be included in the postprocedure assessment (eg, postdischarge telephone call) completed by the perioperative RN or pharmacist. *[5: Benefits Balanced with Harms]*

Including the patient's medication regimen in the postprocedure assessment provides an opportunity to confirm the patient's status, response to medications, actual adverse conditions (eg, nausea, vomiting, ineffective pain control, inability to perform activities of daily living), and knowledge and compliance with the medication regimen.

Recommendation IX

A person designated by the health care organization must provide education regarding the preoperative and postoperative medication regimen to the patient, caregivers, and other individuals involved in the patient's care.[23,132]

Evidence supports patient education and shows patients may not understand their medication regimen.[242] Education is connected with decreasing adverse drug events related to medications improperly self-administered by the patient after discharge[182] and helps decrease readmissions.[117,127]

IX.a. Preprocedure education should include which medications are to be held and which medications are to be taken.[290] *[3: Moderate Evidence]*

IX.b. Postprocedure education should include
  ○ a list of medications to be taken;
  ○ when to discontinue medications;
  ○ when to resume medications that were being taken;
  ○ a list of discontinued medications;
  ○ the method of measurement and self-administration of medications, including injection techniques if injectable medications are prescribed;
  ○ medication safety precautions (eg, medications should be taken only as prescribed, medications should not be shared, medications should be secured);

  ○ when to obtain medication-related laboratory tests;
  ○ potential adverse effects and when to seek medical attention;
  ○ the method of storage and handling;
  ○ the method of disposal for unused medications;
  ○ use of patient-controlled administration devices;
  ○ the importance of keeping a list of current allergies and current medications; and
  ○ sources for additional information and ongoing education.[134,155,242,273,291-298]
  [3: Moderate Evidence]

In addition, evidence suggests that patient education at discharge improves patient satisfaction and medication adherence.[299] Valente and Murray[300] found that after 500 patients returning for care in a physician's office received educational materials on the significance of allergies, 340 of the patients submitted amended forms listing allergies not previously included on their medical records. They concluded that the education resulted in an improvement in the accuracy of the allergies listed on the medical records. Patient education is also supported in the ASHP guidelines on preventing medication errors with chemotherapy and biotherapy.[9]

IX.c. Patient medication instructions should be
  ○ provided verbally and in written format[301]; *[3: Moderate Evidence]*
  ○ tailored to the needs of the patient,[301] including *[3: Moderate Evidence]*
    • age-specific requirements (eg, large print),
    • special population needs (eg, non-English speaking, hearing impaired),
    • readability or level of comprehension (eg, 5th grade, 8th grade, college), and
    • health literacy level;
  ○ provided to the patient, support persons, and any additional care providers[155]; *[2: High Evidence]* and
  ○ documented on the patient record.[154]
  [2: High Evidence]

IX.c.1. Written medication instruction sheets should be standardized and printed electronically.[290] *[3: Moderate Evidence]*

Recommendation X

Precautions should be taken to mitigate the risks related to handling hazardous medications.

The literature contains reports of harmful effects resulting from handling hazardous medications and supports the use of safety measures.[302-308] Absorption of hazardous medications occurs via the dermal route, inhalation, ingestion, accidental injection, and exposure to excreta from patients receiving chemotherapy.[309] In a nonexperimental study, Gulten et al[310] demonstrated that use of personal protective equipment

MEDICATION SAFETY

(PPE) and engineering precautions have preventive effects on genotoxicity caused by handling of antineoplastic drugs.

X.a. The health care organization must create a hazardous medication management plan.[311] *[1: Regulatory Requirement]* Amb

   X.a.1. The plan should include
- a list of hazardous medications administered in the facility[19,312];
- safe work practices, including facility and engineering controls to be used when handling hazardous medications;
- role-specific educational requirements;
- when PPE is to be used and by whom; and
- processes for handling and disposing of waste.[14,309,313,314]

   [2: High Evidence]

   X.a.2. The plan should be reviewed and updated annually and when new hazardous medications are introduced.[309] *[2: High Evidence]*

X.b. The health care organization should provide
- policies and procedures based on the most current evidence related to handling of hazardous medications,
- primary engineering controls (eg, ventilation hood),
- supplemental engineering controls (eg, closed-system transfer devices),
- PPE as applicable to the hazardous medication,
- discipline-specific education as applicable to the hazardous medication,
- instructions for patients and caregivers,
- provisions for hazardous waste disposal, and
- spill kits.[309,312,315,316]

[2: High Evidence]

X.c. The health care organization should provide allowances for personnel of childbearing age (eg, assignments that do not include handling of hazardous medications).[309,312] *[1: Regulatory Requirement]*

   Lawson et al[317] conducted a descriptive study that included 7,482 pregnant nurses, of whom 775 experienced a spontaneous abortion at less than 20 weeks of pregnancy. Of these 775 nurses, 48 (6.1%) had handled antineoplastic medications. Of the 6,707 nurses who gave birth to live infants, 254 (3.8%) had handled antineoplastic medications. After adjusting for age, parity, shift work, and hours worked, the researchers concluded that nurses who were exposed to antineoplastic medications during pregnancy had a two-fold increased risk of spontaneous abortion.

X.d. Hazardous medications should be stored in compliance with USP 800 and applicable regulatory requirements.[313] *[4: Limited Evidence]*

X.e. Hazardous medications should be handled according to manufacturer's instructions for use, regulatory requirements, and advisories from professional organizations (Table 1). *[3: Moderate Evidence]*

   X.e.1. Personal protective equipment must be worn during handling of hazardous medications.[311] *[1: Regulatory Requirement]*

   The collective evidence supports the wearing of PPE.[309,310,312,313,318-320] In a nonexperimental study, Villarini et al[321] found less DNA damage occurred in health care workers involved in preparation, transportation, administration, and disposal of anticancer agents when PPE was worn.

   X.e.2. Personal protective equipment should be selected based on the risk of exposure and the activities to be performed including receipt, storage, transport, compounding, administration, deactivation, spill control, and waste disposal of hazardous medications.[309] *[2: High Evidence]*

   X.e.3. Two pairs of powder-free chemotherapy gloves (or other gloves as described in the manufacturer's instructions for use) that are inspected before use to verify the absence of physical defects should be worn for handling all hazardous medications. *[3: Moderate Evidence]*

   Powder-free gloves help to reduce the potential for work area contamination caused by the dispersal of contaminated powder from the gloves.[312,313,319] Hazardous medications may permeate a single layer of gloves, allowing skin to be exposed to the medication.[309,312,322]

   X.e.4. Gloves should be changed every 30 minutes unless otherwise stated in the glove manufacturer's instructions for use. *[3: Moderate Evidence]*

   Professional guidelines specify changing gloves every 30 minutes when handling chemotherapeutic agents.[309,313,320]

   X.e.5. A single-use chemotherapy gown should be worn during handling of hazardous medications. The gown should be sterile for personnel in the sterile field and nonsterile for personnel not in the sterile field.[323] *[3: Moderate Evidence]*

   Professional guidelines recommend wearing a gown that
- is for single use,
- is lint free,
- is impermeable to hazardous medications,
- is long sleeved,
- fastens in the back,
- has elastic or knit cuffs, and
- does not have seams or closures that are permeable to the medication being handled.[309,312,313]

PATIENT AND WORKER SAFETY

TABLE 1. RESOURCES FOR HANDLING HAZARDOUS MEDICATIONS

Organization	Website
National Institute for Occupational Safety and Health	https://www.cdc.gov/niosh/topics/antineoplastic/ https://www.cdc.gov/niosh/hhe/hheprogram.html
Occupational Safety and Health Administration	https://www.osha.gov/SLTC/hazardousdrugs/index.html
US Pharmacopeial Convention	http://www.usp.org/frequently-asked-questions/hazardous-drugs-handling-healthcare-settings

X.e.6. Goggles or goggles with full face shields must be worn when handling hazardous medications.[309] *[1: Regulatory Requirement]*

Eye glasses or safety glasses with side shields do not provide adequate eye protection. Face shields in combination with goggles provide protection to the face and eyes. Face shields alone do not provide full eye and face protection.[312,313,319]

X.e.7. An N95 respirator or more-protective respirator that meets the Occupational Safety Health Administration requirements for respiratory protection must be worn when there is a risk that airborne powder or aerosol will be generated.[312,313,319,324] *[1: Regulatory Requirement]*

An N95 mask provides protection from aerosolized hazardous medication but provides little or no protection from vapors or gases.[313]

X.e.8. Personal protective equipment worn while handling hazardous medications should be disposed of in a hazardous disposal container.[309] *[2: High Evidence]*

X.e.9. Personnel should wash their hands with soap and water as soon as possible after doffing PPE.[322] *[3: Moderate Evidence]*

X.f. The hazardous medication container should be sealed, leak proof, resistant to breakage, and labeled with the applicable hazard warnings and the same components as any other medication container.[309,312,313,320] *[3: Moderate Evidence]*

X.g. A safety data sheet (SDS) must be present and readily accessible for each hazardous medication present in the facility.[19,309,311,313] *[1: Regulatory Requirement]*

X.h. Hazardous medication spills should be contained and contaminated surfaces cleaned according to the instructions provided in the SDS.[313] *[4: Limited Evidence]*

X.h.1. Spill kits should be accessible in all areas where the potential for a spill exists.[313,322] *[4: Limited Evidence]*

X.h.2. Personal protective equipment appropriate for the type of medication must be worn during the spill cleanup process.[311,313] *[1: Regulatory Requirement]*

X.h.3. Details of the spill, including the name of the medication, time of exposure, and names of those exposed should be documented according to facility policy and procedure.[313] *[4: Limited Evidence]*

X.h.4. Personnel exposed to hazardous medications should seek immediate medical attention.[313] *[4: Limited Evidence]*

X.i. Single-use instruments, if available, should be used for administration of hazardous medications. *[5: Benefits Balanced with Harms]*

The use and disposal of single-use instruments eliminates the need to institute special protocols for deactivation and decontamination and may reduce the risk of exposing personnel to hazardous medications. The process of deactivating the medication and removing the medication from the instrument may be harmful to the instrument.

X.j. Instruments and surfaces contaminated with hazardous medications should be deactivated, cleaned, and decontaminated with agents indicated for the type of contaminant and the surface to be cleaned or decontaminated per the manufacturer's cleaning instructions.[309] *[3: Moderate Evidence]*

The collective evidence shows chemotherapeutic medications are found on many surfaces where hazardous medications are prepared, stored, and administered and supports removal from the surfaces.[310,313,325,326]

X.j.1. Agents for deactivation, cleaning, and decontamination should be selected and used based on the surface and medication manufacturers' instructions for use and the SDS. *[3: Moderate Evidence]*

The efficacy of cleaning agents varies with the surface to be cleaned and the hazardous medication present on the surface.[327-329]

X.j.2. Agents should not be applied with a spray device. *[4: Limited Evidence]*

A spray application may aerosolize the hazardous medication residue.[313]

X.j.3. Personal protective equipment must be worn during the deactivation, cleaning, and decontamination process.[311,313] *[1: Regulatory Requirement]*

X.k. Precautions should be taken in preparation for and during administration of chemotherapeutic medication for hyperthermic intraperitoneal chemotherapy (HIPEC) procedures, including

○ conducting education on the process and potential areas of contamination preprocedure,

○ wearing two pairs of sterile chemotherapy gloves,

○ wearing sterile chemotherapy-protective gowns,

○ minimizing splashing during internal organ manipulation,

○ cleaning up any spilled solution and properly disposing of materials used for cleanup,

○ careful cleaning of the HIPEC device following the manufacturer's instructions for use,

○ wearing an N95 respirator or more-protective respirator, and

○ using infusion bags instead of syringes to inject medication.

[3: Moderate Evidence]

A National Institute for Occupational Safety and Health health hazard evaluation and a descriptive study involving six German hospitals and 19 HIPEC procedures support the recommendations listed above for cisplatin used in intraperitoneal surgical procedures.[330,331] The evidence is limited, and further research is needed, especially related to respiratory protection.

X.l. Personal protective equipment should be worn during handling of excreta from patients who have received hazardous medications within the past 48 hours.[309] *[2: High Evidence]*

X.m. Hazardous medications and associated devices (eg, tubing, syringes, needles, IV bags, drapes contaminated by hazardous medications) must be disposed of according to federal, state, and local regulations.[322,332] *[1: Regulatory Requirement]*

X.m.1. Collection containers should be dedicated for chemotherapy waste.[320] *[3: Moderate Evidence]*

X.n. The health care organization must provide role-specific education related to hazardous medications.[311] *[1: Regulatory Requirement]*

The collective evidence supports the education of personnel who could be exposed to hazardous medications.[9,155,309,312,313,315,318-320,333-338] In a nonexperimental study, Hon et al[339] found there was a lack of knowledge about hazardous medications among all health care personnel, and the lack of knowledge was greater in those who were not responsible for preparing or administering medication. In another nonexperimental study, Hon et al[308] found higher amounts of a chemotherapeutic medication in the urine of personnel who handled hazardous medications but did not receive education regarding the safety measures for handling those medications compared with personnel who did receive the education.

X.n.1. Education on hazardous medication safety practices should include information about

• hazardous medications present and the associated risks,

• the hazardous medication plan,

• the use of PPE and engineering controls,

• hazardous medication exposure response,

• spill management,

• precautions for administration,

• handling of contaminated patient excreta, and

• handling of contaminated waste.

[5: Benefits Balanced with Harms]

X.o. The health care organization must establish and implement policies and procedures for handling hazardous medications.[309,313] *[1: Regulatory Requirement]*

X.o.1. The policies and procedures should define the precautions to be taken during

• receiving;

• storage;

• transport;

• preparation;

• administration;

• spill cleanup;

• waste handling, including deactivation, cleaning, and decontamination including agents to be used, and dilutions if required;

• handling of patient excreta;

• disposal of hazardous medications; and

• use of PPE.[11,309,315,318]

[3: Moderate Evidence]

X.p. A medical surveillance program and followup program should be established for all personnel potentially exposed to hazardous medication. *[3: Moderate Evidence]*

The collective evidence recommends that a medical surveillance program be instituted. A relationship has been established between being exposed to hazardous medications and abnormalities in the blood of those exposed.[304,305,308,309,313,319,336,340,341]

Recommendation XI

Medications must be disposed of according to local, state, and federal regulations and the medication manufacturer's instructions for use.[332,342-344]

Certain medications may be classified as controlled substances or medical hazardous waste, and there may be specific federal, state, or local requirements for disposal.

XI.a. The perioperative team should review the SDS and collaborate with a pharmacist to determine the correct method for disposing of medications. *[5: Benefits Balanced with Harms]*

The SDS provides specific information regarding methods of safe handling and disposal.

XI.a.1. Medications may be disposed of by returning them to the manufacturer; using a third party disposal system; incinerating them, sending them to the landfill, or if permitted, flushing them into the sanitary sewer. *[3: Moderate Evidence]*

Disposal of medications into the sanitary sewer can lead to the presence of medications (eg, controlled substances, chemotherapeutic agents) in hospital waste water. Some of these substances are thought to be ecotoxic, but the definitive effect is unknown.[18,294,345,346] Chiarello et al[345] performed a descriptive study at a Brazilian hospital in which the contents of the hospital sewage was tested for the presence of medications. The researchers found that current methods of sewage treatment only eliminated some medications, and those medications were eliminated with varying success.

XI.b. The perioperative team should collaborate with pharmacy personnel to determine the proper methods for returning unused and unopened medications in medication storage areas to the pharmacy. *[5: Benefits Balanced with Harms]*

Returning medications to the pharmacy increases the accuracy for accounting for unused medications. Returning unopened medications to the pharmacy may increase the chances for exchanging the medications to avoid outdates and consequent waste.

Recommendation XII

The health care organization should provide education and verify competency regarding precautions to be taken to mitigate the risk for medication errors.

Initial and periodic education on safe medication practices provides direction for personnel in providing safe patient care. Additional periodic educational programs provide opportunities to reinforce previous learning and introduce new information on adjunct technology, its use, and potential risks. Competency verification serves as an indicator that personnel have an understanding of safe medication practices. The collective evidence identifies education as a means for decreasing medication errors.[8,9,347-353]

XII.a. Education and competency verification activities should be role specific[9] and include
- the medication use process, including reconciliation;
- pharmacology, including medication intent for use and contraindications;
- medication allergies and treatment;
- medication disposal;
- handling and administering high-alert medications;
- using technology for medication error prevention,[13,30,354,355] and administration[23];
- methods to decrease interruptions;
- methods for handling and preventing near-miss incidents[356];
- calculations[192];
- injection techniques[134];
- tubing types and correct methods for connection;
- use of abbreviations[90];
- review of policies and procedures;
- double-checking processes;
- methods of and significance of reporting adverse drug events;
- medications associated with emergency care;
- use of medication-related education tools for patients and their support persons;
- regulations relevant to safe medication practices;
- identifying distinct pairs for look-alike and sound-alike medications;
- storage requirements for look-alike and sound-alike medications;
- applicable storage requirements (eg, temperature control) for medications;
- rotating stock;
- securing medication inventory (ie, both scheduled and nonscheduled products);
- receiving and processing verbal, written, or electronic orders;
- maintaining preference cards and standing order forms;
- retrieving or returning medications from medication storage areas, including outdated medications;
- age-related requirements when obtaining, preparing, and administering medications;
- using visual and verbal validation when placing a medication on the sterile field;
- labeling medications when outside of their original container (eg, on the sterile field);
- safe dosage limits and dosage calculations;
- use of medication containers, adjunct equipment, and supplies;
- documentation requirements; and
- monitoring patients' responses to medications. *[3: Moderate Evidence]*

The collective evidence establishes that medication errors are reduced when education is provided.[5,7,9,12,18,69,82,91,134,135,140,154,189,192,193,202,223,225,300,350-352,357-370]

XII.b. The health care organization should provide medication reference materials to personnel.[353,371] *[3: Moderate Evidence]*

XII.b.1. Reference materials should
- be readily accessible;
- be current;

- be applicable to the population served; and
- provide information on drug dosing, appropriateness of use, contraindications, adverse effects, drug-drug interactions, drug formula interactions, nursing considerations, and monitoring parameters.[371]

[4: Limited Evidence]

Recommendation XIII

Precautions should be taken to mitigate the risk for errors associated with medication documentation, including during the transcription phase.

Documentation throughout the medication use process is a professional medicolegal standard and provides data for identifying trends and demonstrating compliance with regulatory requirements and accreditation standards. Documentation also facilitates continuity of patient care through clear communication and supports collaboration among health care team members.

The literature contains reports of errors occurring during documentation and transcription. The errors reported include weight-dependent medications ordered without the patient's weight being recorded.[70,150,152,176,372]

XIII.a. Medications administered should be documented in a manner that
- is legible and easily accessible,
- is free of unapproved abbreviations and acronyms, and
- is timely.

[3: Moderate Evidence]

Documentation that occurs in real time has been reported to lower the number of medication errors.[372] Immediate documentation of untoward effects is a medicolegal standard and contributes to planning, intervening, and supporting continuity of care. Documentation also serves as a means for systems review to improve processes related to medication use. In a nonexperimental study, Hartel et al[59] found documentation errors in 3.5% of 1,934 prescriptions. The handwriting readability was rated as being moderate in 42%, poor in 52%, and unreadable in 4% of the prescriptions. The researchers concluded the transcription errors were the result of the poor level of readability.

XIII.a.1. A consistent format should be used for documenting medication administration, including the
- medication name,
- total amount of medication administered when multiple injections of the same medication (eg, lidocaine) are administered during a procedure,
- route of administration,
- administration rate,
- date and time administration began,
- concentration of the medication and solutions administered,
- duration of administration or time that treatment was completed, and
- identity of the person administering the medication.

[1: Strong Evidence]

Requirements for documentation of medication administration are detailed in regulatory requirements[17,23] and professional practice guidelines.[9,16,154]

XIII.a.2. A consistent format should be used for documentation related to medication administration when applicable, including
- patient responses, including any adverse effects observed or reported by the patient during or after administration;
- communications with patients, health care providers, and caregivers, including the dates and times the events occurred, names of persons involved, and steps taken to resolve questions and problems; and
- discharge instructions.

[5: Benefits Balanced with Harms]

XIII.a.3. A consistent format should be used for documenting medication history, including the
- patient's current medications including dosage, frequency, and last dose received;
- patient's allergies[23,132,140] and
- patient's weight in both pounds and kilograms.

[5: Benefits Balanced with Harms]

XIII.b. Medication orders should be verified for accuracy after transcription and before administration to the patient by a second person possessing the competency for managing medications.
[4: Limited Evidence]

Errors have been reported to occur during the transcription phase including transcription into an incorrect patient record, transcription into an incorrect location in the electronic medical record, and transcription of the dosage incorrectly.[164,373]

XIII.c. Precautions should be taken to prevent transmission and receipt of incorrect or partial orders when electronically transmitting or copying, including
- placing only one sheet on the copier screen at a time,
- numbering pages, and
- requesting order confirmation.

[4: Limited Evidence]

A case report describes an error that occurred when an order containing three pages was placed on a fax machine to be transmitted to the pharmacy. The error occurred because only two of the pages were transmitted, and the medications on the page that was not transmitted were not given to the patient.[374]

Recommendation XIV

The health care organization should develop policies and procedures that address all phases of the medication use process in all phases of perioperative care. Policies and procedures should be revised as necessary and should be readily available in the practice setting in which they are used.

Policies and procedures assist in the development of patient safety, quality assessment, and performance improvement activities. Policies and procedures also serve as operational guidelines to minimize patients' risk for injury or complications, standardize practice, and direct personnel. Policies and procedures establish authority, responsibility, and accountability within the practice setting.

XIV.a. Policies and procedures must address
- roles and responsibilities of each discipline (eg, RN, certified RN anesthetist, physician assistant) regarding who may administer medications, the types of medication, routes of administration, and techniques for administration and
- education and training for all personnel who administer medications.[9,23]

[1: Regulatory Requirement]

XIV.b. Policy and procedures related to medication should address
- culturally sensitive medication practices for the communities served, including
  - age-specific populations,
  - special populations (eg, women's practices, ophthalmology, oncology), and
  - ethnically diverse populations;
- handling of hazardous medications[19] (See Recommendation X);
- use of a patient-controlled analgesia device[355];
- prevention of tubing misconnections[225];
- managing medication shortages[14]; and
- the acceptable types of orders, including
  - verbal orders,[23]
  - as needed (PRN) orders,
  - standing orders,
  - automatic stop orders,
  - titrating orders,
  - taper orders,
  - range orders, and
  - signed and held orders;
- medication order content;
- medication disposal;
- labeling;
- storage requirements;
- documentation of all medications administered and postadministration monitoring performed;
- handling of containers from which medication has been removed;
- parameters for monitoring after administration; and
- the medication reconciliation process.

[4: Limited Evidence]

XIV.b.1. The policy and procedure for verbal orders should
- describe when verbal orders may be used,
- provide a means to determine the validity/authenticity of the prescriber,
- list the required contents of a complete verbal order,
- list who may give and receive verbal orders, and
- define criteria for read-back techniques.[162]

[4: Limited Evidence]

Recommendation XV

The health care organization should establish a quality plan that includes evaluation of all phases of the medication use process.

Quality assurance and performance improvement programs can facilitate the identification of problem areas and assist personnel in evaluating and improving the quality of patient care and formulating plans for corrective action. These programs provide data that may be used to determine whether an individual organization is within benchmark goals, and if not, to identify areas that may require corrective action. A quality management program provides a mechanism to evaluate effectiveness of processes and compliance with medication safety policies and procedures. The evidence supports the use of a quality plan to analyze all data collected on medication errors (eg, causes, frequency, severity), and assist with determining corrective interventions.[14,375,376]

XV.a. Health care organizations should use a mechanism to determine and analyze medication errors, near misses, and adverse drug events, which may include
- trigger tools,[377-380]
- self-reporting tools (eg, electronic, paper),[9,176,381]
- direct observation with immediate feedback,[382]
- chart review, and
- a combination of mechanisms.[7,383-385]

[3: Moderate Evidence]

In a nonexperimental retrospective study, Elliot et al[386] compared the use of an electronic reporting tool to a paper method. The researchers found the use of the electronic system resulted in an increase in the number of reported occurrences, and occurrences were reported earlier. The researchers also found that users thought the system was easier to use, was more accessible, and was more consistent than the paper system.

In a systematic literature review, Meyer-Massetti et al[387] identified strengths and weaknesses for all of the mechanisms listed above. The reviewers concluded the trigger tools were the most effective method and required less labor, while the incident report review was the most effective at identifying the severity of the medication events.

XV.b. The quality plan should contain the following components:

- clearly defined quality metrics that address preventable adverse events, medication errors, and technology;
- metrics that can lead to specific interventions (eg, if a stocking error is the metric, the intervention is to change the method of stocking);
- metrics that are applicable to the facility;
- a method for analyzing medication errors (eg, failure mode, effects, and criticality analysis; healthcare failure mode effect analysis; plan, do, check, act; define, measure, analyze, improve, control; audit and feedback process);
- a method to assess technology workarounds and solutions for workarounds if technology is used, and
- a method to identify medication errors that occur during medical emergencies.[9,203,354,388-397]

[3: Moderate Evidence]

The literature contains reports of workarounds that have been created that could interfere with the purpose of the technology[72,369,398,399] or have negative effects on patient safety.

Niazkhani et al[400] conducted a qualitative study in The Netherlands and found that when the labels for the medication administration record did not arrive in a timely manner, the medication information was handwritten in, and this resulted in the medication being administered to patients twice. A descriptive study by Gokhman et al[361] recommends that emergency situations be included in the quality monitoring program.

XV.c. Medication administration errors must be reported immediately to the attending physician and, if appropriate, to the health care organization's quality program.[23,132] *[1: Regulatory Requirement]*

XV.d. Quality data, reports, and action plans should be shared with all involved personnel (eg, pharmacy, physicians, nursing, purchasing, governing board). *[3: Moderate Evidence]*

Sharing the information with all involved personnel can result in interventions occurring at all phases of the medication use process to correct the identified problem areas.[193,401,402]

Glossary

As needed (PRN) orders: Orders acted on based on the occurrence of a specific indication or symptom.

Automatic stop orders: Orders that include a date or time to discontinue a medication.

Compounding: The process of combining two or more different medications. Compounding does not include mixing, reconstituting, or similar acts that are performed in accordance with the directions contained in approved labeling provided by the product's manufacturer or other manufacturer directions consistent with that labeling.

Hazardous drug: Any medication that is identified to meet one of the following criteria: carcinogenicity, teratogenicity, or developmental toxicity; reproductive toxicity in humans; organ toxicity at low doses in humans or animals; and genotoxicity or a new medication that mimics existing hazardous medications in structure or toxicity.

High-alert medication: A medication that has a heightened risk of causing significant patient harm when used in error.

Licensed independent practitioner: Any individual permitted by law and the organization to provide care and services without direction or supervision, within the scope of the individual's license and consistent with individually granted clinical privileges.

Medication error: A preventable event that occurs during any phase of the medication use process including procuring, prescribing, transcribing, dispensing, administering, or monitoring. The event may or may not lead to patient harm or inappropriate medication use.

Medication reconciliation: The process of comparing the patient's current medications at the time of admission or at the time of arrival at the present point of care to the list of medications ordered at the time of transfer of care or discharge. This reconciliation process begins at the point of admission to the perioperative care area and ends at the point of discharge from the perioperative care area.

Multidose vial: Defined by the Safe Injection Practices Coalition as a bottle of injectable medication that contains more than one dose of medication and has a label to indicate approval by the US Food and Drug Administration for use on more than one person.

Near miss: A variation in a normal process that, if continued, could result in negative patient outcome.

Range orders: Medication orders in which the dose or dosing interval varies over a prescribed range, depending on the situation or patient's status.

Signed and held orders: New prewritten (held) medication orders and specific instructions from a licensed independent practitioner to administer medication(s) to a patient in clearly defined circumstances that become active upon the release of the orders on a specific date(s) and time(s).

Standing order: A prewritten medication order and specific instructions from the licensed independent practitioner to administer a medication to a person in clearly defined circumstances.

Tall man lettering: The capitalization of the dissimilar portion of the name of a medication that distinguishes it from a similar drug name (Examples: vinblastine – vinBLAStine; vincristine – vinCRIStine).

Taper order: A medication order in which the dose is decreased by a particular amount with each dosing interval.

Titrating order: A medication order in which the dose is either progressively increased or decreased in response to the patient's status.

Trigger tool: A software tool that reviews a patient's record looking for clues, events, or sentinel words (eg, the ordering of certain drugs, orders for antidotes, certain abnormal laboratory values, abrupt stop orders) to identify potential adverse events. When the program identifies the established clue, event, or sentinel word on a patient's chart, a notice is sent to the designated person to initiate a more detailed chart audit. The messages received may be called alerts or notifications.

References

1. Boeker EB, de Boer M, Kiewiet JJS, Lie-A-Huen L, Dijkgraaf MGW, Boermeester MA. Occurrence and preventability of adverse drug events in surgical patients: a systematic review of literature. *BMC Health Serv Res.* 2013;13:364. [IIIA]

2. ASHP guidelines on preventing medication errors in hospitals. *Am J Hosp Pharm.* 1993;50(2):305-314. [IVC]

3. Hicks RW, Wanzer L, Goeckner B. Perioperative pharmacology: a framework for perioperative medication safety. *AORN J.* 2011;93(1):136-142. [VB]

4. Seidling HM, Stutzle M, Hoppe-Tichy T, et al. Best practice strategies to safeguard drug prescribing and drug administration: an anthology of expert views and opinions. *Int J Clin Pharm.* 2016;38(2):362-373. [IIIB]

5. Adhikari R, Tocher J, Smith P, Corcoran J, MacArthur J. A multi-disciplinary approach to medication safety and the implication for nursing education and practice. *Nurse Educ Today.* 2014;34(2):185-190. [IIIB]

6. Cousins DH, Gerrett D, Warner B. A review of medication incidents reported to the national reporting and learning system in England and Wales over 6 years (2005-2010). *Br J Clin Pharmacol.* 2012;74(4):597-604. [IIIB]

7. Härkänen M, Turunen H, Vehviläinen-Julkunen K. Differences between methods of detecting medication errors: a secondary analysis of medication administration errors using incident reports, the global trigger tool method, and observations. *J Patient Saf.* March 24, 2016. Epub ahead of print. [IIIA]

8. Grou Volpe CR, Moura Pinho DL, Morato Stival M, De Oliveira Karnikowski MG. Medication errors in a public hospital in Brazil. *Br J Nurs.* 2014;23(11):552-559. [IIIC]

9. Goldspiel B, Hoffman JM, Griffith NL, et al. ASHP guidelines on preventing medication errors with chemotherapy and biotherapy. *Am J Health Syst Pharm.* 2015;72(8):e6-e35. [IVC]

10. Anderson P, Townsend T. Preventing high alert medication errors in hospital patients. *Am Nurse Today.* 2015;10(5):18-23. [VC]

11. ASHP guidelines: minimum standard for pharmacies in hospitals. *Am J Health Syst Pharm.* 2013;70(18):1619-1630. [IVC]

12. Sanchez SH, Sethi SS, Santos SL, Boockvar K. Implementing medication reconciliation from the planner's perspective: a qualitative study. *BMC Health Serv Res.* 2014;14:290. [IIIB]

13. Mandrack M, Cohen MR, Featherling J, et al. Nursing best practices using automated dispensing cabinets: nurses' key role in improving medication safety. *Medsurg Nurs.* 2012;21(3):134-144. [VB]

14. Buxton JA, Babbitt R, Clegg CA, et al. ASHP guidelines: minimum standard for ambulatory care pharmacy practice. *Am J Health Syst Pharm.* 2015;72(14):1221-1236. [IVB]

15. Zhao RY, He XW, Shan YM, Zhu LL, Zhou Q. A stewardship intervention program for safe medication management and use of antidiabetic drugs. *Clin Interv Aging.* 2015;10:1201-1212. [VA]

16. Merry AF, Shipp DH, Lowinger JS. The contribution of labelling to safe medication administration in anaesthetic practice. *Best Pract Res Clin Anaesthesiol.* 2011;25(2):145-159. [VB]

17. May SK, Park S. Risk factors and strategies for prevention of medication errors in patients with subarachnoid hemorrhage. *Hosp Pharm.* 2013;48(Suppl 5):S10-S20. [VB]

18. Mankes RF, Silver CD. Quantitative study of controlled substance bedside wasting, disposal and evaluation of potential ecologic effects. *Sci Total Environ.* 2013;444:298-310. [IIIB]

19. ASHP guidelines on handling hazardous drugs. *Am J Health Syst Pharm.* 2006;63(12):1172-1193. [IVC]

20. De Oliveira GSJ, Theilken LS, McCarthy RJ. Shortage of perioperative drugs: implications for anesthesia practice and patient safety. *Anesth Analg.* 2011;113(6):1429-1435. [VB]

21. Golembiewski J. Drug shortages in the perioperative setting: causes, impact, and strategies. *J Perianesth Nurs.* 2012;27(4):286-292. [VB]

22. Engels MJ, Ciarkowski SL. Nursing, pharmacy, and prescriber knowledge and perceptions of high-alert medications in a large, academic medical hospital. *Hosp Pharm.* 2015;50(4):287-295. [IIIA]

23. Centers for Medicare & Medicaid Services (CMS), DHHS. Medicare and Medicaid programs; hospital conditions of participation: requirements for history and physical examinations; authentication of verbal orders; securing medications; and postanesthesia evaluations. Final rule. *Fed Regist.* 2006;71(227):68671-68695.

24. Cohen MR, Smetzer JL. No unlabeled containers anywhere, ever! Where did this come from? *Hosp Pharm.* 2015;50(3):185-188. [VC]

25. Erbe B. Safe medication administration in the operating room. *Tar Heel Nurse.* 2011;73(1):10-13. [VB]

26. Bonkowski J, Carnes C, Melucci J, et al. Effect of barcode-assisted medication administration on emergency department medication errors. *Acad Emerg Med.* 2013;20(8):801-806. [IIB]

27. Bonkowski J, Weber RJ, Melucci J, Pesavento T, Henry M, Moffatt-Bruce S. Improving medication administration safety in solid organ transplant patients through barcode-assisted medication administration. *Am J Med Qual.* 2014;29(3):236-241. [IIB]

28. Sethuraman U, Kannikeswaran N, Murray KP, Zidan MA, Chamberlain JM. Prescription errors before and after introduction of electronic medication alert system in a pediatric emergency department. *Acad Emerg Med.* 2015;22(6):714-719. [IIIB]

29. Ching JM, Williams BL, Idemoto LM, Blackmore CC. Using lean "automation with a human touch" to improve medication safety: a step closer to the "perfect dose." *Jt Comm J Qual Patient Saf.* 2014;40(8):341-350. [IIB]

30. Armada ER, Villamanan E, Lopez-de-Sa E, et al. Computerized physician order entry in the cardiac intensive care unit: effects on prescription errors and workflow conditions. *J Crit Care.* 2014;29(2):188-193. [IIIB]

31. Allison GM, Weigel B, Holcroft C. Does electronic medication reconciliation at hospital discharge decrease prescription medication errors? *Int J Health Care Qual Assur.* 2015;28(6):564-573. [IIIB]

32. Charles K, Cannon M, Hall R, Coustasse A. Can utilizing a computerized provider order entry (CPOE) system prevent hospital medical errors and adverse drug events? *Perspect Health Inf Manag.* 2014;11:1b. [IIB]

33. Connor AJ, Hutton P, Severn P, Masri I. Electronic prescribing and prescription design in ophthalmic practice. *Eur J Ophthalmol.* 2011;21(5):644-648. [IIIB]

34. Fischer JR. The impact of health care technology on medication safety. *S D Med.* 2014;67(7):279-280. [VC]

35. Green RA, Hripcsak G, Salmasian H, et al. Intercepting wrong-patient orders in a computerized provider order entry system. *Ann Emerg Med.* 2015;65(6):679-686. [IIB]

36. Henneman PL, Marquard JL, Fisher DL, et al. Barcode verification: reducing but not eliminating medication errors. *J Nurs Adm.* 2012;42(12):562-566. [IIIB]

37. Hernandez F, Majoul E, Montes-Palacios C, et al. An observational study of the impact of a computerized physician order entry system on the rate of medication errors in an orthopaedic surgery unit. *PLoS One.* 2015;10(7):e0134101. [IIB]

38. Hassink JJM, Jansen MMPM, Helmons PJ. Effects of bar code-assisted medication administration (BCMA) on frequency, type and severity of medication administration errors: a review of the literature. *Eur J Hosp Pharm Sci Pract.* 2012;19(5):489-494. [VB]

39. Khammarnia M, Kassani A, Eslahi M. The efficacy of patients' wristband bar-code on prevention of medical errors: a meta-analysis study. *Appl Clin Inform.* 2015;6(4):716-727. [IIA]

40. Leung AA, Schiff G, Keohane C, et al. Impact of vendor computerized physician order entry on patients with renal impairment in community hospitals. *J Hosp Med.* 2013;8(10):545-552. [IIB]

41. Manias E, Kinney S, Cranswick N, Williams A, Borrott N. Interventions to reduce medication errors in pediatric intensive care. *Ann Pharmacother.* 2014;48(10):1313-1331. [IIIA]

42. Nuckols TK, Smith-Spangler C, Morton SC, et al. The effectiveness of computerized order entry at reducing preventable adverse drug events and medication errors in hospital settings: a systematic review and meta-analysis. *Syst Rev.* 2014;3:56. [IIIA]

43. Roberts DL, Noble B, Wright MJ, Nelson EA, Shaft JD, Rakela J. Impact of computerized provider order entry on hospital medication errors. *J Clin Outcomes Manag.* 2013;20(3):109-115. [IIA]

44. Sanchez Cuervo M, Rojo Sanchis A, Pueyo Lopez C, Gomez De Salazar Lopez De Silanes E, Gramage Caro T, Bermejo Vicedo T. The impact of a computerized physician order entry system on medical errors with antineoplastic drugs 5 years after its implementation. *J Clin Pharm Ther.* 2015;40(5):550-554. [IIA]

45. Shawahna R, Rahman N, Ahmad M, Debray M, Yliperttula M, Decleves X. Electronic prescribing reduces prescribing error in public hospitals. *J Clin Nurs.* 2011;20(21-22):3233-3245. [IIB]

46. Truitt E, Thompson R, Blazey-Martin D, NiSai D, Salem D. Effect of the implementation of barcode technology and an electronic medication administration record on adverse drug events. *Hosp Pharm.* 2016;51(6):474-483. [IIB]

47. Westbrook JI, Li L, Georgiou A, Paoloni R, Cullen J. Impact of an electronic medication management system on hospital doctors' and nurses' work: a controlled pre-post, time and motion study. *J Am Med Inform Assoc.* 2013;20(6):1150-1158. [IIIB]

48. Jozefczyk KG, Kennedy WK, Lin MJ, et al. Computerized prescriber order entry and opportunities for medication errors: comparison to tradition paper-based order entry. *J Pharm Pract.* 2013;26(4):434-437. [IIB]

49. Buus A, Nyvang L, Heiden S, Pape-Haugaard L. Quality assurance and effectiveness of the medication process through tablet computers? *Stud Health Technol Inform.* 2012;180:348-352. [IIIB]

50. McComas J, Riingen M, Chae Kim S. Impact of an electronic medication administration record on medication administration efficiency and errors. *Comput Inform Nurs.* 2014;32(12):589-595. [IIIB]

51. Seibert HH, Maddox RR, Flynn EA, Williams CK. Effect of barcode technology with electronic medication administration record on medication accuracy rates. *Am J Health Syst Pharm.* 2014;71(3):209-218. [IIA]

52. Dwibedi N, Sansgiry SS, Frost CP, et al. Bedside barcode technology: impact on medication administration tasks in an intensive care unit. *Hosp Pharm.* 2012;47(5):360-366. [IIIB]

53. Abbass I, Mhatre S, Sansgiry SS, Tipton J, Frost C. Impact and determinants of commercial computerized prescriber order entry on the medication administration process. *Hosp Pharm.* 2011;46(5):341-348. [IIIA]

54. Stroud D. Preventing medication administration errors: lockable, computerized medication administration carts help hospitals avoid errors and reduce costs. *Health Manag Technol.* 2013;34(11):18-19. [VC]

55. Aziz MT, Ur-Rehman T, Qureshi S, Bukhari NI. Reduction in chemotherapy order errors with computerised physician order entry and clinical decision support systems. *HIM J.* 2015;44(3):13-22. [IIIB]

56. Maat B, Rademaker CMA, Oostveen MI, Krediet TG, Egberts TCG, Bollen CW. The effect of a computerized prescribing and calculating system on hypo- and hyperglycemias and on prescribing time efficiency in neonatal intensive care patients. *JPEN J Parenter Enteral Nutr.* 2013;37(1):85-91. [IIB]

57. Hollister DJ, Messenger A. Implementation of computerized physician order entry at a community hospital. *Conn Med.* 2011;75(4):227-233. [VB]

58. Morley C, McLeod E, McKenzie D, et al. Reducing dose omission of prescribed medications in the hospital setting: a narrative review. *Drugs Ther Perspect.* 2016;32(5):203-208. [VB]

59. Hartel MJ, Staub LP, Roder C, Eggli S. High incidence of medication documentation errors in a Swiss university hospital due to the handwritten prescription process. *BMC Health Serv Res.* 2011;11:199. [IIIB]

60. Albarrak AI, Al Rashidi EA, Fatani RK, Al Ageel SI, Mohammed R. Assessment of legibility and completeness of handwritten and electronic prescriptions. *Saudi Pharm J.* 2014;22(6):522-527. [IB]

61. Abramson EL, Barron Y, Quaresimo J, Kaushal R. Electronic prescribing within an electronic health record reduces ambulatory prescribing errors. *Jt Comm J Qual Patient Saf.* 2011;37(10):470-478. [IIB]

62. Meisenberg BR, Wright RR, Brady-Copertino CJ. Reduction in chemotherapy order errors with computerized physician order entry. *J Oncol Pract.* 2014;10(1):e5-e9. [VA]

63. Al-Rowibah FA, Younis MZ, Parkash J. The impact of computerized physician order entry on medication errors and adverse drug events. *J Health Care Finance.* 2013;40(1):93-102. [IIIB]

64. Fanning L, Jones N, Manias E. Impact of automated dispensing cabinets on medication selection and preparation error rates in an emergency department: a prospective and direct observational before-and-after study. *J Eval Clin Pract.* 2016;22(2):156-163. [IIIB]

65. Cochran GL, Barrett RS, Horn SD. Comparison of medication safety systems in critical access hospitals: combined analysis of two studies. *Am J Health Syst Pharm.* 2016;73(15):1167-1173. [IIIA]

66. Tsao NW, Lo C, Babich M, Shah K, Bansback NJ. Decentralized automated dispensing devices: systematic

review of clinical and economic impacts in hospitals. *Can J Hosp Pharm*. 2014;67(2):138-148. [IIIB]

67. Turchin A, Shubina M, Goldberg S. Unexpected effects of unintended consequences: EMR prescription discrepancies and hemorrhage in patients on warfarin. *AMIA Annu Symp Proc*. 2011;2011:1412-1417. [IIIB]

68. Sparnon E. Spotlight on electronic health record errors: errors related to the use of default values. *Penn Patient Saf Advis*. 2013;10(3):92-95. [IIIB]

69. Rodriguez-Gonzalez CG, Herranz-Alonso A, Martin-Barbero ML, et al. Prevalence of medication administration errors in two medical units with automated prescription and dispensing. *J Am Med Inform Assoc*. 2012;19(1):72-78. [IIIB]

70. Stultz JS, Nahata MC. Preventability of voluntarily reported or trigger tool-identified medication errors in a pediatric institution by information technology: a retrospective cohort study. *Drug Saf*. 2015;38(7):661-670. [IIIB]

71. Wetterneck TB, Walker JM, Blosky MA, et al. Factors contributing to an increase in duplicate medication order errors after CPOE implementation. *J Am Med Inform Assoc*. 2011;18(6):774-782. [IIIB]

72. Van Der Sijs H, Rootjes I, Aarts J. The shift in workarounds upon implementation of computerized physician order entry. *Stud Health Technol Inform*. 2011;169:290-294. [IIIB]

73. Joy A, Davis J, Cardona J. Effect of computerized provider order entry on rate of medication errors in a community hospital setting. *Hosp Pharm*. 2012;47(9):693-699. [VA]

74. Nelson CE, Selbst SM. Electronic prescription writing errors in the pediatric emergency department. *Pediatr Emerg Care*. 2015;31(5):368-372. [IIIA]

75. Schwartzberg D, Ivanovic S, Patel S, Burjonrappa SC. We thought we would be perfect: medication errors before and after the initiation of computerized physician order entry. *J Surg Res*. 2015;198(1):108-114. [IIB]

76. Naunton M, Gardiner HR, Kyle G. Look-alike, sound-alike medication errors: a novel case concerning a Slow-Na, Slow-K prescribing error. *Int Med Case Rep J*. 2015;8:51-53. [VC]

77. Cohen MR, Smetzer JL. ISMP medication error report analysis—tretinoin confused with isotretinoin; death from intravenous nimodipine; incorrect medication names selected during order entry; reduce Ambien dose in order sets; confusion between levothyroxine and liothyronine. *Hosp Pharm*. 2013;48(6):455-457. [VC]

78. Maat B, Au YS, Bollen CW, van Vught AJ, Egberts TCG, Rademaker CMA. Clinical pharmacy interventions in paediatric electronic prescriptions. *Arch Dis Child*. 2013;98(3):222-227. [IIIA]

79. Tully MP. Prescribing errors in hospital practice. *Br J Clin Pharmacol*. 2012;74(4):668-675. [VB]

80. Villamanan E, Larrubia Y, Ruano M, et al. Potential medication errors associated with computer prescriber order entry. *Int J Clin Pharm*. 2013;35(4):577-583. [IIIB]

81. Warrick C, Naik H, Avis S, Fletcher P, Franklin BD, Inwald D. A clinical information system reduces medication errors in paediatric intensive care. *Intensive Care Med*. 2011;37(4):691-694. [IIB]

82. Gimenes FRE, Marques TC, Teixeira TCA, Mota MLS, Silva AE, Cassiani SH. Medication wrong-route administrations in relation to medical prescriptions. *Rev Lat Am Enfermagem*. 2011;19(1):11-17. [IIIB]

83. Redwood S, Rajakumar A, Hodson J, Coleman JJ. Does the implementation of an electronic prescribing system create unintended medication errors? A study of the sociotechnical context through the analysis of reported medication incidents. *BMC Med Inform Decis Mak*. 2011;11:29. [IIIB]

84. Westbrook JI, Reckmann M, Li L, et al. Effects of two commercial electronic prescribing systems on prescribing error rates in hospital in-patients: a before and after study. *PLoS Med*. 2012;9(1):e1001164. [IIA]

85. Hinojosa-Amaya JM, Rodríguez-Garcia FG, Yeverino-Castro SG, Sánchez-Cárdenas M, Villarreal-Alarcón MÁ, Galarza-Delgado DÁ. Medication errors: electronic vs. paper-based prescribing. Experience at a tertiary care university hospital. *J Eval Clin Pract*. 2016;22(5):751-754. [IIA]

86. Electronic prescribing: the risk of errors and adverse effects. *Prescrire Int*. 2016;25(167):24-27. [VB]

87. Leung AA, Keohane C, Amato M, et al. Impact of vendor computerized physician order entry in community hospitals. *J Gen Intern Med*. 2012;27(7):801-807. [IIB]

88. Hoonakker PLT, Carayon P, Walker JM, Brown RL, Cartmill RS. The effects of computerized provider order entry implementation on communication in intensive care units. *Int J Med Inform*. 2013;82(5):e107-e117. [IIIB]

89. Tschannen D, Talsma A, Reinemeyer N, Belt C, Schoville R. Nursing medication administration and workflow using computerized physician order entry. *Comput Inform Nurs*. 2011;29(7):401-410. [IIIB]

90. Samaranayake NR, Cheung DST, Lam MPS, et al. The effectiveness of a "do not use" list and perceptions of healthcare professionals on error-prone abbreviations. *Int J Clin Pharm*. 2014;36(5):1000-1006. [VB]

91. Samaranayake NR, Dabare PRL, Wanigatunge CA, Cheung BMY. The pattern of abbreviation use in prescriptions: a way forward in eliminating error-prone abbreviations and standardisation of prescriptions. *Curr Drug Saf*. 2014;9(1):34-42. [IIIB]

92. Flannery AH, Parli SE. Medication errors in cardiopulmonary arrest and code-related situations. *Am J Crit Care*. 2016;25(1):12-20. [VB]

93. Thomas AN, Taylor RJ. An analysis of patient safety incidents associated with medications reported from critical care units in the north west of England between 2009 and 2012. *Anaesthesia*. 2014;69(7):735-745. [IIIB]

94. Alex S, Adenew AB, Arundel C, Maron DD, Kerns JC. Medication errors despite using electronic health records: the value of a clinical pharmacist service in reducing discharge-related medication errors. *Qual Manag Health Care*. 2016;25(1):32-37. [VA]

95. Abbasinazari M, Hajhossein Talasaz A, Eshraghi A, Sahraei Z. Detection and management of medication errors in internal wards of a teaching hospital by clinical pharmacists. *Acta Med Iran*. 2013;51(7):482-486. [IIIA]

96. Cesarz JL, Steffenhagen AL, Svenson J, Hamedani AG. Emergency department discharge prescription interventions by emergency medicine pharmacists. *Ann Emerg Med*. 2013;61(2):209-214. [IIIB]

97. Ernst AA, Weiss SJ, Sullivan A4, et al. On-site pharmacists in the ED improve medical errors. *Am J Emerg Med*. 2012;30(5):717-725. [IIIB]

98. Ho L, Akada K, Messner H, Kuruvilla J, Wright J, Seki JT. Pharmacist's role in improving medication safety for patients in an allogeneic hematopoietic cell transplant ambulatory clinic. *Can J Hosp Pharm*. 2013;66(2):110-117. [VA]

99. Jiang S, Zheng X, Li X, Lu X. Effectiveness of pharmaceutical care in an intensive care unit from china. A pre- and post-intervention study. *Saudi Med J*. 2012;33(7):756-762. [IIIB]

100. Jiang SP, Zhu ZY, Wu XL, Lu XY, Zhang XG, Wu BH. Effectiveness of pharmacist dosing adjustment for critically ill patients receiving continuous renal

replacement therapy: a comparative study. *Ther Clin Risk Manag.* 2014;10:405-412. [IIIB]

101. Mergenhagen KA, Blum SS, Kugler A, et al. Pharmacist- versus physician-initiated admission medication reconciliation: impact on adverse drug events. *Am J Geriatr Pharmacother.* 2012;10(4):242-250. [IIB]

102. ASHP statement on the pharmacist's role in medication reconciliation. *Am J Health Syst Pharm.* 2013;70(5):453-456. [IVC]

103. Phatak A, Prusi R, Ward B, et al. Impact of pharmacist involvement in the transitional care of high-risk patients through medication reconciliation, medication education, and postdischarge call-backs (IPITCH Study). *J Hosp Med.* 2016;11(1):39-44. [IB]

104. Lenssen R, Heidenreich A, Schulz JB, et al. Analysis of drug-related problems in three departments of a German university hospital. *Int J Clin Pharm.* 2016;38(1):119-126. [IIIB]

105. Ibanez-Garcia S, Rodriguez-Gonzalez CG, Martin-Barbero ML, Sanjurjo-Saez M, Herranz-Alonso A; iPharma. Adding value through pharmacy validation: a safety and cost perspective. *J Eval Clin Pract.* 2016;22(2):253-260. [IIIB]

106. Fernandez-Llamazares CM, Calleja-Hernandez M, Manrique-Rodriguez S, Perez-Sanz C, Duran-Garcia E, Sanjurjo-Saez M. Prescribing errors intercepted by clinical pharmacists in paediatrics and obstetrics in a tertiary hospital in Spain. *Eur J Clin Pharmacol.* 2012;68(9):1339-1345. [IIIA]

107. Zaal RJ, Jansen MMPM, Duisenberg-van Essenberg M, Tijssen CC, Roukema JA, van den Bemt PMLA. Identification of drug-related problems by a clinical pharmacist in addition to computerized alerts. *Int J Clin Pharm.* 2013;35(5):753-762. [IIIB]

108. Kuo GM, Touchette DR, Marinac JS. Drug errors and related interventions reported by United States clinical pharmacists: the American College of Clinical Pharmacy practice-based research network medication error detection, amelioration and prevention study. *Pharmacotherapy.* 2013;33(3):253-265. [IIIB]

109. Caroff DA, Bittermann T, Leonard CE, Gibson GA, Myers JS. A medical resident-pharmacist collaboration improves the rate of medication reconciliation verification at discharge. *Jt Comm J Qual Patient Saf.* 2015;41(10):457-461. [IIA]

110. Graabaek T, Kjeldsen LJ. Medication reviews by clinical pharmacists at hospitals lead to improved patient outcomes: a systematic review. *Basic Clin Pharmacol Toxicol.* 2013;112(6):359-373. [IIIB]

111. Han J, Ah Y, Suh SY, et al. Clinical and economic impact of pharmacists' intervention in a large volume chemotherapy preparation unit. *Int J Clin Pharm.* 2016;38(5):1124-1132. [IIIB]

112. Khalili H, Farsaei S, Rezaee H, Dashti-Khavidaki S. Role of clinical pharmacists' interventions in detection and prevention of medication errors in a medical ward. *Int J Clin Pharm.* 2011;33(2):281-284. [IIIB]

113. Hohmann C, Neumann-Haefelin T, Klotz JM, Freidank A, Radziwill R. Drug-related problems in patients with ischemic stroke in hospital. *Int J Clin Pharm.* 2012;34(6):828-831. [IIIB]

114. Galvin M, Jago-Byrne M, Fitzsimons M, Grimes T. Clinical pharmacist's contribution to medication reconciliation on admission to hospital in Ireland. *Int J Clin Pharm.* 2013;35(1):14-21. [IIIB]

115. Pal A, Babbott S, Wilkinson ST. Can the targeted use of a discharge pharmacist significantly decrease 30-day readmissions? *Hosp Pharm.* 2013;48(5):380-388. [IIB]

116. Reis WCT, Scopel CT, Correr CJ, Andrzejevski VMS. Analysis of clinical pharmacist interventions in a tertiary teaching hospital in Brazil. *Einstein.* 2013;11(2):190-196. [IIIB]

117. Warden BA, Freels JP, Furuno JP, Mackay J. Pharmacy-managed program for providing education and discharge instructions for patients with heart failure. *Am J Health Syst Pharm.* 2014;71(2):134-139. [IIB]

118. Stasiak P, Afilalo M, Castelino T, et al. Detection and correction of prescription errors by an emergency department pharmacy service. *Can J Emerg Med.* 2014;16(3):193-206. [IIIA]

119. Balling L, Erstad BL, Weibel K. Impact of a transition-of-care pharmacist during hospital discharge. *J Am Pharm Assoc.* 2015;55(4):443-448. [IIIC]

120. Tripathi S, Crabtree HM, Fryer KR, Graner KK, Arteaga GM. Impact of clinical pharmacist on the pediatric intensive care practice: an 11-year tertiary center experience. *J Pediatr Pharmacol Ther.* 2015;20(4):290-298. [IIIB]

121. Sebaaly J, Parsons LB, Pilch NAW, Bullington W, Hayes GL, Easterling H. Clinical and financial impact of pharmacist involvement in discharge medication reconciliation at an academic medical center: a prospective pilot study. *Hosp Pharm.* 2015;50(6):505-513. [IIIB]

122. Hamblin S, Rumbaugh K, Miller R. Prevention of adverse drug events and cost savings associated with PharmD interventions in an academic level I trauma center: an evidence-based approach. *J Trauma Acute Care Surg.* 2012;73(6):1484-1490. [IIIB]

123. Cochran GL, Haynatzki G. Comparison of medication safety effectiveness among nine critical access hospitals. *Am J Health Syst Pharm.* 2013;70(24):2218-2224. [IIIC]

124. McCoy AB, Cox ZL, Neal EB, et al. Real-time pharmacy surveillance and clinical decision support to reduce adverse drug events in acute kidney injury: a randomized, controlled trial. *Appl Clin Inform.* 2012;3(2):221-238. [IA]

125. van den Bemt PMLA, van der Schrieck-de Loos EM, van der Linden C, Theeuwes AMLJ, Pol AG; Dutch CBO WHO High 5s Study Group. Effect of medication reconciliation on unintentional medication discrepancies in acute hospital admissions of elderly adults: a multicenter study. *J Am Geriatr Soc.* 2013;61(8):1262-1268. [IIA]

126. Bishop MA, Cohen BA, Billings LK, Thomas EV. Reducing errors through discharge medication reconciliation by pharmacy services. *Am J Health Syst Pharm.* 2015;72(17 Suppl 2):S120-S126. [IIIB]

127. Gardella JE, Cardwell TB, Nnadi M. Improving medication safety with accurate preadmission medication lists and postdischarge education. *Jt Comm J Qual Patient Saf.* 2012;38(10):452-458. [VA]

128. Kramer JS, Stewart MR, Fogg SM, et al. A quantitative evaluation of medication histories and reconciliation by discipline. *Hosp Pharm.* 2014;49(9):826-838. [IIIB]

129. Beckett RD, Crank CW, Wehmeyer A. Effectiveness and feasibility of pharmacist-led admission medication reconciliation for geriatric patients. *J Pharm Pract.* 2012;25(2):136-141. [IB]

130. Aag T, Garcia BH, Viktil KK. Should nurses or clinical pharmacists perform medication reconciliation? A randomized controlled trial. *Eur J Clin Pharmacol.* 2014;70(11):1325-1332. [IA]

131. Zemaitis CT, Morris G, Cabie M, Abdelghany O, Lee L. Reducing readmission at an academic medical center: results of a pharmacy-facilitated discharge counseling and medication reconciliation program. *Hosp Pharm.* 2016;51(6):468-473. [IIIB]

132. Centers for Medicare & Medicaid Services. *State Operations Manual Appendix L—Guidance for Surveyors: Ambulatory Surgical Centers.* Rev. 137; 2015. https://www.cms.gov/Regulations-and-Guidance/Guidance/Manuals/downloads/som107ap_l_ambulatory.pdf. Accessed July 12, 2017.

133. Cole SL, Grubbs JH, Din C, Nesbitt TS. Rural inpatient telepharmacy consultation demonstration for after-hours medication review. *Telemed J E Health.* 2012;18(7):530-537. [IIB]

134. The Joint Commission. Preventing infection from the misuse of vials. *Sentinel Event Alert.* June 16, 2014;52. https://www.jointcommission.org/sea_issue_52/. Accessed July 12, 2017. [VB]

135. Horvath G, MacGregor RL. Is your facility properly managing pharmaceutical waste? *OR Nurse.* 2013;7(5):8-12. [VB]

136. Buck D, Subramanyam R, Varughese A. A quality improvement project to reduce the intraoperative use of single-dose fentanyl vials across multiple patients in a pediatric institution. *Paediatr Anaesth.* 2016;26(1):92-101. [VA]

137. Yadav G, Gupta SK, Bharti AK, Khuba S, Jain G, Singh DK. Case report: syringe swap and similar looking drug containers: a matter of serious concern. *Anaesth Pain Intensive Care.* 2013;17(2):205-207. [VC]

138. Fry RA, Wilton N, Boyes G. Unusual volatile agent switch: implications for checking unsealed volatile agent containers. *Anaesth Intensive Care.* 2015;43(3):419-420. [VC]

139. De Winter S, Vanbrabant P, Vi NTT, et al. Impact of temperature exposure on stability of drugs in a real-world out-of-hospital setting. *Ann Emerg Med.* 2013;62(4):380-387. [IIIB]

140. Grissinger M. Ambulatory surgery facilities: a comprehensive review of medication error reports in Pennsylvania. *Penn Patient Saf Advis.* 2011;8(3):85-93. [IIIB]

141. Tobias JD, Yadav G, Gupta SK, Jain G. Medication errors: a matter of serious concern. *Anaesth Pain Intensive Care.* 2013;17(2):111-114. [VB]

142. Anto B, Barlow D, Oborne CA, Whittlesea C. Incorrect drug selection at the point of dispensing: a study of potential predisposing factors. *Int J Pharm Pract.* 2011;19(1):51-60. [IIIB]

143. Medication safety. *J Pharm Pract Res.* 2011;41(2):139-143. [VC]

144. Medication safety. *J Pharm Pract Res.* 2011;41(1):52-56. [VC]

145. Cote V, Prager JD. Iatrogenic phenol injury: a case report and review of medication safety and labeling practices with flexible laryngoscopy. *Int J Pediatr Otorhinolaryngol.* 2014;78(10):1769-1773. [VC]

146. Cohen MR, Smetzer JL. ISMP medication error report analysis—FDA advise-ERR: FDA approves hydromorphone labeling revisions to reduce medication errors; differentiating penicillin from penicillamine; infusion reconnected to the wrong patient; spell out acetaminophen on. *Hosp Pharm.* 2012;47(1):10-13. [VC]

147. Cohen MR, Smetzer JL. ISMP medication error report analysis—drug stability and compatibility; proper use of single-dose vials; what drugs are present on nursing units?; Arixtra—not a hemostat; Pradaxa-Plavix mix-up. *Hosp Pharm.* 2012;47(8):578-582. [VC]

148. Butala BP, Shah VR, Bhosale GP, Shah RB. Medication error: subarachnoid injection of tranexamic acid. *Indian J Anaesth.* 2012;56(2):168-170. [VC]

149. Koczmara C, Hyland S. Drug name alert: potential for confusion between Pradaxa and Plavix. *Dynamics.* 2011;22(3):25-26. [VB]

150. Vazin A, Zamani Z, Hatam N. Frequency of medication errors in an emergency department of a large teaching hospital in southern Iran. *Drug Healthc Patient Saf.* 2014;6:179-184. [IIIB]

151. Zeraatchi A, Talebian M, Nejati A, Dashti-Khavidaki S. Frequency and types of the medication errors in an academic emergency department in Iran: the emergent need for clinical pharmacy services in emergency departments. *J Res Pharm Pract.* 2013;2(3):118-122. [IIIB]

152. Manias E, Kinney S, Cranswick N, Williams A. Medication errors in hospitalised children. *J Paediatr Child Health.* 2014;50(1):71-77. [IIIB]

153. 21 USC 13: Drug Abuse Prevention and Control. Subchapter I: Control and enforcement (sections 801-904). US Government Publishing Office. https://www.gpo.gov/fdsys/granule/USCODE-2011-title21/USCODE-2011-title21-chap13/content-detail.html. Accessed July 12, 2017.

154. Guideline for patient information management. In: *Guidelines for Perioperative Practice.* Denver, CO: AORN, Inc; 2017:591-616. [IVA]

155. Neuss MN, Polovich M, McNiff K, et al. 2013 updated American society of clinical oncology/oncology nursing society chemotherapy administration safety standards including standards for the safe administration and management of oral chemotherapy. *J Oncol Pract.* 2013;9(2 Suppl):5s-13s. [IVB]

156. Shawahna R, Rahman N, Ahmad M, Debray M, Yliperttula M, Decleves X. Impact of prescriber's handwriting style and nurse's duty duration on the prevalence of transcription errors in public hospitals. *J Clin Nurs.* 2013;22(3-4):550-558. [IIIB]

157. Cohen MR, Smetzer JL. Dangerous close call with wintergreen oil; are 10 mL syringes needed when giving drugs via venous access devices?; use of "NoAC" abbreviation; unsafe frequency notation; 2014-15 targeted medication safety best practices for hospitals. *Hosp Pharm.* 2014;49(4):325-328. [VC]

158. Paul IM, Neville K, Galinkin JL, et al. Metric units and the preferred dosing of orally administered liquid medications. *Pediatrics.* 2015;135(4):784-787. [IVC]

159. ISMP guidelines for standard order sets. Institute for Safe Medication Practices. http://www.ismp.org/Tools/guidelines/StandardOrderSets.asp. Accessed July 12, 2017. [IVC]

160. Sakushima K, Umeki R, Endoh A, Ito YM, Nasuhara Y. Time trend of injection drug errors before and after implementation of bar-code verification system. *Technol Health Care.* 2015;23(3):267-274. [IIIB]

161. Al-Shaiji TF. Achieving detumescence of ischemic priapism with intra-cavernosal injection of fentanyl: an unexpected outcome of miscommunication error. *Curr Drug Saf.* 2011;6(3):194-196. [VC]

162. Recommendations to reduce medication errors associated with verbal medication orders and prescriptions. National Coordinating Council for Medication Error Reporting and Prevention. http://www.nccmerp.org/recommendations-reduce-medication-errors-associated-verbal-medication-orders-and-prescriptions. Adopted February 20, 2001. Revised May 1, 2015. Accessed July 12, 2017. [IVC]

163. Hicks RW, Becker SC, Windle PE, Krenzischek DA. Medication errors in the PACU. *J Perianesth Nurs.* 2007;22(6):413-419. [IIIC]

164. Hicks RW, Becker SC, and Cousins DD. *MEDMARX Data Report: A Chartbook of Medication Error Findings from the Perioperative Settings from 1998-2005.* Rockville, MD: US Pharmacopeia; 2007. [IIIC]

165. Pharmaceutical compounding—sterile preparations (797). In: *USP Compounding Compendium*. Rockville, MD: US Pharmacopeial Convention; 2016:40-85. [IVB]

166. Matousek P, Kominek P, Garcic A. Errors associated with the concentration of epinephrine in endonasal surgery. *Eur Arch Otorhinolaryngol*. 2011;268(7):1009-1011. [VC]

167. Dehmel C, Braune SA, Kreymann G, et al. Do centrally pre-prepared solutions achieve more reliable drug concentrations than solutions prepared on the ward? *Intensive Care Med*. 2011;37(8):1311-1316. [IIIB]

168. Patel S, Loveridge R. Obstetric neuraxial drug administration errors: a quantitative and qualitative analytical review. *Anesth Analg*. 2015;121(6):1570-1577. [IIIB]

169. Cohen MR, Smetzer JL. ISMP medication error report analysis—important change with heparin labels; Benadryl dispensed instead of vitamins for home parenteral nutrition; potassium and sodium acetate injection mix-ups; don't truncate, stem, or shorten drug names. *Hosp Pharm*. 2013;48(4):267-269. [VC]

170. Cohen M, Smetzer J. ISMP medication error report analysis—preventing mix-ups between various formulations of amphotericin B; Arixtra is not a hemostat; measurement mix-up; drug names too close for comfort; new vaccine errors reporting program. *Hosp Pharm*. 2013;48(2):95-98. [VC]

171. Emmerton L, Rizk MFS, Bedford G, Lalor D. Systematic derivation of an Australian standard for tall man lettering to distinguish similar drug names. *J Eval Clin Pract*. 2015;21(1):85-90. [IIIB]

172. Darker IT, Gerret D, Filik R, Purdy KJ, Gale AG. The influence of "tall man" lettering on errors of visual perception in the recognition of written drug names. *Ergonomics*. 2011;54(1):21-33. [IIIB]

173. DeHenau C, Becker MW, Bello NM, Liu S, Bix L. Tallman lettering as a strategy for differentiation in look-alike, sound-alike drug names: the role of familiarity in differentiating drug doppelgangers. *Appl Ergon*. 2016;52:77-84. [IIIB]

174. Or CKL, Chan AHS. Effects of text enhancements on the differentiation performance of orthographically similar drug names. *Work*. 2014;48(4):521-528. [IIIB]

175. Trudeau M, Green E, Cosby R, et al. Key components of intravenous chemotherapy labeling: a systematic review and practice guideline. *J Oncol Pharm Pract*. 2011;17(4):409-424. [IVB]

176. Harkanen M, Turunen H, Saano S, Vehvilainen-Julkunen K. Detecting medication errors: analysis based on a hospital's incident reports. *Int J Nurs Pract*. 2015;21(2):141-146. [IIIB]

177. Barak M, Greenberg Z, Danino J. Delayed awakening following inadvertent high-dose remifentanil infusion in a 13 year old patient. *J Clin Anesth*. 2011;23(4):322-324. [VC]

178. Cohen MR, Smetzer JL. ISMP medication error report analysis—tragedy in the postanesthesia care unit; mix-ups between risperidone and ropinirole. *Hosp Pharm*. 2013;48(7):538-541. [VC]

179. Medication safety. *J Pharm Pract Res*. 2014;44(1):38-43. [VC]

180. Cohen MR, Smetzer JL. ISMP medication error report analysis—leucovorin-levoleucovorin mix-up; two error-reduction principles, one change; syringe pull-back method of verifying IV admixtures is unreliable; fleet enema saline is not just saline; ISMP processes health IT. *Hosp Pharm*. 2013;48(10):803-806. [VC]

181. Cohen MR, Smetzer JL. U-500 insulin safety concerns mount; improved labeling needed for camphor product; cardizem-cardene mix-up; initiative to eliminate tubing misconnections. *Hosp Pharm*. 2014;49(2):117-120. [VC]

182. Cohen MR, Smetzer JL. ISMP medication error report analysis. *Hosp Pharm*. 2015;50(5):347-350. [VC]

183. Shridhar Iyer U, Fah KK, Chong CK, Macachor J, Chia N. Survey of medication errors among anaesthetists in Singapore. *Anaesth Intensive Care*. 2011;39(6):1151-1152. [IIIC]

184. Kanji S, Lam J, Goddard RD, et al. Inappropriate medication administration practices in Canadian adult ICUs: a multicenter, cross-sectional observational study. *Ann Pharmacother*. 2013;47(5):637-643. [IIIA]

185. Zhou L, Dhopeshwarkar N, Blumenthal KG, et al. Drug allergies documented in electronic health records of a large healthcare system. *Allergy*. 2016;71(9):1305-1313. [IIIB]

186. Echeta G, Moffett BS, Checchia P, et al. Prescribing errors in adult congenital heart disease patients admitted to a pediatric cardiovascular intensive care unit. *Congenit Heart Dis*. 2014;9(2):126-130. [IIIB]

187. Modic MB, Albert NM, Sun Z, et al. Does an insulin double-checking procedure improve patient safety? *J Nurs Adm*. 2016;46(3):154-160. [IB]

188. Girard NJ. Vial mistakes involving heparin. *AORN J*. 2011;94(6):644, 554. [VB]

189. Gilbar PJ, Seger AC. Fatalities resulting from accidental intrathecal administration of bortezomib: strategies for prevention. *J Clin Oncol*. 2012;30(27):3427-3428. [VC]

190. Kellett P, Gottwald M. Double-checking high-risk medications in acute settings: a safer process. *Nurs Manag (Harrow)*. 2015;21(9):16-22. [VC]

191. Alsulami Z, Conroy S, Choonara I. Double checking the administration of medicines: what is the evidence? A systematic review. *Arch Dis Child*. 2012;97(9):833-837. [IIIB]

192. Ofosu R, Jarrett P. Reducing nurse medicine administration errors. *Nurs Times*. 2015;111(20):12-14. [VB]

193. Murphy M, While A. Medication administration practices among children's nurses: a survey. *Br J Nurs*. 2012;21(15):928-933. [IIIB]

194. McLeod M, Barber N, Franklin BD. Facilitators and barriers to safe medication administration to hospital inpatients: a mixed methods study of nurses' medication administration processes and systems (the MAPS study). *PLoS One*. 2015;10(6):e0128958. [IIIB]

195. Raban MZ, Westbrook JI. Are interventions to reduce interruptions and errors during medication administration effective?: a systematic review. *BMJ Qual Saf*. 2014;23(5):414-421. [IIA]

196. Williams T, King MW, Thompson JA, Champagne MT. Implementing evidence-based medication safety interventions on a progressive care unit. *Am J Nurs*. 2014;114(11):53-62. [VB]

197. Choo J, Johnston L, Manias E. Nurses' medication administration practices at two Singaporean acute care hospitals. *Nurs Health Sci*. 2013;15(1):101-108. [IIIB]

198. Bower R, Jackson C, Manning JC. Interruptions and medication administration in critical care. *Nurs Crit Care*. 2015;20(4):183-195. [IIIB]

199. Verweij L, Smeulers M, Maaskant JM, Vermeulen H. Quiet please! Drug round tabards: are they effective and accepted? A mixed method study. *J Nurs Scholarsh*. 2014;46(5):340-348. [IIIB]

200. Fore AM, Sculli GL, Albee D, Neily J. Improving patient safety using the sterile cockpit principle during medication administration: a collaborative, unit-based project. *J Nurs Manag*. 2013;21(1):106-111. [VB]

201. Bravo K, Cochran G, Barrett R. Nursing strategies to increase medication safety in inpatient settings. *J Nurs Care Qual.* 2016;31(4):335-341. [IIIB]

202. Pape TM. The effect of a five-part intervention to decrease omitted medications. *Nurs Forum.* 2013;48(3):211-222. [VB]

203. Capasso V, Johnson M. Improving the medicine administration process by reducing interruptions. *J Healthc Manag.* 2012;57(6):384-390. [VC]

204. Craig J, Clanton F, Demeter M. Reducing interruptions during medication administration: the white vest study. *J Res Nurs.* 2014;19(3):248-261. [IIB]

205. Fabbri G, Panico M, Dallolio L, et al. Outbreak of ampicillin/piperacillin-resistant *Klebsiella pneumoniae* in a neonatal intensive care unit (NICU): investigation and control measures. *Int J Environ Res Public Health.* 2013;10(3):808-815. [VC]

206. Branch-Elliman W, Weiss D, Balter S, Bornschlegel K, Phillips M. Hepatitis C transmission due to contamination of multidose medication vials: summary of an outbreak and a call to action. *Am J Infect Control.* 2013;41(1):92-94. [VC]

207. De Smet B, Veng C, Kruy L, et al. Outbreak of Burkholderia cepacia bloodstream infections traced to the use of Ringer lactate solution as multiple-dose vial for catheter flushing, Phnom Penh, Cambodia. *Clin Microbiol Infect.* 2013;19(9):832-837. [VC]

208. Cohen M, Smetzer J. ISMP medication error report analysis—error prevention strategies for strong iodine solution; do not use an insulin pen for multiple patients. *Hosp Pharm.* 2012;47(4):260-263. [VC]

209. Jog M, Sachidananda R, Saeed K. Risk of contamination of lidocaine hydrochloride and phenylephrine hydrochloride topical solution: in vivo and in vitro analyses. *J Laryngol Otol.* 2013;127(8):799-801. [IIIB]

210. Baniasadi S, Dorudinia A, Mobarhan M, Karimi Gamishan M, Fahimi F. Microbial contamination of single- and multiple-dose vials after opening in a pulmonary teaching hospital. *Braz J Infect Dis.* 2013;17(1):69-73. [IIIB]

211. Moore ZS, Schaefer MK, Hoffmann KK, et al. Transmission of hepatitis C virus during myocardial perfusion imaging in an outpatient clinic. *Am J Cardiol.* 2011;108(1):126-132. [VA]

212. Drezner K, Antwi M, Del Rosso P, Dorsinville M, Kellner P, Ackelsberg J. A cluster of methicillin-susceptible Staphylococcus aureus infections at a rheumatology practice, New York City, 2011. *Infect Control Hosp Epidemiol.* 2014;35(2):187-189. [VC]

213. King CA, Ogg M. Safe injection practices for administration of propofol. *AORN J.* 2012;95(3):365-372. [VB]

214. Kundra S, Singh RM, Grewal A, Gupta V, Chaudhary AK. Necrotizing fasciitis after spinal anesthesia. *Acta Anaesthesiol Scand.* 2013;57(2):257-261. [VB]

215. Ersoz G, Uguz M, Aslan G, Horasan ES, Kaya A. Outbreak of meningitis due to *Serratia marcescens* after spinal anaesthesia. *J Hosp Infect.* 2014;87(2):122-125. [VC]

216. Coyle JR, Goerge E, Kacynski K, et al. Hepatitis C virus infections associated with unsafe injection practices at a pain management clinic, Michigan, 2014-2015. *Pain Med.* 2017;18(2):322-329. [VC]

217. Rashid M, Karagama YG. Study of microbial spread when using multiple-use nasal anaesthetic spray. *Rhinology.* 2011;49(3):281-285. [IIIB]

218. Hilliard JG, Cambronne ED, Kirsch JR, Aziz MF. Barrier protection capacity of flip-top pharmaceutical vials. *J Clin Anesth.* 2013;25(3):177-180. [IIIB]

219. Laha B, Hazra A. Medication error report: intrathecal administration of labetalol during obstetric anesthesia. *Indian J Pharmacol.* 2015;47(4):456-458. [VC]

220. Park JC, Herbert EN. Laser goggles alter the perceived colour of drug labels, increasing the risk for drug errors. *Can J Ophthalmol.* 2013;48(2):e27-e28. [VC]

221. Dolan SA, Arias KM, Felizardo G, et al. APIC position paper: safe injection, infusion, and medication vial practices in health care. *Am J Infect Control.* 2016;44(7):750-757. [IVB]

222. Haas RE, Beitz E, Reed A, et al. No bacterial growth found in spiked intravenous fluids over an 8-hour period. *Am J Infect Control.* 2017;45(4):448-450. [IIIB]

223. Preventing catheter/tubing misconnections: much needed help is on the way! *Alta RN.* 2011;67(2):24-25. [VC]

224. Paparella SF, Wollitz A. Mix-ups and misconnections: avoiding intravenous line errors. *J Emerg Nurs.* 2014;40(4):382-384. [VC]

225. Simmons D, Phillips MS, Grissinger M, Becker SC; USP Safe Medication Use Expert Committee. Error-avoidance recommendations for tubing misconnections when using Luer-tip connectors: a statement by the USP safe medication use expert committee. *Jt Comm J Qual Patient Saf.* 2008;34(5):293-296, 245. [VB]

226. Döring M, Brenner B, Handgretinger R, Hofbeck M, Kerst G. Inadvertent intravenous administration of maternal breast milk in a six-week-old infant: a case report and review of the literature. *BMC Res Notes.* 2014;7:17. [VC]

227. Cohen MR, Smetzer JL. ISMP medication error report analysis. *Hosp Pharm.* 2011;46(2):82-86. [VC]

228. Cohen MR, Smetzer JL. ISMP medication error report analysis—avoiding inadvertent intravenous injection of oral liquids; medication within intravenous tubing may be overlooked; searching by drug name gives information on wrong drug. *Hosp Pharm.* 2012;47(11):825-828. [VC]

229. Shenoi AN, Fortenberry JD, Kamat P. Accidental intra-arterial injection of propofol. *Pediatr Emerg Care.* 2014;30(2):136. [VC]

230. Ross MJ, Wise A. Accidental epidural administration of Syntocinon. *Int J Obstet Anesth.* 2012;21(2):203-204. [VC]

231. Kilcup M, Schultz D, Carlson J, Wilson B. Postdischarge pharmacist medication reconciliation: impact on readmission rates and financial savings. *J Am Pharm Assoc.* 2013;53(1):78-84. [IIB]

232. Ghatnekar O, Bondesson A, Persson U, Eriksson T. Health economic evaluation of the Lund Integrated Medicines Management model (LIMM) in elderly patients admitted to hospital. *BMJ Open.* 2013;3(1). [IIB]

233. Feldman LS, Costa LL, Feroli ERJ, et al. Nurse-pharmacist collaboration on medication reconciliation prevents potential harm. *J Hosp Med.* 2012;7(5):396-401. [IIIB]

234. Gimenez Manzorro A, Zoni AC, Rodriguez Rieiro C, et al. Developing a programme for medication reconciliation at the time of admission into hospital. *Int J Clin Pharm.* 2011;33(4):603-609. [IIB]

235. Selcuk A, Sancar M, Okuyan B, Demirtunc R, Izzettin FV. The potential role of clinical pharmacists in elderly patients during hospital admission. *Pharmazie.* 2015;70(8):559-562. [IIIB]

236. Dodds LJ. Optimising pharmacy input to medicines reconciliation at admission to hospital: lessons from a collaborative service evaluation of pharmacy-led medicines reconciliation services in 30 acute hospitals in England. *Eur J Hosp Pharm Sci Pract.* 2014;21(2):95-101. [IIIA]

237. Lee Y, Kuo L, Chiang Y, et al. Pharmacist-conducted medication reconciliation at hospital admission using information technology in Taiwan. *Int J Med Inf.* 2013;82(6):522-527. [IIIA]

238. Marotti SB, Kerridge RK, Grimer MD. A randomised controlled trial of pharmacist medication histories and supplementary prescribing on medication errors in postoperative medications. *Anaesth Intensive Care.* 2011;39(6):1064-1070. [IB]

239. Mekonnen AB, McLachlan AJ, Brien JE. Effectiveness of pharmacist-led medication reconciliation programmes on clinical outcomes at hospital transitions: a systematic review and meta-analysis. *BMJ Open.* 2016;6(2):e010003. [IIB]

240. Becerra-Camargo J, Martinez-Martinez F, Garcia-Jimenez E. The effect on potential adverse drug events of a pharmacist-acquired medication history in an emergency department: a multicentre, double-blind, randomised, controlled, parallel-group study. *BMC Health Serv Res.* 2015;15:337. [IB]

241. Gattari TB, Krieger LN, Hu HM, Mychaliska KP. Medication discrepancies at pediatric hospital discharge. *Hosp Pediatr.* 2015;5(8):439-445. [IIIB]

242. Ziaeian B, Araujo KLB, Van Ness PH, Horwitz LI. Medication reconciliation accuracy and patient understanding of intended medication changes on hospital discharge. *J Gen Intern Med.* 2012;27(11):1513-1520. [IIIB]

243. Wolf O, Aberg H, Tornberg U, Jonsson KB. Do orthogeriatric inpatients have a correct medication list? A pharmacist-led assessment of 254 patients in a Swedish university hospital. *Geriatr Orthop Surg Rehabil.* 2016;7(1):18-22. [IIIB]

244. Yi SB, Shan JCP, Hong GL. Medication reconciliation service in Tan Tock Seng Hospital. *Int J Health Care Qual Assur.* 2013;26(1):31-36. [IIIC]

245. González-García L, Salmerón-García A, García-Lirola M, Moya-Roldán S, Belda-Rustarazo S, Cabeza-Barrera J. Medication reconciliation at admission to surgical departments. *J Eval Clin Pract.* 2016;22(1):20-25. [IIIB]

246. Hohn N, Langer S, Kalder J, Jacobs MJ, Marx G, Eisert A. Optimizing the pharmacotherapy of vascular surgery patients by medication reconciliation. *J Cardiovasc Surg.* 2014;55(2 Suppl 1):175-181. [IIIB]

247. Knez L, Suskovic S, Rezonja R, Laaksonen R, Mrhar A. The need for medication reconciliation: a cross-sectional observational study in adult patients. *Respir Med.* 2011;105(Suppl 1):S60-S66. [IIIB]

248. Mendes AE, Lombardi NF, Andrzejevski VS, Frandoloso G, Correr CJ, Carvalho M. Medication reconciliation at patient admission: a randomized controlled trial. *Pharm Pract.* 2016;14(1):656. [IB]

249. Holland DM. Interdisciplinary collaboration in the provision of a pharmacist-led discharge medication reconciliation service at an Irish teaching hospital. *Int J Clin Pharm.* 2015;37(2):310-319. [IIIB]

250. Belda-Rustarazo S, Cantero-Hinojosa J, Salmeron-Garcia A, Gonzalez-Garcia L, Cabeza-Barrera J, Galvez J. Medication reconciliation at admission and discharge: an analysis of prevalence and associated risk factors. *Int J Clin Pract.* 2015;69(11):1268-1274. [IIIB]

251. Bemt PMLA, Schrieck-de Loos EM, Linden C, Theeuwes AMLJ, Pol AG. Effect of medication reconciliation on unintentional medication discrepancies in acute hospital admissions of elderly adults: a multicenter study. *J Am Geriatr Soc.* 2013;61(8):1262-1268. [IIA]

252. Benson JM, Snow G. Impact of medication reconciliation on medication error rates in community hospital cardiac care units. *Hosp Pharm.* 2012;47(12):927-932. [IIA]

253. Gao T, Gaunt MJ. Breakdowns in the medication reconciliation process. *Penn Patient Saf Advis.* 2013;10(4):125-136. [IIIA]

254. Rubio CB, Garrido PN, Segura BM, Ferrit M, Calderón AC, Catalá PRM. Medication reconciliation at admission in old patients. *Aten Farm.* 2014;16(1):13-22. [IIIB]

255. Gaspar Carreño M, Gavião Prado C, Costa Nogueira J, et al. Medication reconciliation on admission. *Aten Farm.* 2014;16(4):273-281. [IIIB]

256. Hellstrom LM, Bondesson A, Hoglund P, Eriksson T. Errors in medication history at hospital admission: prevalence and predicting factors. *BMC Clin Pharmacol.* 2012;12:9. [IIIA]

257. Young L, Barnason S, Hays K, Do V. Nurse practitioner-led medication reconciliation in critical access hospitals. *J Nurse Pract.* 2015;11(5):511-518. [IIB]

258. Bell CM, Brener SS, Gunraj N, et al. Association of ICU or hospital admission with unintentional discontinuation of medications for chronic diseases. *JAMA.* 2011;306(8):840-847. [IIIB]

259. Magalhães GF, Santos GN, Rosa MB, Noblat Lde A. Medication reconciliation in patients hospitalized in a cardiology unit. *PLoS One.* 2014;9(12):e115491. [IIIB]

260. Hellstrom LM, Hoglund P, Bondesson A, Petersson G, Eriksson T. Clinical implementation of systematic medication reconciliation and review as part of the Lund Integrated Medicines Management model—impact on all-cause emergency department revisits. *J Clin Pharm Ther.* 2012;37(6):686-692. [IIA]

261. Lehnbom EC, Stewart MJ, Manias E, Westbrook JI. Impact of medication reconciliation and review on clinical outcomes. *Ann Pharmacother.* 2014;48(10):1298-1312. [IIIB]

262. Cortelyou-Ward K, Swain A, Yeung T. Mitigating error vulnerability at the transition of care through the use of health IT applications. *J Med Syst.* 2012;36(6):3825-3831. [VB]

263. Treiber LA, Jones JH. Medication errors, routines, and differences between perioperative and non-perioperative nurses. *AORN J.* 2012;96(3):285-294. [IIIB]

264. Gallo E, Pugi A, Lucenteforte E, et al. Pharmacovigilance of herb-drug interactions among preoperative patients. *Altern Ther Health Med.* 2014;20(2):13-17. [IIIA]

265. Lee A, Varma A, Boro M, Korman N. Value of pharmacist medication interviews on optimizing the electronic medication reconciliation process. *Hosp Pharm.* 2014;49(6):530-538. [IIB]

266. Meyer C, Stern M, Woolley W, Jeanmonod R, Jeanmonod D. How reliable are patient-completed medication reconciliation forms compared with pharmacy lists? *Am J Emerg Med.* 2012;30(7):1048-1054. [IIIB]

267. Lu Y, Clifford P, Bjorneby A, et al. Quality improvement through implementation of discharge order reconciliation. *Am J Health Syst Pharm.* 2013;70(9):815-820. [VB]

268. Richards M, Ashiru-Oredope D, Chee N. What errors can be identified by pharmacy-led medicines reconciliation? A prospective study. *Acute Med.* 2011;10(1):18-21. [IIIB]

269. Karapinar-Carkit F, Borgsteede SD, Zoer J, Egberts TCG, van den Bemt PMLA, van Tulder M. Effect of medication reconciliation on medication costs after hospital discharge in relation to hospital pharmacy labor costs. *Ann Pharmacother.* 2012;46(3):329-338. [IIIB]

270. Philbrick AM, Harris IM, Schommer JC, Fallert CJ. Medication discrepancies associated with subsequent pharmacist-performed medication reconciliations in an

ambulatory clinic. *J Am Pharm Assoc.* 2015;55(1):77-80. [IIIB]

271. Leguelinel-Blache G, Arnaud F, Bouvet S, et al. Impact of admission medication reconciliation performed by clinical pharmacists on medication safety. *Eur J Intern Med.* 2014;25(9):808-814. [IIIB]

272. Mekonnen AB, McLachlan AJ, Brien JE. Pharmacy-led medication reconciliation programmes at hospital transitions: a systematic review and meta-analysis. *J Clin Pharm Ther.* 2016;41(2):128-144. [IIA]

273. Deitelzweig S. Care transitions in anticoagulation management for patients with atrial fibrillation: an emphasis on safety. *Ochsner J.* 2013;13(3):419-427. [VB]

274. Zoni AC, Duran Garcia ME, Jimenez Munoz AB, Salomon Perez R, Martin P, Herranz Alonso A. The impact of medication reconciliation program at admission in an internal medicine department. *Eur J Intern Med.* 2012;23(8):696-700. [IIC]

275. Andreoli L, Alexandra J, Tesmoingt C, et al. Medication reconciliation: a prospective study in an internal medicine unit. *Drugs Aging.* 2014;31(5):387-393. [IIIB]

276. Cornu P, Steurbaut S, Leysen T, et al. Effect of medication reconciliation at hospital admission on medication discrepancies during hospitalization and at discharge for geriatric patients. *Ann Pharmacother.* 2012;46(4):484-494. [IIIB]

277. Shiu JR, Fradette M, Padwal RS, et al. Medication discrepancies associated with a medication reconciliation program and clinical outcomes after hospital discharge. *Pharmacotherapy.* 2016;36(4):415-421. [IIIB]

278. Lee KP, Hartridge C, Corbett K, Vittinghoff E, Auerbach AD. "Whose job is it, really?" Physicians', nurses', and pharmacists' perspectives on completing inpatient medication reconciliation. *J Hosp Med.* 2015;10(3):184-186. [IIIB]

279. De Winter S, Vanbrabant P, Spriet I, et al. A simple tool to improve medication reconciliation at the emergency department. *Eur J Intern Med.* 2011;22(4):382-385. [IIA]

280. Cullinan S, O'Mahony D, Byrne S. Application of the structured history taking of medication use tool to optimise prescribing for older patients and reduce adverse events. *Int J Clin Pharm.* 2016;38(2):374-379. [IIIB]

281. Henneman EA, Tessier EG, Nathanson BH, Plotkin K. An evaluation of a collaborative, safety focused, nurse-pharmacist intervention for improving the accuracy of the medication history. *J Patient Saf.* 2014;10(2):88-94. [IIA]

282. Narendra PL, Biradar PA, Rao AN. Vanishing bowl of local anesthetics: a lesson for sterile labeling. *Anesth Essays Res.* 2014;8(3):407-409. [VC]

283. Medication safety. *J Pharm Pract Res.* 2015;45(1):86-92. [VC]

284. Guideline for sterile technique. In: *Guidelines for Perioperative Practice.* Denver, CO: AORN, Inc; 2017:75-104. [IVA]

285. Or CKL, Wang H. A comparison of the effects of different typographical methods on the recognizability of printed drug names. *Drug Saf.* 2014;37(5):351-359. [IIIB]

286. Sakuma M, Ida H, Nakamura T, et al. Adverse drug events and medication errors in Japanese paediatric inpatients: a retrospective cohort study. *BMJ Qual Saf.* 2014;23(10):830-837. [IIIA]

287. Standards for perioperative nursing. In: *Guidelines for Perioperative Practice.* Denver, CO: AORN, Inc; 2015:693-708. [IVC]

288. Cohen MR, Smetzer JL. ISMP medication error report analysis—fatal patient-controlled anesthesia adverse events; name confusion with new cancer drugs; medication safety officer group to become a part of ISMP. *Hosp Pharm.* 2013;48(9):715-724. [VC]

289. Guideline for care of the patient receiving local anesthesia. In: *Guidelines for Perioperative Practice.* Denver, CO: AORN, Inc; 2017:617-628. [IVA]

290. Pfeifer K, Slawski B, Manley A, Nelson V, Haines M. Improving preoperative medication compliance with standardized instructions. *Minerva Anestesiol.* 2016;82(1):44-49. [VA]

291. Chien HY, Ko JJ, Chen YC, et al. Study of medication waste in Taiwan. *J Exp Clin Med.* 2013;5(2):69-72. [IIIB]

292. Warle-van Herwaarden MF, Kramers C, Sturkenboom MC, van den Bemt PMLA, De Smet PAGM; Dutch HARM-Wrestling Task Force. Targeting outpatient drug safety: recommendations of the Dutch HARM-Wrestling Task Force. *Drug Saf.* 2012;35(3):245-259. [IVB]

293. Manworren RCB, Gilson AM. CE: Nurses' role in preventing prescription opioid diversion. *Am J Nurs.* 2015;115(8):34-40. [VB]

294. Strauch KA. Invisible pollution: the impact of pharmaceuticals in the water supply. *AAOHN J.* 2011;59(12):525-533. [VB]

295. Trovato JA, Tuttle LA. Oral chemotherapy handling and storage practices among veterans affairs oncology patients and caregivers. *J Oncol Pharm Pract.* 2014;20(2):88-92. [VA]

296. Perks S, Robertson S, Haywood A, Glass B. Clozapine repackaged into dose administration aids: a common practice in Australian hospitals. *Int J Pharm Pract.* 2012;20(1):4-8. [IIIB]

297. Beckett VL, Tyson LD, Carroll D, Gooding NM, Kelsall AW. Accurately administering oral medication to children isn't child's play. *Arch Dis Child.* 2012;97(9):838-841. [IIIB]

298. Armor BL, Wight AJ, Carter SM. Evaluation of adverse drug events and medication discrepancies in transitions of care between hospital discharge and primary care follow-up. *J Pharm Pract.* 2016;29(2):132-137. [IIIB]

299. Sarangarm P, London MS, Snowden SS, et al. Impact of pharmacist discharge medication therapy counseling and disease state education: pharmacist assisting at routine medical discharge (project PhARMD). *Am J Med Qual.* 2013;28(4):292-300. [IIB]

300. Valente S, Murray LP. Creative strategies to improve patient safety: allergies and adverse drug reactions. *J Nurses Staff Dev.* 2011;27(1):E1-E5. [VB]

301. Borgsteede SD, Karapinar-Carkit F, Hoffmann E, Zoer J, van den Bemt PMLA. Information needs about medication according to patients discharged from a general hospital. *Patient Educ Couns.* 2011;83(1):22-28. [IIIB]

302. Bouraoui S, Brahem A, Tabka F, Mrizek N, Saad A, Elghezal H. Assessment of chromosomal aberrations, micronuclei and proliferation rate index in peripheral lymphocytes from Tunisian nurses handling cytotoxic drugs. *Environ Toxicol Pharmacol.* 2011;31(1):250-257. [IIIB]

303. Connor TH, Lawson CC, Polovich M, McDiarmid MA. Reproductive health risks associated with occupational exposures to antineoplastic drugs in health care settings: a review of the evidence. *J Occup Environ Med.* 2014;56(9):901-910. [IIIB]

304. El-Ebiary AA, Abuelfadl AA, Sarhan NI. Evaluation of genotoxicity induced by exposure to antineoplastic drugs in lymphocytes of oncology nurses and pharmacists. *J Appl Toxicol.* 2013;33(3):196-201. [IIIB]

305. Gomez-Olivan LM, Miranda-Mendoza GD, Cabrera-Galeana PA, et al. Oxidative stress induced in nurses by exposure to preparation and handling of antineoplastic

drugs in Mexican hospitals: a multicentric study. *Oxid Med Cell Longev.* 2014;2014:858604. [IIIB]

306. Hon C, Abusitta D. Causes of health care workers' exposure to antineoplastic drugs: an exploratory study. *Can J Hosp Pharm.* 2016;69(3):216-223. [IIIB]

307. Musak L, Smerhovsky Z, Halasova E, et al. Chromosomal damage among medical staff occupationally exposed to volatile anesthetics, antineoplastic drugs, and formaldehyde. *Scand J Work Environ Health.* 2013;39(6):618-630. [IIIB]

308. Hon C, Teschke K, Shen H, Demers PA, Venners S. Antineoplastic drug contamination in the urine of Canadian healthcare workers. *Int Arch Occup Environ Health.* 2015;88(7):933-941. [IIIB]

309. Controlling occupational exposure to hazardous drugs. Occupational Safety and Health Administration. https://www.osha.gov/SLTC/hazardousdrugs/controlling_occex_hazardousdrugs.html. Accessed July 13, 2017.

310. Gulten T, Evke E, Ercan I, Evrensel T, Kurt E, Manavoglu O. Lack of genotoxicity in medical oncology nurses handling antineoplastic drugs: effect of work environment and protective equipment. *Work.* 2011;39(4):485-489. [IIIB]

311. Occupational Safety and Health Administration. 29 CFR §1910.1200. Hazard communication. US Government Publishing Office. http://www.ecfr.gov/cgi-bin/text-idx?SID=3a88b79bbd5ccb9689a55025239c3ff8&mc=true&node=se29.6.1910_11200&rgn=div8. Accessed July 13, 2017.

312. Easty AC, Coakley N, Cheng R, et al. Safe handling of cytotoxics: guideline recommendations. *Curr Oncol.* 2015;22(1):e27-e37. [IVB]

313. Hazardous drugs—handling in healthcare settings (800). In: *USP Compounding Compendium.* Rockville, MD: US Pharmacopeial Convention; 2016:86-103. [IVC]

314. Bussieres J, Tanguay C, Touzin K, Langlois E, Lefebvre M. Environmental contamination with hazardous drugs in Quebec hospitals. *Can J Hosp Pharm.* 2012;65(6):428-435. [IIIA]

315. Ensuring healthcare worker safety when handling hazardous drugs. *Oncol Nurs Forum.* 2015;42(3):217-218. [IVB]

316. Boiano JM, Steege AL, Sweeney MH. Adherence to precautionary guidelines for compounding antineoplastic drugs: a survey of nurses and pharmacy practitioners. *J Occup Environ Hyg.* 2015;12(9):588-602. [IIIB]

317. Lawson CC, Rocheleau CM, Whelan EA, et al. Occupational exposures among nurses and risk of spontaneous abortion. *Am J Obstet Gynecol.* 2012;206(4):327.e1-327.e8. [IIIA]

318. Leduc-Souville B, Bertrand E, Schlatter J. Risk management of excreta in a cancer unit. *Clin J Oncol Nurs.* 2013;17(3):248-252. [IIIB]

319. Meade E. Avoiding accidental exposure to intravenous cytotoxic drugs. *Br J Nurs.* 2014;23(16):S34. [VA]

320. Vyas N, Yiannakis D, Turner A, Sewell GJ. Occupational exposure to anti-cancer drugs: a review of effects of new technology. *J Oncol Pharm Pract.* 2014;20(4):278-287. [VB]

321. Villarini M, Dominici L, Piccinini R, et al. Assessment of primary, oxidative and excision repaired DNA damage in hospital personnel handling antineoplastic drugs. *Mutagenesis.* 2011;26(3):359-369. [IIIB]

322. Menonna-Quinn D. Safe handling of chemotherapeutic agents in the treatment of nonmalignant diseases. *J Infus Nurs.* 2013;36(3):198-204. [VB]

323. *PB70: Liquid Barrier Performance and Classification of Protective Apparel and Drapes Intended for use in Health Care Facilities.* Arlington, VA: Association for the Advancement of Medical Instrumentation; 2012. [IVC]

324. Occupational Safety and Health Administration. 29 CFR §1910.134. Respiratory protection. https://www.osha.gov/pls/oshaweb/owadisp.show_document?p_table=standards&p_id=12716. Accessed July 13, 2017.

325. Hon C, Teschke K, Chua P, Venners S, Nakashima L. Occupational exposure to antineoplastic drugs: identification of job categories potentially exposed throughout the hospital medication system. *Saf Health Work.* 2011;2(3):273-281. [IIIB]

326. Hon C, Teschke K, Chu W, Demers P, Venners S. Antineoplastic drug contamination of surfaces throughout the hospital medication system in Canadian hospitals. *J Occup Environ Hyg.* 2013;10(7):374-383. [IIIB]

327. Queruau Lamerie T, Nussbaumer S, Decaudin B, et al. Evaluation of decontamination efficacy of cleaning solutions on stainless steel and glass surfaces contaminated by 10 antineoplastic agents. *Ann Occup Hyg.* 2013;57(4):456-469. [IIIB]

328. Walton AML, Mason S, Busshart M, et al. Safe handling: implementing hazardous drug precautions. *Clin J Oncol Nurs.* 2012;16(3):251-254. [VB]

329. Bohlandt A, Groeneveld S, Fischer E, Schierl R. Cleaning efficiencies of three cleaning agents on four different surfaces after contamination by gemcitabine and 5-fluorouracile. *J Occup Environ Hyg.* 2015;12(6):384-392. [IIIB]

330. Schierl R, Novotna J, Piso P, Bohlandt A, Nowak D. Low surface contamination by cis/oxaliplatin during hyperthermic intraperitoneal chemotherapy (HIPEC). *Eur J Surg Oncol.* 2012;38(1):88-94. [IIIB]

331. Couch J, Burr G, Niemeier MT. Evaluation of exposures to healthcare personnel from cisplatin during a mock interperitoneal operation for cancer treatment. *J Assoc Occup Health Prof Healthc.* 2011;31(2):17-19. [VA]

332. Solid Waste Disposal Act [as amended through Pub L No 107-377, December 31, 2002].

333. Souza Oliveira AD, Cãmara Alves AE, Silva JA, Silva Oliveira LF, Medeiros SM. Occupational risks of the nursing team's exposure to chemotherapeutic agents: integrative literature review. *Rev Enferm UFPE.* 2013;7(3):794-802. [IIIB]

334. Hennessy KA, Dynan J. Improving compliance with personal protective equipment use through the model for improvement and staff champions. *Clin J Oncol Nurs.* 2014;18(5):497-500. [VB]

335. Boiano JM, Steege AL, Sweeney MH. Adherence to safe handling guidelines by health care workers who administer antineoplastic drugs. *J Occup Environ Hyg.* 2014;11(11):728-740. [IIIB]

336. Jeong KW, Lee B, Kwon MS, Jang J. Safety management status among nurses handling anticancer drugs: nurse awareness and performance following safety regulations. *Asian Pac J Cancer Prev.* 2015;16(8):3203-3211. [IIIB]

337. Polovich M, Gieseker KE. Occupational hazardous drug exposure among non-oncology nurses. *Medsurg Nurs.* 2011;20(2):79-85. [VA]

338. Hon C, Teschke K, Demers PA, Venners S. Antineoplastic drug contamination on the hands of employees working throughout the hospital medication system. *Ann Occup Hyg.* 2014;58(6):761-770. [IIIB]

339. Hon C, Teschke K, Shen H. Health care workers' knowledge, perceptions, and behaviors regarding antineoplastic drugs: survey from British Columbia, Canada. *J Occup Environ Hyg.* 2015;12(10):669-677. [IIIA]

340. Ladeira C, Viegas S, Padua M, et al. Assessment of genotoxic effects in nurses handling cytostatic drugs. *J Toxicol Environ Health A.* 2014;77(14-16):879-887. [IIIB]

341. Santovito A, Cervella P, Delpero M. Chromosomal damage in peripheral blood lymphocytes from nurses occupationally exposed to chemicals. *Hum Exp Toxicol.* 2014;33(9):897-903. [IIIB]

342. Drug Enforcement Administration (DEA), Department of Justice. Disposal of controlled substances. Final rule. *Fed Regist.* 2014;79(174):53519-53570.

343. Unused Pharmaceuticals in the Health Care Industry: Interim Report. Washington, DC: Environmental Protection Agency; 2008. https://nepis.epa.gov/Exe/ZyPDF.cgi/P100165B.PDF?Dockey=P100165B.PDF. Accessed July 13, 2017. [VB]

344. Federal Water Pollution Control Act [as amended through Pub L No 107-303, November 27, 2002].

345. Chiarello M, Minetto L, Giustina SVD, Beal LL, Moura S. Popular pharmaceutical residues in hospital wastewater: quantification and qualification of degradation products by mass spectroscopy after treatment with membrane bioreactor. *Environ Sci Pollut Res Int.* 2016;23(16):16079-16089. [IIIB]

346. Frédéric O, Yves P. Pharmaceuticals in hospital wastewater: their ecotoxicity and contribution to the environmental hazard of the effluent. *Chemosphere.* 2014;115(1):31-39. [IIIC]

347. Nguyen H, Pham H, Vo D, et al. The effect of a clinical pharmacist-led training programme on intravenous medication errors: a controlled before and after study. *BMJ Qual Saf.* 2014;23(4):319-324. [IIB]

348. Laukaityte E, Bruyere M, Bull A, Benhamou D. Accidental injection of patent blue dye during gynaecological surgery: lack of knowledge constitutes a system error. *Anaesth Crit Care Pain Med.* 2015;34(1):57-60. [VC]

349. Westbrook JI, Rob MI, Woods A, Parry D. Errors in the administration of intravenous medications in hospital and the role of correct procedures and nurse experience. *BMJ Qual Saf.* 2011;20(12):1027-1034. [IIIB]

350. Karavasiliadou S, Athanasakis E. An inside look into the factors contributing to medication errors in the clinical nursing practice. *Health Sci J.* 2014;8(1):32-44. [VB]

351. Zyoud AH, Abdullah NAC. The effect of individual factors on the medication error. *Glob J Health Sci.* 2016;8(12):57756. [IIIB]

352. Thornton P. Medication safety. *J Pharm Pract Res.* 2015;45(4):450-458. [VC]

353. Niemann D, Bertsche A, Meyrath D, et al. A prospective three-step intervention study to prevent medication errors in drug handling in paediatric care. *J Clin Nurs.* 2015;24(1-2):101-114. [IIIB]

354. Samaranayake NR, Cheung STD, Chui WCM, Cheung BMY. Technology-related medication errors in a tertiary hospital: a 5-year analysis of reported medication incidents. *Int J Med Inform.* 2012;81(12):828-833. [IIIB]

355. Hicks RW, Hernandez J, Wanzer LJ. Perioperative pharmacology: patient-controlled analgesia. *AORN J.* 2012;95(2):255-262. [VB]

356. Speroni KG, Fisher J, Dennis M, Daniel M. What causes near-misses and how are they mitigated? *Nursing.* 2013;43(4):19-24. [IIIB]

357. Abbotoy JL, Sessanna L. Hands-on BCMA education for direct care nurses. *Nurs Manage.* 2012;43(11):15-18. [VC]

358. Cleary-Holdforth J, Leufer T. The strategic role of education in the prevention of medication errors in nursing: part 2. *Nurse Educ Pract.* 2013;13(3):217-220. [VB]

359. Leufer T, Cleary-Holdforth J. Let's do no harm: medication errors in nursing: part 1. *Nurse Educ Pract.* 2013;13(3):213-216. [VB]

360. Lu M, Yu S, Chen I, Wang KK, Wu H, Tang F. Nurses' knowledge of high-alert medications: a randomized controlled trial. *Nurse Educ Today.* 2013;33(1):24-30. [IB]

361. Gokhman R, Seybert AL, Phrampus P, Darby J, Kane-Gill SL. Medication errors during medical emergencies in a large, tertiary care, academic medical center. *Resuscitation.* 2012;83(4):482-487. [IIIA]

362. Lap FT, Tak KY, So Yuen AS. How to change nurses' behavior leading to medication administration errors using a survey approach in United Christian Hospital. *J Nuse Educ Pract.* 2014;4(12):17-26. [IIIB]

363. Sears K, Goodman WM. Risk factors for increased severity of paediatric medication administration errors. *Healthc Policy.* 2012;8(1):e109-e126. [IIIB]

364. Abbasinazari M, Zareh-Toranposhti S, Hassani A, Sistanizad M, Azizian H, Panahi Y. The effect of information provision on reduction of errors in intravenous drug preparation and administration by nurses in ICU and surgical wards. *Acta Med Iran.* 2012;50(11):771-777. [IIB]

365. Haw C, Stubbs J, Dickens G. Medicines management: an interview study of nurses at a secure psychiatric hospital. *J Adv Nurs.* 2015;71(2):281-294. [IIIB]

366. Haseeb A, Winit-Watjana W, Bakhsh AR, et al. Effectiveness of a pharmacist-led educational intervention to reduce the use of high-risk abbreviations in an acute care setting in Saudi Arabia: a quasi-experimental study. *BMJ Open.* 2016;6(6):e011401. [IIB]

367. Chedoe I, Molendijk H, Hospes W, Van den Heuvel ER, Taxis K. The effect of a multifaceted educational intervention on medication preparation and administration errors in neonatal intensive care. *Arch Dis Child Fetal Neonatal Ed.* 2012;97(6):F449-F455. [IIB]

368. Lohmann K, Ferber J, Haefeli MF, et al. Knowledge and training needs of nurses and physicians on unsuitable drugs for patients with dysphagia or feeding tubes. *J Clin Nurs.* 2015;24(19-20):3016-3019. [IIIC]

369. Keane K. Reducing medication errors by educating nurses on bar code technology. *Medsurg Nurs.* 2014;23(5 Suppl 1):10-11. [VC]

370. Alsulami Z, Choonara I, Conroy S. Nurses' knowledge about the double-checking process for medicines administration. *Nurs Child Young People.* 2014;26(9):21-26. [IIIB]

371. Dabliz R, Levine S. Medication safety in neonates. *Am J Perinatol.* 2012;29(1):49-56. [VC]

372. Implementing real-time point of care documentation: a QI project to address medication administration errors. *Online J Nurs Inform.* 2014;18(3):1-1. [VB]

373. Bucsi R. Documentation errors related to electronic health records. *Insight.* 2012;37(3):19. [VB]

374. Order scanning systems (and fax machines) may pull multiple pages through the scanner at the same time, leading to drug omissions. *Alta RN.* 2011;67(1):24-25. [VC]

375. Perez-Garcia MdC, Soria-Aledo V, Collantes F. Implementation and evaluation of the medication management in nursing units of a university hospital by means of a quality improvement cycle. *Appl Nurs Res.* 2016;29:148-156. [VB]

376. Nwasor EO, Sule ST, Mshelia DB. Audit of medication errors by anesthetists in north western Nigeria. *Niger J Clin Pract.* 2014;17(2):226-231. [IIIC]

377. Burch KJ. Using a trigger tool to assess adverse drug events in a children's rehabilitation hospital. *J Pediatr Pharm Ther.* 2011;16(3):204-209. [IIIC]

378. Carnevali L, Krug B, Amant F, et al. Performance of the adverse drug event trigger tool and the global trigger tool for identifying adverse drug events: experience in a

Belgian hospital. *Ann Pharmacother.* 2013;47(11):1414-1419. [IIIB]

379. Nobre C, McKay C. Surveillance of adverse drug events in a large tertiary-care hospital. *Conn Med.* 2012;76(2):91-94. [VB]

380. Harkanen M, Kervinen M, Ahonen J, Voutilainen A, Turunen H, Vehvilainen-Julkunen K. Patient-specific risk factors of adverse drug events in adult inpatients—evidence detected using the global trigger tool method. *J Clin Nurs.* 2015;24(3-4):582-591. [IIIC]

381. Kung K, Carrel T, Wittwer B, Engberg S, Zimmermann N, Schwendimann R. Medication errors in a Swiss cardiovascular surgery department: a cross-sectional study based on a novel medication error report method. *Nurs Res Pract.* 2013;2013:671820. [IIIB]

382. Donaldson N, Aydin C, Fridman M, Foley M. Improving medication administration safety: using naive observation to assess practice and guide improvements in process and outcomes. *J Healthc Qual.* 2014;36(6):58-68. [IIIB]

383. Taghon T, Elsey N, Miler V, McClead R, Tobias J. A medication-based trigger tool to identify adverse events in pediatric anesthesiology. *Jt Comm J Qual Patient Saf.* 2014;40(7):326-334. [VB]

384. Erstad BL, Patanwala AE, Theodorou AA. Comparison of methods for the detection of medication safety events in the critically ill. *Curr Drug Saf.* 2012;7(3):238-246. [IIIB]

385. Davies K, Mitchell C, Coombes I. The role of observation and feedback in enhancing performance with medication administration. *J Law Med.* 2015;23(2):316-321. [VB]

386. Elliott P, Martin D, Neville D. Electronic clinical safety reporting system: a benefits evaluation. *JMIR Med Inform.* 2014;2(1):e12. [IIB]

387. Meyer-Massetti C, Cheng CM, Schwappach DLB, et al. Systematic review of medication safety assessment methods. *Am J Health Syst Pharm.* 2011;68(3):227-240. [IIIB]

388. Cronrath P, Lynch TW, Gilson LJ, et al. PCA oversedation: application of healthcare failure mode effect (HFMEA) analysis. *Nurs Econ.* 2011;29(2):79-87. [IIB]

389. Velez-Diaz-Pallares M, Delgado-Silveira E, Carretero-Accame ME, Bermejo-Vicedo T. Using healthcare failure mode and effect analysis to reduce medication errors in the process of drug prescription, validation and dispensing in hospitalised patients. *BMJ Qual Saf.* 2013;22(1):42-52. [IIB]

390. Curatolo N, Gutermann L, Devaquet N, Roy S, Rieutord A. Reducing medication errors at admission: 3 cycles to implement, improve and sustain medication reconciliation. *Int J Clin Pharm.* 2014;37(1):113-120. [IIIB]

391. Ashley L, Dexter R, Marshall F, McKenzie B, Ryan M, Armitage G. Improving the safety of chemotherapy administration: an oncology nurse-led failure mode and effects analysis. *Oncol Nurs Forum.* 2011;38(6):E436-E444. [VB]

392. Cheng C, Chou C, Wang P, Lin H, Kao C, Su C. Applying HFMEA to prevent chemotherapy errors. *J Med Syst.* 2012;36(3):1543-1551. [VB]

393. Nguyen C, Cote J, Lebel D, et al. The AMELIE project: Failure mode, effects and criticality analysis: a model to evaluate the nurse medication administration process on the floor. *J Eval Clin Pract.* 2013;19(1):192-199. [VB]

394. Beckett RD, Yazdi M, Hanson LJ, Thompson RW. Improving medication safety through the use of metrics. *J Pharm Pract.* 2014;27(1):61-64. [IIIA]

395. de Boer M, Ramrattan MA, Boeker EB, Kuks PFM, Boermeester MA, Lie-A-Huen L. Quality of pharmaceutical care in surgical patients. *PLoS One.* 2014;9(7):e101573. [IIIB]

396. Smeulers M, Verweij L, Maaskant JM, et al. Quality indicators for safe medication preparation and administration: a systematic review. *PLoS One.* 2015;10(4):e0122695. [IIIB]

397. Rodriguez-Gonzalez CG, Martin-Barbero ML, Herranz-Alonso A, et al. Use of failure mode, effect and criticality analysis to improve safety in the medication administration process. *J Eval Clin Pract.* 2015;21(4):549-559. [VB]

398. Miller DF, Fortier CR, Garrison KL. Bar code medication administration technology: characterization of high-alert medication triggers and clinician workarounds. *Ann Pharmacother.* 2011;45(2):162-168. [IIIA]

399. Rack LL, Dudjak LA, Wolf GA. Study of nurse workarounds in a hospital using bar code medication administration system. *J Nurs Care Qual.* 2012;27(3):232-239. [IIIB]

400. Niazkhani Z, Pirnejad H, van der Sijs H, Aarts J. Evaluating the medication process in the context of CPOE use: the significance of working around the system. *Int J Med Inf.* 2011;80(7):490-506. [IIIB]

401. Coleman JJ, Hodson J, Brooks HL, Rosser D. Missed medication doses in hospitalised patients: a descriptive account of quality improvement measures and time series analysis. *Int J Qual Health Care.* 2013;25(5):564-572. [VA]

402. Munn Z, Scarborough A, Pearce S, et al. The implementation of best practice in medication administration across a health network: a multisite evidence-based audit and feedback project. *JBI Database System Rev Implement Rep.* 2015;13(8):338-352. [IIB]

Acknowledgements

LEAD AUTHOR
Byron L. Burlingame, MS, RN, BSN, CNOR
Senior Perioperative Practice Specialist
AORN Nursing Department
Denver, Colorado

CONTRIBUTING AUTHOR
Ramona L. Conner, MSN, RN, CNOR, FAAN
Editor-in-Chief, Guidelines for Perioperative Practice
AORN Nursing Department
Denver, Colorado

The authors and AORN thank Janice Neil, PhD, RN, CNE, Associate Professor, College of Nursing, East Carolina University, Greenville, North Carolina; Mary Lamonte, MPH, MSN, RN, CNOR, Staff Nurse, Stamford Surgical Center, Stamford, Connecticut; Rodney W. Hicks, PhD, RN, FNP-BC, FAANP, Professor, Western University of Health Sciences, Pomona, California; Diana L. Wadlund, MSN, ACNP-C, CRNFA, Nurse Practitioner, Paoli Hospital, Paoli, Pennsylvania; Leslie Jeter, MSNA, RN, CRNA, Staff CRNA, Ambulatory Anesthesia of Atlanta, Georgia; Bernard C. Camins, MD, MSc, Associate Professor of Medicine Division of Infectious Diseases, University of Alabama at Birmingham Healthcare Epidemiologist, UAB Health System Medical Director, UAB Hospital Employee Health and UA HSF Employee Health, Birmingham; Jocelyn M. Chalquist, BSN, RN, CNOR, Surgical Services Educator, Aurora Medical Center-Kenosha, Kenosha, Wisconsin;

Judith L. Goldberg, DBA, MSN, RN, CNOR, CSSM, CHL, Director, Patient Care Services, Perioperative and Procedural Services, Lawrence + Memorial Hospital, New London, Connecticut; Lisa Spruce, DNP, RN, CNS-CP, ACNS, ACNP, CNOR, FAAN, Director of Evidence-based Perioperative Practice, AORN Nursing Department, Denver, Colorado; Colleen Peralta, MSN, RN, Professor, College of Nursing, Long Beach City College, Long Beach, California; Vicki Barnett, MSN, RN, CNOR, Executive Director, Department of Surgical Services, Northside Hospital, Atlanta, Georgia; Evangeline (Vangie) Dennis, BSN, RN, CNOR, CMLSO, Director of Patient Care Practice, Emory Healthcare and Ambulatory Surgery Centers, Atlanta, Georgia; Brenda G. Larkin, MS, RN, CNOR, ACNS-BC, Clinical Nurse Specialist for Perioperative Services, Aurora Lakeland Medical Center and Aurora Memorial Hospital Burlington, Elkhorn, Wisconsin; and James (Jay) Bowers, BSN, RN, CNOR, TNCC, Clinical Educator, West Virginia Healthcare, Morgantown; for their assistance in developing this guideline.

PUBLICATION HISTORY

Originally published December 2011 online in *Perioperative Standards and Recommended Practices*.

Reformatted September 2012 for publication in *Perioperative Standards and Recommended Practices*, 2013 edition.

Minor editing revisions made in November 2014 for publication as "Guideline for medication safety" in *Guidelines for Perioperative Practice*, 2015 edition.

Revised September 2017 for publication in *Guidelines for Perioperative Practice* online.

PATIENT AND WORKER SAFETY

AMBULATORY SUPPLEMENT: MEDICATION SAFETY

Recommendation I

The health care organization should establish a multidisciplinary team to be responsible for the oversight of the medication management plan.

I.g.1. The health care organization may contract with a pharmacist to provide consultative services onsite or via telepharmacy.[A1-A3]

The Centers for Medicare & Medicaid Services (CMS) Conditions of Participation states that "Hospitals must provide pharmaceutical services that meet the needs of their patients."[A1] The CMS Conditions for Coverage for ambulatory surgery centers (ASCs) states that a specific licensed health care professional is required to provide direction to the ASC's pharmaceutical service unless the ASC is performing activities that under state law may only be performed by a licensed pharmacist.[A2]

Amb If an on-site pharmacist is not available, pharmaceutical services provided by the organization should be directed and overseen by a licensed pharmacist, or when appropriate, by a physician or dentist who is qualified to assume responsibility for the pharmaceutical services rendered.[A1,A4]

Amb When required by law and regulation or the policy of the organization, if a medication has been recalled there must be a process by which patients are notified that the medication was recalled for safety reasons by the manufacturer or the US Food and Drug Administration.[A5]

Recommendation II

Precautions should be taken to mitigate the risks associated with medication and medication-related supply procurement and storage.

II.d. All Class II, III, IV, and V medications must be stored in a locked location.[A1,A2]

Amb In accordance with the Comprehensive Drug Abuse Prevention and Control Act of 1970, if Class II, III, IV, and V drugs are used, records of receipt and disposition of the drugs must be maintained. Accountability procedures must be in place to ensure control of the distribution, use, and disposition of all scheduled drugs.

Amb Records to trace the movement of scheduled drugs throughout the ASC must be current and maintained, and any discrepancies in count must be reconciled promptly. Scheduled drugs must be tracked from the point of entry into the ASC to the point of departure, either through administration, destruction, or return to the manufacturer.

Amb The ASC must have a system in place to readily identify loss or diversion of all controlled substances, and the system should minimize the time between the actual loss or diversion and the time of detection.[A1]

Amb The ASC must maintain a current medication formulary that includes the strength and dosage for dispensing and administering the medications. The medication formulary must be readily available to those involved in medication management. There must be a process to select and procure medications that are not on the formulary.[A5] Medications on the formulary that are dispensed or administered should be reviewed annually based on emerging safety and efficacy information.

Recommendation III

Precautions should be taken to mitigate the risk for medication errors in the prescribing phase of the medication use process.

III.b.1 Handwritten medication orders should be legible and include a legible signature of the prescriber initiating the order.

Amb Prescription pads should be controlled and secured from unauthorized patient access, and should not be pre-signed and/or postdated.[A4]

Recommendation V

Precautions should be taken to mitigate the risk for errors during medication administration.

V.a All medications should be administered according to the manufacturer's instructions for use.

Amb Records must be maintained to ensure the control and safe dispensing of sample drugs in compliance with federal and state law.[A4]

Recommendation X

Precautions should be taken to mitigate the risks related to handling hazardous medications.

X.a. The health care organization must create a hazardous medication management plan.[A6]

Amb The ASC must identify, in writing, its hazardous medications and its process for managing hazardous medications. This is also applicable to sample medications.[A2]

REFERENCES

A1. Centers for Medicare & Medicaid Services (CMS), DHHS. Medicare and Medicaid programs; hospital conditions of participation: requirements for history and physical examinations; authentication of verbal orders; securing medications; and postanesthesia evaluations. Final rule. *Fed Regist.* 2006;71(227):68671-68695.

A2. Centers for Medicare & Medicaid Services. *State Operations Manual Appendix L—Guidance for Surveyors: Ambulatory Surgical Centers.* Rev. 137; 2015. https://www.cms.gov/Regulations-and-Guidance/Guidance/Manuals/downloads/som107ap_l_ambulatory.pdf. Accessed July 12, 2017.

A3. Cole SL, Grubbs JH, Din C, Nesbitt TS. Rural inpatient telepharmacy consultation demonstration for after-hours medication review. *Telemed J E Health.* 2012;18(7):530-537. [IIB]

A4. ASHP guidelines: minimum standard for pharmacies in hospitals. *Am J Health Syst Pharm.* 2013;70(18):1619-1630. [IVC]

A5. MM.05.01.17. In: *Standards for Ambulatory Care.* Oak Brook Terrace, IL: The Joint Commission; 2017.

A6. Occupational Safety and Health Administration. 29 CFR §1910.1200. Hazard communication. US Government Publishing Office. http://www.ecfr.gov/cgi-bin/text-idx?SID=3a88b79bbd5ccb9689a55025239c3ff8&mc=true&node=se29.6.1910_11200&rgn=div8. Accessed July 13, 2017.

Acknowledgements

CONTRIBUTING AUTHOR
Jan Davidson, MSN, RN, CNOR, CASC
Director, Ambulatory Surgery Division
AORN, Inc
Denver, Colorado

PUBLICATION HISTORY
Originally published in *Perioperative Standards and Recommended Practices,* 2014 edition.

Revised September 2018 for publication in *Guidelines for Perioperative Practice,* 2018 edition.

PATIENT AND WORKER SAFETY

Ambulatory Surgery

Ambulatory Surgery

PATIENT AND **WORKER** SAFETY

GUIDELINE FOR RADIATION SAFETY

The Guideline for Radiation Safety has been approved by the AORN Guidelines Advisory Board. It was presented as a proposed guideline for comments by members and others. The guideline is effective June 15, 2015. The recommendations in the guideline are intended to be achievable and represent what is believed to be an optimal level of practice. Policies and procedures will reflect variations in practice settings and/or clinical situations that determine the degree to which the guideline can be implemented. AORN recognizes the many diverse settings in which perioperative nurses practice; therefore, this guideline is adaptable to all areas where operative or other invasive procedures may be performed.

Purpose

This document provides guidance for preventing patient and health care worker injury from ionizing radiation exposure during therapeutic, diagnostic, or interventional procedures performed in the perioperative environment. Guidance for low-dose-rate and high-dose-rate brachytherapy using ionizing radiation is included. This guidance applies to patients, perioperative team members, and the caregivers of patients who receive brachytherapy or other radioactive therapeutic implants.

A review of the literature provided evidence that perioperative team members and patients are exposed to radiation in nearly all perioperative specialties (eg, general surgery, urology, neurosurgery, peripheral vascular surgery, cardiac surgery, endoscopy, orthopedics).[1,2] These procedures are performed in various settings (eg, operating rooms [ORs], ambulatory surgery centers, inpatient and outpatient endoscopy suites, physician offices). In some situations, such as when a patient has brachytherapy implants, radiation safety practices extend beyond the clinical setting into the community.[3]

Studies have demonstrated that ionizing radiation can have adverse effects on the human body; therefore, patients and personnel should be protected from unsafe levels of ionizing radiation.[4-8] The adverse effects of radiation are classified as *deterministic* or *stochastic*. The deterministic effects of radiation (eg, skin erythema, hair loss, cataract formation, infertility, circulatory disease) appear at various times after the exposure.[9-13] There have been reports of deterministic effects appearing as soon as 24 to 48 hours after the exposure and as long as three to four years after the exposure.[14,15] The deterministic effects frequently appear at the radiation entrance site (eg, back, neck, buttocks, anterior of the chest).[1,4,6] The stochastic effects (eg, cancer, genetic effects) can appear at any time after the exposure, but usually appear after several years.[13,15-17] The stochastic effects occur when radiation causes a mutation within the cell or cell death. For both the deterministic and stochastic classifications, the severity and type of damage are related to the dose received (ie, the greater the dose, the greater the damage). Several factors affect the radiation dose delivered to the patient and personnel, including

- patient positioning,
- image magnification,
- fluoroscopy duration,
- maintenance of a single beam angle,
- use of high-intensity mode,
- dose monitoring,
- x-ray beam angulation, and
- mechanical defects in the radiation source.

When these factors are controlled by the perioperative team, the dose of radiation received by the patient and the team members will be decreased.[4,18]

The potential for some stochastic effects in patients may be low. Based on a 2009 literature review on ovarian radiation sensitivity and the genetic hazards of ionizing radiation in female mammals including humans, Adriaens et al[19] concluded that much of the literature involved irradiated animals and that the probability of genetic effects in humans resulting from exposure to radiotherapy or radiological examinations and accidental exposure is lower than the risk of genetic effects resulting from spontaneous risks (eg, exposure to the sun). The authors reviewed international articles from the 1970s, articles published between 1990 and 2008 identified in a MEDLINE® search, and additional articles acquired from citations in the literature.

The amount of radiation received by perioperative team members is affected by the direction of the beam, the beam quality, the field size, the position of the operator according to the position of the beam originator, and the dose required to produce a clear image.[20] The radiation dose required varies among procedures, among operators, and among patients undergoing the same procedure.[4,6]

Radiation may be generated by various modalities (eg, C-arm [eg, standard, mini], O-arm, computed tomography [CT], mobile or fixed fluoroscopy, portable x-ray machine)[16,21] or by direct delivery methods (eg, brachytherapy using seeds or balloons, intraoperative radiation therapy).[1] The modality or method chosen for delivery of radiation depends on the procedure being performed.

Perioperative team members are exposed to radiation from three different sources, including

- primary radiation, which is emitted directly from the source;
- leakage radiation, which emanates from the x-ray machine housing; and

- scatter radiation, which is reflected off of the patient, table top, and shielding material.[22]

The main source of radiation for personnel in the perioperative setting is frequently scatter radiation, but the source depends on where the person is located in respect to the device generating the radiation.[23]

The effects of radiation have been known for more than 100 years, and this knowledge has led to the creation of practices to help protect patients and personnel, including[5]

- minimizing time spent near a radiation source,[22]
- maximizing distance from a radiation source,[22]
- using effective shielding,[5,22]
- controlling contamination,[22] and
- participating in educational programs.[5,22]

The following subjects are outside the scope of this document:

- management of radioactive specimens (See the AORN Guideline for Specimen Management),[24]
- the informed consent process for examinations or procedures that involve radiation,
- collimation (ie, determining the size of the area of the beam),
- the principles of justification (ie, a risk-benefit assessment completed by the person requesting the exam),
- precautions to be taken during magnetic resonance imaging (MRI) and positron emission tomography (PET)/CT scanning,
- procedural equipment selection, and
- measures to calculate or regulate the patient's dose of radiation.

Evidence Review

A medical librarian conducted a systematic search of the MEDLINE® and CINAHL® databases and the Cochrane Database of Systematic Reviews for meta-analyses, systematic reviews, randomized controlled and non-randomized trials and studies, case reports, letters, reviews, and guidelines. The librarian also searched the Scopus® database, although not systematically. The search was limited to literature published in English from January 2006 through January 2014.

Search terms included *invasive procedures, interventional procedure, interventional radiography, interventional radiology, intraoperative radiotherapy, cardiac catheterization, heart catheterization, abdominal radiography, radiation, ionizing radiation, iodine radioisotopes, radioactive tracer, radiation safety officer, safety management, radiation safety procedures, risk assessment, occupational radiation dose, occupational diseases, occupational exposure, occupational health, occupational hazards, radioprotection, radiation protection, radiation safety precautions, protective clothing, protective gloves, protective devices, eye protective devices, goggles, glasses, lead shield, lead apron, leaded garment, equipment failure, radiation injuries, patient safety, radiation monitoring, radiopharmaceuticals, radioactive pollutants, radioactive waste, medical waste, medical waste disposal, radiation field, storage, handling, transport, hazardous waste, occupational accident, thermoluminescent* dosimetry, dosimeter, radiometry, staff dose, fetus, fertility, gonads, pregnancy, and *pregnancy outcomes.* These terms were searched in combination with terms such as *healthcare facility, health care facility, ambulatory care facility, surgicenter, ambulatory surgery, outpatient surgery, operating room personnel, interventionalist, surgeon, nurse, anesthesiologist, anaesthesiologist, operator, operating room, operating theater, operating suite,* and *surgical suite.*

At the time of the search, the librarian established weekly alerts on the search topics and until July 2014, presented relevant results to the lead author. During the development of this document, the lead author also requested supplementary literature searches and additional literature that either did not fit the original search criteria or was discovered during the evidence-appraisal process. The time restriction was not considered in these subsequent searches. Relevant guidelines from government agencies and standards-setting bodies also were identified.

Inclusion criteria were research and non-research literature in English, complete publications, relevance to the key questions, and publication dates within the time restriction unless none were available. Excluded were non-peer-reviewed publications, literature that examined radiation safety measures that were determined to be beyond the scope of this document (eg, columnation, methods to decrease fluoroscopy time), and literature outside the time restriction when literature within the time restriction was available. Low-quality evidence was excluded when higher-quality evidence was available. In total, 1,397 research and non-research sources of evidence were identified for possible inclusion; of these, 248 were cited in this guidance document (Figure 1).

Articles identified by the search were provided to a project team that consisted of the lead author and four evidence appraisers. The lead author and the evidence appraisers reviewed and critically appraised each article using the AORN Research or Non-Research Evidence Appraisal Tools as appropriate. The literature was independently evaluated and appraised according to the strength and quality of the evidence. Each article was then assigned an appraisal score. The appraisal score is noted in brackets after each reference, as applicable.

The methodology of the research and non-research evidence used to support this guideline was critically evaluated by the authors for validity and generalizability to current practice. The collective evidence supporting each intervention within a specific recommendation was summarized, and the AORN Evidence-Rating Model was used to rate the strength of the collective evidence. Factors considered in the review of the collective evidence were the quality of the evidence, the quantity of similar evidence on a given topic, and the consistency of the evidence supporting a recommendation. The evidence rating is noted in brackets after each intervention.

Note: *The evidence summary table is available at http://www.aorn.org/evidencetables/.*

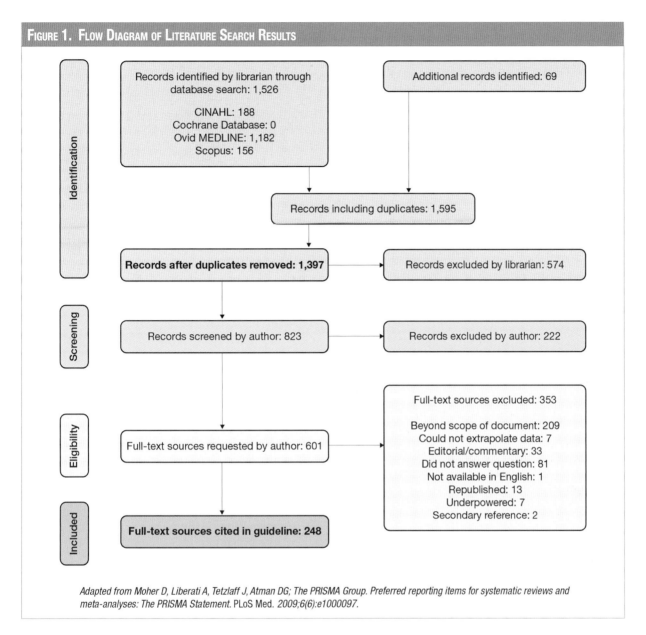

FIGURE 1. FLOW DIAGRAM OF LITERATURE SEARCH RESULTS

Records identified by librarian through database search: 1,526

CINAHL: 188
Cochrane Database: 0
Ovid MEDLINE: 1,182
Scopus: 156

Additional records identified: 69

Records including duplicates: 1,595

Records after duplicates removed: 1,397

Records excluded by librarian: 574

Records screened by author: 823

Records excluded by author: 222

Full-text sources requested by author: 601

Full-text sources excluded: 353

Beyond scope of document: 209
Could not extrapolate data: 7
Editorial/commentary: 33
Did not answer question: 81
Not available in English: 1
Republished: 13
Underpowered: 7
Secondary reference: 2

Full-text sources cited in guideline: 248

Identification · Screening · Eligibility · Included

Adapted from Moher D, Liberati A, Tetzlaff J, Atman DG; The PRISMA Group. Preferred reporting items for systematic reviews and meta-analyses: The PRISMA Statement. PLoS Med. 2009;6(6):e1000097.

In the literature, various metrics were used to report the dose of radiation received; the abbreviations used are listed in Table 1.[25] Additional dose-related definitions are provided in the glossary.

Abbreviations for a number of organizations that author clinical guidelines are used throughout this document. All organization names are spelled out on first reference and the abbreviations are used in subsequent occurrences. Table 2 is provided for easy reference to those organizations that are cited multiple times in the document.

Editor's note: *MEDLINE is a registered trademark of the US National Library of Medicine's Medical Literature Analysis and Retrieval System, Bethesda, MD. CINAHL, Cumulative Index to Nursing and Allied Health Literature, is a registered trademark of EBSCO Industries, Birmingham, AL. Scopus is a registered trademark of Elsevier B.V., Amsterdam, The Netherlands.*

Recommendation I

A radiation safety program must be established in all facilities and health care organizations in which the potential for diagnostic or therapeutic radiation exposure exists. *Amb*

A radiation safety program manages patient and personnel safety by providing guidance on methods to minimize exposure to ionizing radiation to a level that is as low as reasonably achievable (ALARA).[26,27]

The collective evidence, including national regulatory body requirements[27,28] and an article expressing expert opinion,[23] supports the creation of radiation safety programs, which may consist of a series of policies and procedures.[29,30]

I.a. The radiation safety program
   ○ must include a list of the approved equipment operators (See Recommendation I.b.1)[27,31]; *[1: Regulatory Requirement]*

TABLE 1. RADIATION DOSAGE[a] METRICS[1-3]

Term	Abbreviation	Definition
Roentgen equivalents (mammal)	rem	1 roentgen
Millirem	mrem	0.001 rem
Millirad	mrad	0.001 rad
Sievert[b]	Sv	100 rem
Millisievert	mSv	0.001 Sievert
Microsievert	μSv	0.0001 Sievert
Gray[c]	Gy	100 rad
Milligray	mGy	0.001 gray
Microgray	μGy	0.0001 gray

[a] Radiation dose is usually expressed in standard international units (SI).

[b] Effective dose or equivalent dose of radiation received is usually expressed in Sieverts. Equivalent dose may be further defined as deep-dose equivalent or shallow-dose equivalent.

[c] Absorbed dose is usually expressed in Gray.

REFERENCES

1. Lakkireddy D, Nadzam G, Verma A, et al. Impact of a comprehensive safety program on radiation exposure during catheter ablation of atrial fibrillation: a prospective study. J Interv Cardiac Electrophysiol. 2009;24(2):105-112.
2. Weiss EM, Thabit O. Clinical considerations for allied professionals: radiation safety and protection in the electrophysiology lab. Heart Rhythm. 2007;4(12):1583-1587.
3. 29 CFR 1910.1096. Toxic and hazardous substances: Ionizing radiation. Occupational Safety and Health Administration. https://www.osha.gov/pls/oshaweb/owadisp.show_document?p_table=STANDARDS&p_id=10098. Accessed April 13, 2015.

○ must include documentation and record retention requirements (See Recommendation I.e and I.f)[27]; *[1: Regulatory Requirement]*

○ must identify measures for protecting patients and personnel from unnecessary exposure to ionizing radiation, including shielding (eg, aprons, eyewear, fixed and portable barriers, disposable radiation-absorbing sterile patient drapes) (See Recommendations II-VII)[27]; *[1: Regulatory Requirement]*

○ must include procedures for handling and disposing of body fluids and tissue that may be radioactive (See Recommendation VII.f and VII.g)[24,27]; *[1: Regulatory Requirement]* Amb

○ must describe requirements for using radiation monitoring devices (eg, dosimeters) (See Recommendation VI)[27]; *[1: Regulatory Requirement]*

○ should include processes and requirements for selecting equipment at the time of purchase (See Recommendation I.b.2)[26,32]; *[3: Moderate Evidence]*

○ should include requirements for personnel education and competency assessment (See Recommendation I.d)[31,33]; *[1: Strong Evidence]*

○ should contain a quality assurance and improvement program (See Recommendation I.i)[31]; *[4: Limited Evidence]*

○ should describe the frequency of and processes for radiographic testing of protective devices (See Recommendation V.k);

○ should include requirements for patient education (See Recommendation II.f.1 and VII.i); and

○ should include processes for sterilizing radiation seeds when seed sterilization is required (See Recommendation VII.d).

Lakkireddy et al[34] conducted a randomized controlled trial (RCT) to examine patient and operator exposure to radiation during pulmonary vein antral isolation before and after implementation of a comprehensive radiation safety program. The study involved three operators and 41 patients who were randomly assigned to one of two groups. In Group 1 (n = 21), the procedure was performed before implementation of the program; in Group 2 (n = 20), the procedure was performed after implementation of the program. The program consisted of verbal reinforcement of previous fluoroscopy times, effective collimation, minimizing source-intensifier distance, and effective lead shield use. After the implementation of the program, the mean exposure to the operator was decreased by half, and the mean patient skin dose was reduced three to 10 times. The researchers concluded that implementation of the comprehensive safety program measures decreased the radiation exposure of both the patient and the operator.[34]

The use of a radiation safety program is also supported by an expert opinion article published by the Society for Cardiovascular Angiography and Interventions (SCAI) and endorsed by the Asian Pacific Society of Interventional Cardiology, the European Association of Percutaneous Cardiovascular Interventions, and the Latin American Society of Interventional Cardiology.[23]

I.b. The radiation safety program should be established by an interprofessional team composed of

○ a radiation safety officer or administratively designated alternative,[28]

○ a perioperative RN,

TABLE 2. ABBREVIATIONS FOR CLINICAL GUIDELINE AUTHOR ORGANIZATIONS

Abbreviation	Organization
AAPM	American Association of Physicists in Medicine
AAWR	American Association for Women Radiologists
ACR	American College of Radiology
AORN	Association of periOperative Registered Nurses
APDR	Association of Program Directors in Radiology
ASGE	American Society for Gastrointestinal Endoscopy
CIRSE	Cardiovascular and Interventional Radiological Society of Europe
ESGE	European Society of Gastrointestinal Endoscopy
ICRP	International Commission on Radiological Protection
NRC	US Nuclear Regulatory Commission
SCAI	Society for Cardiovascular Angiography and Interventions
SGNA	Society of Gastroenterology Nurses and Associates
SIR	Society of Interventional Radiology
SPR	Society for Pediatric Radiology

○ a radiologist or administratively designated alternative,
○ an anesthesia professional,
○ a scrub person,
○ environmental services personnel,
○ facility administrators,
○ physicians from involved disciplines, and
○ a medical physicist, if available.

[1: Regulatory Requirement]

The interprofessional team members provide information in their areas of expertise (eg, a physicist provides expertise in regulatory compliance, a radiologist provides expertise in optimizing protection, facility administrators provide resources to support the program).[16,26]

I.b.1. The interprofessional team should determine the necessary qualifications for the equipment operator for each type of radiologic device, including the miniature mobile fluoroscopy unit (ie, mini C-arm), based on state regulatory requirements. *[3: Moderate Evidence]*

Legislation has been issued in various states that restricts the use of radiologic equipment to specific personnel who can demonstrate successful completion of formal education and training. These are usually physicians or licensed radiology technicians.[31,35] The Centers for Medicare & Medicaid Services states that only those qualified, as determined by the medical staff, may operate radiologic devices.[29,30]

I.b.2. The interprofessional team should have an integral role in the evaluation and selection of new radiology equipment. *[3: Moderate Evidence]*

The interprofessional team serves to confirm that all aspects of radiation safety (eg, training, requirements for protection, room design, structural components, image quality, ease of use, cost) are considered during purchasing decisions.[16,32,36,37]

I.c. The interprofessional team should determine the unit of measure to be used for monitoring the radiation dose and the peak value for notifying the operator. The unit chosen should be based on the design of the equipment. *[2: High Evidence]*

The units of measure and peak operator notification levels are described by professional guidelines authored by the Society of Interventional Radiology (SIR)[33] and the American College of Radiology (ACR) in collaboration with the American Association of Physicists in Medicine (AAPM)[31] and by experts in the field[38,39] (Table 3).

I.d. Personnel who will potentially be exposed to radiation must be provided with education and competency verification activities as required by state regulations and as applicable to their roles and responsibilities. The education should include
○ risks of radiation exposure,[33]
○ biological effects of radiation,[33]
○ principles of radiation protection (eg, time, distance, shielding),[16]
○ principles of dosimetry (eg, one versus two monitors, location),[16]
○ safe equipment operation,[33] and
○ radiation spill management.[26]

[2: High Evidence]

Education and competency verification of personnel is supported by regulatory requirements27,40; six nonexperimental studies[41-46]; professional guidelines published by the ACR in collaboration with the APPM,[31] the SIR,[33] the Cardiovascular and Interventional Radiological Society of Europe (CIRSE) in collaboration with the SIR,[47] the Society of Gastroenterology Nurses and Associates (SGNA),[48] and the International Commission on Radiological Protection (ICRP)[49]; two quality reports[50,51]; one case report[52]; and two articles expressing expert opinion.[5,23]

The need for education is supported in the results of a Korean survey that involved 27 physicians who were applying to take the final examination to become experts in pain medicine. At the time of the survey, the physicians were practicing in a university setting (n = 25), a general hospital (n = 1), and a local clinic (n = 1). The survey consisted of 12 questions regarding the

RADIATION SAFETY

Ambulatory Surgery

PATIENT AND WORKER SAFETY

TABLE 3. PEAK VALUE UNITS OF MEASURE AND NOTIFICATION POINTS [1-4]

- Peak skin dose
  - first notification: 2,000 mGy
  - second notification: 500 mGy
- Reference point air kerma
  - first notification: 3,000 mGy
  - second notification: 1,000 mGy
- Kerma-area product
  - first notification: 300 Gy/cm2
  - second notification: 100 Gy/cm2
- Fluoroscopy time
  - first notification: 30 minutes
  - second notification: 15 minutes after first notification

REFERENCES

1. ACR–AAPM Technical Standard for Management of the Use of Radiation in Fluoroscopic Procedures. *2013. American College of Radiology.* http://www.acr.org/~/media/f22c9d1ff46f43aab001f9ed0466b7e9.pdf. Accessed April 13, 2015.
2. Stecker MS, Balter S, Towbin RB, et al. Guidelines for patient radiation dose management. *J Vasc Interv Radiol. 2009;20(7 Suppl):S263-S273.*
3. Jaco JW, Miller DL. Measuring and monitoring radiation dose during fluoroscopically guided procedures. *Tech Vasc Interv Radiol. 2010;13(3):188-193.*
4. Vance AZ, Weinberg BD, Arbique GM, Guild JB, Anderson JA, Chason DP. Fluoroscopic sentinel events in neuroendovascular procedures: how to screen, prevent, and address occurrence. *Am J Neuroradiol. 2013;34(8):1513-1515.*

location and type of hospital, the use of C-arm fluoroscopy, radiation safety education, knowledge of the annual permissible radiation dose, use of radiation protection, and efforts to reduce radiation exposure. Based on the survey responses, the participants were categorized into two groups: those who had received (n = 9) and those who had not received (n = 18) radiation safety education. The authors found that the group that had received the education wore radiation protective glasses or goggles and used dosimeters or other radiation monitoring badges at a significantly higher rate than the group that had not received the education. The authors concluded that education is needed to make fluoroscopy safer.[41]

A descriptive study involving 32 Canadian physicians and 30 Canadian medical students also supports education on radiation exposure and associated risks. Ricketts et al[42] found that 28% of the physicians were unaware that mammography used ionizing radiation and 25% were unaware that interventional procedures used ionizing radiation. The researchers found that medical school was the principle location in which the physicians and medical students received their education. Based on these findings, they concluded that the physicians and medical students needed additional education. They recommended that this education be incorporated into the medical school curriculum and that additional seminars or meetings be held on this topic.[42]

In a descriptive study involving 165 US urology residents and fellows, Friedman et al[43] found that 99% of the participants wore body shields but only 73% wore thyroid shields and 70% never used dosimeters. Only 13% of the participants wore lead-lined glasses, and 1.2% wore lead-lined gloves. Fifty-three percent of the participants believed they were adequately educated on the principals of radiation safety. The researchers concluded that radiation safety education was not adequate and should be a mandatory component of residency programs and continuing education for physicians.[43]

Kirkwood et al[44] investigated the effect of education on patient peak skin radiation dose in a descriptive study that measured radiation dose before and after education. Physicians who performed complex fluoroscopically guided procedures attended an education program that focused on significant operating factors that reduce the peak skin radiation dose (eg, table height, collimation, gantry angulation, patient-to-detector distance). The researchers examined 122 fluoroscopically guided procedures that occurred in a single hybrid OR. The procedures were performed by five different physicians with different operating practices and levels of experience. After the education program, peak skin radiation dose was reduced by 16%. The researchers concluded that when physicians received education on the effects of the selected operating factors, the peak skin radiation dose received by the patient was lower.[44]

Vano et al[45] reported on a similar reduction in radiation dose after physician education. The descriptive study involved 325 patients in 2009 and 383 in 2010 who had neurointerventional procedures. The researchers determined the number of patients who were candidates for skin injuries based on the amount of radiation received. In 2009, 19 patients were included. After education on radiation protection was provided to the operators in early 2010, the number of 2010 candidates was only four. The education consisted of a 20-hour course covering methods of radiation protection for fluoroscopy-guided procedures. The researchers concluded that the training reduced the number of candidates for radiation-induced skin injuries.[45]

A similar reduction in peak skin dose after physician education was shown in a Norwegian case report. The investigation was undertaken because of an incident in which a patient suffered a radiation burn during pacemaker implantation. Widmark and Friberg[52] compared the average entrance surface skin radiation dose received by patients during pacemaker insertions before and after physician education. The average entrance surface skin dose before the education was 5.3 Gy (n = 8); after the education, the average dose was 0.4 Gy (n = 6). The authors concluded that competence is a key factor in protecting patients from the harmful effects of radiation.[52]

In a study involving three Greek cardiologists, Abatzoglou et al[50] also found that education on radiation safety decreased the amount of radiation given during interventional cardiac procedures. In this study, the mean monthly dose to the hands of two cardiologists was decreased significantly after they received education on safety practices. The dose reduction ranged from 43.4% to 71.9%. The researchers concluded that the reduction in the radiation dose was a result of the safety practices put in place after the education program.[50]

In a descriptive study, Sheyn et al[46] recorded the frequency of the safety measures used during procedures before (n = 432) and after (n = 616) an educational session covering the ALARA principles. The procedures performed by 11 different operators consisted of uncomplicated peripherally inserted central catheter (PICC) procedures, non-PICC procedures, and complicated PICC procedures. After the education session, the researchers noted a significant increase in the use of leaded eyeglasses and hanging shields and a significant decrease in dose area product and fluoroscopy time for uncomplicated PICC procedures and non-PICC procedures although not for complicated PICC procedures. The researchers concluded that use of radiation safety measures increased after the radiation safety education program.[46]

After conducting a quality improvement initiative, Pitcher et al[51] described the effects of an educational program about the safe use of fluoroscopy on the dose of radiation received by personnel working in an interventional pain management clinic. The cumulative dose received by the personnel was measured before and after completion of a radiation safety education program. The cumulative dose was 18.14 mSv before the program and 9.55 mSv after the program. The authors concluded that the reduction in the dosage received was attributable to the education program. A limitation of this report was that the number of participants was not listed.[51]

I.e. Documentation in the patient's health care record should include the
- diagnostic and therapeutic radiation dose,[16,33,38]
- type and location of patient radiation protection,[31,33,53] and
- pre-radiation and post-radiation exposure patient skin assessment.
[3: Moderate Evidence]
Documentation of the patient's radiation dose is supported by multiple clinical practice guidelines authored by the SIR,[33,54] AORN,[53] the ACR in collaboration with the AAPM,[31] the Society for Atherosclerosis Imaging and Prevention

Tomographic Imaging and Prevention Councils in collaboration with the Society of Cardiovascular Computed Tomography,[55] and the European Society of Gastrointestinal Endoscopy (ESGE)[37] and by expert opinion.[16,39,56-58]

Documentation of the radiation dose provides the information needed to calculate the lifetime patient dose. A high lifetime patient dose has been associated with the appearance of cancer and other adverse effects of radiation that may occur after a prolonged time.[16,38]

In a quality improvement initiative, Steele et al[59] recommended documenting the radiation dose received. The authors found that documentation of the dose provided the data to support changing the threshold for postprocedure follow-up from 3 Gy to 5 Gy. This change decreased personnel administrative time and patients' visits for physician follow-up.[59]

I.f. The health care organization must maintain records of changes to the radiation safety program, program audits, and individual monitoring results as prescribed by regulatory requirements.[27] [1: Regulatory Requirement]

I.g. The radiation safety program must be reviewed at least annually.[27] [1: Regulatory Requirement]

I.h. The radiation safety program should include annual exposure limits. The limits must not exceed those set by the US Nuclear Regulatory Commission (NRC), including the
- total effective dose equivalent (TEDE) to radiation workers—5 rem,
- TEDE to any other individual organ—50 rem,
- TEDE to an embryo or fetus of a declared pregnant woman—0.5 rem,
- dose equivalent to the eye—15 rem,
- shallow dose equivalent to the skin, extremities—50 rem,
- dose to minors—10% of worker limit of 5 rem, and
- dose to members of the public—0.1 rem.[27]
[1: Regulatory Requirement]

I.i. The radiation safety program should include a quality assurance and improvement program.[23] [3: Moderate Evidence]
A quality assurance and improvement program helps provide confidence that optimal levels of quality have been met and provides direction for further action.[16]

I.i.1. The quality assurance and improvement program should include audits of the
- patient outcomes,
- patient dose,
- frequency of when patient dose trigger levels requiring clinical follow-up are exceeded,[16]
- image quality,
- justification for the procedure,
- personal dosimeter values,
- use of and availability of dosimeters,

- use of and availability of radiological protection tools,
- completion of required education on radiological protection (initial and continuing), and
- availability of personnel, such as a medical physicist.[31]

[3: Moderate Evidence]

I.j. Facilities that use therapeutic radionuclides must employ a radiation safety officer. [1: Regulatory Requirement]

The NRC requires that a radiation safety officer be appointed in all facilities in which a radiation by-product is administered to patients (eg, brachytherapy, stereotactic radiosurgery).[28]

I.j.1. The radiation safety officer should
- oversee the radiation safety program;
- monitor compliance with NRC regulations;
- assist in creating and enforcing organizational policies and procedures;
- determine methods for monitoring and recording occupational exposure;
- determine which individuals require monitoring devices;
- identify radiation safety problems[28];
- initiate, recommend, provide, and verify implementation of corrective actions[28];
- stop unsafe practices[28];
- be present before and during radionuclide therapy; and
- be responsible for controlling and maintaining the surveillance program for radionuclides.

[1: Regulatory Requirement]

The roles and responsibilities of the radiation safety officer are described in regulatory documents[28] and professional guidelines.[31,60]

Recommendation II

The perioperative team should implement measures to minimize the patient's exposure to radiation.

Multiple studies confirm that patients are exposed to varying levels radiation while they undergo a variety of procedures (eg, cardiac surgery, neurosurgery, orthopedic procedures). The source of the radiation (eg, C-arm, O-arm, portable or fixed x-ray machine, fixed fluoroscopy unit) is dependent on the procedure and the setting (eg, OR, physician office, interventional radiology, hybrid OR).[61-100]

Minimizing a patient's radiation exposure is supported in professional guidelines published by the ACR in collaboration with the AAPM.[31]

The literature search found several incidents of negative patient outcomes, including radiation burns and radiation dermatitis. These incidents occurred after the patients were exposed to large amounts of radiation during prolonged procedures. The time between the radiation exposure and the appearance of the burn varied greatly.[6,16,101-105]

This literature search also found case reports of radiation burns. The reports describe injuries to the back, neck, buttocks, breasts, and anterior of the chest. The injuries ranged in severity from skin rashes and epilation to necrosis of the skin and its underlying structures.[6,104]

Limitations of the evidence include a small sample size in many of the studies and no recommendations for action related to minimizing patients' exposure to radiation.

The benefits of minimizing a patient's exposure to radiation outweigh any potential harms. The benefits include prevention of the stochastic (ie, short term) and deterministic (ie, long term) effects of radiation. The potential harms created by minimizing the patient's exposure to radiation include the creation of a poor quality image.

II.a. The perioperative RN should assess the pregnancy status of all premenopausal patients. [2: High Evidence]

Assessment of premenopausal women to determine pregnancy status is supported by expert opinion,[35,56] professional association guidelines authored by the ACR in collaboration with the AAPM[31] and the ESGE,[37] and regulatory requirements that state a policy must be in place for identification of patients who are pregnant.[29,30] Radiation to the abdomen and pelvis of a woman who is pregnant poses an increased risk to the fetus and may cause childhood cancers.[16] The *Practice Guideline for Imaging Pregnant or Potentially Pregnant Adolescents and Women with Ionizing Radiation*, authored by the ACR in collaboration with the Society for Pediatric Radiology (SPR), states that the risk to the fetus is uncertain but there is less risk with advanced gestational age. The goal of a screening program is to decrease unexpected exposures to patients who are pregnant, especially during vulnerable stages of gestation.[106]

II.a.1. The perioperative RN should notify the responsible physician when a patient has declared that she could be pregnant.[16,35] [3: Moderate Evidence]

The ACR-SPR guideline states that the physician should perform a risk-benefit analysis before performing a radiologic study.[106]

II.a.2. Lead shielding should be placed between the fetus and the source of radiation when the shielding will not interfere with the performance of the procedure. [3: Moderate Evidence]

Using lead shielding between the fetus and the source of radiation to help protect the fetus when other areas of a pregnant woman's body will receive radiation is supported by professional guidelines authored by the ACR in collaboration with the SPR[106] and the ESGE[37] and by articles expressing expert opinion.[16,35,56,58]

A descriptive study by Kennedy et al[107] also supports the use of lead shielding. The study measured the amount of radiation received by using a sensor placed in the abdominal area of a phantom patient that simulated a pregnant woman. The simulated procedure was a CT scan to rule out pulmonary embolism. The amount of radiation received by the phantom fetus was measured when the edge of the lead shield was moved closer to the radiation source and farther away from the uterus, providing coverage for a greater portion of the abdomen. The fetal dose was decreased from 150 μGy to 50 μGy as the distance between the edge of the lead shielding was increased from 100 mm to 225 mm from the uterus. The researchers concluded that the fetal radiation dose was decreased when shielding was used. They recommended that shielding be placed around the entire patient and up to the caudal edge of the scan area.[107]

II.b. Extraneous body parts should be moved out of the path of the radiation beam. *[1: Strong Evidence]*

The result of extraneous body parts being in the path of the radiation beam is described in a report illustrating the complications of radiation received during fluoroscopically guided complex interventions. The injuries described resulted from increased unintended radiation to the patient's arms and breasts.[6]

Removing extraneous body parts from the path of the radiation beam, especially those located on the x-ray tube side, is supported by professional guidelines authored by the ICRP[108] and the ESGE[37] and by articles expressing expert opinion.[16,109]

An RCT involving 54 women conducted by Foley et al[110] supported the importance of moving extraneous body parts. The study compared the mean breast surface dose of radiation received during coronary CT angiography of the control group in which the breast was not displaced or shielded (n = 22) to a group in which the breast was displaced only (n = 16) and a group in which the breast was displaced and shielded (n = 16). The mean breast surface dose was decreased 23% in the displacement-only group and 36% in the displacement-plus-shielding group. The researchers concluded that breast displacement during coronary CT angiography significantly reduced the radiation dose to the breast surface, and this reduction was enhanced when shielding was used.[110]

II.c. Perioperative team members should collaborate regarding the use and placement of shielding (eg, lead or lead equivalent) over the patient's thyroid, ovaries or testes (ie, gonads), and breasts when these body parts are near the source of radiation. *[2: High Evidence]*

The use of shielding for patients is supported by professional guidelines authored by the ICRP[108] and the ESGE,[37] and one article expressing expert opinion.[58]

The use of shielding is also supported in an Irish study in which the radiation dose received by the gonads of men and women was measured using lateral and anteroposterior projections to the lumbar spine. A phantom was used as a substitute for a patient, and dosimeters were placed in the location of the gonads. The researchers compared the amount of radiation received when no protective apron was used to the amount received when a protective apron was applied to the patient on the tube side, applied on the receptor side, or when a wraparound apron was used. The dose received by the testes was reduced significantly when the tube-side apron and the wraparound apron were used for both projection methods, but no decrease in the radiation received by the ovaries was noted with any of the apron application methods. The researchers recommended using the tube-side apron for both men and women during lumbar spine x-ray studies.[111]

A prospective randomized study by Shortt et al[112] evaluated the effectiveness of thyroid shields on patients undergoing neurointerventional procedures. Patients were randomly assigned to one of two groups. Group 1 participants wore the thyroid shield (n = 34); Group 2 participants did not wear the shield (n = 31). The mean relative thyroid dose reduction in the shielded group was 48% less (3.77 mSv/Gy/cm^2 x 105) than the dose received by the unshielded group (7.23 mSv/Gy/cm^2 x 105). The dose was measured at the collimator. The researchers concluded that thyroid shielding should be used on the patient undergoing a neurointerventional procedure unless placement of the shield interferes with the field of view.[112]

A second study by Shortt et al,[113] in which four-vessel cerebral angiograms were simulated on phantom heads, also supports the use of thyroid shielding. In this study, a total of eight angiograms were simulated on the phantom heads, four with and four without the thyroid shield. The researchers found a 41% to 51% decrease in thyroid radiation dose with the use of thyroid lead shielding. They concluded that thyroid shields should be used for patients having cerebral angiograms.[113]

Sancaktutar et al[114] created a testicular shield from two radiation protective gloves that were placed one inside the other with the fingers turned inside out. The radiation dose was measured by a dosimeter placed within the gloves on the testes and one on the outside of the gloves. The study involved 200 male patients who underwent upper abdominal and pelvic CT

examinations. The results showed that this testes shield decreased the amount of radiation
received by the testes 10-fold. The researchers
concluded that this form of a testes shield was
effective in reducing the radiation received by
the testes and the method was user-friendly,
practical, and inexpensive.[114]

In a review of the literature, Entrikin et al[115]
describe the use of breast shields as highly controversial because although the shields decrease
exposure, they may also decrease the image
quality and increase the image noise, the CT
numbers, and the tube current (ie, the amount
of power required to produce a high-quality
image).

II.c.1.   The shielding should be placed between the
patient and the source of radiation (Figures
2 and 3) but not within the path of the beam
that originates from the x-ray tube. *[4: Limited Evidence]*

The use of a wraparound apron was supported in a study by Jackson and Brennan.[116]
The study used a phantom man and woman
with dosimeters placed in the area of the
ovaries, uterus, and testes. The study compared the dose received by the gonads with
no apron, an apron facing the image receptor, an apron facing the x-ray tube, or a
wraparound apron. The measurements
were taken using posterior-anterior and lateral projections simulating a chest x-ray.
The gonads received the least amount of
exposure with the wraparound apron in
the posterior-anterior projection and in the
lateral projection, except the right ovary,
which received a lower amount with the
apron facing the x-ray tube. The authors
recommend the use of a wraparound apron
for both sexes during chest x-ray.[116]

II.d.   During fluoroscopic procedures, personnel
should keep the patient as close as possible to
the image intensifier side of the fluoroscopic
unit and away from the tube side of the unit. *[3:
Moderate Evidence]*

Positioning the patient close to the image
intensifier is supported by professional guidelines authored by the ACR in collaboration with
the AAPM,[31] the ICRP,[108] and the ESGE[37] and by
articles expressing expert opinion.[58,109,117]

Giordano et al[118] evaluated the dose of radiation received by the patient and the physician
during simulated cervical spine surgery using a
cadaveric cervical spine. The researchers measured the deep-radiation dose to the patient
with the cadaveric cervical spine 2 inches from
the radiation source (16,431 mrem), 10 inches
from the image intensifier (7,628 mrem), and
nearly in contact with the image intensifier
(6,520 mrem). The dosimeters used to measure
the radiation dose were changed at each distance. The researchers found the patient's radi-

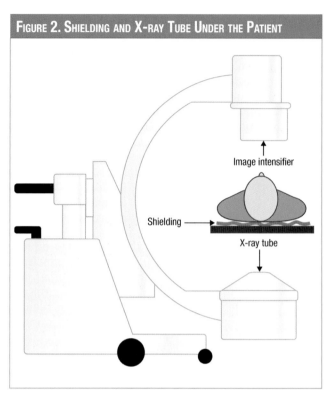

FIGURE 2. SHIELDING AND X-RAY TUBE UNDER THE PATIENT

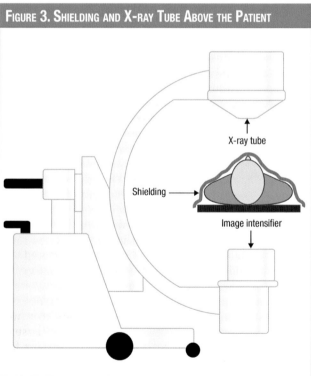

FIGURE 3. SHIELDING AND X-RAY TUBE ABOVE THE PATIENT

ation dose was significantly decreased when
the patient was located closer to the image
intensifier.[118]

II.e.   A perioperative team member (eg, radiation
technologist, nurse, other designated person)
should monitor the radiation dose received by
the patient and inform the operator when the
peak value for notification has been reached. *[3:
Moderate Evidence]*

A perioperative team member is usually needed to do the monitoring because the operator may not be able to see the dosage indicated on the panel of the fluoroscopic device.

Monitoring the radiation dose and reporting the values to the operator is supported in professional guidelines authored by the SIR,[33] a quality improvement initiative,[59] and articles expressing expert opinion.[16,38,39,56,57,59]

II.e.1. Peak values should be expressed using the values recorded by the fluoroscopy unit and not only fluoroscopy time. *[2: High Evidence]*

Sawdy et al[119] compared the incidence of radiation burns identified using fluoroscopy time to the incidence identified using total radiation dose as the method for determining the need for follow-up post procedure. The researchers conducted the study at a single center and used a retrospective chart review to obtain the data (N = 872). When the time-based method was used, the patient would receive brochure and a follow-up telephone call if the fluoroscopy time was greater than 120 minutes. The dose-based method included levels of follow-up based on the dose received. Patients with a radiation dose between 2,000 mGy and 5,499 mGy received an information sheet and a follow-up telephone call at one week. They also received education on the signs and symptoms of radiation burns. Patients with a dose between 5,500 mGy and 8,999 mGy received the information sheet and additional follow-up telephone calls at three and six weeks post procedure. Patients with a dose greater than 9,000 mGy received the same follow-up as above and, in addition, they were scheduled for a clinic visit within six weeks of the procedure.[119]

Using the time-based method as the criteria for follow-up, 0.5% (n = 413) of the patients reported a radiation burn compared with 2% (n = 459) using the radiation dose method. The researchers concluded that the increased number of burns reported was related to use of the total radiation dose as the factor for follow-up because other factors, such as the fluoroscopy time, actually decreased. Based on the results of this study, the researchers recommended using a total radiation dose follow-up program and not a fluoroscopy time-based program.[119]

II.f. The perioperative RN responsible for discharging the patient who has had an image-guided procedure or for transferring the patient to an inpatient bed should consult with the physician regarding the need for post-procedure education and timing of follow-up care.[31,33] *[3: Moderate Evidence]*

Post-procedure patient education provides the patient with the knowledge of the potential for and the cause of a skin reaction, if one occurs. This knowledge may decrease patient anxiety and increase the potential for a correct diagnosis of acute radiation syndrome.[6,16,39] Follow-up care is needed to assess and, if necessary, treat the patient for acute radiation syndrome.

II.f.1. The patient should be provided with education that includes
- signs and symptoms of overexposure to radiation, (eg, gastrointestinal symptoms,[120] radiation burns,[33] potential hair loss[121]),
- the potential time frame for appearance of signs and symptoms,[33] and
- the importance of follow-up with the physician who performed the procedure if questions arise regarding the procedure.[16,31,33,57,122]

[3: Moderate Evidence]

Case reports describe hair loss attributed to the amount of radiation received[121] and gastrointestinal symptoms experienced by a patient after an endovascular abdominal aortic aneurysm repair.[120]

Balter et al[122] reviewed the literature containing descriptions of specific reactions in the skin or hair of patients who had been exposed to radiation. The goal of the review was to determine whether the reactions were caused by a definite dose or a range of doses and whether there was a definite time limit or a range of time before onset of the reaction after exposure. The authors concluded that the dose and times varied, and therefore a set dose or time required for skin or hair damage could not be determined.[122]

Recommendation III

Occupational exposure to radiation should be minimized.

Numerous studies confirm that personnel working in the OR or interventional radiology suite are exposed to varying levels of radiation. This exposure occurs to personnel working in most specialities (eg, trauma, cardiac, neurosurgery, orthopedics, urology). The source of the radiation (eg, C-arm, O-arm, portable or fixed x-ray machine, brachytherapy seeds, fixed fluoroscopy unit) depends on the procedure and the setting (eg, OR, interventional radiology, hybrid OR).[62,73,74,76,78,79,83,87-91,96,97,118,123-145]

Limitations of the evidence include a small sample size in many of the studies and no recommendations for action related to minimizing exposure to radiation. Many of the studies focused on the operator, usually the physician, standing at the sterile field close to the source of radiation; other personnel in the room are frequently excluded from the study data. The benefits of minimizing occupational exposure to radiation outweigh any potential harms. The benefits include preventing stochastic and deterministic effects of radiation. The harms may include orthopedic strain caused by wearing a heavy lead apron for a prolonged period of time.

Radiation that scatters as the x-ray beam passes through the patient is the main source of occupational radiation exposure. The amount of occupational radiation exposure is related to the amount of radiation received by the patient.[16]

The author of a literature review found that modifying risk factors reduced anesthesiologists' radiation exposure. The measures performed to decrease the risk included decreasing the procedure duration, increasing distance from the radiation source, using shielding devices, participating in education programs on radiation safety measures, and using dosimeters. The author concluded that taking these measures would help to ensure that the anesthesia professional is adequately and acceptably protected from exposure to medical radiation.[146]

Vanhavere et al[147] arrived at similar conclusions in a review of the literature published in 2008 that examined extremity dosimetry in diagnostic and therapeutic nuclear medicine and PET, interventional radiology, interventional cardiology, and brachytherapy. They determined that the operator's fingers, which are the body parts closest to the radiation source, frequently receive the highest amount of radiation and that when protective measures were taken, the annual exposure limits were rarely exceeded.[147]

In a literature review that included literature dating back to the 1890s, Linet et al[25] found that the amount of radiation exposure of medical workers who performed diagnostic radiology and fluoroscopically guided procedures decreased with the advent of protective device use. They also reported a decrease in the stochastic effects of radiation in this population. The authors found that the metrics used in the literature varied, which complicated their attempts to summarize trends. Other limitations of much of the literature included a small study population, of which the vast majority were men, and studies that ended before the majority of the population reached an age at which cancer risks are the highest. The authors concluded that more research was needed to evaluate cancer and other serious radiation-related disease risks. They also recommended that this research include large populations, including interventional and noninterventional radiologists and all physicians and other personnel who perform or assist with interventional procedures.

III.a. Personnel should maintain the greatest distance possible from the radiation source and limit the amount of time spent close to the source. *[3: Moderate Evidence]*

The collective evidence, consisting of 14 nonexperimental studies[18,84,148-159]; four professional guidelines authored by the SGNA,[40] the CIRSE and the SIR,[47] the ICRP,[108] and the ESGE[37]; and three articles expressing expert opinion,[14,16,23] establishes that the radiation dose received by the personnel in the room decreases proportionally as the distance between the source of radiation and the person increases.[18,84,148-159]

Radiation dose decreases as the square of the distance between the radiation source and the operator increases. This principle is known as the inverse square law.[16] The inverse square law states that when the distance between the person and the x-ray source is doubled, the exposure is decreased by 25%. When the distance is tripled, the dose is decreased by a factor of nine. The authors of this definition concluded that fluoroscopy operators and staff members can reduce their exposure accordingly by moving away from the x-ray source.[14]

A radius of 6 ft (2 m) from the radiation source is considered the distance at which the radiation is decreased to a safe level, but many state and local regulations require all personnel in the room to use some form of shielding.[160] The ACR and the AAPM recommend that personnel maintain a distance of at least 3 ft (1 m) from the source of the radiation if possible.[31]

III.b. The radiation equipment operator should alert personnel present in the treatment room before activating the equipment. *[4: Limited Evidence]*

Alerting the personnel in the room before activation of the equipment allows them to take protective measures, such as maintaining as great a distance as possible from the source, thereby decreasing the dose of radiation received.

III.c. Personnel involved in fluoroscopic procedures should stand on the image intensifier side of the fluoroscopy unit when procedural considerations allow (Figure 4). *[2: High Evidence]*

Professional guidelines authored by the CIRSE and the SIR[47] and the ICRP,[58] two nonexperimental studies,[135,161] and one article expressing expert opinion[117] support standing on the image intensifier side of the fluoroscopy unit.

von Wrangel et al[161] conducted a comparative study to measure the amount of radiation received by an operator standing on the image intensifier side of the fluoroscope compared with an operator standing on the opposite side. The measurements were conducted using dosimeters placed into phantoms. The phantoms were placed in the standard position for the operator and the patient during a simulated percutaneous vertebroplasty performed on the thoracic or lumbar regions. The dose received by the operator standing on the side opposite the image intensifier was 0.08 mSv/minute, while the dose for the operator standing on the image intensifier side for the thoracic procedure was 0.02 mSv/minute. The doses for the procedure performed on the lumbar area were 0.40 mSv/minute and 0.08 mSv/minute, respectively. The researchers concluded that standing on the same side as the image intensifier decreased the dose of radiation received by a factor of four to five.[161]

PATIENT AND **WORKER** SAFETY

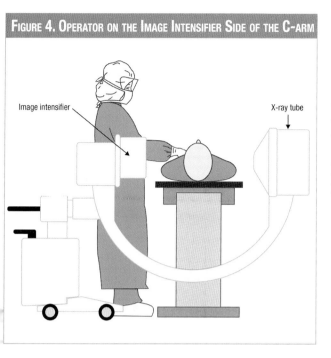

FIGURE 4. OPERATOR ON THE IMAGE INTENSIFIER SIDE OF THE C-ARM

Image intensifier

X-ray tube

A comparative study by Mariscalco et al[135] that involved five surgeons who performed 10 procedures also supports standing on the image intensifier side of the fluoroscopy unit. The researchers measured the radiation dose received at the chest level of a surgeon who stood on the radiation source side of the patient and of a surgeon who stood on the image intensifier side of the patient. Each surgeon performed five minimally invasive lumbar microdiscectomies. The radiation exposure was 5.01 mrad for the surgeon on the radiation source side and 1.14 mrad for the surgeon on the image intensifier side. The researchers concluded that personnel should stand on the image intensifier side of the fluoroscopic unit.

III.d. Slings, traction devices, and sandbags should be used to maintain the patient's position during radiation exposure, and cassette holders should be used to secure films. [3: Moderate Evidence]

The use of devices to hold the patient and cassettes is supported in "Recommendations for occupational radiation protection in interventional cardiology."[23] Holding the patient manually increases the risk of exposure by the direct beam.[23,58] The risks associated with holding the patient during procedures are also explained in two articles expressing expert opinion.[158,109]

Recommendation IV

Personnel with a known or suspected pregnancy must restrict the occupational radiation dose as described in local, state, and federal regulations.

Local, state, and federal regulations determine the radiation precautions to be followed by personnel who are pregnant. State guidelines are based on the regulations established by the NRC. The NRC regulations state the occupational dose to the embryo or fetus of an occupationally exposed health care worker who has declared her pregnancy must not exceed 0.5 rem during the entire gestational period, and should be uniform over time and not received all at once (ie, at one point in the gestational period).[27] The deep-dose equivalent for the worker who has declared a pregnancy is used as the dose to the embryo or fetus.[27]

For recommendations regarding patients who are pregnant see Recommendation II.a.

IV.a. Personnel with a known or suspected pregnancy should declare this condition to the radiation safety officer or through other appropriate facility channels. [2: High Evidence]

Declaration of pregnancy is supported in professional guidelines authored by the ACR in collaboration with the AAPM[31] and the American Association for Women Radiologists (AAWR) in collaboration with the Association for Program Directors in Radiology (APDR).[162] Disclosure of the pregnancy, even if it is obvious, is not legally required.[27]

IV.a.1. A written, voluntary, official declaration that includes the estimated date of conception may be used as a starting point on which to base the total dose limit to the person who is pregnant.[27,162] [2: High Evidence]

IV.b. Pregnant personnel should wear radiation monitors at the waist under shielding during times of exposure to radiation. [2: High Evidence]

The "SCAI consensus document on occupational radiation exposure to the pregnant cardiologist and technical personnel" recommends that the health care worker who is pregnant wear a dosimeter under the apron at the waist level to estimate the amount of radiation received at a level near the level of the fetus.[163]

IV.b.1. Dosimeters of pregnant personnel should be read monthly unless regulatory requirements are more stringent. [4: Limited Evidence]

IV.c. A pregnant health care worker should follow standard radiation protection techniques and, in addition, may wear a maternity or double-thickness apron or a wraparound apron that is large enough to cover the entire abdominal area. [2: High Evidence]

The "SCAI consensus document on occupational radiation exposure to the pregnant cardiologist and technical personnel" supports the pregnant health care worker following standard techniques and wearing additional protection as deemed appropriate by the worker.[163] Wearing of a maternity apron is also supported by the AAWR and the APDR.[162]

The use of aprons was supported in a multi-institutional study by Chandra et al[164] that involved 81 pregnant physicians and radiology technologists. The researchers measured the mothers' whole-body radiation dose and the fetal dose. The whole-body dose was measured by a dosimeter placed above the lead apron and the fetal dose was measured by a dosimeter placed inside the lead apron. The mothers' whole body dose ranged from 21 mrem to 731 mrem. The fetal dose was rounded to zero. The researchers concluded that when standard safety principals were upheld, there was a negligible radiation exposure to the fetus.[164]

Recommendation V

Shielding devices, including architectural (ie, fixed) shielding, equipment-mounted or mobile shields, and personal protective devices should be used with all sources of radiation.

The collective evidence, consisting of one systematic review of the literature[165]; two nonexperimental studies[166,167]; six professional guidelines authored by the ACR in collaboration with the AAPM,[31] the American Society for Gastrointestinal Endoscopy (ASGE),[168] the SGNA,[48] the CIRSE and the SIR,[47] the ICRP,[58] and the ESGE[37]; and eight articles expressing expert opinion,[23,108,109,117,169-172] supports the use of shielding devices.

A limitation of the evidence is a small sample size in some of the studies.

The benefits of using shielding devices outweigh any potential harms. The benefits include preventing the stochastic and deterministic effects of radiation. The harms may include orthopedic strain caused by wearing a heavy lead apron for a prolonged period of time.

In a descriptive study that involved 90 health care personnel who participated in interventional procedures, Basic et al[166] determined that the average amount of radiation received annually by nurses who were not at the sterile field (0.6 mSv) was approximately one-half that received by the physicians at the sterile field (1.1 mSv). The participants practiced at four facilities, with 73% practicing in interventional cardiology. The average measurements were 4.7 mSv above the apron and 0.58 mSv below the apron. This study did not measure the levels received by the scrub person. The researchers recommended using protective garments and wearing dosimeters outside and inside the apron near the neck.[166]

Chida et al[167] used a pinhole camera device and a phantom patient to determine the sources of scatter radiation. They concluded that the primary sources were the patient and the cover of the x-ray beam collimating device. Based on the results, they recommended that those standing close to the patient and to the source of radiation wear radiation protection to decrease their exposure to the scatter radiation.[167]

Kesavachandran et al[165] conducted a systematic review of the literature that included 24 articles published in German or English between January 1990 and October 2011. The inclusion criteria were studies with a cohort or cross-sectional design that involved interventional cardiology staff members and expressed the radiation dose in the workplace as annual and per procedure for different anatomical locations. The authors

concluded that the best method of protecting personnel against radiation exposure was use of shielding devices, including personal protective devices.

V.a. Structural components (eg, walls, windows, control booths, doors, protective cubicles), which frequently have a lead equivalence of 1 mm to 3 mm, should be incorporated into the structure of the building during construction if the radiation source is a fixed feature in the room (eg, hybrid OR, interventional radiology room). *[3: Moderate Evidence]*

The collective evidence, consisting of a nonscientific study,[173] two professional guidelines authored by the FGI[174] and the ESGE,[37] and two articles expressing expert opinion,[175,176] supports the use of structural components for radiation protection based on the anticipated use of the room. Operating rooms frequently do not have these structural components unless they are designed as hybrid ORs.[174,176]

V.b. Shielding devices may be composed of lead or a lead-equivalent material (eg, tungsten antimony, bismuth-antimony). *[3: Moderate Evidence]*

Uthoff et al[177] conducted an RCT of 60 consecutive endovascular procedures performed in an interventional radiology suite during a two-month period. Nine operators performed the procedures. The data set consisted of 70 samples because some of the procedures involved two operators. The study measured the amount of radiation attenuation between

- a 0.5-mm lead-equivalent thyroid shield,
- a bilayer barium sulfate–bismuth oxide composite thyroid shield, and
- a bilayer barium sulfate–bismuth oxide composite hat.

The radiation attenuation was measured by placing one dosimeter outside and one inside the shielding devices. The researchers concluded that the amount of radiation protection provided by the bilayer barium sulfate–bismuth oxide composite thyroid shield (71.9%) was not significantly different than the protection provided by the standard 0.5-mm lead-equivalent thyroid collar (79.7%), and the bilayer barium sulfate–bismuth oxide composite thyroid shield was 27% lighter than the lead shield. The radiation attenuation of the bilayer barium sulfate–bismuth oxide composite hat was 85.4% ± 25.6%.

Mori et al[178] examined the radiation transmission rate of protective aprons. The three-part study compared the effectiveness of

- 0.25-mm lead-equivalent-thickness non-lead aprons to 0.35-mm lead-equivalent-thickness non-lead aprons, which were worn by the first and second operators during abdominal interventional radiology procedures;
- 0.25-mm lead aprons to 0.50-mm lead-equivalent-thickness non-lead aprons, worn

by operators during interventional cardiology procedures; and

○ 0.25-mm lead-equivalent-thickness non-lead aprons to 0.35-mm lead aprons, worn by nurses working in a location where CT scans were performed.

The researchers concluded that 0.25-mm lead-equivalent-thickness aprons were sufficient for operators performing interventional radiology procedures and 0.35-mm thick lead aprons should be worn by the nurses in the location where CT scans are performed. They recommended 0.35-mm thick lead aprons for the nurses because of the high energy x-rays that are encountered during CT scanning compared with those encountered during interventional radiology procedures. The authors did not provide the composition of the lead-equivalent aprons.[178]

Chatterson et al[179] compared the amount of radiation received by a phantom fetus being protected by a lead shield or a bismuth-antimony shield during simulated CT pulmonary angiography. The shields were applied to the abdominal area of the model. The use of the model allowed for repeated radiation exposures beyond that which could be given to a human participant. The protection provided by the bismuth-antimony shield was equivalent to that provided by the lead shield when conservative scanning parameters were used. The researchers found that the bismuth-antimony shield also was lighter and provided for easier manipulation.[179]

The use of a lead-equivalent thyroid shield is supported in a descriptive study that measured the amount of scatter radiation received in the thyroid area of a phantom placed in the location of a physician standing at the sterile field. Lee et al[180] compared the amount of scatter radiation received without a shield, with a lead shield, and with a lead-equivalent shield. The shields were worn tightly, worn loosely, and worn loosely with a bismuth masking reagent. With the lead shield, the phantom received an average of 1.91 μSv/minute, 2.35 μSv/minute, and 1.86 μSv/minute, respectively. With the lead-equivalent shield, the scatter radiation doses were 1.79 μSv/minute, 1.82 μSv/minute, and 1.74 μSv/minute, respectively. The phantom received an average radiation dose of 16.32 μSv/minute when no shielding was provided. The researchers concluded that the lead-equivalent thyroid shield provided greater protection than the lead thyroid shield.[180]

In a descriptive study, Zuguchi et al[181] compared the amount of attenuation of 0.25-mm, 0.35-mm, and 0.475-mm lead aprons and equivalent thickness non-lead aprons. To determine the amount of attenuation, a phantom was x-rayed using a range of settings starting at 60 kilovolts (kV) that increased by increments of 10 kV to 120 kV of radiation. The amount of scatter radiation attenuation was measured 45 cm from the phantom for each thickness of apron. The 0.25-mm lead equivalent provided 98% to 89% attenuation, the 0.35-mm lead equivalent provided 99% to 92% attenuation, and the 0.475-mm lead equivalent provided 100% to 96% attenuation. The decreasing percentage of attenuation occurred in a linear fashion, with the highest percentage occurring at 60 kV and the lowest percentage at 120 kV. The researchers concluded that the non-lead aprons provided sufficient protection for the personnel in the room.[181]

V.c. Equipment-mounted and mobile shields (eg, suspended personal radiation protection systems, mobile hanging shields, under-table skirts, table-mounted side shields, rolling shields, sterile drape shields) should be used in addition to personal shields when personnel are required to remain near the patient or near the sterile field. [2: High Evidence]

The collective evidence, consisting of two RCTs[182,183]; three reports on the European research project Optimization of Radiation Protection of Medical Staff (ORAMED)[184-186]; 13 nonexperimental studies[20,187-198]; six professional guidelines authored by the ACR in collaboration with the AAPM,[31] the ASGE,[168] the SGNA,[48] the CIRSE and the SIR,[47] the ESGE,[37] and the ICRP[108]; and four articles expressing expert opinion,[58,117,171,176] supports the use of equipment-mounted and mobile shields that allow the health care worker to stay close to the patient and provide coverage to parts of the body not otherwise protected by personal protective equipment (PPE) intended for radiation protection.

Behan et al[183] conducted an RCT to compare the radiation dose received by personnel when a mobile shield (ie, a transradial radiation protection board) was used with the dose received when the shield was not used. The measurements were taken during 106 procedures. The staff member participants were randomly assigned to either the control (n = 50) or experimental (n = 56) group. The two groups were not significantly different in respect to age, sex, height, weight, body mass index, or operator experience. The fluoroscopy time, procedure duration, and contrast load were not significantly different between the two groups. The amount of radiation received by the staff members was significantly decreased with the use of the transradial protection board (28 μSV versus 19.5 μSV, $P = .003$).

In an RCT, Ploux et al[182] compared the amount of radiation received by the operator's head, thorax, and back when using a suspended personal radiation protection system (ie, cabin) (n = 30 procedures) to the dose received when wearing leaded glasses, a thyroid collar, and a lead apron (n = 30 procedures). Patients were randomly assigned to each group, and a single operator performed the procedures (eg, placement of pacemaker or cardioverter defibrillators). The mean radiation dose to the operator's thorax and back were similar between the control group and the cabin group. The radiation dose to the operator's head was significantly lower in the cabin group compared with the control group (0.040 µSv and 1.138 µSv, respectively). The researchers concluded that the suspended personal radiation protection system should be used because the operator's head received less radiation, and the use of the suspended personal radiation protection system created less strain on the operator compared with wearing the lead protective devices.

V.d. Personnel may wear protective caps. [1: Strong Evidence]

Uthoff et al[177] conducted an RCT of 60 consecutive endovascular procedures performed in an interventional radiology suite during a two-month period. Nine operators performed the procedures; the data set consisted of 106 samples because some of the procedures involved two operators. The study measured the amount of radiation attenuation of a bilayer barium sulfate–bismuth oxide composite hat. The radiation attenuation was measured by placing one dosimeter outside and one inside the hat. The average radiation attenuation of the bilayer barium sulfate–bismuth oxide composite hat was 85.4%. The researchers recommended that caps for the operators be included in the methods of radiation protection because of the amount of radiation received by the head (at least 15,700 µSv total for the 106 samples in the data set).[177]

In a study involving a single interventionist who wore a radiation protection cap, Karadag et al[199] found the radiation dose on the outside of the cap (0.22 mSv to 2.77 mSV) was greater than the dose inside the cap (< 0.1 mSV). The study was performed during an 18-month period and involved 1,282 procedures. A ceiling-suspended protective shield, used for a portion of the study, resulted in the lower doses of radiation recorded by the dosimeter on the outside of the cap. The researchers concluded that the cap was effective in reducing the radiation dose to the head and that the cap should be used in conjunction with the ceiling-suspended protective shield because the shield decreased the dose to the whole body (7.82 mSv high dose without the shield, 2.69 mSv high dose with the shield) in addition to reducing the dose to the head.[199]

V.e. Radiation protective aprons should be worn by all members of the perioperative team present during procedures when a source of radiation is activated. [2: High Evidence]

Eight nonexperimental studies[18,92,159,187,200-203]; four professional guidelines authored by the ASGE,[168] the SGNA,[48] the CIRSE and the SIR,[47] and the ESGE[37]; and three articles expressing expert opinion[16,58,171] support the use of protective aprons by all members of the perioperative team present during procedures in which radiation is used.

The use of personnel radiation protective equipment was supported in a descriptive study conducted by Carinou et al[187] that involved 1,291 procedures in 34 hospitals located in six European countries. The procedures consisted of 646 interventional cardiac procedures, 441 interventional radiologic procedures, and 204 endoscopic retrograde cholangiopancreatography (ERCP) procedures. The researchers found a reduction in the amount of radiation exposure when PPE was used. The measuring devices were placed on both of the wrists, both legs, and above both eyes. The researchers recommended that PPE be worn by everyone in the room and that lead glasses be worn when ceiling-suspended shields are not available.[187]

In a descriptive study, Steinfort et al[92] measured the amount of radiation received at the sternum inside and outside of the apron on one assistant and one physician. The radiation was measured during 45 consecutive fluoroscopically guided ultrasound bronchoscopies using a mobile C-arm fluoroscopy system. The physician dose was 200 µSv outside the apron and less than 50 µSV inside the apron. The assistant dose was 50 µSv outside the apron and less than 50 µSv inside the apron. The researchers concluded that the dose of radiation received during fluoroscopy-guided bronchoscopies was negligible with the use of shielding, including aprons and thyroid shields.[92]

Ahn et al[200] conducted a prospective study to calculate the number of percutaneous endoscopic lumbar discectomy procedures a surgeon could perform per year before reaching the yearly occupational radiation exposure limit. The study involved three surgeons who performed 30 consecutive percutaneous endoscopic lumbar discectomies. The researchers measured the exposure levels at the surgeons' necks, chests, arms, and both hands. Dosimeters were placed outside and inside the lead apron and the thyroid shield and on the extremities to measure the amount of radiation received. The mean fluoroscopy time was 2.5 minutes per procedure. The calculated average radiation doses for each area outside of the shields were

○ neck, 0.0785 mSv;
○ chest, 0.1718 mSv;
○ right upper arm, 0.0461 mSv;
○ left ring finger, 0.7318 mSv; and
○ right ring finger, 0.6694 mSv.

The amount of radiation received inside the shields was reduced by 96.9% for the apron and 94.2% for the thyroid shield. The researchers concluded that shielding was necessary and that when using whole-body radiation exposure as the measure, 5,379 procedures could be performed per year with use of a lead apron. Only 291 procedures could be performed without use of a lead apron.[200]

In a descriptive study, Parashar et al[201] measured the amount of radiation received by the surgeon, radiation oncologist, surgical assistant, and surgical nurse during implantation of Caesium-131 (^{131}Cs) seeds. The average dosimetry readings were significantly higher for one surgical assistant who did not wear radiation protection than for the other people at the sterile field. The researchers concluded that people at the sterile field should wear lead shields and gloves to decrease the amount of radiation exposure when implanting ^{131}Cs seeds.[201]

Mohapatra et al[18] conducted a descriptive study aimed at determining the amount of radiation exposure to personnel and patients during endovascular surgeries that use fluoroscopy. The data were collected for 39 procedures performed between October 2011 and February 2012. The personnel involved in each procedure included a surgeon, a scrub person, a radiation technologist, and one to three assistants. The exposure for the anesthesia professional was determined by an unshielded dosimeter placed on the anesthesia machine. This method was chosen because the anesthesia professionals were relieved very frequently. The 39 procedures were performed by three different primary surgeons. When the dosimeters were analyzed, the anesthesia machine was found to have the highest dosage, followed by the assistant and the surgeon. The lowest doses were received by the scrub person and radiation technologist. The researchers concluded that the anesthesia machine dose was high because of the absence of shielding.[18]

Ismail et al[202] measured the radiation exposure received by anesthesia professionals during interventional radiological procedures. The prospective study involved anesthesia professionals working in 125 procedures performed in an ERCP suite or cardiac catheterization laboratory. The participants wore dosimeters inside their aprons at the waist level and outside their aprons at the collar level. The amount of radiation received at the collar level was higher than the amount registered at the waist level. The researchers recommended routine use of lead aprons and thyroid shields because the amount of radiation received at the collar level location was 0.25 mSv for ERCP and 1.94 mSv for cardiac catheterization compared with 0.03 mSv for ERCP and 0.11 mSv for cardiac catheterization inside the apron.[202]

Wearing lead aprons during fluoroscopically guided procedures was supported in a descriptive study by van der Merwe.[203] The study involved 17 hand/wrist procedures, 11 foot/ankle procedures, 14 shoulder/tibia/fibula procedures and six femur/hip procedures performed by one orthopedic surgeon. The procedures took place during a two-month period. The x-ray tube was placed either above or under the table as determined by the sterile requirements for each procedure. The study measured the radiation dose to the operator above and below the apron at the level of the pelvis. The dosage received on the outside of the apron was 5.98 mSv and below the apron was 0.34 mSv. The author concluded that wearing the leaded protection is effective in reducing the radiation exposure to the wearer.[203]

Patel et al[159] found that wearing a leaded apron decreased the radiation dose to the operator by 93%. The study measured the dose of radiation on the outside and beneath leaded aprons worn by the operator during 26 infrarenal aortic repairs and 10 elective thoracic aorta repairs. The dose received on the outside of the apron was 65.5 µSv and the dose inside the apron was 5.5 µSv. The authors recommend that leaded aprons be worn.[159]

V.e.1.　Protective aprons should cover the body from the area below the thyroid collar to the knee. *[4: Limited Evidence]*

V.e.2.　Personnel who may expose their backs to the radiation beam should wear wraparound aprons. *[3: Moderate Evidence]*

Alzimami et al[204] conducted a study that measured the mean radiation doses at the chest level (6.4 µGy) (n = 153) and back shoulder (38.7 µGy) (n = 85) of a physician performing therapeutic ERCP procedures. In this study, the physician's back was closer to the source of the radiation because the physician was watching the monitor, which was positioned in a location that required the physician to turn away from the source of radiation. The researchers concluded that the primary physician should wear a wraparound apron because the radiation dose to the back shoulder was higher than the dose to the chest.[204]

V.f.　Thyroid shields should be worn by all personnel present during procedures in which fluoroscopy is used. *[3: Moderate Evidence]*

The collective evidence, consisting of four descriptive studies[154,180,202,205]; four professional guidelines authored by the ASGE,[168] the SGNA,[48] the CIRSE and the SIR,[47] and the ESGE[37]; and two articles expressing expert opinion,[16,171] supports the use of thyroid shields.

Mechlenburg et al[205] measured the radiation dose received by dosimeters located above and below the thyroid shield during 23 periacetabular osteotomy procedures. The median dose received by the single operator was 0.009 mSv below the shield and 0.023 mSv above the shield. The difference in dosage was considered to be significant. The researchers concluded that wearing a thyroid shield significantly reduced the radiation dose to the thyroid.[205]

Lee et al[154] conducted a descriptive study to measure the amount of scatter radiation received in the surgeon's thyroid area during simulated spinal surgery. The study used a phantom physician and a phantom patient exposed to five minutes of continuous radiation from a C-arm. Scatter radiation to the thyroid area was decreased from 15.63 µGy/minute to 1.73 µGy/minute when a thyroid collar was worn. The researchers recommended that thyroid shields be worn to decrease the radiation dose received from scatter radiation.[154]

Ismail et al[202] measured the radiation exposure received by anesthesia professionals during interventional radiology procedures. The prospective study involved anesthesia professionals in 125 procedures performed in an ERCP suite or cardiac catheterization laboratory. The participants wore dosimeters inside their aprons at the waist level and outside their aprons at the collar level. The amount of radiation received at the collar level was higher than the amount registered at the waist level. The researchers recommended routine use of thyroid shields because of the amount of radiation received at the collar level location (0.25 mSv for ERCP and 1.94 mSv for cardiac catheterization compared with 0.03 mSv for ERCP and 0.11 mSv for cardiac catheterization inside the apron).[202]

The use of a thyroid shield is supported in a descriptive study that measured the amount of scatter radiation received in the thyroid area of a phantom placed in the location of a physician standing at the sterile field. The study compared the amount of scatter radiation received without a shield to that received with the physician wearing a shield tightly, loosely, or loosely with a bismuth masking reagent. The average dose measured was 1.91 µSv/minute when the shield was worn tightly, 2.35 µSv/minute when the shield was worn loosely, and 1.86 µSv/minute when the shield was worn loosely with a bismuth masking reagent. The phantom received an average radiation dose of 16.32 µSv/minute when no shielding was provided. The researchers concluded that some form of a thyroid shield should be worn, and the most effective method of wearing a thyroid shield is to wear it tightly or to wear it loosely if combined with a bismuth masking reagent.[180]

V.g. Leaded eye protection (eg, leaded eyeglasses with wraparound side shields, ceiling-suspended shields, clear mobile shields that are taller than the person using them) should be used if the person (eg, the operator) is near the source of the radiation beam. *[3: Moderate Evidence]*

The collective evidence, consisting of two quasi-experimental studies[99,206]; seven nonexperimental studies[20,187,195,207-210]; three professional guidelines authored by the ASGE,[168] the SGNA,[48] and the CIRSE and the SIR[47]; two articles expressing professional opinion[16,171]; and two reviews of the literature,[211,212] supports the use of leaded eye protection. Two descriptive studies state that leaded eye protection is not needed under certain circumstances.[213,214] The studies occurred in a variety of countries, involved the use of leaded eyeglasses with and without mobile or fixed shielding devices, and examined the presence of cataracts in physicians and nurses.

Molyvda-Athanasopoulou et al[99] conducted a quasi-experimental study to measure the eye radiation dose to the operator during 32 interventional radiological examinations. The patients were selected randomly and were assigned to one of the two physicians who shared the workload of the department. There were always two physicians present during the procedures, but at times one of the physicians was a resident. The results of the study showed the mean radiation dose received by the eye was 34.5 mGy for angiographies and 212.3 mGy for angioplasties. This may be a factor limiting the number of procedures a physician can perform in a year. The authors estimated the workload of the department and determined that the annual eye lens dose would be more than 40 mSv and could result in cataract formation if the leaded glasses were not worn to reduce the annual dosage.[99]

A quasi-experimental study by Vano et al[206] supported the use of eye protection during cardiac catheterization. The researchers examined the eyes of 58 physicians and 69 nurses and technicians who worked in interventional radiology and were attending an interventional cardiology convention in South America (ie, the exposure group). They found 50% of the physicians and 41% of the nurses had subcapsular lens changes characteristic of ionizing radiation exposure. The researchers also examined the eyes of 91 non-medical professionals who reported no previous relevant exposure to ionizing radiation in the head and neck region (ie, the control group) and found that less than 10% of this group had subcapsular lens changes. The researchers recommended that radiation protection tools, including protective eyewear, be used during times of radiation exposure.

The use of eye-shielding devices is supported in a descriptive study that determined the radiation received by the first and second operator and the radiographers for 106 interventional cardiology procedures. The second operator was located a short distance from and to the side of the first operator. The researchers concluded that the annual exposure limit of 20 mSv recommended by the ICRP can be achieved in approximately 160 procedures for the first operator,

600 procedures for the second operator, and 1,600 procedures for the radiographer. Based on these data, the researchers recommended that leaded eyeglasses be worn by the first operator if that person will be performing more than 160 procedures per year.[207]

The use of eye-shielding devices was supported in a descriptive study involving 1,291 procedures that occurred in 34 hospitals located in six European countries. The procedures consisted of 646 interventional cardiac procedures, 441 interventional radiologic procedures, and 204 ERCPs. The measuring devices were located above both eyes. The researchers found a reduction in the amount of radiation exposure when PPE was used. As a result of this study, the researchers recommended that lead glasses be worn when ceiling-suspended shields are not available.[187]

Use of leaded eyeglasses by orthopedic surgeons was supported in a descriptive study by Burns et al[208] that used a phantom surgeon and patient. The investigators measured the amount of radiation received at the surgeon's eyes during 16 different fluoroscopic views. The researchers found that the use of leaded eyewear reduced the radiation dose to the surgeon's lens 10-fold. The researchers recommended the use of leaded eyeglasses for orthopedic surgeons who perform procedures that use fluoroscopy.[208]

A descriptive study by Koukorava et al[20] supported the use of leaded eye glasses. The researchers used a phantom patient and operator to determine the radiation dose received by the operator's eye lenses during several simulated interventional radiology and cardiology procedures. The investigators measured the dose of radiation received by the operator's eye lenses with four types of glasses:

○ small glasses with lead equivalent thickness of 0.5 mm,
○ small glasses with 1-mm lead,
○ large glasses with lead equivalent thickness of 0.5 mm, and
○ large glasses with 1-mm lead.

The operator received the least amount of radiation with the large glasses, and the increase in the thickness did not significantly increase the protection. The researchers recommended the use of lead or lead equivalent glasses that completely cover the eyes.[20]

Thornton et al[195] compared the operator eye lens dose received when various protective devices were used (ie, leaded table skirt, nonleaded and leaded eyeglasses, disposable tungsten-antimony drapes, suspended and rolling transparent leaded shields) to the eye lens dose received when no device was in place. They concluded that the use of scatter shielding drapes plus leaded glasses provided greater protection than the other devices used alone, except suspended or mobile leaded shields.[195]

A comparative study by Sturchio et al[210] supported the use of leaded eyeglasses. The researchers compared the amount of protection provided by three different types of radiation-protective glasses and also measured the radiation dose with no glasses. The glasses were described as lightweight, sportwrap, and classic. The primary difference between the three types of glasses was the amount of side shielding provided. The glasses with the greatest amount of side protection provided more protection when the radiation source was to the side of the head. The values obtained at zero degrees were 980 µSv with no protection, 380 µSv for the lightweight glasses, 120 µSv for the sportwrap glasses, and 105 µSv for the classic glasses. The researchers concluded that eye protection was effective and that the style of glasses chosen should be determined by the type of procedure being performed.[210]

Mroz et al[209] conducted a descriptive study that measured the radiation dose to the eye of the operator. The data were gathered using readings from dosimeters placed on the operator during 27 single or multiple level kyphoplasty procedures. A dosimeter located outside the apron on the left side at the chest level was used to calculate the dose received by the eye. The results of the study revealed that the average radiation dose to the eyes of the operator during kyphoplasty was 0.271 mSv per vertebra. The authors concluded that at this dose, the annual occupational limit to the eyes would be exceeded in 300 procedures; therefore, the surgeon should wear leaded glasses. A limitation of this report is that the number of operators was not specified.[209]

Two nonexperimental studies did not find the wearing of leaded eyeglasses to be necessary in all situations. A descriptive study by Taylor et al[213] that included six urologists who performed 28 endourological procedures concluded that the typical urologist did not need to wear eye protection, such as leaded glasses, because the estimated lifetime cumulative dose of radiation to the eye was well below the minimal threshold set by the ICRP. The researchers measured the radiation dose to the eye by placing a dosimeter above the right eye. The protective measures used (eg, thyroid shields, lead-lined aprons, judicious fluoroscopy use, maximum operating distance from the radiation source) may have contributed to the results. None of the participants wore lead-lined eye protection. The researchers noted that a limitation of this study was that extracorporeal shock wave lithotripsy, which may have raised the radiation dose, was not included in the list of procedures.[213]

Penfold et al[214] measured the eye radiation dose for urologists performing only brachytherapy using Iodine-125 (^{125}I) seeds. The descriptive study involved three physicians, each performing only one procedure. The researchers found that if the surgeon performed 60 procedures per year with an average fluoroscopy run time of five minutes per procedure, the cumulative dose of radiation received would not exceed the annual dosage of 20 mSv per year recommended by the ICRP. The researchers concluded that it was unnecessary for the urologist to wear leaded eyeglasses when performing only brachytherapy using ^{125}I seeds. They recommended that the urologist consider the personal total radiation dose received when determining whether leaded glasses are needed.[214]

V.h.   Sterile radiation shield drapes may be used as an alternative to or in addition to equipment-mounted and mobile shields when permitted by the requirements of the invasive procedure. *[1: Strong Evidence]*

The collective evidence, consisting of three RCTs,[215-217] one quasi-experimental study,[218] and one nonexperimental study,[219] supports the use of sterile radiation shield drapes.

An RCT involving 60 cardiac percutaneous coronary intervention procedures at a single facility supported the use of sterile radiation shield drapes. Murphy et al[216] used a 1:1 selection pattern to determine in which procedures the drape would be used. The radiation dose to the primary operator was significantly reduced in the cohort that used the drape compared with the control group. The researchers concluded that the drape significantly reduced the primary operator's radiation dose from scatter radiation.[216]

Politi et al[215] reached the same conclusion after conducting an RCT involving 60 patients undergoing interventional cardiology procedures with radial artery access. The procedures were performed by a single operator. When the drape was used, the radiation dose to the operator was reduced by an average of 23% for all dosimeter locations (ie, the operator's chest, left eye, left wrist, and thyroid).[215]

Iqtidar et al[219] compared the radiation dose received by the primary and secondary operator when a lead drape was placed across the patient just below the umbilicus to the dose received when the lead drape was not used. The measurements were taken during transradial access for cardiac catheterization procedures performed on 137 patients. The radiation doses were measured at the wrist and collar levels of the primary and secondary operators, with a reduction of 17% to 29% at the wrist level and 0% to 17% at the collar level. The researchers concluded that the use of a lead drape placed across the patient just below the umbilicus reduced the radiation exposure to the wrists and to a lesser extent the thyroid for the primary and secondary operator.[219]

Brambilla et al[218] conducted a prospective observational study to determine whether the amount of radiation received by the operator's hand was reduced with the use of a sterile, disposable, bismuth-and-antimony–containing drape. Twenty-two patients who required cardiac resynchronization therapy were randomly assigned to either the control group (n = 11) or the participant group (n = 11). In the participant group, a sterile, disposable, bismuth-and-antimony–containing drape was placed so that it covered the surfaces inferior and lateral to the beam path. The amount of scatter radiation received by the operator's hand was decreased by 54% in procedures for the participant group compared with the control group. The researchers recommended using a sterile, disposable, bismuth-and-antimony–containing drape.[218]

In an RCT, Lange and von Boetticher[217] determined that the operator dose of radiation was significantly decreased when a pelvic lead shield was placed on the patient during a cardiac catheterization procedure using a femoral or radial access. The shield was placed to decrease the radiation dose received by the operator. The study involved 210 patients who were randomly assigned to a group using the shield (n = 101) or a group with no shield (n = 109). The procedures were completed by a single experienced interventional cardiologist in a single facility. The dosage received was decreased 0.55 μSv when the shield was used for both approaches. The researchers concluded that the use of pelvis lead shielding placed on the patient offered effective radiation protection to the operator.[217]

V.i.   Protective gloves may be worn when the wearer's hands are near but not in the primary x-ray beam. *[3: Moderate Evidence]*

The use of radioprotective gloves is supported by one quasi-experimental study,[220] professional guidelines authored by the SGNA,[48] two nonexperimental studies,[161,201] and two articles expressing expert opinion.[16,58]

In a review of the literature, Schueler[221] cautioned that when hands covered with protective gloves are placed in the x-ray beam, the gloves may increase the dose of radiation to the hand because scatter radiation may be trapped within the glove.

The benefits of using protective gloves was demonstrated in a comparative study. von Wrangel et al[161] compared radiation dose measurements taken outside the radiation-protective gloves to measurements taken inside the gloves. The gloves were placed in a realistic working position on the surface of a phantom patient. The position was one that would likely be used during the performance of a percutaneous vertebroplasty. The dose on the inside of the gloves was 30% to 40% lower than the dose on the outside of the gloves. The researchers concluded that wearing radiation-protective gloves would significantly reduce the radiation dose received by the operator.[161]

In a descriptive study, Parashar et al[201] measured the amount of radiation received by the surgeon, radiation oncologist, surgical assistant, and surgical nurse during implantation of [131]Cs seeds. The average dosimetry readings were significantly higher for one surgical assistant who did not wear radiation protection devices than for the other people in the room. The researchers concluded that people at the sterile field should wear lead shields and gloves to decrease the amount of radiation exposure during implantation of [131]Cs seeds.[201]

Synowitz and Kiwit[220] conducted a study that involved two neurosurgeons who performed 41 fluoroscopically assisted vertebroplasties during a six-month period in a single facility. The per-procedure radiation dosage measured on the protected left hand of Surgeon 1 was 0.112 mSv (n = 20 procedures); the dosage for the unprotected left hand of Surgeon 2 was 0.422 mSv (n = 21 procedures). The radiation dose per procedure for the unprotected right hands of both surgeons were similar at 0.138 mSv and 0.142 mSv. The researchers concluded that surgeons should wear radiation-protective gloves.[220]

V.j.   When permitted by the requirements of the invasive procedure, a combination of personal and movable shielding devices should be used.
[3: Moderate Evidence]

A descriptive study involving 50 procedures by a single operator supported the use of the combination of personal and movable shielding devices. Challa et al[222] found that 0.5-mm lead-equivalent personal barriers reduced operator exposure by 72% to 95%; a 1.0-mm leaded personal barrier (ie, overlapping gown) reduced exposure by 96%. A pair of 0.75-mm leaded glasses reduced exposure to the left eye by 67%. The measurements were recorded only on the left eye because that is the eye that is closest to the source. A leaded left-hand glove reduced exposure by only 20%. When the movable shielding devices were used in addition to the personal devices, the researchers noted an incremental decrease in the radiation dose received. The researchers concluded that the use of personal plus movable barriers reduced the theoretical risk of the operator contracting radiation-induced fatal or nonfatal cancer 22-fold and reduced the potential for a severe genetic effect 25-fold when compared with the use of movable barriers alone.[222]

von Boetticher et al[223] conducted a descriptive study on the reduction of the radiation effective dose with the use of an increasing amount of radiation protection. The study compared the reduction of the effective dose received when three different types of radiation

protection were used, with and without thyroid protection. The protective measures included a 0.35-mm or 0.5-mm lead apron, a lead apron plus table-mounted lower-body protection, and a lead apron plus table-mounted upper- and lower-body protection. When compared to the reference dose recommended by the ICRP, the radiation dose was reduced 97.3% with the use of the table-mounted upper- and lower-body protection and a 0.5-mm apron compared with 96.9% for the use of the 0.35-mm apron and table-mounted upper- and lower-body protection. The dosage was further reduced (1.3% to 1.4%) when a thyroid collar was added. The researchers concluded that the greatest amount of protection was received when the apron was worn with the thyroid shield and the table-mounted upper- and lower-body protection was used.[223]

V.k.   Protective devices should be
   ○ visually inspected and x-rayed for defects at the time of purchase,
   ○ visually inspected for defects before use,
   ○ x-rayed at least annually for defects related to wear, and
   ○ x-rayed whenever damage is suspected.
[2: High Evidence]

Routine testing is supported by regulatory requirements.[29,30] Periodic testing of protective devices is supported by professional guidelines authored by the ACR in collaboration with the AAPM,[31] and annual testing is supported by the SGNA[48] and the ESGE.[37]

Oyar and Kislalioglu[224] conducted a descriptive study in Turkey with 85 personal leaded protective devices (ie, aprons). The aprons were worn in multiple departments, including surgical services and interventional radiology. The newest apron was one year old, and the oldest was older than six years, with the majority being less than two years old. The control group consisted of 10 aprons that had never been used. The aprons were x-rayed to determine the condition of the internal protective lead-based material, and the radiation absorption was tested using dosimeters placed under the apron. The researchers determined that all 85 aprons provided an inadequate amount of protection independent of the cleanliness or the appearance of the apron, the length of time the apron had been in use, or the number of users. They concluded that folding may increase the risk for cracks but did not directly decrease the x-ray permeability. They recommended at least annual testing to determine the amount of protection offered by each apron.[224]

The literature search did not identify any similar studies from the United States. It is unclear whether the conditions of use in the United States and Turkey are comparable.

351

V.k.1. Documentation of leaded protective device testing should be maintained in a central location. *[3: Moderate Evidence]*

Maintaining the documentation in a central location helps make the information available to all personnel.[225]

V.k.2. The personnel responsible for testing should be notified when new shielding devices are purchased. *[3: Moderate Evidence]*

Communication between the person ordering and receiving new shielding devices and the person responsible for testing the devices assists with improving testing compliance.[225]

V.k.3. Personal shielding devices should be labeled with the last test date. *[3: Moderate Evidence]*

Labeling of personal shielding devices assists with tracking of the apron and with identification of the department that owns the device.[225]

V.l. Aprons and thyroid shields should be stored flat or hung vertically and should not be folded. *[2: High Evidence]*

Aprons and shields are susceptible to cracking, which can reduce the apron's effectiveness as a shielding barrier.[225] Storage of aprons as described is supported in professional guidelines authored by the ESGE[37] and the SGNA[48] and one article expressing expert opinion.[16]

V.m. Protective devices should be cleaned and disinfected according to the manufacturer's instructions for use.[226] *[1: Strong Evidence]*

A quantitative clinical audit of lead aprons revealed that aprons become contaminated with use and are a potential reservoir for cross-contamination. Boyle and Strudwick[227] measured the colony-forming units on four locations of 19 aprons at a single facility. The microorganisms identified included coagulase-negative staphylococci, *Staphylococcus aureus*, *Bacillus*, *Diphtheroids*, and some fungal spores. The audit revealed that after routine cleaning with detergent and water, the number of microorganisms present was significantly decreased. The researchers recommended establishing a policy and procedure for routine cleaning of aprons.[227]

V.m.1. An interprofessional team (eg, perioperative nurse, radiology technician, infection preventionist) should establish cleaning frequencies for protective devices.[226] *[2: Strong Evidence]*

One nonexperimental study supports weekly cleaning. Grogan et al[228] conducted a descriptive study in a 224-bed trauma center with 12 main ORs. The investigators took 182 swabs from

- vests in the midline at the collar and the bottom hem on both the front and back sides,
- skirts in the midline at the waist and bottom hem front and back, and
- thyroid shields in the midline at the center of the collar front and back.

Five of the 182 swabs exhibited growth of common skin flora. These five swabs were from the lead apron, midline, bottom outer surface (n = 3); lead thyroid shield midline, inner surface (n = 1); and lead skirt, midline, bottom inner surface (n = 1). The researchers concluded that cleaning on a weekly basis with additional spot cleaning as needed after contamination was adequate.[228]

Recommendation VI

Radiation monitors or dosimeters must be worn by personnel as required by regulatory agencies.

The regulations put forth by the NRC state that monitors must be worn by people who meet the following criteria:

(1) Adults likely to receive, in 1 year from sources external to the body, a dose in excess of 10 percent of the limits in § 20.1201(a),

(2) Minors likely to receive, in 1 year, from radiation sources external to the body, a deep dose equivalent in excess of 0.1 rem (1 mSv), a lens dose equivalent in excess of 0.15 rem (1.5 mSv), or a shallow dose equivalent to the skin or to the extremities in excess of 0.5 rem (5 mSv);

(3) Declared pregnant women likely to receive during the entire pregnancy, from radiation sources external to the body, a deep dose equivalent in excess of 0.1 rem (1 mSv); and

(4) Individuals entering a high or very high radiation area.[229(p359-360)]

Use of personal radiation monitoring devices as the principal mechanism for monitoring radiation exposure of personnel on a day-to-day basis is supported by regulatory requirements[29,30,230]; professional guidelines authored by the ACR in collaboration with the AAPM,[31] the SGNA,[48] the CIRSE and the SIR,[47] the ICRP,[108] and the ESGE[37]; and two articles expressing expert opinion.[171,176]

The benefits of using monitoring devices, which include knowledge of the levels of radiation exposure and being able to limit the dosage if the levels are nearing recommended maximum levels, outweigh any potential harms.

VI.a. Dosimeters should be worn in a consistent location. *[4: Limited Evidence]*

The professional guidelines from the ACR and the AAPM recommend wearing monitors consistently and in the same location to achieve accurate readings.[31]

VI.a.1. One dosimeter should be worn inside the lead apron and one outside the lead apron unless state regulations are more stringent. *[3: Moderate Evidence]*

The ICRP recommends using two dosimeters, one inside the apron and the other at the collar or left shoulder region outside the apron.[16] The use of two dosimeters during fluoroscopic procedures is supported by two nonexperimental studies[166,231]; four professional guidelines authored by the ACR in collaboration with the AAPM,[31] the SGNA,[48] the ICRP,[108] and the ESGE[37]; and one article expressing expert opinion.[58]

A descriptive study by Basic et al[166] involved 90 people working in interventional procedures who wore dual dosimeters, one on top of the apron at the neck level and the other one under the apron at the chest level. The dosimeter worn on top of the apron at the neck level provided a better estimation of the dose received by the eye. The participants practiced at four facilities, with 73% practicing in interventional cardiology. The researchers concluded that the use of dual dosimeters provided a better estimation of the effective dose. They recommended using protective garments and wearing dual dosimeters.[166]

A descriptive study by Chida et al[231] also supported the use of dual dosimeters. This study, performed in Japan, evaluated the annual occupational dose for 18 physicians, seven nurses, and eight radiology technologists who worked in an interventional radiology suite. The participants wore two monitoring badges, one outside the lead apron at the neck level and one inside the apron at the chest or waist level. The researchers found that if the results from only the badge worn under the apron were used to calculate the annual occupational dose, the amount calculated was lower than the amount calculated using two dosimeters. The researchers determined that the physician who was closest to the source of radiation received the highest radiation dose, the nurse received the next-highest dose, and the radiation technologist received the least amount because the radiation technologist is the farthest from the source. The researchers recommended using dual dosimeters when calculating the annual occupational dose.[231]

VI.a.2. Finger dosimeters should be worn by personnel who are within 1 m of the primary x-ray beam. *[2: High Evidence]*

Use of finger dosimeters is supported by professional guidelines authored by the ICRP[108] and the ESGE.[37]

In a descriptive study involving two physicians and two radiology technologists, Ginjaume et al[232] found that the finger dose was three times greater than the wrist dose

and 50 times greater than the whole-body dose as calculated by dosimeters worn on fingers, wrist, and under the lead apron, respectively. The study involved 29 diagnostic procedures with a total of approximately 13 hours of fluoroscopy time. Based on the data, the researchers concluded that finger dosimeters should be worn by personnel who are within 1 m of the primary x-ray beam.[232]

The use of a finger dosimeter is supported in a descriptive study by Hausler et al.[233] The partial body radiation dose was recorded for 39 physicians and nine assistants during the performance of 73 interventional procedures in 14 hospitals in Germany. The operators and in some situations the assistants wore dosimeters in multiple locations (eg, forehead, thyroid, sternum, both sides of the trunk, right and left ulna, thumb, middle finger, palm, hip, knee, feet) resulting in a total of 2,200 readings. The average readings from the dosimeters placed on the hands of the operators were greater than 100 μSv in 184 instances, compared with five instances for the forehead and eight instances for the thyroid. Twenty participants had an exposure of more than 1 mSv at the dosimeters located on the hands. The researchers concluded that dosimeters should be worn on the hands.[233]

Sauren et al[196] found that relatively high doses of radiation were received by the hands of the operator during transcatheter aortic valve implantation procedures. The measurements were performed during 22 transcatheter aortic valve implantations. The average hand dose was 1.9 mSv. If the surgeon performed more than 250 procedures, the annual exposure limit (ie, 500 mSv) would be exceeded for the operator's hand. Based on the results, the authors recommended that hand dose measurement for the operator should become a standard procedure during transcatheter aortic valve implantations.[196]

VI.b. Radiation monitoring devices or dosimeters should be stored at the facility in a designated location at the end of every workday. *[4: Limited Evidence]*

Radiation monitoring devices should not be taken home because the device may collect ionizing radiation from other sources (eg, sun, soil, airport scanners). A designated location facilitates collection of the badges for testing.

VI.c. The results of dosimetry reports must be reported to the individual at least annually. *[1: Regulatory Requirement]*

Annual reporting is required by the Occupational Safety and Health Administration.[230] The

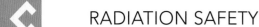

reporting of the results when obtained is supported by professional guidelines authored by the SGNA[48] and the CIRSE and the SIR[47] and by one article expressing expert opinion.[26]

VI.c.1. Dosimetry reports must be kept by the facility or health care organization and the individual for the life of the individual or as determined by regulatory requirements. *[1: Regulatory Requirement]*

Keeping the records for the life of the individual helps determine lifelong radiation exposure levels.[26,27,48]

Recommendation VII

The principles of time, distance, and shielding should be followed by personnel handling therapeutic radionuclides and by personnel caring for patients who have received therapeutic radionuclides.

The collective evidence, including one nonexperimental study[234] and professional guidelines authored by the SGNA,[48] supports use of the principles of time, distance, and shielding during handling of therapeutic radionuclides and during care for patients who have received therapeutic radionuclides.

A limitation of the evidence is a small sample size in many of the studies.

The benefits of using the principles of time, distance, and shielding outweigh any potential harms for the caregiver or facility personnel.

In a descriptive study, Fujii et al[234] measured the radiation dose received by the surgeon (n = 20 procedures), assistant (n = 17 procedures), nurse (n = 19 procedures), radiologist (n = 9 procedures), anesthesiologist (n = 3 procedures), and radiological technologist (n = 1 procedure) during brachytherapy seed implantation procedures. The nurses, radiologist, anesthesiologist, and radiological technologist were behind a protective lead glass and were at a greater distance from the source than the surgeon. The surgeon received a dose of < 100 µGy; the surface doses of the other personnel present were < 10 µGy. The researchers described the difference in values as being related to the variation in distance and the additional protection used by the non-surgeon members of the staff.[234]

VII.a. Therapeutic radiation sources must be handled in accordance with local, state, and federal regulations.[27,235] *[1: Regulatory Requirement]*

VII.a.1. Radioactive sealed sources (eg, capsules, seeds, needles) should be handled with forceps, tongs, or tube racks. *[4: Limited Evidence]*

Coventry et al[236] recommended that forceps be used to handle radioactive materials because when the distance between the health care worker and the radiation source is increased, the dosage is decreased.

VII.b. Radioactive materials must be used under direct supervision of the radiation safety officer or an authorized user. *[1: Regulatory Requirement]*

Using radioactive materials under the direct supervision of a radiation safety officer or an authorized user is supported in the regulations published by the NRC.[27,28,235]

VII.c. Radioactive seeds should be accounted for when present.[237] *[3: Moderate Evidence]*

The NRC recommends accounting for all seeds.[235] A case report by Lamm et al[238] describes a case in which a seed was lost, although no adverse consequences were identified.

VII.c.1. When present, radioactive seeds should be included in the counting procedure.[237] *[2: High Evidence]*

VII.d. Manufacturers' written instructions should be followed for sterilization of radioactive materials. *[1: Strong Evidence]*

Following manufacturers' written instructions is supported by professional guidelines authored by AORN[239] and by a quality report.[240]

VII.e. Precautions should be taken during lymphatic tracing and sentinel lymph node biopsy surgery, including maintaining as great a distance as possible from the irradiated tissue and using long forceps when handling irradiated tissue.[241] *[3: Moderate Evidence]*

Coventry et al[236] conducted a descriptive study of the radiation dose received by personnel involved in 24 procedures using lymphatic mapping and sentinel node biopsy. The researchers found no whole-body dose was detectable for any team member who used dosimetry. The extremity dose for surgeons performing breast cancer procedures was approximately 250 µSv. The dose for pathologists, if the pathological examination was performed on the day of surgery, was approximately 10 µSv. The dose was zero for the radiologist and the courier. The researchers theorized that the dose would be negligible for the perioperative RN because maintaining a distance of 1 m to 2 m from the surgical site decreased the amount of exposure according to the inverse square law. The researchers recommended that the OR staff members maintain as great a distance as possible from the specimen and the irradiated tissue, such as by using a long forceps when handling the tissue.[236] The use of long forceps is also supported in a review of exposure and contamination potentials done by Michel and Hofer.[242]

Klausen et al[243] supported performing sentinel lymph node biopsy surgery without the use of shielding devices. The authors placed dosimeters on the hand and the abdominal wall of surgeons to determine the amount of radiation received by the person closest to the source. The radiation dose was measured for 79 sentinel node biopsies. The doses received by the surgeons was determined to be well below the maximum doses recommended by the ICRP. The researchers also concluded that a surgeon who is pregnant can safely perform as many as 100 procedures during the pregnancy without exceeding the limits set for a pregnant worker.[243]

By using thermoluminescent dosimeters placed on the forehead to measure the amount of radiation received by the scrub person, surgeon, and the assistant during radio-guided sentinel lymph node biopsies, Law et al[244] determined that the mean radiation dose was below the daily background radiation level at the facility. The levels of radiation received by the surgeon and the assistant were low enough that they could perform as many as 2,000 procedures before exceeding the annual dose limit recommended by the ICRP. The researchers concluded that the use of a lead apron during sentinel lymph node biopsies should be optional.[244]

VII.f. Radioactive waste must be disposed of according to local, state, and federal regulations.[27,28,235]

Radioactive waste disposal techniques include
- dilute and disperse (usually used for bodily wastes with low levels of radioactivity, disposed of into the sewer system after flushing twice);
- delay and decay (usually used for bodily wastes with high levels of radioactivity, disposed of into the sewer system after being in a holding tank for the number of days required to decrease the radiation level to a safe level);
- concentrate and contain (used only rarely for items with a very high level of radioactivity; waste is collected into containers and then buried);
- incineration; or
- disposal as routine garbage if the radioactivity of the item does not exceed 1.35 microcuries (eg, syringes, vials, cotton swabs, tissue paper).[245]

[1: Regulatory Requirement]

VII.f.1. Radioactive waste that cannot be disposed of using a dilute-and-disperse technique must be placed in a radioactive waste container in preparation for disposal.[27] *[1: Regulatory Requirement]*

VII.f.2. A radioactive waste label must be placed on radioactive waste and should include the
- radioisotope name,
- amount of radioactivity,
- date of disposal, and
- radiation personnel or authorized user's full name and contact information.[27,229,245,246]

[1: Regulatory Requirement]

VII.g. Perioperative team members (eg, RNs, scrub personnel, sterile processing personnel, environmental services personnel, anesthesia professionals) must receive education regarding handling of therapeutic radiation sources upon hire and annually as applicable to their role and responsibilities. *[1: Regulatory Requirement]*

The educational and annual requirements are supported by regulatory requirements[28] and professional guidelines authored by the ACR in collaboration with the American Society for Radiation Oncology.[60]

VII.g.1. Education and competency verification should include
- minimizing exposure to radiation (ie, ALARA),
- dosimeter use and monitoring,
- care of patients receiving radioactive nuclides,
- handling radioactive nuclides,
- controlling and providing security for the material (ie, constant surveillance), and
- emergency response to spills.[28]

[1: Regulatory Requirement]

VII.h. When transferring patients who received therapeutic radionuclides in the OR, perioperative personnel should notify the personnel who will be receiving the patients of the radiation source and anatomical location before patient transfer. *[4: Limited Evidence]*

Advance communication allows personnel time to protect themselves, other patients, and visitors from unnecessary exposure to radiation.[60]

VII.i. Patients and caregivers must receive instructions regarding precautions to follow after a patient who has received therapeutic radionuclides is discharged. *[1: Regulatory Requirement]*

Regulatory requirements[28] and a descriptive study by Cattani et al[3] support patient and caregiver education. The study measured the levels of radiation exposure in 216 patients with prostate cancer who had radiation seeds implanted in Italy. The researchers stated that the doses received by the caregivers were well below the requirements set by the Italian government. The researchers concluded that education should be provided to patients and caregivers even though the doses received by the caregivers were very low.[3]

VII.i.1. Radiation safety precaution instruction should include
- advising the patient to
  - stay away from crowded places, such as movie theaters;
  - double flush urine and stool;
  - wipe up spills of body fluids immediately; and
  - wear protective clothing (eg, shorts, breast shields)[247,248];
- advising female patients not to breastfeed for one week after treatment[22];
- advising family members, caregivers, and visitors to stay a distance of 3 ft (1 m) from the patient if possible for a period

of time equal to the half life of the radio-nuclide;[3] and

- explaining the length of time the precautions should be continued.

[3: Moderate Evidence]

A descriptive study by Cattani et al[3] measured the mean dose of radiation at the posterior skin surface of 216 patients who received seed implants for prostate carcinoma. Two hundred patients received ^{125}I and 16 patients received Palladium-103 ([103]Pd) seeds. The researchers concluded that if the family members and caregivers maintained a distance of 1 m (3 ft) from the patient, their radiation dose would stay below the European standard of 1 mSv/year. The researchers also recommended that the distance be maintained for the half life of the radionuclide (eg, 60 days for ^{125}I, 15 days for [103]Pd).[3]

In a descriptive study, Keller et al[248] calculated the amount of radiation exposure to family members of 67 female patients who had permanent breast seed implants using [103]Pd between May 2004 and March 2007 at a single facility. The researchers measured exposure by providing the family members (ie, 39 spouses and 28 others) with dosimeters. A control badge was used to measure the atmospheric radiation, and the results of the control dosimeter were subtracted from the family-member dosimeter results. The amount of exposure to the family members was found to be below 5 mSv. The researchers recommended that the patient wear a breast shield in the presence of toddlers and women who are pregnant to provide extra protection.[248]

Glossary

Absorbed dose: The energy imparted to irradiated matter by ionizing radiation to a unit mass of irradiated material at the place of interest. The special units of absorbed dose are the radiation absorbed dose or rad (ie, 0.01 joules per kg) and gray or gy (ie, 1 joule per kg), which is equal to 100 rads. The units for the biological effective dose are the rem and Sievert (Sv).

Deterministic effects: Localized tissue injury caused by an excessive dose of radiation. The amount of injury increases in severity as the dose is increased.

Dosimeter: A device used to determine the external radiation dose that a person has received.

Phantom: An object used as a substitute for live or cadaver subjects. Frequently made to resemble human characteristics such as size and density.

Scatter radiation: Radiation is scattered when an x-ray beam strikes a patient's body, as it passes through the patient's body, and as it strikes surrounding structures (eg, walls, OR furniture).

Shallow dose equivalent: The dose equivalent at a tissue depth of 0.007 cm averaged over an area of 1 cm.

Stochastic effects: The effects of the cumulative dosage of radiation such as malignant diseases and genetic effects. The severity of the effect is not related to a threshold dose.

REFERENCES

1. Chaffins JA. Radiation protection and procedures in the OR. *Radiol Technol.* 2008;79(5):415-428. [VB]

2. Bindal RK, Glaze S, Ognoskie M, Tunner V, Malone R, Ghosh S. Surgeon and patient radiation exposure in minimally invasive transforaminal lumbar interbody fusion. *J Neurosurg Spine.* 2008;9(6):570-573. [IIIC]

3. Cattani F, Vavassori A, Polo A, et al. Radiation exposure after permanent prostate brachytherapy. *Radiother Oncol.* 2006;79(1):65-69. [IIIC]

4. Brown KR, Rzucidlo E. Acute and chronic radiation injury. *J Vasc Surg.* 2011;53(1 Suppl):15S-21S. [VB]

5. Miller DL. Efforts to optimize radiation protection in interventional fluoroscopy. *Health Phys.* 2013;105(5):435-444. [VA]

6. Wagner LK. Radiation injury is potentially a severe consequence of fluoroscopically guided complex interventions. *Health Phys.* 2008;95(5):645-649. [VB]

7. Huda W, Schoepf UJ, Abro JA, Mah E, Costello P. Radiation-related cancer risks in a clinical patient population undergoing cardiac CT. *Am J Roentgenol.* 2011;196(2) W159-W165. [IIIB]

8. Yuan MK, Chien CW, Lee SK, et al. Health effects of medical radiation on cardiologists who perform cardiac catheterization. *J Chin Med Assoc.* 2010;73(4):199-204. [IIIB]

9. O'Connor U, Gallagher A, Malone L, O'Reilly G. Occupational radiation dose to eyes from endoscopic retrograde cholangiopancreatography procedures in light of the revised eye lens dose limit from the International Commission on Radiological Protection. *Br J Radiol.* 2013;86(1022):20120289. [IIIC]

10. Vano E, Kleiman NJ, Duran A, Rehani MM, Echeverri D, Cabrera M. Radiation cataract risk in interventional cardiology personnel. *Radiat Res.* 2010;174(4):490-495. [IIIB]

11. Ciraj-Bjelac O, Rehani M, Minamoto A, Sim KH, Liew HB, Vano E. Radiation-induced eye lens changes and risk for cataract in interventional cardiology. *Cardiology.* 2012;123(3):168-171. [IIIB]

12. Ciraj-Bjelac O, Rehani MM, Sim KH, Liew HB, Vano E, Kleiman NJ. Risk for radiation-induced cataract for staff in interventional cardiology: is there reason for concern? *Catheter Cardiovasc Interv.* 2010;76(6):826-834. [IIIB]

13. Williams PM, Fletcher S. Health effects of prenatal radiation exposure. *Am Fam Physician.* 2010;82(5):488-493. [VB]

14. Killewich LA, Falls G, Mastracci TM, Brown KR. Factors affecting radiation injury. *J Vasc Surg.* 2011;53(1 Suppl):9S-14S. [VB]

15. Health effects of ionising radiation. *Ann ICRP.* 2010;40(6):21-26. [VB]

16. Cousins C, Miller DL, Bernardi G, et al. ICRP Publication 120: Radiological protection in cardiology. *Ann ICRP.* 2013;42(1):1-125. [VB]

17. Saberi A, Salari E, Latifi SM. Cytogenetic analysis in lymphocytes from radiation workers exposed to low level of ionizing radiation in radiotherapy, CT-scan and angiocardiography units. *Mutat Res.* 2013;750(1-2):92-95. [IIIB]

18. Mohapatra A, Greenberg RK, Mastracci TM, Eagleton MJ, Thornsberry B. Radiation exposure to operating room personnel and patients during endovascular procedures. *J Vasc Surg.* 2013;58(3):702-709. [IIIC]

19. Adriaens I, Smitz J, Jacquet P. The current knowledge on radiosensitivity of ovarian follicle development stages. *Hum Reprod Update*. 2009;15(3):359-377. [VB]

20. Koukorava C, Carinou E, Ferrari P, Krim S, Struelens L. Study of the parameters affecting operator doses in interventional radiology using Monte Carlo simulations. *Radiat Measur*. 2011;46(11):1216-1222. [IIIC]

21. Tuohy CJ, Weikert DR, Watson JT, Lee DH. Hand and body radiation exposure with the use of mini C-arm fluoroscopy. *J Hand Surg Am*. 2011;36(4):632-638. [IIIB]

22. Cuaron JJ, Hirsch AE, Medich DC, Hirsch JA, Rosenstein BS. Introduction to radiation safety and monitoring. *J Am Coll Radiol*. 2011;8(4):259-264. [VB]

23. Duran A, Hian SK, Miller DL, Le Heron J, Padovani R, Vano E. Recommendations for occupational radiation protection in interventional cardiology. *Catheter Cardiovasc Interv*. 2013;82(1):29-42. [VB]

24. Guideline for specimen management. In: *Guidelines for Perioperative Practice*. Denver, CO: AORN, Inc; 2015:389-418. [IVA]

25. Linet MS, Kim KP, Miller DL, Kleinerman RA, Simon SL, Berrington de Gonzalez A. Historical review of occupational exposures and cancer risks in medical radiation workers. *Radiat Res*. 2010;174(6):793-808. [VB]

26. Chambers CE, Fetterly KA, Holzer R, et al. Radiation safety program for the cardiac catheterization laboratory. *Catheter Cardiovasc Interv*. 2011;77(4):546-556. [VB]

27. 10 CFR 20. Standards for protection against radiation. 2013. US Government Publishing Office. http://www.gpo.gov/fdsys/pkg/CFR-2013-title10-vol1/pdf/CFR-2013-title10-vol1-part20.pdf. Accessed April 14, 2015.

28. 10 CFR 35. Medical use of byproduct material. 2011. US Government Publishing Office. http://www.gpo.gov/fdsys/pkg/CFR-2011-title10-vol1/pdf/CFR-2011-title10-vol1-part35.pdf. Accessed April 14, 2015.

29. 42 CFR 416.49. Condition for coverage—Laboratory and radiologic services. 2014. US Government Publishing Office. http://www.gpo.gov/fdsys/pkg/CFR-2014-title42-vol3/pdf/CFR-2014-title42-vol3-sec416-49.pdf. Accessed April 14, 2015.

30. 42 CFR 482.26. Condition of participation: Radiologic services. 2011. US Government Publishing Office. http://www.gpo.gov/fdsys/pkg/CFR-2011-title42-vol5/pdf/CFR-2011-title42-vol5-sec482-26.pdf.

31. *ACR–AAPM Technical Standard for Management of the Use of Radiation in Fluoroscopic Procedures*. 2013. American College of Radiology. http://www.acr.org/~/media/f22c9d1ff46f43aab001f9ed0466b7e9.pdf. Accessed April 13, 2015. [IVC]

32. Guideline for product selection. In: *Guidelines for Perioperative Practice*. Denver, CO: AORN, Inc; 2015:179-186. [IVB]

33. Stecker MS, Balter S, Towbin RB, et al. Guidelines for patient radiation dose management. *J Vasc Interv Radiol*. 2009;20(7 Suppl):S263-S273. [IVA]

34. Lakkireddy D, Nadzam G, Verma A, et al. Impact of a comprehensive safety program on radiation exposure during catheter ablation of atrial fibrillation: a prospective study. *J Interv Card Electrophysiol*. 2009;24(2):105-112. [IB]

35. Weiss EM, Thabit O. Clinical considerations for allied professionals: radiation safety and protection in the electrophysiology lab. *Heart Rhythm*. 2007;4(12):1583-1587. [VB]

36. Strauss KJ. Interventional suite and equipment management: cradle to grave. *Pediatr Radiol*. 2006;36(Suppl 2):221-236. [VB]

37. Dumonceau JM, Garcia-Fernandez FJ, Verdun FR, et al. Radiation protection in digestive endoscopy: European Society of Digestive Endoscopy (ESGE) guideline. *Endoscopy*. 2012;44(4):408-421. [IVA]

38. Jaco JW, Miller DL. Measuring and monitoring radiation dose during fluoroscopically guided procedures. *Tech Vasc Interv Radiol*. 2010;13(3):188-193. [VB]

39. Vance AZ, Weinberg BD, Arbique GM, Guild JB, Anderson JA, Chason DP. Fluoroscopic sentinel events in neuroendovascular procedures: how to screen, prevent, and address occurrence. *Am J Neuroradiol*. 2013;34(8):1513-1515. [VC]

40. 10 CFR 71.5. Transportation of licensed material. 2013. http://www.gpo.gov/fdsys/pkg/CFR-2014-title10-vol2/pdf/CFR-2014-title10-vol2-sec71-5.pdf. Accessed April 14, 2015.

41. Park PE, Park JM, Kang JE, et al. Radiation safety and education in the applicants of the final test for the expert of pain medicine. *Korean J Pain*. 2012;25(1):16-21. [IIIC]

42. Ricketts ML, Baerlocher MO, Asch MR, Myers A. Perception of radiation exposure and risk among patients, medical students, and referring physicians at a tertiary care community hospital. *Can Assoc Radiol J*. 2013;64(3):208-212. [IIIB]

43. Friedman AA, Ghani KR, Peabody JO, Jackson A, Trinh QD, Elder JS. Radiation safety knowledge and practices among urology residents and fellows: results of a nationwide survey. *J Surg Educ*. 2013;70(2):224-231. [IIIB]

44. Kirkwood ML, Arbique GM, Guild JB, et al. Surgeon education decreases radiation dose in complex endovascular procedures and improves patient safety. *J Vasc Surg*. 2013;58(3):715-721. [IIIA]

45. Vano E, Fernandez JM, Sanchez RM, et al. Patient radiation dose management in the follow-up of potential skin injuries in neuroradiology. *Am J Neuroradiol*. 2013;34(2):277-282. [IIIB]

46. Sheyn DD, Racadio JM, Ying J, Patel MN, Racadio JM, Johnson ND. Efficacy of a radiation safety education initiative in reducing radiation exposure in the pediatric IR suite. *Pediatr Radiol*. 2008;38(6):669-674. [IIA]

47. Miller DL, Vano E, Bartal G, et al. Occupational radiation protection in interventional radiology: a joint guideline of the Cardiovascular and Interventional Radiology Society of Europe and the Society of Interventional Radiology. *J Vasc Interv Radiol*. 2010;21(5):607-615. [IVA]

48. Kelsey L, Herron-Rice L, Anderson P, et al. SGNA guideline. Radiation safety in the endoscopy setting. *Gastroenterol Nurs*. 2008;31(4):308-311. [IVB]

49. Vano E, Rosenstein M, Liniecki J, Rehani MM, Martin CJ, Vetter RJ. ICRP Publication 113. Education and training in radiological protection for diagnostic and interventional procedures. *Ann ICRP*. 2009;39(5):7-68. [IVC]

50. Abatzoglou I, Koukourakis M, Konstantinides S. Reduction of the radiation dose received by interventional cardiologists following training in radiation protection. *Radiat Prot Dosimet*. 2013;155(1):119-121. [IIIC]

51. Pitcher CD, Melanson MA. The impact of peer-based training on reducing radiation doses from x-ray operations in an interventional pain management clinic. *US Army Med Dep J*. 2010:43-47. [VB]

52. Widmark A, Friberg EG. How "do's" and "dont's" can be of significant importance in radiation protection: a case report. *Radiat Prot Dosimet*. 2011;147(1-2):99-101. [VC]

53. Guideline for perioperative health care information management. In: *Guidelines for Perioperative Practice*. Denver, CO: AORN; 2015:491-512. [IVB]

54. Miller DL, Balter S, Dixon RG, et al. Quality improvement guidelines for recording patient radiation

dose in the medical record for fluoroscopically guided procedures. *J Vasc Interv Radiol.* 2012;23(1):11-18. [IVA]

55. Voros S, Rivera JJ, Berman DS, et al. Guideline for minimizing radiation exposure during acquisition of coronary artery calcium scans with the use of multidetector computed tomography: a report by the Society for Atherosclerosis Imaging and Prevention Tomographic Imaging and Prevention Councils in collaboration with the Society of Cardiovascular Computed Tomography. *J Cardiovasc Comput Tomogr.* 2011;5(2):75-83. [IVB]

56. Marx MV. Interventional radiology: management of the pregnant patient. *Tech Vasc Interv Radiol.* 2010;13(3):154-157. [VC]

57. Miller DL, Balter S, Schueler BA, Wagner LK, Strauss KJ, Vañó E. Clinical radiation management for fluoroscopically guided interventional procedures. *Radiology.* 2010;257(2):321-332. [VA]

58. ICRP; Khong PL, Ringertz H, Donoghue V, et al. ICRP publication 121: radiological protection in paediatric diagnostic and interventional radiology. *Ann ICRP.* 2013;42(2):1-63. [VB]

59. Steele JR, Jones AK, Ninan EP. Quality initiatives: establishing an interventional radiology patient radiation safety program. *Radiographics.* 2012;32(1):277-287. [VB]

60. Erickson BA, Demanes DJ, Ibbott GS, et al. American Society for Radiation Oncology (ASTRO) and America College of Radiology (ACR) practice guideline for the performance of high-dose-rate brachytherapy. *Int J Radiat Oncol Biol Phys.* 2011;79(3):641-649. [IVC]

61. Chen J, Einstein AJ, Fazel R, et al. Cumulative exposure to ionizing radiation from diagnostic and therapeutic cardiac imaging procedures: a population-based analysis. *J Am Coll Cardiol.* 2010;56(9):702-711. [IIIB]

62. Hui CM, MacGregor JH, Tien HC, Kortbeek JB. Radiation dose from initial trauma assessment and resuscitation: review of the literature. *Can J Surg.* 2009;52(2):147-152. [VB]

63. Martinez LC, Vano E, Gutierrez F, Rodriguez C, Gilarranz R, Manzanas MJ. Patient doses from fluoroscopically guided cardiac procedures in pediatrics. *Phys Med Biol.* 2007;52(16):4749-4759. [IIIB]

64. Weiss DJ, Pipinos II, Longo GM, Lynch TG, Rutar FJ, Johanning JM. Direct and indirect measurement of patient radiation exposure during endovascular aortic aneurysm repair. *Ann Vasc Surg.* 2008;22(6):723-729. [VB]

65. Wang W, Zhang M, Zhang Y. Overall measurements of dose to patients in common interventional cardiology procedures. *Radiat Prot Dosimet.* 2013;157(3):348-354. [IIIB]

66. Majewska N, Stanisic MG, Klos MA, et al. Patients' radiation doses during thoracic stent-graft implantation: the problem of long-lasting procedures. *Ann Thorac Surg.* 2012;93(2):465-472. [IIIB]

67. Mancini JG, Raymundo EM, Lipkin M, et al. Factors affecting patient radiation exposure during percutaneous nephrolithotomy. *J Urol.* 2010;184(6):2373-2377. [IIIB]

68. Sandilos P, Tsalafoutas I, Koutsokalis G, et al. Radiation doses to patients from extracorporeal shock wave lithotripsy. *Health Phys.* 2006;90(6):583-587. [IIIB]

69. Stratis AI, Anthopoulos PL, Gavaliatsis IP, et al. Patient dose in cardiac radiology. *Hellenic J Cardiol.* 2009;50(1):17-25. [IIIB]

70. Staton RJ, Williams JL, Arrcola MM, Hintenlang DE, Bolch WE. Organ and effective doses in infants undergoing upper gastrointestinal (UGI) fluoroscopic examination. *Med Phys.* 2007;34(2):703-710. [IIIB]

71. Tsalafoutas IA, Goni H, Maniatis PN, Pappas P, Bouzas N, Tzortzis G. Patient doses from noncardiac diagnostic and therapeutic interventional procedures. *J Vasc Interv Radiol.* 2006;17(9):1489-1498. [IIIB]

72. Sandborg M, Rossitti S, Pettersson H. Local skin and eye lens equivalent doses in interventional neuroradiology. *Eur Radiol.* 2010;20(3):725-733. [IIIA]

73. Beathard GA, Urbanes A, Litchfield T. Radiation dose associated with dialysis vascular access interventional procedures in the interventional nephrology facility. *Semin Dialysis.* 2013;26(4):503-510. [IIIC]

74. Sulieman A, Paroutoglou G, Kapsoritakis A, et al. Reduction of radiation doses to patients and staff during endoscopic retrograde cholangiopancreatography. *Saudi J Gastroenterol.* 2011;17(1):23-29. [IIIB]

75. Thierry-Chef I, Simon SL, Miller DL. Radiation dose and cancer risk among pediatric patients undergoing interventional neuroradiology procedures. *Pediatr Radiol.* 2006;36(Suppl 2):159-162. [IIIA]

76. Ho P, Cheng SW, Wu PM, et al. Ionizing radiation absorption of vascular surgeons during endovascular procedures. *J Vasc Surg.* 2007;46(3):455-459. [IIIB]

77. Peach G, Sinha S, Black SA, et al. Operator-controlled imaging significantly reduces radiation exposure during EVAR. *Eur J Vasc Endovasc Surg.* 2012;44(4):395-398. [IIIB]

78. Joemai RM, Zweers D, Obermann WR, Geleijns J. Assessment of patient and occupational dose in established and new applications of MDCT fluoroscopy. *Am J Roentgenol.* 2009;192(4):881-886. [IIIB]

79. Church CA, Kuhn FA, Mikhail J, Vaughan WC, Weiss RL. Patient and surgeon radiation exposure in balloon catheter sinus ostial dilation. *Otolaryngol Head Neck Surg.* 2008;138(2):187-191. [IIIB]

80. Karthikesalingam A, Markar SR, Weerakkody R, Walsh SR, Carroll N, Praseedom RK. Radiation exposure during laparoscopic cholecystectomy with routine intraoperative cholangiography. *Surg Endosc.* 2009;23(8):1845-1848. [IIIB]

81. Storm ES, Miller DL, Hoover LJ, Georgia JD, Bivens T. Radiation doses from venous access procedures. *Radiology.* 2006;238(3):1044-1050. [IIIB]

82. Tsapaki V, Christou A, Nikolaou N, et al. Radiation doses in a newly founded interventional cardiology department. *Radiat Prot Dosimet.* 2011;147(1-2):72-74. [IIIB]

83. Hidajat N, Wust P, Felix R, Schroder RJ. Radiation exposure to patient and staff in hepatic chemoembolization: risk estimation of cancer and deterministic effects. *Cardiovasc Interv Radiol.* 2006;29(5):791-796. [IIIB]

84. Kirousis G, Delis H, Megas P, Lambiris E, Panayiotakis G. Dosimetry during intramedullary nailing of the tibia. *Acta Orthopaedica.* 2009;80(5):568-572. [IIIC]

85. Kocinaj D, Cioppa A, Ambrosini G, et al. Radiation dose exposure during cardiac and peripheral arteries catheterisation. *Int J Cardiol.* 2006;113(2):283-284. [IIIC]

86. Komiya K, Igarashi T, Suzuki H, Hirabayashi Y, Waechter J, Seo N. In vitro study of patient's and physician's radiation exposure in the performance of epiduroscopy. *Reg Anesth Pain Med.* 2008;33(2):98-101. [IIIB]

87. Safak M, Olgar T, Bor D, Berkmen G, Gogus C. Radiation doses of patients and urologists during percutaneous nephrolithotomy. *J Radiol Prot.* 2009;29(3):409-415. [IIIC]

88. Nishizawa K, Masuda Y, Morinaga K, et al. Surface dose measurement in patients and physicians and effective dose estimation in patients during uterine artery embolisation. *Radiat Prot Dosimet.* 2008;128(3):343-350. [IIIB]

89. Olgar T, Bor D, Berkmen G, Yazar T. Patient and staff doses for some complex x-ray examinations. *J Radiol Prot.* 2009;29(3):393-407. [IIIB]

90. Tsapaki V, Patsilinakos S, Voudris V, et al. Level of patient and operator dose in the largest cardiac centre in Greece. *Radiat Prot Dosimet.* 2008;129(1-3):71-73. [IIIB]

91. Topaltzikis T, Rountas C, Moisidou R, Fezoulidis I, Kappas C, Theodorou K. Radiation dose to patients and staff during angiography of the lower limbs. Derivation of local dose reference levels. *Physica Medica.* 2009;25(1):25-30. [IIIB]

92. Steinfort DP, Einsiedel P, Irving LB. Radiation dose to patients and clinicians during fluoroscopically-guided biopsy of peripheral pulmonary lesions. *Respir Care.* 2010;55(11):1469-1474. [IIIB]

93. Daneault B, Balter S, Kodali SK, et al. Patient radiation exposure during transcatheter aortic valve replacement procedures. *Eurointervention.* 2012;8(6):679-684. [IIIB]

94. Arbique GM, Gilleran JP, Guild JB, Harris JE, Poon CI, Zimmern PE. Radiation exposure during standing voiding cystourethrography in women. *Urology.* 2006;67(2):269-274. [IIIC]

95. Gelfand AA, Josephson SA. Substantial radiation exposure for patients with subarachnoid hemorrhage. *J Stroke Cerebrovasc Dis.* 2011;20(2):131-133. [IIC]

96. Butter C, Schau T, Meyhoefer J, Neumann K, Minden HH, Engelhardt J. Radiation exposure of patient and physician during implantation and upgrade of cardiac resynchronization devices. *Pacing Clin Electrophysiol.* 2010;33(8):1003-1012. [IIIB]

97. Budd H, Patchava A, Khanduja V. Establishing the radiation risk from fluoroscopic-assisted arthroscopic surgery of the hip. *Int Orthop.* 2012;36(9):1803-1806. [IIIC]

98. Noor M, Shekhdar J, Banner NR. Radiation exposure after heart transplantation: trends and significance. *J Heart Lung Transplant.* 2011;30(3):309-314. [IIIA]

99. Molyvda-Athanasopoulou E, Karlatira M, Gotzamani-Psarrakou A, Koulouris Ch, Siountas A. Radiation exposure to patients and radiologists during interventional procedures. *Radiat Prot Dosimet.* 2011;147(1-2):86-89. [IIB]

100. Jamal JE, Armenakas NA, Sosa RE, Fracchia JA. Perioperative patient radiation exposure in the endoscopic removal of upper urinary tract calculi. *J Endourol.* 2011;25(11):1747-1751. [IIIB]

101. Jeskowiak A, Hubmer M, Prenner G, Maechler H. Radiation induced cutaneous ulcer on the back in a patient with congenital anomaly of the upper cava system. *Interact Cardiovasc Thorac Surg.* 2011;12(2):290-292. [VB]

102. Otterburn D, Losken A. Iatrogenic fluoroscopy injury to the skin. *Ann Plast Surg.* 2010;65(5):462-465. [VC]

103. Spiker A, Zinn Z, Carter WH, Powers R, Kovach R. Fluoroscopy-induced chronic radiation dermatitis. *Am J Cardiol.* 2012;110(12):1861-1863. [VB]

104. Takikawa M, Nambu M, Yamamoto N, Azuma R, Kiyosawa T. Radiation-induced skin injury on the upper arm following cardiac interventional radiology: a review and case report. *Wounds.* 2012;24(4):91-98. [VB]

105. Suzuki S, Furui S, Matsumaru Y, et al. Patient skin dose during neuroembolization by multiple-point measurement using a radiosensitive indicator. *Am J Neuroradiol.* 2008;29(6):1076-1081. [IIIB]

106. ACR–SPR Practice Parameter for Imaging Pregnant of Potentially Pregnant Adolescents and Women with Ionizing Radiation. 2013. American College of Radiology. http://www.acr.org/~/media/9e2ed55531fc4b4fa53ef3b6d 3b25df8.pdf. Accessed April 14, 2015. [IVC]

107. Kennedy EV, Iball GR, Brettle DS. Investigation into the effects of lead shielding for fetal dose reduction in CT pulmonary angiography. *Br J Radiol.* 2007;80(956):631-638. [IIIB]

108. Patient and occupational protection. *Ann ICRP.* 2010;40(6):27-39. [IVB]

109. Justino H. The ALARA concept in pediatric cardiac catheterization: techniques and tactics for managing radiation dose. *Pediatr Radiol.* 2006;36(Suppl 2):146-153. [VB]

110. Foley SJ, McEntee MF, Achenbach S, Brennan PC, Rainford LS, Dodd JD. Breast surface radiation dose during coronary CT angiography: reduction by breast displacement and lead shielding. *Am J Roentgenol.* 2011;197(2):367-373. [IB]

111. Clancy CL, O'Reilly G, Brennan PC, McEntee MF. The effect of patient shield position on gonad dose during lumbar spine radiography. *Radiography.* 2010;16(2):131-135. [IIIC]

112. Shortt CP, Fanning NF, Malone L, Thornton J, Brennan P, Lee MJ. Thyroid dose during neurointerventional procedures: does lead shielding reduce the dose? *Cardiovasc Interv Radiol.* 2007;30(5):922-927. [IB]

113. Shortt CP, Malone L, Thornton J, Brennan P, Lee MJ. Radiation protection to the eye and thyroid during diagnostic cerebral angiography: a phantom study. *J Med Imaging Radiat Oncol.* 2008;52(4):365-369. [IIIC]

114. Sancaktutar AA, Bozkurt Y, Onder H, et al. A new practical model of testes shield: the effectiveness during abdominopelvic computed tomography. *J Androl.* 2012;33(5):984-989. [IIIB]

115. Entrikin DW, Leipsic JA, Carr JJ. Optimization of radiation dose reduction in cardiac computed tomographic angiography. *Cardiol Rev.* 2011;19(4):163-176. [VA]

116. Jackson G, Brennan PC. Radio-protective aprons during radiological examinations of the thorax: an optimum strategy. *Radiat Prot Dosimet.* 2006;121(4):391-394. [IIIC]

117. Connolly B, Racadio J, Towbin R. Practice of ALARA in the pediatric interventional suite. *Pediatr Radiol.* 2006;36(Suppl 2):163-167. [VC]

118. Giordano BD, Baumhauer JF, Morgan TL, Rechtine GR. Cervical spine imaging using standard C-arm fluoroscopy: patient and surgeon exposure to ionizing radiation. *Spine.* 2008;33(18):1970-1976. [IIIC]

119. Sawdy JM, Kempton TM, Olshove V, et al. Use of a dose-dependent follow-up protocol and mechanisms to reduce patients and staff radiation exposure in congenital and structural interventions. *Catheter Cardiovasc Interv.* 2011;78(1):136-142. [IIIA]

120. Rahimi SA, Coyle BW, Vogel TR, Haser PB, Graham AM. Acute radiation syndrome after endovascular AAA repair. *Vasc Endovasc Surg.* 2011;45(2):178-180. [VC]

121. Marti N, Lopez V, Pereda C, Martin JM, Montesinos E, Jorda E. Radiation-induced temporary alopecia after embolization of cerebral aneurysms. *Dermatol Online J.* 2008;14(7):19. [VC]

122. Balter S, Hopewell JW, Miller DL, Wagner LK, Zelefsky MJ. Fluoroscopically guided interventional procedures: a review of radiation effects on patients' skin and hair. *Radiology.* 2010;254(2):326-341. [VB]

123. Bor D, Olgar T, Onal E, Caglan A, Toklu T. Assessment of radiation doses to cardiologists during interventional examinations. *Med Phys.* 2009;36(8):3730-3736. [IIIA]

124. Classic KL, Furutani KM, Stafford SL, Pulido JS. Radiation dose to the surgeon during plaque brachytherapy. *Retina.* 2012;32(9):1900-1905. [IIIC]

125. Cohen SA, Rangarajan SS, Chen T, Palazzi KL, Langford JS, Sur RL. Occupational hazard: radiation

exposure for the urologist—developing a reference standard. *Int Braz J Urol.* 2013;39(2):209-213. [IIIC]

126. Sanchez R, Vano E, Fernandez JM, et al. A national programme for patient and staff dose monitoring in interventional cardiology. *Radiat Prot Dosimet.* 2011;147(1-2):57-61. [IIIB]

127. Taher F, Hughes AP, Sama AA, et al. 2013 Young Investigator Award winner: how safe is lateral lumbar interbody fusion for the surgeon? A prospective in vivo radiation exposure study. *Spine.* 2013;38(16):1386-1392. [IIIB]

128. Ingwersen M, Drabik A, Kulka U, et al. Physicians' radiation exposure in the catheterization lab: does the type of procedure matter? *JACC: Cardiovasc Interv.* 2013;6(10):1096-1102. [IIIB]

129. Kim KP, Miller DL, Berrington de Gonzalez A, et al. Occupational radiation doses to operators performing fluoroscopically-guided procedures. *Health Phys.* 2012;103(1):80-99. [IIIA]

130. Sciahbasi A, Romagnoli E, Trani C, et al. Operator radiation exposure during percutaneous coronary procedures through the left or right radial approach: the TALENT dosimetric substudy. *Circ Cardiovasc Interv.* 2011;4(3):226-231. [IIA]

131. Domienik J, Brodecki M, Carinou E, et al. Extremity and eye lens doses in interventional radiology and cardiology procedures: first results of the ORAMED project. *Radiat Prot Dosimet.* 2011;144(1-4):442-447. [IIIA]

132. Singh PJ, Perera NS, Dega R. Measurement of the dose of radiation to the surgeon during surgery to the foot and ankle. *J Bone Joint Surg Br.* 2007;89(8):1060-1063. [IIIC]

133. Vano E, Gonzalez L, Fernandez JM, Haskal ZJ. Eye lens exposure to radiation in interventional suites: caution is warranted. *Radiology.* 2008;248(3):945-953. [IIIB]

134. Lie OO, Paulsen GU, Wohni T. Assessment of effective dose and dose to the lens of the eye for the interventional cardiologist. *Radiat Prot Dosimet.* 2008;132(3):313-318. [IIIB]

135. Mariscalco MW, Yamashita T, Steinmetz MP, Krishnaney AA, Lieberman IH, Mroz TE. Radiation exposure to the surgeon during open lumbar microdiscectomy and minimally invasive microdiscectomy: a prospective, controlled trial. *Spine.* 2011;36(3):255-260. [IIB]

136. Kesavachandran CN, Haamann F, Nienhaus A. Radiation exposure of eyes, thyroid gland and hands in orthopaedic staff: a systematic review. *Eur J Med Res.* 2012;17:28. [IIIB]

137. Radhi AM, Masbah O, Shukur MH, Shahril Y, Taiman K. Radiation exposure to operating theatre personnel during fluoroscopic-assisted orthopaedic surgery. *Med J Malaysia.* 2006;61(Suppl A):50-52. [IIIC]

138. Ubeda C, Vano E, Gonzalez L, et al. Scatter and staff dose levels in paediatric interventional cardiology: a multicentre study. *Radiat Prot Dosimet.* 2010;140(1):67-74. [IIIB]

139. Stavas JM, Smith TP, DeLong DM, Miller MJ, Suhocki PV, Newman GE. Radiation hand exposure during restoration of flow to the thrombosed dialysis access graft. *J Vasc Interv Radiol.* 2006;17(10):1611-1617. [IIIB]

140. Mroz TE, Abdullah KG, Steinmetz MP, Klineberg EO, Lieberman IH. Radiation exposure to the surgeon during percutaneous pedicle screw placement. *J Spinal Disord Tech.* 2011;24(4):264-267. [IIIC]

141. Hammer GP, Scheidemann-Wesp U, Samkange-Zeeb F, Wicke H, Neriishi K, Blettner M. Occupational exposure to low doses of ionizing radiation and cataract development: a systematic literature review and perspectives on future studies. *Radiat Environ Biophys.* 2013;52(3):303-319. [VA]

142. Amoretti N, Lesbats V, Marcy PY, et al. Dual guidance (CT and fluoroscopy) vertebroplasty: radiation dose to radiologists. How much and where? *Skeletal Radiol.* 2010;39(12):1229-1235. [IIIC]

143. Fransen P. Fluoroscopic exposure in modern spinal surgery. *Acta Orthop Belg.* 2011;77(3):386-389. [IIIB]

144. Schiefer H, von Toggenburg F, Seelentag W, et al. Exposure of treating physician to radiation during prostate brachytherapy using iodine-125 seeds: dose measurements on both hands with thermoluminescence dosimeters. *Strahlenther Onkol.* 2009;185(10):689-695. [IIIB]

145. Jindal T. The risk of radiation exposure to assisting staff in urological procedures: a literature review. *Urol Nurs.* 2013;33(3):136-139. [VB]

146. Dagal A. Radiation safety for anesthesiologists. *Curr Opin Anaesthesiol.* 2011;24(4):445-450. [VB]

147. Vanhavere F, Carinou E, Donadille L, et al. An overview on extremity dosimetry in medical applications. *Radiat Prot Dosimet.* 2008;129(1-3):350-355. [VB]

148. Nottmeier EW, Pirris SM, Edwards S, Kimes S, Bowman C, Nelson KL. Operating room radiation exposure in cone beam computed tomography-based, image-guided spinal surgery: clinical article. *J Neurosurg Spine.* 2013;19(2):226-231. [IIIB]

149. Kumari G, Kumar P, Wadhwa P, Aron M, Gupta NP, Dogra PN. Radiation exposure to the patient and operating room personnel during percutaneous nephrolithotomy. *Int Urol Nephrol.* 2006;38(2):207-210. [IIIB]

150. Majidpour HS. Risk of radiation exposure during PCNL. *Urol J.* 2010;7(2):87-89. [IIIB]

151. Haqqani OP, Agarwal PK, Halin NM, Iafrati MD. Defining the radiation "scatter cloud" in the interventional suite. *J Vasc Surg.* 2013;58(5):1339-1345. [IIIB]

152. Abdullah KG, Bishop FS, Lubelski D, Steinmetz MP, Benzel EC, Mroz TE. Radiation exposure to the spine surgeon in lumbar and thoracolumbar fusions with the use of an intraoperative computed tomographic 3-dimensional imaging system. *Spine.* 2012;37(17):E1074-E1078. [IIIC]

153. Efstathopoulos EP, Pantos I, Andreou M, et al. Occupational radiation doses to the extremities and the eyes in interventional radiology and cardiology procedures. *Br J Radiol.* 2011;84(997):70-77. [IIIB]

154. Lee K, Lee KM, Park MS, Lee B, Kwon DG, Chung CY. Measurements of surgeons' exposure to ionizing radiation dose during intraoperative use of C-arm fluoroscopy. *Spine.* 2012;37(14):1240-1244. [IIIC]

155. Sulieman A, Elzaki M, Khalil M. Occupational exposure to staff during endoscopic retrograde cholangiopancreatography in Sudan. *Radiat Prot Dosimet.* 2011;144(1-4):530-533. [IIIB]

156. Mesbahi A, Rouhani A. A study on the radiation dose of the orthopaedic surgeon and staff from a mini C-arm fluoroscopy unit. *Radiat Prot Dosimet.* 2008;132(1):98-101. [IIIC]

157. Schueler BA, Vrieze TJ, Bjarnason H, Stanson AW. An investigation of operator exposure in interventional radiology. *Radiographics.* 2006;26(5):1533-1541. [IIIB]

158. Kim TW, Jung JH, Jeon HJ, Yoon KB, Yoon DM. Radiation exposure to physicians during interventional pain procedures. *Korean J Pain.* 2010;23(1):24-27. [IIIA]

159. Patel AP, Gallacher D, Dourado R, et al. Occupational radiation exposure during endovascular aortic procedures. *Eur J Vasc Endovasc Surg.* 2013;46(4):424-430. [IIIB]

160. Mitchell EL, Furey P. Prevention of radiation injury from medical imaging. *J Vasc Surg.* 2011;53(1 Suppl):22S-27S. [VB]

161. von Wrangel A, Cederblad A, Rodriguez-Catarino M. Fluoroscopically guided percutaneous vertebroplasty: assessment of radiation doses and implementation of procedural routines to reduce operator exposure. *Acta Radiol.* 2009;50(5):490-496. [IIIC]

162. Blake ME, Oates ME, Applegate K, Kuligowska E; American Association for Women Radiologists; Association of Program Directors in Radiology. Proposed program guidelines for pregnant radiology residents: a project supported by the American Association for Women Radiologists and the Association of Program Directors in Radiology. *Acad Radiol.* 2006;13(3):391-401. [IVB]

163. Best PJ, Skelding KA, Mehran R, et al; Women in Innovations (WIN) group of the Society of Cardiac Angiography and Intervention. SCAI consensus document on occupational radiation exposure to the pregnant cardiologist and technical personnel. *Heart Lung Circ.* 2011;20(2):83-90. [IVB]

164. Chandra V, Dorsey C, Reed AB, Shaw P, Banghart D, Zhou W. Monitoring of fetal radiation exposure during pregnancy. *J Vasc Surg.* 2013;58(3):710-714. [IIIC]

165. Kesavachandran CN, Haamann F, Nienhaus A. Radiation exposure and adverse health effects of interventional cardiology staff. *Rev Environ Contam Toxicol.* 2013;222:73-91. [IIIB]

166. Basic B, Beganovic A, Skopljak-Beganovic A, Samek D. Occupational exposure doses in interventional procedures in Bosnia and Herzegovina. *Radiat Prot Dosimet.* 2011;144(1-4):501-504. [IIIB]

167. Chida K, Takahashi T, Ito D, Shimura H, Takeda K, Zuguchi M. Clarifying and visualizing sources of staff-received scattered radiation in interventional procedures. *Am J Roentgenol.* 2011;197(5):W900-W903. [IIIC]

168. ASGE Technology Committee; Pedrosa MC, Farraye FA, Shergill AK, et al. Minimizing occupational hazards in endoscopy: personal protective equipment, radiation safety, and ergonomics. *Gastrointest Endosc.* 2010;72(2):227-235. [IVB]

169. Chida K, Kato M, Kagaya Y, et al. Radiation dose and radiation protection for patients and physicians during interventional procedure. *J Radiat Res.* 2010;51(2):97-105. [VB]

170. Schueler BA. Reducing occupational exposure from fluoroscopy. *J Am Coll Radiol.* 2007;4(5):335-337. [VC]

171. Smilowitz NR, Balter S, Weisz G. Occupational hazards of interventional cardiology. *Cardiovasc Revasc Med.* 2013;14(4):223-228. [VB]

172. Koshy S, Thompson RC. Review of radiation reduction strategies in clinical cardiovascular imaging. *Cardiol Rev.* 2012;20(3):139-144. [VB]

173. Lymperopoulou G, Papagiannis P, Sakelliou L, Georgiou E, Hourdakis CJ, Baltas D. Comparison of radiation shielding requirements for HDR brachytherapy using 169Yb and 192Ir sources. *Med Phys.* 2006;33(7):2541-2547. [IIIB]

174. Facility Guidelines Institute. *Guidelines for Design and Construction of Hospitals and Outpatient Facilities.* Chicago, IL: American Society for Healthcare Engineering; 2014. [IVC]

175. Sabnis RB, Mishra S, Sharma R, Desai MR. Preoperative planning and designing of a fluorocompatible endourology operating room. *J Endourol.* 2009;23(10):1579-1585. [VB]

176. Brusin JH. Radiation protection. *Radiol Technol.* 2007;78(5):378-395. [VB]

177. Uthoff H, Pena C, West J, Contreras F, Benenati JF, Katzen BT. Evaluation of novel disposable, lightweight radiation protection devices in an interventional radiology setting: a randomized controlled trial. *Am J Roentgenol.* 2013;200(4):915-920. [IA]

178. Mori H, Koshida K, Ishigamori O, Matsubara K. Evaluation of the effectiveness of X-ray protective aprons in experimental and practical fields. *Radiol Phys Technol.* 2014;7(1):158-166. [IIIC]

179. Chatterson LC, Leswick DA, Fladeland DA, Hunt MM, Webster ST. Lead versus bismuth-antimony shield for fetal dose reduction at different gestational ages at CT pulmonary angiography. *Radiology.* 2011;260(2):560-567. [IIIC]

180. Lee SY, Min E, Bae J, et al. Types and arrangement of thyroid shields to reduce exposure of surgeons to ionizing radiation during intraoperative use of C-arm fluoroscopy. *Spine.* 2013;38(24):2108-2112. [IIIB]

181. Zuguchi M, Chida K, Taura M, Inaba Y, Ebata A, Yamada S. Usefulness of non-lead aprons in radiation protection for physicians performing interventional procedures. *Radiat Prot Dosimet.* 2008;131(4):531-534. [IIIC]

182. Ploux S, Ritter P, Haissaguerre M, Clementy J, Bordachar P. Performance of a radiation protection cabin during implantation of pacemakers or cardioverter defibrillators. *J Cardiovasc Electrophysiol.* 2010;21(4):428-430. [IB]

183. Behan M, Haworth P, Colley P, et al. Decreasing operators' radiation exposure during coronary procedures: the transradial radiation protection board. *Catheter Cardiovasc Interv.* 2010;76(1):79-84. [IB]

184. Nikodemová D, Brodecki M, Carinou E, et al. Staff extremity doses in interventional radiology. Results of the ORAMED measurement campaign. *Radiat Measur.* 2011;46(11):1210-1215. [IIIA]

185. Vanhavere F, Carinou E, Domienik J, et al. Measurements of eye lens doses in interventional radiology and cardiology: final results of the ORAMED project. *Radiat Measur.* 2011;46(11):1243-1247. [IIIA]

186. Koukorava C, Carinou E, Simantirakis G, et al. Doses to operators during interventional radiology procedures: focus on eye lens and extremity dosimetry. *Radiat Prot Dosimet.* 2011;144(1-4):482-486. [IIIB]

187. Carinou E, Brodecki M, Domienik J, et al. Recommendations to reduce extremity and eye lens doses in interventional radiology and cardiology. *Radiat Measur.* 2011;46(11):1324-1329. [IIIA]

188. Tsapaki V, Paraskeva KD, Mathou N, et al. Patient and endoscopist radiation doses during ERCP procedures. *Radiat Prot Dosimet.* 2011;147(1-2):111-113. [IIIB]

189. Shortt CP, Al-Hashimi H, Malone L, Lee MJ. Staff radiation doses to the lower extremities in interventional radiology. *Cardiovasc Interv Radiol.* 2007;30(6):1206-1209. [IIIB]

190. Jordan RM, Mohammad F, Taylor WB, Cura M, Savage C. Comparison of fluoroscopic operator eye exposures when working from femoral region, side, or head of patient. *Baylor Univ Med Cent Proc.* 2013;26(3):243-246. [IIIB]

191. Marichal DA, Anwar T, Kirsch D, et al. Comparison of a suspended radiation protection system versus standard lead apron for radiation exposure of a simulated interventionalist. *J Vasc Interven Radiol.* 2011;22(4):437-442. [IIIC]

192. Maeder M, Brunner-La Rocca HP, Wolber T, et al. Impact of a lead glass screen on scatter radiation to eyes and hands in interventional cardiologists. *Catheter Cardiovasc Interv.* 2006;67(1):18-23. [IIIB]

193. Mesbahi A, Mehnati P, Keshtkar A, Aslanabadi N. Comparison of radiation dose to patient and staff for two interventional cardiology units: a phantom study. *Radiat Prot Dosimet.* 2008;131(3):399-403. [IIIB]

194. Schulz B, Heidenreich R, Heidenreich M, et al. Radiation exposure to operating staff during rotational flat-panel angiography and C-arm cone beam computed tomography (CT) applications. *Eur J Radiol.* 2012;81(12):4138-4142. [IIIC]

195. Thornton RH, Dauer LT, Altamirano JP, Alvarado KJ, St Germain J, Solomon SB. Comparing strategies for operator eye protection in the interventional radiology suite. *J Vasc Interv Radiol.* 2010;21(11):1703-1707. [IIIC]

196. Sauren LD, van Garsse L, van Ommen V, Kemerink GJ. Occupational radiation dose during transcatheter aortic valve implantation. *Catheter Cardiovasc Interv.* 2011;78(5):770-776. [IIIC]

197. Fetterly KA, Magnuson DJ, Tannahill GM, Hindal MD, Mathew V. Effective use of radiation shields to minimize operator dose during invasive cardiology procedures. *Cardiovasc Interv.* 2011;4(10):1133-1139. [IIIC]

198. Mahnken AH, Sedlmair M, Ritter C, Banckwitz R, Flohr T. Efficacy of lower-body shielding in computed tomography fluoroscopy-guided interventions. *Cardiovasc Interv Radiol.* 2012;35(6):1475-1479. [IIIC]

199. Karadag B, Ikitimur B, Durmaz E, et al. Effectiveness of a lead cap in radiation protection of the head in the cardiac catheterisation laboratory. *EuroIntervention.* 2013;9(6):754-756. [IIIB]

200. Ahn Y, Kim CH, Lee JH, Lee SH, Kim JS. Radiation exposure to the surgeon during percutaneous endoscopic lumbar discectomy: a prospective study. *Spine.* 2013;38(7):617-625. [IIIB]

201. Parashar B, Wernicke AG, Pavese A, et al. Cesium-131 permanent seed brachytherapy: dosimetric evaluation and radiation exposure to surgeons, radiation oncologists, and staff. *Brachytherapy.* 2011;10(6):508-513. [IIIC]

202. Ismail S, Khan F, Sultan N, Naqvi M. Radiation exposure to anaesthetists during interventional radiology. *Anaesthesia.* 2010;65(1):54-60. [IIIB]

203. van der Merwe B. Radiation dose to surgeons in theatre. *S Afr J Surg.* 2012;50(2):26-29. [IIIA]

204. Alzimami K, Sulieman A, Paroutoglou G, Potamianos S, Vlychou M, Theodorou K. Optimisation of radiation exposure to gastroenterologists and patients during therapeutic ERCP. *Gastroenterol Res Pract.* 2013;2013:587574. [IIIB]

205. Mechlenburg I, Daugaard H, Soballe K. Radiation exposure to the orthopaedic surgeon during periacetabular osteotomy. *Int Orthop.* 2009;33(6):1747-1751. [IIIC]

206. Vano E, Kleiman NJ, Duran A, Romano-Miller M, Rehani MM. Radiation-associated lens opacities in catheterization personnel: results of a survey and direct assessments. *J Vasc Interv Radiol.* 2013;24(2):197-204. [IIA]

207. Antic V, Ciraj-Bjelac O, Rehani M, Aleksandric S, Arandjic D, Ostojic M. Eye lens dosimetry in interventional cardiology: results of staff dose measurements and link to patient dose levels. *Radiat Prot Dosimet.* 2013;154(3):276-284. [IIIB]

208. Burns S, Thornton R, Dauer LT, Quinn B, Miodownik D, Hak DJ. Leaded eyeglasses substantially reduce radiation exposure of the surgeon's eyes during acquisition of typical fluoroscopic views of the hip and pelvis. *J Bone Joint Surg Am.* 2013;95(14):1307-1311. [IIIB]

209. Mroz TE, Yamashita T, Davros WJ, Lieberman IH. Radiation exposure to the surgeon and the patient during kyphoplasty. *J Spinal Disord Tech.* 2008;21(2):96-100. [IIIC]

210. Sturchio GM, Newcomb RD, Molella R, Varkey P, Hagen PT, Schueler BA. Protective eyewear selection for interventional fluoroscopy. *Health Phys.* 2013;104(2 Suppl 1):S11-S16. [IIIB]

211. *NCRP Report No. 168, Radiation Dose Management for Fluoroscopically-Guided Interventional Medical Procedures.* Bethesda, MD: National Council on Radiation Protection & Measurements; 2010. [VA]

212. Rehani MM, Vano E, Ciraj-Bjelac O, Kleiman NJ. Radiation and cataract. *Radiat Prot Dosimet.* 2011;147(1-2):300-304. [VB]

213. Taylor ER, Kramer B, Frye TP, Wang S, Schwartz BF, Kohler TS. Ocular radiation exposure in modern urological practice. *J Urol.* 2013;190(1):139-143. [IIIB]

214. Penfold SN, Marcu L, Lawson JM, Asp J. Evaluation of physician eye lens doses during permanent seed implant brachytherapy for prostate cancer. *J Radiol Prot.* 2012;32(3):339-347. [IIIC]

215. Politi L, Biondi-Zoccai G, Nocetti L, et al. Reduction of scatter radiation during transradial percutaneous coronary angiography: a randomized trial using a lead-free radiation shield. *Catheter Cardiovasc Interv.* 2012;79(1):97-102. [IB]

216. Murphy JC, Darragh K, Walsh SJ, Hanratty CG. Efficacy of the RADPAD protective drape during real world complex percutaneous coronary intervention procedures. *Am J Cardiol.* 2011;108(10):1408-1410. [IB]

217. Lange HW, von Boetticher H. Reduction of operator radiation dose by a pelvic lead shield during cardiac catheterization by radial access: comparison with femoral access. *Cardiovasc Interv.* 2012;5(4):445-449. [IB]

218. Brambilla M, Occhetta E, Ronconi M, Plebani L, Carriero A, Marino P. Reducing operator radiation exposure during cardiac resynchronization therapy. *Europace.* 2010;12(12):1769-1773. [IIC]

219. Iqtidar AF, Jeon C, Rothman R, Snead R, Pyne CT. Reduction in operator radiation exposure during transradial catheterization and intervention using a simple lead drape. *Am Heart J.* 2013;165(3):293-298. [IIIB]

220. Synowitz M, Kiwit J. Surgeon's radiation exposure during percutaneous vertebroplasty. *J Neurosurg Spine.* 2006;4(2):106-109. [IIB]

221. Schueler BA. Operator shielding: how and why. *Tech Vasc Interv Radiol.* 2010;13(3):167-171. [VB]

222. Challa K, Warren SG, Danak S, Bates MC. Redundant protective barriers: minimizing operator occupational risk. *J Interv Cardiol.* 2009;22(3):299-307. [IIIB]

223. von Boetticher H, Lachmund J, Hoffmann W. Cardiac catheterization: impact of face and neck shielding on new estimates of effective dose. *Health Phys.* 2009;97(6):622-627. [IIB]

224. Oyar O, Kislalioglu A. How protective are the lead aprons we use against ionizing radiation? *Diagn Interv Radiol.* 2012;18(2):147-152. [IIIB]

225. White T. Management of leaded PPE in the healthcare environment. *Health Phys.* 2013;105(5 Suppl 3):S231-S236. [VB]

226. Guideline for environmental cleaning. In: *Guidelines for Perioperative Practice.* Denver, CO: AORN, Inc; 2014:9-30. [IVA]

227. Boyle H, Strudwick RM. Do lead rubber aprons pose an infection risk? *Radiography.* 2010;16(4):297-303. [IIIC]

228. Grogan BF, Cranston WC, Lopez DM, Furbee C, Murray CK, Hsu JR. Do protective lead garments harbor harmful bacteria? *Orthopedics.* 2011;34(11):861-861. [IIIB]

229. 10 CFR 30.41—Transfer of byproduct material. US NRC. http://www.nrc.gov/reading-rm/doc-collections/cfr/part030/part030-0041.html. Accessed April 14, 2015.

230. 29 CFR 1910.1096. Toxic and hazardous substances: Ionizing radiation. Occupational Safety and Health Administration. https://www.osha.gov/pls/oshaweb/

owadisp.show_document?p_table=STANDARDS&p_id=10098. Accessed April 13, 2015.

231. Chida K, Kaga Y, Haga Y, et al. Occupational dose in interventional radiology procedures. *Am J Roentgenol.* 2013;200(1):138-141. [IIIB]

232. Ginjaume M, Perez S, Ortega X. Improvements in extremity dose assessment for ionising radiation medical applications. *Radiat Prot Dosimet.* 2007;125(1-4):28-32. [IIIC]

233. Hausler U, Czarwinski R, Brix G. Radiation exposure of medical staff from interventional x-ray procedures: a multicentre study. *Eur Radiol.* 2009;19(8):2000-2008. [IIIB]

234. Fujii K, Ko S, Nako Y, et al. Dose measurement for medical staff with glass dosemeters and thermoluminescence dosemeters during 125I brachytherapy for prostate cancer. *Radiat Prot Dosimet.* 2011;144(1-4):459-463. [IIIB]

235. *NRC: Iodine-125 and Palladium-103 Low Dose Rate Brachytherapy Seeds Used for Localization of Non-Palpable Lesions.* US NRC. http://www.nrc.gov/materials/miau/med-use-toolkit/seed-localization.html. Accessed April 14, 2015.

236. Coventry BJ, Collins PJ, Kollias J, et al. Ensuring radiation safety to staff in lymphatic tracing and sentinel lymph node biopsy surgery—some recommendations. *J Nucl Med Radiat Ther.* 2012;S2:008. doi:10.4172/2155-9619.S2-008. [IIIC]

237. Guideline for prevention of retained surgical items. In: *Guidelines for Perioperative Practice.* Denver, CO: AORN, Inc; 2015:347-363.

238. Lamm IL, Horton P, Lehmann W, Lillicrap S. Practical application of suspension criteria scenarios: radiotherapy. *Radiat Prot Dosimet.* 2013;153(2):179-184. [VB]

239. Guideline for sterilization. In: *Guidelines for Perioperative Practice.* Denver, CO: AORN, Inc; 2015:665-692. [IVA]

240. Pavlicek W, Walton HA, Karstaedt PJ, Gray RJ. Radiation safety with use of I-125 seeds for localization of nonpalpable breast lesions. *Acad Radiol.* 2006;13(7):909-915. [VB]

241. Miner TJ, Shriver CD, Flicek PR, et al. Guidelines for the safe use of radioactive materials during localization and resection of the sentinel lymph node. *Ann Surg Oncol.* 1999;6(1):75-82. [IIIB]

242. Michel R, Hofer C. Radiation safety precautions for sentinel lymph node procedures. *Health Phys.* 2004;86(2 Suppl):S35-S37. [VB]

243. Klausen TL, Chakera AH, Friis E, Rank F, Hesse B, Holm S. Radiation doses to staff involved in sentinel node operations for breast cancer. *Clin Physiol Funct Imaging.* 2005;25(4):196-202. [IIIB]

244. Law M, Chow LW, Kwong A, Lam CK. Sentinel lymph node technique for breast cancer: radiation safety issues. *Semin Oncol.* 2004;31(3):298-303. [VB]

245. Khan S, Syed A, Ahmad R, Rather TA, Ajaz M, Jan F. Radioactive waste management in a hospital. *Int J Health Sci.* 2010;4(1):39-46. [VB]

246. 10 CFR 20.1905. Exemptions to labeling requirements. 2013. US Government Publishing Office. http://www.gpo.gov/fdsys/pkg/CFR-2013-title10-vol1/pdf/CFR-2013-title10-vol1-part20.pdf. Accessed April 14, 2015.

247. Kaulich TW, Bamberg M. Radiation protection of persons living close to patients with radioactive implants. *Strahlenther Onkol.* 2010;186(2):107-112. [IIIC]

248. Keller BM, Pignol JP, Rakovitch E, Sankreacha R, O'Brien P. A radiation badge survey for family members living with patients treated with a (103)Pd permanent breast seed implant. *Int J Radiat Oncol Biol Phys.* 2008;70(1):267-271. [IIIB]

Acknowledgements

LEAD AUTHOR
Byron L. Burlingame, MS, BSN, RN, CNOR
Perioperative Nursing Specialist
AORN Nursing Department
Denver, Colorado

CONTRIBUTING AUTHOR
Ramona L. Conner, MSN, RN, CNOR
Editor-in-Chief, Guidelines for Perioperative Practice
AORN Nursing Department
Denver, Colorado

The authors and AORN thank Amy L. Halverson, MD, Associate Professor of Surgery, Northwestern University, Chicago, IL; Nathalie Walker, MBA, RN, CNOR, Metairie, LA; Jennifer Fencl, DNP, RN, CNS-BC, CNOR, Clinical Nurse Specialist, Cone Health, Greensboro, NC; Julia Thompson, PhD, RN, CNOR, CNS-CP, Administrative Director, Harris Health System, Houston, TX; and Janice Neil, PhD, RN, CNE, Associate Professor, College of Nursing, East Carolina University, Greenville, NC, for their assistance in developing this guideline.

PUBLICATION HISTORY

Originally published October 1989, *AORN Journal*, as Recommended Practices: Radiological Safety in the Practice Setting.

Published September 1993, *AORN Journal*, as Proposed Recommended Practices: Reducing Radiological Exposure in the Practice Setting.

Revised and reformatted; published January 2001, *AORN Journal*, as Recommended Practices for Reducing Radiological Exposure in the Practice Setting.

Revised November 2006; published in *Standards, Recommended Practices, and Guidelines*, 2007 edition, as Recommended Practices for Reducing Radiological Exposure in the Perioperative Practice Setting.

Minor editing revisions made to omit PNDS codes; reformatted September 2012 for publication in *Perioperative Standards and Recommended Practices*, 2013 edition.

Minor editing revisions made in November 2014 for publication in *Guidelines for Perioperative Practice*, 2015 edition, as Guideline for Reducing Radiological Exposure.

Revised June 2015 for publication in *Guidelines for Perioperative Practice* online.

Evidence ratings revised in *Guidelines for Perioperative Practice*, 2018 edition, to conform to the current AORN Evidence Rating Model.

AMBULATORY SUPPLEMENT: RADIATION SAFETY

Recommendation I

A radiation safety program must be established in all facilities and health care organizations in which the potential for diagnostic or therapeutic radiation exposure exists.

Amb Certain hospital requirements (related to mandatory provision of radiologic services, supervision of such services by a radiologist, and practitioner signing of radiologic reports) no longer apply to ambulatory surgery centers (ASCs).

---

§416.49 Condition for Coverage: Laboratory and Radiologic Services

(b) Standard: Radiologic services.

(b)(1) Radiologic services may only be provided when integral to procedures offered by the ASC and must meet the requirements specified in §482.26(b), (c)(2), and (d)(2) of this chapter.

(b)(2) If radiologic services are utilized, the governing body must appoint an individual qualified in accordance with State law and ASC policies who is responsible for assuring all radiologic services are provided in accordance with the requirements of this section.

Centers for Medicare and Medicaid Services. Medicare and Medicaid Programs; Regulatory Provisions to Promote Program Efficiency, Transparency, and Burden Reduction; Part II. Final rule. *Fed Regist.* 2014;79(91):27152. http://www.gpo.gov/fdsys/pkg/FR-2014-05-12/html/2014-10687.htm. Accessed April 15, 2015.

---

§482.26 Condition of Participation: Radiologic Services

(b)(1) Proper safety precautions must be maintained against radiation hazards. This includes adequate shielding for patients, personnel, and facilities, as well as appropriate storage, use, and disposal of radioactive materials.

(b)(2) Periodic inspection of equipment must be made and hazards identified must be promptly corrected.

(b)(3) Radiation workers must be checked periodically, by the use of exposure meters or badge tests, for amount of radiation exposure.

(b)(4) Radiologic services must be provided only on the order of practitioners with clinical privileges or, consistent with State law, of other practitioners authorized by the medical staff and the governing body to order the services.

(c)(2) Only personnel designated as qualified by the medical staff may use the radiologic equipment and administer procedures.

(d)(2) The hospital must maintain the following for at least 5 years:

(i) Copies of reports and printouts

(ii) Films, scans, and other image records, as appropriate

---

42 CFR 482.26. Condition of participation: Radiologic services. 2011. US Government Publishing Office. http://www.gpo.gov/fdsys/pkg/CFR-2011-title42-vol5/pdf/CFR-2011-title42-vol5-sec482-26.pdf. Accessed April 14, 2015.

Amb In an ASC, the individual appointed by the governing body to be the radiation safety officer is responsible for ensuring that proper radiation safety precautions are maintained. The radiation safety officer should be someone who currently works in the ASC. This individual is not required to be a radiologist but should be qualified in accordance with state law and ASC policies. As the individual responsible for oversight of the imaging services at the ASC, the radiation safety officer must maintain appropriate exposure records for each employee. In addition, this person is responsible for periodic evaluation and calibration of equipment, including testing the integrity of personal protective devices (eg, lead aprons) in compliance with federal, state, and local laws.[A1]

In an ASC where no radiologist is on staff, the ASC's governing body should verify that the operating surgeon/anesthesiologist is competent in the use of the equipment and interpretation of radiographic images when this is an integral part of the surgical or other invasive procedure. This process should be accomplished through the physician credentialing and privileging process.

I.a.   The radiation safety program
   ○ must include procedures for handling and disposing of body fluids and tissue that may be radioactive.[A2,A3]

   Amb Transport personnel (couriers) may be at some risk of radiation exposure when transporting a sentinel lymph node or melanoma specimen marked with radioactive tracers if the container is improperly handled. Personnel are at risk of radiation exposure if the specimen container is held close to the body. To lessen this risk, it is advised that either the specimen itself or the specimen container be placed inside a standard bucket-type plastic specimen container, and the transport personnel should be instructed to carry the specimen container by the handle.[A4]

I.f.   The health care organization must maintain records of changes to the radiation safety program, program audits, and individual monitoring results as prescribed by regulatory requirements.[A5]

Amb The ASC must have a policy that addresses the storage and retention of diagnostic images in accordance with federal, state, and local laws.[A3]

References

A1. Diagnostic and other imaging services 13(D)(5). In: *Accreditation Handbook for Ambulatory Health Care*. Skokie, IL: Accreditation Association for Ambulatory Health Care, Inc; 2014:65.

A2. Guideline for specimen management. In: *Guidelines for Perioperative Practice*. Denver, CO: AORN, Inc; 2015:389-418. [IVA]

A3. 10 CFR 20. Standards for protection against radiation. 2013. US Government Publishing Office. http://www.gpo.gov/fdsys/pkg/CFR-2013-title10-vol1/pdf/CFR-2013-title10-vol1-part20.pdf. Accessed April 14, 2015.

A4. Coventry BJ, Collins PJ, Kollias J, et al. Ensuring radiation safety to staff in lymphatic tracing and sentinel lymph node biopsy surgery—some recommendations. *J Nucl Med Radiat Ther*. 2012;S2:008. doi:10.4172/2155-9619.S2-008. [IIIC]

A5. 42 CFR 416.49. Condition for coverage—Laboratory and radiologic services. 2014. US Government Publishing Office. http://www.gpo.gov/fdsys/pkg/CFR-2014-title42-vol3/pdf/CFR-2014-title42-vol3-sec416-49.pdf. Accessed April 14, 2015.

Acknowledgements

LEAD AUTHOR, AMBULATORY SUPPLEMENT
Jan Davidson, MSN, RN, CNOR, CASC
Director Ambulatory Surgery Division
AORN, Inc
Denver, CO

PUBLICATION HISTORY

Originally published in *Perioperative Standards and Recommended Practices*, 2014 edition, as Ambulatory Supplement: Reducing Radiological Exposure.

Revised June 2015 for publication in *Guidelines for Perioperative Practice* online.

PATIENT AND WORKER SAFETY

Ambulatory Surgery

365

GUIDELINE FOR PREVENTION OF RETAINED SURGICAL ITEMS

The Guideline for Prevention of Retained Surgical Items has been approved by the AORN Guidelines Advisory Board. It was presented as a proposed guideline for comments by members and others. The guideline is effective January 15, 2016. The recommendations in the guideline are intended to be achievable and represent what is believed to be an optimal level of practice. Policies and procedures will reflect variations in practice settings and/or clinical situations that determine the degree to which the guideline can be implemented. AORN recognizes the many diverse settings in which perioperative nurses practice; therefore, this guideline is adaptable to all areas where operative or other invasive procedures may be performed.

Purpose

This document provides guidance to perioperative team members for prevention of retained surgical items (RSIs) in patients undergoing operative and other invasive procedures. Guidance is provided for implementing a consistent multidisciplinary approach to preventing RSIs, accounting for surgical items (ie, radiopaque soft goods, sharps and miscellaneous items, instruments), preventing retention of device fragments, reconciling count discrepancies, and using adjunct technologies to supplement manual count procedures.

An RSI is a rare but serious preventable error that can result in patient harm. Thus, perioperative team members are ethically and morally obligated to protect patients by preventing RSIs. Case reports of RSIs are documented in the literature, with a case series report dating from as early as 1884.[1] Patient injuries from RSIs vary by the type of item retained (eg, sponge, metal), time to diagnosis, and location of the RSI.[2]

The most common items retained are surgical sponges.[3-7] Other reported RSIs include instruments,[4,5,7,8] needles,[8] and items such as guidewires.[5,7,8]

Time to diagnosis of an RSI can vary greatly. According to Gawande et al,[4] only 6% of RSIs are identified on the operative day. The time to diagnosis ranged from the operative day to 6.5 years, with a median time of 21 days.[4]

The location of an RSI depends on the type of procedure performed. The abdomen and pelvis are reported to be the locations where RSIs are most often found.[3,9] Retained surgical sponges in the abdomen or pelvis can migrate to the intestine, bladder, thorax, or stomach.[10] Other locations for RSIs include the thorax, vagina, and other natural orifices.[3] Retained radiopaque sponges have also been found in the spine, head, neck, and extremities.[4,9]

Retention of items can have disastrous outcomes for patients, such as in the case of a patient's death from myocardial infarction caused by an unintentionally retained pacing wire.[11] In another report, a patient presented with a femur fracture from a retained surgical sponge near the bone.[12] Retained surgical items (ie, guidewires, intravascular devices, broken instruments) in the vascular system can cause complications such as thrombosis, embolization, arrhythmia, tamponade, perforation, or even death.[13-17]

Although patient injury largely depends on variables related to the item retained, overall outcomes are well-documented in the literature. Reported patient outcomes from RSIs include re-operation, readmission or increased length of hospital stay, physical harm, death, and emotional harm.[2,3,18] Re-operation is the most common consequence, reported to occur in 64.8% to 69% of RSI cases.[4,8] Readmission or increased length of stay from an RSI have been reported in 30% to 59% of cases.[4-6]

Physical harm outcomes include infection, fistula development or obstruction, and perforation. Infection is the most reported physical harm, with occurrence ranging from 10% to 43%.[4-6] Development of a fistula or obstruction has been reported to be 15% to 18%, and perforation has been reported to occur in 3% to 7% of RSI cases.[4-6] Mehtsun et al[19] categorized physical harm as being temporary in 78.1% of patients and permanent in 16.3% of patients with an RSI. Death is a less common event, occurring in 2% to 6% of cases.[4,6,19] Although emotional harm has not been uniformly reported, one publication estimated the prevalence to be 1.1%.[19] Further research is needed to assess emotional harm to the patient who has experienced an RSI as this value is likely to be underestimated.

In a survey conducted by Steelman et al,[20] 61% of perioperative nurses identified the prevention of RSIs as one of the top priorities for perioperative patient safety. Avoiding injuries from care that is intended to help patients was identified by the Institute of Medicine as one of six goals to achieve a better health care system.[21] Because an RSI is an event that presents significant risk for patient harm, many states require public reporting when RSI events occur.[22] Federal and state agencies, accrediting bodies, third-party payers, and professional associations consider an unintentionally retained foreign object or RSI to be a serious and largely, if not entirely, preventable event (eg, never event, hospital-acquired condition, sentinel event, serious reportable event).[2,23] Consequently, health care organizations and providers will not be reimbursed for additional care provided as a result of an RSI.[19,24,25] Although the exact costs are highly variable, RSIs can be costly and burdensome to the health care system. Two cost-analysis reports of RSIs in pediatric patients estimated additional hospital charges to be $35,681[26] and $42,077[27] for this complication in 2010 and 2009, respectively.

Current law does not prescribe what methods should be used to prevent RSIs, who should use them, or even that they need to be used. The law does, however, require that surgical items not intended to remain in the patient be removed. The doctrine of *res ipsa loquitur* (ie, "the thing speaks for itself") is most applicable in RSI incidents. Therefore, time and effort in legal tort cases is spent assigning blame or fault for the act because it is not always necessary to prove negligence. Furthermore, the "captain of the ship" doctrine is no longer assumed to be true, and members of the entire surgical team as well as the health care facility can be held liable in RSI litigation.[28-30] Although a review of legal case findings is outside the scope of this document, the evidence review undertaken for the development of this document indicated that legal expenses and settlement payments can vary greatly, adding to the health care costs associated with RSIs. Mehtsun et al[19] estimated the cost of malpractice payments for a surgical retained foreign body to range from $51 to $3,988,829, with a mean of $86,247 and median of $33,953. In 2003, Gawande et al[4] estimated malpractice claim expenses to average $52,581 per case.

Prevention of RSIs requires a multidisciplinary approach that aims to reduce the risks associated with RSIs. The risk for an RSI exists even in the smallest of incisions. The following risk factors have been significantly associated with RSIs:

- incorrect count,[3]
- unexpected change due to intraoperative factors,[3]
- more than one surgical team,[3,31]
- no count (due to inability or emergent situations),[3]
- more than one procedure,[3]
- long procedure,[3,31]
- blood loss > 500 mL,[3]
- high body mass index (BMI),[4,6]
- emergency procedure,[4] and
- occurrence of a safety variance during the procedure.[6]

Unexpected procedure events and equipment failure are specific risk factors that have been significantly associated with intravascular RSIs.[32]

A long-standing and evidence-based strategy for preventing RSIs is to account for all items opened or used during the operative or invasive procedure. Health care organizations are responsible for employing standardized, transparent, verifiable, reliable practices to account for all surgical items used during a procedure. Counts of radiopaque soft goods, sharps, miscellaneous items, and instruments are performed to account for all items used on the surgical field. However, there is a significant potential for inaccurate counts with the use of manual counting practices.[31,33,34] The use of adjunct technology may improve counting accuracy.[8,35-39]

Beyond the count, systems and human factors play a significant role in contributing to RSIs. Therefore, behavioral changes and an understanding of risk-reduction strategies unique to each setting should be employed in the adoption of systems to account for surgical items. Improving system reliability to enhance the performance of human factors may reduce error and improve patient safety.[40] A systems approach to preventing RSIs includes using standardized counting and reconciliation procedures, methodical wound exploration, radiological confirmation, adjunct technology, team training,[41,42] and enhanced communication to promote optimal perioperative patient outcomes.[2,18,43-46]

Further research is needed to determine the incidence of RSIs. Various estimates of RSI incidence have been reported in the literature (Table 1), although RSIs are widely thought to be underreported due to medicolegal consequences. Lack of a universal definition of RSI and varying reporting requirements have limited the ability to interpret RSI data.[19,47] Other issues that complicate the interpretation of RSI incidence include selection bias (eg, severity of cases, patient or payer mix, voluntary reporting), time frames for data collection, varying use of RSI prevention methods, and different procedural settings (eg, hospitals, ambulatory centers).

The limitations of the evidence are that randomized controlled trials of RSI prevention interventions may expose patients to harm and, as such, would not be ethical.[5] Case-control studies of RSI have been conducted and contribute valuable knowledge to the field. However, interpretation of these studies is limited by the nature of this type of research, which can only show association among study variables and cannot determine causation. Because of a lack of research on interventions to prevent RSIs, much of the available evidence is based on generally accepted practices, which were first published in the AORN "Standards for sponge, needle, and instrument procedures" in 1976.

The following topics are outside the scope of this document: retrieval techniques and treatment options for RSIs, management of broken surgical drains during removal, post-procedure management of broken central line catheters, and management of retained endoscopy capsules in the gastrointestinal tract.

Evidence Review

A medical librarian conducted a systematic search of the databases Ovid MEDLINE®, EBSCO CINAHL®, Scopus®, and the Cochrane Database of Systematic Reviews. The search was limited to literature published in English from 2009 through June 2014; editorials, news, and brief items were excluded. The lead author later requested supplementary searches on aspects of inaccuracy in counting and the roles of distraction, noise, and human factors in medical error. Between June 2014 and April 2015, the results of alerts established at the time of the initial search were assessed, and the lead author requested additional articles that either did not fit the original search criteria or were discovered during the evidence appraisal process. Finally, the lead author and the medical librarian identified relevant guidelines from government agencies, professional organizations, and standards-setting bodies.

PATIENT AND WORKER SAFETY

TABLE 1. INCIDENCE OF RETAINED SURGICAL ITEMS (RSIs) BY PUBLICATION YEAR

Author (Year)	RSI Definition	Data Source	Incidence (RSIs per surgeries)
Hempel et al[1] (2015)	Various	Secondary (21 incidence studies)	1:10,000
The Joint Commission[2] (2015)	Unintended retention of a foreign object after surgery (after completion of skin closure)	2004-2014 reports to The Joint Commission	986 RSIs total, surgery data not reported
Moffatt-Bruce et al[3] (2014)	Not provided	Secondary[4,10]	0.3:1,000 to 1:1,000
Stawicki et al[4] (2013)	Unintentionally retained surgical item after final skin or fascial (if skin is left open) wound closure	2003-2009, multicenter	1:6,975
Chen et al[5] (2011)	AHRQ Patient Safety Indicator 5 definition: ICD-9-CM codes 998.4, 998.7, and E891.x	2003-2007 fiscal years, Veterans Affairs hospitals	0.12:1,000
Shah & Lander[6] (2009)	ICD-9-CM codes 998.4 and E871.0	2003, Kids' Inpatient Database	1:32,672
World Health Organization[7] (2009)	Not discussed	Secondary	1:5,000 to 1:19,000 as high as 1:1,000
Cima et al[8] (2008)	Object unintentionally retained at time of final wound closure or end of procedure if no wound	2003-2006, Mayo Clinic Rochester	1:5,500 or 0.178:1,000
Egorova et al[9] (2008)	Retention of surgical instrument, needle, or sponge	2000-2004, Major academic health center and affiliated hospitals	1:7,000
Gawande et al[10] (2003)	Retention of a surgical instrument or sponge	1985-2001 closed claims in Massachusetts	1:8,801 to 1:18,760
Hyslop & Maull[11] (1982)	Retained surgical sponge	Not reported	Celiotomies 1:1,000

REFERENCES
1. Hempel S, Maggard-Gibbons M, Nguyen DK, et al. Wrong-site surgery, retained surgical items, and surgical fires: a systematic review of surgical never events. JAMA Surg. 2015;150(8):796-805. [IIIB]
2. Summary Data of Sentinel Events Reviewed by The Joint Commission. The Joint Commission. http://www.jointcommission.org/assets/1/18/2004_to_2014_4Q_SE_Stats_-_Summary.pdf. Accessed November 10, 2015.
3. Moffatt-Bruce SD, Cook CH, Steinberg SM, Stawicki SP. Risk factors for retained surgical items: a meta-analysis and proposed risk stratification system. J Surg Res. 2014;190(2):429-436. [IIIA]
4. Stawicki SP, Moffatt-Bruce SD, Ahmed HM, et al. Retained surgical items: a problem yet to be solved. J Am Coll Surg. 2013;216(1):15-22. [IIIB]
5. Chen Q, Rosen AK, Cevasco M, Shin M, Itani KM, Borzecki AM. Detecting patient safety indicators: How valid is "foreign body left during procedure" in the Veterans Health Administration? J Am Coll Surg. 2011;212(6):977-983. [IIIB]
6. Shah RK, Lander L. Retained foreign bodies during surgery in pediatric patients: a national perspective. J Pediatr Surg. 2009;44(4):738-742. [IIIA]
7. WHO Guidelines for Safe Surgery 2009. Geneva, Switzerland: WHO Press; 2009. [IVB]
8. Cima RR, Kollengode A, Garnatz J, Storsveen A, Weisbrod C, Deschamps C. Incidence and characteristics of potential and actual retained foreign object events in surgical patients. J Am Coll Surg. 2008;207(1):80-87. [IIIB]
9. Egorova NN, Moskowitz A, Gelijns A, et al. Managing the prevention of retained surgical instruments: what is the value of counting? Ann Surg. 2008;247(1):13-18. [IIIA]
10. Gawande AA, Studdert DM, Orav EJ, Brennan TA, Zinner MJ. Risk factors for retained instruments and sponges after surgery. N Engl J Med. 2003;348(3): 229-235. [IIIA]
11. Hyslop JW, Maull KI. Natural history of the retained surgical sponge. South Med J. 1982;75(6):657-660. [VB]

Search terms included the subject headings *surgical count procedure, surgical instruments, operative surgical procedures, foreign bodies, medical errors, postoperative complications, re-operation, surgical wound infection, accident prevention, documentation, situational awareness, human error, noise,* and *interdisciplinary communication.* Other subject headings and key words were included to address the concepts of specific surgical items, root causes of errors in surgical counts, and methods for preventing RSIs. Complete search strategies are available upon request.

Excluded were non-peer-reviewed publications, evidence from other disciplines when evidence from the perioperative setting was available, and case reports that did not provide recommendations for preventing RSIs. Lower-level or lower-quality evidence was excluded when higher-level or higher-quality evidence was available. Opinion leaders have

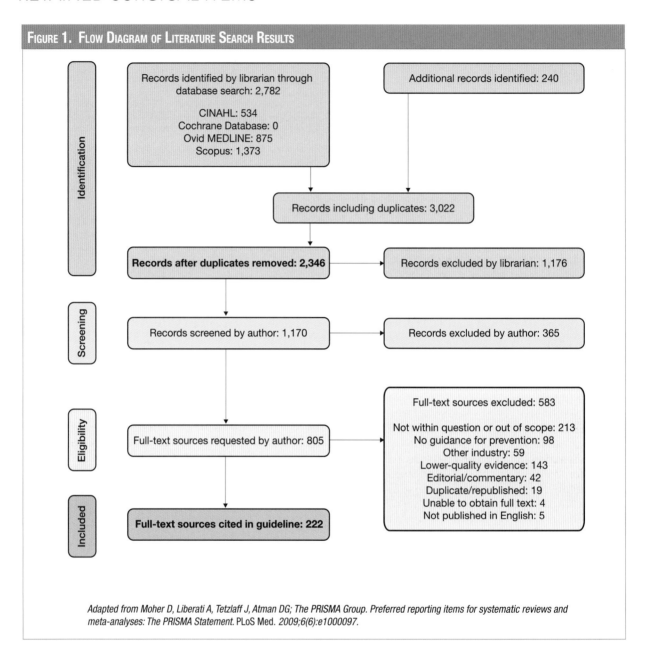

FIGURE 1. FLOW DIAGRAM OF LITERATURE SEARCH RESULTS

Records identified by librarian through database search: 2,782

CINAHL: 534
Cochrane Database: 0
Ovid MEDLINE: 875
Scopus: 1,373

Additional records identified: 240

Records including duplicates: 3,022

Records after duplicates removed: 2,346

Records excluded by librarian: 1,176

Records screened by author: 1,170

Records excluded by author: 365

Full-text sources requested by author: 805

Full-text sources excluded: 583

Not within question or out of scope: 213
No guidance for prevention: 98
Other industry: 59
Lower-quality evidence: 143
Editorial/commentary: 42
Duplicate/republished: 19
Unable to obtain full text: 4
Not published in English: 5

Full-text sources cited in guideline: 222

Identification | Screening | Eligibility | Included

Adapted from Moher D, Liberati A, Tetzlaff J, Atman DG; The PRISMA Group. Preferred reporting items for systematic reviews and meta-analyses: The PRISMA Statement. PLoS Med. 2009;6(6):e1000097.

established accounting protocols for prevention of RSIs that were not published in peer-reviewed literature during the time frame of this systematic literature search, and thus these were excluded from this document (Figure 1).

Articles identified by the search were provided to the project team for evaluation. The team consisted of the lead author and four evidence appraisers. The lead author divided the search results into topics and assigned members of the team to review and critically appraise each article using the AORN Research or Non-Research Evidence Appraisal Tools as appropriate. The literature was independently evaluated and appraised according to the strength and quality of the evidence. Each article was then assigned an appraisal score. The appraisal score is noted in brackets after each reference, as applicable.

The collective evidence supporting each intervention within a specific recommendation was summarized and the AORN Evidence Rating Model was used to rate the strength of the evidence. Factors considered in the review of the collective evidence were the quality of the evidence, the quantity of similar evidence on a given topic, and the consistency of evidence supporting a recommendation. The evidence rating is noted in brackets after each intervention.

Note: *The evidence summary table is available at http://www.aorn.org/evidencetables/.*

Editor's note: *MEDLINE is a registered trademark of the US National Library of Medicine's Medical Literature Analysis and Retrieval System, Bethesda, MD. CINAHL, Cumulative Index to Nursing and Allied Health Literature, is a registered trademark of EBSCO*

PATIENT AND WORKER SAFETY

Industries, Birmingham, AL. Scopus is a registered trademark of Elsevier B.V., Amsterdam, The Netherlands.

Recommendation I

A consistent multidisciplinary approach should be used for preventing RSIs during all surgical and invasive procedures.

The collective evidence and guidance from professional organizations[2,18,40-46,48] support that RSIs are preventable events for which the incidence can be reduced by implementing a consistent multidisciplinary approach. The approach for RSI prevention is multidisciplinary because systems that involve counting and detection are team-based activities that comprise input from multiple perioperative team members.

Establishing a system that accounts for all surgical items opened and used during a procedure constitutes a primary and proactive strategy to prevent patient harm. Reason's model of human error states that errors involve some kind of deviation from routine practice.[49] The ideal RSI prevention measures are standardized, transparent, verifiable, and reliable. Deliberate, consistent application of and adherence to standardized procedures are necessary to prevent the retention of surgical items.

I.a. All perioperative team members should engage in safe practices that support prevention of RSIs.[2,18,43-46,48] *[1: Strong Evidence]*

All perioperative team members are responsible for the prevention of RSIs. Professional organizations[2,18,43-46,48] recommend engaging a multidisciplinary team as part of a systems approach to RSI prevention. Teamwork and communication problems are common areas where failures occur in the prevention of RSIs.[49-53] Improving teamwork and communication in an effort to foster a just culture focused on patient safety is part of a systems approach to reducing surgical errors such as RSIs.[40]

I.a.1. The RN circulator should actively participate in safety measures to prevent RSIs.[54] The RN circulator should

- perform a room survey for open countable items from a previous procedure before conducting an initial count[43,55];
- verify that the count board (eg, whiteboard) and count sheets do not contain information from a previous procedure[43];
- initiate the count;
- view the surgical items being counted;
- record in a visible location (eg, the count board) the counts of soft goods, sharps, miscellaneous items, and items placed in the wound[43,55];
- record instrument counts on pre-printed count sheets;
- observe for items dropped from the sterile field;
- consult with the team about whether any supplies will be needed before initiating the closing count;

- participate in count reconciliation activities;
- report any count discrepancy; and
- document count activities (See Recommendation VIII).

[2: High Evidence]

Accurately accounting for items used during a surgical procedure is a primary responsibility of the RN circulator.[54] The RN circulator plays a leading role in implementing measures to account for surgical items. In an organizational experience study, Yang et al[56] observed 18 cardiovascular procedures for potential and actual errors to conceptualize the role that the RN circulator plays in preventing error. Of 200 errors, 8% were attributed to counting errors. Had the RN circulator not caught these counting errors, they might not have been resolved and could have resulted in RSIs.

The Institute for Clinical Systems Improvement (ICSI)[43] recommends performing a room survey before the baseline count to reduce the risk for error in the count. Loftus et al[55] implemented the room survey as a part of count protocols in a safe surgery program. Loftus et al[55] also recommended documenting the count on a whiteboard that is visible to the surgical team, which is a practice supported by the ICSI.[43]

I.a.2. The scrub person should actively participate in safety measures to prevent RSIs.[54,57] The scrub person should

- maintain an organized sterile field according to the health care organization's policy; there should be minimal variation in how different scrub persons organize the sterile field;
- maintain awareness of the location of soft goods (eg, radiopaque sponges, towels, textiles), sharps, and instruments on the sterile field and in the wound during the course of the procedure;
- know the character and configuration of items that are used by the surgeons and first assistants;
- verify the integrity and completeness of items when they are returned from the surgical site;
- consult with the surgeon about whether any supplies will be needed before performing the closing count;
- count surgical items in a manner that allows the RN circulator to see the surgical items being counted;
- speak up when a discrepancy exists; and
- participate in count reconciliation activities.

[2: High Evidence]

Accurately accounting for items used during a surgical procedure is a primary responsibility of the scrub person.[54,57] Maintaining an organized sterile field facilitates

371

accounting for all items during and after the procedure. Standardized sterile setups established by the health care organization's policy help reduce variation and may lessen the risk for error. Two articles from psychological journals indicated that a random arrangement of objects coupled with distracters increased counting difficulty and errors.[58,59]

I.a.3. Surgeons and surgical first assistants should actively participate in safety measures to prevent RSIs.[44] The surgeon and surgical first assistant should
- use radiopaque surgical items (eg, soft goods) in the wound[18,43,44];
- maintain awareness of the location of items in the surgical wound during the course of the procedure;
- communicate placement of surgical items in the wound to the perioperative team for notation in a visible location (eg, the count board);
- acknowledge awareness of the start of the count process;
- notify the team if any supplies will be needed on the sterile field before the start of the closing count[60];
- remove unneeded counted items from the surgical field at the initiation of the count process;
- perform a methodical wound exploration before closing the wound, using both visualization and touch when feasible[18,43,44];
- notify the scrub person and RN circulator about surgical items returned to the surgical field to complete the final count;
- communicate and document items left intentionally as packing[44];
- participate in count reconciliation activities;
- document actions taken to resolve count discrepancies[44]; and
- verify and document results of the final count.[2,44]

[2: High Evidence]

Accurately accounting for items used during a surgical procedure is a primary responsibility of the surgeon and surgical first assistant. The American College of Surgeons recognizes patient safety as "the highest priority and strongly urges individual hospitals and health care organizations to take all reasonable measures to prevent the retention of foreign bodies in the surgical wound."[44]

Use of radiopaque items in the surgical wound provides a mechanism to locate misplaced items as part of resolving count discrepancies. Not all items are manufactured with radiopaque indicators. The ICSI[43] recommends using only radiopaque items when the product is manufactured in both radiopaque and non-radiopaque forms (eg, soft goods).

I.a.4. Anesthesia professionals should actively participate in safety measures to prevent RSIs. The anesthesia professional should
- plan anesthetic milestone actions (eg, emergence from anesthesia) so that these actions do not pressure the perioperative team to circumvent safe accounting practices[61];
- not use counted items;
- communicate to the perioperative team when throat packs, bite blocks, and other similar devices are inserted in the oropharynx; and
- verify that throat packs, bite blocks, and other similar devices are removed from the oropharynx and communicate to the perioperative team when these items are removed.[62-65]

[2: High Evidence]

Surgical counts and anesthetic milestones, such as emergence from anesthesia, are both critical phases of the procedure during which distractions should be minimized.[61] Planning and coordination will allow the perioperative team to focus on both of these critical portions of the procedure with less distraction and will potentially lessen the risk for errors.

Use of counted items by the anesthesia professional may lead to count discrepancies that could subject the patient to unnecessary radiation exposure and reconciliation procedures. The retention of throat packs has been reported, and the collective evidence[62-65] indicates that measures can be taken to prevent this type of RSI, including communication of the throat pack placement and removal.

I.a.5. Any individual who observes an item dropped from the surgical field should immediately inform the RN circulator and other members of the perioperative team. *[5: Benefits Balanced with Harms]*

I.a.6. Perioperative team members should verbally verify the final count as part of a checklist.[18,66-71] *[2: High Evidence]*

The collective evidence and professional organizations[18,66-71] support using a checklist to increase communication among perioperative team members and improve surgical patient outcomes. In a systematic review with meta-analysis, Lyons and Popejoy[66] examined the effectiveness of implementing a safe surgery checklist on the outcomes of teamwork, communication, morbidity, mortality, and compliance with safety measures in 19 research studies. The authors found that use of the checklist significantly improved all outcomes, although they noted that the generalizability of this meta-analysis is limited and that further research is needed.

In a landmark study, Haynes et al[67] found that implementation of a checklist significantly reduced morbidity and mortality in patients undergoing non-cardiac surgery. Completion of needle, sponge, and instrument counts were part of the checklist. Implementation of the checklist increased compliance with sponge count completion across the multicenter study.[67] Based on the evidence of the effectiveness of checklists in improving surgical patient outcomes for non-cardiac surgery, the American Heart Association (AHA)[71] recommends that checklists be used for every cardiac case.

In a literature review of surgical checklist use in 23 studies from 17 countries, McDowell and McComb[69] found themes of increased communication and enhanced patient safety from checklist use. In a systematic review, Borchard et al[70] also found surgical checklists to be effective in reducing morbidity and mortality and stated that further research is needed to determine the influence of the organization's culture on checklist implementation.

In a literature review, Collins et al[68] examined the impact of culture on checklist implementation by applying Reason's Swiss Cheese Model to the use of checklists. They found that successful use of a checklist for prevention of medical errors included involvement of key perioperative stakeholders, an understanding of error occurrence, recognition of system and individual dynamics, and creation of a just culture in which there is a shared vision of patient safety.

I.b. Perioperative team members should actively participate in team training as a measure to prevent RSIs.[2,41,42,71-77] *[2: High Evidence]*

The collective evidence and professional organizations[2,41,42,71-77] support team training as an effective intervention for improving communication and teamwork in the perioperative setting. Team training may prevent RSIs by reducing the risk for human error (eg, safety omissions) while improving team communication and attitudes.

The Joint Commission[2] recommends team training, including briefings and debriefings, to promote open communication and overcome hierarchal barriers as a measure to prevent RSIs. According to The Joint Commission's most recent analysis of unintended retention of foreign object events from 2004 to 2014, the top root causes of events reviewed (N = 986) were elements of teamwork, including leadership, human factors, and communication.[51]

A statement from the AHA[71] about human factors and teamwork in cardiac operating rooms (ORs) says that poor teamwork contributes to errors and that team training should reduce the incidence of errors. Therefore, the AHA recommends that all cardiac OR team members participate in team training to improve communication, leadership, and situational awareness.[71]

Stawicki et al[6] found that safety omissions, which result from a breakdown in system procedures and team communication, were a risk factor for RSIs. In their post hoc analysis of a multicenter retrospective RSI study, Stawicki et al[42] found that 90% of RSI events were associated with either a team or systems error; they recommended team training as an intervention to prevent these types of errors.

The effectiveness of formal programs for team training has been studied. Crew Resource Management is a team training program widely used in health care. Papaspyros et al[73] implemented an element of Crew Resource Management, the briefing and debriefing, as part of a quality improvement (QI) initiative in their cardiac OR, and found a qualitative improvement in team communication.

The evidence indicates that implementing TeamSTEPPS® in the perioperative setting may improve teamwork as part of QI processes. Weaver et al[75] researched the effect of implementation of a TeamSTEPPS team training program on several outcomes, including trainee reactions, learning, behaviors in the OR, and answers on the Hospital Survey on Patient Safety Culture and the Operating Room Management Attitudes Questionnaire. The researchers found that a group that underwent TeamSTEPPS training significantly improved their briefings, quality of teamwork behavior during procedures, perceptions of patient safety culture, and teamwork attitudes compared with a group that did not undergo TeamSTEPPS training.

Based on the work by Weaver et al, Johnson and Kimsey[77] implemented a team training program focusing on TeamSTEPPS as part of a QI project. Their facility experienced a notable reduction in serious events, including RSIs, as a result of the initiative. Tibbs and Moss[76] also conducted a QI program implementing TeamSTEPPS and recommended that perioperative team members participate in team training to improve communication and team relationships. In yet another QI initiative, Armour Forse et al[72] implemented TeamSTEPPS and found significant improvement in OR staff teamwork and OR communications; however, the authors noted a reduction in improvement after one year of implementation and suggested continued team training to sustain culture improvement.

Medical Team Training is a team training program developed by the Veterans Health Administration that emphasizes communication and teamwork with the use of checklist-driven operative briefings and debriefings.[74] One difference in the Medical Team Training Program compared to other Crew Resource Management-based programs is that the training faculty members work with an implementation team, including surgical personnel, for a two-month planning and preparation phase before implementation. In a retrospective cohort study of 119,383 procedures in 74 Veterans Health Administration facilities, Young-Xu et al[74] found that facilities participating in the Medical Team Training program (n = 42) had a significantly lower surgical morbidity rate than facilities that were not participating in the program (n = 32). This study demonstrated an important link between improvement of teamwork in the OR and improvement of a measurable patient outcome, surgical morbidity.

In another QI project, team training was incorporated, although a formal program was not discussed. Cima et al[41] implemented a multidisciplinary team approach and educational campaign to reduce the incidence of RSIs. As a part of the program, they identified cultural barriers, communication problems, and lack of situational awareness as barriers to implementation, and they refocused their initiative to improve team communication.

I.c. Distractions, noise, and unnecessary interruptions should be minimized during the surgical count.[43,61,78-81] *[1: Strong Evidence]*

The collective evidence[61,78-81] indicates that minimizing distractions, noise, and interruptions in the OR creates a safer environment for patients and perioperative team members. Operative and other invasive procedures are high-risk activities that require vigilance, concentration, and situational awareness.[61] Distractions increase the risk for omission and mental lapse errors by diverting attention from the current task.[61] Noise and interruption are distractions that can affect one's concentration and ability to perform complex tasks, leading to poor task performance and potential for error.[61]

In an observational study performed during 10 surgical procedures, Christian et al[79] recorded 11 events that had the potential to compromise patient safety, including counting errors. The researchers identified communication flow problems, workflow, and competing tasks as possible sources of the events.[79] Rowlands and Steeves[80] conducted a qualitative analysis of incorrect surgical count events and found themes of general chaos in the OR that included loud music, excessive talking, talking during critical moments of the count, fast pace, deafening noise levels, and idle chatter. Steelman and Cullen[81] conducted a healthcare failure mode and effect analysis of surgical sponge management and found that distraction was the potential cause of failures 20.8% of the time, followed closely by multitasking, which was the potential cause of failures 17.9% of the time.

The psychology literature indicates that the task of counting requires attention, and improving attention can improve count accuracy.[82-84] Ortuño et al[82] investigated the relative cerebral blood flow of 10 volunteers in Spain who were given neurocognitive tests during positron emission tomography scans. The results showed that sustained attention was required for counting tasks.[82] Camos and Barrouillet[83] investigated resource demands in 36 psychology student volunteers counting multiple arrays as part of a two-series experiment. The researchers found that adult counting is a resource-demanding activity that requires switching attention between memory and counting.[83] Disruption to attention may affect count accuracy through this pathway.

In 2007, Railo et al[84] conducted a two-series psychology experiment in Finland with 72 and 40 adult volunteer participants, respectively. The researchers determined that even when counting small numbers of items, attentional demands increased as objects to be enumerated increased and that improving attention increased accuracy. Furthermore, they found that only the numbers one and two were counted correctly when attention was reduced, which implies that distraction affected count accuracy.

I.c.1. All perioperative team members should minimize distractions, noise, and interruptions during the surgical count.[43,61,78] *[1: Strong Evidence]*

Reduction of distractions and noise during perioperative patient care requires a multidisciplinary team approach to creating a safe environment for patients and perioperative team members.[61] Factors that contribute to distractions include

- technology (eg, telephones, wireless devices, wireless communication systems, paging systems, computers, music devices, hand-held two-way radio transceivers),
- electronic activities (eg, e-mail, texting, social media, Internet, games),
- patient care activities (eg, medical records, clinical alarms, monitors, medical equipment and devices),
- behavioral activities (eg, conversations, personnel movement in and out of the room), and
- the mechanical (physical) environment (eg, heating, ventilation, and air conditioning systems; metal equipment; powered surgical instruments; moveable equipment; equipment problems; reflective surfaces on floors, walls, and ceilings; pneumatic tube systems).[61,78]

I.c.2. During the surgical count, a no-interruption zone should be created that prohibits non-essential conversation and activities[2,60,61] and prohibits rushing the count.[55,80,81,85] *[2: High Evidence]*

Guidance from an accrediting body[2] and an organizational experience report[60] support creating a no-interruption zone during the surgical count. The Joint Commission[2] supports empowering perioperative team members to call for a "closing time out" to allow for an uninterrupted closing count. Clark[60] reported on a facility that successfully implemented a "Pause for the Counts" campaign to minimize interruptions during surgical counts. As part of the multidisciplinary initiative, the RN circulator notified the team when it was time to count and asked whether any supplies would be needed on the sterile field. This communication to the team was intended to reduce interruptions for supplies during the count.[60]

The collective evidence[80,81,85] also suggests that rushing a count is a form of interruption. Butler et al[85] conducted a descriptive study in seven large ORs in Australia and found that both the RN circulator and scrub person were rushed to complete the required count procedures by the fast pace of the perioperative environment, especially when handling urgent requests of the team. The researchers also identified time pressures from the surgeon or anesthesia professional to quickly finish the surgical procedure and move to the next patient as factors contributing to count errors.[85]

In a qualitative study, Rowlands and Steeves[80] found that themes of chaos and feelings of being rushed contributed to safety variances and incorrect counts. Some participants reported that having difficulty locating equipment for a procedure caused them to rush through the initial count.[80] Steelman and Cullen[81] conducted a health-care failure mode and effect analysis of surgical sponge management and found that time pressure occurred in 13.2% of potential failures. Loftus et al[55] included "no rushed counts" as part of their count protocol in a safe surgery program.

I.c.3. Counts and events that would require a count (eg, relief of the scrub person or RN circulator) should not be performed during critical phases of the procedure,[43] including
- time-out periods,
- critical dissections,
- confirming and opening of implants,
- induction of and the patient's emergence from anesthesia, and
- care and handling of specimens.[61]

[1: Strong Evidence]

I.d. A consistent accounting methodology should be used for all surgical counts.[2,18,44,55,80,86-89] *[2: High Evidence]*

The collective evidence and professional organizations[2,18,44,55,80,86-89] support using a standardized, consistent accounting method to prevent RSIs.

In a retrospective cohort study, Loftus et al[55] implemented a standardized safe surgery program, including a standardized count protocol, with the goal of reducing serious reportable event rates (ie, RSIs; wrong site, wrong patient, wrong procedure surgeries) during a four-year period. Although the researchers did not observe a statistically significant reduction in RSIs alone, there was a marked reduction in RSI rates, and the overall serious reportable event rate was significantly reduced by 52%.

Rowlands and Steeves[80] performed a qualitative analysis of incorrect surgical counts using a cross-sectional, hermeneutic phenomenological method in interviews of 22 RNs and surgical technologists. As part of a general theme of "bad behavior," patterns of inconsistency in manual count procedures were reported by the participants as evidenced by comments such as "the process of counting is different from room to room and sometimes person to person."

Edel[86] described a QI project to improve consistency in count procedures at a large city hospital. The author found variation in numerous counting practices, including the count sheet used, the types of items counted, reconciliation procedures, and even the timing of counts. She also found variation in the use of tools; for example, there was inconsistency in the use of sponge bags for counting and use of needle counters. Edel noted that this variation was a cause for concern because of an increased risk for error when counts are recorded differently among providers. New count procedures were implemented, and audits of those procedures showed that the team members were compliant and count variability practices were reduced, although metrics to measure reduction in count variability were not reported.

Norton et al[87] conducted a QI project to reduce RSIs that involved implementing standardized count practices at a large pediatric hospital. Their activities to standardize counts included policy revision and enforcement, education, standardizing dry-erase boards to document counts, streamlining instrument sets, and updating count sheets. As a result of their multiple-strategy approach, they found a 50% reduction in reported incorrect counts during the one-year project period.

In a case report of a retained surgical sponge, Grant-Orser et al[88] found in their incident analysis that there were communication failures between multiple teams and practices inconsistent with counting protocols. The

PATIENT AND WORKER SAFETY

authors recommended developing standardized protocols for RSI prevention and consistent count policies in addition to increasing communication among team members.

The evidence review included a review of count protocols with varying levels of detail. The evidence was limited by generalizability across institutions due to level of protocol implementation and compliance. The NoThing Left Behind® national surgical patient safety project is a widely referenced standardized program for RSI prevention that includes a counting protocol and is based on the principle of implementing consistent methods.[89] Further research is needed to evaluate the effects of a count protocol on patient outcomes.

I.d.1. A count may be requested by any perioperative team member. *[5: Benefits Balanced with Harms]*

I.d.2. The initial count should be conducted before the patient enters the OR or procedure room, when possible.[43,55,76] When conducting the initial count before the patient enters the room is not possible, a second RN circulator may assist the primary RN circulator.[43,55] *[1: Strong Evidence]*

The collective evidence[55,76] supports conducting the initial count before the patient enters the room as part of count protocols, which is also a practice recommended by the ICSI.[43] Loftus et al[55] explained that this practice allows attention to be given to the count with minimal distraction. Performing the initial count before the patient enters the room gives the perioperative team the benefit of reduced interruption from patient care distractions.

For a count after the patient enters the room, the ICSI[43] recommends a parallel process in which two teams work separately and are not multi-tasking, and in which one RN circulator is dedicated to patient care and one is dedicated to the count process. Loftus et al[55] also described use of a parallel process when counting before the patient enters the room is not feasible; a second RN circulator and scrub person perform an uninterrupted baseline count while the primary team remains focused on patient care.

I.d.3. The health care organization should establish the sequence in which the counts should be conducted. The counting sequence should be in a logical progression (eg, order of standardized count board or sheet, proximal to distal from the patient).[18,43,55,87] *[1: Strong Evidence]*

The collective evidence and guidance from professional organizations[18,43,55,87] support counting in a standardized sequence. When determining the order of items to count, Loftus et al[55] followed the sequence

of the standardized count board (eg, whiteboard) as part of their count protocols, which is also a practice recommended by the ICSI.[43] Norton et al[87] implemented a count protocol that involved counting items in a manner that progressed from proximal to distal from the patient: surgical field, Mayo stand, back table, and sponge receptacle.

I.d.4. Items being counted should be viewed concurrently by two individuals, one of whom should be the RN circulator, and counted audibly.[2,18,43,55,87] When possible, counts during a procedure should be performed by the same two individuals.[18,34] *[1: Strong Evidence]*

The collective evidence and guidance from professional organizations[2,18,43,55,87] recommend that two team members, including the RN circulator, concurrently view and audibly count surgical items. Concurrent verification of counts by two individuals may lessen the risk of inaccurate counts, although further research is needed to evaluate this theory. Loftus et al[55] and Norton et al[87] used verbal counting by two individuals as part of their count protocols. Articles in the psychology literature indicated that verbal counting resulted in fewer errors than nonverbal counting at higher numbers[90] and that suppression of count articulation increased errors.[91]

The World Health Organization (WHO)[18] recommends that the same two individuals conduct the counts during a procedure. As part of a prospective observational study at a large academic medical center, Greenberg et al[34] found that counting activities involving a personnel change of either the RN circulator or scrub person resulted in a threefold higher risk of count discrepancy than in procedures with no personnel changes. The researchers noted that a limitation of the study was a small sample size.[34]

A limitation of the evidence is a lack of studies that have examined whether multiple teams participating in a procedure may contribute to inconsistent counting methods. Although multiple teams being present during a procedure is associated with higher risk for an RSI,[3,31,34] the existing evidence has not associated multiple teams with inconsistent counting methods. Data showing multiple teams and an increased number of personnel as a risk factor for RSIs may be indicative of inconsistent counting methods, but this may be confounded by the length and complexity of the procedure (eg, transplantation), which are also risk factors for RSI.[31] However, in a systematic review with meta-analysis, Moffatt-Bruce et al[3] found that changes in nursing staff were not significantly associated with RSI risk. Further research is needed to determine whether the involvement of multiple teams is a risk factor for an inconsistent counting method.[34]

I.d.5. Items should be separated[18] and pointed out[58] while being audibly counted. *[3: Moderate Evidence]*

Separating items may reduce the risk of miscounting items by omission if an item is not seen. The WHO[18] recommends completely separating all items during counting procedures.

The psychology literature supports that identifying items being counted may affect count accuracy; individuation, or object identification, is required before enumeration can occur.[92-94] Individuation is an important part of counting that is required for tracking and counting multiple objects[95] and for counting each item only once.[96] Furthermore, Camos[58] found that a motor activity, such as pointing, facilitated verbal counting in a psychology experiment in which children and adults counted on a number line. Manual pointing may be a method of individuating objects and keeping track of items being counted.

I.d.6. Packaged items should be counted according to the number that the item is packaged in. Packages containing an incorrect number of items or items with a manufacturing defect (eg, missing marker, tag, or chip) should be
- excluded from the count,
- removed from the field,
- isolated from the rest of the countable items in the OR, and
- labeled.

These may be removed from the room before the patient's entry.[18,43] *[1: Strong Evidence]*

Counting to the number that items are packaged in allows perioperative team members to identify packaging errors and may serve as an indication of a miscount. Professional organizations[18,43] recommend removing defective packaged items from the surgical count. Incorrect numbers of items or product defects within a package occur, although the prevalence has not been reported in the literature. Isolating the entire package containing an incorrect number of items may reduce the potential for error in subsequent counts. Removing packages that contain an incorrect number of items from the room before the patient's entry may decrease confusion and the likelihood for error.

I.d.7. If the count is interrupted, the count for the type of item being counted during the inter-ruption (eg, laparotomy sponge) should be restarted.[18,43,55] *[1: Strong Evidence]*

Professional organizations[18,43] recommend restarting an interrupted count to reduce the risk for a count error. As part of their count protocols, Loftus et al[55] required interrupted counts to be repeated without interruption.

I.d.8. For multiple procedures or sterile fields, all items should be counted together at the final count while sterile technique is maintained. *[5: Benefits Balanced with Harms]*

This evidence review found no literature to support or refute this recommendation. Multiple procedures or sterile fields increase the risk of counted items moving between setups and creating confusion during counting, which may contribute to counting errors if items are missed. Counting items across all sterile fields, while maintaining sterile technique, accounts for all surgical items in the room and validates that the items have not been retained in the patient.

I.e. The RN circulator should record the count
- immediately after each type of item is counted (eg, laparotomy sponges, suture needles),[43,55]
- on a standardized template,[43,55,87]
- in a location that is visible to the surgical team (eg, count board),[43,55,87,97] and
- in agreement with the scrub person.[55]

[1: Strong Evidence]

The collective evidence[55,87,97] and guidance from the ICSI[43] support recording the count in one standardized, visible location. Recording of the count on a count board (eg, whiteboard) in a visible location allows all team members to view the count independently[43] and confirm the accuracy of the counted items. Loftus et al[55] included immediate recording after counting each item in their count protocol, which is a practice also recommended by the ICSI.[43] The psychology literature indicates that counting requires memory to keep a running total[91] and that concurrent memory load increases counting time.[83] Immediate documentation of counted items may reduce the risk of a count error by reducing reliance on memory accuracy and attentional demands that compete with counting tasks. Further research is needed to examine the relationship between counting and memory.

I.e.1. If the RN circulator cannot immediately record the count and concurrently visualize the items being counted, the RN circulator may document the number of counted items on a standardized count sheet and then transfer the information to the count board.[43] *[1: Strong Evidence]*

I.e.2. Countable items added to the field after the initial count should be counted immediately, recorded on the count board in a standardized format as defined by the health care organization, and verified with the scrub person.[55] Any perioperative team member (eg, anesthesia professional, float RN) who assists the surgical team by opening countable items onto the sterile field should also promptly inform the RN circulator about what was added. *[2: High Evidence]*

Opening extra supplies without properly adding them to the count board may lead to a discrepancy at the end of the procedure. Loftus et al[55] included immediate documentation of added items to the count board and confirmation of the number with the scrub person as part of their count protocol. They also recommended holding the added item's package as a memory aid until the item is written on the count board, then discarding the package.

Other team members may be asked to open supplies while the RN circulator is occupied with other patient care activities. Notifying the RN circulator of added items may reduce the risk of a count discrepancy.

I.e.3. The count running total should be maintained in one location.[43] *[1: Strong Evidence]*

Maintaining the running total of the count in one location, as recommended by the ICSI,[43] reduces the risk for errors that may occur with multiple counts. Counting using a count sheet and transferring the information is not an ideal practice, as errors in transcription may occur and multiple count documentation may cause confusion. However, there may be situations, depending on the room configuration for various procedures, in which immediate documentation on the count board would not allow for the RN circulator to visualize the count. In those instances, immediate documentation on the count board may not be feasible and a count sheet may need to be used as a memory aid to avoid memory lapse errors in count documentation; this is also recommended by the ICSI.[43]

I.e.4. If an item is passed or dropped from the sterile field, the RN circulator should retrieve it using standard precautions, show it to the scrub person, isolate it from the field, and include it in the final count.[43] *[1: Strong Evidence]*

I.e.5. Items should not be subtracted or removed from the count. *[5: Benefits Balanced with Harms]*

Removal or subtraction of items from the surgical count may increase the risk of count discrepancy by introducing confusion about which items have or have not been counted. The benefits of saving time by subtracting from the count do not outweigh the risks of a count discrepancy.

Thomas and Adcock[98] analyzed near-miss events at a facility in Australia. They found that the practice of counting sponges twice, placing the sponges in a clear plastic bag, and keeping the bags in the room until the end of the procedure ("bagging off") was a behavior that could contribute to a preventable counting error because relief RNs were not aware of "bagged off" packs in the room.

I.f. All counted items should remain within the OR or procedure room until the counts are completed and reconciled. Linen and waste containers should not be removed from the OR or procedure room until all counts are completed and reconciled and the patient has been transferred out of the room.[18] *[2: High Evidence]*

Confining all counted items to the OR may help eliminate the possibility of a count discrepancy. The WHO[18] also recommends keeping all counted items in the room until the final count is reconciled.

I.g. Used or open counted items should be removed from the OR or procedure room at the end of the procedure after the patient has left the room.[43] *[1: Strong Evidence]*

Removing counted items from the room may prevent count discrepancies for the next patient. The ICSI[43] recommends removing counted items after counts are reconciled. In a healthcare failure mode and effect analysis report, Steelman and Cullen[81] found through focus groups that leaving a sponge in the room from a previous procedure was a potential failure that could contribute to a miscount.

I.h. A structured hand-over communication of accounting procedures should be performed at times of relief of the RN circulator or scrub person.[2,18,43,99] *[1: Strong Evidence]*

Professional organizations[2,18,43] recommend that perioperative team members perform a structured hand over at times of relief to facilitate communication and reduce the risk of a count discrepancy or sharps injury. As part of a QI project to improve consistency in count procedures at a large city hospital, Edel[86] noted variation in numerous counting practices that caused confusion at shift change and variances in levels of communication among team members. To reduce variability in count practices and communication, Edel[86] included streamlining of hand-over communications and consistent use of count tools (eg, count board, count sheet) as part of the initiative. Greenberg et al[34] recommended further research to standardize communication during unavoidable hand overs.

I.h.1.   A complete count should be performed when there is a permanent relief of the RN circulator or scrub person.[2,55] All items should be accounted for, although direct visualization of all items may not be possible.[43] *[1: Strong Evidence]*

I.h.2.   Counted items in use should be accounted for when there is relief of the RN circulator or scrub person for short durations (eg, a break).[43] *[1: Strong Evidence]*

Recommendation II

Surgical soft goods (eg, sponges, towels, textiles) opened onto the sterile field should be accounted for during all procedures in which soft goods are used.

The collective evidence[3-7] suggests that the most common types of RSIs are surgical sponges. The abdomen and pelvis are reported to be the most common locations where RSIs are found.[3,9] There have also been reports of retained radiopaque sponges in the thorax, spine, head and neck, brain, and extremities.[4,9,100] Surgical soft goods can be retained in the smallest of incisions, including in procedures involving natural orifices, such as the vagina or nose,[3,101,102] and in minimally invasive surgeries.[103] Retained surgical sponges also can occur after a vaginal birth, therefore the collective evidence and guidance from professional organizations recommend accounting for surgical items, including soft goods, before and after a vaginal delivery.[48,104-109]

Surgical sponges are fibrous material made from cotton or synthetic fabric.[9] Human tissue responds to a retained surgical sponge with a fibrous response, including adhesions, encapsulation, or granuloma.[10,110,111] If the sponge is not retained in a sterile environment or migrates to an unsterile location, such as the gastrointestinal tract, the tissue may react with an exudative inflammatory response that could result in an abscess or fistula.[10,110,111] These physiological tissue reactions to surgical sponges are reflective of the most common complications reported from retained surgical sponges: adhesion, abscess formation, and fistula.[9,112] In one case report that described a rare outcome, a patient developed a malignant fibrous histiocytoma from a surgical sponge retained for 32 years and later died from metastatic cancer.[113]

Reports have been published of retained surgical sponges migrating from the abdomen or pelvis to the intestine, bladder, thorax, and stomach.[10] In a laboratory animal study, Wattanasirichaigoon[111] described the stages of transmural sponge migration into the intestine:

- Stage 1 is foreign body reaction during which the sponge is encapsulated.
- Stage 2 is secondary infection during which cytolysis occurs from the cotton interacting with enzymes in the intestinal lumen.
- Stage 3 is mass formation during which a thick fibrous wall develops as part of the granuloma to prevent the infection from spreading in the

abdomen and cotton filaments are released into the intestinal lumen.
- Stage 4 is remodeling during which a fibrotic scar forms after the whole surgical sponge enters the intestinal lumen.

This study demonstrated the potential for infection to occur during the process of migration and explains the mechanism of infection in the cases reported in the literature.[10,110] Although retained surgical sponges may migrate transmurally and be expelled through the rectum spontaneously, 93% of cases reported by Zantvoord et al[10] required an intervention for removal.

II.a.   All soft goods used in the surgical wound should be radiopaque and easily differentiated from non-radiopaque soft goods (eg, sponges, towels).[18,43,44] *[1: Strong Evidence]*

Professional organizations, including the WHO,[18] the American College of Surgeons,[44] and the ICSI[43] recommend using radiopaque soft goods in the surgical wound. The American College of Obstetricians and Gynecologists[48] and the ICSI[109] recommend using only radiopaque soft goods during vaginal deliveries. The Society of Interventional Radiology[114] recommends that interventional radiologists in the interventional radiology suite use only sponges with radiopaque markers to pack an incision.

Radiopaque indicators facilitate locating by radiograph an item presumed lost or left in the surgical field when a count discrepancy occurs. Although the literature search did not find published reports of retained non-radiopaque sponges in the United States, there were a number of case reports[115-130] of retained non-radiopaque sponges in patients who had surgery in countries in which radiopaque sponges are not routinely used.

II.a.1.   Non-radiopaque gauze sponges used for skin antisepsis that have a similar appearance to counted radiopaque sponges should be isolated before the procedure begins to avoid possible confusion with the counted radiopaque sponges. *[5: Benefits Balanced with Harms]*

II.a.2.   If gauze sponges are used for vaginal antisepsis, the gauze sponges should be radiopaque[131] and counted. *[4: Limited Evidence]*

In a report of a legal case,[131] a patient experienced discomfort and re-operation two months after an abdominal hysterectomy to remove a retained sponge that was left in her vagina during preoperative vaginal antisepsis. Accounting for radiopaque surgical sponges during vaginal antisepsis provides a mechanism for verifying that the sponge is not left in the patient and for detecting the sponge by radiography in the event of a discrepancy.

II.a.3. Radiopaque sponges should not be used as postoperative wound dressings. *[5: Benefits Balanced with Harms]*

   The use of radiopaque sponges as surface dressings may invalidate subsequent counts if the patient is returned to the OR. Radiopaque surgical sponges used as surface dressings may appear as foreign items on postoperative radiographs and falsely suggest a retained item.

II.a.4. Non-radiopaque towels should not be used in the surgical wound. If use of towels in the surgical wound is necessary, towels with radiopaque markers should be used. *[5: Benefits Balanced with Harms]*

II.a.5. Non-radiopaque gauze dressing materials should be withheld from the field until the surgical wound is closed.[18,43,55] *[1: Strong Evidence]*

   One nonexperimental study[55] and professional organizations[18,43] support withholding non-radiopaque gauze for dressings from the sterile field until the wound is closed. Separating dressing materials from counted radiopaque sponges may help prevent intermingling with the sponges used in the procedure and reduce the risk of a count discrepancy.

II.a.6. Dressing sponges included in custom packs should remain sealed and isolated on the field until the surgical wound is closed.[55] *[2: High Evidence]*

II.b. Counts of radiopaque surgical soft goods should be performed
   - before the procedure to establish a baseline (ie, initial count)[2,18,43,55];
   - when new items are added to the field[2,18,43,55];
   - before closure of a cavity within a cavity (eg, the uterus)[2,18,43];
   - when wound closure begins[2,18,43];
   - when skin closure begins or at the end of the procedure when counted items are no longer in use (ie, final count)[2,18,43];
   - at the time of permanent relief of either the scrub person or the RN circulator, although direct visualization of all items may not be possible[2,43,55]; and
   - any time a discrepancy is suspected.[43]
   [1: Strong Evidence]

II.b.1. The final count should not be considered complete until all surgical soft goods used in closing the wound are removed from the wound and returned to the scrub person. *[5: Benefits Balanced with Harms]*

II.c. Radiopaque surgical soft goods should be completely separated, viewed concurrently by two individuals, one of whom should be the RN circulator, and counted audibly.[2,18,43,55] *[1: Strong Evidence]*

The collective evidence and professional organizations[2,18,43,55] support having two team members, including the RN circulator, concurrently view and audibly count surgical sponges. Concurrent verification of counts by two individuals may lessen the risk of inaccurate counts. Separating radiopaque sponges during the initial baseline count also helps to identify packaging defects, such as a missing radiopaque marker or identification tag. As part of the NoThing Left Behind Sponge ACCOUNTing system protocol, sponges are counted by two individuals using this method, which is described as "See, Separate, Say."[103,105]

II.c.1. Packaged radiopaque sponges should be counted to the number that the item is packaged in (eg, five, 10). *[5: Benefits Balanced With Harms]*

   Counting to the number that sponges are packaged in allows perioperative team members to identify packaging errors and may serve as an indication of a miscount.

II.c.2. Packages containing an incorrect number of sponges or a manufacturing defect (eg, missing marker, tag, or chip) should be
   - excluded from the count,
   - removed from the field,
   - isolated from the rest of the countable items in the OR, and
   - labeled.
   These may be removed from the room before the patient's entry.[18,43] *[1: Strong Evidence]*

   Professional organizations[18,43] recommend removing defective packaged sponges from the surgical count. Incorrect numbers of sponges or product defects within a package occur, although the prevalence has not been reported in the literature. Isolating an entire package that contains the incorrect number of sponges may reduce the potential for error in subsequent counts. Removing packages that contain an incorrect number of sponges from the room before the patient's entry may decrease confusion and the likelihood of error.

II.c.3. If the surgical sponge package is banded, the band should be broken and discarded before counting.[55] *[2: High Evidence]*

   Leaving the package band in place may prevent the ability to completely separate and see each sponge, which may cause one or more sponges to be undetected. Loftus et al[55] included removal of the surgical sponge band as part of count protocols in their safe surgery program.

II.d. Radiopaque surgical soft goods should be left in the original configuration and should not be cut or altered in any way.[18,43] *[1: Strong Evidence]*

The WHO[18] and the ICSI[43] recommend leaving surgical sponges in the original configuration. Altering a sponge by cutting or removing radiopaque portions invalidates counts and increases the risk of a portion being retained in the wound.

II.e. All radiopaque surgical soft goods placed or packed in the surgical wound or other cavities (eg, throat, vagina) should be audibly communicated and recorded in a visible location (eg, count board) on placement and removal.[55,97] *[2: High Evidence]*

The practice of verbalizing and documenting placed or packed radiopaque sponges is supported in a cohort study. In the count protocol implemented by Loftus et al,[55] the surgeons were responsible for verbalizing placement and removal of placed sponges, and the RN circulators wrote the placement of sponges on a standardized count board. In an organizational experience report, Edel[97] shared a count board protocol that included the RN circulator recording the items packed in the surgical wound on a count/time-out board.

The retention of throat packs has been reported, and the collective evidence[62-65] indicates that measures can be taken to prevent this type of RSI. In a case report of a swallowed throat pack after maxillofacial surgery, Iwai et al[62] created a checklist for insertion and removal of the throat pack to prevent retention. At their facility, they also tied a suture to the throat pack and taped it to the patient's cheek, and the surgeon was responsible for removing the pack at the end of the procedure. Iwai et al[62] also discussed other methods of managing throat packs that they found in their literature review, such as

- having the same person place and remove the pack,
- attaching a heavy suture to the throat pack that extends outside the mouth,
- not using multiple packs,
- suturing the throat pack to the endotracheal tube, or
- placing a label in a prominent location, such as on the endotracheal tube or on the main ventilator knob.

Colbert et al[63] suggested in an expert opinion report that the anesthesia professional wear a red allergy band marked "throat pack" as a reminder to remove the throat pack. The authors alternatively suggested either placing a sticker on the patient's forehead or writing on the board that the throat pack is in place, although they discussed that these alternatives could be more prone to removal than the wrist band.

In another expert opinion report, Jennings and Bhatt[64] suggested that affixing a "throat pack in situ" label on the patient's forehead was not feasible. In their experience, the head and neck surgeons placed the throat pack after draping the patient, and the forehead was not visible. As an alternative solution, the label was placed on the surgical assistant's hat and was a visible reminder to the surgeon and anesthesia professional throughout the case. A limitation of this expert opinion report is that the risk of the sticker becoming detached from the assistant's hat and falling into the sterile field was not addressed.

To assess variations in practice for preventing retention of throat packs, Smith et al[65] surveyed 208 members of the Neuroanaesthesia Society of Great Britain and Ireland and received 141 responses (68% response rate). Although some clinicians did not feel that throat packs were indicated or that the risks outweighed the benefits of placing the throat pack (n = 69), the remaining respondents reported the following practices for pack retention:

- following formal protocols, either leaving a portion of the pack outside the mouth or attaching it to the endotracheal tube;
- using pre-printed "throat pack in situ" labels;
- counting the throat pack with the sponge count; and
- documenting removal by checking a box on the anesthesia record.

II.e.1. If feasible, radiopaque surgical soft goods placed in the surgical wound or cavity should have a portion left outside the wound so that the item remains visible. *[3: Moderate Evidence]*

Leaving a portion of a soft good item outside the wound provides a visual reminder that there is an item placed in the wound. In a case report of a retained sponge after septorhinoplasty, Cho and Jin[101] recommended using gauze packing with a thread tie left outside the nose during nasal procedures to help identify the gauze more easily. A clinician experience article from Japan[132] reported use of sponges with attached thread to reduce the number of missing ophthalmic sponges during trabeculectomy procedures.[132] Another clinician experience article from India[133] reported use of laparotomy sponges tied together in packs of five sponges so that no single sponge was in the surgical wound when the peritoneum was open.

II.f. The surgeon should perform a methodical wound exploration (eg, top to bottom, quadrant to quadrant) for radiopaque surgical soft goods before closing the wound, using both visualization and touch when feasible.[18,43,44] *[1: Strong Evidence]*

Professional organizations[18,43,44] recommend that surgeons conduct a methodical wound exploration of the cavity or surgical wound before closing, using both visualization and touch whenever possible. The Society of Interventional Radiology[114] recommends that interventional radiologists in the interventional radiology suite perform a wound exploration using visual and tactile inspection whenever sponges have been used in an incision. Methodical wound exploration may prevent retention of surgical sponges when counts are falsely correct and count discrepancy protocols are not implemented.

Norton et al[87] implemented a wound closure time out as part of the surgical safety checklist sign-out procedure at a large pediatric hospital. The wound closure time out included an announcement from the surgeon for a closing time out, the surgeon's statement of wound exploration completion, audible counts of surgical items, and team acknowledgment of the closing count status.[87] Methodical wound exploration is also part of the Sponge ACCOUNTing System "Pauze for the Gauze" protocol.[105]

II.f.1. For minimally invasive surgery, the surgeon should perform a methodical wound exploration before camera removal.[103] *[3: Moderate Evidence]*

II.g. Counted radiopaque surgical soft goods (ie, 4 x 4 gauze, laparotomy sponges) should be organized after use in a pocketed sponge bag or by a similar system (Figure 2).[18,55,105] *[2: High Evidence]*

The WHO[18] recommends organizing counted sponges in established multiples that are readily visible. Using a pocketed bag or other system for separating used radiopaque sponges facilitates the ability to see the sponges for counting. Placement of the separated sponges in a standardized pocket bag system supports a consistent counting method.

Use of a pocketed sponge holder system is recommended as part of the Sponge ACCOUNTing System protocol.[103,105] Loftus et al[55] used a pocketed sponge bag system as part of the count protocol in their cohort study.

II.g.1. Used sponges should be placed in a standardized location (eg, kick bucket) until transferred to a pocketed bag system.[105] If a sponge is dropped from the sterile field, the RN circulator should retrieve it using standard precautions, show it to the scrub person, and place it in the pocketed bag system. *[3: Moderate Evidence]*

Placing the sponges in a standardized location after use may minimize the risk of miscounts that can occur by having sponges in multiple locations in the room. Placement of used sponges in kick buckets lined with clear bags is recommended in the Sponge ACCOUNTing System protocols.[105] Because the color of a red bag in the kick bucket may obscure visualization of used sponges and lead to a sponge being missed, the use of a clear bag or a bag in a color that

FIGURE 2. POCKETED SPONGE BAG AND KICK BUCKET

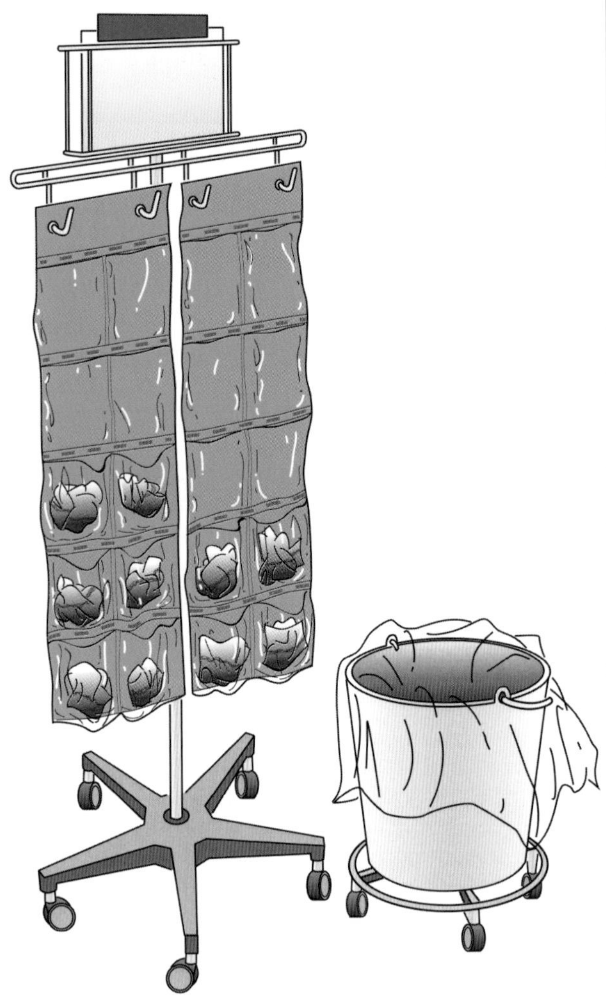

will not obscure white or blood-soaked sponges may reduce the risk of missed sponges. The kick bucket is not the final location of surgical sponge disposal; it serves as a temporary designated location for sponge placement before transfer to a pocketed bag system.

II.g.2. The RN circulator should use standard precautions to retrieve sponges, then completely open and separate each sponge before placing it in a pocketed sponge bag system. *[5: Benefits Balanced with Harms]*

Separating radiopaque sponges after use minimizes errors caused by sponges sticking together.

II.g.3. Sponges should not be draped over the sides of the kick bucket. *[5: Benefits Balanced with Harms]*

Draping used surgical sponges over the sides of the kick bucket is discouraged because it may be difficult for all team members to see each individual sponge. Furthermore, wet used sponges may drip blood and other potentially infectious fluids onto the floor.

II.g.4. Only one sponge should be placed in each pocket of the pocketed sponge bag system. *[5: Benefits Balanced with Harms]*

II.g.5. The radiopaque marker of the sponge should be placed facing forward so that it is readily visible in the pocketed bag system.[105] *[3: Moderate Evidence]*

The radiopaque marker is a visual marker that distinguishes one sponge from another. Having the marker visible in the pocket may facilitate the count process. Placing sponges with the radiopaque marker facing forward is recommended in the Sponge ACCOUNTing System protocol.[105]

II.g.6. The pocketed bag system may be filled from the bottom to the top.[105] *[3: Moderate Evidence]*

Leaving open pockets at the top may provide a more-readily visible indicator of a missing sponge. Filling pocket bag systems from the bottom to top, horizontally, is recommended in the Sponge ACCOUNTing System protocol.[105]

II.g.7. For the final count, unused sponges may be placed in the pocketed sponge bag system to confirm the sponges are not in the patient.[103,105] *[3: Moderate Evidence]*

Placing unused sponges in the pocketed sponge bag system may provide a visual cue that all sponges are accounted for. As part of the Sponge ACCOUNTing System, all sponges are placed in a pocketed bag system at the end of the procedure to verify that the sponges are not retained in the patient and to allow the surgeon to visualize the location of the sponges, which is called the "Show Me" step.[103,105]

II.h. When radiopaque surgical soft goods are used as therapeutic packing (eg, intracavity, oral) and the patient leaves the OR with this packing in place, a standardized procedure should be established and implemented to communicate the location of packing and the plan for eventual removal of the items.[43,44] *[1: Strong Evidence]*

Professional organizations[43,44] recommend communication and documentation of intentionally packed items. In an organizational experience report, McIntyre et al[134] found inconsistency in documentation and changed the health care organization's policy on packed sponges to facilitate a standardized approach to communication of packing.

II.h.1. When radiopaque surgical soft goods are intentionally used as therapeutic packing and the patient leaves the OR with this packing in place, the number and types of

items placed should be documented in the medical record

- as reconciled and confirmed by the surgeon when this information is known with certainty or
- as incorrect if the number and type of sponges used for therapeutic packing is not known with certainty.

[5: Benefits Balanced with Harms]

II.h.2. The number and types of radiopaque surgical soft goods used for therapeutic packing should be communicated as part of the transfer of patient care information and documented in the patient's intraoperative record.[43,99,134] *[1: Strong Evidence]*

II.h.3. When the patient is returned to the OR for a subsequent procedure or to remove therapeutic packing,

- the number and type of radiopaque soft goods to be removed should be determined from the intraoperative record of the surgery during which the packing was placed,
- the number and type of radiopaque soft goods removed should be documented in the medical record,[43]
- the radiopaque sponges removed should be isolated and not included in the counts for the removal procedure,[43]
- the surgeon should perform a methodical wound examination and order an intraoperative radiograph,[43,134] and
- the count on the removal procedure should be noted as reconciled if all radiopaque soft goods have been accounted for.

[1: Strong Evidence]

II.h.4. The surgeon should inform the patient or patient's representative of any surgical soft goods purposely left in the wound at the end of the procedure and the plan for removing these items. *[5: Benefits Balanced with Harms]*

Recommendation III

Sharps and other miscellaneous items that are opened onto the sterile field should be accounted for during all procedures in which sharps and miscellaneous item are used.[2,18,43]

Professional organizations[2,18,43] recommend accounting for sharps and miscellaneous items used in the surgical wound for prevention of RSIs in all procedures, including vaginal deliveries.[48,109]

The collective evidence[8,31,33,34,45] suggests that sharps and miscellaneous items are commonly miscounted and have been retained in patients. Needles are the most likely surgical item to be miscounted,[33] although needles are retained less often than they are miscounted.[8] However, incorrect counts are a concerning risk factor for overall RSI occurrence, although these data are not stratified by type of item retained.[3]

Cima et al[8] found in a retrospective review that needles were miscounted in 76% of the RSI cases, but needles only accounted for 9% of retained items. The Pennsylvania Patient Safety Authority[45] reported that 13% of RSIs were attributed to needles and 40.5% of RSIs were other miscellaneous items, such as guidewires. In other studies of miscount events, Judson et al[31] reported needle miscounts in 48% of events and Greenberg et al[34] reported needle miscounts in 21% of events. The multitude of needles packaged in various amounts and their small size may contribute to miscounts caused by human factors.

A possible explanation for fewer incidents of retained sharp items than surgical soft goods, despite the number of miscounts, is that sharps are often handled in a different manner than surgical sponges. Sharp items are typically exchanged one for one between the surgeon, surgical first assistant, and scrub person and are kept in designated safe locations on the sterile field. Jagger et al[135] reported sharps injuries to perioperative personnel from suture needles to be 43.4% of total sharps injuries and from scalpel blades to be 17% of total sharps injuries. As part of a sharps safety program, awareness and accounting of sharp items may reduce the risk of a sharps injury to perioperative team members,[136] including sterile processing, environmental services, laundry, and morgue personnel.

A limitation of the evidence is that the number of retained sharp and miscellaneous items may be underreported because of the medicolegal implications of an RSI. Underdiagnosis of retained metallic items also may confound the number of reported cases since the body's immune system may not react to metal in the same way it reacts to fibrous material. Retained miscellaneous items may also be under- and misdiagnosed because these objects are often not available in radiopaque forms and may not be visible on radiographic screening.

The benefits of accounting for sharps and miscellaneous items outweigh the harms. Retained miscellaneous surgical items (ie, guidewires, intravascular devices) in the vascular system have been reported to cause complications such as thrombosis, embolization, arrhythmia, tamponade, perforation, and death.[13-16] A patient's death caused by a retained pacing wire in the heart was reported in the literature.[11] Miscellaneous items retained during minimally invasive procedures also have been reported to cause patient injury, including infection from a retained stapler anvil,[137] lung abscess from a retained specimen bag containing bowel,[138] bowel obstruction and biliary obstruction from retained free clips,[139,140] inflammatory response from a retained stapler cover,[141] urinary tract infection caused by bladder obstruction from a retained bulb syringe,[142] and vaginal abscess from a retained bulb syringe.[143]

Further research is needed to describe patient injury from retention of sharp items. A public health notification from the US Food and Drug Administration (FDA)[144] on patient risk for injury from retained unretrieved device fragments is applicable to unintentionally retained sharp and miscellaneous items. Much like device fragments, the patient outcome from a retained sharp or miscellaneous item depends on the biocompatibility of the item's materials, location or potential migration of the item, and the patient's anatomy.[144] Outcomes may include infection, local tissue reaction, perforation or obstruction of blood vessels, and death.[144] If the retained item is metallic, the patient may be at increased risk for injury during magnetic resonance imaging (MRI) procedures because of item migration or internal tissue damage from heating of the object.[144]

III.a. Counts of sharps and miscellaneous items should be performed
- before the procedure to establish a baseline (ie, initial count)[2,18,43,55];
- when new items are added to the field[2,18,43,55];
- before closure of a cavity within a cavity (eg, the uterus)[2,18,43];
- when wound closure begins[2,18,43];
- when skin closure begins or at the end of the procedure when counted items are no longer in use (ie, final count)[2,18,43];
- at the time of permanent relief of either the scrub person or the RN circulator, although direct visualization of all items may not be possible[2,43,55]; and
- any time a discrepancy is suspected.[43]
[1: Strong Evidence]

III.a.1. All suture needles, regardless of size, should be counted for all surgical procedures. *[5: Benefits Balanced with Harms]*

Accounting for all needles during a procedure, including small suture needles, reduces the risk of a needle being retained in the patient and the risk of sharps injuries to personnel. Retained small needles may cause patient injury, depending on the location of retention, such as injury during MRI procedures.[33] A barrier to the practice of counting small needles is the difficulty of reconciling a count discrepancy because needles smaller than 10 mm may be difficult to consistently locate on radiographic screening when retention is suspected.[145-148] Further research is needed to determine more effective and consistent radiographic detection methods for small needles.[149]

III.a.2. Miscellaneous items that should be accounted for include
- catheter sheaths,[43,150]
- electrosurgery scratch pads,[43]
- endostaple reload cartridges,[141]
- guidewires,[16,32,151-154]
- cervical cups,[155]
- specimen bags,[138]
- stapler anvils,[137] bulb syringes (eg, for gynecological procedures),[142,143]
- trocar sealing caps,[43]
- umbilical and hernia tapes,[43]
- vascular inserts,[43]

- vessel clips,[43] and
- vessel loops.[43]

[1: Strong Evidence]

The evidence review included several reports of miscellaneous items retained after minimally invasive procedures, including a stapler anvil, specimen bag, stapler cartridge, cervical cup, bulb syringe, and laser ablation catheter sheath.[137,138,141-143,150,155] The evidence review also found many reports of RSIs from retained guidewires during placement of central line catheters before or during surgical procedures.[16,32,151-154]

Various types of miscellaneous items are used during procedures, and the types of items are heavily dependant on the type of procedure being performed. As such, the selection of miscellaneous items to be counted at the health care organization will depend on the types of procedures performed and the risk for retention of individual items. Items used in the surgical wound are likely to have a higher possibility for retention.

III.a.3. The final count should not be considered complete until all the sharps used in closing the wound are removed from the wound and returned to the scrub person. *[5: Benefits Balanced with Harms]*

III.b. Sharps and miscellaneous items should be viewed concurrently by two individuals, one of whom should be the RN circulator, and counted audibly.[2,18,43,55,87] *[1: Strong Evidence]*

The collective evidence and guidance from professional organizations[2,18,43,55,87] recommend that two team members, including the RN circulator, concurrently view and audibly count surgical items. Concurrent verification of counts by two individuals may lessen the risk for inaccurate counts.

III.c. The scrub person should account for and confine all sharps on the sterile field until the final count is reconciled.[18,136] *[1: Strong Evidence]*

Unconfined sharps that remain on the sterile field may be unintentionally introduced into the incision, may be dropped on the floor, or may penetrate barriers. Confinement and containment of sharps may minimize the risk for injury to personnel as well as reduce the risk for RSIs.[18,136]

III.c.1. Sharps should be confined and contained in specified areas of the sterile field or within a sharps containment device.[18,55] *[2: High Evidence]*

Sharps/needle counting devices protect scrubbed personnel during procedures by segregating sharps in one location until disposal at the end of the procedure.

III.c.2. Sharps/needle counting devices must be
- puncture resistant,

- labeled or color coded in accordance with the bloodborne pathogens standard, and
- leak proof on the sides and bottom.[156]

[1: Regulatory Requirement]

III.c.3. When a sharps container on the sterile field is full, an additional, new container should be used. The full container should be included in the count and should not be removed from the OR until the final count reconciliation is completed and the patient has been taken from the room. *[5: Benefits Balanced with Harms]*

III.c.4. Sharps containers should be securely closed before disposal. *[5: Benefits Balanced with Harms]*

III.d. Sharps and miscellaneous items used in the surgical wound should be accounted for in their entirety immediately on removal from the surgical site.[2,18,43,55,144] *[1: Strong Evidence]*

The collective evidence and guidance from professional organizations[2,18,43,55,144] support the practice of accounting for items used in the surgical wound in their entirety by inspecting for breakage or fragmentation immediately on removal from the surgical site. Inspection will allow for immediate detection of any device fragments and prevent the unintentional retention of fragments.

III.d.1. If a broken or separated item is returned from the surgical site, the scrub person should immediately notify the perioperative team. *[5: Benefits Balanced with Harms]*

III.e. In the event that a needle or miscellaneous item is lost during a minimally invasive procedure, the surgeon should weigh the risks and benefits of retrieving the item.[157,158] *[3: Moderate Evidence]*

The benefits of removing a lost needle or miscellaneous item may not outweigh the harms, depending on the clinical situation. Benefits may include reducing the risk for infection, local tissue reaction, perforation or obstruction of blood vessels, and death.[144] The risk for adverse events caused by an unretrieved surgical item may be affected by the biocompatibility of device materials, the location or potential migration of the item, and the patient's anatomy.[144] Magnetic fields from MRI procedures may increase the risk to the patient by causing migration of the item or internal tissue damage from heating of the object.[144]

The harms of removing the item may include additional injury to tissue and nerve damage, depending on the anatomical location of the item. Retrieving items in laparoscopic procedures may necessitate converting to an open incision procedure,[157] which can increase the patient's risk for infection and pain and increase recovery time. In a survey of surgeons and residents, Ruscher et al[158] reported that 89.4% of respondents believed that converting to laparotomy created a greater risk than the RSI itself. However, 92.6% of the respondents also agreed that an intraperitoneally retained needle put the patient at some degree of future risk.

The evidence review found reports of lost needles during minimally invasive procedures.[157,159] Small et al[160] tested the use of a laparoscopic magnet device in a porcine model and found the tool to be safe and effective for locating lost needles during porcine laparoscopic surgery. In a survey of 305 minimally invasive surgeons, use of a magnetic retriever was reported among successful needle recovery strategies. Using the survey information, Jayadevan et al[161] developed a protocol for recovering lost needles during minimally invasive surgery and recommended using a magnetic device, if one is available. Further research and development is needed to establish the safety and efficacy of using a laparoscopic magnetic tip probe to locate and remove needles lost during minimally invasive surgery. Currently, no laparoscopic magnetic tip probes are cleared by the FDA.

III.e.1. The perioperative team should immediately make an attempt to locate and retrieve the item, depending on the clinical situation.[157,161] *[3: Moderate Evidence]*

The collective evidence[157,161] suggests that delay in retrieval of a lost item may cause the item to become more difficult to remove or inaccessible. Attempting immediate retrieval may reduce the risk of the item being retained.

In a protocol for retrieving lost needles based on a survey of minimally invasive surgeons, Jayadevan et al[161] recommended halting the procedure to survey for the lost needle and conduct a systematic search. In a case report from India of a broken pediatric minimally invasive surgical instrument, Parelkar et al[157] emphasized the importance of retrieving broken instruments without delay. During a laparoscopic inguinal hernia repair with 2-mm instruments, a grasper blade broke but fell within the field of vision. Rather than stopping the repair or inserting another grasper to retrieve the broken instrument, the surgeon completed the hernia repair. When the surgeon attempted to retrieve the broken grasper blade, it had migrated and was no longer visible. After 20 minutes of searching, the broken grasper blade was retrieved, avoiding radiographs and possible conversion to an open procedure.

III.e.2. Free clips (eg, open staples) should be removed from the abdominal cavity when possible.[139,140] *[3: Moderate Evidence]*

The evidence review found reports of two patients who suffered adverse events including bowel and biliary obstructions from free clips retained in the abdomen after minimally invasive surgery.[139,140]

III.f. If a sharp or miscellaneous item is passed or dropped from the sterile field, the RN circulator should retrieve it using standard precautions, show it to the scrub person, isolate it from the field, and include it in the final count.[43] Sharp items should be handled with an instrument and placed in a sharps/needle counting device that is separate from the sterile field.[136] *[1: Strong Evidence]*

The ICSI[43] also recommends isolating dropped items from the sterile field for inclusion in the final count. Handling sharps with an instrument and containing the item in a sharps/needle counting device will reduce the risk of sharps injury and allow the item to be visualized in the final count.[136]

III.f.1. Counted sharp items should not be attached (eg, with tape) to the count board or sheet. *[5: Benefits Balanced with Harms]*

Using tape to attach a sharp item to the count board or sheet increases the risk of bloodborne pathogen exposure and sharps injury.

III.g. Removal of implants in their entirety should be confirmed with the surgeon.[162,163] *[3: Moderate Evidence]*

The evidence review included cases of implants intended to be removed from the patient that were retained and caused the patient harm.[162,163] Kava and Burdick-Will[162] reported four cases of patients with retained penile prostheses that were infected. Due to the complexity of the multi-component penile prosthesis implant, the authors recommended using a removal checklist to confirm that all parts are removed. They also discussed that although complete removal of the implant is the surgeon's responsibility, implementation of an implant-specific checklist may be a rational prevention strategy to prevent unintentionally retained items from causing patient harm.

Felder et al[163] reported a case of a retained gastric band that was intended to be removed during conversion to a sleeve gastrectomy. In this case, the patient experienced recurring sharp abdominal pain and the retained implant was not identified for more than a year until the patient underwent a computed tomography (CT) scan.[163]

III.h. When miscellaneous surgical items (eg, pacing wire, drain) are intentionally left in the surgical wound for postoperative removal, a standardized procedure should be established and implemented to communicate the location and the plan for eventual removal of the item. *[5: Benefits Balanced with Harms]*

The evidence review found one case report of a retained pacing wire. In this report, a 20-year old patient died from myocardial infarction caused by vessel constriction from a retained pacing wire in the heart from a surgery the patient had as a child.[11] A limitation of this report was lack of an explanation of the reason for the retention of the pacing wire from the pediatric heart surgery.

III.h.1.   The number and types of miscellaneous surgical items intentionally placed in the patient should be communicated as part of the transfer of patient care information and documented in the patient's intraoperative record.[99] *[2: High Evidence]*

III.h.2.   The surgeon should inform the patient or patient's representative of any miscellaneous surgical items purposely left in the wound at the end of the procedure and the plan for removing these items. *[5: Benefits Balanced with Harms]*

Recommendation IV

Instruments should be accounted for in all procedures for which the likelihood exists that an instrument could be retained.[2,18,43]

Professional organizations[2,18,43] recommend accounting for instruments when there is a risk for retention. The collective evidence[3-5,8,30,34,45,164-166] indicates that instruments have been retained in patients and are implicated in count discrepancies. In individual retrospective reports, the prevalence of retained instruments has been reported to range from 3% to 43% of RSI cases. Gawande et al[4] reported the percentage of instrument RSIs in their study to be 7%, whereas Lincourt et al[5] found that instruments accounted for 43% of RSIs.[3] The Pennsylvania Patient Safety Authority[45] reported that 16.3% of RSIs were attributed to medical instruments. In a retrospective review, Cima et al[8] reported one retained instrument in 34 cases of retained items. In a study of count discrepancies, Greenberg et al[34] reported that instrument counts were incorrect 34% of the time, although these data were not correlated to actual RSI events.

A limitation of the evidence is that the number of retained instruments may be underreported because of the medicolegal implications of RSI. Underdiagnosis of retained metallic items also may confound the number of reported cases since the body's immune system may not react to metal in the same way it reacts to fibrous material, and the patient may be asymptomatic.

The benefits of accounting for instruments outweigh the harms. The evidence review found reports of patients with retained retractors[30,166] and bulldog clamps.[164,165] Although one patient with a retained bulldog clamp in the heart experienced angina and underwent re-operation for removal of the RSI,[164] another patient with a retained bulldog clamp had not experienced adverse effects at the time of the report.[165] In a legal case description, one patient with a retained rib-bon retractor suffered for nearly six years before the RSI was diagnosed and re-operation was performed.[30] A patient in Italy was reported to have a retained retractor in the abdomen for one month that caused peritonitis and was removed in a subsequent laparotomy procedure.[166]

Information from the FDA on patient outcomes from retained unretrieved device fragments is applicable to patient outcomes from unintentionally retained instruments. The patient outcome from a retained instrument depends on the biocompatibility of the item's materials, the location or potential migration of the item, and the patient's anatomy.[144] Outcomes may include infection, local tissue reaction, perforation or obstruction of blood vessels, and death.[144] Retained metallic items may increase the patient's risk for injury during MRI procedures because of item migration or internal tissue damage from heating of the object.[144]

IV.a.   Instruments should be counted for all procedures in which a body cavity (ie, thorax, abdomen, pelvis) is entered.[4,18,43] *[1: Strong Evidence]*

Professional organizations[18,43] recommend that health care organizations determine which instruments will be counted and which procedures will have instrument counts, to include procedures involving open cavities. Gawande et al[4] recommended counting instruments for every surgical procedure involving an open cavity.

IV.b.   Counts of instruments should be performed
- before the procedure to establish a baseline (ie, initial count)[2,18,43,55];
- when new instruments are added to the field[2,18,43,55];
- when wound closure begins or at the end of the procedure when counted items are no longer in use (ie, final count)[18];
- at the time of permanent relief of either the scrub person or the RN circulator, although direct visualization of all items may not be possible[2,43,55]; and
- any time a discrepancy is suspected.[43]

[1: Strong Evidence]

IV.b.1.   Instruments should be counted when sets are assembled for sterilization. *[5: Benefits Balanced with Harms]*

A count of the instruments at assembly of the instrument set provides a basic inventory reference for the instrument set but is not considered the initial count before the surgical procedure.

IV.b.2.   The final instrument count should not be considered complete until the instruments used in closing the wound (eg, malleable retractors, needle holders, scissors) are removed from the wound and returned to the scrub person.[30] *[4: Limited Evidence]*

Incidents of retention of instruments used in closing the wound have been reported.[30]

IV.c.   Instruments should be viewed concurrently by two individuals, one of whom should be the RN circulator, and counted audibly.[2,18,43,55,87] *[1: Strong Evidence]*

The collective evidence and professional organizations[2,18,43,55,87] support having two team members, including the RN circulator, concurrently view and audibly count surgical items. Concurrent verification of counts by two individuals may lessen the risk for inaccurate counts.

IV.c.1.   Individual pieces of assembled instruments (eg, suction tips, wing nuts, blades, sheaths) should be accounted for separately and documented on the count sheet.[18] *[2: High Evidence]*

Counting individual pieces of assembled instruments before and after a procedure reduces the risk of leaving a piece behind if the instrument becomes disassembled for any reason.[18] Removable instrument parts can be purposefully removed or become loose and fall into the wound or onto or off of the sterile field. In an educational case commentary, Thomas and Moore[167] described a case of a possible RSI from a detached suction tip. The scrub person was concerned that the tip was retained in the patient; however, the tip had actually been placed in irrigation solution.

IV.d.   Preprinted count sheets should be used to record instruments as the count is conducted.[18,43] *[1: Strong Evidence]*

The WHO[18] and the ICSI[43] recommend recording counts on standardized count sheets. Preprinted count sheets provide organization and efficiency, which are key to preventing retained surgical instruments.

IV.d.1.   The RN circulator should record only the number of instruments opened for the procedure. *[5: Benefits Balanced with Harms]*

IV.e.   Instruments used in the surgical wound should be accounted for in their entirety, including any instrument labels, by inspecting for breakage or fragmentation immediately on the instrument's removal from the surgical site.[2,18,43,55,144,168,169] *[1: Strong Evidence]*

The collective evidence and guidance from professional organizations[2,18,43,55,144,168,169] support accounting for instruments used in the surgical wound in their entirety by inspecting instruments for breakage or fragmentation immediately on their removal from the surgical site.

Bansal et al[168] reported a case of a retained outflow cannula fragment found six years after a knee arthroscopy. The patient presented with acute pain, and radiographs showed a retained metallic object in the operative knee. The retained fragment was removed by arthroscopy and the patient subsequently developed deep vein thrombosis. The authors advised diligent inspection of instruments that have been used on a patient, even if the risk for complication is low.

Ipaktchi et al[169] reported a near-miss event in which an instrument label fragment was discovered in the surgical wound during closing. They recommended inspecting instruments after use in their entirety, including the label, to prevent the unintentional retention of instrument label fragments.

IV.f.   All counted instruments should remain within the OR or procedure room during the procedure until all counts are completed and reconciled.[18] *[2: High Evidence]*

The WHO[18] recommends confining all counted instruments to the room to help eliminate the possibility of a count discrepancy.

IV.g.   If an instrument is passed or dropped from the sterile field, the RN circulator should retrieve it using standard precautions, show it to the scrub person, isolate it from the field, and include it in the final count.[43] *[1: Strong Evidence]*

IV.h.   Instrument sets and count sheets should be standardized with the minimum number and variety of instruments needed for the procedure.[18,87] *[2: High Evidence]*

The WHO[18] recommends using standardized instrument sets. Reducing the number and types of instruments and streamlining standardized sets increases the ease and efficiency of counting.

As part of a QI project to standardize count practices, Norton et al[87] streamlined instrument sets to remove obsolete and redundant items and updated instrument count sheets to facilitate the counting process. Instrument stringers were arranged in the same order of the count sheet, and the count sheet was updated to show a total for each instrument group (eg, scissors).[87]

IV.h.1.   Instruments that are not routinely used in procedures should be removed from sets. *[5: Benefits Balanced with Harms]*

Additional or infrequently used instruments can be opened as needed and added to the count.

IV.i.   The health care organization should establish a policy for instrument counting.[18,43] *[1: Strong Evidence]*

The WHO[18] and the ICSI[43] recommend that health care organizations determine which instruments will be counted and which procedures will have instrument counts. The ICSI[43] provides further guidance for health care organizations when determining instrument count protocols, including consideration of the size of the instrument relative to the size of the wound and the visibility of the item throughout the procedure.

IV.i.1. The health care organization's policy should define circumstances in which the instrument count may be waived. *[5: Benefits Balanced with Harms]*

Procedures in which accurate instrument counts may not be achievable or practical include

- complex procedures involving large numbers of instruments (eg, anterior-posterior spinal procedures),
- trauma,[4,170,171]
- procedures that require complex instruments with numerous small parts, and
- procedures for which the width and depth of the incision is too small to retain an instrument.

Recommendation V

Measures should be taken to prevent retention of device fragments.

Serious adverse events associated with unretrieved device fragments have been reported to the FDA.[144] Fragments of devices can cause patient harm during removal or in the event that the item is retained.

The limitations of the evidence are that few reports of device fragmentation are published in peer-reviewed literature. Further research is needed to determine the best methods for preventing retention of device fragments.

The harms associated with retained fragments include local tissue reaction, perforation or obstruction of blood vessels, and death.[144] Harms related to fragment removal include additional injury to tissue, nerve damage, increased operative time, exposure to radiation, and conversion of laparoscopic procedures to open.[157]

V.a. Measures should be taken to prevent instrument breakage,[144] including fragmentation of instrument labels.[169] *[4: Limited Evidence]*

According to the FDA, instrument fragments may cause patient harm on removal or in the event of retention.[144] Ipaktchi et al[169] described a near-miss event in which a plastic instrument label fragment was discovered in the surgical wound. The fragment was retrieved from the wound before closure. The authors recommended considering instrument labels to be part of the instrument and taking measures to prevent fragmentation.

V.a.1. Instruments should be used in accordance with the manufacturer's instructions for use.[144] *[3: Moderate Evidence]*

Using an instrument of inappropriate size or for purposes other than those intended by the manufacturer may increase the likelihood of instrument damage and fragmentation. In a case report from India, Parelkar et al[157] reported breakage of a 2-mm grasper blade inside a pediatric patient during an inguinal hernia repair. Although the cause of breakage was not confirmed, the authors hypothesized that inserting the instrument without a trocar may have exposed the grasper tip to more force than it would have encountered through a cannula.

V.a.2. Instruments, including attached labels,[169] should be inspected before use to identify any defects that may increase the likelihood of fragmentation.[2,18,55,144] Defective instruments should not be used. *[2: High Evidence]*

The collective evidence and guidance from professional organizations[2,18,55,144] support inspecting devices for signs of breakage or fragmentation before use. Inspection will allow for defective items to be removed from use and help prevent risks to the patient associated with a fragmented device. Identifying a broken instrument before use will also prevent the unnecessary consequences of searching for a device fragment that does not exist, such as additional injury to tissue, nerve damage, increased operative time, exposure to radiation, and conversion of a laparoscopic to an open procedure.

V.a.3. Instruments, including labels,[169] should be maintained and serviced in accordance with the device manufacturer's written instructions for use.[172] *[1: Strong Evidence]*

Preventive maintenance performed according to the device manufacturer's instructions for use is necessary to maintain instruments in optimal working order.[172] Ipaktchi et al[169] reported a near-miss event in which an instrument label fragment was discovered in the surgical wound during closing and removed. To prevent the unintentional retention of instrument label fragments, the authors recommended routine inspection and maintenance of labels.

V.b. Items used in the surgical wound should be accounted for in their entirety by inspection for breakage or fragmentation immediately on removal from the surgical site.[2,18,43,55,144] (See Recommendation III.d. and IV.e.) *[1: Strong Evidence]*

The collective evidence and guidance from professional organizations[2,18,43,55,144] support inspecting devices for signs of breakage or fragmentation after use. Inspection will allow for immediate detection of any device fragments and reduce the risk of unintentional retention of fragments.

V.b.1. If a broken item is returned from the surgical site, the scrub person should immediately notify the perioperative team. *[5: Benefits Balanced with Harms]*

V.c. If a broken instrument with a missing fragment is identified during reprocessing, sterile processing personnel should notify the perioperative

389

team immediately.[173] When notified of a missing device fragment, the perioperative team should immediately investigate and follow established count reconciliation procedures. *[3: Moderate Evidence]*

Notification of the perioperative team is supported in a report of an organizational experience. Reece et al[173] described a process for managing broken surgical instruments. If the sterile processing technician identified a damaged or fragmented instrument during the cleaning and assembly process, the technician notified the OR charge nurse. At their facility, Reece et al used a barcode system and sterile processing tracking software to allow a broken instrument with missing fragments to be traced to the patient on whom it was last used. The perioperative team then collaboratively determined whether the item was potentially retained, and a radiograph was obtained to rule out a retained device fragment if indicated.[173]

V.d. Measures should be taken to prevent intravascular device (ie, catheter, guidewire, sheath) fragments.[16,32,174] *[3: Moderate Evidence]*

The collective evidence[32,174] suggests that preventative measures are needed to avoid the complications associated with removal or retention of device fragments from intravascular catheters, guidewires, and sheaths. The evidence review included multiple reports of intravascular RSIs that were caused by device fragments.[13-16,32,153,175,176]

V.d.1. Intravascular devices should be inserted and removed in accordance with the manufacturer's instructions for use.[13,174,175] *[3: Moderate Evidence]*

The collective evidence[13,174,175] indicates that misuse of intravascular devices leading to device fragment retention is a preventable complication and supports following the manufacturer's instructions for use, insertion, and removal. Fischer[174] described a case of guidewire fracture in which the guidewire was weakened by manipulation into a shape for which the device was not designed.

In a Japanese review of intravascular unretrieved device fragments, Tateishi and Tomizawa[13] concluded that many preventable device-fracture complications were related to inappropriate use of intravascular devices, including use of devices for off-label purposes and reuse of single-use devices. Pillarisetti et al[175] described a specific example of failure to follow the device manufacturer's instructions in a case report of femoral vascular sheath breakage during removal. The authors emphasized the importance of following the manufacturer's instructions for use, including using an obturator or dilator when removing the

sheath, to prevent adverse events associated with a retained sheath.

V.d.2. Intravascular devices should be inspected before use to identify any defects that may increase the likelihood of fragmentation.[174] *[3: Moderate Evidence]*

The author of an expert opinion report[174] advised inspecting intravascular devices for breakage or manufacturing defects to minimize the risk for retained device fragments. Inspection will allow for defective items to be identified and removed before use to prevent the risks to the patient associated with a fragmented device. Identifying a broken instrument before use will also prevent unnecessary searching for a device fragment and the associated consequences, such as additional injury to tissue, nerve damage, increased operative time, and exposure to radiation.

V.d.3. Catheters and guidewires should not be withdrawn through a needle. If the catheter or guidewire is replaced, it should be withdrawn simultaneously with the needle.[16,174] *[3: Moderate Evidence]*

The evidence[16,174] indicates that withdrawing a guidewire through a needle increases the risk of guidewire fracture. Fischer[174] described catheter removal through or over a needle as an inappropriate technique that can result in unretrieved device fragments. In a review of guidewire retention during central venous catheterizations reported to the University HealthSystem Consortium Safety Intelligence® Patient Safety Organization database, Williams et al[16] advised withdrawing the guidewire together as a unit with the needle. The authors explained that withdrawing the guidewire through the needle increases the risk of damage to or shearing of the wire on the needle bevel.

V.d.4. Bent guidewires should be replaced immediately.[16] *[3: Moderate Evidence]*

Replacement of bent guidewires was supported in a review of cases of guidewire retention during central venous catheterization reported in the University HealthSystem Consortium Safety Intelligence Patient Safety Organization database.[16] Williams et al[16] found that attempts at recannulation with a bent guidewire could increase the risk of shearing the wire.

V.d.5. Intravascular devices should be accounted for in their entirety by inspection for breakage immediately on removal from the patient.[15,16] *[3: Moderate Evidence]*

The evidence[15,16] suggests that inspection of intravascular devices will allow for immediate detection of any breakage. A review by Williams et al[16] recommended confirming removal of the guidewire and inspecting its integrity. Johnson et al[15] reported a case of a retained introducer sheath radiopaque marker. The patient underwent removal of an inferior vena cava filter, after which the filter and introducer catheters were found to be intact. On a subsequent chest radiograph, a radiopaque foreign body was found and removed from the subcutaneous tissue below the access site. Although this was a rare occurrence and related to device malfunction, the authors advised confirming the position of the radiopaque marker after its removal.

V.e. Measures should be taken to prevent retention of hypodermic needle fragments.[177-181] *[3: Moderate Evidence]*

The collective evidence[177-181] supports taking measures to prevent hypodermic needle fragments during inferior alveolar nerve blocks and subcutaneous injections. The evidence review included several reports of needle fracture occurring during local anesthesia injection in dental procedures.[177-180] A case report of needle breakage during a growth hormone injection suggested similar preventive measures for needle breakage during subcutaneous injections.[181]

The limitations of the evidence are that the generalizability to other types of injections with hypodermic needles may be limited. Further research is needed to determine the risk of hypodermic needle fracture during invasive procedures and to establish optimal prevention measures.

V.e.1. Thin (ie, 30-gauge) and short (ie, 20-mm) needles should not be used unless clinically necessary.[177-179] *[3: Moderate Evidence]*

The evidence review indicated that thin needles may be more prone to fracture. The harm of needle fracture from inappropriate use of a thin needle outweighs the perceived benefit of reducing patient discomfort. Use of smaller gauge needles has not been correlated with reduced patient discomfort during injection.[177-179]

The authors of two literature reviews on dental needle breakage incidence and prevention have advised against using short needles and 30-gauge needles for inferior alveolar nerve blocks.[177,178] According to reports of dental needle breakage, short needles are more likely to be inserted up to the hub, which is a risk factor for needle fracture.[178,179] Augello et al[177] recommended using 25-gauge to 27-gauge and 35-mm length needles for inferior alveolar nerve blocks.

V.e.2. Hypodermic needles should be inspected for defects that may increase the likelihood of fragmentation before use.[177,180,181] Defective hypoder-

mic needles should not be used. *[3: Moderate Evidence]*

Augello et al[177] performed a review of the literature of local anesthesia needle breakage in the oral cavity and found that hypodermic needles may have defects that could pose a risk for fracture. They recommended checking the needle before use. In a case series of four needles broken during dental anesthetic injections, Catelani et al[180] recommended that needles be inspected for manufacturing defects before use.

Inspection of hypodermic needles is also supported in a case report by Kim et al,[181] who reported a case of needle breakage during subcutaneous growth hormone injection. The authors recommended checking the needle before subcutaneous injection for manufacturing defects, checking for dull or deformed needles, and not using the needle if a defect is identified. For growth hormone injections, they also discussed that the common practice of using the same 30-gauge needle to reconstitute and inject the medication subcutaneously can lead to bending the needle tip into a hook shape that can break off and leave a needle fragment in the skin.

V.e.3. Hypodermic needles should not be bent.[177-180] *[3: Moderate Evidence]*

The evidence review found that bending of hypodermic needles is a risk factor for needle fracture. Augello et al[177] stated that dentists should not pre-bend the hub area of the needle before local injection because of the risk for needle fracture. The authors of another literature review and of two case series reports of needle fractures also cautioned dentists not to bend needles before insertion into soft tissue because of the concern for fracture.[178-180]

V.e.4. Hypodermic needles should not be inserted to the hub.[178-180,182] *[3: Moderate Evidence]*

The evidence review indicated that needle fracture was more likely to occur if the needle was inserted in the tissue up to the needle hub, which is the weakest part of the needle.[178-180] The literature also indicates that needle fracture retrieval is more complicated when the hub is buried in the tissue, which places the patient at increased risk for an invasive procedure to remove the fragment.[182]

Because of the risk of fracture and subsequent possible surgical intervention to locate the buried needle fragment, Malamed et al[178] advised dentists not to insert needles to the hub in soft tissue unless this is essential to the success of the injection. In an expert review of oral maxillofacial surgery complications, Alexander and Attia[182] also advised against burying the needle to the hub because of the certainty of difficult retrieval in the event of breakage.

In a case series report of 16 cases of needle fracture at one academic institution, Pogrel[179] found that all cases had needle separation at the hub, not along the needle shaft. He cautioned dentists not to bury the needle in the tissue to the extent that the hub indents the mucosa.

In a case series of four needles broken during dental anesthetic injections, Catelani et al[180] also recommended avoiding pushing the whole length of the needle into the tissue. Augello et al[177] advised leaving at least 5 mm of the needle outside the tissue during dental local anesthesia injection to prevent insertion of the needle to the hub and needle fracture.

V.e.5. The direction of the hypodermic needle should not be changed during the injection.[177,180,181] If changing the needle angle is necessary, the needle should be removed from the tissue and repositioned.[177] *[3: Moderate Evidence]*

The evidence review suggested that changing the direction of the needle during injection is a risk factor for needle fracture.[177,180,181] In a case series of four needles broken during dental anesthetic injections, Catelani et al[180] advised dentists to avoid changing the angle of the needle during injection. In a literature review of dental needle breakage, Augello et al[177] advised taking the needle from the tissue when changing needle angulation during injection, to reduce the risk for needle fracture. Kim et al[181] also reported a case of needle breakage during subcutaneous injection and recommended not changing the direction of the needle during injection because of the risk of bending or breaking the needle.

V.e.6. A patient under local anesthesia or moderate sedation should be advised about possible pain before being given an injection.[177,181] *[3: Moderate Evidence]*

A literature review showed that sudden or unexpected movement by the patient during injection may be a risk factor for needle breakage.[177] Augello et al[177] recommended informing patients about possible abrupt pain and warning them of impending puncture to reduce the risk of needle breakage caused by patient movement. In their report of a broken needle from a subcutaneous growth hormone injection, Kim et al[181] also advised informing the patient about possible pain to prevent needle breakage.

V.e.7. Thin (ie, 30-gauge) hypodermic needles should not be reused on the same patient.[181,182] *[3: Moderate Evidence]*

The evidence review indicated that reuse of needles, even on the same patient, increases the risk for needle fracture.[181,182] The needle gauge size commonly associated with needle breakage was 30 gauge.

In an expert opinion review, Alexander and Attia[182] cautioned that repeated use of the same needle should be avoided because this practice increases the risk for breakage. Kim et al[181] also advised not reusing needles as part of preventive measures to avoid needle breakage during subcutaneous injections.

V.f. In the event that a device fragment is retained, the surgeon should weigh the risks and benefits of retrieving the fragment.[144] *[5: Benefits Balanced with Harms]*

The FDA[144] advises careful consideration, and discussion with the patient if possible, of the risks and benefits of retrieving versus leaving the device fragment in the patient.

The benefits of removing device fragments may not outweigh the harms, depending on the clinical situation. Benefits include reducing the risk for infection, local tissue reaction, perforation or obstruction of blood vessels, and death.[144] The risk for adverse events from an unretrieved device fragment may be affected by biocompatibility of the device materials, the location or potential migration of the fragment, and the patient's anatomy.[144] Magnetic fields from MRI procedures may increase the risk to the patient by causing migration of the device fragment or internal tissue damage from heating of the object.[144]

The harms of removing device fragments may include additional injury to tissue and nerve damage, depending on the anatomical location of the fragment. Retrieving device fragments retained during laparoscopic procedures may necessitate converting to an open incision procedure,[157] which can increase the patient's risk for infection and pain and increase recovery time.

V.f.1. The perioperative team should immediately attempt to locate and retrieve the device fragment, depending on the clinical situation.[17,157,182] *[3: Moderate Evidence]*

The collective evidence[17,157,182] suggests that delay in retrieval of a lost item may cause the device fragment to become more difficult to remove or inaccessible. Immediate retrieval may reduce the risk of the fragment becoming lost or retained.

In an expert review of oral maxillofacial surgery displacement complications, Alexander and Attia[182] advised that the operator immediately discontinue the procedure and attempt to retrieve the material before it becomes inaccessible. In a case report from India of a broken pediatric minimally invasive surgical instrument, Parelkar et

PATIENT AND WORKER SAFETY

al[157] also emphasized the importance of retrieving broken instruments without delay. During a laparoscopic inguinal hernia repair with 2-mm instruments, a grasper blade broke but fell within the field of vision. Rather than stopping the repair or inserting another grasper to retrieve the broken instrument, the surgeon completed the hernia repair. When the surgeon attempted to retrieve the broken grasper blade, it had migrated and was no longer visible. After 20 minutes of searching, the broken grasper blade was retrieved, avoiding radiographs and possible conversion to an open procedure.

Bydon et al[17] reported a more complicated case that illustrates the practical challenges associated with immediate location of a device fragment. During a spine procedure, the surgeon noted that a rongeur tip was missing when the rongeur was withdrawn from the surgical site. An intraoperative C-arm fluoroscopic radiograph showed that the tip had migrated through a vascular injury. After consulting with the vascular team, the surgical team made the decision to complete the spine procedure given the patient's hemodynamic stability. After surgery, the patient underwent an abdominal CT scan, chest radiograph, transthoracic echocardiogram, cardiac catheterization, and thoracic CT scan over the course of two days before the rongeur tip was localized to the left ventricle. The patient then underwent a sternotomy for removal of the rongeur tip and closure of a previously undiagnosed patent foramen ovale. Afterward, the patient recovered in the cardiac intensive care unit in stable condition. Although this is a rare case report of vascular injury from device fragmentation during a spine procedure, the authors emphasized the need for rapid diagnosis and collaboration to treat a potentially devastating complication from a retained device fragment.

V.g. In the event that an unretrieved device fragment is left in the surgical wound, the surgeon should inform the patient or patient's representative of the nature of the item and the risks associated with leaving it in the wound.[144] *[5: Benefits Balanced with Harms]*

V.g.1. Information provided to the patient should include the
- risks and benefits of leaving the device fragment in the wound;
- material composition of the fragment (if known);
- size of the fragment (if known);
- location of the fragment;

- potential mechanisms for injury (eg, migration, infection); and
- procedures or treatments that should be avoided, such as MRI examinations in the case of metallic fragments.[144]

[5: Benefits Balanced with Harms]

V.h. Unretrieved device fragments must be documented in the patient's record.[183,184] Documentation should include the
- material composition of the fragment (if known),
- size of the fragment (if known),
- location (if known),
- manufacturer,
- measures taken to recover the fragment, and
- patient notification.

[1: Regulatory Requirement]

The Centers for Medicare and & Medicaid Services requires surgical complications to be documented in the operative report.[183,184]

V.i. The health care organization should establish mechanisms for documenting and reporting device fragments.[144] *[5: Benefits Balanced with Harms]*

Health care facilities are required to report deaths and serious injuries associated with the use of medical devices to the FDA.[144] The FDA safety communication on unretrieved device fragments advises that reportable adverse events related to unretrieved device fragments be reported through the health care organization's reporting mechanism and encourages reporting of adverse events related to device fragments that do not meet mandatory reporting requirements.[144]

V.i.1. Deaths and serious adverse events associated with device fragments must be reported to the FDA.[144] *[1: Regulatory Requirement]*

V.i.2. The device and fragment should be retained for investigation according to the health care organization's policy.[144,173] *[3: Moderate Evidence]*

Retaining the device and fragment provides information for the health care organization to investigate the cause and to determine appropriate action. The FDA safety communication on unretrieved device fragments advises retaining the device and fragment for investigation of the event by the manufacturer.[144] In an organizational experience report, Reece et al[173] reported that at their facility, sterile processing personnel disinfected and tagged all damaged instruments and stored them for a minimum of one year. The retired instrument was then logged into a database and monitored by the perioperative quality council.[173]

Recommendation VI

Standardized measures for reconciling count discrepancies should be taken during the closing count and before the end of surgery. When a discrepancy in a count is identified, the surgical team should take actions to locate the missing item.[2,3,5,6,18,43] *Amb*

Professional organizations[2,18,43] recommend accounting for surgical items used in the wound for prevention of RSI in all procedures, including vaginal deliveries.[48,109] Accounting for surgical items encompasses reconciling count discrepancies.

The collective evidence[3,5,6,33] indicates that count discrepancies are a risk factor for RSI. In a meta-analysis of three case-control studies, Moffatt-Bruce et al[3] found that patients with an incorrect surgical count were at the highest risk for RSI compared with other risk factors. In one retrospective case-control study included in this meta-analysis, Stawicki et al[6] found that incorrect surgical counts resulted in a higher risk of RSIs, and they recommended using a standardized, goal-oriented approach to resolving count discrepancies, including standardized recounts, wound exploration, and plain radiographs. Lincourt et al[5] also found a significant association between recorded incorrect counts and patients with an RSI. Egorova et al[33] was able to quantify this association, finding that retained items occurred more frequently in discrepant cases (one in 70) compared to all cases (one in 7,000).

Greenberg et al[34] conducted a prospective observational study to further investigate count discrepancy events. They categorized discrepancies as being a result of miscounts (eg, incorrect baseline count, overcount, undercount), documentation errors (eg, addition), or misplaced items (eg, retained). The most common discrepancy was from a misplaced, or retained, item, which occurred in 59% of cases, whereas discrepancies from human error (ie, miscount [3%], documentation [38%]) accounted for 41% of discrepancies.[34] In their study, count discrepancies occurred in one of eight cases, or one per 14 hours of operating time, and took an average of 13 minutes to resolve.[34]

Egorova et al[33] found that the sensitivity of counting was 77.2% and the specificity was 99.2%, but the positive predictive value was only 1.6%, meaning that there were a substantial number of incorrect counts that did not involve a true RSI. Due to the higher frequency of count discrepancies[34] and the less common occurrence of RSI, Stawicki et al[6] suggested that perioperative teams may be desensitized to incorrect counts to explain why they are disregarded. Human factors such as complacency and normalization of deviance may contribute to lack of follow-up on incorrect counts, although further research is needed to confirm this.

The collective evidence indicates that risk factors for count discrepancies include personnel changes,[34,185] the number of providers,[31,185] the length of the procedure,[31] higher surgical risk,[185] a complicated procedure,[185] an unplanned procedure,[185] and a low BMI.[185] Further research is needed to assess causal factors for count discrepancies, as the existing evidence is limited by only being able to demonstrate relationships of association.

VI.a. All perioperative team members should take immediate actions to resolve a count discrepancy (Figure 3).[18,31,41,43] *[1: Strong Evidence]*

The collective evidence and professional organizations[18,31,41,43] support immediate notification of the team in the event of a count discrepancy and team participation in activities to reconcile the count.

VI.a.1. The RN circulator should inform the team and receive verbal acknowledgment from the surgeon, including the type and number of items missing, as soon as a discrepancy in a surgical count is identified.[18,31,41,43] *[1: Strong Evidence]*

The collective evidence and guidance from professional organizations[18,31,41,43] support immediate notification of the team, including verbal acknowledgement, in the event of a count discrepancy. The RN circulator has a responsibility and ethical obligation to speak up promptly when a discrepancy is identified.

VI.a.2. When a discrepancy in the count is identified, the RN circulator should
- call for assistance[31,43];
- search the room, including the area near the sterile field, floor, kick buckets, and linen and trash receptacles[18,31,41,43]; and
- recount with the scrub person.[6,18,41,43]

[1: Strong Evidence]

The collective evidence and guidance from professional organizations[18,31,41,43] support searching the room to locate the missing item and recounting the type of item that is involved in the count discrepancy. Judson et al[31] further recommended that the RN circulator obtain assistance from an additional RN circulator and scrub person to resolve a count discrepancy, which is also recommended by the ICSI.[43] Having a second RN circulator and scrub person may allow the primary team to reconcile the count without distractions.

VI.a.3. When a discrepancy in the count is identified, the scrub person should
- organize the sterile field[31,80];
- search the sterile field, including drapes and tables[18,43]; and
- recount with the RN circulator.[6,18,41,43]

[1: Strong Evidence]

The collective evidence and guidance from professional organizations[18,31,41,43] support searching the sterile field to locate the missing item and recounting the type of item that is involved in the count discrepancy. Judson et al[31] and Rowlands and Steeves[80] recommended organizing the sterile field to facilitate the count process.

FIGURE 3. COUNT RECONCILIATION DECISION TREE

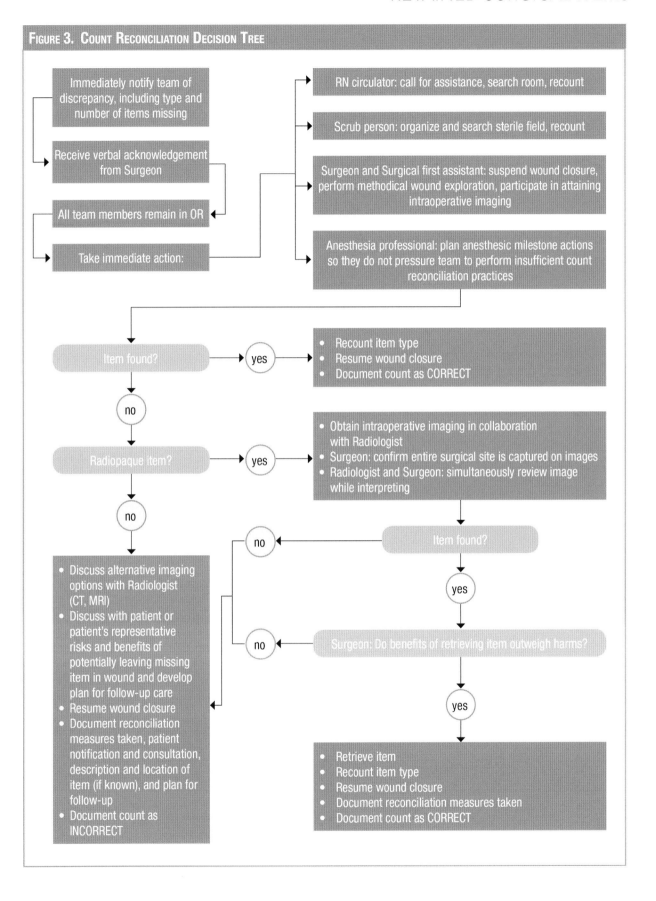

VI.a.4. When a discrepancy in the count is identified, the surgeon and surgical first assistant should

- suspend closure of the wound if the patient's condition permits,[6,41,43]
- perform a methodical wound examination while actively looking for the missing item,[6,41,43]
- participate in the attainment of intraoperative radiographs or other imaging modalities as indicated to find the missing item,[6,41] and
- remain in the OR until the item is found or it is determined not to be in the patient.[6]

[1: Strong Evidence]

The collective evidence[6,41] and the ICSI[43] support the surgeon performing a methodical wound exploration and obtaining radiographs as soon as possible when a count discrepancy is identified, if the patient's condition allows. Stawicki et al[6] suggested that count discrepancies require a hard stop before wound closure, the patient's emergence from anesthesia, or leaving the OR, for reinspection of the surgical site and obtaining radiographic confirmation.

VI.a.5. When a discrepancy in the count is identified, the anesthesia professional should plan anesthetic milestone actions (eg, emergence from anesthesia) so that these actions do not pressure the perioperative team to perform insufficient count reconciliation practices.[61] (See Recommendation I.a.4.) *[2: High Evidence]*

VI.a.6. Nonessential personnel changes (eg, break, relief) should not occur until the count is resolved.[31] *[2: High Evidence]*

Judson et al[31] implemented the practice of a "No Hand-off Zone," which defined a time when no breaks or relief of personnel were permitted until resolution of the count discrepancy.

VI.a.7. Empty packages should not be used to reconcile count discrepancies.[41,43] *[1: Strong Evidence]*

Cima et al[41] recommended not reconciling counts with packages, as the number on the pre-printed package may not be an accurate representation of items counted. The ICSI[43] also recommends this.

VI.b. When the missing item is found, the item type (eg, laparotomy sponges, suture needles) should be recounted.[41,43] *[1: Strong Evidence]*

Cima et al[41] recommended recounting the category of item that was missing as part of count reconciliation procedures. The ICSI[43] also recommends this.

VI.c. If a missing item is not recovered, intraoperative imaging should be performed to rule out a retained item before final closure of the wound, if the patient's condition permits.[6,18,43,44,186] If the patient's condition is unstable, a radiograph should be taken as soon as possible in the next phase of care.[43] *[1: Strong Evidence]*

The collective evidence and guidance from professional organizations[6,18,43,44,186] support obtaining an intraoperative radiograph to find the missing item before final wound closure, if the patient's condition allows. Obtaining a radiograph when all other efforts have failed allows the surgical team to remove a potential RSI before the wound is closed completely. The ICSI[43] recommends performing postoperative imaging in a radiographic room with fixed equipment if the patient's condition does not allow for intraoperative imaging.

VI.c.1. When accurate counting of surgical items is not possible, intraoperative imaging should be performed before the patient is transferred from the OR.[43] *[1: Strong Evidence]*

The ICSI[43] recommends performing intraoperative imaging when there is a concern about the count accuracy or when the patient's condition does not allow for the count process to be followed (eg, may result in a rushed or incomplete count).

VI.c.2. If intraoperative imaging is not available, the health care organization should have a policy and procedure describing the actions and communication required between referring and receiving organizations. *[5: Benefits Balanced with Harms]* Amb

VI.c.3. A radiograph to locate a possible retained item may be waived under certain circumstances as defined in the health care organization's policy and procedure. *[5: Benefits Balanced with Harms]*

There are situations in which it may be medically appropriate for the surgeon to determine that it is not in the individual patient's best interest to undergo an intraoperative radiograph to locate a potential RSI.

VI.c.4. Complete and detailed communication among the perioperative team, radiology technologists, and radiologists should occur during a request for radiological support to prevent an RSI.[2,31,41] The radiology request should include standardized information about the missing surgical item, including

- the room in which the procedure is being performed or the patient is located,[43]
- the patient's status,[43]
- the type of radiograph and views needed,
- a description of the missing surgical item,[43]
- the procedure performed,[43] and
- the surgical site, including involvement of any body cavities (eg, the abdomen).

[1: Strong Evidence]

The collective evidence and guidance from professional organizations[2,31,41,43] support using detailed, standardized communication with the radiologist when ordering radiographs to rule out an RSI. These activities may aid in the radiologist's ability to identify surgical items on the radiograph.

VI.c.5. The radiology technologist should be called promptly and respond expeditiously when an incorrect count occurs in the OR. *[5: Benefits Balanced with Harms]*

VI.c.6. Intraoperative imaging should provide full coverage of the surgical site and should include any views deemed necessary by the surgeon and radiologist to maximize the opportunity to identify a missing surgical item.[2,43] Radiological techniques may include

- use of portable or fixed radiographic equipment,[8]
- portable anterior and posterior and oblique views,[97]
- multiple images for full coverage of the surgical site or body cavity as confirmed by the surgeon,[5,43,88,134]
- fluoroscopy, and
- CT, which may be used postoperatively or intraoperatively (if available) when previous radiographic images are negative and a high suspicion remains for an RSI.

[1: Strong Evidence]

The collective evidence and guidance from professional organizations[2,8,43] support imaging the entire surgical site and any involved body cavity with views deemed necessary by a collaborative decision between the surgeon and radiologist. The ICSI[43] advises that multiple images may be needed depending on the location of the surgical site and recommends that the surgeon confirm full coverage of the surgical site or body cavity on the image before it is read by the radiologist. There are reported incidents of an RSI attributed to failure to capture the full surgical site on radiographic imaging. In a case control study of 30 patients with RSIs, Lincourt et al[5] reported that for four patients, the imaging taken to resolve the count discrepancy did not capture the location of the retained item in the field of view. Grant-Orser et al[88] reported a case of a retained surgical sponge that was missed on imaging because the radiograph of the abdomen did not extend fully from the diaphragm to the pubis. Similarly, McIntyre et al[134] reported a case series of three patients with RSIs at the authors' institution; two of the patients had retained sponges that were missed on intraoperative imaging because of incomplete imaging of the abdomen.

As part of a radiographic screening protocol, Cima et al[8] implemented screening with high-resolution images taken with fixed radiology equipment that was located in a designated room within the surgical suite. As part of this protocol, they identified 34 retained surgical sponges, needles, an instrument, and miscellaneous items with the high-resolution images.

Further research is needed to determine the quality differences and impact on patient care (eg, benefits and harms, cost) of radiographs taken with fixed equipment in a radiology suite compared with images taken with portable equipment in an OR. When considering use of portable intraoperative imaging to resolve a count discrepancy, the ICSI[43] recommends evaluating the patient's condition, size and type of the retained item, placement options for radiograph cassettes, lower tube power, instruments obscuring the view, and availability of portable equipment and personnel. The benefits of portable imaging may outweigh the harms, depending on the clinical situation.

Edel[97] reported one radiology protocol for resolving count discrepancies that included obtaining an anterior and posterior film and a 20-degree view of the surgical site to provide the radiologist with two perspectives of the area.

The evidence review found no literature to support the preference for use of a portable radiograph versus an image intensifier (ie, fluoroscopy unit). Further research is needed to evaluate and compare the benefits and harms of various imaging techniques, such as plain portable radiograph, plain fixed radiograph, fluoroscopy (eg, C-arm),[187] CT imaging (eg, three dimensional [3D]),[149] MRI, ultrasound, and transesophageal echocardiogram[188] for intraoperative identification of radiopaque and non-radiopaque RSIs.

VI.c.7. In addition to imaging of the surgical site, a sample image of an item similar to the missing object may be taken.[31,97,189] *[2: High Evidence]*

The collective evidence[31,97,189] suggests that a visual reference of the missing item may assist the radiologist in locating the item radiographically. Gayer et al[190] explained various imaging presentations of RSIs and the complexity of identifying retained items amid other patient care items, such as packing, drains, and implants. Edel[97] and Judson et al[31] included imaging of a like item in their discrepancy protocols to facilitate the radiologist's review of the images. Hunter and Gimber[189] described a radiograph reference guide that was created for the radiologist reviewing radiograph screening images.

VI.c.8. The radiologist and surgeon should simultaneously review and interpret intraoperative imaging for RSIs.[31,43] When the radiologist is not immediately available, the surgeon should conduct a preliminary interpretation of the image.[43] *[1: Strong Evidence]*

The ICSI[43] recommends that the radiologist and surgeon simultaneously review the intraoperative image verbally and visually to correlate the anatomical coverage of the surgical site and description of the missing item. If the radiologist is not immediately available, the ICSI[43] recommends that the surgeon take primary responsibility to interpret the image. Judson et al[31] implemented this practice in their count discrepancy protocol, requiring that the attending surgeon speak with the attending radiologist either by telephone or in person while concurrently viewing the x-ray.

VI.c.9. The health care organization's policy should define the needle size limits for which radiographs will be used to assist in identifying retained needles. *[5: Benefits Balanced with Harms]*

The collective evidence is inconclusive about how effective radiographs are in detecting small suture needles. Several studies conflict regarding the ability to consistently locate 10-mm to 13-mm needles on radiographic screening when retention is suspected.[145-148] Further research is needed to determine the most effective and consistent radiographic detection method for small needles.

VI.d. Unresolved count discrepancies must be documented in the patient's record,[183,184] including all measures taken to recover the missing item, description and location of the item if known, patient notification and consultation, and the plan for follow-up care.[31,41,43,44] *[1: Regulatory Requirement]*

The Centers for Medicare & Medicaid Services requires surgical complications to be documented in the operative report.[183,184] The collective evidence and guidance from professional organizations[31,41,43,44] support documenting count reconciliation measures and consulting with the patient or patient's representative regarding the plan for follow-up, including additional imaging and possible risks of a potentially retained item. Judson et al[31] integrated their count reconciliation protocols into an electronic health record for documentation.

VI.d.1. Environmental services personnel and the next perioperative team in the room should be notified about items reported missing in an unresolved count discrepancy.[43] *[1: Strong Evidence]*

The ICSI[43] recommends notifying environmental services personnel and the next team in the room after an unresolved count discrepancy. Having an unaccounted surgical item in the OR may effect the validity of subsequent counts. If the item missing is a sharp object, communication to other perioperative team members is important to alert them to the potential risk for a sharps injury.

Recommendation VII

A multidisciplinary team may evaluate adjunct technologies for use as a supplement to manual counting procedures at the health care organization.[2,18,43,44]

Professional organizations[2,18,43,44] recommend considering adjunct technology for use as a supplement to manual counting procedures. Several published nonresearch papers[8,89,103,186,191-194] have discussed the potential benefits of adjunct technology (ie, two-dimensional [2D] matrix, radio-frequency [RF], radio-frequency identification [RFID]) and recommended consideration of this technology as an adjunct to manual counting of surgical soft goods (ie, sponges, towels). Judson et al[31] analyzed miscount events and recommended considering the use of adjunct technology (ie, sponge/instrument barcoding, RF detection) in high-risk cases, such as procedures of long duration and procedures with high numbers of personnel, even when counts are documented as correct. However, the authors noted that further research is needed to define high-risk procedures.[31]

The collective evidence[4,8,33] suggests that the sensitivity and specificity of manual counting and radiograph screening is insufficient to prevent RSI. Egorova et al[33] reported that the manual count sensitivity was 77.2% and the specificity was 99.2%, meaning that patients with retained items were accurately identified 77.2% of the time by manual counting procedures. Cima et al[8] and Gawande et al[4] found that the final count was documented as correct in 62% and 88% of RSI cases, respectively. Erroneously correct counts are falsely reassuring and harmful to the patient because discrepancy reconciliation pathways will not be activated to locate a misplaced item.[4,8] Intraoperative radiographs also are not always effective in identifying RSIs. In a retrospective review, Cima et al[8] reported that 67% of intraoperative radiographs were read as negative when an RSI actually was present. Regenbogen et al[37] predicted the cost-effectiveness of several RSI prevention strategies compared with standard counting procedures. They estimated that standard manual counting prevents 82% of retained sponges, and they found that barcoding may prevent 97.5% of retained sponges.

The collective evidence[34,81] also indicates that manual counting could be affected by human factors that might be improved with technological support. Steelman and Cullen[81] reported 57 potential failures in the manual counting of sponges in elective abdominal surgery and found that the most common failure causes were related to human factors, including distraction, multitasking, not following procedure, and time pressure. The authors recommended that additional technological controls be considered due to the concern that these types of failures are not likely to be improved with educational interventions.[81] Greenberg et al[34] found that human error was attributed to 41% of count discrepancies in their prospective study that was nested in a randomized controlled trial of barcoding technology. They recommended further investigation of technological solutions to improve human performance.

The limitations of the evidence are that research has not confirmed the benefit of widespread implementation of adjunct technology as part of an RSI prevention protocol. Further research is needed to validate the efficacy, safety, and cost-effectiveness of adjunct technology systems.[31]

The benefits of using adjunct technology to supplement manual procedures for counting surgical sponges may outweigh the harms, although further research is needed. Benefits may include timely facilitation of the surgical count and possible improved count accuracy.[37] Some technology (ie, RF, RFID) has the capability of detecting an object within the patient and may also benefit the patient by eliminating the need for a radiograph and thereby reduce exposure to radiation. However, if the adjunct technology device is not used in accordance with the manufacturer's instructions for use or is not validated for efficacy, the benefits may not be fully achieved and the patient could be at risk for an RSI in the event of a false-negative result.

Stawicki et al[6] reported that RSI occurred in two of 32 cases using RF tagged sponges. Although this was less frequent than the occurrence of RSI in 13 of 51 patients who had radiographic screening, the authors noted that technology alone cannot completely prevent RSI and that further research is needed to determine best technology-supported practices for prevention of RSI.[6] A limitation of this report is that the specific type of adjunct technology was not described.

The harms of adjunct technology may also include detachment of the tracking device and potential RSI, which may be minimized by inspecting the product for manufacturing defects before and immediately after use in the surgical wound. However, no published incidents of harm from manufacturing defects were found in the evidence review. Harms to the patient from RFID technology may include the potential to interfere with pacemakers, implantable cardioverter defibrillators, and other electronic medical devices, or the potential hazard of electromagnetic interference (EMI) to electronic medical devices from RF transmitters.[195] No published incidents of patient harm from electronic medical device interference or EMI were found in the evidence review.

Adjunct technology for intraoperative surgical item identification is evolving rapidly. Hadjiiski et al[196] reported an experimental trial of a 3D micro tag for surgical sponges that is designed to have a signature appearance on radiograph from any view. As part of the trial, the researchers embedded 3D micro tags in surgical sponges that were placed in cadavers. The researchers then imaged the cadavers and assessed the sensitivity of detecting the 3D micro tags on radiograph images among surgeons (81.5%) and radiologists (96.1%). This study also presented the application of computer-aided detection technology for detection of the micro tag on radiograph imaging. Further research is needed to establish the safety, efficacy, and cost-effectiveness of emerging micro tag and computer-aided detection technology.

VII.a. A mechanism for evaluating and selecting existing and emerging adjunct technology products should be implemented by the health care organization.[197] *[2: High Evidence]*

Patient safety concerns are the impetus for perioperative personnel as they participate in evaluating and selecting medical devices and products for use in practice settings.

The evidence review included cost-benefit analysis reports comparing various RSI prevention methods.[33,37,198] However, the collective evidence is inconclusive about which technology is the most beneficial and cost-effective. Some of the evidence[35,37] establishes the cost benefits of adjunct technology (ie, barcoding, RF) for RSI prevention; however, one systematic review[198] reported that standard counting is the most economical strategy.

VII.a.1. Perioperative RNs, physicians, and other health care providers involved in the use of products and medical devices for prevention of RSIs should be part of a multidisciplinary product evaluation and selection committee when the health care organization is evaluating the purchase of adjunct technology.[197] *[2: High Evidence]*

VII.a.2. Perioperative personnel should evaluate existing and emerging adjunct technology to determine the application that may be most suitable in their setting. *[5: Benefits Balanced with Harms]*

VII.b. The multidisciplinary team may evaluate FDA-cleared adjunct technology for surgical soft goods as a supplement to manual count procedures.[36,38,39,199-201] *[2: High Evidence]*

The collective evidence supports the use of adjunct technology (eg, 2D matrix,[199,200] RF,[36,38,39,202] RFID[201,203]) to supplement manual count procedures of surgical soft goods. However, further research is needed to validate the efficacy, safety, and cost-effectiveness of adjunct technology systems.

In a randomized controlled trial, Greenberg et al[199] compared a barcoded sponge system (ie, 2D matrix) to a traditional count protocol in 300 general surgery procedures and found that the barcoding system identified significantly more count discrepancies than the traditional manual count protocol, although the system increased the time spent counting. The researchers discussed that the introduction of technology and the associated learning curve may have influenced the study results, as a qualitative survey showed that some personnel struggled while most easily adapted to the technology. A limitation of the study is that it was not statistically powered to detect a reduction in retained surgical sponges, which is a rare event requiring a very large sample size.

In an organizational experience study, Cima et al[200] reported on implementation of a data-matrix-coded (ie, 2D matrix) sponge system at a large health care organization. They initially conducted two trials to assess the system before institution-wide implementation. In an 18-month period during which 87,404 procedures were performed, no RSIs were reported.[200] The first trial measured time spent counting data-matrix-coded sponges (n = 365) and control sponges (n = 335) for colon and rectal procedures. Although the initial time for counting data-matrix-coded sponges was 11 seconds, the time was reduced to five seconds after four days of implementation; the time to count control sponges was four seconds.[200] This report is limited by the nature of an organizational experience report and may not be generalizable to other institutions.

Initial studies in the laboratory setting assessed the feasibility of identifying RF-[202] and RFID-tagged[203] surgical sponges and durability of the device in water and body fluids. Macario et al[201] tested an RFID wand device in eight patients undergoing abdominal surgery as part of an experimental trial with blinding. The RFID wand detected all sponges correctly in less than three seconds. However, the study was limited by a very small sample size.

The evidence review included several clinical trials of RF adjunct technology for managing surgical sponges. In a larger prospective trial, Rupp et al[36] implemented an RF detection system in conjunction with a previously implemented sponge management protocol (ie, Sponge ACCOUNTing System) at a large health care institution. The addition of the RF detection system in 2,285 cases facilitated the resolution of one near-miss event that was not detected by manual counting and the resolution of 35 count discrepancy events. Rupp et al[36] noted that time for use of the detection system was not measured, although it was a negligible amount of time, and that surveys of personnel suggested high confidence in the system for preventing RSI. This study was limited by lack of statistical power to detect errors in the RF detection system.

Steelman[38] conducted a prospective, blinded, crossover study with the participants serving as their own controls. Each participant (N = 210), including 101 participants who were morbidly obese, had four surgical sponges (three RF tagged, one control with no tag) randomly placed behind their torso in assigned abdominal quadrant areas and read with an RF wand. The results showed that the detection of the RF tagged sponges was 100% for both sensitivity and specificity. A limitation of this study was that the readings were done with simulated placement in abdominal quadrants and were not placed within the abdominal cavity.

Steelman and Alasagheirin[39] conducted a similar prospective, double-blinded, crossover study with participants (N = 203) serving as their own controls to evaluate the ability of an RF mat to detect RF tagged sponges. The results showed that the sensitivity of the mat was 98.1% and the specificity was 100%. A second phase of the study in a subset of participants evaluated the effectiveness of the RF wand (n = 117), which showed a sensitivity and specificity of 100%. The subset included participants in whom the mat did not detect a sponge. The researchers concluded that the RF wand was more sensitive than the mat for detecting tagged sponges in individuals who were morbidly obese. This study was also limited by the placement of sponges outside the abdominal cavity.

VII.b.1. Adjunct technology should be used in accordance with the manufacturer's instructions for use. *[5: Benefits Balanced with Harms]*

VII.b.2. Radio-frequency identification technology should be used with caution in patients with pacemakers, implantable cardioverter defibrillators, and other electronic medical devices.[195] *[5: Benefits Balanced with Harms]*

According to the FDA,[195] RFID transmitters may interfere with electronic medical devices. No published incidents of patient harm from electronic medical device interference or EMI were found in the evidence review.

VII.b.3. Adjunct technology equipment should be cleaned and disinfected after each use in accordance with the manufacturer's instructions for use.[204] *[1: Strong Evidence]*

VII.c. The multidisciplinary team may evaluate FDA-cleared adjunct technology for detecting retained surgical instruments as a supplement to manual count procedures.[205,206] *[3: Moderate Evidence]*

The collective evidence[205,206] indicated that RFID tag technology for surgical instruments is an emerging adjunct technology with potential application for prevention of retained surgical instruments. However, further research is needed to validate the efficacy, safety, and cost-effectiveness of adjunct technology (ie, RFID tags) for surgical instrument tracking.

Kranzfelder et al[205] used RFID tagged instruments in 10 laparoscopic cholecystectomies and found that this technology was feasible for real-time, reliable instrument detection. However, some miscounts occurred during continuous application of electrosurgery current.[205] This study is limited by a small sample size. In a simulation environment, Neumuth and Meissner[206] reported use of RFID information fusion technology and correctly identified instrument usage during surgical procedures 97% of the time.

VII.c.1. Radio-frequency identification tags for surgical instruments should be used, cleaned, and sterilized in accordance with the device and instrument manufacturer's validated and written instructions for use.[172,207] *[1: Strong Evidence]*

Items cannot be assumed to be clean, decontaminated, or sterile unless the manufacturer's instructions for use are derived from validation testing and the user has followed those instructions.[172] The device manufacturer has validated the cycle, identified in the instructions for use, that must be used to ensure sterility.[207]

In one study, Yamashita et al[208] evaluated the effectiveness of a washer-disinfector for cleaning surgical instruments with attached RFID tags. After fixation of simulated contaminants (sheep blood treated with heparin and 1% protamine sulfate) on the surgical instrument RFID tag, the researchers cleaned one group of instruments in a washer disinfector and another group in an ultrasonic washer; a third group underwent no cleaning process. Following these interventions, the residual protein was recovered and measured using cleaning appraisal guidelines from Japan and Germany. The results showed that the washer-disinfector was effective in achieving recommended residual protein amounts after cleaning of instruments with RFID tags. Although the researchers concluded that secondary infection risk from surgical instruments with RFID tags attached was low, the study was not designed to assess patient outcomes and infection risk. A major limitation of this study was that the sample size and type of instruments were not reported.

VII.c.2. Radio-frequency identification tags attached to surgical instruments should be accounted for before and immediately after use in a surgical wound. *[5: Benefits Balanced with Harms]*

Detachment of an RFID tag from a surgical instrument in the wound may become a potential RSI. Kranzfelder et al[205] used RFID tagged instruments in 10 laparoscopic cholecystectomies and no RFID tag failures occurred.

Recommendation VIII

Documentation should reflect activities related to prevention of RSIs.

Documentation is a professional medicolegal standard. Documentation related to prevention of RSIs is applicable at the systems level and the patient care level. At the systems level, documentation serves as a basis for monitoring compliance and measuring performance as part of a quality assurance program. At the patient care level, documentation facilitates continuity of patient care through clear communication and supports collaboration among health care team members.

VIII.a. The RN circulator should document soft good, sharp, miscellaneous item, and instrument counts on the patient's intraoperative record.[209] *[2: High Evidence]*

Documentation of nursing activities related to the patient's perioperative care provides an account of the nursing care administered and provides a mechanism for comparing actual versus expected outcomes.[209] Such documentation is considered sound professional practice and demonstrates that all reasonable efforts were made to protect the patient's safety by preventing an RSI.

VIII.b. Documentation of measures taken for the prevention of RSIs should include
- types of counts (eg, radiopaque sponges, sharps, miscellaneous items, instruments);
- number of counts;
- names and titles of personnel performing the counts[18,29];
- results of surgical item counts (ie, correct or incorrect)[2,18,44];
- surgeon notification of count results[44];
- any adjunct technology that was used and any associated records;
- an explanation for any waived counts[18];
- number and location of any instruments intentionally remaining with the patient or radiopaque sponges intentionally retained as therapeutic packing[2,18,43,44];
- actions taken if count discrepancies occurred, including all measures taken to recover the missing item or device fragment and any patient communication regarding the outcome[2,18,43,44];
- rationale if counts were not performed or completed as prescribed by policy[18]; and
- the outcome of actions taken.
[1: Strong Evidence]

Professional organizations[2,18,43,44] recommend documenting RSI prevention activities. In a description of a legal RSI case in the United Kingdom, Brown and Feather[29] noted that three circulating nurses were documented as participating in the surgery but it was not clear who verified the final count. They recommended that the name of each person performing the count be clearly documented.

Extreme patient emergencies and certain individual patient considerations may necessitate waived counts to preserve a patient's life or limb. Documenting the rationale for waived counts and for variation in count procedures provides a record of the occurrence and an alert to subsequent health care providers that the patient may be at an increased risk for an RSI.

Recommendation IX

Policies and procedures for the prevention of RSIs should be developed, reviewed periodically, revised as necessary, and readily available in the practice setting. *Amb*

Policies and procedures assist in the development of patient safety, quality assessment, and performance improvement activities. Policies and procedures establish authority, responsibility, and accountability within the organization. Policies and procedures also serve as operational guidelines that are used to minimize patient risk for injury or complications, standardize practice, direct perioperative personnel, and establish continuous performance improvement programs.

IX.a. A multidisciplinary team should develop policies and procedures for preventing RSIs.[6,18,44] *[2: High Evidence]* *Amb*

Developing and maintaining policies and procedures that guide patient care is a regulatory requirement[183,184] and accreditation agency standard[210] for both hospitals and ambulatory settings. Some accrediting bodies specifically require policies and procedures for surgical counts.[2,211,212]

In addition to regulatory and accreditation requirements, the evidence review also included recommendations for RSI prevention policies and procedures in the literature[6] and from professional organizations.[18,44] Stawicki et al[6] recommended that surgical facilities maintain and enforce a surgical safety policy for RSI prevention.

IX.a.1. The multidisciplinary team should include perioperative nurses, surgeons, anesthesia professionals, sterile processing personnel, risk managers, leaders, and other stakeholders as deemed necessary. *[5: Benefits Balanced with Harms]*

IX.b. Policies and procedures for prevention of RSI should include
- items to be counted,
- directions for performing counts (eg, sequence, item grouping),
- waived count procedures in which baseline and/or subsequent counts may be exempt,
- multidisciplinary team actions and procedures for count discrepancy reconciliation,
- use of radiographic screening,
- use of adjunct technology, and
- documentation and reporting procedures for RSIs and near misses.
[5: Benefits Balanced with Harms]

IX.b.1. A policy and procedure for reporting product packaging defects to manufacturers should be established in collaboration with materials management personnel. *[5: Benefits Balanced with Harms]*

IX.b.2. If intraoperative imaging is not available, the health care organization should have a policy and procedure describing actions necessary and communication required between referring and receiving organizations. *[5: Benefits Balanced with Harms]* *Amb*

IX.c. Based on risk analysis, the health care organization should establish policies that define when additional measures for RSI prevention should be performed or when they may be waived (eg, trauma,[170,171] cystoscopy, ophthalmology).[2,18,43,44] *[1: Strong Evidence]*

The collective evidence[170,171] and guidance from professional organizations[2,18,43,44] indicate that there are situations in which the baseline count may need to be waived for patients in life-threatening situations, such as in trauma cases. This evidence review found no other literature about criteria for waiving of count procedures, including criteria for pediatric patients. The size of a pediatric patient may dictate a correspondingly small incision that may make retention of an instrument in the surgical wound unlikely; however, RSIs can occur in the smallest of incisions. Careful consideration should be given when establishing a policy for waived counts for the pediatric patient based on age, weight, or incision size, because it is difficult to determine risk for an RSI.

The collective evidence[3-6,8,31] and professional organizations[2,18,45] support considering additional measures, such as radiographic screening of high-risk patients, as an adjunct to surgical item accounting procedures. The following risk factors have been significantly associated with RSI:
- incorrect count,[3]
- unexpected change due to intraoperative factors,[3]
- more than one surgical team,[3,31]
- no count (due to inability or emergent situations),[3]
- more than one procedure,[3]
- long procedure,[3,31]
- blood loss > 500 mL,[3]
- high BMI,[4,6]
- emergency procedure,[4] and
- occurrence of a safety variance during the procedure.[6]

Because of these identified risk factors, Lincourt et al[5] recommended routine radiographic screening for emergency procedures and when multiple major procedures are being performed because this indicates the presence of multiple surgical teams. Gawande et al[4] recommended routine intraoperative radiographic screening for select, high-risk patients (ie, emergency procedures, unplanned changes in procedure, high BMI) to detect RSIs.

Moffatt-Bruce et al[3] conducted a meta-analysis of risk factors for RSIs in three case-control studies and proposed a risk stratification system. In this system, patients were stratified by high risk and intermediate risk based on odds ratios with a cut off of 3. The high risk category includes risk factors that are associated with more than a three times greater risk for RSIs: incorrect surgical count, unexpected intraoperative factors, and more than one surgical team. The intermediate category includes risk factors with less than a three times greater risk for RSIs: surgical count not performed, more than one subprocedure, long duration of surgery, and estimated blood loss > 500 mL. The researchers recommended further research to prospectively evaluate interventions on their effectiveness to reduce the risk for RSIs. This systematic review was limited by the retrospective nature of the review and the quality of the included studies.

Professional organizations also recommend radiographic screening of high-risk patients. The WHO[18] recommends intraoperative imaging, when possible, when no counts were performed. The Joint Commission[2] recommends intraoperative imaging when the patient is determined to be at high risk for an RSI, even if the count was correct and a methodical wound exploration was performed. The Pennsylvania Patient Safety Authority[45] recommends intraoperative imaging for high-risk cases, including incorrect counts, emergency procedures, patients with a high BMI, and procedures with unplanned changes.

Further research is needed to evaluate the clinical application of additional measures, including intraoperative imaging, that target risk factors for RSI prevention. Further research is also needed to determine the benefits and harms of universal imaging. Cima et al[8] recommended universal postoperative imaging surveillance for RSIs in a dedicated imaging room located in the surgical suite.

IX.d. Policies and procedures should include RSI prevention measures for organ procurement procedures. *[4: Limited Evidence]*

Counted items that are sent with the donated organ(s) may increase the risk of count discrepancy and RSIs for the organ recipient and could create sharps injury hazards for personnel. Counted sharps and instruments that are retained in the donor may cause injury at autopsy, as reported by Burton,[213] and contribute to inventory loss.

Recommendation X

Perioperative personnel should participate in a variety of quality assurance and performance improvement activities that are consistent with the facility or health care organization plan to improve understanding and compliance with the principles and processes of RSI prevention.

Quality assurance and performance improvement programs assist in evaluating and improving the quality of patient care and formulating plans for corrective action. These programs provide data that may be used to determine whether an individual organization is within benchmark goals and, if not, to identify areas that may require corrective action.

X.a. A systems approach for quality assurance and performance improvement should be used for prevention of RSIs. Health care organizations should value learning and respond to errors with a focus on process improvement rather than individual blame.[40,49,50,214-216] *[3: Moderate Evidence]*

The evidence review indicates that perioperative teams can better understand how adverse events like RSIs occur and learn how to redesign the system to prevent these errors when the interactions between individuals and systems are understood and the location where failure occurs is identified.[40,214,215] The perioperative setting is a highly complex system, and many factors can influence individual performance. Butler et al[85] discussed that in addition to team performance, factors such as the type of surgery, technical complexity of the procedure, unplanned changes, and patient acuity place a high amount of pressure on the perioperative nurse to remain alert, observant, and responsive through the fatigue and stress from the physical and psychological demands of working in this setting. A systems approach targets quality interventions to address cognitive factors, team dynamics, and perceptual biases as part of a systems initiative to decrease RSIs and improve patient safety.[40]

Reason's model of human error distinguishes the systems approach from individual approaches for prevention of medical errors.[49] Focusing on systems for RSI prevention, rather than blaming individuals, aims to reduce the incidence of RSIs by improving systems to prevent predictable human errors.[40,49,214] Accountability also plays a role in systems improvement. Each perioperative team member has an ethical obligation to perform his or her role and responsibilities with appropriate competence and the highest level of personal integrity.[54] However, perioperative team members in a just culture are not only accountable for their own actions but are also accountable to each other in protecting patients.[216] Riley et al[50] discussed that increasing professional accountability may improve patient safety by minimizing the effects of normalization and complacency that may occur during the repetitive task of the surgical count. However, systems improvement is beyond individual accountability and responsibility. According to Reason,[49] dealing with individual errors rather than fixing a broken system will not stop unsafe acts from occurring.

X.a.1. Errors should be evaluated in such a manner that contributing factors are first reviewed and then accountability is determined in relation to actions. *[5: Benefits Balanced with Harms]*

Continuous quality improvement opportunities arise from documented and structured quality processes and measures that can define and resolve problems.

X.a.2. Personnel should identify and respond to opportunities for improvement. *[5: Benefits Balanced with Harms]*

To evaluate the quality of patient care and formulate plans for corrective action, it is necessary to maintain a system of evaluation.

X.b. A multiphase, multidisciplinary process improvement program should be implemented,[212,217-220] including
○ an ongoing risk assessment and review (eg, failure mode and effect analysis);[81]
○ a policy design and review;
○ a review of published evidence, internal data collection, and data analysis; and
○ plans for the ongoing monitoring and analysis of processes, near misses, and adverse events related to the prevention of RSIs.[41,86,87]
[3: Moderate Evidence]

A comprehensive QI program may identify opportunities for minimizing the risk of RSI events. Establishment of a quality and performance improvement program is an accreditation requirement.[212,217-220]

The evidence review found that implementation of comprehensive process improvement programs reduced RSI events and improved count procedures in health care organizations.[41,86,87] As part of an organizational experience report, Cima et al[41] implemented a multidisciplinary, multiphase approach for process improvement that involved defect analysis, policy review, increasing awareness and communication among personnel, and a monitoring and control phase. After implementation of the program, the health care organization experienced a significant and sustained reduction in RSI events during a two-year period, going from an average of one RSI or near miss every 16 days to an average of one RSI or near miss every 69 days.[41]

Edel[86] reported on an organizational experience QI project that involved analysis of surgical count practice variability, policy revision, personnel education, and auditing for compliance. As a result, variability in count practices was reduced although metrics were not reported.[86] In an organizational experience in a pediatric teaching hospital, Norton et al[87] discussed implementation of a quality program to standardize count practices, revise policies, educate personnel, and review every reported count discrepancy. During a one-year period, the hospital reported a 50% reduction in the number of incorrect counts and count discrepancies with sustained results.

The evidence review also indicated that healthcare failure mode and effect analysis can identify potential failures in the counting of surgical sponges.[81] In an organizational experience, Steelman and Cullen[81] conducted a healthcare failure mode and effect analysis that included observation of surgical sponge counting procedures during two elective abdominal procedures, process mapping, focus groups, and healthcare failure mode and effect analysis hazard scoring. The authors found 57 potential failures during the management of surgical sponges, with 106 failure/cause combinations during six stages of surgical sponge management: room preparation, initial count, adding sponges, removing sponges, first closing count, and final closing count. The researchers reported that 50.9% of failures occurred before the final closing count and that the top causes of failures were distraction, multitasking, and time pressure.

X.c. The health care organization should monitor for adherence to policies and procedures for prevention of RSI as part of quality assurance and process improvement initiatives.[4,6] *[2: High Evidence]*

The collective evidence[4,6] supports monitoring for adherence to policies and procedures for RSI prevention. Gawande et al[4] strongly recommended that hospitals actively monitor compliance with policies and procedures for counting, including standard sponge counting in every surgical procedure and instrument counting for every surgery involving an open cavity.

In a retrospective case-control study, Stawicki et al[6] found that policy deviations identified as safety omissions/variations were significantly associated with an increased risk for RSI. The authors recommended that surgical facilities enforce a surgical safety policy for RSI prevention to foster a culture of zero tolerance for policy deviations.[6]

X.d. A critical investigation should be conducted regarding any adverse event or near miss related to RSIs.[2,87] *[2: High Evidence]*

Error and near-miss reporting is the first step to addressing error reduction. As part of the sentinel event policy, The Joint Commission[2] requires a root cause analysis of all sentinel events, including unintended retention of foreign objects. There are a number of analysis methods (eg, root cause analysis, appreciative inquiry) available to health care organizations that may be used to conduct a critical investigation of adverse events.[2,87,221] Agrawal[104] reported a root cause analysis of a retained vaginal sponge. Bell[221] reported a critical incident analysis of a near miss where the sponge was found in the drapes during count reconciliation procedures.

As part of a multiple initiative QI project in a pediatric teaching hospital, Norton et al[87] reviewed every reported count discrepancy by root cause analysis in addition to implementing standardization of count practices, policy revision, and personnel education. During a one-year period, the hospital reported a 50% reduction in the number of incorrect counts and count discrepancies with sustained results.[87]

X.d.1. Multidisciplinary teams should be involved in the review process and address any changes in policy that can improve patient safety. *[5: Benefits Balanced with Harms]*

X.d.2. A human factors analysis may be used in the critical investigation of an RSI event.[40] *[3: Moderate Evidence]*

Use of human factors analysis is supported in an organizational experience report. Thiels et al[40] applied Reason's model to never events, including RSI, and identified four categories of human error: unsafe actions, preconditions for unsafe actions, oversight/supervisory factors, and organizational influences. During a five-year period, they captured reported incidents and near misses of never events, including RSI, at a tertiary-care hospital. Human behaviors in the incident analysis were coded in subcategories of the four main categories with nano-codes. For retained foreign objects, the majority of coded behaviors (n = 221) were in the categories of unsafe actions (n = 102) and preconditions for actions (n = 94). The researchers recommended using the Human Factors Analysis and Classification System to assist in linking human factors by error type to provide targets for intervention and mitigation.

X.e. Reporting mechanisms for adverse events and near misses related to RSIs must be established. *[1: Regulatory Requirement]*

Federal and state agencies, accrediting bodies, third-party payers, and professional associations consider unintentionally retained foreign objects or RSIs to be reportable events that require further investigation.[2,23,222] Many states require public reporting when RSI events occur.[22]

X.e.1. Events that necessitate reopening a wound to retrieve an RSI should be reported in compliance with health care organizational

policy, as well as local, state, and federal regulatory agencies. *[5: Benefits Balanced with Harms]*

Editor's note: *TeamSTEPPS is a registered trademark of the US Department of Defense, Bethesda, MD. NoThing Left Behind is a registered trademark of Verna C. Gibbs, San Francisco, CA. University Health-System Consortium Safety Intelligence is a registered trademark of VHA Inc, Irving, TX.*

Glossary

Radio-frequency identification (RFID): A system that transmits the identity of an object (in the form of a unique serial number) wirelessly, using radio waves.

Root cause analysis: A retrospective process for identifying basic or causal factors underlying variation in performance, including the occurrence or possible occurrence of a sentinel event.

Sentinel event: An unanticipated incident involving death or serious physical or psychological injury, or the risk of serious injury or adverse outcome.

Unretrieved device fragment: A fragment of a medical device that has separated and unintentionally remains in the patient after a procedure.

REFERENCES

1. Wilson C. Foreign bodies left in the abdomen after laparotomy. *Trans Am Gynecol Soc.* 1884;9:94-117. [VC]

2. The Joint Commission. Preventing unintended retained foreign objects. *Sentinel Event Alert.* October 17, 2013;51. http://www.jointcommission.org/sea_issue_51/. Accessed November 10, 2015. [IVB].

3. Moffatt-Bruce SD, Cook CH, Steinberg SM, Stawicki SP. Risk factors for retained surgical items: a meta-analysis and proposed risk stratification system. *J Surg Res.* 2014;190(2):429-436. [IIIA]

4. Gawande AA, Studdert DM, Orav EJ, Brennan TA, Zinner MJ. Risk factors for retained instruments and sponges after surgery. *N Engl J Med.* 2003;348(3):229-235. [IIIA]

5. Lincourt AE, Harrell A, Cristiano J, Sechrist C, Kercher K, Heniford BT. Retained foreign bodies after surgery. *J Surg Res.* 2007;138(2):170-174. [IIIB]

6. Stawicki SP, Moffatt-Bruce SD, Ahmed HM, et al. Retained surgical items: a problem yet to be solved. *J Am Coll Surg.* 2013;216(1):15-22. [IIIB]

7. Chen Q, Rosen AK, Cevasco M, Shin M, Itani KM, Borzecki AM. Detecting patient safety indicators: how valid is "foreign body left during procedure" in the Veterans Health Administration? *J Am Coll Surg.* 2011;212(6):977-983. [IIIB]

8. Cima RR, Kollengode A, Garnatz J, Storsveen A, Weisbrod C, Deschamps C. Incidence and characteristics of potential and actual retained foreign object events in surgical patients. *J Am Coll Surg.* 2008;207(1):80-87. [IIIB]

9. Wan W, Le T, Riskin L, Macario A. Improving safety in the operating room: a systematic literature review of retained surgical sponges. *Curr Opin Anaesthesiol.* 2009;22(2):207-214. [VA]

10. Zantvoord Y, van der Weiden RM, van Hooff MH. Transmural migration of retained surgical sponges: a systematic review. *Obstet Gynecol Surv.* 2008;63(7):465-471. [VB]

11. Cohen SB, Bartz PJ, Earing MG, Sheil A, Nicolosi A, Woods RK. Myocardial infarction due to a retained epicardial pacing wire. *Ann Thorac Surg.* 2012;94(5):1724-1726. [VB]

12. Suh DH, Yoon JR, Kang KB, Han SB, Kim HJ, Lee SJ. A gossypiboma-induced pathological fracture of the proximal femur. *Clin Radiol.* 2009;64(11):1132-1135. [VC]

13. Tateishi M, Tomizawa Y. Intravascular foreign bodies: danger of unretrieved fragmented medical devices. *J Artif Organs.* 2009;12(2):80-89. [VB]

14. Al-Moghairi AM, Al-Amri HS. Management of retained intervention guide-wire: a literature review. *Curr Cardiol Rev.* 2013;9(3):260-266. [VA]

15. Johnson C, Alomari AI, Chaudry G. Detachment of introducer sheath radiopaque marker during retrieval of G2 filter. *Cardiovasc Intervent Radiol.* 2011;34(2):431-434. [VB]

16. Williams TL, Bowdle TA, Winters BD, Pavkovic SD, Szekendi MK. Guidewires unintentionally retained during central venous catheterization. *J Assoc Vasc Access.* 2014;19(1):29-34. [VA]

17. Bydon A, Xu R, Conte JV, et al. Surgical mystery: where is the missing pituitary rongeur tip? *Spine.* 2010;35(17):E867-E872. [VB]

18. *WHO Guidelines for Safe Surgery 2009.* Geneva, Switzerland: WHO Press; 2009. [IVB]

19. Mehtsun WT, Ibrahim AM, Diener-West M, Pronovost PJ, Makary MA. Surgical never events in the United States. *Surgery.* 2013;153(4):465-472. [IIIB]

20. Steelman VM, Graling PR, Perkhounkova Y. Priority patient safety issues identified by perioperative nurses. *AORN J.* 2013;97(4):402-418. [IIIA]

21. Kohn LT, Corrigan JD, Molla S. *To Err Is Human: Building a Safer Health System.* Washington, DC: National Academy Press; 2000.

22. West N, Eng T, Kirk A. *Update on State Government Tracking of Health Care-Acquired Conditions and a Four-State In-Depth Review.* Baltimore, MD: Center for Medicare and Medicaid Innovation, Centers for Medicare & Medicaid Services; 2012. https://www.cms.gov/Medicare/Medicare-Fee-for-Service-Payment/HospitalAcqCond/Downloads/Phase-3-State-Tracking-Report.pdf. Accessed November 10, 2015.

23. FY 2013, FY 2014, and FY 2015 Final HAC List. Centers for Medicare & Medicaid Services. https://www.cms.gov/medicare/medicare-fee-for-service-payment/hospitalacqcond/downloads/fy_2013_final_hacscodelist.pdf. Accessed November 10, 2015.

24. 42 CFR Subchapter C—Medical Assistance Programs. Part 430. Subpart C—Grants; Reviews and Audits; Withholding for Failure To Comply; Deferral and Disallowance of Claims; Reduction of Federal Medicaid Payments. Electronic Code of Federal Regulations. http://www.ecfr.gov/cgi-bin/text-idx?SID=86ae42db45723f0073ecc0d7c2218484&node=sp42.4.430.c&rgn=div6. Accessed November 10, 2015.

25. Ricciardi R, Baxter NN, Read TE, Marcello PW, Schoetz DJ, Roberts PL. Surgeon involvement in the care of patients deemed to have "preventable" conditions. *J Am Coll Surg.* 2009;209(6):707-711. [IIIB]

26. Camp M, Chang DC, Zhang Y, Chrouser K, Colombani PM, Abdullah F. Risk factors and outcomes for foreign body left during a procedure: analysis of 413 incidents after 1,946,831 operations in children. *Arch Surg.* 2010;145(11):1085-1090. [IIIA]

27. Shah RK, Lander L. Retained foreign bodies during surgery in pediatric patients: a national perspective. *J Pediatr Surg.* 2009;44(4):738-742. [IIIA]

28. Murphy EK. "Captain of the ship" doctrine continues to take on water. *AORN J.* 2001;74(4):525-528. [VC]

29. Brown J, Feather D. Surgical equipment and materials left in patients. *Br J Perioper Nurs.* 2005;15(6):259-262. [VB]

30. Retained surgical retractor. November 22, 2013. Texas Medical Liability Trust. https://www.tmlt.org/blog/Closed-Claim-Studies/General-surgery/Retained-surgical-retractor.html. Accessed November 10, 2015. [VC]

31. Judson TJ, Howell MD, Guglielmi C, Canacari E, Sands K. Miscount incidents: a novel approach to exploring risk factors for unintentionally retained surgical items. *Jt Comm J Qual Patient Saf.* 2013;39(10):468-474. [IIIA]

32. Moffatt-Bruce SD, Ellison EC, Anderson HL 3rd, et al; OPUS 12 Foundation, Inc. Multi-Center Trials Group. Intravascular retained surgical items: a multicenter study of risk factors. *J Surg Res.* 2012;178(1):519-523. [IIIC]

33. Egorova NN, Moskowitz A, Gelijns A, et al. Managing the prevention of retained surgical instruments: what is the value of counting? *Ann Surg.* 2008;247(1):13-18. [IIIA]

34. Greenberg CC, Regenbogen SE, Lipsitz SR, Diaz-Flores R, Gawande AA. The frequency and significance of discrepancies in the surgical count. *Ann Surg.* 2008;248(2):337-341. [IIIA]

35. Williams TL, Tung DK, Steelman VM, Chang PK, Szekendi MK. Retained surgical sponges: findings from incident reports and a cost-benefit analysis of radiofrequency technology. *J Am Coll Surg.* 2014;219(3):354-364. [IIIB]

36. Rupp CC, Kagarise MJ, Nelson SM, et al. Effectiveness of a radiofrequency detection system as an adjunct to manual counting protocols for tracking surgical sponges: a prospective trial of 2,285 patients. *J Am Coll Surg.* 2012;215(4):524-533. [IIIB]

37. Regenbogen SE, Greenberg CC, Resch SC, et al. Prevention of retained surgical sponges: a decision-analytic model predicting relative cost-effectiveness. *Surgery.* 2009;145(5):527-535. [IIIB]

38. Steelman VM. Sensitivity of detection of radiofrequency surgical sponges: a prospective, cross-over study. *Am J Surg.* 2011;201(2):233-237. [IIA]

39. Steelman VM, Alasagheirin MH. Assessment of radiofrequency device sensitivity for the detection of retained surgical sponges in patients with morbid obesity. *Arch Surg.* 2012;147(10):955-960. [IIA]

40. Thiels CA, Lal TM, Nienow JM, et al. Surgical never events and contributing human factors. *Surgery.* 2015;158(2):515-521. [IIIB]

41. Cima RR, Kollengode A, Storsveen AS, et al. A multidisciplinary team approach to retained foreign objects. *Jt Comm J Qual Patient Saf.* 2009;35(3):123-132. [VB]

42. Stawicki SP, Cook CH, Anderson HL 3rd, et al. Natural history of retained surgical items supports the need for team training, early recognition, and prompt retrieval. *Am J Surg.* 2014;208(1):65-72. [VA]

43. Card R, Sawyer M, Degnan B, et al. *Perioperative Protocol.* Bloomington, MN: Institute for Clinical Systems Improvement; March 2014. [IVA]

44. Statement on the prevention of retained foreign bodies after surgery. October 1, 2005. American College of Surgeons. https://www.facs.org/about-acs/statements/51-foreign-bodies. Accessed November 10, 2015. [IVB]

45. Martindell D. Update on the prevention of retained surgical items. *Penn Patient Saf Advis*. 2012;9(3):106-110. [IVB]

46. ECRI. Unintentionally retained surgical items. *Operating Room Risk Management*. 2012;2(Surgery):1. [VC]

47. Hempel S, Maggard-Gibbons M, Nguyen DK, et al. Wrong-site surgery, retained surgical items, and surgical fires: a systematic review of surgical never events. *JAMA Surg*. 2015;150(8):796-805. [IIIB]

48. Committee opinion no. 464: patient safety in the surgical environment. *Obstet Gynecol*. 2010;116(3):786-790. [IVB]

49. Reason J. Safety in the operating theatre—Part 2: human error and organisational failure. *Qual Saf Health Care*. 2005;14(1):56-60. [VB]

50. Riley R, Manias E, Polglase A. Governing the surgical count through communication interactions: implications for patient safety. *Qual Saf Health Care*. 2006;15(5):369-374. [IIIB]

51. *Sentinel Event Data: Root Causes by Event Type*, 2004-2014. The Joint Commission. http://www.jointcommission.org/assets/1/18/Root_Causes_by_Event_Type_2004-2014.pdf. Accessed November 10, 2015.

52. Gurses AP, Kim G, Martinez EA, et al. Identifying and categorising patient safety hazards in cardiovascular operating rooms using an interdisciplinary approach: a multisite study. *BMJ Qual Saf*. 2012;21(10):810-818. [IIIB]

53. Gurses AP, Martinez EA, Bauer L, et al. Using human factors engineering to improve patient safety in the cardiovascular operating room. *Work*. 2012;41(Suppl 1):1801-1804. [IIIB]

54. Standards of perioperative nursing. In: *Guidelines for Perioperative Practice*. Denver, CO: AORN, Inc; 2015:693-708. [IVB]

55. Loftus T, Dahl D, OHare B, et al. Implementing a standardized safe surgery program reduces serious reportable events. *J Am Coll Surg*. 2015;220(1):12-17.e3. [IIIA]

56. Yang YT, Henry L, Dellinger M, Yonish K, Emerson B, Seifert PC. The circulating nurse's role in error recovery in the cardiovascular OR. *AORN J*. 2012;95(6):755-762. [VB]

57. *Recommended Standard of Practice for Counts*. 2006. Association of Surgical Technologists. http://www.ast.org/uploadedFiles/Main_Site/Content/About_Us/Standard%20Counts.pdf. Accessed November 10, 2015. [IVC]

58. Camos V. Coordination process in counting. *Int J Psychol*. 2003;38(1):24-36. [IIIB]

59. Camos V. Counting strategies from 5 years to adulthood: adaptation to structural features. *Eur J Psychol Educ*. 2003;18(3):251-265. [IIIA]

60. Clark GJ. Strategies for preventing distractions and interruptions in the OR. *AORN J*. 2013;97(6):702-707. [VB]

61. AORN position statement on managing distractions and noise during perioperative patient care. *AORN J*. 2014;99(1):22-26. [IVB]

62. Iwai T, Goto T, Matsui Y, Tohnai I. Endoscopic removal of throat-packing gauze swallowed during general anesthesia. *J Craniofac Surg*. 2012;23(5):1547-1549. [VC]

63. Colbert S, Jackson M, Turner M, Brennan PA. Reducing the risk of retained throat packs after surgery. *Br J Oral Maxillofac Surg*. 2012;50(7):680-681. [VC]

64. Jennings A, Bhatt V. Throat packs: in your face? *Anaesthesia*. 2010;65(3):312-313. [VC]

65. Smith M, Turnbull D, Andrzejowski J. Throat packs in neuroanaesthesia. *Anaesthesia*. 2012;67(7):804-805. [IIIB]

66. Lyons VE, Popejoy LL. Meta-analysis of surgical safety checklist effects on teamwork, communication, morbidity, mortality, and safety. *West J Nurs Res*. 2014;36(2):245-261. [IIA]

67. Haynes AB, Weiser TG, Berry WR, et al. A surgical safety checklist to reduce morbidity and mortality in a global population. *N Engl J Med*. 2009;360(5):491-499. [IIA]

68. Collins SJ, Newhouse R, Porter J, Talsma A. Effectiveness of the surgical safety checklist in correcting errors: a literature review applying Reason's Swiss Cheese Model. *AORN J*. 2014;100(1):65-79. [VB]

69. McDowell DS, McComb SA. Safety checklist briefings: a systematic review of the literature. *AORN J*. 2014;99(1):125-137. [VB]

70. Borchard A, Schwappach DL, Barbir A, Bezzola P. A systematic review of the effectiveness, compliance, and critical factors for implementation of safety checklists in surgery. *Ann Surg*. 2012;256(6):925-933. [IIIA]

71. Wahr JA, Prager RL, Abernathy JH 3rd, et al; American Heart Association Council on Cardiovascular Surgery and Anesthesia Council on Cardiovascular and Stroke Nursing and Council on Quality of Care and Outcomes Research. Patient safety in the cardiac operating room: human factors and teamwork: a scientific statement from the American Heart Association. *Circulation*. 2013;128(10):1139-1169. [IVB]

72. Armour Forse R, Bramble JD, McQuillan R. Team training can improve operating room performance. *Surgery*. 2011;150(4):771-778. [VB]

73. Papaspyros SC, Javangula KC, Adluri RKP, O'Regan DJ. Briefing and debriefing in the cardiac operating room. Analysis of impact on theatre team attitude and patient safety. *Interact Cardiovasc Thorac Surg*. 2010;10(1):43-47. [VB]

74. Young-Xu Y, Neily J, Mills PD, et al. Association between implementation of a Medical Team Training program and surgical morbidity. *Arch Surg*. 2011;146(12):1368-1373. [IIIA]

75. Weaver SJ, Rosen MA, Diaz Granados D, et al. Does teamwork improve performance in the operating room? A multilevel evaluation. *Jt Comm J Qual Patient Saf*. 2010;36(3):133-142. [IIB]

76. Tibbs SM, Moss J. Promoting teamwork and surgical optimization: combining TeamSTEPPS with a specialty yeam protocol. *AORN J*. 2014;100(5):477-488. [VA]

77. Johnson HL, Kimsey D. Patient safety: break the silence. *AORN J*. 2012;95(5):591-601. [VB]

78. Guideline for a safe environment of care, part 2. In: *Guidelines for Perioperative Practice*. Denver, CO: AORN, Inc; 2015:265-290. [IVA]

79. Christian CK, Gustafson ML, Roth EM, et al. A prospective study of patient safety in the operating room. *Surgery*. 2006;139(2):159-173. [IIIB]

80. Rowlands A, Steeves R. Incorrect surgical counts: a qualitative analysis. *AORN J*. 2010;92(4):410-419. [IIIB]

81. Steelman VM, Cullen JJ. Designing a safer process to prevent retained surgical sponges: a healthcare failure mode and effect analysis. *AORN J*. 2011;94(2):132-141. [VB]

82. Ortuño F, Ojeda N, Arbizu J, et al. Sustained attention in a counting task: normal performance and functional neuroanatomy. *Neuroimage*. 2002;17(1):411-420. [IIIB]

83. Camos V, Barrouillet P. Adult counting is resource demanding. *Br J Psychol*. 2004;95(1):19-30. [IIIB]

84. Railo H, Koivisto M, Revonsuo A, Hannula MM. The role of attention in subitizing. *Cognition.* 2008;107(1):82-104. [IIIA]

85. Butler M, Ford R, Boxer E, Sutherland-Fraser S. Lessons from the field: an examination of count errors in the operating theatre. *ACORN.* 2010;23(3):6-16. [IIIB]

86. Edel EM. Surgical count practice variability and the potential for retained surgical items. *AORN J.* 2012;95(2):228-238. [VB]

87. Norton EK, Martin C, Micheli AJ. Patients count on it: an initiative to reduce incorrect counts and prevent retained surgical items. *AORN J.* 2012;95(1):109-121. [VB]

88. Grant-Orser A, Davies P, Singh SS. The lost sponge: patient safety in the operating room. *CMAJ.* 2012;184(11):1275-1278. [VA]

89. Gibbs VC. Thinking in three's: changing surgical patient safety practices in the complex modern operating room. *World J Gastroenterol.* 2012;18(46):6712-6719. [VB]

90. Boisvert MJ, Abroms BD, Roberts WA. Human nonverbal counting estimated by response production and verbal report. *Psychon Bull Rev.* 2003;10(3):683-690. [IIIB]

91. Logie RH, Baddeley AD. Cognitive processes in counting. *J Exp Psychol Learn Mem Cogn.* 1987;13(2):310-326. [IIIB]

92. Nan Y, Knösche TR, Luo Y-J. Counting in everyday life: discrimination and enumeration. *Neuropsychologia.* 2006;44(7):1103-1113. [IIIB]

93. Trick LM, Pylyshyn ZW. Why are small and large numbers enumerated differently? A limited-capacity preattentive stage in vision. *Psychol Rev.* 1994;101(1):80-102. [VA]

94. Goldfarb L, Levy S. Counting within the subitizing range: the effect of number of distractors on the perception of subset items. *PLoS One.* 2013;8(9):e74152. [IIIB]

95. Watson DG, Maylor EA, Bruce LAM. The efficiency of feature-based subitization and counting. *J Exp Psychol Hum Percept Perform.* 2005;31(6):1449-1462. [IIIB]

96. Mazza V, Pagano S, Caramazza A. Multiple object individuation and exact enumeration. *J Cogn Neurosci.* 2013;25(5):697-705. [IIIB]

97. Edel EM. Increasing patient safety and surgical team communication by using a count/time out board. *AORN J.* 2010;92(4):420-424. [VB]

98. Thomas J, Adcock F. A review of existing count practice in the operating suite to achieve best practice and safe patient care. *ACORN.* 2014;27(1):20-27. [VB]

99. Guideline for transfer of patient care information. In: *Guidelines for Perioperative Practice.* Denver, CO: AORN, Inc; 2015:583-588. [IVB]

100. Peloquin P, Vannemreddy PS, Watkins LM, Byrne RW. Intracranial cotton ball gossypiboma mimicking recurrent meningioma: report of a case with literature review for intentional and unintentional foreign body granulomas. *Clin Neurol Neurosurg.* 2012;114(7):1039-1041. [VC]

101. Cho SW, Jin HR. Gossypiboma in the nasal septum after septorhinoplasty: a case study. *J Oral Maxillofac Surg.* 2013;71(1):e42-e44. [VB]

102. Chang CY, Tsai EM, Wu CH, Wang CL, Liu CM, Long CY. Pelvic floor abscess secondary to gossypiboma following a total Prolift procedure. *Taiwan J Obstet Gynecol.* 2012;51(2):283-284. [VB]

103. Gibbs VC. Retained surgical items and minimally invasive surgery. *World J Surg.* 2011;35(7):1532-1539. [VA]

104. Agrawal A. Counting matters: lessons from the root cause analysis of a retained surgical item. *Jt Comm J Qual Patient Saf.* 2012;38(12):566-574. [VB]

105. Chagolla BA, Gibbs VC, Keats JP, Pelletreau B. A system-wide initiative to prevent retained vaginal sponges. *MCN Am J Matern Child Nurs.* 2011;36(5):312-317. [VB]

106. Garry DJ, Asanjarani S, Geiss DM. Policy for prevention of a retained sponge after vaginal delivery. *Case Rep Med.* 2012;2012:317856. [VB]

107. Healy P. Retained vaginal swabs: review of an adverse event in obstetrics through closed claims analysis. *Br J Midwifery.* 2012;20(9):666-669. [IIIB]

108. Lutgendorf MA, Schindler LL, Hill JB, Magann EF, O'Boyle JD. Implementation of a protocol to reduce occurrence of retained sponges after vaginal delivery. *Mil Med.* 2011;176(6):702-704. [VB]

109. Retained foreign objects during vaginal deliveries. Prevention of unintentionally. 4th ed. 2012. Institute for Clinical Systems Improvement. https://www.icsi.org/guidelines__more/catalog_guidelines_and_more/catalog_guidelines/catalog_patient_safetyreliability_guidelines/rfo/. Accessed November 10, 2015. [IVB]

110. Hyslop JW, Maull KI. Natural history of the retained surgical sponge. *South Med J.* 1982;75(6):657-660. [VB]

111. Wattanasirichaigoon S. Transmural migration of a retained surgical sponge into the intestinal lumen: an experimental study. *J Med Assoc Thai.* 1996;79(7):415-422. [IIB]

112. Gumus M, Gumus H, Kapan M, Onder A, Tekbas G, Bac B. A serious medicolegal problem after surgery: gossypiboma. *Am J Forensic Med Pathol.* 2012;33(1):54-57. [IIIB]

113. Kaplan M, Iyikosker HI. A new complication of retained surgical gauze: development of malignant fibrous histiocytoma—report of a case with a literature review. *World J Surg Oncol.* 2012;10:139. [VC]

114. Statler JD, Miller DL, Dixon RG, et al. Society of interventional radiology position statement: prevention of unintentionally retained foreign bodies during interventional radiology procedures. *J Vasc Interv Radiol.* 2011;22(11):1561-1562. [IVC]

115. Amr AE. A submandibular gossypiboma mimicking a salivary fistula: a case report. *Cases J.* 2009;2:6413. [VB]

116. Baruah BP, Young P, Douglas-Jones A, Mansel R. Retained surgical swab following breast augmentation: a rare cause of a breast mass. *BMJ Case Rep.* 2009;2009. http://www.ncbi.nlm.nih.gov/pmc/articles/PMC3028288/. Accessed November 10, 2015. [VB]

117. Fouelifack FY, Fouogue JT, Fouedjio JH, Sando Z. A case of abdominal textiloma following gynecologic surgery at the Yaounde Central Hospital, Cameroon. *Pan Afr Med J.* 2013;16:147. [VB]

118. Gencosmanoglu R, Inceoglu R. An unusual cause of small bowel obstruction: gossypiboma—case report. *BMC Surg.* 2003;3:6. [VB]

119. Irabor DO. Under-reporting of gossipiboma in a third-world country. A sociocultural view. *Niger J Med.* 2013;22(4):365-367. [VB]

120. Joshi MK, Jain BK, Rathi V, Agrawal V, Mohanty D. Complete enteral migration of retained surgical sponge—report of two cases. *Trop Gastroenterol.* 2011;32(3):229-232. [VC]

121. Kansakar R, Hamal BK. Cystoscopic removal of an intravesical gossypiboma mimicking a bladder mass: a case report. *J Med Case Rep.* 2011;5(1):579. [VC]

122. Karasaki T, Nomura Y, Nakagawa T, Tanaka N. Beware of gossypibomas. *BMJ Case Rep.* 2013;2013. [VC]

123. Kim KS. Changes in computed tomography findings according to the chronicity of maxillary sinus gossypiboma. *J Craniofac Surg.* 2014;25(4):e330-e333. [VC]

124. Kohli S, Singhal A, Tiwari B, Singhal S. Gossypiboma, varied presentations: a report of two cases. *J Clin Imaging Sci.* 2013;3:11. [VC]

125. Lundin K, Allen JE, Birk-Soerensen L. Gossypiboma after breast augmentation. *Case Rep Surg.* 2013;2013:808624. [VC]

126. Naama O, Quamous O, Elasri CA, et al. Textiloma: an uncommon complication of posterior lumbar surgery. *J Neuroradiol.* 2010;37(2):131-134. [VB]

127. Ogundiran T, Ayandipo O, Adeniji-Sofoluwe A, Ogun G, Oyewole O, Ademola A. Gossypiboma: complete transmural migration of retained surgical sponge causing small bowel obstruction. *BMJ Case Rep.* 2011;2011. http://www.ncbi.nlm.nih.gov/pmc/articles/PMC3128338/. Accessed November 10, 2015. [VC]

128. veli Ozkan O, Bas G, Akcakaya A, Sahin M. Transmural migration of a retained sponge through the rectum: a case report. *Balkan Med J.* 2011;28(1):94-95. [VC]

129. Quraishi AH. Beyond a gossypiboma. *Case Rep Surg.* 2012;2012:263841. [VB]

130. Sumer A, Carparlar MA, Uslukaya O, et al. Gossypiboma: retained surgical sponge after a gynecologic procedure. *Case Rep Med.* 2010;2010. http://www.ncbi.nlm.nih.gov/pmc/articles/PMC2929520/. Accessed November 10, 2015. [VC]

131. Nurse Left Sponge in Pt. During Preoperative Procedure: Case on Point: Burke v. AnMedHealth, 4828 SCCA(4/27/2011)-SC. *Nurs Law Regan Rep.* 2011;52(3):4. [VC]

132. Yuki K, Shiba D, Ota Y, Ozeki N, Murat D, Tsubota K. A new method to prevent loss of mitomycin C soaked sponges under the conjunctiva during trabeculectomy. *Br J Ophthalmol.* 2010;94(8):1111-1112. [VC]

133. Srivastava A, Kataria K, Chella VR. Prevention of gossypiboma. *Indian J Surg.* 2014;76(2):169. [VC]

134. McIntyre LK, Jurkovich GJ, Gunn ML, Maier RV. Gossypiboma: tales of lost sponges and lessons learned. *Arch Surg.* 2010;145(8):770-775. [VA]

135. Jagger J, Berguer R, Phillips EK, Parker G, Gomaa AE. Increase in sharps injuries in surgical settings versus nonsurgical settings after passage of national needlestick legislation. *J Am Coll Surg.* 2010;210(4):496-502. [VA]

136. Guideline for sharps safety. In: *Guidelines for Perioperative Practice.* Denver, CO: AORN, Inc; 2015:365-388. [IVA]

137. Kelly RJ, Whipple OC. Retained anvil after laparoscopic gastric bypass. *Surg Obes Relat Dis.* 2011;7(5):e13-e15. [VB]

138. Magalini S, Sermoneta D, Lodoli C, Vanella S, Di Grezia M, Gui D. The new retained foreign body! Case report and review of the literature on retained foreign bodies in laparoscopic bariatric surgery. *Eur Rev Med Pharmacol Sci.* 2012;16(Suppl 4):129-133. [VA]

139. Stephens M, Ruddle A, Young WT. An unusual complication of a dropped clip during laparoscopic cholecystectomy. *Surg Laparosc Endosc Percutan Tech.* 2010;20(3):e103-e104. [VC]

140. Chepla KJ, Wilhelm SM. Delayed mechanical small bowel obstruction caused by retained, free, intraperitoneal staple after laparoscopic appendectomy. *Surg Laparosc Endosc Percutan Techniq.* 2011;21(1):e19-e20. [VB]

141. Ozsoy M, Celep B, Ozsan I, Bal A, Ozkececi ZT, Arikan Y. A retained plastic protective cover mimicking malignancy: case report. *Int J Surg Case Rep.* 2013;4(12):1084-1087. [VC]

142. Toubia T, Sangha R. Retained vaginal foreign body in minimally invasive gynecological surgeries. *CRSLS MIS Case Reports.* 2014; e2014.00240. http://crsls.sls.org/wp-content/uploads/2014/11/13-00240.pdf. Accessed November 10, 2015. [VA]

143. Sakhel K, Hines J. To forget is human: the case of the retained bulb. *J Robotic Surg.* 2009;3(1):45-47. [VB]

144. FDA Public Health Notification: Unretrieved Device Fragments. US Food and Drug Administration. http://www.fda.gov/MedicalDevices/Safety/AlertsandNotices/PublicHealthNotifications/ucm062015.htm. Issued January 15, 2008. Accessed November 10, 2015.

145. Barrow CJ. Use of x-ray in the presence of an incorrect needle count. *AORN J.* 2001;74(1):80-81. [VB]

146. Ponrartana S, Coakley FV, Yeh BM, et al. Accuracy of plain abdominal radiographs in the detection of retained surgical needles in the peritoneal cavity. *Ann Surg.* 2008;247(1):8-12. [IIIB]

147. Use of x-rays for incorrect needle counts. *Pa Patient Saf Advis.* 2004;1(2):5-6. [IVC]

148. Kieval JZ, Walsh M, Legutko PA, Daly MK. Efficacy of portable X-ray in identifying retained suture needles in ophthalmologic cases. *Eye.* 2009;23(8):1731-1734. [IIIB]

149. Hacivelioglu S, Karatag O, Gungor AC, et al. Is there an advantage of three dimensional computed tomography scanning over plain abdominal radiograph in the detection of retained needles in the abdomen? *Int J Surg.* 2013;11(3):278-281. [IIIB]

150. Ren S, Liu P, Wang W, Yang Y. Retained foreign body after laser ablation. *Int Surg.* 2012;97(4):293-295. [VB]

151. Vannucci A, Jeffcoat A, Ifune C, Salinas C, Duncan JR, Wall M. Special article: retained guidewires after intraoperative placement of central venous catheters. *Anesth Analg.* 2013;117(1):102-108. [VB]

152. Song Y, Messerlian AK, Matevosian R. A potentially hazardous complication during central venous catheterization: lost guidewire retained in the patient. *J Clin Anesth.* 2012;24(3):221-226. [VB]

153. Omar HR, Sprenker C, Karlnoski R, Mangar D, Miller J, Camporesi EM. The incidence of retained guidewires after central venous catheterization in a tertiary care center. *Am J Emerg Med.* 2013;31(10):1528-1530. [VB]

154. Horberry T, Teng YC, Ward J, Patil V, Clarkson PJ. Guidewire retention following central venous catheterisation: a human factors and safe design investigation. *Int J Risk Saf Med.* 2014;26(1):23-37. [IIIB]

155. Ellett L, Maher P. Forgotten surgical items: lessons for all to learn: case report and 3-year audit of retained surgical items at a tertiary referral centre. *Gynecol Surg.* 2013;10(4):295-297. [VB]

156. 29 CFR 1910.1030. Occupational exposure. Bloodborne pathogens. 2009. Occupational Safety & Health Administration. https://www.osha.gov/pls/oshaweb/owadisp.show_document?p_table=STANDARDS&p_id=10051. Accessed November 10, 2015.

157. Parelkar SV, Sanghvi BV, Shetty SR, Athawale H, Oak SN. Needle in a haystack: intraoperative breakage of pediatric minimal access surgery instruments. *J Postgrad Med.* 2014;60(3):324-326. [VB]

158. Ruscher KA, Modeste KA, Staff I, Papasavas PK, Tishler DS. Retained needles in laparoscopic surgery: open or observe? *Conn Med.* 2014;78(4):197-202. [IIIB]

159. Barto W, Yazbek C, Bell S. Finding a lost needle in laparoscopic surgery. *Surg Laparosc Endosc Percutan Tech.* 2011;21(4):e163-e165. [IIIB]

160. Small AC, Gainsburg DM, Mercado MA, Link RE, Hedican SP, Palese MA. Laparoscopic needle-retrieval device for improving quality of care in minimally invasive surgery. *J Am Coll Surg.* 2013;217(3):400-405. [IIIB]

161. Jayadevan R, Stensland K, Small A, Hall S, Palese M. A protocol to recover needles lost during minimally invasive surgery. *JSLS.* 2014;18(4). http://www.ncbi.nlm.nih.gov/pmc/articles/PMC4254476/. Accessed November 10, 2015. [IIIB]

162. Kava BR, Burdick-Will J. Complications associated with retained foreign bodies from infected penile implants: proposal for the use of an implant-specific checklist at the time of device removal. *J Sex Med.* 2013;10(6):1659-1666. [VA]

163. Felder SI, Liou DZ, Gangi A. Gastric adjustable band as a retained foreign object: a case report. *Bariatr Surg Patient Care.* 2013;8(4):166-168. [VB]

164. Celkan MA, Bayatli K. A bulldog clamp that was forgotten during a coronary artery bypass operation 8 years ago. *Interact Cardiovasc Thorac Surg.* 2012;15(4):777-778. [VB]

165. Tulmac M, Ozer N, Ebinc H, Simsek V, Dogru MT. Uncomplicated retainment of metal coronary bulldog clips recognized five years after coronary artery bypass graft surgery. *Turk J Thorac Cardiovasc Surg.* 2011;19(3):432-433. [VC]

166. Massimiliano PA, Massimo PS. Retained intra-abdominal surgical instrument: a rare condition of acute abdomen. *ANZ J Surg.* 2010;80(10):758. [VC]

167. Thomas EJ, Moore FA. The missing suction tip. AHRQ WebM&M [serial online]. https://psnet.ahrq.gov/webmm/case/37/the-missing-suction-tip. Accessed November 10, 2015. [VC]

168. Bansal M, Heckl F, English K. Retained broken outflow cannula recovered 6 years post-knee arthroscopy. *Orthopedics.* 2011;34(12):e945-e947. [VB]

169. Ipaktchi K, Kolnik A, Messina M, Banegas R, Livermore M, Price C. Current surgical instrument labeling techniques may increase the risk of unintentionally retained foreign objects: a hypothesis. *Patient Saf Surg.* 2013;7(1):31. [VC]

170. Teixeira PG, Inaba K, Salim A, et al. Retained foreign bodies after emergent trauma surgery: incidence after 2526 cavitary explorations. *Am Surg.* 2007;73(10):1031-1034. [IIIB]

171. Murdock D. Trauma: when there's no time to count. *AORN J.* 2008;87(2):322-328. [VB]

172. Guideline for cleaning and care of surgical instruments. In: *Guidelines for Perioperative Practice.* Denver, CO: AORN, Inc; 2015:615-650. [IVA]

173. Reece M, Troeleman ND, McGowan JE, Furuno JP. Reducing the incidence of retained surgical instrument fragments. *AORN J.* 2011;94(3):301-304. [VB]

174. Fischer RA. Danger: beware of unretrieved device fragments. *Nursing.* 2007;37(11):17. [VB]

175. Pillarisetti J, Biria M, Balda A, Reddy N, Berenbom L, Lakkireddy D. Integrity of vascular access: the story of a broken sheath! *J Vasc Nurs.* 2009;27(3):75-77. [VB]

176. DerDerian T, Ascher E, Hingorani A, Jimenez R. A rare complication of a retained wire during endovascular abdominal aortic aneurysm repair. *Ann Vasc Surg.* 2013;27(8):1183.e11-1183.e15. [VB]

177. Augello M, von Jackowski J, Gratz KW, Jacobsen C. Needle breakage during local anesthesia in the oral cavity—a retrospective of the last 50 years with guidelines for treatment and prevention. *Clin Oral Investig.* 2011;15(1):3-8. [VB]

178. Malamed SF, Reed K, Poorsattar S. Needle breakage: incidence and prevention. *Dent Clin North Am.* 2010;54(4):745-756. [VB]

179. Pogrel MA. Broken local anesthetic needles: a case series of 16 patients, with recommendations. *J Am Dent Assoc.* 2009;140(12):1517-1522. [VA]

180. Catelani C, Valente A, Rossi A, Bertolai R. Broken anesthetic needle in the pterygomandibular space. Four case reports. *Minerva Stomatol.* 2013;62(11-12):455-463. [VB]

181. Kim SH, Huh K, Jee YS, Park MJ. Breakage of growth hormone needle in subcutaneous tissue. *J Spec Pediatr Nurs.* 2011;16(2):162-165. [VC]

182. Alexander G, Attia H. Oral maxillofacial surgery displacement complications. *Oral Maxillofac Surg Clin North Am.* 2011;23(3):379-386. [VA]

183. *State Operations Manual Appendix A: Survey Protocol, Regulations and Interpretive Guidelines for Hospitals.* Rev 116; 2014. Centers for Medicare & Medicaid Services. https://www.cms.gov/Regulations-and-Guidance/Guidance/Manuals/downloads/som107ap_a_hospitals.pdf. Accessed November 10, 2015.

184. *State Operations Manual Appendix L: Guidance for Surveyors: Ambulatory Surgical Centers.* Rev 99;2014. Centers for Medicare & Medicaid Services. https://www.cms.gov/Regulations-and-Guidance/Guidance/Manuals/downloads/som107ap_l_ambulatory.pdf. Accessed November 10, 2015.

185. Rowlands A. Risk factors associated with incorrect surgical counts. *AORN J.* 2012;96(3):272-284. [IIIB]

186. Hariharan D, Lobo DN. Retained surgical sponges, needles and instruments. *Ann R Coll Surg Engl.* 2013; 95(2):87-92. [VB]

187. Sencimen M, Bayar GR, Gulses A. Removal of the retained suture needle under C-arm fluoroscopy: a technical note. *Dent Traumatol.* 2010;26(6):527-529. [VC]

188. Huang J, Bouvette MJ, Chari R, Vuddagiri V, Kraemer MC, Zhou J. The detection of a retained sponge in the aorta by transesophageal echocardiography. *J Cardiothorac Vasc Anesth.* 2010;24(2):314-315. [VC]

189. Hunter TB, Gimber LH. Identification of retained surgical foreign objects: policy at a university medical center. *J Am Coll Radiol.* 2010;7(9):736-738. [VB]

190. Gayer G, Lubner MG, Bhalla S, Pickhardt PJ. Imaging of abdominal and pelvic surgical and postprocedural foreign bodies. *Radiol Clin North Am.* 2014;52(5):991-1027. [VA]

191. Asiyanbola B, Etienne-Cummings R, Lewi JS. Prevention and diagnosis of retained foreign bodies through the years: past, present, and future technologies. *Technol Health Care.* 2012;20(5):379-386. [VA]

192. Berkowitz S, Marshall H, Charles A. Retained intra-abdominal surgical instruments: time to use nascent technology? *Am Surg.* 2007;73(11):1083-1085. [VA]

193. Ellner SJ, Joyner PW. Information technologies and patient safety. *Surg Clin North Am.* 2012;92(1):79-87. [VA]

194. ECRI. Radio-frequency surgical sponge detection: a new way to lower the odds of leaving sponges (and similar items) in patients. *Health Devices.* 2008;37(7):193-203. [VC]

195. Electromagnetic Compatibility (EMC). Radio Frequency Identification (RFID). US Food and Drug Administration. http://www.fda.gov/Radiation-EmittingProducts/RadiationSafety/ElectromagneticCompatibilityEMC/ucm116647.htm. Accessed November 10, 2015.

196. Hadjiiski L, Marentis TC, Chaudhury AR, Rondon L, Chronis N, Chan HP. Computer aided detection of surgical retained foreign object for prevention. *Med Phys.* 2015;42(3):1213. [IIIB]

197. Guideline for product selection. In: *Guidelines for Perioperative Practice.* Denver, CO: AORN, Inc; 2015:179-186. [IVB]

198. Etchells E, Koo M, Daneman N, et al. Comparative economic analyses of patient safety improvement strategies in acute care: a systematic review. *BMJ Qual Saf.* 2012;21(6):448-456. [IIIA]

199. Greenberg CC, Diaz-Flores R, Lipsitz SR, et al. Barcoding surgical sponges to improve safety: a randomized controlled trial. *Ann Surg.* 2008;247(4):612-616. [IB]

200. Cima RR, Kollengode A, Clark J, et al. Using a data-matrix-coded sponge counting system across a surgical practice: impact after 18 months. *Jt Comm J Qual Patient Saf.* 2011;37(2):51-58. [VB]

201. Macario A, Morris D, Morris S. Initial clinical evaluation of a handheld device for detecting retained surgical gauze sponges using radiofrequency identification technology. *Arch Surg.* 2006;141(7):659-662. [IIC]

202. Fabian CE. Electronic tagging of surgical sponges to prevent their accidental retention. *Surgery.* 2005;137(3):298-301. [IIB]

203. Rogers A, Jones E, Oleynikov D. Radio frequency identification (RFID) applied to surgical sponges. *Surg Endosc.* 2007;21(7):1235-1237. [IIIB]

204. Guideline for environmental cleaning. In: *Guidelines for Perioperative Practice.* Denver, CO: AORN, Inc; 2015:9-30. [IVA]

205. Kranzfelder M, Schneider A, Fiolka A, et al. Real-time instrument detection in minimally invasive surgery using radiofrequency identification technology. *J Surg Res.* 2013;185(2):704-710. [IIIB]

206. Neumuth T, Meissner C. Online recognition of surgical instruments by information fusion. *Int J Comput Assist Radiol Surg.* 2012;7(2):297-304. [IIIB]

207. Guideline for sterilization. In: *Guidelines for Perioperative Practice.* Denver, CO: AORN, Inc; 2015:665-692. [IVA]

208. Yamashita K, Kusuda K, Tokuda Y, et al. Validation of cleaning evaluation of surgical instruments with RFID tags attached based on cleaning appraisal judgment guidelines. *Conference Proceedings: Annual International Conference of the IEEE Engineering in Medicine & Biology Society*; 2013:926-929. [IIC]

209. Guideline for health care information management. In: *Guidelines for Perioperative Practice.* Denver, CO: AORN, Inc; 2015:491-512. [IVB]

210. LD.04.01.07: The hospital has policies and procedures that guide and support patient care, treatment, and services. In: *Hospital Accreditation Standards.* Oakbrook Terrace, IL: Joint Commission Resources; 2014.

211. SS.1: Organization. In: *NIAHO Interpretive Guidelines and Surveyor Guidance.* 10.1 ed. Milford, OH: DNV Healthcare Inc; 2012:70-71.

212. *2014 Accreditation Requirements for Acute Care Facilities.* Chicago, IL: Healthcare Facilities Accreditation Program; 2014.

213. Burton JL. Health and safety at necropsy. *J Clin Pathol.* 2003;56(4):254-260. [VC]

214. Karl R, Karl MC. Adverse events: root causes and latent factors. *Surg Clin North Am.* 2012;92(1):89-100. [VB]

215. Elbardissi AW, Sundt TM. Human factors and operating room safety. *Surg Clin North Am.* 2012;92(1):21-35. [VA]

216. Boysen PG 2nd. Just culture: a foundation for balanced accountability and patient safety. *Ochsner J.* 2013;13(3):400-406. [VB]

217. LD.04.04.05 The hospital has an organization-wide, integrated patient safety program within its performance improvement activities. In: *Hospital Accreditation Standards.* Oakbrook Terrace, IL: Joint Commission Resources; 2015.

218. American Association for Accreditation of Ambulatory Surgery Facilities. Quality assessment/quality improvement: quality improvement. In: *Regular Standards and Checklist for Accreditation of Ambulatory Surgery Facilities.* Version 14 ed. Gurnee, IL: American Association for Accreditation of Ambulatory Surgery Facilities; 2014:65.

219. Quality management system. In: *NIAHO Interpretive Guidelines and Surveyor Guidance.* 10.1 ed. Milford, OH: DNV Healthcare Inc; 2012:10-16.

220. Quality management and improvement. In: *2014 Accreditation Handbook for Ambulatory Health Care.* Skokie, IL: Accreditation Association for Ambulatory Health Care; 2014:32-36.

221. Bell R. Hide and seek, the search for a missing swab: a critical analysis. *J Perioper Pract.* 2012;22(5):151-156. [VA]

222. *Serious Reportable Events in Healthcare—2011 Update: A Consensus Report.* Washington, DC: National Quality Forum; 2011.

Acknowledgements

LEAD AUTHOR
Amber Wood, MSN, RN, CNOR, CIC
Senior Perioperative Practice Specialist
AORN Nursing Department
Denver, Colorado

CONTRIBUTING AUTHOR
Ramona L. Conner, MSN, RN, CNOR
Editor-in-Chief, Guidelines for Perioperative Practice
AORN Nursing Department
Denver, Colorado

The authors and AORN thank David L. Feldman, MD, MBA, CPE, FACS, Senior Vice President and Chief Medical Officer, Hospitals Insurance Company, New York, New York; Victoria Steelman, PhD, RN, CNOR, FAAN, Associate Professor, University of Iowa, Iowa City; Amy L. Halverson, MD, Associate Professor of Surgery, Northwestern University, Chicago, Illinois; Judith L. Goldberg, DBA, MSN, RN, CNOR, CSSM, CHL, Director, Patient Care Services, Perioperative and Procedural Services, Lawrence + Memorial Hospital, New London, Connecticut; Barbara L. Nalley, MSN, CRNP, CNOR, Manager, Anne Arundel Medical Group, Annapolis, Maryland; Deborah F. Mulloy, PhD, RN, CNOR, Associate Chief Nurse, Quality & Center for Nursing Excellence, Brigham & Womens Hospital, Newtonville, Massachusetts; Jocelyn M. Chalquist, BSN, RN, CNOR, Surgical Services Educator, Aurora Medical Center-Kenosha, Kenosha, Wisconsin; Janice Neil, PhD, RN, CNE, Associate Professor, College of Nursing, East Carolina University, Greenville, North Carolina; Aileen R. Killen, RN, PhD, CPPS, Director, Patient Safety Program, Memorial Sloan Kettering Cancer Center, New York, New York;

Lisa Spruce, DNP, RN, CNS-CP, ACNS, ACNP, CNOR, FAAN, Director of Evidence-based Perioperative Practice, AORN Nursing Department, Denver, Colorado; Jay Bowers, BSN, RN, CNOR, TNCC, Clinical Educator, WVU Health Care, Morgantown, West Virginia; Sandy Albright, MSHM, BSN, RN, CNOR, Clinical Consultant, Cardinal Health, Dublin, Ohio; and Christine Anderson, PhD, RN, Clinical Assistant Professor, University of Michigan School of Nursing, Division of Health Systems and Effectiveness Science, Ann Arbor, Michigan, for their assistance in developing this guideline..

PUBLICATION HISTORY

Originally published May 1976, *AORN Journal*, as "Standards for sponge, needle, and instrument procedures."

Format revision March 1978, July 1982.

Revised March 1984, March 1990.

Revised November 1995; published October 1996, *AORN Journal*.

Revised; published December 1999, *AORN Journal*.

Reformatted July 2000.

Revised November 2005; published as Recommended Practices for Sponge, Sharp, and Instrument Counts in *Standards, Recommended Practices, and Guidelines*, 2006 edition.

Reprinted February 2006, *AORN Journal*.

Revised July 2010 for online publication in *Perioperative Standards and Recommended Practices*.

Reformatted September 2012 for publication in *Perioperative Standards and Recommended Practices*, 2013 edition.

Minor editing revisions made in November 2014 for publication in *Guidelines for Perioperative Practice*, 2015 edition, as Guideline for Prevention of Retained Surgical Items.

Revised January 2016 for publication in *Guidelines for Perioperative Practice*, 2016 edition.

Minor editing revisions made in October 2016 for publication in *Guidelines for Perioperative Practice*, 2017 edition.

PATIENT AND WORKER SAFETY

AMBULATORY SUPPLEMENT: RETAINED SURGICAL ITEMS

Recommendation VI

Standardized measures for reconciling count discrepancies should be taken during the closing count and before the end of surgery. When a discrepancy in the count is identified, the surgical team should take actions to locate the missing item.[A1-A6]

VI.c.2. If intraoperative imaging is not available, the health care organization should have a policy and procedure describing the actions and communication required between referring and receiving organizations. *[5: Benefits Balanced with Harms]*

Amb The ambulatory surgery facility should have a policy and procedure describing actions to take when on-site radiology services are not available to perform a radiograph and interpret the result.

Amb A surgeon with perioperative radiologic privileges may consider using fluoroscopy to locate the retained item.[A7]

Amb Fluoroscopy may be used and a reading obtained by a surgeon with privileges to interpret radiographic studies.[A7]

Recommendation IX

Policies and procedures for the prevention of RSIs [retained surgical items] should be developed, reviewed periodically, revised as necessary, and readily available in the practice setting.

IX.a. A multidisciplinary team should develop policies and procedures for preventing RSIs.[A4,A5,A8] *[2: High Evidence]*

IX.b.2. If intraoperative imaging is not available, the health care organization should have a policy and procedure describing actions necessary and communication required between referring and receiving organizations. *[5: Benefits Balanced with Harms]*

Amb Policies and procedures should include circumstances in which the patient should be transferred to the postanesthesia care unit and/or a subsequent receiving facility for further radiologic imaging.

References

A1. The Joint Commission. Preventing unintended retained foreign objects. *Sentinel Event Alert.* October 17, 2013;51. http://www.jointcommission.org/sea_issue_51/. Accessed November 10, 2015. [IVB].

A2. Moffatt-Bruce SD, Cook CH, Steinberg SM, Stawicki SP. Risk factors for retained surgical items: a meta-analysis and proposed risk stratification system. *J Surg Res.* 2014;190(2):429-436. [IIIA]

A3. Lincourt AE, Harrell A, Cristiano J, Sechrist C, Kercher K, Heniford BT. Retained foreign bodies after surgery. *J Surg Res.* 2007;138(2):170-174. [IIIB]

A4. Stawicki SP, Moffatt-Bruce SD, Ahmed HM, et al. Retained surgical items: a problem yet to be solved. *J Am Coll Surg.* 2013;216(1):15-22. [IIIB]

A5. *WHO Guidelines for Safe Surgery 2009.* Geneva, Switzerland: WHO Press; 2009. [IVB]

A6. Card R, Sawyer M, Degnan B, et al. *Perioperative Protocol.* Bloomington, MN: Institute for Clinical Systems Improvement; March 2014. [IVA]

A7. §482.26(b)(4). In: Centers for Medicare & Medicaid Services. *State Operations Manual Appendix L—Guidance for Surveyors: Ambulatory Surgical Centers.* Rev 137; 2015. https://www.cms.gov/Regulations-and-Guidance/Guidance/Manuals/downloads/som107ap_l_ambulatory.pdf. Accessed November 19, 2015.

A8. Statement on the prevention of retained foreign bodies after surgery. October 1, 2005. American College of Surgeons. https://www.facs.org/about-acs/statements/51-foreign-bodies. Accessed November 10, 2015. [IVB]

Publication History

Originally published in *Perioperative Standards and Recommended Practices*, 2014 edition.

Revised January 2016 for publication in *Guidelines for Perioperative Practice*, 2016 edition.

PATIENT AND WORKER SAFETY

Ambulatory Surgery

GUIDELINE FOR SHARPS SAFETY

The following Guideline for Sharps Safety has been approved by the AORN Recommended Practices Advisory Board. It was presented as proposed recommendations for comments by members and others. The guideline is effective June 15, 2013. The recommendations in the guideline are intended to be achievable and represent what is believed to be an optimal level of practice. Policies and procedures will reflect variations in practice settings and/or clinical situations that determine the degree to which the guideline can be implemented. AORN recognizes the various settings in which perioperative nurses practice; therefore, this guideline is adaptable to various practice settings. These practice settings include traditional operating rooms (ORs), ambulatory surgery centers, physicians' offices, cardiac catheterization laboratories, endoscopy suites, radiology departments, and all other areas where operative and other invasive procedures may be performed.

Purpose

This document provides guidance to perioperative registered nurses (RNs) in identifying potential sharps hazards and developing and implementing best practices to prevent sharps injuries and reduce bloodborne pathogen exposure to perioperative patients and personnel.

Health care workers are at risk for percutaneous injury, exposure to bloodborne pathogens, and occupational transmission of disease.[1] Annually, an estimated 384,325 hospital health care workers sustain a percutaneous injury.[2] When non-hospital health care workers are included, the number increases to more than 500,000.[3] Percutaneous injuries are associated primarily with occupational transmission of hepatitis B virus (HBV), hepatitis C virus (HCV), and HIV, but also may be implicated in the transmission of other pathogens.[1,3-17] A 2006 review of pathogens transmitted in published cases since 1966 showed transmission of 60 pathogens or species, which included 26 viruses, 18 bacteria or Rickettsia, 13 parasites, and three yeasts.[18]

The occupational risk of HBV transmission is dependent on the level of exposure to blood and the type of hepatitis B antigens.[19] Since the widespread adoption of HBV immunizations, the number of HBV infections in health care workers has declined significantly.[19-23] The reported number of HBV-infected providers in 1983 was 10,000 compared to approximately 100 in 2009.[20,21] The rate of anti-HCV seroconversion after an occupational exposure to HCV positive blood ranges from 0% to 7% with an average rate of 1.8%.[13,19,21,24,25] Although the risk of occupational transmission of HIV depends on the type and severity of the exposure,[19,26-28] the average risk is 0.3%.[12,19,26,28,29]

Percutaneous injuries carry risks not only to perioperative personnel but to patients as well.[20,21,25,30-33] If a health care worker infected with a bloodborne pathogen experiences a percutaneous injury and the object that caused the injury reconnects with the patient or the health care worker's glove perforation is undetected, the patient is at risk for infection.[34] There have been 132 documented cases of health care provider to patient transmission of HBV, HCV, or HIV worldwide.[17,20,31,35-37]

The bloodborne pathogens standard 29 CFR 1910.1030 became effective March 6,1992.[38] The standard includes definitions, an exposure control plan, engineering and work practice controls (eg, personal protective equipment [PPE]), vaccinations, postexposure follow-up, employee training, and record keeping.[38] The purpose of the bloodborne pathogen standard is to limit health care worker exposure to HBV, HCV, HIV, and other potentially infectious materials in the workplace through the implementation of engineering and work practice controls.[39]

The Needlestick Safety and Prevention Act was signed into law on November 6, 2000.[40] The act directs the Occupational Safety and Health Administration (OSHA) to revise the bloodborne pathogens standard. The revisions included adding engineering control definitions; including requirements for technology changes that eliminate or reduce bloodborne pathogen exposure in exposure control plans; including input from frontline, non-managerial employees in the identification, evaluation, and selection of safety-engineered devices and work practice controls; annually documenting the evaluation in the exposure control plan; including employee input in the exposure control plan; and maintaining a sharps injury log.[40-42]

Sharps injury prevention is a concern for all members of the perioperative team. Many perioperative professional associations have developed sharps safety position and guidance statements. AORN adopted its "Position statement on workplace safety" in 2003, identifying bloodborne pathogen exposures from percutaneous injuries as a risk in the perioperative environment.[43] The "AORN guidance statement: Sharps injury prevention in the perioperative setting," published in 2005, assisted perioperative nurses in developing sharps injury prevention programs and provided strategies to overcome compliance obstacles. Risk-reduction strategies included double gloving, using the neutral or hands-free zone, and using safety-engineered devices.[44]

The Association of Surgical Technologists (AST) adopted its "Guideline statement for the implementation of the neutral zone in the perioperative environment" in 2006.[45] The AST "Recommended standards of practice for sharps safety and use of the neutral zone" were developed the same year to provide support for and reinforce sharps safety and the use of a neutral zone.[46]

The American Academy of Orthopaedic Surgeons issued a statement on preventing the transmission of bloodborne pathogens in 2001.[32] Prevention strategies included employers establishing a prevention and treatment-of-exposure plan, providing PPE, and promoting double gloving and the use of a neutral zone.[32]

The American College of Surgeons (ACS) developed and approved its statement on sharps safety [ST-58] in 2007. The ACS recommends the universal adoption of double gloving, using blunt suture needles to close the fascia and muscle, using hands-free techniques, and using sharps injury prevention devices.[47]

The Council on Surgical & Perioperative Safety (CSPS)—a member organization composed of AORN, the American Association of Nurse Anesthetists, the American Association of Surgical Physician Assistants, the ACS, the American Society of Anesthesiologists, the American Society of PeriAnesthesia Nurses, and the AST—endorsed sharps safety measures to prevent injury during perioperative care. Sharps safety measures should include double gloving, using blunt suture needles for closing facia and muscle, and using a neutral zone when appropriate to avoid hand-to-hand passage of sharps. The CSPS sharps statement was adopted in 2007 and modified in 2009.[48]

In November 2010, a consensus statement and call to action was drafted by members of the steering committee at the 10th Anniversary of the Needlestick Safety and Prevention Act: Mapping Progress, Charting a Future Path conference, sponsored by the International Healthcare Worker Safety Center at the University of Virginia. The consensus statement was released in 2012 and endorsed by 20 organizations. It lists improving sharps safety in surgical settings as the number-one priority to reduce percutaneous injuries.[49]

In a joint safety communication, the US Food and Drug Administration (FDA), the National Institute for Occupational Safety and Health (NIOSH), and OSHA encourage health care professionals in surgical settings to use blunt-tip suture needles for suturing muscle and fascia when it is clinically appropriate.[50] Blunt-tip suture needles reduce the risk of needlestick injury and the risk of bloodborne pathogen transmission.[50]

Understanding the etiology of percutaneous injuries in the perioperative setting is paramount to developing a sharps injury prevention program. The perioperative setting is a high-risk environment for exposure to bloodborne pathogens from percutaneous injuries.[51] The International Healthcare Worker Safety Center at the University of Virginia compared percutaneous injury surveillance data of 87 participating hospitals before and after the passage of the Needlestick Safety and Prevention Act of 2000. The analysis showed a 6.5% increase in injuries in the surgical setting compared to a 31.6% decrease in nonsurgical settings.[36,51] There were 7,186 sharps injuries to surgical personnel reported between 1993 and 2006.[51] When surgeons and

surgical residents sustained a sharps injury, they were the original user of the device in 81.9% and 67.3% of the injuries, respectively. Nurses and surgical technologists were injured by devices used by others in 77.2% and 85.1% of the injuries, respectively. The majority of injuries occur to surgeons and surgical residents during use, while the sharps injuries to nurses and surgical technologists occur during passing, disassembling, and disposal.[51] The perioperative environment is unique in health care.[51] Perioperative personnel are at a distinct risk of percutaneous injury because of the presence of large quantities of blood and other potentially infectious body fluids, prolonged exposure to open surgical sites, frequent handling of sharp instruments, and the requirement for coordination between team members while passing sharp surgical instruments.[51,52]

An economic analysis of a retrospective survey estimated the effect of an occupational exposure from a needlestick injury. Associated costs included post-exposure health services, post-exposure testing, post-exposure prophylaxis, missed work days, and loss of productivity. Based on the findings, researchers projected the national economic burden per year at $65 million.[53] A convenience sample of health care facilities provided information on the cost of managing an occupational exposure, including reporting time, follow-up, salaries, and laboratory testing of the source individual and exposed health care worker. Overall costs ranged from $71 to $4,838 per exposure.[54] An analysis of the estimated costs of needlestick injuries and subsequent infections for hospital and non-hospital-based health care workers for testing, prophylaxis, and long-term infection suggests a range of $100.7 million to $405.9 million annually based on 2004 statistics.[55] The emotional burden of an occupationally acquired infection to the health care worker and his or her family members and the time spent waiting and wondering cannot be measured.[56]

Sharps safety is a priority in the perioperative environment and includes considerations for standard precautions, health care worker vaccination, post-exposure protocols and follow-up treatment, and treatment for health care workers infected with a bloodborne pathogen. These topics are addressed in other AORN guidelines, and although they are mentioned briefly where applicable (eg, standard precautions), broader discussions of these topics are outside the scope of this document.

Evidence Review

A medical librarian conducted a systematic review of MEDLINE®, CINAHL®, Scopus®, and the Cochrane Database of Systematic Reviews for meta-analyses, randomized and nonrandomized trials and studies, systematic and nonsystematic reviews, guidelines, case reports, and opinion documents and letters. Search terms included *needlestick injuries, sharps injuries, blood-borne pathogens, occupational accidents, occupational injuries, medical staff, nurses, perioperative nursing, operating room nursing, perioperative nurses, operating room nurses, operating rooms, surgical*

PATIENT AND WORKER SAFETY

procedures, surgical instruments, safety devices, sutures, scalpels, sharps, scalpel injuries, needlesticks, needle sticks, safety scalpels, safety-engineered sharps, blunt-tip needles, hands-free passing, neutral zone, double gloving, and *double-gloving.*

The lead author and medical librarian identified and obtained relevant guidelines from government agencies, other professional organizations, and standards-setting bodies. The lead author assessed additional professional literature, including some that initially appeared in other articles provided to the author.

The initial search was conducted in 2011 and was limited to articles published in English from 1992, when OSHA's Bloodborne Pathogens Final Standard was established. The librarian established continuing alerts on sharps safety-related topics and provided relevant results to the lead author. The lead author and medical librarian also identified relevant guidelines from accreditation organizations, government agencies, and standards-setting bodies. In addition, the lead author requested other articles identified through literature appraisal and other outside sources.

Articles identified by the search were provided to the project team for evaluation. The team consisted of the lead author, three members of the Recommended Practices Advisory Board, two members of the Research Committee, and a doctorally prepared evidence appraiser. The lead author divided the search results into topics and assigned members of the team to review and critically appraise each article using the Johns Hopkins Evidence-Based Practice Model and the Research or Non-Research Evidence Appraisal Tools as appropriate. The literature was independently evaluated and appraised according to the strength and quality of the evidence. Each article was then assigned an appraisal score as agreed upon by consensus of the team. The appraisal score is noted in brackets after each reference, as applicable. The collective evidence supporting each intervention within a specific recommendation was summarized and used to rate the strength of the evidence using the AORN Evidence Rating Model. Factors considered in review of the collective evidence were the quality of research, quantity of similar studies on a given topic, and consistency of results supporting a recommendation. The evidence rating is noted in brackets after each intervention.

Editor's note: *MEDLINE is a registered trademark of the US National Library of Medicine's Medical Literature Analysis and Retrieval System, Bethesda, MD. CINAHL, Cumulative Index to Nursing and Allied Health Literature, is a registered trademark of EBSCO Industries, Birmingham, AL. Scopus is a registered trademark of Elsevier B.V., Amsterdam, Netherlands.*

Recommendation I

Health care facilities must establish a written bloodborne pathogens exposure control plan.[38]

Bloodborne pathogens are pathogenic microorganisms that are present in human blood and can cause disease (eg, HBV, HCV, HIV).[28] Federal and state regulations and organizational standards that mandate bloodborne pathogen guidelines are intended to reduce health care provider exposure and to minimize the risk of infection.[38,57] The bloodborne pathogens standard 29 CFR 1910.1030 includes a requirement for an exposure control plan.[38]

I.a.   The exposure control plan must be reviewed and updated at least annually and whenever new or modified tasks or procedures are implemented.[38] *[1: Regulatory Requirement]*

I.a.1.   The review and update should include changes in technology that reduce or eliminate bloodborne pathogen exposure[38] and should document the annual trial and implementation of effective, commercially available, safer medical devices that are designed to eliminate or minimize bloodborne pathogen exposure.[38]

I.a.2.   The employer must ask for input from non-managerial employees responsible for direct patient care who may potentially be exposed to injuries from contaminated sharps to identify, evaluate, and select effective engineering and work practice controls. The employer must document the process in the exposure control plan.[38]

I.b.   The employer must prepare an exposure determination of any employee with the potential for exposure to bloodborne pathogens.[38] *[1: Regulatory Requirement]*

I.b.1.   The exposure determination must include a list of all job classifications that place any employee in that classification at risk for bloodborne pathogen exposure.[38]

I.b.2.   The exposure determination must be based on the level of risk when the employee is wearing no PPE.[38]

I.c.   As part of the written bloodborne pathogens exposure control plan, the organization's plan to reduce sharps injuries should include
   ○ a profile of how sharps injuries occur,
   ○ the occupational group sustaining the most injuries,
   ○ the location (ie, department, work area) where the injuries occur,
   ○ the sharps devices involved in the injuries,
   ○ the procedures (eg, recapping needles) that most commonly contribute to sharps injuries, and
   ○ the sharps injury reduction devices that have been implemented.[4]
   [1: Strong Evidence]
   Monitoring sharps injury data allows results to be compared to a predetermined level of quality. Reviewing the findings provides information to identify problems and trends, which can be used to improve practice.[4,13]

I.d. The priority of risk-reduction strategies should be determined and should be based on the greatest risk of bloodborne pathogen exposure, frequency of injury, and problem-prone areas with frequent sharps injuries.[4] *[1: Strong Evidence]*

Analysis of sharps injury logs or other sharps surveillance programs aids in identifying the types of injuries, types of devices, frequency of injuries, and work areas where exposure has occurred.[58]

I.d.1. Sharps hazard control methods should be based on a hierarchy of controls to include
- elimination of the hazard,
- engineering controls,
- work practice controls,
- administrative controls, and
- PPE.[13,24,59,60]

Elimination of the hazard includes removing the sharp object from use (eg, using electrosurgery instead of a scalpel for the incision). Engineering controls include using a safety-engineered device (eg, safety scalpel). Work practice controls include using a neutral or safe zone for passing sharp instruments and devices and wearing proper PPE, including double gloving.[24,59,60] Administrative controls include developing policies and procedures, incorporating sharps safety prevention into a new or existing committee structure, implementing an exposure control plan, and providing education and training.

I.e. The health care organization must establish a process for selecting and evaluating sharps safety devices as part of the written bloodborne pathogens exposure control plan.[24,38] *[1: Regulatory Requirement]*

I.e.1. A multidisciplinary committee that includes frontline workers should develop, implement, and evaluate a plan to reduce sharps injuries in the perioperative setting and to evaluate sharps safety devices.[24,61] The multidisciplinary team may include representatives from clinical staff, materials management, infection prevention and control, risk management, administration, occupational health, sterile processing, environmental cleaning services, and waste management, depending on the device being evaluated.[61]

I.e.2. Priorities should be identified and should be based on the mechanism of sharps injuries, frequency of injuries, procedure-specific risks, relative risk of disease transmission, and the devices involved in sharps injuries.[24,61] Highest priority should be given to the device that will have the greatest effect on reducing sharps injuries.[24,61]

I.e.3. Device selection factors should include patient and worker safety, efficiency, user acceptability, and overall performance.[24] Safety features should be simple, reliable, clear, and easily understood.[61]

Safety device design may be passive, active, or integrated, or a safety device may be an accessory.[62] A passive safety device requires no worker action for the safety feature to function. An active safety device requires the worker to take an action to initiate the safety feature.[62] A multicenter study of different types of safety-engineered devices showed that passive devices are associated with fewer sharps injuries.[62] An integrated safety design is an integral part of the device. An accessory safety device is an external feature to the device that is affixed either temporarily or permanently.[61]

I.e.4. Product evaluation should be accomplished by a representative group of frontline users of the safety device who have been educated and trained in the correct use of the device. The length of the evaluation period should be established, and a survey tool that includes the criteria and measures for the evaluation should be used.[24,61]

Factors that may influence product evaluation outcomes include the end user's experience with the safety device and the current device in use, the end user's previous experience in product evaluations, the product evaluation team members' attitudes and involvement, and the end user's peer opinions, as well as time intervals between distribution of the product and the survey, self-selection biases,[61] and the availability of the current product during the evaluation period.

I.e.5. The survey form should be easy to complete and score (eg, a Likert-type scale), limited to a single page, contain established performance criteria, have space for comments, and collect product user information (eg, name, title).[61]

I.e.6. Final product selection should be based on data analysis of the completed product evaluation forms.[61,63]

I.e.7. Final product selection should not be based on cost alone.[63] Cost analysis should include the cost of the sharps safety product, the potential cost savings of reducing or eliminating sharps injuries, and the cost of educating and training personnel.[61]

I.e.8. After the introduction of a new safety device, an assessment should be performed to evaluate acceptance, correct usage, usage rate, device performance, and the effect on the rate of sharps injuries.[24]

I.e.9. Safety-engineered devices must be evaluated annually.[38] Current devices should be evaluated for efficacy in reducing or preventing sharps injuries.[64] If current devices are not preventing sharps injuries, new devices should be evaluated.[42]

I.e.10. The safety-engineered device product evaluation process must be documented as part of the exposure control plan.[38,42]

I.f. The exposure control plan must be accessible to all employees.[38] *[1: Regulatory Requirement]*

Recommendation II

Perioperative personnel must use sharps with safety-engineered devices (ie, engineering controls).[38]

The Needlestick Safety and Prevention Act of 2000 mandates that employers provide safety-engineered devices in the health care setting to prevent sharps injuries.[40] According to OSHA, engineering controls are safety-engineered devices that isolate or remove the risk of a bloodborne pathogen exposure.[38] Safety-engineered devices include sharps with engineered sharps injury protection (SESIP) and needleless systems. A SESIP is a sharp with a built-in safety feature or mechanism that reduces the risk of a bloodborne pathogen exposure, such as safety or sheathed scalpels, blunt suture needles, and safety syringes and needles.

Sharps injuries increase the risk of bloodborne pathogen exposure in the OR. A review of 17 studies that evaluated safety-engineered device implementation and percutaneous injury rates showed a substantial decrease in percutaneous injuries after implementation of safety-engineered devices in all of the studies. The range of percutaneous injury reduction was 22% to 100%.[65] Researchers conducting a multisite survey compared the injury rates of different safety-engineered devices. During the time frame of the study, 22 million safety-engineered devices were purchased and evaluated with the conclusion that passive (ie, automatic) safety-engineered devices are the most effective in preventing percutaneous injuries.[62]

In a quasi-experimental trial with before-and-after intervention evaluations, researchers reported a 93% reduction in relative risk when safety devices were used. The researchers concluded that the proper use of safety-engineered devices is an effective measure to prevent percutaneous injuries.[66]

Researchers conducted a controlled, retrospective, interventional study of safety-engineered device implementation. Percutaneous injuries resulting from a safety-engineered device (ie, an intravenous catheter stylet with a retractable protection shield) were compared to sharp suture needle injuries in the control group. There was a statistically significant decrease in percutaneous injuries from intravenous catheter styli during the 18-month study period. Percutaneous injury rates from sharp suture needles increased from 5.3 to 10.7 per 1,000 health care workers during the same 18-month period.[67]

Researchers using the Massachusetts Sharps Injury Surveillance System examined trends in sharps injury rates by occupation, hospital size, and device. Seventy-six hospitals reported 16,158 sharps injuries to the surveillance system. During the five-year surveillance period, the overall annual sharps injury rate declined by 22%. Injury rates decreased when sharps with engineered sharps injury protection devices were available and used.[68]

The International Healthcare Worker Safety Center at the University of Virginia analyzed 16,871 sharp object injuries using data collected through the EPI-Net™ system. The data analysis found that 94% of the reported injuries were caused by a conventional device and only 6% were caused by a safety-engineered device.[58]

Researchers conducting a retrospective review of 161 injuries found that an estimated 65% of the injuries could have been prevented by using a device with safety-engineered features.[69] A prospective study of 952 health care worker occupational needlestick injuries estimated that 52% could have been prevented by use of a safety-engineered device.[70]

II.a. Blunt suture needles should be used unless clinically contraindicated (eg, scarred or thick fascia). [14,47,48,50,71-74] *[1: Strong Evidence]*

Blunt suture needles may prevent percutaneous injuries. Sharp suture needles account for 51% to 77% of the percutaneous injuries to surgical personnel.[52,75,76] Blunt suture needles decrease the occurrence of glove perforations, percutaneous injuries, and exposure risks to blood and body fluids by reducing the number of needlestick injuries.[52,71,72,76-82] A Cochrane review of 10 randomized controlled trials evaluated blunt versus sharp needles for preventing percutaneous exposure incidents in surgical staff members. Using blunt needles versus sharp suture needles reduced glove perforation risk by 54% as well as reduced the risk of infectious disease transmission.[71]

In a randomized controlled trial that compared blunt tapered and sharp needles in closing abdominal fascia in 200 general surgery patients undergoing laparotomy, the glove perforation rate for blunt suture needles was 12% compared to 28% for sharp needles. The researchers concluded that use of blunt tapered suture needles reduce the incidence of glove perforations.[72]

In a 15-month surveillance study of occupational blood exposures in the ORs of six hospitals, researchers reported 197 suture needle injuries; 59% of the injuries were attributable to suture needles used to suture muscle or fascia. Use of blunt suture needles as a prevention strategy could reduce percutaneous injuries in the OR by 30%.[52]

A randomized controlled study compared wound morbidity after cesarean deliveries using blunt suture needles and sharp suture needles.

The researchers concluded that blunt-tip suture needles do not increase wound morbidity.[83]

The use of blunt suture needles is supported by OSHA, the FDA, NIOSH, and the ACS when clinically indicated.[47,50] Additionally, OSHA has identified blunt suture needles as an acceptable engineering control.[73]

II.a.1. Blunt suture needles should be used for perineal laceration and episiotomy repair.[84-86]

In a survey of obstetricians regarding the use of blunt suture needles for episiotomy and laceration repair, 95% of respondents reported that blunt suture needles were an excellent to good alternative to sharp suture needles. There were no needlestick injuries or glove perforations reported during the time frame of the study.[84]

A randomized, controlled trial compared the number of glove perforations when using blunt-tip needles to sharp needles for suturing perineal tears and episiotomies. Researchers reported that the rate of glove punctures with blunt-tip needles was 8.6% and the rate with sharp needles was 16.5%.[85]

A randomized, prospective trial compared the rate of surgical glove perforations when blunt and sharp suture needles were used to repair obstetrical lacerations. There were five glove perforations in the sharp suture needle group and four glove perforations in the blunt suture group. The difference between the two groups was not statistically significant.[87]

II.b. Safety scalpel devices should be used when clinically feasible.[88] *[1: Regulatory Requirement]*

Scalpel injuries are the second most common injury in the perioperative setting, comprising 17% of injuries.[51,89] Scalpel injuries pose a risk of injury to the skin and underlying tissue and a bloodborne pathogen exposure risk.[4] Scalpel injuries occur to the surgeon or assistant, the original user of the device, as well as to the nurses and surgical technologists when scalpels are passed or blades are removed.[51]

II.b.1. There are several types of safety scalpel devices that may be used in the perioperative setting, each of which has an associated reduced risk of injury.

- Single-use scalpel handles and blades that do not require disassembly (ie, removal of the blade) are associated with 68% fewer percutaneous injuries.[90]
- Retracting scalpel blades withdraw the blade into the handle when they are passed between perioperative team members and when not in use.[91,92] When they are used consistently and correctly, there is the potential to prevent 65% of scalpel injuries.[90]

- Shielded or sheathed scalpel blades allow the blade to be covered by the shield or sheath when passed between perioperative team members and when not in use.[91] When used consistently and correctly, there is the potential to prevent 65% of scalpel injuries.[90]
- Rounded tip scalpel blades[4] may be effective in reducing scalpel injuries. No studies were found in the literature review regarding effectiveness of rounded tip scalpel blades in reducing scalpel injuries.
- Scalpel blade removal devices permit the safe removal of the blade at the conclusion of the procedure.[91] In a retrospective study of a metropolitan hospital's sharps injuries database, chart review, and hypothetical modeling of the data, researchers concluded that 44.5% of scalpel injuries could be prevented by using a combination of hands-free techniques and a scalpel blade removal device.[91]

II.c. Alternative wound closure devices should be used when clinically indicated.[93,94] *[2: High Evidence]*

Alternative skin closure devices reduce the use of sharp suture needles and the incidence of percutaneous injuries.[52,94,95] A systematic review of 14 randomized, controlled trials evaluated the tissue effects on surgical wound healing when tissue adhesives were used for skin closure. Researchers found no significant difference between sutures and adhesives in regard to infection, patient and user satisfaction, and cost. Sutures were better than adhesives for minimizing wound dehiscence in 10 trials, and were significantly faster to use. Adhesive tapes were faster to use than adhesives.[95]

Researchers conducting a single-center, prospective study that compared arthroscopy portal wound closure methods found comparable wound healing with adhesive wound closure strips and nylon suture. Eliminating the suture reduces the possibility of a percutaneous injury.[94] A randomized controlled animal study compared a fascial closure device to traditional suture closure. The researchers evaluated the amount of time needed to close the fascia, accuracy of placement, and abdominal bursting pressures. Fascial closure time was reduced by 24% with the closure device, and both methods had comparable closure integrity. Fascial closure devices may reduce percutaneous injuries by reducing the use of sutures to close the fascial layer.[96]

II.c.1. Alternative closure methods may include
- fascial closure devices,[92,96]
- tissue staplers,[92]
- tissue adhesives,[92] and
- adhesive skin closure strips.

II.d. Perioperative team members should use syringes, needles, and IV catheters that incorporate safety-engineered features. *[1: Regulatory Requirement]*

Appropriate methods to protect health care workers from exposure to bloodborne pathogens and to decrease the risk of disease transmission through sharps injuries are specified in OSHA regulations.[38]

Researchers prospectively monitored needlestick injuries for two years after the introduction of safety-engineered devices (ie, retractable syringes, needle-free IV systems) and compared injury rate to pre-intervention needlestick injury data at a large teaching hospital. All needlestick injuries decreased by 49%. Needlestick injuries related to IV line access decreased 81%. Hollow-bore needlestick injuries were reduced by 57%.[97]

A prospective surveillance study of 76 acute care hospitals examined sharps injuries over time, occupation, hospital size, and device. The sharps injury rates decreased steadily and significantly for hypodermic needles and syringes when safety-engineered devices were available and used. The rate of sharps injury decreased 3.5% per year.[68]

A three-year controlled retrospective interventional study analyzed injury data of health care workers with the potential to be exposed to bloodborne pathogens. Use of an IV catheter with a safety-engineered feature was implemented. Injuries from IV catheters decreased significantly from 2.3 to 2.5 percutaneous injuries per 1,000 health care workers during the pre-intervention period to 0.2 to 1.9 percutaneous injuries per 1,000 health care workers during the post-intervention period.[67]

II.d.1. Safety-engineered syringes and needles that may be used in the perioperative setting include
- a syringe or needle with a sliding sheath that covers the needle after use,
- a hinged needle guard that is attached to the hub of the needle and manually folds over the needle,
- a sliding shield needle guard that moves forward to cover the needle after use, and
- a syringe with a needle that retracts inside the syringe after use.[4]

II.d.2. Needleless systems should be used for
- the collection or withdrawal of bodily fluids after the initial access is established,
- the administration of medications or fluids, and
- any other procedure involving the potential for occupational exposure to bloodborne pathogens because of percutaneous injuries from contaminated sharps.[38]

Needleless systems protect against bloodborne pathogen exposure by eliminating the use of needles. A review of 17 studies evaluated the effect of safety-engineered device implementation on the rate of percutaneous injuries. Researchers evaluated needleless systems in eight of the 17 studies and reported a 22% to 100% reduction in overall percutaneous injuries.[65] In another review of 11 studies, authors concluded that the use of a needleless IV system and surgical assist devices led to a significant reduction in glove perforations.[98]

One study of needlestick injuries at an 800-bed university hospital in Australia indicated that introducing safety-engineered devices (ie, retractable syringes, needle-free IV systems, safety winged butterfly needles) reduced hollow-bore needlestick injuries by 49%.[97] The investigators also noted a 57% reduction in high-risk injuries after introducing retractable syringes and a virtual elimination of needlestick injuries related to accessing IV lines.[97]

II.d.3. A blunt cannula should be used to withdraw medication and fluid from a vial.[99]

Recommendation III

Perioperative personnel must use work practice controls when handling scalpels, hypodermic needles, suture needles, bone fragments, K-wires, burrs, saw blades, drill bits, trocars, razors, bone cutters, towel clips, scissors, electrosurgical tips, skin hooks, retractors, and other sharp devices.[38,100,101]

Work practice controls, as required by OSHA, reduce the likelihood of exposure by changing the method of performing a task to minimize the risk of exposure to blood or other potentially infectious materials.[38,42,101]

III.a. Sharps should be confined and contained in specified areas of the sterile field or within a sharps containment device.[102] *[3: Moderate Evidence]*

III.a.1. The scrub person should account for and confine all sharps on the sterile field until the patient is transferred out of the room.[102]

Unconfined sharps that remain on the sterile field may be unintentionally introduced into the incision, may be dropped on the floor, or may penetrate barriers. Confinement and containment of sharps may minimize the risk of injury to personnel as well as reduce the risk of retained surgical items.

III.a.2. Used sharps on the sterile field should be kept in a puncture-resistant container.

Collecting used sharps (eg, needles, blades) in a puncture-resistant container helps ensure their containment on the sterile field.

III.a.3. When a needle disposal container on the sterile field is full, an additional, new container should be used. Sharps are included in the count and should not be removed from the OR until the final count reconciliation is completed and the patient has been taken from the room.[102]

III.a.4. Needle containers should be securely closed before disposal.

III.b. Surgical team members should use a neutral zone or hands-free technique for passing sharp instruments, blades, and needles.[12,14,46-48,92,103-107] [3: Moderate Evidence]

Analysis of percutaneous injury surveillance data from 87 hospitals in the United States during a 13-year period showed that most sharps injuries occur when suture needles or sharps are passed between perioperative team members.[51] Changes in surgical practice to minimize manual manipulation of sharps (ie, neutral zone or no-touch techniques) can have a major effect on these injuries. Creation of a neutral zone (ie, where instruments are put down and picked up rather than passed hand to hand) may decrease injuries from sharp instruments.[4] In a 2007 standards interpretation letter, OSHA recommends the use of the neutral zone.[108]

The use of a no-touch technique (ie, no two people touch a sharp at the same time) was described in 1988 as a means to minimize the risk of a sharps injury and exposure to HIV.[109] The author advocated the use of a magnetic pad as the neutral zone and for scrubbed team members to provide verbal warnings of sharps in use.

A pre-intervention and post-intervention study investigated whether preventative practice changes (ie, reducing the use of sharp instruments, using a neutral zone, using a no-touch technique) during orthopedic procedures would decrease the risk of blood exposure for the surgical technologist, first assistant, surgeon, and patient. Researchers defined the no-touch technique as using an instrument instead of manually manipulating any sharp (eg, suture needle, scalpel blade). Before the introduction of preventative practice changes, the researchers studied sharps injuries and glove perforations for 347 procedures and 1,068 staff members using traditional working methods that included hand-to-hand passing of sharp instruments. During the pre-intervention phase, there were 24 incidents (ie, 13 injuries, 11 glove perforations) during 6.8% of procedures. After introducing preventative practice changes, researchers studied sharps injuries and glove perforations for 383 orthopedic procedures and 1,058 staff members using the no-touch and neutral zone techniques. During the post-intervention phase, there were 10 incidents (ie, six injuries, four glove perforations) during 2.7% of procedures.[103]

In a pre-intervention and post-intervention study, researchers used a hands-free technique training video as the intervention to increase the use of the hands-free technique and reduce bloodborne pathogen exposures. They found that use of the video and technique were effective in reducing injuries, glove tears, and contaminations.[107]

In a prospective study of 3,765 procedures performed in inpatient and outpatient settings, RN circulators recorded the use of the hands-free technique during each procedure. The rates of incidents (ie, percutaneous injuries, glove tears, contaminations) were compared in procedures during which the technique was and was not used. The effectiveness of the hands-free technique in decreasing percutaneous injuries was evaluated, and researchers found that it was more effective in surgeries with blood loss greater than 100 mL.[110]

In a study evaluating behavioral treatment that combined goal setting, task clarification, and feedback as a means to increase the use of the hands-free technique, researchers found the combined treatment increased use of the hands-free technique from 32% to 64% in the inpatient setting and from 31% to 70% in the outpatient setting. Sharps injuries declined from 10.3 per quarter to six per quarter.[111]

A self-administered questionnaire surveyed the use of the hands-free technique among 158 perioperative nurses in seven different facilities. Data analysis showed a significant association between hands-free technique education and the perceived need for using it. Researchers concluded that increasing education on the hands-free technique could increase its use.[104]

A 1997 randomized, prospective study of the use of a neutral zone during cesarean births showed no statistically significant difference in the number of glove perforations between the control and intervention groups. Based on their findings, the researchers concluded that while there are no proven benefits, there are few adverse effects of using a passing tray.[112]

III.b.1. Use of a neutral zone should include
- identifying the neutral zone in the preoperative briefing[45,46,106,109];
- using a basin, instrument mat, magnetic pad, or designated area on the Mayo stand as the neutral zone[45,46,103,106,109,113,114];
- giving verbal notification when a sharp is in the neutral zone[45,46,109,114];
- placing one sharp at a time in the neutral zone[45,46];
- orienting the sharp for easy retrieval by the surgeon[45,46];
- handling of a sharp item by only one team member at a time[106,109]; and
- placing sharp items in the neutral zone after use.[106]

III.b.2. A modified neutral zone (eg, a limited hands-free passing technique) should be used during procedures that require the use of a microscope. The scrub person should place the sharp in the surgeon's hand. The surgeon should return the sharp to the designated neutral zone.

Low lighting, microscope magnification, and a narrow field of vision contribute to sharps injury risks during microscopic procedures.[115] A retrospective review of reported sharps injuries during ophthalmic procedures in a six-year period showed that most of the sharps injuries occurred while the device was being used or passed between health care workers in the OR.[115] A modified neutral zone (eg, limited hands-free passing technique) may reduce sharps injuries.[115]

III.c. A no-touch technique should be used when handling sharps.[32,103,109,116] [3: Moderate Evidence]

The no-touch technique minimizes manual handling of sharp devices and instruments, reducing the risk of injury to perioperative team members.[103,109]

III.c.1. Suture needles should not be manipulated with gloved hands.[12,103]

Suture needle injuries occur when loading the needle holder or repositioning the needle.

III.c.2. When suture is being loaded on a needle holder, the suture packet should be used to position the suture needle in the needle holder without touching the needle.

III.c.3. A blunt instrument (eg, forceps) should be used to manipulate and guide the suture needle through tissue to avoid finger contact with the suture needle or the tissue being sutured.[103,109,117]

The most common site of percutaneous injuries in the perioperative setting is to the non-dominant hand during suturing. In a randomized clinical trial, the rate of glove perforations of the non-dominant hand occurred in 88% of the procedures for the surgeon and in 78% of the procedures for assistants.[72] The researchers found that the use of a blunt instrument-assisted technique reduced the need for finger contact with the suture needle or the tissue being sutured.

III.c.4. The perioperative team member performing suturing should use a forceps to turn the suture needle 90 degrees toward the box lock of the needle holder before returning the loaded needle holder to the Mayo stand if a hands-free zone is not being used.[103,117,118]

Turning the loaded needle may reduce the risk of sharps injury during instrument passing.[118]

III.c.5. An instrument should be used to pick up sharp items (eg, scalpel blades, suture needles) that have fallen off the sterile field.

III.d. Sharp instruments (eg, retractors, towel clips) should be used only when clinically necessary.[52,114] Sharp devices should be used only when there is no safer alternative available.[52] [2: High Evidence]

A study about the feasibility of performing specific general surgery procedures without sharp instruments (eg, scalpels, sutures) was evaluated. Researchers identified 91 procedures preoperatively as appropriate non-sharp procedures. A total of 86.8% of the procedures were completed without the use of sharp instrumentation, eliminating the risks of sharps injury to perioperative personnel.[93]

III.e. Safe scalpel handling methods should be used when clinically feasible. [3: Moderate Evidence]

Scalpel injuries are the second most common injury in the perioperative setting, comprising 17% of the injuries.[51,89] Scalpel injuries pose a risk of injury to the skin and underlying tissue and a risk of bloodborne pathogen exposure.[4]

Scalpel injuries occur to the surgeon or assistant, the original user of the device, as well as to the nurses and surgical technologists when scalpels are passed or blades are removed.[51]

III.e.1. An instrument should be used for loading a scalpel blade on a knife handle when a safety-engineered device is not available.[103]

III.e.2. A scalpel blade remover or instrument should be used to remove the blade when a safety-engineered device is not available.[103,119]

III.f. Alternative cutting devices (eg, electrosurgery, diathermy, electrosurgical plasma; adapted electrosurgical tips) should be used when clinically indicated. [1: Strong Evidence]

A systematic review and meta-analysis compared cutting diathermy (ie, electrosurgery) to the use of a scalpel for skin incisions. The researchers concluded that skin incisions using electrosurgical instruments were quicker, associated with less blood loss, and resulted in no difference in wound rate complications or pain.[120]

III.f.1. A hand piece that uses electrosurgical plasma induced with pulsed radio-frequency energy to cut tissue may be used as an alternative to scalpels.[121]

A hand piece that uses electrosurgical plasma induced with pulsed radio-frequency energy may reduce the risk of sharps injuries by decreasing the use of sharp instruments.[121]

III.f.2. Specially adapted electrosurgical tips for cutting with power mode may be used as an alternative to scalpels.

III.g. Perioperative team members should use additional sharps safety practices, including
- maintaining situational awareness of all sharps on the sterile field[14,114];
- communicating the location of sharps on the sterile field with other members of the perioperative team during the procedure and at times of personnel change;
- removing suture needles from the suture before tying (eg, cutting, control release);
- retracting tissue with instruments (eg, retractors) rather than hands;
- handling (eg, applying, passing, using, removing) saw blades, sharp K-wires, burrs, and other sharp devices with caution[114]; and
- covering with a protective cap or cutting the exposed ends of sharp pins or K-wires after they have passed through the patient's skin.[32]

[3: Moderate Evidence]

A multi-center surveillance study identified patterns of blood exposure and exposure-prevention strategies. Researchers reported 386 percutaneous exposure events during a 15-month period in six OR suites. Manual tissue retraction accounted for 3.4% of the injuries.[52]

III.h. Perioperative team members should use safe practices when injecting medications or withdrawing bodily fluids.[99] [1: Regulatory Requirement]

Safe injection practices protect health care workers from exposure to bloodborne pathogens and decrease the risk of disease transmission through sharps injuries. These practices are specified in OSHA regulations.[38]

III.h.1. Needles should not be recapped. When a safe needle device is not available and recapping is required, a one-handed scooping recapping technique must be used.[38,122]

Two-handed recapping of hypodermic needles is associated with an increased incidence of injuries.[4] A study comparing the incidence of sharps injuries in medical students before and after a demonstration of the scooping recapping technique and a lecture on the dangers of sharps injuries showed a reduction in the incidence of sharps injuries from 17.4% to 2.8%.[123]

III.h.2. Contaminated needles and other contaminated sharps must not be bent, recapped, or removed unless there is no alternative or the action is required because of a specific medical or dental procedure.[38]

III.h.3. Needleless entry devices should be used whenever possible to withdraw contents from multidose vials.[99]

III.i. Perioperative team members should practice ampule safety to minimize percutaneous injury during or after opening of an ampule.[124] [2: High Evidence]

Safety measures may include
- using a reusable or disposable ampule breaker that covers the neck of the ampule during the breaking process or
- wrapping a sterile gauze pad around the ampule neck before breaking the top.[125]

Opening a glass ampule may produce glass fragments and a jagged or sharp edge. The Centers for Disease Control and Prevention (CDC) estimated that glass devices account for 2% of percutaneous injuries among all health care personnel.[4] A cross-sectional survey of 864 nurses at a large teaching hospital showed that 29% of the injuries were related to use of ampules or vials.[126] A randomly completed survey of all anesthetists at the Bristol Royal Infirmary after an anesthetic session indicated there was a 6% incidence of hand laceration after opening a glass ampule.[127] In one study, researchers used a questionnaire-based methodology to investigate the prevalence and cause of needlestick injuries in a cross-section of 274 nursing students. The results demonstrated an injury rate of 36% when opening an ampule.[128] A multi-center study determined the incidence and causes of anesthesia professionals' hazards by data analysis. Broken glass ampules were the causative factor in 54.2% of the incidents.[129]

Recommendation IV

Perioperative personnel must use PPE.

The use of PPE is required by OSHA where there is a risk of occupational exposure to blood, body fluids, or other potentially infectious materials after engineering and work practice controls are implemented. Personal protective barriers are required when it can be reasonably anticipated that a health care worker will be exposed to bloodborne pathogens or other potentially infectious materials.[42] The use of PPE (eg, gloves) protects health care worker's skin from coming into contact with blood, body fluids, and other potentially infectious materials.[38,130]

IV.a. Health care personnel should use standard precautions when caring for all patients in the perioperative setting.[131] [1: Strong Evidence]

Standard precautions are the foundation for preventing transmission of infectious diseases. Standard precautions apply to all patients across all health care settings (eg, hospitals, ambulatory surgery centers, freestanding specialty care sites, interventional sites).[130,132] Standard precautions include practices for hand hygiene, PPE, patient resuscitation, environmental control, respiratory hygiene/cough etiquette, sharps safety, and textiles and laundry.[130]

IV.b. Scrubbed team members should wear two pairs of surgical gloves, one over the other, during surgical and other invasive procedures that have the potential for exposure to blood, body fluids, or other potentially infectious materials.[12,32,46-48,131,133-135] *[1: Strong Evidence]*

Wearing two pairs of gloves reduces the risk of glove perforation and percutaneous injury. A systematic review of 31 randomized controlled trials of gloving practices demonstrated that double gloving minimizes the risk of exposure to blood during invasive procedures by providing a protective barrier.[136] The studies compared single gloves to double gloves; double gloves to indicator gloves; double gloves to double latex gloves plus a glove liner; double gloves to latex inner gloves with knitted outer gloves; double gloves to latex inner gloves with steel-weave outer gloves; and double gloves to triple gloves.[136] Double gloving (eg, two pairs of gloves, indicator glove with over glove) is more effective than single gloving in reducing glove perforations.[82,136-143]

Double gloving minimizes bloodborne pathogen exposure.[137,144-147] Studies have demonstrated that double gloving reduces contact with blood by a factor of 5.8 to 10.[144,148] When two pairs of gloves are worn (ie, double gloving), in most instances only the outer glove is perforated when punctured by a sharp device. In addition, research demonstrates that when two pairs of gloves are worn and a puncture occurs, the volume of blood on a solid sharp device (eg, suture needle) is reduced by as much as 95%. There is evidence that double gloving can reduce the risk of exposure to blood and body fluids by as much as 87% if the outer glove is punctured.[76,133,149]

A prospective cohort study compared the frequency of glove perforations in single and double gloves by testing 1,000 pairs of gloves after the end of pelvic surgery procedures. Of the single glove sets, 11% had a perforation, and 2% of the double glove sets had a perforation in the inner and outer gloves.[145]

A prospective study investigated the efficacy of double gloving by comparing the frequency of glove perforations from 100 consecutive major and 100 consecutive minor orthopedic procedures. All surgical team members wore double gloves. Researchers examined the gloves for perforations after the procedures. The overall perforation rate was 15.8%. Major procedures had a 21.6% perforation rate while minor procedures had a 3.6% perforation rate. The outer glove perforation rate was 22.7% while the inner glove perforation rate was 3.7%; inner gloves were perforated only in major procedures. The majority of outer glove perforations (72.7%) were not detected by the surgical team members. The most common site of perforation occurred on the dominant thumb. Based on these results, the authors recommended routine double gloving during orthopedic procedures given the integrity of the inner gloves.[150]

A prospective, randomized, controlled trial calculated the rate of barrier breaches when personnel were single and double gloved in 99 procedures. Single gloves were breached at a rate of 35% per procedure and 21% per individual.[151] Only one breach was immediately detected by the wearer. The breach rate in the outer glove of personnel who wore double gloves was similar to those wearing single gloves, but none of the inner gloves were breached, which reduced the risk of bloodborne pathogen exposure.[151]

IV.b.1. When double gloves are worn, perforation indicator systems should be used.[81,152]

A perforation indicator system uses a colored pair of gloves worn beneath a standard pair of gloves. When glove perforation occurs, moisture from the surgical field seeps through the perforation between the layers of gloves, revealing the underlying color and signaling a perforation.[60,81,151,153] Perforations are detected more frequently and reliably with a perforation indicator glove system.[133,136,149,151,153-155]

A double-blind, randomized study evaluated the ability of participants to locate a 30-micron sized hole in various glove configurations (ie, single gloves, double gloves, double gloves using a glove perforation indicator system) during simulated surgery. While wearing the indicator system, participants detected 84% of the perforations with the latex indicator system and 56% of the perforations with the synthetic indicator system.[155]

IV.b.2. When indicated by a clinical need for high tactile sensitivity, a single pair of gloves may be worn.

IV.c. Perioperative personnel should monitor gloves for punctures. *[1: Strong Evidence]*

Careful inspection of glove integrity throughout the procedure may prevent unnoticed glove perforation. Undetected glove perforation during operative or other invasive procedures may present an increased risk for bloodborne pathogen transmission to perioperative team members related to prolonged exposure to blood, body fluids, or other potentially infectious materials.

Intact gloves provide a barrier that reduces the passage of microorganisms from surgical team members' hands to the operative field. Intact gloves also provide a barrier that prevents bloodborne pathogen exposure to the wearer. Glove failures can be caused by punctures, tears by sharp devices, or spontaneous failures. The ASTM Standard Specification for Rubber Surgical Gloves allows for a 1.5% glove hole failure rate.[152,156] A comparison study of

PATIENT AND WORKER SAFETY

single and double gloving analyzed the frequency of glove perforations during surgery. The rate of perforations during surgical procedures that lasted fewer than two hours was 4.21%; the rate of perforations during procedures that were longer than two hours was 11.69%.[149] Researchers calculated the increased perforation risk per additional 10 minutes of operating time to be 1.115 times.[140,149] When single gloves were worn, the detection rate of a perforation was 36.84%. When a double glove puncture indication system was worn, the detection rate for a perforation was 86.52%.[149]

A prospective study assessed glove perforation rates in 130 consecutive orthopedic procedures. A total of 1,452 gloves from all surgical team members were tested. The overall perforation rate was 3.58%. Perforations went unnoticed 61.5% of the time. Single glove perforations occurred at a rate of 10.87% compared to 3.34% when two pairs of gloves were used. When double gloves were used, the inner glove was perforated at a rate of 0.36%.[139]

A study of glove perforations when team members double gloved during hip and knee arthroplasty showed a perforation rate of 18.4% to the outer glove and 8.4% to the inner glove. The most frequent site of perforation was the second finger of the nondominant hand.[157] A prospective study of four brands of latex-free gloves used during arthroplasty showed a higher perforation rate and poorer handling properties than latex gloves.[158] A randomized controlled study of personnel scrubbed on primary cemented total hip replacement surgeries evaluated the incidence of glove perforation and contamination when outer gloves were changed at specific intervals. In the study group, outer gloves were changed every 20 minutes, prior to cementation, and when a visible puncture was detected. In the control group, outer gloves were changed prior to cementation and when a visible puncture was detected. There was a statistically significant lower rate of perforations for surgeons and scrub persons in the study group compared with surgeons and scrub persons in the control group. There also was a statistically significant lower rate of glove contamination in the study group compared to the control group. The researchers found that regular glove changes during a procedure can reduce the incidence of perforation and contamination.[159]

Researchers in a cross sectional study investigated the incidence and recognition of glove perforations during gynecological procedures. Perforations occurred in 24.4% of the procedures and were detected 37.5% of the time by the gynecologist.[160] A randomized study of single and double gloving analyzed glove punctures during major gynecological surgery. When the staff physician and resident were single gloved, the rate of perforation was 22.1%. The

perforation rate was 2.7% when the staff physician and resident were double gloved.[134]

Glove microperforations were studied by testing 180 pairs of gloves with both the water load test and electrical conductance following use in endoscopic, laparoscopic, and open urology procedures. The glove defect rate was 29% in all urologic procedures. The rate of glove perforations was 15% in endoscopy procedures, 25% in laparoscopic procedures, and 30.6% in open urologic procedures. The investigators concluded that double gloving in urologic procedures protects the patient from cross contamination and protects the surgical team from occupational exposure.[161]

A prospective, randomized study compared glove perforations between perioperative nurses who were single and double gloved. Perforations were detected in 8.9% of nurses wearing single gloves and 11.3% in the outer glove of nurses wearing double gloves. No inner gloves were perforated. The average time for a perforation to occur was 69.8 minutes after the beginning of surgery. The researchers concluded that double gloving was effective in preventing exposure to bloodborne pathogens.[141]

IV.c.1.   Gloves should be changed when a suspected or actual perforation occurs or a visible defect is noted.[60]

    Surgical gloves develop microperforations depending on the length of time the gloves are worn. Perforations allow bacteria to pass from the surgical site through the glove.[162]

IV.d.   Virus-inhibiting protective gloves may be worn. *[2: High Evidence]*

    Virus-inhibiting gloves reduce the amount of virus transmitted when a glove is perforated.[163-165] An automatic apparatus was used to study the influence of the puncture and type of glove on the volume of blood transferred during a simulated percutaneous injury with a hollow bore needle. The researchers found an 81% reduction in virus transmission with virus-inhibiting gloves compared to single or double latex glove systems.[164] A study of virus transmission showed a 15-fold or greater reduction in virus transmission with virus-inhibiting gloves compared to standard gloves of the same thickness.[165] The researchers concluded that virus-inhibiting gloves could provide increased protection against HIV and HCV exposures.[165]

A prospective clinical study evaluated the tolerance, ergonomics, and glove barrier value of virus-inhibiting gloves. The researchers examined 834 gloves from 100 procedures and concluded that the virus-inhibiting gloves afforded mechanical protection against punctures and may be recommended in high-risk surgical procedures.[163] In another study, researchers randomly assigned study volunteers into one of three groups: single gloves, double gloves, and antimicrobial gloves. The researchers found a significant reduction in microbial passage with antimicrobial gloves.[166]

Recommendation V

Sharp devices must be contained and disposed of safely.

Containing sharps in an appropriate container can reduce sharps injuries. Causes of container-related injuries include a sharp protruding from disposal container; a sharp piercing the side of a disposal container; a sharp left on or near the disposal container; a sharp left on the floor, table, or other inappropriate place; and a sharp protruding from a trash bag or inappropriate disposal container.[167]

The OSHA bloodborne pathogens standard requires the safe disposal of contaminated sharps devices to minimize the risk of bloodborne pathogen transmission.[38,168] Analysis of data reported to a national surveillance system compared percutaneous injuries from sharps device disposal from two time periods, before and after the regulatory-driven improvements in sharps disposal practices. Between 1992 and 1994, 36.8% of percutaneous injuries were attributed to disposal of sharps devices. Between 2006 and 2007, 19.3% of percutaneous injuries were attributed to disposal of sharps devices.[168] The 53% decline in container-related injuries is attributable to widespread use of point-of-use, puncture-resistant sharps containers.[168,169]

V.a. Selection criteria for sharps containers should include functionality, accessibility, accommodation, and visibility.[169] *[2: High Evidence]*

Sharps disposal injuries have been attributed to inappropriate sharps containment practices by the user, inadequate sharps disposal container design, inappropriate sharps container placement, and over-filling of sharps disposal containers.[169]

V.a.1. Functional selection criteria for a sharps disposal container should include that the container
- is durable (ie, resistant to punctures and chemical or liquid leaks),
- has a mechanism for closing that minimizes exposure to contents and hand injuries during handling and that is resistant to being opened manually,
- is stable (ie, is not prone to tipping), and
- is of a size and shape to accommodate the type of sharps that require disposal.[169]

V.a.2. Accessibility criteria for a sharps disposal container should include that
- the container is placed in close proximity to the point of use,
- there is an obstacle-free pathway between the point of use and the container, and
- the container is reachable by personnel of varied heights.[169]

V.a.3. Accommodation criteria for a sharps disposal container should include that the container requires minimal training to use and provides ease of storage, assembly, and operation.[169]

V.a.4. Visibility criteria for a sharps disposal container should include that the container
- is easily recognizable (eg, has a hazard warning label or container color),
- is visible to the user,
- has a visible fill level, and
- is placed under sufficient illumination.[169]

V.b. All sharps must be handled and disposed of safely.[38] *[1: Regulatory Requirement]*

Safe handling of contaminated sharps protects the original user and environmental services, laundry, sterile processing, and waste disposal personnel. One waste disposal company reported 40 sharps injuries occurring at a rate of one per 29,000 labor hours. Causes of the injuries were improperly closed or overfilled sharps containers and incorrect disposal of sharps into plastic garbage bags.[170]

V.b.1. Disposable sharps contaminated with blood or other potentially infectious materials should be disposed of in a closeable, puncture-resistant container that is leakproof on its sides and bottom and is labeled or color-coded.[38]

V.b.2. Sharps disposal receptacles should be
- appropriately sized with a fill line that is readily visible,
- located close to the point of use,
- maintained upright when in use, and
- routinely replaced and not overfilled.[38]

V.b.3. Container devices with enhanced engineering (eg, counterbalanced tray, one-hand sharp deposit, hand entry restriction, tamper proof locks) should be used.

Researchers conducting a nonrandomized intervention and cohort study from 2006 to 2008 evaluated sharps injury rates during use of an enhanced engineered sharps container compared to during use of an existing sharps container. The enhanced engineering controls included a large horizontal aperture, counterbalanced tray, one-hand sharp deposit, and hand entry restriction. The study device was associated with a 30% reduction in after-procedure sharps injuries; a 57% reduction indisposal-related sharps injuries; and an 81% reduction in container-associated sharps injury. The control group had no significant reductions in sharps injuries.[167]

V.c. Sharps/needle counter devices should be used to contain and isolate sharps on the sterile back table. Sharps/needle counter devices should be
- puncture resistant,

- labeled or color-coded in accordance with the bloodborne pathogens standard, and
- leak proof on the sides and bottom.[38]

[1: Regulatory Requirement]

Sharps/needle counter devices protect scrubbed personnel during procedures by segregating sharps in one location until disposal at the end of the procedure.

V.d. Contaminated, reusable sharps (eg, skin hooks, trocars) should be segregated from non-sharp instruments after use for transport to the decontamination area in a puncture-resistant container that is labeled as biohazardous. *[1: Regulatory Requirement]*

Segregating sharp instruments minimizes the risk of injury to personnel handling the instruments during decontamination. Processes that require employees to place their hands into basins of sharp instruments are prohibited by OSHA because of the risk of percutaneous exposure to bloodborne pathogens.[38]

Recommendation VI

The perioperative RN should demonstrate personal and professional responsibility in preventing sharps injuries and preventing the transmission of bloodborne pathogens.

It is the perioperative RN's responsibility to evaluate his or her practice in context with current professional practice standards, rules, and regulations.[171]

VI.a. The perioperative RN should observe local, state, and federal regulations (eg, OSHA regulations).[171] *[1: Regulatory Requirement]*

It is the perioperative RN's responsibility to practice nursing in accordance with the standards and guidelines of regulatory bodies.[38,171]

VI.b. The perioperative RN and other surgical team members should comply with methods of protection (eg, PPE, HBV immunization) against disease transmission.[13,20,22,23,131] *[1: Strong Evidence]*

Occupational exposure to bloodborne pathogens is a risk for all health care workers.[14] There is potential increased risk in the OR because of the nature of the work, amount of blood exposure, and use of sharp devices.[14,51] There have been 132 documented cases of health care provider to patient transmission of HBV, HCV, or HIV worldwide.[17,31,35,36] Protective barriers contribute to the prevention of occupational and patient exposure.[14]

Since the widespread adoption of HBV immunizations, the number of HBV infections in health care workers has declined significantly.[19-23] The reported number of HBV-infected providers in 1983 was 10,000 compared to approximately 100 in 2009.[20,21]

VI.b.1. Perioperative personnel should be immunized against the hepatitis B virus.[20,131]

Hepatitis B is highly contagious and can be transmitted via percutaneous exposure (eg, needlestick injury) or mucosal exposure to infected blood or body fluids. The risk of acquiring HBV infection from occupational exposure depends on the frequency of percutaneous and mucosal exposure to blood or body fluids that contain the virus. Risks to health care providers from sharps injuries and blood and body fluid exposure have been reduced as a result of widespread HBV immunization.[131] Although rare, health care personnel who have HBV or HCV have transmitted these infections to patients.[17,31,35,36] The HBV vaccine, given in three intramuscular injections, induces a protective antibody response in 90% of healthy recipients.[13] Since 1991, OSHA requires employers of persons at risk for occupational exposure to provide the hepatitis B vaccine at no cost to the employee.[38]

VI.b.2. Perioperative personnel should report sharps injuries immediately.

Reporting facilitates prophylaxis against bloodborne pathogen exposure. Post-exposure prophylactic medication reduces the risk of acquiring HIV, immunoglobulin and vaccination reduces the risk of HBV infection, and surveillance for HCV detects an acquired infection and facilitates prompt treatment.[172]

Researchers examined blood exposure, percutaneous injury, and reporting in a stratified random sample of 5,123 physicians, nurses, and medical technologists. Under-reporting of percutaneous injuries varied by occupation but, overall, 32% did not report an exposure.[173] A questionnaire surveying perioperative personnel showed that 90.4% knew how to report a sharps injury, but 32.4% admitted to not reporting a percutaneous injury.[172] Reasons for not reporting an injury included not considering the patient to be high risk, finding the reporting process to be too difficult, and not having enough time.[172,174,175]

VI.c. Perioperative team members should use devices with safety features that are provided by the employer.[38] *[1: Regulatory Requirement]*

Safety devices are only effective when used (see Recommendation II).

VI.c.1. Perioperative personnel should actively participate in the safety conversion process and help others adapt to the change.

Recommendation VII

Personnel should receive initial and ongoing education and competency verification on their understanding of the principles of and performance of the processes for sharps safety.[176]

Health care organizations are responsible for providing initial and ongoing education and evaluating the competency of perioperative team members in the use of sharps safety devices and the performance of sharps safety measures.

Initial and ongoing education on sharps safety practices facilitates the development of knowledge, skills, and attitudes that affect safe patient care and workplace safety with regard to the prevention of percutaneous injuries.[13,66,82,177-180] Ongoing development of knowledge and skills and documentation of personnel participation is a regulatory and accreditation requirement for both hospitals and ambulatory settings.[181-184]

Periodic education programs provide the opportunity to reinforce the principles of sharps safety as well as explain safety-engineered devices and potential hazards to patients and personnel. Periodic education programs also provide the opportunity to introduce information on technology changes and new applications.[59]

Competency assessment measures individual performance, provides a mechanism for documentation, and verifies that perioperative personnel have an understanding of sharps safety and facility policies. Every nurse is responsible for being personally accountable for maintaining competency validation.[185]

There are no universally accepted or mandated ways to perform or validate competency, and strategies to accomplish this differ among states. The goal of competency strategies is to reassure the public that nurses have the knowledge, skills, and judgment to provide safe and effective care.[186]

VII.a. Perioperative personnel should receive education that addresses sharps safety practices upon orientation to the perioperative setting. Continuing education should be provided when new equipment or processes are introduced. *[3: Moderate Evidence]*

Sharps injuries may be minimized and safety improved with regularly scheduled education, training, and competency demonstrations.[177,187-189]

Residents, students, and personnel with less experience are at an increased risk for percutaneous injuries.[75,175,190-192] A survey of surgeons-in-training at 17 medical centers showed that 83% had a needlestick injury during training. By the end of their five-year training period, 99% had sustained an injury.[75] A retrospective review of the occupational health records of surgical trainees showed that senior and chief residents had a lower exposure rate than junior residents.[193]

VII.a.1. The perioperative RN should participate in education about bloodborne pathogens and follow recommended infection prevention practices.[38,131]

VII.a.2. Perioperative team members should practice using safety devices.

Practice before use will establish familiarity and experience with the device before use in clinical practice.

VII.b. Health care personnel who are occupationally exposed to blood or other potentially infectious materials must receive training before assignment to tasks during which occupational exposure may occur, at least annually thereafter, and when changes to procedures or tasks affect occupational exposure.[36,38] *[1: Regulatory Requirement]*

Employers are responsible for providing training on bloodborne exposure guidelines at no cost to the employee during working hours. Employers are also responsible for ensuring employees participate in the training program and for offering materials in appropriate languages and at appropriate literacy levels.[38]

Providing the basis for the prevention of bloodborne pathogen exposure may instill an understanding of the processes that need to be followed and thereby prevent disease transmission. Education and training efforts are equally important in promoting awareness of hazards and acceptance of safe work practices and material-handling procedures in the workplace.[59,194] Educating employees on safe work practices (eg, using PPE) can help protect staff members, their family members, and the community from disease transmission.

VII.b.1. Education and competency assessment related to sharps safety and injury prevention should include a review of
- exposure control plans,
- safety-engineered devices,
- blunt suture needle use,
- neutral or safe zone concepts,
- no-touch technique,
- double gloving, and
- sharps disposal.

VII.b.2. Sharps safety should be included in the organization's annual bloodborne pathogens training program.[38,131]

Recommendation VIII

Documentation should reflect activities related to sharps safety.[38]

Documentation related to sharps safety is applicable at the systems level. Documentation serves as a basis for monitoring compliance, measuring performance, maintaining employee records, and logging exposure incidents.

VIII.a. Employers must maintain training records for three years. The records must include
- training dates,
- the content or a summary of the training,
- the names and qualifications of the trainer(s), and
- the names and job titles of the trainees.[38]

[1: Regulatory Requirement]

429

VIII.b. Health care facilities must have a documented exposure control plan.[38] *[1: Regulatory Requirement]*

VIII.b.1. As part of the health care facility's written exposure control plan, all incidents of occupational exposure to blood or other potentially infectious materials must be documented.[38,195] Documentation must include

- the employee's name and identification;
- the employee's hepatitis B vaccination status, including vaccination dates, and other relevant medical information for both individuals;
- results of all related examinations, medical tests, and post-exposure evaluation and follow-up procedures;
- a licensed health care professional's written evaluation of the risk of transmission; and
- a copy of the information provided to the employee.[38]

Additional documentation should include

- the route of exposure;
- the circumstances associated with the exposure; and
- the source individual's serological status, if known.

Documenting each exposure incident provides a record of the incident, what follow-through was taken, and the current status of the incident.

VIII.b.2. Input from non-managerial health care workers should be solicited and documented in the exposure control plan with regard to identifying, evaluating, and selecting safety-engineered sharp devices.[38]

VIII.b.3. The employer should document in the exposure control plan that safety-engineered sharps devices and needleless systems have been evaluated and implemented.[38]

VIII.c. Employers must maintain a sharps injury log to document all percutaneous injuries from contaminated sharps and must maintain the log in such a way that an injured employee's identification remains confidential.[38] At a minimum, a sharps injury log must include

- the type and brand of device involved in the incident,
- the department or work area where the exposure incident occurred, and
- an explanation of how the incident occurred. *[1: Regulatory Requirement]*

VIII.c.1. Documentation related to exposure incidents must be maintained for the employee's duration of employment plus 30 years.[38]

Recommendation IX

Policies and procedures for sharps safety processes and practices should be developed, reviewed periodically, revised as necessary, and readily available in the practice setting.

Policies and procedures assist in the development of patient and workplace safety, quality assessment, and performance improvement activities. Policies and procedures establish authority, responsibility, and accountability within the facility. Policies and procedures also serve as operational guidelines that are used to minimize patient and health care worker risks, to standardize practice, and to direct perioperative personnel.

IX.a. Policies and procedures should be developed to guide, support, and monitor adherence to sharps safety and injury prevention practices, including the use of systems that should be used to collect, analyze, and communicate information related to sharps safety.[130] *[1: Strong Evidence]*

Definitive policies and procedures as part of an overall administrative strategy can demonstrate a commitment to preventing sharps injuries by incorporating sharps safety into the organizational objectives for patient and occupational safety.

IX.b. Policies and procedures should be developed and implemented for
- double gloving,
- neutral (hands-free) zone,
- safety-engineered devices (eg, blunt suture needles, scalpels, safety syringes and needles),[196]
- post-exposure protocols,[19,131] and
- safety-engineered device selection and evaluation.[38]
[1: Regulatory Requirement]

IX.c. Policies and procedures designed to minimize or eliminate health care personnel exposure to blood and other potentially infectious materials must be developed and implemented.[38] *[1: Regulatory Requirement]*

A written bloodborne pathogens exposure plan that is consistent with federal, state, and local rules and regulations and that governs occupational exposure to bloodborne pathogens, is reviewed periodically, and is readily available in the practice setting promotes safety with medical devices and blood and body fluids.[38]

IX.d. Policies should be developed in accordance with federal and state guidelines and should be consistent with existing impaired-provider and disability guidelines to define work restrictions for health care personnel who have a transmissible bloodborne infection (eg, HIV, HBV, HCV).[197] The policies should define work restrictions based on whether the employee

- ○ has a viral burden above the recommended threshold for the relevant virus;
- ○ has a medical condition or conditions that result in an inability to perform assigned tasks;
- ○ has experienced documented untoward events (eg, having transmitted HBV, HCV, or HIV);
- ○ refuses or is unable to follow recommended guidelines to prevent transmission of infectious diseases; or
- ○ is unable to perform regular duties, assuming that reasonable accommodation has been offered for the disability.[22]

[1: Strong Evidence]

IX.e.   Policies and procedures should include processes for initial education, training, ongoing competency validation, and annual review for issues related to sharps injury prevention.[183,184]
[1: Regulatory Requirement]

Policies and procedures assist in the development of activities that support patient safety, quality assessment, and the establishment of guidelines for continuous performance improvement. Standardizing processes for performance expectations between perioperative settings facilitates continuity of care and reduces the risk of error when personnel rotate among areas.

Recommendation X

Perioperative team members should participate in a variety of quality improvement activities to monitor and improve the prevention of sharps injuries.

Quality assurance and performance improvement programs assist in evaluating worker safety and formulating plans for corrective actions. These programs provide data that may be used to determine whether an individual organization is within benchmark goals and, if not, identify areas that may require corrective actions. These programs may also provide ongoing feedback regarding whether problems are improving, stabilizing, or worsening.

X.a.   Quality indicators should be developed to measure improvement in sharps injury prevention. Quality indicators for measuring sharps safety in the perioperative setting should include rates of percutaneous injuries and near misses.
[1: Strong Evidence]

Quality indicators are measurable and demonstrate that facilities are using specific interventions to provide safe patient care.[198] According to the Agency for Healthcare Research and Quality (AHRQ), "An adequate quality indicator must have sound clinical or empirical rationale for its use. It should measure an important aspect of quality that is subject to provider or health care system control."[198(p3)] The AHRQ quality indicators are one response to the need for multidimensional, accessible quality measures that can be used to gauge performance in health care. The quality indicators are evidence based and can be used to identify variations in the quality of care provided on both an inpatient and outpatient basis.

X.b.   Process monitoring should be a part of every perioperative setting as part of an overall sharps injury prevention program. Process monitoring should include
- ○ sharps injury data,[4]
- ○ double gloving compliance,
- ○ standard and transmissible infection precaution compliance,
- ○ safety-engineered device compliance, and
- ○ neutral zone implementation.

[1: Strong Evidence]

Monitoring sharps injury data allows results to be compared to a predetermined level of quality. Reviewing the findings provides information to identify problems and trends, which can be used to improve practice.[4,13]

X.b.1.   Perioperative personnel should report all percutaneous injuries according to organizational policy.

Injury reports provide data that can be used to identify problems and trends, and thus used used to improve safety. Health care workers in the perioperative setting under-report percutaneous injuries.[4,30,174] A questionnaire study asked surgeons how often they reported a sharps injury. Only 25.8% reported all of their injuries, 22.5% reported some of their injuries, and 51.7% reported none of their injuries.[199] In a retrospective survey of surgeons' needlestick injuries, only 9% reported the injury.[200]

X.b.2.   Sharps injury logs should be reviewed to identify trends in types and frequency of injuries.

X.b.3.   The organization should perform periodic audits for compliance with policies and use of safety-engineered devices, work practice controls, and barrier protection methods.

X.b.4.   Processes and systems should be evaluated after any sharps injury by using a quality improvement tool (eg, process map, flow chart, fishbone or cause-and-effect diagram, affinity diagram, root cause analysis).[4]

X.c.   The health care organization must conduct a yearly product evaluation and selection of safety-engineered devices.[38] *[1: Regulatory Requirement]*

X.d.   Perioperative nurses should contribute to creating a culture of safety. Health care organizations that support and promote safety may have a reduction in occupational exposures to bloodborne pathogens.[13,126,177,201-206] A culture of safety is created through

○ management initiatives that improve patient and health care personnel safety, [201,207,208]

○ health care personnel participation in safety planning,[4,201,209]

○ the availability of appropriate PPE and safety devices for identified tasks,[4]

○ the influence of group norms regarding appropriate safety practices,[207] and

○ the facility's socialization process for newly hired personnel.[4]

[2: High Evidence]

Glossary

Bloodborne pathogens: Pathogenic microorganisms that are present in human blood and can cause disease in humans. These pathogens include, but are not limited to, hepatitis B virus (HBV), hepatitis C virus (HCV), and human immunodeficiency virus (HIV) as defined by OSHA bloodborne pathogens standard 1910.1030.

Engineering controls: Safety-engineered devices designed to prevent or reduce the incidence of worker injury and the risk of bloodborne pathogen exposure to the worker.

Hands-free technique: Work practice that restricts members of the perioperative team at the sterile field from touching the same sharp instrument at the same time. Synonym, neutral zone.

Neutral zone: A safe work-practice control technique used to ensure that the surgeon and scrubbed person do not touch the same sharp instrument at the same time. This technique is accomplished by establishing a designated neutral zone on the sterile field and placing sharp items within the zone for transfer of the item between scrubbed personnel. Synonym: Hands-free technique.

No-touch technique: Technique that minimizes manual handling of sharp devices and instruments.

Perforation indicator system: A double gloving system comprising a colored pair of surgical gloves worn beneath a standard pair of surgical gloves. When a glove perforation occurs, moisture from the surgical field seeps through the perforation between the layers of gloves, allowing the site of perforation to be more easily seen.

Personal protective equipment (PPE): Specialized equipment or clothing for eyes, face, head, body, and extremities; protective clothing; respiratory devices; and protective shields and barriers designed to protect the worker from injury or exposure to a patient's blood, tissue, or body fluids. Used by health care workers and others whenever necessary to protect themselves from the hazards of processes or environments, chemical hazards, or mechanical irritants encountered in a manner capable of causing injury or impairment in the function of any part of the body through absorption, inhalation, or physical contact.

Potentially infectious material: Blood; all body fluids, secretions, and excretions (except sweat), regardless of whether they contain visible blood; nonintact skin; mucous membranes; and airborne, droplet, and contact-transmitted epidemiologically important pathogens.

Sharps with engineered sharps injury protection (SESIP): A sharp with a built-in safety feature or mechanism intended to reduce the risk of sharps injury.

Sharps: Items with edges or points capable of cutting or puncturing through other items. In the context of surgery, items include, but are not limited to, suture needles, scalpel blades, hypodermic needles, electrosurgical needles and blades, instruments with sharp edges or points, and safety pins.

Standard precautions: The primary strategy for successful infection control and reduction of worker exposure. Precautions used for care of all patients regardless of their diagnosis or presumed infectious status.

Work practice controls: Measures taken to reduce the likelihood of exposure by changing the method of performing a task to minimize the risk of exposure to blood or other potentially infectious materials.

REFERENCES

1. Pruss-Ustun A, Rapiti E, Hutin Y. Estimation of the global burden of disease attributable to contaminated sharps injuries among health-care workers. *Am J Ind Med.* 2005;48(6):482-490. [IVC]

2. Panlilio AL, Orelien JG, Srivastava PU, et al. Estimate of the annual number of percutaneous injuries among hospital-based healthcare workers in the United States, 1997-1998. *Infect Control Hosp Epidemiol.* 2004;25(7):556-562. [VB]

3. Weiss ES, Makary MA, Wang T, et al. Prevalence of blood-borne pathogens in an urban, university-based general surgical practice. *Ann Surg.* 2005;241(5):803-807;discussion 807-809. [VA]

4. *Workbook for Designing, Implementing, and Evaluating a Sharps Injury Prevention Program.* Centers for Disease Control and Prevention. http://www.cdc.gov/sharpssafety/pdf/sharpsworkbook_2008.pdf Accessed April 4, 2013. [IVA]

5. Vigler M, Mulett H, Hausman MR. Chronic Mycobacterium infection of first dorsal web space after accidental Bacilli Calmette-Guerin injection in a health worker: case report. *J Hand Surg Am* Vol. 2008;33(9):1621-1624. [VB]

6. Apisarnthanarak A, Mundy LM. Cytomegalovirus mononucleosis after percutaneous injury in a Thai medical student. *Am J Infect Control.* 2008;36(3):228-229. [VB]

7. Tarantola AP, Rachline AC, Konto C, et al. Occupational malaria following needlestick injury. *Emerg Infect Dis.* 2004;10(10):1878-1880. [VB]

8. Douglas MW, Walters JL, Currie BJ. Occupational infection with herpes simplex virus type 1 after a needlestick injury. *Med J Aust.* 2002;176(5):240. [VB]

9. Cone LA, Curry N, Wuestoff MA, O'Connell SJ, Feller JF. Septic synovitis and arthritis due to Corynebacterium striatum following an accidental scalpel injury. *Clin Infect Dis.* 1998;27(6):1532-1533. [VB]

10. Alweis RL, DiRosario K, Conidi G, Kain KC, Olans R, Tully JL. Serial nosocomial transmission of Plasmodium falciparum malaria from patient to nurse to patient. *Infect Control Hosp Epidemiol.* 2004;25(1):55-59. [VB]

11. Shibuya A, Takeuchi A, Sakurai K, Saigenji K. Hepatitis G virus infection from needle-stick injuries in hospital employees. *J Hosp Infect.* 1998;40(4):287-290. [IIIB]

12. Hidalgo JA, MacArthur RD, Crane LR. An overview of HIV infection and AIDS: etiology, pathogenesis, diagnosis, epidemiology, and occupational exposure. *Semin Thorac Cardiovasc Surg.* 2000;12(2):130-139. [VB]

13. MacCannell T, Laramie AK, Gomaa A, Perz JF. Occupational exposure of health care personnel to hepatitis B and hepatitis C: prevention and surveillance strategies. *Clin Liver Dis.* 2010;14(1):23-36, vii. [VA]

14. Fry DE. Occupational risks of blood exposure in the operating room. *Am Surg.* 2007;73(7):637-646. [VB]

15. Do AN, Ciesielski CA, Metler RP, Hammett TA, Li J, Fleming PL. Occupationally acquired human immunodeficiency virus (HIV) infection: national case surveillance data during 20 years of the HIV epidemic in the United States. *Infect Control Hosp Epidemiol.* 2003;24(2):86-96. [VA]

16. Tomkins S, Ncube F. Occupationally acquired HIV: international reports to December 2002. *Euro Surveill.* 2005;10(3):E050310.2. [VC]

17. Henderson DK. Managing occupational risks for hepatitis C transmission in the health care setting. *Clin Microbiol Rev.* 2003;16(3):546-568. [VA]

18. Tarantola A, Abiteboul D, Rachline A. Infection risks following accidental exposure to blood or body fluids in health care workers: a review of pathogens transmitted in published cases. *Am J Infect Control.* 2006;34(6):367-375. [VA]

19. US Public Health Service. Updated US Public Health Service guidelines for the management of occupational exposures to HBV, HCV, and HIV and recommendations for postexposure prophylaxis. *MMWR Recomm Rep.* 2001;50(RR-11):1-52. [IVA]

20. Centers for Disease Control and Prevention (CDC). Updated CDC recommendations for the management of hepatitis B virus-infected health-care providers and students. *MMWR Recomm Rep.* 2012;61(RR-3):1-12. [IVA]

21. Williams IT, Perz JF, Bell BP. Viral hepatitis transmission in ambulatory health care settings. *Clin Infect Dis.* 2004;38(11):1592-1598. [VA]

22. Advisory Committee on Immunization Practices, Centers for Disease Control and Prevention (CDC). Immunization of health-care personnel: recommendations of the Advisory Committee on Immunization Practices (ACIP). *MMWR Recomm Rep.* 2011;60(RR-7):1-45. [IVA]

23. *Combating the Silent Epidemic of Viral Hepatitis: Action Plan for the Prevention, Care & Treatment of Viral Hepatitis.* 2011. US Department of Health & Human Services. http://www.hhs.gov/ash/initiatives/hepatitis/actionplan_viralhepatitis2011.pdf. Accessed April 4, 2013. [IVA]

24. *NIOSH Alert: Preventing Needlestick Injuries in Health Care Settings.* NIOSH publication no. 2000-108. November 1999. National Institute for Occupational Safety and Health. http://www.cdc.gov/niosh/docs/2000-108/pdfs/2000-108.pdf. Accessed April 4, 2013. [IVB]

25. Mills PR, Thorburn D, McCruden EAB. Occupationally acquired hepatitis C infection. *Rev Med Microbiol.* 2000;11(1):15-22. [VA]

26. Panlilio AL, Cardo DM, Grohskopf LA, Heneine W, Ross CS; US Public Health Service. Updated US Public Health Service guidelines for the management of occupational exposures to HIV and recommendations for postexposure prophylaxis. *MMWR Recomm Rep.* 2005;54(RR-9):1-17. [IVA]

27. Young TN, Arens FJ, Kennedy GE, Laurie JW, Rutherford GW. Antiretroviral post-exposure prophylaxis (PEP) for occupational HIV exposure. *Cochrane Database Syst Rev.* 2007;(1):CD002835 [IA]

28. Cardo DM, Culver DH, Ciesielski CA, et al. A case-control study of HIV seroconversion in health care workers after percutaneous exposure. Centers for Disease Control and Prevention Needlestick Surveillance Group. *N Engl J Med.* 1997;337(21):1485-1490. [IIIB]

29. Regez RM, Kleipool AE, Speekenbrink RG, Frissen PH. The risk of needle stick accidents during surgical procedures: HIV-1 viral load in blood and bone marrow. *Int J STD AIDS.* 2005;16(10):671-672. [IVB]

30. Jagger J, Balon M. Suture needle and scalpel blade injuries: frequent but underreported. *Adv Expo Prev.* 1995;1(3):1-6. [VA]

31. Mallolas J, Gatell JM, Bruguera M. Transmission of HIV-1 from an obstetrician to a patient during a caesarean section [1]. *AIDS.* 2006;20(13):1785. [VB]

32. Information statement: Preventing the transmission of bloodborne pathogens. February 2001. Revised June 2008. Reviewed June 2012. American Academy of Orthopaedic Surgeons. http://www.aaos.org/about/papers/advistmt/1018.asp. Accessed April 4, 2013. [IVB]

33. Ross RS, Viazov S, Roggendorf M. Risk of hepatitis C transmission from infected medical staff to patients: model-based calculations for surgical settings. *Arch Intern Med.* 2000;160(15):2313-2316. [IIIB]

34. Folin AC, Nordstrom GM. Accidental blood contact during orthopedic surgical procedures. *Infect Control Hosp Epidemiol.* 1997;18(4):244-246. [VA]

35. Perry JL, Pearson RD, Jagger J. Infected health care workers and patient safety: a double standard. *Am J Infect Control.* 2006;34(5):313-319. [VB]

36. Jagger J, Perry J, Gomaa A, Phillips EK. The impact of US policies to protect healthcare workers from bloodborne pathogens: the critical role of safety-engineered devices. *J Infect Public Health.* 2008;1(2):62-71. [VA]

37. Fry DE. Hepatitis: risks for the surgeon. *Am Surg.* 2000;66(2):178-183. [VB]

38. 29 CFR 1910.1030. Occupational exposure. Bloodborne pathogens. 2009. http://www.gpo.gov/fdsys/pkg/CFR-2011-title29-vol6/pdf/CFR-2011-title29-vol6-sec1910-1030.pdf. Accessed April 4, 2013.

39. OSHA's bloodborne pathogens standard [risk analysis]. *Healthcare Risk Control.* 2008;4(Infection Control 13.1):1-20. [VA]

40. Needlestick Safety and Prevention Act of 2000. PL 106.430. http://www.gpo.gov/fdsys/pkg/PLAW-106publ430/html/PLAW-106publ430.htm. Accessed April 4, 2013.

41. Enforcement procedures for the occupational exposure to bloodborne pathogens. CPL 02-02-069. 2001. http://www.osha.gov/pls/oshaweb/owadisp.show_document?p_table=directives&p_id=2570. Accessed April 4, 2013.

42. Occupational exposure to bloodborne pathogens; needlestick and other sharps injuries; final rule. Occupational Safety and Health Administration (OSHA), Department of Labor. Final rule; request for comment on the Information Collection (Paperwork) Requirements. *Fed Regist.* 2001;66(12):5318-5325.

43. AORN position statement: workplace safety. AORN, Inc. http://www.aorn.org/uploadedFiles/Main_Navigation/Clinical_Practice/ToolKits/PosStat%20Work place%20Safety.pdf. Accessed April 5, 2013. [IVB]

44. AORN guidance statement: sharps injury prevention in the perioperative setting. In: *Perioperative Standards and Recommended Practices.* Denver, CO: AORN; 2012:711-716. [IVB]

45. Guideline statement for the implementation of the neutral zone in the perioperative environment. 2006. Association of Surgical Technologists. http://www.ast.org/

SHARPS SAFETY

PATIENT AND WORKER SAFETY

pdf/Standards_of_Practice/Guideline_Neutral_Zone.pdf. Accessed April 5, 2013. [IVC]

46. Recommended standards of practice for sharps safety and use of the neutral zone. 2006. Association of Surgical Technologists. http://www.ast.org/pdf/Standards_of_Practice/RSOP_Sharps_Safety_Neutral_Zone.pdf. Accessed April 5, 2013. [IVC]

47. Statement on sharps safety. American College of Surgeons. http://www.facs.org/fellows_info/statements/st-58.html. Accessed April 5, 2013. [IVB]

48. Sharps Safety #5: The CSPS endorses sharps safety measures to prevent injury during perioperative care. Sharps safety measures should include double-gloving, blunt suture needles for fascial closure, and the neutral zone when appropriate to avoid hand to hand passage of sharps. (Adopted 7.15.07, Modified 2.5.09). Council on Surgical & Perioperative Safety. http://cspsteam.org/sharpssafety/sharpssafety.html. Accessed April 5, 2013. [IVA]

49. Moving the sharps safety agenda forward in the United States: concensus statement and call to action. International Healthcare Worker Safety Center at the University of Virginia. http://www.healthsystem.virginia.edu/pub/epinet/ConsensusStatementOnSharpsInjuryPrevention.pdf. Accessed April 5, 2013. [IVA]

50. FDA, NIOSH & OSHA joint safety communication: blunt-tip surgical suture needles reduce needlestick injuries and the risk of subsequent bloodborne pathogen transmission to surgical personnel. US Food and Drug Administration. http://www.fda.gov/downloads/MedicalDevices/Safety/AlertsandNotices/UCM306035.pdf. Accessed April 5, 2013. [IVA]

51. Jagger J, Berguer R, Phillips EK, Parker G, Gomaa AE. Increase in sharps injuries in surgical settings versus nonsurgical settings after passage of national needlestick legislation. J Am Coll Surg. 2010;210(4):496-502. [VA]

52. Jagger J, Bentley M, Tereskerz P. A study of patterns and prevention of blood exposures in OR personnel. AORN J. 1998;67(5):979-987. [IIIA]

53. Lee WC, Nicklasson L, Cobden D, Chen E, Conway D, Pashos CL. Short-term economic impact associated with occupational needlestick injuries among acute care nurses. Curr Med Res Opin. 2005;21(12):1915-1922. [IIIA]

54. O'Malley EM, Scott RD 2nd, Gayle J, et al. Costs of management of occupational exposures to blood and body fluids. Infect Control Hosp Epidemiol. 2007;28(7):774-782. [VB]

55. Leigh JP, Gillen M, Franks P, et al. Costs of needlestick injuries and subsequent hepatitis and HIV infection. Curr Med Res Opin. 2007;23(9):2093-2105. [VA]

56. Lee JM, Botteman MF, Xanthakos N, Nicklasson L. Needlestick injuries in the United States. Epidemiologic, economic, and quality of life issues. AAOHN J. 2005;53(3):117-133. [IIIB]

57. APIC position paper: prevention of device-mediated bloodborne infections to health care workers. Association for Professionals in Infection Control and Epidemiology, Inc. Am J Infect Control. 1998;26(6):578-580. [IVB]

58. Jagger J, Perry J. Using needlestick data to target safety device implementation. Clin Occup Environ Med. 2002;2(3):557-573. [VA]

59. Adams D. Needlestick and sharps injuries: practice update. Nurs Stand. 2012;26(37):49-57; quiz 58. [VA]

60. Rabussay DP, Korniewicz DM. Improving glove barrier effectiveness. AORN J. 1997;66(6):1043-1046. [IVB]

61. Chiarello LA. Selection of needlestick prevention devices: a conceptual framework for approaching product evaluation. Am J Infect Control. 1995;23(6):386-395. [VB]

62. Tosini W, Ciotti C, Goyer F, et al. Needlestick injury rates according to different types of safety-engineered devices: results of a French multicenter study. Infect Control Hosp Epidemiol. 2010;31(4):402-407. [IIIB]

63. Safer medical devices must be selected based on employee feedback and device effectiveness, not Group Purchasing Organizations. November 21, 2002. Occupational Safety and Health Administration. http://www.osha.gov/pls/oshaweb/owadisp.show_document?p_table=INTERPRETATIONS. Accessed April 5, 2013.

64. Employer's responsibility to re-evaluate engineering controls, i.e., safer needle devices, at least annually. January 20, 2004. Occupational Safety and Health Administration. http://www.osha.gov/pls/oshaweb/owadisp.show_document?p_table=INTERPRETATIONS&p_id=24780. Accessed April 5, 2013.

65. Tuma S, Sepkowitz KA. Efficacy of safety-engineered device implementation in the prevention of percutaneous injuries: a review of published studies. Clin Infect Dis. 2006;42(8):1159-1170. [IVA]

66. Valls V, Lozano MS, Yanez R, et al. Use of safety devices and the prevention of percutaneous injuries among healthcare workers. Infect Control Hosp Epidemiol. 2007;28(12):1352-1360. [IIA]

67. Azar-Cavanagh M, Burdt P, Green-McKenzie J. Effect of the introduction of an engineered sharps injury prevention device on the percutaneous injury rate in healthcare workers. Infect Control Hosp Epidemiol. 2007;28(2):165-170. [IIA]

68. Laramie AK, Pun VC, Fang SC, Kriebel D, Davis L. Sharps Injuries among employees of acute care hospitals in Massachusetts, 2002-2007. Infect Control Hosp Epidemiol. 2011;32(6):538-544. [IIIB]

69. Waclawski ER. Evaluation of potential reduction in blood and body fluid exposures by use of alternative instruments. Occup Med (Lond). 2004;54(8):567-569. [VA]

70. Cullen BL, Genasi F, Symington I, et al. Potential for reported needlestick injury prevention among healthcare workers through safety device usage and improvement of guideline adherence: expert panel assessment. J Hosp Infect. 2006;63(4):445-451. [IIIB]

71. Parantainen A, Verbeek JH, Lavoie MC, Pahwa M. Blunt versus sharp suture needles for preventing percutaneous exposure incidents in surgical staff. Cochrane Database Syst Rev. 2011;11:CD009170. [IA]

72. Nordkam RA, Bluyssen SJ, van Goor H. Randomized clinical trial comparing blunt tapered and standard needles in closing abdominal fascia. World J Surg. 2005;29(4):441-445. [IA]

73. Use of blunt-tip suture needles to decrease percutaneous injuries to surgical personnel. DHHS (NIOSH) Publication No. 2008–101. 2008. http://www.cdc.gov/niosh/docs/2008-101/pdfs/2008-101.pdf. Accessed April 5, 2013. [IVA]

74. Miller SS, Sabharwal A. Subcuticular skin closure using a "blunt" needle. Ann R Coll Surg Engl. 1994;76(4):281. [IIIC]

75. Makary MA, Al-Attar A, Holzmueller CG, et al. Needlestick injuries among surgeons in training. N Engl J Med. 2007;356(26):2693-2699. [IIIA]

76. Berguer R, Heller PJ. Preventing sharps injuries in the operating room. J Am Coll Surg. 2004;199(3):462-467. [VA]

77. Sullivan S, Williamson B, Wilson LK, Korte JE, Soper D. Blunt needles for the reduction of needlestick injuries during cesarean delivery: a randomized controlled trial. Obstet Gynecol. 2009;114(2 Pt 1):211-216. [IA]

78. Centers for Disease Control and Prevention (CDC). Evaluation of blunt suture needles in preventing percutaneous injuries among health-care workers

during gynecologic surgical procedures—New York City, March 1993-June 1994. *MMWR Morb Mortal Wkly Rep.* 1997;46(2):25-29. [IIIB]

79. Hartley JE, Ahmed S, Milkins R, Naylor G, Monson JR, Lee PW. Randomized trial of blunt-tipped versus cutting needles to reduce glove puncture during mass closure of the abdomen. *Br J Surg.* 1996;83(8):1156-1157. [IB]

80. Mingoli A, Sapienza P, Sgarzini G, et al. Influence of blunt needles on surgical glove perforation and safety for the surgeon. *Am J Surg.* 1996;172(5):512-516. [IB]

81. Edlich RF, Wind TC, Hill LG, Thacker JG, McGregor W. Reducing accidental injuries during surgery. *J Long Term Eff Med Implants.* 2003;13(1):1-10. [IB]

82. Yang L, Mullan B. Reducing needle stick injuries in healthcare occupations: an integrative review of the literature. *ISRN Nurs.* 2011;2011:315432. doi:10.5402/2011/315432. [VA]

83. Stafford MK, Pitman MC, Nanthakumaran N, Smith JR. Blunt-tipped versus sharp-tipped needles: wound morbidity. *J Obstet Gynaecol.* 1998;18(1):18-19. [IB]

84. Mornar SJ, Perlow JH. Blunt suture needle use in laceration and episiotomy repair at vaginal delivery. *Am J Obstet Gynecol.* 2008;198(5):e14-e15. [IIIB]

85. Ablett JC, Whitten M, Smith JR. Do blunt tipped needles reduce the risk of glove puncture and needlestick injury in the suture of episiotomy and perineal repair? *J Obstet Gynaecol.* 1998;18(5):478-479. [IA]

86. Catanzarite V, Byrd K, McNamara M, Bombard A. Preventing needlestick injuries in obstetrics and gynecology: how can we improve the use of blunt tip needles in practice? *Obstet Gynecol.* 2007;110(6):1399-1403. [IIIB]

87. Wilson LK, Sullivan S, Goodnight W, Chang EY, Soper D. The use of blunt needles does not reduce glove perforations during obstetrical laceration repair. *Am J Obstet Gynecol.* 2008;199(6):641.e1-641.e3. [IA]

88. Limiting factors for implementing the use of engineering controls, i.e., safety scalpels, under the Bloodborne Pathogens standard. September 1, 2004. Occupational Safety and Health Administration. http://www.osha.gov/pls/oshaweb/owadisp.show_document?p_table=INTERPRETATIONS&p_id=25090. Accessed April 5, 2013.

89. Jagger J, Berguer R, Phillips EK, Parker G, Gomaa AE. Increase in sharps injuries in surgical settings versus nonsurgical settings after passage of national needlestick legislation. *AORN J.* 2011;93(3):322-330. [VA]

90. Perry J, Parker G, Jagger J. Scalpel blades: reducing injury risk. *Adv Expo Prev.* 2003;6(4):37-40. [VA]

91. Fuentes H, Collier J, Sinnott M, Whitby M. Scalpel safety: modeling the effectiveness of different safety devices' ability to reduce scalpel blade injuries. *Intern J Risk Safety Med.* 2008;20(1-2):83-89. [IIIC]

92. Dagi TF, Berguer R, Moore S, Reines HD. Preventable errors in the operating room—part 2: retained foreign objects, sharps injuries, and wrong site surgery. *Curr Probl Surg.* 2007;44(6):352-381. [VA]

93. Makary MA, Pronovost PJ, Weiss ES, et al. Sharpless surgery: a prospective study of the feasibility of performing operations using non-sharp techniques in an urban, university-based surgical practice. *World J Surg.* 2006;30(7):1224-1229. [IIIB]

94. Bhattacharyya M, Bradley H. Intraoperative handling and wound healing of arthroscopic portal wounds: a clinical study comparing nylon suture with wound closure strips. *J Perioper Pract.* 2008;18(5):194-196. [IB]

95. Coulthard P, Esposito M, Worthington HV, van der Elst M, van Waes OJ, Darcey J. Tissue adhesives for closure of surgical incisions. *Cochrane Database Syst Rev.* 2010;(5)(5):CD004287. [IA]

96. Williams CP, Rosen MJ, Jin J, McGee MF, Schomisch SJ, Ponsky J. Objective analysis of the accuracy and efficacy of a novel fascial closure device. *Surg Innov.* 2008;15(4):307-311. [IA]

97. Whitby M, McLaws ML, Slater K. Needlestick injuries in a major teaching hospital: the worthwhile effect of hospital-wide replacement of conventional hollow-bore needles. *Am J Infect Control.* 2008;36(3):180-186. [IIA]

98. Rogers B, Goodno L. Evaluation of interventions to prevent needlestick injuries in health care occupations. *Am J Prev Med.* 2000;18(4 Suppl):90-98. [IA]

99. Guideline for medication safety. In: *Guidelines for Perioperative Practice.* Denver, CO: AORN, Inc; 2015:291-329. [IVB]

100. Perry J, Parker G, Jagger JJ. EPINet report: 2003 percutaneous injury rates. *Adv Expo Prev.* 2005;7(4):42-45. [VA]

101. Perry J, Parker G, Jagger J. EPINet report: 2007 percutaneous injury rates. 2009. University of Virginia Health System. http://www.healthsystem.virginia.edu/pub/epinet/epinet-2007-rates.pdf. Accessed April 5, 2013. [VA]

102. Guideline for prevention of retained surgical items. In: *Guidelines for Perioperative Practice.* Denver, CO: AORN, Inc; 2015:347-363. [IVB]

103. Folin A, Nyberg B, Nordstrom G. Reducing blood exposures during orthopedic surgical procedures. *AORN J.* 2000;71(3):573-576. [IIB]

104. Jeong IS, Park S. Use of hands-free technique among operating room nurses in the Republic of Korea. *Am J Infect Control.* 2009;37(2):131-135. [IIIB]

105. Stringer B, Haines AT, Goldsmith CH, Berguer R, Blythe J. Is use of the hands-free technique during surgery, a safe work practice, associated with safety climate? *Am J Infect Control.* 2009;37(9):766-772. [IIIA]

106. Stringer B, Haines T. The hands-free technique: an effective and easily implemented work practice. *Perioper Nurs Clin.* 2010;5(1):45-58. [VC]

107. Stringer B, Haines T, Goldsmith CH, et al. Hands-free technique in the operating room: reduction in body fluid exposure and the value of a training video. *Public Health Rep.* 2009;124(Suppl 1):169-179. [IIB]

108. The use of safety-engineered devices and work practice controls in operating rooms; hospital responsibility to protect independent practitioners under BBP standard. January 18, 2007. Occupational Safety and Health Administration. http://www.osha.gov/pls/oshaweb/owadisp.show_document?p_table=INTERPRETATIONS&p_id=25620. Accessed April 5, 2013.

109. Bessinger CD Jr. Preventing transmission of human immunodeficiency virus during operations. *Surg Gynecol Obstet.* 1988;167(4):287-289. [VA]

110. Stringer B, Infante-Rivard C, Hanley JA. Effectiveness of the hands-free technique in reducing operating theatre injuries. *Occup Environ Med.* 2002;59(10):703-707. [IIIB]

111. Cunningham TR, Austin J. Using goal setting, task clarification, and feedback to increase the use of the hands-free technique by hospital operating room staff. *J Appl Behav Anal.* 2007;40(4):673-677. [IIA]

112. Eggleston MK Jr, Wax JR, Philput C, Eggleston MH, Weiss MI. Use of surgical pass trays to reduce intraoperative glove perforations. *J Matern Fetal Med.* 1997;6(4):245-247. [IC]

113. Stringer B, Haines T, Goldsmith CH, Blythe J, Harris KA. Perioperative use of the hands-free technique: a semistructured interview study. *AORN J.* 2006;84(2):233-248. [IIIB]

114. Lopez RA, Rayan GM, Monlux R. Hand injuries during hand surgery: a survey of intraoperative sharp injuries

435

of the hand among hand surgeons. *J Hand Surg Eur Vol.* 2008;33(5):661-666. [IIIA]

115. Ghauri AJ, Amissah-Arthur KN, Rashid A, Mushtaq B, Nessim M, Elsherbiny S. Sharps injuries in ophthalmic practice. *Eye.* 2011;25(4):443-448. [IIIB]

116. Raahave D, Bremmelgaard A. New operative technique to reduce surgeons' risk of HIV infection. *J Hosp Infect.* 1991;18(Suppl A):177-183. [VB]

117. Wallace CG, Browning GG. A novel technique to reduce curved needlestick injuries. *Ann R Coll Surg Engl.* 2004;86(2):128. [VB]

118. Kunishige J, Wanitphakdeedecha R, Nguyen TH, Chen TM. Surgical pearl: a simple means of disarming the "locked and loaded" needle. *Int J Dermatol.* 2008;47(8):848-849. [VC]

119. Sinnott Michael, Shaban Ramon. "Scalpel Safety," not "Safety Scalpel": A New Paradigm in Staff Safety. *Perioper Nurs Clin.* 2010;5(1):59-67. [VA]

120. Ly J, Mittal A, Windsor J. Systematic review and meta-analysis of cutting diathermy versus scalpel for skin incision. *Br J Surg.* 2012;99(5):613-620. [IA]

121. Vose JG, McAdara-Berkowitz J. Reducing scalpel injuries in the operating room. *AORN J.* 2009;90(6):867-872. [VB]

122. Hutin Y, Hauri A, Chiarello L, et al. Best infection control practices for intradermal, subcutaneous, and intramuscular needle injections. *Bull World Health Organ.* 2003;81(7):491-500. [IVA]

123. Froom P, Kristal-Boneh E, Melamed S, Shalom A, Ribak J. Prevention of needle-stick injury by the scooping-resheathing method. *Am J Ind Med.* 1998;34(1):15-19. [IIIB]

124. Carraretto AR, Curi EF, de Almeida CE, Abatti RE. Glass ampoules: risks and benefits. *Rev Bras Anestesiol.* 2011;61(4):513-521. [VB]

125. Section VI: Chapter 2: Controlling occupational exposure to hazardous drugs. In: *OSHA Technical Manual.* 1999. Occupational Health & Safety Administration. http://www.osha.gov/dts/osta/otm/otm_vi/otm_vi_2.html. Accessed April 5, 2013.

126. Smith DR, Muto T, Sairenchi T, et al. Hospital safety climate, psychosocial risk factors and needlestick injuries in Japan. *Ind Health.* 2010;48(1):85-95. [IIIA]

127. Parker MR. The use of protective gloves, the incidence of ampoule injury and the prevalence of hand laceration amongst anaesthetic personnel. *Anaesthesia.* 1995;50(8):726-729. [IIIB]

128. Smith DR, Leggat PA. Needlestick and sharps injuries among nursing students. *J Adv Nurs.* 2005;51(5):449-455. [IIIB]

129. Pulnitiporn A, Chau-in W, Klanarong S, Thienthong S, Inphum P. The Thai Anesthesia Incidents Study (THAI Study) of anesthesia personnel hazard. *J Med Assoc Thai.* 2005;88(Suppl 7):S141-S144. [IIIB]

130. Siegel JD, Rhinehart E, Jackson M, Chiarello L; Health Care Infection Control Practices Advisory Committee. 2007 Guideline for isolation precautions: preventing transmission of infectious agents in health care settings. *Am J Infect Control.* 2007;35(10 Suppl 2):S65-S164. [IVA]

131. Guideline for prevention of transmissible infections. In: *Guidelines for Perioperative Practice.* Denver, CO: AORN, Inc; 2015:419-451. [IVA]

132. Cicconi L, Claypool M, Stevens W. Prevention of transmissible infections in the perioperative setting. *AORN J.* 2010;92(5):519-527. [VB]

133. Aarnio P, Laine T. Glove perforation rate in vascular surgery—a comparison between single and double gloving. *Vasa.* 2001;30(2):122-124. [IA]

134. Plucknett B, Kaminski PF, Podczaski ES, Sorosky JI, Pees RC. Punctured surgical gloves in major gynecologic

surgery: does surgical experience of the operator make a difference? *J Gynecol Surg.* 1992;8(2):77-80. [IIIC]

135. Guideline for sterile technique. In: *Guidelines for Perioperative Practice.* Denver, CO: AORN, Inc; 2015:67-96. [IVA]

136. Tanner J, Parkinson H. Double gloving to reduce surgical cross-infection. *Cochrane Database Syst Rev.* 2009;3:CD003087. [IA]

137. Kinlin LM, Mittleman MA, Harris AD, Rubin MA, Fisman DN. Use of gloves and reduction of risk of injury caused by needles or sharp medical devices in healthcare workers: results from a case-crossover study. *Infect Control Hosp Epidemiol.* 2010;31(9):908-917. [IIIB]

138. Wittmann A, Kralj N, Kover J, Gasthaus K, Lerch H, Hofmann F. Comparison of 4 different types of surgical gloves used for preventing blood contact. *Infect Control Hosp Epidemiol.* 2010;31(5):498-502. [IIA]

139. Chan KY, Singh VA, Oun BH, To BH. The rate of glove perforations in orthopaedic procedures: single versus double gloving. A prospective study. *Med J Malaysia.* 2006;61(Suppl B):3-7. [IIIB]

140. Tanner J. Surgical gloves: perforation and protection. *J Perioper Pract.* 2006;16(3):148-152. [VB]

141. Guo YP, Wong PM, Li Y, Or PP. Is double-gloving really protective? A comparison between the glove perforation rate among perioperative nurses with single and double gloves during surgery. *Am J Surg.* 2012;204(2):210-215. [IIA]

142. Thomas S, Agarwal M, Mehta G. Intraoperative glove perforation—single versus double gloving in protection against skin contamination. *Postgrad Med J.* 2001;77(909):458-460. [IB]

143. Mansouri M, Tidley M, Sanati KA, Roberts C. Comparison of blood transmission through latex and nitrile glove materials. *Occup Med.* 2010;60(3):205-210. [IB]

144. Wittmann A, Kralj N, Kover J, Gasthaus K, Hofmann F. Study of blood contact in simulated surgical needlestick injuries with single or double latex gloving. *Infect Control Hosp Epidemiol.* 2009;30(1):53-56. [IIA]

145. Lancaster C, Duff P. Single versus double-gloving for obstetric and gynecologic procedures. *Am J Obstet Gynecol.* 2007;196(5):e36-e37. http://www.ajog.org/article/S0002-9378(06)01185-9/fulltext. Accessed April 5, 2013. [VA]

146. Lefebvre DR, Strande LF, Hewitt CW. An enzyme-mediated assay to quantify inoculation volume delivered by suture needlestick injury: two gloves are better than one. *J Am Coll Surg.* 2008;206(1):113-122. [IA]

147. Chapman S, Duff P. Frequency of glove perforations and subsequent blood contact in association with selected obstetric surgical procedures. *Am J Obstet Gynecol.* 1993;168(5):1354-1357. [IIIB]

148. Bennett NT, Howard RJ. Quantity of blood inoculated in a needlestick injury from suture needles. *J Am Coll Surg.* 1994;178(2):107-110. [IB]

149. Laine T, Aarnio P. How often does glove perforation occur in surgery? Comparison between single gloves and a double-gloving system. *Am J Surg.* 2001;181(6):564-566. [IA]

150. Ersozlu S, Sahin O, Ozgur AF, Akkaya T, Tuncay C. Glove punctures in major and minor orthopaedic surgery with double gloving. *Acta Orthop Belg.* 2007;73(6):760-764. [IIIB]

151. Caillot JL, Paparel P, Arnal E, Schreiber V, Voiglio EJ. Anticipated detection of imminent surgeon-patient barrier breaches. A prospective randomized controlled trial using an indicator underglove system. *World J Surg.* 2006;30(1):134-138. [IB]

152. Edlich RF, Long WB 3rd, Gubler K, et al. Reducing accidental injuries during surgery. *J Environ Pathol Toxicol Oncol.* 2010;29(4):317-326. [VB]

153. Edlich RF, Wind TC, Heather CL, Thacker JG. Reliability and performance of innovative surgical double-glove hole puncture indication systems. *J Long Term Eff Med Implants.* 2003;13(2):69-83. [IB]

154. Edlich RF, Wind TC, Hill LG, Thacker JG. Resistance of double-glove hole puncture indication systems to surgical needle puncture. *J Long Term Eff Med Implants.* 2003;13(2):85-90. [IB]

155. Florman S, Burgdorf M, Finigan K, Slakey D, Hewitt R, Nichols RL. Efficacy of double gloving with an intrinsic indicator system. *Surg Infect (Larchmt).* 2005;6(4):385-395. [IIB]

156. ASTM D3577-09e1: Standard specification for rubber surgical gloves. 2009. [IVB]

157. Demircay E, Unay K, Bilgili MG, Alataca G. Glove perforation in hip and knee arthroplasty. *J Orthop Sci.* 2010;15(6):790-794. [IIIA]

158. Thomas S, Aldlyami E, Gupta S, Reed MR, Muller SD, Partington PF. Unsuitability and high perforation rate of latex-free gloves in arthroplasty: a cause for concern. *Arch Orthop Trauma Surg.* 2011;131(4):455-458. [IIIB]

159. Al-Maiyah M, Bajwa A, Mackenney P, et al. Glove perforation and contamination in primary total hip arthroplasty. *J Bone Joint Surg Br.* 2005;87(4):556-559. [IA]

160. Faisal-Cury A, Rossi Menezes P, Kahhale S, Zugaib M. A study of the incidence and recognition of surgical glove perforation during obstetric and gynecological procedures. *Arch Gynecol Obstet.* 2004;270(4):263-264. [IIIB]

161. Feng T, Yohannan J, Gupta A, Hyndman ME, Allaf M. Microperforations of surgical gloves in urology: minimally invasive versus open surgeries. *Can J Urol.* 2011;18(2):5615-5618. [IIIB]

162. Harnoss JC, Partecke LI, Heidecke CD, Hubner NO, Kramer A, Assadian O. Concentration of bacteria passing through puncture holes in surgical gloves. *Am J Infect Control.* 2010;38(2):154-158. [IIA]

163. Caillot JL, Voiglio EJ. First clinical study of a new virus-inhibiting surgical glove. *Swiss Med Wkly.* 2008;138(1-2):18-22. [IIIA]

164. Krikorian R, Lozach-Perlant A, Ferrier-Rembert A, et al. Standardization of needlestick injury and evaluation of a novel virus-inhibiting protective glove. *J Hosp Infect.* 2007;66(4):339-345. [IIB]

165. Bricout F, Moraillon A, Sonntag P, Hoerner P, Blackwelder W, Plotkin S. Virus-inhibiting surgical glove to reduce the risk of infection by enveloped viruses. *J Med Virol.* 2003;69(4):538-545. [IB]

166. Daeschlein G, Kramer A, Arnold A, Ladwig A, Seabrook GR, Edmiston CE Jr. Evaluation of an innovative antimicrobial surgical glove technology to reduce the risk of microbial passage following intraoperative perforation. *Am J Infect Control.* 2011;39(2):98-103. [IIB]

167. Grimmond T, Bylund S, Anglea C, et al. Sharps injury reduction using a sharps container with enhanced engineering: a 28 hospital nonrandomized intervention and cohort study. *Am J Infect Control.* 2010;38(10):799-805. [IIB]

168. Perry J, Jagger J, Parker G, Phillips EK, Gomaa A. Disposal of sharps medical waste in the United States: impact of recommendations and regulations, 1987-2007. *Am J Infect Control.* 2011;40(4):354-358.

169. Selecting, evaluating, and using sharps disposal containers. NIOSH publication no. 97-111. 1998. National Institute for Occupational Safety and Health. http://www.cdc.gov/niosh/pdfs/97-111.pdf. Accessed April 5, 2013. [IVB]

170. Blenkharn JI, Odd C. Sharps injuries in healthcare waste handlers. *Ann Occup Hyg.* 2008;52(4):281-286. [IIIC]

171. Standards of perioperative nursing. In: *Perioperative Standards and Recommended Practices.* Denver, CO: AORN, Inc; 2012:2-20. [IVB]

172. Cutter J, Jordan S. Uptake of guidelines to avoid and report exposure to blood and body fluids. *J Adv Nurs.* 2004;46(4):441-452. [IIIB]

173. Doebbeling BN, Vaughn TE, McCoy KD, et al. Percutaneous injury, blood exposure, and adherence to standard precautions: are hospital-based health care providers still at risk? *Clin Infect Dis.* 2003;37(8):1006-1013. [IIIB]

174. Kennedy R, Kelly S, Gonsalves S, Mc Cann PA. Barriers to the reporting and management of needlestick injuries among surgeons. Ir *J Med Sci.* 2009;178(3):297-299. [IIIB]

175. Kessler CS, McGuinn M, Spec A, Christensen J, Baragi R, Hershow RC. Underreporting of blood and body fluid exposures among health care students and trainees in the acute care setting: a 2007 survey. *Am J Infect Control.* 2011;39(2):129-134. [IIIB]

176. Kak N, Burkhalter B, Cooper M-A. *Measuring the Competence of Healthcare Providers.* Operations Research Issue Paper 2(1). Bethesda, MD: Quality Assurance Project for the US Agency for International Development; 2001. http://www.hciproject.org/sites/default/files/Measuring%20the%20Competence%20of%20HC%20Providers_QAP_2001.pdf. Accessed April 5, 2013. [VA]

177. Vaughn TE, McCoy KD, Beekmann SE, Woolson RE, Torner JC, Doebbeling BN. Factors promoting consistent adherence to safe needle precautions among hospital workers. *Infect Control Hosp Epidemiol.* 2004;25(7):548-555. [IIA]

178. Holodnick CL, Barkauskas V. Reducing percutaneous injuries in the OR by educational methods. *AORN J.* 2000;72(3):461-476. [VB]

179. Brusaferro S, Calligaris L, Farneti F, Gubian F, Londero C, Baldo V. Educational programmes and sharps injuries in health care workers. *Occup Med (Oxford).* 2009;59(7):512-514. [IIB]

180. Bakaeen F, Awad S, Albo D, et al. Epidemiology of exposure to blood borne pathogens on a surgical service. *Am J Surg.* 2006;192(5):e18-e21. [VA]

181. HR.01.05.03: Staff participate in ongoing education and training. In: *Comprehensive Accreditation Manual for Ambulatory Care.* Oakbrook Terrace, IL: The Joint Commission; 2012.

182. HR.01.05.03: Staff participate in ongoing education and training. In: *Comprehensive Accreditation Manual: CAMH for Hospitals.* Oakbrook Terrace, IL: The Joint Commission; 2012.

183. State Operations Manual. Appendix A: Survey protocol, regulations and interpretive guidelines for hospitals. Rev 78;2011. Centers for Medicare & Medicaid Services. http://www.cms.gov/Regulations-and-Guidance/Guidance/Manuals/downloads/som107ap_a_hospitals.pdf. Accessed April 5, 2013.

184. State Operations Manual. Appendix L: Guidance for surveyors: ambulatory surgical centers. Rev 76;2011. Centers for Medicare & Medicaid Services. http://www.cms.gov/Regulations-and-Guidance/Guidance/Manuals/downloads/som107ap_l_ambulatory.pdf. Accessed April 5, 2013.

185. Sportsman S. Competency education and validation in the United States: what should nurses know? *Nurs Forum.* 2010;45(3):140-149. [VA]

186. Jordan C, Thomas MB, Evans ML, Green A. Public policy on competency: how will nursing address this complex issue? *J Contin Educ Nurs.* 2008;39(2):86-91. [VA]

187. Yang YH, Liou SH, Chen CJ, et al. The effectiveness of a training program on reducing needlestick injuries/

sharp object injuries among soon graduate vocational nursing school students in southern Taiwan. *J Occup Health.* 2007;49(5):424-429. [IIIB]

188. Ling ML, Wee M, Chan YH. Sharps and needlestick injuries: the impact of hepatitis B vaccination as an intervention measure. *Ann Acad Med Singap.* 2000;29(1):86-89. [IIB]

189. Elliott SK, Keeton A, Holt A. Medical students' knowledge of sharps injuries. *J Hosp Infect.* 2005;60(4):374-377. [IIIB]

190. Hambridge K. Needlestick and sharps injuries in the nursing student population. *Nurs Stand.* 2011;25(27):38-45. [VB]

191. Blackwell L, Bolding J, Cheely E, et al. Nursing students' experiences with needlestick injuries. *J Undergrad Nurs Scholarsh.* 2007;9(1). http://www.juns.nursing.arizona.edu/articles/Fall%202007/Nursing%20Students'%20Experiences%20with%20Needlestick%20Injuries.pdf. Accessed April 5, 2013. [IIIB]

192. Salzer HJ, Hoenigl M, Kessler HH, et al. Lack of risk-awareness and reporting behavior towards HIV infection through needlestick injury among European medical students. *Int J Hyg Environ Health.* 2011;214(5):407-410. [IIIB]

193. Brasel KJ, Mol C, Kolker A, Weigelt JA. Needlesticks and surgical residents: who is most at risk? *J Surg Educ.* 2007;64(6):395-398. [VB]

194. Protecting workers' families: a research agenda. Report of the Workers' Family Protection Task Force. DHHS (NIOSH) Publication No. 2002–113. 2002. National Institute for Occupational Safety and Health. http://www.cdc.gov/niosh/docs/2002-113/pdfs/2002-113.pdf. Accessed April 5, 2013. [VA]

195. 29 CFR 1904.8. Recording criteria for needlestick and sharps injuries. 2010. US Government Printing Office. http://www.gpo.gov/fdsys/granule/CFR-2010-title29-vol5/CFR-2010-title29-vol5-sec1904-8/content-detail.html. Accessed April 5, 2013.

196. Self-assessment questionnaire: bloodborne pathogens policies and procedures. *Operating Room Risk Management.* 2010;1-28. [VB]

197. Hubbard A. The rights of healthcare professionals with blood-borne illnesses under the Americans with Disabilities Act. *Clin Occup Environ Med.* 2002;2(3):593-608. [VA]

198. Farquhar M, Hughes R, Hughes RF. AHRQ quality indicators. In: Hughes RF, ed. *Patient Safety and Quality: An Evidence-based Handbook for Nurses.* Rockville MD: Agency for Healthcare Research and Quality; 2008:41-67. http://www.ahrq.gov/qual/nurseshdbk/. Accessed April 5, 2013. [IA]

199. Kerr HL, Stewart N, Pace A, Elsayed S. Sharps injury reporting amongst surgeons. *Ann R Coll Surg Engl.* 2009;91(5):430-432. [VB]

200. Thomas WJ, Murray JR. The incidence and reporting rates of needle-stick injury amongst UK surgeons. *Ann R Coll Surg Engl.* 2009;91(1):12-17. [VB]

201. Hooper J, Charney W. Creation of a safety culture: reducing workplace injuries in a rural hospital setting. *AAOHN J.* 2005;53(9):394-398. [IIIB]

202. McIntosh KR, Rever-Moriyama SD. Using a systems approach in developing a survey to assess the contributing factors to needlestick injuries. *Proc Hum Fact Ergon Soc Annu Meet.* 1997;41(2):782-786. [IIIB]

203. McIntosh KR. Taking the blame off of health care workers: using a systems approach to determine the contributing factors to needlestick injuries. *Proc Hum Fact Ergon Soc Annu Meet.* 1998;42(14):1033-1037. [IIIB]

204. Taylor JA, Dominici F, Agnew J, Gerwin D, Morlock L, Miller MR. Do nurse and patient injuries share common antecedents? An analysis of associations with safety climate and working conditions. *BMJ Qual Saf.* 2012;21(2):101-111. [IIIB]

205. Blouin AS, McDonagh KJ. Framework for patient safety, part 1: culture as an imperative. *J Nurs Adm.* 2011;41(10):397-400. [VB]

206. Mark BA, Hughes LC, Belyea M, et al. Does safety climate moderate the influence of staffing adequacy and work conditions on nurse injuries? *J Saf Res.* 2007;38(4):431-446. [IIIA]

207. Gershon RR, Karkashian CD, Grosch JW, et al. Hospital safety climate and its relationship with safe work practices and workplace exposure incidents. *Am J Infect Control.* 2000;28(3):211-221. [IIIB]

208. Hunt J, Murphy C. Measurement of nursing staff occupational exposures in the operating suite following introduction of a prevention programme. *Aust Infect Control.* 2004;9(2):57. [IIB]

209. Blouin AS, McDonagh KJ. A framework for patient safety, part 2: resilience, the next frontier. *J Nurs Adm.* 2011;41(11):450-452. [VA]

Acknowledgements

LEAD AUTHOR
Mary J. Ogg, MSN, RN, CNOR
Perioperative Nursing Specialist
AORN Nursing Department
Denver, Colorado

CONTRIBUTING AUTHOR
Ramona Conner, MSN, RN, CNOR
Manager, Standards and Guidelines
AORN Nursing Department
Denver, Colorado

The authors and AORN thank George D. Allen, PhD, MS, RN, CNOR, CIC, Director, Infection Control, Downstate Medical Center, and Clinical Assistant Professor, SUNY College of Health Related Professions, Brooklyn, NY; Amy L. Halverson, MD, American College of Surgeons; Rodney W. Hicks, PhD, ARNP, RN, FAANP, FAAN, Professor, Western University of Health Science, Pomona, CA; Elayne Kornblatt Phillips, PhD-BSN, MPH, RN, International Healthcare Worker Safety Center, University of Virginia, Charlottesville; Rev Donna S. Nussman, PhD, RN, Surgical Health Care Consultant, and Adjunct Professor, College of Mechanical Engineering/BioEngineering Department, University of North Carolina - Charlotte; and Lisa Spruce, DNP, RN, ACNS, ACNP, ANP, CNOR, Director of Evidence-based Nursing Practice, AORN, Inc, Denver, CO, for their assistance in developing this guideline.

PUBLICATION HISTORY
Originally published June 2013 online in *Perioperative Standards and Recommended Practices.*

Evidence ratings revised 2013 to conform to the AORN Evidence Rating Model.

Minor editing revisions made in November 2014 for publication in *Guidelines for Perioperative Practice,* 2015 edition.

Evidence ratings revised in *Guidelines for Perioperative Practice,* 2018 edition, to conform to the current AORN Evidence Rating Model.

GUIDELINE FOR SPECIMEN MANAGEMENT

The Guideline for Specimen Management has been approved by the AORN Guidelines Advisory Board. It was presented as a proposed guideline for comments by members and others. The guideline is effective May 15, 2014. The recommendations in the guideline are intended to be achievable and represent what is believed to be an optimal level of practice. Policies and procedures will reflect variations in practice settings and/or clinical situations that determine the degree to which the guideline can be implemented. AORN recognizes the many diverse settings in which perioperative nurses practice; therefore, this guideline is adaptable to all areas where operative and other invasive procedures may be performed.

Purpose

This document provides guidance for management of surgical specimens in the perioperative practice setting, including guidance for the handling of body parts being reattached to the patient, forensic and radioactive specimens, and explanted medical devices and orthopedic hardware. Surgical techniques for resection of specimens is outside the scope of this guideline. This document does not address clinical laboratory specimens obtained for diagnostic or other screening procedures performed on blood, body fluids, or other potentially infectious materials. The reader should refer to 42 CFR 493, Laboratory Requirements, for guidance in this area.[1]

Specimen management is a multifaceted, multidisciplinary process that includes
- needs assessment,
- site identification,
- collection and handling,
- transfer from the sterile field,
- containment,
- specimen identification and labeling,
- preservation,
- transport,
- disposition of the specimen, and
- documentation.

Accurate specimen management requires effective multidisciplinary communication, minimized distractions, and awareness of the potential opportunities for error. An error is an unintended act of omission (ie, failing to perform an action) or commission (ie, performing an action that results in harm).[2] Errors in specimen management leading to inaccurate or incomplete diagnosis, the need for additional procedures, and physical and psychological injury have been reported.[3-5]

In a survey commissioned by the Association of Directors of Anatomic and Surgical Pathology to assess perceptions and definitions of errors in surgical pathology and to examine and measure the frequency of errors among its members, researchers randomly surveyed pathologists in 40 academic pathology laboratories in the United States and one in Canada (N = 41). When asked to indicate where most errors in surgical pathology occurred, 53% of respondents indicated the preanalytical phase (ie, before the specimen reaches the pathology laboratory for analysis and processing), 38% indicated the analytical phase (ie, within the pathology laboratory while the specimen is being analyzed and processed), and 6% indicated the postanalytical phase (ie, after the specimen has been analyzed and processed in the pathology laboratory).[6]

Examples of errors that may occur during the preanalytical phase include incorrect
- pathology request,
- order entry,
- patient identification,
- specimen identification,
- specimen (or no specimen) in the container,
- collection or handling methods,
- container or preservative, and
- transport methods or destination.

Examples of errors that may occur during the analytical phase include
- equipment malfunction,
- specimen mix-ups, and
- undetected failure in quality control.

Examples of errors that may occur during the postanalytical phase include
- confirmation of erroneous data,
- failure or delay in pathology reporting or addressing the pathology report,
- excessive turnaround time, and
- improper data entry and manual transcription.

Errors that may have occurred during the preanalytical phase are often detected during the analytical phase because the histology visualized under the microscope does not correspond to the biopsy site specified in the accompanying documentation or clinical history.[7] There are many points in the analytical phase during which an error can occur. Errors occurring during the analytical phase have the potential to cause great patient harm because the results of the examination by the pathologist may be critical for effective patient care.[7]

Errors in specimen management may be classified as
- near misses (ie, the error has the potential to harm the patient, but does not, either by chance or because the error was detected before harm resulted),[7,8]
- adverse events (ie, the error causes the patient either inconvenience or harm),[7] or
- sentinel events (ie, the error results in significant harm to the patient).[8]

Specimen management errors may be attributed to human factors (eg, poor communication, fatigue, inadequate education or competency verification), the environment, equipment failure, or inadequate policies and procedures.[7] The causes of specimen management errors may be determined through a process of root cause analysis in which knowledgeable individuals and other persons involved in the event make a critical analysis and a determination as to the factor(s) that contributed to the error.[7]

Most errors in specimen management are a result of human errors caused by slips, lapses, and mistakes.[7]

- Slips are unintended actions[9] (eg, placing an incorrect label on a specimen container).
- Lapses are omissions of intended actions[9] (eg, omitting the last letter of a patient's name and writing "Smith" rather than "Smithe").
- Mistakes are errors of conscious thought[9] (eg, choosing to disregard known policies and procedures).

Most errors in specimen management are classified as slips and lapses. Errors caused by slips and lapses are the result of automatic actions and are therefore difficult to prevent.[7] These type of errors are often not noticed at the time they occur.[7] The result of the error may not become apparent until hours or days after it has occurred.[7]

The true frequency of errors in specimen management is difficult to quantify. Most estimates are based on studies conducted in single institutions. Estimates based on multi-institutional studies suggest that the number of errors in specimen management varies widely among institutions and is likely associated with specimen identification practices unique to the institution.[7]

Reducing errors in specimen management requires a careful examination of the preanalytical, analytical, and postanalytical phases for system flaws that may contribute to errors and be responsive to analysis and correction. The simple application of redundancy to various portions of the specimen management cycle (ie, double-checking steps of the process that may be subject to slips and lapses) has the potential to significantly reduce errors.[7,10]

Evidence Review

A medical librarian conducted a systematic search of the databases MEDLINE, CINAHL, and the Cochrane Database of Systematic Reviews for meta-analyses, systematic reviews, randomized controlled and nonrandomized trials and studies, case reports, reviews, and guidelines. Scopus was also consulted, although not searched systematically. Search terms included *specimen handling, surgical specimen, specimen type, fresh specimen, fresh tissue, anticoagulants, explant, bone screws, bone plates, bone nails, calculi, gallstones, urinary calculi, kidney stones, renal calculi, surgical pathology, clinical pathology, cell biology, cytology, stone analysis, gross examination, gross evaluation, fixatives, additives, tissue preservatives, preservative, saline solution, paraffin, formaldehyde, formalin, cryoultramicrotomy, freezing, time factors, transportation, chain of custody, container, transfer, handling, mishandling, delivery, storage, organizational policy, documentation, clinical information, name, patient information, patient identification systems, labels, labeling, mislabeling, suture tags, tissue markers, medical errors, diagnostic errors, equipment contamination, specimen contamination, safety precautions, occupational health, occupational accidents, radioactive, radioactivity, forensic, wounds, gunshot, forensic pathology, law enforcement, religion, cross-cultural comparison, cultural diversity, funeral rites, radiologic health, occupational accidents, occupational health, perioperative nursing, nurse's role, intraoperative care, intraoperative period, perioperative care, surgical procedures,* and *operating rooms.*

The search was originally limited to literature published in English between January 2007 and October 2012. The medical librarian conducted the first database search on October 11, 2012. Older articles were included when there were no articles within this time period. Additional articles not identified in the original search were obtained after a review of the reference lists of the articles obtained originally. In addition, between October 2012 and January 2014, the results of alerts established at the time of the initial searches were considered. During the development of the document, the lead author requested supplementary searches and requested additional articles that either did not fit the original search criteria or were discovered during the evidence appraisal process. Finally, the lead author and the medical librarian identified relevant guidelines from government agencies and standards-setting bodies.

More than 374 articles or documents were reviewed in preparation for writing this guideline. Approximately 120 were ultimately selected for inclusion as suitable references. Articles were rejected primarily because they addressed surgical techniques for specimen resection or procedures for processing of specimens in the pathology laboratory.

As relevant research and other evidence was located, it was independently evaluated and critically appraised according to the strength and quality of the evidence using the AORN Evidence Appraisal Tools (Research and Non-Research) by the lead author and an independent reviewer. The reviewers participated in conference calls to discuss their individual appraisal scores and to establish consensus. Each article or study was assigned an appraisal score as agreed upon by the reviewers. The appraisal scores are noted in brackets at the end of each citation in the references list at the end of the document.

After the evidence was reviewed and appraised, the collective evidence supporting each intervention within a specific recommendation was rated using the AORN Evidence Rating Model. Ratings include Strong Evidence, Regulatory Requirement, Moderate Evidence, Limited Evidence, Benefits Balanced With Harms, and No Evidence. Factors considered when applying the AORN Evidence Rating Model to the collective body of evidence included the quality of research, quantity of similar studies on a given topic, consistency of results supporting a recommendation, and whether the potential benefits of following the recommendation outweigh the harms. The evidence rating is noted in brackets following each intervention.

Editor's note: *MEDLINE is a registered trademark of the US National Library of Medicine's Medical Literature Analysis and Retrieval System, Bethesda, MD. CINAHL, Cumulative Index to Nursing and Allied Health Literature, is a registered trademark of EBSCO Industries, Birmingham, AL. Scopus is a registered trademark of Elsevier B.V., Amsterdam, Netherlands.*

Recommendation I

The perioperative registered nurse (RN) should incorporate specimen management needs when developing the plan of care.

Early assessment of specimen management needs may help improve processes and decrease or prevent errors related to specimen management.

I.a.   Assessment of specimen management needs should begin when the need for obtaining a specimen is identified and should include
   ○ personnel to be notified (eg, pathologist for frozen section),
   ○ requirements for specimen collection and handling (eg, keeping the specimen moist until transfer from the sterile field),
   ○ method of transfer (eg, using sterile technique),
   ○ requirements for containment (eg, size of the container),
   ○ method of preservation, (eg, type of solution),
   ○ transport needs (eg, availability of personnel),
   ○ disposition of the specimen (eg, disposal, returned to the patient), and
   ○ documentation (eg, noting the location of suture tags).
   [5: Benefits Balanced with Harms]
   Conducting an assessment that begins when the need for obtaining a specimen is identified may help to improve efficiency and ensure identified needs are met.
   Evidence addressing the need for assessment of specimen management needs was not identified during the evidence review for this guideline. Further research is warranted.

I.a.1.   When on-site pathology, laboratory, or courier services are not available and the need for these services is identified, services may be contracted with a third party.

I.b.   The cultural and personal preferences of the patient should be assessed preoperatively to determine special needs for collecting, handling, or disposing of specimens. *[3: Moderate Evidence]*
   Specimen management may be influenced by a patient's beliefs about his or her body that are derived from both cultural and religious contexts.[11] For example, a Vietnamese patient may be extremely fearful of operative or other invasive procedures involving blood loss.[12] The patient may refuse to have blood drawn, believing that any body tissue or fluid removed cannot be replaced and that the body suffers the loss of the removed tissue or fluid in this life and in the afterlife.[12]
   According to Jewish law, blood and limbs are considered part of the human being, and therefore, should be buried.[13] Limbs that are amputated require burial in the patient's future gravesite.[13] If the amputated limb is donated for medical research, burial is required when the limb is no longer in use.[13] Muslim patients also may request that amputated limbs be made available for burial.[14]
   In a qualitative study conducted to explore the cultural attitudes of 94 Hmong Americans about placental specimen disposition, Helsel and Mochel found there was a strong persistence in the traditional belief that placentas should be buried at home. The Hmong believe that after death, the spirit returns to the place the placenta is buried. The placenta is necessary for the soul to be able to rejoin ancestors in the spirit world. Hmong patients were reluctant to ask health care providers for permission to take placentas home for burial. The researchers suggested that health care providers develop an awareness of cultural practices and the reluctance of some patients to verbalize their wishes.[15]
   Incorporating an approach to specimen management that acknowledges the value of cultural beliefs and encourages increasing cultural knowledge and expertise may improve the quality of perioperative nursing care related to specimen management.[11]

I.b.1.   Policies and procedures should be developed to address patient requests for nontraditional specimen management.
   The patient's cultural or personal preferences may require that specimens be handled in a nontraditional manner.
   Baergen et al conducted a nonexperimental study to review the practices and experiences of perinatal and placental pathologists surrounding placental release, to discuss the reasons for release, and to determine problems that have been encountered. They found that requests for release of the placenta to patients had increased; however, no statistical data were provided as to the number of increased requests. The most common reason for this request was to bury the placenta. No adverse consequences or legal ramifications related to placental release were reported by any of the survey respondents. The researchers recommended that health care organizations create a multidisciplinary team that includes personnel from obstetrics, infection control, pathology, and administration to develop a policy

to follow when requests for placental release are received.[16]

I.c. Specimen management should be assessed and planned among surgical team members during the preoperative briefing before operative or other invasive procedures. *[3: Moderate Evidence]*

Management of specimens is a multidisciplinary process. Collaborative preprocedure assessment and planning may improve efficiency and communication among team members and may help to reduce or eliminate potential errors[17] in specimen management.

Recommendation II

The perioperative RN should complete a preoperative assessment that confirms the site identification of specimens to be collected.

Site identification may be necessary to confirm the location of tissue, foreign objects, or body substances to be removed from the patient and sent for pathology examination or study. Accurate preoperative identification of the site from which specimens are to be collected may help prevent wrong site surgery.

Implementing error prevention strategies for the identification and verification of the correct site of specimens to be collected may reduce the risk for error.[18]

II.a. Photographs of dermatologic lesions that will be excised or biopsied during the surgical procedure, if available, should be labeled with the patient's identification and displayed in the procedure room. *[3: Moderate Evidence]*

Photographs help to identify and verify the location of dermatologic lesions to be removed and reduce the risk of wrong site dermatological surgery.[19-22]

In an online survey of 722 members of the American College of Mohs Surgery conducted to quantify the problem of biopsy site identification on the day of surgery, Nemeth and Lawrence found that accurate biopsy site identification is a problem encountered by Mohs surgeons. The majority (89%) responded that a high-quality photograph would provide the most useful information for accurate identification of the biopsy site.[19]

McGinness and Goldstein conducted a nonexperimental study of 271 surgical sites to determine the value of preoperative biopsy site photography. Patients with preoperative biopsy-site photography of cutaneous malignancies and their physicians were asked to identify the surgical sites on the day of the procedure. The patients were not given any help in locating the lesion. The physicians were then asked to identify the lesion using only a diagram of the location of the biopsy site. The patients incorrectly identified 45 of 271 surgical sites (16.6%). The physicians incorrectly identified 16 of 271 sur-

gical sites (5.9%). Twelve of the 271 surgical sites were incorrectly identified by both the patient and the physician (4.4%). When the patients and physicians used the preoperative biopsy site photographs, they correctly identified all sites. The results of this study support the use of preoperative photography to help reduce the incidence of wrong site surgery for removal of cutaneous lesions.[20]

In another prospective, nonexperimental study of 329 patients representing 333 skin cancers primarily located on the head and neck, Rossy and Lawrence evaluated the difficulty associated with surgical site identification. Preoperatively, patients were asked to identify and confirm the surgical site. Thirty patients (9.1%) were unable to do so. There was a statistically significant difference in the percentage of patients able to identify lesions located in an area that was visible to them versus those patients with lesions in an area not easily seen. The results of this study demonstrate the need for accurate documentation and prebiopsy site photography of skin cancers, especially those that are not visible to the patient, as a means to reduce the possibility of wrong site surgery.[21]

In an observational study of 34 biopsy sites conducted in a university-based dermatological surgery clinic, Ke et al compared the reliability of patient and blinded dermatologist surgical site identification with identification based on biopsy site photography. On the day of the procedure, the patient was asked to identify the biopsy site. The physician was then given the general body location (eg, ear, cheek) and asked to identify the site. The photograph of the biopsy site taken during the patient's previous visit to the clinic was then reviewed to verify the surgical site. The patients and the dermatologist incorrectly identified four biopsy sites (11.8%). The patients alone incorrectly identified an additional six biopsy sites, for a total of 10 sites (29.4%) incorrectly identified by patients. The results of this study support the need for preoperative biopsy site photography to prevent wrong site surgery during removal of cutaneous skin malignancies.[22]

II.a.1. The preoperative photographs should accurately depict the biopsy site, physical features, and anatomical landmarks of the area.[19,20]
- The photograph should be in focus and taken from a distance that allows for accurate identification of the biopsy site.[20]
- Additional photographs taken from a greater distance may be helpful for identification of anatomic landmarks.[20]
- Photographs including anatomic landmarks such as the lip, ear, nose, or eyebrow, or a ruler or other measuring device showing the distance to the anatomical

PATIENT AND WORKER SAFETY

landmarks may be helpful for identification of the biopsy site.[20]

- Circling the biopsy site with a surgical marker before taking the photograph may help to distinguish the biopsy site from other cutaneous lesions in the biopsy site area.[20]
- Photographs taken close up may be helpful for identification of nearby cutaneous lesions or skin surface changes in the biopsy site area.[20]

Recommendation III

Specimens should be collected and handled in a manner that protects and preserves the integrity of the specimen.

Specimen collection refers to the act or process of obtaining a biopsy or resecting a specimen. Specimen handling involves holding, securing, moving, or manipulating a specimen.

Incorrect collection and handling may compromise specimens and lead to inaccurate or incomplete diagnosis or the need for additional procedures or unnecessary surgeries.

III.a.   Specimens of breast tissue to be examined for cancer should be collected and handled in a manner that preserves the molecular and genetic signatures of the specimen. *[2: High Evidence]*

Mishandling of specimens may compromise the accuracy of the pathology data and result in the loss of valuable histological information.

Tissue sent for pathology examination for cancer also may be used for molecular assays of nucleic acids or proteins.[23] Cancer therapy may involve limited and individualized selection and use of a drug or biologic when the targeted tumor is expressing a biological marker.[24] Current methods of tissue handling and specimen preparation are not standardized, and this lack of standardization may result in variability of the quality of the samples and the biomarkers that can be recovered from the tissue.[23,25,26]

The time required for arterial ligation and specimen removal (ie, warm ischemic time) can vary depending on the complexity of the surgical procedure. As the sample is excised, the reduction or elimination of blood flow causes progressive tissue ischemia, hypoxia, and tissue degradation.[23,25,26] Likewise, the period of time between the removal of the specimen and its placement into fixative (ie, cold ischemic time) can vary.[25,26]

During these ischemic periods, nucleic acid and protein changes occur that can negatively affect accurate histological and biomolecular evaluation of the sample;[23-26] however, these changes cease when the fixation process begins.[25,26] Keeping both the warm and cold ischemic times as short as possible and verifying that the biomarker levels are attributable to the underlying tumor and not to artifacts related to delays in fixation may help to prevent false results (positive or negative). Individualized therapy may eliminate the use of an agent that may be costly and provide little benefit to the patient.[24] False results may lead to therapeutic consequences with the potential to harm the patient and affect outcomes, as well as the inability to elicit accurate molecular and genetic signatures that are valuable for targeted treatment.[23-26]

Levels of human epidermal growth factor receptor 2 (HER2) are increased in a percentage of breast cancers.[27] In 2007, an expert panel commissioned by the American Society of Clinical Oncology (ASCO) and the College of American Pathologists (CAP) performed a systematic review of the literature to develop recommendations for improving the accuracy of HER2 testing and its usefulness as a predictive marker for therapeutic decision making for patients with breast cancer.[27,28] In 2012, an Update Committee was convened to review literature published since 2006 and to revise and update the guidelines as necessary.[29] Current recommendations of the ASCO/CAP panel include

- establishing HER2 status for all primary, recurrent, and metastatic breast cancers;
- keeping the time to specimen fixation as short as possible (ie, less than one hour); and
- recording the time to fixation for each sample.[27-29]

Estrogen receptor status in breast cancer is an important predictive biomarker for determining breast cancer prognosis after treatment with endocrine therapy.[30] In 2008, an ad hoc committee of expert pathologists, laboratory scientists, and technical experts developed consensus recommendations for standardized procedures for estrogen receptor testing in breast cancer by immunohistochemistry for the purpose of reducing what was believed to be an unacceptably high rate of false positives.[30] The committee recommended

- sectioning and placing breast resection specimens in an adequate volume of fixative (ie, one part tissue to 20 parts fixative) within a maximum time of one hour;
- processing and fixing breast core biopsies in the same manner as resected specimens;
- placing needle core biopsies immediately into fixative and recording the time of fixative placement;
- recording both the time of specimen removal and the time of placement into fixative when specimen x-rays are required;
- keeping specimens being examined for calcifications moist on saline-soaked gauze to prevent drying of the specimen before placement in fixative;
- using only 10% phosphate-buffered formalin as the fixative for breast tissue specimens to

allow for more accurate correlation of data on estrogen receptor status; and

○ recording the time between removal of the specimen and placement into fixative, as well as the length of fixation time.[30]

In 2010, the ASCO/CAP panel supported the 2008 consensus recommendations of the ad hoc committee and also recommended that estrogen and progesterone receptor status be determined on all invasive breast cancers and breast cancer reoccurrences.[28] Additional studies with larger numbers of patients are needed to fully determine the effects of extended cold ischemia time on breast samples.

Nkoy et al conducted a retrospective study to test the variability in estrogen and progesterone negativity among hospitals using a single laboratory and to examine the association between prolonged specimen conditions and estrogen and progesterone receptor negativity. They studied the records of 5,077 women with breast cancers who had undergone breast surgery and estrogen- and progesterone-receptor testing between 1997 and 2003 at seven different hospitals within a single health care system. The results showed that estrogen- and progesterone-receptor negativity varied greatly among the different hospitals even when a single laboratory was used, and the negativity levels were significantly associated with prolonged specimen handling. The researchers concluded that estrogen- and progesterone-receptor expressions can be altered by prolonged exposure to room temperature before fixation, the length of the fixation, and the type of fixation.[31]

In a study conducted by Khoury et al to determine the effects of progressive delay to formalin fixation on breast cancer biomarkers, 10 palpable breast cancers were resected. Each specimen was divided into eight portions and fixed in formalin at consecutive intervals of zero, 10, and 30 minutes, and one, two, four, and eight hours. One section was placed in saline and stored at 39.2° F (4° C) as a control. The results showed that estrogen receptors began to decline at two hours and progesterone receptors at one hour. Compromise to interpretation of HER2 began at one hour and became statistically significant at two hours. The researchers recommended that specimens be placed in fixative within one hour of resection.[32]

Some researchers have argued that cold ischemia time longer than one hour may not detrimentally effect HER2 levels. In a study conducted to assess the effect of prolonged ischemic time, a modified radical mastectomy specimen with a 10-cm grade 3 invasive ductal carcinoma was processed immediately after resection. More than 80% of the specimen was removed and stored at 39.2° F (4° C) without any fixative. The unfixed specimen was cut into 97 equal samples and placed into 20 mL of one

of six different preservative solutions (ie, 10% formalin, 15% formalin, Pen-Fix®, Bouin solution, Sakura® molecular fixative, zinc formalin) for zero, one, two, three, four, five, six, seven, eight, nine, 10, 11, 12, 24, 48, 72, or 168 hours. Immunohistochemical studies and fluorescence in situ hybridization were performed. The researchers found that HER2 results remained accurate beyond the ASCO/CAP recommended one hour to fixation time.[33]

In a study conducted between August 2008 and August 2009 to address the effect of cold ischemia time on HER2 levels, Portier et al identified and collected breast resection specimens from 92 patients for which the time the specimen was handed off the sterile field and the time the sample was placed in fixative had been recorded. The samples were divided into four groups representing cold ischemic times:

○ < 1 hour (n = 45),
○ 1 to 2 hours (n = 27),
○ > 2 to 3 hours (n = 6), and
○ > 3 hours (n = 6).

Each group of samples was then evaluated using two different US Food and Drug Administration (FDA)-approved methods and an immunohistochemistry assay. The researchers found that cold ischemia time up to three hours had no detrimental effect on the HER2 levels.[34]

III.a.1. The time from excision to fixation of breast cancer specimens should be less than one hour.[27-29]

Long delays between excision and fixation of the specimen may result in a decreased ability to detect breast biomarkers in samples.[30] The current ASCO/CAP recommendations include keeping the time to fixation less than one hour.[27-29]

In a study to determine the difficulty of achieving the recommended one-hour time for breast biopsies and excised breast samples to be placed in fixative, researchers implemented a rapid tissue acquisition program in which the collection time, laboratory receipt time, and fixation start time were recorded for each sample. Results showed that meeting the one-hour time was achievable but required a commitment of personnel and resources to meet this goal.[25,26]

III.a.2. Excised breast specimens should be kept moist until transfer from the sterile field and should not be placed on dry, absorbent surfaces or materials.

Air exposure can lead to desiccation of tissue.[35] Keeping specimens moist helps to prevent drying of the specimen before placement in fixative.[30] Dry, absorbent surfaces or materials may adhere to the tissue, which may result in the loss of portions of the resection margins.[35]

III.a.3.   The time of excision of breast cancer specimens and the time of fixation should be recorded.

The ASCO/CAP recommendations include recording the time of removal of tissue from the patient and the time of fixation for each sample.[28] Accurate recording of times can be helpful for verification that the testing was performed during a period of time when the biomarkers were stable.[23,26]

III.b.   Amputated digits to be reimplanted should be collected and handled in a manner to protect and preserve the integrity of the specimen and the potential for replantation survival. *[3: Moderate Evidence]*

Cooling of recently amputated digits may help to preserve tissue and increase the chance of replantation survival.[36-38]

In a retrospective study of 211 patients who underwent replantation surgery following complete fingertip amputation between August 1990 and March 2006, Li et al evaluated 17 independent variables to determine primary causes of unsuccessful replantation. A total of 172 patients (81.5%) had a successful replantation. The researchers found the primary factors associated with failed replantation were mechanism of injury, high platelet count, postoperative smoking, incorrect preservation of the amputated part, and the use of vein grafting. The amputated fingertips were preserved either dry at room temperature, dry at cool temperature (35.6° F to 42.8° F [2° C to 6° C]), or immersed in a preservative fluid (ie, saline or ethanol). Immersion of the digit in fluid had a higher rate of failure (43%) compared with dry storage at room temperature (20%) or dry storage at a cooler temperature (12%). The difference in survival rates of digits stored in saline versus ethanol was not calculated; however, this study demonstrated that cooling the amputated digit improved survival by 88%.[36]

Partlin et al conducted a prospective study during May and June of 2006 to compare the efficacy of six different cooling methods for preserving amputated digits for replantation, using chicken feet as surrogate tissue because of the similarity in tissue structure to a human digit. The chicken feet were trimmed to approximate a human finger and wrapped in two layers of room-temperature, sterile, saline-soaked gauze. A digital thermometer probe was inserted into each of the six surrogate tissue samples. Three samples were placed into lidded plastic specimen containers and three samples were placed into sealable plastic specimen bags. The samples were contained in a manner that allowed viewing of the temperature probe display. The temperature of each sample was measured and the contained, and bagged samples were then placed into

- a second plastic specimen bag containing 300 mg of ice cubes and 200 mL of tap water,
- a plastic kidney bowl containing 300 mg of ice cubes and 200 mL of tap water, or
- a lidded plastic denture cup containing 80 mg of ice cubes and 60 mL of tap water.

The tissue temperature was measured at the time of placement of the specimen and then measured again when the ice was completely melted. Each of the six methods was tested 12 times, resulting in 72 sets of measurements. The results showed that all methods tested achieved the target temperature of 39.2° F + 3.6° F (4° C ± 2° C); however, the most effective method for maintaining the surrogate tissue at the target temperature for the longest duration of time was wrapping the tissue in saline-soaked gauze, placing it in a lidded specimen container, and placing the container into a sealed specimen bag of ice and water.[37]

III.b.1.   Care of the amputated digit specimen should include the following:
- Preoperatively,
  - dressing the wound with sterile saline-moistened gauze[38];
  - gently wrapping the amputated digit in saline-moistened gauze and placing it into an impervious lidded or sealable container[38] (eg, specimen container, sealable plastic bag)[37];
  - placing the sealed container in a bag of ice water, keeping warm ischemic time to a minimum[37,38]; and
  - replacing the ice and water mixture approximately every four hours or sooner as needed to maintain a target temperature of 39.2° F ± 3.6° F (4° C ± 2° C).[37]
- Intraoperatively,
  - filling a sterile irrigation basin with ice[38];
  - covering the basin with a sterile plastic adhesive drape to provide a barrier[38];
  - placing a moist, sterile towel on top of the plastic barrier to the unsterile ice[38]; and
  - prepping the amputated digit and placing it on the moist towel for preliminary debridement and dissection.[38]
- Postoperatively,
  - checking the temperature of the replanted digit every hour by taping a temperature probe to the pulp of the replanted digit,
  - notifying the surgeon if the temperature drops more than 3.6° F (2° C) from the previous reading,[38] and
  - monitoring the replanted digit for engorgement.[38]

III.b.2. Education and competency verification activities related to best practices for management of amputated digits for replantation should be provided for perioperative or other health care personnel who may be involved in collecting or handling amputated digit specimens or caring for patients undergoing replantation procedures.

In a descriptive telephone survey of 50 respondents in 18 emergency departments in Wales conducted in September 2007 to ascertain perceptions of how amputated digits should be packaged and transported for reimplantation, only nine (18%) of the respondents described the recommended process correctly and sequentially. The results of this study are limited by the small sample size; however, the results indicated the need for education on best practices for correctly managing amputated digits for reimplantation.[39]

III.c. Amputated limbs to be reimplanted should be collected and handled in a manner to protect and preserve the integrity of the specimen and increase the potential for replantation survival. *[3: Moderate Evidence]*

Functional recovery of the replanted limb is dependent on reduced ischemia time and rapid revascularization.[40] Cooling of the amputated limb is beneficial for maintaining optimal muscle viability.[40]

III.c.1. Preoperative management of the amputated limb specimen should include
- handling the limb as gently as possible to avoid crushing or contaminating tissue[40];
- retaining any fragments of tissue to provide tissue for skin, nerve, or bone grafting[40];
- wrapping the limb in sterile gauze moistened with saline, then wrapping the limb again in plastic and placing it in an insulating chest containing crushed ice and water;
- preventing direct contact of the limb with ice to minimize cell damage that may hinder replantation; and
- cannulating the most proximal artery of the cooled limb with an 18-gauge cannula, infusing 1 L of tissue perfusion fluid (eg, ViaSpan) at a temperature of 50° F (10° C) and 120 cm hydrostatic pressure,[40] and leaving the infusion running continuously to help ensure a complete washout of stagnant blood from the amputated limb.[40]

III.d. Forensic specimens should be collected and handled in a manner that preserves and protects the condition of the evidence and verifies that the evidence has been in secure possession at all times. *[3: Moderate Evidence]*

Items such as bullets and bloodstained clothing may be potential evidence in a criminal investigation.[41-43] Evidence that is not correctly collected and handled may be inadmissible as evidence during a criminal investigation.[41-43] As patient advocates, perioperative nurses are responsible for identifying, collecting, preserving, and securing evidence and verifying that potential evidence of a crime is not compromised[41,42] while also protecting the patient's right to privacy and confidentiality of health care information.[43,44]

Guidelines for forensic specimen management from other professional organizations were not identified in the evidence review for this guideline.

III.d.1. When collecting, preserving, and securing potential evidence, perioperative personnel should
- don personal protective equipment (eg, gloves, eye protection)[42];
- handle all potential evidence with gloved hands[41,43];
- place each item in a separate paper bag or envelope to avoid cross contamination[41-43];
- avoid the use of plastic bags because they may trap moisture and facilitate the growth of mold, which could destroy evidence[41,43];
- keep evidence from each wound separate if there are two or more wounds[42];
- secure all of the patient's clothes and belongings, including footwear, as evidence, regardless of the condition[43];
- cut along the seams or around bullet or stab wound holes when removing clothing from the patient[41-43];
- contain and document physical evidence, such as pills or other items found in clothing[43];
- exercise caution because needles or other sharp objects may be present in pockets[43];
- handle clothing as little as possible and avoid shaking clothing to prevent important forensic evidence such as hair, fibers, blood, or DNA from being lost[41,43];
- collect and secure the transfer sheet from the preoperative stretcher to capture evidence that may have fallen from the patient's clothing onto the sheet[43];
- collect, preserve, and secure fabric or other debris removed from the wound or around the wound edges[43];
- not handle bullets with metal instruments that may scratch the bullet surface[41,43] and use instruments with rubber shods if possible[41,43];
- be aware that bullets may have sharp edges that may tear surgical gloves[43];
- handle bullets, bullet fragments, knives, or other projectiles or penetrating devices as little as possible and not wipe them[41-43];

- not handle knives or penetrating devices in the same manner as the perpetrator would have handled them, if possible[43];
- rinse bullets, bullet fragments, knives, or other projectiles or penetrating devices that have been removed surgically in water to prevent destruction of microscopic markings[41,43];
- place rinsed bullets, bullet fragments, knives, or other projectiles or penetrating devices in a nonmetal container and sealed evidence envelope and submit bullets according to local and state law enforcement regulations[41];
- for patient care, remove bags that have been placed over the hands of the patient to prevent removal of gunshot residue and use cotton swabs to recover gunpowder residue[42];
- place collected body fluids (eg urine, gastric contents) into dry containers[42];
- place collected tissue (eg, bone) into a dry container and preserve it according to the facility or health care organization's policy and procedure[42];
- place the evidence directly into a designated and sealed envelope or paper bag labeled with the patient's identification, collection date and time, and name of the collector[41]; and
- submit all evidence collected according to local and state law enforcement regulations. The sealed evidence should be given directly to the responsible law enforcement officer.[41,43] If the law enforcement officer is not immediately available, personnel should follow the facility's or health care organization's policies and procedure for securing sealed evidence.

III.d.2. Documentation to establish the chain of custody and identification of persons in possession of the evidence (ie, tissue specimens, personal clothing, other personal items) should be completed from the point of evidence removal to the point of evidence examination according to facility or health care organization policies and procedures and local, state, and federal regulations.[41] Perioperative RNs should
- document informational evidence (eg, patient statements, appearance, behavior, bodily marks, blood stains, unusual odors) in detail[42,43];
- if possible, use photographs to document wounds (eg, bruises, abrasions, lacerations) and other potential evidence[41];
- if possible and applicable, take photographs before the skin prep because the prep solution may remove evidence such as bloodstains or bloody fingerprints[43];
- if possible, include a ruler or other item (eg, coin) in the photograph to indicate scale[41];
- label each photograph with patient information and place it in a sealed evidence envelope.[41]

III.d.3. Perioperative personnel should receive initial and ongoing education and complete competency verification activities on identifying, collecting, and securing evidence, and maintaining the chain of custody.[41]

Initial and ongoing education of perioperative personnel will help to develop the necessary knowledge and skills for correctly identifying, collecting, and securing evidence and maintaining the chain of custody.

Competency verification activities measure individual performance, provide a mechanism for documentation, and may verify that perioperative personnel have an understanding of the processes for correctly identifying, collecting, and securing evidence and maintaining the chain of custody.

III.d.4. Policies and procedures for identifying, collecting, and securing evidence and maintaining the chain of custody should be developed, reviewed periodically, revised as necessary, and readily available in the practice setting.[42]

Policies and procedures establish authority, responsibility, and accountability within the organization. Policies and procedures also serve as operational guidelines that are used to standardize practice, direct perioperative personnel, and establish continuous performance improvement programs. Policies and procedures should address
- criminal cases requiring investigation;
- personnel responsibilities;
- evidence collection protocols;
- documentation requirements;
- chain of custody protocols; and
- care of victims, suspected perpetrators, and family members or designated support persons.[42]

III.e. Radioactive specimens must be collected and handled according to facility or health care organization policies and procedures and local, state, and federal regulations.[45,46] *[1: Regulatory Requirement]*

Occupational doses of radiation must be maintained as low as is reasonably achievable (ALARA).[45,46] Developing policies and procedures for maintaining occupational doses of radiation ALARA is a regulatory requirement.[45]

The maximum occupational radiation exposure limit for radiation workers is 5,000 millirem (mrem) per year or 50,000 mrem per year for skin or extremities.[45] The exposure limit for women who are pregnant or for nonradiation personnel (eg, pathology personnel) is 500 mrem per year, provided that the facility or health care organization has policies and procedures in place to maintain the dose ALARA.[45]

Although radiation exposure from procedures such as radioactive seed localization and sentinel node biopsy is low, policies and procedures for specimen and seed handling are required to prevent unnecessary exposure of personnel.[47,48] The seed(s) may be removed from the tissue specimen in surgery, or the tissue specimen containing the seed may be sent to the pathology laboratory for removal of the seed and analysis of the tissue.[49] The CAP recommends having separate policies for tissues obtained during sentinel lymph node biopsy and procedures involving radiation implant devices that may have higher radiation levels.[50]

In a study by Miner et al conducted at a military medical center, researchers obtained 318 lymph nodes during 57 sentinel lymph node procedures (37 breast cancer, 20 melanoma) and determined the amount of radiation in each node at 24 and 72 hours. Specimens with readings consistent with background radiation were considered nonradioactive. The radiation dose to the hands of the surgical team members was evaluated by placing sterilized thermoluminescent dosimeter chips in the glove of the left ring finger of both the primary surgeon and first assistant.[51]

All specimens were found to be radioactive at the first reading. The radioactivity of the breast specimens was higher than the radioactivity of the melanoma specimens. All specimens were nonradioactive at the second reading. There was no radioactivity in any of the waste materials produced by the procedures. There was no significant difference noted in the radiation levels obtained from the surgeon or the first assistant or between the levels obtained during breast or melanoma procedures. The mean radiation dose to the surgeon's hand was found to be 9.6 ± 3.6 mrem of radiation per surgery. The researchers theorized that exposure to the rest of the surgeon's body would be considerably less because the surgeon's body is farther away from the surgical site than the surgeon's hands. They concluded that a surgeon could perform more than 5,000 procedures each year without approaching the regulatory exposure limits.[51]

To quantify the occupational radiation exposure of personnel performing or assisting with sentinel lymph node biopsy procedures at a university medical center, Law et al measured whole-body and finger radiation doses of surgical and pathology personnel using high-sensitivity thermoluminescent dosimeters and then compared the results with the annual dose limits recommended by the International Commission of Radiological Protection. Results showed the surgeons' left index fingers received the highest doses. The researchers suggested that this was because the surgeons' left hands were in close contact with the injection site during the radio-guided search for the lymph node basins. All other doses were measured to be less than the daily background radiation level in the institution.[52]

In a study to explore the perception of personnel that the level of radiation in sentinel node procedures was higher than in the past, Renshaw et al reviewed records of radiation levels of 2,902 specimens from sentinel node procedures performed between 2003 and 2009. Results showed that the percentage of specimens with greater than background radiation (ie, ≥ 0.2 mrem/hour) rose from 6.3% in 2003 to 34.8% in 2009. Specimens with more than 10 mrem/hour rose from 0.0% to 9.3%. The researchers theorized that the higher levels were likely a result of higher doses of radiopharmaceuticals being administered to patients, but they also considered that the higher levels could be a result of specimens being transported more rapidly to the pathology laboratory. The researchers recommended measuring radiation levels of sentinel node and primary resection specimens upon receipt in the pathology laboratory.[53]

To evaluate radiation exposure levels of the hands and whole body and establish safe work practices for personnel involved in melanoma and breast sentinel lymph node biopsy procedures, Coventry et al measured cumulative data collected from personnel dosimeters worn during melanoma and breast sentinel lymph node biopsy procedures. Results showed the extremity dose to the surgeon was measurably higher for breast cancer procedures than for melanoma procedures, despite a longer average exposure time for melanoma procedures. The researchers theorized that this was likely caused by the shorter distance of the sentinel nodes from the primary tumor in breast cancer procedures, which increased the surgeon's working time close to the injection site. However, the data showed the whole-body dose to the surgeon was negligible for either procedure.[54]

Likewise, the whole-body doses to the radiologist, pathologist, and transport personnel were negligible. The radiation dose to the perioperative RN was not measured. The researchers theorized that the dose would also be negligible for the perioperative RN because a distance of 3.3 ft to 6.6 ft (1 m to 2 m) from the surgical site is generally maintained. In addition, exposure is reduced by using forceps or other instruments to transfer radioactive specimens into specimen containers.[54]

The researchers concluded that radiation doses for all personnel were low, but good radiation handling practices should be implemented and followed to ensure that exposure is ALARA. Results of this study also confirmed the finding of Miner et al[51] that a surgeon would have to perform thousands of sentinel node biopsy procedures each year to exceed the regulatory exposure limit.[54]

III.e.1. Policies and procedures for radioactive seed localization procedures where the seed is resected with the specimen must align with 10 CFR 35.1000, Medical Use of Byproduct Material[46]; guidance documents provided by the US Nuclear Regulatory Commission (NRC)[49]; and local and state regulations.

The use of radioactive seed localization is considered an "other medical use of byproduct material" by the NRC.[46] The NRC oversees the use of radioactive materials in clinical practice and has provided guidance documents for the performance of radioactive seed localization procedures, including the safe handling of radioactive seeds.[49]

III.e.2. Policies and procedures for managing radioactive specimens should be developed by a multidisciplinary team including representatives from the pathology laboratory; a radiation safety officer; personnel from radiology, perioperative services, and risk management; and other involved perioperative team members (eg, a scrub person).

Specimen management is a multidisciplinary process. Including the radiation safety officer and representative personnel from all involved areas will help to facilitate the development of safe and effective policies and procedures.

III.e.3. Facility or health care organization policies and procedures should define when personal shielding and exposure monitoring is required.

Personnel radiation exposure monitoring devices and shielding may not be needed for the surgical team if low levels of radioactivity have been found and exposure time is limited.[45,51]

III.e.4. Personnel performing or participating in radioactive seed localization or sentinel lymph node biopsy procedures should use standard precautions.[47,48,50]

The radiopharmaceuticals used for sentinel lymph node procedures become bound to the tissue and therefore do not produce high levels of radiation.[48] For this reason, only standard precautions are required, and these precautions will also prevent any uptake of radiation by those handling the specimens.[48]

III.e.5. Forceps or other instruments should be used to place radioactive specimens that have been removed from the patient into sealed containers.[48]

III.e.6. When a radioactive seed is retrieved, the seed should be immediately placed in a sealed specimen container and labeled with patient and specimen identifiers,[47,55] the date and time the specimen was collected, and the name of the isotope (eg, ^{99m}technetium-sulfur colloid [^{99m}Tc]).[48] The container of radioactive material must be labeled, "Caution— Radioactive Material" if the container holds more than 1.0 millicuries (mCi) of ^{99m}Tc.[45] The container need not be labeled if it holds less than 1.0 mCi of ^{99m}Tc[56] or specimens are attended by individuals taking the necessary precautions (ie, standard precautions) to prevent exposure, only authorized personnel have access to the specimen containers, and the containers are accompanied with written documentation that identifies the contents.[56]

Labeling requirements are dependent on the amount of radioactive material in the specimen.[56] Doses of 0.4 mCi to 1.0 mCi of ^{99m}Tc are typically used in sentinel lymphadenectomy for melanoma or breast cancer.[50] If the facility or health care organization policies and procedures specify that only authorized personnel are permitted to handle specimens, warning labels that identify radioactive material are not required.[56]

III.e.7. The presence of a radioactive seed should be documented on the pathology requisition slip and also communicated verbally to pathology personnel at the time of specimen delivery.[47,55]

III.e.8. Specimens containing radioactive material should be promptly transported to the pathology laboratory in sealed, labeled containers.[50] Specimens should not be left unattended or in unsecured areas.[50]

III.e.9. Radioactive specimens containing more than 1 mCi of iodine-125 or 100 mCi of palladium-103 that are transferred to an outside pathology laboratory must be transferred to an NRC or Agreement State-licensed laboratory authorized to receive radioactive contaminated tissue or seed.[57]

- Specimens must be packaged and prepared in accordance with 10 CFR 71.5, Transportation of Licensed Material, or an equivalent Agreement State regulation for shipping.[58]
- Specimens may also require "Caution— Radioactive Material" labeling when
  ○ specimens are not attended by individuals taking the necessary precautions (ie, standard precautions) to prevent exposure[56] and

449

◦ unauthorized personnel may have access to the specimen containers.[56]

III.e.10. When the operative or other invasive procedure is completed, all instruments (eg, forceps, scissors) that had contact with the radioactive specimen should be processed using standard precautions.[48]

III.e.11. The seed should be transported to facility or health care organization nuclear medicine or radiation safety personnel for disposal.[47,55]

Nuclear medicine or radiation safety personnel should

• examine the seed before disposal to verify that radiation is at background radiation levels[48] and

• remove any "Caution—Radioactive Materials" labels that have been attached to the container before disposal.[45]

III.e.12. Radiation safety education addressing routine radiation monitoring and emergency procedures (eg, broken or leaking seed) must be provided at least annually to personnel involved in radiation seed localization procedures.[46,49]

Annual safety instruction on routine monitoring and emergency procedures for personnel involved in radiation seed localization procedures is a regulatory requirement.[46,49]

III.f. Explanted medical devices should be collected and handled according to the facility's or health care organization's policies and procedures; manufacturers' instructions; and local, state, and federal regulations. *[1: Regulatory Requirement]*

Hospitals and other health care facilities that implant medical devices are considered final distributors (ie, any person or entity that distributes a tracked device to the patient, including licensed practitioners, retail pharmacies, hospitals, and other facilities).[59] Final distributors are subject to medical device tracking requirements and are responsible for providing information to the manufacturer about explanted devices.[60]

Medical device tracking is required if the FDA issues an order to the manufacturer and the device meets one of the following criteria:

◦ the failure of the device (ie, failure to perform or function as intended) would likely have serious adverse health consequences (ie, significant events that are life-threatening or involve permanent or long-term injury or illness);

◦ the device is intended to be implanted in the human body (ie, placed into a surgically or naturally formed human body cavity to continuously assist, restore, or replace the function of an organ system or structure) for more than one year; or

◦ the device is a life-sustaining or life-supporting device (ie, essential to the restoration or contin-

uation of a bodily function) used outside of the device user facility (ie, intended for use outside a hospital, nursing home, ambulatory surgery facility, or diagnostic or outpatient treatment facility).[59]

III.f.1. Explanted medical devices that are subject to medical device tracking regulation must be reported to the manufacturer.[61] Information that must be provided to the manufacturer includes the

• date the device was explanted;

• name, mailing address, and telephone number of the explanting physician; and

• date of the patient's death or the date the device was returned to the manufacturer, permanently retired from use, or otherwise disposed of permanently.[61]

The FDA has issued orders to manufacturers that require tracking of the following of implantable devices:

• temporomandibular joint prosthesis

• glenoid fossa prosthesis

• mandibular condyle prosthesis

• implantable pacemaker pulse generator

• cardiovascular permanent implantable pacemaker electrode

• replacement heart valve (mechanical only)

• automatic implantable cardioverter/defibrillator

• implanted cerebellar stimulator

• implanted diaphragmatic/phrenic nerve stimulator

• implantable infusion pumps

• abdominal aortic aneurysm stent grafts

• silicone gel-filled breast implants

• cultured epidermal autografts

• thoracic aortic aneurysm stent grafts

• transcatheter pulmonary valve prosthesis[60]

III.f.2. Manufacturers' instructions for packaging and shipping should be followed when the explanted device is returned to the manufacturer. If the manufacturer of the explanted device cannot be determined, facility personnel must attempt to locate the manufacturer and report the explant.[60] If facility personnel are unable to locate the manufacturer, a record of the explantation and an attempt to locate the manufacturer must be maintained in the facility's implant tracking records.[60]

III.f.3. Deaths related to an implanted medical device must be reported to both the FDA and the manufacturer.[61,62] Serious injury related to an implanted medical device must be reported to the device manufacturer.[61,62] If the medical device manufacturer cannot be identified, the injury should be reported to the FDA.[61,62]

Implanted medical device malfunctions are not required to be reported; however, the facility or health care organization may use the voluntary MedWatch program[63] to advise the FDA of potential problems with an implanted medical device.[61,62]

III.f.4. Explanted orthopedic hardware (eg, plates, screws) to be returned to the manufacturer should be collected, handled, packaged, and shipped according to the manufacturers' instructions.

III.f.5. Explanted orthopedic hardware to be returned to the patient should be collected, handled, decontaminated, labeled, packaged, and documented according to the facility or health care organization policies and procedures.[64]

- Before returning the explanted hardware to the patient, facility or health care organization personnel should verify that the explanted hardware has not been recalled and does not need to be returned to the manufacturer.[64]
- Return of the explanted hardware should be documented in the patient's health record, including the
  - patient's request for return of the explanted hardware and
  - personnel returning the explanted hardware to the patient.[64]

III.f.6. Explanted orthopedic hardware may be excluded from submission to the pathologist for examination, provided there is an alternative policy in place for documentation of surgical removal.[65]

In a study conducted between September 2, 2004, and December 16, 2005, to evaluate the cost and effectiveness of sending explanted internal fixation hardware to the pathologist for examination, Davidovitch et al prospectively followed and analyzed 46 consecutive patients who underwent elective hardware removal after internal fixation. In all cases, it was determined that the residual pain at the fracture site was completely hardware-related and not a result of fracture disunion or infection. The researchers reviewed pathology reports for all patients. All reports had the same basic structure and content. The only information that could be discerned from the report was that the hardware had been removed from a specific location.[66]

Pathology examination of explanted hardware is costly and provides no benefit to the patient or physician. In lieu of pathologic examination, the researchers recommended a single radiographic view of the explanted hardware and documentation in the postoperative report to verify removal of the hardware.[66]

III.f.7. Explanted orthopedic hardware that is not submitted to the pathologist, returned to the manufacturer, or returned to the patient should be disposed of according to the facility or health care organization policies and procedures.

III.f.8. Policies and procedures related to collecting and handling of explanted medical devices should be developed by a multidisciplinary team including personnel from administration, risk management, pathology, infection prevention, materials management, sterile processing, and perioperative services. Policies and procedures should be in compliance with local, state, and federal regulations and should address collection and handling of explanted

- medical devices subject to medical device tracking,
- medical devices related deaths or serious injuries,[62] and
- devices to be returned to the patient.

Recommendation IV

Specimens should be transferred from the sterile field in a manner that maintains the integrity of the specimen.

Specimen transfer refers to the process of moving a specimen from the sterile field to a containment device.

Specimens that are incorrectly transferred from the sterile field may be compromised, which may lead to inaccurate or incomplete diagnostic information resulting in the need for additional procedures.

IV.a. Specimens should be passed off the sterile field as soon as possible. *[5: Benefits Balanced with Harms]*

Passing the specimen off the sterile field as soon as possible reduces the potential for the integrity of the specimen to be compromised or for the specimen to be misplaced or lost.

Evidence addressing the need for passing the specimen off the sterile field as soon as possible was not identified during the evidence review for this guideline.

IV.b. Specimens kept on the sterile field before transfer should be sequestered, identified, and monitored. *[5: Benefits Balanced with Harms]*

Sequestering, identifying, and monitoring specimens kept on the sterile field reduces the possibility for the specimen to be compromised or lost.

Evidence addressing the need for sequestering, identifying, and monitoring specimens kept on the sterile field was not identified during the evidence review for this guideline.

IV.c. Specimens should be kept moist until transfer from the sterile field and should not be placed on dry, absorbent surfaces or materials. *[2: High Evidence]*

Air exposure can lead to desiccation of tissue.[35] Keeping specimens moist helps to prevent drying of the specimen before placement in fixative.[29] Dry, absorbent surfaces or materials may adhere to the tissue, which may result in the loss of portions of the resection margins.[35]

IV.d. Patient and specimen identification should be verified before transfer from the sterile field. Specimens transferred from the sterile field should be verbally identified by the surgeon and verified by the perioperative RN using a "write down, read back" technique.[67] *[3: Moderate Evidence]*

Verifying identification of the specimen during the transfer process minimizes opportunities for error and helps prevent misidentification of the specimen.

IV.e. Specimens should be transferred from the sterile field by personnel using standard precautions. *[1: Strong Evidence]*

Standard precautions represent the minimum infection prevention strategy to be applied during all patient care activities (regardless of suspected or confirmed infection status of the patient) in any setting in which health care is delivered.[68] Implementing standard precautions when specimens are transferred from the sterile field helps prevent exposure of personnel to blood, body fluids, or other potentially infectious materials.[68]

IV.f. Specimens should be transferred from the sterile field by personnel using sterile technique. *[5: Benefits Balanced with Harms]*

Using sterile technique when specimens are transferred from the sterile field helps to prevent microbial contamination of the specimen.

Evidence addressing the need for transferring specimens from the sterile field using sterile technique was not identified during the evidence review for this guideline.

IV.g. The cellular structure of the specimen should be maintained during the transfer process by not crushing, twisting, or otherwise damaging the integrity of the tissue. *[5: Benefits Balanced with Harms]*

Maintaining the cellular structure of the specimen reduces the potential for inaccurate or incomplete diagnostic information.

Evidence addressing the need for maintaining the cellular structure of the specimen during transfer from the sterile field was not identified during the evidence review for this guideline.

Recommendation V

Containment of the specimen should be completed in a manner that protects and secures the specimen and prevents exposure of health care personnel to blood, body fluids, or other potentially infectious materials.

Specimen containment involves securing the specimen by placing it in an item used for storage and transport.

Containing the specimen in a manner that protects and secures the specimen may help to prevent damage to or loss of the specimen. Containing the specimen in a manner that prevents exposure of health care personnel to blood, body fluids, or other infectious materials is a regulatory requirement.[69]

V.a. Containers and collection devices needed for specimen management during the procedure should be determined and obtained before the procedure. *[5: Benefits Balanced with Harms]*

Determining and obtaining specimen containers before the procedure may help to improve process efficiency and prevent damage to or loss of the specimen.

Evidence addressing the need for determining and obtaining containers and collection devices necessary for specimen management before the procedure was not identified during the evidence review for this guideline.

V.b. Containers must be leak proof and puncture resistant.[69] *[1: Regulatory Requirement]*

Using specimen containers that are leak proof and puncture resistant is a regulatory requirement.[69]

V.b.1. Containers should be of the correct size and type and should be large enough to fully secure the specimen and preservative fluids.

Verifying that specimen containers are of the correct size and type to fully secure the specimen and preservative fluids used may help prevent damage to the specimen. This can also prevent leakage and help protect perioperative personnel or others handling the container or its contents from unnecessary exposure to blood, body fluids, or other infectious materials.

V.b.2. The container or collection device should be large enough to allow the preservative solution, if used, to contact all surfaces of the specimen.

V.b.3. Specimen collection containers may be sterile or clean, depending on collection requirements.

V.c. The specimen should be contained and labeled immediately after transfer from the sterile field. *[3: Moderate Evidence]*

Containing specimens immediately after transfer from the sterile field may prevent damage to or loss of the specimen.

In a study to evaluate the incidence and cause of tissue biopsy loss, Sandbank et al tracked the biopsy specimens taken by a single plastic surgeon at an outpatient clinic between October 2001 and April 2005. A total of 4,400 tissue biopsy specimens were submitted, and a total of five specimens were reported as lost during the study period. Two of the specimens were located. After formal review of the remaining three lost specimens, the researchers determined that one specimen had been lost in the pathology laboratory during processing, and two specimens had been lost because they had not been inserted into the specimen container. The researchers recommended inserting the specimen into the container immediately after excision and verifying that the specimen is in the container at the end of the procedure.[70]

Recommendation VI

Specimens containers should be labeled to communicate patient, specimen, preservative,[71] and biohazard[69] information.

Specimen identification and labeling is the process of affixing to a container information that establishes or indicates the specifications or characteristics of the enclosed sample.

Misidentification of a specimen, its margins, or other information (eg, location of suture tags) could result in errors or delay in diagnosis or treatment or the need for additional procedures.

Labeling to communicate chemical preservative and biohazard information is a regulatory requirement.[69,71] Failure to communicate preservative and biohazard information could result in exposure or injury to personnel handling the contained specimen.

Evidence related to specimen identification and labeling identified during the evidence review for this guideline. revealed a number of studies and quality improvement initiatives conducted for the purpose of reducing errors in specimen identification[72-78]; however, there are variances in terminology,[77,78] quality indicators,[72,75,76] and organizational practices,[7] and there is no clear solution for eliminating errors.[7,72,77]

Makary et al conducted a prospective cohort study designed to measure the incidence and type of specimen identification errors occurring in the surgical patient population during the preanalytical phase. The study included all surgical patients (ie, outpatient and inpatient) for whom a pathology specimen was sent between October 2004 and April 2005. The researchers analyzed a total of 21,351 specimens for identification errors (ie, any discrepancy between information on the specimen requisition form and the accompanying labeled specimen received in the pathology laboratory). There were a total of 91 specimen identification errors, including

- specimen not labeled (n = 18),
- empty specimen container (n = 16),
- incorrect laterality (n = 16),
- incorrect tissue site (n = 14),
- incorrect patient (n = 11),
- no patient name (n = 9), and
- no tissue site (n = 7).[72]

Identification errors occurred in 4.3 per 1,000 surgical specimens. This translates to approximately 182 mislabeled specimens per year. These events occurred in 53 patients from outpatient clinics and 38 patients from hospital operating rooms (ORs). The most com-

mon identification errors occurred in biopsy procedures (n = 54), followed by excisional procedures (n = 24), and resection procedures (n = 3). The most common mislabeled specimens included breast tissue (n = 11), skin (n = 10), and colon (n = 8). The researchers concluded that surgical specimen identification errors are common and present an important safety risk for patients. Strategies to reduce the rate of errors should therefore be a research priority.[72]

Quillen and Murphy conducted a study of 49,955 specimens obtained between January 1, 2004, and September 30, 2005, in a university hospital, to determine the number of specimen mislabeling events, specifically major mislabeling events, and to design and implement a corrective plan of action for reducing specimen mislabeling. They recorded and classified all mislabeling events into two categories:

- minor mislabeling: truncated name or medical record number, misspelled name, missing information (eg, date, signature) or
- major mislabeling: unlabeled specimen, mismatched information on specimen and requisition, wrong blood in the tube.[73]

The overall incidence of specimen mislabeling events during the 21-month study period was 0.5% (n = 243 of 49,955). Of the mislabeling events, 47% (n = 114) were defined as major events. The researchers noted that the highest proportion of mislabeling events came from the emergency department. Weekly feedback was provided to address the mislabeling events, and within one year, the number of mislabeling events in the emergency department was reduced from 47% (n = 23 of 49) to 14% (n = 4 of 29). The researchers concluded that collecting and reviewing data on mislabeled specimens and providing timely feedback can change practice and reduce specimen mislabeling.[73]

In early 2005, the CAP conducted a survey of 120 institutions to determine the

- frequency of identification errors detected before and after verification of results,
- frequency of adverse events caused by specimen misidentification, and
- factors associated with low error rates and detection of errors.

Participants tracked data on identification errors related to all types of anatomic (ie, examining and processing of surgical specimens) and clinical (ie, laboratory testing) errors related to all inpatients and outpatients for five weeks. The term *specimen identification error* was considered to represent any result reported for the wrong specimen (or one that would have been reported for the wrong specimen without some intervention).[74]

The researchers reviewed information from a total of 6,705 identification errors. The majority (85.5%) were detected before verification, with the remaining portion (14.5%) detected after results were released. More than 50% of the identification errors resulted from specimen labeling errors, with 22% resulting from registration or order entry errors. Approximately one in 18 identification errors resulted in an adverse event, with more than 70% of adverse events resulting in patient inconvenience rather than a change in treatment or outcome. The researchers concluded that identification errors are common, but most are detected before results are released, and only a fraction are associated with adverse patient events.[74]

In April 2003, a multidisciplinary team from a statewide children's hospital and clinics system performed an intense scrutiny of specimen labeling methods to identify areas in the current processes that might lead to potential errors. The labeling process was critically observed, recorded, and reviewed during interviews with involved personnel. The preanalytical phase was identified as the primary focus area because it was revealed that nearly two-thirds of the labeling errors occurred during this phase.[75]

The team decided to have laboratory personnel reject all specimens that were not correctly labeled. Personnel submitting the specimen could challenge the rejection by following a procedure that involved a discussion with the ordering clinician, the health care worker who collected and labeled the specimen, and the pathologist. The discussion could result in labeling or relabeling of the specimen in question. The rejection and discussion process resulted in a 75% decrease in the number of mislabeled or unlabeled specimens received in the pathology laboratory.[75]

In a study conducted during the fall of 2009 to quantify the rates of mislabeled cases, specimens, blocks, and slides; identify the sources of error; and review the ways specimen labeling errors are discovered, Nakhleh et al prospectively reviewed voluntarily submitted surgical pathology data from 136 participating institutions for eight weeks or until 30 errors (ie, mislabeled cases, specimens, blocks, slides) were identified. Study participants used the following definitions for defining mislabeling errors:

- mislabeled case: wrong patient or case number applied to the entire case
- mislabeled specimen: wrong specimen labeling (eg, right versus left)
- mislabeled block: histological block labeled with the wrong patient or case number
- mislabeled slide: histological slide labeled with the wrong patient or case number

Information collected on each labeling error included the

- work location where the defect occurred,
- item that was mislabeled,
- number of items affected,
- point of detection, and
- consequences of the mislabeling error.[76]

The rates of mislabeled cases, specimens, blocks, and slides were also tested for association with institutional demographics and practice variables. Results from a total of 1,811 mislabeling occurrences showed the overall mislabeling rates to be 27.1% of cases, 19.8% of specimens, 25.5% of blocks, and 27.7% of slides. Mislabeling of specimens most often occurred during the preanalytical or analytical phases. In most cases, the errors were detected during the steps immediately following the error. Errors were corrected before the pathology report was issued 96.7% of the time, with a corrected report necessary for only 3.2% of errors. Study participants estimated that patient care was affected for 1.3% of error occurrences.

The researchers pointed out that the results of this study failed to show a detectable benefit associated with the use of technology (eg, bar codes) or the use of processes designed to promote continuous improvement and reduce wasted resources. They concluded that there is a need for quality checks throughout the system to reduce errors in specimen labeling.[76]

Bixenstine et al convened an expert panel to develop and pilot test a tool of standardized measures and definitions to evaluate the quality of surgical specimen identification during the preanalytical phase. The panel included physicians, nurses, students, and administrators with expertise in pathology or quality improvement. The preanalytical phase was chosen because specimen identification processes in this phase are completely preventable. A literature review was conducted to identify published surgical specimen identification defects.[77]

Group consensus was achieved on a set of surgical specimen identification quality measures and also on procedures for collecting and measuring data. Quality measures included the following container and requisition defects:

- Container defects included
  - no specimen in the container or requisition received without a container,
  - no identifying label or misplaced label,
  - no patient name or incorrect patient name,
  - no numeric patient identifier or incorrect numeric patient identifier,
  - no specimen type or source or incorrect specimen type or source, and
  - no specimen laterality or incorrect specimen laterality.
- Requisition defects included
  - no requisition or a blank requisition received with the specimen container,
  - no date and time or incorrect date and time,
  - no patient name or incorrect patient name,
  - no numeric patient identifier or incorrect numeric patient identifier,
  - no specimen type or source or incorrect specimen type or source, and
  - no specimen laterality or incorrect specimen laterality.[77]

A total of 69 diverse hospitals in Michigan and one in Iowa submitted prospectively collected data during a three-month period in 2009. The results showed an average specimen identification defect rate of nearly 3%. During the three-month study period, the identified specimen identification defects involved 1,780 patients. The overall container defect rate was about 1%, with the most common container defects being omitted or incorrect specimen source or type. The overall requisition defect rate was more than 2%, with the most common requisition defect being omitted or incorrect date and time. The consequences of these defects represent a significant risk to patient safety.[77]

SPECIMEN MANAGEMENT

The researchers contended that without standardized definitions, quality measures, and methodology, it is difficult to accurately estimate and compare the incidence of defects and to identify the most common defects in specimen identification. Additional research is needed to determine whether these measures can be used to reduce the frequency of surgical specimen identification errors and improve patient safety.[77]

In a systematic study of amended pathology reports from 2001 to 2004 conducted by a university health system to determine the types of errors and the effectiveness of efforts to improve surgical pathology processes, researchers classified amended pathology reports by four root causes:

- misidentifications (ie, wrong patient, tissue, laterality, or anatomic location),
- specimen defects (ie, lost, inadequate size or volume, missing or discrepant critical measurements),
- misinterpretations (ie, diagnosis not justified by available evidence [eg, false positives]), and
- report defects (ie, transmission of erroneous information not related to misidentification, specimen defects, or misinterpretations).

Three specific interventions designed to promote continuous improvement and reduce wasted resources were applied and assessed between 2005 and 2008, including

- clinician education to reduce identification defects,
- redesign of specimen processing to reduce specimen defects, and
- double review of breast and prostate specimens before sign-out to decrease interpretation defects.[78]

During the four-year period, misidentification defects decreased from 16% to 9%; specimen defects remained variable, ranging from 2% to 11%; misinterpretations decreased from 18% to 3%; and report defects increased from 64% to 83%. The researchers concluded that misidentification, specimen defects, and misinterpretations were relatively resistant to the applied educational interventions. This finding also underscores the multiple places misidentification errors can occur during the preanalytical and analytical phases and supports the need to double check the processes that occur in these phases.[78]

Specimen defect rates remained variable because the redesign of specimen processing only reduced specimen defects during the analytical phase. The applied interventions markedly decreased specimen misinterpretations. This finding suggests that double review of specimens by pathologists to resolve discrepancies during the analytical phase may be a valuable practice. The increase in report defects demonstrates the effectiveness of capturing data when amended reports are monitored for specific root causes and also demonstrates the need to apply consistent and specific terminology.[78]

VI.a. Patient identification should be confirmed using two unique identifiers according to facility or health care organization policy at the time the specimen is removed from the patient

and placed into the container. *[3: Moderate Evidence]*

Using two patient identifiers reduces the risk for misidentification. The CAP recommends two or more patient identifiers (neither of which is the patient's room number) on specimen labels.[79]

VI.b. Specimen identification should be confirmed verbally between the surgeon and the perioperative RN circulator and documented accurately, legibly, and completely using a "read back" verification of the information provided for specimen labeling. *[3: Moderate Evidence]*

Using a "write down, read back" process to confirm the communication provided for specimen labeling minimizes the risk of communication errors.[67]

In a descriptive retrospective study to develop and prioritize strategies for preventing communication breakdowns that result in surgical patient injury, Greenberg et al identified and reviewed 60 cases involving error and patient injury related to communication breakdowns. Results showed the majority of communication breakdowns were verbal (92%) and involved a single transmitter and a single receiver (64%). The most common error was failure to transmit the information followed by inaccurate communication of the information.[67]

After a qualitative assessment of the communication breakdowns, the researchers developed a set of strategic interventions to reduce communication breakdowns based on the patterns observed in the study. Strategies included identifying trigger events that require immediate communication with the physician, the standard use of read backs, and the use of structured protocols for transfer of care. The cases were reviewed a second time to determine whether the errors could have been prevented by implementing the strategies developed by the researchers. The researchers concluded that the standard use of identified triggers, read backs, and standardized protocols for transfer of care could improve communication and patient safety.[67]

VI.b.1. Specimen identification that should be confirmed and documented includes
- facility or health care organization-defined unique patient identifiers (eg, patient name and medical record number);
- originating source of the specimen including laterality, if applicable;
- type of tissue;
- clinical diagnosis, and
- additional pertinent clinical information (eg, location of suture tags).

VI.c. Specimens must be labeled to communicate chemical preservative[71] and biohazard information.[69] *[1: Regulatory Requirement]*

SPECIMEN MANAGEMENT

Labeling to communicate chemical preservative and biohazard information is a regulatory requirement.[69,71] Failure to communicate preservative and biohazard information could result in exposure or injury to personnel handling the contained specimen.

VI.d. Specimen identification labels should be securely affixed to the container, not the lid. *[3: Moderate Evidence]*

Placing the label on the container instead of the lid may help prevent loss of specimen information after the lid is removed from the container or if the lid becomes detached from the container.[79]

VI.d.1. Information on the label should include
- facility or health care organization-defined unique identifiers (eg, patient name and medical record number);
- specimen type and site including laterality, if applicable; and
- date of resection and preservation.

VI.d.2. Dark, indelible ink should be used on labels.

Using dark ink improves visibility of both handwritten and electronic labels. Using indelible ink helps prevent ink from being removed from the label.

VI.d.3. Unused printed or handwritten labels should be discarded or removed from the OR or procedure room at the end of each procedure.

Disposal or removal of unused printed or handwritten labels helps prevent the risk of an incorrect label being secured to a specimen container, pathology requisition, or other document intended for another patient.

VI.e. Specimen identification and labeling should be confirmed among surgical team members during the debriefing at the end of the operative or other invasive procedure. Confirmation should include
- visual confirmation that the specimen is in the container;
- verification that the patient information on the label and requisition are correct and legible;
- verification that the number and type of specimens are correct, including laterality as applicable;
- verification that the specimens have been correctly fixed, as applicable; and
- confirmation of other pertinent information (eg, documentation of suture tags).

[3: Moderate Evidence]

Management of specimens is a multidisciplinary process. Postprocedure confirmation of the specimen identification and labeling can improve communication among team members and may help to reduce or eliminate potential errors[80] in specimen management.

VI.f. A point-of-care bar coding or radio-frequency identification (RFID) patient and specimen labeling system may be used. *[3: Moderate Evidence]*

The CAP recommends using a bar-code patient and specimen labeling system.[79] Using point-of-care bar-coding or RFID technology has the potential to significantly reduce identification errors.[7,79,81,82]

Manual entry of patient identification has an error rate of approximately one character per 300 characters entered.[7] Bar-code technology has a substitution rate of only one per 1 million characters.[7] Most bar-code systems also have a first-read rate of 95% or better, making the acquisition of patient identifying information faster and more accurate than manual methods.[7] Although bar-code technology reduces transcription errors, it does not guarantee accurate patient or specimen identification.[7] After bar codes are printed on labels, the label could be applied to the wrong specimen container, particularly when specimen containers are labeled in advance of specimen collection.[7] Using point-of-care bar-code label printers and scanners minimizes the potential for labels to be applied to the wrong container.[7]

In a quality improvement initiative conducted in December 2002 designed to reduce patient identification errors and unidentified blood glucose results for point-of-care glucose testing, manual steps involved in patient identification were automated using armbands and bar-code scanners. The process changes resulted in a gradual decrease in patient identification errors from 12.4% to 4.9%, and a reduction in the number of unidentified blood glucose results from between 400 and 500 to 274.[83]

In March 2003, the bar-code width was reduced and the wristband was placed in a protective pouch to increase ease of scanning. Data collected after the implementation of the new wristband showed a decrease in patient identification errors from 4.9% to 1.7%, and a reduction in the number of unidentified blood glucose results from 274 to 102. Additional education and nonpunitive feedback was provided to individuals with high error rates. By December 2003, patient identification errors had decreased to 0.7%, and the number of unidentified blood glucose results was reduced to 25.[83]

In a quality improvement project conducted in 2008 in the emergency department of a medical center treating more than 42,000 patients per year, the rate of mislabeled specimens (ie, two per week) was determined to be unacceptable. A multidisciplinary team was brought together to explore options, and use of a bar-coding device designed for use with bedside computers and printers was implemented in 2010. Use of

456

PATIENT AND WORKER SAFETY

the bar-coding device, in combination with dual identification of the patient, eliminated specimen labeling errors.[84]

In an integrated health care delivery system composed of three large acute care hospitals and a reference laboratory where more than 1 million point-of-care tests are performed annually, a performance improvement initiative was prompted by a number of identification errors occurring with glucose and blood gas point-of-care testing devices. Nichols et al approached the goal of reducing identification errors associated with point-of-care testing by applying two strategies. They conducted an analysis of the identification processes to determine the various ways that identification errors could occur. Data entry was determined to be the primary source of error because of the need to enter 14 digits with every test. The first strategy involved holding clinical operators accountable for mistakes in data entry. This strategy led to only partial improvements in error rates.[85]

The investigators theorized that bar coding would be the most effective means of addressing the data entry problem. Bar coding was implemented as a second strategy in November 2002. The rates of identification errors decreased significantly for both glucose and blood gas devices; however, identification errors still occurred because operators resorted to manual entry when they encountered a bar code that was difficult to scan. Errors also occurred when patients were found to have incorrect information on bar-coded wristbands. The investigators concluded that bar-coding technology significantly reduced identification errors with point-of-care testing, improved patient care, and enhanced interdisciplinary communication, but additional steps are needed to verify that patient wristbands contain accurate information.[85]

Francis et al conducted a study in a high-volume gastroenterology and colorectal surgery outpatient endoscopy unit that yields more than 30,000 specimens annually, for the purpose of eliminating the paper requisitions that accompanied tissue specimens sent for pathologic evaluation and creating a system that would automate specimen bottle tracking. The study was undertaken as an initiative to reduce specimen-labeling errors in response to a wrong site surgery that was performed as the result of a mislabeled pathology specimen. The researchers applied RFID technology to specimen bottles and initiated dual confirmation of the correct site and patient for each specimen by both the endoscopy RN and the endoscopist.

The researchers reviewed and compared the number of specimen labeling errors that occurred in the unit during January through March 2007, before the initiative, and during January through March 2008, after the initiative. Errors were categorized as

- class 1 (ie, typographical errors with no potential clinical consequences),
- class 2 (ie, minor errors unlikely to have clinical consequences), or
- class 3 (ie, significant errors with the potential to detrimentally affect patient care).[82]

During 2007, there were 646 class 1 errors (7.85%), 112 class 2 errors (1.36%), and seven class 3 errors (0.09%) for 8,229 specimens. In 2008, there were 35 class 1 errors (0.41%), 10 class 2 errors (0.12%), and two class 3 errors (0.02%) for 8,536 specimens. The researchers concluded that the dual confirmation of patient and surgical site and the initiation of an electronic requisition and RFID technology significantly reduced specimen labeling errors in every class.[82]

VI.g. Perioperative RNs responsible for specimen management should receive education and complete competency verification activities related to reducing errors in specimen identification and labeling.[10] *[3: Moderate Evidence]*

O'Neill et al conducted a retrospective study to investigate the combined effect of an educational campaign and strict enforcement of specimen labeling policy for the purpose of reducing the incidence of mislabeled and wrong blood in the tube specimens detected by blood bank personnel. The researchers calculated and compared the incidence of mislabeled and wrong blood in the tube specimens from October 1, 2001, through September 30, 2004, preceding the education and policy enforcement, and then from October 1, 2004, through September 30, 2007, after the education and policy enforcement. Results showed that following the educational campaign and strict policy enforcement, the incidence of mislabeling errors decreased by 86.4%. The incidence of wrong blood in the tube decreased by 73.5%. The researchers concluded that education and policy enforcement can lead to statistically significant decrease in the incidence of specimen mislabeling and wrong blood in the tube.[86]

VI.h. Facility or health care organization policies and procedures should provide guidance for specimen
- collection and handling,
- identification and labeling, and
- transport.[79]
[3: Moderate Evidence]

Policies and procedures provide guidance and detail responsibilities for specimen identification and labeling.[10]

In 2006, personnel at a major university hospital noted that the number of specimen identification errors was greater than desired and represented a risk to patient safety. Between 2007

457

and 2011, a collaborative effort between nursing and laboratory personnel was initiated to improve performance and reduce the number of errors involving inpatient, ambulatory, and surgical services areas. The improvement process began with a review of current practices to determine how the errors were occurring. The types of errors also were reviewed and categorized; they included

- unlabeled specimen,
- lack of patient identification on the request form,
- no request form,
- specimen labeled with only one patient identifier (ie, patient name), and
- specimen and request form unmatched (ie, specimen labeled with the wrong patient or request form labeled with the wrong patient).

Applied strategies for improvement included

- establishing clear expectations for specimen identification by reviewing and updating all policies and procedures related to specimen identification,
- providing education to all clinical personnel who collect specimens,
- providing individualized feedback to each employee involved in an incorrect specimen identification event, and
- addressing the process when specific types of errors occurred repeatedly.

The applied performance improvement interventions successfully reduced the number of errors from 128 per year to 30 per year (77%).[87]

Recommendation VII

Specimens should be preserved in a manner that protects the integrity of the specimen and prevents exposure of health care personnel to chemicals, blood, body fluids, or other potentially infectious materials.

Specimen preservation involves the act of protecting a specimen to preserve morphology, reduce the loss of molecular components into solution, prevent decomposition and autolysis, and prevent microbial growth.[88]

Unpreserved or incorrectly preserved specimens may be compromised and lead to inaccurate or incomplete diagnostic information or the need for additional procedures.

Containing the specimen in a manner that prevents exposure of health care personnel to chemicals, blood, body fluids, or other infectious materials is a regulatory requirement.[69,71]

A full discussion of safe practices for handling formalin or other preservative solutions or chemicals is outside of the scope of this guideline. The reader should refer to the AORN Guideline for a Safe Environment of Care: Part 1[89] for additional guidance.

VII.a. The use of preservatives or chemical additives for tissue preservation should be confirmed with the physician. *[5: Benefits Balanced with Harms]*

Verifying the use of preservatives or chemical additives with the physician may help to prevent errors in tissue preservation.

Evidence addressing the need for confirming the use of chemical additives for preservation with the physician was not identified during the evidence review for this guideline.

VII.b. Formalin should be dispensed and stored in an area other than the OR or procedure room unless ignition sources are not used and the regulatory requirements for locations where formalin is used and stored are met. *[1: Regulatory Requirement]*

Formalin is a combustible liquid.[90] Storage and use of formalin is regulated by the Occupational Safety and Health Administration and other federal and state health regulatory agencies.[71,91]

Locations where formalin is used must have

- posted signs warning of formaldehyde use,
- eyewash stations available within the immediate area, and
- ventilation systems with adequate capacity to maintain levels below the permissible exposure limits (ie, eight-hour total weighted average of 0.75 ppm or 15-minute short-term exposure limit of 2.0 ppm).[71]

VII.b.1. Eyewash stations should be located

- so that travel time is no greater than 10 seconds from the location of chemical use or storage, or immediately next to or adjoining the area of chemical use or storage if the chemical is caustic or a strong acid and
- on the same level as the hazard, with the path of travel free of obstructions (eg, doors) that may inhibit immediate use of an eyewash station.[92]

When walking at a normal pace, the average person covers a distance of 55 feet in 10 seconds; however, a person who has experienced a chemical splash to the eyes or face may be visually impaired, in discomfort or pain, and in a state of panic. For this reason, it is prudent to consider the physical and emotional state of the person as well as the availability of assistive personnel in the immediate area when determining the location of eyewash stations.[92]

VII.c. Personnel handling formalin must wear personal protective equipment including face and eye shields, gloves, and other protective garments.[71,90,93] *[1: Regulatory Requirement]*

Formaldehyde, the active ingredient in formalin, is a potential carcinogen. It may cause acute and chronic health conditions, including sensitization leading to asthma and contact dermatitis. Formalin can be absorbed through the skin and nasal passages, splashed in the eyes, or ingested. Exposure can result in irritation, burns, or allergic reactions.[71,90,91,93]

VII.d. Specimens should be fully immersed in a ratio of fixative volume to specimen volume determined by the pathologist or receiving pathology laboratory personnel. *[2: High Evidence]*

The volume of formalin required for tissue fixation is not generally agreed upon.[94] The literature is inconclusive regarding the amount of solution that should be used for specimen preservation and the suggested amounts vary.[30,88,94,95]

In a review of the literature conducted in 2007 on function and management of the pathology laboratory, common specimen types, biohazard exposure and safety, and collection of tissue for research, Bell et al recommended a volume of at least 10 times the volume of the specimen for effective fixation.[88]

In 2008, an ad hoc committee of expert pathologists, laboratory scientists, and technical experts who developed consensus recommendations for standardized procedures for estrogen-receptor testing in breast cancer recommended placing breast resection specimens in a volume of fixative that is one part tissue to 20 parts fixative.[30]

In a study published in 2010 that examined the use of under-vacuum sealing as an alternative to fixing specimens in formalin, Di Novi et al recommended a volume of fixative that is 20 times the weight of the specimen.[95]

Fixative-to-tissue volume ratios of 1:20 have been advocated because of the consideration that fixatives are poor buffers; however, this is not the case with neutral buffered formalin.[94] In addition, it has been argued that large amounts of fixative are needed to prevent dilution of the fixative, but this is primarily applicable to fixatives that do not contain water, which is not the case with neutral buffered formalin.[94]

In a study to determine the smallest amount of neutral buffered formalin to provide adequate tissue fixation, Buesa and Peshkov fixed a total of 60 tissue samples from human breast, uterus, liver, skin, and abdominal fat for eight, 24, and 48 hours at room temperature (ie, 68° F to 71.6° F [20° C to 22° C]), with neutral buffered formalin at fixative-to-tissue volume ratios of 1:1. 2:1, 5:1, and 10:1. After processing, nine pathologists from three different histopathology institutions evaluated the slides. Results showed that the fixation process is more time and temperature dependent and less related to the volume of fixative used. Preserving tissues with a fixative-to-tissue volume of 2:1 for 48 hours at room temperature was enough to ensure proper fixation and infiltration of the tissue samples, and the researchers anticipated that other tissues would show similar results. The researchers concluded that using formalin in fixative-to-tissue ratios of lower than 10:1 will improve health care worker safety while still allowing for the use of formalin as a tissue fixative solution.[94]

VII.e. Specimens and chemicals used for preservation of specimens must be disposed of according to local, state, and federal regulations.[69,71] *[1: Regulatory Requirement]*

Disposal of pathology waste and chemicals is regulated by multiple entities and jurisdictions.[69,71]

VII.f. Alternatives to formalin may be used for tissue fixation or preservation. *[3: Moderate Evidence]*

Formalin is widely used for tissue fixation; however, concerns regarding its toxicity and potential carcinogenicity in combination with the need for more effective preservation of nucleic acids have led to attempts to find a safer alternative.[95-103]

To address concerns associated with personnel exposure to formalin during fixation of surgical specimens in a university hospital, Bussolati et al purchased an under-vacuum sealing device. The under-vacuum sealing process was tested on a variety of tissue and organs (ie, colon, gallbladder, spleen, kidney) to verify histological preservation, and then the device was transferred to the hospital surgical area where it was used successfully for more than one year. The process involved placing large surgical specimens (eg, thyroid, breast, colon) into plastic bags immediately after removal from the patient and then sealing them using the under-vacuum sealing device. The sealing process takes approximately 15 seconds. The labeled specimen was then placed into a refrigerator or taken directly to the pathology laboratory. In most cases, the specimen was kept in the refrigerator for only a few hours, but in some cases specimens were kept in the refrigerator for as long as one to two days.[96]

Under-vacuum sealing decreases the autolytic processes and enhances specimen cooling because of the absence of insulating air. Under-vacuum sealing of surgical specimens results in a lightweight bag that is easier to carry than a formalin-filled plastic container. More than 2,000 specimens were processed using the under-vacuum sealing method without any problems related to morphological preservation or immunohistochemical reactivity. Although refrigeration of specimens for longer periods was not optimal, it did not in any case prevent histopathology processing and reading.[96]

Personnel found the under-vacuum sealing process to be easy and preferable to fixing specimens in formalin. One additional benefit of the under-vacuum sealing process is that because the tissues are not exposed to formalin, material can be provided for tissue banking and research. Previously, the amount of formalin used in the surgical area in this hospital was approximately 15 L per week; currently, no formalin is used.[96]

In an attempt to limit the use of formalin to the pathology laboratory where it is handled under a hood in safe environmental conditions and avoid its use in less-protected areas of the hospital, such as the surgical operating theaters, Di Novi et al proposed an alternative procedure of under-vacuum sealing specimens in plastic bags and refrigerating the sealed, labeled bags at 39.2° F (4° C) until transfer to the pathology laboratory. The under-vacuum sealing process was used successfully for more than two years in a single surgical theater and then extended to an entire teaching hospital with 1,162 beds and approximately 54,560 admissions and 40,000 histopathology examinations per year. In a study conducted between October 2008 and April 2009 to compare the feasibility of the new procedure and compliance of personnel, the researchers used surveys and interviews with all involved personnel (ie, nurses, technicians, pathologists [N = 177]) who specifically dealt with the various steps of the under-vacuum sealing process. Data analysis showed the under-vacuum sealing process to be superior in terms of both personnel satisfaction and gross anatomic preservation. No problems with histopathology preservation were encountered. The use of formalin is now confined to the pathology laboratory and its use on hospital premises is greatly reduced.[95]

In a separate study to quantify the effect of formalin on hospital workers' respiratory systems, Berton and Di Novi used data collected from the previous study and found that only 4.3% of the respondents using the under-vacuum sealing process for containing surgical specimens suffered from respiratory symptoms (eg, cough, chest pain, shortness of breath, wheezing). This figure was approximately 30 percentage points higher for respondents using formalin for fixation of surgical specimens. The researchers concluded that the effect of formalin on the short-term probability of displaying respiratory symptoms is robust and significantly positive, and the substitution of formalin fixation with the under-vacuum sealing process would markedly improve the health of personnel.[97]

In a study to compare the effect of under-vacuum sealing to the effect of cooling alone, Kristensen et al collected tissue samples from five different organs (ie, spleen, breast, kidney, liver, colon). The collected samples underwent one of four treatments:

○ under-vacuum sealing and storage at room temperature (vacuum effect),
○ no under-vacuum sealing and storage at 39.2° F (4° C) (cooling effect),
○ under-vacuum sealing and storage at 39.2° F (4° C) (vacuum and cooling effect), or
○ no under-vacuum sealing and storage at room temperature (no treatment control).[104]

The samples were tested at seven time points: one, two, four, eight, 20, 44, and 92 hours. The results showed no preserving effect of under-vacuum sealing with respect to cellular morphology, immunohistochemical reactivity, or nucleic acid integrity. Storage at cooled temperatures was found to preserve tissue to a higher degree than storage at room temperature, independent of whether the tissue was subjected to under-vacuum sealing. The researchers concluded that under-vacuum sealing is not an alternative to cooling.[104]

Al-Maaini and Bryant conducted a study in 2006 at a university college of medicine to determine the effectiveness of honey as a substitute for formalin in the histological fixation of tissue. The researchers fixed rat liver and kidney tissues at 98.6° F (37° C) and at room temperature, with and without agitation, in concentrations of honey ranging from 10% to 100% diluted with distilled water. The tissues were processed, examined, and compared with tissues fixed in 10% neutral buffered formalin. Results showed that the tissues fixed in 10% and 20% honey concentrations at room temperature with and without agitation provided comparable results to the control tissues fixed in formalin. Honey concentrations greater than 20% were less successful and resulted in slower penetration times, hardening of tissues, and difficulty in sectioning. The researchers recommended additional studies with different brands of honey and a wider range of tissues and fixation times.[98]

In a study to determine the effectiveness of pine honey for tissue fixation and to compare it to other fixatives used for histopathology, Ozkan et al obtained eight different fresh tissue samples (endometrium, breast, placenta, uterus, omentum, suprarenal, stomach, lung). Each tissue sample was divided and placed into one of three fixative solutions:

○ 10% honey in distilled water,
○ 10% neutral buffered formalin, or
○ alcoholic formalin.[99]

All tissues were fixed for 24 hours at room temperature and then processed and examined. Results showed similar tissue histomorphology for all solutions; however, there were minor histomorphological differences among the various tissues fixed in the honey solution. The differences did not influence correct diagnostic conclusions. The researchers concluded that honey can be used as a safe alternative to formalin in histopathology.[99]

In a study that used a systematic approach to evaluate the biomolecular status of a large number of clinical tissue specimens processed using a non-formalin fixation method, Gillespie et al reviewed tissue processed with several fixatives in a major teaching university pathology laboratory to determine whether the various fixatives were sufficient to provide a clinical diagnosis. Results showed that 70% ethanol was acceptable for clinical and molecular analysis.[100]

In the second phase of the study, the researchers fixed 50 radical prostatectomy specimens in 70% ethanol and studied them during a two-year period. The researchers had no difficulty in making a clinical diagnosis in any of the samples and also determined that ethanol fixation was consistently comparable to formalin fixation. The researchers noted, however, that 70% ethanol penetrates prostate tissue at a slower rate than 10% neutral buffered formalin. The researchers concluded that specimens fixed in 70% ethanol permitted recovery of nucleic acids and proteins sufficient for molecular analysis.[100]

In a study to determine the effect of two alcohol-based fixatives on various tissues, van Essen et al fixed a wide range of fresh tissue samples in BoonFix, RCL2®, and 4% neutral buffered formalin. The tissue was stored at room temperature and processed after fixation. A blinded evaluation was conducted by two experienced pathologists. Results showed that the formalin provided significantly better staining results (84%) than RCL2 (66%) or BoonFix (60%). Omission of pepsin pretreatment was found to be important to retain morphology of immunostained tissues preserved in alcohol-based fixatives; however, alcohol-based fixatives may have advantages for molecular techniques because they cause less degradation of nucleic acids.[101]

Prento and Lyon compared the performance of six commercial fixatives (ie, HistoChoice®, Kryofix, Mirsky's Fixative™, NoTox, Omnifix II, Tissue-Tek®) with the performance of neutral buffered formalin on tissue samples of rat liver, small intestine, and kidney, to determine the

○ rate of penetration,
○ mode of fixation,
○ extent of protein and structural immobilization,
○ quality of histology and cellular structure following routine processing, and
○ performance as a fixative.[103]

Results showed that only neutral buffered formalin worked equally well on all tissues tested. The researchers noted prominent histological distortion, cell shrinkage, and vacuolization when formalin substitutes or ethanol was used. The researchers concluded that none of the proposed substitutes for neutral buffered formalin was adequate for critical histology or histopathology.[103]

In a blinded study to assess histomorphology using different formalin substitute fixatives, four experienced, board-certified, surgical pathologists examined seven tissue specimens (ie, hepatocellular carcinoma, ovarian sex cord/stromal tumor, myxoid liposarcoma, uterine endometrioid adenocarcinoma, splenic follicular hyperplasia, infiltrating mammary carcinoma, cecal signet ring carcinoma) fixed with

neutral buffered formalin and five proprietary formalin substitutes (ie, Glyo-Fixx™, STF-Streck®, Omnifix, HistoChoice, Histofix). In each case, the pathologists evaluated
○ cellular outlines,
○ cytoplasmic detail,
○ nuclear detail,
○ erythrocyte integrity,
○ lymphocyte integrity,
○ overall morphology, and
○ overall staining.

The results showed that formalin fixation provided the highest morphologic quality. The researchers concluded that when discontinuing the use of formalin, pathologists should familiarize themselves with the microscopic details of the replacement fixative.[105]

Recommendation VIII

Specimens should be transported in a manner that protects the integrity of the specimen; prevents exposure of health care personnel to chemicals, blood, body fluids, or other potentially infectious materials; and maintains the confidentiality of protected patient information.[69,71]

Specimen transport refers to carrying or conveying a specimen from one location to another. Specimens that are not safely transported may be compromised, which can lead to inaccurate or incomplete diagnostic information or the need for additional procedures.

Transporting the specimen in a manner that prevents exposure of health care personnel to chemicals, blood, body fluids, or other infectious materials and ensures confidentiality of personal health information is a regulatory requirement.[69,71]

VIII.a. Clean secondary packaging or containment devices should be used to prevent contamination of personnel and the environment during transport of specimens. [5: Benefits Balanced with Harms]

Containing the specimen in a manner that prevents exposure of health care personnel to chemicals, blood, body fluids, or other infectious materials is a regulatory requirement.[69,71]

VIII.a.1. Accompanying documents (eg, pathology requisition) should be protected from contamination.

VIII.b. Patient and specimen information should be verified by transport personnel at each point of exchange. [5: Benefits Balanced with Harms]

Misidentification of the patient or specimen could result in errors or delay in diagnosis or treatment or the need for additional procedures.

Evidence addressing the need for transport personnel to verify patient and specimen information at each point of exchange was not identified during the evidence review for this guideline.

VIII.c. Specimens that will not be transported immediately to the pathology laboratory must be temporarily stored in a manner that maintains specimen integrity for examination.[106] [1: Regulatory Requirement]

Maintaining optimal integrity of patient specimens and ensuring the specimen is stored properly (eg, refrigerated, kept at room temperature) is a regulatory requirement.[106]

VIII.c.1. Until transport can take place, equipment (eg, refrigerators) used for temporary storage or devices used for transport or storage should maintain specimens at the temperature established in accordance with local, state, and federal regulations by a multidisciplinary team that includes pathology laboratory representatives, facility or health care organization physicians,[65,107] and perioperative RNs.

VIII.d. Devices intended for transport of specimens must be labeled to communicate chemical[71] and biohazard information.[69] [1: Regulatory Requirement]

Labeling to communicate chemical preservative and biohazard information is a regulatory requirement.[69,71] Failure to communicate preservative and biohazard information could result in exposure or injury to personnel handling the contained specimen.

VIII.e. Specimens must be transported in a manner that helps ensure confidentiality of personal health information[44] and minimizes visibility of the specimen. [1: Regulatory Requirement]

Maintaining confidentiality of protected health information is a regulatory requirement and a standard of perioperative nursing care.[44,108,109]

Recommendation IX

Policies and procedures for disposition of specimens should be established in accordance with local, state, and federal regulations by a multidisciplinary team that includes pathology laboratory representatives, facility or health care organization physicians,[65,107] and perioperative RNs.

The pathologist's report is often the key factor in accurate clinical diagnosis and management of patient care.[107]

The CAP and the Royal College of Pathologists recommend that disposition of specimens for each facility or health care organization be determined by the pathologist in collaboration with facility representatives or health care organization physicians.[65,107] Some explanted medical devices are subject to regulatory tracking or reporting requirements.[59-62]

IX.a. Policies and procedures for disposition of specimens should
- state that a pathologist will perform an examination of the specimen when requested by the physician or licensed independent practitioner or when the pathologist determines a pathology examination is indicated;
- address the diagnostic needs of medical personnel, including the potential for discovery

of significant findings in specimens that are typically exempted from pathology examination, and address the potential for medicolegal implications; and
- include an alternative procedure for documenting the removal and disposition of any specimens or devices not submitted to the pathologist for examination.[65]

[2: High Evidence]

IX.a.1. A pathology report should be generated for every specimen submitted to the pathologist for examination.[65]

IX.a.2. The facility or health care organization should develop policies and procedures for
- receipt of laboratory testing or pathology reporting results,
- communication of laboratory testing or pathology reporting results to the physician, and
- verification that laboratory testing or pathology reporting results are added to the patient's health record.

IX.b. Policies and procedures should be developed to identify tissues or other specimens that require only gross identification or disposal.[65,107] [2: High Evidence]

In some instances, a gross examination and documentation of the submitted specimen by the pathologist without histological examination is sufficient.[107]

The CAP recommends that each facility or health care organization develop a written policy that addresses which specimens do not need to be submitted to the pathologist and which specimens are exempted from microscopic examination.[65]

IX.b.1. Policies and procedures may be developed in accordance with CAP guidelines.[65] The CAP suggests creating two lists:
- specimens exempt from pathology examination and
- specimens to be submitted for gross examination only.[65]

IX.b.2. The following specimens may be excluded from submission to the pathologist for examination, provided there is a procedure for documenting removal and disposition:
- bone donated to the bone bank;
- bone fragments removed during corrective or reconstructive orthopedic procedures (eg, rotator cuff repair), excluding large specimens (eg, femoral heads) and knee, ankle, or elbow reconstructions;
- cataracts removed by phacoemulsification;
- dental appliances;
- fat removed by liposuction;
- foreign bodies (eg, bullets) or other medicolegal evidence given directly to law enforcement personnel;

- foreskin from circumcision of a newborn;
- intrauterine contraceptive devices without attached tissue;
- medical devices (eg, catheters, gastrostomy tubes, myringotomy tubes, stents, sutures) that have not contributed to patient illness, injury, or death;
- middle ear ossicles;
- orthopedic hardware and other radiopaque medical devices, provided there is a policy for documentation of surgical removal;
- placentas from uncomplicated pregnancies that do not meet the facility or health care organization criteria for pathology examination and appear normal at the time of delivery;
- rib segments or other tissues removed for the purpose of gaining surgical access, provided the patient does not have a history of malignancy;
- saphenous vein segments harvested for coronary artery bypass;
- skin or other normal tissue removed during a cosmetic or reconstructive procedure (eg, blepharoplasty, abdominoplasty, rhytidectomy), provided it is not contiguous with a lesion and the patient does not have a history of malignancy;
- teeth when there is no attached tissue;
- therapeutic radioactive materials; and
- normal toenails and fingernails that are incidentally removed.[65]

IX.b.3. The following specimens may be submitted for gross examination only, with exceptions at the discretion of the pathologist or physician:
- accessory digits,
- bunions and hammertoes,
- extraocular muscle from corrective surgical procedures (eg, strabismus),
- inguinal hernia sacs (with specific age requirements determined by the facility or health care organization),
- nasal bone and cartilage from rhinoplasty or septoplasty,
- prosthetic breast implants,
- tonsils and adenoids (with specific age requirements determined by the facility or health care organization),
- torn meniscus,
- umbilical hernia sacs (with specific age requirements determined by the facility or health care organization), and
- varicose veins.[65]

Recommendation X

Nursing activities related to specimen management should be documented in a manner consistent with facility or health care organization policies and procedures and regulatory and accrediting agency requirements.

Documentation of nursing activities serves as the legal record of care delivery. Documentation of nursing activities is dictated by the facility or health care organization policy and regulatory and accrediting agency requirements and is necessary to inform other health care professionals involved in the patient's care. Highly reliable data collection is not only necessary to chronicle patients' responses to nursing interventions, but also to demonstrate the facility or health care organization's progress toward quality care outcomes.[108]

X.a. Documentation related to specimen management should include
- patient identification,
- specimen identification,
- additional information pertinent to the specimen or source (eg, location of suture tags),
- pathology examination required (eg, gross only, frozen section),
- final disposition of tissue and explanted devices,
- requests for special handling (eg, return of explanted orthopedic hardware),
- date and time of specimen collection,
- physician identification and contact information, and
- perioperative RN identification.
[2: High Evidence]

Perioperative documentation that accurately reflects the patient's experience is essential for the continuity of outcome-focused nursing care and for effective comparison of realized versus anticipated patient outcomes.[108]

Inaccurate, illegible, or incomplete documentation of specimen management may lead to incomplete or erroneous diagnostic information or the need for additional procedures.

Effective management and collection of health care information that accurately reflects the patient's care, treatment, and services is a regulatory and accreditation requirement for both hospitals and ambulatory settings.[110-121]

X.a.1. Specimen requisition forms and other relevant documentation should accompany the specimen, be secured to the container, and be protected from contamination.

X.b. Documentation should be completed using standardized printed tools or electronic technology. When handwriting is required, it should be legible. *[3: Moderate Evidence]*

Using a standardized printed tool assists in achieving accuracy and consistency when documenting. Studies of human error have shown that many errors involve a deviation from routine practice.[9] Common reasons for errors related to specimen management include unlabeled containers, insufficient patient identification, and incomplete or illegible information.[7] Using electronic tools minimizes errors related to handwriting.[7]

X.c. Verbal communication from the pathologist related to diagnosis or specific information about the specimen (eg, results of frozen section) should be provided directly to the physician (ie, not through a third party). *[5: Benefits Balanced with Harms]*

Using direct verbal communication minimizes the risk of communication errors.

Evidence addressing the need for providing verbal communication related to diagnosis or specific information about the specimen directly to the physician was not identified during the evidence review for this guideline.

X.c.1. If direct verbal communication between physicians is not possible, the communication should be received by the perioperative RN and documented in the patient's health record using a "read back" verification of the information provided.

The date and time of the indirect communication should be recorded along with the signature and title of the perioperative RN receiving the communication. Using a "write down, read back" process to confirm the communication provided minimizes the risk of communication errors.[67]

Editor's note: *Pen-Fix is a registered trademark of Richard-Allen Scientific Co, Kalamazoo, MI. Sakura and Tissue-Tek are registered trademarks of Sakura Finetek, Inc, Torrance, CA. RCL2 is a registered trademark of Alphelys, Plaisir, France. HistoChoice is a registered trademark of Amresto, LLC, Solon, OH. Mirsky's Fixative is a trademark of National Diagnostics, Atlanta, GA. Glyo-Fixx is a trademark of Thermo Fisher Scientific Inc, Waltham, MA. STF-Streck is a registered trademark of Streck Laboratories, Inc, Omaha, NE.*

Glossary

Agreement State: Any state with which the Nuclear Regulatory Commission or the Atomic Energy Commission has entered into a covenant under the Atomic Energy Act of 1954.

Analytical phase: Processes for specimen analysis that occur within the pathology laboratory (eg, gross examination, microscopic examination).

Assay: A procedure for measuring the presence or amount of a drug or biochemical substance in a sample. The substance being measured is considered the target of the assay.

Autolysis: The destruction of cells or tissue of an organism by substances produced within the organism.

Background radiation: Radiation from naturally occurring sources of radioactive material and global fallout as it exists in the environment that is not subject to control.

Biomarker: A biological molecule found in blood or other body fluids that is indicative of a particular condition or disease. Biomarker levels may be used to evaluate a patient's response to treatment.

Chain of custody: A process used to maintain, secure, and document the chronological history and persons in possession of evidence in order for the evidence to be legally accepted in court.

Cold ischemic time: The period of time between removal of the specimen and placement into fixative.

Forensic evidence: Evidence for use in legal or criminal proceedings.

Gross examination: The inspection of surgical specimens by a pathologist using only visual examination to obtain diagnostic information.

Point-of-care testing: Testing conducted at or close to the location where clinical care is delivered.

Postanalytical phase: Processes that occur after the specimen has been analyzed in the pathology laboratory (eg, recording and relaying the interpretation to the clinician).

Preanalytical phase: Processes that occur before the specimen reaches the pathology laboratory for analysis (eg, transfer of information from the physician to the perioperative RN during the procedure, and subsequent labeling, containment, and transport).

Radio-frequency identification (RFID): A system that transmits the identity (in the form of a unique serial number) of an object wirelessly using radio waves.

Root cause analysis: A retrospective process for identifying basic or causal factor(s) underlying variation in performance, including the occurrence or possible occurrence of a sentinel event.

Sentinel event: An unacticipated incident involving death or serious physical or psychological injury, or the risk of serious injury or adverse outcome.

Site identification: The act or process of positively establishing or confirming the location of tissue, foreign objects, or body substances to be removed from the patient and sent for pathology examination.

Specimen: Tissue, foreign objects, or body substances removed from a patient and sent for pathology examination.

Specimen collection: The act or process of obtaining a biopsy or resecting a specimen.

Specimen containment: The act or process of securing a specimen by placing it in a container used for storage or transport.

Specimen disposition: The act of positioning or distributing tissue, foreign bodies, explanted items, or body fluids removed from a patient for pathology examination.

Specimen handling: The act or process of holding, securing, moving, or manipulating a specimen.

Specimen identification and labeling: The process of affixing information to a container that establishes or indicates the specifications or characteristics of the enclosed sample.

Specimen preservation: The act or process of protecting a specimen to maintain morphology, reduce the loss of molecular components, prevent decomposition and autolysis, and prevent microbial growth.

Specimen transfer: The process of moving a specimen from the sterile field to the containment device.

Specimen transport: The act of carrying or conveying a specimen from one location to another.

Warm ischemic time: The time required for arterial ligation and removal of a specimen.

REFERENCES

1. 42 CFR 493. Laboratory Requirements. 2013. http://www.gpo.gov/fdsys/pkg/CFR-2013-title42-vol5/pdf/CFR-2013-title42-vol5-part493.pdf. Accessed April 7, 2014.

2. Leape LL. Error in medicine. *JAMA.* 1994;272(23):1851-1857. [VA]

3. Medal of Justice Award, May 24, 2012: Molly Akers. Center for Justice & Democracy. http://centerjd.org/content/cjd-medal-justice-award-may-24-2012-molly-akers. Accessed April 7. 2014.

4. Fischer B. U of C hospitals sued for error that resulted in removal of breast. *Chicago Sun-Times.* May 11, 2005. [VC]

5. Velasco A. St Vincent's settles suits over fetal remains. *The Birmingham News.* October 24, 2009:1A-2A. [VC]

6. Cooper K. Errors and error rates in surgical pathology: an Association of Directors of Anatomic and Surgical Pathology survey. *Arch Pathol Lab Med.* 2006;130(5):607-609. [IIIC]

7. Valenstein PN, Sirota RL. Identification errors in pathology and laboratory medicine. *Clin Lab Med.* 2004;24(4):979-996, vii. [VB]

8. Smith ML, Wilkerson T, Grzybicki DM, Raab SS. The effect of a lean quality improvement implementation program on surgical pathology specimen accessioning and gross preparation error frequency. *Am J Clin Pathol.* 2012;138(3):367-373. [VB]

9. Reason J. Safety in the operating theatre—part 2: human error and organisational failure. *Qual Saf Health Care.* 2005;14(1):56-60. [VA]

10. Novis DA. Detecting and preventing the occurrence of errors in the practices of laboratory medicine and anatomic pathology: 15 years' experience with the College of American Pathologists' Q-PROBES and Q-TRACKS programs. *Clin Lab Med.* 2004;24(4):965-978. [VA]

11. Metzger LK. An existential perspective of body beliefs and health assessment. *J Religion Health.* 2006; 45(1):130-146. [VB]

12. Purnell LD. Traditional Vietnamese health and healing. *Urol Nurs.* 2008;28(1):63-67. [VC]

13. Lamm M. The interment. Chabad.org. http://www.chabad.org/library/article_cdo/aid/281565/jewish/The-Interment.htm. Accessed April 7, 2014. [VB]

14. Ehman J. Religious diversity: practical points for health care providers. Penn Medicine: Pastoral Care & Education. http://www.uphs.upenn.edu/pastoral/resed/diversity_points.html. Accessed April 8, 2014. [VB]

15. Helsel DG, Mochel M. Afterbirths in the afterlife: cultural meaning of placental disposal in a Hmong American community. *J Transcult Nurs.* 2002;13(4):282-286. [IIIB]

16. Baergen R, Thaker HM, Heller DS. Placental release or disposal? Experiences of perinatal pathologists. *Pediatr Dev Pathol.* 2013;16(5):327-330. [IIIC]

17. Makary MA, Holzmueller CG, Thompson D, et al. Operating room briefings: working on the same page. *Jt Comm J Qual Patient Saf.* 2006;32(6):351-355. [VB]

18. *AORN Position Statement: Preventing Wrong-Patient, Wrong-Site, Wrong-Procedure Events.* https://www.aorn.org/PracticeResources/AORNPositionStatements/. AORN, Inc. Accessed April 8, 2014. [IVB]

19. Nemeth SA, Lawrence N. Site identification challenges in dermatologic surgery: a physician survey. *J Am Acad Dermatol.* 2012;67(2):262-268. [IIIB]

20. McGinness JL, Goldstein G. The value of preoperative biopsy-site photography for identifying cutaneous lesions. *Dermatol Surg.* 2010;36(2):194-197. [IIIB]

21. Rossy KM, Lawrence N. Difficulty with surgical site identification: what role does it play in dermatology? *J Am Acad Dermatol.* 2012;67(2):257-261. [IIIB]

22. Ke M, Moul D, Camouse M, et al. Where is it? The utility of biopsy-site photography. *Dermatol Surg.* 2010;36(2):198-202. [IIIC]

23. Hewitt SM, Lewis FA, Cao Y, et al. Tissue handling and specimen preparation in surgical pathology: issues concerning the recovery of nucleic acids from formalin-fixed, paraffin-embedded tissue. *Arch Pathol Lab Med.* 2008;132(12):1929-1935. [VB]

24. Balch CM. Reexamining our routines of handing surgical tissue in the operating room. *J Natl Cancer Inst Monogr.* 2011;2011(42):39-40. [VB]

25. Hicks DG, Kushner L, McCarthy K. Breast cancer predictive factor testing: the challenges and importance of standardizing tissue handling. *J Natl Cancer Inst Monographs.* 2011;2011(42):43-45. [VB]

26. Hicks DG, Boyce BF. The challenge and importance of standardizing pre-analytical variables in surgical pathology specimens for clinical care and translational research. *Biotechnic Histochem.* 2012;87(1):14-17. [VB]

27. Wolff AC, Hammond ME, Schwartz JN, et al. American Society of Clinical Oncology/College of American Pathologists guideline recommendations for human epidermal growth factor receptor 2 testing in breast cancer. *Arch Pathol Lab Med.* 2007;131(1):18-43. [IVB]

28. Hammond ME, Hayes DF, Dowsett M, et al. American Society of Clinical Oncology/College of American Pathologists guideline recommendations for immunohistochemical testing of estrogen and progesterone receptors in breast cancer. *J Clin Oncol.* 2010; 28(16):2784-2795. [IVB]

29. Wolff AC, Hammond ME, Hicks DG, et al. Recommendations for human epidermal growth factor receptor 2 testing in breast cancer: American Society of Clinical Oncology/College of American Pathologists clinical practice guideline update. *Arch Pathol Lab Med.* 2014;138(2):241-256. [IVB]

30. Yaziji H, Taylor CR, Goldstein NS, et al. Consensus recommendations on estrogen receptor testing in breast cancer by immunohistochemistry. *Appl Immunohistochem Mol Morphol.* 2008;16(6):513-520. [IVB]

31. Nkoy FL, Hammond ME, Rees W, et al. Variable specimen handling affects hormone receptor test results in women with breast cancer: a large multihospital retrospective study. *Arch Pathol Lab Med.* 2010;134(4):606-612. [IIIB]

32. Khoury T, Sait S, Hwang H, et al. Delay to formalin fixation effect on breast biomarkers. *Mod Pathol.* 2009;22(11):1457-1467. [IIB]

33. Moatamed NA, Nanjangud G, Pucci R, et al. Effect of ischemic time, fixation time, and fixative type on HER2/neu immunohistochemical and fluorescence in situ hybridization results in breast cancer. *Am J Clin Pathol.* 2011;136(5):754-761. [IIB]

34. Portier BP, Wang Z, Downs-Kelly E, et al. Delay to formalin fixation "cold ischemia time": effect on ERBB2 detection by in-situ hybridization and immunohistochemistry. *Mod Pathol.* 2013;26(1):1-9. [IIB]

35. Lagios MD. Pathology procedures for evaluation of the specimen with potential or documented ductal carcinoma in situ. *Semin Breast Dis.* 2000;3:42-49. [VB]

36. Li J, Guo Z, Zhu Q, et al. Fingertip replantation: determinants of survival. *Plast Reconstr Surg.* 2008;122(3):833-839. [IIIB]

37. Partlin MM, Chen J, Holdgate A. The preoperative preservation of amputated digits: an assessment of proposed methods. *J Trauma.* 2008;65(1):127-131. [IIB]

38. Allen DM, Levin LS. Digital replantation including postoperative care. *Tech Hand Up Extrem Surg.* 2002; 6(4):171-177. [VA]

39. Azzopardi EA, Whitaker IS, Laing H. Perceptions of correct preoperative storage and transfer of amputated digits: a national survey of referring emergency departments. *J Plast Reconstr Aesthet Surg.* 2008;61(11):1418-1419. [IIIC]

40. Lloyd MS, Teo TC, Pickford MA, Arnstein PM. Preoperative management of the amputated limb. *Emerg Med J.* 2005;22(7):478-480. [VB]

41. Evans MM, Stagner PA, Rooms R. Maintaining the chain of custody—evidence handling in forensic cases. *AORN J.* 2003;78(4):563-569. [VA]

42. Carrigan M, Collington P, Tyndall J. Forensic perioperative nursing. Advocates for justice. *Can Oper Room Nurs J.* 2000;18(4):12-16. [VA]

43. Porteous J. Don't tip the scales! Care for patients involved in a police investigation. *Can Oper Room Nurs J.* 2005;23(3):12-16. [VA]

44. Modifications to the HIPAA privacy, security, enforcement, and breach notification rules under the Health Information Technology for Economic and Clinical Health Act and the Genetic Information Nondiscrimination Act; other modifications to the HIPAA rules. *Fed Regist.* 2013;78(17 Part 2):5566-5702. http://www.gpo.gov/fdsys/pkg/FR-2013-01-25/pdf/2013-01073.pdf. Accessed April 8, 2014.

45. 10 CFR 20. Standards for Protection Against Radiation. 2013. http://www.gpo.gov/fdsys/pkg/CFR-2013-title10-vol1/pdf/CFR-2013-title10-vol1-part20.pdf. Accessed April 8, 2014.

46. 10 CFR 35. Medical Use of Byproduct Material. 2011. http://www.gpo.gov/fdsys/pkg/CFR-2011-title10-vol1/pdf/CFR-2011-title10-vol1-part35.pdf. Accessed April 8, 2014.

47. Graham RP, Jakub JW, Brunette JJ, Reynolds C. Handling of radioactive seed localization breast specimens in the pathology laboratory. *Am J Surg Pathol.* 2012;36(11):1718-1723. [VB]

48. Michel R, Hofer C. Radiation safety precautions for sentinel lymph node procedures. *Health Phys.* 2004;86(2 Suppl):S35-S37. [VB]

49. Iodine-125 and palladium-103 low dose rate brachytherapy seeds used for localization of non-palpable lesions. US Nuclear Regulatory Commission. http://www.nrc.gov/materials/miau/med-use-toolkit/seed-localization.html. Accessed on April 8, 2014.

50. Fitzgibbons PL, LiVolsi VA. Recommendations for handling radioactive specimens obtained by sentinel lymphadenectomy. Surgical Pathology Committee of the College of American Pathologists and the Association of Directors of Anatomic and Surgical Pathology. *Am J Surg Pathol.* 2000;24(11):1549-1551. [IVB]

51. Miner TJ, Shriver CD, Flicek PR, et al. Guidelines for the safe use of radioactive materials during localization and resection of the sentinel lymph node. *Ann Surg Oncol.* 1999;6(1):75-82. [IIB]

52. Law M, Chow LW, Kwong A, Lam CK. Sentinel lymph node technique for breast cancer: radiation safety issues. *Semin Oncol.* 2004;31(3):298-303. [VB]

53. Renshaw AA, Kish R, Gould EW. Increasing radiation from sentinel node specimens in pathology over time. *Am J Clin Pathol.* 2010;134(2):299-302. [IIIB]

54. Coventry BJ, Collins PJ, Kollias J, et al. Ensuring radiation safety to staff in lymphatic tracing and sentinel lymph node biopsy surgery—some recommendations. *J Nuclear Med Rad Ther.* 2012:1-5. http://www.omicsonline.org/ensuring-radiation-safety-to-staff-in-lymphatic-tracing-and-sentinel-lymph-node-biopsy-surgery-some-recommendations-2155-9619.S2-008.php?aid=6937. Accessed April 8, 2014. [IIIC]

55. Pavlicek W, Walton HA, Karstaedt PJ, Gray RJ. Radiation safety with use of I-125 seeds for localization of nonpalpable breast lesions. *Acad Radiol.* 2006;13(7):909-915. [VB]

56. 10 CFR 20.1905. Exemptions to Labeling Requirements. 2013. http://www.gpo.gov/fdsys/pkg/CFR-2013-title10-vol1/pdf/CFR-2013-title10-vol1-part20.pdf. Accessed April 8, 2014.

57. 10 CFR 30.41. Transfer of Byproduct Material. 2013. US Nuclear Regulatory Commission. http://www.nrc.gov/reading-rm/doc-collections/cfr/part030/part030-0041.html. Accessed April 8, 2014.

58. 10 CFR 71.5 Transportation of Licensed Material. 2013. US Nuclear Regulatory Commission. http://www.nrc.gov/reading-rm/doc-collections/cfr/part071/part071-0005.html. Accessed April 8, 2014.

59. 21 CFR 821. Medical Device Tracking Requirements. 2013. US Food and Drug Administration. http://www.accessdata.fda.gov/scripts/cdrh/cfdocs/cfcfr/CFRSearch.cfm?CFRPart=821. Accessed April 8, 2014.

60. Medical device tracking; guidance for industry and FDA staff. US Food and Drug Administration. http://www.fda.gov/medicaldevices/deviceregulationandguidance/guidancedocuments/ucm071756.htm. Accessed April 8, 2014.

61. 21 CFR 803 Subpart C. User Facility Reporting Requirements. 2013. http://www.accessdata.fda.gov/scripts/cdrh/cfdocs/cfCFR/CFRSearch.cfm?CFRPart=803&showFR=1&subpartNode=21:8.0.1.1.3.3. Accessed April 8, 2014

62. Medical device reporting. US Food and Drug Administration. http://www.fda.gov/medicaldevices/safety/reportaproblem/default.htm. Accessed April 8, 2014.

63. MedWatch: The FDA Safety Information and Adverse Event Reporting Program. US Food and Drug Administration. http://www.fda.gov/Safety/MedWatch/. Accessed April 8, 2013.

64. Burlingame B. Tracking and documenting implants; Returning explants to patients. [Clinical Issues]. *AORN J.* 2012;95(2):288-296. [VA]

65. Policy on surgical specimens to be submitted to pathology for examination. Appendix M. 2007. College of American Pathologists. http://www.cap.org/apps/docs/laboratory_accreditation/build/pdf/surgical_specimens.pdf. Accessed April 8, 2014. [IVB]

66. Davidovitch RI, Temkin S, Weinstein BS, Singh JR, Egol KA. Utility of pathologic evaluation following removal of explanted orthopaedic internal fixation hardware. *Bull NYU Hosp Joint Dis.* 2010;68(1):18-21. [IIIC]

67. Greenberg CC, Regenbogen SE, Studdert DM, et al. Patterns of communication breakdowns resulting in injury to surgical patients. *J Am Coll Surg.* 2007;204(4):533-540. [IIIB]

68. Siegel JD, Rhinehart E, Jackson M, Chiarello L; the Healthcare Infection Control Practices Advisory Committee. 2007 guideline for isolation precautions: preventing transmission of infectious agents in healthcare settings. Centers for Disease Control and Prevention. http://www.cdc.gov/hicpac/pdf/isolation/isolation2007.pdf. Accessed April 8, 2014. [IVA]

69. 29 CFR 1910.1030. Hazardous Substances. Bloodborne Pathogens. 2013. Occupational Safety and

Health Administration. https://www.osha.gov/pls/oshaweb/owadisp.show_document?p_id=10051&p_table=STANDARDS. Accessed April 8, 2014. [Regulatory]

70. Sandbank S, Klein D, Westreich M, Shalom A. The loss of pathological specimens: incidence and causes. *Dermatol Surg.* 2010;36(7):1084-1086. [VB]

71. CFR 1910.1048: Hazardous substances. Formaldehyde. Occupational Safety and Health Administration. https://www.osha.gov/pls/oshaweb/owadisp.show_document?p_id=10075&p_table=STANDARDS. Accessed April 8. 2014. [Regulatory]

72. Makary MA, Epstein J, Pronovost PJ, Millman EA, Hartmann EC, Freischlag JA. Surgical specimen identification errors: a new measure of quality in surgical care. *Surgery.* 2007;141(4):450-455. [IIIA]

73. Quillen K, Murphy K. Quality improvement to decrease specimen mislabeling in transfusion medicine. *Arch Pathol Lab Med.* 2006;130(8):1196-1198. [VB]

74. College of American Pathologists; Valenstein PN, Raab SS, Walsh MK. Identification errors involving clinical laboratories: a College of American Pathologists Q-Probes study of patient and specimen identification errors at 120 institutions. *Arch Pathol Lab Med.* 2006;130(8):1106-1113. [IIIB]

75. Dock B. Improving the accuracy of specimen labeling. *Clin Lab Sci.* 2005;18(4):210-212. [VB]

76. Nakhleh RE, Idowu MO, Souers RJ, Meier FA, Bekeris LG. Mislabeling of cases, specimens, blocks, and slides: a College of American Pathologists study of 136 institutions. *Arch Pathol Lab Med.* 2011;135(8):969-974. [IIIB]

77. Bixenstine PJ, Zarbo RJ, Holzmueller CG, et al. Developing and pilot testing practical measures of preanalytic surgical specimen identification defects. *Am J Med Qual.* 2013;28(4):308-314. [IIIB]

78. Meier FA, Varney RC, Zarbo RJ. Study of amended reports to evaluate and improve surgical pathology processes. *Adv Anat Pathol.* 2011;18(5):406-413. [VB]

79. When a rose is not a rose: the problem of mislabeled specimens. Lab Med DirecTIPs. 2009. College of American Pathologists. http://www.cap.org/apps/portlets/contentViewer/show.do?printFriendly=true&contentReference=practice_management%2Fdirectips%2Fmislabeled_specimens.html. Updated February 23, 2010. Accessed April 14, 2014. [VB]

80. Makary MA, Holzmueller CG, Sexton JB, et al. Operating room debriefings. *Jt Comm J Qual Patient Saf.* 2006;32(7):407-410, 357. [VB]

81. Trask L, Tournas E. Barcode specimen collection improves patient safety. *Mlo: Medical Laboratory Observer.* 2012;44(4):42. [VB]

82. Francis DL, Prabhakar S, Sanderson SO. A quality initiative to decrease pathology specimen-labeling errors using radiofrequency identification in a high-volume endoscopy center. *Am J Gastroenterol.* 2009;104(4):972-975. [IIIB]

83. Colard D. Reduction of patient identification errors using technology. *Point of Care.* 2005;4(1):61-63. [VB]

84. Granata J. Getting a handle on specimen mislabeling. *J Emerg Nurs.* 2011;37(2):167-168. [VC]

85. Nichols JH, Bartholomew C, Brunton M, et al. Reducing medical errors through barcoding at the point of care. *Clin Leadersh Manag Rev.* 2004;18(6):328-334. [VB]

86. O'Neill E, Richardson-Weber L, McCormack G, Uhl L, Haspel RL. Strict adherence to a blood bank specimen labeling policy by all clinical laboratories significantly reduces the incidence of "wrong blood in tube." *Am J Clin Pathol.* 2009;132(2):164-168. [VB]

87. Rees S, Stevens L, Mikelsons D, Quam E, Darcy T. Reducing specimen identification errors. *J Nurs Care Qual.* 2012;27(3):253-257. [VB]

88. Bell WC, Young ES, Billings PE, Grizzle WE. The efficient operation of the surgical pathology gross room. *Biotechnic Histochem.* 2008;83(2):71-82. [VB]

89. Guideline for a safe environment of care, part 1. In: *Guidelines for Perioperative Practice.* Denver, CO: AORN; 2015:239-263. [IVA]

90. *NIOSH Pocket Guide to Chemical Hazards.* DHHS (NIOSH) Publication No. 2005-149 ed. Cincinnati, OH: National Institute for Occupational Safety and Health; 2007.

91. OSHA FactSheet: Formaldehyde. 2011. Occupational Safety and Health Administration. http://www.osha.gov/OshDoc/data_General_Facts/formaldehyde-factsheet.pdf. Accessed April 8, 2014. [Regulatory]

92. *ANSI/ISEA Z358.1-2009: American National Standard for Emergency Eyewash and Shower Equipment.* New York, NY: American National Standards Institute; 2009. [IVC]

93. Material Safety Data Sheet—Formalin 10%. 2013. American Master Tech. http://www.americanmastertech.com/PDF/SSFXBFO.PDF. Accessed April 8, 2014.

94. Buesa RJ, Peshkov MV. How much formalin is enough to fix tissues? *Ann Diagn Pathol.* 2012;16(3):202-209. [IIB]

95. Di Novi C, Minniti D, Barbaro S, Zampirolo MG, Cimino A, Bussolati G. Vacuum-based preservation of surgical specimens: an environmentally-safe step towards a formalin-free hospital. *Sci Total Environ.* 2010;408(16):3092-3095. [VB]

96. Bussolati G, Chiusa L, Cimino A, D'Armento G. Tissue transfer to pathology labs: under vacuum is the safe alternative to formalin. *Virchows Arch.* 2008;452(2):229-231. [VB]

97. Berton F, Di Novi C. Occupational hazards of hospital personnel: assessment of a safe alternative to formaldehyde. *J Occup Health.* 2012;54(1):74-78. [IB]

98. Al-Maaini R, Bryant P. The effectiveness of honey as a substitute for formalin in the histological fixation of tissue. *J Histotechnol.* 2006;29:173-176. [IIC]

99. Ozkan N, Salva E, Cakalagaoglu F, Tuzuner B. Honey as a substitute for formalin? *Biotechnic Histochem.* 2012;87(2):148-153. [IIC]

100. Gillespie JW, Best CJ, Bichsel VE, et al. Evaluation of non-formalin tissue fixation for molecular profiling studies. *Am J Pathol.* 2002;160(2):449-457. [IIB]

101. van Essen HF, Verdaasdonk MA, Elshof SM, de Weger RA, van Diest PJ. Alcohol based tissue fixation as an alternative for formaldehyde: influence on immunohistochemistry. *J Clin Pathol.* 2010;63(12):1090-1094. [IIB]

102. Buesa RJ. Histology without formalin? *Ann Diagn Pathol.* 2008;12(6):387-396. [VA]

103. Prento P, Lyon H. Commercial formalin substitutes for histopathology. *Biotechnic Histochem.* 1997;72(5):273-282. [IIB]

104. Kristensen T, Engvad B, Nielsen O, Pless T, Walter S, Bak M. Vacuum sealing and cooling as methods to preserve surgical specimens. *Appl Immunohistochem Mole Morphol.* 2011;19(5):460-469. [IIB]

105. Titford ME, Horenstein MG. Histomorphologic assessment of formalin substitute fixatives for diagnostic surgical pathology. *Arch Pathol Lab Med.* 2005;129(4):502-506. [IIB]

106. 42 CFR 493 Subpart K. Quality system for nonwaived testing. 2013. http://www.gpo.gov/fdsys/pkg/CFR-2013-title42-vol5/pdf/CFR-2013-title42-vol5-part493-subpartK.pdf. Accessed April 8, 2014.

107. *Histopathology and Cytopathology of Limited or No Clinical Value.* 2nd ed. London: Royal College of Pathologists; 2005. [IVB]

108. Guideline for perioperative health care information management. In: *Guidelines for Perioperative Practice.* Denver, CO: AORN, Inc; 2015:491-512. [IVB]

109. Standards of perioperative nursing. In: *Perioperative Standards and Recommended Practices.* Denver, CO: AORN, Inc; 2014:3-42. [IVB]

110. *State Operations Manual Appendix A: Survey Protocol, Regulations and Interpretive Guidelines for Hospitals.* Rev 84. 2013. Centers for Medicare & Medicaid Services. http://www.cms.gov/Regulations-and-Guidance/Guidance/Manuals/downloads/som107ap_l_ambulatory.pdf. Accessed April 8, 2014.

111. *State Operations Manual Appendix L: Guidance for Surveyors: Ambulatory Surgical Centers.* Rev 89. 2013. Centers for Medicare & Medicaid Services. http://www.cms.gov/Regulations-and-Guidance/Guidance/Manuals/downloads/som107ap_l_ambulatory.pdf. Accessed April 8, 2014.

112. RC.01.01.01: The hospital maintains complete and accurate medical records for each individual patient. In: *Hospital Accreditation Standards 2013.* Oakbrook Terrace, IL: Joint Commission Resources; 2013.

113. RC.02.01.03: The patient's medical record documents operative or other high-risk procedures and the use of moderate or deep sedation or anesthesia. In: *Joint Commission Comprehensive Accreditation and Certification Manual. Hospital.* e-dition release 5.1 ed. Oakbrook Terrace, IL: Joint Commission Resources; 2013.

114. RC.01.01.01: The organization maintains complete and accurate clinical records. In: *Standards for Ambulatory Care 2013: Standards, Elements of Performance Scoring Accreditation Policies.* Oakbrook Terrace, IL: The Joint Commission; 2013.

115. RC.02.01.03: The patient's clinical record documents operative or other high-risk procedures and the use of moderate or deep sedation or anesthesia. In: *Joint Commission Comprehensive Accreditation and Certification Manual. Ambulatory.* e-dition release 5.1 ed. Oakbrook Terrace, IL: Joint Commission Resources; 2013.

116. Clinical records and health information. In: *2013 Accreditation Handbook for Ambulatory Health Care.* Skokie, IL: Accreditation Association for Ambulatory Health Care; 2013:35-37.

117. Medical records: procedure room records. In: *Procedural Standards and Checklist for Accreditation of Ambulatory Surgery Facilities.* Version 3 ed. Gurnee, IL: American Association for Accreditation of Ambulatory Surgery Facilities; 2011:64-66.

118. Medical records: operating room records. In: *Regular Standards and Checklist for Accreditation of Ambulatory Surgery Facilities.* Version 13 ed. Gurnee, IL: American Association for Accreditation of Ambulatory Surgery Facilities; 2011:64-66.

119. Medical records: general. In: *Procedural Standards and Checklist for Accreditation of Ambulatory Surgery Facilities.* Version 3 ed. Gurnee, IL: American Association for Accreditation of Ambulatory Surgery Facilities; 2011:60-61.

120. Medical records: general. In: *Regular Standards and Checklist for Accreditation of Ambulatory Surgery Facilities.* Version 13 ed. Gurnee, IL: American Association for Accreditation of Ambulatory Surgery Facilities; 2011:61.

121. Medical records: pre-operative medical record. In: *Regular Standards and Checklist for Accreditation of Ambulatory Surgery Facilities.* Version 13 ed. Gurnee, IL: American Association for Accreditation of Ambulatory Surgery Facilities; 2011:62-63.

Acknowledgements

LEAD AUTHOR
Sharon A. Van Wicklin, MSN, RN, CNOR, CRNFA, CPSN, PLNC
Perioperative Nursing Specialist
AORN Nursing Department
Denver, Colorado

CONTRIBUTING AUTHOR
Ramona Conner, MSN, RN, CNOR
Manager, Standards and Guidelines
AORN Nursing Department
Denver, Colorado

The authors and AORN thank Marie A. Bashaw, DNP, RN, NEA-BC, CNOR, Clinical Assistant Professor, Wright State University College of Nursing and Health, Dayton, OH; Patricia Graybill-D'Ercole, MSN, RN, CNOR, CHL, CRCST, Clinical Specialist, Integra Life Science, York, PA; Deborah Farina Mulloy, PhD, RN, Associate Chief Nurse Quality and Center for Nursing Excellence, Brigham and Women's Hospital, Boston, MA for their assistance in developing this guideline.

PUBLICATION HISTORY
Originally approved November 2005, AORN Board of Directors. Published in *Standards, Recommended Practices, and Guidelines*, 2006 edition.

Reprinted March 2006, *AORN Journal.*

Minor editing revisions made to omit PNDS codes; reformatted September 2012 for publication in *Perioperative Standards and Recommended Practices*, 2013 edition.

Revised January 2014 for online publication in *Perioperative Standards and Recommended Practices.*

Minor editing revisions made in November 2014 for publication in *Guidelines for Perioperative Practice*, 2015 edition.

Evidence ratings revised in *Guidelines for Perioperative Practice*, 2018 edition, to conform to the current AORN Evidence Rating Model.

GUIDELINE FOR SURGICAL SMOKE SAFETY

The Guideline for Surgical Smoke Safety has been approved by the AORN Guidelines Advisory Board. It was presented as a proposed guideline for comments by members and others. The guideline is effective December 15, 2016. The recommendations in the guideline are intended to be achievable and represent what is believed to be an optimal level of practice. Policies and procedures will reflect variations in practice settings and/or clinical situations that determine the degree to which the guideline can be implemented. AORN recognizes the many diverse settings in which perioperative nurses practice; therefore, this guideline is adaptable to all areas where operative or other invasive procedures may be performed.

Purpose

This document provides guidance on surgical smoke safety precautions to help the perioperative team establish a safe environment for the surgical patient and team members through consistent use of control measures.

Surgical smoke is the by-product of use of energy-generating devices (eg, electrosurgery units, lasers, powered instruments).[1] When surgical energy devices raise intracellular temperatures to 100° C (212° F) or higher, the tissue vaporizes, producing surgical smoke.[2] This gaseous by-product is visible and malodorous.[3] Surgical smoke may contain gaseous toxic compounds (eg, hydrogen cyanide, toluene, benzene), bio-aerosols, viruses (eg, human papilloma virus [HPV], human immunodeficiency virus [HIV]),[3] viable cancer cells, non-viable particles (ie, lung damaging dust of 0.5 µm to 5.0 µm), carbonized tissue,[3] blood fragments, and bacteria. The water vapor content of surgical smoke ranges from 1% to 11%[4] and serves as a carrier for the compounds, viruses, and other substances. Researchers began analyzing the contents of surgical smoke in the early 1980s. In a 1981 study, Tomita et al[5] found that the contents of surgical smoke are similar to the contents of cigarettes, with known and suspected carcinogens and mutagens.

Electrosurgical devices use radio-frequency current to cut and coagulate. Heat is generated in the body tissue through which the current passes. The heat causes cell walls to explode, releasing the cellular fluid as steam and the cell contents into the air, forming surgical smoke. Lasers produce an intense, coherent, directional beam of light and also produce high heat, which raises the temperature within the cell, vaporizing the contents and releasing steam and cell contents.[1] Ultrasonic devices remove tissue by rapid mechanical action. Ultrasonic aspirators produce a fine mist, and ultrasonic scalpels produce a vapor.[1] High-speed electrical devices (eg, bone saws,

drills) cut, dissect, and resect tissue. The mechanical action of the saw or drill combined with irrigation fluid used to cool the device produces aerosols that may contain viable bloodborne pathogens.[1]

The Occupational Safety and Health Administration (OSHA) has estimated that more than 500,000 health care workers are exposed to surgical smoke every year.[6] Perioperative nurses report twice the incidence of many respiratory problems compared to the general population.[7,8] Case reports have established the link between inhalation of surgical smoke during excision of anogenital condylomata procedures to transmission of HPV to health care providers.[9-11] For example, a laser surgeon developed laryngeal papillomatosis of the same virus type as his patient,[10] and experts at a virological institute confirmed a high probability of occupational exposure in a gynecologic perioperative nurse who developed recurrent and histologically proven laryngeal papillomatosis.[9]

Surgical smoke exposure is also hazardous to patients. Risks to patients include loss of visibility in the surgical field during minimally invasive procedures[12-18] with potential to delay the procedure,[19-22] port site metastasis,[23] exposure to carbon monoxide,[22,24,25] and increased levels of carboxyhemoglobin.[22,24]

AORN, the National Institute for Occupational Safety and Health (NIOSH),[26] and other professional organizations[27-31] have recommended surgical smoke evacuation for more than 20 years. Perioperative team members continue to demonstrate a lack of knowledge of the hazards of surgical smoke[32-34] and a lack of compliance in evacuating surgical smoke.[8,32,33,35] Even though smoke generated by electrosurgery[5] is more hazardous than laser-generated surgical smoke, there is greater compliance with smoke evacuation for laser procedures.[36,37]

Surgical smoke is often referred to as *surgical plume, smoke plume, bio-aerosols, laser-generated airborne contaminants,* and *lung-damaging dust.* For the purpose of this document, the term *surgical smoke* will be used unless another term has been specifically used in a reference source.

Evidence Review

A medical librarian conducted systematic searches of the databases MEDLINE®, CINAHL®, Scopus®, and the Cochrane Database of Systematic Reviews. Results were limited to literature published in English from January 1985 to November 2015. During the development of the guideline, the lead author requested additional articles that either did not fit the original search criteria or were discovered during the evidence appraisal process, and the lead author and the medical librarian identified relevant guidelines

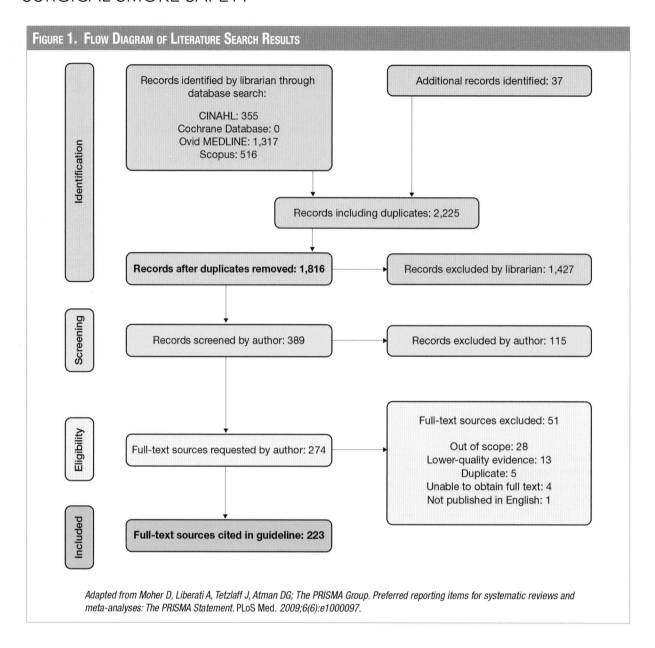

FIGURE 1. FLOW DIAGRAM OF LITERATURE SEARCH RESULTS

Records identified by librarian through database search:

CINAHL: 355
Cochrane Database: 0
Ovid MEDLINE: 1,317
Scopus: 516

Additional records identified: 37

Records including duplicates: 2,225

Records after duplicates removed: 1,816

Records excluded by librarian: 1,427

Records screened by author: 389

Records excluded by author: 115

Full-text sources requested by author: 274

Full-text sources excluded: 51

Out of scope: 28
Lower-quality evidence: 13
Duplicate: 5
Unable to obtain full text: 4
Not published in English: 1

Full-text sources cited in guideline: 223

Identification
Screening
Eligibility
Included

Adapted from Moher D, Liberati A, Tetzlaff J, Atman DG; The PRISMA Group. Preferred reporting items for systematic reviews and meta-analyses: The PRISMA Statement. PLoS Med. 2009;6(6):e1000097.

from government agencies and standards-setting bodies. Updated searches were completed in January 2016.

Search terms related to procedures included the subject headings and keywords *diathermy, cautery, laser, electrosurgery,* and *surgical procedures, operative.* Search terms and keywords related to by-products included *smoke, plume, fume, exhaust, mist, particulate matter, bioaerosols, aerosols, smoke evacuation, smoke extractor,* and *occupational air pollutants.*

Inclusion criteria were research and non-research literature in English, complete publications, and publication dates within the time restriction unless none were available. Excluded were non-peer-reviewed publications and literature on surgical smoke safety. Letters and editorials were excluded. Low-quality evidence was excluded when higher-quality evidence was available, and literature outside the time restriction was excluded when literature within the time restriction was available (Figure 1).

Articles identified in the search were provided to the project team for evaluation. The team consisted of the lead author and two evidence appraisers. The lead author divided the search results into topics and assigned members of the team to review and critically appraise each article using the AORN Research or Non-Research Evidence Appraisal Tools as appropriate. The literature was independently evaluated and appraised according to the strength and quality of the evidence. Each article was then assigned an appraisal score. The appraisal score is noted in brackets after each reference, as applicable.

The collective evidence supporting each intervention within a specific recommendation was summarized, and the AORN Evidence Rating Model was used to rate the strength of the evidence. Factors considered in the review of the collective evidence were the quality of the evidence, the quantity of similar evidence on a given topic, and the consistency of evidence supporting a recommendation. The evidence rating is noted in brackets after each intervention.

Note: *The evidence summary table is available at* http://www.aorn.org/evidencetables/.

Editor's note: *MEDLINE is a registered trademark of the US National Library of Medicine's Medical Literature Analysis and Retrieval System, Bethesda, MD. CINAHL, Cumulative Index to Nursing and Allied Health Literature, is a registered trademark of EBSCO Industries, Birmingham, AL. Scopus is a registered trademark of Elsevier, B.V., Amsterdam, The Netherlands.*

Recommendation I

The health care organization should provide a surgical smoke-free work environment.

Under the General Duty Clause, Section 5(a)(1) of the Occupational Safety and Health Act of 1970, employers are required to provide their employees with a place of employment that is "free from recognizable hazards that are causing or likely to cause death or serious harm to employees."[38,39]

A court interpretation of the Occupational Safety and Health Administration (OSHA) General Duty Clause is that the employer has a legal obligation to provide a workplace free of conditions or activities that either the employer or industry recognizes as hazardous and that cause or are likely to cause death or serious physical harm to employees when there is a feasible method to abate the hazard.[40]

I.a. The health care organization should assess the perioperative team's risk of exposure to surgical smoke. *[2: High Evidence]*

The collective evidence describes the contents of surgical smoke and demonstrates the exposure risks and hazards to the perioperative team. Surgical smoke contains many components that are recognized health hazards. The identified contents of surgical smoke include

- aromatic hydrocarbons[41] (eg, benzene,[41-52] toluene,[41,43,45-49,50-58] xylene[41,46,51,52,57,58]),
- volatile organic compounds,[59-61]
- polycyclic aromatic hydrocarbons[41,62,63] (eg, benzo[a]pyrene, dibenzo[a,h]anthracene, anthracene[64]),
- hydrogen cyanide,[41,49,61,64]
- inorganic gases[60] (eg, carbon monoxide[19,20,46,49,65]),
- nitriles[66] (eg, acetonitrile, acrylonitrile[43,46,47]),
- aldehydes[52,60] (eg, acetaldehyde,[53,54,56,60] formaldehyde[41,46,49,53,54,56,64]),
- particles,[19,67-79]
- viruses[3,80-87] (eg, HPV,[88-95] HIV[96,97]),
- bacteria,[87,98-104]
- blood,[100,105-110] and
- cancer cells.[23,111-113]

Chemicals

The collective evidence establishes the presence of harmful chemicals in surgical smoke, with an estimated 150 chemical compounds[114,115] discovered using gas chromatography,[50,57,63] a combination of gas chromatography and mass spectrometry,[45-47,51,52,55,57,58-62,116-118] and laser spectroscopy[43,44,48,119-121] (Table 1). The content of surgical smoke varies by the type of tissue treated (eg, muscle, fat),[19,44,47,48,55,57,60,61,122,123] type of energy-generating device (eg, laser,[49] electrosurgical unit [ESU]) used,[19,60,118,123] duration of the procedure,[55] and the amount of time the energy-generating device was activated.[19,43,48,57]

Näslund Andréasson et al[63] collected personal and stationary samplings of polycyclic aromatic hydrocarbons (PAHs) in electrocautery smoke during 40 peritonectomy procedures for *pseudomyxoma peritonei* (n = 22), colorectal cancer (n = 11), appendiceal cancer (n = 5), and ovarian cancer (n = 2). The primary aim of the study was to identify and quantify the US Environmental Protection Agency's 16 priority pollutant PAHs (Table 2). All 16 PAHs were detected in personal and stationary samples. Personal samplings were collected using a 40-mm absorbent filter cassette fixed near the surgeon's breathing zone to absorb organic compounds. The stationary samplings were collected with a 20-mm smoke evacuator hose connected to a smoke evacuator system. The absorbent filter cassette tubing was inserted in a small slit 5 cm from the tip of the electrocautery device.

Naphthalene, a possible human carcinogen, was the most abundant PAH and was found in all but one of the samples (97.5%). In addition to naphthalene, phenanthrene (93%), florene (63.3%), acenaphthene (40%), and acenaphthylene (36.7%) were detected in the personal samplings. Acenaphthylene (93.3%), phenanthrene (90%), acenaphthene (90%), and florene (83.3%) were detected in the stationary samplings. The researchers postulated that long-term exposure to PAHs could lead to high cumulative levels of PAHs in perioperative team members, and consideration should be given to the possibility that simultaneous exposure to particles, PAHs, and volatile organic compounds may have synergistic and additive effects. More studies are needed to evaluate the possible risk of PAH exposure in the OR.[63]

Petrus et al[44] used laser photoacoustic spectroscopy to quantitatively analyze the trace gas concentrations in surgical smoke produced in vitro in nitrogen or synthetic air atmospheres. The researchers used a carbon dioxide (CO_2) laser to generate surgical smoke by irradiating fresh animal tissue, then measured the levels of ethylene, benzene, ammonia, and methanol. Benzene was detected in high concentrations in all smoke samples at a level hundreds of time higher than the recommended exposure limit established by OSHA and NIOSH. Ammonia also exceeded the exposure limit. Methanol and

TABLE 1. CHEMICAL CONTENTS OF SURGICAL SMOKE[1]

- Acetonitrile
- Acetylene
- Acroloin
- Acrylonitrile
- Alkyl benzene
- Benzaldehyde
- Benzene
- Benzonitrile
- Butadiene
- Butene
- 3-Butenenitrile
- Carbon monoxide
- Creosol
- 1-Decene
- 2,3-Dihydro indene
- Ethane
- Ethyl benzene
- Ethylene
- Formaldehyde
- Furfural
- Hexadecanoic acid
- Hydrogen cyanide
- Indole
- Methane
- 3-Methyl butenal
- 6-Methyl indole
- 4-Methyl phenol
- 2-Methyl propanol
- Methyl pyrazine
- Phenol
- Propene
- 2-Propylene nitrile
- Pyridine
- Pyrrole
- Styrene
- Toluene
- 1-Undecene
- Xylene

REFERENCE
1. Barrett WL, Garber SM. Surgical smoke: a review of the literature. Business Briefing: Global Surgery. 2004:1-7.

From Ulmer BC. The hazards of surgical smoke. AORN J. 2008;87(4):721-734. Reprinted with permission.

ethylene were detected in the smoke but were within recommended exposure limits. The researchers concluded that additional factors to consider are the cumulative effect of all volatile organic compounds released during laser surgery and the harmful effects to the surgical team of continuous exposure by surgical smoke inhalation.

In a subsequent study, Petrus et al[43] used the laser photoacoustic spectroscopy technique to quantitatively analyze the concentrations of acetonitrile, acrolein, ammonia, benzene, and toluene in surgical smoke in vitro. A CO_2 laser was used to irradiate fresh animal tissue to generate surgical smoke. The researchers found that all of the gases were present in the surgical smoke, with an average gas concentration of acetonitrile 190 ppm, acrolein 35 ppm, ammonia 25 ppm, benzene 20 ppm, ethylene 0.410 ppm, and toluene 45 ppm.

Particles

The collective evidence indicates that the particles in surgical smoke generated by surgical energy-generating devices (eg, monopolar and bipolar electrosurgery, lasers) are within the respirable range.[67-75,77] Electrosurgery generates the smallest aerodynamic size particles (< 0.07 μm to 0.1 μm); laser tissue ablation creates larger particles (~ 0.31 μm); and ultrasonic scalpels create the largest particles (0.35 μm to 6.5 μm).[19]

Ragde et al[77] conducted a study to assess the exposure of surgical personnel to ultrafine particles (UFPs), to identify the predictors of exposure, and to characterize the particle size distribution of surgical smoke. The researchers measured personal exposures for the surgeon, assistant, scrub nurse, and anesthetic nurse during five different procedures (ie, nephrectomy, breast reduction, abdominoplasty, hip replacement, transurethral resection of the prostate) using spectrometry to assess the exposure to UFPs and characterize the particle distribution. Possible predictors of exposure were investigated using linear mixed effects models.

Exposure to UFPs was highest during abdominoplasty and lowest during hip replacement surgeries. Seventy percent or more of the measured particles were in the ultrafine range. The use of electrosurgery resulted in short-term, high-peak exposure with a maximum peak exposure of 272,000 particles cm^{-3} during a breast reduction surgery. The peaks corresponded to the use of the electrosurgery unit. Nephrectomy, transurethral resection of the prostate, and hip replacement surgeries produced the smallest size particles (9 nm) and also had the highest percentages of UFPs. Breast reduction surgery and abdominoplasty produced larger sized particles (70 nm and 81 nm, respectively) and had a lower percentage of

TABLE 2.   US ENVIRONMENTAL PROTECTION AGENCY PRIORITY POLLUTANTS POLYCYCLIC AROMATIC HYDROCARBONS[1]

- Benzo[a]anthracene
- Benzo[a]pyrene
- Benzo[b]fluoranthene
- Benzo[k]fluoranthene
- Chrysene/triphenylene
- Dibenzo[a,h]anthracene
- Indenol[1,2,3-cd]pyrene
- Acenaphthene
- Acenaphthylene
- Anthracene
- Benzo[ghi]perylene
- Phenanthrene
- Fluoranthene
- Fluorene
- Naphthalene
- Pyrene

REFERENCE

1.   Näslund Andréasson S, Mahteme H, Sahlberg B, Anundi H. Polycyclic aromatic hydrocarbons in electrocautery smoke during peritonectomy procedures. J Environ Public Health. 2012;2012:929053.

UFPs. There were no significant differences in exposure among the team members. The researchers concluded that the use of electrosurgery resulted in short-term, high-peak exposures to UFPs and recommended the correct use of smoke evacuators, the use of a built-in smoke evacuator tubing on the electrosurgery pencil, and the use of two smoke evacuators if two electrosurgery pencils are required.[77]

Wang et al[73] conducted a prospective study to analyze fine particles < 2.5 μm ($PM_{2.5}$) in surgical smoke by time and distance during urology procedures. The three types of surgeries included in the study were open surgeries, laparoscopic partial nephrectomy, and transurethral resection of bladder tumor. Three subtypes of the open surgery group, according to surgery depth, were inguinal lymph node dissection for penile cancer (superficial), partial nephrectomy (abdominal), and radical prostatectomy (pelvic). The sample size of each group was five patients per surgery. All procedures were performed in the same laminar airflow room. An instrument using a laser light scattering technique measured the number of particles. Particle counts were expressed as a concentration per 0.01 feet[3]. The instrument calculated an adjusted measurement of $PM_{2.5}$ mass (μg/m[3]). Particle counts were

measured at 40 cm, 60 cm, and 120 cm during open and laparoscopic surgeries to simulate the positions of the surgeon, assistant, and scrub person and were measured at 40 cm during the transurethral surgeries.

During the open surgeries, $PM_{2.5}$ was measured with and without wall suction for smoke evacuation. To evaluate the air quality, the researchers used the AIR Quality Index (AQI), the National Ambient Air Quality Standards for Particle Pollution revised by the US Environmental Protection Agency. Background particle measurements in the OR before the surgeries were nearly 5 μg/m[3]. The AQI of the air 40 cm from the open surgery incisions turned to unhealthy and very unhealthy in 3 to 6 seconds. In laparoscopic surgeries, the AQI 40 cm from the trocar reached hazardous levels in 3 seconds after the trocar valve was opened, releasing the surgical smoke. In the transurethral surgeries, the AQI was moderate 40 cm from the resectoscope. Use of wall suction decreased the inhalation dose of fine particles 48% in superficial surgeries and 52% in abdominal surgeries. The main finding of this study was that the concentration of fine particles of a single smoke plume could become very unhealthy for the surgeon. The researchers concluded that increasing the distance to the incision site decreased the concentration and inhalation of fine particles, and the use of smoke evacuation can reduce the concentration of fine particles.[73]

HPV

The evidence regarding the presence of HPV in surgical smoke is inconclusive. Human papillomavirus has been detected in the surgical smoke generated by lasers and ESUs during treatment of genital infections,[88-91,124] verrucae,[93,94] laryngeal papillomavirus,[92] and bovine papillomavirus-induced cutaneous fibropapillomas.[81] However, some studies have found no detectable HPV in laser plume generated during treatment of laryngeal papillomas.[125-127]

Kashima et al[92] conducted a prospective study to determine whether HPV DNA was in the smoke plume after CO_2 laser treatment of recurrent respiratory papillomatosis (RRP). Twenty-two patients with diagnoses of adult-onset RRP (n = 7), juvenile-onset RRP (n = 12), laryngeal carcinoma (n = 2), and nonspecific laryngitis (n = 1) participated in the study. The researchers collected 30 paired tissue and smoke samples during microlaryngoscopy with CO_2 laser excision under general anesthesia. To avoid contamination, the samples were processed separately with a polymerase chain reaction (PCR) assay for amplification of HPV-6 and HPV-11 sequences. Seventeen of the 30 smoke samples were positive for HPV DNA; three of the samples were identified as HPV-6 and 14 samples as HPV-11. Only the RRP specimens

SURGICAL SMOKE SAFETY

were HPV positive. The DNA types HPV-6 and HPV-11 are recognized as etiological agents in RRP. The researchers concluded that the consequences of HPV in smoke plume are unknown. To reduce the risk of potential infection to the patient and perioperative team members, they recommended using personal protective equipment (PPE) (eg, masks, gowns, gloves) and a gas-scavenging system whenever viral-infected lesions are treated with a CO_2 laser.

In a prospective study, Hughes and Hughes[126] collected and evaluated the laser plume of erbium:YAG laser-treated human warts to determine the presence or absence of HPV DNA in the plume. The researchers excised half of five patients' *verrucae vulgaris* and submitted the specimens for histopathological diagnosis and HPV DNA detection (HPV-1 and HPV-2) with in situ hybridization for HPV. The remaining half of the *verrucae vulgaris* were ablated with the erbium:YAG laser. A smoke evacuator collected the plume for evaluation of HPV DNA by PCR with consensus primers for the HPV previously detected in the *verruca vulgaris* specimens. The histopathological diagnosis of all five specimens was *verruca vulgaris*. All of the specimens with in situ hybridization contained HPV-2 DNA. Using PCR with consensus primers for HPV-2, the researchers did not detect HPV-2 in the laser plume of the same specimens. They concluded that the negative HPV plume results with the erbium:YAG laser were contradictory to the positive HPV plume findings in two other studies[93,94] in which CO_2 laser and electrosurgical excision and CO_2 laser excision were used. Hughes and Hughes postulated that the negative results could be a result of the radical explosive ejection of the erbium:YAG laser disrupting the HPV and rendering it undetectable.

Studies by Bergbrant et al,[124] Sood et al,[88] and Sawchuck et al[93] describe the risks of HPV exposure from ESU-generated smoke.

HIV

Johnson and Robinson[97] conducted a study to determine whether infectious HIV-1 could be isolated from aerosols generated from human blood containing HIV-1 during orthopedic and other surgical procedures that generate aerosols. The researchers prepared a mixture of human packed red blood cells negative for cytomegalovirus and HIV antibodies, a culture medium, and a culture medium containing a 10^5 tissue culture infectious dose of HIV-1. Individually, samples of the mixture were subjected to electrocautery in the coagulation and cutting modes, a high-speed bone cutting router, an oscillating bone saw, and a wound irrigation syringe jet. The cool aerosol or smoke plume generated by the procedures was suctioned and cultured.

Cultures positive for HIV-1 developed from the cool aerosols generated by the effects of the high-speed router tip and the oscillating bone saw on the blood mixture containing HIV-1. Cultures negative for HIV-1 developed from the cool aerosols generated by the wound irrigation syringe jet. Negative culture results were also obtained from six experiments of cutting and six experiments of coagulation with the electrocautery. The researchers concluded that infectious HIV-1 could be isolated from cool aerosols created from HIV-1 positive blood exposed to orthopedic routers and oscillating saws but that the high temperature of the electrocautery may inactivate HIV-1.[97]

Blood

Jewett et al[107] conducted a study to characterize the hemoglobin content by particle size of blood-containing aerosols generated by surgical power tools. Part of this study extends the work of Johnson and Robinson[97] described earlier. The researchers used two different protocols to generate aerosols. In a laboratory simulation of an operating room (OR), an oscillating bone saw, a high-speed air-driven drill, and a high-speed irrigating drill were used to "operate" on bone, and an ESU was used to cut and coagulate tendons. To simulate the blood present during surgery, blood was dripped onto the working area. The researchers collected a sampling from each test condition in addition to a control sampling using distilled water instead of blood. The second protocol was the same as that described by Johnson and Robinson[97] except the blood was not infected with HIV.

All of the instrumentation tested produced blood-containing aerosol particles in the respirable size range (< 5 μm). The researchers concluded that hemoglobin is an adequate marker of blood and therefore of bloodborne pathogens. The results suggest there is potential for breathing-zone exposure to respirable blood-containing particles during surgery performed with similar instrumentation. Additional research is needed in clinical settings.[107]

In a prospective, single-center trial, Ishihama et al[106] investigated whether blood-contaminated aerosols were present in a room where oral surgery procedures (N = 100) were performed with a high-speed drill. The sampling results were 76% positive in blood presumptive tests at 20 cm (7.9 inches) from the surgical site and 57% positive at 100 cm (39.4 inches) from the surgical site. The researchers concluded that these results suggest a risk for floating blood particles with the potential to cause airborne infection during use of high-speed instruments in oral surgery procedures.

In a subsequent study, Ishihama et al[105] used two protocols to investigate the presence of blood-contaminated aerosols in ORs during oral

PATIENT AND WORKER SAFETY

surgery procedures. For both protocols, the exhaust ducts of the central air-conditioning system were covered with a filter to collect the atmospheric samples. In the accumulation protocol, the researchers left the filters in place for 1, 2, and 4 weeks in one OR. In the second protocol, to analyze contributing factors, the test filters were changed after each surgical procedure. A leucomalachite green presumptive test for blood was used to test each filter. The researchers also collected additional data (ie, the type of procedure, the use of a high-speed rotating instrument or electric coagulator device, blood loss volume, and length of the procedure).

In the accumulation protocol, the positive sites for blood increased from 26 after 1 week to 92 and 143 after 2 and 4 weeks, respectively. Following the individual procedures, there were positive sites for blood in 21 of 33 procedures. Contributing factors to a positive result for blood included use of a high-speed instrument (9 of 10 surgeries), use of an electric coagulator (16 of 17 surgeries), and use of a high-speed instrument or electric coagulator (20 of 21 surgeries). Contributing factors to a negative result for blood included use of no device (11 of 12 surgeries). The researchers discussed the lack of evidence of infection risk from inhalation of floating infectious materials. Most health care workers who contract an occupational infection cannot pinpoint a causative injury such as a mucous membrane exposure. The researchers recommended using caution, especially for personnel who remain in the OR for long periods of time (eg, anesthesia providers, surgical assistants).[105]

I.a.1. The health care organization should determine the hazard exposure to the perioperative team by the
- job classifications that place team members at risk,[128]
- number of procedures where surgical smoke is generated,[128]
- percentage of surgical procedures where surgical smoke is not evacuated,
- type of energy-generating devices used,
- number of smoke evacuators available,
- number of ORs needing smoke evacuators, and
- current usage of smoke evacuation soft goods (ie, smoke evacuator tubing, smoke evacuator filters, in-line filters, laparoscopic filters).[128]
[5: Benefits Balanced with Harms]

I.b. The health care organization should use OSHA's hierarchy of controls[40] to reduce the perioperative team's exposure to surgical smoke and establish safe practices. The hierarchy of controls includes
- eliminating the hazard,
- using engineering controls (eg, room ventilation[115] of 20 total air exchanges per hour[42,129,130]),
- using work practice controls (eg, smoke evacuation[53,54,56,115]),
- using administrative controls (eg, policies and procedures, education and training), and
- using PPE.[131]
[3: Moderate Evidence]

Controlling exposures to hazards and toxic substances is the fundamental method of protecting workers. A hierarchy of controls is used as a means of determining how to implement feasible and effective controls. The OSHA hierarchy of controls is a systematic approach that can be used to identify the most effective method of risk reduction. Where possible, elimination or substitution is the most effective approach followed by use of engineering controls. Engineering controls are physical changes to the work environment that will minimize the health care worker's exposure to the hazard. Work practice controls establish efficient processes and procedures. Administrative controls (eg, policies and procedures) are used in conjunction with the other controls that more directly reduce or eliminate exposure to the hazard. Personal protective equipment reduces exposure to the risks and is the last line of defense against exposure to surgical smoke when exposure cannot be reduced through a higher level of control.[40]

I.b.1. When possible, the perioperative team should use the highest level of control.[39] If the hazard (eg, surgical smoke) cannot be eliminated, the team should employ the next level in the hierarchy. *[1: Regulatory]*

I.b.2. Smoke evacuation should be used in addition to room ventilation. *[2: High Evidence]*

The National Institute for Occupational Safety and Health recommends using a combination of ventilation techniques to control the airborne contaminants of surgical smoke. Because general room ventilation of 20 air exchanges per hour is insufficient to capture the contaminants, smoke evacuation (ie, local exhaust ventilation) is also necessary.[115]

I.c. Perioperative team members should wear PPE (ie, respiratory protection) as secondary protection against residual surgical smoke. *[2: High Evidence]*

Standards,[130,132,133] regulations,[128,130] and guidance from professional organizations[27-31,41] recommend using PPE (eg, a fit-tested surgical N95 respirator[128]) as a secondary defense against the inhalation of surgical smoke. General room ventilation and smoke evacuation (ie, local exhaust ventilation) are the first lines of protection against the hazards of surgical smoke.[115] When respiratory protection is required, the minimum respiratory protection device is a filtering face piece respirator (eg, an N95 respirator).[134]

A fit-tested surgical N95 filtering face piece respirator is a personal protective device that is worn on the face, covers the nose and mouth, and is used to reduce the wearer's risk of inhaling hazardous airborne particles including infectious agents.[76] The NIOSH respirator approval regulation defines the term N95 as a filter class that removes at least 95% of airborne particles during "worse case" testing using a "most-penetrating" sized particle.[135] Filters meeting the criteria are given a 95 rating. Many filtering face piece respirators have an N95 class filter, and those meeting this filtration performance are often referred to simply as "N95 respirators."[135] A surgical N95 respirator is fluid resistant on the outside to protect the wearer from splashes or sprays of body fluids.[40]

A surgical mask is not considered respiratory protection.[40] A surgical mask is a loose-fitting face mask intended to prevent the release of potential contaminants from the user into his or her immediate environment.[40,76] A surgical mask is fluid resistant, providing protection from large droplets, sprays, and splashes of body fluids,[76] but does not give the wearer a reliable level of protection from inhaling small airborne particles.[40] A high-filtration surgical face mask is designed to filter particulate matter that is 0.1 µm in size and larger. Similar to a surgical mask, a high-filtration mask does not create a seal between the face and the mask and may allow dangerous contaminants to enter the health care worker's breathing zone.[41,76,136]

The collective evidence[76,137-141] demonstrates the measurable superiority in protection provided by a surgical N95 respirator compared with high-filtration and surgical masks.

Gao et al[137] investigated the performance of surgical masks (n = 2) and surgical N95 respirators (n = 2) during exposure to surgical smoke. Ten participants were fit tested for the N95 respirators before the experiment. The participants performed surgical dissections on animal tissue in a simulated OR with an electrocautery device to generate surgical smoke. Each of the participants wore all four types of masks or respirators in random order. The generated surgical smoke was sampled in the breathing zone directly outside the mask or respirator to represent the inhalation exposure of an unprotected individual and inside the mask or respirator to represent the inhalation exposure of a protected wearer. The aerosol concentrations and particle size distribution of the inside- and outside-sampled aerosols were measured for 12 minutes each with a particle size spectrometer in combination with an optical particle counter. The simulated workplace protection factor (SWPF) was calculated for the masks and respirators. The SWPF values for both surgical masks were close to 1, indicat-

ing essentially no protection. The SWPF values for both N95 masks exceeded 100, the OSHA fit test passing level. The results suggest that surgical masks cannot protect health care workers against surgical smoke but that N95 NIOSH-certified respiratory protection devices can.

The collective evidence demonstrates that surgical masks have inadequate filter performance for aerosols[142,143] and submicron particles[136,144-147] (1 micron = 1 micrometer [µm]).

Rengasamy et al[136] investigated the filtration performance of surgical masks for a wide size range of submicron particles, including the size of many viruses. US Food and Drug Administration (FDA)-cleared masks can be categorized into three barrier types: high, moderate, and low. High and moderate barrier masks are cleared with > 98% filtration efficiency for bacterial filtration efficiency and particle filtration efficiency. Low barrier masks require > 95% for bacterial filtration efficiency only. The researchers tested five models of FDA-cleared surgical masks of all barrier types (n = 1 high barrier type, n = 2 moderate barrier type, and n = 2 low barrier type) for room air particle penetrations under constant and cyclic flow conditions. The following tests were performed:

- room air particle penetration at constant flow condition,
- room air particle penetration as a function of particle size,
- particle penetration measurement at cyclic flow conditions,
- polydisperse sodium chloride aerosol penetration measurement,
- monodisperse aerosol test method, and
- effect of isopropanol treatment on monodisperse aerosol penetrations.

Results of this study showed a wide variation in filtration performance. The researchers concluded that the wide variation in penetration levels for room air particles, which included particles in the viruses size range, confirms that surgical masks should not be used as respiratory protection.[136]

Oberg and Brosseau[148] evaluated nine types of surgical masks for filtration performance and facial fit. The types included surgical, laser, and procedure masks that were cupped, flat, and duckbilled with ties and ear loops. The masks' filter efficiency varied widely from very low to high. Facial fit was evaluated quantitatively and qualitatively. When filter performance and facial fit were evaluated, none of the surgical masks met the qualifications of respiratory protection devices.

I.c.1. A fit-tested surgical N95 filtering face piece respirator should be used during higher-risk, aerosol-generating procedures and procedures on patients with known or suspected aerosol transmissible diseases

PATIENT AND WORKER SAFETY

(eg, tuberculosis, varicella, rubeola).[134] *[1: Strong Evidence]*

Respiratory protection for aerosol transmissible diseases is based on the pathogen and the anticipated risk associated with the specific procedure.[40] Aerosol-generating procedures (eg, endotracheal intubation, bronchoscopy) generate higher concentrations of airborne particles and aerosol transmissible disease pathogens.[40] The Centers for Disease Control and Prevention[134] recommends that all team members present during cough-inducing or aerosol-generating procedures on patients with suspected or confirmed tuberculosis use respiratory protection.

Chen et al[149] measured the filtration efficiencies of a single-use submicron surgical mask and three types of respirators against aerosolized mycobacteria. In a specially designed enclosed test apparatus, an aerosol was generated with a known concentration of *Mycobacterium chelonae*, a surrogate for *Mycobacterium tuberculosis*. The researchers used Andersen samplers to measure aerosol concentrations upstream and downstream of the test masks and respirators. Mean percentage efficiencies for *Mycobacterium chelonae* ranged from 97% for the molded surgical mask and one type of respirator to 99.99% for the high-efficiency particulate air (HEPA) respirator. An analysis of variance demonstrated that the effect of mask or respirator type was significant. The researchers concluded that their evaluations could lead to development of an effective and practical device that would protect the health care worker without compromising patient care or safety.

I.c.2. In disease transmissible cases (eg, HPV),[10,81,94] the perioperative team may use a fit-tested surgical N95 filtering face piece respirator in conjunction with smoke evacuation. *[3: Moderate Evidence]*

A fit-tested surgical N95 filtering face piece respirator does not replace the need to use a smoke evacuation system as the first line of protection against the hazards of surgical smoke.

Recommendation II

The perioperative team should evacuate all surgical smoke.

The collective evidence[3,17,18,52,61,77,80,82,92,110,111,133,150-165]; standards[132,133]; regulations[128,130]; and guidance from NIOSH,[42,53,54,56,64,115] the Healthcare Infection Control Practices Advisory Committee,[166] and professional organizations[27-31] indicates that evacuating surgical smoke protects patients and health care workers from the hazards of surgical smoke (Table 3).

II.a. The perioperative team should use a smoke evacuation system (eg, smoke evacuator, in-line filter) to evacuate all surgical smoke. *[2: High Evidence]*

The National Institute for Occupational Safety and Health recommends using smoke evacuation systems to reduce potential acute and chronic health risks to health care personnel and patients.[115] The hazards of surgical smoke exposure to the perioperative team are respiratory, chemical, biologic (eg, blood, virus, bacteria), carcinogenic, mutagenic, and cytotoxic. Repeated exposure to the contents of surgical smoke may be cumulative[7,8,50] and increases the possibility of developing adverse effects.[44,52] Surgical smoke exposure risks to patients during minimally invasive procedures[12-18] include loss of visibility in the surgical field with potential to delay the procedure,[19-22] port site metastasis,[23] exposure to carbon monoxide,[22,24,25] and increased levels of carboxyhemoglobin,[22,24] and risks during open procedures include potential respiratory inflammation[165] and postoperative refractive errors.[167]

In Zgierz, Poland, Dobrogowski et al[52] conducted a study to identify and quantitatively measure selected chemical substances in surgical smoke and to assess the risk of the chemicals to medical personnel. The researchers collected air samples in the OR during laparoscopic cholecystectomy procedures. A complete qualitative and quantitative analysis of the samples showed the presence of aldehydes, benzene, toluene, ethylbenzene, xylene, ozone, and dioxins in concentrations lower than the hygienic standards used in the European Union. The researchers noted that the synergistic and antagonistic interactions of these substances have not been studied and are difficult to predict, and they concluded that surgical smoke should be evacuated to protect the OR team from the toxic and possibly carcinogenic, mutagenic, and genotoxic effects.

Moot et al[61] used selected ion flow tube mass spectrometry to analyze the composition of volatile organic compounds in diathermy plume produced during abdominal surgery. The researchers identified hydrogen cyanide, acetylene, and 1,3-butadiene in the plume. They concluded that although there is no evidence of adverse health effects from volatile organic compounds in surgical smoke plume, there is no evidence to indicate that it is safe to breathe smoke plume; thus, they recommended using smoke evacuators.

Respiratory Hazards

The size (ie, aerodynamic diameter) of the particles in the surgical smoke directly influences the type of adverse respiratory health effects experienced by the perioperative team.[19,41,66,69,73,76,102,123,168-171] Particle size depends on the type of surgical device generating the surgical smoke.[1,19,20] The ESU creates particles with the mean aerodynamic size

SURGICAL SMOKE SAFETY

TABLE 3. HEALTH EFFECTS OF CHEMICALS IN SURGICAL SMOKE[1,2]

Chemical	Health Effects
Acetaldehyde	Eye, skin, and respiratory irritation; eye and skin burns; dermatitis; conjunctivitis; cough; central nervous system (CNS) depression; delayed pulmonary edema; carcinogenic effects (nasal cancer)
Acetonitrile	Eye, skin, and nose irritation; cyanosis; cardiac and respiratory arrest
Acetylene	Headache, dizziness, reduced visual acuity, poor judgment, weakness, unconsciousness, rapid pulse and respiration, cyanosis, cardiac and respiratory symptoms related to oxygen deficiency
Acrolein	Eye, skin, and upper respiratory irritation; decreased pulmonary function; delayed pulmonary edema; chronic respiratory disease; possible increased blood clotting time; liver and kidney damage
Acrylonitrile	Eye and skin irritation, asphyxia, headache, sneezing, nausea, vomiting, lassitude, dizziness, skin vesicles, scaling dermatitis, CNS impairment, potential carcinogenic effects (brain tumors, lung and bowel cancer)
Anthracene	Skin damage, burning, itching, edema, headaches, nausea, loss of appetite, stomach and intestinal swelling, slowed reaction time, weakness, reduced serum immunoglobulins
Benzaldehyde	Acute eye and skin irritation and redness
Benzene	Eye, skin, nose, and respiratory irritation; dizziness; headache; nausea; staggered gait; anorexia; weakness; fatigue; dermatitis; bone marrow depression; potential carcinogenic effects (leukemia)
Benzonitrile	Eye and skin irritation
Butadiene (1,3 Butadiene)	Eye, nose, and throat irritation; drowsiness; dizziness; carcinogenic effects (leukemia and lymphoma)
Carbon monoxide	Headache, tachypnea, nausea, vomiting, fatigue, dizziness, confusion, hallucinations, cyanosis, cardiac dysrhythmias, myocardial ischemia, lactic acidosis, syncope, convulsion, coma Symptoms depend on the degree of exposure and susceptibility of the individual.
Creosol	Respiratory, eye, and skin irritation; cytotoxic effects; corrosive effects
Cyclohexanone	Respiratory irritation (potent irritant)
Decane	Eye, skin, and respiratory irritation; headache; dizziness; stupor; incoordination; loss of appetite; nausea; dermatitis
1-Decene (hydrocarbon)	Eye and respiratory irritation; may be a slight anesthetic at high concentrations
Ethane	Asphyxiation (simple asphyxiant)
Ethanol	Eye, skin, and nose irritation; headache; drowsiness; lassitude; narcosis; cough; liver damage; anemia; reproductive and teratogenic effects
Ethylene	Headache, muscular weakness, drowsiness, dizziness, unconsciousness
Ethyl benzene	Eye, throat, skin, and mucous membrane irritation; dizziness; dermatitis; narcosis; coma
Formaldehyde	Eye, nose, throat, and respiratory irritation; coughing; bronchospasm; lacrimation; cough; wheezing; potential carcinogenic effects (nasal cancer)
Furfural	Eye, skin, and upper respiratory irritation; sore throat; cough; bronchospasm; shortness of breath; headache; vomiting; dermatitis
Hydrogen cyanide	Asphyxiation, lassitude, headache, confusion, nausea, vomiting, increased rate and depth of respirations, slow and gasping respirations, thyroid and blood changes
Isobutene	Dizziness, drowsiness, dullness, nausea, unconsciousness, vomiting
Isopropanol	Eye, nose, and throat irritation; drowsiness; dizziness; headache
Methane	CNS depression, cardiac sensitization

continued on next page

PATIENT AND WORKER SAFETY

Table 3 continued. Health Effects of Chemicals in Surgical Smoke[1,2]

Chemical	Health Effects
4-Methyl phenol (p-cresol)	Eye, skin, and mucous membrane irritation; CNS effects; confusion; depression; respiratory failure; dyspnea; irregular rapid respiration; weak pulse; eye and skin burns; dermatitis; lung, liver, kidney, and pancreatic damage
2-Methyl propanol	Eye, skin, and throat irritation; headaches; drowsiness
Phenol	Eye, nose, and throat irritation; anorexia; weight loss; lassitude; muscle ache; pain; dark urine; cyanosis; liver and renal damage; skin burns; dermatitis; tremor; convulsions; twitching
Polycyclic aromatic hydrocarbons	Eye and respiratory irritation, dermatitis, conjunctivitis, increased risk of certain cancers
Propylene	Drowsiness, dizziness, unconsciousness
Pyridine	Eye irritation, headache, anxiety, dizziness, insomnia, nausea, anorexia, dermatitis, liver and kidney damage
Styrene	Eye, nose, and respiratory irritation; headache; lassitude; dizziness; confusion; malaise; drowsiness; unsteady gait; defatting dermatitis; possible liver injury; reproductive effects
Toluene	Eye and nose irritation, lassitude, confusion, euphoria, dizziness, headache, dilated pupils, lacrimation, anxiety, muscle fatigue, insomnia, paresthesia, dermatitis, liver and kidney damage
Xylene	Eye, skin, nose, and throat irritation; dizziness; excitement; drowsiness; incoordination; staggering gait; anorexia; nausea; vomiting; abdominal pain; dermatitis

REFERENCES
1. Pierce JS, Lacey SE, et al. An assessment of the occupational hazards related to medical lasers. J Occup Environ Med. 2011;53(11):1302-1309.
2. Okoshi K, Kobayashi K, et al. Health risks associated with exposure to surgical smoke for surgeons and operating room personnel. Surg Today. 2015;45(8):957-965.

of < 0.1 µm, laser particles are ~ 0.31 µm, and ultrasonic scalpel particles are 0.35 µm to 6.5 µm.[1,19,144] Particle size affects how far the particle can travel in the respiratory system.[19,76] Particles that are 5 µm or larger settle in the walls of the nose and pharynx; particles 3 µm to 5 µm settle in the trachea; particles 1 µm to 3 µm settle in the bronchus and bronchioles; and particles smaller than 1 µm can penetrate to the alveoli (Figure 2).[112,123,145] Particles smaller than 5 µm are categorized as lung-damaging dust,[172] as they can penetrate to the deepest areas of the lung and obstruct gas exchange.[19,76,168]

Näslund Andréasson et al[67] compared the amount of airborne particles and UFPs generated during peritonectomy with the amount of airborne particles and UFPs generated during colon and rectal cancer surgery. Personal and stationary samplings of UFPs were taken during peritonectomy procedures (n = 14) and colon and rectal cancer surgeries (n = 11). The median, maximum, and cumulative UFP levels for personal and stationary samplings were higher during the peritonectomy procedures than during the colon and rectal cancer surgeries. The mean cumulative levels were statistically significant for both the personal and stationary samplings. In discussing the results, the researchers compared the cumulative concentrations of UFP to smoking cigarettes or frying beef. They concluded that high levels of UFPs generated by electrocautery devices can be a health risk, and this warrants further investigation.

Chemical Hazards

The chemical content of surgical smoke varies by the type of tissue treated (eg, muscle, fat),[19,44,47,48,55,57,60,61,122,123] type of device (eg, laser,[49] ESU) used,[1,19,43,48,57,60,118,123] and duration of the procedure.[55]

Hollman et al[119] conducted an assay of surgical smoke generated during a reduction mammoplasty procedure. Monopolar electrocautery was used for dissection and resection, which resulted in intense smoke production. The researchers collected smoke samples (N = 25) whenever the electrocautery was in use. Laser spectroscopy was used to determine the gas components and corresponding concentration in the smoke samples collected. Eleven gases (ie, 1-ethenyl-3-methyl-benzene; 1,3-butadiene; propanenitrile; toluene; thiocyanic acid, methyl ester; 1-heptene; ethylene; ammonia; 1-decene; 2-furancarbox aldehyde; methylpropene) were identified and quantified. The researchers concluded that there is no doubt that surgical smoke generated by electrocautery is a potential health danger to the OR team. The degree of the threat is unclear. Follow-up studies are needed to determine particulate material, biological impurities, and gaseous components.

Hassan et al[150] conducted a prospective study to quantify the exposure of the surgeon and the patient to known chemical toxins in electrocautery smoke, and to determine whether there were qualitative or quantitative differences in exposure

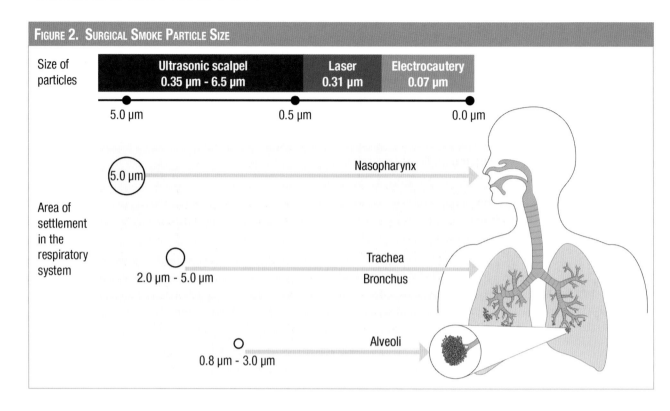

FIGURE 2. SURGICAL SMOKE PARTICLE SIZE

Size of particles

| Ultrasonic scalpel 0.35 μm - 6.5 μm | Laser 0.31 μm | Electrocautery 0.07 μm |

5.0 μm   0.5 μm   0.0 μm

Area of settlement in the respiratory system

5.0 μm — Nasopharynx

2.0 μm - 5.0 μm — Trachea / Bronchus

0.8 μm - 3.0 μm — Alveoli

during laparoscopic or open ileal loop pouch anastomosis. The researchers measured the surgeon's exposure to benzene, toluene, xylene, acetone, and styrene. They tested the patient's blood preoperatively within 6 hours of surgery and at the end of the procedure for benzene, ethyl benzene, toluene, xylene, carboxyhemoglobin, and cyanide. During the laparoscopic procedures, a smoke filter was used to maintain visibility, and during the open procedures, the electrocautery smoke was suctioned by the first assistant. The samplings of the surgeon's exposure were all negative. The patients' preoperative and postoperative levels of cyanide, carbon monoxide, benzene, ethyl benzene, toluene, and xylene were below standard detectable levels in the laparoscopic and open procedures. The researchers concluded that the methods (ie, suction devices) used to remove smoke from the surgical field and the OR air exchanges of the HVAC system were effective and minimized exposure of the health care team and the patient to the chemicals in surgical smoke. Additional qualitative and quantitative studies of the contents of electrocautery smoke are needed as well as technology that more efficiently and effectively evacuates surgical smoke from the surgical site and the OR environment.

In a study to determine the chemical composition of surgical smoke, Sagar et al[45] collected samples of surgical smoke generated by electrocautery during colorectal surgery. The sampling tube was attached near the end of the electrocautery pencil or held in the plume above the pencil. The researchers analyzed the collected smoke samples for PAHs, nitrosamines, nitrates,

nitrites, and volatile organic compounds by using high-performance liquid chromatography, gas chromatography with a thermal energy analyzer, ion chromatography, and mass spectrometry. The electrocautery smoke contained significant levels of benzene, ethyl benzene, styrene, carbon disulphide, and toluene. Benzene, a known carcinogen, was detected in significant quantities (71 μg/m³). The substances detected cause eye irritation, dermatitis, central nervous system effects, and hepatic and renal toxicity. The researchers concluded that additional studies are needed to determine the extent of exposure to the entire OR team and to develop methods to reduce the health risks.

Petrus et al[43] quantitatively analyzed surgical smoke produced in vitro by vaporization of fresh animal tissue with a CO_2 laser in a closed nitrogen atmosphere. The concentrations of acetonitrile, acrolein, ammonia, benzene, ethylene, and toluene in surgical smoke were determined with laser photoacoustic spectroscopy. The researchers investigated different types of tissue (ie, pig kidney, muscle, skin, heart) at a laser vaporization power of 10 watts and 15 watts with exposure times of 5 seconds and 15 seconds. Several smoke samples were collected, and the average gas concentrations were measured. The concentrations of the six gases measured were acetonitrile 190 ppm, acrolein 35 ppm, ammonia 25 ppm, benzene 20 ppm, ethylene 0.410 ppm, and toluene 45 ppm. The researchers concluded that the concentrations of all six gases increased depending on the laser power, exposure time, and type of tissue and that the laser photoacoustic spectroscopy system was efficient in analyzing a multicomponent gas mixture.

Carcinogenic Hazards

The evidence is inconclusive as to whether exposure to surgical smoke places perioperative team members at increased risk of developing cancer.[23,62,111-113,173-175]

Tseng et al[62] investigated particle number concentrations, size distribution, and gaseous and particle phase PAHs as the tracers of surgical smoke in the OR. Through their investigation of PAH concentrations for different surgical personnel, the potential cancer risk can be estimated for OR team members exposed to electrosurgery smoke. The researchers chose mastectomy procedures because of procedure length and high electrocautery use. During 14 mastectomy procedures, samples from the breathing zones of the surgeon and anesthesia provider were collected at 5-minute intervals. The majority of the airborne particles (70%) were 0.3 µm in size.

The downward flow of air (ie, positive pressure) from the OR ceiling distributed the smoke into the surrounding environment, exposing all personnel in the room instantaneously. The particle and gaseous PAH concentrations for the surgeon and anesthesia provider increased 40 to 100 times over the initial baseline measurements. The surgeon was exposed to the highest level of PAHs, approximately 1.5 times higher than the anesthesia provider. Although the anesthesia provider's levels were less than the surgeon's, longer hours working in the OR increased the risk. The researchers concluded that the submicron particles in the smoke contained carcinogenic chemicals and could threaten the health of the OR team through respiration of the particles. Using the toxicity equivalency factor, the average cancer risk in a 70-year lifetime for the surgeons and the anesthesia provider was calculated to be 117×10^{-6} and 270×10^{-6}, respectively, which are significantly higher the World Health Organization recommendation of 1×10^{-6}.[62]

In et al[111] conducted a two-part in vitro experiment to determine whether viable cells were present in surgical smoke. If viable tumor cells were found, the in vivo study portion evaluated their carcinogenicity. Viable cells were identified in the smoke at 5 cm from the ultrasonic scalpel. No viable cells were detected in the smoke from the ESU or radio-frequency ablation device. The viable cells were injected on both sides of the lower back of 20 mice. After 2 weeks, there was tumor growth in 16 of the 40 injection sites. Biopsies for morphological assessment showed highly mitotic cells, including irregularly shaped nuclei consistent with malignant tumors. The results suggest that malignant cells can be aerosolized when the ultrasonic scalpel is used on tumor-bearing tissue and may be the reason for tumor recurrence at a port site remote from the original tumor. The researchers concluded that smoke from an ultrasonic scalpel may contain viable tumor cells, and there is a theoretical risk of transfer of the viable tumor cells to anyone close to the surgical procedure.

Mowbray et al[112] conducted a systematic review of the literature to evaluate the properties of surgical smoke and the evidence of the harmful effects to OR team. The authors reviewed 20 studies that met the inclusion criteria for documentation of the contents of surgical smoke during human surgical procedures, methods to analyze the smoke, implication of smoke exposure, and type of energy device. The authors concluded that their review confirmed surgical smoke contains potentially carcinogenic compounds small enough to be respirable and reach the lower airways. The potential for harm is present, but the risk to the OR personnel remains unproven.

Mutagenic Hazards

Several studies[5,147,155,176,177] have demonstrated the mutagenicity of surgical smoke. Gatti et al[146] collected multiple air samples in the OR during reduction mammoplasty procedures using electrocautery for dissection and excision of the breast tissue. The OR samples were collected approximately 2.5 ft to 3 ft above the surgical field. Control air samples were taken in a separate room. All of the samples were tested for mutagenic activity in standard tester strains TA98 and TA100 of *Salmonella typhimurium* using the *Salmonella* microsomal microsuspension test. The results showed the air samples were mutagenic to the TA98 strain of *Salmonella typhimurium*. The TA100 strain of *Salmonella typhimurium* did not appear to be significantly altered by the smoke. The researchers concluded from this preliminary study that the smoke produced by the electrocautery during reduction mammoplasty is mutagenic. Mutagenic potential may vary among patients. Safe levels of ambient mutagens have not been determined.

To test the mutagenic activity of surgical smoke condensates, Tomita et al[5] used a CO_2 laser to irradiate and an ESU to cauterize excised canine tongue. The researchers tested the generated smoke with the microbial strains TA98 and TA100 of *Salmonella typhimurium*. The laser condensates showed mutagenicity on TA98 in the presence of S9 mix. The S9 mix contained 50 µmoles sodium phosphate buffer, 4 µmoles magnesium chloride, 16.5 µmoles potassium chloride, 2.5 µmoles glucose-6 phosphate, 2 µmoles nicotinamide adenine dinucleotide phosphate, and 150 µL of S9 fraction (prepared from rat liver pretreated with polychlorobiphenyl) in a total volume of 0.5 mL. The ESU condensates exhibited mutagenic activity on both strains in the presence of S9 mix. The mutagenic ability of laser condensates was one-half that of the ESU condensates for the microbial strain TA98. The microbial strain TA98 of *Salmonella typhimurium* was 10 times more sensitive than microbial strain TA100 of *Salmonella typhimurium* to the condensates.

The ESU may be more favorable for the generation of mutagens than laser irradiation. The mutagenic potency of the laser condensates was comparable to that of cigarette smoke. The researchers collected about 40 mg of laser and ESU condensates from 1 g of vaporized or cauterized tissue. This amount of laser condensate was equivalent to that from three cigarettes, and this amount of ESU condensate was equivalent to that from six cigarettes. The researchers concluded that more research is needed to evaluate the hazards of laser and ESU smoke on human health and, unless proven otherwise, there is a potential health risk to surgeons, anesthesia providers, nurses, and patients.[5]

Hill et al[154] studied six human and 78 porcine tissue samples to find the mass of tissue ablated during 5 minutes of monopolar ESU use. They also recorded electronically the total daily duration of ESU use in a plastic surgery OR during a 2-month period. An initial pilot study compared a human tissue sample with the animal model. No difference was found between the two tissue types. Porcine tissue is the most physiologically similar tissue to human tissue. For the human tissue, the mass of the ESU tissue ablation after 5 minutes of continuous cutting ablation was 2.4132 g and the mass after coagulation ablation was 1.5817 g. For the porcine tissue, the mass of the ESU tissue ablation after 5 minutes of continuous cutting ablation was 2.3721 g and the mass after coagulation ablation was 1.5406 g. The mean daily ESU activation time was 12 minutes 43 seconds. Using Tomita's results that 1 g of tissue equals six unfiltered cigarettes,[5] the researchers quantified the environmental OR air pollution. They concluded that the equivalent of 27 to 30 unfiltered cigarettes would need to be smoked in the OR on a daily basis to generate a passive air pollution with an equivalent mutagenicity. The long-term effects of chronic surgical smoke exposure remains unproven. It is known that surgical smoke is mutagenic and contains the same carcinogens as tobacco smoke. The dangers of passive exposure to tobacco smoke are well documented. The researchers recommended using smoke evacuators.

Cytotoxic Hazards

There is limited evidence regarding the cytotoxic effects of surgical smoke.[177-180]

Hensman et al[178] exposed cultured cells for a short period of time to smoke produced in a confined space in vitro to determine whether significant toxicity can occur. The smoke was produced in helium, carbon dioxide, and air-saturated environments. The toxic, infective, and mutagenic risks of surgical smoke during open surgeries are known. In minimally invasive surgery, it is unknown whether the smoke produced in a carbon dioxide-saturated environment may have a different composition. The chemical contents identified in the smoke produced in helium, carbon dioxide, and air were similar in composition. The researchers concluded the ESU smoke generated in a closed environment produced several toxic chemicals. The effect of the toxic chemicals on cell viability, macrophage, and endothelial cell activation is unknown. Until the effects of these toxic chemicals is known, smoke evacuation is recommended during minimally invasive surgery.

Viral Hazards

Several studies[95,181-185] demonstrated a low risk of HPV transmission and subsequent infection.

Kofoed et al[183] investigated the prevalence of mucosal HPV types in medical personnel employed in the gynecology and dermato-venereology departments of multiple Denmark hospitals in relation to occupational exposure to HPV. The participants (N = 287) completed a questionnaire with demographic data, their previous and current work-related HPV exposure, and history of HPV-related disease. The researchers collected oral and nasal mucosa samples from the participants and analyzed the samples using HPV genotyping. In relation to exposure, a mucosal HPV type was found in

- 5.8% of employees with experience in treating genital warts with a laser compared to 1.7% of the participants who did not have this experience;
- 6.5% of participants with experience in treating genital warts with electrosurgery compared to 2.8% of the participants who did not have this experience; and
- 4.7% of participants with experience in treating genital warts with loop electrode excision procedure compared to 4.6% of the participants who did not have this experience.

Physician and non-physician laser personnel who had treated patients with genital warts for at least 5 years had a significantly higher prevalence of mucosal HPV types than personnel who had less than 5 years of experience or no experience treating genital wards with a laser. The researchers found that participating in CO_2 laser or electrosurgical evaporation of genital warts or loop electrode excision of cervical dysplasia did not significantly increase the prevalence of nasal or oral HPV. Mucosal HPV types are infrequent in the oral and nasal cavities of health care personnel.

Despite the low risk of transmission and subsequent infection with HPV, there have been reported cases of occupational transmission of HPV.[9-11] In 1991, Hallmo and Naess[10] reported the case of a 44-year-old laser surgeon who presented with a large, confluent papillomatous mass in the anterior commissure and along the right vocal cord and four smaller, discrete, smooth papillomas on the left vocal cord. Biopsies of the laryngeal lesions showed squamous papillomas with moderate focal dysplasia. Types HPV-6 and HPV-11 DNA were identified in groups of tumor cells. The surgeon had no known source of infection other than that he had used the Nd:YAG laser for therapeutic procedures involving anogenital condyloma acuminata. Anogenital condylomas harbor HPV types 6 and 11. The authors concluded that any of the surgeon's patients with anogenital warts could have been the source of the surgeon's HPV contamination, and there is a similar risk for laser procedure team members.

Calero and Brusis[9] reported the case of a 28-year-old OR nurse who developed recurrent and histologically proven laryngeal papillomatosis. The nurse's occupational history included assisting on electrosurgical and laser surgical excisions of anogenital condylomas. After a virological institute confirmed the high probability of correlation between the occupational exposure and laryngeal papillomatosis, the nurse's condition was accepted as an occupational disease. Hallmo and Naess[10] and Calero and Brusis[9] concluded that the occupational transmission risk of HPV is low when recommended protective measures (eg, smoke evacuation) are employed.

Rioux et al[11] described the cases of HPV-16 positive oropharyngeal squamous cell carcinomas in two surgeons with long-term histories of occupational laser plume exposure to HPV. A 53-year-old gynecologist sought consultation for a lesion on his right tonsil and a lump in the right side of his neck. The biopsy of the right tonsil confirmed invasive squamous cell carcinoma of moderate to poor differentiation. The lesion was positive for HPV-16 by hybrid capture assay. The patient was a non-smoker who consumed alcohol occasionally, was in a monogamous relationship, and whose partner tested negative for HPV. The only identifiable risk factor for oropharyngeal cancer and HPV was occupational exposure to HPV-positive laser plume. The surgeon performed more than 3,000 laser ablations and loop electrosurgical excisions for dysplastic cervical and vulvar lesions over 20 years.

The second case was a 62-year-old gynecologist who sought consultation for a foreign body sensation in his throat. A biopsy of the base of his tongue was positive for squamous cell carcinoma and HPV-16. The surgeon was a non-smoker who consumed alcohol occasionally and had been married twice. The surgeon's occupational history consisted of performing weekly laser ablations with a CO_2 laser for 15 years and performing loop electrosurgical excision procedures for 15 years. The authors suggested prophylactic HPV vaccination against oncogenic HPV strains to prevent infection and reduce the risk of oropharyngeal cancer.

In a university laboratory research center, Garden et al[81] investigated whether laser-generated plume from infected animal tissue (ie, bovine papillomavirus [BPV]-induced cutaneous fibropapilloma) can reproduce disease. The researchers evaluated three laser settings, suctioned and collected the laser plume at each setting, and re-inoculated the laser plume onto the skin of three calves. All of the laser plume samples at the three laser settings contained BPV DNA. Two calves developed marked lesions at the sites of BPV inoculum, and the third calf developed minimal growth. The histological evaluation of the excised laser-plume induced lesions was typical of BPV fibropapillomas. The DNA extracts from each of the three induced tumors contained high levels of BPV DNA, thus confirming that the lesions resulted from the BPV infection. The researchers found the lesions induced by the laser plume were identical to the original lesions based on the histopathological and viral typing.

The evidence conflicts on whether pathogenic virus transfer occurs during excimer laser treatment of corneal tissue.[85,186,187]

Hagen et al[187] developed a model system to test the possibility of virus transmission during excimer laser treatment through airborne excimer laser debris. An excimer laser was used to ablate a culture plate infected with psuedorabies virus. Psuedorabies virus is a porcine enveloped herpes virus, similar in structure and life cycle to HIV and the herpes simplex virus. In vitro transfer of viable psuedorabies virus by excimer laser plume did not appear to occur. The researchers concluded that the surgeon and team members are at low risk of infection by enveloped viruses (eg, HIV, herpes simplex) transmitted by the excimer laser plume.

In 1997, Taravella et al[186] used an excimer laser to ablate fibroblasts infected with attenuated varicella-zoster virus. The researchers collected the laser plume for PCR analysis and viral cultures. Their results suggested that viral DNA fragments remain intact after ablation but the virus particles capable of causing infection in the fibroblast culture do not. They concluded that attenuated varicella-zoster virus does not seem to survive excimer laser ablation, and further research is needed to determine whether other viruses could remain infectious after exposure to excimer laser radiation.

In a subsequent experimental study in 1999, Taravella et al[85] used an excimer laser to ablate fibroblasts infected with oral polio vaccine virus. The researchers collected the laser plume for viral cultures. The cultures were positive for the virus. The researchers also analyzed the role of virus size and its ability to remain infectious after excimer laser ablation. The oral polio virus is approximately 30 nm in size compared with 200 nm for the herpes virus family. The results suggested that smaller viruses might be able to escape ablation, whereas larger viruses may not. The researchers concluded that the oral polio virus can survive excimer laser ablation and that whether other viruses, such as HIV, can withstand ablation and remain infectious needs to be determined.

Bacterial Hazards

Capizzi et al[98] conducted a prospective study to analyze the potential bacterial and viral exposure to OR personnel from the laser smoke plume generated by CO_2 laser resurfacing. During 13 consecutive laser resurfacing procedures, the researchers captured the smoke plume using a smoke evacuator with a HEPA filter. Before the resurfacing procedures, the room air was filtered with the smoke evacuator. The HEPA filter served as the control. Two bacterial and two viral cultures were collected per filter. Bacterial cultures were incubated for 14 days if results were negative, and the viral cultures were incubated for 28 days if the results were negative. There was no growth from any of the viral cultures. Five patients had a bacterial culture that grew +1 coagulase-negative *Staphylococcus*. Two of these five patients also had a concomitant bacterial growth of either *Corynebacterium* or *Neisseria*. The researchers concluded that viable bacteria exist within the laser smoke plume generated during laser resurfacing. Additional research is needed to define the exposure risk associated with patients who have hepatitis, HIV, and antibiotic-resistant bacteria.

Patient Health Effects

Two studies[165,167] report potential hazardous effects to patients from surgical smoke exposure.

Freitag et al[165] investigated the harmful effects of surgical smoke inhalation for the patient and the OR team in an animal study. To simulate a single patient exposure of the respiratory system during a procedure, the researchers measured the effects of one 10-minute exposure on airway resistance, gas exchange, and mucociliary clearance rate in the trachea. To simulate the repetitive exposures of surgical smoke inhalation by the OR team, the researchers measured the effects of three separate 10-minute exposures on airway resistance, gas exchange, and mucociliary clearance rate in the trachea. They found a decrease in arterial partial pressure of oxygen after smoke inhalation. Tracheal mucous velocity was significantly depressed in a dose-dependent manner with increasing smoke exposure. Results of bronchoalveolar lavages showed smoke inhalation induced a severe inflammation with increases of inflammatory cells. The researchers concluded that the surgeon should be aware that inhalation of laser-generated smoke may cause transient hypoxia, depression of lung defense mechanisms, and delayed airway inflammation.

Charles[167] retrospectively studied the effects of laser plume evacuation on laser in-situ keratomileusis (LASIK) outcomes in 199 patients (n = 82 with no evacuation, n = 117 with plume evacuation). There were no statistical differences in the frequency of corneal abrasion, flap slippage, or the level of postoperative debris. A significant difference was noted in postoperative residual refractive error and uncorrected visual acuity. In the no evacuation group, 90% had uncorrected visual acuity of 20/40 or better, 68% saw 20/25 or better, and 59% saw 20/20 or better. In the plume evacuation group 96% had uncorrected visual acuity of 20/40 or better, 89% saw 20/25 or better, and 74% saw 20/20 or better. Charles concluded that using plume evacuation for LASIK procedures improved refractive and uncorrected visual acuity outcomes following the procedure.

II.a.1. The decision to evacuate or not evacuate surgical smoke should not be made at the discretion of an individual practitioner.[32] *[3: Moderate Evidence]*

The patient and other perioperative team members are continually exposed to the hazards of surgical smoke.[32]

II.a.2. A smoke evacuator with a 0.1 µm filter (eg, ultra-low particulate air [ULPA]) should be used when surgical smoke is anticipated.[27,30,31,115,128,132] *[2: High Evidence]*

Electrosurgery generates the smallest aerodynamic size particles (< 0.07 µm to 0.1 µm); laser tissue ablation creates larger particles (~ 0.31 µm); and ultrasonic scalpels create the largest particles (0.35 µm to 6.5 µm).[19] An ULPA filter has an a 99.999% efficiency.[188]

II.a.3. When using a medical-surgical vacuum system, a 0.1 µm in-line filter (eg, ULPA) should be in place between the suction wall connection and the suction cannister.[30,31,115,128,130,132,133] *[2: High Evidence]*

An in-line 0.1 µm filter captures airborne contaminants in surgical smoke.[115]

II.a.4. A medical-surgical vacuum system (ie, wall suction) may be used to evacuate small amounts[188] of surgical smoke as defined by the health care organization's policy and procedures. *[5: Benefits Balanced with Harms]*

Low suction flow rates[128] associated with medical-surgical vacuum systems limit their efficiency in evacuating surgical smoke, making them suitable only for the evacuation of small amounts of smoke.[130,188]

II.a.5. Preventative maintenance for a centralized stationary smoke evacuation system should include flushing of the smoke evacuator lines according to the manufacturer's instructions.[130] *[4: Limited Evidence]*

A centralized stationary smoke evacuation system is permanently installed in mechanical spaces and provides evacuation to several points of use.[128] The scavenged, filtered air is exhausted outside of the building.[128] Regular maintenance of the smoke evacuator lines prevents particulate matter buildup or contamination of the suction line.

II.a.6. Smoke evacuation units and accessories should be used according to manufacturers' written instructions (eg, filter change, distance of the capture device from the generation of surgical smoke).[30,31,115,130] *[2: High Evidence]*

II.b. The capture device (eg, wand, tubing) of a smoke evacuation system should be positioned as close to the surgical site as necessary to effectively collect all traces of surgical smoke. *[2: High Evidence]*

Standards[130,132] and guidance from NIOSH[115] and professional organizations[27,30,31] recommend that the surgical smoke capture device be kept as close as possible to the surgical site; NIOSH[115] recommends that the device be kept within 2 inches (5.08 cm) of the surgical site. Capture performance is affected by the smoke evacuator flow rate,[188,189] distance of the evacuator nozzle to the surgical site,[188-190] tubing size, and amount of smoke generated.[189]

If there is a detectable odor when a smoke evacuation system is in use, it is a signal that
- smoke is not being captured at the site where it is being generated,
- there is inefficient air movement through the suction or smoke evacuation wand, or
- the filter has exceeded its usefulness and should be replaced.[191]

In a preliminary study to simulate smoke production conditions during CO_2 laser surgery, Smith et al[190] measured smoke concentrations at 6 inches, 3 feet, and 4 feet from the site of the laser interaction with the tissue. The 6-inch distance represented the location of the surgeon and other personnel performing the surgery. The 3- and 4-feet distances were used to monitor the areas in which other personnel might be present

in the room and to estimate background concentrations of the smoke in various parts of the room. The nozzle of the smoke evacuator was located at 2 inches, 6 inches, and 12 inches to measure the relative effectiveness of the smoke evacuation system. The researchers used aerosol and dust monitors to measure the relative concentration of the smoke with a scale of zero to 20. When the smoke was not evacuated, the relative concentration of smoke at 6 inches was high, ranging from 10 to 20, compared to the background relative concentration of zero to 1, demonstrating a clear indication to use a smoke evacuator. When the smoke evacuator nozzle was 2 inches from the laser interaction site, the nozzle completely collected the smoke when the evacuator was activated. At 6 inches, the smoke collection was not complete and the relative concentrations rose as high as 8. The results at 12 inches was qualitatively similar to the results at 6 inches except that background smoke levels increased. The researchers concluded that positioning the nozzle of the smoke evacuator at a distance of 2 inches is adequate for smoke capture. Distances greater than 2 inches may result in exposure to high concentrations of smoke for personnel working near the surgical site and are likely to an increase the background concentrations in the room.

In a randomized controlled trial, Pillinger et al[162] investigated whether a suction clearance device would reduce the amount of smoke reaching the surgeon's mask compared to no smoke evacuation. All of the patients underwent either thyroid or parathyroid surgery with a standard anterior cervical collar incision and division of the strap muscles. The amount of smoke reaching the level of the surgeon's mask was measured with an aerosol monitor. Smoke evacuation was used for the patients in the experimental group (n = 15), and no smoke evacuation was used for the patients in the control group (n = 15). Baseline measurements were taken before the patients entered the OR, continuously during surgery, and postoperatively after the patient left the OR for the postanesthesia care unit.

Use of smoke extraction resulted in a significant reduction in the mean amount of smoke detected at the level of the surgeon's mask. In surgeries that used no smoke evacuation, the mean amount of smoke detected at the surgeon's mask was 137 µg/m³. In surgeries that used smoke evacuation, the mean amount of smoke detected at the surgeon's mask was 12 µg/m³. Use of smoke extraction resulted in a significant reduction in the maximum amount of smoke detected at the level of the surgeon's mask (control group 2411 µg/m³; experimental group 255 µg/m³). Clearing the smoke improved visibility of the surgical field and reduced the characteristic diathermy smell. The researchers concluded that evacuation of surgical plume resulted in a significant reduction in the amount of smoke reaching the level of the surgeon's mask and that the use of smoke evacuation is advisable.[162]

II.b.1. The smoke evacuation system (eg, smoke evacuator, medical-surgical vacuum with in-line filter) should be activated at all times while surgical smoke is being generated.[115] *[2: High Evidence]*

II.c. The perioperative team should use a smoke evacuation system during minimally invasive procedures. *[3: Moderate Evidence]*

The use of a smoke evacuation system during minimally invasive procedures protects the patient and personnel from the hazards of surgical smoke.[19,24,65,130,192-194] The collective evidence demonstrates that the risks of surgical smoke exposure to the patient are reduced visibility of the surgical site during the procedure,[12-15,17-20,22,195] potential delays during the procedure,[19-22] absorption and excretion of smoke by-products (eg, carbon monoxide,[22,24,25] benzene),[193,196] carboxyhemoglobinemia,[22,24] and port site metastasis.[23,108,197]

Dobrogowski et al[196] assessed patient exposure to organic substances produced and identified in surgical smoke generated during laparoscopic cholecystectomy procedures. The researchers collected urine samples of 69 patients undergoing laparoscopic cholecystectomy procedures before and after surgery and analyzed them for benzene, toluene, ethylbenzene, and xylene. Samples of the gases in the abdominal cavity were obtained from the trocar for identification of the main chemical compounds. The researchers identified about 40 substances, such as aldehydes, unsaturated and saturated hydrocarbons, aromatic hydrocarbons, and dioxins. The concentrations of benzene and toluene were significantly higher in the urine samples after surgery compared with preoperative levels. This is direct evidence that the compounds were produced intraoperatively and absorbed into the blood. The postoperative levels of benzene, a known human carcinogen, were three times higher than before surgery. The researchers concluded that the concentrations of the compounds in the urine were only a small percentage of the total absorbed dose. The mixture of the toxic compounds in the urine can significantly increase the overall toxicity potential caused by the interaction of the compounds. There is also a potential threat from carcinogenic compounds (eg, benzene) despite a short exposure time and low concentrations.

Takahashi et al[17] used an industrial smoke-detection device to evaluate the efficacy of an automatic smoke evacuator in eliminating surgical smoke, including harmful substances, in experimental laparoscopic surgery. Surgical smoke was generated with either a high-frequency ESU or laparoscopic coagulating shears. The participants were divided into a smoke evacuation group and a control group with no smoke evacuation. Ten laparoscopic surgeons independently and subjectively evaluated the laparoscopic field of view. The composition of the smoke was analyzed by mass spectrometry. More than 40 chemical compounds were identified in the smoke. The subjective evaluations indicated a superior field of view in the evacuation group compared with the control group at 15 seconds after activation of the ESU. The estimated volume of residual intra-abdominal smoke after activation of the ESU was significantly lower in the smoke evacuation group. The researchers concluded that the use of an automatic smoke evacuator enhanced the field of view and reduced smoke exposure in experimental laparoscopic surgery.

The evidence conflicts regarding elevated blood[16,22,24,65,194] or intraperitoneal[16,22,65] levels of carbon monoxide posing a patient risk.

In a prospective study, Nezhat et al[194] analyzed the blood samples of patients undergoing laparoscopic procedures with accompanying laser and bipolar ESU smoke generation. Carboxyhemoglobin concentrations were measured with gas chromatography. Preoperatively, the mean carboxyhemoglobin levels were $0.70 \pm 0.15\%$, and postoperatively, the levels were $0.58 \pm 0.20\%$. The decrease was statistically significant. The researchers concluded that carbon monoxide poisoning is not associated with laparoscopic procedures. They attributed the results to aggressive smoke evacuation that minimized patient exposure to carbon monoxide and to active elimination by ventilation with high oxygen concentrations.

To determine the absorption of carbon monoxide from the peritoneal cavity, Ott[24] measured patients' preoperative, intraoperative, and postoperative levels of carboxyhemoglobin. In the control group (n = 25), no lasers or smoke-generating devices were used during the laparoscopic procedure. In the experimental group (n = 25), lasers were used during the laparoscopic procedures. Patients were screened preoperatively for environmental or occupational sources of elevated carbon monoxide. The patients were evaluated for carbon monoxide levels before induction of anesthesia, periodically during the procedure, and postoperatively at 2, 3, 6, 12, and 24 hours. The control group showed no statistical change of preoperative, intraoperative, or postoperative levels of carboxyhemoglobin. Significant elevation of carboxyhemoglobin was found in all 25 of the experimental group members at 10 minutes. The carboxyhemoglobin levels ranged from 2.8% to 18.5% saturation of whole blood and were elevated for as long as 16 hours after the end of the procedure. The patients with the

PATIENT AND WORKER SAFETY

highest postoperative levels had symptoms of carbon monoxide poisoning (eg, dizziness, nausea, headache, weakness). Ott concluded that patients having laparoscopic procedures with a CO_2 laser were exposed to high levels of carbon monoxide and that smoke evacuation reduces the hazards of carbon monoxide absorption, decreases carboxyhemoglobin formation, and reduces the consequences of acute iatrogenic surgical carbon monoxide exposure resulting from laser-generated smoke during laparoscopic surgery.

II.d. Used smoke evacuator filters, tubing, and wands must be handled using standard precautions, and disposed of as biohazardous waste.[28,30,31,96,115,128,132,198] *[1: Regulatory Requirement]*

Surgical smoke contains potentially hazardous (infectious) material, including viruses[3,80-86] (eg, HPV,[88-95] HIV[96,97]), bacteria,[98-102] blood,[100,105-110] particles,[19,67-77] and cancer cells.[23,111-113]

II.e. A multidisciplinary team that includes perioperative RNs, surgeons, and scrub personnel should select surgical smoke safety equipment to be used in the perioperative setting. Additional team members may include an infection preventionist, engineers (eg, biomedical, HVAC systems), and a materials manager. *[5: Benefits Balanced with Harms]*

Involvement of a multidisciplinary committee allows input from all departments in which the product will be used and from personnel with expertise beyond clinical end users (eg, infection preventionists, materials management personnel). The perioperative RN has a professional responsibility to consider "factors related to safety, effectiveness, efficiency, and the environment, as well as the cost in planning, delivering, and evaluating patient care."[199(p702)] Perioperative RNs play a crucial role in providing practical insight and expertise in the use and evaluation of surgical products.

II.e.1. The multidisciplinary team should evaluate smoke evacuators before purchase.[130] *[3: Moderate Evidence]*

Manufacturers use various technological approaches to achieve smoke evacuation. Items to evaluate may include the type of filters used (eg, ULPA, carbon),[128,188] whether the system has a variable flow rate to accommodate different levels of smoke,[128] noise level, whether the system has automatic remote activation, the type of filter monitoring system,[128] compatibility of products, and equipment effectiveness and efficiency.[188,200] The ULPA filter captures particles in surgical smoke, whereas the carbon filter absorbs the gases in surgical smoke. A noise level of 60 A-weighted decibels (dBA) or less facilitates communication during the procedure.[188]

II.e.2. In collaboration with the perioperative team, the surgical specialists (eg, generalist, otorhinolaryngologist, plastic surgeon, urologist) should evaluate alternative energy-generating devices. *[5: Benefits Balanced with Harms]*

The collective evidence indicates that bipolar instruments,[12,157,201] ultrasonic instruments,[12,50,110,201-207] certain surgical techniques,[208,209] and alternative devices[21,161,185,210-215] generate low amounts of surgical smoke.

Recommendation III

Perioperative team members should receive initial and ongoing education and competency verification on surgical smoke safety.

Initial and ongoing education of perioperative team members facilitates the development of knowledge, skills, and attitudes that affect safe patient care and workplace safety. The health care organization is responsible for providing initial and ongoing education and verifying the competency of its personnel[199]; however, the primary responsibility for maintaining ongoing competency remains with the individual.[216]

Competency verification activities provide a mechanism for competency documentation and help verify that perioperative team members understand the hazards of surgical smoke, evacuation methods, proper equipment usage, and disposal of used tubing and filters.

III.a. The health care organization should establish education and competency verification activities for its personnel and determine intervals for education and competency verification related to surgical smoke safety practices. *[5: Benefits Balanced with Harms]*

III.b. Education and competency verification activities related to surgical smoke safety should include
- defining surgical smoke (ie, the gaseous products of burning organic material created as a result of the destruction of tissue),
- describing critical factors for managing surgical smoke for all procedures that generate surgical smoke,
- identifying sources of surgical smoke (eg, lasers, ESUs, ultrasonic devices, high-speed drills, burrs, saws),
- explaining the effect of particle size on the speed[217] and distance smoke travels,
- describing the health effects of smoke exposure on patients and health care workers,[160]
- selecting smoke evacuation systems and supplies (eg, ESU pencils with incorporated evacuation tubing, in-line filters, smoke evacuator units) in accordance with the procedure being performed,
- testing smoke evacuation equipment before the procedure,
- connecting equipment correctly,
- using smoke evacuation equipment correctly during the procedure,

○ using standard precautions to handle used smoke evacuation supplies and discarding biohazardous waste,

○ reviewing policies and procedures related to smoke evacuation, and

○ participating in quality improvement programs related to the management of surgical smoke as assigned.

[5: Benefits Balanced with Harms]

The evidence indicates there is a lack of knowledge among perioperative team members regarding surgical smoke. Steege et al[32] conducted a web-based survey of members of professional organizations representing health care occupations in which there is routine contact with selected chemical agents, including surgical smoke. Laser surgery and electrosurgery were addressed in separate submodules of the survey. Eligible respondents (N = 4,533) worked within 5 ft of surgical smoke generation during electrosurgery (99%) or laser surgery (31%). The respondents were nurse anesthetists (33%), perioperative nurses (19%), anesthesiologists (21%), surgical technologists (16%), and others (11%). In response to questions on training, 49% of the respondents to the survey laser submodule and 44% of the respondents to the electrosurgery submodule reported that they had never received training on the hazards of surgical smoke.

III.c. Personnel should receive education and complete competency verification activities before new smoke evacuators and accessories are introduced. *[5: Benefits Balanced with Harms]*

Receiving education and completing competency verification activities in advance of changes helps ensure safe practice.

Recommendation IV

Policies and procedures for surgical smoke safety should be developed, reviewed periodically, revised as necessary, and readily available in the practice setting in which they are used.

Policies and procedures regarding surgical smoke safety provide guidance to perioperative team members for creating an environment that reduces the exposure of patients and the perioperative team to surgical smoke. Policies and procedures assist in the development of patient safety, workplace safety, quality assessment, and performance improvement activities. Policies and procedures also serve as operational guidelines used to minimize patients' and perioperative team members' risk for injury or complications, standardize practice, direct personnel, and establish continuous performance improvement programs. Policies and procedures establish authority, responsibility, and accountability within the practice setting. Having policies and procedures in place that guide and support patient care, treatment, and services is a regulatory requirement.[218-221]

IV.a. Policies and procedures for surgical smoke safety should include

○ evacuating all surgical smoke generated by energy-generating devices (eg, ESUs, lasers, ultrasonic scalpels/dissectors) during operative or other invasive procedures;

○ selecting a smoke evacuation system and supplies (eg, ESU pencils with smoke evacuator tubing, in-line filters, smoke evacuator units) based on the procedure being performed;

○ using a smoke evacuator with a 0.1 μm filter (eg, ULPA filter) or a medical-surgical vacuum system with a 0.1 μm in-line filter in place between the suction wall connection and the suction canister to evacuate small amounts of surgical smoke;

○ positioning the smoke capture device (eg, wand, tubing) as close to the surgical site as necessary to effectively collect surgical smoke;

○ activating the smoke evacuator at all times when surgical smoke is produced during surgical procedures;

○ using a smoke evacuation system during minimally invasive procedures;

○ handling used smoke evacuator filters, tubing, and wands as potentially infectious waste by using standard precautions and disposing of these items as biohazardous waste;

○ wearing respiratory protective equipment as secondary protection against residual surgical smoke;

○ wearing a fit-tested surgical N95 filtering face piece respirator during higher-risk, aerosol-generating procedures and procedures on patients with known or suspected aerosol transmissible diseases (eg, tuberculosis, varicella, rubeola);

○ knowing the criteria (eg, procedure type) for use of a suction tubing with an in-line filter to evacuate a small amount of surgical smoke and the indications to convert to using a smoke evacuator with larger tubing and suction capacity; and

○ meeting education and competency verification requirements.

[5: Benefits Balanced with Harms]

IV.b. The policy should include procedures for reporting instances of health symptoms and effects associated with surgical smoke exposure (eg, reporting to the occupational health department). *[3: Moderate Evidence]*

The potential hazards of surgical smoke exposure to the perioperative team are respiratory, biologic (eg, blood, virus, bacteria), carcinogenic, chemical, cytotoxic, and mutagenic. Repeated exposure to the contents of surgical smoke increases the possibility of developing adverse effects (See Recommendation II.a.) (Table 4).

TABLE 4. HEALTH EFFECTS OF SURGICAL SMOKE EXPOSURE[1]

- Acute and chronic inflammatory respiratory changes (eg, emphysema, asthma, chronic bronchitis)
- Anemia
- Anxiety
- Carcinoma
- Cardiovascular dysfunction
- Colic
- Dermatitis
- Eye irritation
- Headache
- Hepatitis
- HIV
- Hypoxia or dizziness
- Lacrimation
- Leukemia
- Lightheadedness
- Nasopharyngeal lesions
- Nausea or vomiting
- Sneezing
- Throat irritation
- Weakness

REFERENCE
1. Alp E, Bijl D, Bleichrodt RP, Hansson B, Voss A. Surgical smoke and infection control. J Hosp Infect. 2006;62(1):1-5.

From Ulmer BC. The hazards of surgical smoke. AORN J. 2008;87(4): 721-734. Adapted with permission.

At the request of several health care organizations,[42,53,54,56,64] the Hazard Evaluation and Technical Assistance Branch of NIOSH conducted field investigations of possible health hazards associated with surgical smoke in the workplace. At the Laser Institute at the University of Utah Health Sciences Center in Salt Lake City[64]; Inova Fairfax Hospital in Falls Church, Virginia[53]; Morton Plant Hospital in Dunedin, Florida[54]; and Carolinas Medical Center in Charlotte, North Carolina,[56] NIOSH tested the air for chemicals commonly found in surgical smoke and surveyed employees about heath symptoms associated with surgical smoke exposure. At Inova Fairfax Hospital, Morton Plant Hospital, and the Carolinas Medical Center, formaldehyde, acetaldehyde, and toluene were present in the air. The levels of the compounds were below the relevant criteria for occupational exposure.

Of the employees surveyed at the hospitals, the range of at least one symptom associated with surgical smoke exposure was 36% to 52%.

In the hospitals tested, 33% to 46% of the employees described eye and upper respiratory irritation. The National Institute for Occupational Safety and Health recommended that the health care organization's management team implement engineering controls during smoke-producing procedures and that the employees report instances of health symptoms associated with surgical smoke exposure to the organization's occupational health personnel. At the Laser Institute at the University of Utah Health Sciences Center, the investigators found detectable levels of ethanol, isopropanol, anthracene, formaldehyde, cyanide, and airborne mutagenic substances. The National Institute for Occupational Safety and Health recommended the use of smoke evacuators to minimize the potential for health effects and improve visualization of the surgical field.[53,54,56,64]

Ball's[7] research indicated that perioperative nurses report having twice the incidence of some respiratory problems compared to the general population.

Recommendation V

Perioperative personnel should participate in a variety of quality assurance and performance improvement activities that are consistent with the health care organization's plan to improve understanding and compliance with the principles and processes of surgical smoke evacuation.

Quality assurance and performance improvement programs assist in evaluating and improving the quality of patient care and workplace safety and in formulating plans for corrective action. These programs provide data that may be used to determine whether an organization is within its benchmark goals and, if not, to identify areas that may require corrective action.

V.a.   The quality assurance and performance improvement program for surgical smoke safety should include assessment of compliance with surgical smoke evacuation. Compliance indicators include
- surgical smoke is evacuated with a smoke evacuator, a laparoscopic filter, or suction with an in-line filter during all smoke-generating procedures;
- the smoke evacuation capture device is positioned as close as possible to the generation of surgical smoke to effectively collect all traces of the smoke;
- an additional standard suction is used to evacuate fluid;
- smoke evacuation filters are used according to manufacturer's instructions for use (eg, single use, all day);
- perioperative team members wear PPE (eg, gloves) when disposing of contaminated filters and smoke supplies; and
- perioperative team members adhere to policies and procedures for smoke evacuation.

[3: Moderate Evidence]

The evidence indicates there is a lack of compliance with surgical smoke evacuation.[8,32-34,36,37,222] Steege et al[32] conducted a web-based survey of members of professional organizations representing health care occupations in which there is routine contact with selected chemical agents including surgical smoke. Laser surgery and electrosurgery were addressed in separate submodules of the survey. Eligible respondents (N = 4,533) worked within 5 ft of surgical smoke generation during electrosurgery (99%) or laser surgery (31%). The respondents were nurse anesthetists (33%), perioperative nurses (19%), anesthesiologists (21%), surgical technologists (16%), and others (11%). Only 47% of the respondents reported always using local exhaust ventilation during laser procedures and 14% reported always using local exhaust ventilation during electrosurgery. Reasons reported for not using local exhaust ventilation included that it was not provided by the employer, the smoke exposure was minimal, and use of local exhaust ventilation was not part of the facility's protocol. Respondents also wrote in answers in the "other" category, and the majority responded that they did not know why local exhaust ventilation was not used and that they had no control over the decision to use local exhaust ventilation. The authors concluded that the decision to use local exhaust ventilation should not be made at the discretion of an individual practitioner when others (eg, anesthesia personnel, nurses) will be exposed to surgical smoke. The survey results provide a valuable snapshot of existing practices and can be used to raise awareness of surgical smoke controls.

V.a.1.   Smoke evacuation practices should be measured by direct observation. Other measures to evaluate smoke evacuation practices may include product usage or documentation of smoke evacuation in the perioperative patient record. [5: Benefits Balanced with Harms]

V.b.   Barriers to evacuating surgical smoke in the perioperative setting should be identified and addressed through interventions to improve smoke safety practices. [3: Moderate Evidence] Barriers include

- no smoke evacuator available,[223]
- smoke accessories (eg, tubing, laparoscopic filter) not available,
- surgeon refusal to evacuate surgical smoke,[223]
- the smoke evacuator being too noisy,[223]
- the smoke evacuator tubing being too cumbersome,[223]
- evacuation of surgical smoke interfering with the procedure, and
- competency deficits (eg, equipment, use).

Identifying barriers to smoke safety practices allows the health care organization to develop relevant interventions to improve surgical smoke evacuation.

Glossary

Aldehydes: Organic compounds containing the CHO radical. Examples are acetaldehyde and formaldehyde.

Aromatic hydrocarbon: Any of a class of hydrocarbon molecules that have multiple carbon rings and that include carcinogenic substances and environmental pollutants.

Hydrogen cyanide: A poisonous, usually gaseous compound, also known as hydrocyanic acid (HCN), that has the odor of bitter almonds and boils at 25.6° C (78.1° F).

Inorganic gases: Gases that do not contain carbon and hydrogen as the principle elements (eg, carbon monoxide, carbon dioxide, sulphur dioxide, nitrous oxide, nitrogen dioxide).

Laser-generated airborne contaminants: Particles, toxins, and steam produced by vaporization of target tissues.

Lung-damaging dust: Categorization of particles smaller than 5 μm that can penetrate to the deepest areas of the lung and obstruct gas exchange.

Nitrile: An organic compound containing a cyanide group —CN bound to an alkyl group.

Smoke: The visible vapor and gases given off by a burning or smoldering substance, especially of organic origin, made visible by the presence of small particles of carbon.

Surgical smoke: The gaseous products of burning organic material created as a result of the destruction of tissue by lasers, electrosurgical units, ultrasonic devices, power instruments, and other heat-producing surgical tools. Surgical smoke can contain toxic gases and vapors such as benzene, hydrogen cyanide, formaldehyde, bioaerosols, dead and live cellular material including blood fragments, and viruses. At high concentrations, surgical smoke causes ocular and upper respiratory tract irritation in health care workers and creates obstructive visual problems for the surgeon. Surgical smoke has unpleasant odors and has been shown to have mutagenic potential.

Ultra low particulate air (ULPA) filter: Theoretically, an ULPA filter can remove from the air 99.9999% of bacteria, dust, pollen, mold, and particles with a size of 120 nm or larger.

Volatile organic compounds: Carbon-based chemicals that evaporate easily.

REFERENCES

1. Ulmer BC. The hazards of surgical smoke. *AORN J.* 2008;87(4):721-734. [VB]

2. Ott DE. Proposal for a standard for laser plume filter technology. *J Laser Appl.* 1994;6(2):108-110. [IIB]

3. Stephenson DJ, Allcott DA, Koch M. The presence of P22 bacteriophage in electrocautery aerosols. In: *Proceedings of the National Occupational Research Agenda Symposium.* Salt Lake City, UT; 2004. [IIB]

4. Bratu AM, Petrus M, Patachia M, Dumitras DC. Carbon dioxide and water vapors detection from surgical smoke by laser photoacoustic spectroscopy. *UPB*

Scientific Bulletin, Series A: Applied Mathematics and Physics. 2013;75(2):139-146. [IIB]

5. Tomita Y, Mihashi S, Nagata K, et al. Mutagenicity of smoke condensates induced by CO_2-laser irradiation and electrocauterization. *Mutat Res.* 1981;89(2):145-149. [IIB]

6. Safety and Health Topics: Laser/Electrosurgery Plume. Occupational Safety and Health Administration. https://www.osha.gov/SLTC/laserelectrosurgeryplume/. Accessed September 20, 2016. [VA]

7. Ball K. Compliance with surgical smoke evacuation guidelines: implications for practice. *AORN J.* 2010;92(2):142-149. [IIIB]

8. Ball K. Compliance with surgical smoke evacuation guidelines: implications for practice. *ORNAC J.* 2012;30(1):14-16. [IIIB]

9. Calero L, Brusis T. Laryngeal papillomatosis—first recognition in Germany as an occupational disease in an operating room nurse. *Laryngorhinootologie.* 2003;82(11):790-793. [VB]

10. Hallmo P, Naess O. Laryngeal papillomatosis with human papillomavirus DNA contracted by a laser surgeon. *Eur Arch Otorhinolaryngol.* 1991;248(7):425-427. [VB]

11. Rioux M, Garland A, Webster D, Reardon E. HPV positive tonsillar cancer in two laser surgeons: case reports. *J Otolaryngol Head Neck Surg.* 2013;42:54. [VB]

12. Weld KJ, Dryer S, Ames CD, et al. Analysis of surgical smoke produced by various energy-based instruments and effect on laparoscopic visibility. *J Endourol.* 2007;21(3):347-351. [IIB]

13. Khoder WY, Stief CG, Fiedler S, et al. In-vitro investigations on laser-induced smoke generation mimicking the laparoscopic laser surgery purposes. *J Biophotonics.* 2015;8(9):714-722. [IIA]

14. Loukas C, Georgiou E. Smoke detection in endoscopic surgery videos: a first step towards retrieval of semantic events. *Int J Med Robot.* 2015;11(1):80-94. [IIIA]

15. da Silva RD, Sehrt D, Molina WR, Moss J, Park SH, Kim FJ. Significance of surgical plume obstruction during laparoscopy. *JSLS.* 2014;18(3). [VB]

16. Wu JS, Monk T, Luttmann DR, Meininger TA, Soper NJ. Production and systemic absorption of toxic byproducts of tissue combustion during laparoscopic cholecystectomy. *J Gastrointest Surg.* 1998;2(5):399-405. [IIB]

17. Takahashi H, Yamasaki M, Hirota M, et al. Automatic smoke evacuation in laparoscopic surgery: a simplified method for objective evaluation. *Surg Endosc.* 2013;27(8):2980-2987. [IIB]

18. Divilio LT. Improving laparoscopic visibility and safety through smoke evacuation. *Surg Laparosc Endosc.* 1996;6(5):380-384. [VB]

19. Alp E, Bijl D, Bleichrodt RP, Hansson B, Voss A. Surgical smoke and infection control. *J Hosp Infect.* 2006;62(1):1-5. [VB]

20. Barrett WL, Garber SM. Surgical smoke: a review of the literature. *Business Briefing: Global Surgery.* 2004:1-7. [VA]

21. Ansell J, Warren N, Wall P, et al. Electrostatic precipitation is a novel way of maintaining visual field clarity during laparoscopic surgery: a prospective double-blind randomized controlled pilot study. *Surg Endosc.* 2014;28(7):2057-2065. [IB]

22. Wu JS, Luttmann DR, Meininger TA, Soper NJ. Production and systemic absorption of toxic byproducts of tissue combustion during laparoscopic surgery. *Surg Endosc.* 1997;11(11):1075-1079. [IIB]

23. Fletcher JN, Mew D, Descôteaux J-G. Dissemination of melanoma cells within electrocautery plume. *Am J Surg.* 1999;178(1):57-59. [IIB]

24. Ott DE. Carboxyhemoglobinemia due to peritoneal smoke absorption from laser tissue combustion at laparoscopy. *J Clin Laser Med Surg.* 1998;16(6):309-315. [IIB]

25. Esper E, Russell TE, Coy B, Duke BE 3rd, Max MH, Coil JA. Transperitoneal absorption of thermocautery-induced carbon monoxide formation during laparoscopic cholecystectomy. *Surg Laparosc Endosc.* 1994;4(5):333-335. [IIB]

26. Control of smoke from laser/electric surgical procedures. National Institute for Occupational Safety and Health. *Appl Occup Environ Hyg.* 1999;14(2):71.

27. IFPN guideline on risks, hazards, and management of surgical plume. 2015. International Federation of Perioperative Nurses. http://www.ifpn.org.uk/guidelines/Surgical_Plume_-_Risks_Hazards_and_Management.pdf. Accessed September 20, 2016. [IVB]

28. Standard: surgical plume. In: *2014-2015 ACORN Standards for Perioperative Nursing: Including Nurses Roles, Guidelines, Position Statements, Competency Standards.* Adelaide, SA: Australian College of Operating Room Nurses; 2014:149-153. [IVB]

29. *ORNAC Standards for Perioperative Registered Nursing Practice.* 12 ed. Kingston, ON: Operating Room Nurses Association of Canada; 2015. [IVB]

30. *AST Standards of Practice for Use of Electrosurgery.* 2012. Association of Surgical Technologists. http://www.ast.org/uploadedFiles/Main_Site/Content/About_Us/Standard%20Electrosurgery.pdf. Accessed September 20, 2016. [IVB]

31. *AST Standards of Practice for Laser Safety.* 2010. Association of Surgical Technologists. http://www.ast.org/uploadedFiles/Main_Site/Content/About_Us/Standard%20Laser%20Safety.pdf. Accessed September 20, 2016. [IVB]

32. Steege AL, Boiano JM, Sweeney MH. Secondhand smoke in the operating room? Precautionary practices lacking for surgical smoke. *Am J Ind Med.* June 10, 2016. Epub ahead of print. doi: 10.1002/ajim.22614. [IIIA]

33. Steege AL, Boiano JM, Sweeney MH. NIOSH health and safety practices survey of healthcare workers: training and awareness of employer safety procedures. *Am J Ind Med.* 2014;57(6):640-652. [IIIB]

34. Spearman J, Tsavellas G, Nichols P. Current attitudes and practices towards diathermy smoke. *Ann R Coll Surg Engl.* 2007;89(2):162-165. [IIIB]

35. Lopiccolo MC, Balle MR, Kouba DJ. Safety precautions in Mohs micrographic surgery for patients with known blood-borne infections: a survey-based study. *Dermatol Surg.* 2012;38(7 Part 1):1059-1065. [IIIA]

36. Edwards BE, Reiman RE. Comparison of current and past surgical smoke control practices. *AORN J.* 2012;95(3):337-350. [IIIB]

37. Edwards BE, Reiman RE. Results of a survey on current surgical smoke control practices. *AORN J.* 2008;87(4):739-749. [IIIB]

38. PL 91–596. Occupational Safety and Health Act of 1970. December 29, 1970, as amended through January 1, 2004. Occupational Safety and Health Administration. http://www.osha.gov/pls/oshaweb/owadisp.show_document?p_table=OSHACT&p_id=2743. Accessed September 21, 2016.

39. OSHA General Duty Clause. Occupational Safety and Health Administration. https://www.osha.gov/pls/oshaweb/owadisp.show_document?p_table=OSHACT&p_id=3359. Accessed September 21, 2016.

40. US Department of Labor, Occupational Safety and Health Administration, Department of Health and Human Services, Centers for Disease Control and Prevention, National Institute of Occupational Safety and Health. *Hospital Respiratory Protection Program Toolkit: Resources for Respirator Program Administrators.* May 2015. Occupational Safety and Health Administration. https://www.osha.gov/Publications/OSHA3767.pdf. Accessed September 21, 2016. [VA]

41. Eickmann U, Falcy M, Fokuhl I, Rüegger M, Bloch M, Merz B. *Surgical Smoke: Risks and Preventive Measures.* Hamburg, Germany: International Social Security Association Section on Prevention of Occupational Risks in Health Services; 2011. [VA]

42. HHE report no. HETA-85-126-1932. Bryn Mawr Hospital, Bryn Mawr, Pennsylvania. September 1, 1988. National Institute for Occupational Safety and Health. http://www.cdc.gov/niosh/nioshtic-2/00184451.html. Accessed September 21, 2016. [VA]

43. Petrus M, Bratu AM, Patachia M, Dumitras DC. Spectroscopic analysis of surgical smoke produced in vitro by laser vaporization of animal tissues in a closed gaseous environment. *Romanian Reports in Physics.* 2015;67(3):954-965. [IIA]

44. Petrus M, Matei C, Patachia M, Dumitras DC. Quantitative in vitro analysis of surgical smoke by laser photocoustic spectroscopy. *J Optoelectron Adv M.* 2012;14(7-8):664-670. [IIA]

45. Sagar PM, Meagher A, Sobczak S, Wolff BG. Chemical composition and potential hazards of electrocautery smoke. *Br J Surg.* 1996;83(12):1792. [IIB]

46. Weston R, Stephenson RN, Kutarski PW, Parr NJ. Chemical composition of gases surgeons are exposed to during endoscopic urological resections. *Urology.* 2009;74(5):1152-1154. [IIB]

47. Zhao C, Kim MK, Kim HJ, Lee SK, Chung YJ, Park JK. Comparative safety analysis of surgical smoke from transurethral resection of the bladder tumors and transurethral resection of the prostate. *Urology.* 2013;82(3):744.e9-744.e14. [IIB]

48. Bratu AM, Petrus M, Patachia M, et al. Quantitative analysis of laser surgical smoke: targeted study on six toxic compounds. *Rom Journ Phys.* 2015;60(1-2):215-227. [IIA]

49. Lippert JF, Lacey SE, Jones RM. Modeled occupational exposures to gas-phase medical laser-generated air contaminants. *J Occup Environ Hyg.* 2014;11(11):722-727. [IIA]

50. Fitzgerald JE, Malik M, Ahmed I. A single-blind controlled study of electrocautery and ultrasonic scalpel smoke plumes in laparoscopic surgery. *Surg Endosc.* 2012;26(2):337-342. [IIA]

51. Shewale SB, Briggs RD. Gas chromatography-mass spectroscopy analysis of emissions from cement when using ultrasonically driven tools. *Acta Orthopaedica.* 2005;76(5):647-650. [IIB]

52. Dobrogowski M, Wesolowski W, Kucharska M, et al. Health risk to medical personnel of surgical smoke produced during laparoscopic surgery. *Int J Occup Med Environ Health.* 2015;28(5):831-840. [IIIB]

53. NIOSH Health Hazard Evaluation Report: HETA-2000-0402-3021. Inova Fairfax Hospital, Falls Church, Virginia. November 2006. National Institute for Occupational Safety and Health. https://www.cdc.gov/niosh/hhe/reports/pdfs/2000-0402-3021.pdf. Accessed September 21, 2016. [VA]

54. NIOSH Health Hazard Evaluation Report: HETA-2001-0066-3019. Morton Plant Hospital, Dunedin, Florida. October 2006. National Institute for Occupational

Safety and Health. https://www.cdc.gov/niosh/hhe/reports/pdfs/2001-0066-3019.pdf. Accessed September 21, 2016. [VA]

55. Lin YW, Fan SZ, Chang KH, Huang CS, Tang CS. A novel inspection protocol to detect volatile compounds in breast surgery electrocautery smoke. *J Formosan Med Assoc.* 2010;109(7):511-516. [IIIB]

56. NIOSH Health Hazard Evaluation Report: HETA-2001-0030-3020. Carolinas Medical Center, Charlotte, North Carolina. November 2006. National Institute for Occupational Safety and Health. https://www.cdc.gov/niosh/hhe/reports/pdfs/2001-0030-3020.pdf. Accessed September 21, 2016. [VA]

57. Wu YC, Tang CS, Huang HY, et al. Chemical production in electrocautery smoke by a novel predictive model. *Eur Surg Res.* 2011;46(2):102-107. [IIB]

58. Al Sahaf OS, Vega-Carrascal I, Cunningham FO, McGrath JP, Bloomfield FJ. Chemical composition of smoke produced by high-frequency electrosurgery. *Ir J Med Sci.* 2007;176(3):229-232. [IIB]

59. Choi SH, Kwon TG, Chung SK, Kim TH. Surgical smoke may be a biohazard to surgeons performing laparoscopic surgery. *Surg Endosc.* 2014;28(8):2374-2380. [IIB]

60. Krones CJ, Conze J, Hoelzl F, et al. Chemical composition of surgical smoke produced by electrocautery, Harmonic scalpel, and argon beaming—a short study. *Eur Surg.* 2007;39(2):118-121. [IIA]

61. Moot AR, Ledingham KM, Wilson PF, et al. Composition of volatile organic compounds in diathermy plume as detected by selected ion flow tube mass spectrometry. *ANZ J Surg.* 2007;77(1-2):20-23. [IIB]

62. Tseng HS, Liu SP, Uang SN, et al. Cancer risk of incremental exposure to polycyclic aromatic hydrocarbons in electrocautery smoke for mastectomy personnel. *World J Surg Oncol.* 2014;12:31. [IIB]

63. Näslund Andréasson S, Mahteme H, Sahlberg B, Anundi H. Polycyclic aromatic hydrocarbons in electrocautery smoke during peritonectomy procedures. *J Environ Public Health.* 2012;2012:929053. [IIA]

64. HHE report no. HETA-88-101-2008. University of Utah Health Sciences Center, Salt Lake City, Utah. February 1990. National Institute for Occupational Health and Safety. https://www.cdc.gov/niosh/hhe/reports/pdfs/1988-0101-2008.pdf. Accessed September 21, 2016. [VA]

65. Beebe DS, Swica H, Carlson N, Palahniuk RJ, Goodale RL. High levels of carbon monoxide are produced by electro-cautery of tissue during laparoscopic cholecystectomy. *Anesth Analg.* 1993;77(2):338-341. [IIB]

66. Fan JK, Chan FS, Chu KM. Surgical smoke. *Asian J Surg.* 2009;32(4):253-257. [VA]

67. Andréasson SN, Anundi H, Sahlberg B, et al. Peritonectomy with high voltage electrocautery generates higher levels of ultrafine smoke particles. *Eur J Surg Oncol.* 2009;35(7):780-784. [IIB]

68. Taravella MJ, Viega J, Luiszer F, et al. Respirable particles in the excimer laser plume. *J Cataract Refract Surg.* 2001;27(4):604-607. [IIB]

69. Pierce JS, Lacey SE, Lippert JF, Lopez R, Franke JE. Laser-generated air contaminants from medical laser applications: a state-of-the-science review of exposure characterization, health effects, and control. *J Occup Environ Hyg.* 2011;8(7):447-466. [VB]

70. Bruske-Hohlfeld I, Preissler G, Jauch KW, et al. Surgical smoke and ultrafine particles. *J Occup Med Toxicol.* 2008;3:31. [IIB]

71. DesCoteaux JG, Picard P, Poulin EC, Baril M. Preliminary study of electrocautery smoke particles produced

in vitro and during laparoscopic procedures. *Surg Endosc.* 1996;10(2):152-158. [IIB]

72. Farrugia M, Hussain SY, Perrett D. Particulate matter generated during monopolar and bipolar hysteroscopic human uterine tissue vaporization. *J Minim Invasive Gynecol.* 2009;16(4):458-464. [IIA]

73. Wang HK, Mo F, Ma CG, et al. Evaluation of fine particles in surgical smoke from an urologist's operating room by time and by distance. *Int Urol Nephrol.* 2015;47(10):1671-1678. [IIB]

74. Lopez R, Lacey SE, Jones RM. Application of a two-zone model to estimate medical laser-generated particulate matter exposures. *J Occup Environ Hyg.* 2015;12(5):309-313. [IIB]

75. Lopez R, Lacey SE, Lippert JF, Liu LC, Esmen NA, Conroy LM. Characterization of size-specific particulate matter emission rates for a simulated medical laser procedure—a pilot study. *Ann Occup Hyg.* 2015;59(4):514-524. [IIIA]

76. Benson SM, Novak DA, Ogg MJ. Proper use of surgical N95 respirators and surgical masks in the OR. *AORN J.* 2013;97(4):457-467. [VA]

77. Ragde SF, Jorgensen RB, Foreland S. Characterisation of exposure to ultrafine particles from surgical smoke by use of a fast mobility particle sizer. *Ann Occup Hyg.* 2016;60(7):860-874. [IIIA]

78. Brace MD, Stevens E, Taylor SM, et al. "The air that we breathe": assessment of laser and electrosurgical dissection devices on operating theater air quality. *J Otolaryngol Head Neck Surg.* 2014;43(1):39-57. [IIA]

79. Norris BK, Goodier AP, Eby TL. Assessment of air quality during mastoidectomy. *Otolaryngol Head Neck Surg.* 2011;144(3):408-411. [IIB]

80. Ziegler BL, Thomas CA, Meier T, Müller R, Fliedner TM, Weber L. Generation of infectious retrovirus aerosol through medical laser irradiation. *Lasers Surg Med.* 1998;22(1):37-41. [IIB]

81. Garden JM, Kerry O'Banion M, Bakus AD, Olson C. Viral disease transmitted by laser-generated plume (aerosol). *Arch Dermatol.* 2002;138(10):1303-1307. [IIB]

82. Price JA, Yamanashi W, McGee JM. Bacteriophage phi X-174 as an aerobiological marker for surgical plume generated by the electromagnetic field focusing system. *J Hosp Infect.* 1992;21(1):39-50. [IIB]

83. Matchette LS, Faaland RW, Royston DD, Ediger MN. In vitro production of viable bacteriophage in carbon dioxide and argon laser plumes. *Lasers Surg Med.* 1991;11(4):380-384. [IIB]

84. Matchette LS, Vegella TJ, Faaland RW. Viable bacteriophage in CO2 laser plume: aerodynamic size distribution. *Lasers Surg Med.* 1993;13(1):18-22. [IIB]

85. Taravella MJ, Weinberg A, May M, Stepp P. Live virus survives excimer laser ablation. *Ophthalmology.* 1999;106(8):1498-1499. [IIB]

86. Ediger MN, Matchette LS. In vitro production of viable bacteriophage in a laser plume. *Lasers Surg Med.* 1989;9(3):296-299. [IIB]

87. Mellor G, Hutchinson M. Is it time for a more systematic approach to the hazards of surgical smoke?: reconsidering the evidence. *Workplace Health Saf.* 2013;61(6):265-270. [IIA]

88. Sood AK, Bahrani-Mostafavi Z, Stoerker J, Stone IK. Human papillomavirus DNA in LEEP plume. *Infect Dis Obstet Gynecol.* 1994;2(4):167-170. [IIB]

89. Andre P, Orth G, Evenou P, Guillaume JC, Avril MF. Risk of papillomavirus infection in carbon dioxide laser treatment of genital lesions. *J Am Acad Dermatol.* 1990;22(1):131-132. [IIB]

90. Ferenczy A, Bergeron C, Richart RM. Carbon dioxide laser energy disperses human papillomavirus deoxyribonucleic acid onto treatment fields. *Am J Obstet Gynecol.* 1990;163(4 Part 1):1271-1274. [IIB]

91. Ferenczy A, Bergeron C, Richart RM. Human papillomavirus DNA in CO2 laser-generated plume of smoke and its consequences to the surgeon. *Obstet Gynecol.* 1990;75(1):114-118. [IIB]

92. Kashima HK, Kessis T, Mounts P, Shah K. Polymerase chain reaction identification of human papillomavirus DNA in CO_2 laser plume from recurrent respiratory papillomatosis. *Otolaryngol Head Neck Surg.* 1991;104(2):191-195. [IIB]

93. Sawchuk WS, Weber PJ, Lowy DR, Dzubow LM. Infectious papillomavirus in the vapor of warts treated with carbon dioxide laser or electrocoagulation: detection and protection. *J Am Acad Dermatol.* 1989;21(1):41-49. [IIB]

94. Garden JM, O'Banion MK, Shelnitz LS, et al. Papillomavirus in the vapor of carbon dioxide laser-treated verrucae. *JAMA.* 1988;259(8):1199-1202. [IIB]

95. Weyandt GH, Tollmann F, Kristen P, Weissbrich B. Low risk of contamination with human papilloma virus during treatment of condylomata acuminata with multilayer argon plasma coagulation and CO_2 laser ablation. *Arch Dermatol Res.* 2011;303(2):141-144. [IIB]

96. Baggish MS, Poiesz BJ, Joret D, Williamson P, Refai A. Presence of human immunodeficiency virus DNA in laser smoke. *Lasers Surg Med.* 1991;11(3):197-203. [IIA]

97. Johnson GK, Robinson WS. Human immunodeficiency virus-1 (HIV-1) in the vapors of surgical power instruments. *J Med Virol.* 1991;33(1):47-50. [IIA]

98. Capizzi PJ, Clay RP, Battey MJ. Microbiologic activity in laser resurfacing plume and debris. *Lasers Surg Med.* 1998;23(3):172-174. [IIC]

99. McKinley IB Jr, Ludlow MO. Hazards of laser smoke during endodontic therapy. *J Endod.* 1994;20(11):558-559. [IIIB]

100. Nogler M, Lass-Florl C, Wimmer C, Mayr E, Bach C, Ogon M. Contamination during removal of cement in revision hip arthroplasty. A cadaver study using ultrasound and high-speed cutters. *J Bone Joint Surg Br.* 2003;85(3):436-439. [IIA]

101. Rautemaa R, Nordberg A, Wuolijoki-Saaristo K, Meurman JH. Bacterial aerosols in dental practice—a potential hospital infection problem? *J Hosp Infect.* 2006;64(1):76-81. [IIIC]

102. Cukier J, Price MF, Gentry LO. Suction lipoplasty: biohazardous aerosols and exhaust mist—the clouded issue. *Plast Reconstr Surg.* 1989;83(3):494-497. [IIB]

103. Schultz L. Can efficient smoke evacuation limit aerosolization of bacteria? *AORN J.* 2015;102(1):7-14. [IIB]

104. Lewin JM, Brauer JA, Ostad A. Surgical smoke and the dermatologist. *J Am Acad Dermatol.* 2011;65(3):636-641. [VB]

105. Ishihama K, Sumioka S, Sakurada K, Kogo M. Floating aerial blood mists in the operating room. *J Hazard Mater.* 2010;181(1-3):1179-1181. [IIC]

106. Ishihama K, Koizumi H, Wada T, et al. Evidence of aerosolised floating blood mist during oral surgery. *J Hosp Infect.* 2009;71(4):359-364. [IIB]

107. Jewett DL, Heinsohn P, Bennett C, Rosen A, Neuilly C. Blood-containing aerosols generated by surgical techniques: a possible infectious hazard. *Am Ind Hyg Assoc J.* 1992;53(4):228-231. [IIB]

108. Champault G, Taffinder N, Ziol M, Riskalla H, Catheline JM. Cells are present in the smoke created during laparoscopic surgery. *Br J Surg.* 1997;84(7):993-995. [IIB]

109. Collins D, Rice J, Nicholson P, Barry K. Quantification of facial contamination with blood during orthopaedic procedures. *J Hosp Infect.* 2000;45(1):73-75. [IIC]

110. Ott DE, Moss E, Martinez K. Aerosol exposure from an ultrasonically activated (Harmonic) device. *J Am Assoc Gynecol Laparosc.* 1998;5(1):29-32. [IIB]

111. In SM, Park DY, Sohn IK, et al. Experimental study of the potential hazards of surgical smoke from powered instruments. *Br J Surg.* 2015;102(12):1581-1586. [IIA]

112. Mowbray N, Ansell J, Warren N, Wall P, Torkington J. Is surgical smoke harmful to theater staff? A systematic review. *Surg Endosc.* 2013;27(9):3100-3107. [IIIA]

113. Nahhas WA. A potential hazard of the use of the surgical ultrasonic aspirator in tumor reductive surgery. *Gynecol Oncol.* 1991;40(1):81-83. [VA]

114. Pierce JS, Lacey SE, Lippert JF, Lopez R, Franke JE, Colvard MD. An assessment of the occupational hazards related to medical lasers. *J Occup Environ Med.* 2011;53(11):1302-1309. [VB]

115. Control of Smoke from Laser/Electric Surgical Procedures (DHHS [NIOSH] Pub No 96-128). National Institute for Occupational Safety and Health. http://www.cdc.gov/niosh/docs/hazardcontrol/hc11.html. Accessed September 21, 2016. [IVB]

116. Chung YJ, Lee SK, Han SH, et al. Harmful gases including carcinogens produced during transurethral resection of the prostate and vaporization. *Int J Urol.* 2010;17(11):944-949. [IIB]

117. Park SC, Lee SK, Han SH, Chung YJ, Park JK. Comparison of harmful gases produced during Green-Light High-Performance System laser prostatectomy and transurethral resection of the prostate. *Urology.* 2012;79(5):1118-1124. [IIB]

118. Rey JM, Schramm D, Hahnloser D, Marinov D, Sigrist MW. Spectroscopic investigation of volatile compounds produced during thermal and radiofrequency bipolar cautery on porcine liver. *Meas Sci Technol.* 2008;19(7):075602. [IIB]

119. Hollmann R, Hort CE, Kammer E, Naegele M, Sigrist MW, Meuli-Simmen C. Smoke in the operating theater: an unregarded source of danger. *Plast Reconstr Surg.* 2004;114(2):458-463. [IIB]

120. Gianella M, Hahnloser D, Rey JM, Sigrist MW. Quantitative chemical analysis of surgical smoke generated during laparoscopic surgery with a vessel-sealing device. *Surg Innov.* 2014;21(2):170-179. [IIB]

121. Gianella M, Sigrist MW. Infrared spectroscopy on smoke produced by cauterization of animal tissue. *Sensors.* 2010;10(4):2694-2708. [IIB]

122. Lindsey C, Hutchinson M, Mellor G. The nature and hazards of diathermy plumes: a review. *AORN J.* 2015;101(4):428-442. [IIIB]

123. Okoshi K, Kobayashi K, Kinoshita K, Tomizawa Y, Hasegawa S, Sakai Y. Health risks associated with exposure to surgical smoke for surgeons and operation room personnel. *Surg Today.* 2015;45(8):957-965. [VB]

124. Bergbrant IM, Samuelsson L, Olofsson S, Jonassen F, Ricksten A. Polymerase chain reaction for monitoring human papillomavirus contamination of medical personnel during treatment of genital warts with CO_2 laser and electrocoagulation. *Acta Derm Venereol.* 1994;74(5):393-395. [IIIB]

125. Abramson AL, DiLorenzo TP, Steinberg BM. Is papillomavirus detectable in the plume of laser-treated laryngeal papilloma? *Arch Otolaryngol Head Neck Surg.* 1990;116(5):604-607. [IIB]

126. Hughes PS, Hughes AP. Absence of human papillomavirus DNA in the plume of erbium:YAG laser-treated warts. *J Am Acad Dermatol.* 1998;38(3):426-428. [IIB]

127. Kunachak S, Sithisarn P, Kulapaditharom B. Are laryngeal papilloma virus-infected cells viable in the plume derived from a continuous mode carbon dioxide laser, and are they infectious? A preliminary report on one laser mode. *J Laryngol Otol.* 1996;110(11):1031-1033. [IIB]

128. Guideline: Work Health and Safety—Controlling Exposure to Surgical Plume (Document Number GL2015_002). January 19, 2015. New South Wales Ministry of Health. http://www0.health.nsw.gov.au/policies/gl/2015/pdf/GL2015_002.pdf. Accessed September 21, 2016.

129. Guideline for a Safe Environment of Care, Part 2. In: *Guidelines for Perioperative Practice.* Denver, CO: AORN, Inc; 2016:263-288. [IVA]

130. *Z305.13-13: Plume Scavenging in Surgical, Diagnostic, Therapeutic, and Aesthetic Settings.* Toronto, ON: Canadian Standards Association; 2013.

131. Safety and Health Management Systems eTool. Occupational Safety and Health Administration. https://www.osha.gov/SLTC/etools/safetyhealth/comp3.html. Accessed September 21, 2016. [VA]

132. American National Standards Institute. Laser Institute of America. *American National Standard for Safe Use of Lasers in Health Care.* Orlando, FL: Laser Institute of America; 2011. [IVB]

133. American Association of Physics in Medicine, American College of Medical Physics. *Medical Lasers: Quality Control, Safety Standards, and Regulations.* Joint Report Task Group No 6. Madison, WI: Medical Physics Publishing; 2001. [IVB]

134. Guidelines for Preventing the Transmission of Mycobacterium tuberculosis in Health-Care Settings, 2005. Centers for Disease Control and Prevention. http://www.cdc.gov/mmwr/preview/mmwrhtml/rr5417a1.htm. Accessed September 21, 2016. [IVA]

135. Respirator Trusted-Source Information. The National Personal Protective Technology Laboratory. http://www.cdc.gov/niosh/npptl/topics/respirators/disp_part/respsource.html. Accessed September 21, 2016. [IVB]

136. Rengasamy S, Miller A, Eimer BC, Shaffer RE. Filtration performance of FDA-cleared surgical masks. *J Int Soc Respir Prot.* 2009;26:54-70. [IIB]

137. Gao S, Koehler RH, Yermakov M, Grinshpun SA. Performance of facepiece respirators and surgical masks against surgical smoke: simulated workplace protection factor study. *Ann Occup Hyg.* 2016;60(5):608-618. [IIIA]

138. Davidson C, Green CF, Panlilio AL, et al. Method for evaluating the relative efficiency of selected N95 respirators and surgical masks to prevent the inhalation of airborne vegetative cells by healthcare personnel. *Indoor and Built Environment.* 2011;20(2):265-277. [IIB]

139. Derrick JL, Li PT, Tang SP, Gomersall CD. Protecting staff against airborne viral particles: in vivo efficiency of laser masks. *J Hosp Infect.* 2006;64(3):278-281. [IIA]

140. Eninger RM, Honda T, Adhikari A, Heinonen-Tanski H, Reponen T, Grinshpun SA. Filter performance of N99 and N95 facepiece respirators against viruses and ultrafine particles. *Ann Occup Hyg.* 2008;52(5):385-396. [IIB]

141. Redmayne AC, Wake D, Brown RC, Crook B. Measurement of the degree of protection afforded by respiratory protective equipment against microbiological aerosols. *Ann Occup Hyg.* 1997;41(Suppl 1):636-640. [IIB]

142. Chen CC, Willeke K. Aerosol penetration through surgical masks. *Am J Infect Control.* 1992;20(4):177-184. [IIB]

143. Weber A, Willeke K, Marchioni R, et al. Aerosol penetration and leakage characteristics of masks

used in the health care industry. *Am J Infect Control.* 1993;21(4):167-173. [IIB]

144. Nezhat C, Winer WK, Nezhat F, Nezhat C, Forrest D, Reeves WG. Smoke from laser surgery: is there a health hazard? *Lasers Surg Med.* 1987;7(4):376-382. [IIIB]

145. Kunachak S, Sobhon P. The potential alveolar hazard of carbon dioxide laser-induced smoke. *J Med Assoc Thai.* 1998;81(4):278-282. [IIB]

146. Gatti JE, Bryant CJ, Noone RB, Murphy JB. The mutagenicity of electrocautery smoke. *Plast Reconstr Surg.* 1992;89(5):781-784. [IIB]

147. Barrett WL, Garber SM. Surgical smoke: a review of the literature. Is this just a lot of hot air? *Surg Endosc.* 2003;17(6):979-987. [VA]

148. Oberg T, Brosseau LM. Surgical mask filter and fit performance. *Am J Infect Control.* 2008;36(4):276-282. [IIB]

149. Chen SK, Vesley D, Brosseau LM, Vincent JH. Evaluation of single-use masks and respirators for protection of health care workers against mycobacterial aerosols. *Am J Infect Control.* 1994;22(2):65-74. [IIB]

150. Hassan I, Drelichman ER, Wolff BG, Ruiz C, Sobczak SC, Larson DW. Exposure to electrocautery toxins: understanding a potential occupational hazard. *Prof Saf.* 2006;51(4):38-41. [IIB]

151. Wenig BL, Stenson KM, Wenig BW, Tracey D. Effects of plume produced by the Nd:YAG laser and electrocautery on the respiratory system. *Lasers Surg Med.* 1993;13(2):242-245. [IIB]

152. Baggish MS, Elbakry M. The effects of laser smoke on the lungs of rats. *Am J Obstet Gynecol.* 1987;156(5):1260-1265. [IIA]

153. Baggish MS, Baltoyannis P, Sze E. Protection of the rat lung from the harmful effects of laser smoke. *Lasers Surg Med.* 1988;8(3):248-253. [IIB]

154. Hill DS, O'Neill JK, Powell RJ, Oliver DW. Surgical smoke—a health hazard in the operating theatre: a study to quantify exposure and a survey of the use of smoke extractor systems in UK plastic surgery units. *J Plast Reconstr Aesthet Surg.* 2012;65(7):911-916. [IIB]

155. Wollmer W. Problems caused by laser plume, especially considering laser microlaryngoscopy. *Adv Otorhinolaryngol.* 1995;49:20-22. [VB]

156. Hou M-F, Lin G-T, Tang C-S, et al. Reducing dust using the electrocautery pencil with suction combined with the infusion catheter in mastectomy. *Am Surg.* 2002;68(9):808-811. [IB]

157. Hubner M, Sigrist MW, Demartines N, Gianella M, Clavien PA, Hahnloser D. Gas emission during laparoscopic colorectal surgery using a bipolar vessel sealing device: a pilot study on four patients. *Patient Saf Surg.* 2008;2:22. [IIB]

158. Janda P, Leunig A, Sroka R, Betz CS, Rasp G. Preliminary report of endolaryngeal and endotracheal laser surgery of juvenile-onset recurrent respiratory papillomatosis by Nd:YAG laser and a new fiber guidance instrument. *Otolaryngol Head Neck Surg.* 2004;131(1):44-49. [IIB]

159. Khajuria A, Maruthappu M, Nagendran M, Shalhoub J. What about the surgeon? *Int J Surg.* 2013;11(1):18-21. [VB]

160. OSH Answers Fact Sheets: Laser Plumes—Health Care Facilities. Canadian Center for Occupational Health and Safety. https://www.ccohs.ca/oshanswers/phys_agents/laser_plume.html. Accessed September 21, 2016. [VB]

161. Mattes D, Silajdzic E, Mayer M, et al. Surgical smoke management for minimally invasive (micro) endoscopy: an experimental study. *Surg Endosc.* 2010;24(10):2492-2501. [IIB]

162. Pillinger SH, Delbridge L, Lewis DR. Randomized clinical trial of suction versus standard clearance of the diathermy plume. *Br J Surg.* 2003;90(9):1068-1071. [IB]

163. Makama GJ, Ameh EA. Hazards of surgical diathermy. *Niger J Med.* 2007;16(4):295-300. [VB]

164. Nori S, Greene MA, Schrager HM, Falanga V. Infectious occupational exposures in dermatology—a review of risks and prevention measures: I. For all dermatologists. *J Am Acad Dermatol.* 2005;53(6):1010-1019. [VA]

165. Freitag L, Chapman GA, Sielczak M, Ahmed A, Russin D. Laser smoke effect on the bronchial system. *Lasers Surg Med.* 1987;7(3):283-288. [IIB]

166. Guidelines for Environmental Infection Control in Health-Care Facilities. Atlanta, GA: US Department of Health and Human Services, Centers for Disease Control and Prevention; 2003. http://www.cdc.gov/hicpac/pdf/guidelines/eic_in_hcf_03.pdf. Accessed September 21, 2016. [IVA]

167. Charles K. Effects of laser plume evacuation on laser in situ keratomileusis outcomes. *J Refract Surg.* 2002;18(3 Suppl):S340-S342. [IIIB]

168. Born H, Ivey C. How should we safely handle surgical smoke? *Laryngoscope.* 2014;124(10):2213-2215. [VB]

169. Sanderson C. Surgical smoke. *J Perioper Pract.* 2012;22(4):122-128. [VB]

170. O'Grady KF, Easty AC. Electrosurgery smoke: hazards and protection. *J Clin Eng.* 1996;21(2):149-155. [VB]

171. Fader DJ, Ratner D. Principles of CO2/erbium laser safety. *Dermatol Surg.* 2000;26(3):235-239. [VB]

172. Bargman H. Laser-generated airborne contaminants. *J Clin Aesthet Dermatol.* 2011;4(2):56-57. [VC]

173. Gates MA, Feskanich D, Speizer FE, Hankinson SE. Operating room nursing and lung cancer risk in a cohort of female registered nurses. *Scand J Work Environ Health.* 2007;33(2):140-147. [IIIA]

174. Voorhies RM, Lavyne MH, Strait TA, Shapiro WR. Does the CO2 laser spread viable brain-tumor cells outside the surgical field? *J Neurosurg.* 1984;60(4):819-820. [IIB]

175. Oosterhuis JW, Verschueren RC, Eibergen R, Oldhoff J. The viability of cells in the waste products of CO2-laser evaporation of Cloudman mouse melanomas. *Cancer.* 1982;49(1):61-67. [IIB]

176. Stocker B, Meier T, Fliedner TM, Plappert U. Laser pyrolysis products: sampling procedures, cytotoxic and genotoxic effects. *Mutat Res.* 1998;412(2):145-154. [IIA]

177. Plappert UG, Stocker B, Helbig R, Fliedner TM, Seidel HJ. Laser pyrolysis products-genotoxic, clastogenic and mutagenic effects of the particulate aerosol fractions. *Mutat Res.* 1999;441(1): 29-41. [IIA]

178. Hensman C, Baty D, Willis RG, Cuschieri A. Chemical composition of smoke produced by high-frequency electrosurgery in a closed gaseous environment: an in vitro study. *Surg Endosc.* 1998;12(8):1017-1019. [IIB]

179. Hensman C, Newman EL, Shimi SM, Cuschieri A. Cytotoxicity of electro-surgical smoke produced in an anoxic environment. *Am J Surg.* 1998;175(3):240-241. [IIB]

180. Gonzalez-Bayon L, Gonzalez-Moreno S, Ortega-Perez G. Safety considerations for operating room personnel during hyperthermic intraoperative intraperitoneal chemotherapy perfusion. *Eur J Surg Oncol.* 2006;32(6):619-624. [VA]

181. Wisniewski PM, Warhol MJ, Rando RF, Sedlacek TV, Kemp JE, Fisher JC. Studies on the transmission of viral disease via the CO2 laser plume and ejecta. *J Reprod Med.* 1990;35(12):1117-1123. [IIB]

182. Ilmarinen T, Auvinen E, Hiltunen-Back E, Ranki A, Aaltonen L-M, Pitkäranta A. Transmission of human papillomavirus DNA from patient to surgical masks, gloves and oral mucosa of medical personnel during treatment of laryngeal papillomas and genital warts. *Eur Arch Otorhinolaryngol.* 2012;269(11):2367-2371. [IIB]

183. Kofoed K, Norrbom C, Forslund O, et al. Low prevalence of oral and nasal human papillomavirus in employees performing CO_2-laser evaporation of genital warts or loop electrode excision procedure of cervical dysplasia. *Acta Derm Venereol.* 2015;95(2):173-176. [IIIB]

184. Gloster HM Jr, Roenigk RK. Risk of acquiring human papillomavirus from the plume produced by the carbon dioxide laser in the treatment of warts. *J Am Acad Dermatol.* 1995;32(3):436-441. [IIIB]

185. Manson LT, Damrose EJ. Does exposure to laser plume place the surgeon at high risk for acquiring clinical human papillomavirus infection? *Laryngoscope.* 2013;123(6):1319-1320. [VB]

186. Taravella MJ, Weinberg A, Blackburn P, May M. Do intact viral particles survive excimer laser ablation? *Arch Ophthalmol.* 1997;115(8):1028-1030. [IIB]

187. Hagen KB, Kettering JD, Aprecio RM, Beltran F, Maloney RK. Lack of virus transmission by the excimer laser plume. *Am J Ophthalmol.* 1997;124(2):206-211. [IIB]

188. *Smoke Evacuation Systems, Surgical.* Plymouth Meeting, PA: ECRI Institute; 2015. [VA]

189. Smith JP, Topmiller JL, Shulman S. Factors affecting emission collection by surgical smoke evacuators. *Lasers Surg Med.* 1990;10(3):224-233. [IIB]

190. Smith JP, Moss CE, Bryant CJ, Fleeger AK. Evaluation of a smoke evacuator used for laser surgery. *Lasers Surg Med.* 1989;9(3):276-281. [IIB]

191. ECRI. Surgical smoke evacuation systems. *Healthcare Risk Control.* 2000;4(Surgery and Anesthesia 17.1):1-7. [VA]

192. Watson DS. Surgical smoke evacuation during laparoscopic surgery. *AORN J.* 2010;92(3):347-350. [VB]

193. Ott D. Smoke production and smoke reduction in endoscopic surgery: preliminary report. *Endosc Surg Allied Technol.* 1993;1(4):230-232. [IIB]

194. Nezhat C, Seidman DS, Vreman HJ, Stevenson DK, Nezhat F, Nezhat C. The risk of carbon monoxide poisoning after prolonged laparoscopic surgery. *Obstet Gynecol.* 1996;88(5):771-774. [IIB]

195. Ulmer BC. Best practices for minimally invasive procedures. *AORN J.* 2010;91(5):558-575. [VB]

196. Dobrogowski M, Wesolowski W, Kucharska M, Sapota A, Pomorski LS. Chemical composition of surgical smoke formed in the abdominal cavity during laparoscopic cholecystectomy—assessment of the risk to the patient. *Int J Occup Med Environ Health.* 2014;27(2):314-325. [IIIB]

197. Bigony L. Risks associated with exposure to surgical smoke plume: a review of the literature. *AORN J.* 2007;86(6):1013-1020. [VA]

198. 29 CFR §1910.1030: Bloodborne Pathogens. Occupational Safety and Health Administration. http://www.osha.gov/pls/oshaweb/owadisp.show_document?p_table=STANDARDS&p_id=10051. Accessed September 21, 2016.

199. Standards of perioperative nursing practice. In: *Guidelines for Perioperative Practice.* Denver, CO: AORN, Inc; 2015:693-708. [IVB]

200. Scott H, Mustard P, Cooper H, Hayde C. Development of a plume evacuation policy—a health and safety issue. *Dissector.* 2014;41(4):10-14. [VB]

201. Edelman DS, Unger SW. Bipolar versus monopolar cautery scissors for laparoscopic cholecystectomy: a randomized, prospective study. *Surg Laparosc Endosc.* 1995;5(6):459-462. [IB]

202. Kim FJ, Sehrt D, Pompeo A, Molina WR. Laminar and turbulent surgical plume characteristics generated from curved- and straight-blade laparoscopic ultrasonic dissectors. *Surg Endosc.* 2014;28(5):1674-1677. [IIB]

203. Kim FJ, Sehrt D, Pompeo A, Molina WR. Comparison of surgical plume among laparoscopic ultrasonic dissectors using a real-time digital quantitative technology. *Surg Endosc.* 2012;26(12):3408-3412. [IIA]

204. Sherman JA, Davies HT. Ultracision: the Harmonic scalpel and its possible uses in maxillofacial surgery. *Br J Oral Maxillofac Surg.* 2000;38(5):530-532. [VC]

205. Shabbir A, Dargan D. Advancement and benefit of energy sealing in minimally invasive surgery. *Asian J Endosc Surg.* 2014;7(2):95-101. [VA]

206. Schneider A, Doundoulakis E, Can S, Fiolka A, Wilhelm D, Feuner H. Evaluation of mist production and tissue dissection efficiency using different types of ultrasound shears. *Surg Endosc.* 2009;23(12): 2822-2826. [IIB]

207. Devassy R, Gopalakrishnan S, De Wilde RL. Surgical efficacy among laparoscopic ultrasonic dissectors: are we advancing safely? A review of literature. *J Obstet Gynecol India.* 2015;65(5):293-300. [VA]

208. Bui MH, Breda A, Gui D, Said J, Schulam P. Less smoke and minimal tissue carbonization using a thulium laser for laparoscopic partial nephrectomy without hilar clamping in a porcine model. *J Endourol.* 2007;21(9):1107-1111. [IIB]

209. Kisch T, Liodaki E, Kraemer R, et al. Electrocautery devices with feedback mode and Teflon-coated blades create less surgical smoke for a quality improvement in the operating theater. *Medicine (United States).* 2015;94(27):e1104. [IIB]

210. Wagner JA, Bodendorf MO, Grunewald S, Simon JC, Paasch U. Circular directed suction technique for ablative laser treatments. *Dermatol Surg.* 2013;39(8):1184-1189. [IIB]

211. Liang JH, Pan YL, Kang J, Qi J. Influence of irrigation on incision and coagulation of 2.0-μm continuous-wave laser: an ex vivo study. *Surg Laparosc, Endosc Percutan Tech.* 2012;22(3):e122-e125. [IIB]

212. Liang J-H, Xu C-L, Wang L-H, Hou J-G, Gao X-F, Sun Y-H. Irrigation eliminates smoke formation in laser laparoscopic surgery: ex vivo results. *Surg Laparosc Endosc Percutan Tech.* 2008;18(4):391-394. [IIB]

213. Nicholson G, Knol J, Houben B, Cunningham C, Ashraf S, Hompes R. Optimal dissection for transanal total mesorectal excision using modified CO2 insufflation and smoke extraction. *Colorectal Dis.* 2015;17(11):O265-O267. [VB]

214. Vavricka SR, Tutuian R, Imhof A, et al. Air suctioning during colon biopsy forceps removal reduces bacterial air contamination in the endoscopy suite. *Endoscopy.* 2010;42(9):736-741. [IB]

215. Schultz L. An analysis of surgical smoke plume components, capture, and evacuation. *AORN J.* 2014;99(2):289-298. [VB]

216. Jordan C, Thomas MB, Evans ML, Green A. Public policy on competency: how will nursing address this complex issue? *J Contin Educ Nurs.* 2008;39(2):86-91. [VA]

217. Nicola JH, Nicola EMD, Vieira R, Braile DM, Tanabe MM, Baldin DHZ. Speed of particles ejected from animal skin by CO2 laser pulses, measured by laser Doppler velocimetry. *Phys Med Biol.* 2002;47(5):847-856. [IIA]

218. 42 CFR §482. Conditions of participation for hospitals. Centers for Medicare & Medicaid Services. Department of Health and Human Services. https://www.gpo.

gov/fdsys/granule/CFR-2011-title42-vol5/CFR-2011-title42-vol5-part482/content-detail.html. Accessed September 21, 2016.

219. 42 CFR §416. Ambulatory surgical services. Centers for Medicare & Medicaid Services. Department of Health and Human Services. https://www.cms.gov/Regulations-and-Guidance/Legislation/CFCsAndCoPs/ASC.html. Accessed September 21, 2016.

220. State Operations Manual Appendix A: Survey Protocol, Regulations and Interpretive Guidelines for Hospitals. Rev 151; 2015. Centers for Medicare & Medicaid Services. https://www.cms.gov/Regulations-and-Guidance/Guidance/Manuals/downloads/som107ap_a_hospitals.pdf. Accessed September 21, 2016.

221. State Operations Manual Appendix L: Guidance for Surveyors: Ambulatory Surgical Centers. Rev 137; 2015. Centers for Medicare & Medicaid Services. https://www.cms.gov/Regulations-and-Guidance/Guidance/Manuals/downloads/som107ap_l_ambulatory.pdf. Accessed September 21, 2016.

222. Oganesyan G, Eimpunth S, Kim SS, Jiang SI. Surgical smoke in dermatologic surgery. *Dermatol Surg.* 2014;40(12):1373-1377. [IIIB]

223. Ball K. Surgical smoke evacuation guidelines: compliance among perioperative nurses. *AORN J.* 2010;92(2):e1-e23. [IIIB]

Acknowledgements

LEAD AUTHOR
Mary J. Ogg, MSN, RN, CNOR
Senior Perioperative Practice Specialist
AORN Nursing Department
Denver, Colorado

The author and AORN thank Brenda Ulmer, MSN, RN, CNOR, Consultant, Snellville, Georgia; Debra A. Novak, PhD, RN, Senior Service Fellow, National Personal Protective Technology Lab, NIOSH, CDC, Pittsburgh, Pennsylvania; Melanie Sandoval, PhD, RN, ACNP, Assistant Professor of Research, University of Colorado-Denver, School of Medicine, Aurora; Lisa Spruce, DNP, RN, CNS-CP, CNOR, ACNS, ACNP, FAAN, Director, Evidence-based Perioperative Practice, Denver, Colorado; Jocelyn M. Chalquist, BSN, RN, CNOR, Surgical Services Educator, Aurora Medical Center, Kenosha, Wisconsin; Michelle R. Dempsey-Evans, MSN, RN, CNOR, CRCST, Orthopaedic Program Coordinator, Bon Secours Mary Immaculate Hospital, Newport News, Virginia; and Nathalie Walker, MBA, RN, CNOR, Louisiana Nursing Supply and Demand Center, Metairie, Louisiana, for their assistance in developing this guideline.

PUBLICATION HISTORY
Originally published December 2016 in *Guidelines for Perioperative Practice* online.

PATIENT AND WORKER SAFETY

GUIDELINE FOR PREVENTION OF TRANSMISSIBLE INFECTIONS

The Guideline for Prevention of Transmissible Infections was approved by the AORN Recommended Practices Advisory Board. It was presented as proposed recommendations for comments by members and others. The guideline is effective December 15, 2012. The recommendations in the guideline are intended to be achievable and represent what is believed to be an optimal level of practice. Policies and procedures will reflect variations in practice settings and/or clinical situations that determine the degree to which the guideline can be implemented. AORN recognizes the various settings in which perioperative nurses practice; therefore, this guideline is adaptable to various practice settings. These practice settings include traditional operating rooms (ORs), ambulatory surgery centers, physicians' offices, cardiac catheterization laboratories, endoscopy suites, radiology departments, and all other areas where operative and other invasive procedures may be performed.

Purpose

The rapidly changing health care environment presents health care personnel with continual challenges in the form of newly recognized pathogens and well-known microorganisms that have become more resistant to today's therapeutic modalities. Protecting patients and health care practitioners from potentially infectious agent transmission continues to be a primary focus of perioperative registered nurses (RNs). The prevention and control of multidrug-resistant organisms (MDROs) requires that all health care organizations implement, evaluate, and adjust efforts to decrease the risk of transmission.

There are three principal elements required for an infection to occur:

- a source or reservoir,
- a susceptible host with a portal of entry to receive the infectious agent, and
- a method of transmission.[1]

This document provides guidance to perioperative RNs in implementing standard precautions and transmission-based precautions (ie, contact, droplet, airborne) to prevent infection in the perioperative practice setting. Additional guidance is provided for bloodborne pathogens; personal protective equipment (PPE); health care-associated infections and multidrug-resistant organisms (MDROs); immunization; and activities of health care workers with infections, exudative lesions, and nonintact skin. Finally, the document includes guidance for ongoing education and competency evaluation, documentation requirements, policies and procedures, and quality assurance and performance improvement processes.

Prevention of transmissible infections is a priority in the perioperative environment and includes considerations for environment of care, sharps safety and safe injection practices, hand hygiene, sterile technique, and sterilization. These topics are addressed in separate AORN guidelines and although they are mentioned briefly where applicable (eg, standard precautions), the broader discussions are outside the scope of this document.

Evidence Review

A medical librarian conducted a systematic search of the databases MEDLINE®, CINAHL®, Scopus®, and the Cochrane Database of Systematic Reviews for meta-analyses, systematic reviews, randomized controlled trials, guidelines, and additions to the *Morbidity and Mortality Weekly Report*. The report was also regularly consulted for newly added, relevant entries. Search terms included *infectious disease transmission, infectious skin diseases, soft tissue infections, blood-borne pathogens, gram-negative bacteria, gram-positive bacteria, gram-negative bacterial infections, gram-positive bacterial infections, viral hepatitis, viral meningitis, viral skin diseases, HIV infections, disease outbreaks, infectious disease transmission, needlestick injuries, occupational accidents, occupational health, occupational diseases, droplet precautions, standard precautions, isolation precautions, airborne precautions, patient isolation, microbial drug resistance, methicillin-resistant* Staphylococcus aureus, *methicillin resistance,* Staphylococcus aureus, *vancomycin resistance, vaccination, immunization, disaster planning, emergency preparedness, bioterrorism,* and *chemical terrorism*.

The search was limited to articles published in English between 1989 and 2011. The librarian established continuing alerts on the transmissible infection topics. The authors and medical librarian identified relevant guidelines from government agencies and standards-setting bodies. In addition, the authors requested articles that highlight the causes, identification, and treatment of transmissible infection, including some that were beyond the scope of this search.

Articles identified by the search were provided to the project team for evaluation. The team consisted of the lead author, three members of the Recommended Practices Advisory Board, and a doctorally prepared evidence appraiser. The lead author divided the search results into topics and assigned members of the team to review and critically appraise each article using the Johns Hopkins Evidence-Based Practice Model and the Research or Non-Research Evidence Appraisal Tools as appropriate. The literature was independently evaluated and appraised according to the strength and quality of the evidence. Each article was then assigned an appraisal score as agreed upon by consensus of the team. The appraisal score is noted in brackets after each reference, as applicable.

The collective evidence supporting each intervention within a specific recommendation was summarized and used to rate the strength of the evidence using the AORN Evidence Rating Model. Factors considered in review of the collective evidence were the quality of research, quantity of similar studies on a given topic, and consistency of results supporting a recommendation. The evidence rating is noted in brackets after each intervention.

Editor's note: MEDLINE is a registered trademark of the US National Library of Medicine's Medical Literature Analysis and Retrieval System, Bethesda, MD. CINAHL, Cumulative Index to Nursing and Allied Health Literature, is a registered trademark of EBSCO Industries, Birmingham, AL. Scopus is a registered trademark of Elsevier B.V., Amsterdam, Netherlands.

Recommendation I

Health care workers should use standard precautions when caring for all patients in the perioperative setting.

Standard precautions are the foundation for preventing transmission of infectious diseases. They apply to all patients and across all health care settings (eg, hospitals, ambulatory surgery centers, free-standing specialty care sites, interventional sites). Standard precautions include practices for hand hygiene, PPE, patient resuscitation, environmental control, respiratory hygiene/cough etiquette, sharps safety, and textiles and laundry.[1]

I.a. All personnel in the health care organization should follow established hand hygiene practices.[1,2] *[1: Strong Evidence]*

Hand hygiene is one of the most effective ways to prevent disease transmission and control infections in health care settings.[3]

I.b. Perioperative personnel should wear PPE whenever the possibility exists for exposure to blood or other potentially infectious materials. *[1: Regulatory Requirement]*

The use of PPE protects the health care provider's mucous membranes, airway, skin, and clothing from coming into contact with blood, body fluids, and other potentially infectious materials.[1,4] (See Recommendation VI.)

I.c. The health care provider should use a mouthpiece, resuscitation bag, or other ventilation device during resuscitation. *[1: Strong Evidence]*

Respiratory droplets are generated during cardiopulmonary resuscitation (CPR),[1] and if CPR is given to a patient with a transmissible infection, disease transfer is possible.[5-7] Mouthpieces, resuscitation bags, pocket masks with one-way valves, and other ventilation devices allow caregivers to perform CPR without exposing their nose and mouth to oral and respiratory fluids.[1]

I.d. The patient should be provided a clean, safe environment.[8-11] *[1: Strong Evidence]*

Hospital surfaces are often contaminated with health care-associated pathogens and may be responsible for cross-transmission.[12] Infections have been associated with surface contamination in hospital rooms, and the level of patient-to-patient transmission has been directly related to the level of environmental contamination.[13] In one case of an adenovirus outbreak in a military facility, during which 15 trainees were hospitalized for pneumonia, investigators recovered the infection serotype from several hospital surfaces.[14] The researchers concluded that there was a need to reinforce infection control guidelines.

Improved cleaning and disinfection of environmental surfaces can reduce the spread of numerous pathogens (eg, methicillin-resistant *Staphylococcus aureus* [MRSA], vancomycin-resistant *Enterococcus* spp [VRE], norovirus, *Clostridium difficile*, *Acinetobacter* spp).[13] Research has demonstrated that by consistently cleaning frequently touched items in the patient care environment (eg, toilet handholds, light switches, door knobs, nurse call devices, bedside rails), infections can be reduced.[10]

I.e. All people who enter the health care facility should practice respiratory hygiene and cough etiquette. *[1: Strong Evidence]*

Following an outbreak of severe acute respiratory syndrome (SARS) in 2003, the Centers for Disease Control and Prevention (CDC) expanded its guideline for infection prevention to include respiratory hygiene and cough etiquette.[1] Transmission of the virus was believed to occur because simple hygienic measures were not followed in health care facilities. Failure to use respiratory hygiene and cough etiquette may result in transmission of a respiratory tract infection.[1,15]

I.e.1. Respiratory hygiene and cough etiquette should include
- covering the mouth and nose with a tissue or a sleeve rather than the hand when coughing or sneezing;
- disposing of used tissues quickly;
- performing hand hygiene after coming into contact with respiratory secretions;
- having the person who exhibits signs of respiratory infection wear a surgical mask if he or she is able; and
- separating those who have a respiratory infection from others by more than 3 feet when possible.[1]

I.e.2. Health care organizations should promote proper respiratory hygiene and cough etiquette by
- providing resources and instructions for performing hand hygiene in or near waiting areas,
- placing alcohol-based hand rub dispensers in convenient locations,
- keeping supplies for hand washing where sinks are available,
- offering surgical masks to coughing patients during periods of increased community respiratory infections (eg, as indicated by increased school absences or patients seeking care for such infections),
- encouraging patients who exhibit signs of respiratory infection to stay at least 3 feet away from others in common areas when possible, and
- posting signs at entrances and in strategic places within ambulatory and inpatient settings in all languages that are applicable to the population served and that provide instructions for proper respiratory hygiene and cough etiquette.[1]

I.e.3. Perioperative nurses should promote compliance with respiratory hygiene and cough etiquette by educating health care personnel, patients, and visitors to cover their mouth or nose with tissue or to sneeze or cough into the crook of their arm, especially during seasonal community outbreaks of viral respiratory infections (eg, influenza, adenovirus), and by providing products (eg, tissues, surgical masks, no-touch waste receptacles, hand hygiene products) as control measures for minimizing contact with respiratory secretions.[1,15]

I.f. Perioperative team members should use safe injection practices (eg, one syringe and one needle, complying with sharps safety measures).[1,16] *[1: Strong Evidence]*

Using needles and syringes more than once increases the risk of infection, and unsafe medication injection practices have been implicated in outbreaks of hepatitis B and hepatitis C.[1,17-19] The CDC conducted investigations of four large outbreaks in ambulatory surgery facilities and found there is a need to reinforce safe injection practices.[19] The breaks in infection control practices were reinserting used needles into a multidose vial or solution container (eg, saline bag) and using a single needle or syringe to administer IV medication to multiple patients.

Appropriate methods to protect health care workers from exposure to hazardous materials or bloodborne pathogens and to decrease the risk of disease transmission through sharps injuries are specified in US Occupational Safety and Health Administration (OSHA) regulations.[4]

I.f.1. A syringe and needle should be used only once to administer a medication to a single patient, after which the syringe and needle should be discarded. When administering incremental doses to a single patient from the same syringe is an integral part of the procedure, the same syringe and needle may be reused, with strict adherence to aseptic technique, for the same patient as part of a single procedure. The syringe should never be left unattended and should be discarded immediately at the end of the procedure.[16]

I.f.2. Perioperative RNs should collaborate with pharmacists to procure and store single-dose vials rather than multidose vials.[16]

Reuse of multidose vials of medication is a concern as a cause of iatrogenic bloodborne pathogen infection.[18,20] Outbreaks of hepatitis B and C viruses in New York, Oklahoma, and Nebraska were attributed to unsafe injection practices that led to patient-to-patient transmission, including contamination of multidose medication vials and reuse of syringes and needles.[19]

HIV can be transmitted either parenterally or across mucous membranes. The risk of transmission from mucocutaneous exposure is estimated at 0.03%, and the risk of infection as a result of intact skin exposure is below detection.[20] Health care providers are among at-risk populations for occupational exposure to HIV, and transmission is significantly associated with procedures involving a needle placed in the source patient's blood vessel.[21]

Following fundamental infection-control principles (eg, safe injection practices, appropriate aseptic techniques) helps reduce the risk of bloodborne pathogen transmission.[18,19]

I.g. Reusable health care textiles should be changed and laundered after each patient use or when soiled. Health care textiles should be laundered in a health care-accredited laundry facility.[22] *[2: High Evidence]*

Health care textiles (eg, patient gowns, bed linens, privacy curtains, washcloths) may become contaminated by bacteria and fungi during wear or use, and microbes can survive on textiles for extended periods.[23,24] Contaminated textiles could contaminate the environment or health care providers' hands or clothing.[1]

Recommendation II

Contact precautions should be used when providing care to patients who are known or suspected to be infected or colonized with microorganisms that are transmitted by direct contact or indirect contact.

Contact precautions are in addition to standard precautions, including PPE (eg, gloves, gowns, masks, face protection). Additional precautions include flushing mucous membranes and washing skin that is exposed to blood or other potentially infectious materials, taking special considerations for patient transport, increasing environmental cleaning, adequate cleaning and disinfection of patient care equipment and items, and coordinating with an infection preventionist.

Contact with infected patients or contaminated surfaces leads to pathogen transmission 45% of the time, according to a review of 1,022 health care-associated infection outbreaks.[25] Health care providers are at risk of spreading health care-associated infections (eg, *S aureus,* VRE) through contact, according to a study in which researchers saw positive cultures from imprints of health care providers' hands after contact with surfaces near 34 out of 64 patients.[26] Adherence to contact precautions helps prevent transmission of infectious agents, including MDROs.[1,27-29]

Clostridium difficile is known to be transmitted by contact with contaminated people or environmental surfaces,[12] and skin contamination and environmental shedding of the pathogen can persist after symptoms resolve for up to four weeks after therapy.[30] An outbreak of staphylococcal bullous impetigo during a five-month period in a maternity ward was caused by contact with an auxiliary nurse, who was an asymptomatic nasal carrier of the strain.[31] In a study of VRE transmission, researchers cultured the intact skin of 22 colonized patients and sites in the patients' rooms before and after care by 98 health care providers.[32] The health care providers touched 151 VRE-negative sites after touching a VRE-positive site. The researchers found that VRE was transferred via health care providers' hands or gloves 10.6% of the time.

Contact precautions, as part of an overall infection control program, have been shown to decrease MRSA infection and transmission[33,34] and multidrug resistant *Acinetobacter baumannii* infection.[35]

II.a.   Personal protective equipment should be worn in the perioperative setting as part of contact precautions. *[1: Regulatory Requirement]*

The use of PPE protects the health care provider's mucous membranes, airway, skin, and clothing from coming into contact with blood, body fluids, and other potentially infectious materials.[1,4] (See Recommendation VI.)

II.a.1.   Perioperative personnel should don PPE upon room entry and discard PPE upon exiting the room when caring for a patient who requires contact precautions.[1]

Donning a gown and gloves when treating a patient who requires contact precautions and discarding them when leaving the patient's room helps contain pathogens, especially those that can be transmitted through environmental contamination (eg, VRE, *C difficile,* norovirus).[1]

Although PPE as part of contact precautions may help contain pathogens, there is some conflicting evidence. One cluster-randomized trial in an intensive care unit setting indicated that contact precautions (ie, gloves, gowns, hand hygiene) were not significantly more effective in preventing transmission of MRSA or VRE than universal gloving.[36] In six months, there were 5,434 admissions to 10 intervention intensive care units compared with 3,705 admissions to eight control intensive care units, and the rate of colonization or infection per 1,000 patient-days at risk did not differ significantly between the intervention and control sites. However, the providers did not use contact precautions as often as required: when contact precautions were specified, gloves were used for a median of 82% of contacts, gowns for 77% of contacts, and hand hygiene after 69% of contacts.[36]

II.b.   Health care providers must wash their hands and skin with soap and water or flush their mucous membranes with water immediately or as soon as possible after coming into direct contact with blood or other potentially infectious materials.[1,4] *[1: Regulatory Requirement]*

Exposure to environmental pathogens (eg, *Aspergillus* spp, *Legionella* spp) can cause illness among health care providers and adverse patient outcomes.[9] There is a risk of bloodborne disease transmission from splash injuries during endourology and other minimally invasive procedures, according to a study of 118 procedures performed by five surgeons.[37] The researchers noted that mucocutaneous and transconjunctival exposure are important portals for transmission. In a study of 25 consecutive patients who were undergoing dental surgery for impacted mandibular third molars, investigators concluded that surgeons were exposed to possible bloodborne infections by splashing in nearly 90% of the procedures.[38]

II.c.   When patient transport is necessary, precautions should be taken to reduce the opportunity for transmission of microorganisms to other patients, personnel, and visitors and to reduce contamination of the environment.[1] *[1: Strong Evidence]*

II.c.1.   Patient transport should be limited to essential diagnostic and therapeutic procedures that cannot be performed in the patient's room.[1]

II.c.2.   When transport is necessary, appropriate barriers should be used on the patient to cover affected areas if infectious skin lesions or drainage are present. These barriers should be consistent with the route and risk of transmission.[1]

II.c.3.   When a patient who requires contact precautions is transported from one area to another, the nurse should notify the receiving team members that the patient is coming and what precautions should be taken to prevent transmission.[1]

II.d. Environmental cleaning should be included as part of a program to control the transmission of MDROs.[27] *[1: Strong Evidence]*

Environmental reservoirs have been implicated in transmission of VRE and other MDROs. Thorough cleaning and disinfection practices, including of frequently touched surfaces (eg, bedrails, charts, bedside commodes, doorknobs), can help control the spread of MDROs.[27] Improved environmental cleaning can reduce the transmission of multidrug-resistant *A baumannii*, MRSA, VRE, *Acinetobacter* spp, and *C difficile*.[13,39-41]

II.d.1. Patient care areas of patients infected with *C difficile* should be cleaned with a 10% bleach solution and allowed to air dry.

Contamination of environmental surfaces contributes to the spread of *C difficile*.[42] *Clostridium difficile* is a spore that can survive for months in the environment and is not killed by standard processes for environmental cleaning.[39]

Educating housekeeping personnel on environmental cleaning practices significantly reduces the amount of contamination, according to a prospective, six-week before-and-after study.[42] When housekeeping personnel used 10% bleach solution to disinfect frequently touched surfaces (eg, bed rails, bedside tables, call buttons, telephones, toilet seats, door handles), contamination was significantly reduced, from nine rooms with positive cultures before cleaning to two rooms with positive cultures after cleaning.

II.e. All noncritical equipment (eg, commodes, IV pumps, ventilators, computers, personal electronic devices) should be cleaned and disinfected before use on another patient and should be handled in a manner to prevent health care provider or environmental contact with potentially infectious materials.[1] *[1: Strong Evidence]*

II.e.1. Dedicated noncritical equipment such as stethoscopes, blood pressure cuffs, and electronic thermometers may be used.[1,43]

II.f. Routine cleaning of environmental surfaces (eg, floors, walls) should be performed according to facility policy and more frequently when necessary.[11] *[2: High Evidence]*

Surface cleaning and disinfection practices are recommended to manage outbreaks caused by *Acinetobacter* spp, *C difficile*, MRSA, norovirus, and VRE.[13] Cleaning may need to be more thorough or performed more frequently depending on the patient's level of hygiene, the degree of environmental contamination, and the type of infectious agent (eg, if the infectious reservoir is the intestinal tract).[1]

II.g. An infection preventionist should be consulted for guidance when measures are indicated to prevent the spread of highly transmissible or epidemiologically important pathogens.[1] *[1: Strong Evidence]*

II.h. Perioperative nurses should evaluate and manage any negative patient outcomes that may be caused by using contact precautions. *[1: Strong Evidence]*

Studies have shown that health care providers are half as likely to enter the rooms of or examine patients who require contact precautions.[44,45] Patients may experience increased anxiety and depression and decreased levels of satisfaction under isolation precautions.[27,46]

A systematic review of 15 studies from 1989 to 2008[46] indicated four adverse outcomes related to contact precautions:
- less patient-to-health care provider contact,
- changes to systems of care that produce delays and more noninfectious adverse events,
- increased symptoms of depression and anxiety, and
- decreased satisfaction with care.

Although the majority of patients believe that contact precautions protect them and others, it is important to carefully consider whether contact precautions are necessary and to communicate the primary function of using contact precautions to the patient.[47]

By educating a patient who requires contact precautions and his or her family members, the perioperative nurse may be able to minimize feelings of isolation, depression, and anxiety. Nurses are in a position to evaluate patients for negative feelings, improve social contact, and provide education and frequent communication to the patient.

Recommendation III

Droplet precautions should be used throughout the perioperative environment (ie, preoperative, intraoperative, postoperative) when providing care to patients who are known or suspected to be infected with microorganisms that can be transmitted by large droplets.[1] *Amb*

Droplet precautions in addition to standard precautions reduce the risk of pathogens that spread through close respiratory or mucous membrane contact (eg, adenovirus, group A streptococcus, influenza, *Neisseria meningitides*, pertussis, rhinovirus).[1] Droplet precautions include donning PPE, considering patient placement to minimize contact with other patients, consulting with an infection preventionist, and placing a mask on the patient during transport.

Droplets in exhaled breath (ie, mouth or nose breathing, coughing, talking) may carry microorganisms that can be transmitted over short and long distances,[48] and infected droplets may originate during certain procedures (eg, suctioning, endotracheal induction, CPR).[1,5] During the 2003 SARS outbreak in Toronto, Canada, 26 health care providers contracted the virus from seven patients. Researchers concluded that close contact with the ill patients' airways (eg, during intubation, transportation) and failure to prevent exposure to respiratory secretions through infection control practices were associated with transmission.[49]

III.a. When a patient believed to have mumps, rubella, or pertussis enters the health care facility, droplet precautions should be implemented and followed, and only health care providers with presumptive immunity should be exposed to the patient.[50] *[1: Strong Evidence]*

III.b. Personal protective equipment should be worn in the perioperative setting as part of droplet precautions. *[1: Regulatory Requirement]*

The use of PPE protects the health care provider's mucous membranes, airway, skin, and clothing from coming into contact with blood, body fluids, and other potentially infectious materials.[1,4] (See Recommendation VI.)

III.b.1. Perioperative personnel should don surgical masks when in close contact with a patient who requires droplet precautions.[1]

Surgical masks prevent the transmission of large droplets (ie, greater than 5 microns) and, worn correctly, protect health care providers who are within close proximity of a patient who requires droplet precautions.[1] Masks serve as protection from infectious microorganisms from patients (eg, respiratory secretions, blood spatters, body fluid).

III.b.2. Health care providers should change PPE and clothing when they are exposed to patient secretions or droplets.

Changing PPE can help prevent cross-contamination of influenza viruses.[51]

III.c. Patients who require droplet precautions should be placed in a single-patient room before and after surgery. *[1: Strong Evidence]*

Single-patient placement in an isolation room helps prevent the spread of infection from patient to patient.[1,27,52] Special air handling and ventilation are not required as a part of droplet precautions.[1]

III.c.1. If single patient placement is not possible, the perioperative nurse should collaborate with the facility infection preventionist to establish optimal preoperative and postoperative placement for a patient who requires droplet precautions.[1]

The infection preventionist can help assess and mitigate the risks associated with non-isolation placement options (eg, cohorting, keeping the patient with an existing roommate) to minimize the potential for cross-contamination.

III.c.2. Patients who require droplet precautions should be placed at least 3 feet away from other patients.[1]

The defined risk area (ie, > 3 feet) around the patient is based on epidemiologic and simulated infection studies.[1]

III.c.3. If possible, draw curtains or close doors.

Curtains and doors help to separate the patients and reduce transmission of infectious organisms.

III.d. When transporting the patient from one area to another, the patient should wear a mask.[1] *[1: Strong Evidence]*

Masks prevent possible spread of infectious respiratory secretions from the patient to other individuals.

Recommendation IV

Airborne precautions should be used when providing care to patients who are known or suspected to be infected with microorganisms that can be transmitted by the airborne route.

Some procedures performed in the perioperative setting require access to the airway; therefore, special infection-control considerations for preventing transmission of airborne disease are necessary.[53] Airborne precautions in addition to standard precautions for the OR include consultation with an infection preventionist, respiratory protection, PPE, patient placement and transport precautions, administrative controls, and environmental controls.[9,53]

Airborne transmission can occur when small particles that contain infectious agents that remain infective over time and distance are inhaled.[1] This is specific to particles that are approximately 1 μm to 5 μm and that remain airborne for prolonged periods by normal air currents, which allow them to spread throughout a room or building.[53] The use of airborne precautions can help minimize transfer of diseases that are spread by the airborne route[54] (eg, *Mycobacterium tuberculosis* [TB], rubeola, Varicella zoster[1]).

IV.a. An infection preventionist should be consulted to determine necessary supplemental controls for patients requiring airborne isolation.[53] *[1: Strong Evidence]*

IV.b. When a patient suspected of measles infection enters the health care facility, all health care personnel should use respiratory protection, regardless of presumptive immunity, when providing care to the patient. *[1: Strong Evidence]*

Measles vaccination can fail and is ineffective for preventing measles about 1% of the time. Measles is highly contagious and transmission can occur anywhere from four days before presentation of a rash to four days after the rash resolves.[50]

IV.c. When a patient with confirmed or suspected varicella infection enters the health care facility, airborne and contact precautions should be implemented and followed, and only health care providers with evidence of immunity should provide care to the patient.[50] *[1: Strong Evidence]*

IV.d. Personal protective equipment should be worn in the perioperative setting as part of airborne precautions. *[1: Regulatory Requirement]*

The use of PPE protects the health care provider's mucous membranes, airway, skin, and clothing from coming into contact with blood, body fluids, and other potentially infectious materials.[1,4] (See Recommendation VI.)

IV.d.1. Perioperative personnel should don a surgical mask or N95 or higher level respirator, depending on disease-specific recommendations, before entering the room of a patient who requires airborne precautions.[1]

Wearing an N95 or higher level respirator, or a mask if a respirator is not available, reduces the risk of airborne transmission.[1]

IV.d.2. Respiratory protective devices worn during care of a patient with TB should be
- certified by the CDC/US National Institute for Occupational Safety and Health (NIOSH) as a nonpowered particulate filter respirator (N-, R-, or P-95, 99, or 100), including a disposable respirator or powered air-purifying respirator with high efficiency filters,[55] and
- available in different sizes and models to accommodate the different facial sizes and characteristics of health care providers.[53]

IV.e. An airborne infection isolation room should be used if available for patients who require airborne precautions, including during surgery and postoperative recovery.[1,53] *[1: Strong Evidence]*

Use of special air handling and ventilation systems such as an airborne infection isolation room helps prevent the spread of airborne pathogens, particularly TB, rubeola, and varicella zoster, and is recommended during procedures that can generate infectious aerosols (eg, endotracheal intubation, bronchoscopy, suctioning, autopsy procedures involving oscillating saws).[1(p31)]

IV.e.1. If no airborne infection isolation room is available, a portable anteroom system (PAS)-high-efficiency particulate air (HEPA) combination unit may be used.

A pilot study comparing freestanding HEPA filter units placed inside the OR with a novel PAS-HEPA combination unit that was placed outside the OR showed that the PAS-HEPA unit was more effective.[56] The PAS-HEPA unit achieved a downward evacuation of plume, away and toward the main entry door from the sterile field. Compara-

tively, the portable freestanding HEPA unit inside the OR moved the plume vertically upward and directly into the breathing zone where the surgical team would be during a procedure. Results indicated that the PAS-HEPA system effectively removed more than 94% of an initial release of at least 500,000 submicron particles per cubic foot within 20 minutes after release.

IV.f. When transporting the patient from an airborne infection isolation room to the OR, the patient should wear a mask if clinically appropriate.[1] Patients should be transported directly to the OR, bypassing the preoperative area, and transferred directly to an airborne infection isolation room in the postanesthesia care unit or other part of the hospital at the end of the procedure. *[1: Strong Evidence]*

IV.g. After cough-inducing procedures are performed in the OR, sufficient time should be allowed for 99% or more of airborne particles to be removed before sterile supplies are opened for subsequent patients. *[1: Strong Evidence]*

Performing cough-inducing procedures such as intubation, extubation, and bronchoscopy increases the likelihood that droplet nuclei will be expelled into the air.[53] For example, by waiting to place another patient in the room, the risk of airborne transmission of TB is reduced. The length of time required to expel more than 99% of airborne contaminants varies by the efficiency of the ventilation or filtration system.

IV.h. Elective surgery should be postponed for patients who have suspected or confirmed TB until the patient is determined to be noninfectious. If surgery cannot be postponed, perioperative personnel should follow airborne precautions and consult with an infection preventionist.[9,53] *[1: Strong Evidence]* **Amb**

Postponing elective surgery may prevent transmission of TB.

IV.h.1. A single-use, disposable bacterial filter should be placed between the anesthesia circuit and the patient's airway.

Placing a bacterial filter between the anesthesia circuit and the patient's airway prevents contamination of the anesthesia equipment and release of tubercle bacilli into the room.[9,53] The preferred filter will filter particles 0.3 µm or larger in size in both loaded and unloaded states and will have a filter efficiency of 95% (ie, filter penetration of < 5%) at the maximum design flow rates of the ventilator for the service life of the filter.[53]

IV.h.2. The patient should be intubated and extubated and placed for recovery in an airborne infection isolation room. If intubation or extubation must be performed in the OR, a portable, industrial-grade HEPA filter should be used to supplement air cleaning in the following manner:

- position the unit near the patient's breathing zone,
- obtain engineering consultation to determine the appropriate placement,
- switch the portable unit off during the surgical procedure, and
- provide fresh air according to ventilation standards for the OR.[9]

Switching the unit off during the procedure is recommended because after the patient is intubated, the airway is circulating in a closed system; therefore, the portable units do not serve any purpose while the patient is intubated. Fresh air must be provided because portable units do not meet the requirements for the number of fresh air changes per hour.[9]

IV.h.3. If the patient is intubated or extubated in the OR, the OR doors should remain closed until adequate time has passed for air changes per hour to clean 99% of airborne particles from the air (eg, 15 air exchanges per hour for 28 minutes to remove 99.9% of airborne contaminants).[9]

IV.h.4. Standard cleaning and disinfection procedures should be followed after surgery on a patient who has TB, and should only be performed after the appropriate amount of time for air ventilation. Personal respiratory protective equipment is not necessary for cleaning an OR if the appropriate ventilation time is allowed. If room cleaning activities begin before the appropriate amount of time for air ventilation, cleaning personnel should wear N95 respirators or powered air-purifying respirators.[53]

IV.i. Administrative controls should be established to reduce the risk of TB exposure to patients and personnel. Administrative controls should include

- implementing work practices for managing patients with suspected or confirmed TB;
- ensuring potentially contaminated equipment (eg, endoscopes) is properly cleaned and sterilized or disinfected;
- training and educating health care providers about TB prevention, transmission, and symptoms;
- establishing a TB screening program to screen and evaluate health care providers who are at risk for TB or who might be exposed to *M tuberculosis*; and
- implementing a respiratory protection program for personnel requiring fit testing and certification to use an N95 respirator.[53]

[1: Strong Evidence]

IV.j. Environmental controls should be established to prevent the spread of airborne diseases. Environmental controls should include

- controlling the source of infection by using local exhaust ventilation (eg, hoods, tents, booths),[53]
- diluting and removing contaminated air with general ventilation,[53]
- controlling airflow to prevent contamination of air in areas adjacent to the source,[53]
- cleaning the air using HEPA filtration or ultraviolet germicidal irradiation,[53]
- using central wall suction units with inline filters to evacuate minimal surgical smoke,[9,57] and
- using a mechanical smoke evacuation system with HEPA filtration to manage large amounts of surgical smoke.[9]

[1: Strong Evidence]

The CDC recommends environmental controls to prevent the spread of airborne infections (eg, TB)[53] and to minimize exposure to laser plume that may contain infectious material (eg, human papilloma virus).[9]

Recommendation V

Health care personnel must follow the OSHA bloodborne pathogens standard when there is a risk of exposure to blood or other potentially infectious materials.[4]

Bloodborne pathogens are pathogenic microorganisms that are present in human blood and can cause disease (eg, hepatitis B, HIV).[4] Federal and state regulations and organizational standards[58,59] mandating bloodborne pathogen guidelines are intended to reduce health care provider exposure to bloodborne pathogens and to minimize the risk of infection.

There has been a focus on preventing bloodborne transmission of hepatitis B, hepatitis C, and HIV in particular.[1,19,60-62] These viruses are more easily transmitted parenterally or across mucous membranes.[20]

Methods for preventing bloodborne pathogen exposure include using PPE, implementing engineering and work practice controls, following infection prevention precautions, and establishing and following an infection control plan.

V.a. Health care personnel must wear PPE in the perioperative setting as part of the bloodborne pathogens standard.[4] *[1: Regulatory Requirement]*

The use of PPE protects the health care provider's mucous membranes, airway, skin, and clothing from coming into contact with blood, body fluids, and other potentially infectious materials.[1,4] Appropriate PPE does not permit blood or other potentially infectious materials to pass through to or reach the employee's work clothes, street clothes, undergarments, skin, eyes, mouth, or other mucous membranes under normal conditions of use and for the duration that the PPE is used.[4] (See Recommendation VI.)

V.a.1. If a garment is penetrated by blood or other potentially infectious materials, the health care provider must remove the garment immediately or as soon as possible.[4]

V.a.2. Health care personnel must wear gloves when hand contact with blood, other potentially infectious materials, mucous membranes, or non-intact skin can be reasonably anticipated; when performing vascular access procedures; and when handling or touching contaminated items or surfaces.[4]

V.a.3. Health care personnel must wear masks in combination with eye protection devices whenever splashes, spray, spatter, or droplets of blood or other potentially infectious materials may be generated and eye, nose, or mouth contamination can be reasonably anticipated.[4]

Eye protection devices include goggles, glasses with solid side shields, and chin-length face shields.

V.a.4. Health care personnel must wear gowns, aprons, and other protective body clothing when exposure to blood or other potentially infectious materials is anticipated.[4]

V.a.5. Health care personnel must wear surgical caps or hoods and shoe covers or boots when gross contamination can be reasonably anticipated (eg, orthopedic surgery).[4]

V.b. Food and drink must not be taken into the semirestricted or restricted areas of the perioperative suite. Food and drink must not be kept in refrigerators, freezers, shelves, or cabinets or on counter tops or work spaces where blood or other potentially infectious materials are present.[4] [1: Regulatory Requirement]

V.c. Perioperative personnel must use engineering and work practice controls.[4] [1: Regulatory Requirement]

Engineering controls isolate or remove the risk of exposure, and work practice controls reduce the likelihood of exposure by changing the method of performing a task.[4]

Engineering controls include
○ needleless systems,[4,63,64]
○ self-sheathing needles,[4] and
○ sharps storage and disposal containers.[4]
Work practice controls include
○ prohibiting risky handling of needles and sharps,
○ prohibiting recapping of needles by a two-handed technique,[4]
○ using a neutral zone or hands-free technique for passing sharps,[4,65] and
○ double gloving during all surgical procedures (See Recommendation VI.b.).

V.d. Health care organizations must establish a written exposure control plan, make it accessible to employees, and review and update it at least annually.[4] [1: Regulatory Requirement]

Recommendation VI

Perioperative personnel must wear PPE when exposure to blood or other potentially infectious materials is anticipated.[4]

The OSHA standard requires employers to provide appropriate PPE to health care providers at no cost to reduce the risk of skin and mucous membrane exposure to blood, body fluids, and other potentially infectious materials.[4]

All health care providers are responsible for ensuring the safety of patients, other health care providers, their own family members, and the community.[66] According to the Workers' Family Protection Task Force, there are limited data to quantify household exposures to potentially infectious organisms; however, workers who may not exhibit negative effects from workplace exposure still may expose their family members by taking infectious pathogens home (eg, occupationally acquired hepatitis C or HIV). Existing standards that require employers and employees to reduce occupational risks (eg, using PPE, engineering controls) protect the workers' families as well.

It is the employer's responsibility to ensure that PPE is available and readily accessible, alternatives are available for employees with allergies, and that personnel use the appropriate PPE. Personal protective equipment includes gloves, gowns, eye protection, masks, and respirators.

VI.a. Gloves must be worn when hand contact with blood or other potentially infectious materials, mucous membranes, or non-intact skin can be reasonably anticipated,[4] including when
○ performing vascular access procedures[3,4];
○ coming into direct contact with patients who are colonized or infected with pathogens (eg, VRE, MRSA, respiratory syncytial virus)[27]; and
○ handling or touching contaminated patient care items or environmental surfaces.[4]
[1: Regulatory Requirement]

Gloves help prevent health care providers' hands from becoming contaminated by patient blood, body fluids, and other potentially infectious materials.[3,4,26,32,67,68] Gloves have been found to protect health care providers' hands from VRE contamination[69] and to reduce the risks of sharps injuries.[70]

VI.a.1. Unsterile gloves should be visually inspected upon donning, before contact with potentially contaminated surfaces, and periodically throughout use.[71] After use, perioperative personnel should remove gloves, discard them, and perform hand hygiene.

VI.a.2. Sterile gloves should be visually inspected immediately upon donning and before contact with sterile supplies or the sterile field.

507

Gloves may have perforations or tears that occur in the manufacturing process or as gloves are donned.

VI.a.3. Sterile gloves should be changed
- after each patient contact;
- when a visible defect is noted;
- when suspected or actual contamination occurs; and
- when a suspected or actual perforation occurs.[4,72,73]

Breaches in the glove barrier pose a risk for transmission of bloodborne pathogens during surgical procedures. Glove perforation also increases the risk of surgical site infection (SSI).[74]

Depending on the duration of wear, surgical gloves can develop microperforations that are not immediately recognizable to the wearer.[75-77] These perforations allow bacteria from the surgical site to pass through to the wearer's hands. One method for preventing this is to mandate regular glove changes in organizational policy. Changing gloves at regular intervals may decrease the incidence of glove perforation and bacterial contamination during surgical procedures.[73,77,78]

VI.a.4. Use of polyvinyl chloride or vinyl gloves should be limited to brief, low-risk exposures.

Research has shown that vinyl and polyvinyl gloves have a higher failure rate in use than nitrile or latex gloves.[71,79-81] In a study of 137 procedures, researchers noted higher microbial contamination of the health care providers' hands and a higher frequency of leaks with vinyl gloves compared to latex.[71] Similarly, a study of 886 examination gloves showed vinyl gloves were much more likely to leak than latex (51.3% vs 19.7%) as demonstrated by a standardized clinical protocol designed to mimic patient care activities.[79] Research also has indicated polyvinyl chloride gloves fail to protect against virus exposure 22% of the time.[82]

Comparisons of different glove types have supported the decreased durability of vinyl and polyvinyl chloride gloves. Researchers evaluated 2,000 gloves (ie, 800 latex, 800 vinyl, 400 nitrile) and tested them immediately out of the box and after manipulations designed to simulate in-use conditions.[81] Vinyl gloves failed 12% to 61% of the time, whereas latex and nitrile had failure rates of 0% to 4% and 1% to 3%, respectively.

Another comparison involving 5,510 medical examination gloves (1,464 nitrile, 1,052 latex, 1,006 copolymer, 1,988 vinyl) showed that vinyl and copolymer (ie, polyvinyl chloride) gloves were less effective barriers than latex and nitrile.[80] Results showed 8.2% failure rates for the vinyl and copolymer gloves compared to 1.3% for nitrile and 2.2% for latex.

VI.b. Perioperative team members should wear two pairs of surgical gloves, one over the other, during surgical and other invasive procedures with the potential for exposure to blood, body fluids, or other potentially infectious materials. When double gloves are worn, perforation indicator systems should be used. *[1: Strong Evidence]*

Glove barrier failure is a common occurrence in the perioperative setting. Glove failures can be caused by punctures, tears by sharp devices, or spontaneous failures. Breaches in the glove barrier pose a risk of transmission of bloodborne pathogens during surgery. Wearing double gloves helps prevent SSI and protect health care providers' hands.[83-89]

According to a study of 155 surgeons and residents in Canada, double gloving is an effective means to reduce the risk of percutaneous injury.[90] Double gloving also minimizes the amount of blood that is transferred to the health care provider's hands during a needlestick injury,[91] reduces the risk of glove perforation associated with lengthy surgical procedures,[92] and reduces the risk of perforation of the innermost glove.[85]

Double gloving or double gloving with an indicator glove system may increase the wearer's awareness of a perforation and thereby protect against exposure to bloodborne pathogens during surgery.[86,89,93,94] In one 24-month study,[86] researchers investigated the effects of double gloving with inner indicator gloves and found that the frequency of seeing blood on the hand after surgery was higher with single gloving than double gloving. They also noted that surgical team members were more likely to change their gloves during surgery when they double gloved with an indicator system compared with double gloving alone.

VI.b.1. When the invasive procedure is completed, perioperative personnel should remove both pairs of gloves, discard them, and perform hand hygiene.[2]

VI.c. Perioperative personnel must wear fluid-resistant attire during activities that generate splashes, spatter, sprays, or aerosols of blood or other potentially infectious materials.[4] *[1: Regulatory Requirement]*

The CDC recommends wearing fluid-resistant gowns for all patient contact.[1] Fluid-resistant attire protects health care providers' skin from being exposed to blood, body fluids, and other potentially infectious materials. Surgical scrub attire, laboratory coats, or jackets worn over personal clothing are not considered PPE.[1]

VI.d. Health care personnel must wear eye protection when splashes, spray, spatter, or droplets of blood or other potentially infectious materials can be reasonably anticipated.[4] *[1: Regulatory Requirement]*

The CDC recommends eye protection as part of standard precautions[1] and when there is a risk of infectious materials entering the eye.[95] Using eye protection helps prevent exposure to bloodborne pathogens and other diseases (eg, SARS, TB, *Neisseria meningitidis*) during aerosol-generating procedures, including bronchoscopy, endotracheal intubation, and open suctioning of the respiratory tract.[1]

Infectious diseases, including adenovirus, herpes simplex, *S aureus*, hepatitis B, hepatitis C, and HIV, can be transmitted through the mucous membranes of the eye (ie, conjunctiva).[95] These infectious agents can be introduced directly to the eye by blood splashes or respiratory droplets that are generated during coughing or suctioning or from touching the eyes with contaminated fingers or other objects.[95]

The type of eye protection that is necessary depends on the circumstances of exposure, other PPE that is being used, and personal vision needs; however, regular prescription eyeglasses and contact lenses are not considered eye protection.[95] Appropriate eye protection includes goggles, face shields, and full-face respirators. The CDC recommends selecting eye protection based on other PPE requirements to ensure proper fit and optimal protection.[95]

VI.d.1. Goggles should fit snugly, especially at the corners of the eye and across the brow, be indirectly vented, and have anti-fog properties.

Fitted, indirectly vented goggles with a manufacturer's anti-fog coating are the most reliable and practical means of protecting health care providers' eyes from splashes, sprays, and respiratory droplets. They can be fit over prescription glasses. Safety glasses do not provide splash or droplet protection and are not recommended for infection control purposes.[95]

VI.d.2. Face shields should be selected for circumstances where eye protection alone is not sufficient.

Face shields provide protection to the eyes and other areas of the face. Face shields that have crown and chin protection and wrap around the face to the point of the ear allow for the best face and eye protection from splashes and sprays. Although disposable face shields that fit loosely and are made of light-weight films with attached surgical masks are available, these may not provide complete protection.[95]

VI.d.3. Full facepiece elastomeric respirators and powered air-purifying respirators should be selected based on the respiratory hazard in an infection control situation.[95]

Full facepiece elastomeric respirators and powered air-purifying respirators provide highly effective eye protection in addition to respiratory protection.[95] These devices require prescription inserts for health care providers who wear glasses to avoid compromising the seal around the face. Another option for health care providers who wear prescription glasses is a powered air-purifying respirator that is designed with a loose-fitting face piece or with a hood that completely covers the head and neck.

VI.d.4. Eye protection should be removed by handling only the portion of the equipment that secures the device to the head.

By removing eye protection by the plastic temples, elasticized band, or ties rather than handling the front or sides, health care providers can minimize the risk of contamination of their hands.[95]

VI.d.5. Non-disposable eye protection should be placed in a designated receptacle for subsequent cleaning and disinfection, and health care providers should each be given their own eye protection when possible.[95]

VI.e. Perioperative personnel must wear surgical masks when splashes, spray, spatter, or droplets of blood or other potentially infectious materials may be generated and nose or mouth contamination can be reasonably anticipated.[4] *[1: Regulatory Requirement]*

Masks protect the mucous membranes of the nose and mouth, which are susceptible to infectious agents.[1,4] Masks are used to prevent contact with respiratory secretions or sprays of blood and body fluid as part of standard and droplet precautions.[1]

Splash injuries are common during endoscopic and laparoscopic urologic procedures, a fact that has implications for all minimally invasive procedures, according to a four-month study of 118 endoscopy procedures.[37] The investigators collected 236 masks from surgeons, surgical assistants, and perioperative nurses and analyzed them for blood macroscopically and using forensic techniques. Results indicated 48.5% of the surgeons' masks, 29.5% of the assistants' masks, and 31.8% of the nurses' masks were splashed with blood.

Masks also are used as part of sterile technique to protect patients from exposure to infectious agents that may be carried in the health care provider's mouth or nose.[1] Surgical masks have been shown to reduce bacterial contamination produced by dispersal of organisms from the wearer's upper airway[96] and are believed to protect the surgical site from becoming contaminated.[97] During cataract surgery, for example, there is significantly less bacterial contamination of the surgical site when the surgeon wears a face mask.[98] Visor masks are recommended as a standard practice during oral surgery when high-speed rotary instruments are used because these procedures result in splashing nearly 90% of the time.[38]

The Society for Cardiovascular Angiography and Interventions recommends wearing a mask to protect patients during cardiac catheterization procedures.[99] The Society noted that mask use has become more important with increased use of the catheterization laboratory as an interventional suite for device implantation. Significantly less bacterial contamination of the operative field during cardiac catheterization occurs when health care providers wear full masks compared to no masks, and there is a nonsignificant trend of increased bacterial colony counts when masks are worn below the nose as opposed to above the nose.[100]

The two types of masks available in health care settings are surgical masks and procedure masks. Surgical masks, which are evaluated by the US Food and Drug Administration for fluid resistance, bacterial filtration efficacy, differential pressure, and flammability, are appropriate for use as PPE in the perioperative setting.[1]

Whether to wear a mask or respirator depends on disease-specific recommendations,[101] but the CDC notes that it is good practice to don a mask within 6 to 10 feet of a patient or on entry to the patient's room when exposure to an "emerging or highly virulent pathogen" is likely.[1]

VI.e.1.   Employers should provide masks in a variety of shapes (eg, molded, non-molded), sizes, filtration efficiencies, and methods of attachment (eg, ties, elastic, ear loops).

Providing several varieties may be necessary to meet individual health care providers' needs.[1]

VI.f.   Perioperative personnel should wear N95 or higher level respirators during aerosol-generating procedures involving patients who have TB, SARS, or avian or pandemic influenza viruses.[1] *[1: Strong Evidence]*

Wearing an N95 or higher level respirator when caring for a patient who requires airborne precautions reduces the likelihood of airborne infection transmission.[1]

One review of 21 studies indicated that N95 respirators are more protective against influenza and similarly sized particles than surgical masks.[102] However, the investigators noted that additional research is needed to support the World Health Organization guidelines for wearing surgical masks for all patient care and N95 respirators for aerosol-generating procedures. In another review of 45 articles, researchers were unable to determine which specific hygienic measures were most effective in reducing MRSA rates, but they noted that a combination of measures—masks, gloves, gowns, and hand hygiene—are effective together.[103]

VI.g.   Perioperative personnel must replace PPE and clothing as soon as possible after exposure to blood or other potentially infectious materials.[4] *[1: Regulatory Requirement]*

Replacing PPE and clothing after exposure to secretions and droplets that contain viruses is effective for preventing cross-infection.[51]

VI.h.   Perioperative personnel must remove all PPE before leaving the work area and must place used PPE in an appropriately designated area or container for storage, washing, decontamination, or disposal.[4] After removing PPE, hand hygiene should be performed.[2] *[1: Regulatory Requirement]*

VI.h.1.   Perioperative personnel should stand 3 feet away from the disposal container when removing soiled gloves.

One study of glove removal procedures indicated that when personnel stood 3 feet away from the garbage bin as opposed to 2 feet, there was less contamination on the cover of the bin and the front of the removed gloves.[104] There was no significant difference in hand contamination levels based on distance to the disposal container.

Recommendation VII

Perioperative personnel should take action to prevent the transmission of health care-acquired infections.

Several types of infections may be acquired in the perioperative setting and are affected by perioperative care, including SSIs, MDROs, central line-associated blood stream infections, and catheter-associated urinary tract infections. The entire perioperative team is responsible for collaborating to prevent these types of infections.

VII.a.   Perioperative team members should adopt a systematic approach for reducing the risk of surgical site infections.[97] *[1: Strong Evidence]*

Despite advances in infection control practices (eg, improved OR ventilation, sterilization methods, barriers, surgical technique, antimicrobial prophylaxis), SSIs remain a substantial cause of morbidity and mortality among hospitalized patients.[97] Surgical site infections occur in 2% to 5% of US patients who undergo surgery in inpatient facilities for a total of approximately 500,000 SSIs each year, at a cost of up to $10 billion annually.[105] Furthermore, these infections are associated with seven to 10 additional postoperative days per SSI and increase the risk of death by as much as 11 times.

According to the Hospital Infection Control Practices Advisory Committee Guideline, SSI is the third most frequently reported health care–associated infection and accounts for between 14% and 16% of all health care-associated infections in hospitalized patients.[97] Among surgical patients, SSIs account for 38% of health care-associated infections, and 77% of deaths in surgical patients who develop an SSI are related to the infection.[97,105]

The pathogens that contribute most frequently to SSI include *S aureus*, coagulase-negative staphylococci, *Enterococcus* spp, and *Escherichia coli*, and increasingly include *Candida albicans* and MRSA.[97] Most SSIs are caused by the patient's endogenous flora (eg, gram-positive cocci, anaerobic bacteria, gram-negative aerobes), but they also can be caused by exogenous sources of pathogens such as members of the surgical team; the OR environment and air; and all devices, instruments, and materials that are brought to the sterile field.[97]

Surgical site infection prevention measures (ie, an action or a set of actions taken to reduce the risk of SSI) focus on reducing opportunities for microbial contamination of the patient's tissues or sterile surgical instruments. Specific methods for preventing SSI include adhering to sterile technique, implementing environmental cleaning protocols, using appropriate barriers and surgical attire, performing proper skin antisepsis and hand hygiene, minimizing traffic in the OR during surgical procedures, using adequate sterilization methods, treating carriers of *S aureus* preoperatively, and using preoperative antimicrobial prophylaxis.[97]

VII.a.1. Perioperative personnel should implement sterile technique when preparing, performing, or assisting with invasive procedures.[11,73,106]

Sterile technique performed by all perioperative team members is the foundation of SSI prevention.[97] Failure to adhere to the principles of asepsis is independently related to the risk of SSI.[1,73,107]

VII.a.2. A clean environment should be maintained.[11,97]

VII.a.3. Perioperative personnel should wear clean surgical attire.[22]

Although few controlled trials have evaluated whether the use of surgical attire has an effect on reducing SSIs, the Hospital Infection Control Practices Advisory Committee recommends the use of barriers (eg, scrub suits, masks, surgical caps, hoods, shoe covers, sterile gloves, gowns, drapes) to minimize the patient's exposure to the skin, mucous membranes, and hair of surgical team members.[97]

Wound infections may result when pathogens that adhere to the hair or scalp (eg, *S aureus*, Group A streptococcus, *Staph-ylococcus epidermidis*) are released into the operative air and settle into the surgical incision.[108-110]

VII.a.4. Preoperative skin antisepsis of the surgical site should be performed.[111]

Antiseptic skin preparation of the surgical site is intended to reduce the risk of postoperative SSI by removing soil and transient microorganisms from the skin; reducing the resident microbial count to subpathogenic levels in a short period and with the least amount of tissue irritation; and inhibiting rapid, rebound growth of microorganisms.

VII.a.5. Perioperative personnel should follow proper hand hygiene practices.[2]

Hand hygiene helps reduce the bacterial colony count on perioperative team members' hands and is believed to reduce the risk of SSI.[97,112] In one study, the introduction of a hand sanitizer with 70% isopropyl alcohol and 0.5% chlorhexidine gluconate and training perioperative team members on its use reduced SSI overall and superficial SSI in particular among patients undergoing neurosurgery.[113]

VII.a.6. Traffic in and out of the OR should be minimized during surgical procedures.[114]

The air in the OR may contain microbe-laden dust, lint, skin squames, or respiratory droplets, and the microbial level in the air is directly related to the number of people who are moving around in the room.[97]

VII.a.7. Perioperative personnel should provide reusable surgical items that are free of contamination at the time of use. Reusable surgical items should be subjected to cleaning and decontamination, followed by a disinfection or sterilization process.[115]

Inadequate sterilization of surgical instruments can contribute to SSI outbreaks.[97]

VII.a.8. Perioperative nurses should collaborate with medical colleagues to evaluate testing or decolonizing patients preoperatively for carriage of *S aureus* and using preoperative prophylaxis on carriers.

S aureus is carried in the nasal nares of 20% to 30% of healthy individuals, and this carriage has been found to be "the most powerful independent risk factor for SSI" in patients undergoing cardiothoracic surgery.[97] Among 135 orthopedic surgeons at a teaching hospital, 1.5% tested positive for MRSA and 35.7% tested positive for methicillin-sensitive *S aureus*.[116]

Mupirocin ointment may be an effective topical therapy for removing *S aureus* from the nares of colonized patients and health care providers, and the ointment can lower the risk of SSI when it is used on patients regardless of carrier status.[97,117] The evidence is conflicting, however. Another study failed to demonstrate an overall reduction in SSI when intranasal mupirocin was administered to carriers of *S aureus* preoperatively, and the study only showed a trend for decreased health care-associated infections caused by *S aureus*.[118]

Researchers in the Netherlands found that decontaminating endogenous microorganisms in the nasopharynx and oropharynx with chlorhexidine gluconate preoperatively reduces health care-associated infection after cardiac surgery.[119]

VII.a.9. Perioperative nurses should verify that preoperative antimicrobial prophylaxis is administered according to health care organization policy.

Surgical antimicrobial prophylaxis is a critically timed adjunct therapy intended to reduce the microbial burden of surgical contamination to a level that cannot overwhelm the patient's defenses.[97] The surgeon decides which antimicrobial agent to use by anticipating the surgical wound class for a given procedure. Comparisons of various antibiotics for short-term treatment have been shown to be equally effective against SSI in patients undergoing elective implant surgery[120] and orthopedic surgery.[121] To maximize the benefits of antimicrobial prophylaxis, the Hospital Infection Control Practices Advisory Committee[97] recommends

- using an antimicrobial agent for all procedures or classes of procedures for which use has been shown to reduce SSI rates or for procedures from which incisional or organ/space SSI would be catastrophic;
- using a medication that is safe, inexpensive, and bactericidal with an in vitro spectrum that covers the most probable intraoperative contaminants for the surgery;
- timing the initial dose of the medication so that a bactericidal concentration is established in serum and tissues by the time of the incision; and
- maintaining therapeutic antimicrobial levels in both serum and tissues during the procedure and until a few hours after the incision is closed.

The Society for Healthcare Epidemiology of America/Infectious Diseases Society of America practice recommendations[105] include

- delivering IV prophylaxis within one hour before the incision is made, or two hours for vancomycin and fluoroquinolones;

- using an antimicrobial agent that is consistent with published guidelines; and
- discontinuing use of the antimicrobial agent within 24 hours after surgery, or 48 hours for cardiothoracic procedures in adult patients.

VII.b. To limit or slow the spread of MDROs, perioperative personnel should collaborate with an infection preventionist to determine the best and safest plan for surgical patients who are diagnosed with an MDRO. *[1: Strong Evidence]*

Methicillin-resistant *S aureus* and VRE are not the only MDROs that present an infection prevention challenge. Other MDROs continue to emerge as a public health concern. Carbapenem-resistant Enterobacteriaceae has become a serious threat to public health. These organisms have the potential to spread and are associated with high mortality rates, and they often carry genes that cause high levels of resistance to many antimicrobial agents, leaving extremely limited options for treatment.[122,123]

When MDROs are introduced into a health care setting, several factors determine the likelihood of transmission and persistence of the resistant strain:

- vulnerability of patients (ie, patients in the hospital are more likely to get an infection because their immunity is weakened from the disease state),
- numbers of colonized patients,
- increased antimicrobial use, and
- effect of and adherence to prevention efforts.[27]

Successful approaches to preventing and controlling MDROs are often a combination of strategies,[27,124] including

- garnering administrative support (eg, commitment of fiscal and staffing resources, implementation of system changes, expert consultation, laboratory support, adherence monitoring, data analysis)[27,125];
- following and improving hand hygiene practices[13,27,34,41,69,126-130];
- using contact precautions until patients are culture negative[27,34,41,127];
- performing enhanced environmental cleaning[13,27,32,41,127];
- managing vascular and urinary catheters[27];
- preventing lower respiratory tract infection in intubated patients[27];
- accurately diagnosing infectious etiologies[27];
- following the recommendations of the CDC Campaign to Prevent Antimicrobial Resistance[27,131];
- limiting and carefully selecting antimicrobial agents[27,121,132-136];
- conducting MDRO surveillance as part of an MDRO control program[27,41,127,137,138];
- using active surveillance cultures[27,34,126];

- educating staff members to encourage behavior change through better understanding of MDROs[27,41,139]; and
- improving communication about patients with MDROs within and between health care facilities.[27]

Several studies also promote cohorting patients,[140,141] using designated beds or units, universal screening,[142] and closing units when necessary to control transmission of MDROs.[27]

VII.c. Perioperative personnel should implement CDC guidelines to prevent central line infections, including using sterile technique and maximal sterile barrier precautions (ie, hair covering, mask, sterile gown, sterile gloves, a sterile full body drape) when inserting central catheters.[143] *[1: Strong Evidence]*

Central line infections cause significant problems for patients and health care facilities in terms of increased length of stay and increased cost. It is a national imperative to eliminate central line-associated blood stream infection among patients, and the CDC Healthcare Infection Control Practices Advisory Committee has specific recommendations for all health care providers who insert central catheters, which includes anesthesia professionals. It is the perioperative nurses' responsibility to make sure this evidence-based guideline is followed to promote safety in all perioperative patients.[143]

One study from the United Kingdom demonstrated that 39% of hospital-acquired MRSA bacteremia cases were caused by a central line. The researchers recommended a focus of infection prevention efforts should be on improving insertion and care of central lines.[144]

Intraoperative stopcock contamination increases the rate of patient mortality, and patient and provider reservoirs contribute to 30-day postoperative infections, according to a multicenter study.[145] Researchers observed stopcock transmission events in 274 ORs and collected reservoir bacterial cultures. They identified stopcock contamination in 23% of procedures and concluded that although patients, provider hands, and the environment may have contributed to the transmission events, the environment was the most likely source. The researchers recommended designing multimodal programs to target each reservoir in parallel and introducing a comprehensive approach to reducing intraoperative bacterial contamination.

VII.d. Perioperative nurses should follow the CDC guidelines for the prevention of catheter-associated urinary tract infections[146] and the health care organization's policies and procedures for urinary catheter insertion to prevent urinary tract infections. *[1: Strong Evidence]*

Catheter-associated urinary tract infections are considered health care-associated infections. They are preventable by following evidence-based recommendations.[146]

One UK study showed that 51% of hospital-acquired MRSA bacteremia cases were caused by urinary catheters. The researchers recommended focusing infection prevention efforts on improving the insertion and care of urinary catheters.[144]

VII.d.1. Perioperative personnel should
- insert catheters only for medically indicated conditions;
- use urinary catheters for surgical patients only as necessary as opposed to routinely;
- document the date and time of catheter insertion and remove the catheter as soon as possible postoperatively, preferably within 24 hours;
- strictly follow sterile technique when placing a urinary catheter; and
- allow only trained persons who are familiar with correct sterile technique and maintenance to insert urinary catheters.[146]

Recommendation VIII

Health care personnel should be immunized against vaccine-preventable diseases.

The CDC Advisory Committee for Immunization Practices recommends that health care providers receive immunizations if they come into contact with patients or infectious material from patients that may put them at risk for exposure and possible transmission of vaccine-preventable disease.[50] Including vaccinations as part of an organizational infection control and prevention program reduces the risk of occupationally acquired infections and, therefore, harm to patients from vaccine-preventable diseases.[4,50]

The CDC recommends that health care providers receive vaccinations for diseases for which routine vaccination or documentation of immunity is recommended because of risks in the workplace (ie, hepatitis B, seasonal influenza, measles, mumps, rubella, pertussis, varicella).[50]

VIII.a. Employers must make the hepatitis B vaccination series available to all perioperative employees whose work involves a reasonable risk of exposure to blood or other potentially infectious materials and must provide post-exposure evaluation and follow-up to all employees who have an exposure incident.[4,50] *[1: Regulatory Requirement]*

Hepatitis B is highly contagious and is transmitted via percutaneous exposure (eg, needlestick injury) or mucosal exposure to infected blood or body fluids. The risk of acquiring hepatitis B infection from occupational exposure depends on the frequency of percutaneous and mucosal exposure to blood or body fluids that contain the virus.[50] Risks to health care providers from sharps injuries and blood and body fluid exposure has been reduced as a result of widespread hepatitis B vaccination.[17]

Although rare, health care personnel who have hepatitis B or hepatitis C can transmit them to patients.[147]

VIII.a.1. Serologic testing should be repeated after hepatitis B vaccination for health care personnel who are at "high risk" of occupational percutaneous or mucosal exposure to blood or body fluids. If antibody levels are too low (< 10 mIU/mL), the health care provider should be revaccinated and tested again after completing the series.[50]

Performing serologic testing one to two months after the last dose of the vaccine helps determine whether there is a need for revaccination and guides post-exposure prophylaxis in the event of an exposure incident.[50]

VIII.a.2. In the event of blood or body fluid exposure (ie, percutaneous, ocular, mucous membrane, nonintact skin), the need for post-exposure prophylaxis should be evaluated immediately based on the hepatitis B surface antigen status of the source and the health care provider's vaccination history and vaccine-response status.[50]

VIII.b. All health care personnel who have no contraindications should receive annual influenza vaccinations. *[1: Strong Evidence]*

Health care providers are exposed to patients who have influenza and are therefore at risk of occupationally acquired influenza and transmitting the disease to patients and other providers.[50]

VIII.b.1. Health care organizations should implement strategies to improve influenza vaccination rates among perioperative personnel.

Strategies that can improve vaccination rates include

- establishing evidence-based educational and promotional programs to communicate about the disease and the vaccine,[50,148,149]
- capitalizing on the belief in ethical responsibility and protecting patients,[150]
- running a campaign that emphasizes the benefits of vaccination for personnel and patients,[50,151]
- implementing a vaccine declination policy,[50]
- encouraging senior medical staff members or opinion leaders to get vaccinated,[50]
- removing administrative barriers (eg, costs),[50,151]
- providing incentives for getting vaccinated,[50,151]
- providing the vaccine in locations and at times that are easily accessible to health care providers,[50,151] and
- monitoring and reporting provider vaccination rates.[50]

In January 2007, the Joint Commission began requiring accredited facilities to provide staff members, including volunteers and licensed independent practitioners, with influenza vaccinations and to report coverage levels.[50] As of January 2013, the Centers for Medicare & Medicaid Services will require acute care hospitals to report vaccination rates among providers as part of its hospital inpatient quality reporting program.[50]

Despite the fact that annual vaccination has been recommended for health care providers and is a high priority for reducing morbidity associated with the virus in health care settings, vaccination rates among health care providers still need to improve.[50,148,152]

According to a survey of 304 health care personnel at a German tertiary care university hospital, concern about adverse effects was a primary reason to avoid vaccination.[148] Health care providers who are less likely to get vaccinated include

- women[152];
- nurses, technicians, and administrative workers[152]; and
- those who did not receive a vaccine the previous year.[152]

According to a survey conducted across eight university medical centers in the Netherlands,[153] health care providers are more likely to get an influenza vaccination if they

- are older than 40 years of age,
- have a chronic illness,
- are aware of personal risk or the risk of infecting patients,
- trust that the vaccine is effective for reducing the risk of infecting patients,
- believe in the health care provider's responsibility to "do no harm" and ensure continuity of care, and
- have convenient access to the vaccine.

Social pressure for vaccination also increased the likelihood of health care providers getting vaccinated.

Health care personnel are more likely to accept the influenza vaccine if they have a desire to protect themselves or patients or have a perception that the vaccine is effective.[50]

Establishing a mandatory vaccination program is feasible and leads to high vaccination rates, as demonstrated by a five-year study conducted at a tertiary care center in Seattle, Washington.[154] In the first year of the program, 4,588 of 4,703 health care providers (97.6%) were vaccinated, and rates stayed above 98% for the subsequent four years. Of those who declined vaccination, 0.7% did so for religious reasons and were required to wear a mask during influenza season, and less than 0.2% opted to leave the facility. Although 72% of survey respondents at another facility in which mandatory vaccination was implemented reported feeling that the policy was "coercive," more than 90% agreed that the policy was ethically responsible and important for protecting patients and staff members.[150]

VIII.c. Perioperative personnel should have presumptive evidence of immunity to measles, mumps, and rubella, and this information should be documented and readily available in the health care setting.[50] *[1: Strong Evidence]*

Presumptive evidence includes written documentation of vaccination with two doses of measles-mumps-rubella vaccine administered at least 28 days apart, laboratory evidence of immunity, laboratory confirmation of disease, or birth before 1957.

Measles and mumps are highly contagious and can have serious consequences. Rubella was declared eliminated from the United States in 2004, but there is a risk of resurgence from importation.[50]

Exposure to measles, mumps, or rubella in the health care setting can be expensive and disruptive because of containment measures, necessary personnel furloughs or reassignments, and potential closures.[50]

VIII.d. Health care personnel should receive a single dose of tetanus toxoid, reduced diphtheria toxoid, and acellular pertussis (Tdap) as soon as feasible upon hire if they have not been vaccinated previously.[50] *[1: Strong Evidence]*

Pertussis (ie, whooping cough) is a highly contagious bacterial infection and is transmitted via contact and droplet routes.[50] Pertussis outbreaks in health care facilities can be costly in terms of personnel, testing, treatment, and prophylaxis, but adult vaccination may reduce the disease burden.[155] The Tdap vaccine protects against pertussis and reduces the risk of transmission to patients, other health care providers, family members, and the community.[50]

In October 2010, the CDC Advisory Committee for Immunization Practices recommended expanding the use of the Tdap vaccine.[156] According to CDC, although there is a high rate of coverage for pertussis vaccination in children, the disease is "poorly controlled in the United States;" Tdap coverage is 56% among adolescents and less than 6% among adults.[156]

VIII.d.1. Health care organizations should establish programs to increase Tdap vaccination among personnel, including providing convenient access to the vaccination, giving the vaccination free of charge, and educating health care providers about the benefits of vaccination.[50]

VIII.e. Health care organizations should ensure that all health care personnel have evidence of immunity to varicella, and providers who have no evidence of immunity should receive the varicella vaccine. This information should be documented and readily available in the health care setting.[50] *[1: Strong Evidence]*

Varicella is highly infectious and is transmitted via contact, droplet, and airborne routes. Primary infection usually results in lifetime immunity, and the US vaccination program that began in 1995 has led to greater than 85% declines in varicella incidence, hospitalizations, and deaths.[50]

Despite the reduced incidence, health care-associated transmission is still a risk and the disease can be fatal. Varicella is more likely to spread in hospital settings and long-term care facilities.[50] Varicella exposure among patients and health care providers can disrupt patient care and cost the facility in terms of identifying susceptible patients and staff members, managing those who are exposed, and mandating furloughs for exposed staff members.

VIII.e.1. When a patient with confirmed or suspected varicella infection enters the health care facility, airborne and contact precautions should be implemented and followed, and only health care providers with evidence of immunity should provide care to the patient.[50]

VIII.f. Health care organizations should review health care provider vaccination and immunity status at the time of hire and at least annually thereafter. *[1: Strong Evidence]*

Regularly reviewing vaccination and immunity status helps ensure that health care providers are up to date with respect to the recommended vaccines.[50]

VIII.f.1. All health care personnel should receive baseline TB screening upon hire. Follow-up testing should be performed in the case of exposure to TB.[53]

Recommendation IX

Activities of health care personnel with infections, exudative lesions, and nonintact skin should be restricted when these activities pose a risk of transmission of infection to patients and other health care providers. State, federal, and professional guidelines and strategies should be followed to determine the need for work restrictions for health care personnel with bloodborne infections.[20,28]

Restricting activities of personnel who have transmissible infections reduces transmission between providers and patients depending on the mode of transmission and epidemiology of the disease.[28] Infections that may require restrictions from providing direct patient care, entering the patient's environment, or handling instruments or devices that may be used during a surgical or invasive procedure include

- viral respiratory infections (eg, influenza, respiratory syncytial virus),[28]
- keratoconjunctivitis or purulent conjunctivitis caused by other microorganisms,[28]
- acute gastrointestinal illnesses (ie, vomiting or diarrhea with or without nausea, fever, or abdominal pain),[28,157]
- diphtheria (ie, identification as an asymptomatic carrier),[28]
- exudative lesions that cannot be contained (eg, eczema, impetigo, smallpox),[28,29,31,109]
- herpes simplex infections of the fingers or hands (ie, herpetic whitlow),[28]
- pediculosis,[28]
- scabies,[28] and
- meningococcal infection (ie, until 24 hours after the start of effective therapy).[28]

Work restrictions for health care personnel with bloodborne infections who provide direct patient care depend on several factors, including circulating viral burden and category of clinical activities.[20]

IX.a.   An employee health nurse, infection preventionist, or physician should assess any health care provider with an infection, exudative lesions, or nonintact skin before he or she is allowed to return to work providing direct patient care or handling medical devices that are used in surgical or other invasive procedures. *[1: Strong Evidence]*

    Medical clearance is necessary before health care providers who have an infection, exudative lesions, or nonintact skin can return to work with patients or other health care providers.[28]

IX.b.   Health care personnel should report exposures as soon as they occur and infections as soon as the disease process is noted. *[1: Strong Evidence]*

    Early self-reporting of exposures and infections helps prevent transmission to patients and other health care providers. Health care providers can be encouraged to self-report exposures or infections when facility policies are designed to prevent judgement or penalty (eg, loss of wages, benefits, job status) for self-reporting.[28,97]

IX.c.   The health care organization should have a written policy regarding health care personnel who have a potentially transmissible infection. The policy should establish responsibility for reporting the condition, work restrictions, and guidelines for clearing the employee for work after an illness that required a restriction.[28,97] *[1: Strong Evidence]*

Recommendation X

Perioperative personnel should receive initial and ongoing education and complete competency verification of their understanding of the principles of infection prevention and the performance of standard, contact, droplet, and airborne precautions for prevention of transmissible infections and MDROs. `Amb`

Education and competency verification are prerequisites for ensuring standard and transmission-based precautions are understood and followed.[158] Ongoing development of knowledge and skills and documentation of personnel participation is a regulatory and accreditation requirement for both hospitals and ambulatory settings.[159-162]

Initial and ongoing education on infection prevention practices facilitate the development of knowledge, skills, and attitudes that affect safe patient care. Periodic education programs provide the opportunity to reinforce the principles of infection prevention, the necessary precautions to take when providing care to a patient who has a transmissible infection (eg, standards, contact, droplet, airborne), and the actions to take when a health care provider has a transmissible infection.

Competency verification measures individual performance; provides a mechanism for documentation; and verifies that perioperative personnel have an understanding of infection prevention, MDROs, and facility policies. Every nurse is personally accountable for maintaining competency validation.[163]

There are no universally accepted or mandated ways to perform or verify competency, and strategies differ between states. Some states mandate specific topics that affect public health (eg, bioterrorism) or that are specific to certain areas of nursing. The goal of competency verification is to reassure the public that nurses have the knowledge, skills, and judgment to provide safe and effective care.[164]

X.a.   Education, training, and competency verification should address
- standard precautions;
- contact precautions;
- airborne precautions;
- droplet precautions;
- MDROs;
- procedures for transporting patients who require infection precautions;
- use of N95 or powered air-purifying respirators;
- bloodborne pathogens;
- double gloving;
- sharps safety; and
- perioperative considerations to prevent central line-associated blood stream infections, catheter-associated urinary tract infections, SSIs, and carbapenem-resistant Enterobacteriaceae.

[3: Moderate Evidence]

Standard precautions are used for all patients in the perioperative setting, and transmission-based precautions can be modified depending on local conditions and patient characteristics (Table 1). Including each topic in education and training helps ensure appropriate follow-through in the event of a suspected or identified case of infection. Understanding the scientific premise of these precautions allows health care providers to follow and modify the precautions safely based on identified changes, resources, and health care settings.

X.b. Health care personnel who are occupationally exposed to blood or other potentially infectious materials must receive training before assignment to tasks where occupational exposure may occur, at least annually thereafter, and when changes to procedures or tasks affect occupational exposure.[4] *[1: Regulatory Requirement]*

Employers are responsible for providing training on the bloodborne pathogens standard during working hours at no cost to the employee. Employers are also responsible for ensuring employees participate in the training program and for offering materials in appropriate languages and at appropriate literacy levels.[4]

Providing the basis for the prevention of bloodborne pathogen exposure may instill an understanding of the processes that need to be followed and thereby prevent disease transmission. Education and training efforts are equally important in promoting awareness of hazards and acceptance of safe work and material-handling procedures in the workplace.[66] Educating employees on safe work practices (eg, using PPE) can help protect personnel, their family members, and the community from take-home transmissions.

X.b.1. Employee education must include
- an explanation of the modes of transmission of bloodborne pathogens and an explanation of the employer's exposure control plan;
- an explanation of the use and limitations of methods for reducing exposure (eg, engineering controls, work practices, PPE); and
- information on the hepatitis B vaccine, its efficacy and safety, the method of administration, and the benefits of vaccination.[4]

X.c. Perioperative personnel should receive education and competency validation on preventing the spread of MDROs as part of the health care organization's infection prevention program. Education should include
○ mechanisms of infection transmission,
○ case-based scenarios for managing infected patients,

○ participatory decision-making exercises about the implementation of precautions in addition to standard precautions, and
○ practice in the use of PPE for patients who require additional precautions.
[2: High Evidence]

Implementing a mandatory, organization-wide infection-control program can significantly improve the rate of health care-associated MRSA infections.[139]

X.d. Perioperative personnel should participate in programs to educate health care personnel about the importance of being immunized against epidemiologically important pathogens. *[3: Moderate Evidence]*

Programs that deliver educational and promotional messages about the benefits of vaccination can improve vaccination rates among health care personnel.[151]

X.e. Health care personnel should be educated on the benefits of reporting infections, exudative lesions, and nonintact skin in a timely manner and on related work restrictions. *[1: Strong Evidence]*

Institutional policies and procedures that guide work restrictions because of infections are designed to protect patients. Health care providers have an ethical responsibility to promote their own health and well being, and a responsibility to remove themselves from care situations if it is clear that there is a significant risk to patients despite appropriate preventive measures.[20]

X.f. Health care personnel should receive education and training on the facility emergency preparedness plan. *[1: Strong Evidence]*

It is important for health care personnel to be prepared to respond to threats of intentionally released pathogens and to treat patients who are exposed to biological agents.[165]

X.g. Perioperative personnel should participate in educational programs to improve infection control practices. *[3: Moderate Evidence]*

Surgical teams at a large UK teaching hospital implemented a "clean practice protocol" that increased adherence to overall infection control practices from 63% to 89% in three months, as demonstrated by undisclosed infection-control audits held before and after the education protocol.[166] The protocol combined the use of a reminder poster and auditing several surgical units for activities related to hand decontamination, correct use of gloves, instrument cleaning, garment contamination, and notes contamination. After the audits and education, hand decontamination and the correct use of gloves and aprons improved significantly.

TABLE 1. GUIDE FOR PERIOPERATIVE PERSONNEL CARING FOR PATIENTS WITH TRANSMISSIBLE INFECTIONS[1]

Type of precaution	Type of organism/ disease	Transport	Protection for unscrubbed personnel*	Preoperative area	Environmental measures
Contact	Draining abscess, infectious wounds, *Clostridium difficile*, acute viral infection, methicillin-resistant *Staphylococcus aureus* (MRSA), vancomycin-resistant Enterococci (VRE), vancomycin-intermediate/resistant *S aureus* (VISA/VRSA), extended-spectrum beta-lactamase (ESBL), multidrug-resistant pneumonia	Cover or contain the infected or colonized areas of the patient's body. Remove and dispose of contaminated personal protective equipment (PPE) and perform hand hygiene before transporting the patient. Don clean PPE to handle the patient at the transport destination.	Standard precautions plus the following: Wear gloves whenever touching the patient's skin or items that are in close proximity to the patient. Wear a gown when it can be anticipated that clothing will come into contact with the patient or contaminated environmental surfaces. Don a gown upon entry into the room, remove and perform hand hygiene before exiting.	Hold the patient in a single patient room if possible; otherwise keep ≥ 3 ft separation between patients.	Clean the room (eg, OR, airborne infection isolation room [AIIR]) immediately after patient use. Focus on frequently touched surfaces.
Droplet	Diphtheria, haemophilus influenza type b, seasonal influenza, pandemic influenza, meningococcal disease, mumps, mycoplasma pneumonia, group A streptococcus, pertussis, adenovirus, rubella	Instruct the patient to wear a mask and follow respiratory hygiene and cough etiquette. The transporter is not required to wear a mask.	Standard precautions plus the following: Wear a mask upon entry into the room.	Hold the patient in a single patient room if possible; otherwise keep ≥ 3 ft separation between patients. Draw a privacy curtain between beds to minimize the opportunity for close contact.	Routine
Airborne	Tuberculosis, disseminated herpes zoster, rubeola, monkeypox, smallpox, varicella zoster, chicken pox	Instruct the patient to wear a mask and follow respiratory hygiene and cough etiquette. Cover and contain affected skin lesions. The transporter is not required to wear a mask.	Standard precautions plus the following: Wear a fit-tested N95 or higher level respirator that is approved by the National Institute for Occupational Safety and Health.	Place the patient in an AIIR, if possible. Provide at least six (existing facility) or 12 (new construction/renovation) air changes per hour.	Consult an infection preventionist before patient placement to determine the safety of an alternative room that does not meet AIIR requirements. If an AIIR is not available, the OR should remain vacant postoperatively for the appropriate time to allow for a full exchange of air, generally one hour.

* "Unscrubbed personnel" include anesthesia professionals, the circulating RN, and preoperative and postanesthesthia care personnel.

Infection control professionals should modify or adapt this table according to local conditions and special patient considerations.

REFERENCE
1. Siegel JD, Rhinehart E, Jackson M, Chiarello L; the Healthcare Infection Control Practices Advisory Committee. 2007 Guideline for Isolation Precautions: Preventing Transmission of Infectious Agents in Health Care Settings. Am J Infect Control. 2007;35(10 Suppl 2):S65-S164.

PATIENT AND WORKER SAFETY

Recommendation XI

Documentation should reflect activities related to infection prevention. *Amb*

Documentation is a professional medicolegal standard.[167] Documentation related to infection prevention is applicable at the systems level and the patient care level. At the systems level, documentation serves as a basis for monitoring compliance, measuring performance, maintaining employee records, and logging exposure incidents. At the patient care level, documentation facilitates continuity of patient care through clear communication and supports collaboration between health care team members.

XI.a. Employers must maintain training records related to bloodborne pathogens for three years.[4] The records must include
- training dates,
- content or a summary of the training,
- names and qualifications of trainer(s), and
- names and job titles of trainees.

[1: Regulatory Requirement]

XI.b. All incidents of occupational exposure to blood or other potentially infectious materials must be documented.[4] Documentation should include
- the route of exposure;
- the circumstances associated with the exposure;
- the source individual's serological status, if known;
- the employee's name and social security number;
- the employee's hepatitis B vaccination status and other relevant medical information for both individuals, including vaccination dates and any medical records related to the employee's ability to receive vaccinations;
- results of all related examinations, medical tests, and post-exposure evaluation and follow-up procedures;
- a licensed health care professional's written opinion; and
- a copy of the information provided to the employee.

[1: Regulatory Requirement]

Documenting each exposure incident provides a record of the incident, what follow-through was taken, and the current status of the incident.

XI.b.1. Employers must maintain a sharps injury log to document all percutaneous injuries from contaminated sharps and must maintain the log in such a way that an injured employee's identification remains confidential.[4] At a minimum, a sharps injury log must include
- the type and brand of device involved in the incident,
- the department or work area where the exposure incident occurred, and
- an explanation of how the incident occurred.

Some health care employers may be exempt from maintaining a sharps injury log. The requirement to establish and maintain a sharps injury log applies to any employer who is required to maintain a log of occupational injuries and illnesses under 29 CFR §1904.[4]

XI.b.2. Documentation related to exposure incidents must be maintained for the employee's duration of employment plus 30 years.[4]

XI.c. Records and results of TB screening should be maintained for each employee in the employee's health record.[53] If an employee has symptoms of TB, the symptoms should be recorded in the employee health record or medical record.[53] *[1: Strong Evidence]*

XI.d. Vaccination records should be maintained for each employee. All employee vaccinations should be documented in each employee's health record. Records of any vaccinations administered during employment should include
- the type of vaccine given;
- the date on which the vaccine is given;
- the name of the vaccine manufacturer and the lot number;
- any documented episodes of adverse reactions to a vaccination;
- the name, address, and title of the person who administered the vaccination; and
- the edition and distribution date of the language-appropriate vaccine information statement provided to the employee at the time of vaccination.[50]

[1: Strong Evidence]

Accurate vaccination records make it possible to quickly identify health care personnel who are susceptible to infection during an outbreak and can reduce costs and disruptions to health care operations.[50]

XI.d.1. Each employee's immunity status for vaccine-preventable diseases, including documented disease, vaccination history, and serology results, should be recorded in the employee's record.[50]

XI.d.2. The health care organization should use a secure computerized system to manage vaccination records for health care personnel.[50]

Computerized systems allow records to be retrieved easily and as needed.[50]

XI.e. Wound class should be documented according to the CDC Surgical Wound Classification system at the conclusion of the procedure.[97] *[1: Strong Evidence]*

The surgical wound classification system has been shown to be a predictor of the relative probability that a wound infection will

PATIENT AND WORKER SAFETY

occur.[97,168] In addition, the classification allows for comparison of wound infection rates associated with different surgical techniques, surgeons, and facilities. The comparison may be useful for research and also may serve to alert infection prevention personnel to wounds at increased risk for infection, enabling health care providers to implement appropriate surveillance and preventative measures.[97,168]

The definitions of the four CDC wound classifications are

○ Class 1—Clean wounds: These are uninfected operative wounds in which no inflammation is encountered, and the respiratory, alimentary, genital, or uninfected urinary tracts are not entered. In addition, clean wounds are primarily closed, and, if necessary, drained with closed drainage (eg, Jackson-Pratt). Operative incisional wounds that follow nonpenetrating (blunt) trauma should be included in this category if they meet the criteria.

○ Class 2—Clean-contaminated wounds: These are operative wounds in which the respiratory, alimentary, genital, or urinary tract is entered under controlled conditions and without unusual contamination. Specifically, operations involving the biliary tract, appendix, vagina, and oropharynx are included in this category, provided no evidence of infection or major break in technique is encountered (eg, spillage from the gastrointestinal tract).

○ Class 3—Contaminated wounds: These include open, fresh, accidental wounds; operations with major breaks in sterile technique (eg, a procedure performed with unsterile instruments) or gross spillage from the gastrointestinal tract; and incisions in which acute, nonpurulent inflammation is encountered.

○ Class 4—Dirty or infected wounds: These include old traumatic wounds with retained devitalized tissue and those that involve existing clinical infection or perforated viscera. This definition suggests that the organisms causing postoperative infection were present in the operative field before the operation.

XI.e.1. Perioperative nurses should use educational tools to assist in accurately identifying surgical wounds.

The AORN Surgical Wound Classification Decision Tree can help perioperative nurses accurately identify surgical wounds (Figure 1).

XI.f. Breaks in sterile technique should be documented per organization policy in consultation with infection prevention personnel.[73] *[1: Strong Evidence]*

Thoughtful assessment, collaboration with the surgeon and surgical team members, and the application of informed clinical judgment is required when determining whether contamination resulting from a break in sterile technique is significant enough for an infection to occur and the wound classification to be changed.

XI.g. Results of documented surveillance should be shared with perioperative personnel. *[1: Strong Evidence]*

Sharing documented surveillance can help to reduce morbidity and mortality.[169] Monitoring performance helps in assessing the effectiveness of quality improvement interventions, and sharing surveillance strategies and results helps in identifying best practices for implementing evidence-based guidelines for preventing health care-associated infections.

Surveillance of both process measures and the infection rates to which they are linked are important for evaluating how effective infection prevention efforts are and identifying what needs to be changed. Surveillance is an ongoing, systematic collection, analysis, interpretation, and dissemination of data based on infections occurring in the health care facility.[1]

Recommendation XII

Policies and procedures for the prevention and control of transmissible infections and MDROs should be developed, reviewed periodically, revised as necessary, and readily available within the practice setting. *Amb*

Policies and procedures assist in the development of patient safety, quality assessment, and performance improvement activities. Policies and procedures establish authority, responsibility, and accountability within the facility. They also serve as operational guidelines that are used to minimize patient risk factors for complications, standardize practice, direct perioperative personnel, and establish continuous performance improvement programs.

XII.a. Policies and procedures should be developed to guide, support, and monitor adherence to standard and transmission-based precautions, including systems that should be used to collect, analyze, and communicate information related to transmissible infections.[1] *[1: Strong Evidence]*

Definitive policies and procedures as part of an overall administrative strategy can demonstrate a commitment to preventing transmissible infections by incorporating infection control into the organizational objectives for patient and occupational safety.[1] Policies and procedures that guide and support patient care, treatment, and services are a regulatory and accreditation requirement for both hospitals and ambulatory settings.[1,161,162,170-173]

FIGURE 1. SURGICAL WOUND CLASSIFICATION DECISION TREE

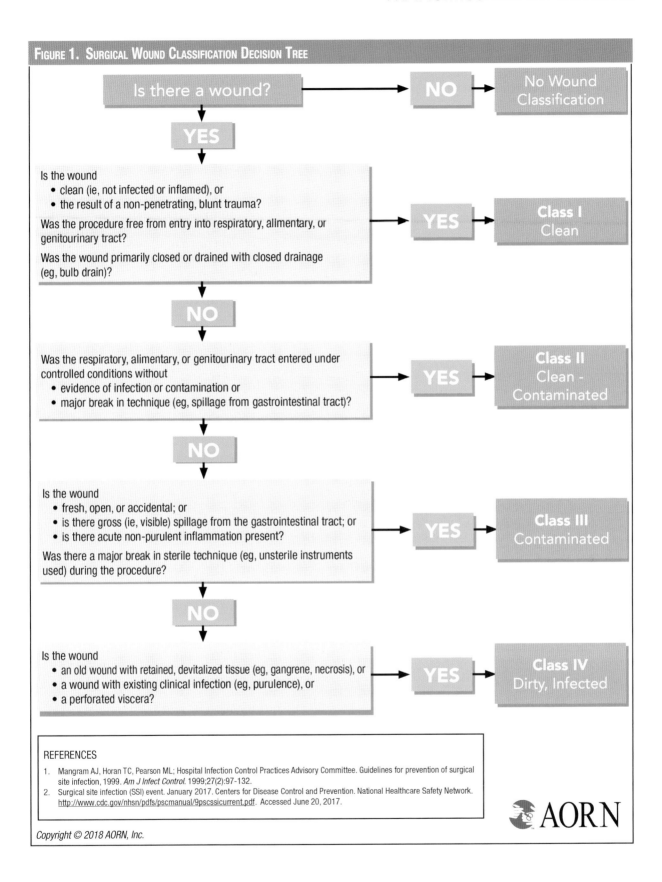

Is there a wound? → **NO** → No Wound Classification

↓ **YES**

Is the wound
- clean (ie, not infected or inflamed), or
- the result of a non-penetrating, blunt trauma?

Was the procedure free from entry into respiratory, alimentary, or genitourinary tract?

Was the wound primarily closed or drained with closed drainage (eg, bulb drain)?

→ **YES** → **Class I** Clean

↓ **NO**

Was the respiratory, alimentary, or genitourinary tract entered under controlled conditions without
- evidence of infection or contamination or
- major break in technique (eg, spillage from gastrointestinal tract)?

→ **YES** → **Class II** Clean - Contaminated

↓ **NO**

Is the wound
- fresh, open, or accidental; or
- is there gross (ie, visible) spillage from the gastrointestinal tract; or
- is there acute non-purulent inflammation present?

Was there a major break in sterile technique (eg, unsterile instruments used) during the procedure?

→ **YES** → **Class III** Contaminated

↓ **NO**

Is the wound
- an old wound with retained, devitalized tissue (eg, gangrene, necrosis), or
- a wound with existing clinical infection (eg, purulence), or
- a perforated viscera?

→ **YES** → **Class IV** Dirty, Infected

REFERENCES

1. Mangram AJ, Horan TC, Pearson ML; Hospital Infection Control Practices Advisory Committee. Guidelines for prevention of surgical site infection, 1999. *Am J Infect Control.* 1999;27(2):97-132.
2. Surgical site infection (SSI) event. January 2017. Centers for Disease Control and Prevention. National Healthcare Safety Network. http://www.cdc.gov/nhsn/pdfs/pscmanual/9pscssicurrent.pdf. Accessed June 20, 2017.

 AORN

XII.a.1. Policies and procedures should be developed and implemented to address specific perioperative interventions to prevent SSIs, MDROs, central line-associated blood stream infections, and catheter-associated urinary tract infections.

XII.b. Policies and procedures designed to eliminate or minimize health care personnel exposure to blood and other potentially infectious materials must be developed and implemented.[4] *[1: Regulatory Requirement]*

A written exposure control plan that is consistent with federal, state, and local rules and regulations and that governs occupational exposure to bloodborne pathogens, is reviewed periodically, and is readily available in the practice setting promotes safety with medical devices and blood and body fluids.[4]

XII.c. Policies should be developed in accordance with federal and state guidelines and should be consistent with existing impaired-provider and disability guidelines to define work restrictions for health care providers who have infections, exudative lesions, and nonintact skin. The policies should include whether the employee

- has a viral burden above the recommended threshold for the relevant virus,
- has a medical condition or conditions that result in an inability to perform assigned tasks,
- has documented untoward events (eg, having transmitted hepatitis B, hepatitis C, or HIV),
- refuses or is unable to follow recommended guidelines to prevent transmission of infectious diseases, or
- is unable to perform regular duties, assuming that reasonable accommodation has been offered for the disability.[50]

[1: Strong Evidence]

XII.d. A comprehensive vaccination policy for all health care personnel should be developed and implemented.[50] The vaccination policy should include a method to ensure that

- all health care personnel are up to date with recommended vaccines,
- health care personnel vaccination and immunity status is reviewed at the time of hire and at least annually thereafter, and
- necessary vaccines are offered to employees in conjunction with routine annual disease-prevention measures (eg, influenza vaccination, TB testing).

[1: Strong Evidence]

XII.e. Policies and procedures should be developed based on federal and state guidelines to define emergency response to threats of intentionally released pathogens (eg, anthrax, botulism, plague, smallpox). *[1: Strong Evidence]*

Establishing policies and procedures for emergency preparedness guides health care providers in responding to intentionally released pathogens and treating patients who are exposed to biological agents.[165]

XII.f. Policies and procedures should include processes for initial education, training, ongoing competency verification, and annual review of issues dealing with infection transmission. *[5: Benefits Balanced with Harms]*

Policies and procedures assist in the development of activities that support patient safety, quality assessment, and the establishment of guidelines for continuous performance improvement. Standardizing processes for performance expectations between perioperative settings facilitates continuity of care and reduces the risk of error when personnel rotate between areas.

Recommendation XIII

Perioperative team members should participate in a variety of quality assurance and performance improvement activities to monitor and improve the prevention of infections and MDROs. *Amb*

Quality assurance and performance improvement programs assist in evaluating the quality of patient care and the formulation of plans for corrective actions. These programs provide data that may be used to determine whether an individual organization is within benchmark goals and, if not, identify areas that may require corrective actions.

XIII.a. Process monitoring should be a part of every perioperative setting as part of an overall infection prevention program. Process monitoring should include[174]

- hand hygiene compliance,
- standard and transmissible infection precaution compliance,
- influenza vaccinations for personnel and patients,
- environmental cleaning practices, and
- central line and urinary catheter insertion practices.

[3: Moderate Evidence]

XIII.a.1. Perioperative nurses should assess and monitor cleaning and disinfection practices.

Monitoring cleaning and disinfection practices to ensure adherence can help control transmission of MDROs and other pathogens that may be residing in the environment.[11,175] The information obtained from assessments can be used to develop focused administrative and educational interventions that incorporate ongoing feedback to the environmental services personnel, to improve cleaning and disinfection practices in health care institutions.[10]

Compliance and adjunct monitoring after terminal cleaning can help prevent cross-contamination of areas that have or have had patients with MDROs.[27,175]

XIII.a.2. Perioperative nurses should participate in quality improvement initiatives that promote understanding of and adherence to the principles of sterile technique.[73]

XIII.a.3. A quality improvement program for the use of indwelling urinary catheters and central lines should be developed and implemented.

Monitoring the use of indwelling catheters can reduce catheter-associated urinary tract infections.[146]

Quality improvement initiatives in which various strategies are "bundled" together may improve compliance with evidence-based recommended practices and reduce the incidence of central line-associated blood stream infections.[143]

XIII.a.4. A quality improvement program for the use of indwelling catheters should be developed and implemented.[143]

XIII.b. Quality indicators should be developed to measure improvement in the control and transmission of infectious diseases, including MDROs. Quality indicators for measuring the provision of safe patient care with regard to transmissible infections in the perioperative setting should include
- the rate of SSIs,
- the selection of antibiotics that are appropriate for surgery,
- the timing of antibiotic administration, and
- immunization rates of patients and personnel.

[1: Strong Evidence]

Quality indicators are measurable and demonstrate that facilities are using specific interventions to provide safe patient care.[176] According to the Agency for Healthcare Research and Quality, "An adequate quality indicator must have a sound clinical or empirical rationale for its use. It should measure an important aspect of quality that is subject to provider or health care system control."[176(p3)] Quality indicators are one response to the need for multidimensional, accessible quality measures that can be used to gauge performance in health care. The quality indicators are evidence-based and can be used to identify variations in the quality of care provided on both an inpatient and outpatient basis.

XIII.b.1. Perioperative personnel who contract an infection or have a communicable disease should report it to the designated responsible person.

Prompt reporting enables employers to provide timely and confidential evaluation, intervention, and testing, or appropriate prophylaxis.[1,28]

XIII.b.2. All exposure incidents (eg, needlesticks, blood exposures) must be reported according to health care organization policy and based on the OSHA bloodborne pathogens standard.[4]

Documenting all exposure incidents provides the employer with feedback regarding the circumstances of employee exposures. This information can be used to focus efforts on decreasing or eliminating specific circumstances or routes of exposures.[60]

XIII.b.3. Perioperative nurses should contribute to ongoing surveillance of proper use of PPE.

By monitoring the proper use of PPE, perioperative nurses can contribute to community safety by helping limit take-home transmissions of infectious and toxic agents.[66] To gather data on take-home transmissions, NIOSH has recommended expanding current surveillance programs, such as building on the existing NIOSH Sentinel Event Notification Surveillance for Occupational Risks programs for lead and pesticides, which would require prioritizing toxic agents and targeting surveillance in areas where workplace exposure is relatively common.

The NIOSH Task Force recommends, at a minimum,
- develop surveillance programs to document the effectiveness of control measures being used, including an assessment of the feasibility and effectiveness of alternative measures;
- assess the performance of existing protective clothing (eg, single-use disposable clothing, clothing that can be laundered) as barriers for chemical, biological, thermal, and physical hazards;
- assess the use and acceptance of PPE by workers;
- research and develop new types of materials for protective clothing and gloves, including evaluating performance and characteristics; and
- ensure that protective clothing is made available and designed to fit all workers.

XIII.c. Rates of transmissible infections and MDROs should be monitored, documented, and reported to the designated infection preventionist and quality assurance improvement manager and any other personnel deemed appropriate by the health care organization. Surveillance should include monitoring
- use of standard precautions, contact precautions, droplet precautions, and airborne precautions;
- outbreak-specific pathogens (eg, N meningitides);
- isolation precautions for MDROs, surveillance practices, and practitioner adherence[177];
- bloodborne pathogen exposures;
- use of PPE; and

○ health care personnel immunization rates. *[1: Strong Evidence]*

Surveillance is a critical component of any MDRO control program because it allows for the detection of newly emerging pathogens, helps identify epidemiologic trends (eg, single patient, clusters of patients), and measures the effectiveness of interventions.[27] Surveillance is important for follow-up with health care personnel who may have an infection or be colonized.[1]

XIII.d. Perioperative nurses should participate in surveillance programs for SSI. *[1: Strong Evidence]*

Routine review and interpretation of SSI rates may help detect significant increases or outbreaks and identify areas where additional resources might be needed to improve SSI rates.[105]

A successful surveillance program includes using epidemiologically sound infection definitions, surveillance methods, stratification of SSI rates according to risk factors associated with SSI development, and data feedback.[97] Using consistent definitions as part of an SSI surveillance program helps ensure accurate interpretation and reporting. The CDC's National Nosocomial Infections Surveillance system has developed standardized surveillance criteria for defining SSIs.[97]

Knowing what patient and surgery characteristics may influence the risk of SSI allows the surveillance team to stratify surgeries, makes surveillance data more comprehensible, and allows for targeted prevention measures.[97] According to the Hospital Infection Control Practices Advisory Committee, patient characteristics that may be associated with an increased risk of SSI include diabetes, cigarette smoking, systemic steroid use, obesity (ie, > 20% ideal body weight), extremes of age, poor nutritional status, and perioperative transfusion of certain blood products. Surgery characteristics that affect SSI incidence include preoperative antiseptic showering, preoperative hair removal, skin prep practices, preoperative hand and forearm antisepsis, management of infected or colonized perioperative team members, and antimicrobial prophylaxis.

XIII.d.1. Perioperative nurses should implement and record the measures related to Surgical Care Improvement Project (SCIP) initiatives according to health care organization policy.

As a national quality improvement initiative, SCIP is supported by more than 10 national organizations with the goal of improving surgical outcomes and significantly reducing surgical complications. Surgical Care Improvement Project measures are part of the Joint Commission's accountability measures.[178]

One study that involved Surgical Care Improvement Project initiatives showed the importance of following these standard guidelines to decrease the number of patients who experience an SSI.[179] Perioperative nurses can take an active role in implementing Surgical Care Improvement Project measures and reporting data to identify areas where improvements can be made.

XIII.d.2. The choice of which procedures to monitor should be made jointly by surgeons and infection prevention personnel. SSI surveillance should target high-risk procedures.[97]

XIII.d.3. When a cluster of SSIs involves an unusual organism, a formal epidemiologic investigation should be conducted.[97] *Amb*

Outbreaks and clusters of SSIs that involved unusual organisms (eg, *Clostridium perfringens*, *Legionella pneumophila*, *Legionelle dumoffii*, *Nocardia farcinica*, *Pseudomonas multivorans*, *Rhizopus oryzae*, *Rhodococcus bronchialis*) have been attributed to contaminated adhesive dressings, elastic bandages, colonized surgical personnel, tap water, and disinfectant solutions.[97]

XIII.e. Perioperative nurses should contribute to creating a culture of safety. *[1: Strong Evidence]*

A culture of safety is created through
○ management initiatives that improve patient and health care personnel safety,
○ health care personnel participation in safety planning,
○ the availability of appropriate PPE for the identified tasks,
○ the influence of group norms regarding appropriate safety practices, and
○ the facility's socialization process for new hires.[1]

A culture of safety has a direct effect on preventing transmissible infections.[1]

Glossary

Airborne infection isolation: The isolation of patients infected with organisms spread via airborne droplet nuclei < 5 μm in diameter.

Airborne precautions: Precautions that reduce the risk of an airborne transmission of infectious airborne droplet nuclei (ie, small particle residue 5 microns or smaller). Airborne transmission refers to contact with infectious airborne droplet nuclei that can remain suspended in the air for extended periods of time or infectious dust particles that can be circulated by air currents.

Contact precautions: Precautions designed to reduce the risk of transmission of epidemiologically important microorganisms by direct or indirect contact.

PATIENT AND WORKER SAFETY

Direct contact: Person-to-person contact resulting in physical transfer of infectious microorganisms between an infected or colonized person and a susceptible host.

Droplet precautions: Precautions that reduce the risk of large particle droplet (ie, 5 microns or larger) transmission of infectious agents.

Enhanced environmental cleaning: Environmental cleaning practices implemented to prevent the spread of infections or outbreaks, enhanced cleaning practices promote consistent and standardized cleaning procedures that extend beyond routine cleaning.

Exposure incident: A specific eye, mouth, other mucous membrane, non-intact skin, or parenteral contact with blood or other potentially infectious materials that results from the performance of an employee's duties.

Indirect contact: Contact of a susceptible host with a contaminated object (eg, instruments, hands).

Infection preventionist: A health care professional specializing in leading and directing infection prevention and control programs.

Isolation precautions: Special precautionary measures, practices, and procedures used in the care of patients with contagious or communicable diseases.

Personal protective equipment (PPE): Specialized equipment or clothing for eyes, face, head, body, and extremities; protective clothing; respiratory devices; and protective shields and barriers designed to protect the worker from injury or exposure to a patient's blood, tissue, or body fluids. Used by health care workers and others whenever necessary to protect themselves from the hazards of processes or environments, chemical hazards, or mechanical irritants encountered in a manner capable of causing injury or impairment in the function of any part of the body through absorption, inhalation, or physical contact.

Powered air-purifying respirator: A respirator that uses a battery-powered blower to move the air flow through the filters.

Procedure mask: A mask that covers the nose and mouth and is intended for use in general patient care situations. These masks generally attach to the face with ear loops rather than ties or elastic. Unlike surgical masks, procedure masks are not regulated by the US Food and Drug Administration.

Respirator: A personal protective device that is worn on the face, covers at least the nose and mouth, and is used to reduce the wearer's risk of inhaling hazardous airborne particles (including dust particles and infectious agents), gases, or vapors. Source: What is a respirator? NIOSH. http://www.cdc.gov/niosh/npptl/topics/respirators/disp_part/RespSource1.html. Accessed October 2, 2012.

Standard precautions: The primary strategy for successful infection control and reduction of worker exposure. Precautions used for care of all patients regardless of their diagnosis or presumed infectious status.

Surgical mask: A device worn over the mouth and nose by perioperative team members during surgical procedures to protect both the surgical patient and perioperative team members from transfer of microorganisms and body fluids. Surgical masks are also used to protect health care providers from contact with large infectious droplets (>5 mcm in size). According to draft guidance issued by the US Food and Drug Administration on May 15, 2003, surgical masks are evaluated using standardized testing procedures for fluid resistance, bacterial filtration efficiency, differential pressure (air exchange), and flammability to mitigate the risks to health associated with the use of surgical masks. These specifications apply to any masks that are labeled surgical, laser, isolation, or dental or medical procedure.

Transmission-based precautions: Precautions designed to be used with patients known or suspected to be infected or colonized with highly transmissible or epidemiologically important pathogens for which additional precautions are needed to prevent transmission in the practice setting.

REFERENCES

1. Siegel JD, Rhinehart E, Jackson M, Chiarello L; Health Care Infection Control Practices Advisory Committee. 2007 Guideline for Isolation Precautions: Preventing Transmission of Infectious Agents in Health Care Settings. *Am J Infect Control.* 2007;35(10 Suppl 2): S65-S164. doi:10.1016/j.ajic.2007.10.007. [IVA]

2. Recommended practices for hand hygiene in the perioperative setting. In: *Perioperative Standards and Recommended Practices.* Denver, CO: AORN, Inc; 2012:73-86. [IVB]

3. World Health Organization. WHO Guidelines on Hand Hygiene in Health Care. Geneva, Switzerland: World Health Organization; 2009. [IVA]

4. Occupational Safety and Health Standards, Toxic and Hazardous Substances: Bloodborne Pathogens, 29 CFR §1910.1030 (2012). Occupational Safety and Health Administration. http://www.osha.gov/pls/oshaweb/owadisp.show_document?p_table=STANDARDS&p_id=10051. Accessed October 18, 2012.

5. Valenzuela TD, Hooton TM, Kaplan EL, Schlievert P. Transmission of "toxic strep" syndrome from an infected child to a firefighter during CPR. *Ann Emerg Med.* 1991;20(1):90-92. [VC]

6. Yu IT, Xie ZH, Tsoi KK, et al. Why did outbreaks of severe acute respiratory syndrome occur in some hospital wards but not in others? *Clin Infect Dis.* 2007;44(8):1017-1025. [IIB]

7. Stuart JM, Gilmore AB, Ross A, et al. Preventing secondary meningococcal disease in health care workers: recommendations of a working group of the PHLS meningococcus forum. *Commun Dis Public Health.* 2001;4(2):102-105. [IVA]

8. *Practice Guidance for Healthcare Environmental Cleaning.* Chicago, IL: American Society for Healthcare Environmental Services; 2008. [IVC]

9. Sehulster L, Chinn RY; CDC, HICPAC. Guidelines for environmental infection control in health-care facilities. Recommendations of CDC and the Healthcare Infection Control Practices Advisory Committee (HICPAC) [published correction appears in *MMWR Morb Mortal Wkly Rep.* 2003;52(42):1025-1026]. *MMWR Recomm Rep.* 2003;52(RR-10):1-42. [IVA]

10. Carling PC, Parry MF, Von Beheren SM; Healthcare Environmental Hygiene Study Group. Identifying opportunities to enhance environmental cleaning in 23 acute care hospitals. *Infect Control Hosp Epidemiol.* 2008;29(1):1-7. doi:10.1086/524329. [IIIB]

11. Recommended practices for environmental cleaning in the perioperative setting. In: *Perioperative Standards*

and *Recommended Practices*. Denver, CO: AORN, Inc; 2012:237-250. [IVB]

12. Mutters R, Nonnenmacher C, Susin C, Albrecht U, Kropatsch R, Schumacher S. Quantitative detection of *Clostridium difficile* in hospital environmental samples by real-time polymerase chain reaction. *J Hosp Infect.* 2009;71(1):43-48. doi:10.1016/j.jhin.2008.10.021. [IIIB]

13. Weber DJ, Rutala WA, Miller MB, Huslage K, Sickbert-Bennett E. Role of hospital surfaces in the transmission of emerging health care-associated pathogens: norovirus, *Clostridium difficile*, and Acinetobacter species. *Am J Infect Control.* 2010;38(5 Suppl 1):S25-S33. [VA]

14. Lessa FC, Gould PL, Pascoe N, et al. Health care transmission of a newly emergent adenovirus serotype in health care personnel at a military hospital in Texas, 2007. *J Infect Dis.* 2009;200(11):1759-1765. [IIIA]

15. Boyce JM, Pittet D; Healthcare Infection Control Practices Advisory Committee, HICPAC/SHEA/APIC/IDSA Hand Hygiene Task Force. Guideline for Hand Hygiene in Health-Care Settings. Recommendations of the Healthcare Infection Control Practices Advisory Committee and the HICPAC/SHEA/APIC/IDSA Hand Hygiene Task Force. Society for Healthcare Epidemiology of America/Association for Professionals in Infection Control/Infectious Diseases Society of America. *MMWR Recomm Rep.* 2002;51(RR-16):1-45. [IVA]

16. Guideline for medication safety. In: *Guidelines for Perioperative Practice*. Denver, CO: AORN, Inc; 2015:291-329. [IVB]

17. Perz JF, Thompson ND, Schaefer MK, Patel PR. US outbreak investigations highlight the need for safe injection practices and basic infection control. *Clin Liver Dis.* 2010;14(1):137-151. doi:10.1016/j.cld.2009.11.004. [VA]

18. Williams IT, Perz JF, Bell BP. Viral hepatitis transmission in ambulatory health care settings. *Clin Infect Dis.* 2004;38(11):1592-1598. doi:10.1086/420935. [VA]

19. Centers for Disease Control and Prevention (CDC). Transmission of hepatitis B and C viruses in outpatient settings—New York, Oklahoma, and Nebraska, 2000-2002. *MMWR Morb Mortal Wkly Rep.* 2003;52(38):901-906. [VA]

20. Henderson DK, Dembry L, Fishman NO, et al. SHEA guideline for management of healthcare workers who are infected with hepatitis B virus, hepatitis C virus, and/or human immunodeficiency virus. *Infect Control Hosp Epidemiol.* 2010;31(3):203-232. [IVA]

21. Young TN, Arens FJ, Kennedy GE, Laurie JW, Rutherford G. Antiretroviral post-exposure prophylaxis (PEP) for occupational HIV exposure. *Cochrane Database Syst Rev.* 2012;5. [IA]

22. Recommended practices for surgical attire. In: *Perioperative Standards and Recommended Practices*. Denver, CO: AORN, Inc; 2012:57-72. [IVB]

23. Neely AN, Maley MP. Survival of enterococci and staphylococci on hospital fabrics and plastic. *J Clin Microbiol.* 2000;38(2):724-726. [IIB]

24. Neely AN, Orloff MM. Survival of some medically important fungi on hospital fabrics and plastics. *J Clin Microbiol.* 2001;39(9):3360-3361. [IIIB]

25. Gastmeier P, Stamm-Balderjahn S, Hansen S, et al. How outbreaks can contribute to prevention of nosocomial infection: analysis of 1,022 outbreaks. *Infect Control Hosp Epidemiol.* 2005;26(4):357-361. doi:10.1086/502552. [VA]

26. Bhalla A, Pultz NJ, Gries DM, et al. Acquisition of nosocomial pathogens on hands after contact with environmental surfaces near hospitalized patients. *Infect Control Hosp Epidemiol.* 2004;25(2):164-167. doi:10.1086/502369. [IIB]

27. Siegel JD, Rhinehart E, Jackson M, Chiarello L; Healthcare Infection Control Practices Advisory Committee. *Management of Multidrug-Resistant Organisms in Healthcare Settings, 2006*. Atlanta, GA: Centers for Disease Control and Prevention; 2006. [IVA] 28. Bolyard EA, Tablan OC, Williams WW, Pearson ML, Shapiro CN, Deitchmann SD. Guideline for infection control in healthcare personnel, 1998. Hospital Infection Control Practices Advisory Committee. *Infect Control Hosp Epidemiol.* 1998;19(6):407-463. [IVA]

29. Wharton M, Strikas RA, Harpaz R, et al. Recommendations for using smallpox vaccine in a pre-event vaccination program. Supplemental recommendations of the Advisory Committee on Immunization Practices (ACIP) and the Healthcare Infection Control Practices Advisory Committee (HICPAC). *MMWR Recomm Rep.* 2003;52(RR-7):1-16. [IVA]

30. Sethi AK, Al-Nassir WN, Nerandzic MM, Bobulsky GS, Donskey CJ. Persistence of skin contamination and environmental shedding of *Clostridium difficile* during and after treatment of *C difficile* infection. *Infect Control Hosp Epidemiol.* 2010;31(1):21-27. [IIA]

31. Occelli P, Blanie M, Sanchez R, et al. Outbreak of staphylococcal bullous impetigo in a maternity ward linked to an asymptomatic healthcare worker. *J Hosp Infect.* 2007;67(3):264-270. [IIIB]

32. Duckro AN, Blom DW, Lyle EA, Weinstein RA, Hayden MK. Transfer of vancomycin-resistant enterococci via health care worker hands. *Arch Intern Med.* 2005;165(3):302-307. doi:10.1001/archinte.165.3.302. [IIIB]

33. Edgeworth JD. Has decolonization played a central role in the decline in UK methicillin-resistant *Staphylococcus aureus* transmission? A focus on evidence from intensive care. *J Antimicrob Chemother.* 2011;66(Suppl 2):ii41-ii47. [VA]

34. Boyce JM, Havill NL, Kohan C, Dumigan DG, Ligi CE. Do infection control measures work for methicillin-resistant *Staphylococcus aureus*? *Infect Control Hosp Epidemiol.* 2004;25(5):395-401. doi:10.1086/502412. [IIIB]

35. Mastoraki A, Douka E, Kriaras I, Stravopodis G, Saroglou G, Geroulanos S. Preventing strategy of multidrug-resistant *Acinetobacter baumanii* susceptible only to colistin in cardiac surgical intensive care units. *Eur J Cardiothorac Surg.* 2008;33(6):1086-1090. [IIIB]

36. Huskins WC, Huckabee CM, O'Grady NP, et al. Intervention to reduce transmission of resistant bacteria in intensive care. *N Engl J Med.* 2011;364(15):1407-1418. [IA]

37. Wines MP, Lamb A, Argyropoulos AN, Caviezel A, Gannicliffe C, Tolley D. Blood splash injury: an underestimated risk in endourology. *J Endourol.* 2008;22(6):1183-1187. [IIIB]

38. Ishihama K, Iida S, Koizumi H, et al. High incidence of blood exposure due to imperceptible contaminated splatters during oral surgery. *J Oral Maxillofac Surg.* 2008;66(4):704-710. [IIIB]

39. Vonberg RP, Kuijper EJ, Wilcox MH, et al. Infection control measures to limit the spread of *Clostridium difficile*. *Clin Microbiol Infect.* 2008;14(Suppl 5):2-20. doi:10.1111/j.1469-0691.2008.01992.x. [VA]

40. Datta R, Platt R, Yokoe DS, Huang SS. Environmental cleaning intervention and risk of acquiring multidrug-resistant organisms from prior room occupants. *Arch Intern Med.* 2011;171(6):491-494. doi:10.1001/archinternmed.2011.64. [IIB]

41. Rodríguez-Baño J, García L, Ramírez E, et al. Long-term control of hospital-wide, endemic multidrug-resistant *Acinetobacter baumannii* through a comprehensive

"bundle" approach. *Am J Infect Control.* 2009;37(9):715-722. [IIA]

42. Eckstein BC, Adams DA, Eckstein EC, et al. Reduction of *Clostridium difficile* and vancomycin-resistant Enterococcus contamination of environmental surfaces after an intervention to improve cleaning methods. *BMC Infect Dis.* 2007;7:61. [IIIA]

43. Jernigan JA, Siegman-Igra Y, Guerrant RC, Farr BM. A randomized crossover study of disposable thermometers for prevention of *Clostridium difficile* and other nosocomial infections. *Infect Control Hosp Epidemiol.* 1998;19(7):494-499. [IA]

44. Kirkland KB. Taking off the gloves: toward a less dogmatic approach to the use of contact isolation. *Clin Infect Dis.* 2009;48(6):766-771. doi:10.1086/597090. [VB]

45. Saint S, Higgins LA, Nallamothu BK, Chenoweth C. Do physicians examine patients in contact isolation less frequently? A brief report. *Am J Infect Control.* 2003;31(6):354-356. [IVA]

46. Morgan DJ, Diekema DJ, Sepkowitz K, Perencevich EN. Adverse outcomes associated with contact precautions: a review of the literature. *Am J Infect Control.* 2009;37(2):85-93. doi:10.1016/j.ajic.2008.04.257. [VA]

47. Zastrow RL. Emerging infections: the contact precautions controversy. *Am J Nurs.* 2011;111(3):47-53. [VB]

48. Papineni RS, Rosenthal FS. The size distribution of droplets in the exhaled breath of healthy human subjects. *J Aerosol Med.* 1997;10(2):105-116. [IIB]

49. Raboud J, Shigayeva A, McGeer A, et al. Risk factors for SARS transmission from patients requiring intubation: a multicentre investigation in Toronto, Canada. *PLoS ONE* [Electronic Resource]. 2010;5(5):e10717. [IIIA]

50. Advisory Committee on Immunization Practices; Centers for Disease Control and Prevention (CDC). Immunization of health-care personnel: recommendations of the Advisory Committee on Immunization Practices (ACIP). *MMWR Recomm Rep.* 2011;60(RR-7):1-45. [IVA]

51. Sakaguchi H, Wada K, Kajioka J, et al. Maintenance of influenza virus infectivity on the surfaces of personal protective equipment and clothing used in healthcare settings. *Environ Health Prev Med.* 2010;15(6):344-349. [IIIB]

52. Kilpatrick C, Prieto J, Wigglesworth N. Single room isolation to prevent the transmission of infection: Development of a patient journey tool to support safe practice. *Br J Infect Control.* 2008;9(6):19-25. [VB]

53. Centers for Disease Control and Prevention (CDC). Guidelines for preventing the transmission of *Mycobacterium tuberculosis* in health-care settings, 2005. *MMWR Morb Mortal Wkly Rep.* 2005;54(RR-17):1-140. [IVA]

54. Bassetti S, Bischoff WE, Walter M, et al. Dispersal of *Staphylococcus aureus* into the air associated with a rhinovirus infection. *Infect Control Hosp Epidemiol.* 2005;26(2):196-203. doi:10.1086/502526. [IIB]

55. Respirator trusted-source information. Centers for Disease Control and Prevention. http://www.cdc.gov/niosh/npptl/topics/respirators/disp_part/RespSource.html. Accessed October 26, 2012.

56. Olmsted RN. Pilot study of directional airflow and containment of airborne particles in the size of *Mycobacterium tuberculosis* in an operating room. *Am J Infect Control.* 2008;36(4):260-267. doi:10.1016/j.ajic.2007.10.028. [IIB]

57. Guideline for electrosurgery. In: *Guidelines for Perioperative Practice.* Denver, CO: AORN, Inc; 2015:121-138. [IVB]

58. Preventing the transmission of bloodborne pathogens information statement. American Academy of Orthopaedic Surgeons. http://www.aaos.org/about/papers/advistmt/1018.asp. Updated June 2008. Accessed October 26, 2012. [VA]

59. Association for Professionals in Infection Control and Epidemiology, Inc. APIC position paper: prevention of device-mediated bloodborne infections to health care workers. *Am J Infect Control.* 1998;26(6):578-580. [VA]

60. OSHA's bloodborne pathogens standard: analysis and recommendations. *Health Devices.* 1993;22(2):35-92.

61. Aarnio P, Laine T. Glove perforation rate in vascular surgery—a comparison between single and double gloving. *Vasa.* 2001;30(2):122-124. [IIIC]

62. Wilburn SQ. Needlestick and sharps injury prevention. *Online J Issues Nurs.* 2004;9(3):5. [VA]

63. Jagger J, Perry J, Gomaa A, Phillips EK. The impact of U.S. policies to protect healthcare workers from bloodborne pathogens: the critical role of safety-engineered devices. *J Infect Public Health.* 2008;1(2):62-71. doi:10.1016/j.jiph.2008.10.002. [VA]

64. Tuma S, Sepkowitz KA. Efficacy of safety-engineered device implementation in the prevention of percutaneous injuries: a review of published studies. *Clin Infect Dis.* 2006;42(8):1159-1170. doi:10.1086/501456. [IVA]

65. Vose JG, McAdara-Berkowitz J. Reducing scalpel injuries in the operating room. *AORN J.* 2009;90(6):867-872. doi:10.1016/j.aorn.2009.07.025. [VB]

66. Protecting workers' families: a research agenda report of the Workers' Family Protection Task Force [DHHS (NIOSH) publication number 2002-113]. http://www.cdc.gov/niosh/docs/2002-113. Accessed October 26, 2012. [VA]

67. Tenorio AR, Badri SM, Sahgal NB, et al. Effectiveness of gloves in the prevention of hand carriage of vancomycin-resistant enterococcus species by health care workers after patient care. *Clin Infect Dis.* 2001;32(5):826-829. doi:10.1086/319214. [IIB]

68. Daeschlein G, Kramer A, Arnold A, Ladwig A, Seabrook GR, Edmiston CE Jr. Evaluation of an innovative antimicrobial surgical glove technology to reduce the risk of microbial passage following intraoperative perforation. *Am J Infect Control.* 2011;39(2):98-103. doi:10.1016/j.ajic.2010.05.026. [IIB]

69. Hayden MK, Blom DW, Lyle EA, Moore CG, Weinstein RA. Risk of hand or glove contamination after contact with patients colonized with vancomycin-resistant enterococcus or the colonized patients' environment. *Infect Control Hosp Epidemiol.* 2008;29(2):149-154. [IIIA]

70. Kinlin LM, Mittleman MA, Harris AD, Rubin MA, Fisman DN. Use of gloves and reduction of risk of injury caused by needles or sharp medical devices in healthcare workers: results from a case-crossover study. *Infect Control Hosp Epidemiol.* 2010;31(9):908-917. doi:10.1086/655839. [IIIB]

71. Olsen RJ, Lynch P, Coyle MB, Cummings J, Bokete T, Stamm WE. Examination gloves as barriers to hand contamination in clinical practice. *JAMA.* 1993;270(3):350-353. [IIB]

72. Eklund AM, Ojajarvi J, Laitinen K, Valtonen M, Werkkala KA. Glove punctures and postoperative skin flora of hands in cardiac surgery. *Ann Thorac Surg.* 2002;74(1):149-153. [IIB]

73. Guideline for sterile technique. In: *Guidelines for Perioperative Practice.* Denver, CO: AORN, Inc; 2015:67-96. [IVA]

74. Misteli H, Weber WP, Reck S, et al. Surgical glove perforation and the risk of surgical site infection. *Arch Surg.* 2009;144(6):553-558. doi:10.1001/archsurg.2009.60. [IIIA]

75. Harnoss JC, Partecke LI, Heidecke CD, Hubner NO, Kramer A, Assadian O. Concentration of bacteria passing

PATIENT AND WORKER SAFETY

through puncture holes in surgical gloves. *Am J Infect Control.* 2010;38(2):154-158. [IIA]

76. Hubner NO, Goerdt AM, Stanislawski N, et al. Bacterial migration through punctured surgical gloves under real surgical conditions. *BMC Infect Dis.* 2010;10:192. [IIC]

77. Partecke LI, Goerdt AM, Langner I, et al. Incidence of microperforation for surgical gloves depends on duration of wear. *Infect Control Hosp Epidemiol.* 2009;30(5):409-414. [IIIA]

78. Al-Maiyah M, Bajwa A, Mackenney P, et al. Glove perforation and contamination in primary total hip arthroplasty. *J Bone Joint Surg Br.* 2005;87(4):556-559. [IA]

79. Korniewicz DM, Kirwin M, Cresci K, et al. Barrier protection with examination gloves: double versus single. *Am J Infect Control.* 1994;22(1):12-15. [IIB]

80. Korniewicz DM, El-Masri M, Broyles JM, Martin CD, O'connell KP. Performance of latex and nonlatex medical examination gloves during simulated use. *Am J Infect Control.* 2002;30(2):133-138. [IIB]

81. Rego A, Roley L. In-use barrier integrity of gloves: latex and nitrile superior to vinyl. *Am J Infect Control.* 1999;27(5):405-410. [IIB]

82. Klein RC, Party E, Gershey EL. Virus penetration of examination gloves. *Biotechniques.* 1990;9(2):196-199. [IIB]

83. Tulipan N, Cleves MA. Effect of an intraoperative double-gloving strategy on the incidence of cerebrospinal fluid shunt infection. *J Neurosurg.* 2006;104(1 Suppl):5-8. doi:10.3171/ped.2006.104.1.5. [IIA]

84. Tanner J, Parkinson H. Surgical glove practice: the evidence. *J Perioper Pract.* 2007;17(5):216-218, 220-222, 224-225. [IA]

85. Tanner J, Parkinson H. Double gloving to reduce surgical cross-infection. *Cochrane Database Syst Rev.* 2009;1. [IA]

86. Korniewicz D, El-Masri M. Exploring the benefits of double gloving during surgery. *AORN J.* 2012;95(3):328-336. doi:10.1016/j.aorn.2011.04.027. [IIIB]

87. Berguer R, Heller PJ. Preventing sharps injuries in the operating room. *J Am Coll Surg.* 2004;199(3):462-467. doi:10.1016/j.jamcollsurg.2004.04.018. [VA]

88. Lancaster C, Duff P. Single versus double-gloving for obstetric and gynecologic procedures. *Am J Obstet Gynecol.* 2007;196(5):e36-e37. doi:10.1016/j.ajog.2006.08.045. [VA]

89. Laine T, Kaipia A, Santavirta J, Aarnio P. Glove perforations in open and laparoscopic abdominal surgery: the feasibility of double gloving. *Scand J Surg.* 2004;93(1):73-76. [IA]

90. Haines T, Stringer B, Herring J, Thoma A, Harris KA. Surgeons' and residents' double-gloving practices at 2 teaching hospitals in Ontario. *Can J Surg.* 2011;54(2):95-100. [IIIB]

91. Wittmann A, Kralj N, Kover J, Gasthaus K, Hofmann F. Study of blood contact in simulated surgical needlestick injuries with single or double latex gloving. *Infect Control Hosp Epidemiol.* 2009;30(1):53-56. doi:10.1086/593124. [IIA]

92. Myers DJ, Epling C, Dement J, Hunt D. Risk of sharp device-related blood and body fluid exposure in operating rooms. *Infect Control Hosp Epidemiol.* 2008;29(12):1139-1148. doi:10.1086/592091. [VA]

93. Florman S, Burgdorf M, Finigan K, Slakey D, Hewitt R, Nichols RL. Efficacy of double gloving with an intrinsic indicator system. *Surg Infect (Larchmt).* 2005;6(4):385-395. [IIB]

94. Duron JJ, Keilani K, Elian NG. Efficacy of double gloving with a coloured inner pair for immediate detection of operative glove perforations. *Eur J Surg.* 1996;162(12):941-944. [VB]

95. Eye safety: eye protection for infection control. NIOSH workplace safety and health topic. Centers for Disease Control and Prevention. http://www.cdc.gov/niosh/topics/eye/eye-infectious.html. Accessed October 26, 2012. [IVB]

96. Philips BJ, Fergusson S, Armstrong P, Anderson FM, Wildsmith JA. Surgical face masks are effective in reducing bacterial contamination caused by dispersal from the upper airway. *Br J Anaesth.* 1992;69(4):407-408. [IIC]

97. Mangram AJ, Horan TC, Pearson ML, Silver LC, Jarvis WR; Hospital Infection Control Practices Advisory Committee. Guideline for prevention of surgical site infection, 1999. *Infect Control Hosp Epidemiol.* 1999;20(4):250-278. doi:10.1086/501620. [IVA]

98. Alwitry A, Jackson E, Chen H, Holden R. The use of surgical facemasks during cataract surgery: is it necessary? *Br J Ophthalmol.* 2002;86(9):975-977. [IB]

99. Chambers CE, Eisenhauer MD, McNicol LB, et al. Infection control guidelines for the cardiac catheterization laboratory: society guidelines revisited. *Catheter Cardiovasc Interv.* 2006;67(1):78-86. doi:10.1002/ccd.20589. [IVA]

100. Berger SA, Kramer M, Nagar H, Finkelstein A, Frimmerman A, Miller HI. Effect of surgical mask position on bacterial contamination of the operative field. *J Hosp Infect.* 1993;23(1):51-54. [IIB]

101. Lipp A. The effectiveness of surgical face masks: what the literature shows. *Nurs Times.* 2003;99(39):22-24. [VB]

102. Gralton J, McLaws ML. Protecting healthcare workers from pandemic influenza: N95 or surgical masks? *Crit Care Med.* 2010;38(2):657-667. [VA]

103. Korczak D, Schöffmann C. Medical and health economic evaluation of prevention- and control measures related to MRSA infections or -colonisations at hospitals. *GMS Health Technol Assess.* 2010;6:Doc04. [IIIB]

104. Lai JY, Guo YP, Or PP, Li Y. Comparison of hand contamination rates and environmental contamination levels between two different glove removal methods and distances. *Am J Infect Control.* 2011;39(2):104-111. doi:10.1016/j.ajic.2010.06.007. [IIB]

105. Anderson DJ, Kaye KS, Classen D, et al. Strategies to prevent surgical site infections in acute care hospitals. *Infect Control Hosp Epidemiol.* 2008;29(Suppl 1):S51-S61. doi:10.1086/591064. [IVA]

106. Recommended practices for cleaning and care of surgical instruments and powered equipment. In: *Perioperative Standards and Recommended Practices.* Denver, CO: AORN, Inc; 2012:513-536. [IVB]

107. Beldi G, Bisch-Knaden S, Banz V, Muhlemann K, Candinas D. Impact of intraoperative behavior on surgical site infections. *Am J Surg.* 2009;198(2):157-162. [IA]

108. Dineen P, Drusin L. Epidemics of postoperative wound infections associated with hair carriers. *Lancet.* 1973;2(7839):1157-1159. [VA]

109. Mastro TD, Farley TA, Elliott JA, et al. An outbreak of surgical-wound infections due to group A streptococcus carried on the scalp. *N Engl J Med.* 1990;323(14):968-972. [IIIB]

110. Mase K, Hasegawa T, Horii T, et al. Firm adherence of *Staphylococcus aureus* and *Staphylococcus epidermidis* to human hair and effect of detergent treatment. *Microbiol Immunol.* 2000;44(8):653-656. [IIB]

111. Recommended practices for preoperative patient skin antisepsis. In: *Perioperative Standards and Recommended Practices.* Denver, CO: AORN, Inc; 2012:445-464. [IVB]

112. Carro C, Camilleri L, Traore O, et al. An in-use microbiological comparison of two surgical hand disinfection techniques in cardiothoracic surgery: hand rubbing versus hand scrubbing. *J Hosp Infect.* 2007;67(1):62-66. [IIIA]

113. Le TA, Dibley MJ, Vo VN, Archibald L, Jarvis WR, Sohn AH. Reduction in surgical site infections in neurosurgical patients associated with a bedside hand hygiene program in Vietnam. *Infect Control Hosp Epidemiol.* 2007;28(5):583-588. doi:10.1086/516661. [IIA]

114. Recommended practices for traffic patterns in the perioperative practice setting. In: *Perioperative Standards and Recommended Practices.* Denver, CO: AORN, Inc; 2012:95-98. [IVB]

115. Guideline for sterilization. In: *Guidelines for Perioperative Practice.* Denver, CO: AORN, Inc; 2015:665-692. [IVB]

116. Schwarzkopf R, Takemoto RC, Immerman I, Slover JD, Bosco JA. Prevalence of *Staphylococcus aureus* colonization in orthopaedic surgeons and their patients: a prospective cohort controlled study. *J Bone Joint Surg Am.* 2010;92(9):1815-1819. doi:10.2106/JBJS.I.00991. [IIA]

117. Ammerlaan HS, Kluytmans JA, Wertheim HF, Nouwen JL, Bonten MJ. Eradication of methicillin-resistant *Staphylococcus aureus* carriage: a systematic review. *Clin Infect Dis.* 2009;48(7):922-930. doi:10.1086/597291. [IA]

118. Konvalinka A, Errett L, Fong IW. Impact of treating *Staphylococcus aureus* nasal carriers on wound infections in cardiac surgery. *J Hosp Infect.* 2006;64(2):162-168. [IA]

119. Segers P, Speekenbrink RG, Ubbink DT, van Ogtrop ML, de Mol BA. Prevention of nosocomial infection in cardiac surgery by decontamination of the nasopharynx and oropharynx with chlorhexidine gluconate: a randomized controlled trial. *JAMA.* 2006;296(20):2460-2466. [IA]

120. Yinusa W, Onche II, Thanni LO. Short-term antibiotic prophylaxis in implant surgery: a comparison of three antibiotics. *Niger Postgrad Med J.* 2007;14(2):90-93. [IB]

121. Kato D, Maezawa K, Yonezawa I, et al. Randomized prospective study on prophylactic antibiotics in clean orthopedic surgery in one ward for 1 year. *J Orthop Sci.* 2006;11(1):20-27. doi:10.1007/s00776-005-0970-0. [IIB]

122. Centers for Disease Control and Prevention (CDC). Carbapenem-resistant Enterobacteriaceae containing New Delhi metallo-beta-lactamase in two patients – Rhode Island, March 2012. *MMWR Morb Mortal Wkly Rep.* 2012;61:446-448. [VA]

123. Healthcare-associated infections (HAIs). 2012 CRE toolkit – Guidance for control of carbapenem-resistant Enterobacteriaceae (CRE). Part 2: Regional CRE prevention. Centers for Disease Control and Prevention. http://www.cdc.gov/hai/organisms/cre/cre-toolkit/rCRE prevention-AppendixC.html. Accessed October 26, 2012. [IVA]

124. Fairclough SJ. Why tackling MRSA needs a comprehensive approach. *Br J Nurs.* 2006;15(2):72-75. [VA]

125. Larson EL, Quiros D, Giblin T, Lin S. Relationship of antimicrobial control policies and hospital and infection control characteristics to antimicrobial resistance rates. *Am J Crit Care.* 2007;16(2):110-120. [IIIA]

126. Ellingson K, Muder RR, Jain R, et al. Sustained reduction in the clinical incidence of methicillin-resistant *Staphylococcus aureus* colonization or infection associated with a multifaceted infection control intervention. *Infect Control Hosp Epidemiol.* 2011;32(1):1-8. [IIB]

127. Griffin FA. 5 Million Lives Campaign. Reducing methicillin-resistant *Staphylococcus aureus* (MRSA) infections. *Jt Comm J Qual Patient Saf.* 2007;33(12):726-731. [IVA]

128. Sroka S, Gastmeier P, Meyer E. Impact of alcohol hand-rub use on methicillin-resistant *Staphylococcus aureus*: an analysis of the literature. *J Hosp Infect.* 2010;74(3):204-211. doi:10.1016/j.jhin.2009.08.023. [VC]

129. Miyachi H, Furuya H, Umezawa K, et al. Controlling methicillin-resistant *Staphylococcus aureus* by stepwise implementation of preventive strategies in a university hospital: impact of a link-nurse system on the basis of multidisciplinary approaches. *Am J Infect Control.* 2007;35(2):115-121. [IIIB]

130. Hsu J, Abad C, Dinh M, Safdar N. Prevention of endemic healthcare-associated Clostridium difficile infection: reviewing the evidence. *Am J Gastroenterol.* 2010;105(11):2327-2339. doi:10.1038/ajg.2010.254. [IVA]

131. Salgado CD, O'Grady N, Farr BM. Prevention and control of antimicrobial-resistant infections in intensive care patients. *Crit Care Med.* 2005;33(10):2373-2382. [VA]

132. Tyllianakis ME, Karageorgos ACh, Marangos MN, Saridis AG, Lambiris EE. Antibiotic prophylaxis in primary hip and knee arthroplasty: comparison between cefuroxime and two specific antistaphylococcal agents. *J Arthroplasty.* 2010;25(7):1078-1082. doi:10.1016/j.arth.2010.01.105. [IB]

133. Zilberberg MD, Chen J, Mody SH, Ramsey AM, Shorr AF. Imipenem resistance of Pseudomonas in pneumonia: a systematic literature review. *BMC Pulm Med.* 2010;10:45. doi:10.1186/1471-2466-10-45. [VA]

134. Tacconelli E. Antimicrobial use: risk driver of multidrug resistant microorganisms in healthcare settings. *Curr Opin Infect Dis.* 2009;22(4): 352-358. doi:10.1097/QCO.0b013e32832d52e0. [VA]

135. Tacconelli E, De Angelis G, Cataldo MA, Pozzi E, Cauda R. Does antibiotic exposure increase the risk of methicillin-resistant *Staphylococcus aureus* (MRSA) isolation? A systematic review and meta-analysis. *J Antimicrob Chemother.* 2008;61(1):26-38. [VB]

136. Davey P, Brown E, Fenelon L, et al. Interventions to improve antibiotic prescribing practices for hospital inpatients. *Cochrane Database Syst Rev.* 2009;1. [IA]

137. Rodríguez-Baño J, García L, Ramírez E, et al. Long-term control of endemic hospital-wide methicillin-resistant *Staphylococcus aureus* (MRSA): the impact of targeted active surveillance for MRSA in patients and healthcare workers. *Infect Control Hosp Epidemiol.* 2010;31(8):786-795. [IIA]

138. Warren DK, Guth RM, Coopersmith CM, Merz LR, Zack JE, Fraser VJ. Impact of a methicillin-resistant *Staphylococcus aureus* active surveillance program on contact precaution utilization in a surgical intensive care unit. *Crit Care Med.* 2007;35(2):430-434. [IIA]

139. Lee TC, Moore C, Raboud JM, et al. Impact of a mandatory infection control education program on nosocomial acquisition of methicillin-resistant *Staphylococcus aureus*. *Infect Control Hosp Epidemiol.* 2009;30(3):249-256. [IIA]

140. Rosenberger LH, Hranjec T, Politano AD, et al. Effective cohorting and "superisolation" in a single intensive care unit in response to an outbreak of diverse multi-drug-resistant organisms. *Surg Infect (Larchmt).* 2011;12(5):345-350. doi:10.1089/sur.2010.076. [IIIB]

141. Curran ET, Hamilton K, Monaghan A, McGinlay M, Thakker B. Use of a temporary cohort ward as part of an intervention to reduce the incidence of methicillin-resistant *Staphylococcus aureus* in a vascular surgery ward. *J Hosp Infect.* 2006;63(4):374-379. doi:10.1016/j.jhin.2006.02.017. [IIIA]

142. Murthy A, De Angelis G, Pittet D, Schrenzel J, Uckay I, Harbarth S. Cost-effectiveness of universal MRSA

screening on admission to surgery. *Clin Microbiol Infect.* 2010;16(12):1747-1753. [IIIB]

143. O'Grady NP, Alexander M, Burns LA, et al. Guidelines for the prevention of intravascular catheter-related infections. *Am J Infect Control.* 2011;39(4 Suppl 1):S1-S34. doi:10.1016/j.ajic.2011.01.003. [IVA]

144. Carnicer-Pont D, Bailey KA, Mason BW, Walker AM, Evans MR, Salmon RL. Risk factors for hospital-acquired methicillin-resistant *Staphylococcus aureus* bacteraemia: a case-control study. *Epidemiol Infect.* 2006;134(6):1167-1173. [IIB]

145. Loftus RW, Brown JR, Koff MD, et al. Multiple reservoirs contribute to intraoperative bacterial transmission. *Anesth Analg.* 2012;114(6):1236-1248. doi:10.1213/ANE.0b013e31824970a2. [IIA]

146. Gould CV, Umscheid CA, Agarwal RK, Kuntz G, Pegues DA; Healthcare Infection Control Practices Advisory Committee. Guideline for prevention of catheter-associated urinary tract infections 2009. *Infect Control Hosp Epidemiol.* 2010;31(4):319-326. doi:10.1086/651091. [VA]

147. Carlson AL, Perl TM. Health care workers as source of hepatitis B and C virus transmission. *Clin Liver Dis.* 2010;14(1):153-168. [VA]

148. Ehrenstein BP, Hanses F, Blaas S, Mandraka F, Audebert F, Salzberger B. Perceived risks of adverse effects and influenza vaccination: A survey of hospital employees. *Eur J Public Health.* 2010;20(5):495-499. [IIIB]

149. Pearson ML, Bridges CB, Harper SA; Healthcare Infection Control Practices Advisory Committee (HICPAC), Advisory Committee on Immunization Practices (ACIP). Influenza vaccination of health-care personnel: recommendations of the Healthcare Infection Control Practices Advisory Committee (HICPAC) and the Advisory Committee on Immunization Practices (ACIP) [published correction appears in *MMWR Recomm Rep.* 2006;10;55(9):252]. *MMWR Recomm Rep.* 2006;55(RR-2):1-16. [IVA]

150. Feemster KA, Prasad P, Smith MJ, et al. Employee designation and health care worker support of an influenza vaccine mandate at a large pediatric tertiary care hospital. *Vaccine.* 2011;29(9):1762-1769. [IIIB]

151. Llupia A, Garcia-Basteiro AL, Olive V, et al. New interventions to increase influenza vaccination rates in health care workers. *Am J Infect Control.* 2010;38(6):476-481. [IIB]

152. Amodio E, Anastasi G, Marsala MGL, Torregrossa MV, Romano N, Firenze A. Vaccination against the 2009 pandemic influenza A (H1N1) among healthcare workers in the major teaching hospital of Sicily (Italy). *Vaccine.* 2011;29(7):1408-1412. [IIIB]

153. Hopman CE, Riphagen-Dalhuisen J, Looijmans-van den Akker I, et al. Determination of factors required to increase uptake of influenza vaccination among hospital-based healthcare workers. *J Hosp Infect.* 2011;77(4):327-331. [IIIB]

154. Rakita RM, Hagar BA, Crome P, Lammert JK. Mandatory influenza vaccination of healthcare workers: a 5-year study. *Infect Control Hosp Epidemiol.* 2010;31(9):881-888. [IIIB]

155. Leekha S, Thompson RL, Sampathkumar P. Epidemiology and control of pertussis outbreaks in a tertiary care center and the resource consumption associated with these outbreaks. *Infect Control Hosp Epidemiol.* 2009;30(5):467-473. [IIIB]

156. Centers for Disease Control and Prevention (CDC). Updated recommendations for use of tetanus toxoid, reduced diphtheria toxoid and acellular pertussis (Tdap) vaccine from the Advisory Committee on Immunization Practices, 2010. *MMWR Morb Mortal Wkly Rep.* 2011;60(1):13-15. [IVA]

157. Johnston CP, Qiu H, Ticehurst JR, et al. Outbreak management and implications of a nosocomial norovirus outbreak. *Clin Infect Dis.* 2007;45(5):534-540. [IIIB]

158. Kak N, Burkhalter B, Cooper M-A. Measuring the competence of healthcare providers [Issue paper]. Bethesda, MD: US Agency for International Development; 2001. http://www.hciproject.org/sites/default/files/Measuring%20the%20Competence%20of%20HC%20Providers_QAP_2001.pdf. Accessed October 26, 2012. [VA]

159. HR.01.05.03: Staff participate in ongoing education and training. In: *Comprehensive Accreditation Manual: CAMH for Hospitals.* Oakbrook Terrace, IL: The Joint Commission; 2012.

160. HR.01.05.03: Staff participate in ongoing education and training. In: *Comprehensive Accreditation Manual for Ambulatory Care.* Oakbrook Terrace, IL: Joint Commission; 2012.

161. Centers for Medicare & Medicaid Services. *State Operations Manual Appendix A—Survey Protocol, Regulations and Interpretive Guidelines for Hospitals.* Rev. 78; 2011.

162. Centers for Medicare & Medicaid Services. *State Operations Manual Appendix L: Guidance for Surveyors: Ambulatory Surgical Centers.* Rev. 76; 2011.

163. Sportsman S. Competency education and validation in the United States: what should nurses know? *Nurs Forum.* 2010;45(3):140-149. doi:10.1111/j.1744-6198.2010.00183.x. [VA]

164. Jordan C, Thomas MB, Evans ML, Green A. Public policy on competency: how will nursing address this complex issue? *J Contin Educ Nurs.* 2008;39(2):86-91. [VA]

165. Bioterrorism agents/diseases: emergency preparedness and response. Centers for Disease Control and Prevention. http://www.bt.cdc.gov/agent/agentlist.asp. Accessed October 26, 2012. [IVA]

166. Howard DP, Williams C, Sen S, et al. A simple effective clean practice protocol significantly improves hand decontamination and infection control measures in the acute surgical setting. *Infection.* 2009;37(1):34-38. [IIB]

167. Guideline for perioperative health care information management. In: *Guidelines for Perioperative Practice.* Denver, CO: AORN, Inc; 2015:491-512. [IVB]

168. Simmons BP. Guideline for prevention of surgical wound infections. *Am J Infect Control.* 1983;11(4):133-143. [IVB]

169. Yokoe DS, Classen D. Improving patient safety through infection control: a new healthcare imperative. *Infect Control Hosp Epidemiol.* 2008;29(Suppl 1):S3-S11. doi:10.1086/591063. [IVA]

170. Governance. In: *2012 Accreditation Handbook for Ambulatory Health Care.* Skokie, IL: Accreditation Association for Ambulatory Health Care; 2012:20-27.

171. Personnel: personnel records. In: *Procedural Standards and Checklist for Accreditation Ambulatory Facilities.* Version 1. Gurnee, IL: American Association for Accreditation of Ambulatory Facilities; 2008:51-52.

172. LD.04.01.07: The hospital has policies and procedures that guide and support patient care, treatment, and services. In: *Hospital Accreditation Standards 2012.* Oakbrook Terrace, IL: Joint Commission on Resources; 2012.

173. LD.04.01.07: The organization has policies and procedures that guide and support patient care, treatment, or services. In: *Standards for Ambulatory Care 2012: Standards, Elements of Performance Scoring Accreditation*

Polices. Oakbrook Terrace, IL: The Joint Commission; 2012.

174. National action plan to prevent healthcare-associated infections: roadmap to elimination. US Department of Health & Human Services. http://www.hhs.gov/ash/initiatives/hai/actionplan/. Accessed October 26, 2012. [VA]

175. Carling PC, Bartley JM. Evaluating hygienic cleaning in health care settings: what you do not know can harm your patients. *Am J Infect Control.* 2010;38(5 Suppl 1):S41-S50. doi:10.1016/j.ajic.2010.03.004. [IIB]

176. Farquhar M. AHRQ quality indicators. In: Hughes RG, ed. *Patient Safety and Quality: An Evidence-Based Handbook for Nurses.* Rockville MD: Agency for Healthcare Research and Quality; 2008:41-67. http://purl.access.gpo.gov/GPO/LPS93676. Accessed October 26, 2012. [IA]

177. Larson EL, Cohen B, Ross B, Behta M. Isolation precautions for methicillin-resistant *Staphylococcus aureus*: electronic surveillance to monitor adherence. *Am J Crit Care.* 2010;19(1):16-26. doi:10.4037/ajcc2009467. [IVA]

178. Accountability measures. Joint Commission. http://www.jointcommission.org/accountability_measures.aspx. Accessed October 26, 2012.

179. Rosenberger LH, Politano AD, Sawyer RG. The surgical care improvement project and prevention of post-operative infection, including surgical site infection. *Surg Infect (Larchmt).* 2011;12(3):163-168. doi:10.1089/sur.2010.083. [VA]

Acknowledgments

LEAD AUTHOR
Lisa Spruce, DNP, RN, ACNS, ACNP, ANP, CNOR
Director of Evidence-based Perioperative Practice
AORN Nursing Department
Denver, Colorado

CONTRIBUTING AUTHORS
Ramona Conner, MSN, RN, CNOR
Manager, Standards and Guidelines
AORN Nursing Department
Denver, Colorado

Kimberly J. Retzlaff
Managing Editor
AORN Publications Department
Denver, Colorado

The authors and AORN thank George Allen, PhD, MS, RN, CNOR, CIC, Director Infection Control, Downstate Medical Center and Clinical Assistant Professor, SUNY College of Health Related Professions, Brooklyn, New York; Hudson Garret, Jr., PhD, MSN, MPH, FNP-BC, Senior Director, Clinical Affairs, PDI Healthcare, Atlanta, Georgia; Marcia R. Patrick, MSN, RN, CIC, Association for Professionals in Infection Control and Epidemiology liaison to the AORN Recommended Practices Advisory Board and Independent Consultant, Tacoma, Washington; and Rebecca Saxton, PhD, RN, CNOR, CNE, Associate Professor, Research College of Nursing, Director, Center for Nursing Research and Innovation, Kansas City, Missouri, for their assistance in developing this guideline.

PUBLICATION HISTORY
Originally published February 1993, *AORN Journal*, as "Recommended practices for universal precautions in the perioperative practice setting."

Revised November 1998 as "Recommended practices for standard and transmission-based precautions in the perioperative practice setting"; published February 1999, *AORN Journal.* Reformatted July 2000.

Approved June 2006, AORN Board of Directors, as "Recommended practices for prevention of transmissible infections in perioperative practice settings." Published in *Standards, Recommended Practices, and Guidelines*, 2007 edition.

Revised and reformatted December 2012 for online publication in *Perioperative Standards and Recommended Practices.*

Evidence ratings revised 2013 to conform to the AORN Evidence Rating Model.

Minor editing revisions made in November 2014 for publication in *Guidelines for Perioperative Practice*, 2015 edition.

Evidence ratings revised in *Guidelines for Perioperative Practice*, 2018 edition, to conform to the current AORN Evidence Rating Model.

AMBULATORY SUPPLEMENT: TRANSMISSIBLE INFECTIONS

Recommendation III

Droplet precautions should be used throughout the perioperative environment (ie, preoperative, intraoperative, postoperative) when providing care to patients who are known or suspected to be infected with microorganisms that can be transmitted by large droplets.[A1]

Amb The facility should screen individuals for infectious agents (eg, influenza, pertussis) transmitted by droplets.[A1] Identification of infected individuals before their admission to the ambulatory surgery center (ASC) may prevent infection transmission.[A1]

Recommendation IV

Airborne precautions should be used when providing care to patients who are known or suspected to be infected with microorganisms that can be transmitted by the airborne route.

IV.h. Elective surgery should be postponed for patients who have suspected or confirmed [tuberculosis] TB until the patient is determined to be noninfectious. If surgery cannot be postponed, perioperative personnel should follow airborne precautions and consult with an infection preventionist.

Amb Personnel in an ASC that provides care to patients with confirmed or suspected TB should follow recommendation IV.

Amb Unless the facility has the capability of establishing a negative pressure room, patients with suspected or confirmed cases of TB should be transferred to or re-scheduled at a facility with a negative pressure room. A negative pressure airborne infection isolation room and a respiratory protection program are needed for airborne infection isolation. Airborne infection isolation is needed for any patient with suspected or confirmed active pulmonary TB.[A1-A3]

Recommendation X

Perioperative personnel should receive initial and ongoing education and competency validation of their understanding of the principles of infection prevention and the performance of standard, contact, droplet, and airborne precautions for prevention of transmissible infections and [multidrug-resistant organisms] MDROs.

Amb An ASC that is certified by the Centers for Medicare & Medicaid Services (CMS) must designate a staff member trained in infection prevention to lead the facility's infection prevention program.[A4]

Interpretive Guidelines: §416.51(b)(1)

The ASC must designate in writing, a qualified licensed health care professional who will lead the facility's infection control program. The ASC must determine that the individual has had training in the principles and methods of infection control.

Interpretative Guidelines: §416.51(b)(1). In: Centers for Medicare & Medicaid Services. *State Operations Manual Appendix A—Survey Protocol, Regulations and Interpretive Guidelines for Hospitals.* Rev. 89; 2013.

Amb Ambulatory surgery center personnel, including
- medical personnel,
- nursing personnel,
- personnel responsible for on-site sterilization/high-level disinfection processes, and
- environmental services personnel

should receive infection prevention education.[A5]

Amb Infection prevention education should be conducted
- upon hire,
- annually, and
- periodically as needed.[A5]

Recommendation XI

Documentation should reflect activities related to infection prevention.

Amb A CMS-certified facility's infection prevention program must document the process of consideration, selection, and implementation of a nationally recognized infection control guideline,[A4] such as the AORN *Perioperative Standards and Recommended Practices.*[A6]

Amb Supporting documentation for the surgical site infection tracking and surveillance program should be maintained.[A5]

Amb Infection prevention education records should be maintained for all personnel.[A7]

Recommendation XII

Policies and procedures for the prevention and control of transmissible infections and MDROs should be developed, reviewed periodically, revised as necessary, and readily available within the practice setting.

Amb The infection prevention policy and procedure must comply with the state's reporting requirements for notifiable diseases.[A5,A8]

Recommendation XIII

Perioperative team members should participate in a variety of quality assurance and performance improvement activities to monitor and improve the prevention of infections and MDROs.

Amb A risk assessment should be conducted as part of the infection prevention plan. There are diverse floor plans and environmental controls in ASCs that may present challenges to supporting current infection prevention practices.

Amb The patient population and community served should be part of the risk assessment.

Amb The ASC must have a program to control and investigate infectious and communicable diseases.[A8]

Amb The infection prevention program should include surgical site infection (SSI) surveillance.[A8]

Amb A CMS-certified facility is required to have a process to follow up on each patient after discharge to identify and track infections associated with the patient's stay in the ASC.[A9]

The information should include
- a report of any SSI,
- identification details (eg, culture),
- symptoms,
- treatment, and
- prescribed antibiotics.[A5]

XIII.d.3. When a cluster of SSIs involves an unusual organism, a formal epidemiologic investigation should be conducted.[A10]

Amb An outbreak investigation should be conducted if there is an unexpected increase in infections.[A11]

Amb A multidisciplinary team should be assembled to conduct the investigation.

Amb Resources for conducting an investigation may include
- an infectious disease physician,
- the state department of health, and
- the Centers for Disease Control and Prevention.

Amb A facility participating in the CMS Ambulatory Surgical Quality Reporting Program must report influenza vaccination data for health care personnel (eg, employees, licensed independent practitioners, students, volunteers).[A12]

Glossary

Surveillance: The ongoing collection of data that pertains to occurrence of a specific disease or health care concern of interest (eg, surgical site infection, hand hygiene compliance) and the analysis, interpretation, and then dissemination of this data analysis to those who are responsible for implementing measures to control the disease or health problem.

References

A1. Siegel JD, Rhinehart E, Jackson M, Chiarello L; Health Care Infection Control Practices Advisory Committee. 2007 Guideline for Isolation Precautions: Preventing Transmission of Infectious Agents in Health Care Settings. *Am J Infect Control.* 2007;35(10 Suppl 2): S65-S164. doi:10.1016/j.ajic.2007.10.007. [IVA]

A2. Bennett G, Kassai M. Isolation precautions: special applications in ambulatory surgery settings. In: *Infection Prevention Manual for Ambulatory Surgery Centers.* Rome, GA: ICP Associates, Inc; 2011:Section 4:15.

A3. Jensen PA, Lambert LA, Iademarco MF, Ridzon R; CDC. Guidelines for preventing the transmission of *Mycobacterium tuberculosis* in health-care settings, 2005. *MMWR Recomm Rep.* 2005;54(RR17):1-141. http://www. cdc.gov/mmwr/preview/mmwrhtml/rr5417a1.htm?s_cid=rr5417a1_e. Accessed October 24, 2013.

A4. §416.51(b) Standard: Infection control program. In: Centers for Medicare & Medicaid Services. *State Operations Manual Appendix L—Guidance for Surveyors: Ambulatory Surgical Centers.* Rev. 89; 2013. http://www.cms.gov/ Regulations-and-Guidance/Guidance/Manuals/downloads/ som107ap_l_ambulatory.pdf. Accessed October 18, 2013.

A5. Exhibit 351: ASC Infection Control Surveryor Worksheet (Rev. 84, Issued: 06-07-13, Effective: 06-07-13, Implementation: 06-07-13). Centers for Medicare & Medicaid Services. http://www.cms.gov/Regulations-and-Guidance/Guidance/Manuals/downloads/som107_exhibit_351.pdf. Accessed October 18, 2013.

A6. *Perioperative Standards and Recommended Practices.* Denver, CO: AORN, Inc; 2013.

A7. Occupational Safety and Health Standards, Toxic and Hazardous Substances: Bloodborne Pathogens, 29 CFR §1910.1030. Occupational Safety and Health Administration. https://www.osha.gov/pls/oshaweb/ owadisp.show_document?p_table=standards&p_ id=10051. Accessed October 18, 2013.

A8. Interpretative Guidelines: §416.51(b)(3). In: Centers for Medicare & Medicaid Services. *State Operations Manual Appendix L—Guidance for Surveyors: Ambulatory Surgical Centers.* Rev. 89; 2013. http://www. cms.gov/Regulations-and-Guidance/Guidance/Manuals/ downloads/som107ap_l_ambulatory.pdf. Accessed October 18, 2013.

A9. Survey Procedures: §416.51(b)(3). In: Centers for Medicare & Medicaid Services. *State Operations Manual Appendix L—Guidance for Surveyors: Ambulatory Surgical Centers.* Rev. 89; 2013. http://www.cms.gov/ Regulations-and-Guidance/Guidance/Manuals/downloads/ som107ap_l_ambulatory.pdf. Accessed October 18, 2013.

A10. Mangram AJ, Horan TC, Pearson ML, Silver LC, Jarvis WR; Hospital Infection Control Practices Advisory Committee. Guideline for prevention of surgical site infection, 1999. Infect Control Hosp Epidemiol. 1999;20(4):250-278. doi:10.1086/501620. [IVA]

A11. *APIC Text of Infection Control & Epidemiology.* 3rd ed. Vol 1. Essential Elements. Washington, DC: Association for Professionals in Infection Control & Epidemiology, Inc; 2009.

A12. Centers for Medicare & Medicaid Services. *Ambulatory Surgical Center Quality Reporting Program Quality Measures Specifications Manual.* Version 3. July 2013. QualityNet. http://qualitynet.org/dcs/ContentServer?c= Page&pagename=QnetPublic%2FPage%2FQnetTier2& cid=1228772475754. Accessed October 18, 2013.

PATIENT AND WORKER SAFETY

Ambulatory Surgery

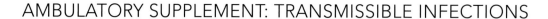
RESOURCES

Outbreak Database. http://www.outbreak-database.com. Accessed October 18, 2013.

Steps of an outbreak investigation. Centers for Disease Control and Prevention. http://www.cdc.gov/excite/classroom/outbreak/steps.htm. Accessed October 18, 2013.

Ambulatory Surgery

PATIENT AND **WORKER** SAFETY

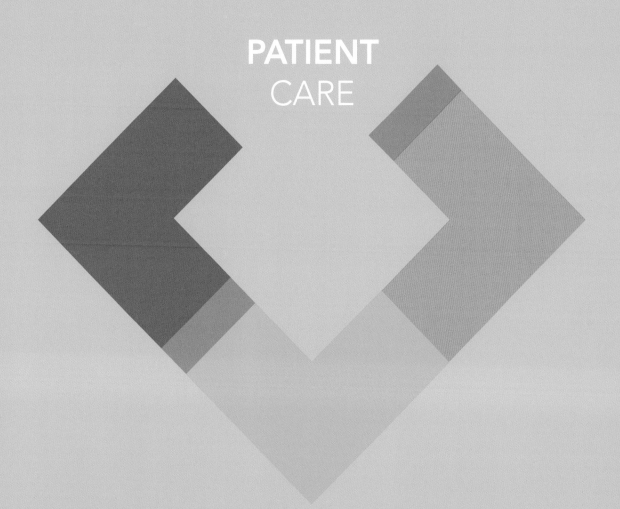

PATIENT
CARE

GUIDELINE FOR COMPLEMENTARY CARE INTERVENTIONS

The Guideline for Complementary Care Interventions has been approved by the AORN Guidelines Advisory Board. It was presented as a proposed guideline for comments by members and others. The guideline is effective January 15, 2015. The recommendations in this guideline are intended to be achievable and represent what is believed to be an optimal level of practice. Policies and procedures will reflect variations in practice settings and/or clinical situations that determine the degree to which the guideline can be implemented. AORN recognizes the many diverse settings in which perioperative nurses practice; therefore, this guideline is adaptable to all areas where operative and other invasive procedures may be performed.

Purpose

This document provides guidance for perioperative registered nurses (RNs) when complementary care interventions are implemented in the perioperative setting. This document includes guidance for music therapy, hypnosis, massage, acupuncture and acupressure, aromatherapy, Reiki, and guided imagery for patients before, during, or after surgery. The goal of complementary care interventions is to minimize the anxiety and pain of the perioperative patient.

Surgical patients experience high levels of anxiety.[1] Reasons for this anxiety include fear of surgery, anesthesia, loss of control, and disease.[2] The percentage of adult surgical patients who experience anxiety ranges from 11% to as high as 80%.[2] Anxiety can have negative effects on pain management.[3-5] An anxious patient may require more anesthetics and more opioids to relieve pain.[2]

Mitchell[6,7] surveyed 214 surgical outpatients to evaluate the effect of the clinical environment on the anxiety of patients who are scheduled to receive local or regional anesthesia. Seventy-seven percent of the patients surveyed reported that they experienced some degree of anxiety, as rated on a 5-point Likert-type scale that ranged from "feeling a little anxious" to "extremely anxious," on the day of their procedure. The highest percentage of patients (47%) reported feeling a little anxious.

The ability to provide complementary care interventions depends on several factors, including the patient's acceptance and engagement; the clinical experience, education, and competency of the perioperative team to provide complementary care interventions; and procedural and facility constraints. Complementary care may not be feasible or appropriate for every patient.

The topics of animal therapy, natural hormones, and dietary supplements as complementary care interventions are outside the scope of this document.

Evidence Review

On April 15, 2013, a medical librarian conducted a systematic search of the databases MEDLINE®, CINAHL®, and the Cochrane Database of Systematic Reviews for meta-analyses, systematic reviews, randomized controlled and non-randomized trials and studies, case reports, reviews, and guidelines from government agencies and standards-setting bodies. The librarian also searched the Scopus® database, although not systematically. Searches were limited to literature published in English since January 2006. At the time of the initial searches, the librarian established weekly alerts on the search topics and until July 2014, presented relevant results to the lead author. During the development of this guideline, the author requested supplementary literature searches and additional literature that either did not fit the original search criteria or was discovered during the evidence-appraisal process.

The lead author's original search request for literature related to moderate sedation and local anesthesia yielded 862 sources deemed appropriate for consideration in guidelines on those topics. Of these, 59 were identified as relevant to complementary care interventions (Figure 1). Search terms that yielded these results included *sedation, conscious sedation, moderation sedation, topical anesthesia, local anesthesia, local infiltration, anxiety, anti-anxiety agents, analgesia, surgical procedures, perioperative nursing,* and *nurse's role.* The literature scope was not expanded to the terms *complementary care, integrative medicine, complementary alternative medicine, healing touch, therapeutic touch, reflexology, herbal medicine, nausea,* or *vomiting.* Future review and update of this document will include a literature search that includes these terms.

Excluded were non-peer-reviewed publications and studies on the topics of pet therapy, natural hormones, and dietary supplements. Low-quality evidence was excluded when higher-quality evidence was available.

Included articles were independently evaluated and critically appraised according to the strength and quality of the evidence. Articles identified by the search were provided to the project team for evaluation. The team consisted of the lead author and four evidence appraisers. The lead author divided the search results and assigned members of the team to review and critically appraise each article using the AORN Research or Non-Research Evidence Appraisal Tools as appropriate. The literature was independently evaluated and appraised according to the strength and quality of the evidence. Each article was

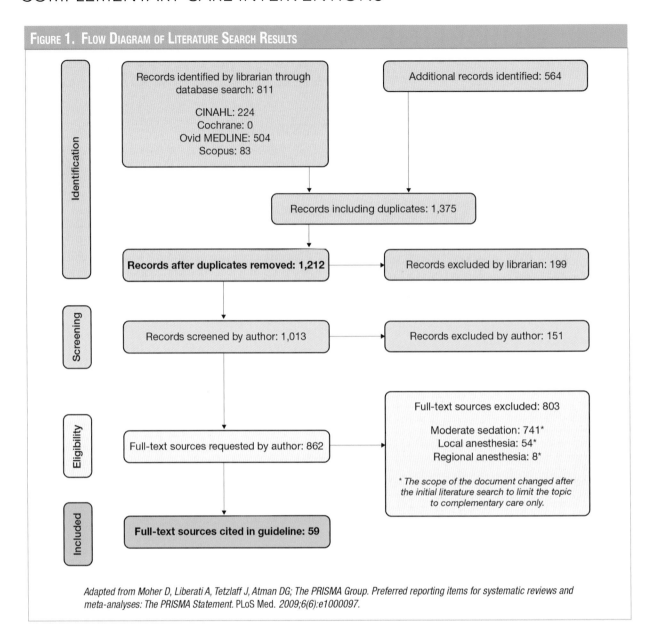

FIGURE 1. FLOW DIAGRAM OF LITERATURE SEARCH RESULTS

Identification

Records identified by librarian through database search: 811

CINAHL: 224
Cochrane: 0
Ovid MEDLINE: 504
Scopus: 83

Additional records identified: 564

Records including duplicates: 1,375

Records after duplicates removed: 1,212

Records excluded by librarian: 199

Screening

Records screened by author: 1,013

Records excluded by author: 151

Eligibility

Full-text sources requested by author: 862

Full-text sources excluded: 803

Moderate sedation: 741*
Local anesthesia: 54*
Regional anesthesia: 8*

* The scope of the document changed after the initial literature search to limit the topic to complementary care only.

Included

Full-text sources cited in guideline: 59

Adapted from Moher D, Liberati A, Tetzlaff J, Atman DG; The PRISMA Group. Preferred reporting items for systematic reviews and meta-analyses: The PRISMA Statement. PLoS Med. 2009;6(6):e1000097.

then assigned an appraisal score. The appraisal score is noted in brackets after each reference, as applicable.

The collective evidence supporting each intervention within a specific recommendation was summarized, and the AORN Evidence-Rating Model was used to rate the strength of the evidence. Factors considered in review of the collective evidence were the quality of the evidence, the quantity of similar evidence on a given topic, and the consistency of evidence supporting a recommendation. The evidence rating is noted in brackets after each intervention.

Note: The evidence summary table is available at http://www.aorn.org/evidencetables/.

Editor's note: MEDLINE is a registered trademark of the US National Library of Medicine's Medical Literature Analysis and Retrieval System, Bethesda, MD. CINAHL, Cumulative Index to Nursing and Allied Health Literature, is a registered trademark of EBSCO Industries, Bir-

mingham, AL. Scopus is a registered trademark of Elsevier B.V., Amsterdam, The Netherlands.

Recommendation I

The perioperative team can implement music interventions.

The collective body of evidence strongly supports the use of music to relieve anxiety during surgical and other invasive procedures.[1,3,8-34]

Sixteen studies,[3,10-16,18,19,21,24-26,34,35] three systematic reviews,[8,23,36] an integrative review,[1] and five literature reviews[27-29,31,33] evaluated the ability of music interventions to reduce patient anxiety, pain, and stress before, during, and after operative and other invasive procedures. Thirteen studies found that music was an effective intervention to reduce anxiety levels in the surgical and invasive procedure areas. Three studies found that a music intervention did not have a significant effect on anxiety levels but that music contributed to an overall favorable patient experience.[15,19,25]

The limitations of the evidence are that few studies have explored the feasibility of incorporating music into everyday practice. Further research is needed to define feasibility of using music therapy in the perioperative area.

The benefits of using music therapy outweigh the harms. The benefits include a possible reduction in the patient's anxiety.

I.a. The perioperative team can implement music interventions across the perioperative continuum of care. *[1: Strong Evidence]*

The collective evidence indicates that music is effective in decreasing patient anxiety and pain in all phases of perioperative care.

Nilsson[8] conducted a systematic review of the anxiety- and pain-reducing effects of music interventions. In the 42 randomized controlled trials (RCTs) reviewed, 3,936 patients had elective surgeries of various types (eg, gynecological, orthopedic, general, cardiac, urologic). The timing of the music intervention was preoperative, intraoperative, postoperative, a combination of two of these periods, or a combination of all three periods. The author concluded that music interventions could reduce anxiety, pain, the use of sedatives and analgesics, heart rate, blood pressure, respiratory rate, and blood cortisol levels.

Johnson et al[16] evaluated the anxiety levels of 119 female patients undergoing outpatient gynecological surgery in an experimental three-group design of music with headphones, headphones only, and usual care. The researchers measured preoperative and postoperative anxiety levels using the Rapid Assessment Anxiety tool. The music-with-headphones and headphones-only interventions continued from the preoperative area, through surgery, and into the postanesthesia care unit until the patient's Aldrete level of consciousness equaled 2. After surgery, the music group experienced the lowest anxiety scores among the patients who had reported moderate to high anxiety levels before surgery. The researchers concluded that music is an easy and inexpensive intervention to reduce anxiety.

In an RCT, Hook et al[18] examined the effect of music on reducing preoperative and postoperative anxiety and postoperative pain and distress in 102 female surgical patients. The researchers used a pretest-posttest design to measure anxiety with the State-Trait Anxiety Inventory (STAI) and a visual analog scale (VAS). The researchers also used the VAS to measure postoperative pain sensation and pain distress (Figure 2).

The control and experimental groups received standard preoperative and postoperative nursing and medical care. The experimental group listened to 30 minutes of music twice before and six times after surgery at defined intervals. The experimental music group had a significant change in postoperative anxiety and postoperative pain. The findings suggested that music is a nonpharmacological, complementary, noninvasive intervention to reduce anxiety and postoperative pain.[18]

Binns-Turner et al[3] evaluated the effect of music provided throughout the preoperative, intraoperative, and postoperative periods on anxiety, pain, heart rate, and mean arterial pressure (MAP). A convenience sample of 30 women

FIGURE 2. PAIN AND ANXIETY MEASUREMENT INSTRUMENTS

The State-Trait Anxiety Inventory (STAI)
- Psychological inventory that measures two types of anxiety:
  - state measures anxiety about an event
  - trait measures anxiety as a characteristic
- Based on a 4-point Likert scale
- Consists of 40 items on a self-report basis
- Total scores range from 20 to 80
  - High anxiety: 60-80
  - Moderate anxiety: 40-59
  - Mild anxiety: 20-39

Visual Analog Score (VAS)
- A measurement instrument that assesses a characteristic that cannot be directly measured and that ranges across a continuum.
- An example is the amount of pain a patient experiences—it can range from no pain to extreme pain.
- The VAS is a horizontal line 100 mm in length with "no pain" at one end and "extreme pain" at the other end.

Examples of a VAS

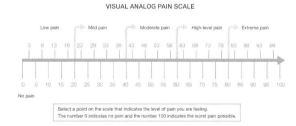

A variation is the use of faces to gauge the level of pain.

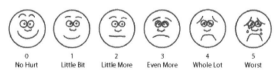

Wong-Baker FACES Pain Rating Scale. In: Hockenberry MJ, Wilson D. Wong's Essentials of Pediatric Nursing. 8th ed. St Louis, MO: Mosby; 2009. Used with permission. Copyright Mosby.

undergoing a mastectomy for a breast malignancy were randomly assigned to either a control group or a music therapy group. The control group received standard care and the intervention group listened to music with earphones throughout the perioperative period. The researchers measured anxiety, pain, heart rate, and MAP before and after surgery. Anxiety was measured using the Spielberger State Anxiety Scale, and pain was measured with a VAS. The findings included a statistically significant difference in MAP, anxiety scores, and pain scores between the control group and the music intervention groups. The intervention group's anxiety, pain, and MAP were significantly lower or improved after surgery. Limitations of the study included that the sample was a small, convenience sample.

A systematic Cochrane review,[23] six RCTs,[10-12,14,26,35] and an integrative review[1] evaluated the effect of music in reducing anxiety levels in the preoperative area.

In an RCT, Bringman et al[14] studied the preoperative anxiety levels of 327 patients undergoing elective surgery. In the preoperative area, a music therapist randomly assigned patients to either listen to relaxing music with earphones or receive an oral dose of midazolam 0.05 mg/kg to 0.1 mg/kg. Patients completed the STAI before and after the interventions. The STAI scale ranges from 20 to 80. The mean STAI anxiety score of the control group ranged from 37.63 to 44.43. The anxiety scores of the music intervention group decreased by 5.72 units on the STAI compared with the scores of the standard care control group. The researchers concluded that relaxing music decreased preoperative anxiety to a greater extent than oral midazolam and that listening to music has no adverse effects. The authors concluded that the use of preoperative, relaxing music should be supported to reduce preoperative anxiety.

Lee et al[11] conducted an RCT that compared the effectiveness of music played via headphones, music broadcast via room speakers, or no music to reduce preoperative patients' anxiety while they waited for surgery. The sample size was 167 patients. The researchers used the VAS to measure anxiety subjectively on a scale of "not anxious" to "extremely anxious." The heart rate variability (HRV) tool was used to measure anxiety objectively by identifying the effect of mental stress on the autonomic control of the heart rate. There was not a significant difference in the HRV in the three groups. The VAS levels for the two music groups were reduced after the music interventions. The researchers concluded that music via either headphones or speakers was effective in reducing preoperative anxiety.

Lee et al[26] conducted another RCT of 140 patients that compared listening to relaxing music via headphones for 10 minutes with listening to no music in the preoperative area. Anxiety levels were measured with VAS scores and HRV monitoring. The experimental group's VAS scores were significantly decreased after they listened to the music. The control group's VAS scores increased after 10 minutes of rest. The heart rate decrease in the experimental group was significantly greater than that in the control group. The researchers concluded that listening to music was an effective way to decrease the anxiety of preoperative patients. In addition, the researchers concluded the HRV assessment is an objective way for nurses to measure patient's preoperative anxiety when a patient cannot express subjective feelings.

El-Hassan et al[12] conducted a prospective RCT of 180 endoscopy patients to determine whether music reduced their preoperative anxiety. The anxiety levels of the music intervention group were measured with the STAI before and after the intervention (ie, listening to music for 15 minutes). The anxiety levels of the control group receiving standard care with no music were measured with the STAI after admission to the pre-endoscopy area and 15 minutes later. The intervention group listened to self-selected music for 15 minutes with headphones before the endoscopy procedure. The control group received the same care as the intervention group with the exception of listening to music. The researchers found a significant reduction in the postintervention anxiety scores of the group that listened to self-selected music. The researchers concluded that music is a simple way to improve well-being in preprocedure patients.

Ni et al[35] randomly assigned 172 adult surgical outpatients into one of two groups to evaluate the effect of music on preoperative anxiety and vital signs. The experimental group listened to music through headphones for 20 minutes before surgery and the control group received routine nursing care. Vital signs (ie, blood pressure, heart rate) and STAI anxiety levels were measured before and after the interventions. The STAI score of the music group decreased by 5.83 units. The STAI score of the control group decreased by 1.72 units. The difference between the music group's postintervention STAI scores for anxiety and the control's group's scores was statistically significant. Blood pressure and heart rate decreased in both groups. The researchers concluded that a music intervention might lower preoperative anxiety levels, blood pressure, and heart rate.

A Cochrane systematic review by Bradt et al[23] evaluated the effects of music interventions on preoperative patient anxiety. The review included 26 randomized and quasi-randomized trials with 2,051 participants and compared music interventions with standard preoperative

PATIENT CARE

care to standard care alone. The anxiety scores of the music intervention group decreased by 5.72 units on the STAI compared with the scores of the standard care group. The researchers concluded that listening to music might decrease preoperative patient anxiety. These findings are consistent with three other Cochrane reviews[37-39] that evaluated the use of music to reduce medical patients' anxiety.

Using an RCT design, Arslan et al[10] studied preoperative anxiety levels in men undergoing urogenital surgery. The experimental group participants listened to their choice of music through earphones for 30 minutes before surgery. The control group received routine preoperative care and 30 minutes of rest. Anxiety levels were measured with the STAI preintervention and postintervention. The experimental group had significantly lower postintervention anxiety scores and the control group had significantly increased postintervention anxiety scores. The researchers concluded that offering music to preoperative patients is an independent nursing intervention that may reduce anxiety levels.

An integrative review by Pittman and Kridli[1] analyzed 11 experimental and nonexperimental research studies that compared listening to music to no music and used the STAI preintervention and postintervention to measure anxiety levels. After a review of the 11 studies, the authors found that in three studies listening to music lowered blood pressure; three studies demonstrated a relationship between listening to music and decreased heart rates; and two studies provided evidence of a decreased respiratory rate after participants listened to music. The reviewers concluded that nurses can use music interventions to establish a calm, relaxing preoperative environment that supports reducing anxiety.

Seven RCTs,[13,15,17,19,21,34,40] a systematic review with meta-analysis,[9] and one quasi-experimental study[24] examined the effect of music on anxiety levels during surgery (ie, peripheral vascular, gynecological, urological, plastic, gastroenterological) and invasive procedures (ie, interventional radiology, angiography).

In a prospective RCT of 40 patients, Jiménez-Jiménez et al[17] compared patients undergoing peripheral vascular surgery who received routine intraoperative care with patients who listened to music through headphones during the procedure. The researchers used the STAI to measure anxiety before and after surgery. The anxiety and stress feelings scores were significantly lower in the music therapy group after surgery.

In a systematic review with meta-analysis of eight studies with 722 patients who underwent colonoscopy, Tam et al[9] examined the effect of listening to music during surgery. They concluded that listening to music reduced anxiety,

procedure time, and the amount of sedation used.

Zhang et al[40] assessed male patient anxiety and pain during flexible cystoscopy procedures. The patients were randomly assigned to either the experimental group that listened to music of their choice or the control group that did not listen to music. The researchers measured anxiety levels with the STAI-state (STAI-s) before and after the procedure. Pain levels were assessed postoperatively using the VAS. The difference in the mean pain and postprocedure anxiety levels were statistically significant in the experimental group. The researchers concluded that patients listening to music experienced less discomfort and anxiety and that music was a simple, nonpharmocological intervention to increase patient satisfaction.

Yeo et al[21] randomly assigned 70 male patients undergoing rigid cystoscopy into one of two groups. The experimental group listened to classical music during the procedure and the control group did not listen to music. Before and after surgery, anxiety levels were measured with the STAI, and pain and satisfaction were measured with a VAS. The music group had significantly less anxiety and pain, higher satisfaction scores, and lower postprocedure pulse rates and systolic blood pressures. Limitations of the study were a small sample size and that the study was not blinded to the patient or the surgeon.

Sadideen et al[24] studied anxiety and satisfaction levels in patients undergoing plastic surgery under local anesthesia. The intervention group listened to music via speakers in the OR. The control group did not have music played in the OR. Objective measures of anxiety were VAS scores and respiratory rate. The researchers quantified patients' satisfaction using a 5-point Likert scale. Measurements were taken before the procedure started and on completion. After surgery, the music group had lower VAS scores and respiratory rates. The difference in the satisfaction scores between the two groups was not statistically significant.

Two RCTs studied the effect of music on anxiety levels of patients undergoing coronary angiography procedures.[13,34] Weeks and Nilsson[34] randomly assigned 98 patients to one of three groups. Patients listened to music through an audio pillow, music through the loud speaker, or no music. Patients in the two music groups had a significant reduction in anxiety levels compared with the control group.

Doğan and Senturan[13] randomly assigned 100 patients to an experimental group that listened to music during the procedure and 100 patients to a control group that received standard care. The anxiety levels of the experimental group decreased more significantly than those of the control group.

McLeod[25] studied the effectiveness of music on patient anxiety levels during minor plastic surgery procedures. The Speilberger STAI questionnaire was used to assess the anxiety of 80 patients before and after surgery. Forty patients in the experimental group listened to self-selected music during surgery, and the 40 patients in the control group received standard care with no music. Statistical analysis of the STAI scores demonstrated that there was not a significant difference in the anxiety scores between the experimental group that listened to music and the control group. The researchers reported that the patients seemed to enjoy the music.

Nilsson et al[19] and Kulkarni et al[15] evaluated the effect of music on patient anxiety during interventional radiology procedures. Both studies found that there was not a significant difference in the anxiety levels between the music intervention groups or the control groups.

I.a.1. The perioperative RN should assess the patient's acceptance of and willingness to use music as a complementary intervention and should obtain consent. *[5: Benefits Balanced with Harms]*

I.a.2. The perioperative RN should solicit the patient's music preference (eg classical, easy listening). *[5: Benefits Balanced with Harms]*

I.a.3. When music therapy is used, the patient should use personal listening devices (eg, head phones, ear buds) when feasible. *[5: Benefits Balanced with Harms]*

The use of personal listening devices limits noise and distraction in the perioperative setting.

Recommendation II

The perioperative team can implement preoperative or postoperative massage therapy.

The collective body of evidence supports the use of massage to relieve anxiety during surgical and other invasive procedures.[41-43] Two RCTs and one quasi-experimental study investigated massage as an intervention to reduce patient anxiety.[41-43]

The limitations of the evidence are that few studies have explored the feasibility of incorporating massage into everyday practice and the competency of perioperative nurses to implement massage techniques. Further research is needed.

The benefits of using massage outweighs the harms. The benefits include a potential reduction in the patient's anxiety.

II.a. Massage therapy techniques can be used. *[2: High Evidence]*

Wentworth et al[41] assessed the effect of a 20-minute massage session on patients' pain, anxiety, and tension before an invasive cardio-vascular procedure. The study method was an experimental pretest-posttest design with random assignment of 130 patients. The control group received standard care with relaxation time and the intervention group received hands-on massage 30 minutes before the procedure. The researchers measured pain, anxiety, and tension levels with a VAS before the intervention and after the procedure. Mean results for patients in the massage intervention group indicated a significant decrease in pain, muscle tension, and anxiety from before the massage therapy to after the massage therapy. The mean results for patients in the standard care group indicated an insignificant change in pain, muscle tension, and anxiety before and after standard care. The researchers' findings suggest that massage therapy can be delivered to patients before an invasive procedure and that massage is an effective technique for reducing pain, tension, and anxiety.

In an RCT, Rosen et al[43] studied the effectiveness of massage therapy to reduce pain and anxiety in patients with cancer undergoing surgical placement of a vascular access device. The intervention group received massage therapy for two 20-minute sessions, one before and one after surgery. The control group received structured attention. Anxiety and pain were measured with the STAI before surgery and after each intervention. The massage group had a statistically significant decrease in anxiety after the first massage compared with the control group.

Using a quasi-experimental design with pretest and posttest evaluations and non-random assignment, Brand et al[42] studied the effect of hand massage in reducing preoperative patient anxiety in an ambulatory surgery center. Anxiety levels were measured using a VAS. A certified massage therapist trained three nurses to perform the hand massage procedure. The intervention group received a five-minute massage on each hand, and the control group received standard care. The intervention group had a significant decrease in postintervention anxiety scores. The control group's anxiety scores decreased, but the decrease was not statistically significant. An unexpected finding of this study was that the hand massage facilitated the IV start.

II.a.1. The perioperative RN should assess the patient's acceptance of and willingness to use massage as a complementary intervention and should obtain consent. *[5: Benefits Balanced with Harms]*

II.a.2. Perioperative RNs who provide massage interventions (eg, hand rubs) should receive education and complete competency verification activities on the principles and techniques of massage therapy that are in compliance with state regulation. *[5: Benefits Balanced with Harms]*

Licensure may be required by the state for providers of some massage therapies.

Recommendation III

The perioperative team can implement preoperative acupuncture and acupressure.

The collective body of evidence supports the use of acupuncture and acupressure to relieve anxiety during surgical and other invasive procedures.[44-47]

The limitations of the evidence are that few studies have explored the feasibility of incorporating acupuncture and acupressure into everyday practice and the competency of perioperative nurses to implement these holistic measures. Further research is needed.

The benefits of using acupressure and acupuncture outweigh the harms. The benefits include a potential reduction in the patient's anxiety.

III.a.   Acupuncture can be implemented before surgery. *[3: Moderate Evidence]*

Two RCTs investigated the effect of acupuncture on preoperative patient anxiety levels.[44,46] Acar et al[44] investigated the effect of ear-press needle acupuncture on the Yintang point to decrease preoperative anxiety in a prospective randomized single-blind controlled study. Patient anxiety was measured before and after the interventions with the STAI and the bispectral index (BIS). The BIS uses electroencephalogram-derived data intraoperatively to monitor the depth of anesthesia. The BIS is also used to monitor sedation in the intensive care unit and during monitored anesthesia care and has been used preoperatively to assess anxiety.

The experimental group received acupuncture at the Yintang point, which is at the root of the nose and between the eyebrows. The control group received sham acupuncture at a nonacupoint 2 cm lateral to the distal end of the right eyebrow. The BIS values were significantly lower in the acupuncture group at two minutes to 20 minutes compared with the sham site group. The mean STAI-s scores decreased in the acupuncture group. The researchers concluded that the lower BIS and STAI scores indicated the patients were calmer and more relaxed and that acupuncture at the Yintang point significantly decreased preoperative patient anxiety.[44]

Wu et al[46] compared the effectiveness of body acupuncture to auricular acupuncture on preoperative patient anxiety in a blinded RCT. Ambulatory surgery patients were randomly assigned to either the body acupuncture intervention or the ear acupuncture intervention. The researchers measured anxiety levels using the ZUNG Self-Rating Anxiety Scale before and after the interventions. Both acupuncture methods decreased the anxiety of the preoperative patients, but the reductions did not reach statistical significance.

III.a.1.   The perioperative RN should assess the patient's acceptance of and willingness to use acupuncture as a complementary intervention and should obtain consent. *[5: Benefits Balanced with Harms]*

III.a.2.   Acupuncture should be performed by licensed acupuncturist as required by state regulation. *[5: Benefits Balanced with Harms]*

III.b.   Acupressure can be implemented before surgery. *[2: High Evidence]*

Use of acupressure before surgery is supported by one RCT.[45] Valiee et al[45] investigated the effect of acupressure on preoperative patient anxiety levels. Anxiety levels were measured using a standard VAS and vital signs (ie, blood pressure, heart rate, respiratory rate). The experimental group received acupressure on the correct acupoints, and the control group received acupressure on sham points. The postintervention anxiety levels decreased 21% for the acupressure group and 6.1% for the placebo group. The researchers concluded that results of the study support the use of acupressure to reduce preoperative anxiety. The acupressure intervention on the third eye and Shen Men points can be performed by a trained patient or a health care professional.

III.b.1.   The perioperative RN should assess the patient's acceptance of and willingness to use acupressure as a complementary intervention and should obtain consent. *[5: Benefits Balanced with Harms]*

III.b.2.   Acupressure practitioners should receive education and complete competency verification activities on the principles and techniques of acupressure. *[5: Benefits Balanced with Harms]*

Recommendation IV

The perioperative team can implement preoperative aromatherapy.

Aromatherapy is based on the use of oils extracted from aromatic plants with medicinal qualities.[2] The collective body of evidence supports the use of aromatherapy to relieve anxiety during surgical and other invasive procedures.[2,36,48,49]

Four RCTs studied aromatic agents (ie, essential oil of lavandin, lavandula, essential oil of lavender, neroli oil) to reduce preoperative anxiety levels.[2,36,48,49]

The limitations of the evidence are that few studies have explored the feasibility of incorporating aromatherapy into everyday practice and the competency of perioperative nurses to use aromatherapy. Further research is needed.

The benefits of using aromatherapy outweigh the harms. The benefits include a potential reduction in the patient's anxiety.

IV.a. Aromatic essential oils can be used. *[2: High Evidence]*

Braden et al[48] evaluated the ability of the essential oil lavandin to reduce preoperative anxiety. Anxiety levels were measured with the VAS on admission and before the patient was taken to the operating room (OR). A total of 150 patients were randomly assigned to one of three groups. The control group received standard care. The jojoba oil group received the oil on a cotton ball for olfactory application; the oil was applied to the pedal pulse point and covered with a bandage for absorption. The undiluted lavandin group received the oil on a cotton ball for olfactory application; the oil was applied to the pedal pulse point and covered with a bandage for absorption. The anxiety scores of the lavandin oil group were lower at the time of transfer to the OR but the difference was not statistically significant.

Fayazi et al[2] investigated the effect of inhalation aromatherapy to reduce patients' preoperative anxiety. The aromatherapy intervention was two drops of lavandula oil on a handkerchief that was inhaled for 20 minutes. The placebo group inhaled two drops of water on the handkerchief for 20 minutes. Anxiety levels were measured with the STAI before and after the interventions. The mean level of anxiety in the experimental group was 51 before the intervention of inhaling the lavandula oil and 38.61 after the intervention. The mean level of anxiety in the control group was 50.67 before the placebo intervention and 49.53 after the intervention. The mean difference in the STAI scores before and after the interventions was 12.34 for the lavandula group and 2.42 for the control group. The lavandula group's anxiety decreased from moderate to mild anxiety. The placebo group's anxiety level remained at a moderate level. The difference between the two groups was statistically significant. The researchers concluded that nurses could use aromatherapy as an intervention to reduce patients' preoperative anxiety.

Two RCTs studied aromatherapy to reduce patient anxiety levels in gastroenterology procedures.[36,49] Hoya et al[36] studied the optimal soothing environment (OSE) as a nonpharmacological intervention to reduce anxiety before gastroscopy procedures. The OSE intervention included an essential oil burner with lavender essential oil and a DVD with soothing natural environmental images and sounds. The control group received standard care. Anxiety levels of both groups were measured on arrival, before the procedure, and after the procedure with the FACES Scale, a type of VAS. The anxiety level of the control group increased before the gas-

troscopy procedure. The anxiety level of the OSE group did not increase before the gastroscopy. The researchers concluded that the OSE intervention was effective for reducing anxiety and that nurses could use this therapy to promote health and wellness.

Hu et al[49] investigated the effect of aromatherapy on anxiety, stress, and physiological parameters of patients undergoing colonoscopy. Anxiety levels were measured with the STAI-s before aromatherapy and after the colonoscopy. Pain levels were measured with a VAS. Heart rate, respiratory rate, and blood pressure were measured before aromatherapy and after the colonoscopy. The experimental group inhaled 50 mL of neroli oil on a piece of gauze in a hand-held nebulizer. The control group inhaled 50 mL of sunflower oil on a piece of gauze in a hand-held nebulizer. The STAI scores of the aromatherapy group decreased 11 points which was statistically significant. The STAI scores of the control group decreased 7 points which was not statistically significant. The difference between the anxiety scores of the two groups was not a significant. The researchers concluded that aromatherapy before colonoscopy procedures can have an effect on anxiety and physiological parameters (eg, blood pressure), and aromatherapy is a safe and inexpensive pre-procedure technique.

IV.a.1. Aromatherapy should be provided in a manner that will limit exposure of the aromatic essential oils to the intended patient. *[5: Benefits Balanced with Harms]*

Other occupants (eg, patients, visitors, personnel) of the area may be sensitive to the aromatic essential oils.

IV.a.2. The perioperative RN should assess the patient's acceptance of and willingness to use aromatherapy as a complementary intervention and should obtain consent. *[5: Benefits Balanced with Harms]*

IV.a.3. Perioperative RNs who implement aromatherapy should receive education and complete competency verification activities on the principles and techniques of aromatherapy. *[5: Benefits Balanced with Harms]*

Recommendation V

The perioperative team can implement patient hypnosis before, during, and after the surgical procedure.

The collective body of evidence supports the use of hypnosis to relieve anxiety and pain during surgical and other invasive procedures.[50-54] Three RCTs[50,51,54] and a case-controlled study[52] evaluated the use of hypnosis to reduce anxiety and pain.

The limitations of the evidence are that few studies have explored the feasibility of incorporating hypnosis into everyday practice and the competency of perioperative nurses to implement hypnosis. Further research is needed.

The benefits of using hypnosis outweigh the harms. Benefits include a potential reduction in the patient's anxiety and pain.

V.a.   Patient hypnosis therapy can be used. *[2: High Evidence]*

In an RCT, Lang et al[51] studied the use of self-hypnotic relaxation to reduce anxiety and pain during percutaneous tumor treatment by transcatheter embolization or radio-frequency ablation in 201 patients. The self-hypnotic relaxation treatment was compared to standard care, and empathetic attention. The standard care group consisted of 70 patients, the empathy group consisted of 65 patients, and the hypnosis group consisted of 66 patients. The hypnosis group had less pain and anxiety and used less medication than the standard care and empathy groups. The researchers concluded that procedural hypnosis that included empathetic attention reduced pain, anxiety, and medication use. Empathetic attention without hypnosis did not help the patients with self-coping strategies and could result in more adverse events.

Schnur et al[54] used an RCT design to study 90 patients undergoing excisional breast biopsy. Patients received either a 15-minute hypnosis session before surgery or a 15-minute attention control session before surgery. The VAS and the short version of the Profile of Mood States (SV-POMS) were used to measure patients' distress before and after surgery. The hypnosis intervention group experienced significantly lower mean values of emotional upset measured by the VAS before surgery. After hypnosis, compared with the control group, the patients in the hypnosis group had significantly lower mean levels of emotional upset and depressed mood as measured by the VAS, significantly lower levels of anxiety as measured by the SV-POMS, and significantly higher levels of relaxation as measured by the VAS. The researchers concluded that a brief hypnosis session before surgery is an effective technique to decrease patient distress before an excisional breast biopsy when many patients have a high level of anxiety.

In an RCT, Marc et al[50] studied women's satisfaction with using a hypnotic intervention to reduce anxiety and pain during an outpatient gynecology procedure. A total of 350 patients were randomly assigned to either a short, standardized hypno-analgesia intervention or standard care. Ninety-seven percent of the hypnosis group reported that they would recommend the technique to a friend having a similar procedure. All but one patient in the 172-patient intervention group appreciated the hypnosis experience. The hypnosis group required less pain medication than the control group. The researchers did not comment on postprocedure anxiety levels.

Abdeshahi et al[52] conducted a case-controlled study to evaluate the effect of hypnosis on pain, anxiety, and hemorrhage during the extraction of third molars. The patients served as their own control group by undergoing extraction of the molars on one side under hypnosis and the opposite side under local anesthesia. There was a significant difference in pain scores at five and 12 hours after surgery, with the hypnosis group taking less analgesic medications. There was significantly greater hemorrhage in the local anesthetic group (41.7%) compared with the hypnosis group (20.8%) at five hours after surgery. Anxiety scores were not reported. The researchers concluded that hypnosis is an adjunct technique to treat anxious patients when conventional methods cannot be used and the practitioner is experienced in the technique.

V.a.1.   The perioperative RN should assess the patient's acceptance of and willingness to use hypnosis as a complementary intervention and should obtain consent. *[5: Benefits Balanced with Harms]*

V.a.2.   Perioperative RNs who implement hypnosis therapy should receive education and complete competency verification activities on the principles and techniques of hypnosis. *[5: Benefits Balanced with Harms]*

Recommendation VI

The perioperative team can implement preoperative Reiki therapy.

Reiki is an ancient Tibetan technique and healing practice.[55] The Reiki practitioner gently lays his or her hands on or above 12 strategic areas on the patient's body.[55] The Reiki practitioner's energy is thought to promote healing and bring harmony to the patient's energy field.[56]

The collective body of evidence supports that Reiki has a minimal effect in relieving anxiety.[55,56] Two studies investigated the use of Reiki in the gastroenterology procedure area.[55,56]

The limitations of the evidence are that few studies have explored the feasibility of incorporating Reiki by competent practitioners into everyday practice. Further research is needed.

The benefits of using Reiki outweigh the harms. Benefits include a potential reduction in the patient's anxiety and pain.

VI.a.   Reiki therapy performed by a Reiki practitioner can be used. *[4: Limited Evidence]*

Bourque et al[56] conducted a pilot study to determine whether the use of Reiki before a surgical procedure would decrease the amount of meperidine required during the procedure. To determine the average dose of meperidine used during the procedure, the investigators conducted a chart review of 30 patients undergoing screening colonoscopy. The average dose of meperidine was 50 mg. The control group were patients in the chart review. The experimental group of 25 patients received Reiki 10 minutes before the start of the colonoscopy. Five patients were randomly chosen to receive placebo Reiki which did not involve the proper hand positions, symbols, or energy transfers.

There was not a significant difference in the amount of meperidine used by the Reiki group, the placebo Reiki group, or the chart review group. Four patients in the Reiki group received less than the average 50 mg dose. No patients in the chart review group or the placebo Reiki group received less than 50 mg of meperidine. The researchers concluded that Reiki could potentially reduce the amount of medication needed during screening colonoscopy.[56]

Hulse et al[55] conducted a pilot study to investigate the use of Reiki before colonoscopy to reduce anxiety and medication use during the procedure. A prospective nonblinded partially randomized patient preference design was used in the study. The study was partially randomized because patients assigned to the control group asked to be part of the Reiki group.

The experimental group received 15 minutes of a modified Reiki intervention by a Reiki-trained nurse. The control group received standard care. Baseline, postintervention, and post-colonoscopy measures of pain and anxiety were collected with a self-report instrument developed by the nurse principal investigator. The Reiki group did not have statistically significant reductions in pain and blood pressure. The Reiki group did have statistically significant reductions in heart rate, respirations, and self-reported anxiety after the intervention compared with baseline values. The researchers concluded that anxious people are more likely to participate in adjunctive therapies. Limitations of this pilot study were that the principal investigator was not blinded to the group assignments; the sample size was small; and a non-validated pain and anxiety instrument was used.

VI.a.1.   The perioperative RN should assess the patient's acceptance of and willingness to use Reiki as a complementary intervention and should obtain consent. *[5: Benefits Balanced with Harms]*

VI.a.2.   Reiki practitioners should receive education and complete competency verification activities on the principles and techniques of Reiki therapy. *[5: Benefits Balanced with Harms]*

Recommendation VII

Additional complementary care interventions can be used.

Three studies of other holistic interventions (eg, guided imagery,[57] relaxation tapes,[58] essential oils[59])

evaluated measures to reduce surgical patients' anxiety and pain. The collective body of evidence supports the use of these holistic care interventions to relieve anxiety during surgical and other invasive procedures.[57-59]

The limitations of the evidence are that few studies have explored the feasibility of incorporating holistic measures into everyday practice and the competency of perioperative nurses to implement holistic measures. Further research is needed.

The benefits of using holistic interventions outweigh the harms. Benefits include a potential reduction in the patient's anxiety and pain.

VII.a.   Guided imagery can be used. *[2: High Evidence]*

In a randomized single-blinded study, Gonzales et al[57] evaluated the effect of guided imagery on the anxiety and pain of adult patients undergoing same-day surgery. Patients were randomly assigned to one of two groups. Patients in the experimental group listened to a guided imagery compact disc with headphones for 28 minutes before surgery and throughout induction. Patients in the control group had 28 minutes of quiet before surgery and no intervention.

Baseline anxiety was measured using the Amsterdam Preoperative Anxiety and Information Scale (APAIS) and the vertical VAS (vVAS). The APAIS and vVAS data collection continued after surgery with measurements at one and two hours after surgery in the postanesthesia care unit and the ambulatory procedure unit until discharge. There was a significant decrease in the postoperative anxiety levels of the experimental group. The reduction in the pain levels of the experimental group approached statistical significance. The researchers concluded that guided imagery could be useful in the ambulatory surgery area to reduce preoperative anxiety and postoperative pain but that further research is needed.[57]

VII.a.1.   The perioperative RN should assess the patient's acceptance of and willingness to use guided imagery as a complementary intervention and should obtain consent. *[5: Benefits Balanced with Harms]*

VII.a.2.   Perioperative RNs who implement guided imagery should receive education and complete competency verification activities on the principles and techniques of guided imagery. *[5: Benefits Balanced with Harms]*

VII.b.   Relaxation tapes can be used. *[4: Limited Evidence]*

Ko and Lin[58] used a pretest-posttest design to evaluate the effects of a relaxation tape on the anxiety levels of 80 surgical patients. Before surgery, the patients listened to a 10-minute tape that included a five-minute preparation period of deep breathing followed by a five-minute period of guided imagery, meditation, and recovery. The researchers used the STAI to measure anxiety before and after the patients listened to the tape. The pretest-posttest STAI scores changed significantly, with female patients having a greater reduction in anxiety than the male patients. The results indicated that relaxation tapes could reduce the anxiety levels of surgical patients. A limitation of the study was the use of a convenience sample with no matched control group.

VII.b.1. The perioperative RN should assess the patient's acceptance of and willingness to use relaxation tapes as a complementary intervention and should obtain consent. *[5: Benefits Balanced with Harms]*

VII.c. Oral essential oils can be used. *[1: Strong Evidence]*

Akhlaghi et al[59] studied 60 minor surgery patients using a double-blind design. A psychologist measured the baseline anxiety using the STAI and the APAIS. The patients received an oral premedication two hours before surgery. The experimental group received Citrus aurantium blossom distillate 1 mL/kg. The control group received a placebo of saline solution 1 mL/kg. A psychologist measured anxiety levels two hours after administration of the premedication and before induction of anesthesia. The researchers analyzed both the STAI-s and APAIS scores and concluded that the experimental group had significantly less anxiety than the control group. The researchers concluded Citrus aurantium blossom distillate may reduce outpatient preoperative anxiety and that there may be a role for herbal medicine as a premedication.

VII.c.1. The perioperative RN should assess the patient's acceptance of and willingness to use oral essential oils as a complementary intervention and should obtain consent. *[5: Benefits Balanced with Harms]*

VII.c.2. Perioperative RNs who provide oral essential oils should receive education and complete competency verification activities on the principles and techniques of essential oils. *[5: Benefits Balanced with Harms]*

Glossary

State-Trait Anxiety Inventory (STAI): A tool used to measure anxiety. The state score measures how a person feels at a specific moment in time. The trait score measures how a person feels generally.

Visual analog scale (VAS): A measure of pain intensity that consists of a line 100 mm long, with two descriptors representing extremes of pain intensity from no pain to extreme pain at each end of the scale. Patients rate their pain intensity by making a mark somewhere on the line that represents their pain intensity, and the VAS is scored by measuring the distance from the "no pain" end of the line. A variation is the use of six different faces that represent a pain level from zero to 10.

REFERENCES

1. Pittman S, Kridli S. Music intervention and preoperative anxiety: an integrative review. *Int Nurs Rev.* 2011;58(2):157-163. [IIB]

2. Fayazi S, Babashahi M, Rezaei M. The effect of inhalation aromatherapy on anxiety level of the patients in preoperative period. *Iran J Nurs Midwifery Res.* 2011;16(4):278-283. [IB]

3. Binns-Turner PG, Wilson LL, Pryor ER, Boyd GL, Prickett CA. Perioperative music and its effects on anxiety, hemodynamics, and pain in women undergoing mastectomy. *AANA J.* 2011;79(4 Suppl):S21-S27. [IIB]

4. Sadati L, Pazouki A, Mehdizadeh A, Shoar S, Tamannaie Z, Chaichian S. Effect of preoperative nursing visit on preoperative anxiety and postoperative complications in candidates for laparoscopic cholecystectomy: a randomized clinical trial. *Scand J Caring Sci.* 2013;27(4):994-998. [IB]

5. Pinto PR, McIntyre T, Nogueira-Silva C, Almeida A, Araujo-Soares V. Risk factors for persistent postsurgical pain in women undergoing hysterectomy due to benign causes: a prospective predictive study. *J Pain.* 2012;13(11):1045-1057. [IIIA]

6. Mitchell M. Patient anxiety and conscious surgery. *J Perioper Pract.* 2009;19(6):168-173. [IIIB]

7. Mitchell M. Conscious surgery: influence of the environment on patient anxiety. *J Adv Nurs.* 2008;64(3):261-271. [IIIB]

8. Nilsson U. The anxiety- and pain-reducing effects of music interventions: a systematic review. *AORN J.* 2008;87(4):780-807. [IA]

9. Tam WW, Wong EL, Twinn SF. Effect of music on procedure time and sedation during colonoscopy: a meta-analysis. *World J Gastroenterol.* 2008;14(34):5336-5343. [IA]

10. Arslan S, Özer N, Özyurt F. Effect of music on preoperative anxiety in men undergoing urogenital surgery. *Aust J Adv Nurs.* 2008;26(2):46-54. [IA]

11. Lee KC, Chao YH, Yiin JJ, Chiang PY, Chao YF. Effectiveness of different music-playing devices for reducing preoperative anxiety: a clinical control study. *Int J Nurs Stud.* 2011;48(10):1180-1187. [IB]

12. El-Hassan H, McKeown K, Muller AF. Clinical trial: music reduces anxiety levels in patients attending for endoscopy. *Aliment Pharmacol Ther.* 2009;30(7):718-724. [IA]

13. Dogan MV, Leman S. The effect of music therapy on the level of anxiety in the patients undergoing coronary angiography. *Open J Nurs.* 2012;2(3):165-169. [IB]

14. Bringman H, Giesecke K, Thorne A, Bringman S. Relaxing music as pre-medication before surgery: a randomised controlled trial. *Acta Anaesthesiol Scand.* 2009;53(6):759-764. [IA]

15. Kulkarni S, Johnson PC, Kettles S, Kasthuri RS. Music during interventional radiological procedures, effect on sedation, pain and anxiety: a randomised controlled trial. *Br J Radiol.* 2012;85(1016):1059-1063. [IB]

16. Johnson B, Raymond S, Goss J. Perioperative music or headsets to decrease anxiety. *J PeriAnesth Nurs.* 2012;27(3):146-154. [IA]

17. Jiménez-Jiménez M, Garcia-Escalona A, Martin-Lopez A, De Vera-Vera R, De Haro J. Intraoperative stress and anxiety reduction with music therapy: a controlled randomized clinical trial of efficacy and safety. *J Vasc Nurs.* 2013;31(3):101-106. [IA]

18. Hook L, Sonwathana P, Petpichetchian W. Music therapy with female surgical patients: effect on anxiety and pain. *Thai J Nurs Res.* 2008;12(4):259-271. [IA]

19. Nilsson U, Lindell L, Eriksson A, Kellerth T. The effect of music intervention in relation to gender during coronary angiographic procedures: a randomized clinical trial. *Eur J Cardiovasc Nurs.* 2009;8(3):200-206. [IB]

20. Ottaviani S, Bernard JL, Bardin T, Richette P. Effect of music on anxiety and pain during joint lavage for knee osteoarthritis. *Clin Rheumatol.* 2012;31(3):531-534. [IB]

21. Yeo JK, Cho DY, Oh MM, Park SS, Park MG. Listening to music during cystoscopy decreases anxiety, pain, and dissatisfaction in patients: a pilot randomized controlled trial. *J Endourol.* 2013;27(4):459-462. [IC]

22. Wu J, Chaplin W, Amico J, et al. Music for surgical abortion care study: a randomized controlled pilot study. *Contraception.* 2012;85(5):496-502. [IC]

23. Bradt J, Dileo C, Shim M. Music interventions for preoperative anxiety. *Cochrane Database Syst Rev.* 2013;6:006908. [IIA]

24. Sadideen H, Parikh A, Dobbs T, Pay A, Critchley PS. Is there a role for music in reducing anxiety in plastic surgery minor operations? *Ann R Coll Surg Engl.* 2012;94(3):152-154. [IIB]

25. Mcleod Roddy. Evaluating the effect of music on patient anxiety during minor plastic surgery. *J Perioper Pract.* 2012;22(1):14-18. [IIC]

26. Lee KC, Chao YH, Yiin JJ, Hsieh HY, Dai WJ, Chao YF. Evidence that music listening reduces preoperative patients' anxiety. *Biol Res Nurs.* 2012;14(1):78-84. [IB]

27. Moris DN, Linos D. Music meets surgery: two sides to the art of "healing." *Surg Endosc.* 2013;27(3):719-723. [VA]

28. Beccaloni AM. The medicine of music: a systematic approach for adoption into perianesthesia practice. *J Peri-Anesth Nurs.* 2011;26(5):323-330. [VB]

29. Wakim JH, Smith S, Guinn C. The efficacy of music therapy. *J PeriAnesth Nurs.* 2010;25(4):226-232. [VC]

30. Selimen D, Andsoy II. The importance of a holistic approach during the perioperative period. *AORN J.* 2011;93(4):482-490. [VB]

31. Gooding L, Swezey S, Zwischenberger JB. Using music interventions in perioperative care. *South Med J.* 2012;105(9):486-490. [VB]

32. Kim YK, Kim SM, Myoung H. Musical intervention reduces patients' anxiety in surgical extraction of an impacted mandibular third molar. *J Oral Maxillofac Surg.* 2011;69(4):1036-1045. [IB]

33. Matsota P, Christodoulopoulou T, Smyrnioti ME, et al. Music's use for anesthesia and analgesia. *J Altern Complement Med.* 2013;19(4):298-307. [VA]

34. Weeks BP, Nilsson U. Music interventions in patients during coronary angiographic procedures: a randomized controlled study of the effect on patients' anxiety and well-being. *Eur J Cardiovasc Nurs.* 2011;10(2):88-93. [IC]

35. Ni CH, Tsai WH, Lee LM, Kao CC, Chen YC. Minimising preoperative anxiety with music for day surgery patients—a randomised clinical trial. *J Clin Nurs.* 2012;21(5):620-625. [IA]

36. Hoya Y, Matsumura I, Fujita T, Yanaga K. The use of nonpharmacological interventions to reduce anxiety in patients undergoing gastroscopy in a setting with an optimal soothing environment. *Gastroenterol Nurs.* 2008;31(6):395-399. [IC]

37. Bradt J, Dileo C, Grocke D. Music interventions for mechanically ventilated patients. *Cochrane Database Syst Rev.* 2010;(12):CD006902. [IIA]

38. Bradt J, Dileo C, Grocke D, Magill L. Music interventions for improving psychological and physical outcomes in cancer patients. *Cochrane Database Syst Rev.* 2011;(8):CD006911. [IIA]

39. Bradt J, Dileo C, Potvin N. Music for stress and anxiety reduction in coronary heart disease patients. *Cochrane Database Syst Rev.* 2013;12:CD006577. [IIA]

40. Zhang ZS, Wang XL, Xu CL, et al. Music reduces panic: an initial study of listening to preferred music improves male patient discomfort and anxiety during flexible cystoscopy. *J Endourol.* 2014;28(6):739-744. [IA]

41. Wentworth LJ, Briese LJ, Timimi FK, et al. Massage therapy reduces tension, anxiety, and pain in patients awaiting invasive cardiovascular procedures. *Prog Cardiovasc Nurs.* 2009;24(4):155-161. [IB]

42. Brand LR, Munroe DJ, Gavin J. The effect of hand massage on preoperative anxiety in ambulatory surgery patients. *AORN J.* 2013;97(6):708-717. [IIB]

43. Rosen J, Lawrence R, Bouchard M, Doros G, Gardiner P, Saper R. Massage for perioperative pain and anxiety in placement of vascular access devices. *Adv Mind Body.* 2013;27(1):12-23. [IB]

44. Acar HV, Cuvas O, Ceyhan A, Dikmen B. Acupuncture on Yintang point decreases preoperative anxiety. *J Altern Complement Med.* 2013;19(5):420-424. [IA]

45. Valiee S, Bassampour SS, Nasrabadi AN, Pouresmaeil Z, Mehran A. Effect of acupressure on preoperative anxiety: a clinical trial. *J PeriAnesth Nurs.* 2012;27(4):259-266. [IB]

46. Wu S, Liang J, Zhu X, Liu X, Miao D. Comparing the treatment effectiveness of body acupuncture and auricular acupuncture in preoperative anxiety treatment. *J Res Med Sci.* 2011;16(1):39-42. [IC]

47. Liodden I, Norheim AJ. Acupuncture and related techniques in ambulatory anesthesia. *Curr Opin Anaesthesiol.* 2013;26(6):661-668. [VB]

48. Braden R, Reichow S, Halm MA. The use of the essential oil lavandin to reduce preoperative anxiety in surgical patients. *J PeriAnesth Nurs.* 2009;24(6):348-355. [IA]

49. Hu PH, Peng YC, Lin YT, Chang CS, Ou MC. Aromatherapy for reducing colonoscopy related procedural anxiety and physiological parameters: a randomized controlled study. *Hepatogastroenterology.* 2010;57(102-103):1082-1086. [IC]

50. Marc I, Rainville P, Masse B, et al. Women's views regarding hypnosis for the control of surgical pain in the context of a randomized clinical trial. *J Womens Health.* 2009;18(9):1441-1447. [IB]

51. Lang EV, Berbaum KS, Pauker SG, et al. Beneficial effects of hypnosis and adverse effects of empathic attention during percutaneous tumor treatment: when being nice does not suffice. *J Vasc Interv Radiol.* 2008;19(6):897-905. [IA]

52. Abdeshahi SK, Hashemipour MA, Mesgarzadeh V, Shahidi Payam A, Halaj Monfared A. Effect of hypnosis on induction of local anaesthesia, pain perception, control of haemorrhage and anxiety during extraction of third molars: a case-control study. *J Craniomaxillofac Surg.* 2013;41(4):310-315. [IIB]

53. Flory N, Martinez Salazar GM, Lang EV. Hypnosis for acute distress management during medical procedures. *Int J Clin Exp Hypn.* 2007;55(3):303-317. [VB]

54. Schnur JB, Bovbjerg DH, David D, et al. Hypnosis decreases presurgical distress in excisional breast biopsy patients. *Anesth Analg.* 2008;106(2):440-444. [IB]

55. Hulse RS, Stuart-Shor EM, Russo J. Endoscopic procedure with a modified Reiki intervention: a pilot study. *Gastroenterol Nurs.* 2010;33(1):20-26. [IC]

56. Bourque AL, Sullivan ME, Winter MR. Reiki as a pain management adjunct in screening colonoscopy. *Gastroenterol Nurs.* 2012;35(5):308-312. [IIC]

PATIENT CARE

57. Gonzales EA, Ledesma RJ, McAllister DJ, Perry SM, Dyer CA, Maye JP. Effects of guided imagery on postoperative outcomes in patients undergoing same-day surgical procedures: a randomized, single-blind study. *AANA J.* 2010;78(3):181-188. [IB]

58. Ko YL, Lin PC. The effect of using a relaxation tape on pulse, respiration, blood pressure and anxiety levels of surgical patients. *J Clin Nurs.* 2012;21(5-6):689-697. [IIIB]

59. Akhlaghi M, Shabanian G, Rafieian-Kopaei M, Parvin N, Saadat M, Akhlaghi M. Citrus aurantium blossom and preoperative anxiety. *Rev Bras Anestesiol.* 2011;61(6):702-712. [IA]

Acknowledgements

LEAD AUTHOR
Mary J. Ogg, MSN, RN, CNOR
Perioperative Nursing Specialist
AORN Nursing Department
Denver, Colorado

CONTRIBUTING AUTHOR
Ramona L. Conner, MSN, RN, CNOR
Manager, Standards and Guidelines
AORN Nursing Department
Denver, Colorado

The authors and AORN thank Lisa Spruce, DNP, RN, ACNS, ACNP, ANP, CNOR, Director of Evidence-based Perioperative Practice, AORN, Inc, Denver, Colorado; Elayne Kornblatt Phillips, PhD-BSN, MPH, RN, Clinical Associate Professor, University of Virginia, Charlottesville; Melanie F. Sandoval, PhD, RN, Research Nurse Scientist, Perioperative Services, University of Colorado, Aurora; and Deborah S. Hickman, MS, RN, CNOR, CRNFA, Director, Renue Plastic Surgery, Brunswick, Georgia, for their assistance in developing this guideline.

PUBLICATION HISTORY
Originally published in *Guidelines for Perioperative Practice*, 2015 edition.

Evidence ratings revised in *Guidelines for Perioperative Practice*, 2018 edition, to conform to the current AORN Evidence Rating Model.

GUIDELINE FOR PREVENTION OF UNPLANNED PATIENT HYPOTHERMIA

The Guideline for Prevention of Unplanned Patient Hypothermia has been approved by the AORN Guidelines Advisory Board. It was presented as a proposed guideline for comments by members and others. The guideline is effective November 15, 2015. The recommendations in the guideline are intended to be achievable and represent what is believed to be an optimal level of practice. Policies and procedures will reflect variations in practice settings and/or clinical situations that determine the degree to which the guideline can be implemented. AORN recognizes the many diverse settings in which perioperative nurses practice; therefore, this guideline is adaptable to all areas where operative or other invasive procedures may be performed.

Purpose

This document provides guidance for assessing patients for factors associated with unplanned intraoperative hypothermia, monitoring patient temperatures, preventing unplanned perioperative patient hypothermia, and developing policies and procedures and education for perioperative personnel related to maintaining patient normothermia.

Core body temperature is normally tightly regulated by the body, but this regulatory mechanism is altered by general, epidural, and other regional anesthetic agents and by environmental factors during the perioperative experience that can result in unintentional hypothermia.[1-3] Unplanned patient hypothermia may contribute to patient complications (See Recommendation III).

General anesthesia inhibits tonic vasoconstriction of the peripheral vasculature, causing vasodilation and loss of core warming. During the first hour after induction of general anesthesia, the core temperature can decrease from 0.5° C to 1.5° C (0.9° F to 2.7° F).[1,4-6] Epidural and spinal anesthesia cause vasoconstriction and shivering to a slightly lesser degree, depending on the level of the anesthetic block.[1,4,6]

Environmental factors that contribute to unplanned intraoperative hypothermia include low perioperative room temperatures, less clothing, and other factors unique to surgery that promote excessive heat loss (eg, administration of room temperature IV and irrigation fluids, evaporation of skin-preparation solutions, air movement).[1,6] These environmental factors contribute to heat loss through four types of mechanisms: radiant, conductive, evaporative, or convective.[7-9]

The temperature value used to define hypothermia varies among sources, but it is frequently stated as lower than 35° C or 36° C (95° F or 96.8° F) and may be further defined as mild (32° C to 35° C [89.6° F to 95° F]), moderate (28° C to 32° C [82.4° F to 89.6° F]),

or severe (< 28° C [< 82.4° F]).[8] Hypothermia occurs during many types of surgical procedures.[10,11]

In a descriptive study, Steelman et al[12] identified prevention of hypothermia as one of the top 10 patient safety concerns for perioperative RNs. In this study, AORN members employed in ambulatory and hospital settings (N = 37,022) received an electronic survey. Of the 3,137 returned surveys that contained complete information, 966 respondents (30.8%) identified prevention of hypothermia as a high priority.

Professional guidelines authored by the Best Practice in General Surgery Committee, University of Toronto[13]; the American Society of PeriAnesthesia Nurses (ASPAN)[14]; the Enhanced Recovery After Surgery Society[15-17]; and the National Institute for Health and Clinical Excellence (NICE)[18] also recognize the importance of preventing perioperative hypothermia. Hypothermia may cause multiple complications, such as adverse myocardial outcomes, altering the pharmacodynamics of anesthetics and other medications, thermal discomfort, increased length of stay in the postanesthesia care unit (PACU), and shivering.[2]

The following topics are outside the scope of this guideline:
- planned, intentional, or therapeutic hypothermia;
- rewarming after an intentional or accidental hypothermic event;
- pharmacological agents used for prevention of hypothermia (eg, amino acids, fructose, carbohydrates);
- cost-benefit analyses of treatment methods;
- treatment for shivering;
- treatment for accidental or extreme hypothermia related to trauma or conditions outside of a health care facility; and
- care and treatment for patients experiencing a malignant hyperthermia crisis. For guidance in treating malignant hyperthermia, readers should contact the Malignant Hyperthermia Association of the United States (MHAUS) Hotline at (800) 644-9737.

Evidence Review

A medical librarian conducted a systematic literature search of the Ovid MEDLINE® and EBSCO CINAHL® databases on August 23 and September 4, 2013, respectively, and limited results to meta-analyses, systematic reviews, randomized controlled and nonrandomized trials and studies, reviews, and guidelines. The librarian also conducted a non-systematic search of Scopus® on September 13, 2013. All searches were limited to literature published in English between January 2007 and the search date. At the time of the initial search, the librarian also established weekly alerts on the topics included in the initial search. The librarian later added terms

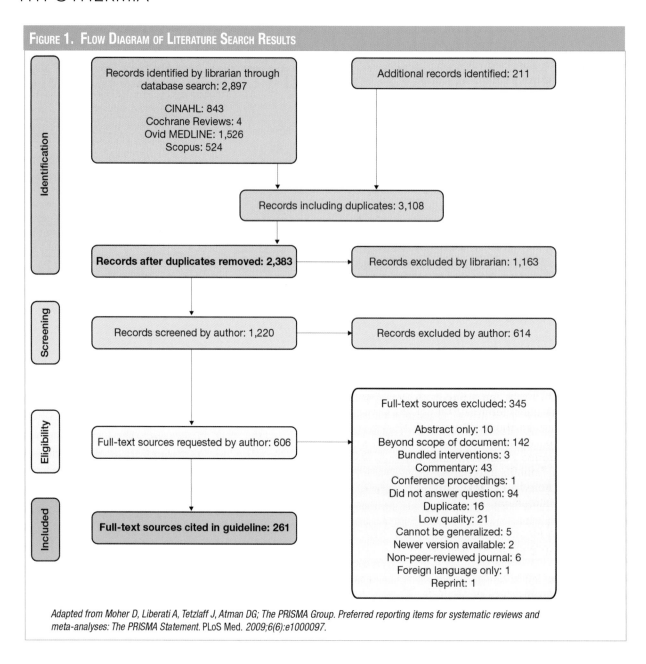

Figure 1. Flow Diagram of Literature Search Results

Adapted from Moher D, Liberati A, Tetzlaff J, Atman DG; The PRISMA Group. Preferred reporting items for systematic reviews and meta-analyses: The PRISMA Statement. PLoS Med. 2009;6(6):e1000097.

from subsequent supplementary searches to the alerts and presented relevant results to the lead author. On March 7, 2014, the librarian conducted supplementary searches and on February 2015, reconducted searches to identify articles that had been published since the original searches but that were not captured in the established alerts. The alerts were terminated in April 2015.

Broad search terms included *perioperative period, perioperative nursing, normothermia; accidental, unplanned, inadvertent, unintentional, core,* and *redistribution hypothermia; shivering; operative surgical procedures; anesthesia; heat loss; heat distribution; body temperature regulation; thermal management; thermoregulatory response threshold; thermoregulatory vasoconstriction;* and *hypothermia.* Terms related to rewarming included *heat loss; preoperative, intraoperative,* and *comfort warming; warming technique;*

warming blanket; energy transfer and thermal pad; forced-air and convective warming; negative pressure rewarming; circulating water garment; cutaneous warming system; resistive heating; inspired gas humidification; intravenous infusing warming; warming irrigation; and brand names of warming devices. Temperature-monitoring terms included *intraoperative monitoring; thermography; skin-surface temperature gradient;* and types of temperature and thermometers (eg, *skin, esophageal, tympanic, temporal artery, oral, axillary*). Other search terms included *intraoperative and perioperative complications; risk factors* (eg, *blood transfusion, obesity, diabetic neuropathies, pneumatic tourniquet*); *pressure ulcers; decubitus ulcers;* and *burns.*

Inclusion criteria were research and non-research literature in English, complete publications, relevance to the key questions, and publication dates within the time restriction unless none were available.

Excluded were non-peer-reviewed publications; literature that examined shivering, traumatic hypothermia, intentional or therapeutic hypothermia, anesthesia techniques to manage hypothermia, malignant hyperthermia, and bundling of treatment or preventative measures. Low-quality evidence was excluded when higher quality evidence was available, and literature outside the time restriction was excluded when literature within the time restriction was available (Figure 1).

Articles identified in the search were provided to the lead author and evidence reviewers for review and critical appraisal using the AORN Research or Non-Research Evidence Appraisal Tools as appropriate. The literature was independently evaluated and appraised according to the strength and quality of the evidence. Each article was then assigned an appraisal score. The appraisal score is noted in brackets after each reference, as applicable.

The evidence supporting each intervention and activity statement within a specific recommendation was summarized, and the AORN Evidence-Rating Model was used to rate the strength of the collective evidence. Factors considered in the review of the collective evidence were the quality of the evidence, the quantity of similar evidence on a given topic, the consistency of evidence supporting a recommendation, and the potential benefits and harms. The assigned evidence rating is noted in brackets after each intervention and activity statement.

Note: *The evidence summary table is available at http://www.aorn.org/evidencetables/.*

Editor's note: *MEDLINE is a registered trademark of the US National Library of Medicine's Medical Literature Analysis and Retrieval System, Bethesda, MD. CINAHL, Cumulative Index to Nursing and Allied Health Literature, is a registered trademark of EBSCO Industries, Birmingham, AL. Scopus is a registered trademark of Elsevier B.V., Amsterdam, The Netherlands.*

Recommendation I

The perioperative registered nurse (RN) should perform a preoperative nursing assessment to determine the presence of factors that could contribute to unplanned hypothermia.

Patient assessment before an intervention is a standard of perioperative nursing practice.[19] The American Nurses Association's *Nursing: Scope and Standards of Practice*[20] and the AORN "Standards of perioperative nursing"[19] direct the RN to collect health data that are relevant to the patient's care.

I.a. The preoperative patient assessment should include factors that may contribute to unplanned hypothermia, such as
- type and duration of the surgical procedure[21-28];

- ambient operating room (OR) temperature lower than 20° C (68° F)[25,29,30];
- type and duration of planned anesthesia[2,6,9,14, 22,24,30-34];
- procedure-related devices (eg, tourniquet, sequential compression devices)[6,21,35]; and
- patient-related factors, including
  - age (eg, premature and other low-birth-weight infants, > 65 years),[8,14,22,24, 25,29,34,36-39]
  - sex (ie, female),[14,36,40]
  - low body-surface area or weight,[6,14,22,26,29, 30,34,36,40]
  - congestive heart failure,[36]
  - higher ventricular function,[36]
  - preexisting medical conditions (eg, hypothyroidism, hypoglycemia, malnourishment, burns, trauma, infantile neuronal ceroid lipofuscinosis, neurologic disorders),[25,40-42]
  - cardiac vessel disease,[36]
  - previous cardiac surgery,[36]
  - hypotension,[14,26] and
  - history of organ transplant.[36]
  [2: High Evidence]

I.a.1. The assessment should be shared with all members of the perioperative team.[9,14,43] *[1: Strong Evidence]*

I.b. Policies and procedures related to the components of the preoperative, intraoperative, and postoperative nursing assessments that are applicable to the maintenance of normothermia should be developed, reviewed periodically, revised as necessary, and readily available in the practice setting. *[5: Benefits Balanced with Harms]*

Recommendation II

The patient's temperature should be measured and monitored in all phases of perioperative care.

The evidence[9,13-15,24,31,35,44-54] establishes the importance of monitoring the patient's temperature.

A randomized controlled trial (RCT) conducted by Huh et al[35] involved 47 patients undergoing laparoscopic resection for colorectal cancer. The study compared the temperatures in a group for which no sequential compression devices were used to the temperatures in a group wearing calf- or thigh-length sequential compression devices on both legs. The researchers found that the temperature drop in the group wearing the sequential compression devices was significantly greater than in the group without the devices. They recommended temperature monitoring because of the core temperature drop noted in the group wearing the sequential compression devices.

Arshad et al[45] performed an observational study that involved 300 patients receiving general anesthesia. They found that 75 of the patients developed hypothermia. Based on the rate of hypothermia, the researchers recommended taking a temperature reading every 15 minutes for patients undergoing general anesthesia.

HYPOTHERMIA

II.a. The method of temperature monitoring should be selected based on the requirements of the procedure (eg, accessibility of the route, invasiveness of the route, anesthesia type, anesthesia delivery method). Temperature may be measured using core temperature sites (eg, tympanic membrane [via thermistor], distal esophagus, cutaneous [via zero-heat-flux thermometry], nasopharynx, pulmonary artery) or "near-core" sites (eg, mouth, axilla, bladder, rectum, skin, tympanic membrane [via infrared sensor]).[2,4,14,55-57] *[1: Strong Evidence]*

The collective evidence[2,22,29,46,52,53,57-90] is inconclusive regarding a preferred method for temperature monitoring but supports making the choice based on the clinical situation. The evidence review revealed basic agreement that the distal esophagus, nasopharynx, and pulmonary artery are reliable locations for monitoring core body temperature. There is disagreement regarding the reliability of tympanic membrane probe temperature measurement. There is general agreement that using the bladder temperature as representative of core body temperature is an acceptable practice when a less-invasive measure is needed and the patient has an indwelling urinary catheter for reasons other than for monitoring temperature. For noninvasive temperature measures, there is general agreement that oral temperatures are reliable and that tympanic membrane infrared monitoring devices may not be reliable. There is general agreement that noninvasive temperature measures are reliable when patients are within a normothermic range, but not reliable for indicating early signs of hypothermia or hyperthermia.

The ASPAN guidelines for promotion of perioperative normothermia[14] state that temperatures taken at the near-core sites are approximately equivalent to core temperatures but should not be relied on for extreme values (eg, < 35° C [< 95° F], or > 39° C [> 102.2° F]). The guidelines also state that the temporal artery temperature approximates core temperature but should not be used for measuring extreme values.

The American College of Critical Care Medicine and the Infectious Diseases Society of America recommend choosing "the most accurate and reliable method to measure temperature based on the clinical circumstances of the patient."[51(p1332)]

A clinical evidenced-based guideline endorsed by the Canadian Association of General Surgeons recommends esophageal or oral temperature monitoring in all surgical patients and recommends that infrared tympanic membrane thermometry not be used if a more reliable method is available.[13]

In an RCT, Sato et al[58] compared the difference between urinary bladder temperatures and distal esophageal temperatures in patients receiving a high IV fluid volume (10 mL/kg/hour) versus low fluid volume (3 mL/kg/hour). Each group consisted of 12 participants who were undergoing tympanoplasty and had an American Society of Anesthesiologists physical status classification of I or II. The researchers concluded that urinary bladder temperatures correlate more closely to the distal esophageal temperatures when urinary flow rates are high and that urinary bladder temperature is an alternative to distal esophageal temperature for clinical use at a high urine flow rate but not at a low urine flow rate.

II.a.1. The same method of temperature measurement should be used throughout the perioperative period when clinically feasible. *[2: High Evidence]*

The collective evidence[9,14,52,67] supports using the same method of temperature measurement throughout the entire perioperative period if clinically possible. A limitation of the evidence is that no studies were found that examined a consistent method of temperature measurement in all three phases of perioperative care.

Washington and Matney[67] conducted a quasi-experimental study to determine the correlation or agreement between oral and axillary temperature measurements. They found there was no agreement between core temperature and either device. Based on these findings, the researchers recommended using just one device for temperature measurement during the patient's entire length of stay.

II.a.2. The selected temperature monitoring device should be calibrated according to the manufacturer's written instructions for use.[51] *[2: High Evidence]*

II.b. The temperature and the site of temperature measurement should be documented in the patient's record.[51] *[2: High Evidence]*

Documentation serves as a method of communication among all care providers involved in planning, implementing, and evaluating patient care. Documenting nursing activities provides a description of the perioperative nursing care administered and the status of patient outcomes on transfer of care.[91]

II.c. Patient temperature results should be communicated
  ○ before surgery,
  ○ to the perioperative team during surgery when the temperature is outside the range of normothermia, and
  to the responsible caregiver after surgery.[92]
  [2: High Evidence]

II.d. Policies and procedures describing when to measure the patient's temperature preoperatively,

PATIENT CARE

intraoperatively, and postoperatively should be developed, reviewed periodically, revised as necessary, and readily available in the practice setting. *[2: High Evidence]*

The evidence is inconclusive regarding the length of procedures that require temperature monitoring. The literature includes recommendations for temperature monitoring in procedures longer than 15, 30, and 60 minutes.[2,4,8,45,50,52,53,93,94]

Recommendation III

In all phases of perioperative care, the perioperative RN should develop an individualized plan of care and implement the interventions chosen for prevention of unplanned hypothermia.

The collective evidence conflicts in regard to the relationship between hypothermia and specific surgical complications. The majority of the evidence establishes a correlation between hypothermia and surgical complications, including increased bleeding, myocardial events, wound infections, postoperative pain, increased PACU length of stay, mortality, increased peripheral vascular resistance, left shift of the hemoglobin-oxygen saturation curve, reversible coagulopathy (platelet dysfunction), postoperative protein catabolism and stress-response-altered mental status, impaired renal function, decreased drug metabolism, poor wound healing, other cellular level effects, pressure ulcers, increased incidence of infection, increased need for transfusion, and prolonged hospitalization.[2,3,8,9,11,13-18,22,24,25,28,31,36,42,44,46,52-54,95-122] However, a number of researchers found no relationship between hypothermia and surgical site infection, blood loss, wound complications, mortality, increased length of hospitalization, or increased length of time in the PACU.[120,123-136]

A limitation of the evidence is that the method of temperature monitoring used is often inconsistent among the studies, and the temperature end point used to define hypothermia is stated at < 35° C (< 95° F) or < 36° C (< 96.8° F), making the incidence and impact of hypothermia difficult to determine.

Schmied et al[95] conducted an RCT in which 60 patients undergoing total hip arthroplasty were randomly assigned to either a normothermia group (n = 30) or a mild hypothermia group (n = 30). The temperature in the normothermia group was maintained near 36.5° C (97.7° F) with the use of a forced-air warming device and warm IV fluids. The temperature in the mild hypothermia group was allowed to drop to approximately 35° C (95° F), and this group did not receive the warming measures. The blood loss in the hypothermic group was significantly greater than in the normothermic group. The researchers concluded that blood loss is decreased by maintaining normothermia.

Kurz et al[115] conducted an RCT that involved 200 patients undergoing colorectal surgery. The participants were randomly assigned to either a hypothermic group (n = 96) or a normothermic group (n = 104). The normothermic group received additional warming methods. The researchers found surgical site infections were present in 19% of the hypothermic group but only 6% of the normothermic group. The researchers concluded that hypothermia may delay healing, which may lead to an increased incidence of surgical site infections.

Frank et al[116] conducted an RCT with 270 surgical patients scheduled for admission to the intensive care unit after surgery (n = 143 in the control group, n = 127 in the experimental group). The patients in the experimental group were warmed using a forced-air warming device. The researchers found that the frequency of cardiac events was lower in the warmed group. They concluded that maintenance of normothermia is associated with a decrease in the frequency of cardiac events including ventricular tachycardia.

Rajagopalan et al[96] conducted a systematic review with meta-analysis that included 18 RCTs that investigated the connection between hypothermia and blood loss. The authors concluded that blood loss is increased with even mild hypothermia, which leads to an increased risk for transfusion.

Scott and Buckland[44] conducted a systematic review of 26 RCTs. They concluded that a hypothermic patient has a greater risk of shivering, experiencing a cardiac event, requiring a blood transfusion, developing a wound infection, and developing pressure ulcers.

An RCT conducted by Smith et al[129] included 383 surgical patients in an ambulatory surgery center. The researchers randomly assigned the participants to either a non-warmed group (n = 192) or a warmed group (n = 191). They found no significant difference between the groups with respect to the time spent in the PACU and concluded that warming the patient did not decrease the time spent in the PACU.

Salazar et al[130] conducted an RCT that revealed a possible negative effect of maintaining normothermia in patients older than 65 years who underwent total hip arthroplasty. The researchers investigated postoperative cognitive dysfunction using a longitudinal study design. A total of 125 patients were assigned to either a control group (n = 63) or a warmed group (n = 62). The researchers concluded that there was a higher incidence of cognitive dysfunction in the warmed group on the fourth postoperative day, but after three months, cognitive functioning was equal between the groups. The researchers concluded that more research should be performed and assumptions regarding the association between patient temperatures and prognosis should be reevaluated.

In a descriptive study, Melton et al[123] found no significant correlation between surgical site infection and patient temperature in 1,008 patients undergoing colorectal surgery.

Geiger et al[124] reviewed the records of 79 patients who had an elective segmental colectomy without a stoma. They found that patients with intraoperative and immediate postoperative temperatures of < 36° C (< 96.8° F) had a lower rate of surgical site infections, shorter length of stay, and fewer anastomosis leaks in the postoperative period than patients with intraoperative temperatures > 36° C (> 96.8° F). The authors concluded that intraoperative patient temperatures > 36° C (> 96.8° F) increased these postoperative complications and that temperatures < 36° C (< 96.8° F) may protect the patient from complications.

Linam et al[125] compared the intraoperative temperatures of 44 pediatric patients who developed infections after posterior spinal fusion procedures to 132 patients who had the same procedure but did not develop an infection. The researchers found that the patients who developed postoperative infections had an intraoperative temperature of > 35.5° C (> 95.9° F) and those who did not develop infections had a temperature < 35.5° C (< 95.9° F). The researchers concluded that an intraoperative temperature < 35.5° C (< 95.9° F) may be protective against surgical site infection in the pediatric population and that more research should be conducted to examine this relationship.

In a descriptive study, Long et al[126] found that intraoperative hypothermia alone was not associated with the development of postoperative complications. The study involved 297 women undergoing cytoreductive surgery for advanced ovarian cancer. The researchers concluded that the use of intraoperative vasopressors, epidural anesthesia, transfusion of fresh frozen plasma, and blood loss were associated with intraoperative hypothermia, but hypothermia was not associated with postoperative complications in general.

Tedesco et al[127] studied the relationship between blood loss and hypothermia in 160 patients undergoing lumbar spine surgery. They found that blood loss was associated with surgery time and surgery type but not intraoperative core body temperature. After controlling for covariates, they concluded that hypothermia did not affect the amount of intraoperative blood loss.

Karalapillai et al[128] investigated the relationship between hypothermia and increased hospital mortality. They reviewed the records of 50,689 patients of whom 23,165 had experienced intraoperative hypothermia. The researchers found that hypothermia was not associated with an increased rate of hospital mortality.

III.a. Methods of warming (ie, active, passive, a combination of methods) should be chosen and implemented by the perioperative team after a collaborative discussion among the team members.[2] *[1: Strong Evidence]*

Active warming methods (eg, conductive, convective) include
- increased ambient room temperature,
- radiant warming,
- forced-air warming (eg, blanket, gown),
- water-filled mattresses,
- circulating water garments,
- warmed IV and irrigation fluids,
- electric warming blankets,
- carbon-fiber blankets,
- resistive polymer blankets,
- electric heating pads,
- thermal exchange chambers, and
- negative pressure warming systems.[137]

Passive warming methods are insulating devices, including
- cotton blankets,
- surgical drapes,
- plastic sheeting, and
- blankets or garments made of reflective composite fabric (eg, space blankets).[2]

The collective evidence[2,10,13,14,16,17,22,29,31,35,37,39,53,121,137-150] establishes the importance of perioperative warming but is inconclusive regarding the preferred warming method.

Benson et al[138] conducted an RCT that involved 30 patients undergoing total knee arthroplasty. The patients were randomly and equally assigned to a control group or a group that was warmed using a patient-controlled, forced-air warming gown. The researchers found that the warmed group required less opioid medication, had higher temperatures on admission to the PACU, and were more satisfied with their thermal comfort than the control group. They recommended that all patients, especially those with compromised thermoregulatory systems, receive warming methods.

An RCT by Huh et al[35] involved 47 patients undergoing laparoscopic resection for colorectal cancer. The study compared the temperatures in a group with no sequential compression devices (n = 23) to a group wearing calf-thigh-length sequential compression devices on both legs (n = 24). The researchers found the temperature drop in the group wearing the sequential compression devices was significantly greater than in the group without the devices. The researchers recommended using active warming methods.

Guedes Lopes et al[151] systematically reviewed seven studies and concluded that using active warming methods was more effective in maintaining normothermia than using passive methods. They found that forced-air warming and circulating water devices were the most effective of the active methods.

Warming of insufflation gases is not included in the list of active warming methods because it was found to be ineffective in a Cochrane review of the available literature.[152] The review included 16 RCTs, five of which demonstrated a benefit and nine of which did not, and many of the trials were considered to have a risk for bias.

III.a.1. The method of warming, should be selected based on
- the planned procedure,
- patient positioning,
- IV access sites, and
- warming equipment constraints (eg, access to the surgical site, skin surface area contact).[137]

[3: Moderate Evidence]

III.a.2. A combination of active and passive warming methods may be used. *[2: High Evidence]*

The collective evidence[129,153-155] suggests that using a combination of methods for

PATIENT CARE

patient warming may be the most effective approach.

In an RCT that included a total of 160 patients undergoing abdominal surgery, Shao et al[153] compared the temperatures of a control group (n = 32) to those of groups receiving a combination of warming methods. The combined warming methods were

- body wrapping and a heating blanket (n = 32);
- body wrapping, heated moist dressings, and a heating blanket (n = 32);
- body wrapping, heated moist dressings, warmed irrigation and IV fluids, and a heating blanket (n = 32); and
- body wrapping, heated moist dressings, and warmed irrigation and IV fluids without a heating blanket (n = 32).

The researchers found that the warmed groups had significantly higher temperatures than the unwarmed group. They concluded that using a combination of body wrapping and a heating blanket was more effective than the other combinations.

Pagnocca et al[154] conducted an RCT that involved 43 patients undergoing exploratory laparotomy. The patients were randomly assigned to either a group that was warmed with a circulating water mattress (n = 24) or a group that was warmed with a circulating water mattress and a forced-air warming device (n = 19). The researchers found that the group that received the combined warming method had a higher temperature than the control group at the end of anesthesia and the end of surgery. The researchers concluded that the combined warming method was more effective in maintaining normothermia than the circulating water mattress alone.

III.a.3. Warming devices should be used, cleaned, and maintained according to the manufacturer's written instructions for use. *[5: Benefits Balanced with Harms]*

III.b. A period of preoperative warming may be instituted as determined by the individual patient's needs. *[1: Strong Evidence]*

The collective evidence conflicts in regard to the benefits of preoperative patient warming and the time frame required. The majority of the evidence[2,9,13,14,16-18,24,25,38,52,53,142,148,156-173] establishes the benefit of preoperative patient warming. However, some of the evidence[132,174-177] indicates that there is not any benefit to preoperative warming.

Andrzejowski et al[157] conducted an RCT with 68 adult patients undergoing spinal surgery under general anaesthesia. The participants were assigned to either a group that received prewarming with a forced-air warming system (n = 31) or a control group that did not receive

the prewarming measures (n = 37). The researchers found that temperatures were maintained above 36° C (96.8° F) in 21 patients in the prewarmed group but in only 16 patients in the control group. The researchers concluded that 60 minutes of prewarming lessened the decrease in intraoperative core temperature.

De Witte et al[158] conducted an RCT in which 27 patients undergoing laparoscopic colorectal surgery were randomly and equally assigned to one of three groups: no prewarming, prewarming using a carbon-fiber total body cover, or prewarming using a forced-air heating device. The researchers found a significant difference in the end-of-surgery temperatures between the group prewarmed by the resistive heating method and the control group. A difference was also found between the control group and the group prewarmed with a forced-air heating device, but the difference was not statistically significant. The researchers concluded that prewarming should be performed when patients are at risk for developing postoperative hypothermia.

Chung et al[159] conducted an RCT to determine the effects of prewarming with either forced-air devices or warmed IV fluids on patients undergoing cesarean delivery. The study included 45 women randomly and equally assigned to one of three groups. The first group was prewarmed with a forced-air warming device for 15 minutes before administration of the anesthetic, the second group received IV fluids warmed to 40° C (104° F) for 15 minutes, and the third group did not receive any form of prewarming. The researchers found that the groups that received prewarming by either method maintained a higher temperature at 45 minutes into the procedure than did the control group, and the group that received the forced-air warming method maintained a higher temperature than the group that received warm IV fluids. The researchers concluded that prewarming using either method helped prevents hypothermia in patients undergoing cesarean deliveries.

The efficacy of prewarming is also supported by an RCT conducted by Horn et al.[160] The study involved 200 surgical patients randomly assigned to one of four groups, the control group (n = 55) and three experimental groups that received prewarming with a forced-air warming device for different amounts of time: 10 minutes (n = 52), 20 minutes (n = 43), or 30 minutes (n = 50). The researchers found a significant difference in the rate of hypothermia in the control group compared with the warmed groups but no significant differences between the warmed groups. The researchers concluded that prewarming for at least 10 or 20 minutes helped reduce the rate of hypothermia.

An RCT by Cassey et al[161] supports prewarming of pediatric patients ages six weeks to 15 years by raising the ambient temperature. The study involved children scheduled for elective surgery lasting at least 20 minutes. The ambient temperature for the control group (n = 30) was set at 21° C (69.8° F); the ambient temperatures for the experimental group (n = 30) was set at 26° C (78.8° F). The researchers found that the warmed group had a significantly higher core temperature compared with the control group. They concluded there was an advantage to prewarming by increasing the ambient temperature from 21° C (69.8° F) to 26° C (78.8° F) for the population studied.

Wong et al[162] found that a two-hour period of prewarming using a conductive carbon-polymer mattress decreased blood loss and complications in patients undergoing major abdominal surgery. The RCT included 103 patients (n = 56 in the control group, n = 47 in the experimental group). The researchers concluded that prewarming with a conductive carbon-polymer mattress was beneficial.

Wasfie et al[163] conducted an RCT that involved 94 patients randomly assigned to a control group (n = 48) or a group that was prewarmed using a warming garment (n = 46). They found a 48% lower rate of hypothermia in the warmed group, but the lower rate was not statistically significant. The researchers concluded that the incidence of hypothermia was decreased when patients were prewarmed.

Vanni et al[164] conducted an RCT to compare the effects of warming on 30 patients undergoing lower abdominal surgery who were randomly and equally assigned to one of the three groups: prewarming for 45 minutes plus intraoperative warming, intraoperative warming only, or no warming. The researchers found that the prewarmed group had significantly higher temperatures before anesthesia, but all the patients were hypothermic on admission to the PACU. The prewarmed group and the intraoperative warming-only group had significantly higher temperatures at the end of surgery compared to the no-warming group. The researchers concluded that 45 minutes of prewarming combined with intraoperative warming minimized hypothermia but did not eliminate it.

Perl et al[165] compared the efficacy of two prewarming methods in an RCT that involved patients assigned to one of three groups: group one (n = 30) received only a hospital duvet cover (ie, the standard insulation), group two (n = 20) received a commercial heat-reflective prewarming suit, and group three (n = 18) received prewarming using a forced-air warmer connected to the same prewarming suit. The researchers found a significantly lower incidence of hypothermia in groups two and three compared with group one. They also found a greater decrease in the rate of hypothermia in group three (zero of 18) compared with group

two (four of 20). The researchers concluded that of the methods studied, a forced-air warmer connected to a commercial prewarming suit was the most effective method for decreasing the incidence of hypothermia.

An RCT conducted by Shukry et al[174] involved 49 pediatric patients (ages six months to 3.5 years) undergoing surgery lasting less than 130 minutes. The participants were randomly assigned to either a control group (n = 25) that was not warmed or an experimental group (n = 24) that was warmed using cotton blankets and a forced-air warming device applied after the patients entered the OR and before induction of anesthesia. The researchers found that the mean core body temperature in the two groups did not differ significantly at induction or at the end of surgery. They concluded that covering and actively warming children during anesthesia induction may not affect core body temperature at the end of surgery.

Nicholson et al[175] also concluded that prewarming did not decrease the number of patients experiencing hypothermia after 15 minutes in the PACU. This RCT involved 66 patients undergoing colon surgery. The patients in the experimental group (n = 34) were prewarmed for 30 minutes before arrival in the OR; the patients in the control group (n = 32) did not receive any prewarming. The researchers found no significant difference in the incidence of hypothermia between the experimental group and the control group.

III.c.   When hypothermia is identified preoperatively, interventions to normalize the patient's core temperature should be initiated before the patient's transfer to the OR, if possible. *[2: High Evidence]*

The collective evidence[9,14,18,34,53] recommends that the patient be normothermic before surgery.

In a nonexperimental study involving 147 patients, Kim et al[34] identified a low preoperative body temperature as a risk factor for intraoperative hypothermia. The patients in this study all underwent abdominal surgery under general anesthesia. The researchers found a significant relationship between a low preoperative core body temperature and the incidence of hypothermia at one hour after the administration of anesthesia.

III.d.   Forced-air warming methods (eg, blankets, warm-air gowns) may be used. *[1: Strong Evidence]*

The collective evidence regarding the benefits and superiority of forced-air warming systems conflicts. A majority of the evidence[2,8,9,13-18,25,47,52,53,117,140-143,148,178-195] indicates that forced-air warming devices are effective. However, some the evidence[151,196-198] indicates that other products may be equally effective at maintaining normothermia when compared with forced-air warming devices, and another portion of the evidence[140,199-202] indicates that other products may be more effective at maintaining normothermia than forced-air warming devices.

In a single-blind RCT, Kim et al[178] included 24 older adult patients (> 65 years old) undergoing unilateral total knee replacements, with 12 patients receiving only a warmed cotton blanket and no active warming and 12 patients receiving forced-air warming. The authors found that the core body temperature increased in the group that received forced-air warming. The researchers concluded that using active warming resulted in better maintenance of patient temperature at the time of tourniquet deflation.

Pu et al[179] conducted an RCT of 110 patients undergoing laparoscopic abdominal surgery who were randomly and equally assigned to either a control group or an experimental group. The experimental group was warmed by an underbody forced-air warming device. Fifty-two percent of the control group and 5.5% of the experimental group experienced intraoperative hypothermia. The researchers concluded that use of an underbody forced-air warming system was both feasible and effective in decreasing the incidence of hypothermia.

Yoo et al[180] conducted an RCT to determine the efficacy of forced-air warming devices compared with cotton blankets in patients undergoing shoulder arthroscopy. The 44 participants were randomly and equally assigned to either a group receiving the forced-air warming device or a group receiving only cotton blankets. The intraoperative drop in temperature at 90 minutes after induction was significantly less in the forced-air warming group than in the cotton blanket group. The researchers concluded that use of the forced-air warming device was more effective in preventing hypothermia than were cotton blankets only. A limitation of this study is that the researchers did not specify whether the cotton blankets were room temperature or warmed.

Trentman et al compared the equivalence of a forced-air warming device to a conductive warming device consisting of circulating warm water in a pad wrapped around a single extremity together with a vacuum applied to the limb.[181] The RCT involved 55 patients undergoing unilateral total knee arthroplasty. The participants were randomly assigned to receive intraoperative warming with either the forced-air warming device (n = 25) or the conductive device (n = 30). The researchers found the temperatures in the group using the conductive system were more than 0.5° C (0.9° F) lower than in the forced-air warming device group. The temperatures were taken within 10 minutes of the patients' arrival in the PACU. The researchers concluded that the conductive system did not

meet the established non-inferiority limits they had set (ie, a difference of < 0.5° C [< 0.9° F]).

Calcaterra et al[199] compared the amount of blood loss during use of a forced-air warming device to the amount of blood loss during use of a disposable gel pad circulating water device. The RCT included 50 patients having off-pump coronary artery bypass procedures who were randomly and equally assigned to one of two groups. The group that used the circulating water device had significantly less blood loss and shorter overall hospital stays. The researchers concluded that the blood loss and lengths of hospital stay were decreased with the use of the disposable gel pad circulating water device compared with the forced-air warming device.

Galvao et al[200] performed a systematic review of 14 RCTs published between January 2000 and the end of April 2007. They concluded that carbon-fiber blankets and a forced-air warming system were equally effective in decreasing the rate of hypothermia but were less effective than circulating water garments.

Tanaka et al[196] conducted an RCT that included 64 patients undergoing major abdominal surgery. The control group was warmed using a forced-air warming system (n = 31) and the experimental group was warmed using a carbon-fiber resistive heating blanket (n = 33). The researchers found the time-weighted core temperatures in the experimental group were not inferior to those in the control group. The researchers concluded that the resistive warming system was not inferior to the forced-air warming system.

Rathinam et al[197] found similar results in an RCT comparing a forced-air warming device to a passive warming blanket (ie, a heat-reflective, non-linting wrap). The study included 30 patients who were randomly assigned to be warmed by a forced-air warming unit (n = 14) or warmed by a passive warming device (n = 16). The researchers concluded that the passive warming device used in the study was as effective as forced-air warming in maintaining normothermia during the intraoperative period.

In an RCT, Ng et al[198] randomly and equally assigned 60 patients to either a group using a forced-air warming device or a group using an electric heating pad. The researchers found no differences in temperature between the two groups. They concluded that the two methods were equally effective in preventing hypothermia.

An RCT by Butwick et al[203] refuted the benefits of using a forced-air warming device. The study involved 30 women undergoing cesarean deliveries. The participants were randomly and equally assigned to either a group that was warmed using a lower-body forced-air warming device or a group that did not receive the device. The researchers found no difference between the groups in the number of patients who became hypothermic. They concluded that lower-body forced-air warming did not help prevent hypothermia.

The collective evidence regarding the effect of forced-air warming on surgical site infections is inconclusive. One portion of the evidence[204-213] supports that use of a forced-air warming device may increase the risk of contamination. In contrast, other evidence[81,214-218] indicates there is no correlation between forced-air warming and sterile field or environmental contamination.

Legg and Hamer[204] conducted a quasi-experimental study using a simulated patient to measure the particle count concentration with and without an operational forced-air warming device. They found a 1,000-fold increase in the air particle count when the forced-air warming device was operational. The researchers concluded that the use of a forced-air warming device can significantly disrupt unidirectional airflow and draw particles from below the sterile field.

In a quasi-experimental study, Belani et al[205] examined the effects of the heat generated by a forced-air warming device on the ventilation airflow. The authors used a mannequin as a substitute for a patient and neutrally buoyant detergent bubbles to simulate the airflow patterns. They found that the exhaust from the forced-air warming device generated hot air convection currents that mobilized bubbles over the anesthesia drape and into the surgical site. The researchers concluded there was disruption in the ventilation airflows over the surgical site when the forced-air warming device was in use.

Legg et al[206] conducted a quasi-experimental study to determine the number of particles in the air over the surgical site during use of a forced-air warming device, a radiant warmer, and no warming device. The researchers used a volunteer to simulate the patient and prepared the room for a lower-limb arthroplasty procedure. They found that during use of the forced-air warming device, there were approximately five times as many particles in the air than during the use of the radiant warmer. They postulated that with the increase in the number of particles, there may be an increase in the number of bacteria in the surgical site because particles are needed to transport bacteria.

Moretti et al[219] conducted a quasi-experimental study in which the bacterial counts at three places on the surgical field were taken with a forced-air warming device in place, with the room unoccupied, and during the procedure without the forced-air warmer activated. They found a lower bacterial load at the test points when the forced-air warming device was in use than when it was not in use. They concluded that the forced-air warming device did not

increase the risk for health care-associated infections.

In a quasi-experimental study, Sessler et al[220] also determined that use of a forced-air warming device did not decrease the air quality in the OR when laminar flow ventilation was in use. The researchers measured background tracer particle concentrations and used smoke as a visual tracer in an OR with a volunteer to simulate a patient and a heated mannequin to represent the surgeon. The researchers found that use of a forced-air warming device did not create an upward air draft or interfere with the function of the laminar flow system.

Zink et al[215] conducted a quasi-experimental study to determine whether the number of bacterial colonies on the skin surface of eight healthy volunteers increased when they were warmed using a forced-air warming device. The results did not show an increase in the number of bacterial colonies on the skin surface of the volunteers. The researchers concluded that use of a forced-air warming device did not increase the bacterial contamination of the surgical site.

Rein et al[202] compared the effectiveness of an upper-body forced-air warming device to a device using warm water and pulsating negative pressure. The RCT involved 20 patients undergoing prolonged laparotomy for gastric surgery. The patients were randomly and equally assigned to either a control group that was warmed using the forced-air warming device or an experimental group that was warmed using the warm water and pulsating negative pressure device. The researchers found that the temperature of the group warmed by the warm water and pulsating negative pressure device returned to baseline (37° C [98.6° F]) faster than the temperature for the group warmed using the forced-air warming device. The researchers concluded that using warm water and a pulsating negative pressure device was significantly better than using the forced-air warming device.

III.d.1. Forced-air warming devices should be used with the manufacturer-designated blanket attached to the hose and according to the manufacturer's instructions for use.[212,221,222] *[3: Moderate Evidence]*

Using a forced-air warming device attached to the manufacturer-designated blanket is necessary because the temperature at the hose can range from 41.5° C to 47.7° C (106.7° F to 117.9° F), which may cause burns. The temperature of the air leaving the blanket is 2.5° C to 16.9° C (4.5° F to 30.4° F) lower.[223]

III.d.2. When using a forced-air warming blanket with a head drape, the drape should be vented or placed in a manner that allows the air to flow freely from under the drape, and the blower should be turned on whenever the drape is in place.[224,225] *[1: Strong Evidence]*

A quality study by Chapp and Lange[224] supported placement of the drape in a manner that allows the air to flow freely from under the drape. The authors measured the amount of oxygen that accumulated under the head drape of a forced-air warming device. The source of the oxygen was a leak in the anesthesia tubing. The researchers found that an oxygen-enriched atmosphere was created under a tucked forced-air warming device head drape in five to 10 minutes. They also noted that the time was decreased when the oxygen flow was higher, the drape was tucked tightly, and the blower was turned off. The authors concluded the head drape should not be tucked tightly or a hole should be made in the drape and the blower should be on at all times when the drape is used.

III.e. Warm water circulating devices may be used. *[1: Strong Evidence]*

The collective evidence[2,9,14,17,47,53,140,141,151,181,187,191,199,201,202,226-228] supports the use of warm water circulating devices as an effective measure to decrease the risk of hypothermia.

Calcaterra et al[199] compared the amount of blood loss with use of a forced-air warming device to that with use of a disposable gel pad circulating water device. The RCT involved 50 patients undergoing off-pump coronary artery bypass who were randomly and equally assigned to either a control group warmed with a forced-air warming device or an experimental group warmed with a disposable gel pad circulating water device. The group warmed with the circulating water device had significantly higher core body temperatures, less blood loss, and shorter overall hospital stays than the group warmed with a forced-air warming device. The researchers concluded that the patient outcomes (ie, normothermia, less blood loss, decreased length of stay) were improved with the use of the disposable gel pad circulating water device.

An RCT by Wagner et al[226] supports the use of a circulating warm water gel pad mattress. The study involved 95 patients undergoing elective electrophysiology surgery in a cardiac catheterization laboratory. The patients were randomly assigned to either an experimental group that was warmed with a gel pad (n = 48) or a control group that was placed on a gel pad that was not warmed (n = 47). The researchers found that the warmed group was significantly less likely to be hypothermic at the end of the procedure compared with the control group. They concluded that the circulating warm water gel pad mattress was an effective means for preventing hypothermia.

In a systematic literature review of 14 RCTs published between January 2000 and the end of April 2007, Galvao et al[200] concluded that circulating water garments were the most effective method for maintaining normothermia when compared with carbon-fiber blankets and forced-air warming devices.

Trentman et al[181] tested a conductive warming device that used circulating warm water in a pad wrapped around a single extremity together with a vacuum applied to the limb compared with a forced-air warming device. The RCT involved 55 patients undergoing unilateral total knee arthroplasty who were randomly assigned to receive either intraoperative warming using the conductive system (n = 30) or the forced-air warming device (n = 25). The researchers found the temperatures of patients using the conductive system were more than 0.5° C (0.9° F) lower than those using the forced-air warming device. The temperatures were taken taken within 10 minutes of arrival in the PACU. The researchers concluded that the conductive system did not meet the established non-inferiority limits they had set (ie, a difference of < 0.5° C [< 0.9° F]).

Rein et al[202] compared the effectiveness of an upper-body forced-air warming device to a device using warm water and pulsating negative pressure. The RCT involved 20 patients undergoing prolonged laparotomy for gastric surgery. The patients were randomly and equally assigned to either a control group that was warmed using the forced-air warming device or an experimental group that was warmed using the warm water and pulsating negative pressure device. The researchers found that the temperature of the group warmed by the warm water and pulsating negative pressure device returned to baseline (37° C [98.6° F]) faster than the temperature for the group warmed using the forced-air warming device. The researchers concluded that using warm water and a pulsating negative pressure device was significantly better than using the forced-air warming device.

Perez-Protto et al[227] conducted an RCT to determine whether a circulating water garment alone was more effective than a circulating water mattress used in combination with a forced-air warming device. The study included 36 patients undergoing abdominal surgery who were randomly assigned to either a group warmed with a circulating water garment (n = 16) or a group warmed with a circulating water mattress and a forced-air warming device (n = 20). The researchers found the core temperatures increased significantly in both groups during the first three hours of surgery. They concluded that the circulating water garment was comparably effective to the combination of the circulating water mattress and forced-air warming device.

III.e.1. Warm saline-circulating central venous catheters may be used.[229,230] *[3: Moderate Evidence]*

Davis et al[229] conducted a quasi-experimental study to determine the effectiveness of a warm saline-circulating catheter. The participants were burn patients (N = 62) who were assigned to one of two groups. Group one (n = 23) was warmed using the warm saline-circulating catheter and group two (n = 39) was warmed using traditional temperature-conserving interventions (ie, increasing the ambient air temperature, warming IV fluids, applying a forced-air warming unit). The researchers found that the deviation in the patient temperatures was almost equal in both groups, but the perioperative team was more satisfied with the warm saline-circulating catheter because the ambient temperature of the OR was not increased. The researchers also found that the patients could tolerate a longer procedure with use of the catheter compared to the traditional methods. The procedure was halted if the patient's temperature dropped below a determined amount. The authors concluded that warming burn patients with the catheter may be more effective than using traditional methods.

III.f. Conductive/resistive devices (eg, electric heating pads, carbon-fiber resistive heating blanket, conductive warming mattresses) may be used. *[1: Strong Evidence]*

The majority of the evidence[52,186,188-190,196, 198,200,206,231-235] establishes conductive/resistive devices as effective for preventing hypothermia. One quasi-experimental study found other methods of warming to be more effective than conductive/resistive warming methods.[201]

Paris et al[231] conducted an RCT that involved patients giving birth by cesarean delivery who were randomly assigned to either a control group (n = 76) or a group warmed with a conductive underbody warming mattress (n = 77). The researchers found that the warmed group had higher temperatures in the PACU. They concluded that use of an underbody conductive warming mattress decreased the occurrence of hypothermia in patients undergoing cesarian delivery.

In an RCT, Chakladar et al[232] randomly assigned 119 patients undergoing cesarian delivery to either a control group (n = 58) or a group warmed by a resistive warming mattress (n = 58). The rate of hypothermia in the warmed group was 5.2% and the rate in the control group was 19%. The researchers concluded that use of a resistive warming mattress should be considered for patients undergoing cesarean delivery.

Perl et al[233] investigated the effectiveness of a conductive warming mattress plus insulation compared with insulation alone. The RCT involved 30 patients undergoing elective head or neck surgery who were randomly and equally assigned to one of two groups. The control group received insulation only with a standard hospital duvet and the experimental group received the same insulation plus a conductive warming mattress. The researchers found a significantly higher core temperature in the experimental group at 45, 60, 75, 90, 105, and 120 minutes. The experimental group also had a significantly lower rate of hypothermia. The researchers concluded that the use of insulation plus a conductive warming mattress was effective in reducing perioperative hypothermia.

In an RCT, Sharma et al[234] randomly assigned 70 patients undergoing day surgery in the supine position in procedures scheduled to last less than 40 minutes to either a group that received standard care (n = 37), consisting of the application of blankets and sheets, or a group that received standard care plus an electric carbon-polymer warming blanket (n = 33). The researchers found that 24% of the warming blanket group was hypothermic at the end of the surgical procedure compared with 39% of the standard care group. They concluded that use of an electric carbon-polymer warming blanket may reduce the incidence of unplanned intraoperative hypothermia.

In a systematic review of the literature, Galvao et al[200] concluded that carbon-fiber blankets and forced-air warming blankets were equally effective in decreasing the rate of hypothermia but less effective than circulating water garments. The authors reviewed 14 RCTs published between January 2000 and the end of April 2007.

Tanaka et al[196] conducted and RCT involving 64 patients undergoing major abdominal surgery. The control group was warmed using a forced-air warming system (n = 31), and the experimental group was warmed using a carbon-fiber resistive warming device (n = 33). The researchers found that the time-weighted core temperatures of the experimental group were not inferior to those of the control group. They concluded that the resistive warming system was not inferior to the forced-air warming system.

Ng et al[198] conducted an RCT to compare the efficacy of a forced-air warming device to an electric heating pad. The study involved 60 patients who were randomly and equally assigned to either a group using the forced-air warming device or a group using an electric heating pad. The researchers found no differences between the temperatures of the two groups. They concluded that the two methods were equally effective in preventing hypothermia.

A systematic review of the literature performed by Munday et al[235] involved a total of 719 participants in 12 studies. The authors found that underbody carbon-polymer mattresses were effective in preventing hypothermia, and the effectiveness of this device was increased when it was applied before surgery. The authors concluded that preoperative warming strategies including underbody carbon-polymer mattresses should be used when possible.

A quasi-experimental study by Hasegawa et al[201] compared the effectiveness of circulating-water leg wraps combined with a full-length circulating-water mattress set at 42° C (107.6° F), a lower-body forced-air blanket set on high (43° C [109.4° F]), and a carbon-fiber resistive-heating blanket set at 42° C (107.6° F). The study involved 36 patients randomly and equally assigned to one of the three warming systems. The researchers found that the temperature two hours after anesthesia induction and at the end of the procedure was significantly higher in the group warmed with the circulating-water leg wraps combined with a full-length circulating-water mattress set at 42° C (107.6° F). They concluded that the combination of circulating-water leg wraps and a mattress was more effective than the other two systems.

III.g. Passive warming methods (eg, thermal clothing, cotton blankets, plastic sheeting, heat-reflective, non-linting wrap, blankets or garments made of reflective composite fabric) may be used. [1: Strong Evidence]

The majority of the evidence[2,8,9,14,25,52,53,197,236] supports the use of passive warming methods. However, one study found passive warming methods to be ineffective at maintaining normothermia.[237]

In an RCT, Hirvonen et al[236] randomly assigned 39 patients undergoing transurethral resection of the prostate under spinal anesthesia to either a group that wore a thermal suit (n = 19) or a group that did not wear the thermal suit (n = 20). The researchers found that significantly fewer patients experienced hypothermia in the group that wore the suit. They concluded that use of a thermal suit is an effective alternative to conventional measures of warming (ie, pajama trousers and jackets made of a one-layer cotton textile).

Rathinam et al[197] compared a forced-air warming device to a passive heat-reflective, non-linting wrap in an RCT that included 30 patients undergoing thoracotomy procedures. The patients were randomly assigned to either a group that was warmed using a forced-air warming device (n = 14) or a group that was warmed using a passive heat-reflective, non-linting wrap (n = 16). The researchers found the intraoperative core temperature was maintained equally well in both groups. They concluded that the passive warming device used in this study was as effective as forced-air warming in maintaining normothermia during the intraoperative period.

Koeter et al[237] conducted an RCT of 58 patients undergoing unilateral total hip or knee arthroplasty. The experimental group (n = 29) had a reflective blanket applied, and the control group (n = 29) had two cotton blankets applied. The researchers found that the mean of the lowest core temperatures did not differ significantly between the two groups. They concluded that the use of a reflective thermal blanket is not effective in decreasing the incidence of hypothermia when compared with the use of two cotton blankets.

III.h. Anesthesia gases may be warmed intraoperatively using an active warming method. [1: Strong Evidence]

The collective evidence[238-241] supports active warming of anesthesia gases.

Han et al[238] conducted an RCT of 34 patients undergoing liver transplantation who were assigned equally to one of two groups. The anesthesia gases for the control group were warmed and humidified using a heat-and-moisture exchanger (ie, passive warming). In the experimental group, the gases were warmed using a heated humidifier (ie, active warming). The rate and duration of hypothermia in the active warming group was significantly less than in the passive warming group. The researchers concluded that the anesthesia gases should be warmed using an active method, such as heated humidification.

Jo et al[239] concluded that active warming and humidification of anesthesia gases did not eliminate hypothermia but did decrease the degree of hypothermia. The RCT involved 40 patients undergoing arthroscopic shoulder surgery. The participants were equally and randomly assigned to either an experimental group that received actively warmed and humidified anesthesia gases or a control group that received room-temperature anesthesia gases. The researchers found that all of the patients were hypothermic at the end of the procedure, but the degree of hypothermia was significantly greater in the control group.

Lee et al[240] found similar results in a RCT involving 80 patients undergoing posterior lumbar spinal fusion. The patients were randomly and equally assigned to either an experimental group that received anesthesia gases warmed using an electrically heated humidifier or a control group for which the anesthesia gases were not warmed. The researchers found that the group receiving the warmed gases had a smaller temperature drop and less blood loss than the group that did not receive the warmed anesthesia gases. The researchers recommended using an active anesthesia gas-warming device.

III.i. Warmed intravenous fluids should be administered as indicated by individual patient needs. [1: Strong Evidence]

The collective evidence[2,8,9,13,14,18,25,38,47,52,53,195,231,235,242-248] establishes the benefits of warming IV fluids.

Kim et al[242] conducted an RCT that involved 53 women undergoing short, ambulatory urological procedures. The participants were randomly assigned to either a control group (n = 26) that received room-temperature fluids or an experimental group (n = 27) that received IV fluids warmed to approximately 41° C (105.8° F) in a warming cabinet. Forty-two percent of the control group and 15% of the experimental group were hypothermic (ie, core temperature < 36° C [< 96.8° F]) in the PACU. The researchers concluded that administering warmed IV fluids decreased the incidence of hypothermia.

Paris et al[231] conducted an RCT of women giving birth by cesarian delivery. The patients were randomly assigned to either a control group (n = 76) or a group receiving IV fluids warmed to 41° C (105.8° F) (n = 73). The researchers found that the group receiving the warmed IV fluids had higher intraoperative temperatures. They concluded that use of warmed IV fluids significantly decreased the rate of intraoperative hypothermia in patients undergoing cesarian delivery.

Xu et al[243] conducted an RCT involving patients undergoing abdominal surgery. The 30 patients were assigned equally to either a group receiving IV fluids warmed to 37° C (98.6° F) or a group receiving room-temperature fluids. The mean core temperature in the control group was 35.5° C (95.9° F) and the core temperature in the group that received warmed IV fluids was 36.5° C (97.7° F). The researchers concluded that the use of warmed IV fluids decreased the level of hypothermia in patients undergoing abdominal surgery.

Yokoyama et al[244] conducted an RCT that included 30 women undergoing cesarean delivery. The experimental group (n = 15) received IV fluids warmed to 41° C (105.8° F) and the control group (n = 15) received room-temperature IV fluids. The researchers found that the core temperature in the group receiving the warmed fluids was significantly higher than the group receiving the room-temperature fluids.

Similar results were found in an RCT involving 75 women undergoing cesarean delivery. Woolnough et al[245] assigned the participants randomly to one of three equal groups. One group received IV fluids at room temperature, one group received IV fluids warmed in a cabinet to 45° C (113° F) and one group received fluids warmed with an IV fluid-warming device. The researchers found that the patient temperature decrease at 60 minutes was similar in both warming groups, but the temperature decrease in the room-temperature group was significantly greater. The researchers concluded that IV fluids

should be warmed and that warming using a cabinet or an IV fluid-warming device was equally effective.

In an RCT, Hasankhani et al[246] randomly and equally assigned 30 patients undergoing orthopedic surgery to an experimental group that received warmed IV fluids or a control group that did not. The researchers found a significantly lower drop in the temperature of the experimental group compared with the control group. They concluded that warmed IV fluids should be administered.

Munday et al[235] performed a systematic review of 12 studies with a total of 719 participants. Intravenous fluid warming was found to be effective in decreasing the rate of hypothermia. The authors recommended warming IV fluid by any method in all cesarean deliveries and applying preoperative warming strategies when possible.

In an RCT, De Mattia et al[247] assigned 60 adult surgical patients to one of two equal groups; one group received IV fluids warmed to 40° C (104° F) and the other group received room-temperature fluids. Twenty-two patients in each group developed hypothermia. The researchers concluded that warming IV fluids alone was not effective in preventing hypothermia and that IV fluid warming should be performed in conjunction with other warming methods.

A quasi-experimental study by Andrezjowski et al[248] included 76 patients undergoing day surgery procedures lasting less than 30 minutes. The patients were assigned to one of three groups. Group one (n = 25) received IV fluids at room temperature, group two (n = 25) received IV fluids warmed in a warming cabinet set at 41° C (105.8° F), and group three (n = 26) received fluids warmed using an in-line IV fluid warmer. The researchers found that the groups that received warmed IV fluids had higher temperatures than the group that received room-temperature IV solutions. Patients who received the IV fluids warmed by the in-line IV fluid warming device had comparable temperatures to those receiving the solution warmed in the warming cabinet.

III.i.1. IV fluids should be warmed using technology designed for this purpose and cleared by the US Food and Drug Administration for this purpose. The technology should be used according to the manufacturer's written instructions for use.[52,137] [1: Strong Evidence]

III.j. Irrigation solutions warmed to 33° C to 40° C (91.4° F to 104° F) may be used. [1: Strong Evidence]

The majority of the collective evidence[5,9,14,18,25,26,52,53,249-252] indicates that the use of warmed irrigation solutions is effective in reducing the incidence or degree of hypothermia. However, one RCT did not find a benefit in the use of warmed irrigation fluids.[253]

In an RCT, Tekgul et al[249] assigned 60 patients undergoing percutaneous nephrolithotomy to one of two equal groups; one group received warmed irrigation fluids (37° C [98.6° F]) and the other group received room-temperature irrigation fluids 21° C (69.8° F). Nineteen patients in the warmed fluid group and 27 in the room-temperature fluid group experienced hypothermia. The researchers concluded that using warmed irrigation fluids decreased the rate of hypothermia.

In an RCT, Kim et al[250] randomly assigned 46 patients undergoing arthroscopic surgery to either a control group (n = 23) or a group receiving warmed irrigation fluids (n = 23). The researchers concluded that using irrigation fluids warmed to 37° C to 39° C (98.6° F to 102.2° F) decreased the incidence of intraoperative hypothermia. The rate of hypothermia was 91.3% in the control group and 17.4% in the group receiving the warmed solution.

Jin et al[251] performed a systematic review of 13 RCTs that compared the rate of hypothermia in patients receiving room-temperature irrigation solution to those receiving warmed solution. The studies included a total of 686 patients undergoing endoscopic surgery. The authors found that those groups receiving warmed solution had a lower rate of hypothermia compared with those receiving room-temperature solution. The authors concluded that irrigation solution should be warmed to between 33° C and 40° C (91.4° F and 104° F).

Oh et al[253] found no difference in the rate of hypothermia between patients who received warmed irrigation fluids (36° C [96.8 °F]) and those who received room-temperature fluids. The study involved 72 patients undergoing arthroscopic shoulder surgery. The participants were assigned equally and randomly to one of two groups. The experimental group received warmed irrigation fluids and the control group received room-temperature fluids. The researchers concluded that using warmed irrigation fluids did not decrease the rate of hypothermia in patients having arthroscopic shoulder surgery.

III.j.1. Before instillation, the temperature of warmed irrigation solution should be measured with a US Food and Drug Administration-cleared device at the point of use. *[5: Benefits Balanced with Harms]*

III.k. Ambient room temperatures may be increased in certain clinical situations and used in combination with other measures to maintain normothermia. *[1: Strong Evidence]*

The collective evidence[2,8,14,53,161,254-256] supports increasing the room temperature to maintain normothermia.

Deren et al[254] conducted an RCT in which 66 patients undergoing elective knee or minimally invasive hip arthroplasty were randomly and equally assigned to a group for which the OR was prewarmed to a temperature of 24° C (75.2° F) or a group for which the OR temperature was set at 17° C (62.6° F). The researchers found no significant difference between the groups for the last recorded temperatures. They concluded that prewarming the OR had minimal effect on preventing intraoperative hypothermia. A limitation of this study is that the researchers examined the effect of prewarming and not an increase in the ambient temperature for the entire procedure.

Cassey et al[161] conducted an RCT that involved children six weeks to 15 years of age scheduled for elective surgery lasting at least 20 minutes. The ambient temperature for the control group (n = 30) was set at 21° C (69.8° F) and for the experimental group (n = 30) was set at 26° C (78.8° F). The researchers found that the experimental group had a significantly higher core temperature compared with the control group. They concluded that there were advantages to prewarming pediatric patients by increasing the ambient temperature.

III.l. Radiant warming devices may be used.[9,257] *[3: Moderate Evidence]*

In a quasi-experimental study, Yang et al[257] compared the time required for rewarming by applying warm cotton blankets to the time required for rewarming with the application of a radiant warming device for 130 hypothermic patients in the PACU. They found that the time required for rewarming was shorter for the radiant warmer group (n = 65) than for the warm blankets group (n = 65). The researchers concluded that the radiant warmer was more effective than warm cotton blankets for warming hypothermic patients.

III.m. When hypothermia is identified on admission to the PACU, methods of warming (eg, forced-air warming, radiant warming devices, passive thermal measures, ambient room temperature at or above 24° C [75.2° F], warmed IV fluids, warmed oxygen) should be initiated. *[1: Strong Evidence]*

The collective evidence[9,14,25,52,183,257] establishes the benefits of using warming methods in the PACU.

III.n. Measures taken to maintain patient normothermia, including the warming method used, warming device identifier, and temperature settings when applicable, should be documented in the patient's medical record. *[2: High Evidence]*

Documentation serves as a method of communication among all care providers involved in planning, implementing, and evaluating patient care. Documenting nursing activities provides a description of the perioperative nursing care administered and the status of patient outcomes on transfer of care.[91]

III.o. Policies and procedures should be developed, reviewed periodically, revised as necessary, and readily available in the practice setting. *[5: Benefits Balanced with Harms]*

The policies and procedure should address
- when warming equipment should be used in the preoperative, intraoperative, and postoperative phases of patient care;
- time frames and methods for cleaning and maintaining warming equipment; and
- competency requirements related to hypothermia prevention.

Recommendation IV

A quality improvement (QI)/management program should be in place to identify and respond to opportunities for improvement related to unplanned perioperative hypothermia.

The benefits of a QI program are illustrated in a quality report by Al-Qahtani and Messahel.[258] The authors performed a QI project in which they benchmarked the facility policy on management of hypothermia to the guidance provided by the NICE guidelines on hypothermia prevention. The authors found many discrepancies between the guidelines and the policy. Their findings resulted in the policy being changed to reflect the NICE guidelines. Three months later, the authors performed a quality check and found that the rate of hypothermia had dropped from 1.5% to 0.3%. The authors concluded that benchmarking policies against best practice should be a facet of a quality program.

IV.a. Quality monitoring activities should measure
- compliance with the use of consistent temperature measurement throughout all phases of perioperative care,
- compliance with including temperature and thermoregulation interventions in the handover or transfer-of-care report,
- compliance with documenting the patient care provided related to thermoregulation,
- the incidence of unplanned hypothermia,
- adverse events related to thermoregulation, and
- compliance with using temperature measurement and normothermia maintenance devices according to the manufacturer's instructions for use. *[3: Moderate Evidence]*

Lynch et al[148] conducted a QI project to evaluate methods of intraoperative warming to achieve optimal patient temperatures, minimize patient risks, and meet the patient safety requirements of governing agencies. The authors randomly chose 112 patients and assigned them to one of four groups of 28 patients each. The groups included
- a control group for which only warm blankets were used to cover the patient in the intraoperative and postoperative periods,

- an intervention group for which warmed laparoscopic irrigation fluids were the only means of warming,
- an intervention group for which force-air warming was used in the intraoperative and postoperative periods, and
- a follow-up group for retrospective review of patients who had received forced-air warming preoperatively, intraoperatively, and postoperatively.

The first three groups of patients underwent laparoscopic cholecystectomy procedures, which represented the largest volume of procedures performed at the facility. The follow-up group underwent procedures from various surgical specialties. Using a tympanic membrane thermometer in all phases of perioperative care, the researchers reported that 75% of the patients who received forced-air warming had temperatures that were normothermic within 15 minutes of leaving the OR, which was their benchmark. The results of this QI project prompted a practice change to using forced-air warming for all surgical patients.

Recommendation V

Health care personnel should receive education about hypothermia as applicable to the person's job responsibilities. [3: Moderate Evidence]

The collective evidence[8,43,259-261] establishes the importance of education specific to patient thermoregulation.

Hegarty et al[259] conducted a quantitative, descriptive study to measure nurses' knowledge of hypothermia. The study involved 130 participants at a national nursing meeting in Ireland. The researchers found that the nurses' knowledge about the characteristics and effects of hypothermia, definitions of hypothermia and normothermia, and treatment methods was limited. The researchers concluded that education should be offered on prevention of patient hypothermia.

V.a. Education related to prevention and treatment of hypothermia should include
- clinical signs and symptoms of hypothermia and
- measures for preventing hypothermia.

Glossary

Active warming method: A method that warms the patient by application of heat to the surface of the skin, blood, or internal structures (eg, forced-air warming, IV or irrigation fluid warming, warming of anesthesia gases).

Conductive heat loss: Body heat that is transferred from the body to another object by direct physical contact.

Conductive warming method: A warming method that uses electricity passing through a conductor that generates heat. Synonym: Resistive warming method.

Convective heat loss: Body heat lost when air moves across the skin.

Convective warming method: A device used to transfer heat to the body by warming the air surrounding the patient.

Evaporative heat loss: Body heat lost through water evaporation from the skin and mucous membranes.

Hypothermia: A decrease in core body temperature below 36° C (96.8° F).

Malignant hyperthermia: A rare genetic condition characterized by a severe hypermetabolic state and rigidity of the skeletal muscles that can occur when affected individuals are exposed to a triggering agent such as inhalation anesthetics and succinylcholine, a depolarizing muscle relaxant.

Normothermia: Normal core body temperature between 36° C to 38° C (96.8° F to 100.4° F).

Passive warming methods: A device used to prevent patient heat loss (eg, insulating garments, warm blankets).

Radiant heat loss: Body heat transferred to the environment when the environment is cooler than the body.

Reflective composite fabric: A fabric that reduces the amount of body heat lost through radiation and convection.

REFERENCES

1. Kurz A. Physiology of thermoregulation. *Best Pract Res Clin Anaesthesiol.* 2008;22(4):627-644. [VA]

2. Kurz A. Thermal care in the perioperative period. *Best Pract Res Clin Anaesthesiol.* 2008;22(1):39-62. [VA]

3. Sessler DI. Thermoregulatory defense mechanisms. *Crit Care Med.* 2009;37(7 Suppl):S203-S210. [VA]

4. Sessler DI. Temperature monitoring and perioperative thermoregulation. *Anesthesiology.* 2008;109(2):318-338. [VA]

5. Board TN, Srinivasan MS. The effect of irrigation fluid temperature on core body temperature in arthroscopic shoulder surgery. *Arch Orthop Trauma Surg.* 2008;128(5):531-533. [IIC]

6. Sessler DI. Perioperative heat balance. *Anesthesiology.* 2000;92(2):578-590. [VA]

7. Lantry J, Dezman Z, Hirshon JM. Pathophysiology, management and complications of hypothermia. *Br J Hosp Med.* 2012;73(1):31-37. [VB]

8. Mitchell JC, D'Angelo M. Implications of hypothermia in procedural areas. *J Radiol Nurs.* 2008;27(2):70-73. [VC]

9. Hart SR, Bordes B, Hart J, Corsino D, Harmon D. Unintended perioperative hypothermia. *Ochsner J.* 2011;11(3):259-270. [VB]

10. Rozentsveig V, Neulander EZ, Roussabrov E, et al. Anesthetic considerations during percutaneous nephrolithotomy. *J Clin Anesth.* 2007;19(5):351-355. [IIIC]

11. Sun Z, Honar H, Sessler DI, et al. Intraoperative core temperature patterns, transfusion requirement, and hospital duration in patients warmed with forced air. *Anesthesiology.* 2015;122(2):276-285. [IIIA]

12. Steelman VM, Graling PR, Perkhounkova Y. Priority patient safety issues identified by perioperative nurses. *AORN J.* 2013;97(4):402-418. [IIIB]

13. Forbes SS, Eskicioglu C, Nathens AB, et al; Best Practice in General Surgery Committee, University of Toronto. Evidence-based guidelines for prevention of perioperative hypothermia. *J Am Coll Surg.* 2009;209(4):492-503.e1. [IVA]

14. Hooper VD, Chard R, Clifford T, et al. ASPAN's evidence-based clinical practice guideline for the promotion of perioperative normothermia: second edition. *J Perianesth Nurs.* 2010;25(6):346-365. [IVA]

15. Nygren J, Thacker J, Carli F, et al; Enhanced Recovery After Surgery Society. Guidelines for perioperative care in elective rectal/pelvic surgery: Enhanced Recovery After Surgery (ERAS®) Society recommendations. *Clin Nutr.* 2012;31(6):801-816. [IVA]

16. Lassen K, Soop M, Nygren J, et al. Consensus review of optimal perioperative care in colorectal surgery: Enhanced Recovery after Surgery (ERAS) Group recommendations. *Arch Surg.* 2009;144(10):961-969. [IVA]

17. Lassen K, Coolsen MM, Slim K, et al; ERAS® Society; European Society for Clinical Nutrition and Metabolism; International Association for Surgical Metabolism and Nutrition. Guidelines for perioperative care for pancreaticoduodenectomy: Enhanced Recovery After Surgery (ERAS®) Society recommendations. *Clin Nutr.* 2012;31(6):817-830. [IVA]

18. National Collaborating Centre for Nursing and Supportive Care. *The Management of Inadvertent Perioperative Hypothermia in Adults* [NICE Clinical Guidelines No. 65]. London, United Kingdom: Royal College of Nursing; 2008. [IVA]

19. Standards of perioperative nursing. In: *Guidelines for Perioperative Practice.* Denver, CO: AORN, Inc; 2015:693-708. [IVB]

20. American Nurses Association. *Nursing: Scope and Standards of Practice.* Silver Spring, MD: American Nurses Association; 2010. [IVB]

21. Chon JY, Lee JY. The effects of surgery type and duration of tourniquet inflation on body temperature. *J Int Med Res.* 2012;40(1):358-365. [IIIA]

22. Holtzclaw BJ. Managing inadvertent and accidental hypothermia. *Online J Clin Innov.* 2008;10(2):1-58. [IIIA]

23. Leijtens B, Koeter M, Kremers K, Koeter S. High incidence of postoperative hypothermia in total knee and total hip arthroplasty: a prospective observational study. *J Arthroplasty.* 2013;28(6):895-898. [IIIB]

24. Journeaux M. Peri-operative hypothermia: implications for practice. *Nurs Stand.* 2013;27(45):33-38. [VB]

25. Paulikas CA. Prevention of unplanned perioperative hypothermia. *AORN J.* 2008;88(3):358-365. [VC]

26. Parodi D, Tobar C, Valderrama J, et al. Hip arthroscopy and hypothermia. *Arthroscopy.* 2012;28(7):924-928. [IIIB]

27. Khan SA, Aurangzeb M, Zarin M, Khurshid M. Temperature monitoring and perioperative heat loss. *Journal of Postgraduate Medical Institute (Peshawar - Pakistan).* 2010;24(2):85-90. [IIIC]

28. Pearce B, Christensen R, Voepel-Lewis T. Perioperative hypothermia in the pediatric population: prevalence, risk factors and outcomes. *J Anesth Clin Res.* 2010;1(1):1-4. [VB]

29. Winslow EH, Cooper SK, Haws DM, et al. Unplanned perioperative hypothermia and agreement between oral, temporal artery, and bladder temperatures in adult major surgery patients. *J Perianesth Nurs.* 2012;27(3):165-180. [IIIA]

30. de Brito Poveda V, Galvao CM, dos Santos CB. Factors associated to the development of hypothermia in the intraoperative period. *Rev Lat Am.* 2009;17(2):228-233. [IIIB]

31. Hernandez M, Cutter TW, Apfelbaum JL. Hypothermia and hyperthermia in the ambulatory surgical patient. *Clin Plast Surg.* 2013;40(3):429-438. [VB]

32. Lenhardt R. The effect of anesthesia on body temperature control. *Front Biosci.* 2010;2:1145-1154. [VA]

33. Hoyle J, Andrzejowski J. An audit of perioperative temperature management in a day case surgery unit. *J One Day Surg.* 2008;18(3):76-78. [IIIC]

34. Kim EJ, Yoon H. Preoperative factors affecting the intraoperative core body temperature in abdominal surgery under general anesthesia: an observational cohort. *Clin Nurse Spec.* 2014;28(5):268-276. [IIIB]

35. Huh J, Cho YB, Yang MK, Yoo YK, Kim DK. What influence does intermittent pneumatic compression of the lower limbs intraoperatively have on core hypothermia? *Surg Endosc.* 2013;27(6):2087-2093. [IA]

36. Hannan EL, Samadashvili Z, Wechsler A, et al. The relationship between perioperative temperature and adverse outcomes after off-pump coronary artery bypass graft surgery. *J Thorac Cardiovasc Surg.* 2010;139(6):1568-1575.e1. [IIIA]

37. Araz C, Pirat A, Unlukaplan A, et al. Incidence and risk factors of intraoperative adverse events during donor lobectomy for living-donor liver transplantation: a retrospective analysis. *Exp Clin Transplant.* 2012;10(2):125-131. [IIIA]

38. Yang R, Wolfson M, Lewis MC. Unique aspects of the elderly surgical population: an anesthesiologist's perspective. *Geriatr Orthop Surg Rehabil.* 2011;2(2):56-64. [VA]

39. Talley HC, Talley CH. AANA Journal course update for nurse anesthetists—part 5: evaluation of older adults. *AANA J.* 2009;77(6):451-460. [VB]

40. Han SB, Gwak MS, Choi SJ, et al. Risk factors for inadvertent hypothermia during adult living-donor liver transplantation. *Transplant Proc.* 2014;46(3):705-708. [IIIB]

41. Miao N, Levin SW, Baker EH, et al. Children with infantile neuronal ceroid lipofuscinosis have an increased risk of hypothermia and bradycardia during anesthesia. *Anesth Analg.* 2009;109(2):372-378. [IIA]

42. Billeter AT, Hohmann SF, Druen D, Cannon R, Polk HC Jr. Unintentional perioperative hypothermia is associated with severe complications and high mortality in elective operations. *Surgery.* 2014;156(5):1245-1252. [IIIA]

43. Seifert PC, Wahr JA, Pace M, Cochrane AB, Bagnola AJ. Crisis management of malignant hyperthermia in the OR. *AORN J.* 2014;100(2):189-202. [VC]

44. Scott EM, Buckland R. A systematic review of intraoperative warming to prevent postoperative complications. *AORN J.* 2006;83(5):1090-1113. [IA]

45. Arshad M, Qureshi WA, Ali A, Haider SZ. Frequency of hypothermia during general anaesthesia. *Pak J Med Health Sci.* 2011;5(3):549-552. [IIIC]

46. Flaifel HA, Ayoub F. Esophageal temperature monitoring. *Middle East J Anesthesiol.* 2007;19(1):123-147. [IIIB]

47. Gustafsson UO, Scott MJ, Schwenk W, et al. Guidelines for perioperative care in elective colonic surgery: Enhanced Recovery After Surgery (ERAS®) Society recommendations. *Clin Nutr.* 2012;31(6):783-800. [IVA]

48. *Standards for Basic Anesthetic Monitoring.* 2010. American Society of Anesthesiologists. http://www.asahq.org/~/media/Sites/ASAHQ/Files/Public/Resources/standards-guidelines/standards-for-basic-anesthetic-monitoring.pdf. Accessed September 21, 2015. [IVC]

49. *Standards for Nurse Anesthesia Practice.* 2013. American Association of Nurse Anesthetists. http://www.aana.com/resources2/professionalpractice/Documents/PPM%20Standards%20for%20Nurse%20Anesthesia%20Practice.pdf. Accessed September 21, 2015. [IVC]

50. *Temperature Monitoring During Surgical Procedures.* Malignant Hyperthermia Association of the United States. http://www.mhaus.org/healthcare-professionals/mhaus-recommendations/temperature-monitoring. Accessed September 21, 2015. [IVB]

51. O'Grady NP, Barie PS, Bartlett JG, et al. Guidelines for evaluation of new fever in critically ill adult patients: 2008 update from the American College of Critical Care Medicine and the Infectious Diseases Society of America. *Crit Care Med.* 2008;36(4):1330-1349. [IVB]

52. Torossian A, Brauer A, Hocker J, Bein B, Wulf H, Horn EP. Preventing inadvertent perioperative hypothermia. *Dtsch Arztebl Int.* 2015;112(10):166-172. [IVA]

53. Torossian A. Thermal management during anaesthesia and thermoregulation standards for the prevention of inadvertent perioperative hypothermia. *Best Pract Res Clin Anaesthesiol.* 2008;22(4):659-668. [VB]

54. Sessler DI. Temperature monitoring: the consequences and prevention of mild perioperative hypothermia. *South Afr J Anaesth Analg.* 2014;20(1):25-31. [VB]

55. Bridges E, Thomas K. Noninvasive measurement of body temperature in critically ill patients. *Crit Care Nurse.* 2009;29(3):94-97. [VB]

56. Lawson L, Bridges EJ, Ballou I, et al. Accuracy and precision of noninvasive temperature measurement in adult intensive care patients. *Am J Crit Care.* 2007;16(5):485-496. [IIIB]

57. Eshraghi Y, Nasr V, Parra-Sanchez I, et al. An evaluation of a zero-heat-flux cutaneous thermometer in cardiac surgical patients. *Anesth Analg.* 2014;119(3):543-549. [IIIB]

58. Sato H, Yamakage M, Okuyama K, et al. Urinary bladder and oesophageal temperatures correlate better in patients with high rather than low urinary flow rates during non-cardiac surgery. *Eur J Anaesthesiol.* 2008;25(10):805-809. [IB]

59. Kimberger O, Saager L, Egan C, et al. The accuracy of a disposable noninvasive core thermometer. *Can J Anaesth.* 2013;60(12):1190-1196. [IIB]

60. Barringer LB, Evans CW, Ingram LL, Tisdale PP, Watson SP, Janken JK. Agreement between temporal artery, oral, and axillary temperature measurements in the perioperative period. *J Perianesth Nurs.* 2011;26(3):143-150. [IIB]

61. Frommelt T, Ott C, Hays V. Accuracy of different devices to measure temperature. *Medsurg Nurs.* 2008;17(3):171-174. [IIA]

62. Langham GE, Maheshwari A, Contrera K, You J, Mascha E, Sessler DI. Noninvasive temperature monitoring in postanesthesia care units. *Anesthesiology.* 2009;111(1):90-96. [IIB]

63. McConnell E, Senseney D, George SS, Whipple D. Reliability of temporal artery thermometers. *Medsurg Nurs.* 2013;22(6):387-392. [IIB]

64. Stelfox HT, Straus SE, Ghali WA, Conly J, Laupland K, Lewin A. Temporal artery versus bladder thermometry during adult medical-surgical intensive care monitoring: an observational study. *BMC Anesthesiology.* 2010;10:13. [IIIA]

65. Sahin SH, Duran R, Sut N, Colak A, Acunas B, Aksu B. Comparison of temporal artery, nasopharyngeal, and axillary temperature measurement during anesthesia in children. *J Clin Anesth.* 2012;24(8):647-651. [IIB]

66. Hocker J, Bein B, Bohm R, Steinfath M, Scholz J, Horn EP. Correlation, accuracy, precision and practicability of perioperative measurement of sublingual temperature in comparison with tympanic membrane temperature in awake and anaesthetised patients. *Eur J Anaesthesiol.* 2012;29(2):70-74. [IIB]

67. Washington GT, Matney JL. Comparison of temperature measurement devices in post anesthesia patients. *J Perianesth Nurs.* 2008;23(1):36-48. [IIA]

68. Moran JL, Peter JV, Solomon PJ, et al. Tympanic temperature measurements: are they reliable in the critically ill? A clinical study of measures of agreement. *Crit Care Med.* 2007;35(1):155-164. [IIA]

69. Gasim GI, Musa IR, Abdien MT, Adam I. Accuracy of tympanic temperature measurement using an infrared tympanic membrane thermometer. *BMC Res Notes.* 2013;6:194. [IIB]

70. Jay O, Molgat-Seon Y, Chou S, Murto K. Skin temperature over the carotid artery provides an accurate noninvasive estimation of core temperature in infants and young children during general anesthesia. *Paediatr Anaesth.* 2013;23(12):1109-1116. [IIB]

71. Masamune T, Yamauchi M, Wada K, et al. The usefulness of an earphone-type infrared tympanic thermometer during cardiac surgery with cardiopulmonary bypass: clinical report. *J Anesth.* 2011;25(4):576-579. [IIB]

72. Opatz O, Trippel T, Lochner A, et al. Temporal and spatial dispersion of human body temperature during deep hypothermia. *Br J Anaesth.* 2013;111(5):768-775. [IIB]

73. Kiya T, Yamakage M, Hayase T, Satoh J, Namiki A. The usefulness of an earphone-type infrared tympanic thermometer for intraoperative core temperature monitoring. *Anesth Analg.* 2007;105(6):1688-1692. [IIIB]

74. Fetzer SJ, Lawrence A. Tympanic membrane versus temporal artery temperatures of adult perianesthesia patients. *J Perianesth Nurs.* 2008;23(4):230-236. [IIB]

75. Kimberger O, Thell R, Schuh M, Koch J, Sessler DI, Kurz A. Accuracy and precision of a novel non-invasive core thermometer. *Br J Anaesth.* 2009;103(2):226-231. [IIB]

76. Farnell S, Maxwell L, Tan S, Rhodes A, Philips B. Temperature measurement: comparison of non-invasive methods used in adult critical care. *J Clin Nurs.* 2005;14(5):632-639. [IIB]

77. Calonder EM, Sendelbach S, Hodges JS, et al. Temperature measurement in patients undergoing colorectal surgery and gynecology surgery: a comparison of esophageal core, temporal artery, and oral methods. *J Perianesth Nurs.* 2010;25(2):71-78. [IIB]

78. Apa H, Gözmen S, Bayram N, et al. Clinical accuracy of tympanic thermometer and noncontact infrared skin thermometer in pediatric practice: an alternative for axillary digital thermometer. *Pediatr Emerg Care.* 2013;29(9):992-997. [IIIB]

79. Hooper VD, Andrews JO. Accuracy of noninvasive core temperature measurement in acutely ill adults: the state of the science. *Biol Res Nurs.* 2006;8(1):24-34. [IIIA]

80. Kimberger O, Cohen D, Illievich U, Lenhardt R. Temporal artery versus bladder thermometry during perioperative and intensive care unit monitoring. *Anesth Analg.* 2007;105(4):1042-1047. [IIIB]

81. Tan GM, Galinkin JL, Pan Z, Polaner DM. Laryngeal view and temperature measurements while using the perilaryngeal airway (Cobra-PLUS) in children. *Paediatr Anaesth.* 2013;23(12):1180-1186. [IIA]

82. Lefrant JY, Muller L, de La Coussaye JE, et al. Temperature measurement in intensive care patients: comparison of urinary bladder, oesophageal, rectal, axillary, and inguinal methods versus pulmonary artery core method. *Intensive Care Med.* 2003;29(3):414-418. [IIIB]

83. Eyelade OR, Orimadegun AE, Akinyemi OA, Tongo OO, Akinyinka OO. Esophageal, tympanic, rectal, and skin temperatures in children undergoing surgery with general anesthesia. *J Perianesth Nurs.* 2011;26(3):151-159. [IIB]

84. Drake-Brockman TFE, Hegarty M, Chambers NA, Von Ungernsternberg BS. Monitoring temperature in children undergoing anaesthesia: a comparison of methods. *Anaesth Intensive Care.* 2014;42(3):315-320. [IIIA]

85. Gobolos L, Philipp A, Ugocsai P, et al. Reliability of different body temperature measurement sites during aortic surgery. *Perfusion.* 2014;29(1):75-81. [IIIB]

86. Pawley MD, Martinsen P, Mitchell SJ, et al. Brachial arterial temperature as an indicator of core temperature: proof of concept and potential applications. *J Extra Corpor Technol.* 2013;45(2):86-93. [IIIB]

87. Fallis WM. Monitoring bladder temperatures in the OR. *AORN J.* 2002;76(3):467-489. [VA]

88. Smith J. Methods and devices of temperature measurement in the neonate: a narrative review and practice recommendations. *Newborn Infant Nurs Rev.* 2014;14(2):64-71. [VA]

89. Asher C, Northington LK. Position statement for measurement of temperature/fever in children. *J Pediatr Nurs.* 2008;23(3):234-236. [IVC]

90. *Clinical Practice Guideline: Non-invasive Temperature Measurement in the Emergency Department.* 2011; title revised 2013. Emergency Nurses Association. https://www.ena.org/practice-research/research/CPG/Documents/TemperatureMeasurementCPG.pdf. Accessed September 21, 2015. [IVA]

91. Guideline for health care information management. In: *Guidelines for Perioperative Practice.* Denver, CO: AORN, Inc; 2015:491-511. [IVB]

92. Guideline for transfer of patient care information. In: *Guidelines for Perioperative Practice.* Denver, CO: AORN, Inc; 2015:583-588. [IVB]

93. Putzu M, Casati A, Berti M, Pagliarini G, Fanelli G. Clinical complications, monitoring and management of perioperative mild hypothermia: anesthesiological features. *Acta Biomed Ateneo Parmense.* 2007;78(3):163-169. [VB]

94. Collins JB, Verheyden CN, Mahabir RC. Core measures: implications for plastic surgery. *Plast Reconstr Surg.* 2013;131(6):1266-1271. [VB]

95. Schmied H, Kurz A, Sessler DI, Kozek S, Reiter A. Mild hypothermia increases blood loss and transfusion requirements during total hip arthroplasty. *Lancet.* 1996;347(8997):289-292. [IB]

96. Rajagopalan S, Mascha E, Na J, Sessler DI. The effects of mild perioperative hypothermia on blood loss and transfusion requirement. *Anesthesiology.* 2008;108(1):71-77. [IA]

97. Kiekkas P, Theodorakopoulou G, Stefanopoulos N, Tsotas D, Baltopoulos GI. Postoperative hypothermia and mortality in critically ill adults: review and meta-analysis. *Aust J Adv Nurs.* 2011;28(4):60-67. [IIIB]

98. Jeyadoss J, Thiruvenkatarajan V, Watts RW, Sullivan T, van Wijk RM. Intraoperative hypothermia is associated with an increased intensive care unit length-of-stay in patients undergoing elective open abdominal aortic aneurysm surgery: a retrospective cohort study. *Anaesth Intensive Care.* 2013;41(6):759-764. [IIIC]

99. Karalapillai D, Story DA, Calzavacca P, Licari E, Liu YL, Hart GK. Inadvertent hypothermia and mortality in postoperative intensive care patients: retrospective audit of 5050 patients. *Anaesthesia.* 2009;64(9):968-972. [IIIA]

100. Liu CK, Liao CH, Wan KS, et al. Change in intraoperative rectal temperature influencing erectile dysfunction following transurethral resection of the prostate. *J Formosan Med Assoc.* 2012;111(6):320-324. [IIIB]

101. Moslemi-Kebria M, El-Nashar SA, Aletti GD, Cliby WA. Intraoperative hypothermia during cytoreductive

surgery for ovarian cancer and perioperative morbidity. *Obstet Gynecol.* 2012;119(3):590-596. [IIIA]

102. Yamasaki H, Tanaka K, Funai Y, et al. The impact of intraoperative hypothermia on early postoperative adverse events after radical esophagectomy for cancer: a retrospective cohort study. *J Cardiothorac Vasc Anesth.* 2014;28(4):955-959. [IIIA]

103. Sumer BD, Myers LL, Leach J, Truelson JM. Correlation between intraoperative hypothermia and perioperative morbidity in patients with head and neck cancer. *Arch Otolaryngol Head Neck Surg.* 2009;135(7):682-686. [IIIB]

104. Quiroga E, Tran NT, Hatsukami T, Starnes BW. Hypothermia is associated with increased mortality in patients undergoing repair of ruptured abdominal aortic aneurysm. *J Endovasc Ther.* 2010;17(3):434-438. [IIIB]

105. Oda J, Kasai K, Noborio M, Ueyama M, Yukioka T. Hypothermia during burn surgery and postoperative acute lung injury in extensively burned patients. *J Trauma.* 2009;66(6):1525-1529. [IIIB]

106. Coon D, Michaels J 5th, Gusenoff JA, Chong T, Purnell C, Rubin JP. Hypothermia and complications in postbariatric body contouring. *Plast Reconstr Surg.* 2012;130(2):443-448. [IIIA]

107. Morehouse D, Williams L, Lloyd C, et al. Perioperative hypothermia in NICU infants: its occurrence and impact on infant outcomes. *Adv Neonatal Care.* 2014;14(3):154-164. [IIIB]

108. Reynolds L, Beckmann J, Kurz A. Perioperative complications of hypothermia. *Best Pract Res Clin Anaesthesiol.* 2008;22(4):645-657. [VA]

109. Burke S, Hanani M. The actions of hyperthermia on the autonomic nervous system: central and peripheral mechanisms and clinical implications. *Autonomic Neurosci.* 2012;168(1-2):4-13. [VB]

110. Vanamoorthy P, Pandia MP, Bithal PK, Valiaveedan SS. Refractory hypotension due to intraoperative hypothermia during spinal instrumentation. *Indian J Anaesth.* 2010;54(1):56-58. [VA]

111. Dickinson A, Qadan M, Polk HC Jr. Optimizing surgical care: a contemporary assessment of temperature, oxygen, and glucose. *Am Surg.* 2010;76(6):571-577. [VB]

112. Qadan M, Gardner SA, Vitale DS, Lominadze D, Joshua IG, Polk HC Jr. Hypothermia and surgery: immunologic mechanisms for current practice. *Ann Surg.* 2009;250(1):134-140. [IIIC]

113. Fred C, Ford S, Wagner D, Vanbrackle L. Intraoperatively acquired pressure ulcers and perioperative normothermia: a look at relationships. *AORN J.* 2012;96(3):251-260. [IIIB]

114. Diaz M, Becker DE. Thermoregulation: physiological and clinical considerations during sedation and general anesthesia. *Anesth Prog.* 2010;57(1):25-32. [VC]

115. Kurz A, Sessler DI, Lenhardt R. Perioperative normothermia to reduce the incidence of surgical-wound infection and shorten hospitalization. Study of Wound Infection and Temperature Group. *N Engl J Med.* 1996;334(19):1209-1215. [IA]

116. Frank SM, Fleisher LA, Breslow MJ, et al. Perioperative maintenance of normothermia reduces the incidence of morbid cardiac events. A randomized clinical trial. *JAMA.* 1997;277(14):1127-1134. [IB]

117. Mahoney CB, Odom J. Maintaining intraoperative normothermia: a meta-analysis of outcomes with costs. *AANA J.* 1999;67(2):155-163. [IIIB]

118. Seamon MJ, Wobb J, Gaughan JP, Kulp H, Kamel I, Dempsey DT. The effects of intraoperative hypothermia on surgical site infection: an analysis of 524 trauma laparotomies. *Ann Surg.* 2012;255(4):789-795. [IIIB]

119. Romlin B, Petruson K, Nilsson K. Moderate superficial hypothermia prolongs bleeding time in humans. *Acta Anaesthesiol Scand.* 2007;51(2):198-201. [IIIB]

120. Lista F, Doherty CD, Backstein RM, Ahmad J. The impact of perioperative warming in an outpatient aesthetic surgery setting. *Aesthet Surg J.* 2012;32(5):613-620. [VB]

121. Esnaola NF, Cole DJ. Perioperative normothermia during major surgery: is it important? *Adv Surg.* 2011;45:249-263. [VB]

122. Lau AW, Chen CC, Wu RS, Poon KS. Hypothermia as a cause of coagulopathy during hepatectomy. *Acta Anaesthesiol Taiwan.* 2010;48(2):103-106. [VA]

123. Melton GB, Vogel JD, Swenson BR, Remzi FH, Rothenberger DA, Wick EC. Continuous intraoperative temperature measurement and surgical site infection risk: analysis of anesthesia information system data in 1008 colorectal procedures. *Ann Surg.* 2013;258(4):606-612; discussion 612-613. [IIIA]

124. Geiger TM, Horst S, Muldoon R, et al. Perioperative core body temperatures effect on outcome after colorectal resections. *Am Surg.* 2012;78(5):607-612. [IIIB]

125. Linam WM, Margolis PA, Staat MA, et al. Risk factors associated with surgical site infection after pediatric posterior spinal fusion procedure. *Infect Control Hosp Epidemiol.* 2009;30(2):109-116. [IIIA]

126. Long KC, Tanner EJ, Frey M, et al. Intraoperative hypothermia during primary surgical cytoreduction for advanced ovarian cancer: risk factors and associations with postoperative morbidity. *Gynecol Oncol.* 2013;131(3):525-530. [IIIA]

127. Tedesco NS, Korpi FP, Pazdernik VK, Cochran JM. Relationship between hypothermia and blood loss in adult patients undergoing open lumbar spine surgery. *J Am Osteopath Assoc.* 2014;114(11):828-838. [IIIA]

128. Karalapillai D, Story D, Hart GK, et al. Postoperative hypothermia and patient outcomes after major elective non-cardiac surgery. *Anaesthesia.* 2013;68(6):605-611. [IIIB]

129. Smith CE, Sidhu RS, Lucas L, Mehta D, Pinchak AC. Should patients undergoing ambulatory surgery with general anesthesia be actively warmed? *Internet J Anesthesiol.* 2007;12(1):18p. [IB]

130. Salazar F, Donate M, Boget T, et al. Intraoperative warming and post-operative cognitive dysfunction after total knee replacement. *Acta Anaesthesiol Scand.* 2011;55(2):216-222. [IA]

131. Silva AB, Peniche Ade C. Perioperative hypothermia and incidence of surgical wound infection: a bibliographic study. *Einstein (Sao Paulo).* 2014;12(4):513-517. [IIIB]

132. Constantine RS, Kenkel M, Hein RE, et al. The impact of perioperative hypothermia on plastic surgery outcomes: a multivariate logistic regression of 1062 cases. *Aesthet Surg J.* 2015;35(1):81-88. [IIIB]

133. Lehtinen SJ, Onicescu G, Kuhn KM, Cole DJ, Esnaola NF. Normothermia to prevent surgical site infections after gastrointestinal surgery: holy grail or false idol? *Ann Surg.* 2010;252(4):696-704. [IIIA]

134. Young H, Bliss R, Carey JC, Price CS. Beyond core measures: identifying modifiable risk factors for prevention of surgical site infection after elective total abdominal hysterectomy. *Surg Infect (Larchmt).* 2011;12(6):491-496. [IIIB]

135. Baucom RB, Phillips SE, Ehrenfeld JM, et al. Defining intraoperative hypothermia in ventral hernia repair. *J Surg Res.* 2014;190(1):385-390. [IIIA]

136. Fecho K, Lunney AT, Boysen PG, Rock P, Norfleet EA. Postoperative mortality after inpatient surgery: incidence

and risk factors. *Ther Clin Risk Manag.* 2008;4(4):681-688. [IIIA]

137. John M, Ford J, Harper M. Peri-operative warming devices: performance and clinical application. *Anaesthesia.* 2014;69(6):623-638. [IB]

138. Benson EE, McMillan DE, Ong B. The effects of active warming on patient temperature and pain after total knee arthroplasty. *Am J Nurs.* 2012;112(5):26-33. [IC]

139. Sajid MS, Shakir AJ, Khatri K, Baig MK. The role of perioperative warming in surgery: a systematic review. *Sao Paulo Med J.* 2009;127(4):231-237. [IB]

140. Galvao CM, Liang Y, Clark AM. Effectiveness of cutaneous warming systems on temperature control: meta-analysis. *J Adv Nurs.* 2010;66(6):1196-1206. [IB]

141. Poveda Vde B, Martinez EZ, Galvao CM. Active cutaneous warming systems to prevent intraoperative hypothermia: a systematic review. *Rev Lat Am.* 2012;20(1):183-191. [IB]

142. Moola S, Lockwood C. Effectiveness of strategies for the management and/or prevention of hypothermia within the adult perioperative environment. *Int J Evid Based Healthc.* 2011;9(4):337-345. [IB]

143. Alderson P, Campbell G, Smith AF, Warttig S, Nicholson A, Lewis SR. Thermal insulation for preventing inadvertent perioperative hypothermia. *Cochrane Database Syst Rev.* 2014;6:CD009908. [IIA]

144. Shorrab AA, El-Sawy ME, Othman MM, Hammouda GE. Prevention of hypothermia in children under combined epidural and general anesthesia: a comparison between upper- and lower-body warming. *Paediatr Anaesth.* 2007;17(1):38-43. [IIB]

145. Yokoe DS, Anderson DJ, Berenholtz SM, et al. A compendium of strategies to prevent healthcare-associated infections in acute care hospitals: 2014 updates. *Infect Control Hosp Epidemiol.* 2014;35(8):967-977. [IVB]

146. Colwell AS, Borud LJ. Optimization of patient safety in postbariatric body contouring: a current review. *Aesthet Surg J.* 2008;28(4):437-442. [VA]

147. Munday J, Hines SJ, Chang AM. Evidence utilisation project: management of inadvertent perioperative hypothermia. The challenges of implementing best practice recommendations in the perioperative environment. *Int J Evid Based Healthc.* 2013;11(4):305-311. [VB]

148. Lynch S, Dixon J, Leary D. Reducing the risk of unplanned perioperative hypothermia. *AORN J.* 2010;92(5):553-562. [VB]

149. Aksu C, Ku A, Gürkan Y, Solak M, Toker K. Survey on postoperative hypothermia incidence in operating theatres of Kocaeli university. *Turk Anesteziyoloji ve Reanimasyon Dernegi Dergisi.* 2014;42(2):66-70. [IIIB]

150. Fleisher LA, Fleischmann KE, Auerbach AD, et al. 2014 ACC/AHA guideline on perioperative cardiovascular evaluation and management of patients undergoing noncardiac surgery: a report of the American College of Cardiology/American Heart Association Task Force on Practice Guidelines. *Circulation.* 2014;130(24):2215-2245. [IVA]

151. Guedes Lopes Inês, Sousa Magalhães António Manuel, Abreu de Sousa, Batista de Ara. Preventing perioperative hypothermia: an integrative literature review. *Revista de Enfermagem Referência.* 2015;8(1):147-155. [IIA]

152. Birch DW, Manouchehri N, Shi X, Hadi G, Karmali S. Heated CO(2) with or without humidification for minimally invasive abdominal surgery. *Cochrane Database Syst Rev.* 2011;(1):007821. [IA]

153. Shao L, Zheng H, Jia FJ, et al. Methods of patient warming during abdominal surgery. *PLoS One.* 2012;7(7):e39622. [IC]

154. Pagnocca ML, Tai EJ, Dwan JL. Temperature control in conventional abdominal surgery: comparison between conductive and the association of conductive and convective warming. *Rev Bras Anestesiol.* 2009;59(1):56-66. [IB]

155. Kim P, Taghon T, Fetzer M, Tobias JD. Perioperative hypothermia in the pediatric population: a quality improvement project. *Am J Med Qual.* 2013;28(5):400-406. [VA]

156. Melling AC, Ali B, Scott EM, Leaper DJ. Effects of preoperative warming on the incidence of wound infection after clean surgery: a randomised controlled trial. *Lancet.* 2001;358(9285):876-880. [IB]

157. Andrzejowski J, Hoyle J, Eapen G, Turnbull D. Effect of prewarming on post-induction core temperature and the incidence of inadvertent perioperative hypothermia in patients undergoing general anaesthesia. *Br J Anacsth.* 2008;101(5):627-631. [IB]

158. De Witte JL, Demeyer C, Vandemaele E. Resistive-heating or forced-air warming for the prevention of redistribution hypothermia. *Anesth Analg.* 2010;110(3):829-833. [IA]

159. Chung SH, Lee BS, Yang HJ, et al. Effect of preoperative warming during cesarean section under spinal anesthesia. *Korean J Anesthesiol.* 2012;62(5):454-460. [IB]

160. Horn EP, Bein B, Bohm R, Steinfath M, Sahili N, Hocker J. The effect of short time periods of pre-operative warming in the prevention of peri-operative hypothermia. *Anaesthesia.* 2012;67(6):612-617. [IB]

161. Cassey JG, King RA, Armstrong P. Is there thermal benefit from preoperative warming in children? *Paediatr Anaesth.* 2010;20(1):63-71. [IB]

162. Wong PF, Kumar S, Bohra A, Whetter D, Leaper DJ. Randomized clinical trial of perioperative systemic warming in major elective abdominal surgery. *Br J Surg.* 2007;94(4):421-426. [IB]

163. Wasfie TJ, Barber KR. Value of extended warming in patients undergoing elective surgery. *Int Surg.* 2015;100(1):105-108. [IB]

164. Vanni SMD, Castiglia YMM, Ganem EM, et al. Preoperative warming combined with intraoperative skin-surface warming does not avoid hypothermia caused by spinal anesthesia in patients with midazolam premedication. *Sao Paulo Med J.* 2007;125(3):144-149. [IB]

165. Perl T, Peichl LH, Reyntjens K, Deblaere I, Zaballos JM, Brauer A. Efficacy of a novel prewarming system in the prevention of perioperative hypothermia. A prospective, randomized, multicenter study. *Minerva Anestesiol.* 2014;80(4):436-443. [IA]

166. Minchin I. Management of temperature & major abdominal surgery. *Dissector.* 2009;37(3):13-15. [IIC]

167. Llewellyn L. Effect of pre-warming on reducing the incidence of inadvertent peri-operative hypothermia for patients undergoing general anaesthesia: a mini-review. *Br J Anaesth Recovery Nurs.* 2013;14(1-2):3-10. [IA]

168. de Brito Poveda V, Clark AM, Galvao CM. A systematic review on the effectiveness of prewarming to prevent perioperative hypothermia. *J Clin Nurs.* 2013;22(7-8):906-918. [IA]

169. Roberson MC, Dieckmann LS, Rodriguez RE, Austin PN. A review of the evidence for active preoperative warming of adults undergoing general anesthesia. *AANA J.* 2013;81(5):351-356. [IIB]

170. Gorges M, Ansermino JM, Whyte SD. A retrospective audit to examine the effectiveness of preoperative warming on hypothermia in spine deformity surgery patients. *Paediatr Anaesth.* 2013;23(11):1054-1061. [IIIB]

171. Kiekkas P. Prewarming critically ill patients. *AORN J.* 2012;96(4):409-411. [VB]

172. Roth JV. Some unanswered questions about temperature management. *Anesth Analg.* 2009;109(5):1695-1699. [VB]

173. Bitner J, Hilde L, Hall K, Duvendack T. A team approach to the prevention of unplanned postoperative hypothermia. *AORN J.* 2007;85(5):921-923. [VB]

174. Shukry M, Matthews L, de Armendi AJ, et al. Does the covering of children during induction of anesthesia have an effect on body temperature at the end of surgery? *J Clin Anesth.* 2012;24(2):116-120. [IA]

175. Nicholson M. A comparison of warming interventions on the temperatures of inpatients undergoing colorectal surgery. *AORN J.* 2013;97(3):310-322. [IC]

176. Adriani MB, Moriber N. Preoperative forced-air warming combined with intraoperative warming versus intraoperative warming alone in the prevention of hypothermia during gynecologic surgery. *AANA J.* 2013;81(6):446-451. [IIA]

177. Fettes S, Mulvaine M, Van Doren E. Effect of preoperative forced-air warming on postoperative temperature and postanesthesia care unit length of stay. *AORN J.* 2013;97(3):323-328. [VA]

178. Kim YS, Jeon YS, Lee JA, et al. Intra-operative warming with a forced-air warmer in preventing hypothermia after tourniquet deflation in elderly patients. *J Int Med Res.* 2009;37(5):1457-1464. [IA]

179. Pu Y, Cen G, Sun J, et al. Warming with an under-body warming system reduces intraoperative hypothermia in patients undergoing laparoscopic gastrointestinal surgery: a randomized controlled study. *Int J Nurs Stud.* 2014;51(2):181-189. [IA]

180. Yoo HS, Park SW, Yi JW, Kwon MI, Rhee YG. The effect of forced-air warming during arthroscopic shoulder surgery with general anesthesia. *Arthroscopy.* 2009;25(5):510-514. [IB]

181. Trentman TL, Weinmeister KP, Hentz JG, Laney MB, Simula DV. Randomized non-inferiority trial of the vitalHEAT temperature management system vs the Bair Hugger warmer during total knee arthroplasty. *Can J Anaesth.* 2009;56(12):914-920. [IB]

182. Fleisher LA, Metzger SE, Lam J, Harris A. Perioperative cost-finding analysis of the routine use of intraoperative forced-air warming during general anesthesia. *Anesthesiology.* 1998;88(5):1357-1364. [IB]

183. Pikus E, Hooper VD. Postoperative rewarming: are there alternatives to warm hospital blankets. *J Perianesth Nurs.* 2010;25(1):11-23. [IIIB]

184. Leung KK, Lai A, Wu A. A randomised controlled trial of the electric heating pad vs forced-air warming for preventing hypothermia during laparotomy. *Anaesthesia.* 2007;62(6):605-608. [IIA]

185. Moyses AM, Trettene Ados S, Navarro LH, Ayres JA. Hypothermia prevention during surgery: comparison between thermal mattress and thermal blanket. *Rev Esc Enferm USP.* 2014;48(2):228-235. [IIB]

186. Egan C, Bernstein E, Reddy D, et al. A randomized comparison of intraoperative PerfecTemp and forced-air warming during open abdominal surgery. *Anesth Analg.* 2011;113(5):1076-1081. [IIB]

187. Ruetzler K, Kovaci B, Guloglu E, et al. Forced-air and a novel patient-warming system (vitalHEAT vH2) comparably maintain normothermia during open abdominal surgery. *Anesth Analg.* 2011;112(3):608-614. [IIB]

188. Brandt S, Oguz R, Hüttner H, et al. Resistive-polymer versus forced-air warming: comparable efficacy in orthopedic patients. *Anesth Analg.* 2010;110(3):834-838. [IIB]

189. Fanelli A, Danelli G, Ghisi D, Ortu A, Moschini E, Fanelli G. The efficacy of a resistive heating under-patient blanket versus a forced-air warming system: a randomized controlled trial. *Anesth Analg.* 2009;108(1):199-201. [IIB]

190. Kadam VR, Moyes D, Moran JL. Relative efficiency of two warming devices during laparoscopic cholecystectomy. *Anaesth Intensive Care.* 2009;37(3):464-468. [IIB]

191. Ihn CH, Joo JD, Chung HS, et al. Comparison of three warming devices for the prevention of core hypothermia and post-anaesthesia shivering. *J Int Med Res.* 2008;36(5):923-931. [IIB]

192. Sato H, Yamakage M, Okuyama K, et al. Forced-air warming effectively prevents midazolam-induced core hypothermia in volunteers. *Eur J Anaesthesiol.* 2009;26(7):566-571. [IIB]

193. Witt L, Dennhardt N, Eich C, et al. Prevention of intraoperative hypothermia in neonates and infants: results of a prospective multicenter observational study with a new forced-air warming system with increased warm air flow. *Paediatr Anaesth.* 2013;23(6):469-474. [IIIB]

194. Panossian C, Simoes CM, Milani WR, Baranauskas MB, Margarido CB. The intraoperative use of warming blankets in patients undergoing radical prostatectomy is related with a reduction in post-anesthetic recovery time. *Rev Bras Anestesiol.* 2008;58(3):220-226. [IIIC]

195. Carpenter L, Baysinger CL. Maintaining perioperative normothermia in the patient undergoing cesarean delivery. *Obstet Gynecol Surv.* 2012;67(7):436-446. [VA]

196. Tanaka N, Ohno Y, Hori M, Utada M, Ito K, Suzuki T. A randomised controlled trial of the resistive heating blanket versus the convective warming system for preventing hypothermia during major abdominal surgery. *J Perioper Pract.* 2013;23(4):82-86. [IB]

197. Rathinam S, Annam V, Steyn R, Raghuraman G. A randomised controlled trial comparing Mediwrap heat retention and forced air warming for maintaining normothermia in thoracic surgery. *Interact Cardiovasc Thorac Surg.* 2009;9(1):15-19. [IA]

198. Ng V, Lai A, Ho V. Comparison of forced-air warming and electric heating pad for maintenance of body temperature during total knee replacement. *Anaesthesia.* 2006;61(11):1100-1104. [IIB]

199. Calcaterra D, Ricci M, Lombardi P, Katariya K, Panos A, Salerno TA. Reduction of postoperative hypothermia with a new warming device: a prospective randomized study in off-pump coronary artery surgery. *J Cardiovasc Surg.* 2009;50(6):813-817. [IA]

200. Galvao CM, Marck PB, Sawada NO, Clark AM. A systematic review of the effectiveness of cutaneous warming systems to prevent hypothermia. *J Clin Nurs.* 2009;18(5):627-636. [IA]

201. Hasegawa K, Nakagawa F, Negishi C, Ozaki M. Core temperatures during major abdominal surgery in patients warmed with new circulating-water garment, forced-air warming, or carbon-fiber resistive-heating system. *J Anesth.* 2012;26(2):168-173. [IIA]

202. Rein EB, Filtvedt M, Walloe L, Raeder JC. Hypothermia during laparotomy can be prevented by locally applied warm water and pulsating negative pressure. *Br J Anaesth.* 2007;98(3):331-336. [IC]

203. Butwick AJ, Lipman SS, Carvalho B. Intraoperative forced air-warming during cesarean delivery under spinal anesthesia does not prevent maternal hypothermia. *Anesth Analg.* 2007;105(5):1413-1419. [IC]

204. Legg AJ, Hamer AJ. Forced-air patient warming blankets disrupt unidirectional airflow. *Bone Joint J.* 2013;95-B(3):407-410. [IIB]

205. Belani KG, Albrecht M, McGovern PD, Reed M, Nachtsheim C. Patient warming excess heat: the effects on orthopedic operating room ventilation performance. *Anesth Analg.* 2013;117(2):406-411. [IIB]

206. Legg AJ, Cannon T, Hamer AJ. Do forced air patient-warming devices disrupt unidirectional downward airflow? *J Bone Joint Surg Br*. 2012;94(2):254-256. [IIC]

207. Reed M, Kimberger O, McGovern PD, Albrecht MC. Forced-air warming design: evaluation of intake filtration, internal microbial buildup, and airborne-contamination emissions. *AANA J*. 2013;81(4):275-280. [IIIB]

208. Dasari KB, Albrecht M, Harper M. Effect of forced-air warming on the performance of operating theatre laminar flow ventilation. *Anaesthesia*. 2012;67(3):244-249. [IIB]

209. Albrecht M, Gauthier RL, Belani K, Litchy M, Leaper D. Forced-air warming blowers: an evaluation of filtration adequacy and airborne contamination emissions in the operating room. *Am J Infect Control*. 2011;39(4):321-328. [IIIB]

210. Albrecht M, Gauthier R, Leaper D. Forced-air warming: a source of airborne contamination in the operating room? *Orthop Rev (Pavia)*. 2009;1(2):e28. [IIIB]

211. McGovern PD, Albrecht M, Belani KG, et al. Forced-air warming and ultra-clean ventilation do not mix: an investigation of theatre ventilation, patient warming and joint replacement infection in orthopaedics. *J Bone Joint Surg Br*. 2011;93(11):1537-1544. [IIIC]

212. Wu X. The safe and efficient use of forced-air warming systems. *AORN J*. 2013;97(3):302-308. [VB]

213. Wood AM, Moss C, Keenan A, Reed MR, Leaper DJ. Infection control hazards associated with the use of forced-air warming in operating theatres. *J Hosp Infect*. 2014;88(3):132-140. [VB]

214. Tumia N, Ashcroft GP. Convection warmers—a possible source of contamination in laminar airflow operating theatres? *J Hosp Infect*. 2002;52(3):171-174. [IIC]

215. Zink RS, Iaizzo PA. Convective warming therapy does not increase the risk of wound contamination in the operating room. *Anesth Analg*. 1993;76(1):50-53. [IIC]

216. Kellam MD, Dieckmann LS, Austin PN. Forced-air warming devices and the risk of surgical site infections. *AORN J*. 2013;98(4):354-366. [IIIB]

217. Huang JK, Shah EF, Vinodkumar N, Hegarty MA, Greatorex RA. The Bair Hugger patient warming system in prolonged vascular surgery: an infection risk? *Crit Care*. 2003;7(3):R13-R16. [IIIB]

218. Forced-air warming and surgical site infections. Our review finds insufficient evidence to support changes in current practice. *Health Devices*. 2013;42(4):122-125. [VB]

219. Moretti B, Larocca AM, Napoli C, et al. Active warming systems to maintain perioperative normothermia in hip replacement surgery: a therapeutic aid or a vector of infection? *J Hosp Infect*. 2009;73(1):58-63. [IIB]

220. Sessler DI, Olmsted RN, Kuelpmann R. Forced-air warming does not worsen air quality in laminar flow operating rooms. *Anesth Analg*. 2011;113(6):1416-1421. [IIB]

221. Chung K, Lee S, Oh SC, Choi J, Cho HS. Thermal burn injury associated with a forced-air warming device. *Korean J Anesthesiol*. 2012;62(4):391-392. [VC]

222. Sikka RS, Prielipp RC. Forced air warming devices in orthopaedics: a focused review of the literature. *J Bone Joint Surg Am*. 2014;96(24):e200. [VB]

223. Brauer A, Quintel M. Forced-air warming: technology, physical background and practical aspects. *Curr Opin Anaesthesiol*. 2009;22(6):769-774. [VA]

224. Chapp K, Lange L. Warming blanket head drapes and trapped anesthetic gases: understanding the fire risk. *AORN J*. 2011;93(6):749-760. [VB]

225. Guideline for a safe environment of care, part 1. In: *Guidelines for Perioperative Practice*. Denver, CO: AORN, Inc; 2015:239-264. [IVA]

226. Wagner K, Smith CE, Quan KJ. Prevention of hypothermia during interventional cardiology procedures in adults. *Internet J Anesthesiol*. 2010;23(2):14p. [IB]

227. Perez-Protto S, Sessler DI, Reynolds LF, et al. Circulating-water garment or the combination of a circulating-water mattress and forced-air cover to maintain core temperature during major upper-abdominal surgery. *Br J Anaesth*. 2010;105(4):466-470. [IC]

228. Wadhwa A, Komatsu R, Orhan-Sungur M, et al. New circulating-water devices warm more quickly than forced-air in volunteers. *Anesth Analg*. 2007;105(6):1681-1687. [IIC]

229. Davis JS, Rodriguez LI, Quintana OD, et al. Use of a warming catheter to achieve normothermia in large burns. *J Burn Care Res*. 2013;34(1):191-195. [IIB]

230. Corallo JP, King B, Pizano LR, Namias N, Schulman CI. Core warming of a burn patient during excision to prevent hypothermia. *Burns*. 2008;34(3):418-420. [VB]

231. Paris LG, Seitz M, McElroy KG, Regan M. A randomized controlled trial to improve outcomes utilizing various warming techniques during cesarean birth. *J Obstet Gynecol Neonatal Nurs*. 2014;43(6):719-728. [IA]

232. Chakladar A, Dixon MJ, Crook D, Harper CM. The effects of a resistive warming mattress during caesarean section: a randomised, controlled trial. *Int J Obstet Anesth*. 2014;23(4):309-316. [IA]

233. Perl T, Rhenius A, Eich CB, Quintel M, Heise D, Bräuer A. Conductive warming and insulation reduces perioperative hypothermia. *Cent Eur J Med*. 2012;7(3):284-289. [IA]

234. Sharma M, Dixon M, Eljelani F, Crook D, Harper M. A randomised controlled trial to determine the influence of carbon-polymer warming blankets on the incidence of perioperative hypothermia during and after short, day-case operations. *J One Day Surg*. 2014;24(4):92-99. [IB]

235. Munday J, Hines S, Wallace K, Chang AM, Gibbons K, Yates P. A systematic review of the effectiveness of warming interventions for women undergoing cesarean section. *Worldviews Evid Based Nurs*. 2014;11(6):383-393. [IA]

236. Hirvonen EA, Niskanen M. Thermal suits as an alternative way to keep patients warm peri-operatively: a randomised trial. *Eur J Anaesthesiol*. 2011;28(5):376-381. [IB]

237. Koeter M, Leijtens B, Koeter S. Effect of thermal reflective blanket placement on hypothermia in primary unilateral total hip or knee arthroplasty. *J Perianesth Nurs*. 2013;28(6):347-352. [IA]

238. Han SB, Gwak MS, Choi SJ, et al. Effect of active airway warming on body core temperature during adult liver transplantation. *Transplant Proc*. 2013;45(1):251-254. [IB]

239. Jo YY, Kim HS, Chang YJ, Yun SY, Kwak HJ. The effect of warmed inspired gases on body temperature during arthroscopic shoulder surgery under general anesthesia. *Korean J Anesthesiol*. 2013;65(1):14-18. [IA]

240. Lee HK, Jang YH, Choi KW, Lee JH. The effect of electrically heated humidifier on the body temperature and blood loss in spinal surgery under general anesthesia. *Korean J Anesthesiol*. 2011;61(2):112-116. [IA]

241. Lee Y, Kim H. The effects of heated humidified gases on body temperature and shivering in patients under general anesthesia. *Int J Biosci Biotechnol*. 2013;5(4):61-72. [IIB]

242. Kim G, Kim MH, Lee SM, Choi SJ, Shin YH, Jeong HJ. Effect of pre-warmed intravenous fluids on perioperative hypothermia and shivering after ambulatory surgery under monitored anesthesia care. *J Anesth*. 2014;28(6):880-885. [IA]

243. Xu HX, You ZJ, Zhang H, Li Z. Prevention of hypothermia by infusion of warm fluid during abdominal surgery. *J Perianesth Nurs.* 2010;25(6):366-370. [IB]

244. Yokoyama K, Suzuki M, Shimada Y, Matsushima T, Bito H, Sakamoto A. Effect of administration of pre-warmed intravenous fluids on the frequency of hypothermia following spinal anesthesia for cesarean delivery. *J Clin Anesth.* 2009;21(4):242-248. [IB]

245. Woolnough M, Allam J, Hemingway C, Cox M, Yentis SM. Intra-operative fluid warming in elective caesarean section: a blinded randomised controlled trial. *Int J Obstet Anesth.* 2009;18(4):346-351. [IB]

246. Hasankhani H, Mohammadi E, Moazzami F, Mokhtari M, Naghgizadh MM. The effects of intravenous fluids temperature on perioperative hemodynamic situation, post-operative shivering, and recovery in orthopaedic surgery. *Can Oper Room Nurs J.* 2007;25(1):20-24. [IB]

247. De Mattia AL, Barbosa MH, de Freitas Filho JP, Rocha Ade M, Pereira NH. Warmed intravenous infusion for controlling intraoperative hypothermia. *Rev Lat Am.* 2013;21(3):803-810. [IA]

248. Andrzejowski JC, Turnbull D, Nandakumar A, Gowthaman S, Eapen G. A randomised single blinded study of the administration of pre-warmed fluid vs active fluid warming on the incidence of peri-operative hypothermia in short surgical procedures. *Anaesthesia.* 2010;65(9):942-945. [IA]

249. Tekgul ZT, Pektas S, Yildirim U, et al. A prospective randomized double-blind study on the effects of the temperature of irrigation solutions on thermoregulation and postoperative complications in percutaneous nephrolithotomy. *J Anesth.* 2014;29(2):165-169. [IA]

250. Kim YS, Lee JY, Yang SC, Song JH, Koh HS, Park WK. Comparative study of the influence of room-temperature and warmed fluid irrigation on body temperature in arthroscopic shoulder surgery. *Arthroscopy.* 2009;25(1):24-29. [IB]

251. Jin Y, Tian J, Sun M, Yang K. A systematic review of randomised controlled trials of the effects of warmed irrigation fluid on core body temperature during endoscopic surgeries. *J Clin Nurs.* 2011;20(3-4):305-316. [IB]

252. Parodi D, Valderrama J, Tobar C, et al. Effect of warmed irrigation solution on core body temperature during hip arthroscopy for femoroacetabular impingement. *Arthroscopy.* 2014;30(1):36-41. [IIA]

253. Oh JH, Kim JY, Chung SW, et al. Warmed irrigation fluid does not decrease perioperative hypothermia during arthroscopic shoulder surgery. *Arthroscopy.* 2014;30(2):159-164. [IIA]

254. Deren ME, Machan JT, DiGiovanni CW, Ehrlich MG, Gillerman RG. Prewarming operating rooms for prevention of intraoperative hypothermia during total knee and hip arthroplasties. *J Arthroplasty.* 2011;26(8):1380-1386. [IA]

255. Ozer AB, Tosun F, Demirel I, Unlu S, Bayar MK, Erhan OL. The effects of anesthetic technique and ambient temperature on thermoregulation in lower extremity surgery. *J Anesth.* 2013;27(4):528-534. [IIB]

256. Cheng KW, Wang CH, Chen CL, et al. Decreased fresh gas flow cannot compensate for an increased operating room temperature in maintaining body temperature during donor hepatectomy for living liver donor hepatectomy. *Transplant Proc.* 2010;42(3):703-704. [IIIB]

257. Yang HL, Lee HF, Chu TL, Su YY, Ho LH, Fan JY. The comparison of two recovery room warming methods for hypothermia patients who had undergone spinal surgery. *J Nurs Scholarsh.* 2012;44(1):2-10. [IIB]

258. Al-Qahtani AS, Messahel FM. Benchmarking inadvertent perioperative hypothermia guidelines with the National Institute for Health and Clinical Excellence. *Saudi Med J.* 2011;32(1):27-31. [VB]

259. Hegarty J, Walsh E, Burton A, Murphy S, O'gorman F, McPolin G. Nurses' knowledge of inadvertent hypothermia. *AORN J.* 2009;89(4):701-704. [IIIB]

260. Gurunluoglu R, Swanson JA, Haeck PC; ASPS Patient Safety Committee. Evidence-based patient safety advisory: malignant hyperthermia. *Plast Reconstr Surg.* 2009;124(4 Suppl):68S-81S. [IVA]

261. Litman RS, Joshi GP. Malignant hyperthermia in the ambulatory surgery center: how should we prepare? *Anesthesiology.* 2014;120(6):1306-1308. [VB]

Acknowledgements

LEAD AUTHOR
Byron L. Burlingame, MS, BSN, RN, CNOR
Senior Perioperative Nursing Specialist
AORN Nursing Department
Denver, Colorado

CONTRIBUTING AUTHOR
Ramona L. Conner, MSN, RN, CNOR
Editor-in-Chief, Guidelines for Perioperative Practice
AORN Nursing Department
Denver, Colorado

The authors and AORN thank Armin Schubert, MD, MBA, Anesthesiologist, Ochsner Medical Center, New Orleans, Louisiana; Donna Ford, MSN, RN-BC, CNOR, CRCST, Staff Registered Nurse, Mayo Clinic, Rochester, Minnesota; Christine Anderson, PhD, RN, Clinical Assistant Professor, University of Michigan School of Nursing, Ypsilanti; George Allen, PhD, MS, RN, CNOR, CIC, Director Infection Control, Downstate Medical Center, and Clinical Assistant Professor, SUNY College of Health Related Professions, Brooklyn, New York; Janice Neil, PhD, RN, CNE, Associate Professor, College of Nursing, East Carolina University, Greenville, North Carolina; Lisa Spruce, DNP, RN, CNS-CP, CNOR, ACNS, ACNP, Director of Evidence-based Perioperative Practice, AORN Nursing Department, Denver, Colorado; Mary Lamonte, MPH, MSN, RN, CNOR, Staff Nurse, Stamford Surgical Center, Stamford, Connecticut; and Leslie Ann Jeter, RN, CRNA, MSNA, Staff CRNA, American Association of Nurse Anesthetists, Atlanta, Georgia, for their assistance in developing this guideline.

PUBLICATION HISTORY
Originally published as Recommended Practices for the Prevention of Unplanned Perioperative Hypothermia in *Perioperative Standards and Recommended Practices*, 2008 edition.

Minor editing revisions made to omit PNDS codes; reformatted September 2012 for publication in *Perioperative Standards and Recommended Practices*, 2013 edition.

Minor editing revision made in November 2014 for publication as Guideline for Prevention of Unplanned Perioperative Hypothermia in *Guidelines for Perioperative Practice*, 2015 edition.

Revised November 2015 for publication in *Guidelines for Perioperative Practice* online.

GUIDELINE FOR PATIENT INFORMATION MANAGEMENT

The Guideline for Patient Information Management has been approved by the AORN Guidelines Advisory Board. It was presented as a proposed guideline for comments by members and others. The guideline is effective July 1, 2016. The recommendations in the guideline are intended to be achievable and represent what is believed to be an optimal level of practice. Policies and procedures will reflect variations in practice settings and/or clinical situations that determine the degree to which the guideline can be implemented. AORN recognizes the many diverse settings in which perioperative nurses practice; therefore, this guideline is adaptable to all areas where operative or other invasive procedures may be performed.

Purpose

This document provides guidance to assist perioperative nurses in documenting and managing patient care information within the perioperative practice setting. Highly reliable data collection is not only necessary to chronicle the patient's response to nursing interventions, but also to demonstrate the health care organization's progress toward improving health care outcomes. Health care data collection and retention is rapidly transitioning from traditional paper formats to standardized electronic applications that incorporate criteria from statutes and regulations, accreditation requirements, and standards-setting bodies. Whether patient data are captured using paper or electronic formats, the nursing process should be completed for each surgical or procedural intervention performed.[1,2]

The nursing process is a formalized systematic approach to providing and documenting patient care that is embedded within perioperative patient care workflow (ie, clinical workflow). Comprehensive perioperative documentation accurately reflects the patient experience and is essential for the continuity of goal-directed nursing care and for effective comparison of realized versus anticipated patient outcomes.[3,4]

This document should be viewed as a conceptual outline that can be used to create a comprehensive documentation platform. It is not inclusive of all documentation elements, nor should it be seen as the only guideline that may be used when developing or revising a clinical documentation system.

The following topics are outside the scope of this document: electronic health record (EHR) adoption, accreditation requirements for health information technology criteria, EHR certification, EHR human factors science, establishing health information exchanges and interoperability requirements, submission of mandatory quality reporting criteria, hand-off communication requirements, perioperative team communications, requirements to complete data analytics, and patient access to personal health information.

Evidence Review

A medical librarian conducted a systematic search of the databases MEDLINE®, CINAHL®, and the Cochrane Database of Systematic Reviews. The librarian also conducted a non-systematic search of the Scopus® database. Results were limited to literature published in English from January 2011 to June 2015. During the development of the guideline, the lead author requested additional articles that either did not fit the original search criteria or were discovered during the evidence appraisal process, and the lead author and the medical librarian identified relevant guidelines from government agencies and standards-setting bodies. At the time of the initial search, the librarian established weekly alerts on the search topics and until October 2015, presented relevant alert results to the lead author.

Search terms included the subject headings and keywords *medical informatics, nursing informatics, documentation, information management, medical records, electronic health records, computerized patient records, information storage and retrieval, forms and records control, computer-assisted decision making, operating room information systems, hospital information systems, health information exchange, clinical decision support systems, interoperability, systems integration, data mining,* and *informed consent.* The concepts of standardized terminologies were included with a broad subject-heading controlled vocabulary as well as individual headings and keywords for relevant standardized terminologies. Subject headings and keywords related to government regulations included *government regulation, meaningful use, Health Insurance Portability and Accountability Act, HIPAA, Health Information Technology for Economic and Clinical Health, American Recovery and Reinvestment Act, Affordable Care Act,* and *Medicare and Medicaid Electronic Health Care Record.* The keywords *big data, electronic signature, charting by exception, variance charting, electronic medical record, EHR, Health Level Seven International, HL7,* and *EMR* also were included in the search, as were terms related to the concepts of data collection, retention, storage, and governance.

Articles identified by the search were provided to the lead author and an evidence appraiser. Excluded were non-peer-reviewed publications and evidence from other disciplines when evidence from the perioperative setting was available (Figure 1). The lead author and the evidence appraiser reviewed and critically appraised each article using the AORN Research or Non-Research Evidence Appraisal Tools

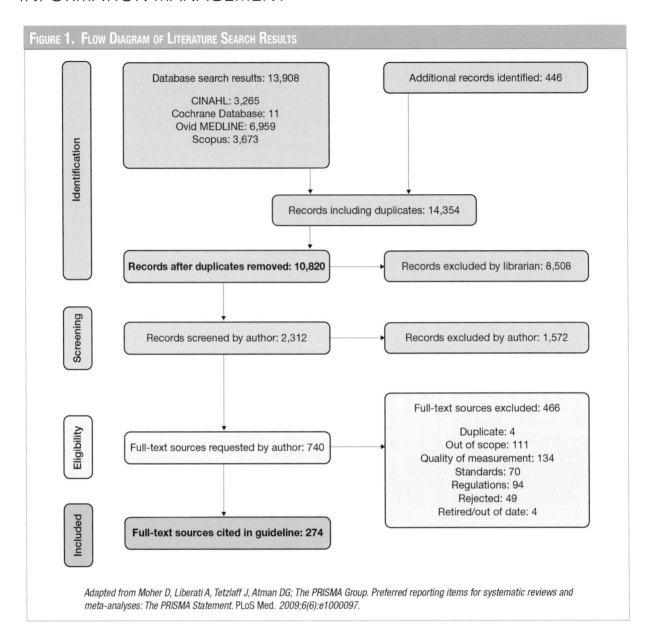

FIGURE 1. FLOW DIAGRAM OF LITERATURE SEARCH RESULTS

Database search results: 13,908

CINAHL: 3,265
Cochrane Database: 11
Ovid MEDLINE: 6,959
Scopus: 3,673

Additional records identified: 446

Records including duplicates: 14,354

Records after duplicates removed: 10,820

Records excluded by librarian: 8,508

Records screened by author: 2,312

Records excluded by author: 1,572

Full-text sources requested by author: 740

Full-text sources excluded: 466

Duplicate: 4
Out of scope: 111
Quality of measurement: 134
Standards: 70
Regulations: 94
Rejected: 49
Retired/out of date: 4

Full-text sources cited in guideline: 274

Identification · Screening · Eligibility · Included

Adapted from Moher D, Liberati A, Tetzlaff J, Atman DG; The PRISMA Group. Preferred reporting items for systematic reviews and meta-analyses: The PRISMA Statement. PLoS Med. 2009;6(6):e1000097.

as appropriate. The literature was independently evaluated and appraised according to the strength and quality of the evidence. Each article was then assigned an appraisal score. The appraisal score is noted in brackets after each reference, as applicable.

The collective evidence supporting each intervention within a specific recommendation was summarized and the AORN Evidence Rating Model was used to rate the strength of the evidence. Factors considered in the review of the collective evidence were the quality of the evidence, the quantity of similar evidence on a given topic, and the consistency of the evidence supporting a recommendation. The evidence rating is noted in brackets after each intervention.

Note: The evidence summary table is available at http://www.aorn.org/evidencetables/.

Editor's note: *MEDLINE is a registered trademark of the US National Library of Medicine, Bethesda, MD.*

CINAHL, Cumulative Index to Nursing and Allied Health Literature, is a registered trademark of EBSCO Industries, Birmingham, AL. Scopus is a registered trademark of Elsevier B.V., Amsterdam, The Netherlands.

Recommendation I

As part of the legal health record, the perioperative patient health care record should reflect the plan of care, including assessment, nursing diagnosis, outcome identification, planning, implementation of interventions, and evaluation of progress toward the expected outcome.[3-6]

The nursing process provides the guiding framework for documenting perioperative nursing care. When the nursing process is used in perioperative practice settings, it demonstrates the critical-thinking skills practiced by the registered nurse (RN) in caring for the patient undergoing operative or other invasive procedures.[3-5,7,8] Documentation includes information about the patient's current and past health status, nursing diagnoses and interventions, expected outcomes, and evaluation of the patient's response to perioperative nursing care.[7,9-11]

I.a. The perioperative RN should record the assessment findings (eg, physical, psychosocial, cultural, spiritual) in the patient health care record before the operative or other invasive procedure. *[1: Strong Evidence]*

The patient assessment forms a baseline for identifying the patient's health status, developing nursing diagnoses, and establishing an individualized plan of care. Recurring assessments throughout the patient's perioperative experience contribute to continuity in the delivery of care.[5,11-13]

Intraoperative nursing interventions are embedded within the delivery of care but are not consistently reflected in clinical documentation.[8,14,15] In a systematic review of nursing documentation literature, Wang et al[16] found that inadequacies in the use of nursing process structure within clinical documentation resulted in one or more deficiencies in the application of the assessment process. In a subsequent qualitative content analysis of nursing communication and documentation patterns, Keenan et al[17] identified that inconsistent nursing documentation practices contributed to discrepancies in the transfer of information, causing vulnerabilities for serious and undetectable clinical errors.

I.b. The health care record should include the nursing interventions performed, the time at which they were performed, the location of care, and the name and role of the person performing the care.[4,6,12] *[1: Strong Evidence]*

Clinical judgments are based on actual or potential patient problems (eg, nursing diagnoses) that determine the nursing interventions to be implemented to achieve expected perioperative patient outcomes.[4,5,11] Documenting nursing interventions promotes continuity of patient care and improves the exchange of patient care information between health care team members. Researchers who conducted a qualitative study of eight medical-surgical settings across four hospitals identified discrepancies in interdisciplinary information exchange and what nurses documented about patient care. They recommended capturing core patient information to increase consistency in care planning and accessibility of information for the patient care team.[17]

I.c. The perioperative RN should record expected and interim patient outcomes in the patient health care record.[3,5,11] *[1: Strong Evidence]*

The goals for nursing interventions are to prevent potential patient injury or complications and treat actual patient problems (eg, nursing diagnoses). Identified nursing diagnoses

contribute to interim and expected patient outcomes for the planned surgical or procedural intervention.[9] Expert consensus indicates that nurses who associate the patient diagnoses with planned interventions are more outcome focused than task oriented.[18]

I.d. The patient health care record should reflect continuous reassessment and evaluation of perioperative nursing care and the patient's response to implemented nursing interventions.[3,5,12,13,19] *[1: Strong Evidence]*

The nursing process directs perioperative nurses to evaluate the effectiveness of nursing interventions toward attaining desired patient outcomes. Reassessment throughout the patient's perioperative experience contributes to continuity in the delivery of care.[3,5,11]

The evaluation process provides information for continuity of care, performance improvement activities, perioperative nursing research, and management of risk. Professional nursing associations have determined that documentation provides a mechanism for comparing actual versus expected outcomes.[3,5,9]

I.d.1. Patient data must be collected concurrently with each assessment, reassessment, or evaluation and recorded in the patient health care record.[20,21] *[1: Regulatory Requirement]*

Continuous evaluation of the patient's condition establishes a baseline to determine fluctuations in the patient's status.[5,3,12] Appropriately captured patient data contribute to a centralized repository that members of the health care team can use to monitor the patient's status, coordinate prescribed treatments, and evaluate the effectiveness of care rendered.[19,22-25]

Recommendation II

Perioperative nursing documentation should be synchronized with the nursing workflow.[26-29]

Nursing workflow represents the cognitive process of nursing care activities and establishes the approach for patient care data collection. Documentation of nursing activities is dictated by health care organization policy and by regulatory and accrediting agency requirements and is necessary to inform other health care professionals involved in the patient's care. To accurately represent the patient's experience and promote quality delivery of care, data aggregation should be coordinated with clinical workflow.[4,14,26,30] Hayrinen et al[31] conducted a retrospective, descriptive study in which they examined 489 nursing care plans. They found that the incorporation of nursing process workflow into the framework of clinical documentation platforms improved documentation completeness and compliance with regulatory requirements.

II.a. Clinical documentation should facilitate data capture using a format designed to support clinical workflow activities while eliminating redundancy in data entry.[2,27,29,32,33] *[2: High Evidence]*

The collective evidence indicates that work inefficiencies, such as the format or the location where clinical data are captured within documentation systems, have a negative correlation on clinical reasoning and decision making.[30,34-38]

The burden of clinical documentation has been associated with decreased nursing attention to patient care activities, which has been shown to adversely affect patient safety. In a time-motion study spanning 274 health systems in 15 states, Hendrich et al[39] found that when nursing time was divided between patient care responsibilities and transferring patient information between different information systems, the frequency of transcription errors, fragmentation of care, and duplication of effort increased and resulted in an inefficient measurement of nursing care quality.

Several studies have shown that interruption during established clinical processes results in competition for cognitive resources and may contribute to an adverse event or patient harm by reducing situational awareness.[40-42] Redundancy in the design of documentation activities further reduces the nurse's ability to focus on the clinical environment and may create a risk for error.[33,43] The authors of a Cochrane Review on the effects of using nursing record systems on nursing practice and health care outcomes identified that when processes are simplified and data capture is standardized and organized, there is a reduction in the reliance on memory to complete tasks, thereby potentially eliminating harmful events.[15]

In a single-site observational study on nursing workflow, Cornell et al[43] examined the percentage of time nurses dedicated to patient care and documentation activities. They found that nursing time was focused primarily on patient care (eg, assessment, interventions) with documentation being completed in intervals and not concurrently with patient care. This, along with frequent switching between patient care and documentation, was correlated with nursing cognitive disruption, which resulted in slower performance and increased the potential for error.

In a subsequent follow-up observational and randomized investigation, Cornell et al[44] examined the effect of new electronic documentation implementation on nursing activities and workflow. Findings indicated that the repeated clustering of patient care and documentation activities, evenly distributed, affected nursing workflow by increasing the amount of time dedicated to electronic documentation without negatively affecting direct patient care time.

II.a.1. Clinical documentation should reflect patient-focused care.[45-48] *[3: Moderate Evidence]*

Clinical (eg, nursing) documentation systems often do not support health care personnel in accommodating the specific needs of the individual (eg, teaching needs, age-specific criteria, self-care requirements).[45,49,50] Health care currently relies on the technology-centered medical model of care, and patient-centric, evidence-based care is often not represented within documentation platforms. Researchers have identified discrepancies between care delivered and what is captured in patient care documentation; thus, efforts to improve and ensure the accuracy of patient care data capture are necessary.[51,52]

II.a.2. All necessary patient care data important to ongoing and transitional care should be incorporated into the patient's health care record. *[2: High Evidence]*

Despite the efficiencies in the quality and quantity of patient care information captured by electronic documentation systems, the reliance on asynchronous information transfer to communicate continuing patient care needs means critical elements necessary to ensure a comprehensive treatment plan are often lacking. A recent systematic literature review that explored the role that electronic patient records have on shift hand over (ie, hand off) identified that omissions of detailed care information and communication errors occurred frequently during the hand-over period.[53] The authors concluded that the completion of documentation fields resulted in less missing data and the quality of information was more accurate and current, resulting in improved clinician synchronous communications and care continuity.

The quality of information available to clinicians affects the quality of care provided. Nurse scientists conducted an exploratory study on the characteristics of clinical health care decision making as influenced by data collection and information processing.[54] Findings from this small qualitative study of patient records at one hospital suggest that the type of data captured in the clinical documentation produced the necessary information for therapeutic interventions.

A comparative study of nursing verbal communications and related documentation for care transitions revealed that synchronous oral exchanges during hand overs incorporated more contextual information related to the current and future needs of the patient, while associated documentation reflected only the clinical observations of care interventions.[55]

II.a.3. Perioperative RNs should evaluate perioperative electronic documentation systems for their effect on clinical workflow and patient safety and their ability to accommodate the organization's objectives for the implementation site. Perioperative RNs should provide input and recommendations for improvement to the information technology team.[15,16,26,27,56]

Clinical information systems should address

- clinical workflow,[26,27,57-61]
- information needs of the patient care environment,[46,58,60]
- patient population characteristics,[45,47,49,60] and
- clinician and provider usability requirements.[40,42,58,59,62]

[1: Strong Evidence]

The collective evidence indicates that effective information systems collect, store, and organize patient information to allow real-time updates and support clinical decision making and are accessible to health care professionals when needed.[61,63,64] Research on the effect of health information technology implementation has shown that changes in contextual clinical work processes made to accommodate clinical information systems have both positive and negative influences on clinical workflow and patient safety.[37,42,50,58,65] Technology can more positively affect clinical workflow, data availability, patient outcomes, and health care provider satisfaction when clinicians are involved in the selection and implementation of the information system.[15,51,66]

Recommendation III

Electronic perioperative nursing documentation should use the Perioperative Nursing Data Set (PNDS) and other structured vocabularies inclusive of the nursing process workflow with discrete representation of each phase of the perioperative patient care continuum (ie, preadmission, preoperative, intraoperative, postoperative).[31,67,68]

The use of a structured vocabulary facilitates the capture of expressed observations, treatments, and patient responses within the clinical domain of care. A structured vocabulary describes patient care using controlled (ie, standardized) and unambiguous terms that are interpreted with consistent meaning by health care clinicians.[31,69,70] Patient information gathered from the collection of standardized data creates the knowledge perioperative RNs use to provide individualized patient care. The synthesis of knowledge for patient care interventions is in turn documented, resulting in the wisdom of perioperative nursing practice.[70,71]

Using structured nursing data elements (eg, the PNDS) that include nursing diagnoses, interventions, and outcomes in clinical documentation demonstrates perioperative nursing contributions to patient outcomes and represents professional nursing practice.[4,8,72,73]

III.a. The PNDS should be incorporated into the documentation platform.[8,9,72] *[1: Strong Evidence]*

The PNDS is a controlled, structured, and coded nursing language that describes perioperative nursing influence on the effectiveness and safety of patient care delivery and the contributions of perioperative nursing to patient outcomes. Although a gap exists in the current literature regarding clinical application of the PNDS, the existing evidence demonstrates that clinical documentation systems that incorporate standardized language provide patient care data that can be aggregated and analyzed to determine clinical efficiencies, examine operational metrics, and create new evidence for sustainable improvements in health care quality.[9,11,26,68]

III.a.1. Each phase of perioperative nursing documentation should incorporate nursing process workflow and require unambiguous representation of the patient experience.[74-76] *[2: High Evidence]*

The phases of perioperative patient care collectively represent the unique domain of perioperative nursing. Standardization of patient care information improves the quality of the data[77] and can be used to support the extraction and interpretation of data for

- clinical decision support,[78-80]
- improved quality metrics,[31,80,81]
- information exchange,[80,81]
- research,[81,82]
- policy making,[31,81] and
- nursing visibility.[4,8,9,31,67,69,74,83,84]

III.b. The health care organization should implement a documentation system that includes a standardized perioperative electronic framework. *[1: Strong Evidence]*

Standardization in documentation platforms promotes uniformity in comprehensive patient care data capture among health care organizations and creates a foundation for sharing health care data.[85,86] The burgeoning cost of health care and the drive for improved quality have created urgency for implementation of electronic medical records (EMRs) and interoperable electronic health record (EHR) systems.[87-89] Adoption of EHR systems is a component of the American Recovery and Reinvestment Act (ARRA) of 2009[22] to facilitate access to quality care and improve patient safety[79,86] through high-reliability processes using data analysis to evaluate performance and outcomes.[90] Data quality facilitated by the adoption of an EHR and established by compliance with laws, clinical practice standards, and national quality measures adds to the relevance of efficiency benchmarks. Experts agree that the adoption of EHR technology also will lead to quantifiable improvements in reducing the time required for patient care data capture by nurses.[77,81,88,91]

Inpatient and ambulatory EHR implementation has been stimulated by the ARRA incentives for EHR adoption and subsequent analysis and dissemination of performance metrics.[86] Achieving success with the national Health Information Technology for Economic and Clinical Health (HITECH)[86] agenda for comparative analysis among health care organizations can be accomplished by implementing an electronic documentation framework (eg, AORN Syntegrity®) embedded with standardized sets of documentation values applicable across multiple perioperative settings to increase the confidence in data quality and research validity.[77,81,92]

III.b.1. The health care documentation system must incorporate the standardized clinical terminologies identified by the US government to promote interoperability of health care data.[80,93,94] *[1: Regulatory Requirement]*

To accomplish the national health care strategy of promoting the availability of patient care data between and across health care organizations and providers, the Health Information Technology Standards Committee established by the Office of the National Coordinator for Health Information Technology (ONC) has identified clinical terminologies to standardize EHR data for interoperability (Table 1).[80,95] Experts assert that the standardization of EHR data allows the electronic sharing of vital patient care information and thereby supports the continuity of uninterrupted ongoing care.[85]

The PNDS is incorporated into the ONC clinical vocabulary standards through the Systematized Nomenclature of Medicine–Clinical Terms (SNOMED-CT®).[9] The incorporation of the PNDS into the US government vocabulary standards enables measurement of the perioperative nursing contribution to the quality and outcomes of population health.

III.b.2. Structured data collected using a standardized perioperative electronic framework should allow for data aggregation and be extractable for use in research and analytics. *[2: High Evidence]*

The ability to mine standardized clinical data fuels the development of new knowledge to transform practice and improve patient outcomes.[96] Structured data made available for direct import into statistical applications expands the capacity to generate and analyze observational evidence that can be generalizable to all perioperative settings.[96,97] Standardized data are more easily integrated into larger data sets, facilitating the reuse of de-identified clinical data for predictive analytics that improve the detection of disease processes and facilitate earlier interventions and improvements in the quality and efficiency of health care delivery.[98,99]

Recommendation IV

Perioperative nursing documentation should be structured to meet professional and regulatory compliance requirements for a comprehensive representation of patient care.[20,21,100-102]

Patient care information collected and entered into the health care record is a tool for monitoring and evaluating the patient's health status and response to care, a resource for evaluating compliance with regulatory requirements, and a method for aligning provision of services with reimbursement.[4,103,104]

IV.a. Perioperative nursing documentation must correspond to the elements of regulatory statutes, health care accreditation measures, national practice standards, and mandatory quality and reimbursement for quality performance criteria.[20,105] *[1: Regulatory Requirement]*

Clinical documentation serves as the legal record of care delivery (ie, legal health record) and assists with cross-disciplinary patient care coordination.[21,103,106]

IV.a.1. The components for clinical documentation should include
- assessments;
- clinical problems;
- communications with other health care professionals regarding the patient;
- communication with and education of the patient, the patient's family members, the patient's designated support person, and other third parties;
- medication records;
- order acknowledgement, implementation, and management;
- patient care interventions;
- patient clinical parameters;
- patient responses and outcomes, including changes in the patient's status; and
- plans of care that reflect the social and cultural framework of the patient.[4]

[1: Strong Evidence]

IV.a.2. Perioperative nursing documentation frameworks should correspond to professional guidelines and standards. *[1: Strong Evidence]*

Organizations that provide guidelines and standards relevant to perioperative practice settings include the
- Association of periOperative Registered Nurses,
- American Association of Blood Banks,

TABLE 1. OFFICE OF THE NATIONAL COORDINATOR FOR HEALTH INFORMATION TECHNOLOGY CLINICAL VOCABULARY STANDARDS FOR INTEROPERABILITY

Vocabulary	Data Type
CVX Codes for Vaccines Administered	Vaccines (administered)
CPT Current Procedural Terminology	Medical, surgical, and diagnostic services rendered for claims
CDC PHIN/VADS Centers for Disease Control and Prevention Public Health Information Network/Vocabulary Access and Distribution System	Patient characteristic (administrative gender, date of birth)
HCPCS* Healthcare Common Procedure Coding System	Medical, surgical, and diagnostic services rendered for claims
ICD-9 CM* International Statistical Classification of Diseases and Related Health Problems—Clinical Modification (9th ed)	Diagnoses and assessments
ICD-9 PCS* International Statistical Classification of Diseases and Related Health Problems—Procedural Coding System (9th ed)	Diagnoses and assessments
ICD-10 CM International Statistical Classification of Diseases and Related Health Problems—Clinical Modification (10th ed)	Diagnoses and assessments
ICD-10 PCS International Statistical Classification of Diseases and Related Health Problems—Procedural Coding System (10th ed)	Diagnoses and assessments
ICF International Classification of Functioning, Disability, and Health	Functional status
ISO-639 International Organization for Standardization – Standard 639	Representation of languages and language groups
LOINC® Logical Observation Identifiers, Names, and Codes	Outcomes and assessments
RxNORM	Normalized clinical drug names
SNOMED-CT® Systematized Nomenclature of Medicine Clinical Terms	Diagnoses, interventions, and outcomes
UCUM The Unified Code for Units of Measure	Units of measure for results

LOINC is a registered trademark of Regenstrief Institute, Inc, Indianapolis, IN. SNOMED-CT is a registered trademark of the International Health Terminology Standards Development Organisation, Copenhagen, Denmark.

* ICD-9 is being discontinued from US mandatory quality reporting beginning calendar year 2017.

Adapted from A Blueprint for the CMS Measures Management System. Version 11.1 ed. Washington, DC: Centers for Medicare & Medicaid Services; August 2015. https://www.cms.gov/Medicare/Quality-Initiatives-Patient-Assessment-Instruments/MMS/Downloads/Blueprint111.pdf. Accessed April 20, 2016.

- American Association of Nurse Anesthetists,
- American Health Information Management Association,
- Agency for Healthcare Research and Quality,
- American National Standards Institute,
- American Society of Anesthesiologists,
- Association for the Advancement of Medical Instrumentation,
- Association of PeriAnesthesia Nurses,
- Institute for Safe Medication Practices,
- Malignant Hyperthermia Association of the United States,
- National Fire Protection Agency,
- National Institute for Occupational Safety and Health,
- National Quality Forum,
- US Pharmacopeia, and
- United Network for Organ Sharing.

Examples of guidance from professional standards-setting agencies that may be considered for incorporation into perioperative documentation include

- national patient safety guidelines,

579

- organ and tissues tracking guidelines,
- perioperative recommendations for safe patient care,
- safe medication administration guidelines, and
- timing of clinical events.

As licensed health care professionals, perioperative RNs have a responsibility to maintain the established standards of perioperative nursing care. The standards of nursing practice require documentation to be based on the patient's condition or needs and the relationship to the proposed intervention and to be relevant to the period of patient care (eg, preadmission testing, preoperative, intraoperative, postoperative care).[4,5,107] National practice standards cross all disciplines of nursing care and are applicable to perioperative nursing practice.

IV.a.3. Perioperative nursing documentation should correspond to established guidelines and practices for perioperative nursing care.[107] Elements of perioperative guidelines that should be incorporated into clinical documentation include
- aseptic technique maintenance[76,108-111];
- local anesthesia administration[23,101,112-122];
- medication administration practices (eg, use of abbreviations)[23,112,113,115,118,123-126];
- moderate sedation/analgesia administration[23,101-121,127-129];
- patient care considerations (eg, latex allergy, implanted electronic device, dentures)[20,76,100,113,118,130-137];
- patient positioning[76,101,114,118,132,138];
- patient information exchanged[3,100-102,118,120,121,136,139-143];
- safety precautions, including
  - electrical safety precautions,[118,136,142-147]
  - equipment use precautions (eg, laser, pneumatic tourniquet, magnetic resonance imaging),[133,147-151]
  - fire prevention,[76,100,118,124,130,141,144,146,150,152-154]
  - human tissue procurement, processing, and preservation precautions,[76,118,120-122,155-160]
  - infection prevention,[76,112,114,118,124,125,142,152,161-168]
  - tissue protection,[30,114,118,124,150,152,169-172]
  - radiation exposure prevention,[170]
  - retained surgical items prevention,[115,118,173,174]
  - correct site, side, person surgery processes,[76,88,100,116,120,121,124,135,136,138,145,175-181] and
  - skin preparation and antisepsis[23,76,101,114,115,117,118,124,128,142,153,164,168,182,183];
- specimen and tissue management[20,76,114,118,121,122,155,158,174,180];
- sterilization/disinfection practices[76,114,118,128,130,131,145,146,153,166,179,180,184-188]; and

- traffic control measures.[76,130,141,152,153,166] *[1: Strong Evidence]*

The AORN guidelines for perioperative nursing practice are nationally recognized as the standard of care for all operative or invasive procedure patient care settings. Perioperative recommendations for practice are not mandatory nursing care criteria but have been incorporated into regulatory and other standards-setting agencies' guidelines and have been used to support judicial decisions.[189-195]

IV.a.4. Perioperative nursing documentation must correspond to local, state, and federal regulatory requirements. *[1: Regulatory Requirement]*

State and federal regulations are a collection of general and permanent rules (ie, laws) established to protect the welfare of the public and fortify the guiding principles of the nation. Many statutes or laws are established at the national level and may be amplified at the state level. The amplified statute would become the mandatory authority for the state. An example of this would be document retention requirements that vary among states. Failure to comply with the final law-making authority could result in monetary penalties for the offending organization or monetary penalties or incarceration for the offending individual. Agencies with regulatory authority include the
- Centers for Disease Control and Prevention,
- Centers for Medicare & Medicaid Services (CMS),
- Department of Health and Human Services,
- Occupational Safety and Health Administration, and
- US Food and Drug Administration.

Criteria identified by regulatory agencies for patient care documentation include
- allergies,[21,76,100,102,106,182,196]
- cultural variables,[21,100,106,116,135,197]
- equipment used for patient care (eg, type, model number),[76,100-102,115,134,135,144,145,174,182,196,198]
- names of legal guardian(s) and patient support person(s),[76,102,116,135,196]
- nutritional considerations,[20,100,102,196]
- ordered tests and services provided,[76,100,134,199]
- patient and family education and engagement,[21,100,106,135,165,196,200]
- patient identifiers and demographics,[20,76,100,134,174]
- patient attributes and status (eg, immunizations, disabilities)[20-22,76,100,101,106,135,176,177,196,201]
- safety precautions,[21,76,106,144,163,199]
- surgical consent(s),[76,100,135,177] and

- surgical implants and explants, including unique identifiers.[21,76,100,106,134,157,198,201-204]

IV.a.5. Perioperative nursing documentation must correspond to health care accreditation organization requirements. *[1: Regulatory Requirement]*

Compliance with state or national health care accreditation agency criteria is mandatory for organizations seeking CMS reimbursement or striving to meet established patient safety goals.[20,105] Accrediting bodies review documentation for compliance to the minimum standards for an element of performance. The following accreditation agencies currently have deemed status:

- the American Association for Accreditation of Ambulatory Surgery Facilities, Inc[143];
- the Accreditation Association for Ambulatory Health Care, Inc[142];
- State CMS[205];
- DNV-GL[206];
- the Healthcare Facilities Accreditation Program[207]; and
- The Joint Commission.[208,209]

Elements of performance identified by accreditation agencies may include evidence of[20,105]

- blood and tissue tracking;
- compliance with The Joint Commission's National Patient Safety Goals;
- elimination of nationally identified unacceptable abbreviations, acronyms, and symbols;
- hand-over communications;
- identification of implantable objects;
- identification of designated support person(s);
- infection control practices;
- medication reconciliation;
- patient care elements (eg, care plans, tests, services provided);
- pain management interventions;
- education of the patient, the patient's family members, and the patient's designated support person;
- patient demographics; and
- the presence of a current history and physical.

IV.a.6. Perioperative nursing documentation must incorporate mandatory reporting criteria for quality performance reimbursement. *[1: Regulatory Requirement]*

To improve population health, the US government is coordinating evidence-based standards development to be incorporated into the national agenda on health care reform. These efforts are incentivized through inclusion within the CMS reimbursement programs and made public through national reporting forums (eg, Hospital Compare[210]). Agencies responsible for national standards development or reimbursement for quality performance criteria include, but are not limited to, the

- Centers for Disease Control and Prevention,
- National Quality Forum, and
- Agency for Healthcare Research and Quality.

Measurement criteria for quality performance reimbursement are included in the following regulations and reporting requirements:

- Ambulatory Surgical Center Payment System,[211]
- Deficit Reduction Act of 2005,[174]
- Hospital Inpatient Prospective Payment System,[211]
- Hospital Outpatient Prospective Payment System,[211]
- National quality reporting metrics,[211] including the
  - Hospital Inpatient Quality Reporting Program, inclusive of the Surgical Care Improvement Project measures,
  - Hospital Acquired Condition Reduction Program,
  - Hospital Value-based Purchasing Program,
  - Hospital Outpatient Quality Reporting Program, and
  - Ambulatory Surgical Center Quality Reporting Program.

IV.b. Perioperative documentation must include all patient care orders given in the perioperative patient care setting.[20,100] *[1: Regulatory Requirement]*

The CMS requires that patient care orders be documented.

IV.b.1. Patient care orders should be entered into the clinical documentation system close to the time when the order is communicated or the intervention is initiated. *[5: Benefits Balanced with Harms]*

IV.b.2. All orders, including verbal orders, standing orders, orders included on surgeon preference cards, and order sets must be dated, timed, and authenticated by the ordering health care practitioner with prescriptive authority.[100,208,209,212-215] *[1: Regulatory Requirement]*

IV.b.3. To prevent patient harm from occurring as a result of outdated, incomplete, or erroneous entries, standing orders and preprinted order sets in the documentation framework should[216-219]

- not use unacceptable abbreviations,
- not use trailing zeros in medication dosages,

- use standardized names and terms to describe treatments and interventions (eg, brand names versus generic names for medications, device instructions), and
- be reviewed by the attending surgeon for accuracy of information for the intended procedure.

[2: High Evidence]

The use of preprinted standing orders that have been updated and do not have any of the problems in the bulleted list above has been shown to reduce medication errors and improve documentation compliance.[220]

IV.b.4. Verbal orders should be documented when they are communicated and verified using a read-back process that involves the ordering health care practitioner.[215-218,221] *[2: High Evidence]*

IV.c. The patient care record must include a complete and accurate informed patient consent for each operative or invasive procedure to be performed.[100,116,177,213] The informed consent process must be documented for procedures and treatments that are identified in the health care facility's medical staff policies as requiring informed consent.[21,100,177] Unless designated as an emergency situation in the health care facility's informed consent policy, a "properly executed informed consent"[116] must include[20,21,106]

- the name of the health care facility providing the surgery or invasive procedure;
- the specific name of the intervention to be performed;
- indications for the proposed intervention;
- the name of the responsible health care provider performing the intervention;
- a statement identifying the risks and benefits associated with the proposed intervention and indication of discussion with the patient or patient's legal representative;
- the signature of the patient or the patient's legal representative;
- the date and time the patient or the patient's legal representative signed the informed consent document;
- the date and time and the signature of the person who witnessed the patient or the patient's legal representative signing the informed consent document; and
- the signature of the responsible health care provider who executed the informed consent discussion with the patient or the patient's legal representative.

[1: Regulatory Requirement]

The patient or the patient's legal representative is entitled to participate in the informed decision-making process for planning care and treatment, including the right to request or refuse treatment.[116,213]

IV.c.1. Additional content that may be identified on the informed consent document and may be regulated by state statutes and administrative rules includes[20,21,106]

- identification of assisting physicians including, but not limited to, medical residents who will be contributing significantly to the proposed intervention and
- identification of assisting health care personnel who are not physicians but who are performing within their scope of practice (eg, RN first assistant, nurse practitioner) and who will be contributing significantly to the proposed intervention.

[1: Regulatory Requirement]

IV.d. The names, roles, and credentials of individuals participating in the patient's perioperative care, as well as those not directly involved in the scheduled surgical or procedural intervention, must be recorded in the patient health care record.[21,106] *[1: Regulatory Requirement]*

Individuals participating in the patient's perioperative care experience may include

- surgical or procedural patient care team members,
- identified legal representatives,
- identified patient support person(s),
- recipients of patient care information on behalf of the patient,
- health care professionals contributing to the patient's care (eg, pathologist, x-ray technician, approved health care student),
- industry representatives,
- law enforcement officers (eg, prison guards), or
- approved observers.

A comprehensive patient-centric record of care reflects interactions between the patient's health care team and those individuals legally representing or providing physical, spiritual, or other support services to the patient.[21,106] Documentation of interactions provides the groundwork for transparency in care planning through effective representation of the patient's involvement in the plan of care and contributions made toward the treatment plan.

IV.e. Clinical documentation platforms (ie, paper, electronic) should support the collection of tailored health care information using a format that accommodates and is customized to the clinical environment.[49] *[2: High Evidence]*

Tailoring patient health information allows the collection of unique patient care data (eg, communicable diseases, responses to medications, psychosocial considerations) that may affect the planned operative or other invasive procedure. The collection of tailored health care information is standardized to the clinical setting (eg, surgical versus interventional radiology) but may vary by the requirements of the environment where perioperative care is delivered (eg, pediatric hospital, cancer treatment center, ambulatory surgery center).[49,50]

IV.e.1. Formats selected for the collection of tailored patient care information should be established based on nationally recognized standards of practice that outline the nurse's responsibilities to the patient.[4,104] *[2: High Evidence]*

IV.e.2. Charting by exception processes should be formatted and reviewed by the health care organization's risk management and legal representatives.[222,223] *[3: Moderate Evidence]*

The minimum criteria for charting by exception should include

- identifying objective physical assessment criteria for the patient population being served (eg, endoscopy patients, orthopedic patients);
- identifying and defining what constitutes normal findings;
- describing the process for documenting normal findings (eg, "within normal limits");
- describing the process for identifying, describing, and documenting objective abnormal or key findings;
- listing the practice standards, care guidelines, and clinical pathways used to guide patient care;
- listing a rationale, including decisions and interventions, for deviations from established guidance for patient care;
- setting the frequency of documentation entries; and
- adhering to state or national statutory requirements (eg, record authentication).[104,194,224]

Short[225] reported that charting by exception, also known as variance charting, was successfully implemented at one medical center. When charting by exception, the nurses' documentation time was significantly reduced when used with a comprehensively designed documentation system.

A well-designed documentation system corresponds to the health care organization's policy for charting by exception and allows for an indisputable description of the patient's condition. Charting by exception may lead to litigious situations when organizational policy has not been well formulated or updated for changes in statutory requirements or when the nurse has not followed the established guidance for charting by exception.[104,194,222]

IV.f. Cognitive processes used in patient care should be supported by clinical support technologies (eg, AORN Syntegrity) that are embedded within electronic clinical documentation systems.[37,226,227] *[3: Moderate Evidence]*

The processes within perioperative patient care are classified as cognitive performance or the intellectual processing of information to complete a finite task.[226] Multitasking, environmental stimulation, and availability of information contribute to the nurse's ability or inability to accommodate needed adjustments in patient care activities. The collective evidence indicates that use of poorly designed clinical information systems, those not conforming to national data standards, or those that do not incorporate clinical workflow and work process requirements may contribute to patient harm.[30,37,56,226-229] Alternately, clinical information systems that incorporate technology innovations (eg, order entry, decision support, clinical alerts) and support the cognitive processes of patient care have been found to enhance health care worker performance and result in improved patient safety and quality patient outcomes.[30,37,63,226-229]

Recommendation V

Patient information must be secure, held confidential, and protected from unauthorized disclosure.[230]

The Health Insurance Portability and Accountability Act (HIPAA) of 1996 guarantees the privacy of individuals receiving health services and the confidentiality of "individually identifiable health information."[230] Updated to correspond with the HITECH Act, HIPAA now includes security standards for protecting electronic health information (ie, Security Rule) and regulations that specify compliance, investigation, payments, and penalties (ie, Enforcement Rule) that were established in 1996.[230,231]

V.a. Access to patient health information must be limited to authorized individuals based on the health care role (eg, surgeon, RN, perfusionist), responsibility, and function (eg, postanesthesia care unit RN assisting in the endoscopy unit).[20,230-232] *[1: Regulatory Requirement]*

Controlling access to the patient's health information prevents privacy and security breaches for HIPAA-covered entities.[230-232] The health care organization has a legal responsibility to establish procedures to prevent unauthorized access to sensitive patient health information and to execute a plan for data breach notification practices should a breach occur.[230,231,233]

V.a.1. Risk-reduction strategies to proactively mitigate potential access violations should include[224,232]

- establishing perioperative information management policies that include remote access protocols, on-/off-site information storage practices, and employee exit strategies that are reviewed and updated as the environment changes (eg, new regulations, transitions from paper to electronic documentation platforms);
- identifying procedures for the use of organizational and personal mobile devices (eg, cell phones, tablet technologies, video

imaging) within the perioperative care environment;

- establishing awareness and sensitivity to data security and privacy by reinforcing the existing health care organization's information security policy for monitoring and auditing access to patient health information;
- restricting access to electronic health information to users with individualized, unique authorization credentials that are associated with time-sensitive passwords using alphanumeric-symbol combinations; and
- holding competency-based education programs on information access and sharing for all employees upon hire, when changes are made for documentation practices, and when problems are identified within the perioperative care environment.

[3: Moderate Evidence]

V.a.2. Ambulatory surgery centers must have a person designated to oversee the protection of clinical records. This individual is responsible not only for the confidentiality, security, and physical safety of the clinical records, but also for maintaining a method of tracking who has access to the records and identifying designated locations of paper records throughout the facility in an effort to prevent unauthorized access.[20,230,231,234] *[1: Regulatory Requirement]*

V.a.3. Any significant medical advice given to a patient via text, e-mail, or telephone must be permanently entered in the patient's clinical record and signed and dated.[20,234] *[1: Regulatory Requirement]*

V.b. Perioperative health care personnel should comply with the health care organization's information policies for sharing electronic patient information. The organization's information policies should include[224,235,236] processes for

- determining that electronic patient health information, either to or from outside organizations or shared with the patient, meets current requirements for information exchange and security (eg, malware protection);
- validating original source authenticity and the accuracy of transmitted information; and
- evaluating electronically transmitted content (eg, e-mail, text, file transfer protocol [FTP]) for potential corruption.

[1: Strong Evidence]

Electronic transmission of patient health information is held to the same privacy and security criteria as facility-based EHRs. Sensitive patient information in paper, electronic text, or image formatting can be exposed to unintended or unauthorized disclosure if effective sharing safeguards are not in place.[230,231,236]

Authors of a systematic review of the literature on the security and privacy of EHRs found that compliance with the standards and federal regulations for sharing protected patient information has been accomplished by using interchange script language, using multi-agent hierarchical architecture, adding precision access control with on-demand revocation to access control processes, and employing systems that gather disparate patient data while preserving patient anonymity during communications.[232] Electronic transmission of patient health information by e-mail, mobile storage media, or other formats may introduce malicious software into the health care information system.

V.b.1. Health care organizations should establish policies and procedures for verifying electronic patient health information for authenticity and accuracy and for evaluating content for potential corruption.[224,231,236,237] *[1: Strong Evidence]*

V.b.2. The patient must have a signed consent for release of information in the health care record before graphic imaging takes place and before the release of patient-specific information, including remote access to and relocation of health information from the treating organization.[177,230,231,238,239] Non-consented disclosure of sensitive patient health information requires execution of the data breach notification process by the health care organization.[230,231,237,240] *[1: Regulatory Requirement]*

V.b.3. To complete full disclosure and reporting, the organization's information technology and risk management personnel should collaborate to discover all patient care records that were involved in a non-consented disclosure.[240,241] *[2: High Evidence]*

V.c. Documentation entries made into the patient health care record must include an authentication process at the completion of the documentation process or according to the organization's established policies.[80,86,100,101,224,242,243] Health care records must accurately reflect the patient care experience, be completed promptly, and be associated with an author identification procedure to ensure the integrity of the content.[20,100,105] *[1: Regulatory Requirement]*

Authentication identifies the author of the documentation entry and indicates responsibility for the interventions performed and patient information collected. Authentication legally binds the owner of the signature with the responsibility for the accuracy of the content within the document.[224]

V.c.1. The authentication process may include, but is not limited to,[224,233,244]

- using an electronic or digital signature or a code key in the format designated by

Table 2. US Federal Minimum Retention Guidelines

Source	Retention Period
Ambulatory surgical services[1]	Not specified
Hospitals[2]	5 years from the date of discharge
Hospitals, critical access[3]	6 years from date of last entry or longer as mandated by state statutory guidelines or as necessary for legal proceedings
Department of Veterans Affairs operation log file (including type of surgery, date, patient's name, surgeon, assistant scrub person, anesthetist, agent, method, sponge count, preoperative and postoperative diagnoses, complications, and other information)[4]	Destroy after 20 years
Department of Veterans Affairs (date surgery was performed, members of the surgical and nursing teams, and other information pertaining to the surgery of a patient)[4]	Destroy after 3 years

REFERENCES

1. 42 CFR §416.47. Condition of participation: medical records. Centers for Medicare & Medicaid Services. Department of Health and Human Services. https://www.gpo.gov/fdsys/granule/CFR-2007-title42-vol3/CFR-2007-title42-vol3-sec416-47. Accessed April 20, 2016.

2. 42 CFR §482.24. Condition of participation: medical record services. Centers for Medicare & Medicaid Services. Department of Health and Human Services. https://www.gpo.gov/fdsys/granule/CFR-2011-title42-vol5/CFR-2011-title42-vol5-sec482-24/content-detail.html. Accessed April 20, 2016.

3. 42 CFR §485.638. Conditions of participation: clinical records. Centers for Medicare & Medicaid Services. Department of Health and Human Services. https://www.gpo.gov/fdsys/granule/CFR-2011-title42-vol5/CFR-2011-title42-vol5-sec485-638. Accessed April 21, 2016.

4. Department of Veterans Affairs Records Control Schedule 10-1. Washington, DC: Veterans Health Administration; 2016. http://www1.va.gov/vhapublications/RCS10/rcs10-1.pdf. Accessed April 21, 2016.

the health care organization as the legal representation of an individual's written signature for the EHR.

- completing a pen-to-paper signature, using initials with a signature legend on the same document, or a rubber signature stamp for paper-based documentation platforms (eg, faxed, scanned documents) and as permitted by the health care organization's policy.
  - Initials with a signature legend should be avoided on narrative documentation (eg, comments, patient quotes, consultation), assessment data collection, or when a signature is required by law (eg, patient informed consent).
  - Digitized inked signatures (ie, signature image) should only be used when deemed acceptable by the health care organization and allowed by state or federal reimbursement regulations.
- using a countersignature demonstrating accuracy of content entered into a patient health care record; once countersigned, the content is legally considered the cosigner's entry (eg, cosigned nursing student entry).

[1: Regulatory Requirement]

V.c.2. Authentication of verbal orders must occur within the time frame specified by state statutory guidelines. If state law does not specify a time frame, the federal mandate applies for verbal orders to be authenticated by the responsible physician within 48 hours of entering the order.[100] *[1: Regulatory Requirement]*

V.d. The patient care record must be retained in the original or a legally reproducible format for the minimum allocation of time dictated by federal regulations and state statutes of limitations. Organizational policies may address other time frames for record retention based on the patient population served (eg, pediatric patients, oncology patients), facility demographics (eg, research, trauma, academic), media used to store patient data (eg, paper, microfilm, optical disc), or operational requirements (eg, regulatory compliance).[20,76,105,215,224,245,246] *[1: Regulatory Requirement]*

The American Health Information Management Association recommends retaining operative indexes for a minimum of 10 years and the register of surgical procedures permanently.[215] The minimum retention guidelines for perioperative information according to US federal regulations are detailed in Table 2.

V.e. Electronic documentation platforms should have an alternate data entry and backup process.[247-250] Perioperative services should formalize a complete downtime process that addresses hardware, operating system, and network disruptions to preserve data accuracy and uninterrupted health care processes. Downtime planning should incorporate strategies to

- facilitate an uninterrupted patient care schedule (eg, paper forms, documentation backup media),
- identify changes to existing workflows (eg, how new orders are communicated, clinical resources),
- recover potential loss of patient care data, and
- incorporate patient care data that are captured using alternate documentation platforms (eg, paper forms) into the electronic information system.[41,247,251]

[1: Strong Evidence]

Backup processes will mitigate interruptions in patient care that could result from technology failures. Dependence on technology can significantly influence the effectiveness and efficiency of patient care delivery when systems are interrupted.[41,247,251]

V.e.1.   Perioperative personnel with system access responsibilities should receive education on the policies, procedures, and alternate workflows associated with the downtime or technology performance issues.[41,247,251] *[1: Strong Evidence]*

Recommendation VI

Modifications to existing content in the patient health care record should comply with federal and state regulations, health care accreditation requirements, and national practice guidelines.[4,224]

The patient care record is a legal representation of services provided by the health care organization. Perioperative nurses are obligated to accurately represent the patient's care within the health care record.[100,105,230]

VI.a.   Amendments, corrections, or addendums to the patient care record should only be made to present an accurate description of the care provided or to protect the patient's interest.[252,253] *[2: High Evidence]*

Using inappropriate methods to correct, clarify, or change existing entries in the patient health care record may expose the health care organization or clinicians to liability for falsification of patient care information.[4,19] After conducting a meta-study of the essentials of quality nursing documentation, Jefferies et al[104] recommended recording patient care activities as they occur and avoiding late entries, duplication of events, unnecessary information, or controversial information that could lead to modifications of the patient care record.

VI.b.   The health care organization's information management policy should outline the processes for making legally acceptable modifications to the patient care record.[224,252] *[2: High Evidence]*

Corrections, amendments, and addendums are limited by the functionality of the documentation platform used.

VI.b.1.   Amendments or addendums to the patient care record should follow established organizational policies and procedures. Corrections, amendments, and addendums in paper records should be performed by[6,12,224,254]

- placing a single line through the incorrect entry, being careful not to obliterate the inaccurate information;
- writing "error," "mistaken entry," or "omit" next to the incorrect text as determined by organizational policy;
- providing the rationale for the correction above the inaccurate entry if room is available or adding it to the margin of the document;
- signing and dating the entry; and
- entering the correct information in the next available space or adjacent to the acknowledged inaccurate information.

[3: Moderate Evidence]

VI.b.2.   Corrections, amendments, and addendums in EHRs should[224,252]

- have a versioning or "track corrections" function (eg, an electronic strike-through with a time stamp) to identify the alterations made to an entry that has been authenticated;
- automatically date-, time-, and author-stamp each entry;
- generate a symbol or other notation to identify when an alteration has been made to existing content that creates a new version of the document;
- retain and link the original document version to the newly created version; and
- reflect corrections made to the EHR on the paper copy.

[2: High Evidence]

VI.b.3.   Corrections completed after a final signature or authentication process has occurred should be consistent with the functionality of the information system and established organizational policies and procedures. *[5: Benefits Balanced with Harms]*

VI.b.4.   Corrections completed before the final signature or authentication process might not be classified as a "correction" according to organizational policy and the information system in place. *[5: Benefits Balanced with Harms]*

VI.b.5.   Addendums should be completed within the original document created using the source information system when available and should be reflected in the permanent patient care record or data repository system. *[5: Benefits Balanced with Harms]*

VI.b.6. Deletions and retractions of content from a closed EHR system should be made according to organizational policies and procedures and the functionality of the information system in place. *[5: Benefits Balanced with Harms]*

Recommendation VII

Perioperative personnel should receive initial and ongoing education and competency verification on their understanding of the principles and performance of the processes for documenting patient care and of best practices for maintaining the security of patient care information.[4,255,256]

Initial and periodic competency-based education programs to maintain proficiency in the application of knowledge and use of the documentation platform improve the effectiveness of documentation practices and reinforce strategies to avert unintentional disclosure of patient care information.[257] In a non-experimental study conducted in the United Kingdom, fewer than half of the responding clinicians (n = 141) reported having received any form of data protection training. The researchers suggested that this could increase the risk for mishandling patient data.[258] Bruylands et al[259] conducted a mixed-method study on the quality of nursing care with the use of electronic nursing documentation. They identified that skill in using documentation tools deteriorated without subsequent education and reinforcement of practices.

VII.a. The health care organization's policies for information management and the procedures for documentation processes and activities should be incorporated into orientation and ongoing education for personnel in the perioperative care environment.[5,107,260] *[1: Strong Evidence]*

Perioperative personnel who receive ongoing education and participate in periodic review of policies and procedures develop the knowledge, skills, and attitudes that affect patient outcomes.[107]

VII.a.1. Perioperative RNs should receive education on the significance and use of structured vocabularies for clinical documentation. At a minimum, education on structured terminologies should include[4,9,31,68,72]
- the value structured terminology brings to clinical documentation;
- an overview of the PNDS;
- the contributions of the PNDS to perioperative nursing practice and patient outcomes; and
- how standardized documentation facilitates benchmarking, comparative analysis, predictive analytics, and efficiency reporting.

[1: Strong Evidence]

VII.a.2. Education and competency verification for perioperative RNs should include reviewing[261-263]
- national and organizational documentation standards, guidelines, and requirements;
- procedures for completing amendments, addendums, and corrections;
- procedures for sharing patient information securely while maintaining patient privacy;
- procedures for initiating breach notification;
- compliance requirements for health care data capture; and
- legal implications for failure to comply with documentation standards.

[3: Moderate Evidence]

VII.a.3. Education and competency verification for users of perioperative information systems, a component of the EHR, should also incorporate the following minimum skills by demonstrating[261,263,264]
- accessing and closing the patient care record;
- the information system's functionality (eg, data entry, order acknowledgment);
- the authentication processes;
- downtime procedures including alternate workflows to accommodate patient care; and
- compliance requirements for health care data capture.

[3: Moderate Evidence]

Recommendation VIII

Policies and procedures for perioperative information management should be developed, reviewed periodically, revised as necessary, and readily available in the practice setting. As new evidence emerges, policies and procedures should evolve to accommodate best practices and technology developments.[260]

Policies and procedures establish authority, responsibility, and accountability and serve as operational guidelines that are used to minimize patient risk factors, standardize practice, direct health care personnel, and establish guidelines for continuous performance improvement activities.

VIII.a. The perioperative services information management policy should be developed and established by a multidisciplinary team, complement and reinforce existing organization-wide policies (ie, risk management, quality improvement, health information privacy and security), and include the unique considerations of the perioperative care environment.[260] *[2: High Evidence]*

A collaborative approach to policy development and the provision of access to policies for all health care personnel results in improved communication and compliance with established practices within the health care organization.

VIII.a.1. Information management policies and documentation procedures for EHR systems should include guidance on[252,253,260,265]

- forwarding addendums to each destination where patient information is retained,
- editing content before a final signature or authentication process occurs,
- using cut-copy-paste and "carry forward" functionality to populate the patient care record,
- completing corrections in an active or locked patient care record,
- rectifying a misidentification of patient health information (ie, wrong name association),
- amending clinical content in an active or locked patient care record,
- completing a delayed entry and updating the long-term record or data repository,
- deleting or retracting information from a locked patient care record while maintaining the integrity of the record, and
- defining components that are required for record completion.

[2: High Evidence]

VIII.b. Policies and procedures must include information on data privacy and security and identify risk-reduction strategies to proactively mitigate potential violations of patient health information access.[230,231] *[1: Regulatory Requirement]*

VIII.b.1. Risk-reduction strategies should include[224,235,253,262]

- establishing remote access protocols, on-site/off-site information storage practices, and employee exit strategies to protect patient health information;
- frequently reviewing and updating policies as the health care information environment changes (eg, new regulations, transitions from paper to electronic documentation platforms);
- identifying procedures for using mobile devices (eg, cell phone, tablet technologies, video imaging) within the perioperative care environment;
- reinforcing the existing health care organization's information security policy for monitoring and auditing access to patient health information within the perioperative care environment;
- restricting access to electronic health information by user type with individualized unique authorization credentials associated with time-sensitive passwords using alpha-numeric-symbol combinations; and
- holding annual competency-based education programs on information access and sharing for all employees in the perioperative care environment.

[2: High Evidence]

Recommendation IX

A quality management program should be developed and implemented, and should focus on the integrity of the data within the patient health care record.[260]

Regularly monitoring and validating documentation processes is necessary for variance reporting, which supports process and performance measurement to quantify organizational effectiveness and nursing influence on patient outcomes.[4,107]

IX.a. Perioperative personnel should participate in the organization-wide clinical documentation improvement (CDI) program. *[2: High Evidence]*

Participation in a CDI program facilitates data and documentation analysis while providing a structured framework to achieve consistency in quality processes that affect patient satisfaction, accreditation standing, and reimbursement status.[261] Representation of perioperative RNs in the CDI program will allow concerns specific to perioperative practice to be addressed and areas for improvement identified.

IX.a.1. A perioperative CDI program should be reviewed for[16,224,255]

- use of acceptable abbreviations,
- timeliness and chronology of patient information,
- legibility,
- use of clear and specific language,
- blank spaces or data fields,
- content omissions (eg, missing informed consent),
- delayed entries (eg, next day entry),
- inconsistencies (eg, conflicting assessment findings, procedure start times),
- inappropriate information (eg, communications with attorneys),
- authentication of verbal orders,
- absence of signatures or countersignature,
- approved documentation practices (eg, charting by exception/variance charting), and
- alterations to clinical content.

[2: High Evidence]

IX.b. Validation procedures for the perioperative information system should be incorporated into the quality management program and comprehensive strategies for EHR system security and maintenance.[250,266] Data quality may be determined by periodic validation of the information system for the integrity of[224,250,252]

- collected patient care information,
- report generation,
- file storage and retrieval,
- data security, and
- control for document versioning.

[2: High Evidence]

Perioperative information systems are complex systems that contribute to improved care or may add to error-prone documentation processes.[250,267-269] Validation procedures help to maintain the integrity of patient health information.

IX.b.1. Health care organizations should establish audits performed as a part of a quality-driven information management program. Audit trails should be retained and placed on a retention schedule following the state statute of limitations and needs of the health care organization.[224,270] Audit trails may include[224,270,271]

- paper-based sign-out processes,
- logbook activities,
- EHR access and operations performed,
- EHR metadata,
- electronic tracking system, and
- data mining activities.

[2: High Evidence]

Auditing procedures help to establish user and organizational accountability for the legal integrity of the patient health care record.

IX.b.2. Perioperative information systems should be included in the organizational information technology risk mitigation plan.[250,268,272] In collaboration with the organization's risk manager, information services department, and engineering department, perioperative nursing leaders should coordinate efforts to plan for[250,268,272-274]

- perioperative information system upgrades and maintenance;
- system redundancies (eg, remote patient care record access, backup generators);
- unanticipated access to and theft of patient health care information; and
- organizational information technology network infrastructure maintenance, upgrades, and conversions to the perioperative information system.

[3: Moderate Evidence]

Proactive multidisciplinary contingency planning for information system failures and disaster response procedures will help maintain continuity in patient care activities.

Editor's note: *AORN Syntegrity is a registered trademark of AORN, Inc, Denver, CO. SNOMED-CT is a registered trademark of the International Health Terminology Standards Development Organisation, Copenhagen, Denmark.*

Glossary

Addendum: New documentation used to add information to an original documentation entry of patient health information.

Amendment: Additional documentation completed to clarify a preexisting entry of patient health information.

American Recovery and Reinvestment Act (ARRA): An economic stimulus package enacted by the US Congress in 2009 with a defined purpose of stimulating jobs, investments, and consumer spending. The ARRA contains provisions for improving health care quality through the use of health information technology.

Authentication: A security measure to establish the validity of an electronic transmission, message, or original source (eg, author) or to verify the authorization of an individual to receive specific information. Authentication is used to confirm that an individual or system is who or what it claims to be.

Clinical information systems: Computer technology used in the patient care environment for collecting patient health care information.

Clinical support technologies: Assorted technologies used in the patient care environment to facilitate the clinician's ability to provide safe, comprehensive interventions for the delivery of quality health care.

Code key: A computer code used to authenticate entries in an electronic health record as permitted by state, federal, and reimbursement regulations.

Controlled terminology: Terminology developed according to specific characteristics so that each data element is expressed as a single, clear and unambiguous concept. Controlled terminology concepts maintain their meaning permanently.

Correction: A change made to the documented patient health information meant to clarify the entry after the document has been authenticated.

Customize: To specifically select or set preferences or options for health care information.

Data mining: The process of extracting and analyzing data for usable information from relationships, patterns, information clusters, and data trends. The new information may be used for predictive modeling in decision support processes for clinical, operational, and research utilization.

Data quality: Data remaining unchanged from their original meaning; data are complete, correct, comprehensive, and consistent for the intended use.

Data repository: A central location where health care data (eg, clinical, financial, operational) and files are stored and maintained for later retrieval and use.

Decision support: An interactive computer-based program that provides reminders, advice, or interpretation of patient data at a specific point in time.

Deemed status: The "deeming" authority granted to national accreditation organizations (eg, The Joint Commission, DNV-GL) by the Centers for Medicare & Medicaid Services (CMS) to determine, on CMS's behalf, whether a health care provider organization is in compliance with the regulations to provide and receive payment for Medicare services. Six areas are deemable: quality assurance, antidiscrimination, access to services, confidentiality and accuracy of enrollee records, information on advance directives, and provider participation rules.

Digital signature: A cryptographic signature (ie, digital key) used to authenticate the user, provide legal ownership, and ensure integrity of the unit of information.

Digitized inked signature: A handwritten signature using a pen pad to create an electronic representation of the actual signature.

Downtime: Periods of time when the clinical information system (ie, electronic health record) is unavailable because of scheduled maintenance or upgrades or technology failure, power outage, or another unscheduled event.

Electronic health record: An electronic record of health-related information for an individual that conforms to nationally recognized interoperability standards and that can be created, managed, and consulted by authorized clinicians and staff members across more than one health care organization.

Electronic medical record: An electronic record of health-related information for an individual that can be created, gathered, managed, and consulted by authorized clinicians and staff members within one health care organization.

Electronic signature: The technology-neutral electronic process used to sign (ie, attest) content for authorship and legal responsibility for a section of information. The electronic signature format is determined by the technology used to collect or create the signature.

Health Information Technology for Economic and Clinical Health (HITECH): A component of the American Recovery and Reinvestment Act of 2009 that addresses the use of electronic health information technology to improve health care quality, coordination of care, and health information privacy and security.

Integrity: The accuracy, consistency, and reliability of information content, processes, and systems.

Interoperable: The ability for health information systems to exchange or share health information within and across organizational boundaries.

Legal health record: The medical record generated at or for a health care organization as its business record or released upon request, which represents an exact duplicate of the original record.

Malware: Software considered harmful to a computer system including but not limited to viruses, worms, Trojan horses, spyware, and unauthorized adware.

Metadata: The descriptive data that characterizes other data to create a clearer understanding of their meaning and to achieve greater reliability and quality of information (eg, name, address, and telephone number of a patient)

Signature legend: A document that identifies an author's full signature and title when initials are used to authenticate entries in the health care record.

Tailored health care information: The unique patient characteristics based on multiple factors influencing health status and health behaviors and collected to inform individualized nursing interventions.

Versioning: The process of assigning a unique version name or number to an electronic heath record and used to identify revisions occurring to previously documented content.

REFERENCES

1. Chow M, Beene M, O'Brien A, et al. A nursing information model process for interoperability. *J Am Med Inform Assoc.* 2015;22(3):608-614. [VB]

2. Gugerty B, Maranda MJ, Beachley M, et al. *Challenges and Opportunities in Documentation of the Nursing Care of Patients.* Baltimore, MD: Maryland Nursing Workforce Commission, Documentation Work Group; 2007. [IIIB]

3. Standards of perioperative nursing. In: *Guidelines for Perioperative Practice.* Denver, CO: AORN, Inc, 2015:693-708. [IVA]

4. *ANA Principles for Documentation.* Silver Spring, MD: American Nurses Association; 2010. [IVA]

5. *Nursing: Scope and Standards of Practice.* Silver Spring, MD: American Nurses Association; 2010. [IVA]

6. Peterson AM. Medical record as a legal document part 2: meeting the standards. *J Legal Nurse Consult.* 2013;24(1):4-10. [VA]

7. *Nursing's Social Policy Statement: The Essence of the Profession.* Silver Spring, MD: American Nurses Association; 2010. [IVA]

8. Beyea SC. Describing professional nursing through a universal record in perioperative settings. *Int J Nurs Terminol Classif.* 2003;14(S4):23. [IIIB]

9. Petersen C, ed. *Perioperative Nursing Data Set.* 3rd ed. Denver, CO: AORN; 2011. [IVA]

10. Kuc JA, Iyer PW, Levin BL, Shea MA. Perioperative records. In: Iyer PW, Levin BL, Shea MA, eds. *Medical Legal Aspects of Medical Records.* Tucson, AZ: Lawyers & Judges Publishing Company; 2006:657-677. [IVA]

11. Junttila K, Hupli M, Salanterä S. The use of nursing diagnoses in perioperative documentation. *Int J Nurs Terminol Classif.* 2010;21(2):57-68. [IIIB]

12. Guido GW. *Legal & Ethical Issues in Nursing.* 5th ed. Boston, MA: Pearson; 2010. [VA]

13. Exhibit B: Perioperative explications for the *ANA Code of Ethics for Nurses.* In: *Guidelines for Perioperative Practice.* Denver, CO: AORN, Inc; 2015:711-732. [IVB]

14. Staggers N, Clark L, Blaz JW, Kapsandoy S. Why patient summaries in electronic health records do not provide the cognitive support necessary for nurses' handoffs on medical and surgical units: insights from interviews and observations. *Health Informatics J.* 2011;17(3):209-223. [IIIB]

15. Urquhart C, Currell R, Grant MJ, Hardiker NR. Nursing record systems: effects on nursing practice and healthcare outcomes. *Cochrane Database Syst Rev.* 2009;(1):CD002099. [IA]

16. Wang N, Hailey D, Yu P. Quality of nursing documentation and approaches to its evaluation: a mixed-method systematic review. *J Adv Nurs.* 2011;67(9):1858-1875. [IIA]

17. Keenan G, Yakel E, Dunn Lopez K, Tschannen D, Ford YB. Challenges to nurses' efforts of retrieving, documenting, and communicating patient care information. *J Am Med Inform Assoc.* 2013;20(2):245-251. [IIIA]

18. Micek WT, Berry L, Gilski D, Kallenbach A, Link D, Scharer K. Patient outcomes: the link between nursing diagnoses and interventions. *J Nurs Adm.* 1996;26(11):29-35. [VA]

19. Monarch K. Documentation, part 1: principles for self-protection. Preserve the medical record—and defend yourself. *Am J Nurs.* 2007;107(7):58-60. [VB]

20. 42 CFR §416.47. Condition of participation: medical records. Centers for Medicare & Medicaid Services. Department of Health and Human Services. https://www.gpo.gov/fdsys/granule/CFR-2007-title42-vol3/CFR-2007-title42-vol3-sec416-47. Accessed April 20, 2016. [IA]

PATIENT CARE

21. 42 CFR §482. Conditions of participation for hospitals. Centers for Medicare & Medicaid Services. Department of Health and Human Services. https://www.gpo.gov/fdsys/granule/CFR-2011-title42-vol5/CFR-2011-title42-vol5-part482/content-detail.html. Accessed April 20, 2016. [IA]

22. 42 USC § 18001. Patient Protection and Affordable Care Act. January 7, 2011. https://www.gpo.gov/fdsys/granule/USCODE-2010-title42/USCODE-2010-title42-chap157-subchapI-sec18001. Accessed April 20, 2016. [IA]

23. Guideline for medication safety. In: *Guidelines for Perioperative Practice.* Denver, CO: AORN, Inc; 2016:289-332. [IVB]

24. Barney L, Jackson JJ, Ollapally VM, Savarise MT, Senkowski CK. Documentation of services provided in the postoperative global period. *Bull Am Coll Surg.* 2013;98(5):48-51. [IVB]

25. Ammenwerth E, Rauchegger F, Ehlers F, Hirsch B, Schaubmayr C. Effect of a nursing information system on the quality of information processing in nursing: an evaluation study using the HIS-monitor instrument. *Int J Med Inf.* 2011;80(1):25-38. [IIA]

26. Whittenburg L. Workflow viewpoints: analysis of nursing workflow documentation in the electronic health record. *J Healthc Inf Manag.* 2010;24(3):71-75. [VB]

27. Lee S, McElmurry B. Capturing nursing care workflow disruptions: comparison between nursing and physician workflows. *Comput Inform Nurs.* 2010;28(3):151-599. [IIIB]

28. *Better EHR: Usability, Workflow and Cognitive Support in Electronic Health Records.* Houston, TX: National Center for Cognitive Informatics & Decision Making; 2014. [IVA]

29. Colligan L, Potts HW, Finn CT, Sinkin RA. Cognitive workload changes for nurses transitioning from a legacy system with paper documentation to a commercial electronic health record. *Int J Med Inf.* 2015;84(7):469-476. [IIA]

30. Institute of Medicine; Page A, eds. Keeping Patients Safe: *Transforming the Work Environment of Nurses.* Washington, DC: National Academies Press; 2004. [IVA]

31. Hayrinen K, Lammintakanen J, Saranto K. Evaluation of electronic nursing documentation—nursing process model and standardized terminologies as keys to visible and transparent nursing. *Int J Med Inform.* 2010;79(8):554-564. [IIIB]

32. Keohane CA, Bane AD, Featherstone E, et al. Quantifying nursing workflow in medication administration. *J Nurs Adm.* 2008;38(1):19-26. [IIIB]

33. Capuano T, Bokovoy J, Halkins D, Hitchings K. Work flow analysis: eliminating non-value-added work. *J Nurs Adm.* 2004;34(5):246-256. [IIIA]

34. Roberson D, Connell M, Dillis S, et al. Cognitive complexity of the medical record is a risk factor for major adverse events. *Permanente J.* 2014;18(1):4-8. [IB]

35. Ahmed A, Chandra S, Herasevich V, Gajic O, Pickering BW. The effect of two different electronic health record user interfaces on intensive care provider task load, errors of cognition, and performance. *Crit Care Med.* 2011;39(7):1626-1634. [IB]

36. Potter P, Boxerman S, Dunagan C, et al. An analysis of nurses' cognitive work: a new perspective for understanding medical errors. *Adv Patient Saf.* 2005;1:39-51. [IIA]

37. Karsh BT, Holden RJ, Alper SJ, Or CK. A human factors engineering paradigm for patient safety: designing to support the performance of the healthcare professional. *Qual Saf Health Care.* 2006;15(Suppl 1):i59-i65. [VB]

38. Benner P, Sheets V, Uris P, Malloch K, Schwed K, Jamison D. Individual, practice, and system causes of errors in nursing: a taxonomy. *J Nurs Adm.* 2002;32(10):509-523. [IIIB]

39. Hendrich A, Chow M, Skierczynski BA, Lu Z. A 36-hospital time and motion study: how do medical-surgical nurses spend their time? *Permanente J.* 2008;12(3):25-34. [IIIA]

40. Ash JS, Berg M, Coiera E. Some unintended consequences of information technology in health care: the nature of patient care information system-related errors. *J Am Med Inform Assoc.* 2004;11(2):104-112. [IIIA]

41. Bloomrosen M, Starren J, Lorenzi NM, Ash JS, Patel VL, Shortliffe EH. Anticipating and addressing the unintended consequences of health IT and policy: a report from the AMIA 2009 Health Policy Meeting. *J Am Med Inform Assoc.* 2011;18(1):82-90. [IVB]

42. Harrison MI, Koppel R, Bar-Lev S. Unintended consequences of information technologies in health care—an interactive sociotechnical analysis. *J Am Med Inform Assoc.* 2007;14(5):542-549. [VA]

43. Cornell P, Herrin-Griffith D, Keim C, et al. Transforming nursing workflow, part 1: the chaotic nature of nurse activities. *J Nurs Adm.* 2010;40(9):366-373. [IIIB]

44. Cornell P, Riordan M, Herrin-Griffith D. Transforming nursing workflow, part 2: the impact of technology on nurse activities. *J Nurs Adm.* 2010;40(10):432-439. [IIB]

45. Irwin RS, Richardson ND. Patient-focused care: using the right tools. *Chest.* 2006;130(1 Suppl):73S-82S. [VA]

46. Allan J, Englebright J. Patient-centered documentation: an effective and efficient use of clinical information systems. *J Nurs Adm.* 2000;30(2):90-95. [VB]

47. Nailon RE. The assessment and documentation of language and communication needs in healthcare systems: current practices and future directions for coordinating safe, patient-centered care. *Nurs Outlook.* 2007;55(6):311-317. [VA]

48. Institute of Medicine. *Crossing the Quality Chasm: A New Health System for the 21st Century.* Washington, DC: National Academies Press; 2001. [IVA]

49. Spooner SA; Council on Clinical Information Technology American Academy of Pediatrics. Special requirements of electronic health record systems in pediatrics. *Pediatrics.* 2007;119(3):631-637. [IVB]

50. Park EJ, McDaniel A, Jung MS. Computerized tailoring of health information. *Comput Inform Nurs.* 2009;27(1):34-43. [VA]

51. Payne TH, tenBroek AE, Fletcher GS, Labuguen MC. Transition from paper to electronic inpatient physician notes. *J Am Med Inform Assoc.* 2010;17(1):108-111. [VC]

52. Korst LM, Eusebio-Angeja AC, Chamorro T, Aydin CE, Gregory KD. Nursing documentation time during implementation of an electronic medical record. *J Nurs Adm.* 2003;33(1):24-30. [IIIB]

53. Flemming D, Hübner U. How to improve change of shift handovers and collaborative grounding and what role does the electronic patient record system play? Results of a systematic literature review. *Int J Med Inf.* 2013;82(7):580-592. [IIIA]

54. Andreia Neves da Mota L, Soares Pereira FM, Ferreira de Sousa PA. Nursing information systems: exploration of information shared with physicians. *Refencia.* 2014;4(1):83-89. [IIIB]

55. Jefferies D, Johnson M, Nicholls D. Comparing written and oral approaches to clinical reporting in nursing. *Contemp Nurse.* 2012;42(1):129-138. [IIIA]

56. Ammenwerth E, Eichstadter R, Haux R, Pohl U, Rebel S, Ziegler S. A randomized evaluation of a

computer-based nursing documentation system. *Methods Inf Med.* 2001;40(2):61-68. [IA]

57. Harrington L. Electronic health record workflow: why more work than flow? *AACN Adv Crit Care.* 2015;26(1):5-9. [VC]

58. Asaro PV, Boxerman SB. Effects of computerized provider order entry and nursing documentation on workflow. *Acad Emerg Med.* 2008;15(10):908-915. [IIB]

59. Ay F, Polat Ş. The belief and opinions of nurses on the electronic patient record system. *Int J Caring Sci.* 2014;7(1):258-268. [IIIB]

60. Mahler C, Ammenwerth E, Wagner A, et al. Effects of a computer-based nursing documentation system on the quality of nursing documentation. *J Med Syst.* 2007;31(4):274-282. [IIA]

61. Stead WW, Lin HS, eds. *Computational Technology for Effective Health Care: Immediate Steps and Strategic Directions.* Washington, DC: National Academies Press; 2009. [IVA]

62. Poissant L, Pereira J, Tamblyn R, Kawasumi Y. The impact of electronic health records on time efficiency of physicians and nurses: a systematic review. *J Am Med Inform Assoc.* 2005;12(5):505-516. [IIA]

63. Amarasingham R, Plantinga L, Diener-West M, Gaskin DJ, Powe NR. Clinical information technologies and inpatient outcomes: a multiple hospital study. *Arch Intern Med.* 2009;169(2):108-114. [IIB]

64. Shojania KG, Jennings A, Mayhew A, Ramsay CR, Eccles MP, Grimshaw J. The effects of on-screen, point of care computer reminders on processes and outcomes of care. *Cochrane Database Syst Rev.* 2009;(3):CD001096. [IA]

65. Harrington L, Kennerly D, Johnson C. Safety issues related to the electronic medical record (EMR): synthesis of the literature from the last decade, 2000-2009. *J Healthc Manag.* 2011;56(1):31-43. [IIIB]

66. *ANA Position Statement: Electronic Health Record.* December 11, 2009. http://nursingworld.org/MainMenu-Categories/Policy-Advocacy/Positions-and-Resolutions/ANAPositionStatements/Position-Statements-Alphabetically/Electronic-Health-Record.html. Accessed April 20, 2016. [IVB]

67. Kim H, Dykes P, Mar P, Goldsmith D, Choi J, Goldberg H. Towards a standardized representation to support data reuse: representing the ICNP semantics using the HL7 RIM. *Stud Health Technol Inform.* 2009;146:308-313. [IIIB]

68. Lundberg C, Warren J, Brokel J, et al. Selecting a standardized terminology for the electronic health record that reveals the impact of nursing on patient care. *Online J Nurs Inform.* 2008;12(2). [IVA] 69. Zielstorff RD. Characteristics of a good nursing nomenclature from an informatics perspective. *Online J Nurs Inform.* 1998;3(2). [VC]

70. Tastan S, Linch GC, Keenan GM, et al. Evidence for the existing American Nurses Association-recognized standardized nursing terminologies: a systematic review. *Int J Nurs Stud.* 2014;51(8):1160-1170. [IIIA]

71. Graves JR, Corcoran S. The study of nursing informatics. *Image J Nurs Sch.* 1989;21(4):227-231. [IVB]

72. Beyea SC. Standardized language—making nursing practice count. *AORN J.* 1999;70(5):831-838. [IVB]

73. Carrington JM. The usefulness of nursing languages to communicate a clinical event. *Comput Inform Nurs.* 2012;30(2):82-88. [IIIA]

74. Saba VK, Taylor SL. Moving past theory: use of a standardized, coded nursing terminology to enhance nursing visibility. *Comput Inform Nurs.* 2007;25(6):324-331. [IVB]

75. Dykes PC, DaDamio RR, Goldsmith D, Kim HE, Ohashi K, Saba VK. Leveraging standards to support patient-centric interdisciplinary plans of care. *AMIA Annual Symp Proc.* 2011;2011:356-363. [IIIB]

76. 42 CFR §482.51. Condition of participation: surgical services. Centers for Medicare & Medicaid Services. Department of Health and Human Services. https://www.gpo.gov/fdsys/granule/CFR-2010-title42-vol5/CFR-2010-title42-vol5-sec482-51. Accessed April 20, 2016. [IA]

77. Westra BL, Subramanian A, Hart CM, et al. Achieving "meaningful use" of electronic health records through the integration of the Nursing Management Minimum Data Set. *J Nurs Adm.* 2010;40(7-8):336-343. [IVB]

78. Mangalmurti SS, Murtagh L, Mello MM. Medical malpractice liability in the age of electronic health records. *N Engl J Med.* 2010;363(21):2060-2067. [IVA]

79. Centers for Medicare & Medicaid Services (CMS) HHS. Medicare and Medicaid programs; changes in provider and supplier enrollment, ordering and referring, and documentation requirements; and changes in provider agreements. Final rule. *Fed Regist.* 2012;77(82):25284-25318. [IA]

80. 42 CFR Part 495 Medicare and Medicaid programs; Electronic Health Record Incentive Program—modifications to meaningful use in 2015 through 2017. Proposed rule. *Fed Regist.* 2015;80(72):20346-20399. [IA]

81. Hayrinen K, Saranto K, Nykanen P. Definition, structure, content, use and impacts of electronic health records: a review of the research literature. *Int J Med Inform.* 2008;77(5):291-304. [IIIA]

82. Hyun S, Bakken S. Toward the creation of an ontology for nursing document sections: mapping section names to the LOINC semantic model. *AMIA Annu Symp Proc.* 2006;2006:364-368. [IIIB]

83. National Quality Forum. Executive summary. In: *Health Information Technology Automation of Quality Measure: Quality Data Set and Data Flow.* Washington, DC: NQF;2009:iii-vi. [IA]

84. Goossen WT, Ozbolt JG, Coenen A, et al. Development of a provisional domain model for the nursing process for use within the Health Level 7 reference information model. *J Am Med Inform Assoc.* 2004;11(3):186-194. [IIIB]

85. Adler-Milstein J, Jha AK. Sharing clinical data electronically: a critical challenge for fixing the health care system. *JAMA.* 2012;307(16):1695-1696. [VA]

86. Centers for Medicare & Medicaid Services (CMS) HHS. Medicare and Medicaid programs; electronic health record incentive program—stage 2. Final rule. *Fed Regist.* 2012;77(171):53967-54162. [IA]

87. Jha AK, DesRoches CM, Campbell EG, et al. Use of electronic health records in US hospitals. *N Engl J Med.* 2009;360(16):1628-1638.

88. Brown DS, Donaldson N, Burnes Bolton L, Aydin CE. Nursing-sensitive benchmarks for hospitals to gauge high-reliability performance. *J Healthc Qual.* 2010;32(6):9-17. [IVB]

89. US Department of Health and Human Services. *Report to Congress: Medicare Ambulatory Surgical Center Value-Based Purchasing Implementation Plan.* Washington, DC: Centers for Medicare & Medicaid Services; 2011. https://www.cms.gov/Medicare/Medicare-Fee-for-Service-Payment/ASCPayment/Downloads/C_ASC_RTC-2011.pdf. Accessed April 20, 2016. [IA]

90. *Becoming a High Reliability Organization: Operational Advice for Hospital Leaders.* Rockville, MD: Agency for Healthcare Research and Quality; 2008. [IVB]

PATIENT CARE

91. Thompson D, Johnston P, Spurr C. The impact of electronic medical records on nursing efficiency. *J Nurs Adm.* 2009;39(10):444-451. [VB]

92. Shekelle PG, Morton SC, Keeler EB. *Costs and Benefits of Health Information Technology.* Evidence Report/Technology Assessment No. 132. (Prepared by the Southern California Evidence-based Practice Center under Contract No. 290-02-0003.). Rockville, MD: Agency for Healthcare Research and Quality; 2006. [IVA]

93. Department of Veterans Affairs. Sharing information between the Department of Veterans Affairs and the Department of Defense. Interim final rule. *Fed Regist.* 2011;76(203):65133-65135.

94. Office of the National Coordinator for Health Information Technology (ONC) Department of Health and Human Services. 2014 Edition Release 2 Electronic Health Record (EHR) certification criteria and the ONC HIT Certification Program; regulatory flexibilities, improvements, and enhanced health information exchange. Final rule. *Fed Regist.* 2014;79(176):54429-54480. [IA]

95. *A Blueprint for the CMS Measures Management System.* Version 11.1 ed. Washington, DC: Centers for Medicare & Medicaid Services; August 2015. https://www.cms.gov/Medicare/Quality-Initiatives-Patient-Assessment-Instruments/MMS/Downloads/Blueprint111.pdf. Accessed April 20, 2016. [IA]

96. Murdoch TB, Detsky AS. The inevitable application of big data to health care. *JAMA.* 2013;309(13):1351-1352. [VA]

97. Al-Rawajfah OM, Aloush S, Hewitt JB. Use of electronic health-related datasets in nursing and health-related research. *West J Nurs Res.* 2015;37(7):952-983. [IIIA]

98. *Transforming Health Care Through Big Data.* New York, NY: Institute for Health Technology Transformation; 2013. [VB]

99. Sun J, Hu J, Luo D, et al. Combining knowledge and data driven insights for identifying risk factors using electronic health records. *AMIA Annu Symp Proc.* 2012;2012:901-910. [IIA]

100. 42 CFR §482.24. Condition of participation: medical record services. Centers for Medicare & Medicaid Services. Department of Health and Human Services. https://www.gpo.gov/fdsys/granule/CFR-2011-title42-vol5/CFR-2011-title42-vol5-sec482-24/content-detail.html. Accessed April 20, 2016. [IA]

101. 42 CFR §482.23. Condition of participation: nursing services. Centers for Medicare & Medicaid Services. Department of Health and Human Services. https://www.gpo.gov/fdsys/granule/CFR-2011-title42-vol5/CFR-2011-title42-vol5-sec482-23/content-detail.html. Accessed April 20, 2016. [IA]

102. 42 CFR §416.46. Condition for Coverage—Nursing services. Centers for Medicare & Medicaid Services. Department of Health and Human Services. https://www.gpo.gov/fdsys/granule/CFR-2007-title42-vol3/CFR-2007-title42-vol3-sec416-46. Accessed April 20, 2016. [IA]

103. Scruth EA. Quality nursing documentation in the medical record. *Clin Nurse Spec.* 2014;28(6):312-314. [VC]

104. Jefferies D, Johnson M, Griffiths R. A meta-study of the essentials of quality nursing documentation. *Int J Nurs Pract.* 2010;16(2):112-124. [IIIA]

105. 42 CFR §485.638. Conditions of participation: clinical records. Centers for Medicare & Medicaid Services. Department of Health and Human Services. https://www.gpo.gov/fdsys/granule/CFR-2011-title42-vol5/CFR-2011-title42-vol5-sec485-638. Accessed April 21, 2016. [IA]

106. 42 CFR §416. Ambulatory surgical services. Centers for Medicare & Medicaid Services. Department of Health and Human Services. https://www.cms.gov/Regulations-and-Guidance/Legislation/CFCsAndCoPs/ASC.html. Accessed April 21, 2016. [IA]

107. *Guidelines for Perioperative Practice.* Denver, CO: AORN, Inc; 2016. [IVA]

108. 42 CFR §416.51. Conditions for coverage: infection control. Centers for Medicare & Medicaid Services. Department of Health and Human Services. https://www.gpo.gov/fdsys/granule/CFR-2012-title42-vol3/CFR-2012-title42-vol3-sec416-51. Accessed April 21, 2016. [IA]

109. NPSG.07.05.01: Implement evidence-based practices for preventing surgical site infections. In: *Comprehensive Accreditation Manual for Hospitals.* Oakbrook Terrace, IL: The Joint Commission; 2015. [IVA]

110. IC.01.05.01: The hospital has an infection prevention and control plan. In: *Comprehensive Accreditation Manual for Hospitals.* Oakbrook Terrace, IL: The Joint Commission; 2015. [IVA]

111. IC.02.01.01: The hospital implements its infection prevention and control plan. In: *Comprehensive Accreditation Manual for Hospitals.* Oakbrook Terrace, IL: The Joint Commission; 2015. [IVA]

112. Guideline for care of the patient receiving local anesthesia. In: *Guidelines for Perioperative Practice.* Denver, CO: AORN, Inc; 2016:577-588. [IVB]

113. Krenzischek DA, Wilson L; ASPAN. ASPAN pain and comfort clinical guideline. *J Perianesth Nurs.* 2003;18(4):232-236. [IVC]

114. ASPAN. 2015-2017 *Perianesthesia Nursing Standards, Practice Recommendations and Interpretive Statements.* Cherry Hill, NJ: American Society of PeriAnesthesia Nurses; 2015. [IVB]

115. 42 CFR §416.48. Condition for coverage: pharmaceutical services. Centers for Medicare & Medicaid Services. Department of Health and Human Services. https://www.gpo.gov/fdsys/granule/CFR-2007-title42-vol3/CFR-2007-title42-vol3-sec416-48/content-detail.html. Accessed April 21, 2016. [IA]

116. Centers for Medicare & Medicaid Services. Department of Health and Human Services. Condition of participation: patient's rights. 42 CFR §482.13. http://www.ecfr.gov/cgi-bin/text-idx?rgn=div5;node=42:5.0.1.1.1;cc=ecfr. Accessed April 21, 2016. [IA]

117. Medication management. In: *Comprehensive Accreditation Manual for Hospitals.* Oakbrook Terrace, IL: The Joint Commission; 2015. [IVA]

118. Provision of care, treatment, and services. In: *Comprehensive Accreditation Manual for Hospitals.* Oakbrook Terrace, IL: The Joint Commission; 2015. [IVA]

119. Medical records: 600.040.010. In: *Medicare Standards and Checklist for Accreditation of Ambulatory Surgery Facilities.* 6.5 ed. Gurnee, IL: American Association for Accreditation of Ambulatory Surgery Facilities; 2014:89. [IVA]

120. Clinical records and health information. In: *Accreditation Handbook for Ambulatory Health Care.* Skokie, IL: Accreditation Association for Ambulatory Health Care Inc; 2015:49-51. [IVA]

121. Quality of care provided. In: *Accreditation Handbook for Ambulatory Health Care.* Skokie, IL: Accreditation Association for Ambulatory Health Care Inc; 2015:42-43. [IVA]

122. 29 CFR §1910.1030. Bloodborne pathogens. US Department of Labor, Occupational Safety and Health Standards. http://www.osha.gov/pls/oshaweb/owadisp.show_document?p_table=standards&p_id=10051. Accessed April 21, 2016. [IA]

123. *AORN Position Statement: Preventing Wrong-Patient, Wrong-Site, Wrong-Procedure Events.* AORN, Inc. https://www.aorn.org/guidelines/clinical-resources/position-statements. Accessed April 20, 2016. [IVB]

124. Guideline for preoperative patient skin antisepsis. In: *Guidelines for Perioperative Practice.* Denver, CO: AORN, Inc; 2016:41-64. [IVA]

125. Rights and responsibilities of the individual. In: *Comprehensive Accreditation Manual for Hospitals.* Oakbrook Terrace, IL: The Joint Commission; 2015. [IVA]

126. NPSG.03.06.01: Maintain and communicate accurate patient medication information. In: *Comprehensive Accreditation Manual for Hospitals.* Oakbrook Terrace, IL: The Joint Commission; 2015. [IVA]

127. Guideline for prevention of transmissible infections. In: *Guidelines for Perioperative Practice.* Denver, CO: AORN, Inc; 2016:471-506. [IVA]

128. Postanesthetic care unit (PACU). In: *Regular Standards and Checklist for Accreditation of Ambulatory Surgery Facilities.* 14.4 ed. Gurnee, IL: American Association for Accreditation of Ambulatory Surgery Facilities; 2016:43-45. [IVB]

129. Guideline for care of the patient receiving moderate sedation/analgesia. In: *Guidelines for Perioperative Practice.* Denver, CO: AORN, Inc; 2016:617-648. [IVB]

130. Guideline for a safe environment of care, part 1. In: *Guidelines for Perioperative Practice.* Denver, CO: AORN, Inc; 2016:237-262. [IVA]

131. Guideline for prevention of unplanned patient hypothermia. In: *Guidelines for Perioperative Practice.* Denver, CO: AORN, Inc; 2016:531-554. [IVB]

132. Guideline for prevention of deep vein thrombosis. In: *Guidelines for Perioperative Practice.* Denver, CO: AORN, Inc; 2016:521-530. [IVB]

133. Guideline for positioning the patient. In: *Guidelines for Perioperative Practice.* Denver, CO: AORN, Inc; 2016:649-668. [IVB]

134. 42 CFR §482.27. Condition of participation: laboratory services. Centers for Medicare & Medicaid Services. Department of Health and Human Services. https://www.gpo.gov/fdsys/granule/CFR-2011-title42-vol5/CFR-2011-title42-vol5-sec482-27/content-detail.html. Accessed April 21, 2016. [IA]

135. 42 CFR §416.52. Conditions for coverage: patient admission, assessment and discharge. Centers for Medicare & Medicaid Services. Department of Health and Human Services. https://www.gpo.gov/fdsys/granule/CFR-2011-title42-vol3/CFR-2011-title42-vol3-sec416-52. Accessed April 21, 2016. [IA]

136. Record of care, treatment, and services. In: *Comprehensive Accreditation Manual for Hospitals.* Oakbrook Terrace, IL: The Joint Commission; 2015. [IVA]

137. Guideline for complementary care interventions. In: *Guidelines for Perioperative Practice.* Denver, CO: AORN, Inc; 2016:507-520. [IVA]

138. Universal Protocol. In: *Comprehensive Accreditation Manual for Hospitals.* Oakbrook Terrace, IL: The Joint Commission; 2015. [IVA]

139. Quality and performance improvement standards for perioperative nursing. In: *Guidelines for Perioperative Practice.* Denver, CO: AORN, Inc; 2015:761-770. [IVB]

140. Guideline for transfer of patient care information. In: *Guidelines for Perioperative Practice.* Denver, CO: AORN, Inc; 2016:669-674. [IVB]

141. Surgical and related services. In: *Accreditation Handbook for Ambulatory Health Care.* Skokie, IL: Accreditation Association for Ambulatory Health Care Inc; 2015:64-71. [IVA]

142. Accreditation Association for Ambulatory Health Care. *Accreditation Handbook for Ambulatory Health Care.* Skokie, IL: The Association; 2015. [IVA]

143. *Regular Standards and Checklist for Accreditation of Ambulatory Surgery Facilities.* Version 14.4. Gurnee, IL: American Association for Accreditation of Ambulatory Surgery Facilities; 2016. [IVA]

144. 42 CFR §482.41. Condition of participation: physical environment. Centers for Medicare & Medicaid Services. Department of Health and Human Services. https://www.gpo.gov/fdsys/granule/CFR-2011-title42-vol5/CFR-2011-title42-vol5-sec482-41. Accessed April 21, 2016. [IA]

145. 42 CFR §416.44. Condition for coverage: environment. Centers for Medicare & Medicaid Services. Department of Health and Human Services. https://www.gpo.gov/fdsys/granule/CFR-2012-title42-vol3/CFR-2012-title42-vol3-sec416-44. Accessed April 21, 2016. [IA]

146. Environment of care. In: *Comprehensive Accreditation Manual for Hospitals.* Oakbrook Terrace, IL: The Joint Commission; 2015. [IVA]

147. Guideline for electrosurgery. In: *Guidelines for Perioperative Practice.* Denver, CO: AORN, Inc; 2016:119-136. [IVB]

148. Guideline for care of patients undergoing pneumatic tourniquet-assisted procedures. In: *Guidelines for Perioperative Practice.* Denver, CO: AORN, Inc; 2016:151-176. [IVA]

149. Guideline for minimally invasive surgery. In: *Guidelines for Perioperative Practice.* Denver, CO: AORN, Inc; 2016:589-616. [IVB]

150. Guideline for laser safety. In: *Guidelines for Perioperative Practice.* Denver, CO: AORN, Inc; 2016:137-150. [IVB]

151. Guideline for sharps safety. In: *Guidelines for Perioperative Practice.* Denver, CO: AORN, Inc; 2016:417-440. [IVA]

152. Guideline for a safe environment of care, part 2. In: *Guidelines for Perioperative Practice.* Denver, CO: AORN, Inc; 2016:263-288. [IVA]

153. Infection prevention and control. In: *Comprehensive Accreditation Manual for Hospitals.* Oakbrook Terrace, IL: The Joint Commission; 2015. [IVA]

154. *ANSI/AAMI ST79:2010, A1, A2, A3 & A4:2013: Comprehensive Guide to Steam Sterilization and Sterility Assurance in Health Care Facilities.* Arlington, VA: Association for the Advancement of Medical Instrumentation; 2013. [IVA]

155. Medical records: 600.010.060. In: *Medicare Standards and Checklist for Accreditation of Ambulatory Surgery Facilities.* 6.5 ed. Gurnee, IL: American Association for Accreditation of Ambulatory Surgery Facilities; 2014:79. [IVA]

156. Guideline for autologous tissue management. In: *Guidelines for Perioperative Practice.* Denver, CO: AORN, Inc; 2016:185-236. [IVA]

157. 24 CFR §482.45. Condition of participation: organ, tissue, and eye procurement. Centers for Medicare & Medicaid Services. https://www.gpo.gov/fdsys/granule/CFR-2011-title42-vol5/CFR-2011-title42-vol5-sec482-45. Accessed April 21, 2016. [IA]

158. Guideline for specimen management. In: *Guidelines for Perioperative Practice.* Denver, CO: AORN, Inc; 2016. [IVA]

159. *Policy on Standardized Packaging of Human Organs and Tissue Typing Materials.* Richmond, VA: Organ Procurement and Transplantation Network; 2010. [IA]

160. Transplant safety. In: *Comprehensive Accreditation Manual for Hospitals.* Oakbrook Terrace, IL: The Joint Commission; 2015. [IVA]

161. Guideline for processing flexible endoscopes. In: *Guidelines for Perioperative Practice.* Denver, CO: AORN, Inc; 2016:675-758. [IVB]

162. Guideline for cleaning and care of surgical instruments. In: *Guidelines for Perioperative Practice.* Denver, CO: AORN, Inc; 2016:773-808. [IVA]

163. Quality Indicators. Agency for Healthcare Research and Quality. http://www.qualityindicators.ahrq.gov/. Accessed April 21, 2016. [IA]

164. Mangram AJ, Horan TC, Pearson ML, Silver LC, Jarvis WR. Guideline for prevention of surgical site infection, 1999. Hospital Infection Control Practices Advisory Committee. *Infect Control Hosp Epidemiol.* 1999;20(4):247-278. [IVA]

165. 42 CFR §482.43. Condition of participation: discharge planning. Centers for Medicare & Medicaid Services. Department of Health and Human Services. https://www.gpo.gov/fdsys/granule/CFR-2011-title42-vol5/CFR-2011-title42-vol5-sec482-43/content-detail.html. Accessed April 21, 2016. [IA]

166. National Patient Safety Goal 7: Reduce the risk of health care-associated infections. In: *Comprehensive Accreditation Manual for Hospitals.* Oakbrook Terrace, IL: The Joint Commission; 2015. [IVA]

167. SCIP-Inf-4: Cardiac surgery patients with controlled 6 a.m. postoperative blood glucose. In: *The Specifications Manual for National Hospital Inpatient Quality Measures.* Version 3.3. Washington, DC: Centers for Medicare & Medicaid Services and Joint Commission; 2011. http://www.wicheckpoint.org/Docs/STK_Q2-11_Manual_CMSTJC.pdf. Accessed April 21, 2016.

168. SCIP-Inf-6: Surgery patients with appropriate hair removal. In: *The Specifications Manual for National Hospital Inpatient Quality Measures.* Version 3.3. Washington, DC: Centers for Medicare & Medicaid Services and Joint Commission; 2011. http://www.wicheckpoint.org/Docs/STK_Q2-11_Manual_CMSTJC.pdf. Accessed April 21, 2016. [IA]

169. General safety in the facility. General. In: *Regular Standards and Checklist for Accreditation of Ambulatory Surgery Facilities.* 14.4 ed. Gurnee, IL: American Association for Accreditation of Ambulatory Surgery Facilities; 2016:45-50. [IVB]

170. Guideline for radiation safety. In: *Guidelines for Perioperative Practice.* Denver, CO: AORN, Inc; 2016:333-368. [IVB]

171. *ANSI Z136.4-2010: American National Standard Recommended Practice for Laser Safety Measurements for Hazard Evaluation.* Orlando, FL: Laser Institute of America; 2010. [IVA]

172. *ANSI Z136.7-2008: American National Standard for Testing and Labeling of Laser Protective Equipment.* Orlando, FL: Laser Institute of America; 2008. [IVA]

173. Guideline for prevention of retained surgical items. In: *Guidelines for Perioperative Practice.* Denver, CO: AORN, Inc; 2016:369-416. [IVA]

174. 109th US Congress. Deficit Reduction Act of 2005. Pub L 109-171. February 8, 2006. https://www.gpo.gov/fdsys/pkg/PLAW-109publ171/html/PLAW-109publ171.htm. Accessed April 21, 2016. [IA]

175. *AORN Position Statement: Creating a Practice Environment of Safety.* AORN, Inc. http://www.aorn.org/guidelines/clinical-resources/position-statements. Accessed April 20, 2016. [IVB]

176. 42 CFR §482.22. Condition of participation: medical staff. Centers for Medicare & Medicaid Services. Department of Health and Human Services. http://www.gpo.gov/fdsys/pkg/CFR-2010-title42-vol5/pdf/CFR-2010-title42-vol5-sec482-22.pdf. Accessed April 21, 2016. [IA]

177. 42 CFR §416.42. Condition for coverage: surgical services. Centers for Medicare & Medicaid Services. Department of Health and Human Services. https://www.gpo.gov/fdsys/granule/CFR-2007-title42-vol3/CFR-2007-title42-vol3-sec416-42/content-detail.html. Accessed April 21, 2016. [IA]

178. 42 CFR §416.49. Condition for coverage: laboratory and radiologic services. Centers for Medicare & Medicaid Services. Department of Health and Human Services. https://www.gpo.gov/fdsys/granule/CFR-2010-title42-vol3/CFR-2010-title42-vol3-sec416-49. Accessed April 21, 2016. [IA]

179. Anesthesia. Pre-anesthesia care. In: *Regular Standards and Checklist for Accreditation of Ambulatory Surgery Facilities.* 14.4 ed. Gurnee, IL: American Association for Accreditation of Ambulatory Surgery Facilities; 2016:79-81. [IVB]

180. General environment—additional Medicare standards. In: *Medicare Standards and Checklist for Accreditation of Ambulatory Surgery Facilities.* 6.5 ed. Gurnee, IL: American Association for Accreditation of Ambulatory Surgery Facilities; 2014:37. [IVA]

181. Operating suite: 200.010.005. In: *Medicare Standards and Checklist for Accreditation of Ambulatory Surgery Facilities.* 6.5 ed. Gurnee, IL: American Association for Accreditation of Ambulatory Surgery Facilities; 2014:9. [IVA]

182. 42 CFR §482.25. Condition of participation: pharmaceutical services. Centers for Medicare & Medicaid Services. Department of Health and Human Services. https://www.gpo.gov/fdsys/granule/CFR-2011-title42-vol5/CFR-2011-title42-vol5-sec482-25. Accessed April 21, 2016. [IA]

183. National Patient Safety Goal 2: Improve the effectiveness of communication among caregivers. In: *Comprehensive Accreditation Manual for Hospitals.* Oakbrook Terrace, IL: The Joint Commission; 2015. [IVA]

184. Operating room policy, environment and procedures. Sterilization. In: *Medicare Standards and Checklist for Accreditation of Ambulatory Surgery Facilities.* 6.5 ed. Gurnee, IL: American Association for Accreditation of Ambulatory Surgery Facilities; 2014:13-15. [IVA]

185. Quality control. In: *ANSI/AAMI ST79:2010, A1, A2, A3 & A4:2013: Comprehensive Guide to Steam Sterilization and Sterility Assurance in Health Care Facilities.* Arlington, VA: Association for the Advancement of Medical Instrumentation; 2013:97-138. [IVA]

186. Guideline for high-level disinfection. In: *Guidelines for Perioperative Practice.* Denver, CO: AORN, Inc; 2016:759-772. [IVA]

187. Clinical practice guideline 1: ASPAN's evidence-based clinical practice guideline for the promotion of perioperative normothermia. In: *Perianesthesia Nursing Standards and Practice Recommendations 2010-2012.* Cherry Hill, NJ: American Society of PeriAnesthesia Nurses; 2010:24-45. [IVA]

188. Operating room policy, environment and procedures. Procedures—sterilization. In: *Regular Standards and Checklist for Accreditation of Ambulatory Surgery Facilities.* 14.4 ed. Gurnee, IL: American Association for Accreditation of Ambulatory Surgery Facilities; 2016:27-28. [IVA]

189. Beyond the count: preventing the retention of foreign objects during interventional radiology procedures. *Pa Patient Saf Advis.* 2008;5(1):24-27. [IVB]

190. ECRI Institute. Sales representatives and other outsiders in the OR. *Operating Room Risk Management.* 2013;1. [IVB]

191. Use of blunt-tip suture needles to decrease percutaneous injuries to surgical personnel: safety and health information bulletin. National Institute for Occupational Safety and Health. http://www.cdc.gov/niosh/docs/2008-101/. Accessed April 20, 2016. [IA]

192. Rutala WA, Weber DJ; Healthcare Infection Control Practices Advisory Committee (HICPAC). *Guideline for Disinfection and Sterilization in Healthcare Facilities, 2008.* Atlanta, GA: Centers for Disease Control and Prevention; 2008.

193. *Pommier v ABC Insurance Company*, 715 So2d 1270, 1297-1342 (La.App.3dCir. 1998). [IA]

194. *Lama v Borras*, 1994 16 F3d 473 (United States Court of Appeals, First Circuit, February 25, 1994). http://law.justia.com/cases/federal/appellate-courts/F3/16/473/491880/. Accessed April 21, 2016. [IA]

195. *Ledesma v Shashoua*, 2007 WL 2214650 (Tex App, August 3, 2007). [IA]

196. 42 CFR §482.52. Condition of participation: anesthesia services. Centers for Medicare & Medicaid Services. Department of Health and Human Services. https://www.gpo.gov/fdsys/granule/CFR-2011-title42-vol5/CFR-2011-title42-vol5-sec482-52/content-detail.html. Accessed April 21, 2016. [IA]

197. 42 CFR §482.28. Condition of participation: food and dietetic services. Centers for Medicare & Medicaid Services. Department of Health and Human Services. https://www.gpo.gov/fdsys/granule/CFR-2011-title42-vol5/CFR-2011-title42-vol5-sec482-28. Accessed April 21, 2016. [IA]

198. 21 CFR §821. Medical device tracking requirements. US Food and Drug Administration. Department of Health and Human Services. https://www.gpo.gov/fdsys/granule/CFR-2011-title21-vol8/CFR-2011-title21-vol8-part821. Accessed April 21, 2016. [IA]

199. 42 CFR §482.26. Condition of participation: radiologic services. Centers for Medicare & Medicaid Services. Department of Health and Human Services. https://www.gpo.gov/fdsys/granule/CFR-2011-title42-vol5/CFR-2011-title42-vol5-sec482-26. Accessed April 21, 2016. [IA]

200. Andreae C, Ekstedt M, Snellman I. Patients' participation as it appears in the nursing documentation, when care is ruled by standardized care plans. *ISRN Nurs.* 2011;2011:707601. [IIIB]

201. Social Security Act, 42 USC 1396d §1905, Pub L No. 74-271. [IA]

202. Medical device tracking; guidance for industry and FDA staff. US Food and Drug Administration. http://www.fda.gov/MedicalDevices/DeviceRegulationandGuidance/GuidanceDocuments/ucm071756.htm. Accessed April 21, 2016. [IA]

203. Food and Drug Administration Modernization Act of 1997, S 830, 105th Cong, 1st Sess (1997), Pub L No 105-115. [IA]

204. *UDI Compliance Initiative Summary.* Scituate, MA: Strategic Marketplace Initiative; 2015. [VC]

206. Survey & Certification—certification & compliance. Centers for Medicare & Medicaid Services. https://www.cms.gov/Medicare/Provider-Enrollment-and-Certification/CertificationandComplianc/index.html. Accessed April 21, 2016. [IA]

206. *NIAHO Interpretive Guidelines and Surveyor Guidance.* 10.1 ed. Milford, OH: DNV Healthcare Inc; 2012. [IVA]

207. Overview. Healthcare Facilities Accreditation Program. http://www.hfap.org/about/overview.aspx. Accessed April 21, 2016. [IVA]

208. *Comprehensive Accreditation Manual for Ambulatory Care.* Oakbrook Terrace, IL: The Joint Commission; 2015. [IVA]

209. *Comprehensive Accreditation Manual for Hospitals.* Oakbrook Terrace, IL: The Joint Commission; 2015. [IVA]

210. Hospital compare. Medicare.gov. https://www.medicare.gov/hospitalcompare/search.html?. Accessed April 21, 2016. [IA]

211. Centers for Medicare & Medicaid Services (CMS) HHS. Medicare and Medicaid programs: hospital outpatient prospective payment and ambulatory surgical center payment systems and quality reporting programs; Hospital Value-Based Purchasing Program; organ procurement organizations; quality improvement organizations; Electronic Health Records (EHR) Incentive Program; provider reimbursement determinations and appeals. Final rule with comment period and final rules. *Fed Regist.* 2013;78(237):74825-75200. [IA]

212. Straube BM. Letter to David T. Tayloe Jr. [written communication]. Baltimore, MD: Department of Health & Human Services; 2010. [IA]

213. 42 CFR §416.50. Condition for coverage: patient rights. Centers for Medicare & Medicaid Services. US Department of Health and Human Services. https://www.gpo.gov/fdsys/granule/CFR-2011-title42-vol3/CFR-2011-title42-vol3-sec416-50. Accessed April 21, 2016. [IA]

214. RC.02.03.07: Qualified staff receive and record verbal orders. In: *Comprehensive Accreditation Manual for Ambulatory Care.* Oakbrook Terrace, IL: The Joint Commission; 2015. [IVA]

215. Bryant G, DeVault K, Ericson C, et al. Guidance for clinical documentation improvement programs. *J AHIMA.* 2010;81(5):45-50. [IVB]

216. Dawson A, Orsini MJ, Cooper MR, Wollenburg K. Medication safety—reliability of preference cards. *AORN J.* 2005;82(3):399-407. [IIB]

217. MM.04.01.01: Medication orders are clear and accurate. In: *Comprehensive Accreditation Manual for Hospitals.* Oakbrook Terrace, IL: The Joint Commission; 2015. [IVA]

218. Cole LM. Med report. Documenting to reduce medication errors. *OR Nurse.* 2008;2(7):17-19. [IVC]

219. Brunetti L, Santell JP, Hicks RW, Stevenson JG. USP Medication Safety Forum. The impact of abbreviations on patient safety. *Jt Comm J Qual Patient Saf.* 2007;33(9):576-583. [IIIA]

220. Broussard M, Bass PF 3rd, Arnold CL, McLarty JW, Bocchini JA Jr. Preprinted order sets as a safety intervention in pediatric sedation. *J Pediatr.* 2009;154(6):865-868. [IIB]

221. MM.04.01.01: Medication orders are clear and accurate. In: *Comprehensive Accreditation Manual for Ambulatory Care.* Oakbrook Terrace, IL: The Joint Commission; 2015. [IVA]

222. Murphy EK. Charting by exception. *AORN J.* 2003;78(5):821-823. [VA]

223. Kerr N. "Creating a protective picture": a grounded theory of RN decision making when using a charting-by-exception documentation system. *Medsurg Nurs.* 2013;22(2):110-118. [IIIA]

224. AHIMA e-HIM Work Group on Maintaining the Legal EHR. Maintaining a legally sound health record: paper and electronic. *J AHIMA.* 2005;76(10):64A-64L. [IVB]

225. Short MS. Charting by exception on a clinical pathway. *Nurs Manage.* 1997;28(8):45-46. [IIIB]

226. Holden RJ. Cognitive performance-altering effects of electronic medical records: an application of the human factors paradigm for patient safety. *Cogn Technol Work.* 2011;13(1):11-29. [IIIB]

227. *Driving Quality and Performance Measurement—A Foundation for Clinical Decision Support: A Consensus Report.* Washington, DC: NQF; 2010.

228. Committee on Data Standards for Patient Safety Board on Health Care Services Institute of Medicine of the National Academies. *Key Capabilities of an Electronic Health Record System. Letter Report.* Washington, DC: National Academies Press; 2003. [IVA]

229. Institute of Medicine. *Digital Infrastructure for the Learning Health System: The Foundation for Continuous Improvement in Health and Health Care: Workshop Series Summary.* Washington, DC: The National Academies Press; 2011. [IVA]

230. Health Insurance Portability and Accountability Act of 1996, 42 USC §201 (1996), Pub L No. 104-191, 110 Stat 1936. [IA]

231. Modifications to the HIPAA Privacy, Security, Enforcement, and Breach Notification rules under the Health Information Technology for Economic and Clinical Health Act and the Genetic Information Nondiscrimination Act; other modifications to the HIPAA rules. *Fed Regist.* 2013;78(17):5565-5702. [IA]

232. Fernandez-Aleman JL, Senor IC, Lozoya PA, Toval A. Security and privacy in electronic health records: a systematic literature review. *J Biomed Inform.* 2013;46(3):541-562. [IIB]

233. 21 CFR §11. Electronic records; electronic signatures. US Food and Drug Administration. Department of Health and Human Services. http://www.ecfr.gov/cgi-bin/text-idx?SID=801a6a66afbc46f404bcd011da79ab5e&mc=true&tpl=/ecfrbrowse/Title21/21cfrv1_02.tpl#0. Accessed April 21, 2016. [IA]

234. Accreditation Association for Ambulatory Health Care. Clinical records and health information. In: *Accreditation Handbook for Ambulatory Health Care.* Skokie, IL: The Association; 2015:49-51.

235. US Department of Health and Human Services. *Nationwide Privacy and Security Framework for Electronic Exchange of Individually Identifiable Health Information.* Washington, DC: Office of the National Coordinator for Health Information Technology; 2008. https://www.healthit.gov/sites/default/files/nationwide-ps-framework-5.pdf. Accessed April 21, 2016. [IA]

236. Connecting for Health Work Group on Consumer Access Policies for Networked Personal Health Information. *Security and Systems Requirements.* New York, NY: Markle Foundation; 2008. [IVA]

237. 16 CFR §318. Health breach notification rule. US Federal Trade Commission. https://www.ftc.gov/enforcement/rules/rulemaking-regulatory-reform-proceedings/health-breach-notification-rule. Accessed April 21, 2016. [IA]

238. RI.01.03.03: The hospital honors the patient's right to give or withhold informed consent to produce or use recordings, films, or other images of the patient for purposes other than his or her care. In: *Comprehensive Accreditation Manual for Hospitals.* Oakbrook Terrace, IL: The Joint Commission; 2015. [IVA]

239. RI.01.03.01: The hospital honors the patient's right to give or withhold informed consent. In: *Comprehensive Accreditation Manual for Hospitals.* Oakbrook Terrace, IL: The Joint Commission; 2015. [IVA]

240. The AMA Code of Medical Ethics' opinion on computerized medical records. *Virtual Mentor.* 2011;13(3):161-162. [IVB]

241. *Nursing Informatics: Scope and Standards of Practice.* 2nd ed. Silver Spring, MD: American Nurses Association; 2014. [IVA]

242. RC.01.02.01. Entries in the clinical record are authenticated. In: *Comprehensive Accreditation Manual for Ambulatory Care.* Oakbrook Terrace, IL: The Joint Commission; 2015. [IVA]

243. RC.01.04.01: The hospital audits its medical records. In: *Comprehensive Accreditation Manual for Hospitals.* Oakbrook Terrace, IL: The Joint Commission; 2015. [IVA]

244. Public Law 106-229: Electronic Signatures in Global and National Commerce Act. https://www.gpo.gov/fdsys/pkg/PLAW-106publ229/content-detail.html. Accessed April 21, 2016. [IA]

245. RC.01.05.01: The hospital retains its medical records. In: *Comprehensive Accreditation Manual for Hospitals.* Oakbrook Terrace, IL: The Joint Commission; 2015. [IVA]

246. RC.01.05.01: The organization retains its clinical records. In: *Comprehensive Accreditation Manual for Ambulatory Care.* Oakbrook Terrace, IL: The Joint Commission; 2015. [IVA]

247. Campbell EM, Sittig DF, Guappone KP, Dykstra RH, Ash JS. Overdependence on technology: an unintended adverse consequence of computerized provider order entry. *AMIA Annu Symp Proc.* 2007: 94-98. [IIIB]

248. Drass R, Free J. Planning for the unknown: maintaining your network infrastructure during a disaster. *Health Manag Technol.* 2014;35(2):18-20.

249. Rector M. Improving disaster recovery outcomes. Healthcare data must be protected to conform to HIPAA requirements, which active archive supports through the expanded role of tape. *Health Manag Technol.* 2012;33(3):16-17. [VB]

250. *SAFER Guide: High Priority Practices.* HealthIT.gov. http://www.healthit.gov/sites/safer/files/guides/safer_highprioritypractices_sg001_form_0.pdf. Accessed April 20, 2016. [IA]

251. Agrawal A, Glasser AR. Barcode medication. Administration implementation in an acute care hospital and lessons learned. *J Healthc Inf Manag.* 2009;23(4):24-29. [VA]

252. *Amendments, Corrections, and Deletions in the Electronic Health Record Toolkit.* Chicago, IL: American Health Information Management Association; 2009. [IVB]

253. Weis JM, Levy PC. Copy, paste, and cloned notes in electronic health records; prevalence, benefits, risks, and best practice recommendations. *Chest.* 2014;145(3):632-638. [VA]

254. Peterson AM. Medical record as a legal document part 1: setting the standards. *J Legal Nurse Consult.* 2012;23(2):9-17. [VA]

255. Medical records. *Operating Room Risk Management.* 2008;1(Medical Records 3). [IVB]

256. Bredfeldt CE, Awad EB, Joseph K, Snyder MH. Training providers: beyond the basics of electronic health records. *BMC Health Serv Res.* 2013;13:503. [IIB]

257. Sittig DF, Singh H. Rights and responsibilities of users of electronic health records. *CMAJ.* 2012;184(13):1479-1483. [IVB]

258. Tahim A, Sabharwal S, Dhokia R, Bajekal R, Kyriacou S. Data protection training improves data handling. *Clinical Teacher.* 2012;9(6):403-407. [IIIB]

259. Bruylands M, Paans W, Hediger H, Muller-Staub M. Effects on the quality of the nursing care process through an educational program and the use of electronic nursing documentation. *Int J Nurs Knowl.* 2013;24(3):163-170. [IIA]

260. Clark JS, Delgado VA, Demorsky S, et al. Assessing and improving EHR data quality (updated). *J AHIMA.* 2013;84(3):48-53. [IVB]

261. Russo R; American Health Information Management Association. *Clinical Documentation Improvement.* Chicago, IL: AHIMA, American Health Information Management Association; 2010. [IVB]

262. Agaku IT, Adisa AO, Ayo-Yusuf OA, Connolly GN. Concern about security and privacy, and perceived control over collection and use of health information are related to withholding of health information from healthcare providers. *J Am Med Inform Assoc.* 2014;21(2):374-378. [IIIA]

263. Gajanayake R, Iannella R, Sahama T. Privacy oriented access control for electronic health records. *Electronic Journal of Health Informatics.* 2014;8(2):e15. [IIIB]

264. Berretoni A, Bochantin F, Brown T, et al. HIM functions in healthcare quality and patient safety. *J AHIMA.* 2011;82(8):42-45. [IVB]

265. Hersh W. Copy and paste. *AHRQ WebM&M* [serial online]. https://psnet.ahrq.gov/webmm/case/157. Published July/August 2007. Accessed April 21, 2016. [VA]

266. Singh H, Ash JS, Sittig DF. Safety Assurance Factors for Electronic Health Record Resilience (SAFER): study protocol. *BMC Med Inform Decis Mak.* 2013;13:46. [VA]

267. Clancy CM. Nursing, system design, and health care quality. *AORN J.* 2009;90(4):581-583. [VA]

268. *SAFER Guide: Organizational Responsibilities.* HealthIT.gov. https://www.healthit.gov/safer/guide/sg002. Accessed April 21, 2016. [IA]

269. Magrabi F, Ong M-S, Runciman W, Coiera E. An analysis of computer-related patient safety incidents to inform the development of a classification. *J Am Med Inform Assoc.* 2010;17(6):663-670. [IIA]

270. Nunn S. Managing audit trails. *J AHIMA.* 2009;80(9):44-45. [VC]

271. Haugen MB, Herrin B, Slivochka S, Tolley LM, Warner D, Washington L. Rules for handling and maintaining metadata in the EHR. *J AHIMA.* 2013;84(5):50-54. [IVB]

272. *SAFER Guide: Contingency Planning.* HealthIT.gov. https://www.healthit.gov/safer/guide/sg003. Accessed April 21, 2016. [IA]

273. *SAFER Guide: System Interfaces.* HealthIT.gov. https://www.healthit.gov/safer/guide/sg005. Accessed April 21, 2016. [IA]

274. Zoraster RM, Burkle CM. Disaster documentation for the clinician. *Disaster Med Public Health Prep.* 2013;7(4):354-360. [VA]

Acknowledgements

LEAD AUTHOR
Sharon Giarrizzo-Wilson, MS, RN-BC, CNOR
President and CEO
SymQuality Consulting, LLC
Denver, Colorado

CONTRIBUTING AUTHOR
Ramona L. Conner, MSN, RN, CNOR
Editor-in-Chief, Guidelines for Perioperative Practice
AORN Nursing Department
Denver, Colorado

The authors and AORN thank Janice Neil, PhD, RN, CNE, Associate Professor, College of Nursing, East Carolina University, Greenville, North Carolina; Lisa Spruce, DNP, RN, CNS-CP, ACNS, ACNP, CNOR, FAAN, Director of Evidence-based Perioperative Practice, AORN Nursing Department, Denver, Colorado; Martha Stratton, MSN, MHSA, RN, CNOR, NEA-BC, Vice President of Perioperative Services, Doctors Hospital, Augusta, Georgia; Missi Merlino, MHA, RN-BC, CNOR, Staff Nurse II, Baylor Scott & White Health, Temple, Texas; and Nathalie Walker, MBA, BS, RN, CNOR, Member of the Louisiana Nursing Supply and Demand Commission, a subcommittee of the Health Works Commission of Louisiana, Metairie, for their assistance in developing this guideline.

PUBLICATION HISTORY
Originally published March 1982, *AORN Journal*, as "Recommended practices for documentation of perioperative nursing care."

Format revision July 1982.

Revised March 1987; revised September 1991; revised November 1995; published June 1996.

Revised; published January 2000, *AORN Journal*.
Reformatted July 2000.

Revised November 2011; published online as "Recommended practices for perioperative health care information management" in *Perioperative Standards and Recommended Practices*.

Reformatted September 2012 for publication in *Perioperative Standards and Recommended Practices*, 2013 edition.

Minor editing revisions made in November 2014 for publication as "Guideline for health care information management" in *Guidelines for Perioperative Practice*, 2015 edition.

Revised July 2016 for publication in *Guidelines for Perioperative Practice* online.

PATIENT CARE

GUIDELINE FOR CARE OF THE PATIENT RECEIVING LOCAL ANESTHESIA

he Guideline for Care of the Patient Receiving Local Anesthesia has been approved by the AORN Guidelines Advisory Board. It was presented as a proposed guideline for comments by members and others. The guideline is effective January 15, 2015. The recommendations in this guideline are intended to be achievable and represent what is believed to be an optimal level of practice. Policies and procedures will reflect variations in practice settings and/or clinical situations that determine the degree to which the guideline can be implemented. AORN recognizes the many diverse settings in which perioperative nurses practice; therefore, this guideline is adaptable to all areas where operative and other invasive procedures may be performed.

Purpose

This document provides guidance for the perioperative registered nurse (RN) caring for a patient who is receiving local anesthesia by injection, infiltration, or topical application. This document includes guidance for patient assessment, patient monitoring, recognition and treatment of local anesthetic systemic toxicity (LAST), assessment for local anesthetic allergies, and documentation of patient care. It is not the intent of this guideline to address situations that require the services of an anesthesia professional or to substitute the services of a perioperative RN in those situations that require the services of an anesthesia professional.

The goal of the perioperative team is to provide safe care without causing undue pain and anxiety to the patient receiving local anesthesia. Local anesthesia is safe and effective although, rarely, a patient may have a toxic systemic or allergic reaction to the local anesthetic. Local anesthetic systemic toxicity occurs as serum levels of the local anesthetic increase. The symptoms of LAST may present as central nervous system (CNS) or cardiovascular system (CVS) complications or both.[1-7] Although the incidence of LAST is rare,[8-11] the consequences may be severe, potentially resulting in death. Allergic reactions to local anesthetics are also rare, occurring in less than 1% of all patients who receive a local anesthetic.[12,13]

Moderate sedation analgesia and regional anesthesia are outside the scope of this document.

Evidence Review

On April 15, 2013, a medical librarian conducted a systematic search of the databases MEDLINE®, CINAHL®, and the Cochrane Database of Systematic Reviews for meta-analyses, systematic reviews, randomized controlled and non-randomized trials and studies, case reports, reviews, and guidelines from government agencies and standards-setting bodies. The librarian also searched the Scopus® database, although not systematically. The search was limited to literature published in English since January 2006. At the time of the initial search, the librarian established weekly alerts on the search topics and until July 2014, presented relevant results to the lead author. During the development of this guideline, the author requested supplementary literature searches and additional literature that either did not fit the original search criteria or was discovered during the evidence-appraisal process.

Although the lead author's original search request encompassed both moderate sedation and local anesthesia, only literature relevant to the care and management of patients receiving local anesthesia was considered for inclusion in this document. Of the 862 sources deemed appropriate for consideration in the areas of moderate sedation and local anesthesia, 63 were identified as relevant to local anesthesia (Figure 1). Germane search terms included *surgical procedures, analgesia, local anesthesia, topical anesthesia, local infiltration, lidocaine, bupivacaine, anxiety, anti-anxiety agents, drug hypersensitivity, allergy, anaphylaxis, risk assessment, physical examination, vital signs, blood pressure, blood pressure determination, pulse, physiologic monitoring, advanced cardiac life support, ACLS, nurse's role,* and *perioperative nursing.*

Excluded were non-peer-reviewed publications and studies that addressed moderate sedation, regional anesthesia, pediatric patients, or pregnant patients. Low-quality evidence was excluded when higher-quality evidence was available.

Articles identified in the search were provided to the lead author and divided and assigned to four evidence reviewers for review and critical appraisal using the AORN Research or Non-Research Evidence Appraisal Tools as appropriate. The lead author and the evidence reviewers independently evaluated and appraised the literature according to the strength and quality of the evidence. Each article was then assigned an appraisal score determined by consensus. The appraisal score is noted in brackets after each reference, as applicable.

The evidence supporting each intervention and activity statement within a specific recommendation was summarized, and the AORN Evidence-Rating Model was used to rate the strength of the collective evidence. Factors considered in review of the collective evidence were the quality of evidence, the quantity of similar evidence on a given topic, and the consistency of evidence supporting a recommendation. The evidence rating is noted in brackets after each intervention.

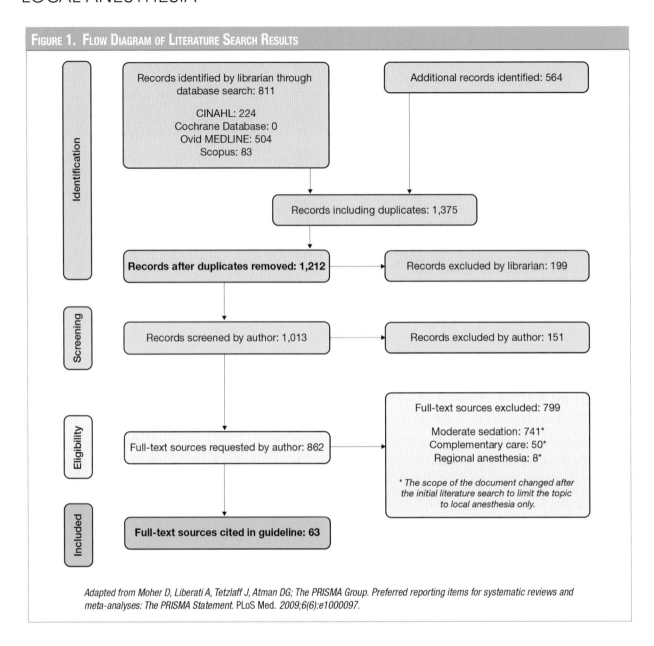

FIGURE 1. FLOW DIAGRAM OF LITERATURE SEARCH RESULTS

Identification

Records identified by librarian through database search: 811

CINAHL: 224
Cochrane Database: 0
Ovid MEDLINE: 504
Scopus: 83

Additional records identified: 564

Records including duplicates: 1,375

Records after duplicates removed: 1,212

Records excluded by librarian: 199

Screening

Records screened by author: 1,013

Records excluded by author: 151

Eligibility

Full-text sources requested by author: 862

Full-text sources excluded: 799

Moderate sedation: 741*
Complementary care: 50*
Regional anesthesia: 8*

The scope of the document changed after the initial literature search to limit the topic to local anesthesia only.

Included

Full-text sources cited in guideline: 63

Adapted from Moher D, Liberati A, Tetzlaff J, Atman DG; The PRISMA Group. Preferred reporting items for systematic reviews and meta-analyses: The PRISMA Statement. PLoS Med. 2009;6(6):e1000097.

Note: *The evidence summary table is available at* http://www.aorn.org/evidencetables/.

Editor's note: *MEDLINE is a registered trademark of the US National Library of Medicine's Medical Literature Analysis and Retrieval System, Bethesda, MD. CINAHL, Cumulative Index to Nursing and Allied Health Literature, is a registered trademark of EBSCO Industries, Birmingham, AL. Scopus is a registered trademark of Elsevier B.V., Amsterdam, The Netherlands.*

Recommendation I

The perioperative RN should perform a preoperative nursing assessment for the patient who will receive local anesthesia.

Patient assessment before an intervention is a standard of perioperative nursing practice.[14] The American Nurses Association's *Nursing: Scope and Standards of Practice*[15] and the AORN "Standards of perioperative

nursing"[14] direct the RN to collect patient health data that are relevant to the patient's care.

The collective evidence suggests that the preoperative patient assessment should include of a review of the patient's history that includes the cardiac, renal, and hepatic systems.[7,10,16] In addition to the total dose of the local anesthetic, cardiac, renal, or hepatic dysfunction are factors to consider when calculating local anesthetic plasma levels.[1,7,10,16]

The benefits of performing a nursing assessment outweigh the harms. Benefits include the ability to identify allergies and comorbid conditions that might affect the absorption of the local anesthetic; obtain baseline measures of vital signs, pain, and anxiety; and evaluate the patient's level of consciousness.

A limitation of the evidence is that no research studies were found that addressed preoperative nursing assessment of the patient receiving local anesthesia. Research is needed to define the exact elements that should be assessed before surgery.

I.a. The preoperative nursing assessment should include a review of the patient's
- allergies and sensitivities (eg, medications, tape, latex)[17];
- age;
- height, weight, and body mass index;
- current medications and use of alternative/complementary therapies[18];
- NPO status[19];
- medical history (eg, history and physical, progress note)[7,19];
- laboratory test results[17];
- diagnostic test results[17];
- baseline cardiac status (eg, heart rate, blood pressure)[6,17];
- baseline respiratory status (eg, rate, rhythm, blood oxygen level [SpO_2])[17];
- baseline skin condition for integrity (eg, rash, breaks, ecchymosis)[17];
- baseline neurological status[6,17];
- sensory impairments (eg, visual, auditory)[17];
- ability to tolerate the required operative position with draping for the duration of the procedure[17];
- level of anxiety[17];
- level of pain[17];
- perceptions of surgery[17]; and
- need for intravenous access.

[2: High Evidence]

The collective evidence indicates that preoperative patient assessment provides important information regarding underlying conditions (eg, cardiac,[1,3,6,7,8,10,20,21] hepatic,[1,3,6,8,20] renal[3,20]) that may affect the patient's ability to metabolize the local anesthetic and place him or her at risk for developing LAST.[6] Preoperative vital signs provide a baseline reference for comparison if there is an adverse reaction to the local anesthetic. A systematic review[8] and seven literature reviews[1,3,6,7,10,20,21] describe underlying conditions that place a patient at increased risk for developing LAST.

I.b. The perioperative RN should use a physical acuity assessment tool (eg, the American Society of Anesthesiologists Physical Status Classification [Table 1][19,22] to determine patient acuity. *[3: Moderate Evidence]*

Use of a physical assessment tool with interrater reliability provides an objective and consistent means for assessing the patient's acuity.

I.b.1. If the perioperative RN identifies a concern regarding the patient's acuity, the RN should consult with the physician to determine the plan of care. *[5: Benefits Balanced with Harms]*

I.c. Based on the patient assessment (ie, acuity, anxiety level), the type of procedure,[23,24] and the health care organization policy,[14] the perioperative RN should identify the personnel needed to implement the plan of care (eg, an additional RN to monitor). At a minimum, one perioperative RN circulator should be dedicated to each patient undergoing an operative or other invasive procedure and should be present during that patient's entire intraoperative experience.[25] *[3: Moderate Evidence]*

AORN is committed to the provision of safe perioperative nursing care by ensuring that every patient undergoing an operative or other invasive procedure is cared for by minimum of one RN in the circulating role. The perioperative RN works collaboratively with other perioperative professionals (eg, surgeons, anesthesia professionals, surgical technologists) to meet patient needs, the perioperative RN is accountable for the patient's outcomes resulting from the nursing care provided during the operative or other invasive procedure. Using clinical knowledge, judgment, and clinical-reasoning skills based on scientific principles, the perioperative RN plans and implements nursing care to address the physical, psychological, and spiritual responses of the patient undergoing an operative or other invasive procedure.[25]

TABLE 1. PHYSICAL STATUS CLASSIFICATION

Status	Definition of patient status	Example
P1	A normal healthy patient	No physiologic, psychological, biochemical, or organic disturbance.
P2	A patient with mild systemic disease	Cardiovascular disease, asthma, chronic bronchitis, obesity, or diabetes mellitus.
P3	A patient with severe systemic disease	Cardiovascular or pulmonary disease that limits activity; severe diabetes with systemic complications; history of myocardial infarction, angina pectoris, or poorly controlled hypertension.
P4	A patient with severe systemic disease that is a constant threat to life	Severe cardiac, pulmonary, renal, hepatic, or endocrine dysfunction.
P5	A moribund patient who is not expected to survive without the operation	Surgery is done as a last recourse or resuscitative effort; major multi-system or cerebral trauma, ruptured aneurysm, or large pulmonary embolus.
P6	A declared brain-dead patient whose organs are being removed for donor purposes	

Reproduced with permission from the American Society of Anesthesiologists, Park Ridge, IL.

A practice guideline by the American Society of Anesthesiologists (ASA)[23] and one literature review[24] support the need for adequate staffing. The number and qualifications of nurses are not delineated in the literature for the care of the patient receiving a local anesthetic. This issue warrants further research. The ASA practice guideline states that there should be an adequate number of personnel (eg, licensed and qualified nurses) to meet the patient's needs for all procedures performed.[23] The literature review supports the practice guideline and recommends adequate staffing levels.[24]

Recommendation II

The perioperative RN should monitor and document the patient's physiological and psychological responses, identify nursing diagnoses based on assessment of the data, and implement the plan of care.

Patient assessment, diagnosis, and implementation are standards of perioperative nursing practice.[14] The American Nurses Association's *Nursing: Scope and Standards of Practice*[15] and the AORN "Standards of perioperative nursing"[14] direct the RN to collect patient health data that are relevant to the patient's situation (eg, surgical or invasive procedure), analyze the assessment data, and implement nursing interventions.

Monitoring of the patient's physiological and psychological status may lead to early detection of potential complications.[19] Changes in the patient's cardiac rhythm and rate, blood pressure, and mental status may be early manifestations of LAST.

Monitoring parameters and frequency are unresolved issues that warrant further research. Clark[6] advocated for monitoring vital signs before the procedure and then at five-minute intervals. Kosh et al[28] recommended taking the vital signs before patient discharge.

The collective evidence supports monitoring and interpreting the patient's physiological and psychological responses while he or she is receiving a local anesthetic during a procedure. One practice guideline[16] and nine literature reviews[1,4,5,7,11,20,26-28] describe the signs and symptoms of LAST.

The limitations of the evidence are that no studies were found that identify the parameters that should be monitored or the optimal frequency for monitoring. Further research is needed.

The benefits of patient monitoring outweigh the harms. Benefits include early detection of symptoms of LAST or allergic reaction, pain, and anxiety.

II.a. The perioperative RN should determine data collection priorities based on the patient's condition and needs and the procedure to be performed. Data collection should include the parameters to be monitored (eg, heart rate and rhythm, blood pressure, level of consciousness), the frequency (eg, baseline,[6] after local anesthetic administration, every five[6] to 15 minutes,

postprocedure,[28] before discharge[29]), and documentation. *[3: Moderate Evidence]*

In the case of *Messer v Martin,* the court upheld the standard of care to monitor the patient's vital signs during and after a procedure performed with the patient under local anesthesia. In this case, a patient underwent a surgical procedure with local anesthesia and then fainted in the elevator after leaving the clinic. The patient filed suit against the physician, the clinic, and the professional liability carrier for neglecting to monitor the patient's postoperative vital signs and was granted summary judgment. An expert RN witness stated in a deposition that the standard of care was to monitor the patient's vital signs. The assigned nurse failed to monitor the vital signs during or after the procedure.[29]

II.a.1. Baseline patient monitoring[7] and documentation should include
- pulse,
- blood pressure,[6,28]
- respiratory rate,[19]
- SpO_2 by pulse oximetry,[6,19]
- pain level,
- anxiety level, and
- level of consciousness.[6,28]
[3: Moderate Evidence]

II.a.2. Intraoperative and postoperative patient monitoring[7] and documentation should include
- pain level,
- anxiety level, and
- level of consciousness.[6,28]
[3: Moderate Evidence]

II.a.3. Intraoperative and postoperative patient monitoring[7] and documentation may include
- pulse,
- blood pressure,[6,28]
- heart rhythm and rate,
- respiratory rate,[19] and
- SpO_2 by pulse oximetry.[6,19]
[3: Moderate Evidence]

Recommendation III

The perioperative RN should receive initial and ongoing education and competency verification on his or her understanding of local anesthesia pharmacology, calculation of total dose, contraindications, desired effects, adverse effects, and resuscitation.

The collective evidence supports that perioperative RNs should have knowledge of the local anesthetic medication's indications for use, contraindications, desired effects, and adverse effects. Local anesthetics produce the desired effect of pain relief by preventing the generation and conduction of nerve impulses by the peripheral nervous system and the CNS.[1,11,30] Although LAST and allergic reactions are rare events, early detection and treatment can lead to a better outcome for the patient. Early recognition of an adverse

TABLE 2. LOCAL ANESTHETIC CLASSIFICATION, ONSET, AND DURATION

Local Anesthetic	Classification	Onset	Duration
Bupivacaine[1]	Aminoamide	Slow	Long
Lidocaine[1]	Aminoamide	Fast	Medium
Mepivacaine[1]	Aminoamide	Fast	Medium
Prilocaine[2]	Aminoamide	Fast	Medium
Procaine[2]	Aminoester	Slow	Short
Ropivacaine[1]	Aminoamide	Slow	Long
Tetracaine[1]	Aminoester	Slow	Long

REFERENCES

1. Culp Jr WC, Culp WC. Practical application of local anesthetics. J Vasc Interv Radiol. 2011;22(2):111-118.
2. Jackson T, McLure HA. Pharmacology of local anesthetics. Ophthalmol Clin North Am. 2006;19(2):155-161.

reaction that could lead to LAST,[16] cessation of the local anesthetic injection, and treatment may prevent symptom progression.[4,10]

The limitations of the evidence are that no studies were found that have investigated the perioperative RN's knowledge of local anesthetics as a risk factor for the patient's development of LAST or allergic reaction. Further research is needed to define the role of the perioperative RN in early detection of LAST and adverse medication reactions (eg, allergy).

The benefits of the perioperative RN knowing the local anesthetic medication's indications for use, contraindications, desired effects, and adverse effects outweigh the harms. Benefits include the potential for early detection and treatment of LAST and allergic reactions.

III.a. The perioperative RN should receive initial and ongoing education and competency verification on the local anesthetic recommended dose, onset, and duration of action.[18] [3: Moderate Evidence]

Four literature reviews[1,4,11,30] describe local anesthetic duration and onset. Local anesthetics have different durations of action depending on their affinity for protein and the length of time the local anesthetic is near the neural fibers.[1,30] Constriction of the blood vessels in the area delays absorption. Adding a vasopressor (eg, epinephrine) to the local anesthetic will delay absorption and prolong the effect.[4,30]

Local anesthetics can be classified into two groups: aminoamide and aminoester.[1,11] The local anesthetic's molecular structure determines its classification.[1,11] The aminoamide group includes lidocaine, bupivacaine, mepivacaine, and prilocaine.[11] The aminoester group includes tetracaine[1] and procaine.[11] Local anesthetics differ in the time to onset of action and duration (Table 2).[1,11]

III.a.1. Before administration of the local anesthetic, the perioperative RN should verify the correct dosing parameters and identify the patient-specific maximum dose by consulting either the health care organization's medication formulary, a pharmacist, a physician, or the product information sheet or other published reference material.[18] [3: Moderate Evidence]

Estimating the maximum dosage before administration of the local anesthetic,[7] using the smallest amount of local anesthetic to achieve the desired effect,[16] injecting the medication incrementally,[1,10,16,31] avoiding intravascular injection, and frequent aspiration[1,10] are important safety measures to decrease the risk of LAST.[7]

Tanawuttiwat et al[32] reported the case of a patient undergoing implantation of a cardioverter defibrillator under local anesthesia. The surgical site at the left infraclavicular area was infiltrated with 20 mL 2% lidocaine followed by another 10 mL to relieve the patient's discomfort. A contrast venogram showed an obstruction in the axillary-subclavian system. The team switched to the right side and infiltrated this site with 30 mL 2% lidocaine. While the surgeon was closing the site, the patient suffered a tonic-clonic seizure followed by pulseless electrical activity. The patient was successfully revived.

The result of the lidocaine level drawn during resuscitation was 8.7 mcg/mL. The normal value at this organization was 1.5 mcg/mL to 5.0 mcg/mL. Contributing factors were the patient's advanced heart failure and age and mixed metabolic and respiratory acidosis. The authors recommended that risk factors for lidocaine toxicity be identified before surgery.[32]

III.a.2. The perioperative RN should document the local anesthetic administered, including the
- medication,
- strength,

- total amount administered,
- route,
- time,
- expiration date,
- lot number,
- response, and
- adverse reactions.[18]

  [3: Moderate Evidence]

III.b.   The perioperative RN should know the symptoms of LAST, including

- metallic taste,[4,11,16,28]
- numbness of the tongue and lips,[1,4,11,16,20,26,28]
- auditory changes (eg, tinnitus),[4,7,11,16,20,26,28]
- light-headedness,[1,4,7,11,20,26]
- dysarthria (eg, slurred speech),[4,11,26]
- shivering,[5]
- tremors,[5]
- confusion,[11,20,26,28]
- agitation,[11,16,26]
- syncope,[20,26]
- seizures,[1,4,7,11,20,16,26,27]
- coma,[4,7,11,16]
- tachycardia/hypertension (initially),[5,7,16,20,26]
- bradycardia/hypotension (with increased toxicity),[11,16,27,28]
- ventricular arrhythmias,[4,5,16,20,26,28]
- asystole,[4,26,27] and
- respiratory arrest.[4,16,20]

[1: Strong Evidence]

Local anesthetic systemic toxicity is well documented in the literature. The evidence review included a systematic review,[8] a retrospective nonexperimental study,[9] a clinical practice guideline,[16] and 12 literature reviews that describe the signs and symptoms of LAST.[1,7,10,11,20,26,27,30,31,33-35] The collective evidence indicates that the incidence of LAST is rare[8-11] and that LAST occurs as serum levels of the local anesthetic increases, presenting as CNS and CVS complications.[1-7] No randomized controlled trials (RCTs) have studied LAST in humans, and conducting RCTs with human participants raises ethical concerns.[16,36,37]

The CNS signs and symptoms of LAST can be divided into three phases: initial, excitation, and depression. During the initial phase, patients may experience tinnitus, confusion, lightheadedness, dizziness, drowsiness, an abnormal sense of taste (eg, metallic taste), and numbness or tingling of the lips and tongue.[20] During the excitation phase, patients may experience tonic-clonic convulsions. During the depression phase, patients may experience unconsciousness, CNS depression, and respiratory arrest.[20]

The CVS signs and symptoms of LAST also can be divided into three phases. The initial phase includes hypertension and tachycardia during the CNS excitation phase. The intermediate phase includes myocardial depression, decreased cardiac output, and mild to moderate hypertension. The third, terminal phase, includes peripheral vasodilation,[20] hypotension,[7] sinus bradycardia,[20] conduction defects,[20] ventricular dysrhythmias,[20] cardiovascular collapse,[20,7] and death.[7]

Liu et al[8] conducted a systematic review of adverse drug reactions to local anesthetics. Studies included in the review were RCTs, nonrandomized controlled trials, and cross-sectional studies. The 101 articles reviewed contained 1,645 events. Lidocaine was involved in 43.17% of the events and bupivacaine was involved in 16.32% of the events. In 1,645 events, there were seven deaths.

Fuzier et al,[9] in a retrospective review, studied adverse drug reactions to local anesthetics reported to the French Pharmacovigilance System from 1995 to 2006. There were 210,017 reported adverse events. Local anesthetics were suspected in 727 reports, representing 0.3% of the total. The second most common type of adverse event from local anesthetics was neurological (eg, seizures), numbering 161 reports (22.1% of the cases). Cardiovascular events were the fourth most frequently reported at 111 (15.3% of the cases). Ropivacaine was used in 10 of the procedures. The cardiovascular events included chest discomfort, hypotension, cardiac arrest, bradycardia, tachycardia, and circulatory shock. Three of the 22 patients who experienced cardiac arrest died. Respiratory events (eg, dyspnea, bronchoconstriction, respiratory arrest) occurred in 2.8% of the cases.

In the practice advisory of the American Society of Regional Anesthesia and Pain Medicine (ASRA), Neal et al[16] reviewed human and animal experimental studies. In the classic presentation, LAST CNS excitement precedes cardiac toxicity. Examination of published case reports showed variability in the onset, signs, symptoms, and duration of LAST in nearly 40% of the cases. The authors concluded that it is critical for health care practitioners to recognize the early signs of LAST, be aware of the variability, and consider LAST for unexplained agitation, CNS depression or progressive hypotension, or bradycardia or ventricular arrhythmias. Analysis of LAST case reports demonstrated that one-third of the patients with cardiac and CNS toxicity had preexisting cardiac, neurologic, or metabolic disease (eg, diabetes, renal failure). Symptoms occurred in as little as 56 seconds to more than five minutes after injection.

Di Gregorio et al[26] retrospectively reviewed 93 published reports of LAST during a 30-year period from 1979 to 2009. The cases were analyzed for onset of toxicity and signs and symptoms. The onset of LAST generally occurred after a single injection of a local anesthetic. Onset occurred in less than one minute in more than 50% of the cases and less than five minutes in 75% of the cases. The median time for onset of signs of toxicity was 52.5 seconds. In 25% of the

TABLE 3. TREATMENT FOR LOCAL ANESTHETIC SYSTEMIC TOXICITY

- Suppress seizures (eg, with benzodiazepines)[1,2]

- Avoid vasopressin, calcium channel blockers, beta blockers, or local anesthetics[1]

- Reduce individual epinephrine doses to < 1mcg/kg[1]

- Infuse a 20% lipid emulsion[1,3]
  - Administer an IV bolus 1.5 mL/kg (lean body mass) longer than 1 minute (approximately 100 mL).[1-3]
  - Infuse at 0.25 mL/kg/minute (approximately 18 mL/minute; adjust by roller clamp)[1]
  - Repeat the bolus once or twice for persistent cardiovascular collapse.[1]
  - Double the infusion rate to 0.5 m/kg/minute if blood pressure remains low.[1]
  - Continue infusion for at least 10 minutes after attaining circulatory stability.[1]
  - The recommended upper limit is approximately 10 mL/kg lipid emulsion during the first 30 minutes.[1]

- Avoid propofol in patients showing signs of cardiovascular instability[1,4]

- Alert the nearest facility with cardiopulmonary bypass capability[1]

REFERENCES

1. Neal JM, Bernards CM, Butterworth JF 4th, et al. ASRA practice advisory on local anesthetic systemic toxicity. Reg Anesth Pain Med. 2010;35(2):152-161.
2. AAGBI Safety Guideline: Management of Severe Local Anaesthetic Toxicity. 2010. Association of Anaesthetists of Great Britain & Ireland. http://www.aagbi.org/sites/default/files/la_toxicity_2010_0.pdf. Accessed October 15, 2014.
3. Vanden Hoek TL, Morrison LJ, Shuster M, et al. Part 12: Cardiac arrest in special situations: 2010 American Heart Association guidelines for cardiopulmonary resuscitation and emergency cardiovascular care. Circulation. 2010;122(18 Suppl 3):S829-61.
4. Mercado P, Weinberg GL. Local anesthetic systemic toxicity: prevention and treatment. Anesthesiol Clin. 2011;29(2):233-242.

cases, symptoms occurred five minutes or more after initial injection. In a single case, the symptoms of LAST occurred at 60 minutes. Central nervous system symptoms were the most common manifestation of LAST, occurring in 44% of the reports; CVS symptoms occurred in 11% of the reports, and a combination of CNS and CVS symptoms occurred in 45% of the reports.

In a review of the mechanisms and toxicity of LAST, Wolfe and Butterworth[38] concluded that short-acting and lower-potency local anesthetics (eg, lidocaine, mepivacaine) depressed cardiac contractility without causing cardiac arrhythmias. The authors further concluded that longer-acting and higher-potency local anesthetics (eg, bupivacaine, levobupivacaine, ropivacaine) produced conduction defects and cardiac arrhythmias with or without reduced contractile function. A lower ratio dose of bupivacaine, levobupivacaine, and ropivacaine can produce cardiovascular toxicity versus CNS toxicity. Treatment of CNS toxicity from local anesthetics is easier and provides better chances for recovery than treatment of cardiovascular toxicity. The outcomes of cardiovascular toxicity from local anesthetics may be serious injury or death.

Byrne and Engelbrecht[20] conducted a review of the toxicity of local anesthetic agents and concluded that no dose of local anesthetic is safe if administered incorrectly (eg, intravascularly, intra-arterially). The authors found that toxicity is dependent on the absolute plasma level and the rate of the rise in the plasma level. Most incidences of toxicity are caused by intravascular injection of local anesthetic, and an intra-arterial injection is more dangerous than an IV injection. Bupivacaine, levobupivacaine, and ropivacaine are more toxic than lidocaine and prilocaine. In 17 of 20 case reports of LAST, the local anesthetic used was ropivacaine or bupivacaine.

III.c. The perioperative RN should receive initial and ongoing education and competency verification of the treatment of LAST. *[3: Moderate Evidence]*

The collective evidence indicates that early recognition of LAST symptoms and treatment are very important.[4,21,39] Initial treatment should focus on airway management.[4] Hypoxemia and acidosis intensify the effects of LAST.[4,36] Four articles describe the importance of early recognition, airway management with oxygenation, and treatment.[4,21,36,39]

III.c.1. If LAST occurs, the perioperative RN should
- call for help (eg, anesthesia professional, code team, 911),[1,10,16,40]
- help maintain the airway,[10,16,40]
- ventilate with 100% oxygen,[1,10,16,40]
- assist with basic or advanced cardiac life support,[6]
- be prepared to establish or assist with IV access,[6,16,40] and
- be prepared to assist with the administration of 20% lipid emulsion therapy.[16]

[1: Strong Evidence]

The "ASRA practice advisory on local anesthetic systemic toxicity,"[16] the Association of Anesthetists of Great Britain and Ireland's *AAGBI Safety Guideline: Management* of Severe Local Anaesthetic Toxicity,[40] and the American Heart Association's guidelines for cardiac arrest in special situations[41] provide guidance for treating LAST (Table 3).

The collective evidence indicates that early recognition and treatment of LAST symptoms with a focus on airway management are important because hypoxemia and acidosis potentiate the effects of LAST.[4,36,39]

The use of lipid emulsion therapy for the treatment of LAST started with animal testing in 1998, and the first clinical use was in 2006.[36] Current recommendations have evolved from the laboratory studies and case reports of lipid emulsion treatment for LAST.[36,42]

Although case reports[43-45] of using lipid emulsion therapy have limitations (eg, reporting only favorable outcomes; underreporting of unfavorable outcomes; variability in dosing and timing), they provide the best evidence available for the treatment of LAST.[3,36,39] Ozcan and Weinberg[39] reviewed 10 case reports in which lipid emulsion was used for bupivacaine-related LAST. The symptoms of all 10 patients resolved after treatment with lipid emulsion. The authors reviewed seven case reports that used lipid emulsion for non-bupivacaine-related LAST. The symptoms of six of the seven patients resolved after treatment. The authors concluded there is mounting clinical evidence that suggests early administration of lipid emulsion with effective cardiopulmonary resuscitation might restore circulation without the use of large doses of vasopressors.

III.c.2.   The perioperative RN should monitor the patient with LAST for signs of cardiovascular instability after the patient receives lipid emulsion therapy. *[3: Moderate Evidence]*

The recommended action is supported by a case study. After the successful resuscitation with cardiopulmonary resuscitation and lipid emulsion of a patient who received an accidental intravascular injection of bupivacaine, Marwick et al[44] reported cardiac toxicity 40 minutes after the cessation of lipid emulsion therapy. The authors attributed the cardiovascular instability to a recurrence of LAST after lipid rescue.

III.d.   The perioperative RN should receive initial and ongoing education and competency verification on recognition of the signs and symptoms of an allergic reaction to a local anesthetic, including
- anxiety,[13,46]
- bronchospasm,[46,47]
- dizziness,[13,46]
- dyspnea,[46]
- erythema,[13,48]
- edema,[13,46-48]
- heart arrhythmias (ie, tachycardia, bradycardia),[46]
- hypotension,[46-48]
- nausea,[46]
- pallor,[46]
- palpitations,[46,48]
- pruritus,[13,46-48]
- rash,[13,46,47]
- syncope,[13,46,48] and
- urticaria.[13,46-48]

[3: Moderate Evidence]

Allergic reactions to local anesthetics are rare, occurring in less than 1% of all patients who receive a local anesthetic.[12,13] The primary symptoms of an immediate allergic reaction to a local anesthetic are cutaneous and occur within a few minutes of the injection, although symptoms may occur as late as one month after the injection.[47] The evidence review included five retrospective reviews,[13,46-49] nine case reports,[50-58] and a literature review.[12] The retrospective reviews investigated the prevalence of a true local anesthetic allergy among patients who reported a hypersensitivity reaction and sought evaluation.[13,46-49]

Batinac et al[13] retrospectively reviewed and analyzed the medical records of 331 patients who were referred to the dermatology department for evaluation of their local anesthetic hypersensitivity. The aim of the study was to quantify the prevalence of a true local anesthetic allergy among the referred patients. The patients' skin was tested, and three patients (0.91%) had an allergic reaction. Most of the patients' reported adverse reactions to local anesthetics were determined not to be immune related and may have been vasovagal or anxiety reactions. Psychological stress, fear of the procedure, or fear of the injection may cause psychological symptoms that alter blood levels of stress hormones. These symptoms included altered heart rate, generalized weakness, dizziness, fainting, anxiety, and fear. The researchers concluded that allergic reactions to local anesthetics comprise less than 1% of the adverse drug reactions to local anesthetics. The true allergic reactions are type IV immune reactions.

Harboe et al[46] retrospectively reviewed the medical records of 135 patients referred to the allergy department for evaluation of adverse reactions to local anesthetics. Evaluation included a case history review, skin testing, a subcutaneous challenge test, and *in vitro* IgE analysis. Sensitivity tests were also conducted for latex, chlorhexidine, and relevant medications based on the referral information. The researchers found 1.5% of the patients had a hypersensitivity to local anesthetics and concluded that this rate was consistent with the findings of other studies. They also found that 7% of the patients had allergic reactions to the other substances tested. These results indicate that other substances should be investigated as a cause of hypersensitivity reactions to local anesthetics. Psychological reactions were common during the testing.

Saito et al[49] used the leukocyte migration test (LMT) to evaluate 43 patients who had a suspected allergy to amide-type local anesthetic agents (eg, lidocaine, bupivacaine). Twenty patients had a positive LMT for lidocaine hydrochloride. The researchers tested 15 of the positive patients with lidocaine that contained antiseptic agents (eg, parabens, sodium pyrosulfite) and found a 100% positive reaction. When tested with lidocaine hydrochloride alone, only 20% tested positive, indicating that 80% of the reactions were caused by the antiseptic not the lidocaine. Paraben additives are also in cosmetics and hair products, which may lead to sensitization from daily use.

The researchers postulated that there is a risk of a local anesthetic allergy during first-time administration because of the daily paraben sensitization by cosmetic and hair products. Another key finding was the relationship between an amide-type local anesthetic allergy and history of a medication allergy. Patients with a history of a medication allergy had a twentyfold risk of developing an amide-type local anesthetic allergy compared with patients who had no medication allergies. Based on the prevalence of antiseptic allergies, the researchers suggested that using local anesthetic agents with no antiseptics is preferred.[49]

Amado et al[59] patch tested 1,143 patients using the North American Contact Dermatitis Group Standard Allergen Tray. There were 16 cases of allergic contact dermatitis and delayed hypersensitivity to lidocaine. A patient's previous exposure to lidocaine was a factor in determining lidocaine hypersensitivity. The authors concluded that over-the-counter lidocaine products could be the source of exposure and sensitization to lidocaine. Anti-hemorrhoidal products are the most common cause of allergic contact dermatitis. Other commonly used products that contain lidocaine are antiseptics, sunburn relief gels, and pain relief preparations (eg, creams, patches, sprays).

Fuzier et al[47] analyzed documented adverse drug reactions to amide local anesthetics (ie, lidocaine, bupivacaine, ropivacaine, levobupivicaine, mepivacaine) reported to two French databases during a 12-year period. Documentation included a clear and detailed medical history with a positive skin test (eg, patch test, prick test, intradermal injection). The aim of the study was to define the clinical, allergic, and pharmacological components of the adverse drug reactions. The main symptom was skin eruptions (eg, urticaria). The symptoms occurred in as little as a few minutes to as late as one month. Six patients demonstrated cross-reactivity between amide-type local anesthetics.

Bhole et al[12] conducted a review of local allergy reactions that were a type 1 or IgE-mediated immediate hypersensitivity. They identified and analyzed 23 case series involving 2,978 patients. A true IgE-mediated allergy to a local anesthetic was demonstrated in 29 patients, which is a prevalence rate of less than 1%. Seventy-five percent of these patients were allergic to amide local anesthetics. The researchers postulated that the higher rate of allergy to amide agents compared to aminoester agents was a result of the preferred use of amide agents.

There are numerous case reports of local anesthetic allergies confirmed with the patient's medical history and patch testing.[50-58] Reported symptoms include redness,[50-52] swelling,[50,51,54,56] blistering,[50] vesicular dermatitis,[51] eczematous dermatitis,[58] urticaria,[57] itching,[57] conjunctivitis,[56] bronchospasm,[55] lightheadedness,[54] wheezing,[54] and perianal dermatitis.[51,53]

Recommendation IV

The perioperative RN should provide patient education regarding perioperative care of patients undergoing local anesthesia.

One of nursing's primary responsibilities is patient education.[14]

A limitation of the evidence is a lack of studies investigating the benefits of teaching the patient about the local anesthesia care experience.

The benefits of educating the patient outweigh the harms. Benefits include the potential for increased patient cooperation, compliance with postoperative instructions, and anxiety and pain management.

IV.a. Education information for local anesthesia patients should include
- the expected sequence of events before, during,[60] and immediately after the procedure[61];
- instructions on completing a pain level assessment (eg, visual analog scale);
- requesting additional pain relief measures during and after the procedure; and
- postoperative signs and symptoms that should be reported to a designated health care provider.
[3: Moderate Evidence]

Two literature reviews support explaining the intraoperative[60] or postoperative[61] sequence of events to the patient. Mitchell[60] suggested that patient education about the intraoperative experience may reduce anxiety. A literature review by Davis[61] suggests that explaining the sequence of perioperative events may reduce patient anxiety and help the patient establish realistic expectations.

IV.a.1. Teaching strategies should be appropriate to the patient's learning needs, language preference, culture, cognitive ability, and developmental level.[14] *[3: Moderate Evidence]*

IV.a.2. The perioperative RN should assess the patient's comprehension of new information.[17] *[2: High Evidence]*

Recommendation V

Policies and procedures for the care of the patient receiving local anesthesia should be developed, reviewed periodically, revised as necessary, and readily available in the practice setting.

Policies and procedures assist in the development of patient safety, quality assessment, and performance improvement activities. Policies and procedures establish authority, responsibility, and accountability within the organization. Policies and procedures also serve as operational guidelines that are used to minimize patient risk for injury or complications, standardize practice, direct perioperative personnel, and establish continuous performance improvement programs.

The Centers for Medicare & Medicaid Services (CMS) requires health care organizations that provide care to patients covered by Medicare and Medicaid to establish policies and procedures for patient care.[62,63] The evidence review for this guideline included the CMS regulatory requirements for policies and procedures[62,63] and two literature reviews.[6,28]

V.a. A multidisciplinary team should develop policies and procedures regarding the care of the patient receiving local anesthesia without monitoring by an anesthesia professional. *[5: Benefits Balanced with Harms]*

The evidence review found no research evidence to support or refute this recommendation. Development of policies and procedures that guide and support patient care, treatment, and services is a regulatory requirement for both hospitals and ambulatory settings.[62,63]

V.a.1. The multidisciplinary team should include representatives from perioperative nursing, surgery, anesthesia, and other health care departments as deemed necessary. *[5: Benefits Balanced with Harms]*

V.b. Policies and procedures regarding the care of the patient receiving local anesthesia should include
- patient assessment criteria;
- personnel qualifications, competencies, and certifications (eg, certified basic life support, certified advanced cardiovascular life support)[16,40];
- staffing requirements[23];
- monitoring (ie, parameters, frequency);
- risk assessment and criteria for consultation with an anesthesia professional;
- recovery and discharge criteria;
- documentation requirements (eg, vital signs, anxiety level, medication response);
- medication supplies[23] (eg, lipid emulsion, resuscitation medications);
- emergency equipment (eg, supplemental oxygen, suction apparatus, resuscitation)[23,62];

- emergency procedures[16,40]; and
- emergency transfer protocols.[16,62]

[3: Moderate Evidence]

Three clinical practice guidelines[16,23,40] and CMS requirements[62] support portions of the policy and procedure recommendations.

V.b.1. At a minimum, personnel should be competent in basic life support.[16,40] *[1: Strong Evidence]*

Serious cardiac or respiratory complications can occur abruptly after the administration of local anesthetic medications. If the medication enters the bloodstream directly, seizures, circulatory and respiratory distress, cardiovascular collapse, or even death can result. The initial treatment of LAST is maintaining an airway and basic life support.[16,40]

Glossary

Local anesthetic systemic toxicity (LAST): An uncommon, potentially fatal, toxic reaction that occurs when the threshold blood levels of a local anesthetic are exceeded by an inadvertent, intravascular injection or slow systemic absorption of a large, extravascular volume of local anesthetic.

REFERENCES

1. Culp WC Jr, Culp WC. Practical application of local anesthetics. *J Vasc Intervent Radiol.* 2011;22(2):111-118. [VA]

2. Bern S, Akpa BS, Kuo I, Weinberg G. Lipid resuscitation: a life-saving antidote for local anesthetic toxicity. *Curr Pharm Biotechnol.* 2011;12(2):313-319. [VA]

3. Ciechanowicz S, Patil V. Lipid emulsion for local anesthetic systemic toxicity. *Anesthesiol Res Pract.* 2012;2012:131784. [VA]

4. Morau D, Ahern S. Management of local anesthetic toxicity. *Int Anesthesiol Clin.* 2010;48(4):117-140. [VB]

5. Khatri KP, Rothschild L, Oswald S, Weinberg G. Current concepts in the management of systemic local anesthetic toxicity. *Adv Anesth.* 2010;28(1):147-159. [VA]

6. Clark MK. Lipid emulsion as rescue for local anesthetic-related cardiotoxicity. *J Perianesth Nurs.* 2008;23(2):111-117. [VB]

7. Bourne E, Wright C, Royse C. A review of local anesthetic cardiotoxicity and treatment with lipid emulsion. *Local Reg Anesth.* 2010;3:11-19. [VA]

8. Liu W, Yang X, Li C, Mo A. Adverse drug reactions to local anesthetics: a systematic review. *Oral Surg, Oral Med, Oral Pathol Oral Radiol.* 2013;115(3):319-327. [IIIB]

9. Fuzier R, Lapeyre-Mestre M, Samii K, Montastruc JL; French Association of Regional Pharmacovigilance Centres. Adverse drug reactions to local anaesthetics: a review of the French pharmacovigilance database. *Drug Saf.* 2009;32(4):345-356. [IIIB]

10. Mercado P, Weinberg GL. Local anesthetic systemic toxicity: prevention and treatment. *Anesthesiol Clin.* 2011;29(2):233-242. [VA]

11. Jackson T, McLure HA. Pharmacology of local anesthetics. *Ophthalmol Clin North Am.* 2006;19(2):155-161. [VB]

12. Bhole MV, Manson AL, Seneviratne SL, Misbah SA. IgE-mediated allergy to local anaesthetics: separating

fact from perception: a UK perspective. *Br J Anaesth.* 2012;108(6):903-911. [VA]

13. Batinac T, Sotosek Tokmadzic V, Peharda V, Brajac I. Adverse reactions and alleged allergy to local anesthetics: analysis of 331 patients. *J Dermatol.* 2013;40(7):522-527. [IIIA]

14. Standards of perioperative nursing. In: *Perioperative Standards and Recommended Practices.* Denver, CO: AORN, Inc; 2014:3-18. [IVB]

15. American Nurses Association. *Nursing: Scope and Standards of Practice.* Silver Spring, MD: American Nurses Association; 2010. [IVB]

16. Neal JM, Bernards CM, Butterworth JF 4th, et al. ASRA practice advisory on local anesthetic systemic toxicity. *Reg Anesth Pain Med.* 2010;35(2):152-161. [IVA]

17. Petersen C. *Perioperative Nursing Data Set: The Perioperative Nursing Vocabulary.* 3rd ed. Denver, CO: AORN, Inc; 2011. [IVB]

18. Guideline for medication safety. In: *Guidelines for Perioperative Practice.* Denver, CO: AORN, Inc; 2015:291-329. [IVB]

19. Treasure T, Bennett J. Office-based anesthesia. *Oral Maxillofac Surg Clin North Am.* 2007;19(1):45-57. [VB]

20. Byrne K, Engelbrecht C. Toxicity of local anaesthetic agents. *Trends Anaesth Crit Care.* 2013;3(1):25-30. [VB]

21. Weinberg GL. Current concepts in resuscitation of patients with local anesthetic cardiac toxicity. *Reg Anesth Pain Med.* 2002;27(6):568-575. [VB]

22. ASA Physical Status Classification System. American Society of Anesthesiologists. http://www.asahq.org/Home/For-Members/Clinical-Information/ASA-Physical-Status-Classification-System. Accessed October 15, 2014. [VA]

23. American Society of Anesthesiologists. Guidelines for Ambulatory Anesthesia and Surgery. American Society of Anesthesiologists. http://www.asahq.org/formembers/~/media/For%20Members/documents/Standards%20Guidelines%20Stmts/Ambulatory%20Anesthesia%20and%20Surgery.ashx. Accessed October 15, 2014. [IVC]

24. Kataria T, Cutter TW, Apfelbaum JL. Patient selection in outpatient surgery. *Clin Plast Surg.* 2013;40(3):371-382. [VB]

25. *AORN Position Statement on One Perioperative Registered Nurse Circulator Dedicated to Every Patient Undergoing an Operative or Other Invasive Procedure.* AORN, In.c http://www.aorn.org/Clinical_Practice/Position_Statements/Position_Statements.aspx. Accessed October 15, 2014.

26. Di Gregorio G, Neal JM, Rosenquist RW, Weinberg GL. Clinical presentation of local anesthetic systemic toxicity: a review of published cases, 1979 to 2009. *Reg Anesth Pain Med.* 2010;35(2):181-187. [VA]

27. Fuzier R, Lapeyre-Mestre M. Safety of amide local anesthetics: new trends. *Expert Opin Drug Saf.* 2010;9(5):759-769. [VA]

28. Kosh MC, Miller AD, Michels JE. Intravenous lipid emulsion for treatment of local anesthetic toxicity. *Ther Clin Risk Manag.* 2010;6:449-451. [VC]

29. Failure to monitor local anesthesia pt. before discharge. Case on point: Messer v. Martin, 2004 WL 1171736 N.W.2d -WI(2004). *Nurs Law Regan Rep.* 2004;45(1):2. [VB]

30. Becker DE, Reed KL. Local anesthetics: review of pharmacological considerations. *Anesth Prog.* 2012;59(2):90-101. [VA]

31. Mulroy MF, Hejtmanek MR. Prevention of local anesthetic systemic toxicity. *Reg Anesth Pain Med.* 2010;35(2):177-180. [VB]

32. Tanawuttiwat T, Thisayakorn P, Viles-Gonzalez JF. LAST (Local Anesthetic Systemic Toxicity) but not least: systemic lidocaine toxicity during cardiac intervention. *J Invasive Cardiol.* 2014;26(1):E13-E15. [VB]

33. Butterworth JF 4th. Models and mechanisms of local anesthetic cardiac toxicity: a review. *Reg Anesth Pain Med.* 2010;35(2):167-176. [VA]

34. Mather LE. The acute toxicity of local anesthetics. *Expert Opin Drug Metab Toxicol.* 2010;6(11):1313-1332. [VA]

35. Conroy PH, O'Rourke J. Tumescent anaesthesia. *Surgeon.* 2013;11(4):210-221. [VA]

36. Weinberg GL. Lipid emulsion infusion: resuscitation for local anesthetic and other drug overdose. *Anesthesiology.* 2012;117(1):180-187. [VB]

37. Manavi MV. Lipid infusion as a treatment for local anesthetic toxicity: a literature review. *AANA J.* 2010;78(1):69-78. [VB]

38. Wolfe JW, Butterworth JF. Local anesthetic systemic toxicity: update on mechanisms and treatment. *Curr Opin Anaesthesiol.* 2011;24(5):561-566. [VB]

39. Ozcan MS, Weinberg G. Update on the use of lipid emulsions in local anesthetic systemic toxicity: a focus on differential efficacy and lipid emulsion as part of advanced cardiac life support. *Int Anesthesiol Clin.* 2011;49(4):91-103. [VA]

40. AAGBI Safety Guideline: Management of Severe Local Anaesthetic Toxicity. 2010. Association of Anaesthetists of Great Britain & Ireland. http://www.aagbi.org/sites/default/files/la_toxicity_2010_0.pdf. Accessed October 15, 2014. [IVC]

41. Vanden Hoek TL, Morrison LJ, Shuster M, et al. Part 12: cardiac arrest in special situations: 2010 American Heart Association Guidelines for Cardiopulmonary Resuscitation and Emergency Cardiovascular Care. *Circulation.* 2010;122(18 Suppl 3): S829-S861. [IVA]

42. Burch MS, McAllister RK, Meyer TA. Treatment of local-anesthetic toxicity with lipid emulsion therapy. *Am J Health Syst Pharm.* 2011;68(2):125-129. [VB]

43. Gallagher C, Tan JM, Foster C-G. Lipid rescue for bupivacaine toxicity during cardiovascular procedures. *Heart Int.* 2010;5(1):20-21. [VB]

44. Marwick PC, Levin AI, Coetzee AR. Recurrence of cardiotoxicity after lipid rescue from bupivacaine-induced cardiac arrest. *Anesth Analg.* 2009;108(4):1344-1346. [VA]

45. Litz RJ, Roessel T, Heller AR, Stehr SN. Reversal of central nervous system and cardiac toxicity after local anesthetic intoxication by lipid emulsion injection. *Anesth Analg.* 2008;106(5):1575-1577. [VB]

46. Harboe T, Guttormsen AB, Aarebrot S, Dybendal T, Irgens A, Florvaag E. Suspected allergy to local anaesthetics: follow-up in 135 cases. *Acta Anaesthesiol Scand.* 2010;54(5):536-542. [IIIB]

47. Fuzier R, Lapeyre-Mestre M, Mertes PM, et al. Immediate- and delayed-type allergic reactions to amide local anesthetics: clinical features and skin testing. *Pharmacoepidemiol Drug Saf.* 2009;18(7):595-601. [IIIC]

48. Grzanka A, Misiolek H, Filipowska A, Miśkiewicz-Orczyk K, Jarzab J. Adverse effects of local anaesthetics—allergy, toxic reactions or hypersensitivity. *Anestezjol Intens Ter.* 2010;42(4):175-178. [IIIB]

49. Saito M, Abe M, Furukawa T, et al. Study on patients who underwent suspected diagnosis of allergy to amide-type local anesthetic agents by the leukocyte migration test. *Allergol Int.* 2014;63(2):267-277. [IIIA]

50. Levy J, Lifshitz T. Lidocaine hypersensitivity after subconjunctival injection. *Can J Ophthalmol.* 2006;41(2):204-206. [VB]

51. Gunson TH, Greig DE. Allergic contact dermatitis to all three classes of local anaesthetic. *Contact Derm.* 2008;59(2):126-127. [VB]

52. Timmermans MW, Bruynzeel DP, Rustemeyer T. Allergic contact dermatitis from EMLA cream: concomitant sensitization to both local anesthetics lidocaine and prilocaine. *J Deutschen Dermatologischen Gesellschaft [Journal of the German Society of Dermatology].* 2009;7(3):237-238. [VA]

53. Yuen WY, Schuttelaar ML, Barkema LW, Coenraads PJ. Bullous allergic contact dermatitis to lidocaine. *Contact Derm.* 2009;61(5):300-301. [VA]

54. Haugen RN, Brown CW. Case reports: type I hypersensitivity to lidocaine. *J Drugs Dermatol.* 2007;6(12):1222-1223. [VA]

55. Caron AB. Allergy to multiple local anesthetics. *Allergy Asthma Proc.* 2007;28(5):600-601. [VC]

56. Fellinger C, Wantke F, Hemmer W, Sesztak-Greinecker G, Wohrl S. The rare case of a probably true ige-mediated allergy to local anaesthetics. *Case Rep Med.* 2013;2013:201586. [VA]

57. Gonzalez-Delgado P, Anton R, Soriano V, Zapater P, Niveiro E. Cross-reactivity among amide-type local anesthetics in a case of allergy to mepivacaine. *J Investig Allergol Clin Immunol.* 2006;16(5):311-313. [VB]

58. Wobser M, Gaigl Z, Trautmann A. The concept of "compartment allergy": prilocaine injected into different skin layers. *Allergy Asthma Clin Immunol.* 2011;7(1):7. [VB]

59. Amado A, Sood A, Taylor JS. Contact allergy to lidocaine: a report of sixteen cases. *Dermatitis.* 2007;18(4):215-220. [VB]

60. Mitchell M. Conscious surgery: influence of the environment on patient anxiety. *J Adv Nurs.* 2008;64(3):261-271. [IIIB]

61. Davis-Evans Chassidy. Alleviating anxiety and preventing panic attacks in the surgical patient. *AORN J.* 2013;97(3): 355-363. [VB]

62. *State Operations Manual Appendix L: Guidance for Surveyors: Ambulatory Surgical Centers.* Rev 99; 2014. Centers for Medicare & Medicaid Services. http://www.cms.gov/Regulations-and-Guidance/Guidance/Manuals/downloads/som107ap_l_ambulatory.pdf. Accessed October 15, 2014.

63. *State Operations Manual Appendix A: Survey Protocol, Regulations and Interpretive Guidelines for Hospitals.* Rev 105;2014. Centers for Medicare & Medicaid Services. https://www.cms.gov/Regulations-and-Guidance/Guidance/Transmittals/Downloads/R105SOMA.pdf. Accessed October 15, 2014.

Acknowledgements

LEAD AUTHOR
Mary J. Ogg, MSN, RN, CNOR
Perioperative Nursing Specialist
AORN Nursing Department
Denver, Colorado

CONTRIBUTING AUTHOR
Ramona L. Conner, MSN, RN, CNOR
Manager, Standards and Guidelines
AORN Nursing Department
Denver, Colorado

The authors and AORN thank Lisa Spruce, DNP, RN, ACNS, ACNP, ANP, CNOR, Director of Evidence-based Perioperative Practice, AORN, Inc, Denver, CO; Elayne Kornblatt Phillips, PhD-BSN, MPH, RN, Clinical Associate Professor, University of Virginia, Charlottesville, VA; Melanie F. Sandoval, PhD, RN, Research Nurse Scientist, Perioperative Services, University of Colorado, Aurora, CO; and Deborah S. Hickman, MS, RN, CNOR, CRNFA, Director, Renue Plastic Surgery, Brunswick, GA, for their assistance in developing this guideline.

PUBLICATION HISTORY
Originally published May 1984, *AORN Journal.*
Revised September 1989. Revised August 1993.
Revised November 1997; published February 1998.
Reformatted July 2000.
Revised November 2001; published April 2002, *AORN Journal.*
Revised 2006; published in *Standards, Recommended Practices, and Guidelines,* 2007 edition.
Minor editing revisions made to omit *Perioperative Nursing Data Set* codes; reformatted September 2012 for publication in *Perioperative Standards and Recommended Practices,* 2013 edition.
Revised October 2014; published in *Guidelines for Perioperative Practice,* 2015 edition.
Evidence ratings revised in *Guidelines for Perioperative Practice,* 2018 edition, to conform to the current AORN Evidence Rating Model.

GUIDELINE FOR MINIMALLY INVASIVE SURGERY

The Guideline for Minimally Invasive Surgery has been approved by the AORN Guidelines Advisory Board. It was presented as a proposed guideline for comments by members and others. The guideline is effective December 15, 2016. The recommendations in the guideline are intended to be achievable and represent what is believed to be an optimal level of practice. Policies and procedures will reflect variations in practice settings and/or clinical situations that determine the degree to which the guideline can be implemented. AORN recognizes the many diverse settings in which perioperative nurses practice; therefore, this guideline is adaptable to all areas where operative or other invasive procedures may be performed.

Purpose

This document provides guidance for creating a safe environment of care for patients undergoing minimally invasive surgical procedures. The guideline addresses distention media used during endoscopic procedures, hybrid operating rooms (ORs), magnetic resonance imaging (MRI) hybrid ORs, navigation-guided procedures, and robotic-assisted surgery. The document provides guidance to

- perioperative personnel to reduce risks to patients and perioperative team members during minimally invasive surgery (MIS) and computer-assisted technology procedures;
- perioperative registered nurses (RNs) to assist in managing distention media (eg, gas, fluid) and irrigation fluid; and
- health care organizations for incorporating advancements in technology with consideration for workplace safety and ergonomics.

Minimally invasive surgery is a technique used in most surgical specialties. This guideline was initially developed to provide guidance during the emergence of endoscopic procedures in the 1990s but has been expanded to include other emerging technologies. Computer science development has led to advances in computer software and hardware for medical devices that allow the surgeon to perform surgery through smaller incisions or no incisions by using digital images and data. Use of these new technologies requires multidisciplinary teams and departments to merge knowledge and skill mix in new environments to enhance patient outcomes. *Digital OR* is a new term used to describe the complex environment of endoscopic suites, hybrid ORs, and computer-assisted surgeries. The technological enhancements allow for improved efficiencies and management of surgical areas.

The following topics are outside the scope of this document:

- flexible endoscopic gastrointestinal procedures,
- care and cleaning of instruments and related equipment (See the AORN Guideline for Processing Flexible Endoscopes[1] and the AORN Guideline for Cleaning and Care of Surgical Instruments[2]),
- design of the physical environment (See the AORN Guideline for a Safe Environment of Care, Part 2[3]),
- surgical smoke safety (See the AORN Guideline for Surgical Smoke Safety[4]),
- fluid warming (See the AORN Guideline Prevention of Unplanned Patient Hypothermia[5] and the AORN Guideline for a Safe Environment of Care, Part 1[6]),
- patient positioning (See the AORN Guideline for Patient Positioning[7]),
- energy-generating devices (See the AORN Guideline for Safe Use of Energy-Generating Devices[8]), and
- surgical technique (eg, trocar entry techniques).

Evidence Review

In January 2016, a medical librarian conducted systematic searches of the databases MEDLINE®, CINAHL®, and Scopus® and the Cochrane Database of Systematic Reviews, limiting the results to articles published in English after 2009. During the development of this guideline, the lead author requested supplementary searches for topics not included in the original search as well as articles and other sources that were discovered during the evidence appraisal process. The lead author and the medical librarian also identified relevant guidelines from government agencies and standards-setting bodies.

Search terms included the subject headings and keywords *minimally invasive surgical procedures, robotic surgical procedures, angioscopy, morcellation, interventional magnetic resonance imaging, interventional radiography, interventional ultrasonography, angioplasty, endoscopy, cholangiography,* and *hybrid operating room,* as well as headings and keywords identifying specific procedures. Patient monitoring and procedural complications were addressed by headings and keywords that included *nursing assessment, intraoperative and postoperative complications, intraoperative and physiologic monitoring, fluid monitoring, insufflation, extravasation, pneumoperitoneum, intraabdominal pressure, TUR syndrome,* and *compartment syndrome.* Occupational risks related to minimally invasive surgery were included in the search with terms such as *human engineering, occupational injuries, ergonomics, musculoskeletal injuries,* and *occupational accidents.*

Excluded were non-peer-reviewed publications and lower-level or lower-quality evidence when higher-level or higher-quality evidence was available.

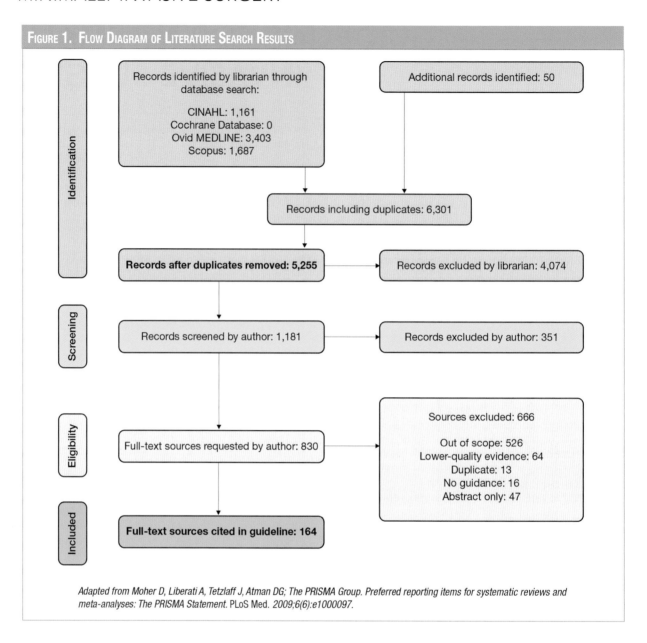

FIGURE 1. FLOW DIAGRAM OF LITERATURE SEARCH RESULTS

Records identified by librarian through database search:

CINAHL: 1,161
Cochrane Database: 0
Ovid MEDLINE: 3,403
Scopus: 1,687

Additional records identified: 50

Records including duplicates: 6,301

Records after duplicates removed: 5,255

Records excluded by librarian: 4,074

Records screened by author: 1,181

Records excluded by author: 351

Full-text sources requested by author: 830

Sources excluded: 666

Out of scope: 526
Lower-quality evidence: 64
Duplicate: 13
No guidance: 16
Abstract only: 47

Full-text sources cited in guideline: 164

Identification

Screening

Eligibility

Included

Adapted from Moher D, Liberati A, Tetzlaff J, Atman DG; The PRISMA Group. Preferred reporting items for systematic reviews and meta-analyses: The PRISMA Statement. PLoS Med. 2009;6(6):e1000097.

Surgical techniques (eg, open versus closed technique, trocar insertion, natural orifice technique, single-incision laparoscopic surgery) and anesthesia techniques (eg, goal-directed fluid therapy), endoclip migration, future product development and applications, equipment prototypes, enhanced recovery after surgery, dental navigation-guided surgery, and gastrointestinal endoscopy procedures also were excluded (Figure 1).

Articles identified in the search were provided to the project team for evaluation. The team consisted of the lead author and four evidence appraisers. The lead author divided the search results into topics and assigned members of the team to review and critically appraise each article using the AORN Research or Non-Research Evidence Appraisal Tools as appropriate. The literature was independently evaluated and appraised according to the strength and quality of the evidence. Each article was then assigned an appraisal score. The appraisal score is noted in brackets after each reference, as applicable.

The collective evidence supporting each intervention within a specific recommendation was summarized and the AORN Evidence Rating Model was used to rate the strength of the evidence. Factors considered in the review of the collective evidence were the quality of the evidence, the quantity of similar evidence on a given topic, and the consistency of evidence supporting a recommendation. The evidence rating is noted in brackets after each intervention.

Note: *The evidence summary table is available at http://www.aorn.org/evidencetables/.*

Editor's note: *MEDLINE is a registered trademark of the US National Library of Medicine's Medical Literature Analysis and Retrieval System, Bethesda, MD. CINAHL, Cumulative Index to Nursing and Allied Health Literature, is a registered trademark of EBSCO Industries, Birmingham, AL. Scopus is a registered trademark of Elsevier B.V., Amsterdam, The Netherlands.*

PATIENT CARE

Recommendation I

Health care organizations should establish a multidisciplinary team to create an efficient, safe environment for minimally invasive procedures.

Experts agree on the need for a multidisciplinary team to plan the design and workflow of the minimally invasive OR environment.[3,9-12]

Strong et al[13] described creating a committee composed of representatives from hospital administration and physician and nursing leadership to review ethical considerations for implementing new technologies and new techniques in surgery. In an effort to improve quality, this committee reviewed new devices and procedures, approved the introduction of new devices into the health care system, provided uniform credentialing standards, and reviewed early patient outcomes.

I.a. The multidisciplinary team, including perioperative RNs, physicians, surgical technologists, infection preventionists, biomedical engineers, and other members of the health care team, should plan the room configuration. *[5: Benefits Balanced With Harms]*

In describing their experience with developing an endoscopic surgical suite at the International Neuroscience Institute in Hanover, Germany, Samii and Gerganov[9] stated that "a dedicated endoscopic OR should provide work flow optimization, ergonomics, and highest safety standards for the patient."

In a literature review regarding endourology ORs, Sabnis et al[10] provided a description of an optimal endoscopy suite. The review authors recommended a surgical suite 60 m² to 70 m² in size to provide adequate space for multiple ceiling booms, fluoroscopy equipment, an ultrasonography machine, a laser machine, irrigation pumps, and an integrated technologies system to record and archive data from cameras and imaging equipment. The authors described advances in data relay systems that create a seamless two-way communication between the ORs and electronic medical records, a radiological picture archiving and communication system, and classrooms or auditoriums anywhere in the world. The authors recommended installing ceiling-mounted equipment booms to improve efficiency, reduce clutter, and interconnect equipment. They also recommended reducing tripping hazards by providing electrical outlets close to the location of the equipment stored on the shelves and providing video display monitors in all four quadrants of the room for nurses, assistants, surgical technologists, and anesthesiologists to keep the team focused on the surgical procedure.

I.a.1. The room configuration plan should include
- access to the patient and surgical field;
- placement of equipment booms, video monitors, and overhead lights to reduce distractions[11] and ergonomic hazards specific to MIS (ie, slips, trips, falls in low lighting, collisions);
- an adequate quantity of dedicated electrical circuits and appropriate placement and connection of power cords and cables;
- systems to evacuate and filter surgical smoke during the MIS procedure and at the end of the procedure when the pneumoperitoneum is released;
- methods to control and minimize traffic; and
- collaboration with vendors to achieve medical device intraoperability.

[5: Benefits Balanced With Harms]

Equipment booms provide shelving, electrical outlets, and medical gas ports to improve ergonomics and safety related to the multiple cords and tubing required to perform minimally invasive procedures. Installation of overhead ceiling-mounted arms to support the video monitors improves the ability of the surgical team to view the endoscopic images. Integration systems used for routing and switching images to and from the OR environment also provide archiving capabilities that can be used for patient teaching, remote viewing, and creating educational materials for the health care team members. The focus of the multidisciplinary team is to use these technologies to enhance the quality and safety of surgery.[9,10]

Problems with equipment may be a source of distraction for the surgical team. In a facility observation of endourological procedures, Persoon et al[11] measured the level of observed interference with the main task of the surgical team. The authors also interviewed eight urologists and seven residents on the effects of distracting factors. During the 78 procedures that were observed, a median of 20 distracting events occurred per procedure. The researchers calculated that there was one distraction every 1.8 minutes during the procedure. Equipment problems (ie, availability and failure) were the most frequently observed distraction and were identified by the physicians as a source of distraction. The problem of equipment failure in endoscopic surgery demonstrates the need for education, policies, and programs to introduce new technologies to the perioperative team.

The collective evidence identified the need to improve ergonomics in laparoscopic procedures.[14-16]

Choi[14] performed a literature review of the ergonomic challenges of laparoscopic surgery. Surgical personnel encounter physical stress in the head, neck, and shoulders caused by static postures and awkward body positions. Items that create ergonomic challenges include the OR bed position, the position of monitor(s), hand held instruments, the position of foot pedal(s), cognitive challenges (eg, lack of direct viewing of the surgical field and interpretation of the camera angle to images on the video monitor), and the position of equipment cart(s). The author provided a table summarizing the literature on ergonomic considerations for the laparoscopic OR. This review highlighted the need to understand the effects of advanced technology in the OR.

Stavroulis et al[15] conducted a cross sectional survey of 27 theatre personnel at a tertiary referral hospital in the United Kingdom about their experiences with working in integrated and nonintegrated operating theatres. The respondents rated survey items from 1 (poor) to 10 (excellent) regarding everyday tasks, interaction with the medical team, perception of teamwork, stress, and overall satisfaction. The theatre team members had high satisfaction scores related to working in the integrated theatre and believed that this environment resulted in greater efficiency, better teamwork, and reduced stress levels. The limitations of this study were a small sample size and that the questionnaire was not a validated tool.

I.b.   A representative of the health care organization's information technology department should be consulted and should identify information system requirements before new technologies are purchased. *[4: Limited Evidence]*

The American Society of Gastrointestinal Endoscopy (ASGE) Technology Committee reviewed existing, new, and emerging endoscopic technologies.[17] The review featured information about image quality, storage and retrieval systems, ease of use, and safety considerations. The authors recommended that hospitals assess device compatibility with existing systems, type of image capture (eg, standard definition versus high definition), integration with electronic medical record systems, and centralized storage and archiving systems when purchasing an image management system.

Medical devices usually have proprietary interfaces, and it can be a challenge to manage a system that contains components from multiple manufacturers. Rockstroh et al[18] developed a concept for a data storage system to address the inability to easily retrieve data collected from multiple sources in the intraoperative environment. The researchers developed a surgical data recorder prototype to be used in neurosurgical procedures for removal of brain tumors. Data were transmitted and collected from the microscope, navigation equipment, intraoperative ultrasound, and electrophysio-

logical workstation for measurement of evoked potentials. The surgical data recorder was able to store the generated data correctly, completely, and quickly even when more data than expected were sent to the system. The data could be stored in one location for easier retrieval and analysis. Working with the information technology representative for the health care facility early in the product selection process can provide insight into the compatibility of the equipment within the existing system.

I.b.1.   The image capture system must comply with Health Insurance Portability and Accountability Act requirements.[19-21] *[1: Regulatory Requirement]*

I.b.2.   Remote telecommunications technology requirements should be identified that meet the health care organization strategic plan. *[3: Moderate Evidence]*

The collective evidence describes the benefits of telecommunication and telementoring in training, mentoring, and teaching.[17,22-25]

Anderson et al[22] described the use of integrated endourology suites for remote monitoring and supervision of urology residents. The researchers surveyed 100 patients on their satisfaction after surgery in which a junior urology resident performed the procedure and the attending surgeon observed the procedure in a control room equipped with live visual, audio, and telestration communication. The patient satisfaction mean scores were 9.5 out of 10 (ie, highly satisfied) regarding their comfort with having the procedure performed under remote monitoring and supervision. The researchers reported that most patients scored their satisfaction as greater than 7 for comfort with hearing the conversation between the supervising surgeon and resident over the speakers, having a urology resident perform the procedure, having a video camera in the room, and having other residents and medical students watch the procedure and with the privacy provided during the procedure. The researchers proposed using an integrated endourology suite and remote monitoring and supervision as an option to meet training criteria for residents and to promote efficiency, regulatory compliance, safety, and productivity.

Telecommunication has emerged as an alternative to physical presence as a mentoring tool. Santomauro et al[23] studied the use of teleconferencing for proctoring and mentoring surgeons. The authors proposed a pathway for adoption of a telementoring system for surgeon learning. They described the benefits of this technology in providing support and increasing surgeon confidence.

They reported that extensive evidence demonstrated that surgeon volume affected outcomes (ie, a surgeon who performs a high volume of a procedure will have fewer complications). Allowing the high-volume surgeon access to an integrated OR via video and two-way communication provides support to and promotes confidence in a surgeon who may perform fewer procedures (eg, robotic-assisted prostatectomy). Current limitations in telecommunication systems include lag time of signals, insufficient virtual private network bandwidth, inaccuracy of telestration marks on tissue, and medicolegal issues. Improvement in these areas could widen the adoption of a telementoring system.

I.c. The multidisciplinary team should create a room layout with equipment positions for MIS systems based on procedure type(s), physical configuration, and recommendations by the equipment manufacturers. *[2: High Evidence]*

The increase in equipment needed to provide minimally invasive procedures presents challenges to the perioperative team. The collective evidence reflects a need to standardize room setups to improve efficiency, decrease distractions, and improve the safety of patient care.[9-11,14-17,26-34]

The use of ceiling-mounted booms and video monitors is one solution. Nocco and del Torchio[27] conducted a survey of 17 surgeons and nine nurses at one facility in Italy before and after the installation of an integrated OR. The participants agreed that the features of the integrated OR improved quality, reduced risk, and reduced surgical time.

Al-Hakim[29] observed MIS surgeries (N = 17) in one facility and recorded all events that disrupted the operative time. The researchers divided the disruptive events into general categories: prerequisite requirements, work design, communication, and other. Work design events included problems with the OR bed and patient positioning, arrangement of instrumentation and materials, poor lighting, visual quality of monitors, and clothing (eg, lead aprons). The analysis showed that disruptions in the work design, such as an incorrect patient position or equipment failure, prolonged operative time and were recorded most frequently as disruptions to the procedure. The operative time was affected 15% of the time from personnel failure to follow work design protocols.

Klein et al[35] conducted a two-part randomized controlled trial to examine coping strategies associated with the performance of laparoscopic skills. *Strain coping* was defined as straining to use cognitive resources under stressful conditions. The researchers enlisted 48 undergraduate students as participants to help ensure an adequate sample size and variability (n = 24 men, n = 24 women). The students were tasked with performing a laparoscopic maneuver using a simulator. The researchers studied the coping skills of one group of students during a 45-minute peg-transfer task under a low-strain condition with a top camera view of 90 degrees. The second group worked under a high-strain condition with the camera view was rotated to 135 degrees. The 135-degree view created distortion and increased the difficulty of completing the peg maneuver in the specified time frame. Participants experienced strain coping in the group that worked with the extreme camera angle.

In the second part of the study, the researchers assessed the effects of monitoring displayed vital signs on the ability to complete the peg maneuver in the specified time frame. Three 33.02-cm monitors were located 59 cm behind the trainer box, 104.14 cm above the ground, and approximately 124 cm from the participant's eyes. The students were randomly assigned into groups of four men and four women to one of three different display conditions: control, split screen, and separated monitor screens. The control group performed the wood peg maneuver as in Part I, whereas the other groups were introduced to vital sign information.[35]

In the split-screen group, all information was displayed on the middle monitor with the simulator wooden box displayed on the top left, the oxygen value on the bottom left, and the heart rate value on top right quadrant of the screen. The third group saw the information in the same sequence but with each image displayed on a separate screen. Visual scanning by participants in the split screen view required minimal head movement whereas the participants in the separated monitor group were required to move their heads 65 degrees to see the vital signs on the different monitors. Monitoring critical signals resulted in slowed peg transfer compared with no monitoring.[35]

The researchers recommended that displays showing fluctuating information be positioned close together to minimize the effects of visual scanning. The participants using the split screen display did not differ statistically in performance from the participants using separated displays but the results showed a correlation in increased straining and frustration for the group using separated monitors. Using-split screen technology may reduce the number of monitors required. The researchers concluded that the laparoscopic environment induces strain coping and that visual scanning can impair detection of a critical signal (eg, vital sign data).[35]

Further research is needed on the positioning of equipment to enhance the performance of perioperative personnel during minimally invasive procedures.

I.d.   The perioperative team should prepare endoscopic equipment (eg, camera, light source, insufflation device) and instrumentation according to the manufacturer's instructions for use and physician preference. *[5: Benefits Balanced with Harms]*

I.d.1.   The perioperative team should inspect MIS equipment and instrumentation before use, remove defective items from service, and send the item for repair or replacement according to the health care organization's policy and procedures. Items should be inspected for
  - cleanliness;
  - function and alignment of instrumentation;
  - corrosion, pitting, burrs, nicks, and cracks;
  - sharpness of cutting edges;
  - wear and chipping of instruments and plated surfaces;
  - missing parts;
  - integrity of insulation on insulated devices;
  - integrity of cables;
  - clarity of lenses;
  - integrity of seals and gaskets; and
  - other defects.[2,36,37]
  [1: Strong Evidence]

I.e.   The perioperative team should be prepared to convert a laparoscopic procedure to an open procedure. *[5: Benefits Balanced with Harms]*

A systematic review of the literature and a case series article[38,39] reported complications of vessel or organ injury caused by obtaining access during laparoscopic procedures. Evidence is limited about best practices in preparing for these emergencies. In a literature review of bowel injury in gynecological procedures, Llarena et al[38] reported that the overall incidence of bowel injury is one in 769 but the rate increases with surgical complexity. Levy et al[39] reported the incidence of iatrogenic injuries in laparoscopic surgeries to be low and described six case studies of bladder injury in laparoscopic procedures performed under urgent conditions (ie, three cases of appendicitis, two diagnostic laparoscopies for abdominal pain, and one ectopic pregnancy). Research is needed to determine best practices for preparing for emergent conversion to an open procedure.

Recommendation II

Potential patient injuries and complications associated with gas insufflation media used during MIS procedures should be identified, and practices that reduce the risk for injuries and complications should be established.

Gas distention media is used during MIS procedures for creating a pneumoperitoneum or space to visualize the surgical field with the endoscope. Carbon dioxide (CO_2) is the most commonly used gas, but other gases can be used, such as air, nitrogen, nitrous oxide (N_2O),

argon, and helium.[40,41] The gas distention media is chosen based on the properties of the gas media, the procedure, and the patient's history.

Carbon dioxide is colorless, odorless, inexpensive, nonflammable, and easily dissolved in the bloodstream.[40,42,43] It is most frequently used to create a pneumoperitoneum, but is also used in other procedures, such as endovein harvest procedures,[40,44] esophageal endoscopic submucosal dissections,[45] robotic-assisted endoscopic thyroidectomy,[46] and diagnostic hysteroscopy in physician offices.[47] Carbon dioxide has been reported to have metabolic, hemodynamic, and cardiovascular adverse effects, especially among older adults and patients with preexisting medical conditions. The collective evidence indicates that the use of CO_2 for insufflation is safe but can result in hypercarbia, acidosis, peritoneal irritation, gas emboli, and cardiac arrhythmias. However, these complications occur at a rate of less than 1%.[40,42,43,48]

Nitrous oxide has many of the same benefits as CO_2, but its use has historically been considered a safety concern because of fear of combustion. Rammohan et al[49] conducted a randomized controlled trial of 77 patients undergoing laparoscopic surgery during an 8-week period and randomly assigned them to one of two groups. For group I (n = 38), the gas distention medium was N_2O, and for group II (n = 39), the gas distention medium was CO_2. The researchers found that there were significant differences between the two groups in heart rate changes and mean arterial pressure changes during the pneumoperitoneum. The N_2O group did not experience the same initial rise in these vital signs that the CO_2 group did. The patients in the N_2O insufflation group had lower pain scores than the patients in the CO_2 insufflation group.

A Cochrane review conducted by Cheng et al[41] compared CO_2 pneumoperitoneum with N_2O pneumoperitoneum in a review of three randomized controlled trials with a total of 100 participants and found no significant differences between the groups in any surgical outcomes. None of the trials reported any serious adverse events in the N_2O group; however, none of the studies had the statistical power to establish the safety of N_2O in pneumoperitoneum. In this same Cochrane review, the authors compared CO_2 and helium for creating a pneumoperitoneum. There were no significant differences in outcomes related to cardiopulmonary complication or morbidity. The safety of helium is still a large concern due to reports of serious adverse events related to subcutaneous emphysema in the scrotum, face, and cervical areas.

Air, helium, and N_2O are less soluble in blood than CO_2 and, therefore, it takes longer for a gas embolism to absorb in the bloodstream, which makes use of these gases less optimal for managing serious adverse effects.

II.a.   Precautions should be taken to mitigate the risk for injury associated with gas insufflation during MIS. *[5: Benefits Balanced with Harms]*

II.a.1.   Insufflation flow rate should be set according to the surgeon's specification and the

PATIENT CARE

manufacturer's instructions for use.[50] *[3: Moderate Evidence]*

The manufacturer's instructions for use provide specification for flow rate and trocar, filter, and tubing diameter for achieving best insufflation results. The gas flow rate is dependent on the smallest diameter in the insufflation system. Doubling the radius in the lumen of the system will increase gas flow rates. Decreasing the radius will increase resistance. Placing a 10-mm laparoscope in a 10-mm sheath that is also delivering the insufflation gas will decrease the diameter and increase the resistance to insufflation gas flow, which may result in inadequate insufflation. In situations where high gas flow is required, a system with low resistance and a large diameter will improve the gas flow rate.[50]

II.a.2. Manufacturers' instructions for use of insufflation equipment should be reviewed, followed, and readily available to users.[50] *[3: Moderate Evidence]*

II.a.3. The insufflator should be elevated above the level of the surgical cavity if possible. *[3: Moderate Evidence]*

Elevating the insufflator and tubing decreases the risk of body fluids backing up into the insufflator device.[50]

II.a.4. The insufflator and insufflation tubing should be flushed with the selected gas before the tubing is connected to the cannula (eg, Verres needle). *[3: Moderate Evidence]*

Flushing the tubing removes room air from the tubing. Filling the insufflation tubing with the selected insufflation gas reduces the risk for an air embolism.[50,51]

II.a.5. The perioperative RN should verify that a hydrophobic filter is in place between the insufflator and the insufflation tubing. The filter should be compatible with the insufflator. *[3: Moderate Evidence]*

A filter helps prevent contaminants from flowing through the insufflator into the surgical cavity, prevents backflow of abdominal fluids and particulates that could contaminate the insufflator, and prevents cross contamination. When the filter is compatible with the insufflator, it does not interfere with the flow rate.[50]

II.a.6. During a hysteroscopy, insufflators designed and intended for hysteroscopy should be used. *[2: High Evidence]*

The American College of Obstetricians and Gynecologists recommends that insufflators designed for use in laparoscopic procedures not be used for hysteroscopy procedures. The small uterine cavity requires an insufflator that insufflates at high pressures

with low volume. Laparoscopic insufflators insufflate at low pressures with large volumes and are therefore not recommended for hysteroscopy procedures.[47]

II.a.7. Endoscopic gas insufflator alarms should be turned on and sufficiently audible to be heard above competing noise.[3] *[3: Moderate Evidence]*

II.b. When a gas cylinder is used, the perioperative RN should check the cylinder to verify that it contains the selected gas and that it is not empty before the procedure begins. A second full cylinder should be readily available for immediate replacement of an empty cylinder. *[5: Benefits Balanced with Harms]*

II.c. Insufflation pressure should be maintained at the lowest level necessary to achieve pneumoperitoneum within the specification of the surgeon. *[3: Moderate Evidence]*

The collective evidence[52-60] supports maintaining a pneumoperitoneum pressure of less than 15 mmHg. In a randomized controlled trial, Eryilmaz et al[53] tested the liver function of patients during laparoscopic cholecystectomy procedures. The patients were randomly assigned to either a group with a pneumoperitoneum at 10 mmHg (n = 20) or a group with a pneumoperitoneum at 14 mmHg (n = 23). The researchers found that the group with pneumoperitoneum at 14 mmHg had decreased blood flow to the liver and increased postoperative first hour serum aspartate aminotransferase. The researchers concluded that using a 10 mmHg pneumoperitoneum in laparoscopic cholecystectomy procedures is safe.

II.c.1. The perioperative team should monitor gas insufflation pressures for maintenance of pressure at the desired level. *[5: Benefits Balanced with Harms]*

II.d. The perioperative team should be prepared to detect and implement interventions to manage a gas embolism. *[3: Moderate Evidence]*

The occurrence of gas embolism in laparoscopic surgery is rare and is rapidly reversed due to the high gaseous solubility of CO_2.[40,57] The increased intraabdominal pressure and open blood vessels in abdominal laparoscopic surgery increase the chances for gas entrapment into an injured vein, artery, or solid organ. A gas embolus becomes a life-threatening event when large volumes of gas are introduced into the system and migrate to the right ventricle or pulmonary artery.[40] Incidents of gas embolism have been reported in procedures using CO_2 insufflation, such as abdominal laparoscopic procedures,[55] endoscopic vein harvesting,[40] and endoscopic thyroidectomy.[61]

Park et al[40] performed a review of the literature and described the incidence, pathophysiology, clinical signs, diagnosis, prevention, and treatment of CO_2 embolism during all types of laparoscopic surgery. The authors reported varied rates of embolism occurrence in laparoscopic surgeries using CO_2 insufflation.

II.d.1. In the event of a gas embolism, the RN circulator should assist with immediate treatment. *[4: Limited Evidence]*

Treatment to prevent the embolus from blocking circulation to vital organs may include

- discontinuation of the insufflation gas[40];
- discontinuation of the anesthetic agents and ventilation of the patient with 100% oxygen in an attempt to wash out the insufflation gas from the lungs and improve ventilation perfusion mismatch and hypoxemia;
- hyperventilation to assist in the removal of a CO_2 embolus[62];
- changing the patient's position (eg, from supine to Trendelenburg or left lateral position) to favor permanence of air in the appendage of the right atrium, therefore allowing blood flow under the air bubble[62];
- infusion of large amounts of IV fluids in an attempt to push the blocked airlock into the lungs where it can be absorbed (volume expansion will increase the central venous pressure and may reduce further gas entry)[40,62];
- administration of inotropes, vasopressors, and vasodilators specific to pulmonary circulation[40,62];
- cardiopulmonary resuscitation.[40]

Recommendation III

The perioperative RN should identify potential injuries and complications associated with fluid used for irrigation or as distention media during MIS and computer-assisted procedures.

Fluid media is used in MIS procedures for distention to improve visualization of the cavity or irrigation in a joint. The fluid may be instilled under gravity or pressure or with an infusion pump. Complications from fluid extravasation or intravasation are rare but can be life threatening. Fluid extravasation can lead to edema in the surrounding tissue, abdominal distention, or intraabdominal compartment syndrome.[63] Fluid intravasation occurs when the irrigation fluid is absorbed into the patient's bloodstream, leading to physiological changes such as hyponatremia, hypervolemia, and cardiovascular and pulmonary complications. This is also referred to as transurethral resection (TUR) syndrome because it was first reported during transurethral resection of the prostate (TURP) procedures.[47,64]

Fluid distention-related complications occur in less than 1% of procedures but the risks increase with the length of the procedure and the degree of dissection of the surrounding tissues. For example, a diagnostic hys-

terectomy has a lower risk of fluid absorption than a resectoscopic myomectomy.[65]

The collective evidence[47,63-75] indicates that complications in the use of fluid media used to distend the cavity or improve visualization can result in intravasation or extravasation of the fluid. The use of improper or excessive amounts of fluid for irrigation or distention media can lead to hypervolemia and hyponatremia.

Several authors have reported cases of airway compromise caused by extravasation of irrigation fluid during shoulder arthroscopy procedures.[66,68,69] Cases have also been reported of complications in hysteroscopy procedures from irrigation fluid, including fluid overload,[74] hypotonic hyponatremia, heart failure, and cerebral and pulmonary edema.[65,67,70-72]

Kocher et al[63] conducted a survey of hip arthroscopists in the Multicenter Arthroscopy of the Hip Outcomes Research Network to evaluate the incidence of intraabdominal fluid extravasation (IAFE) in patients undergoing hip arthroscopies. Fifteen arthroscopists (88%) responded to the survey. The respondents provided a retrospective review of patient medical records to answer the survey questions related to the number of hip arthroscopies performed and symptomatic IAFE cases they encountered. A total of 25,648 procedures performed between 1984 and 2010 were reported, and 40 patients (0.16%) were reported to have an IAFE complication occur during the procedure.

Prevention of IAFE includes close observation for abdominal distention, a decrease in core body temperature, and hemodynamic instability. Higher arthroscopic fluid pump pressure and iliopsoas tenotomy had a significant correlation as risk factors in the patients who experienced IAFE. The mean pump pressures for reported cases of symptomatic IAFE were 45 mmHg to 90 mmHg. The 15 survey respondents stated they generally used a pump pressures of 30 mmHg to 80 mmHg. Iliopsoas tenotomy was reported to be performed only 25% of the time during hip arthroscopy. In the 40 IAFE cases, 25 patients had an iliopsoas tenotomy performed. The authors recommended early detection of intraabdominal fluid with computed tomography (CT) or ultrasound to prevent adverse outcomes and provided an algorithm for treatment after intraabdominal or retroperitoneal fluid extravasation has been established after hip arthroscopy.[63]

III.a. The RN circulator should select the irrigation or distention fluid in consultation with the surgeon based on procedure type, patient assessment, and instruments to be used (eg, energy-generating devices). *[2: High Evidence]*

The collective evidence[36,37,47,64,65,75-78] indicates that fluid distention media should be selected based on the medium least likely to cause complications in the event of excess fluid absorption and on compatibility with energy-generating devices. Table 1 provides information about fluids used for irrigation or distention media in MIS procedures.

Nonelectrolyte and low viscosity media, such as 1.5% glycine, 3% sorbitol, or 5% mannitol,

Table 1. Fluids Used for Irrigation or Distension Media

Solution	Electrolyte Solution	Uses	Potential Contraindications	Adverse Reactions
0.9% Sodium chloride[1]	Yes	General irrigation, hysteroscopy, use with laser and bipolar electrosurgery, urologic procedures[2,3]	Monopolar electrosurgery	Hypervolemia, pulmonary edema, abdominal cramping, nausea and vomiting, diarrhea
Ringer's lactate[4]	Yes	General irrigation	Monopolar electrosurgery	Fluid shift from intracellular to extracellular compartment, hypervolemia
Dextran[5]	No	Hysteroscopy; volume generally limited to 300 mL and not to exceed 500 mL[5]	Hypersensitivity to dextran or any component of the formulation, hemostatic defects (eg, thrombocytopenia, hypofibrinogenemia), cardiac decompensation, renal disease with severe oliguria or anuria, hepatic impairment[2]	Plasma expander leading to fluid or solute overload; disseminated intravascular coagulation; overdose, marked by pulmonary edema, increased bleeding time, and decreased platelet function[2]
Glycine 1.5%[6]	No	Urologic irrigation, hysteroscopy, and resectoscopy with monopolar electrosurgery[3]	Severe cardiopulmonary or renal dysfunction, decreased liver function; additives may be incompatible, consult with a pharmacist	Aggravated pre-existing hyponatremia caused by shifts from intracellular to extracellular compartment; fluid and electrolyte disturbances (eg, edema, marked diuresis, pulmonary congestion); impaired liver function leading to accumulation of ammonia in the blood; allergic reactions, which are rare[2]
Mannitol 5%[7]	No	Urologic irrigation, hysteroscopy, and resectoscopy with monopolar electrosurgery[2,8]	Severe cardiopulmonary or renal dysfunction	Aggravated pre-existing hyponatremia caused by shifts from intracellular to extracellular compartment, fluid and electrolyte disturbances (eg, edema, marked diuresis, pulmonary congestion), hypernatremia caused by loss of water and excess of electrolytes from continuous administration
Sorbitol 3%[9]	No	Urological irrigation	Severe cardiopulmonary or renal dysfunction, fructose intolerance	Aggravated pre-existing hyponatremia caused by shifts from intracellular to extracellular compartment, hypernatremia caused by loss of water and excess of electrolytes from continuous administration hyperglycemia in patients with diabetes mellitus, allergic reactions (eg, urticaria)[8]

continued on next page

TABLE 1 CONTINUED. FLUIDS USED FOR IRRIGATION OR DISTENSION MEDIA

Solution	Electrolyte Solution	Uses	Potential Contraindications	Adverse Reactions
Sorbitol 3% / Mannitol 0.5%[10]	No	Urologic irrigation	Severe cardiopulmonary or renal dysfunction, fructose intolerance	Aggravated pre-existing hyponatremia caused by shifts from intracellular to extracellular compartment, hypernatremia caused by loss of water and excess of electrolytes from continuous administration, hyperglycemia in patients with diabetes mellitus, hyperlactatemia in patients who are metabolically compromised caused by metabolism of sorbitol[8,10]
Sterile water[11]	No	General irrigation, washing, rinsing, and dilution purposes; transurethral resection of the prostate[11]	Continuous irrigation, as a distention medium; additives may be incompatible, consult with a pharmacist	Hemolysis when absorbed into the bloodstream

Editor's note: This table presents irrigation solutions that are in common use; however, it is not all inclusive. Use of other irrigation solutions may be indicated in certain patient populations and for certain conditions.

REFERENCES

1. *Sodium chloride for irrigation [package insert]. Bethlehem, PA: B. Braun Medical, Inc; 2014.*
2. *AAGL Advancing Minimally Invasive Gynecology Worldwide; Munro MG, Storz K, Abbott JA, et al. AAGL Practice Report: Practice Guidelines for the Management of Hysteroscopic Distending Media: (replaces Hysteroscopic Fluid Monitoring Guidelines. J Am Assoc Gynecol Laparosc. 2000;7:167-168.). J Minim Invasive Gynecol. 2013;20(2):137-148.*
3. *Darwish AM, Hassan ZZ, Attia AM, Abdelraheem SS, Ahmed YM. Biological effects of distension media in bipolar versus monopolar resectoscopic myomectomy: a randomized trial. J Obstet Gynaecol Res. 2010;36(4):810-817.*
4. *Lactated Ringers for irrigation [package insert]. Lake Forrest, IL: Hospira; 2014.*
5. *Dextran [package insert]. Lake Forrest, IL: Hospira; 2014.*
6. *1.5% glycine irrigation [package insert]. Irvine, CA: B. Braun Medical, Inc; 2014.*
7. *5% mannitol irrigation [package insert]. Irvine, CA: B. Braun Medical, Inc; 2014.*
8. *Park JT, Lim HK, Kim S, Um DJ. A comparison of the influence of 2.7% sorbitol-0.54% mannitol and 5% glucose irrigating fluids on plasma serum physiology during hysteroscopic procedures. Korean J Anesthesiol. 2011;61(5):394-398.*
9. *Sorbitol - sorbitol irrigant. Irvine, CA: B. Braun Medical, Inc; 2010.*
10. *Sorbitol - mannitol irrigation [package insert]. Lake Forrest, IL: Hospira; 2009.*
11. *Sterile water for irrigation [package insert]. Lake Forest, IL: Hospira; 2004.*

are most often selected when monopolar instrumentation is required for gynecological and urologic endoscopic procedures. These hypotonic solutions without electrolytes can cause TUR syndrome, although healthy adults typically can accommodate the fluid and electrolyte imbalance created by excess absorption of these solutions. Age and comorbidities, such as cardiovascular and renal dysfunction, may increase a patient's risk for developing hyponatremia and fluid overload.[47,65]

The American Association of Gynecologic Laparoscopists (AAGL) notes that new evidence has led to careful consideration of use of these fluids in premenopausal women. Hyponatremia occurs after surgeries using these solutions with equal frequency in men and women, but premenopausal women who develop hyponatremia and encephalopathy are 25 times more likely to die or have permanent brain damage than men or postmenopausal women.[47]

Normal saline 0.9% is most frequently selected as the distention fluid and can be used in procedures during which bipolar instrumentation will be used. This is an isotonic solution containing electrolytes and can be safer when large amounts of fluid are absorbed. The AAGL recommends using normal saline for hysteroscopy procedures in which bipolar resection is used, to reduce the risk of hyponatremia and hypo-osmolality.[47]

High-viscosity fluid media, such as 32% dextran 70, does not mix or blend with blood, so it is better for visibility in the presence of bleeding during endoscopic procedures. However, dextran can draw six times its own volume into the bloodstream, resulting in vascular overload and subsequent heart failure and pulmonary edema. Munro and Christianson[65] reported limiting the infusion amount of this fluid to between 300 mL and 500 mL. The high sugar content of dextran requires immediate rinsing of the instrumentation to decrease the damage that can occur from the use of this fluid media.[47,65]

Yousef et al[64] compared glycine 1.5%, glucose 5%, and normal saline 0.9% as irrigating solutions during TURP procedures in 360 patients enrolled in a randomized prospective controlled trial. Patients were randomly assigned to one of three groups of 120 patients. The medical and nursing personnel involved in the postoperative care of the patient were blinded to the type of irrigation used during the procedure. Seventeen patients in the glycine group developed TUR syndrome, which occurs when there is excessive absorption of irrigating fluid. The researchers defined TUR syndrome as a sodium level of 125 mmol/L or less after a TURP and two or more symptoms including nausea, vomiting, bradycardia, hypotension, chest pain, mental confusion, anxiety, paresthesia, and visual disturbance.

Traditionally, glycine 1.5% has been used for TURP because it is a nonelectrolyte fluid and is safe to use with monopolar energy-generating devices. Because of the advancement of bipolar resection devices, normal saline can now be used during TURP procedures. The researchers concluded that bipolar resection with saline and monopolar resection with glucose 5% resulted in fewer complications than monopolar resection with glycine 1.5%.[64]

III.a.1. The preoperative nursing risk assessment related to fluid management should include, but not be limited to, the patient's
- skin color and turgor,
- weight and age,
- allergies and sensitivities to medications,
- conditions or diseases that may predispose or exacerbate the seriousness of hyponatremia or hypervolemia, and
- medications that may predispose or exacerbate the seriousness of hyponatremia or hypervolemia.[47,79]

[5: Benefits Balanced with Harms]

The use of improper or excessive amounts of fluid for irrigation or distention media can lead to hypervolemia and hyponatremia. Patients who have congestive heart failure, liver cirrhosis, or renal diseases are more susceptible to hypervolemia and hyponatremia. The main causes of hyponatremia in hypo-osmolar patients are inappropriate antidiuretic hormone secretion, renal disorders, endocrine deficiencies, and certain medications.[47,79]

III.b. The perioperative RN, in collaboration with the anesthesia professional, should monitor the amount of fluid dispensed and collected during the procedure. *[3: Moderate Evidence]*

The collective evidence suggests that intravasation[47,64,65,67,70-72,80,81] or extravasation[63,66,68,69,82-85] of irrigation and distention fluid used during MIS procedures can occur rapidly with only subtle warning signs. Monitoring the amount of fluid infused and collected during the procedure helps determine whether the patient is at risk for complications.

Kumar and Kumar[81] studied the differences between intravasation rates and fluid deficit rates. Intravasation of fluid occurs from the pressure of the irrigation fluid entering the systemic circulation through the cut ends of the traumatized blood vessels. It is influenced by cavity pressure and hemostatic mechanisms, which can change frequently during a procedure and vary from patient to patient. Fluid deficit is the amount of irrigation fluid in milliliters already absorbed by the patient.

The researchers studied 41 hysteroscopic procedures used a controller-operated pump to measure the intravasation rate. When there was a sudden rise in the intravasation rate, the pressure was lowered in the uterine cavity. In some cases, the fluid deficit was within normal limits, but the intravasation rate increased. The researchers suggested that patient safety is increased if intravasation rate monitoring is performed along with conventional fluid deficit monitoring.[81]

The evidence review found only one study that examined all endoscopic procedures (ie, endoscopic prostate surgery, hysteroscopy, bladder, knee and shoulder arthroscopy). Silva et al[79] conducted a cohort study on endoscopic procedures performed at one facility in Brazil. The researchers reviewed 142 patient records and completed a three-part questionnaire collecting data about the preoperative, intraoperative, and postoperative phases of patient care. They reported a 21.8% complication rate. In their analysis of the factors associated with complications, they found age, sodium level at the end of the procedure, and total fluid administered to be statistically correlated with complications in cardiovascular, respiratory, neurological, gastrointestinal, and kidney function. This study is limited by the size and the observational nature of the data collection.

Kocher et al[63] reported that 15 arthroscopists who were members of the Multicenter Arthroscopy of the Hip Outcomes Research Network completed a survey to retrospectively collect data on hip arthroscopies they had performed. Forty cases of IAFE were reported out of the overall 25,648 hip arthroscopies reviewed by the senior author. Preventative measures suggested by the arthroscopists surveyed included lowering the pump settings, maintaining core temperature, monitoring pH and cardiac function, and periodically monitoring intraoperative abdominal distention.

III.b.1. The RN circulator should report fluid deficit to the anesthesia professional and surgeon at regular intervals throughout the procedure. *[3: Moderate Evidence]*

The AAGL practice guideline for the management of hysteroscopic distending media recommends that an automated fluid management system and media management protocol be in place to assist with assessment of risk factors leading to complications from fluid overload. The collective evidence supports the team monitoring the fluid deficit and establishing criteria for treatment and termination of a procedure.[47,63,70]

III.b.2. The patient should be monitored for physiologic changes, including core temperature, laboratory test results (eg electrolytes, coagulation studies), and potential fluid retention in the abdomen, face, and neck. *[3: Moderate Evidence]*

Multiple cases have been reported of complications from fluid intravasation and extravasation in MIS procedures using fluid for irrigation and distention media.[66,68,69,82,84-87] The authors collectively reported early detection through monitoring electrolyte levels, physiologic responses, and core temperature in prevention of these complications. Transurethral resection syndrome is well documented in the literature as a complication from excessive absorption of nonelectrolyte fluid during TURP. Transurethral resection syndrome is used as a common term to describe fluid overload[47] and is identified when the patient experiences more than two of these symptoms: hyponatremia (serum sodium of 125 mmol/L or less), nausea, vomiting, bradycardia, hypotension, chest pain, mental confusion, anxiety, paraesthesia, or visual disturbance.[86] This syndrome is rare but can be life threatening.[47,64,86]

Patients undergoing hip and shoulder arthroscopy procedures are at risk for fluid extravasation and complications of compression to surrounding tissue. Verma and Sekiya[85] reported a case of fluid extravasation in hip arthroscopy in a healthy 21-year-old patient who presented with shortness of breath 24 hours after surgery. An abdominal CT revealed fluid in the patient's abdomen. In their literature review, the authors of this report found three other case studies with similar complications. They suggested five early warning signs: inability to distend the joint, increase in fluid required to distend the joint, frequent cut-off of the pump, abdominal and thigh distention, and acute hypothermia.

Stafford et al[84] reviewed 36 patients undergoing hip arthroscopy performed by one physician in one facility. The volume of irrigation fluid infused, operating time, fluid pressures, and volumes of fluid recovered were measured in all 36 procedures. They found the mean loss of fluid into the peri-articular tissues was 1,132 mL. There was a correlation between the volume of extravasated fluid and both the length of surgery and the volume of infused fluid used. The authors concluded that reduced operative times (< 90 minutes) and fluid pressure at low rates (< 50 mmHg) reduced the risk of fluid extravasation.

Reported cases of fluid leaking into surrounding tissue during shoulder arthroscopy are common, and this generally does not cause harm to the patient. Airway compromise from edema and tracheal compression have been reported.[66,68]

Wegmuller et al[70] described a case of a patient experiencing life-threatening laryngeal edema during a hysteroscopy. When the patient became symptomatic, it was discovered that 76 L of fluid was used, which exceeded the normal amount of 4 L to 7 L. An exact fluid balance was not available during the procedure. The authors calculated a fluid overload of 11 L. Their recommendation from this experience was to ensure there is good communication on clinical observations between the patient (when regional anesthesia is used), anesthesia professional, nurse, and surgeon. An agreement should be determined for measurement of fluid balance and termination of the procedure if fluid absorption reaches 1,000 mL. Based on their literature search and experience, they also recommended keeping resection time to less than 60 minutes to reduce the risk for fluid overload.

Jo et al[67] published a case report of a 34-year-old woman who had elective hysteroscopy and suffered extreme hyponatremia caused by an electrolyte-free sorbitol/mannitol solution used as distention irrigation fluid. During the procedure, 2 L sorbitol/mannitol solution were infused. The author reported difficulty in measuring the fluid absorption rate due to the large amount of fluid leakage through the uterine cervix. The patient's temperature dropped, her pulse oximetry declined to 85%, and her end-tidal CO_2 decreased to 22 mmHg. The surgeon stopped the procedure, and the patient was managed for fluid overload and transferred to the intensive care unit. The patient suffered mild brain swelling without pontine myelinolysis and pulmonary edema. She was discharged on postoperative day four and remained asymptomatic at the 6-month follow-up appointment. The authors concluded that intraoperative fluid balance should be maintained, and early detection and prompt management of suspected fluid absorption are important.

III.b.3. The perioperative team should monitor patients for adverse reactions when medications are added to fluids used for irrigation or distention media.[88] *[3: Moderate Evidence]*

III.c. Fluids used for irrigation or as distention media should be contained. *[3: Moderate Evidence]*
The AAGL recommends that the surgical team account for all fluid used as distention media.[47] The team should accurately monitor all input and output, including fluid returned from the hysteroscope, spilled from the vagina, and lost to the floor.
The collective evidence[47,63,81,89] suggests that a measurement system should be used for accurate monitoring of input and output of fluids in MIS procedures.

III.c.1. Drapes should be used that capture as much fluid return as possible. *[3: Moderate Evidence]*
Drapes designed for collection facilitate the accurate measurement of fluid. Fluid absorption is determined by subtracting the amount of fluid recovered from the amount of fluid instilled. The volumetric calculation does not take into consideration extraneous fluid losses (eg, fluid loss on the floor, on the drape), which cannot be accurately quantified; nor does it consider additives, such as blood.[47,63,89]

III.c.2. As much irrigation or distention fluid as possible should be collected in a closed-container system. *[3: Moderate Evidence]*
Estimating the fluid deficit can be very difficult for the surgical team. Boyd and Stanley[89] studied the accuracy of fluid measurement by the surgical team. Four RN circulators were asked to estimate the initial volume of fluid in the irrigating fluid bag, the remaining volume of irrigating fluid in the bag, fluid volume in kick buckets, fluid lost on the floor, and fluid in the suction canister for gynecological procedures in a simulated OR. The researchers found that fluid collected in rigid suction canisters was most consistently measured accurately. Partially emptied bags, fluid on the floor, and fluid in kick buckets were measured inaccurately.
The researchers also measured the fluid in eleven 3-L bags of 1.5% glycine and found all were overfilled by 2.8% (mean of 84 mL, range 62 mL to 125 mL), which the authors stated was consistent with other research demonstrating that 3-L bags of commonly used media may be overfilled by 2.8% to 6%. The authors concluded that

surgical team members' estimates of the level of fluid left in a bag can vary, which also compounds the problem of fluid measurement inaccuracy. Fluids can also be lost in the drapes and on the floor, making it difficult to estimate output.[89]

III.c.3. Fluids used for irrigation or as distention media should be prevented from coming into contact with electrical equipment. *[5: Benefits Balances with Harm]*
Containing fluid used during a procedure prevents contact with electrical outlets, switches, and the internal components of electrical equipment, including electrosurgical electrodes. Preventing fluid contact with electrical equipment minimizes the risk of burns, fires, and damage to the equipment.[8,36]

III.d. Automated fluid management systems should be used in a manner that minimizes the potential for injury. *[3: Moderate Evidence]*
Automated fluid management systems calculate the amount of fluid dispensed to the patient and compare this with the amount returned to the system. The deficit is measured, and an alarm alerts the user to potential fluid overload. This timely notification of a deficit provides an opportunity to take corrective action before physiologic compromise of the patient.[47,79,81,89]

III.d.1. The fluid selected for the distention media should be consistent with the fluid management system and the endoscope manufacturer's instructions for use.[36] *[5: Benefits Balanced With Harms]*

III.d.2. Accessories (eg, tubing, collection canisters) should be compatible with the fluid management system.[36] *[3: Moderate Evidence]*

III.d.3. Fluid management equipment safety features should include
- clearly labeled control settings,
- a quick setting reference chart attached to the equipment,
- audible alarms,
- a display with measurement of fluid instilled and returned to the regulator (ie, fluid deficit), and[81]
- a display of measurement of cavity pressure.[47]
[3: Moderate Evidence]

III.d.4. The perioperative RN should verify the fluid pump settings for fluid distention with the surgeon before administration and continually monitor the settings throughout the procedure.[47] *[3: Moderate Evidence]*
The collective evidence[47,63,65,79,81] supports monitoring pump pressures, inflow volumes, and outflow volumes of fluids used during MIS procedures.

623

III.d.5. The perioperative team should initiate corrective action in response to audible alarms from the fluid management system and notify the surgeon and anesthesia professional if corrective actions do not result in a reduction of the fluid volume deficit to a safe level. *[5: Benefits Balanced with Harms]*

III.e. The perioperative RN should report, investigate, and take corrective action when an adverse event or near miss related to fluid management equipment occurs. *[5: Benefits Balances with Harms]*

Reporting adverse events and near misses through an adverse event reporting and investigation system provides a mechanism to determine trends and potential risk factors and evaluate the effectiveness of corrective actions.[90]

Recommendation IV

Precautions should be taken to mitigate the risk for injury associated with the use of energy-generating devices during MIS.

The use of bipolar versus monopolar electrosurgery is a physician preference guided by the procedure, tissue type, and choice of distention media.[91-102] Risk for thermal injury from active electrodes has been reported in the literature.[93,95,103] Carbon dioxide is the most commonly used gas distention media because it is nonflammable and presents the least risk for complications from air embolism.[40]

Culp et al[94] studied the clinical implications of CO_2 and air as insufflation media by measuring the spark gap in a biological model. The researchers did not find a difference in the electrocautery function between CO_2 and air. They recommended the use CO_2 over the use of air as an insufflation gas in electrosurgery due to the favorable properties of CO_2 gas as insufflation media.

Fluid distention media can be either conductive or nonconductive. The use of a monopolar active electrode in conductive fluid, such as sodium chloride, has been shown to cause heat transfer and damage to surrounding tissue.[93,95,97] Glycine 1.5%, mannitol 5%, and sorbitol 3% are nonconductive fluids that are most frequently used in urologic and hysteroscopic procedures; however, these fluids have a high risk of producing TUR syndrome.[78]

IV.a. Safety precautions for reducing the risk for injury when using energy-generating devices during MIS should include
- selection of the lowest power setting that achieves the desired result,
- activation of the active electrode only when it is in close proximity to the tissue, and
- activation of the energy-generating device foot pedal only by the person in control of the energy-delivering hand piece (eg, ESU active electrode, laser hand piece, ultrasonic wand).[8,37]

[3: Moderate Evidence]

IV.b. Electrosurgical unit-activated instrumentation (ie, active electrodes) and accessories should be selected to include technology that minimizes or eliminates the risk for insulation failure and capacitive-coupling injuries.[8,37,76] *[3: Moderate Evidence]*

IV.b.1. Conductive trocar systems should be used.[8] *[3: Moderate Evidence]*

IV.b.2. Active electrodes should be examined by the perioperative team for impaired insulation before and after use and, if reusable, during decontamination and package assembly.[2,37] *[3: Moderate Evidence]*

IV.c. The perioperative RN should verify the properties of the selected distention media to minimize risks related to electrosurgery. *[3: Moderate Evidence]*

Collateral tissue injury secondary to increased fluid temperatures can occur if the distention media is conductive.[8,95]

IV.c.1. Nonflammable insufflation gas should be used.[94] *[3: Moderate Evidence]*

IV.c.2. Nonelectrolyte distention fluids should be used when monopolar electrosurgery is used.[47,65,73] *[2: High Evidence]*

Recommendation V

The perioperative team should identify potential risks for injury and complications associated with computer-assisted surgical procedures and should implement safe practices.

Computer-assisted robotic surgery began with research conducted by the National Aeronautics and Space Administration in the 1980s to investigate providing surgical care in remote locations through surgeon-directed controls on Earth.[104] The evolution of robotic technology has been similar to the advancement of endoscopic surgery. Both began in urology and gynecology with a steep learning curve and longer surgical times compared with routine procedures. These technologies later began to be used in general, cardiothoracic,[105] colorectal, pediatric,[106] and head and neck procedures.[104,107] The robotic system provides three-dimensional (3D), high-definition views of the surgical field. Wristed laparoscopic instruments allow the surgeon 7 degrees of freedom of movement. The system eliminates hand tremors and provides motion scaling and improved ergonomics for the surgeon.[23,104,108-111]

Computer-assisted navigation procedures provide a means for the surgical team to navigate with digital 3D images through minimally invasive techniques.[112-117] Navigation can be done with CT-based systems, fluoroscopy-based systems, or imageless systems. Computed tomography-based navigation is performed by scanning an area of the body and using the data to construct a 3D image. Scans can be performed preoperatively or intraoperatively in a hybrid room with a CT scanner or in an OR with a portable CT scanner.

Fluoroscopy-based navigation uses markers based on anatomic landmarks on the patient. The portable fluoroscopy unit can take arbitrary images during the procedure that are sent to the navigation unit by a computer program that relates the images to the surgical field in space and identifies the position of the surgical instruments.

An imageless system is a computer platform with a tracking system (usually an optical camera) and infrared markers on anatomical landmarks; a probe acquires surface points to create triangulation for navigation.[116,118,119] The radiologic 3D images provide the surgical team with the ability to visualize the internal structures for planning the operative approach and navigating with surgical instrumentation. This technology is similar to global positioning systems for orientation and direction. The use of navigation in MIS procedures may improve accuracy and reduce radiation exposure. Navigational minimally invasive approaches are used in neurosurgical, orthopedic, otorhinolaryngology, liver resection, thoracic, and maxillofacial surgical procedures. The registration and planning can be time consuming but promotes accuracy and decreases the invasiveness of surgery.[116] Research is needed on the complications and risks associated with using advanced technologies for all surgical specialties.

V.a.   The patient should be safely positioned in a manner that will facilitate the use of the computer-assisted equipment. *[2: High Evidence]*

Positioning the patient for computer-assisted procedures requires using the extreme Trendelenburg or reverse Trendelenburg position. The gravitational effect of these positions allows the patient's organs to move away from the surgical field. The Trendelenburg position increases venous return and increases the risk for cardiac or respiratory congestion. The reverse Trendelenburg position reduces venous return and cardiac output, increases peripheral and pulmonary resistance, and has the potential to result in misalignment of the patient's extremities.[36,105,108,120-123] (See the AORN Guideline for Positioning the Patient[7] for additional guidance).

V.b.   The perioperative RN circulator should delegate, supervise, and evaluate the activities for setting up the computer-assisted equipment. *[2: High Evidence]*

Computer-assisted robotic equipment consists of a
○ patient cart,
○ surgeon console, and
○ vision cart.

The computer-assisted robotic system is complex, necessitating coordination by the team members to reduce the risk of error and potential injury. The robotic patient cart consists of robotic arms to which instruments are attached, and these instruments are inserted into the body cavity through trocars. The instruments mimic the surgeon's hand movement, with wristed servant tools connected to the robotic arms. An endoscope that provides 3D images to the surgeon console and vision cart is also connected to the robotic arms. "Docking" the patient cart refers to moving the system over the sterile field and attaching the instruments to the robotic arms. This maneuver requires two perioperative personnel, a nonsterile person to move the cart and a sterile person to guide the equipment and prevent a collision with surrounding equipment.[121,124,125]

Computer-assisted surgical navigation equipment includes[116]
○ infrared cameras,
○ advanced digital images of the patient for use with the navigation software, and
○ interactive display monitors.

V.b.1.   The perioperative team should follow the manufacturers' instructions for use for all equipment used in computer-assisted robotic minimally invasive procedures. *[5: Benefits Balanced with Harms]*

V.b.2.   The RN circulator should assist the surgeon with the registration process, which consists of[112,116,117]
• ensuring the preoperative radiologic studies are available,
• positioning the patient,
• positioning the navigation system so that the surgical field is in view of the tracking system (eg, infrared camera),
• attaching the patient antenna,
• collect data points from anatomical landmarks or fiducial markers,
• registering additional instruments if needed, and
• verifying the accuracy of the registration.
[3: Moderate Evidence]

Patient registration is the most important step in ensuring the accuracy of the navigation system. Kaduk et al[116] reported on a facility experience with the use of surgical navigation in maxillofacial surgery. The authors recommend using checklists to help ensure all steps are followed to improve the accuracy of the navigation system. They developed five checklists: preoperative, preoperative planning, OR, intraoperative imaging, and postoperative. These checklists define what is needed in each phase of the process and help ensure the correct images are available on the day of surgery.

V.b.3.   The perioperative team should notify the surgeon if the patient is moved after registration in computer-assisted navigation or after the robotic arms have been docked, and should coordinate corrective action.[105,121] *[3: Moderate Evidence]*

Recommendation VI

The health care organization should determine the requirements for the design and operation of the hybrid OR for surgical or invasive procedures.

Advancements in technology have led to changes and enhancements in OR design and equipment. One development has been the creation of the hybrid OR. The Facilities Guidelines Institute (FGI) defines a hybrid OR as "a room that meets the definition of an operating room and is also equipped to enable diagnostic imaging before, during and after surgical procedures."[126] The room design combines surgical environmental requirements and imaging equipment to accommodate patient care in one location for diagnostic and surgical procedures. The FGI notes that the use of portable imaging technology in an OR does not make the room a hybrid OR.

The collective evidence[76,127-135] supports the use of hybrid OR designs as defined by the FGI guidelines. Imaging equipment is selected based on the types of procedures that will be done in the hybrid OR. Permanently fixed imaging equipment may be single-plane, bi-plane multiaxial rotational angiography systems, CT equipment, or MRI equipment.[133] Fixed radiologic equipment requires that the hybrid OR have lead-lined shielding. Generally, there are four to six flat-screen monitors for projecting digital images to all four quadrants in the room. A large 40-inch to 56-inch flat-panel monitor is also used to show the digital data acquired from the imaging system and monitoring other vital signs.[132,135]

The hybrid OR may be located outside the traditional surgical suite. An OR is designated as a restricted area that can only be accessed through a semi-restricted area.[126] Hybrid ORs have been developed in cardiac catheterization suites, interventional suites, and surgical suites; regardless of location, the design requirements are the same. Meeting the requirements for installing fixed imaging equipment within a surgical environment can be challenging in an existing room or in conversion of an existing area because it requires additional space, equipment, and ceiling supports. A multidisciplinary team that collaborates with imaging personnel and perioperative personnel is key to creating a successful workflow design and a safe patient care environment.

The hybrid OR concept may optimize efficiency by decreasing transport of the patient and minimizing the number of patient hand overs.[133] Combining the efforts of cardiologists, interventional radiologists, and cardiac surgeons has benefitted patients who were not candidates for open heart surgery but were candidates for a less-invasive, lower-risk intervention, such as a transcatheter aortic valve replacement procedure.[131,133] Trauma patients can be sent straight to the hybrid OR, where angiography can be done to assess the extent of the injury and initiate treatment more quickly.[128,136] The hybrid OR is used by practitioners in all specialties (eg, cardiovascular, peripheral vascular, neurovascular, interventional radiology, cardiac catheterization, electrophysiology, orthopedic, trauma). Traditional models provide care separately for each procedure, and patients are transported from the interventional radiology suite or catheterization laboratory to the OR. The construction of the hybrid OR may be new construction or conversion of an existing interventional room or OR. The hybrid OR can be located in the surgical department, cardiac catheterization laboratory, or interventional radiology department. Combining these work areas can be challenging for health care providers, but creates a more efficient treatment option for the patient.[76,127,129-132,134]

VI.a. The health care organization should establish a multidisciplinary team including perioperative and radiology RNs, interventional radiologists, surgeons, first assistants, surgical technologists, anesthesia professionals, infection preventionists, and other involved personnel to develop the design of new construction or renovation of existing space to create a hybrid OR. *[3: Moderate Evidence]*

Organizational experience reports have identified challenges of high cost, complex planning among multiple specialties, space requirements, schedule coordination, location, personnel training, team development, and credentialing criteria in designing a hybrid OR.[127,129,131-133,135,137,138]

Hybrid OR construction and design can be complicated by locating the room outside the surgical suite. Table 2 shows the various procedures reported in the literature to be performed in a hybrid OR. Aston[127] described organizational experiences from various hospitals in which a hybrid OR had recently been installed. One facility described the need to reduce silos developed in traditional care where patients are scheduled for procedures in separate departments. The need to eliminate traditional silos of care by merging personnel and technologies into one location can create an unsettled culture.[129,133] Elimination of multiple hand overs, transportation delays, and possibly multiple anesthetic events benefits the patient.

In an expert opinion article, Schaadt and Landau[135] addressed planning, design, and use of the hybrid OR and suggested that the design should meet the strategic vision and budget and maximize operational efficiencies to promote the same standard of care for all patients.

VI.a.1. The multidisciplinary team should
- develop the design of new construction or renovation of existing space in compliance with federal, state, and local building regulatory requirements;
- identify and define the roles and responsibilities of team members; and
- establish safe processes and practices for working in the hybrid OR.
[5:Benefits Balanced with Harms]

Organizational experiences describe various approaches to creating a hybrid OR and

TABLE 2. EXAMPLES OF PROCEDURES PERFORMED IN A HYBRID OR

Cardiovascular	Cardiothoracic	Neurovascular	Other
Abdominal aortic aneurysm repair[1]	Transcatheter valve replacement (TAVR)[1-3]	Coil embolization or microsurgical clipping of cerebral aneurysms[1,5]	Hemorrhage control in trauma patients[10-12]
Aortic stent grafting[1]	Percutaneous removal of cardiac device leads[1]	Intracranial stenting of cerebral arteries[1,5]	High-risk obstetric procedures[13]
Carotid stent grafting[1]	Minimally invasive endoscopic bypass surgery[3]	Cerebral balloon angioplasty[1,6]	Orthopedic trauma[13,14]
Endovascular aortic repair (EVAR)[2,3]	Minimally invasive direct coronary artery bypass grafting[1,3]	Microneurosurgical resection of brain tumors[1,7]	
Thoracic endovascular aortic repair (TEVAR)[2,3]	Robotically enhanced minimally invasive direct coronary artery bypass[3]	Combined carotid surgical cutdown followed by endovascular coiling for bypass of tortuous anatomy[1,8]	
	Pediatric aortic and pulmonary stenosis[1,3]	Combined arteriovenous malformation embolization followed by microneurosurgical resection.[1,5,9]	
	Hypoplastic left heart syndrome treatment[1]	Cerebral vascular tumors[6]	
	Off-pump coronary artery bypass[1]	Spinal vascular tumors[6]	
	Atrial fibrillation/flutter abalation[3]		
	Hybrid maze procedure[3,4]		

REFERENCES

1. Odle TG. Managing transition to a hybrid operating room. Radiol Technol. 2011;83(2):165-181.
2. Kaneko T, Davidson MJ. Use of the hybrid operating room in cardiovascular medicine. Circulation. 2014;130(11):910-917.
3. Kpodonu J. Hybrid cardiovascular suite: the operating room of the future. J Card Surg. 2010;25(6):704-709.
4. Los-Meyer A. Navigating the mini-maze procedure. Nurse Pract. 2010;35(5):7-10.
5. Murayama Y, Arakawa H, Ishibashi T, et al. Combined surgical and endovascular treatment of complex cerebrovascular diseases in the hybrid operating room. J Neurointerv Surg. 2013;5(5):489-493.
6. Gemmete JJ, Chaudhary N, Pandey AS, et al. Initial experience with a combined multidetector CT and biplane digital subtraction angiography suite with a single interactive table for the diagnosis and treatment of neurovascular disease. J Neurointerv Surg. 2013;5(1):73-80.
7. Childs S, Bruch P. Successful management of risk in the hybrid OR. AORN J. 2015;101(2):223-234.
8. Miguel K, Hirsch JA, Sheridan RM. Team training: a safer future for neurointerventional practice. J Neurointerv Surg. 2011;3(3):285-287.
9. Kotowski M, Sarrafzadeh A, Schatlo B, et al. Intraoperative angiography reloaded: a new hybrid operating theater for combined endovascular and surgical treatment of cerebral arteriovenous malformations: a pilot study on 25 patients. Acta Neurochir (Wien). 2013;155(11):2071-2078.
10. D'Amours SK, Rastogi P, Ball CG. Utility of simultaneous interventional radiology and operative surgery in a dedicated suite for seriously injured patients. Curr Opin Crit Care. 2013;19(6):587-593.
11. Kirkpatrick AW, Vis C, Dube M, et al. The evolution of a purpose designed hybrid trauma operating room from the trauma service perspective: the RAPTOR (resuscitation with angiography percutaneous treatments and operative resuscitations). Injury. 2014;45(9):1413-1421.
12. Tan H, Zhang LY, Guo QS, et al. "One-stop hybrid procedure" in the treatment of vascular injury of lower extremity. Indian J Surg. 2015;77(1):75-78.
13. Clark A, Farber MK, Sviggum H, Camann W. Cesarean delivery in the hybrid operating suite: a promising new location for high-risk obstetric procedures. Anesth Analg. 2013;117(5):1187-1189.
14. Richter PH, Yarboro S, Kraus M, Gebhard F. One year orthopaedic trauma experience using an advanced interdisciplinary hybrid operating room. Injury. 2015;46(Suppl 4):S129-S134.

personnel from multiple disciplines working together.[127-129,131-133,135,139-141] Collectively, the authors describe the hybrid OR project to be the first time interventional or cardiac catheterization laboratory personnel have worked with OR personnel. Each team member provides valuable knowledge of his or her normal workflow and, by describing their experience of aseptic technique, traffic flow, wire management, contrast injector placement, movement of the imaging system, and bed controls, the team members create a new workflow within the hybrid OR environment. The members of this team develop the collaborative culture required for the new environment.

Kirkpatrick et al[128] described creating a mock-up space before construction, where the team could visualize and walk through the normal routine of a surgical procedure. Creating cardboard screens and bringing in movable surgical equipment allowed the team to determine the best placement for ceiling-mounted imaging equipment, monitors, shields, and equipment booms. A mock-up bed with the dimensions and fixed table mounts helped determine how the team would position the patient during procedures. The mocked up space also provided a means to test the length of the boom arms and collision factors for reaching optimal locations. The fixed floor mount of imaging equipment is a factor in designing the bed location relative to placement of anesthesia equipment.[127,135]

VI.a.2. The multidisciplinary team should select the imaging system and adjunct technologies that meet the identified requirements associated with the scope of services. *[3: Moderate Evidence]*

Input from physicians and health care personnel is important when making the decision about the type of imaging system to install in a hybrid OR. The imaging system is the most expensive component of building a hybrid OR.[135] New technologies in the digital manipulation of the images acquired by the system should be considered. Adjunct technologies in the hybrid OR may be 3D imaging reconstruction, echocardiography, intravascular ultrasound, digital subtraction angiography, video integration systems with picture archiving, and audio-visual recording systems.

Angiography is the most common imaging modality used in a hybrid OR. Single-plane, bi-plane, and multi-axial robotic angiography are options for the imaging system. The system may be ceiling mounted or floor mounted. Cardiac and peripheral vascular hybrid procedures require only a single-plane image. Bi-plane systems have two C-arms, one mounted on the floor and one on tracks in the ceiling. A bi-plane system is capable of acquiring images from two reference point at the same time. This system is most often used for smaller vessel angiography in pediatrics and neuroangiography. Using the two C-arms reduces the amount of radiation exposure and contrast media use. The multi-axial robotic angiography system is a single-plane, floor-mounted system with eight rotational axes that can provide more images at different angles without using the biplane technology.[135]

Computed tomography and MRI are other imaging systems that may be installed in a hybrid OR. Odle[133] described the use of CT scanners in an intermittent mode to decrease radiation exposure during CT-guided interventional procedures. Magnetic resonance imaging hybrid ORs may house the scanner between two rooms, allowing it to be brought into the room via a track system. The scanner can be used in conjunction with angiography to assist in planning the surgery or to determine during the procedure whether further resection is needed.

Childs and Bruch[142] described the benefits of an MRI hybrid OR as allowing practitioners to perform preoperative scans in the diagnostic room or in the MRI/OR suite for planning neurosurgical navigation, performing real-time monitoring of laser thermocoagulation of tumors, performing vessel wall imaging studies requiring embolization and operative intervention, and avoiding repeated same-day intubation of pediatric patients.

VI.b. The perioperative team should establish standardized room setups. *[3: Moderate Evidence]*

Standardized room setups may assist in preventing collisions with the imaging system and other equipment (eg, monitors, lead shielding, equipment booms).

Standardized room setups for each procedure will assist personnel in positioning monitors, overhead lights, lead shields, and booms in the appropriate location for each procedure. Standardized room setup eliminates delays caused by team members having differing opinions about equipment placement. The positioning of the patient or side of the approach will also determine the location of bed controls, monitors, and equipment. The location of the imaging controls on the table side or on a remote trolley is determined by physician preference.[127,129,135,143,144]

VI.b.1. The perioperative team should establish the no-fly zone according to the imaging system manufacturer recommendation, patient position, room configuration, and region of body being imaged.[135] *[3: Moderate Evidence]*

Schaadt and Landau[135] described the need for personnel knowledge of the imaging system and required clearances as important in the anticipation and prevention of potential serious collisions that can occur when people or equipment cross over into areas designated as no-fly zones while the imaging equipment is in operation. Some imaging systems have collision-detection devices and will stop moving if a possible collision is detected.

VI.b.2. The perioperative team should assign responsibility for moving or securing equipment before initiation of the imaging system. *[3: Moderate Evidence]*

In combination procedures with open surgical incisions and interventions requiring imaging, equipment booms and OR lights may have been moved into the no-fly zone. When imaging acquisition is required, all equipment should be moved out of the no-fly zone.[135]

VI.b.3. The imaging bed control should be positioned in an accessible location.[135] *[3: Moderate Evidence]*

VI.c. An RN circulator should be assigned to every patient undergoing an operative or other invasive procedure in a hybrid OR. *[3: Moderate Evidence]*

Staffing for the perioperative setting is dynamic in nature and depends on clinical judgment, critical thinking, and the administrative skills of the perioperative RN administrator. Patients undergoing operative and other invasive procedures require perioperative nursing care provided by a perioperative RN, regardless of the setting.

AORN maintains that every surgical patient deserves a perioperative RN for the duration of any operative or other invasive procedure and actively promotes laws and regulation to ensure the supervisory presence of the professional RN in the perioperative setting. A minimum of one perioperative RN circulator dedicated to each patient undergoing an operative or other invasive procedure facilitates the provision of safe, quality patient care in the perioperative setting.[145]

VI.c.1. Additional personnel should be assigned depending on the type of procedure and the skill mix required. *[3: Moderate Evidence]*

The collective evidence[133,139,144,146-150] reflects the complexity of the patient care provided for the combined interventional and surgical procedures. The skill mix required is dependent on the procedure and requires unique coordination of ensuring the right personnel are in the room at the correct time due to the phasing of most procedures. More research is needed in this area.

The perioperative team in a hybrid room may include a
• perioperative circulating RN,
• radiology circulating RN,
• surgical scrub person (ie, RN or surgical technologist),
• radiology technologist,
• surgeon,
• surgical first assistant,
• anesthesia professional,
• radiology technician,
• interventional cardiologist, and
• perfusionist.

Katzen et al[147] described the facility experience at Baptist Cardiac and Vascular Institute after 16 years of having a hybrid OR located in the interventional lab area. A multidisciplinary team was convened to evaluate the program. Review of operating expenses revealed that labor cost was high because of the historic staffing pattern of two OR staff members and two interventional radiology staff members for every endovascular aortic repair procedure. The multidisciplinary team proposed a cross-training program for existing interventional radiology (IR) nurses and technologists to perform the function of the OR staff members.

To understand the scope of practice for each specialty, a team of OR and IR directors, managers, and educators met to perform a crosswalk of roles and responsibilities. The facility created a 15-week training program based on AORN guidelines and trained the IR nurses to achieve competence in traffic patterns, environmental cleaning, aseptic technique, and surgical attire. More studies are needed to review the cross training of roles to provide highly collaborative work team where personnel can work within their scopes of practice and maximize operational efficiencies.[147]

The Department of Veteran Affairs (VA) evaluated the complexities of developing a transthoracic aortic valve replacement (TAVR) program in their system. Since the approval of the TAVR procedure by the US Food and Drug Administration in 2002, more than 20,000 TAVR procedures have been performed, and there is minimal guidance on where the procedure is performed and who is directing the care of the TAVR program.[144] The VA, as a system, decided to develop a standardized approach to review applications for implementation of a structural heart program at any one of their facilities. A centralized team and the use of the Health Failure Mode and Effects Analysis (HFMEA) provided a systematic approach to help ensure room readiness and personnel competency for this complex program. The HFMEA provides a mechanism for identifying high-risk situations and hazard analysis. The personnel in the hybrid room provided unique understanding of roles and the ability to accurately perform their jobs during critical events. They performed drills to identify areas of crossover between roles and the skill level of each role.[144]

D'Amours et al[146] addressed the challenge of working in hybrid rooms on evening, nights, and weekends in a literature review. They described a Canadian study that demonstrated that 78% of major traumas occur in the evening, at nights, and on weekends. The resources required for staffing and coordinating the call schedules can be labor intensive. Clear understanding of clinical leadership and each team member's role is key to the coordination of care for a trauma patient in the hybrid room.

VI.d. The perioperative team should determine what emergency supplies and equipment should be available before the procedure begins (eg, crash cart, supplies for converting to an open procedure, fire extinguisher, gas shutoff valves) based on the location of the hybrid OR and procedure. *[3: Moderate Evidence]*

Evidence about the emergencies associated with combination procedures in a hybrid OR is limited. Research is needed about coordinating the care of patients in the complex hybrid OR environment. The hybrid OR can create efficiencies by decreasing the number of patient transfers and hand overs, but the multiple disciplines involved in the procedure can also create delays in treatment if the team is not well orchestrated.[128]

Kirkpatrick et al[128] and D'Amours et al[146] reported on the use of the hybrid OR for trauma procedures. The authors suggest that using the RAPTOR (resuscitation with angiography percutaneous treatments and operative resuscitations) concept in a hybrid OR provides a safer and more efficient environment for care of trauma patients. Kirkpatrick et al[128] described the design, build, and operation of the RAPTOR hybrid OR. In their facility, this suite was designed to serve the needs in caring for exsanguinating patients. The authors stated that the future is development of resuscitative ORs where patients can be transported to one location for evaluation and treatment without wasting critical time coordinating transport and patient care hand overs. The patient can have the diagnostic angiography to determine the extent of damage and bleeding. A minimally invasive repair may be adequate, but if more extensive surgery is required, the team can quickly move to an open procedure in the hybrid OR.[146]

VI.e. Radiation safety policies and procedures should be established, implemented, and reviewed periodically (See the AORN Guideline for Radiation Safety[151]). *[2: High Evidence]*

VI.f. Structure, process, and clinical outcomes performance measures should be identified for procedures performed in the hybrid OR. *[3: Moderate Evidence]*

Patel et al[139] compared the error rate during the open phase versus the endovascular phase in the repair of aortic aneurysms in a hybrid OR. Two independent observers recorded errors that were defined as having potential to cause harm (ie, danger) or potential to disrupt the procedure (ie, delay). After observing nine procedures and recording the error rate, the researchers determined that more errors occurred during the endovascular phase of the procedure than during the open phase of the procedure (7.6/hour versus 3.75/hour, respectively).

A focus group was convened that devised a structured mental rehearsal to be performed at the beginning of each procedure. The error rate was then observed with the same tool during six procedures in which the mental rehearsal strategy was used. The error rate was significantly lower after the intervention (2.5/hour after the intervention versus 7.6/hour before the mental rehearsal). Danger and delay errors also decreased after the intervention, with 1.2 danger errors/total errors and 1.3 delay errors/total errors after the intervention compared to 1.75 danger errors/total errors and 2.0 delay errors/total errors before the intervention. The mental rehearsal requires all team members (eg, surgeon, anesthesia professional, radiologist, radiographer, nurses) to be present at the start of the radiological phase of combined procedures. The lead endovascular specialist summarizes the main steps of the radiologic phase and equipment needs for each stage. The nurse verbally confirms that equipment is available and present, and if not, it is retrieved from the supply cart. The lead endovascular specialist confirms that all team members understand and agree to proceed.[139]

A limitation of this study was that it included only a small population (N = 15 procedures) in one facility. Randomization is difficult to achieve because of the ethical dilemma of not providing the same intervention to all patients. A partial solution suggested by the researchers is to include multiple centers and randomly assign individual centers to either have the intervention or not. Further research in error prevention and patient safety will improve the coordination of care in this complex environment.[139]

Using change management strategies in the development of the team working in a hybrid room can be beneficial to the success of the program. The multidisciplinary team can assist in the development of and adherence to standards to help ensure that everyone is aware of the new structure for clinical, infection control, and radiation protocols.[133,152,153]

Recommendation VII

The health care organization should identify risks for injury and complications associated with intraoperative MRI procedures and establish safe practices regardless of magnet format or field strength.

The collective evidence describes the MRI hybrid OR as creating specific challenges for the perioperative team and requiring the following considerations:

- magnetic resonance imaging-compatible equipment to provide safety to personnel and the patient,

- safety training before any team member (eg, clinical personnel, custodial workers, engineers, building maintenance personnel) is assigned to work in the environment,
- a safety checklist and time-out procedures to help ensure proper preparation of the environment, and
- screening tools for MRI personnel and patients to help prevent adverse events.[142,154-160]

The magnetic field can cause metal implants in the body to heat up or induce current, causing patient burns, twisting of implant wires, or even malfunction of the implant.[155]

VII.a. Zones and signs denoting the presence of an MRI scanner should be prominently displayed and be posted outside the MRI suite and on the door leading to the scanner room. [3: Moderate Evidence]

The MRI area is usually divided into four zones. Zone I is uncontrolled and can be accessed by the public or if in the surgical suite, can be accessed by all personnel. Zone II is the interface between zones I and III. Zone III is a strictly controlled area containing the control room or vestibule for screened patients and personnel. Zone IV is the scanner room and is restricted to all screened personnel and patients because of the strong magnetic force in this zone.[142,154,155,157]

VII.b. An MRI director should be appointed and responsible for ensuring
- policy development and review,
- consistent practice for MRI safety in all locations,
- review of reported adverse events, and
- continuous quality improvement.[155]
[3: Moderate Evidence]

The American College of Radiology (ACR) published guidance on MRI safe practices developed by a multidisciplinary team of experts in 2013.[155] The MRI director provides consistency in safety practices in all areas where an MRI scanner is present.[155]

VII.c. Every procedure requiring MRI imaging should have an MRI technician assigned who also functions as the MRI safety officer during the procedure. [3: Moderate Evidence]

The ACR described personnel working in an MRI scanner environment as Level 1 and 2. Level 1 MRI personnel have minimal safety training and work within zones I to III. Level 2 MRI personnel (eg, MRI technicians) have more extensive training and supervise all non-MRI personnel in zones III and IV.[155]

VII.d. All patients and personnel wishing to enter Zone III should first pass an MRI safety screening process.[155] [3: Moderate Evidence]

VII.d.1. Personnel with cardiac devices, stents, filters, grafts, cochlear implants, pumps, nerve stimulaters, or metal foreign bodies (ie, bullets, pellets, shrapnel) should be screened

for MRI safety. A screening checklist should be documented for personnel working in zones III and IV.[155] [3: Moderate Evidence]

VII.d.2. Patients with cardiac devices, stents, filters, grafts, cochlear implants, pumps, nerve stimulaters, or metal foreign bodies (ie, bullets, pellets, shrapnel) should be screened for MRI safety. A screening checklist should be documented for every patient scheduled for surgery in the MRI hybrid OR.[155] [3: Moderate Evidence]

VII.d.3. The MRI director should establish a process for further investigation and approval for scanning a patient screened with any implants, foreign bodies, or other devices that are identified as MRI incompatible.[155] [3: Moderate Evidence]

VII.e. Magnetic resonance imaging-safe (eg, non-ferromagnetic) equipment, including
- cardiac and respiratory monitoring devices,
- oxygen tanks and fire extinguishers,
- room equipment (eg, chairs, gurneys, IV poles),
- instruments, and
- positioning equipment
should be used in all procedures.[154,155,157] [3: Moderate Evidence]

Items such as oxygen tanks, IV poles, and anesthesia machines can become lethal projectiles, causing harm to personnel and patients or damage to the scanner.[154,155]

VII.e.1. A safety checklist that confirms that MRI-incompatible equipment has been moved outside the 5 gauss line should be used before the scanner is moved into the hybrid OR. [3: Moderate Evidence]

Childs and Bruch[142] described the design of two hybrid ORs with a shared MRI system, where the magnet is housed between them in the diagnostic room (ie, a garage). The MRI system is brought into the hybrid OR via a track system. The room was designed with markings on the floor to designate the 5 gauss line to alert personnel to where the magnetic force is strongest when the magnet is in the room. All MRI-incompatible equipment is located outside this circle. The authors described the challenges for the team in performing an intraoperative scan and maintaining the integrity of the sterile field for neurosurgical procedures. The authors provided samples of safety checklists used for patient screening, room check before opening the garage door, and a compatibility check of all items before draping.

VII.f. In the event of an emergency, basic cardiopulmonary resuscitation should be initiated and the patient should be moved out of zone IV to prevent an MRI-incompatible device from entering the room.[157] *[3: Moderate Evidence]*

The collective evidence[142,154,155,157] describes the risk of resuscitating any person in zone IV. The consensus of experts is to initiate basic cardiopulmonary resuscitation and then move the patient to a designated location to run the code. Moving the MRI scanner into the holding bay will also eliminate the risk and allow other personnel to enter the room.[142]

VII.f.1. All persons who respond to an emergency situation should be trained in MRI safety, including police and fire responders.[154,155] *[3: Moderate Evidence]*

VII.f.2. A procedure should be established and implemented for using the quench button that includes defining situations for use. *[3: Moderate Evidence]*

A quench button is located in the control room and will turn off the magnet. Quenching the MRI machine can cause damage because the superconduction coils are no longer being cooled by the system. Use of the quench button should be limited and situations for its use should be defined in the procedure.[142,155,157]

VII.f.3. Drills may be used to help the team define and rehearse emergency response protocols. *[5: Benefits Balanced with Harms]*

Recommendation VIII

Perioperative personnel should receive education and complete competency verification activities in the perioperative nursing care of patients who undergo MIS and computer-assisted procedures.

Minimally invasive surgery and computer-assisted systems are complex, can pose a safety risk, and require a steep learning curve for the surgeon and the perioperative team. The collective evidence supports education and competency verification of the perioperative personnel participating in MIS and computer-assisted surgical procedures and credentialing of physician and surgical assistants.[90,106,111,121,161]

VIII.a. Perioperative RNs should receive initial and ongoing education and complete competency verification activities related to MIS procedures, including
- selection criteria, contraindications, and risks related to distention media;
- knowledge of the use and location of instrumentation and specialized equipment;
- preparation for and response to emergency events (eg, air embolism, conversion to an open procedure); and
- reporting of adverse events.
[5: Benefits Balanced with Harms]

Initial and ongoing education of perioperative personnel facilitates the development of knowledge, skills, and attitudes that affect safe patient care. Competency validation measures individual performance and provides a mechanism for documentation. Error may be minimized with education, training, and competency demonstration.

VIII.b. Perioperative team members participating in computer-assisted robotic procedures should receive education and complete competency verification activities. *[3: Moderate Evidence]*

The collective evidence supports that a comprehensive training program and dedicated perioperative personnel are required for safe robotic programs.[106,109,111,118,161-163] Training programs include manufacturer-sponsored or private programs and include opportunities to practice on cadaveric tissue as well as in simulation trainers.

Seder et al[164] developed a triphasic model for a training program with cardiothoracic residents in robotic surgery. They studied the use of a basic algorithm that started with individual preclinical learning (ie, a module and simulation lab for practicing instrument manipulation and suturing), followed by mentored preclinical exercises (ie, cadaveric experiences and a simulation lab), and ending in progressive clinical responsibilities (ie, table-side assisting and second-console assisting with guidance from a trained surgeon). The researchers measured surgical outcomes and reported a 20% complication rate with no 90-day mortality. They discussed the need to look at different outcomes that could more appropriately assess individual competency, such as by measuring the time required for proper port placement, docking, instrument insertion, taking down the inferior pulmonary ligament, or isolating the pulmonary veins. Measuring these specific competencies can help the surgeon assess the area of difficulty and decrease the surgeon's and surgical team's frustration during the steep learning period for computer-assisted procedures.

Larson et al[111] described five ethical considerations concerning safety in robotic-assisted surgery credentialing guidelines: knowledge of laparoscopic physiology, access and management of minimally invasive complications, case selection for robotic skill mix, conversion to an open procedure as an acceptable solution by the facility with a plan for conversion to an open procedure, and having industry representatives advise only on equipment functioning and not make clinical decisions.

Expert opinion and facility experience reports describe the challenges of training, credentialing, and maintenance of competencies for a robotics program.[90,106,111,121,161] In a Pennsylvania Patient Safety Advisory reviewing the complications reported to the Pennsylvania Patient Safety Authority team training, education, and credentialing were identified as key strategies for implementing a robotic surgery program. Of 722 safety concerns reported in relation to robotic-assisted surgery, 545 (75.5%) were categorized as incidents that may or may not have reached the patient but did not result in harm, and 131 (24.0%) were attributed to equipment, supplies, or devices. Serious events were defined as resulting in patient injury (n = 177) including death (n = 10). Hospitals also provided information about contributing factors from their review of the incident. In two of the reported serious events, inexperienced staff members or issues of staff proficiency were identified as a contributing factor. Education and training of personnel were recommended for prevention of serious events.[90]

VIII.b.1. Education and competency verification for computer-assisted procedures should include
- care, handling, and proper use of the robot and accompanying consoles and video equipment;
- troubleshooting equipment problems (eg, emergency shut off, equipment failure); and
- docking and undocking the robot.

[3: Moderate Evidence]

Corrigan[106] described the development of a pediatric robotic program in which a multidisciplinary team of nurses, surgeons, and anesthesiologists were provided with online education modules and simulation training. After several years of using the program, the team developed standardized protocols and a competency checklist for the perioperative personnel at their facility.

Ramsey[161] also described using standardized training and protocols to enhance efficiency and safety in a robotic program. At her facility, the perioperative team was able to demonstrate a reduced turnover time by standardizing preference cards, standardizing positioning, and creating a dedicated team for the robotic program. The author reported that turnover time for gynecologic robotic surgery was reduced to 23.2 minutes from an average of 24.8 minutes, Implementation of this process improvement allowed this facility to schedule an additional robotic procedure per day, and as many as six procedures could be completed by a single surgeon per day.

Zender and Thell[121] described the importance of educating personnel in maintaining safety in the care of patients undergoing robotic surgery. They emphasized the importance of the proficiency of the perioperative nurses in setup, connection, and positioning of the robotic patient cart. Steenwyk and Lyerly[105] recommended that the thoracic robotic team at their facility be able to perform the emergency undocking procedure in less than 60 seconds so they could quickly perform advanced cardiac life support if required.

VIII.b.2. The perioperative RN should complete education and competency training and verification in assisting in the registration of the patient to the computer-assisted navigation system. *[5: Benefits Balanced with Harms]*

VIII.c. Perioperative team members should receive education and complete competency verification activities for radiation safety[151] and operating the imaging table, controls, and accessories in the hybrid OR. *[3: Moderate Evidence]*

Fixed imaging system table tops are mounted on a fixed base. The isocenter and collision detectors are determined from the fixed base. The table tops can be changed to meet the needs of the procedure. They have different weight tolerances and two additional positioning capabilities: transverse and longitudinal. Schaadt and Landau[135] describe "driving the bed" as terminology used in the imaging departments to describe the movement of the table top during the procedure with the bed controls. Determining who drives the bed is dependent on physician preference, the equipment being used, and how the equipment and bed are configured.

There are advances in table top designs that now provide for flexible positioning with breaks in the table top, rails for bed attachments, and varying pad thicknesses.[135]

VIII.d. Personnel (eg, RN circulators, scrub personnel, housekeeping personnel, surgeons, anesthesia providers, MRI technologists) should receive education about working in and managing a hybrid OR with MRI imaging equipment. Education should include
- MRI safety procedures,
- emergency procedures, and
- screening protocols.[142,154,155]

[3: Moderate Evidence]

Recommendation IX

Policies and procedures for MIS and computer-assisted procedures should be developed, reviewed periodically, revised as necessary, and readily available in the practice setting in which they are used.

Policies and procedures assist in the development of patient safety, quality assessment, and improvement activities. Policies and procedures also serve as operational guidelines used to minimize patients' risk for injury or complications, standardize practice, direct personnel, and establish continuous performance improvement programs. Policies and procedures establish authority, responsibility, and accountability within the practice setting.

IX.a. Policies regarding MIS and computer-assisted equipment should include

- required qualifications and credentials for operating specific equipment or devices (eg, radiologic equipment, MRI equipment) and
- procedure scheduling related to equipment availability.

[5: Benefits Balances with Harms]

Compromised patient safety, delay in care, or cancelation of the procedure may result when required equipment or qualified personnel are not available.

IX.a.1. Policies and procedures for managing loaned MIS and computer-assisted equipment or instruments should be developed and implemented.[2] [1: Strong Evidence]

Glossary

Active electrode: An electrosurgical unit accessory that directs current flow to the surgical site (eg, pencil, various pencil tips).

Capacitive coupling: The transfer of electrical current from the active electrode through intact insulation to adjacent conductive items (eg, tissue, trocars).

Computer-assisted technologies: Robotic, interventional radiology, voice-recognition, or other computer technologies used to enhance minimally invasive surgery.

Endoscopic surgery: Surgical procedures performed using endoscopic instrumentation inserted through a natural orifice or through one or more small incisions.

Extravasation: To pass by infiltration or effusion from a proper vessel or channel (eg, a blood vessel) into surrounding tissue.

Fluoroscopy: Observation of the internal features of an object by means of the fluorescence produced on a screen by x-rays transmitted through the object.

Hybrid OR: An operating room designed with numerous imaging technologies (eg, 3-D angiography, computed tomography, magnetic resonance imaging, positron-emission tomography, intravascular ultrasound) to support surgical procedures that require multiple care providers with varied expertise to provide patient care in one location.

Insufflation: The act of blowing gas into a body cavity for the purpose of visual examination.

Intravasation: The entrance of foreign material or solution into a blood vessel.

Isocenter: The point in space through which the central ray of radiation beams pass.

Minimally invasive surgery: Surgical procedures performed through one or more small incisions using endoscopic instruments, radiographic and magnetic resonance imaging, computer-assisted devices, robotics, and other technologies.

No-fly zone: A zone defined by the imaging manufacturer that refers to workflow and the restriction of positioning dynamic equipment into this space during the operation of the imaging equipment.

Pneumoperitoneum: The presence of air or gas within the peritoneal cavity of the abdomen, often induced for diagnostic purposes.

Restricted area: Includes the OR and procedure room, the clean core, and scrub sink areas. People in this area are required to wear full surgical attire and cover all head and facial hair, including sideburns, beards, and necklines.

Semi-restricted area: Includes the peripheral support areas of the surgical suite and has storage areas for sterile and clean supplies, work areas for storage and processing of instruments, and corridors leading to the restricted areas of the surgical suite.

Telestration: A freehand sketch over a video image.

Transurethral resection (TUR) syndrome: A mild to moderately severe absorption of nonelectrolye solution following transurethral resection.

References

1. Guideline for processing flexible endoscopes. In: *Guidelines for Perioperative Practice*. Denver, CO: AORN, Inc; 2016:675-758. [IVA]

2. Guideline for cleaning and care of surgical instruments. In: *Guidelines for Perioperative Practice*. Denver, CO: AORN, Inc; 2016:773-808. [IVB]

3. Guideline for a safe environment of care, part 2. In: *Guidelines for Perioperative Practice*. Denver, CO: AORN, Inc; 2016:263-288. [IVB]

4. Guideline for surgical smoke safety. In: *Guidelines for Perioperative Practice*. Denver, CO: AORN, Inc; 2016:e77-e106. [IVA]

5. Guideline for prevention of unplanned patient hypothermia. In: *Guidelines for Perioperative Practice*. Denver, CO: AORN, Inc; 2016:531-554. [IVA]

6. Guideline for a safe environment of care, part 1. In: *Guidelines for Perioperative Practice*. Denver, CO: AORN, Inc; 2016:237-262. [IVB]

7. Guideline for positioning the patient. In: *Guidelines for Perioperative Practice*. Denver, CO: AORN, Inc; 2016:649-668. [IVB]

8. Guideline for safe use of energy-generating devices. In: *Guidelines for Perioperative Practice*. Denver, CO: AORN, Inc; 2016:e49-e76. [IVA]

9. Samii A, Gerganov VM. The dedicated endoscopic operating room. *World Neurosurg*. 2013;79(2 Suppl):S15.e19-e22. [VB]

10. Sabnis R, Ganesamoni R, Mishra S, Sinha L, Desai MR. Concept and design engineering: endourology operating room. *Curr Opin Urol*. 2013;23(2):152-157. [VB]

11. Persoon MC, Broos HJ, Witjes JA, Hendrikx AJ, Scherpbier AJ. The effect of distractions in the operating room during endourological procedures. *Surg Endosc*. 2011;25(2):437-443. [VA]

12. Koninckx PR, Stepanian A, Adamyan L, Ussia A, Donnez J, Wattiez A. The digital operating room and the surgeon. *Gynecol Surg*. 2013;10(1):57-62. [VB]

13. Strong VE, Forde KA, MacFadyen BV, et al. Ethical considerations regarding the implementation of new technologies and techniques in surgery. *Surg Endosc*. 2014;28(8):2272-2276. [VB]

14. Choi SD. A review of the ergonomic issues in the laparoscopic operating room. *J Healthc Eng*. 2012;3(4):587-603. [IIB]

15. Stavroulis A, Cutner A, Liao L-M. Staff perceptions of the effects of an integrated laparoscopic theatre environment on teamwork. *Gynecol Surg*. 2013;10(3):177-180. [IIIB]

16. Tjiam IM, Goossens RH, Schout BM, et al. Ergonomics in endourology and laparoscopy: an overview

of musculoskeletal problems in urology. *J Endourol.* 2014;28(5):605-611. [IIIA]

17. Murad FM, Banerjee S, Barth BA, et al. Image management systems. *Gastrointest Endosc.* 2014;79(1):15-22. [VA]

18. Rockstroh M, Franke S, Neumuth T. Requirements for the structured recording of surgical device data in the digital operating room. *Int J Comput Assist Radiol Surg.* 2014;9(1):49-57. [IIIC]

19. 45 CFR 162 Subpart F—Standard Unique Employer Identifier. 2016. US Government Publishing Office. http://www.ecfr.gov/cgi-bin/text-idx?SID=cae9c2c6e308e3d431bcaaf2c5a1207a&mc=true&node=sp45.1.162.f&rgn=div6. Accessed October 26, 2016.

20. 45 CFR 160 Subpart C—Compliance and Investigations. 2016. US Government Publishing Office. http://www.ecfr.gov/cgi-bin/text-idx?SID=60c2bd4a007fc0d54110ea2f89d6dab9&mc=true&node=pt45.1.160&rgn=div5#sp45.1.160.c. Accessed October 26, 2016.

21. 45 CFR 162 Subpart D—Standard Unique Health Identifier for Health Care Providers. 2016. US Government Publishing Office. http://www.ecfr.gov/cgi-bin/text-idx?SID=60c2bd4a007fc0d54110ea2f89d6dab9&mc=true&node=pt45.1.162&rgn=div5#sp45.1.162.d. Accessed October 26, 2016.

22. Anderson SM, Kapp BB, Angell JM, et al. Remote monitoring and supervision of urology residents utilizing integrated endourology suites—a prospective study of patients' opinions. *J Endourol.* 2013;27(1):96-100. [IIIC]

23. Santomauro M, Reina GA, Stroup SP, L'Esperance JO. Telementoring in robotic surgery. *Curr Opin Urol.* 2013;23(2):141-145. [VB]

24. Haidegger T, Sándor J, Benyó Z. Surgery in space: the future of robotic telesurgery. *Surg Endosc.* 2011;25(3):681-690. [VB]

25. Nalugo M, Craner DR, Schwachter M, Ponsky TA. What is "telemedicine" and what does it mean for a pediatric surgeon? *Eur J Pediatr Surg.* 2014;24(4):295-302. [VB]

26. Buzink SN, van Lier L, de Hingh IHJT, Jakimowicz JJ. Risk-sensitive events during laparoscopic cholecystectomy: the influence of the integrated operating room and a preoperative checklist tool. *Surg Endosc.* 2010;24(8):1990-1995. [IIB]

27. Nocco U, del Torchio S. The integrated OR: efficiency and effectiveness evaluation after two years use, a pilot study. *Int J Comput Assist Radiol Surg.* 2011;6(2):175-186. [VA]

28. Schmitz PM, Gollnick I, Modemann S, Rothe A, Niegsch R, Strauss G. An improved instrument table for use in functional endoscopic sinus surgery. *Med Sci Monit Basic Res.* 2015;21:131-134. [IIC]

29. Al-Hakim L. The impact of preventable disruption on the operative time for minimally invasive surgery. *Surg Endosc.* 2011;25(10):3385-3392. [IIIC]

30. Held RT, Hui TT. A guide to stereoscopic 3D displays in medicine. *Acad Radiol.* 2011;18(8):1035-1048. [VB]

31. Kong SH, Oh BM, Yoon H, et al. Comparison of two- and three-dimensional camera systems in laparoscopic performance: a novel 3D system with one camera. *Surg Endosc.* 2010;24(5):1132-1143. [IIIA]

32. Kranzfelder M, Schneider A, Gillen S, Feussner H. New technologies for information retrieval to achieve situational awareness and higher patient safety in the surgical operating room: the MRI institutional approach and review of the literature. *Surg Endosc.* 2011;25(3):696-705. [VB]

33. Pluyter JR, Buzink SN, Rutkowski AF, Jakimowicz JJ. Do absorption and realistic distraction influence performance of component task surgical procedure? *Surg Endosc.* 2010;24(4):902-907. [IIA]

34. Shukla PJ, Maharaj R, Fingerhut A. Ergonomics and technical aspects of minimal access surgery in acute surgery. *Eur J Trauma Emerg Surg.* 2010;36(1):3-9. [VB]

35. Klein MI, DeLucia PR, Olmstead R. The impact of visual scanning in the laparoscopic environment after engaging in strain coping. *Hum Factors.* 2013;55(3):509-519. [IIA]

36. Morton PJ. Implementing AORN recommended practices for MIS: Part II. *AORN J.* 2012;96(4):378-392. [VA]

37. Ulmer BC. Best practices for minimally invasive procedures. *AORN J.* 2010;91(5):558-572. [VB]

38. Llarena NC, Shah AB, Milad MP. Bowel injury in gynecologic laparoscopy: a systematic review. *Obstet Gynecol.* 2015;125(6):1407-1417. [IIA]

39. Levy BF, De Guara J, Willson PD, Soon Y, Kent A, Rockall TA. Bladder injuries in emergency/expedited laparoscopic surgery in the absence of previous surgery: a case series. *Ann R Coll Surg Engl.* 2012;94(3):e118-e120. [VC]

40. Park EY, Kwon JY, Kim KJ. Carbon dioxide embolism during laparoscopic surgery. *Yonsei Med J.* 2012;53(3):459-466. [VB]

41. Cheng Y, Lu J, Xiong X, et al. Gases for establishing pneumoperitoneum during laparoscopic abdominal surgery. *Cochrane Database Syst Rev.* 2013(1):CD009569. [IA]

42. Binda MM. Humidification during laparoscopic surgery: overview of the clinical benefits of using humidified gas during laparoscopic surgery. *Arch Gynecol Obstet.* 2015;292(5):955-971. [VA]

43. Lee KC, Kim JY, Kwak HJ, Lee HD, Kwon IW. The effect of heating insufflation gas on acid-base alterations and core temperature during laparoscopic major abdominal surgery. *Korean J Anesthesiol.* 2011;61(4):275-280. [IA]

44. Najam O, Krishnamoorthy B, Kadir I, et al. Scrotal distension after endoscopic harvesting of the saphenous vein in patients with inguinal hernia. *Ann Thorac Surg.* 2011;92(2):733-735. [VC]

45. Maeda Y, Hirasawa D, Fujita N, et al. A pilot study to assess mediastinal emphysema after esophageal endoscopic submucosal dissection with carbon dioxide insufflation. *Endoscopy.* 2012;44(6):565-571. [IA]

46. Kim JA, Kim JS, Chang MS, Yoo YK, Kim DK. Influence of carbon dioxide insufflation of the neck on intraocular pressure during robot-assisted endoscopic thyroidectomy: a comparison with open thyroidectomy. *Surg Endosc.* 2013;27(5):1587-1593. [IIIB]

47. AAGL Advancing Minimally Invasive Gynecology Worldwide; Munro MG, Storz K, Abbott JA, et al. AAGL Practice Report: Practice Guidelines for the Management of Hysteroscopic Distending Media: (replaces Hysteroscopic Fluid Monitoring Guidelines. *J Am Assoc Gynecol Laparosc.* 2000;7:167-168.). *J Minim Invasive Gynecol.* 2013;20(2):137-148. [IVB]

48. Hayden P, Cowman S. Anaesthesia for laparoscopic surgery. *Contin Educ Anaesth Crit Care Pain.* 2011;11(5):177-180. [VC]

49. Rammohan A, Manimaran AB, Manohar RR, Naidu RM. Nitrous oxide for pneumoperitoneum: no laughing matter this! A prospective single blind case controlled study. *Int J Surg.* 2011;9(2):173-176. [IA]

50. Jacobs VR, Morrison JE Jr, Kiechle M. Twenty-five simple ways to increase insufflation performance and patient safety in laparoscopy. *J Am Assoc Gynecol Laparosc.* 2004;11(3):410-423. [VA]

51. Olsen M, Avery N, Khurana S, Laing R. Pneumoperitoneum for neonatal laparoscopy: how safe is it? *Paediatr Anaesth.* 2013;23(5):457-459. [VC]

52. Aran T, Unsal MA, Guven S, Kart C, Cetin EC, Alver A. Carbon dioxide pneumoperitoneum induces systemic oxidative stress: a clinical study. Eur J Obstet Gynecol Reprod Biol. 2012;161(1):80-83. [IIIB]

53. Eryilmaz HB, Memis D, Sezer A, Inal MT. The effects of different insufflation pressures on liver functions assessed with LiMON on patients undergoing laparoscopic cholecystectomy. *The Scientific World Journal.* 2012;2012:172575. [IA]

54. Kim HY, Kim TY, Lee KC, et al. Pneumothorax during laparoscopic totally extraperitoneal inguinal hernia repair—a case report. *Korean J Anesthesiol.* 2010;58(5):490-494. [VC]

55. Otsuka Y, Katagiri T, Ishii J, et al. Gas embolism in laparoscopic hepatectomy: what is the optimal pneumoperitoneal pressure for laparoscopic major hepatectomy? *J Hepatobiliary Pancreat Sci.* 2013;20(2):137-140. [VB]

56. Liu F, Zhu S, Ji Q, Li W, Liu J. The impact of intra-abdominal pressure on the stroke volume variation and plethysmographic variability index in patients undergoing laparoscopic cholecystectomy. *Biosci Trends.* 2015;9(2):129-133. [IIIB]

57. Lasersohn L. Anaesthetic considerations for paediatric laparoscopy. *S Afr J Surg.* 2011;49(1):22-26. [VB]

58. Mura P, Cossu AP, Musu M, et al. Pituitary apoplexy after laparoscopic surgery: a case report. *Eur Rev Med Pharmacol Sci.* 2014;18(22):3524-3527. [VC]

59. Hackethal A, Brennan D, Rao A, et al. Consideration for safe and effective gynaecological laparoscopy in the obese patient. *Arch Gynecol Obstet.* 2015;292(1):135-141. [VB]

60. Meftahuzzaman SM, Islam MM, Chowdhury KK, et al. Haemodynamic and end tidal CO_2 changes during laparoscopic cholecystectomy under general anaesthesia. *Mymensingh Med J.* 2013;22(3):473-477. [IIIB]

61. Kim SH, Park KS, Shin HY, Yi JH, Kim DK. Paradoxical carbon dioxide embolism during endoscopic thyroidectomy confirmed by transesophageal echocardiography. *J Anesth.* 2010;24(5):774-777. [VC]

62. Pandey V, Varghese E, Rao M, et al. Nonfatal air embolism during shoulder arthroscopy. *Am J Orthop (Belle Mead NJ).* 2013;42(6):272-274. [VC]

63. Kocher MS, Frank JS, Nasreddine AY, et al. Intra-abdominal fluid extravasation during hip arthroscopy: a survey of the MAHORN group. *Arthroscopy.* 2012;28(11):1654-1660. [IIIB]

64. Yousef AA, Suliman GA, Elashry OM, Elsharaby MD, Elgamasy AEK. A randomized comparison between three types of irrigating fluids during transurethral resection in benign prostatic hyperplasia. *BMC Anesthesiol.* 2010;10:7. [IB]

65. Munro MG, Christianson LA. Complications of hysteroscopic and uterine resectoscopic surgery. *Clin Obstet Gynecol.* 2015;58(4):765-797. [VB]

66. Edwards DS, Davis I, Jones NA, Simon DW. Rapid tracheal deviation and airway compromise due to fluid extravasation during shoulder arthroscopy. *J Shoulder Elbow Surg.* 2014;23(7):e163-e165. [VC]

67. Jo YY, Jeon HJ, Choi E, Choi YS. Extreme hyponatremia with moderate metabolic acidosis during hysteroscopic myomectomy—a case report. *Korean J Anesthesiol.* 2011;60(6):440-443. [VC]

68. Khan F, Padmanabha S, Shantaram M, Aravind M. Airway compromise due to irrigation fluid extravasation following shoulder arthroscopy. *J Anaesthesiol Clin Pharmacol.* 2013;29(4):578-579. [VC]

69. Manjuladevi M, Gupta S, Upadhyaya KV, Kutappa AM. Postoperative airway compromise in shoulder arthroscopy: a case series. *Indian J Anaesth.* 2013;57(1):52-55. [VC]

70. Wegmuller B, Hug K, Meier Buenzli C, Yuen B, Maggiorini M, Rudiger A. Life-threatening laryngeal edema and hyponatremia during hysteroscopy. *Crit Care Res Pract.* 2011;2011:140381. [VC]

71. Woo YC, Kang H, Cha SM, et al. Severe intraoperative hyponatremia associated with the absorption of irrigation fluid during hysteroscopic myomectomy: a case report. *J Clin Anesth.* 2011;23(8):649-652. [VC]

72. Yang BJ, Feng LM. Symptomatic hyponatremia and hyperglycemia complicating hysteroscopic resection of intrauterine adhesion: a case report. *Chin Med J.* 2012;125(8):1508-1510. [VC]

73. Stocker L, Umranikar A, Moors A, Umranikar S. An overview of hysteroscopy and hysteroscopic surgery. *Obstet Gynaecol Reprod Med.* 2013;23(5):146-153. [VB]

74. Van Kruchten PM, Vermelis JMFW, Herold I, Van Zundert AAJ. Hypotonic and isotonic fluid overload as a complication of hysteroscopic procedures: two case reports. *Minerva Anestesiol.* 2010;76(5):373-377. [VC]

75. Rademaker BMP, van Kesteren PJM, de Haan P, Rademaker D, France C. How safe is the intravasation limit in hysteroscopic surgery? *J Minim Invasive Gynecol.* 2011;18(3):355-361. [IIIB]

76. Morton PJ. Implementing AORN recommended practices for minimally invasive surgery: part I. *AORN J.* 2012;96(3):295-314. [VA]

77. Darwish AM, Hassan ZZ, Attia AM, Abdelraheem SS, Ahmed YM. Biological effects of distension media in bipolar versus monopolar resectoscopic myomectomy: a randomized trial. *J Obstet Gynaecol Res.* 2010;36(4):810-817. [IB]

78. Park JT, Lim HK, Kim SG, Um DJ. A comparison of the influence of 2.7% sorbitol-0.54% mannitol and 5% glucose irrigating fluids on plasma serum physiology during hysteroscopic procedures. *Korean J Anesthesiol.* 2011;61(5):394-398. [IIC]

79. Silva JM Jr, Barros MA, Chahda MAL, Santos IM, Marubayashi LY, Malbouisson LM. Risk factors for perioperative complications in endoscopic surgery with irrigation. *Braz J Anesthesiol.* 2013;63(4):327-333. [IIIA]

80. Bergeron ME, Ouellet P, Bujold E, et al. The impact of anesthesia on glycine absorption in operative hysteroscopy: a randomized controlled trial. *Anesth Analg.* 2011;113(4):723-728. [IA]

81. Kumar A, Kumar A. New hysteroscopy pump to monitor real-time rate of fluid intravasation. *J Minim Invasive Gynecol.* 2012;19(3):369-375. [VA]

82. Ladner B, Nester K, Cascio B. Abdominal fluid extravasation during hip arthroscopy. *Arthroscopy.* 2010;26(1):131-135. [VC]

83. Cavaignac E, Pailhe R, Reina N, Chiron P, Laffosse JM. Massive proximal extravasation as a complication during arthroscopic anterior cruciate ligament reconstruction. *Knee Surg Rel Res.* 2013;25(2):84-87. [VC]

84. Stafford GH, Malviya A, Villar RN. Fluid extravasation during hip arthroscopy. *Hip Int.* 2011;21(6):740-743. [VA]

85. Verma M, Sekiya JK. Intrathoracic fluid extravasation after hip arthroscopy. *Arthroscopy.* 2010;26(9 Suppl):S90-S94. [VC]

86. Hermanns T, Fankhauser CD, Hefermehl LJ, et al. Prospective evaluation of irrigation fluid absorption during pure transurethral bipolar plasma vaporisation of the prostate using expired-breath ethanol measurements. *BJU Int.* 2013;112(5):647-654. [IIIB]

87. Lee KC, Kim HY, Lee MJ, Koo JW, Lim JA, Kim SH. Abdominal compartment syndrome occurring due to uterine perforation during a hysteroscopy procedure. *J Anesth.* 2010;24(2):280-283. [VC]

88. Guideline for medication safety. In: *Guidelines for Perioperative Practice.* Denver, CO: AORN, Inc; 2016:289-332. [IVA]

89. Boyd HR, Stanley C. Sources of error when tracking irrigation fluids during hysteroscopic procedures. *J Am Assoc Gynecol Laparosc.* 2000;7(4):472-476. [VA]

90. Dubeck D. Robotic-assisted surgery: focus on training and credentialing. *Penn Patient Saf Advis.* 2014;11(3):93-101. [VA]

91. Aubé C, Schmidt D, Brieger J, et al. Influence of NaCl concentrations on coagulation, temperature, and electrical conductivity using a perfusion radiofrequency ablation system: an ex vivo experimental study. *Cardiovasc Intervent Radiol.* 2007;30(1):92-97. [IIA]

92. Brace CL, Laeseke PF, Prasad V, Lee FT. Electrical isolation during radiofrequency ablation: 5% dextrose in water provides better protection than saline. *Conf Proc IEEE Eng Med Biol Soc.* 2006;1:5021-5024. [IIB]

93. Closon F, Tulandi T. Future research and developments in hysteroscopy. *Best Pract Res Clin Obstet Gynaecol.* 2015;29(7):994-1000. [VA]

94. Culp WC Jr, Kimbrough BA, Luna S, Maguddayao AJ, Eidson JL, Paolino DV. Use of the electrosurgical unit in a carbon dioxide atmosphere. *J Med Eng Technol.* 2016;40(2):29-34. [IIB]

95. Curtin B, Friebe I. Dermal burn during hip arthroscopy. *Orthopedics.* 2014;37(8):e746-e749. [VA]

96. Deffieux X, Gauthier T, Menager N, Legendre G, Agostini A, Pierre F. Hysteroscopy: guidelines for clinical practice from the French College of Gynaecologists and Obstetricians. *Eur J Obstet Gynecol Reprod Biol.* 2014;178:114-122. [IVA]

97. Faul P, Schlenker B, Gratzke C, Stief CG, Reich O, Gustaw Hahn R. Clinical and technical aspects of bipolar transurethral prostate resection. *Scand J Urol Nephrol.* 2008;42(4):318-323. [VB]

98. Groenman FA, Peters LW, Rademaker BMP, Bakkum EA. Embolism of air and gas in hysteroscopic procedures: pathophysiology and implication for daily practice. *J Minim Invasive Gynecol.* 2008;15(2):241-247. [VA]

99. Huang S, Gateley D, Moss ALH. Accidental burn injury during knee arthroscopy. *Arthroscopy.* 2007;23(12):1363.e1-1363.e3. [VB]

100. Laeseke PF, Sampson LA, Brace CL, Winter TC III, Fine JP, Lee FT Jr. Unintended thermal injuries from radiofrequency ablation: protection with 5% dextrose in water. *Am J Roentgenol.* 2006;186(5 Suppl):S249-S254. [IIA]

101. Ubee SS, Philip J, Nair M. Bipolar technology for transurethral prostatectomy. *Expert Rev Med Devices.* 2011;8(2):149-154. [VA]

102. Vilos GA, Newton DW, Odell RC, Abu-Rafea B, Vilos AG. Characterization and mitigation of stray radiofrequency currents during monopolar resectoscopic electrosurgery. *J Minim Invasive Gynecol.* 2006;13(2):134-140. [VA]

103. Craciunas L, Sajid MS, Howell R. Carbon dioxide versus normal saline as distension medium for diagnostic hysteroscopy: a systematic review and meta-analysis of randomized controlled trials. *Fertil Steril.* 2013;100(6):1709-1714. [IA]

104. Mandapathil M, Teymoortash A, Güldner C, Wiegand S, Mutters R, Werner JA. Establishing a transoral robotic surgery program in an academic hospital in Germany. *Acta Otolaryngol.* 2014;134(7):661-665. [VC]

105. Steenwyk B, Lyerly R 3rd. Advancements in robotic-assisted thoracic surgery. *Anesthesiol Clin.* 2012;30(4):699-708. [VB]

106. Corrigan K. Pediatric robotic surgery program requires multidisciplinary team collaboration. *AORN J.* 2014;99(3):7-8. [VB]

107. Pandey R, Garg R, Chandralekha, et al. Robot-assisted thoracoscopic thymectomy: perianaesthetic concerns. *Eur J Anaesthesiol.* 2010;27(5):473-477. [VA]

108. Best J, Day L, Ingram L, Musgrave B, Rushing H, Schooley B. Comparison of robotic vs standard surgical procedure on postoperative nursing care of women undergoing total abdominal hysterectomy. *Medsurg Nurs.* 2014;23(6):414-421. [IIIA]

109. Nayeemuddin M, Daley SC, Ellsworth P. Modifiable factors to decrease the cost of robotic-assisted procedures. *AORN J.* 2013;98(4):343-352. [VB]

110. Yuh B. The bedside assistant in robotic surgery—keys to success. *Urol Nurs.* 2013;33(1):29-32. [VB]

111. Larson JA, Johnson MH, Bhayani SB. Application of surgical safety standards to robotic surgery: five principles of ethics for nonmaleficence. *J Am Coll Surg.* 2014;218(2):290-293. [VB]

112. Christie S. Electromagnetic navigational bronchoscopy and robotic-assisted thoracic surgery. *AORN J.* 2014;99(6):750-763. [VB]

113. Kawachi H, Kawachi Y, Ikeda C, Takagi R, Katakura A, Shibahara T. Oral and maxillofacial surgery with computer-assisted navigation system. *Bull Tokyo Dent Coll.* 2010;51(1):35-39. [VC]

114. Metz P, Adam J, Gerken M, Jalali B. Compact, transmissive two-dimensional spatial disperser design with application in simultaneous endoscopic imaging and laser microsurgery. *Appl Opt.* 2014;53(3):376-382. [VA]

115. Muns A, Meixensberger J, Arnold S, et al. Integration of a 3D ultrasound probe into neuronavigation. *Acta Neurochir.* 2011;153(7):1529-1533. [VA]

116. Kaduk WMH, Podmelle F, Louis PJ. Surgical navigation in reconstruction. *Oral Maxillofac Surg Clin North Am.* 2013;25(2):313-333. [VB]

117. Young PS, Findlay H, Patton JTS, Mahendra A. (iii) Computer assisted navigation in musculoskeletal oncology. *Orthop Trauma.* 2014;28(5):294-302. [VB]

118. Mavrogenis AF, Savvidou OD, Mimidis G, et al. Computer-assisted navigation in orthopedic surgery. *Orthopedics.* 2013;36(8):631-642. [VA]

119. Kenngott HG, Wagner M, Gondan M, et al. Real-time image guidance in laparoscopic liver surgery: first clinical experience with a guidance system based on intraoperative CT imaging. *Surg Endosc.* 2014;28(3):933-940. [VA]

120. Zullo MD, McCarroll ML, Mendise TM, et al. Safety culture in the gynecology robotics operating room. *J Minim Invasive Gynecol.* 2014;21(5):893-900. [IIA]

121. Zender J, Thell C. Developing a successful robotic surgery program in a rural hospital. *AORN J.* 2010;92(1):72-86. [VB]

122. Gkegkes ID, Karydis A, Tyritzis SI, Iavazzo C. Ocular complications in robotic surgery. *Int J Med Robot.* 2015;11(3):269-274. [VA]

123. Hung CF, Yang CK, Cheng CL, Ou YC. Bowel complication during robotic-assisted laparoscopic radical prostatectomy. *Anticancer Res.* 2011;31(10):3497-3501. [VA]

124. Sarmanian JD. Robot-assisted thoracic surgery (RATS): perioperative nursing professional development program. *AORN J.* 2015;102(3):241-253. [VB]

125. Quinn D, Moohan J. Optimal laparoscopic ergonomics in gynaecology. *Obstet Gynaecol.* 2015;17(2):77-82. [VB]

126. Facility Guidelines Institute; American Society for Healthcare Engineering. *Guidelines for Design and Construction of Hospitals and Outpatient Facilities*. Chicago, IL: American Society for Healthcare Engineering; 2014. [IVA]

127. Aston G. The hybrid OR. *Hosp Health Netw*. 2014;88(3):34-37. [VC]

128. Kirkpatrick AW, Vis C, Dube M, et al. The evolution of a purpose designed hybrid trauma operating room from the trauma service perspective: the RAPTOR (resuscitation with angiography percutaneous treatments and operative resuscitations). *Injury*. 2014;45(9):1413-1421. [VB]

129. Baillie J. Dual hybrid suite "a first" for the UK. *Health Estate*. 2014;68(7):53-58. [VC]

130. Kleiman N. Room considerations with TAVR. *Methodist Debakey Cardiovasc J*. 2012;8(2):19-21. [VC]

131. Knudson L. Hybrid ORs set the stage for cutting-edge care. *AORN J*. 2012;96(2):C1, C8-C9. [VC]

132. Kpodonu J. Hybrid cardiovascular suite: the operating room of the future. *J Card Surg*. 2010;25(6):704-709. [VB]

133. Odle TG. Managing transition to a hybrid operating room. *Radiol Technol*. 2011;83(2):165-181. [VB]

134. Tsagakis K, Konorza T, Dohle DS, et al. Hybrid operating room concept for combined diagnostics, intervention and surgery in acute type A dissection. *Eur J Cardiothorac Surg*. 2013;43(2):397-404. [VB]

135. Schaadt J, Landau B. Hybrid OR 101: a primer for the OR nurse. *AORN J*. 2013;97(1):81-100. [VB]

136. Richter PH, Yarboro S, Kraus M, Gebhard F. One year orthopaedic trauma experience using an advanced interdisciplinary hybrid operating room. *Injury*. 2015;46(Suppl 4):S129-S134. [VB]

137. Klein LW, Miller DL, Balter S, et al. Occupational health hazards in the interventional laboratory: time for a safer environment. *J Radiol Nurs*. 2010;29(3):75-82. [VA]

138. Lauck S, Achtem L, Boone RH, et al. Implementation of processes of care to support transcatheter aortic valve replacement programs. *Eur J Cardiovasc Nurs*. 2013;12(1):33-38. [VB]

139. Patel SR, Gohel MS, Hamady M, et al. Reducing errors in combined open/endovascular arterial procedures: influence of a structured mental rehearsal before the endovascular phase. *J Endovasc Ther*. 2012;19(3):383-389. [IIA]

140. Shunk KA, Zimmet J, Cason B, Speiser B, Tseng EE. Development of a Veterans Affairs hybrid operating room for transcatheter aortic valve replacement in the cardiac catheterization laboratory. *JAMA Surg*. 2015;150(3):216-222. [VC]

141. Urbanowicz JA. The hybrid suite—sweet. *J Radiol Nurs*. 2011;30(2):62-66. [VB]

142. Childs S, Bruch P. Successful management of risk in the hybrid OR. *AORN J*. 2015;101(2):223-234. [VB]

143. Varu VN, Greenberg JI, Lee JT. Improved efficiency and safety for EVAR with utilization of a hybrid room. *Eur J Vasc Endovasc Surg*. 2013;46(6):675-679. [VA]

144. Speiser B, Dutra-Brice C. Transcatheter aortic valve replacement. *Dimens Crit Care Nurs*. 2014;33(5):262-274. [VB]

145. *AORN Position Statement on One Perioperative Registered Nurse Circulator Dedicated to Every Patient Undergoing an Operative or Other Invasive Procedure*. AORN, Inc. http://www.aorn.org/guidelines/clinical-resources/position-statements. Accessed October 26, 2016.

146. D'Amours SK, Rastogi P, Ball CG. Utility of simultaneous interventional radiology and operative surgery in a dedicated suite for seriously injured patients. *Curr Opin Crit Care*. 2013;19(6):587-593. [VB]

147. Katzen BT, Kiah J, Smith D, Denny D, Stoia M. Hybrid interventional radiology. *Perioper Nurs Clin*. 2010;5(2):215-227. [VB]

148. Karkos CD, Menexes GC, Patelis N, Kalogirou TE, Giagtzidis IT, Harkin DW. A systematic review and meta-analysis of abdominal compartment syndrome after endovascular repair of ruptured abdominal aortic aneurysms. *J Vasc Surg*. 2014;59(3):829-842. [IIA]

149. Contrera P, Cushing M. Transcatheter aortic valve replacement. *AANA J*. 2013;81(5):399-408. [VB]

150. Smeltzer HG, Scott JR, Frey SA, et al. Collaboration between interventional neurosurgery and vascular surgery in the hybrid operating room. *J Radiol Nurs*. 2014;33(3):127-131. [VC]

151. Guideline for radiation safety. In: *Guidelines for Perioperative Practice*. Denver, CO: AORN, Inc; 2016:333-368. [IVA]

152. Mason SL, Kuruvilla S, Riga CV, et al. Design and validation of an error capture tool for quality evaluation in the vascular and endovascular surgical theatre. *Eur J Vasc Endovasc Surg*. 2013;45(3): 248-254. [IIIA]

153. Robbins DA. Current modalities for abdominal aortic aneurysm repair: implications for nurses. *J Vasc Nurs*. 2010;28(4):136-146. [IIB]

154. Practice advisory on anesthetic care for magnetic resonance imaging: an updated report by the American Society of Anesthesiologists task force on anesthetic care for magnetic resonance imaging. *Anesthesiology*. 2015;122(3):495-520. [VA]

155. ACR guidance document on MR safe practices: 2013. *J Magn Reson Imaging*. 2013;37(3):501-530. [VA]

156. Zhao Y, Chen X, Wang F, et al. Integration of diffusion tensor-based arcuate fasciculus fibre navigation and intraoperative MRI into glioma surgery. *J Clin Neurosci*. 2012;19(2):255-261. [VA]

157. Ocazionez D, Dicks DL, Favinger JL, et al. Magnetic resonance imaging safety in cardiothoracic imaging. *J Thorac Imaging*. 2014;29(5):262-269. [VB]

158. Henrichs B, Walsh RP. Intraoperative MRI for neurosurgical and general surgical interventions. *Curr Opin Anaesthesiol*. 2014;27(4):448-452. [VB]

159. Hemingway M, Kilfoyle M. Safety planning for intraoperative magnetic resonance imaging. *AORN J*. 2013;98(5):508-524. [VB]

160. Oluigbo CO, Rezai AR. Magnetic resonance imaging safety of deep brain stimulator devices. *Handb Clin Neurol*. 2013;116:73-76. [VB]

161. Ramsey R. Robotic gynecologic surgery: trends and nurse involvement at a regional hospital. *OR Nurse*. 2012;6(2):41-44. [VC]

162. Korb W, Geisler N, Straus G. Solving challenges in inter- and trans-disciplinary working teams: lessons from the surgical technology field. *Artif Intell Med*. 2015;63(3):209-219. [VA]

163. Taylor D. The implementation of a da Vinci Surgical System at The Royal Wolverhampton NHS Trust. *J Perioper Pract*. 2014;24(3):4-12. [VC]

164. Seder CW, Cassivi SD, Wigle DA. Navigating the pathway to robotic competency in general thoracic surgery. *Innovations (Phila)*. 2013;8(3):184-189. [VC]

Acknowledgements

LEAD AUTHOR
Mary C. Fearon, MSN, RN, CNOR
AORN Department of Nursing
Perioperative Practice Specialist
Denver, Colorado

CONTRIBUTING AUTHOR
Ramona Conner, MSN, RN, CNOR, FAAN
Editor-in-Chief, Guidelines for Perioperative Practice
AORN Department of Nursing
Denver, Colorado

The authors and AORN thank Barbara L. Nalley, MSN, CRNP, CNOR, Manager, Jackson Surgical Assistants, Crofton, Maryland; David R. Urbach, MD, Clinical Epidemiology MSc, University Health Network, Toronto, Canada; James (Jay) Bowers, BSN, RN, CNOR, TNCC, Clinical Educator, West Virginia University Healthcare, Morgantown; Janice A. Neil, PhD, CNE, RN, Associate Professor, East Carolina College of Nursing, Greenville, North Carolina; Lisa Spruce, DNP, RN, CNS-CP, CNOR, ACNS, ACNP, FAAN, Director, Evidence-based Perioperative Practice, Department of Nursing, AORN, Denver, Colorado; and Sharon A. Van Wicklin, MSN, RN, CNOR, CRNFA(E), CPSN-R, PLNC, Senior Perioperative Practice Specialist, Department of Nursing, AORN, Denver, Colorado, for their assistance in developing this guideline.

PUBLICATION HISTORY

Originally published as proposed recommended practices February 1994, *AORN Journal.*

Revised November 1998; published February 1999, *AORN Journal.* Reformatted July 2000.

Revised November 2004; published as Recommended Practices for Endoscopic Minimally Invasive Surgery in *Standards, Recommended Practices, and Guidelines,* 2005 edition. March 2005, *AORN Journal.*

Revised October 2009 for online publication in Perioperative Standards and Recommended Practices.

Editorial revision July 2012. Recommendation IV.j revised and approved by the Recommended Practices Advisory Board. Reformatted September 2012 for publication in *Perioperative Standards and Recommended Practices,* 2013 edition.

Minor editing revisions made in November 2014 for publication in *Guidelines for Perioperative Practice,* 2015 edition, as Guideline for Minimally Invasive Surgery.

Revised December 2016 for publication in *Guidelines for Perioperative Practice* online.

GUIDELINE FOR CARE OF THE PATIENT RECEIVING MODERATE SEDATION/ANALGESIA

The Guideline for Care of the Patient Receiving Moderate Sedation/Analgesia has been approved by the AORN Guidelines Advisory Board. It was presented as a proposed guideline for comments by members and others. The guideline is effective December 15, 2015. The recommendations in the guideline are intended to be achievable and represent what is believed to be an optimal level of practice. Policies and procedures will reflect variations in practice settings and/or clinical situations that determine the degree to which the guideline can be implemented. AORN recognizes the many diverse settings in which perioperative nurses practice; therefore, this guideline is adaptable to all areas where operative or other invasive procedures may be performed.

Purpose

This document provides guidance for care of the patient receiving moderate sedation/analgesia provided by a registered nurse (RN) in the perioperative practice setting. Guidance is provided for determining the scope of nursing practice related to administration of moderate sedation/analgesia, patient selection criteria, pre-sedation patient assessment (eg, airway, difficult mask ventilation, obstructive sleep apnea), intraoperative sedation assessment, staffing, monitoring, medication administration, and postoperative discharge criteria.

The goal of moderate sedation/analgesia is drug-induced, mild depression of consciousness achieved with the use of sedatives or a combination of sedatives and analgesic medications, most often administered intravenously, and titrated to achieve a desired effect. The primary goal of moderate sedation/analgesia is to reduce the patient's anxiety and discomfort. Moderate sedation also can facilitate cooperation between the patient and care providers. Moderate sedation produces a condition in which the patient exhibits a mildly depressed level of consciousness and an altered perception of pain but retains the ability to respond appropriately to verbal or tactile stimulation. The patient maintains protective reflexes and may experience some degree of amnesia.[1]

The desired effect is a level of sedation with or without analgesia that enables the patient to tolerate diagnostic, therapeutic, and invasive procedures through relief from anxiety and pain. The four distinct characteristics of moderate sedation/analgesia are the following:

- The patient is able to respond purposefully to verbal commands or light tactile stimulation.
- The patient maintains his or her protective reflexes and is able to communicate verbally.
- The patient maintains adequate, spontaneous ventilation.
- There are minimal variations in the patient's vital signs.[1]

Depth of sedation occurs across a continuum from minimal sedation to moderate sedation/analgesia, deep sedation/analgesia, and finally general anesthesia. Patients' responses to the medications for moderate sedation/analgesia are unpredictable. The patient may slip into a deeper level of sedation than intended; therefore, practitioners who administer moderate sedation/analgesia should be able to rescue a patient who enters deep sedation/analgesia.[1]

This following topics are outside the scope of this document: local anesthesia, local monitored anesthesia care, general anesthesia, regional anesthesia (eg, spinal, epidural), total intravenous anesthesia, minimal sedation, deep sedation, endotracheal intubation, laryngoscopy, awake intubation, dental office procedures, fospropofol, etomidate, propofol administration in the emergency room and intensive care unit, sedation for intubated and mechanically ventilated patients, palliative care, premedication for general anesthesia, pain management following discharge from the postanesthesia care unit (PACU), and proceduralist techniques. It is not the intent of this guideline to address situations that require the services of an anesthesia professional or to substitute the services of a perioperative RN in those situations that require the services of an anesthesia professional.

Moderate sedation/analgesia may be referred to as moderate sedation, conscious sedation, nurse-administered procedural sedation, nurse-administered propofol sedation, or procedural sedation and analgesia. The term moderate sedation/analgesia is used throughout this document in the recommendations, interventions, and activities. Other terms may be seen in the rationales if the cited literature refers to moderate sedation/analgesia by another term.

Evidence Review

A medical librarian conducted systematic searches of the databases MEDLINE®, CINAHL®, and the Cochrane Database of Systematic Reviews in April 2013 and November 2014, and limited results to meta-analyses, systematic reviews, randomized and nonrandomized trials and studies, reviews, and guidelines. The librarian also conducted a non-systematic search of the Scopus® database. The searches were limited to literature published in English between

FIGURE 1. FLOW DIAGRAM OF LITERATURE SEARCH RESULTS

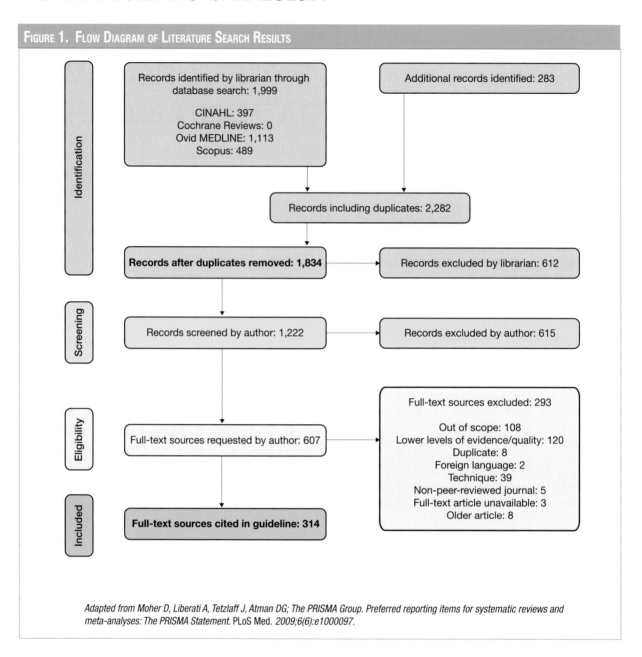

Records identified by librarian through database search: 1,999

CINAHL: 397
Cochrane Reviews: 0
Ovid MEDLINE: 1,113
Scopus: 489

Additional records identified: 283

Identification

Records including duplicates: 2,282

Records after duplicates removed: 1,834

Records excluded by librarian: 612

Screening

Records screened by author: 1,222

Records excluded by author: 615

Eligibility

Full-text sources requested by author: 607

Full-text sources excluded: 293

Out of scope: 108
Lower levels of evidence/quality: 120
Duplicate: 8
Foreign language: 2
Technique: 39
Non-peer-reviewed journal: 5
Full-text article unavailable: 3
Older article: 8

Included

Full-text sources cited in guideline: 314

Adapted from Moher D, Liberati A, Tetzlaff J, Atman DG; The PRISMA Group. Preferred reporting items for systematic reviews and meta-analyses: The PRISMA Statement. PLoS Med. 2009;6(6):e1000097.

2006 and November 2014. At the time of the initial searches, the librarian established weekly alerts on the search topics and until April 2015, presented relevant alert results to the lead author.

During the development of this guideline, the lead author requested supplementary literature searches and additional literature that either did not fit the original search criteria or was discovered during the evidence-appraisal process. Finally, the lead author and the medical librarian identified relevant guidelines from government agencies, professional organizations, and standards-setting bodies.

Although the lead author's original search request encompassed both moderate sedation and local anesthesia, only literature relevant to the care of patients receiving moderate sedation/analgesia was considered for inclusion in this document. Search terms included *conscious sedation, anti-anxiety agents, flu-*

mazenil, naloxone, propofol, midazolam, fentanyl, drug hypersensitivity, risk assessment, sleep apnea syndromes, continuous positive airway pressure, modified Mallampati test, thyromental distance test, bispectral index, airway management, and *patient discharge.* Other key words were included to address the concepts of patient assessment, sedation scales, risk factors, patient monitoring, and tools and methods for predicting difficult mask ventilation. The complete search strategies are available upon request.

Inclusion criteria were research and non-research literature in English, complete publications, relevance to the key questions, and publication dates within the time restriction unless none was available.

Excluded were non-peer-reviewed publications and literature that examined local anesthesia, local monitored anesthesia care, general anesthesia, regional anesthesia (eg, spinal, epidural), total intravenous anesthesia, minimal sedation, deep sedation, endotracheal intubation, laryngoscopy, awake intubation, dental office procedures, fospropofol, etomidate, propofol administration in the emergency room and intensive care unit, sedation for intubated and mechanically ventilated patients, palliative care, premedication for general anesthesia, pain management following discharge from the PACU, and proceduralist techniques. Low-quality evidence was excluded when higher quality evidence was available, and literature outside the time restriction was excluded when literature within the time restriction was available (Figure 1).

Articles identified by the search were provided to the lead author and evidence reviewers for review and critical appraisal using the AORN Research or Non-Research Evidence Appraisal Tools as appropriate. The literature was independently evaluated and appraised according to the strength and quality of the evidence. Each article was then assigned an appraisal score. The appraisal score is noted in brackets after each reference as applicable.

The evidence supporting each intervention and activity statement within a specific recommendation was summarized, and the AORN Evidence Rating Model was used to rate the strength of the collective evidence. Factors considered in the review of the collective evidence were the quality of the evidence, the quantity of similar evidence on a given topic, the consistency of evidence supporting a recommendation, and the potential benefits and harms. The assigned evidence rating is noted in brackets after each intervention and activity statement.

Note: *The evidence summary table is available at http://www.aorn.org/evidencetables.*

Editor's note: *MEDLINE is a registered trademark of the US National Library of Medicine's Medical Literature Analysis and Retrieval System, Bethesda, MD. CINAHL, Cumulative Index to Nursing and Allied Health Literature, is a registered trademark of EBSCO Industries, Birmingham, AL. Scopus is a registered trademark of Elsevier B.V., Amsterdam, The Netherlands.*

Recommendation I

The perioperative RN administering moderate sedation/analgesia must practice within the scope of nursing practice as defined by his or her state board of nursing and should comply with state advisory opinions, declaratory rules, and other regulations that direct the practice of the registered nurse.

The RN's scope of practice is determined by the state's nurse practice act and the state board of nursing. All states and territories have enacted a nurse practice act passed by the state's legislature. Each state's nurse practice act establishes a board of nursing. The board of nursing develops specific rules, regulations, and other guidance such as declaratory rulings and advisory opinions that clarify the law.[2] The state board of nursing grants a license to practice nursing to a competent individual with the skills necessary to perform within a specified scope of practice.[3-6] The state's nurse practice act and its rules protect individuals receiving nursing care from licensed practitioners.[2]

I.a. The perioperative RN should consult with his or her state board of nursing for declaratory rulings and other guidelines that relate to the RN's role as a provider of moderate sedation/analgesia. *[2: High Evidence]*

The professional obligation of the perioperative RN to safeguard patients is grounded in the ethical obligation to the patient, the profession, society, the American Nurses Association (ANA) *Nursing: Scope and Standards of Practice,*[4] AORN's Standards of Perioperative Nursing,[5] AORN's Perioperative Explications for the *ANA Code of Ethics for Nurses,*[7] and state nurse practice acts.

I.a.1. The perioperative RN should verify that administering the medications for moderate sedation/analgesia is within the scope of nursing practice as defined by his or her state board of nursing, state advisory opinions, declaratory rules, and other regulations that direct the practice of the RN. *[1: Strong Evidence]*

Each state board of nursing regulates which medications (eg, propofol, etomidate, nitrous oxide) are within the scope of practice for non-anesthesia providers to administer. The collective evidence conflicts regarding the medications that RNs can safely administer. The American Association of Nurse Anesthetists and the American Society of Anesthesiologists (ASA) issued a joint statement[8] in 2004 that states,

Because sedation is a continuum, it is not always possible to predict how an individual patient will respond. Due to the potential for rapid, profound changes in sedative/analgesia depth and the lack of antagonistic medications, agents such as propofol require special attention.

Whenever propofol is used for sedation/anesthesia, it should be administered only by persons trained in the administration of general anesthesia, who are not simultaneously involved in these surgical or diagnostic procedures. This restriction is concordant with specific language in the propofol insert, and failure to follow these recommendations could put patients at increased risk of significant injury or death.

Similar concerns apply when other intravenous induction agents are used for sedation, such as thiopental, methohexital or etomidate.

The AORN Board of Directors endorsed this statement in 2005.

The ASA amended its *Statement on Safe Use of Propofol*[9] in 2014. If an anesthesiologist is not caring for the patient,

non-anesthesia personnel who administer propofol should be qualified to rescue patients whose level of sedation becomes deeper than initially intended and who enter, if briefly, a state of general anesthesia.

The statement additionally delineates the roles and responsibilities of the physician responsible for moderate sedation/analgesia and the practitioner administering propofol as well as education, training, airway management, cardiovascular management, monitoring, and staffing requirements.

In a systematic review, Singh et al[10] identified, analyzed, and summarized randomized controlled trials (RCTs) that compared the relative effectiveness, patient acceptance, and safety of using propofol for colonoscopy compared with traditional sedatives of narcotics and benzodiazepines. The authors concluded that use of propofol can lead to faster recovery, earlier discharge, and increased patient satisfaction without an increase in adverse effects. Secondarily, one study included in the systematic review compared propofol administration by anesthesiologists to administration by non-anesthesiologists and found no difference in procedure time or patient satisfaction. They concluded that there is insufficient high-quality evidence comparing propofol administration by anesthesiologists to administration by non-anesthesiologists.

The collective evidence[11-34] demonstrates the safety of nurse-administered propofol. The majority of the studies are from the gastroenterology literature. In a prospective, randomized, single-blind study, Lee et al[13] compared two sedation protocols in patients undergoing therapeutic esophagogastroduodenoscopy (EGD) or endoscopic retrograde cholangiopancreatography (ERCP). Registered nurses with advanced cardiac life support certification administered the sedatives and analgesics under the supervision of the endoscopist. The RNs were dedicated to the administration of the medications and patient monitoring. The control group (n = 107) received IV midazolam and intramuscular meperedine. The intervention group (n = 107) received midazolam and meperedine in addition to IV propofol. There were no significant differences between the intervention and control groups in the rates of cardiopulmonary complications (8.8% versus 5.8%, respectively) and transient interruption of procedures (2.9% versus 0%, respectively). No patient required assisted ventilation or premature termination of a procedure. The authors concluded that their study demonstrated that all of the cardiopulmonary complications related to the addition of propofol were minor.

The collective evidence[18,35-69] demonstrates the safety and efficacy of RN-administered sedation/analgesia medications (eg, midazolam, fentanyl, ketamine, dexmedetomidine) alone or in combination. McQuaid and Laine[35] conducted a systematic review and meta-analysis of 36 RCTs containing 3,918 patients undergoing EGD or colonoscopy to compare efficacy, safety, and efficiency of benzodiazepines (eg, midazolam, diazepam), narcotics (fentanyl, meperedine), and propofol used alone or in combination. The authors concluded that sedation for routine EGD and colonoscopy with any currently available agents presented a low risk for clinically significant events. Patients reported higher satisfaction and less frequent memory loss with midazolam than with diazepam. The authors concluded that controlled trials are needed to examine the role of lower doses of propofol in combination with midazolam or narcotics compared with propofol alone or benzodiazepines plus narcotics.

I.b.   A licensed independent practitioner qualified by education,[1,70] training,[1,70] and licensure to administer moderate sedation should supervise the RN administering moderate sedation/analgesia.[71-73] *[2: High Evidence]*

The ASA recommends that a non-anesthesiologist sedation practitioner who supervises administration of medications for moderate sedation satisfactorily complete a formal training program in the safe administration of sedative and analgesic medications and rescue of patients who may slip into a deeper level of sedation (eg, deep sedation, general anesthesia).[71]

Recommendation II

The perioperative RN should perform and document a patient nursing assessment before administering moderate sedation/analgesia.

The collective evidence[1,72,74-76] establishes the benefits of a preprocedure patient assessment. A nursing assessment determines whether a patient is at risk for adverse outcomes[1] related to sedation[74] and is an appropriate candidate for RN-administered moderate sedation and thus reduces the risks for an adverse event[1,74] during moderate sedation.[72,74,75] Patient safety is increased when the perioperative RN identifies potential areas of risk for an adverse event during the preoperative assessment and, in consultation with an anesthesia professional, implements measures to minimize the identified risks.[76]

The ASA Task Force on Sedation and Analgesia by Non-Anesthesiologists[1] found evidence to suggest there may be a relationship between some preexisting conditions and adverse outcomes in patients receiving moderate sedation. The benefits of performing a presedation nursing assessment outweigh the harms. Benefits include the ability to identify patients who meet the selection criteria for moderate sedation/analgesia and to identify allergies, comorbid conditions, obstructive sleep apnea, and a potentially difficult mask ventilation. The assessment provides baseline measures of vital signs, pain, anxiety, and level of consciousness for comparison during the procedure. There are no identifiable harms of performing a nursing assessment.

II.a. The nursing assessment[1] should include a review of the patient's
   o allergies[77,78] and sensitivities (eg, medications,[1,76,79-85] adhesives, chemical agents, food,[79,81,82,86-91] tape, latex[1,70,76,79,81,92,93];
   o age[74,76,77,79];
   o height,[70,76,83] weight,[70,76-78,81,83,85,94] and body mass index (BMI);
   o medical history[81,82,84] (eg, history and physical,[1,80,85] progress note)[1,70,74,76];
   o current medications[1,70,76-85,92-94] (eg, prescribed, over-the-counter,[76] alternative/complementary therapies,[76,77] supplements)[95], dosage, last dose, and frequency;
   o drug use (eg, marijuana, street drugs, nonprescribed prescription drugs)[1,77,80-82];
   o tobacco and alcohol use[1,76,80-82,84,92];
   o laboratory test results[1,96];
   o diagnostic test results[96];
   o baseline cardiac status (eg, heart rate, blood pressure)[1,70,76,77,79,83,85,93,96];
   o baseline respiratory status (eg, rate, rhythm, blood oxygen level [SpO_2])[1,70,76,77,79,83,85,93,96];
   o baseline neurological status[70,76,80,85,93];
   o airway (eg, obstructive sleep apnea, difficult mask ventilation)[77,78,85,94];
   o sensory impairment (eg, visual, auditory)[81];
   o level of anxiety[97];
   o level of pain[70,76,81];
   o pregnancy test results[70,80,84,93] when applicable[81];
   o NPO status[1,70,76,78,81-85,92,93,96,98];
   o previous adverse experiences with anesthesia or moderate sedation, including[1,77,78,84]
      • delayed emergence from anesthesia or sedation,
      • postprocedure nausea and/or vomiting,
      • reported adverse effects from anesthetic or sedative medications, and
      • airway or breathing problems;
   o need for IV access[1];
   o consent explaining the risks, benefits, and alternatives to sedation[1,70,77,78,81,93,96,99]; and
   o arrangement for a responsible adult caregiver to escort him or her home.[70,93]
   [1: Strong Evidence]
   The collective evidence suggests that the preoperative patient assessment should include a review of the patient's history. Campbell et al[100] retrospectively reviewed the use of an automated before-procedure advanced electronic

health record tool to assess 1,682 patients for their appropriateness as candidates for sedation. The tool had an alert function based on clinical guidelines to notify the health care provider of any condition or clinical history that could affect patient management during sedation. Based on the alert function, changes to patient management occurred in 4.2% (n = 70) of eligible procedures (ie, adult outpatient endoscopy procedures with moderate sedation/analgesia). The researchers concluded that use of this type of tool could improve provider efficiency and patient outcomes.

In a retrospective matched case-controlled study, Conway et al[101] examined patient risk factors for impaired respiratory function during nurse-administered procedural sedation in the cardiac catheterization laboratory. The researchers analyzed data from 573 procedures (eg, electrophysiology, coronary, vascular) and found 21 cases of impaired respiratory function. The cases were matched to 113 controls from a consecutive cohort. Patients with each indicator of acute illness (eg, chronic pulmonary disease, chronic heart failure, renal failure, smoking history, sleep apnea) were nearly twice as likely as their controls to experience impaired respiratory function. The researchers identified several factors that predicted the likelihood of impaired respiratory function and concluded that patients with acute illness probably had underlying conditions that affected their cardiopulmonary function. The authors concluded that the results of their study could be used to develop future prospective studies to research the effectiveness of interventions for impaired respiratory function during moderate sedation/analgesia.

Because sedation occurs along a continuum, moderate sedation may become unintended deep sedation or general anesthesia.[102] Patient compliance with ASA fasting guidelines is important to decrease the risk of aspiration, regurgitation, and morbidity.[98]

II.a.1. The need for IV access should be assessed and will vary depending on the level of sedation intended; the route of medication administration (eg, intravenous, intranasal, oral); and organizational policy, procedure, and protocol. [1: Strong Evidence]
   Intravenous administration of both a sedative to reduce anxiety and an analgesic to manage pain increases the probability of satisfactory moderate sedation. Intravenous access provides a route for administration of rescue medications if needed.[1]

II.b. The perioperative RN should use a physical status classification tool (eg, the ASA Physical Status Classification [Table 1])[103] to determine patient acuity. [3: Moderate Evidence]

The collective evidence[103-105] establishes the importance of using the ASA Physical Status Classification system to determine patient acuity.[103]

Tantri et al[104] conducted a retrospective review of 270 cataract surgeries performed with patients under local anesthesia and with moderate sedation provided by an RN under the direction of an ophthalmologist. Anesthesia consultation was requested for 24 patients (8.9%). Five of these patients (3.3%) were classified as ASA II and 19 (16%) were classified as ASA III. The authors concluded that cataract surgery performed under local anesthesia with monitoring and moderate sedation performed by an RN was associated with a low rate of intraoperative anesthesia consultation. The patients classified as ASA III were more likely than those classified as ASA II to require anesthesia consultation.

Patients classified as ASA I, ASA II, and medically stable ASA III are normally considered to be appropriate candidates for RN-administered moderate sedation.[105]

II.c. The perioperative RN should assess the patient for characteristics that may indicate difficulty with mask ventilation, including

- age > 55 years[106-108];
- BMI ≥ 30 kg/m^2 [1,107-109];
- a history of snoring[108], stridor[109], or sleep apnea[1,106-108];
- missing teeth[106-109];
- presence of a beard[106-109];
- short neck[1,109];
- limited neck extension[1,109];
- small mouth opening[1];
- jaw abnormalities (eg, micrognathia, retrognathia)[1];
- macroglossia[1];
- nonvisible uvula[1];
- history of problems with anesthesia or sedation[1];
- advanced rheumatoid arthritis[1];
- chromosomal abnormality (eg, trisomy 21)[1]; and
- tonsillar hypertrophy.[1]

[1: Strong Evidence]

The respiratory depressive effects of moderate sedation medications may compromise respiration,[1] and the ability to ventilate a patient with a mask is vital if there is an unanticipated compromised airway.[107] There is no standard definition of a difficult mask ventilation based on objective criteria. The ASA's 1993 practice guidelines for management of a difficult airway defined elements of a difficult mask ventilation as the inability to maintain oxygen saturation greater than 90% using 100% oxygen and positive pressure ventilation.[110] The ASA's 2013 updated practice guidelines for management of a difficult airway included the problems of inadequate mask seal, excessive gas leak, and excessive resistance to the ingress or egress of

TABLE 1. ASA PHYSICAL STATUS CLASSIFICATION SYSTEM		
Classification	Definition	Examples, including but not limited to:
ASA I	A normal healthy patient	Healthy, non-smoking, no or minimal alcohol use
ASA II	A patient with mild systemic disease	Mild diseases only without substantive functional limitations. Examples include (but not limited to): current smoker, social alcohol drinker, pregnancy, obesity (30 < BMI < 40), well-controlled DM/HTN, mild lung disease
ASA III	A patient with severe systemic disease	Substantive functional limitations; One or more moderate to severe diseases. Examples include (but not limited to): poorly controlled DM or HTN, COPD, morbid obesity (BMI ≥ 40), active hepatitis, alcohol dependence or abuse, implanted pacemaker, moderate reduction of ejection fraction, ERSD undergoing regularly scheduled dialysis, premature infant PCA < 60 weeks, history (> 3 months) of MI, CVA, TIA, or CAD/stents
ASA IV	A patient with severe systemic disease that is a constant threat to life	Examples include (but not limited to): recent (< 3 months) MI, CVA, TIA, or CAD/stents, ongoing cardiac ischemia or severe valve dysfunction, severe reduction of ejection fraction, sepsis, DIC, ARD or ERSD not undergoing regularly scheduled dialysis
ASA V	A moribund patient who is not expected to survive without the operation	Examples include (but not limited to): ruptured abdominal/thoracic aneurysm, massive trauma, intracranial bleed with mass effect, ischemic bowel in the face of significant cardiac pathology or multiple organ/system dysfunction
ASA VI	A declared brain-dead patient whose organs are being removed for donor purposes	

Reproduced with permission from the American Society of Anesthesiologists, Schaumburg, IL.

gas.[111] The collective evidence supports using predictive factors to anticipate a difficult or impossible mask ventilation.[106-109,112-114]

Kheterpal et al[107] conducted a prospective, observational study of adult surgical patients to determine the incidence and predictors of difficult mask ventilation. In reviewing 22,660 cases in which there was an attempt to ventilate with a mask, they found 313 patients (1.4%) were difficult to ventilate and 37 patients (0.16%) were impossible to ventilate. The researchers identified limited or severely limited mandibular protrusion, thick/obese neck anatomy, history of sleep apnea, history of snoring, presence of a beard, age ≥ 57 years, and BMI ≥ 30 kg/m² as independent predictors of a difficult mask ventilation. They concluded that the presence of beard was the only modifiable risk factor and that the mandibular protrusion test may be an essential element of the airway examination.

Lee et al[115] conducted a systematic review and meta-analysis of 42 prospective observational studies of patients undergoing general anesthesia who had a preoperative Mallampati test assessment. They compared the results with the subsequent assessment rate of a difficult airway. The authors concluded that the Mallampati assessment was accurate in predicting difficult laryngoscopy and intubation but was not accurate in predicting difficult mask ventilation.

II.d. The perioperative RN should assess the patient for risk of obstructive sleep apnea. *[1: Strong Evidence]*

The collective body of evidence[116-144] establishes the importance of assessment and screening for obstructive sleep apnea.

Obstructive sleep apnea is a sleep-related breathing disorder characterized by periodic, partial, or complete obstruction of the upper airway during sleep.[116,117] The repeated arousals from sleep to restore airway patency[116] may cause

○ daytime sleepiness,
○ neurocognitive dysfunction (eg, attention/vigilance, delayed long-term visual and verbal memory),
○ cardiovascular disorders (eg, hypertension, ischemic heart disease, arrhythmia, pulmonary hypertension, congestive heart failure), and
○ metabolic dysfunction.[117]

The estimated incidence of obstructive sleep apnea ranges from 2% to 26% and affects men more frequently than women.[118] The undiagnosed range of moderate to severe obstructive sleep apnea is estimated at 82% for men and 92% for women.[140] The number of patients with obstructive sleep apnea is likely to increase[117] as the population ages and becomes more obese,[116] and surgical patients have a reported higher incidence than the general population.[117]

Complications associated with obstructive sleep apnea during perioperative care include cardiac dysrhythmias (eg, bradycardia, atrial fibrillation, premature ventricular contractions), myocardial infarction, severe oxygen desaturation, episodic hypoxemia, hypercapnia, respiratory arrest, airway obstruction, hypoventilation, unplanned intensive care unit admission, impaired arousal from sedation, and sudden death.[145] Moderate sedation medications that affect the central nervous system may interfere with the normal respiratory compensatory mechanisms of hypoxemia and hypercarbia, and depressant medications may facilitate pharyngeal collapse in patients with obstructive sleep apnea.[141]

II.d.1. A screening tool should be used to assess the patient for obstructive sleep apnea. *[2: High Evidence]*

Examples of obstructive sleep apnea screening tools include the

• STOP questionnaire,[118,119,122,131]
• STOP-Bang questionnaire,[117,118,120,121,123,125,126,128,129,131-134,146]
• Berlin questionnaire,[118,122,124,127,130,131]
• Wisconsin sleep questionnaire,[118] and
• ASA checklist for the identification and assessment of obstructive sleep apnea.[116,118,122]

Obstructive sleep apnea screening tools classify patients based on clinical symptoms and risk factors to determine high-risk patients who may need a referral to a higher level of care (eg, an anesthesia professional) or additional diagnostic testing (ie, polysomnography).[118] Representative questions in the screening tools ask about BMI, hypertension, loud snoring, apnea during sleep, tiredness during the day, and neck size.[118]

In a prospective cohort study, Lockhart et al[131] screened surgical patients with four different obstructive sleep apnea tools (ie, STOP questionnaire, STOP-Bang questionnaire, Berlin questionnaire, Flemmons index). They found the most common characteristics of high-risk obstructive sleep apnea patients were male sex, older age, being overweight, and comorbid conditions.

Joshi et al[117] conducted a systematic review to develop the Society for Ambulatory Anesthesia (SAMBA) consensus statement on preoperative selection of adult patients with obstructive sleep apnea scheduled for ambulatory surgery. The SAMBA recommends use of the STOP-Bang questionnaire for obstructive sleep apnea screening because it is easy to administer and has a high sensitivity.

Abrishami et al[118] conducted a systematic review to identify and evaluate the available screening questionnaires for obstructive sleep apnea. The review included an analysis of nine prospective studies and one retrospective study with a total of 1,484 patients in the 10 studies. The authors found that the Wisconsin and the Berlin questionnaires had the highest sensitivity and specificity for predicting the existence of obstructive sleep apnea. The STOP and the STOP-Bang questionnaires had the highest methodological validity, reasonable accuracy, and easy-to-use features. Based on these findings, the authors recommend the use of the STOP and STOP-Bang question-naires to screen surgical patients for obstructive sleep apnea.

II.d.2. Obstructive sleep apnea screening assessment for pediatric patients may include
- weight (ie, 95th percentile for age and sex)[111];
- intermittent vocalization during sleep[111];
- parental report of restless sleep, difficulty breathing, or struggling respiratory effort during sleep[111];
- night terrors[111];
- unusual sleep positions[111];
- new onset enuresis[111];
- somnolence (eg, appears sleepy during the day, is difficult to arouse at usual awakening time)[111];
- being easily distracted[111];
- being overly aggressive[111];
- irritability[111]; and
- difficulty concentrating.[111]
[1: Strong Evidence]

II.d.3. The perioperative RN should consult with an anesthesia professional if the patient presents with a history of severe obstructive sleep apnea. *[1: Strong Evidence]*

Administration of sedatives to the patient with central sleep apnea may inhibit the brain's signal to wake up and breathe.[1,116]

II.d.4. Additional precautions (eg, non-invasive positive pressure ventilation[147] with continuous positive airway pressure [CPAP][117] or bilevel positive airway pressure,[117] careful titration of opioids,[1] non-opioid analgesia techniques,[117,148] multimodal pain management[1,117]) should be taken for patients with sleep apnea who will undergo moderate sedation/analgesia. *[1: Strong Evidence]*

Moderate sedation medications may cause relaxation of the oropharyngeal structures resulting in partial or total airway obstruction.[1,116]

II.e. The perioperative RN should consult with an anesthesia professional and develop a perioperative plan of care if a patient presents with any of the following:
- known history of respiratory[77] or hemodynamic instability,[85,149]
- history of coagulation abnormality,
- history of neurologic or cardiac disease that may be affected by medications administered for moderate sedation/analgesia,
- history of renal or liver disease that may affect metabolism of medications administered for moderate sedation/analgesia,
- previous difficulties with anesthesia or sedation,[1,82,85,149,150]
- severe sleep apnea or other airway related issues,[1,79,85,94,149,150]
- one or more significant comorbidities,[1,85]
- pregnancy,[1]
- inability to communicate (eg, aphasic),
- inability to cooperate,[1]
- multiple drug allergies,
- multiple medications with potential for drug interaction with sedative analgesics,[1]
- current substance abuse (eg, street drugs, alcohol, non-prescribed prescription drugs[151]),[82]
- ASA physical status classification of unstable ASA III,[77,80,83] or
- ASA physical status classification of ASA IV or above.[80,82-84,152]

[1: Strong Evidence]

II.e.1. If an anesthesia professional is not available for consultation, the perioperative RN should consult with the licensed independent practitioner.

II.f. The perioperative RN should determine the patient's suitability for moderate sedation/analgesia based on the selection criteria developed by the collaboration of the interdisciplinary team (eg, perioperative RNs, anesthesia professionals, surgeons, quality and risk managers). *[2: High Evidence]*

The collective evidence[153-156] establishes the importance of proper patient selection. Hassan et al[153] retrospectively studied all patients undergoing neuroendovascular procedures at two academic centers during a four-year period. The authors determined the rate of failure of conscious sedation (ie, moderate sedation/analgesia) and compared the outcomes of patients who converted from conscious sedation to general anesthesia with those of patients whose procedures were initiated with general anesthesia. The study population consisted of patients having general anesthesia (n = 387), conscious sedation (n = 520), and emergent conversion to general anesthesia from conscious sedation (n = 9). Cardiovascular risk factors were similar in all the groups. The researchers concluded that patient selection is important for procedures performed with the patient under conscious sedation. The procedure type, anticipated length of the procedure, and patient characteristics are important in identifying appropriate candidates for conscious sedation.

II.g. The perioperative RN should collaborate with the licensed independent practitioner (eg, physician, podiatrist, dentist) in developing and documenting the sedation plan. The sedation plan should include the medications and route of administration, predetermined depth of sedation to complete the procedure, length of the procedure and sedation, and recovery time.[70] *[3: Moderate Evidence]*

Recommendation III

The perioperative RN administering moderate sedation/analgesia should continuously care for the patient throughout the procedure.

The collective evidence[1,155,157-159] establishes the risk of moderate sedation/analgesia from complications associated with the respiratory system (eg, hypoxia, hypercapnia, impaired airway reflexes, loss of airway patency, airway obstruction, respiratory depression) and cardiovascular system (eg, hypotension, cardiac arrhythmias). Continuous monitoring and observation of the patient's physiological and psychological status can lead to early detection of potential complications.

The benefits of continuously caring for the patient receiving moderate sedation/analgesia outweigh the harms. The benefits include the early identification of respiratory and cardiovascular complications.

III.a. The RN caring for the patient receiving moderate sedation/analgesia should have no competing responsibilities that would compromise continuous monitoring and assessment of the patient during the administration of moderate sedation.[70,99,147,160-163] *[1: Strong Evidence]*

The consensus of professional guidelines and expert opinion supports the perioperative RN having no competing responsibilities.[70,99,147,160-162] The care of the patient receiving moderate sedation/analgesia requires constant vigilance and monitoring to allow for an immediate response to any adverse reaction or complication.[160]

III.a.1. Two perioperative RNs should be assigned to care for the patient receiving moderate sedation/analgesia. One RN should administer the sedation medication and monitor the patient and the other RN should perform the circulating role. *[2: High Evidence]*

AORN maintains that every surgical patient deserves a perioperative RN for the duration of any operative or other invasive procedure and actively promotes laws and regulations to ensure the supervisory presence of the professional RN in the perioperative setting. A minimum of one perioperative RN circulator dedicated to each patient undergoing an operative or other invasive procedure facilitates the provision of safe, quality patient care in the perioperative setting.[164,165]

Twenty-three states have laws or regulations in place that require an RN to serve as the circulator in hospitals, and 16 states have similar language for ambulatory surgical centers. The Center for Medicare & Medicaid Services (CMS) also has regulations and guidance addressing the RN circulator. The CMS interpretive guidelines in §482.51(a)(3) state, "The circulating nurse must be an RN."[166]

Studies have demonstrated that higher nurse-to-patient ratios are associated with lower mortality rates, fewer incidents of failure to rescue, shorter lengths of stay, fewer medication errors, and reduced incidences of pressure ulcers and pneumonia.[167-171] Better outcomes equal lower costs for the health care system.[172,173] Improved patient outcomes have been demonstrated with higher nurse-to-patient ratios, enhanced work environment, and better-educated nurses.[174]

III.b. The perioperative RN providing moderate sedation/analgesia should be in constant attendance with unrestricted immediate visual and physical access to the patient.[1,70] *[1: Strong Evidence]*

III.b.1. The perioperative RN caring for the patient receiving moderate sedation/analgesia may perform short, interruptible tasks (eg, opening additional suture, tying a gown) to assist the perioperative team while remaining within the operating or procedure room.[1,73,77,80,175] *[1: Strong Evidence]*

The collective evidence is inconclusive about whether the perioperative RN caring for the patient receiving moderate sedation may perform brief interruptible tasks. Professional guidelines and position statements[1,73,77,79,175] state that the practitioner administering moderate sedation/analgesia is allowed to perform brief, interruptible tasks. However, two professional nursing associations[147,160] have the divergent opinion that the RN caring for a patient receiving moderate sedation should have no other responsibilities during the procedure.[160]

Hausman and Reich[93] support allowing the sedation practitioner to perform brief interruptible tasks but additionally describe activities that would not be considered brief and interruptible, such as performing biopsies and collecting specimens.

III.b.2. The RN providing moderate sedation/analgesia should not perform short interruptible tasks when propofol is used. The RN should monitor the patient without interruption, assessing the level of consciousness and identifying early signs of hypotension, bradycardia, apnea, airway obstruction, and oxygen desaturation.[9,80] *[1: Strong Evidence]*

Propofol has a narrow therapeutic window, and there is potential for respiratory and cardiopulmonary complications if it is administered inappropriately.[80]

III.c. The RN should monitor and document the patient's physiological and psychological responses, identify nursing diagnoses based on assessment of the data, and implement the plan of care. *[5: Benefits Balanced with Harms]*

The perioperative RN can detect the early signs of potential cardiorespiratory complications by continuously monitoring and observing the patient's physiological and psychological status. Early recognition and management of cardiac or respiratory depression may prevent hypoxic brain damage, cardiac arrest, or death.[1] The primary causes of morbidity associated with moderate sedation are drug-induced respiratory depression and airway obstruction.[1]

III.c.1. Baseline patient monitoring and documentation should include
- pulse,[1,70,73,76,77,79,83,85,93,96,163]
- blood pressure,[1,70,73,76,77,79,83,85,93,96]
- respiratory rate,[70,73,77,83,85]
- SpO$_2$ by pulse oximetry,[70,73,77,85,163]
- end-tidal carbon dioxide (CO_2) by capnography,
- pain level,[70,76,81]
- anxiety level,[97] and
- level of consciousness.[70,76,80,85,93]

[1: Strong Evidence]

Baseline preoperative vital signs provide a reference for comparison if the patient experiences any changes (eg, cardiac depression, respiratory depression)[1] in response to the administration of medications for moderate sedation.

III.c.2. Intraoperative patient monitoring and documentation should include
- cardiac rate and rhythm,[1,73,77,160,176,177]
- blood pressure,[1,73,77,80,160,177]
- respiratory rate,[1,77,78,160]
- SpO$_2$ by pulse oximetry,[1,73,77,78,160,176,177]
- end-tidal CO_2 by capnography,[24,77,80,176-189]
- depth of sedation assessment (Table 2),[77,78,102,190,191]
- pain level,[78,192-195]
- anxiety level, and
- level of consciousness.[1,77,160]

[1: Strong Evidence]

The collective evidence[1,73,160,176,177] supports monitoring and documenting the patient's vital signs (eg, heart rate, blood pressure, SpO$_2$) when the patient is receiv-

ing moderate sedation. The early signs of cardiac and respiratory depression can be recognized by monitoring and documenting cardiac rate and rhythm, blood pressure, respiratory rate, oxygen saturation, end-tidal CO_2, depth of sedation, pain level, anxiety level, and level of consciousness.[196]

The collective evidence[77,80,176-179,182-189,197] supports monitoring end-tidal CO_2 when the patient is receiving moderate sedation. Beitz et al[180] conducted an RCT to determine whether the use of capnographic monitoring reduced the incidence of arterial oxygen desaturation during propofol sedation. Adult patients classified as ASA I to ASA III scheduled to undergo colonoscopy were randomly assigned to either a control group or an intervention group. The control group (n = 376) received standard monitoring of noninvasive blood pressure measured every three minutes, electrocardiogram (ECG), heart rate, and pulse oximetry. The intervention group (n = 384) received the same standard monitoring in addition to capnography.

An independent observer monitored the patients' respiratory activity. Any sign of apnea, altered ventilation, or oxygen desaturation triggered an intervention (ie, patient stimulation, withholding of medications, chin lift or jaw thrust maneuver, increased oxygen supplementation). The primary study outcome of oxygen desaturation occurred in 149 patients in the intervention group and 199 patients in the control group. The authors defined arterial oxygen desaturation as a decrease of $\geq 5\%$ SaO$_2$ compared with baseline or a decrease of SaO$_2 < 90\%$. Secondary study outcomes of apnea, altered ventilation, hypoxemia (SaO$_2 < 90\%$) or severe hypoxemia (SaO$_2 \leq 85\%$) were detected in 217 patients in the intervention group and eight patients in the control group. The differences between

TABLE 2. CONTINUUM OF DEPTH OF SEDATION				
	Minimal sedation anxiolysis	Moderate sedation/analgesia ("conscious sedation")	Deep sedation/analgesia	General anesthesia
Responsiveness	Normal response to verbal stimulation	Purposeful response to verbal or tactile stimulation	Purposeful response following repeated or painful stimulation	Unarousable even with painful stimulation
Airway	Unaffected	No intervention required	Intervention may be required	Intervention often required
Spontaneous ventilation	Unaffected	Adequate	May be inadequate	Frequently inadequate
Cardiovascular function	Unaffected	Usually maintained	Usually maintained	May be impaired

Reproduced with permission from the American Society of Anesthesiologists, Schaumburg, IL.

650

the intervention and control groups for the primary and secondary study outcomes were statistically significant. The researchers concluded that early intervention based on the additional capnographic monitoring of ventilatory activity reduced the incidence of oxygen desaturation and hypoxemia during sedation.

Researchers who conducted a prospective RCT reached a different conclusion that whereas capnography seemed to reduce the number and duration of hypoxic events, it was of limited clinical benefit to increase safety and there were associated additional costs. Slagelse et al[24] studied the role of capnography in 540 adult endoscopy patients undergoing nurse-administered propofol sedation. The control group (n = 277) received standard monitoring of ECG, pulse oximetry, heart rate, blood pressure, and visual assessment of respiration. The intervention group (n = 263) received the same standard monitoring and capnography. In the intervention group, there were 17 hypoxic events among 13 patients and in the control group, there were 28 hypoxic events among 16 patients. The lower number of hypoxic events in the capnography intervention group was not statistically significant. The duration of the hypoxic events was 17.2 seconds in the capnography intervention group and 21.8 seconds in the control group. The researchers concluded that capnography is not necessary during nurse-administered propofol sedation.

III.c.3. Postoperative assessment, monitoring, and documentation should include
- cardiac rate and rhythm,[147]
- blood pressure,[147]
- respiratory rate,[147]
- SpO$_2$,[147]
- pain level,[147]
- sedation level,[147]
- level of consciousness,[147]
- intravenous line (eg, patency, site, type of fluid),[147]
- condition of dressing and wound,[147] and
- type and patency of drainage tubes.[147]
[2: High Evidence]

III.c.4. Monitoring equipment (eg, pulse oximetry,[70,73,198] ECG,[70,73,198] capnography, blood pressure measurement devices[70,73,198]); oxygen source[70,160]; masks and cannulas; suction source,[70,73,160] tubing, and tips[70]; and oral and nasal airways[70,160] should be working properly, and immediately available in the room where the procedure is being performed. *[2: High Evidence]*

III.c.5. Clinical alarms of automatic monitoring devices should be audible and set to alert the perioperative RN to critical changes in the patient's status.[1,80,199] *[1: Strong Evidence]*

A clinical alarm (eg, cardiac monitor, capnography, pulse oximetry) is patient specific and used for the purpose of alerting team members to critical changes in the patient's condition. Patients have experienced injuries and near misses because of alarms being turned off or inaudible.[200-202]

III.c.6. The perioperative RN should assess and document depth of sedation using an objective scale (eg, ASA Continuum of Sedation Scale,[92,102] Ramsay Sedation Scale,[203] Modified Ramsay Sedation Scale,[92] Modified Observer's Assessment of Alertness/Sedation Scale).[191,204,205] *[2: High Evidence]*

The collective evidence[102,191,203-207] establishes the benefits of assessing and documenting the depth of sedation with an objective scale. Using the ASA Continuum of Sedation Scale[102] a patient is moderately sedated when there is a purposeful response to verbal or tactile stimulation, no intervention is required to maintain the airway, ventilations are adequate, and cardiovascular function is usually maintained.

Nisbet and Mooney-Cotter[206] conducted a descriptive, survey-based study to determine validity and reliability of several sedation scales. They concluded that because sedation occurs on a continuum that is unknowable and unpredictable, it must be measured as accurately as possible. Changes in a patient's condition can be communicated with a valid, reliable, and easy-to-use sedation scale (eg, the Pasero Opioid-Induced Sedation Scale). Use of an objective scale facilitates timely recognition of advancing sedation and appropriate nursing actions of dose reduction, escalation of care, team communication, and management of treatment options.

III.c.7. The perioperative RN should assess the patient's level of consciousness by evaluating the patient's ability to respond purposefully to verbal commands either alone or with light tactile stimulation.[1,198] *[1: Strong Evidence]*

Assessing the patient's level of consciousness by his or her verbal responses at regular intervals during the procedure allows for quick determination of whether the patient is also breathing well. In addition, verbally reassuring the patient can divert his or her attention and assist in reducing anxiety.[1]

III.c.8. Bispectral index (BIS) monitoring may be used as adjunct technology to measure the patient's level of sedation. *[2: High Evidence]*

TABLE 3. BISPECTRAL (BIS) INDEX VALUES[1-3]

Value*	Description
0	Coma, absence of cerebral electrical activity
0-40	Deep hypnotic state
40-60	General anesthesia
60-90	Varying levels of conscious sedation (ie, minimal to deep sedation)
90-100	Awake

The BIS is a direct measure of the effects of anesthetics and sedatives on the brain. The BIS is an integrated measure of cerebral electrical activity, derived from the electroencephalogram. Values for BIS range on a scale of zero to 100, with the numbers correlated to level of sedation.

REFERENCES

1. Baysal A, Polat TB, Yalcin Y, Celebi A. Can analysis of the bispectral index prove helpful when monitoring titration of doses of midazolam and ketamine for sedation during paediatric cardiac catheterization. Cardiol Young. 2008;18(1):51-57. [IB]
2. Kang KJ, Min BH, Lee MJ, et al. Efficacy of bispectral index monitoring for midazolam and meperidine induced sedation during endoscopic submucosal dissection: a prospective, randomized controlled study. Gut Liver. 2011;5(2):160-164. [IA]
3. DeWitt JM. Bispectral index monitoring for nurse-administered propofol sedation during upper endoscopic ultrasound: a prospective, randomized controlled trial. Dig Dis Sci. 2008;53(10):2739-2745. [IC]

The collective evidence is inconclusive about whether BIS monitoring provides any additional benefit in monitoring the patient receiving moderate sedation/analgesia. Several studies[208-219] support the use of BIS monitoring to measure the patient's level of sedation (Table 3).

Baysal et al[210] conducted a prospective RCT of 126 pediatric patients scheduled for cardiac catheterization. The control group (n = 66) received sedation without the use of BIS monitoring. The intervention group (n = 60) received sedation with BIS monitoring. The difference in the amount of midazolam and ketamine used was significantly less in the one- to three-year-old age group that received BIS monitoring and in the three- to six-year-old age group that received BIS monitoring. The requirement for respiratory support and the adverse events were significantly lower in the intervention group. The researchers concluded the use of BIS monitoring during sedation for pediatric catheterization decreased the need for midazolam and ketamine, lowered the need for respiratory support, and decreased the number of adverse events.

However, several studies[212,220-226] have drawn a contradictory conclusion that BIS monitoring does not provide additional benefit during moderate sedation/analgesia. In an RCT, von Delius et al[212] evaluated whether BIS monitoring would contribute to improved oxygenation and a reduced rate of cardiopul-

monary complication during endoscopy. The control group (n = 72) received standard monitoring, and the intervention group (n = 72) received standard monitoring in addition to BIS monitoring. The mean oxygen saturation per patient was 97.7% in the intervention group and 97.6% in the control group. The total rates of cardiopulmonary complications; hypoxemic, bradycardic, and hypotensive events; mean medication doses; and quality of sedation demonstrated no statistical significance between the groups. The intervention group did have a faster recovery (eg, shorter time to eye opening and first verbal response). The authors concluded that the addition of BIS monitoring did not improve oxygenation or reduce cardiopulmonary complications, and the clinical benefit of a shorter recovery time in daily practice may be limited.

III.d. A licensed independent practitioner (eg, surgeon, anesthesiologist, dentist, podiatrist) should directly supervise the perioperative RN who is monitoring the patient and administering medications.[71-73] *[2: High Evidence]*

Professional guidelines[71-73,80,227,228] recommend that the practitioner directly supervise the perioperative RN caring for the patient receiving moderate sedation/analgesia. The recommendation in the ASA guideline[71] is that the perioperative RN trained to administer medications and monitor the patient receiving moderate sedation is under the direct supervision of the non-anesthesiologist sedation practitioner or anesthesiologist. The non-anesthesiologist sedation practitioner is qualified by education, training, and licensure to administer moderate sedation or supervise the administration of moderate sedation. The practitioner performs the diagnostic or therapeutic procedure, and the RN cares for the patient (eg, monitoring, administering medications). The practitioner cannot simultaneously perform the procedure, administer medications, and monitor the patient.

III.d.1. The licensed independent practitioner should be physically present and immediately available in the procedure suite for diagnosis, treatment, and management of complications while the patient is sedated.[70,72,73] *[2: High Evidence]*

The collective evidence supports the continued presence of the supervising physician.[70,72,73] The non-anesthesiologist sedation practitioner is responsible for all aspects of the sedated patient's care before, during, and after the surgical procedure.[72]

III.e. Emergency resuscitation equipment and supplies should be immediately available in every location in which moderate sedation is administered.[70,73,74,77,78,80,160] *[1: Strong Evidence]*

Although careful titration of sedation and analgesics to obtain the desired effect during the use of short-acting agents can be very safe, respiratory depression, hypotension, or impaired cardiovascular function are common sequelae of sedation and analgesia.[1]

III.e.1. Emergency equipment and supplies should include age- and size-appropriate
- resuscitation medications,[73,77,80,160]
- opioid and benzodiazepine antagonists,
- airway and ventilatory equipment (eg, laryngoscopes,[73] endotracheal tubes, laryngeal mask airway, oral and nasal airways, mechanical positive bag-valve mask device[73]),[77,160]
- defibrillators,[73,77,160] and
- IV fluids and access equipment.[77]

[2: High Evidence]

Recommendation IV

The perioperative RN should know the recommended dose, recommended dilution, onset, duration, effects, potential adverse reactions, drug compatibility, and contraindications for each medication used during moderate sedation.[95]

Safe administration of medications requires knowledge of the intended purpose, potential adverse effects, recommended dose, recommended dilution, onset, duration, effects, drug compatibility, and contraindications for each medication used for moderate sedation.[1,95]

IV.a. Before administrating medications, the perioperative RN should verify the licensed independent practitioner's order, verify the correct dosing parameters, and identify the patient-specific maximum dose by consulting either the health care organization's medication formulary, a pharmacist, a physician, or the product information sheet or other published reference material.[77,95] [2: High Evidence]

IV.a.1. The perioperative RN should adjust doses of sedatives and analgesics when caring for an older adult, as directed by the licensed independent practitioner. [2: High Evidence]

The collective evidence[229-233] establishes the importance of adjusting medication dosages for elderly patients. Akhtar and Padda[230] conducted a retrospective review of 1,530 patients who underwent colonoscopy procedures during a nine-year period. The patients were stratified into two groups: ≤ 65 years of age (n = 750) and > 65 years of age (n = 780). The patients ≤ 65 years of age served as the control group. The authors collected and analyzed the total dose of medications used for moderate sedation. The results demonstrated that the group > 65 years required lower doses of medication for moderate sedation.

IV.b. Intravenous medications should be administered one at a time, in incremental doses, and titrated to desired effect (ie, moderate sedation that enables the patient to maintain his or her protective reflexes, airway patency, and spontaneous ventilation).[1] [1: Strong Evidence]

The incremental administration of agents decreases the risk for overdose and respiratory or circulatory depression because the person administrating the agents can better observe the patient's response to the medications given.[1]

IV.c. Computer-assisted personalized sedation (CAPS) technology may be used to administer moderate sedation/analgesia. [2: High Evidence]

Computer-assisted personalized sedation is an emerging technology designed to administer propofol and maintain moderate sedation/analgesia based on the patients physiological response and patient monitoring to achieve and maintain minimal to moderate sedation/analgesia.[234] The collective evidence[234-239] supports the use of CAPS technology to administer moderate sedation/analgesia.

In a nonblinded multicenter randomized comparative study, Pambianco et al[235] compared the safety and effectiveness of CAPS (ie, a computer-assisted sedation system integrating propofol delivery with patient monitoring) to sedation using the current standard of care (ie, a combination of benzodiazepine and opioid). The eight study sites included an academic center, four ambulatory surgery centers, and three ambulatory endoscopy centers. One thousand patients classified as ASA I to ASA III were randomly assigned to receive sedation either with the CAPS system (n = 496) or with standard care (n = 504) while undergoing routine EGD or colonoscopy procedures. The CAPS group received an IV bolus of fentanyl adjusted for the patient's age and frailty, followed by propofol three minutes later. The endoscopist determined the rate and titration of the propofol to maintain minimal to moderate sedation. The standard care group received an intermittent IV bolus dose of an opioid (ie, meperedine or fentanyl) and benzodiazepine (ie, midazolam) to achieve and maintain the desired level of sedation. The CAPS technology was used to monitor both groups to capture similar data. Eighteen patients did not complete the study, leaving 489 patients in the CAPS group and 493 in the standard care group.[235]

The primary endpoint of the study was the area under the curve of oxygen desaturation (AUCDesat), which is a composite safety measure comprising the incidence, depth, and duration of oxygen desaturation events. Thirty-eight patients in the CAPS group experienced oxygen desaturation compared with 84 patients in the standard care group. The patients in the CAPS group had a significantly lower mean AUCDesat (23.6%) compared with the standard care group (88%).[235]

Secondary endpoints were the level of sedation measured by the Modified Observer's Assessment of Alertness/Sedation scale, patient satisfaction, clinician satisfaction, and recovery time. Patients in both groups were minimally to moderately sedated. Patients in both groups were satisfied with the sedation they received, but the mean satisfaction score was significantly higher in the CAPS group. The endoscopists were more satisfied with using CAPS versus standard care. The CAPS group recovered significantly faster than the standard care group; 99% of the CAPS group recovered within 10 minutes compared with 75% of the standard care group. The authors concluded that the CAPS system could provide the team of endoscopist and nurse with a safe and effective means to administer propofol for routine colonoscopy and EGD under minimal to moderate sedation. All of the authors disclosed a financial relationship with the manufacturer of the device.

IV.c.1. When the CAPS system is used, an anesthesia professional must be immediately available for assistance or consultation.[234,240] The health care organization should define and determine immediate availability of an anesthesia professional.[234] [1: Regulatory]

The ASA Guidance for Directors of Anesthesia Service for Computer-Assisted Personalized Sedation Devices states

"Immediate availability" as it relates to the FDA restriction on the use of CAPS devices could mean a code team or rapid response team which includes an anesthesia professional at a minimum.[234]

IV.c.2. The CAPS device should be used according to the manufacturer's instructions for use and the US Food and Drug Administration labeling.[234,240] [2: High Evidence]

IV.d. When administering medications by a nonintravenous route (eg, oral, rectal, intramuscular, intranasal, transmucosal), the perioperative RN should allow sufficient time for drug absorption and onset before considering additional medication.[1] [1: Strong Evidence]

The absorption rate of nonintravenous medications may be unpredictable.[1]

The collective evidence[241-247] establishes the benefit and safety of using nonintravenous medications (eg, oral chloral hydrate, intranasal dexmedetomidine, intranasal or oral midazolam) for moderate sedation/analgesia.

IV.e. Supplemental oxygen should be immediately available for the patient receiving moderate sedation/analgesia.[1,70,160,248] [1: Strong Evidence]

Professional guidelines and expert opinion[1,70,160,248] support the immediate availability of a supplemental oxygen source. Supplemental oxygen can decrease the patient's risk of oxygen desaturation during moderate sedation.[1]

IV.e.1. The perioperative RN, under the direction of the supervising licensed independent practitioner, should determine the necessity, method, and flow rate of oxygen administration based on the patient's optimal level of oxygen saturation as measured with pulse oximetry. [1: Strong Evidence]

The collective evidence[1,80,249] establishes the benefit of using supplemental oxygen during moderate sedation/analgesia procedures. Rozario et al[249] conducted a prospective, randomized, non-blinded study to evaluate the use of supplemental oxygen before and during endoscopic procedures with moderate sedation and the occurrence of clinically significant desaturation events. Patients in the experimental group (n = 194) received low-flow oxygen at 2 L/minute before the administration of moderate sedation. The patients in the control group (n = 195) did not routinely receive oxygen unless an episode of desaturation (ie, oxygen saturation ≤ 95%) occurred. In the control group, 138 (70.8%) of the patients experienced a desaturation event compared with 24 (12.4%) in the experimental group. The experimental group was 98% less likely to experience any episode of desaturation than the control group. The researchers concluded that their results supported the routine use of supplemental oxygen at 2 L/minute to prevent desaturation during endoscopy procedures with moderate sedation.

IV.f. The perioperative RN should document the moderate sedation/analgesia medications administered including the
- medication,[77]
- strength,
- total amount administered,[77]
- route,[77]
- time,[77]
- patient response,[77] and
- adverse reactions.[95]
[2: High Evidence]

IV.g. Opioid antagonists (ie, naloxone) and benzodiazepine antagonists (ie, flumazenil) should be readily available whenever opioids and benzodiazepines are administered.[1] [1: Strong Evidence]

There is evidence[250-252] of paradoxical reactions to benzodiazepines (eg, midazolam) necessitating the use of flumazenil. In a prospective review of 4,140 adult endoscopy patients, Tae et al[250] found 1.4% of the patients experienced a paradoxical reaction to midazolam. An indication for the administration of flumazenil was if the reaction was limiting the performance of the scheduled procedure. After administration of flumazenil, 93.3% of the procedures were completed successfully. The author's multivariate analysis of the independent predictors of a paradoxical reaction include male sex, unsuccessful sedation during a previous procedure, upper endoscopy, a higher dose of midazolam, and a lower dose of meperidine.

Recommendation V

The perioperative RN should evaluate the patient for discharge readiness based on specific discharge criteria.

Medications used for moderate sedation/analgesia affect cognition, memory, and motor function.[253-255] The patient's recovery time will depend on the type and amount of sedation/analgesia administered, the procedure performed, and the heath care organization's discharge criteria policy.

V.a. Medical supervision of patient recovery and discharge after moderate sedation/analgesia should be the responsibility of the operating practitioner or a licensed independent practitioner.[1] *[1: Strong Evidence]*

The patient's risk for developing complications may extend into the postoperative period and may require the intervention of the medical practitioner.

V.a.1. A qualified provider defined by and authorized under the health care organization's guidelines and policies should be available in the facility to discharge the patient in accordance with the health care organization's discharge criteria.[160] *[2: High Evidence]*

V.b. The health care organization should create a multidisciplinary team (eg, perioperative RNs, anesthesia professionals, surgeons, other licensed independent practitioners) to collaboratively develop discharge criteria for patients receiving moderate sedation/analgesia. *[1: Strong Evidence]*

Decreased procedural stimulation, delayed absorption of medications administered by nonintravenous routes, and slow drug elimination are contributing factors to residual sedation and cardiorespiratory depression in the postoperative phase of care after moderate sedation/analgesia.[1] Establishing discharge criteria minimizes the risk of an adverse outcome (eg, cardiorespiratory depression) after the patient has been discharged.[1,77,256,257]

V.b.1. Discharge readiness criteria should include
- return to preoperative baseline mental status (eg, alert and oriented),[1,77,81,94,213]
- stable vital signs,[1,77,78,81,94]
- sufficient time interval (eg, two hours) since the last administration of an antagonist (eg, naloxone, flumazenil),[1,163]
- use of an objective patient assessment discharge scoring system (eg, Aldrete Recovery Score, Post-Anesthetic Discharge Scoring System),[1,81,147,258]
- absence of protracted nausea,[94]
- intact protective reflexes,[77,78,163]
- adequate pain control,[78,81,94]
- return of motor/sensory control,[77,81]
- ability to remain awake for at least 20 minutes,[213] and
- arrangement for safe transport from the facility.[1,81,147,253-255]

[1: Strong Evidence]

The collective evidence[1,147,213,258,259] establishes the benefit of using an objective patient discharge readiness scoring system. In a prospective nonrandomized study, Trevisani et al[258] evaluated the safety of a scoring system compared with clinical discharge criteria to determine patient discharge readiness. In the control group (n = 110), patient discharge was based on clinical assessment (ie, age, clinical conditions, dosage of administered drugs, sedation degree). In the study group (n = 110), patient discharge was based on the modified Post-Anesthetic Discharge Scoring System (PADSS). The PADSS is measured on a numerical scale of zero to 10. The five categories in PADSS are vital signs, activity, nausea and vomiting, pain, and surgical bleeding, scored zero, 1, or 2 for a total score. All patients were scheduled for elective colonoscopy and received conscious sedation with midazolam and meperidine to obtain sedation ranging from 2 to 4 on the Ramsay scale. The study group was scored 20 minutes after completion of the procedure and re-scored every 20 minutes until achieving two consecutive PADSS scores of ≥ 9. For the study group, recovery time was 58.75 ± 18.67 minutes versus 95.14 ±10.85 minutes for the control group, and 39 patients in the study group recovered in 60 minutes or less compared with no patients in the control group. There were no early complications in either group. The authors concluded that using the PADSS is as safe as clinical evaluation to assess discharge readiness, and using the PADSS allowed for earlier patient discharge.

Horiuchi et al[255] conducted a prospective, consecutive study of 48 patients to assess patient clinical features, psychomotor recovery, and blood concentration of propofol following a colonoscopy procedure with nurse-administered propofol sedation. Psychomotor recovery was assessed before the procedure and at one and two hours after the procedure using the number connection test and a driving simulator test. All number connection test results were within normal limits one hour after the colonoscopy procedure. Driving skills had recovered to

PATIENT CARE

baseline levels within one hour. The authors concluded that although there were consistent findings in the number connection test and the driving simulation (ie, psychomotor recovery) as early as one hour after propofol sedation, additional studies with more patients and a different patient population are needed before these results can be used to recommend when a patient may drive after propofol sedation.

The current evidence is insufficient to determine the length of time a patient should be monitored after receiving a dose of flumazenil. The ASA guideline[1] recommends that patient be observed until the effect of the antagonist has dissipated and the patient shows no signs of resedation or cardiorespiratory depression. The effects of flumazenil may wear off before a long-acting benzodiazepine is completely cleared from the body. If a patient shows no signs of resedation two hours after a 1-mg dose of flumazenil, resedation is unlikely. Resedation is less likely when flumazenil is administered to reverse a low dose of a short-acting benzodiazepine (eg, less than 10 mg of midazolam). Use of flumazenil is not a substitute for an adequate period of postprocedure monitoring. The use of flumazenil does not reduce the risks associated with the use of large doses of benzodiazepines for sedation.[260]

One study[261] suggests that a shortened recovery period following a dose of flumazenil is safe. Mathus-Vliegen et al[261] used a quasi-experimental design to study the length of recovery time after flumazenil was administered on the patient's arrival in the recovery area. Endoscopy patients (N = 1,506) received 5 mg of midazolam during the procedure and received a median dose of 0.2 mg of flumazenil on arrival in the recovery area. Patients were discharged 65 minutes after the last dose of midazolam. The majority of the patients (n = 1,246, 82.7%) were alert on their way home. Three patients reported an incidence of fainting, fall, or near-fall without consequences. The authors concluded that administering flumazenil shortened the recovery phase, which could potentially offer a substantial savings in time, space, and nursing resources.

V.b.2.   Discharge may be delayed when the patient
● has obstructive sleep apnea,[117,136,138,141]
● receives morphine,[262]
● receives dexmedetomidine,[263]
● receives an antagonist,[1,163] or
● experiences postoperative nausea and vomiting.[264]
[1: Strong Evidence]
Professional guidelines and expert opinions[116,117,138,141] recommend increased post-

operative monitoring and longer stay in the PACU for patients with obstructive sleep apnea. The ASA "Practice guidelines for perioperative management of patients with obstructive sleep apnea"[116] recommends a median length of stay in the PACU of three hours longer for obstructive sleep apnea patients compared with patients who do not have obstructive sleep apnea. Outpatient discharge criteria include a return to baseline oxygen saturation while breathing room air and no hypoxemic events or clinical airway obstruction when left undisturbed in the recovery area. A patient with obstructive sleep apnea may be discharged to an unmonitored situation either at home or in a hospital bed after the patient is no longer at risk for postoperative respiratory depression.

In a retrospective study, Neville et al[265] reviewed charts of 118 adult patients with previously diagnosed sleep apnea treated with pressure-emitting machines (eg, CPAP machines) who underwent outpatient procedures with moderate sedation. The policy of the study hospital was for an obstructive sleep apnea patient to be monitored and observed for a minimum of three hours after surgery. Against medical advice, 92 (78%) of the patients left before three hours of care. The authors concluded that in their sample, the recommended three-hour recovery was not necessary. The exact time for a safe recovery has not been established, and additional research is needed.

In a prospective, observational study, Basu et al[262] compared recovery times of patients receiving morphine (n = 50) with those of patients receiving non-morphine analgesia. Recovery times were significantly greater in the morphine group, and 58% had a delayed discharge compared with 14% in the non-morphine group. The authors concluded that morphine use is associated with increased recovery times and higher rates of delayed discharge.

Makary et al[263] performed a prospective pilot study to determine the feasibility of using dexmedetomidine as a sole sedative agent for office-based maxillofacial surgery procedures. Sixteen patients received a loading dose of dexmedetomidine followed by maintenance doses based on the patient's response to the medication. Sedation level was assessed using the Ramsay sedation scale. Recovery time was prolonged (82.2 ± 24.3 minutes) compared with total procedure time (44.6 ± 27.9 minutes). Patient and surgeon satisfaction scores for sedation with dexmedetomidine were high. The authors concluded that because of the prolonged recovery time, dexmedetomidine was not a suitable sedation medication for a busy office practice at which procedures of short duration were performed.

V.b.3. Pediatric patient discharge may be prolonged when
- the child receives a medication with a long half-life (eg, chloral hydrate)[213,256] and
- only one responsible adult is accompanying a child recovering from moderate sedation/analgesia.[77]

[2: High Evidence]

A guideline published by the American Academy of Pediatrics and the American Academy of Pediatric Dentistry[77] recommends a longer period of observation before discharge of a child who has received a medication with a long half-life and before discharge of a child into the care of only one adult who is driving and thus has limited ability to observe the child.

V.b.4. Discharge instructions given to the adults responsible for the care of an infant or toddler riding home in a car safety seat after receiving moderate sedation/analgesia should include
- careful observation of the child's head position to avoid airway obstruction and
- care of two responsible adults (ie, driver and observer).[77,163]

[1: Strong Evidence]

The collective evidence[77,163,247] establishes the importance of special instructions for observing the child's airway and of having two or more adults accompanying the child in the motor vehicle upon discharge. The American Academy of Pediatrics and the American Academy of Pediatric Dentistry[77] recommend special discharge instructions regarding prevention of airway obstruction after moderate sedation/analgesia for infants and toddlers riding home in a car safety seat. The position of the child's head may cause airway obstruction when the head flexes forward on the body, leading to narrowing of the upper airway. Infants who have received medications with a long half-life (eg, chloral hydrate) are at risk for airway obstruction when riding in a car safety seat.

V.c. The perioperative RN must give the patient and his or her caregiver verbal and written discharge instructions.[77,81,163,266,267] *[1: Regulatory]*

Moderate sedation/analgesia medications may affect cognitive function, reducing the patient's ability to recall events during the perioperative period.[268-270] Veselis et al[268] conducted an RCT to study the effects of moderate sedation medications on conscious memory processes. The researchers randomly assigned healthy volunteers (N = 55) to five experimental groups

that received sequential doses of a placebo, thiopental, propofol, midazolam, or dexmedetomidine. Continuous recognition task, delayed recognition task, and electroencephalogram testing occurred at specified intervals throughout the test period of 424 minutes. The medications increased reaction times and impaired memory on the continuous recognition task equally, except for midazolam which had a greater effect. Via different mechanisms, both propofol and midazolam impair familiarity and recollection processes in recognition from long-term memory. The authors concluded that propofol and midazolam impaired recognition of event-related potentials from long-term memory but not working memory.

V.c.1. A copy of the written discharge instructions must be given to the patient and a copy should be placed in the patient's medical record.[266,267] *[1: Regulatory]*

V.c.2. The patient or a responsible adult should be able to verbalize an understanding of the discharge instructions. *[5: Benefits Balanced with Harms]*

Recommendation VI

The health care organization should provide the perioperative RN with initial and ongoing education and competency verification on his or her understanding of the principles and performance of the skills related to nursing care of the patient receiving moderate sedation/analgesia.

It is the responsibility of the health care organization to provide initial and ongoing education and to verify the competency of perioperative team members to deliver safe care to patients undergoing operative or other invasive procedures.[5] Initial and ongoing education of perioperative personnel on the principles and skills related to the nursing care of the patient receiving moderate sedation/analgesia facilitates the development of knowledge, skills, and attitudes that affect safe patient care. Periodic education programs provide the opportunity to reinforce the principles and skills related to the nursing care of the patient receiving moderate sedation/analgesia and to introduce relevant new equipment or practices.

Competency verification measures individual performance and provides a mechanism for documentation and may verify that perioperative personnel have an understanding of the principles and skills related to nursing care of the patient receiving moderate sedation/analgesia. This knowledge is essential to minimize the risks of moderate sedation and to provide safe patient care.

VI.a. The perioperative RN must receive education and competency verification that addresses specialized knowledge and skills related to administering moderate sedation.[78,266,267] *[1: Regulatory]*

Specialized knowledge includes empirical knowledge (eg, technical understanding), practical knowledge (eg, clinical experience), and aesthetic knowledge (eg, patient advocacy).

Ongoing development of knowledge and skills and documentation of personnel participation is a regulatory and accreditation requirement for both hospitals and ambulatory settings.[266,267]

VI.a.1. Competencies related to administration of moderate sedation/analgesia should include
- patient selection[92,271] and assessment criteria[85] (eg, ASA Physical Status Classification,[78,271] sedation scale,[271] difficult airway, obstructive sleep apnea);
- selection, function, interpretation of measurements, and proficiency in use of physiological monitoring equipment[78,85,92,272];
- pharmacology of the medications (eg, opioids, benzodiazepines, antagonists for opioids and benzodiazepines)[1,70,85,92,271,272];
- compromised airway management[85,272] (eg, head-tilt,[271] jaw-thrust,[271] placement of oral and nasal airways,[271] bag-mask ventilation[271]);
- basic dysrhythmia recognition and management[92];
- emergency response and management;
- advanced cardiac life support (ACLS)[70,271,272] and pediatric advanced life support (PALS)[77] according to the patients served;
- recognition and management of complications[85,92,272] associated with sedation/analgesia (eg, hypoxia,[271] apnea,[271] ability to rescue a patient whose level of sedation progresses to deep sedation)[1];
- review of moderate sedation/analgesia policies and procedures; and
- knowledge of airway anatomy and physiology.[92,271,272]

[1: Strong Evidence]

VI.a.2. Education and competency verification methods may include
- didactic content (eg, lectures,[92,271] computer-based training modules[272-274]),[78,275]
- simulation,[274-280]
- validation of skills[281] (eg, assessment tool,[279,282] return demonstration,[283] observation[92]), and
- examination (eg, written, online).[271]

[1: Strong Evidence]

The collective evidence[92,271-279,281,283] establishes the benefits of various education and competency verification methods. Using a pre-test/post-test quasi-experimental study design, Tobin et al[275] evaluated a moderate sedation course. Before attending the simulation course, the participants (N = 19) completed a pre-test and 12 online training modules (eg, cardiopulmonary considerations, pharmacological review, patient monitoring). During the simulation course,

the participants completed multiple, scripted moderate sedation scenarios for patients displaying sensitive, resistant, and normal reactions to opioids and benzodiazepines. The researchers administered a post-test to the participants with questions from the same question bank as the pre-test after completion of the scenario. The pre-course and post-course cognitive and simulation tests evaluated the educational impact of the course. All participants demonstrated an increase in their cognitive examination performance. The authors concluded that the initial data demonstrated a significant increase in knowledge, skills, and clinical judgment. Further research is needed to examine the validity and reliability of scenario scoring and the impact of training on clinical practice.

VI.b. Relative to the principles and skills related to the nursing care of the patient receiving moderate sedation/analgesia the perioperative RN should
- participate in ongoing educational activities[5];
- identify personal learning needs[5];
- seek experiences to acquire, maintain, and augment personal knowledge and skill proficiency[5];
- share knowledge and skills[5];
- communicate pertinent information to perioperative team members[5,85];
- contribute to a healthy work environment by using appropriate and courteous verbal and nonverbal communication techniques[5]; and
- develop and implement conflict-resolution skills to manage difficult behavior, promote positive working relationships, and advocate for patient safety.[5]

[2: High Evidence]

Education, collegiality, and collaboration are standards of perioperative nursing and a primary responsibility of the perioperative RN who practices in the perioperative setting.[5,284]

VI.c. Competencies should reflect current regulations, nurse practice acts, standards, recommended practices, and guidelines related to the administration of moderate sedation/analgesia.

[5: Benefits Balanced with Harms]

Regulations, nurse practice acts, standards, recommended practices, and guidelines affecting the administration of moderate sedation/analgesia are evolving and may change over time.

VI.d. The perioperative RN who provides moderate sedation/analgesia to pediatric patients should have the additional knowledge and skills (eg, PALS) necessary to provide pediatric care.[77,94]

[2: High Evidence]

Recommendation VII

The health care organization's interdisciplinary team should develop moderate sedation/analgesia policies and procedures based on the state's medical and nurse practice acts, regulatory requirements, practice guidelines, professional organizations' statements, and accreditation requirements.

The collective evidence[1,9,71,72,80,94,98,99,111,147,160,175,190,227,228,248,266,267] establishes the benefit of following established criteria to develop safe practices for moderate/sedation analgesia policy and procedures. These criteria are in the state's medical and nurse practice acts, regulatory requirements, practice guidelines, professional organizations' statements, and accreditation requirements. Policies and procedures assist in the development of patient safety, quality assessment, and performance improvement activities. Policies and procedures establish authority, responsibility, and accountability within the organization. Policies and procedures also serve as operational guidelines used to minimize patient risk for injury or complications, standardize practice, direct perioperative personnel, and establish continuous performance improvement programs.

VII.a. The multidisciplinary team should include representatives from all disciplines (eg, anesthesia, nursing, surgery, risk management, quality, pharmacy) with a role in the processes of moderate sedation/analgesia.[99] [3: Moderate Evidence]

Involvement of a multidisciplinary team allows input from individuals in various disciplines and with varying points of view. Inclusion of individuals with a shared role in the care of patients receiving moderate sedation/analgesia in the development of policy and procedures facilitates the delivery of patient-centered, safe moderate sedation/analgesia.

VII.a.1. The director of anesthesia services in hospitals must be responsible for all anesthesia services including topical or local anesthesia, minimal sedation, moderate sedation/analgesia, and rescue capacity throughout the hospital, including all departments, all campuses, and all off-site locations in Medicare/Medicaid-participating organizations.[166] [1: Regulatory]

Anesthesia services span the spectrum from local anesthesia to general anesthesia. The Centers for Medicare & Medicaid Services include topical, local, minimal, and moderate sedation in the range of anesthesia services under the supervision of a qualified physician.[166]

VII.b. Policies and procedures for moderate sedation/analgesia should include
- assessment parameters[1];
- patient selection criteria[1];
- patient risk assessment and criteria for consultation (eg, anesthesia)[1];
- fasting guidelines[98,285];
- IV access requirements[1,160];
- monitoring[1];
- permitted moderate sedation/analgesia medications and dosage guidelines[85];
- recovery and discharge criteria[1,85];
- documentation[1,85] (eg, parameters, frequency);
- emergency equipment,[1,160] medications, and procedures;
- staffing requirements[1];
- licensed independent practitioner's qualifications, education,[277,286] and competency requirements[71,85] for administering or supervising moderate sedation/analgesia;
- RN qualification, education,[160] and competency requirements[160] for administering moderate sedation/analgesia[85]; and
- alternative care arrangements when the patient's acuity or level of care required is outside the perioperative RN's capabilities or scope of practice.[287]

[1: Strong Evidence]

VII.b.1. Preoperative fasting requirements in the policy and procedure should include duration, type, and volume of permitted intake.[285] [1: Strong Evidence]

Following fasting requirements that restrict food and fluid intake reduces the volume and pH of gastric contents.[285] Fasting reduces the risk of regurgitation, pulmonary aspiration, and pulmonary damage.[98,285] In a Cochrane review, Brady et al[285] systematically reviewed 38 RCTs that compared different preoperative fasting regimens for adult surgical patients and their effects on patient well-being (eg, thirst, hunger, aspiration, regurgitation, pain, nausea, vomiting, anxiety) and postoperative complications. The authors concluded there was no evidence to suggest that decreasing the amount of time that fluids were allowed before surgery increased the risk of aspiration, regurgitation, or morbidity compared with the traditional fasting policy of nothing by mouth after midnight. Drinking water before surgery resulted in significantly lower gastric volumes. The authors concluded that the health care organizational fasting policy should be based on an appraisal of the evidence and a patient risk assessment (eg, history of gastrointestinal disease, autonomic neuropathy, pregnancy, older age).

The ASA practice guidelines for preoperative fasting[98,288] recommend verifying compliance with the fasting requirements during the assessment. The guideline defines preoperative fasting as a "prescribed period of time before a procedure when patients are not allowed the oral intake of liquids or solids."[98(p495)] The prescribed fasting periods allow clear liquids up to two hours; breast milk up to four hours; infant formula up to six hours; a light meal or non-human milk up to six hours; and fatty foods eight hours or more before an elective procedure.[98]

The evidence review found two studies[289] that demonstrated the safety of not fasting for patients receiving intravenous sedation. In a prospective, non-randomized observational study, Manchikanti et al[289] assessed the need for preoperative fasting in patients undergoing 18,472 interventional pain management procedures (eg, epidural injections, facet joint interventions) with intravenous sedation. The patients did not fast, had solid food up to two hours before the procedure, and drank liquids up to 15 minutes before the procedure. The researchers found that postoperative nausea, vomiting, and respiratory depression were rare and that aspiration was almost nonexistent. They concluded that sedation without preoperative fasting is safe for patients receiving interventional pain procedures.

In a larger retrospective cohort chart review of 47,748 outpatient gynecological procedures, Wiebe et al[288] found no complications related to intravenous sedation in non-fasting patients. The researchers concluded that eliminating the fasting requirement decreased stress and unpleasant symptoms without increasing anesthesia-related complications (eg, aspiration).

The benefits of preoperative fasting outweigh the harms. The benefits include a reduction in aspiration, lung damage, death, nausea, and vomiting. The harms of preoperative fasting include the patient experiencing thirst, hunger, aspiration, regurgitation, pain, nausea, vomiting, anxiety, and stress.

Recommendation VIII

Perioperative personnel should participate in quality assurance and performance improvement activities that are consistent with the health care organization's plan to improve understanding of and compliance with the principles and skills of moderate sedation/analgesia administration.

Quality assurance and performance improvement programs assist in evaluating and improving the quality of patient care and formulating plans for corrective action. These programs provide data that may be used to determine whether an individual organization is within benchmark goals and, if not, to identify areas that may require corrective action.

VIII.a. The quality assurance and performance improvement program for moderate sedation/analgesia should include
   o periodically reviewing and evaluating activities to verify compliance or identify the need for improvement,

   o identifying corrective actions directed toward improvement priorities, and
   o taking additional actions when improvement is not achieved or sustained.
[5: Benefits Balanced with Harms]

Reviewing and evaluating quality assurance and performance improvement activities may identify failure points that contribute to errors in moderate sedation/analgesia and help define actions for improvement and increased competency. Taking corrective actions may improve patient safety by enhancing understanding of the principles of and compliance with the processes of moderate sedation/analgesia.

VIII.a.1. Process measures related to moderate sedation/analgesia may include
   • informed consent for the sedation and procedure,[99]
   • NPO status confirmed,
   • history and physical completed,
   • airway assessment completed,
   • requirements for anesthesia consultation identified,
   • adherence to required physiological monitoring, and
   • providers credentialed for procedure/sedation and practice in compliance with facility policy and procedure.
[5: Benefits Balanced with Harms]

VIII.a.2. Patient outcome measures related to moderate sedation/analgesia may include
   • death,[290,291]
   • aspiration,[291-293]
   • adverse reaction to a medication,[291,294-298]
   • antagonist (ie, reversal agent) used,[291-293]
   • unplanned transfer to a higher level of care,[290-293]
   • cardiac or respiratory arrest,[291-293,299]
   • use of a nonapproved sedation agent (eg, use of an anesthetic agent by a non-anesthesia provider),
   • inability to complete the procedure as planned, and
   • emergency procedure without a licensed independent practitioner present.
[2: High Evidence]

The collective evidence[290,294-313] establishes the risks related to moderate sedation/analgesia, as well as the management and minimization of an associated adverse event. In a retrospective study, Sharma et al[300] reviewed the Clinical Outcomes Research Initiative database for cardiopulmonary unplanned events during 324,737 procedures using conscious sedation. The data analysis demonstrated the report of unplanned events in 1.4% of the procedures, and 0.9% of these events were cardiopulmonary in nature. The authors concluded that during gastrointestinal endoscopy with conscious sedation, a higher incidence of cardiopulmonary unplanned events is associated with patient age, ASA classification, inpatient status, trainee participation, and routine use of oxygen.

VIII.a.3. The health care organization must report, track,[266,267] and investigate adverse events through the quality review process (eg, root cause analysis).[266,267] *[1: Regulatory]*

The evidence[291-293] establishes the benefit of reporting, tracking, and investigating adverse events. The International Sedation Task Force of the World Society of Intravenous Anesthesia[291] developed a consensus document and a tool to standardize adverse event reporting and tracking. The authors defined an adverse event as

> *Unexpected and undesirable response(es) to medication(s) and medical intervention used to facilitate procedural sedation and analgesia that threaten or cause patient injury or discomfort.*[291]

The tool characterizes the adverse event across three domains: description, intervention, and outcome. The tool is a five-step process requiring the identification of a sedation event and description of the adverse event, the intervention performed, the outcome, and the severity of the event. The tool has clear definitions to facilitate accurate identification and tracking, providing benchmark data for the number of adverse events and the severity.[291]

VIII.a.4. Adverse events may require reporting to the appropriate regulatory agency or accrediting organization. *[5: Benefits Balanced with Harms]*

VIII.b. Performance improvement activities for moderate sedation/analgesia administration must include monitoring perioperative RNs for understanding of the principles of and compliance with the processes of moderate sedation/analgesia administration. *[1: Regulatory]*

Collecting data to monitor and improve patient care, treatment, and services is a regulatory and accreditation requirement for both hospitals and ambulatory settings.[266,267]

VIII.c. Perioperative RNs should participate in ongoing quality assurance and performance improvement activities related to moderate sedation/analgesia administration by
   - identifying processes that are important for quality monitoring,
   - developing strategies for compliance,
   - establishing benchmarks to evaluate quality indicators,
   - collecting data related to the levels of performance and quality indicators,
   - evaluating practice based on the cumulative data that are collected,
   - taking action to improve compliance, and
   - assessing the effectiveness of the actions taken.

[2: High Evidence]

Participating in ongoing quality assurance and performance improvement activities is a standard of perioperative nursing and a primary responsibility of the perioperative RN who is engaged in practice in the perioperative setting.[5]

Glossary

Benzodiazepine: A pharmacologic agent that has sedative, anxiolytic, amnesic, muscle relaxant, and anticonvulsant properties.

Deep sedation/analgesia: A medication-induced depression of consciousness that allows patients to respond purposefully only after repeated or painful stimulation. The patient cannot be aroused easily, the ability to independently maintain a patent airway may be impaired, and spontaneous ventilation may be inadequate. Cardiovascular function usually is adequate and maintained.

Licensed independent practitioner: A physician, dentist, nurse practitioner, nurse midwife, or any other individual permitted by law and the organization to provide care and services without direction or supervision, within the scope of the individual's license and consistent with individually granted clinical privileges.

Older adult: A person age 65 years or older. Further subdivided into
   - *Young old:* age 65 to 74 years;
   - *Middle old:* age 75 to 84 years;
   - *Old old:* age 85 years and older.

Opioid: A pharmacologic agent that produces varying degrees of analgesia and sedation and relieves pain. Fentanyl, morphine, and hydromorphone are opioid analgesic medications that may be used for moderate sedation/analgesia.

REFERENCES

1. American Society of Anesthesiologists Task Force on Sedation and Analgesia by Non-Anesthesiologists. Practice guidelines for sedation and analgesia by non-anesthesiologists. *Anesthesiology.* 2002;96(4):1004-1017. [IVA]

2. Russell KA. Nurse practice acts guide and govern nursing practice. *J Nurs Regul.* 2012;3(3):36-42. [VA]

3. About nursing licensure. National Council of State Boards of Nursing. https://www.ncsbn.org/licensure.htm. Accessed October 22, 2015. [VA]

4. American Nurses Association. Nursing: *Scope and Standards of Practice.* Silver Spring, MD: American Nurses Association; 2015. [IVB]

5. Standards of perioperative nursing. In: *Guidelines for Perioperative Practice.* Denver, CO: AORN, Inc; 2015:693-710. [IVB]

6. Nurse practice act, rules & regulations. National Council of State Boards of Nursing. https://www.ncsbn.org/nurse-practice-act.htm. Accessed October 22, 2015. [VA]

7. Perioperative explications for the *ANA Code of Ethics for Nurses*. In: *Guidelines for Perioperative Practice*. Denver, CO: AORN, Inc; 2015:711-732. [IVB]

8. *AANA-ASA Joint Position Statement Regarding Propofol Administration*. 2004. American Association of Nurse Anesthetists. https://www.aana.com/resources2/professionalpractice/Documents/PPM%20PS%20Joint%20AANA-ASA%20Propofol.pdf. Accessed October 22, 2015. [IVB]

9. *Statement on Safe Use of Propofol*. 2014. American Society of Anesthesiologists. http://www.asahq.org/~/media/Sites/ASAHQ/Files/Public/Resources/standards-guidelines/statement-on-safe-use-of-propofol.pdf. Accessed October 22, 2015. [IVB]

10. Singh H, Poluha W, Cheung M, Choptain N, Baron KI, Taback SP. Propofol for sedation during colonoscopy. *Cochrane Database Syst Rev*. 2008;(4):CD006268. [IA]

11. Vargo JJ, Cohen LB, Rex DK, et al. Position statement: nonanesthesiologist administration of propofol for GI endoscopy. *Gastroenterology*. 2009;137(6):2161-2167. [IVA]

12. Sethi S, Wadhwa V, Thaker A, et al. Propofol versus traditional sedative agents for advanced endoscopic procedures: a meta-analysis. *Dig Endosc*. 2014;26(4):515-524. [IA]

13. Lee CK, Lee S, Chung I, et al. Balanced propofol sedation for therapeutic GI endoscopic procedures: a prospective, randomized study. *Gastrointest Endosc*. 2011;73(2):206-214. [IB]

14. Yamamoto H, Gotoda T, Nakamura T, et al. Clinical impact of gastroenterologist-administered propofol during esophagogastroduodenoscopy: a randomized comparison at a single medical clinic. *Gastric Cancer*. 2015;18(2):382-389. [IB]

15. Molina-Infante J, Duenas-Sadornil C, Mateos-Rodriguez JM, et al. Nonanesthesiologist-administered propofol versus midazolam and propofol, titrated to moderate sedation, for colonoscopy: a randomized controlled trial. *Dig Dis Sci*. 2012;57(9):2385-2393. [IB]

16. Schilling D, Rosenbaum A, Schweizer S, Richter H, Rumstadt B. Sedation with propofol for interventional endoscopy by trained nurses in high-risk octogenarians: a prospective, randomized, controlled study. *Endoscopy*. 2009;41(4):295-298. [IC]

17. Dewitt J, McGreevy K, Sherman S, Imperiale TF. Nurse-administered propofol sedation compared with midazolam and meperidine for EUS: a prospective, randomized trial. *Gastrointest Endosc*. 2008;68(3):499-509. [IIB]

18. Manjrekar AU, Kane D, Dewoolkar L, Shroff P. Conscious sedation in interventional radiology. *Internet J Anesthesiol*. 2008;18(1):9p-9p. [IC]

19. Sieg A, Beck S, Scholl SG, et al. Safety analysis of endoscopist-directed propofol sedation: a prospective, national multicenter study of 24,441 patients in German outpatient practices. *J Gastroenterol Hepatol*. 2014;29(3):517-523. [IIIA]

20. Lucendo AJ, Olveira A, Friginal-Ruiz AB, et al. Nonanesthesiologist-administered propofol sedation for colonoscopy is safe and effective: a prospective Spanish study over 1000 consecutive exams. *Eur J Gastroenterol Hepatol*. 2012;24(7):787-792. [IIIB]

21. Mao W, Wei XQ, Tao J, Zhen FP, Wen ZF, Wu B. The safety of combined sedation with propofol plus fentanyl for endoscopy screening and endoscopic variceal ligation in cirrhotic patients. *J Dig Dis*. 2014;15(3):124-130. [IIIB]

22. Bosslet GT, Devito ML, Lahm T, Sheski FD, Mathur PN. Nurse-administered propofol sedation: feasibility and safety in bronchoscopy. *Respiration*. 2010;79(4):315-321. [IIIB]

23. Sayfo S, Vakil KP, Alqaqa'a A, et al. A retrospective analysis of proceduralist-directed, nurse-administered propofol sedation for implantable cardioverter-defibrillator procedures. *Heart Rhythm*. 2012;9(3):342-346. [IIIB]

24. Slagelse C, Vilmann P, Hornslet P, Jorgensen HL, Horsted TI. The role of capnography in endoscopy patients undergoing nurse-administered propofol sedation: a randomized study. *Scand J Gastroenterol*. 2013;48(10):1222-1230. [IA]

25. Tohda G, Higashi S, Wakahara S, Morikawa M, Sakumoto H, Kane T. Propofol sedation during endoscopic procedures: safe and effective administration by registered nurses supervised by endoscopists. *Endoscopy*. 2006;38(4):360-367. [IIIB]

26. Morse JW, Fowler SA, Morse AL. Endoscopist-administered propofol: a retrospective safety study. *Can J Gastroenterol*. 2008;22(7):617-620. [IIIC]

27. Sipe BW, Scheidler M, Baluyut A, Wright B. A prospective safety study of a low-dose propofol sedation protocol for colonoscopy. *Clin Gastroenterol Hepatol*. 2007;5(5):563-566. [IIIB]

28. Fatima H, DeWitt J, LeBlanc J, Sherman S, McGreevy K, Imperiale TF. Nurse-administered propofol sedation for upper endoscopic ultrasonography. *Am J Gastroenterol*. 2008;103(7):1649-1656. [IIIB]

29. Frieling T, Heise J, Kreysel C, Kuhlen R, Schepke M. Sedation-associated complications in endoscopy—prospective multicentre survey of 191142 patients. *Z Gastroenterol*. 2013;51(6):568-572. [IIIB]

30. Garcia-Suarez C, Lopez-Roses L, Olivencia P, et al. Sedation with propofol controlled by endoscopists during percutaneous endoscopic gastrostomy. *Rev Esp Enferm Dig*. 2010;102(4):249-256. [IIIC]

31. Garewal D, Powell S, Milan SJ, Nordmeyer J, Waikar P. Sedative techniques for endoscopic retrograde cholangiopancreatography. *Cochrane Database Syst Rev*. 2012;(6):CD007274. [IIA]

32. Kulling D, Orlandi M, Inauen W. Propofol sedation during endoscopic procedures: how much staff and monitoring are necessary? *Gastrointest Endosc*. 2007;66(3):443-449. [IIIA]

33. Adler DG, Kawa C, Hilden K, Fang J. Nurse-administered propofol sedation is safe for patients with obstructive sleep apnea undergoing routine endoscopy: a pilot study. *Dig Dis Sci*. 2011;56(9):2666-2671. [IIIA]

34. Van Beek EJAH, Leroy PLJM. Safe and effective procedural sedation for gastrointestinal endoscopy in children. *J Pediatr Gastroenterol Nutr*. 2012;54(2):171-185. [IIB]

35. McQuaid KR, Laine L. A systematic review and meta-analysis of randomized, controlled trials of moderate sedation for routine endoscopic procedures. *Gastrointest Endosc*. 2008;67(6):910-923. [IA]

36. Mollica G, Mirabella L, Spadaro S, et al. Prospective, randomized comparative study of respiratory and hemodynamic monitoring during colonoscopy using remifentanyl versus propofol/fentanyl. *J Anesth Clinical Res*. 2014;5(1). http://www.omicsonline.org/open-access/a-prospective-randomized-comparative-study-of-respiratory-and-hemodynamic-monitoring-during-colonoscopy-using-remifentanyl-versus-propofolfentanyl-2155-6148.1000381.php?aid=23270. Accessed October 21, 2015. [IB]

37. Terui T, Inomata M. Administration of additional analgesics can decrease the incidence of paradoxical reactions in patients under benzodiazepine-induced sedation during endoscopic transpapillary procedures: prospective

PATIENT CARE

randomized controlled trial. *Dig Endosc.* 2013;25(1):53-59. [IB]

38. Khajavi M, Emami A, Etezadi F, Safari S, Sharifi A, Shariat Moharari R. Conscious sedation and analgesia in colonoscopy: ketamine/propofol combination has superior patient satisfaction versus fentanyl/propofol. *Anesth Pain Med.* 2013;3(1):208-213. [IA]

39. Tu RH, Grewall P, Leung JW, et al. Diphenhydramine as an adjunct to sedation for colonoscopy: a double-blind randomized, placebo-controlled study. *Gastrointest Endosc.* 2006;63(1):87-94. [IA]

40. Welchman S, Cochrane S, Minto G, Lewis S. Systematic review: the use of nitrous oxide gas for lower gastrointestinal endoscopy. *Aliment Pharmacol Ther.* 2010;32(3):324-333. [VB]

41. Levitzky BE, Lopez R, Dumot JA, Vargo JJ. Moderate sedation for elective upper endoscopy with balanced propofol versus fentanyl and midazolam alone: a randomized clinical trial. *Endoscopy.* 2012;44(1):13-20. [IA]

42. Sakurai S, Fukunaga A, Ichinohe T, Kaneko Y. IV ATP potentiates midazolam sedation as assessed by bispectral index. *Anesth Prog.* 2014;61(3):95-98. [IB]

43. Sun GC, Hsu MC, Chia YY, Chen PY, Shaw FZ. Effects of age and gender on intravenous midazolam premedication: a randomized double-blind study. *Br J Anaesth.* 2008;101(5):632-639. [IIB]

44. Dal T, Sazak H, Tunc M, Sahin S, Yilmaz A. A comparison of ketamine-midazolam and ketamine-propofol combinations used for sedation in the endobronchial ultrasound-guided transbronchial needle aspiration: a prospective, single-blind, randomized study. *J Thorac Dis.* 2014;6(6):742-751. [IIB]

45. Bassett K, Smith SW, Cardiff K, Bergman K, Aghajanian J, Somogyi E. Nurse anaesthetic care during cataract surgery: a comparative quality assurance study. *Can J Ophthalmol.* 2007;42(5):689-694. [IIB]

46. Khalil MA, Ebade AA, Abdel Azeem MS. The role of intravenous paracetamol in conscious sedation during Internal Cardioverter Defibrillator (ICD) insertion in geriatric patients. *Egypt J Anaesth.* 2013;29(1):41-45. [IB]

47. Conway A, Page K, Rolley JX, Worrall-Carter L. Nurse-administered procedural sedation and analgesia in the cardiac catheter laboratory: an integrative review. *Int J Nurs Stud.* 2011;48(8):1012-1023. [IIIA]

48. Schaufele MK, Marín DR, Tate JL, Simmons AC. Adverse events of conscious sedation in ambulatory spine procedures. *Spine J.* 2011;11(12):1093-1100. [IIIB]

49. Kezerashvili A, Fisher JD, Delaney J, et al. Intravenous sedation for cardiac procedures can be administered safely and cost-effectively by non-anesthesia personnel. *J Intervent Card Electrophysiol.* 2008;21(1):43-51. [IIIB]

50. Backman ES, Triant VA, Ehrenfeld JM, et al. Safety of midazolam for sedation of HIV-positive patients undergoing colonoscopy. *HIV Med.* 2013;14(6):379-384. [IIIB]

51. Cakmak H, Kocaturk T, Dundar SO, Kaan N, Ozbagcivan M, Erkan E. The effects of diazepam on blood pressure levels in cataract surgery. *Saudi Med J.* 2014;35(7):669-673. [IIIB]

52. Nayar DS, Guthrie WG, Goodman A, et al. Comparison of propofol deep sedation versus moderate sedation during endosonography. *Dig Dis Sci.* 2010;55(9):2537-2544. [IIB]

53. Zaidi N, Scoccia B, Leach RE, Jain T. Moderate conscious sedation for in vitro fertilization oocyte retrieval procedures in an office setting. *Internet J Anesthesiol.* 2007;12(1):7p-7p. [IIIB]

54. Wortman M, Daggett A, Ball C. Operative hysteroscopy in an office-based surgical setting: review of patient safety and satisfaction in 414 cases. *J Minim Invasive Gynecol.* 2013;20(1):56-63. [IIIB]

55. Steinfort DP, Irving LB. Patient satisfaction during endobronchial ultrasound-guided transbronchial needle aspiration performed under conscious sedation. *Respir Care.* 2010;55(6):702-706. [IIIC]

56. Sabbatani P, Mantovan R. Electrical cardioversion of atrial fibrillation: evaluation of sedation safety with midazolam by means of EtCO2 and IPI algorithm analysis. *Int J Cardiol.* 2013;169(6):430-432. [IIIB]

57. Cinar K, Yakut M, Ozden A. Sedation with midazolam versus midazolam plus meperidine for routine colonoscopy: a prospective, randomized, controlled study. *Turk J Gastroenterol.* 2009;20(4):271-275. [IB]

58. Eberl S, Polderman JAW, Preckel B, Kalkman CJ, Fockens P, Hollmann MW. Is "really conscious" sedation with solely an opioid an alternative to every day used sedation regimes for colonoscopies in a teaching hospital? Midazolam/fentanyl, propofol/alfentanil, or alfentanil only for colonoscopy: a randomized trial. *Tech Coloproctol.* 2014;18(8):745-752. [IB]

59. Hutson P. Is the use of intravenous opioids essential to control pain during colonoscopy? *Gastrointest Nurs.* 2009;7(3):15-23. [IIA]

60. Judah JR, Collins D, Gaidos JK, Hou W, Forsmark CE, Draganov PV. Prospective evaluation of gastroenterologist-guided, nurse-administered standard sedation for spiral deep small bowel enteroscopy. *Dig Dis Sci.* 2010;55(9):2584-2591. [IIIC]

61. Kan P, Jahshan S, Yashar P, et al. Feasibility, safety, and periprocedural complications associated with endovascular treatment of selected ruptured aneurysms under conscious sedation and local anesthesia. *Neurosurgery.* 2013;72(2):216-220. [IIIB]

62. Kim YH, Kim JW, Lee KL, et al. Effect of midazolam on cardiopulmonary function during colonoscopy with conscious sedation. *Dig Endosc.* 2014;26(3):417-423. [IIA]

63. Jirapinyo P, Abu Dayyeh BK, Thompson CC. Conscious sedation for upper endoscopy in the gastric bypass patient: prevalence of cardiopulmonary adverse events and predictors of sedation requirement. *Dig Dis Sci.* 2014;59(9):2173-2177. [IIIA]

64. Mador MJ, Abo Khamis M, Nag N, Mreyoud A, Jallu S, Mehboob S. Does sleep apnea increase the risk of cardiorespiratory complications during endoscopy procedures? *Sleep Breath.* 2011;15(3):393-401. [IIIB]

65. Gill J, Vidyarthi G, Kulkarni P, Anderson W, Boyd W. Safety of conscious sedation in patients with sleep apnea in a veteran population. *South Med J.* 2011;104(3):185-188. [IIIB]

66. Svrakic M, Pollack A, Huncke TK, Roland JT Jr. Conscious sedation and local anesthesia for patients undergoing neurotologic and complex otologic procedures. *Otol Neurotol.* 2014;35(10):e277-2285. [IIIB]

67. Mason KP, Robinson F, Fontaine P, Prescilla R. Dexmedetomidine offers an option for safe and effective sedation for nuclear medicine imaging in children. *Radiology.* 2013;267(3):911-917. [IIIA]

68. AB, AS, AS, AD, VG. Cardiorespiratory compromise under conscious sedation during upper gastrointestinal endoscopy. *J Coll Physicians Surg Pak.* 2006;16(9):585-589. [IB]

69. Sethi P, Mohammed S, Bhatia PK, Gupta N. Dexmedetomidine versus midazolam for conscious sedation in endoscopic retrograde cholangiopancreatography: An open-label randomised controlled trial. *Indian J Anaesth.* 2014;58(1):18-24. [IA]

70. Hurford WE, Staubach KC. A hospital policy for procedural sedation in the nonintubated patient. *Int Anesthesiol Clin.* 2013;51(2):1-22. [VB]

71. *Statement on Granting Privileges for Administration of Moderate Sedation to Practitioners Who Are Not Anesthesia Professionals.* 2011. American Society of Anesthesiologists. http://www.asahq.org/~/media/Sites/ASAHQ/Files/Public/Resources/standards-guidelines/statement-on-granting-privileges-for-administration-of-moderate-sedation-to-non-anesthesiologist.pdf. Accessed October 22, 2015. [IVB]

72. *Statement on the Anesthesia Care Team.* 2013. American Society of Anesthesiologists. http://www.asahq.org/~/media/Sites/ASAHQ/Files/Public/Resources/standards-guidelines/statement-on-the-anesthesia-care-team.pdf. Accessed October 22, 2015. [IVB]

73. Heneghan S, Myers J, Fanelli R, Richardson W; Society of American Gastrointestinal Endoscopic Surgeons. Society of American Gastrointestinal Endoscopic Surgeons (SAGES) guidelines for office endoscopic services. *Surg Endosc.* 2009;23(5):1125-1129. [IVC]

74. Chapman W. Administration of sedation in endoscopy: guidance, risks and skill requirements. *Gastrointest Nurs.* 2010;8(2):14-17. [VC]

75. Gupta A. Preoperative screening and risk assessment in the ambulatory surgery patient. *Curr Opin Anaesthesiol.* 2009;22(6):705-711. [VB]

76. Odom-Forren J. Perioperative patient safety and procedural sedation. *Perioper Nurs Clin.* 2008;3(4):355-366. [VA]

77. Coté CJ, Wilson S. Guidelines for monitoring and management of pediatric patients during and after sedation for diagnostic and therapeutic procedures: an update. Clinical report. *Pediatrics.* 2006;118(6):2587-2602. [IVB]

78. Sury M, Bullock I, Rabar S, Demott K; Guideline Development Group. Sedation for diagnostic and therapeutic procedures in children and young people: summary of NICE guidance. *BMJ.* 2010;341:c6819. [VA]

79. Makkad B. Procedural sedation for interventional cardiology procedures. *Int Anesthesiol Clin.* 2013;51(2):112-126. [VB]

80. Standards of Practice Committee of the American Society for Gastrointestinal Endoscopy; Lichtenstein DR, Jagannath S, et al. Sedation and anesthesia in GI endoscopy. *Gastrointest Endosc.* 2008;68(5):815-826. [IVA]

81. Voynarovska M, Cohen LB. The role of the endoscopy nurse or assistant in endoscopic sedation. *Gastrointest Endosc Clin N Am.* 2008;18(4):695-705. [VB]

82. Cohen LB, Delegge MH, Aisenberg J, et al. AGA Institute review of endoscopic sedation. *Gastroenterology.* 2007;133(2):675-701. [IVB]

83. Bui AH, Urman RD. Clinical and safety considerations for moderate and deep sedation. *J Med Pract Manage.* 2013;29(1):35-41. [VA]

84. Mitty RD, Wild DM. The pre- and postprocedure assessment of patients undergoing sedation for gastrointestinal endoscopy. *Gastrointest Endosc Clin North Am.* 2008;18(4):627-640. [VB]

85. Caperelli-White L, Urman RD. Developing a moderate sedation policy: essential elements and evidence-based considerations. *AORN J.* 2014;99(3):416-430. [VA]

86. Molina-Infante J, Arias A, Vara-Brenes D, et al. Propofol administration is safe in adult eosinophilic esophagitis patients sensitized to egg, soy, or peanut. *Allergy.* 2014;69(3):388-394. [IIIB]

87. Murphy A, Campbell DE, Baines D, Mehr S. Allergic reactions to propofol in egg-allergic children. *Anesth Analg.* 2011;113(1):140-144. [IIIC]

88. Tashkandi J. My patient is allergic to eggs, can I use propofol? A case report and review. *Saudi J Anaesth.* 2010;4(3):207-208. [VA]

89. Audicana Berasategui MT, Barasona Villarejo MJ, Corominas Sánchez M, et al; Drug Allergy Committee of the Spanish Society of Allergology and Clinical Immunology (Sociedad Española de Alergologia eInmunologfa Clinica SEAIC). Potential hypersensitivity due to the food or food additive content of medicinal products in Spain. *J Investig Allergol Clin Immunol.* 2011;21(7):496-506. [VA]

90. Cochico SG. Propofol allergy: assessing for patient risks. *AORN J.* 2012;96(4):398-405. [VB]

91. Dewachter P, Mouton-Faivre C, Castells MC, Hepner DL. Anesthesia in the patient with multiple drug allergies: are all allergies the same? *Curr Opin Anaesthesiol.* 2011;24(3):320-325. [VB]

92. Dumonceau J-M, Riphaus A, Beilenhoff U, et al. European curriculum for sedation training in gastrointestinal endoscopy: position statement of the European Society of Gastrointestinal Endoscopy (ESGE) and European Society of Gastroenterology and Endoscopy Nurses and Associates (ESGENA). *Endoscopy.* 2013;45(6):496-504. [IVB]

93. Hausman LM, Reich DL. Providing safe sedation/analgesia: an anesthesiologist's perspective. *Gastrointest Endosc Clin N Am.* 2008;18(4):707-716. [VB]

94. National Institute for Health and Care Excellence. *Sedation in Children and Young People: Sedation for Diagnostic and Therapeutic Procedures in Children and Young People.* [NICE Clinical Guidelines, No 112] London, United Kingdom: Royal College of Physicians; 2010. [IVB]

95. Guideline for medication safety. In: *Guidelines for Perioperative Practice.* Denver, CO: AORN; 2015:291-334. [IVB]

96. Halliday AB. CE Shades of sedation: learning about moderate sedation and analgesia. *Nursing.* 2006;36(4):36-41. [VC]

97. Petersen C. *Perioperative Nursing Data Set.* 3rd ed. Denver, CO: AORN, Inc; 2011. [IVB]

98. American Society of Anesthesiologists Committee. Practice guidelines for preoperative fasting and the use of pharmacologic agents to reduce the risk of pulmonary aspiration: application to healthy patients undergoing elective procedures: an updated report by the American Society of Anesthesiologists Committee on Standards and Practice Parameters. *Anesthesiology.* 2011;114(3):495-511. [IVA]

99. Antonelli MT, Seaver D, Urman RD. Procedural sedation and implications for quality and risk management. *J Healthc Risk Manag.* 2013;33(2):3-10. [VB]

100. Campbell EJ, Krishnaraj A, Harris M, Saini S, Richter JM. Automated before-procedure electronic health record screening to assess appropriateness for GI endoscopy and sedation. *Gastrointest Endosc.* 2012;76(4):786-792. [IIIB]

101. Conway A, Page K, Rolley J, Fulbrook P. Risk factors for impaired respiratory function during nurse-administered procedural sedation and analgesia in the cardiac catheterisation laboratory: a matched case-control study. *Eur J Cardiovasc Nurs.* 2013;12(4):393-399. [IIIA]

102. *Continuum of Depth of Sedation: Definition of General Anesthesia and Levels of Sedation/Analgesia.* 2014. American Society of Anesthesiologists. http://www.asahq.org/~/media/Sites/ASAHQ/Files/Public/Resources/standards-guidelines/continuum-of-depth-of-sedation-definition-of-general-anesthesia-and-levels-of-sedation-analgesia.pdf. Accessed October 22, 2015. [IVB]

103. ASA Physical Status Classification System. American Society of Anesthesiologists. https://www.asahq.org/resources/clinical-information/asa-physical-status-classification-system. Accessed October 22, 2015. [VB]

104. Tantri A, Clark C, Huber P, et al. Anesthesia monitoring by registered nurses during cataract surgery: assessment of need for intraoperative anesthesia consultation. *J Cataract Refract Surg.* 2006;32(7):1115-1118. [IIIB]

105. Knape JT, Adriaensen H, van Aken H, et al. Guidelines for sedation and/or analgesia by non-anaesthesiology doctors. *Eur J Anaesthesiol.* 2007;24(7):563-567. [VB]

106. Langeron O, Masso E, Huraux C, et al. Prediction of difficult mask ventilation. *Anesthesiology.* 2000;92(5):1229-1236. [IIIA]

107. Kheterpal S, Han R, Tremper KK, et al. Incidence and predictors of difficult and impossible mask ventilation. *Anesthesiology.* 2006;105(5):885-891. [IIIA]

108. El-Orbany M, Woehlck HJ. Difficult mask ventilation. *Anesth Analg.* 2009;109(6):1870-1880. [VB]

109. Phero JC, Rosenberg MB, Giovannitti JA. Adult airway evaluation in oral surgery. *Oral Maxillofac Surg Clin North Am.* 2013;25(3):386-399. [VA]

110. American Society of Anesthesiologists Task Force on Management of the Difficult Airway. Practice guidelines for management of the difficult airway: an updated report by the American Society of Anesthesiologists Task Force on Management of the Difficult Airway. *Anesthesiology.* 2003;98(5):1269-1277. [IVA]

111. Apfelbaum JL, Hagberg CA, Caplan RA, et al. Practice guidelines for management of the difficult airway: an updated report by the American Society of Anesthesiologists Task Force on Management of the Difficult Airway. *Anesthesiology.* 2013;118(2):251-270. [IVA]

112. Leoni A, Arlati S, Ghisi D, et al. Difficult mask ventilation in obese patients: analysis of predictive factors. *Minerva Anestesiol.* 2014;80(2):149-157. [IIIB]

113. Magalhaes E, Marques FO, Goveia CS, Ladeira LC, Lagares J. Use of simple clinical predictors on preoperative diagnosis of difficult endotracheal intubation in obese patients. *Braz J Anesthesiol.* 2013;63(3):262-266. [IIIA]

114. Saghaei M, Shetabi H, Golparvar M. Predicting efficiency of post-induction mask ventilation based on demographic and anatomical factors. *Adv Biomed Res.* 2012;1:10. [IIIB]

115. Lee A, Fan LT, Gin T, Karmakar MK, Ngan Kee WD. A systematic review (meta-analysis) of the accuracy of the Mallampati tests to predict the difficult airway. *Anesth Analg.* 2006;102(6):1867-1878. [IIIA]

116. Gross JB, Apfelbaum JL, Caplan RA, et al. Practice guidelines for the perioperative management of patients with obstructive sleep apnea: an updated report by the American Society of Anesthesiologists Task Force on Perioperative Management of patients with obstructive sleep apnea. *Anesthesiology.* 2014;120(2):1-19. [IVA]

117. Joshi GP, Ankichetty SP, Gan TJ, Chung F. Society for Ambulatory Anesthesia consensus statement on preoperative selection of adult patients with obstructive sleep apnea scheduled for ambulatory surgery. *Anesth Analg.* 2012;115(5):1060-1068. [IVA]

118. Abrishami A, Khajehdehi A, Chung F. A systematic review of screening questionnaires for obstructive sleep apnea. *Can J Anaesth.* 2010;57(5):423-438. [IIIA]

119. Chung F, Yegneswaran B, Liao P, et al. STOP questionnaire: a tool to screen patients for obstructive sleep apnea. *Anesthesiology.* 2008;108(5):812-821. [IIIA]

120. Chung F, Subramanyam R, Liao P, Sasaki E, Shapiro C, Sun Y. High STOP-Bang score indicates a high probability of obstructive sleep apnoea. *Br J Anaesth.* 2012;108(5):768-775. [IIIA]

121. Kulkarni GV, Horst A, Eberhardt JM, Kumar S, Sarker S. Obstructive sleep apnea in general surgery patients: is it more common than we think? *Am J Surg.* 2014;207(3):436-440. [IIIB]

122. Chung F, Yegneswaran B, Liao P, et al. Validation of the Berlin questionnaire and American Society of Anesthesiologists checklist as screening tools for obstructive sleep apnea in surgical patients. *Anesthesiology.* 2008;108(5):822-830. [IIA]

123. Chung F, Yang Y, Liao P. Predictive performance of the STOP-Bang score for identifying obstructive sleep apnea in obese patients. *Obes Surg.* 2013;23(12):2050-2057. [IIIA]

124. Mador MJ, Nadler J, Mreyoud A, et al. Do patients at risk of sleep apnea have an increased risk of cardiorespiratory complications during endoscopy procedures? *Sleep Breath.* 2012;16(3):609-615. [IIIB]

125. Corso RM, Petrini F, Buccioli M, et al. Clinical utility of preoperative screening with STOP-Bang questionnaire in elective surgery. *Minerva Anestesiol.* 2014;80(8):877-884. [IIIA]

126. Singh M, Liao P, Kobah S, Wijeysundera DN, Shapiro C, Chung F. Proportion of surgical patients with undiagnosed obstructive sleep apnoea. *Br J Anaesth.* 2013;110(4):629-636. [IIIB]

127. Boese ML, Ransom RK, Roadfuss RJ, Todd A, McGuire JM. Utility of the Berlin Questionnaire to screen for obstructive sleep apnea among patients receiving intravenous sedation for colonoscopy. *AANA J.* 2014;82(1):38-45. [IIIA]

128. Vasu TS, Doghramji K, Cavallazzi R, et al. Obstructive sleep apnea syndrome and postoperative complications: clinical use of the STOP-BANG questionnaire. *Arch Otolaryngol Head Neck Surg.* 2010;136(10):1020-1024. [IIIB]

129. Luo JM, Huang R, Zhong X, Xiao Y, Zhou J. STOP-Bang questionnaire is superior to Epworth sleepiness scales, Berlin questionnaire, and STOP questionnaire in screening obstructive sleep apnea hypopnea syndrome patients. *Chin Med J.* 2014;127(17):3065-3070. [IIIB]

130. Khiani VS, Salah W, Maimone S, Cummings L, Chak A. Sedation during endoscopy for patients at risk of obstructive sleep apnea. *Gastrointest Endosc.* 2009;70(6):1116-1120. [IIIB]

131. Lockhart EM, Willingham MD, Abdallah AB, et al. Obstructive sleep apnea screening and postoperative mortality in a large surgical cohort. *Sleep Med.* 2013;14(5):407-415. [IIIB]

132. Mehta PP, Kochhar G, Kalra S, et al. Can a validated sleep apnea scoring system predict cardiopulmonary events using propofol sedation for routine EGD or colonoscopy? A prospective cohort study. *Gastrointest Endosc.* 2014;79(3):436-444. [IIIB]

133. Ganesh BR, Kulkarni Maitreyi K, Noronha Melita G. Screening of sleep apnoea in middle-aged hypertensive subjects using Stop-Bang questionnaire—an observational study. *Indian J Physiother Occup Ther.* 2014;8(2):13-16. [IIIC]

134. Chia P, Seet E, Macachor JD, Iyer US, Wu D. The association of pre-operative STOP-BANG scores with postoperative critical care admission. *Anaesthesia.* 2013;68(9):950-952. [IIIC]

135. Ankichetty S, Chung F. Considerations for patients with obstructive sleep apnea undergoing ambulatory surgery. *Curr Opin Anaesthesiol.* 2011;24(6):605-611. [VC]

136. Seet E, Chung F. Obstructive sleep apnea: preoperative assessment. *Anesthesiol Clin.* 2010;28(2):199-215. [VB]

137. Becker DE, Rosenberg MB, Phero JC. Essentials of airway management, oxygenation, and ventilation: part 1: basic equipment and devices. *Anesth Prog.* 2014;61(2):78-83. [VB]

138. Porhomayon J, Nader ND, Leissner KB, El-Solh AA. Respiratory perioperative management of patients with obstructive sleep apnea. *J Intensive Care Med.* 2014;29(3):145-153. [VA]

139. Moos DD. Obstructive sleep apnea and sedation in the endoscopy suite. *Gastroenterol Nurs.* 2006;29(6):456-463. [VB]

140. Chung F, Elsaid H. Screening for obstructive sleep apnea before surgery: why is it important? *Curr Opin Anesthesiol.* 2009;22(3):405-411. [VB]

141. Moos DD, Cuddeford JD. Implications of obstructive sleep apnea syndrome for the perianesthesia nurse. *J Perianesth Nurs.* 2006;21(2):103-115. [VA]

142. Auckley D, Bolden N. Preoperative screening and perioperative care of the patient with sleep-disordered breathing. *Curr Opin Pulm Med.* 2012;18(6):588-595. [VB]

143. Pace N. Sedating the patient with underlying sleep apnea. *J Radiol Nurs.* 2008;27(3):107-111. [VB]

144. Sharara AI, El Zahabi L, Maasri K, et al. Persistent snoring under conscious sedation during colonoscopy is a predictor of obstructive sleep apnea. *Gastrointest Endosc.* 2010;71(7):1224-1230. [IIIB]

145. Ead H. Meeting the challenge of obstructive sleep apnea: developing a protocol that guides perianesthesia patient care. *J Perianesth Nurs.* 2009;24(2):103-110. [VA]

146. Chung F, Yang Y, Brown R, Liao P. Alternative scoring models of STOP-bang questionnaire improve specificity to detect undiagnosed obstructive sleep apnea. *J Clin Sleep Med.* 2014;10(9):951-958. [IIA]

147. American Society of PeriAnesthesia Nurses Standards and Guidelines Committee. 2015-2017 *Perianesthesia Nursing Standards, Practice Recommendations and Interpretive Statements.* Cherry Hill, NJ: American Society of PeriAnesthesia Nurses; 2015. [IVB]

148. Blake DW, Yew CY, Donnan GB, Williams DL. Postoperative analgesia and respiratory events in patients with symptoms of obstructive sleep apnoea. *Anaesth Intensive Care.* 2009;37(5):720-725. [IC]

149. Gorospe EC, Oxentenko AS. Preprocedural considerations in gastrointestinal endoscopy. *Mayo Clin Proc.* 2013;88(9):1010-1016. [VA]

150. LÜ F, Lin J, Benditt DG. Conscious sedation and anesthesia in the cardiac electrophysiology laboratory. *J Cardiovasc Electrophysiol.* 2013;24(2):237-245. [VB]

151. Braunstein ED, Rosenberg R, Gress F, Green PH, Lebwohl B. Development and validation of a clinical prediction score (the SCOPE score) to predict sedation outcomes in patients undergoing endoscopic procedures. *Aliment Pharmacol Ther.* 2014;40(1):72-82. [IIIA]

152. DeLegge MH. When to call the anesthesiologist for assistance with sedation. *Gastrointest Endosc.* 2011;74(6):1377-1379. [VB]

153. Hassan AE, Akbar U, Chaudhry SA, et al. Rate and prognosis of patients under conscious sedation requiring emergent intubation during neuroendovascular procedures. *AJNR Am J Neuroradiol.* 2013;34(7):1375-1379. [IIIA]

154. Chawla S, Katz A, Attar BM, Go B. Endoscopic retrograde cholangiopancreatography under moderate sedation and factors predicting need for anesthesiologist directed sedation: a county hospital experience. *World J Gastrointest Endosc.* 2013;5(4):160-164. [IIIB]

155. Amornyotin S. Sedation-related complications in gastrointestinal endoscopy. *World J Gastrointest Endosc.* 2013;5(11):527-533. [VB]

156. Guimaraes ES, Campbell EJ, Richter JM. The safety of nurse-administered procedural sedation compared to anesthesia care in a historical cohort of advanced endoscopy patients. *Anesth Analg.* 2014;119(2):349-356. [IIIB]

157. Cabrini L, Nobile L, Cama E, et al. Non-invasive ventilation during upper endoscopies in adult patients. A systematic review. *Minerva Anestesiol.* 2013;79(6):683-694. [IIIB]

158. Hession PM, Joshi GP. Sedation: not quite that simple. *Anesthesiol Clin.* 2010;28(2):281-294. [VB]

159. Kauling AL, Locks Gde F, Brunharo GM, da Cunha VJ, de Almeida MC. Conscious sedation for upper digestive endoscopy performed by endoscopists. *Rev Bras Anestesiol.* 2010;60(6):577-583. [IIIB]

160. *Registered Nurses Engaged in the Administration of Sedation and Analgesia.* 2005. American Association of Nurse Anesthetists. http://www.aana.com/resources2/professionalpractice/Pages/Registered-Nurses-Engaged-in-the-Administration-of-Sedation-and-Analgesia.aspx. Accessed October 22, 2015. [IVB]

161. Du Rand IA, Blaikley J, Booton R, et al. British Thoracic Society guideline for diagnostic flexible bronchoscopy in adults: accredited by NICE. *Thorax.* 2013;68(Suppl 1):1-44. [IVA]

162. De Vito A, Carrasco Llatas M, Vanni A, et al. European position paper on drug-induced sedation endoscopy (DISE). *Sleep Breath.* 2014;18(3):453-465. [IVB]

163. Lee KK, Anderson MA, Baron TH, et al. Modifications in endoscopic practice for pediatric patients. *Gastrointest Endosc.* 2008;67(1):1-9. [IVA]

164. *AORN Position Statement on One Perioperative Registered Nurse Circulator Dedicated to Every Patient Undergoing an Operative or Other Invasive Procedure.* 2014. AORN, Inc. http://www.aorn.org/Clinical_Practice/Position_Statements/Position_Statements.aspx. Accessed October 22, 2015. [IVB]

165. *AORN Position Statement on Perioperative Safe Staffing and On-Call Practices.* 2014. AORN, Inc. http://www.aorn.org/Clinical_Practice/Position_Statements/Position_Statements.aspx. Accessed October 22, 2015. [IVB]

166. Centers for Medicare & Medicaid Services. 42 CFR 482.51. Condition of participation: surgical services. 2011. http://www.gpo.gov/fdsys/granule/CFR-2011-title42-vol5/CFR-2011-title42-vol5-sec482-51. Accessed October 22, 2015.

167. Kane RL, Shamliyan T, Mueller C, Duval S, Wilt TJ. Nurse staffing and quality of patient care. *Evid Rep Technol Assess (Full Rep).* 2007;(151):1-115. [IIIA]

168. Thungjaroenkul P, Cummings GG, Embleton A. The impact of nurse staffing on hospital costs and patient length of stay: a systematic review. *Nurs Econ.* 2007;25(5):255-265. [IIIA]

169. McGillis Hall L, Doran D, Pink GH. Nurse staffing models, nursing hours, and patient safety outcomes. *J Nurs Adm.* 2004;34(1):41-45. [IVB]

170. Newhouse RP, Johantgen M, Pronovist PJ, Johnson E. Perioperative nurses and patient outcomes: mortality, complications, and length of stay. *AORN J.* 2005;81(3):508-528. [IIIA]

171. Kane RL, Shamliyan TA, Mueller C, Duval S, Wilt TJ. The association of registered nurse staffing levels and patient outcomes: systematic review and meta-analysis. *Med Care.* 2007;45(12):1195-1204. [IIIA]

172. Needleman J, Buerhaus P, Pankratz VS, Leibson CL, Stevens SR, Harris M. Nurse staffing and inpatient hospital mortality. *N Engl J Med.* 2011;364(11):1037-1045. [IIIA]

173. McHugh MD, Berez J, Small DS. Hospitals with higher nurse staffing had lower odds of readmissions

penalties than hospitals with lower staffing. *Health Aff (Millwood).* 2013;32(10):1740-1747. [IIIB]

174. Aiken LH, Cimiotti JP, Sloane DM, Smith HL, Flynn L, Neff DF. Effects of nurse staffing and nurse education on patient deaths in hospitals with different nurse work environments. *Med Care.* 2011;49(12):1047-1053. [IIIA]

175. SGNA Practice Committee. Statement on the use of sedation and analgesia in the gastrointestinal endoscopy setting. *Gastroenterol Nurs.* 2008;31(3):249-251. [IVB]

176. Cohen LB. Patient monitoring during gastrointestinal endoscopy: why, when, and how? *Gastrointest Endosc Clin North Am.* 2008;18(4):651-663. [VA]

177. Eichhorn V, Henzler D, Murphy MF. Standardizing care and monitoring for anesthesia or procedural sedation delivered outside the operating room. *Curr Opin Anaesthesiol.* 2010;23(4):494-499. [VB]

178. *Standards for Basic Anesthetic Monitoring.* 2011. American Society of Anesthesiologists. http://www.asahq.org/~/media/sites/asahq/files/public/resources/standards-guidelines/standards-for-basic-anesthetic-monitoring.pdf. Accessed October 22, 2015. [IVB]

179. Friedrich-Rust M, Welte M, Welte C, et al. Capnographic monitoring of propofol-based sedation during colonoscopy. *Endoscopy.* 2014;46(3):236-244. [IA]

180. Beitz A, Riphaus A, Meining A, et al. Capnographic monitoring reduces the incidence of arterial oxygen desaturation and hypoxemia during propofol sedation for colonoscopy: a randomized, controlled study (ColoCap Study). *Am J Gastroenterol.* 2012;107(8):1205-1212. [IB]

181. Qadeer MA, Lopez AR, Dumot JA, Vargo JJ. Hypoxemia during moderate sedation for gastrointestinal endoscopy: causes and associations. *Digestion.* 2011;84(1):37-45. [IB]

182. Waugh JB, Epps CA, Khodneva YA. Capnography enhances surveillance of respiratory events during procedural sedation: a meta-analysis. *J Clin Anesth.* 2011;23(3):189-196. [IIA]

183. Cacho G, Pérez-Calle JL, Barbado A, Lledó JL, Ojea R, Fernández-Rodríguez CM. Capnography is superior to pulse oximetry for the detection of respiratory depression during colonoscopy. *Rev Esp Enferm Dig.* 2010;102(2):86-89. [IIA]

184. Schlag C, Worner A, Wagenpfeil S, Kochs EF, Schmid RM, von Delius S. Capnography improves detection of apnea during procedural sedation for percutaneous transhepatic cholangiodrainage. *Can J Gastroenterol.* 2013;27(10):582-586. [IIIB]

185. Yarchi D, Cohen A, Umansky T, Sukhotnik I, Shaoul R. Assessment of end-tidal carbon dioxide during pediatric and adult sedation for endoscopic procedures. *Gastrointest Endosc.* 2009;69(4):877-882. [IIIB]

186. Restrepo RD, Nuccio P, Spratt G, Waugh J. Current applications of capnography in non-intubated patients. *Expert Rev Respir Med.* 2014;8(5):629-639. [VA]

187. Welliver M. Why capnography for procedural sedation? *Gastroenterol Nurs.* 2012;35(6):423-425. [VB]

188. Lightdale JR, Goldmann DA, Feldman HA, Newburg AR, DiNardo JA, Fox VL. Microstream capnography improves patient monitoring during moderate sedation: a randomized, controlled trial. *Pediatrics.* 2006;117(6):e1170-e1178. [IB]

189. Langhan ML, Chen L, Marshall C, Santucci KA. Detection of hypoventilation by capnography and its association with hypoxia in children undergoing sedation with ketamine. *Pediatr Emerg Care.* 2011;27(5):394-397. [IIIB]

190. *Distinguishing Monitored Anesthesia Care ("MAC") from Sedation/Analgesia (Conscious Sedation).* 2009. American Society of Anesthesiologists. http://www.asahq.org/~/media/Sites/ASAHQ/Files/Public/Resources/standards-guidelines/distinguishing-monitored-anesthesia-care-from-moderate-sedation-analgesia.pdf. Accessed October 22, 2015. [VB]

191. Sheahan CG, Mathews DM. Monitoring and delivery of sedation. *Br J Anaesth.* 2014;113(Suppl 2):ii37-ii47. [VA]

192. Munson GW, Van Norstrand MD, O'Donnell JJ, Hammes NL, Francis DL. Intraprocedural evaluation of comfort for sedated outpatient upper endoscopy and colonoscopy: the La Crosse (WI) intra-endoscopy sedation comfort score. *Gastroenterol Nurs.* 2011;34(4):296-301. [IIIB]

193. Frölich MA, Zhang K, Ness TJ. Effect of sedation on pain perception. *Anesthesiology.* 2013;118(3):611-621. [IA]

194. Heuss LT, Sughanda SP, Degen LP. Endoscopy teams' judgment of discomfort among patients undergoing colonoscopy: "How bad was it really?" *Swiss Med Wkly.* 2012;142:w13726. [IIIB]

195. Goodyear D, Velanovich V. Measuring pain in outpatient surgical patients: variation resulting from instrument choice. *Am Surg.* 2012;78(11):1292-1296. [IIIB]

196. Froehlich F, Harris JK, Wietlisbach V, et al. Current sedation and monitoring practice for colonoscopy: an international observational study (EPAGE). *Endoscopy.* 2006;38(5):461-469. [IIIB]

197. Qadeer MA, Vargo JJ, Dumot JA, et al. Capnographic monitoring of respiratory activity improves safety of sedation for endoscopic cholangiopancreatography and ultrasonography. *Gastroenterology.* 2009;136(5):1568-1576. [IIB]

198. ASGE Technology Committee; Gottlieb KT, Banerjee S, et al. Monitoring equipment for endoscopy. *Gastrointest Endosc.* 2013;77(2):175-180. [IVB]

199. Guideline for a safe environment of care, part 1. In: *Guidelines for Perioperative Practice.* Denver, CO: AORN, Inc; 2015:239-264. [IVA]

200. Impact of clinical alarms on patient safety: a report from the American College of Clinical Engineering Healthcare Technology Foundation. *J Clin Eng.* 2007;32(1):22-33. [VB]

201. Schmid F, Goepfert MS, Kuhnt D, et al. The wolf is crying in the operating room: patient monitor and anesthesia workstation alarming patterns during cardiac surgery. *Anesth Analg.* 2011;112(1):78-83. [IIIB]

202. *Clinical Alarms: 2011 Summit Report.* Fairfax, VA: Association for the Advancement of Medical Instrumentation; 2011. [VC]

203. Dawson R, von Fintel N, Nairn S. Sedation assessment using the Ramsay scale. *Emerg Nurse.* 2010;18(3):18-20. [VB]

204. Moline B, Roberts M, Houser J. Validity and interrater reliability of the Moline-Roberts Pharmacologic Sedation Scale. *Clin Nurse Spec.* 2012;26(3):140-148. [IIIB]

205. Greenhalgh DL, Kumar CM. Sedation during ophthalmic surgery. *Eur J Anaesthesiol.* 2008;25(9):701-707. [VB]

206. Nisbet AT, Mooney-Cotter F. Comparison of selected sedation scales for reporting opioid-induced sedation assessment. *Pain Manag Nurs.* 2009;10(3):154-164. [IIIB]

207. Newton T, Pop I, Duvall E. Sedation scales and measures—a literature review. *SAAD Dig.* 2013;29:88-99. [VB]

208. Lo Y-L, Lin T-Y, Fang Y-F, et al. Feasibility of bispectral index-guided propofol infusion for flexible bronchoscopy sedation: a randomized controlled trial. *PLoS One.* 2011;6(11):e27769. [IB]

209. Sasaki T, Tanabe S, Azuma M, et al. Propofol sedation with bispectral index monitoring is useful for endoscopic submucosal dissection: a randomized prospective phase II clinical trial. *Endoscopy.* 2012;44(6):584-589. [IC]

210. Baysal A, Polat TB, Yalcin Y, Celebi A. Can analysis of the bispectral index prove helpful when monitoring titration of doses of midazolam and ketamine for sedation during paediatric cardiac catheterization. *Cardiol Young.* 2008;18(1):51-57. [IB]

211. Imagawa A, Fujiki S, Kawahara Y, et al. Satisfaction with bispectral index monitoring of propofol-mediated sedation during endoscopic submucosal dissection: a prospective, randomized study. *Endoscopy.* 2008;40(11):905-909. [IC]

212. von Delius S, Salletmaier H, Meining A, et al. Bispectral index monitoring of midazolam and propofol sedation during endoscopic retrograde cholangiopancreatography: a randomized clinical trial (the EndoBIS study). *Endoscopy.* 2012;44(3):258-264. [IA]

213. Malviya S, Voepel-Lewis T, Ludomirsky A, Marshall J, Tait AR. Can we improve the assessment of discharge readiness?: a comparative study of observational and objective measures of depth of sedation in children. *Anesthesiology.* 2004;100(2):218-224. [IIB]

214. Yang KS, Habib AS, Lu M, et al. A prospective evaluation of the incidence of adverse events in nurse-administered moderate sedation guided by sedation scores or bispectral index. *Anesth Analg.* 2014;119(1):43-48. [IIIB]

215. Hata K, Andoh A, Hayafuji K, et al. Usefulness of bispectral monitoring of conscious sedation during endoscopic mucosal dissection. *World J Gastroenterol.* 2009;15(5):595-598. [IIB]

216. Yamamoto S, Igarashi T, Tetsuka K, Endo S. Bispectral index monitoring of midazolam sedation during flexible bronchoscopy. *J Bronchology Interv Pulmonol.* 2009;16(4):241-244. [IIIC]

217. Haberland CM, Baker S, Liu H. Bispectral index monitoring of sedation depth in pediatric dental patients. *Anesth Prog.* 2011;58(2):66-72. [IIIC]

218. Wehrmann T. Extended monitoring of the sedated patient: bispectral index, Narcotrend and automated responsiveness monitor. *Digestion.* 2010;82(2):90-93. [VB]

219. Malviya S, Voepel-Lewis T, Tait AR, Watcha MF, Sadhasivam S, Friesen RH. Effect of age and sedative agent on the accuracy of bispectral index in detecting depth of sedation in children. *Pediatrics.* 2007;120(3):e461-e470. [IIIC]

220. Yu YH, Han DS, Kim HS, et al. Efficacy of bispectral index monitoring during balanced propofol sedation for colonoscopy: a prospective, randomized controlled trial. *Dig Dis Sci.* 2013;58(12):3576-3583. [IB]

221. Drake LM, Chen SC, Rex DK. Efficacy of bispectral monitoring as an adjunct to nurse-administered propofol sedation for colonoscopy: a randomized controlled trial. *Am J Gastroenterol.* 2006;101(9):2003-2007. [IC]

222. DeWitt JM. Bispectral index monitoring for nurse-administered propofol sedation during upper endoscopic ultrasound: a prospective, randomized controlled trial. *Dig Dis Sci.* 2008;53(10):2739-2745. [IC]

223. Kang KJ, Min BH, Lee MJ, et al. Efficacy of bispectral index monitoring for midazolam and meperidine induced sedation during endoscopic submucosal dissection: a prospective, randomized controlled study. *Gut Liver.* 2011;5(2):160-164. [IA]

224. Qadeer MA, Vargo JJ, Patel S, et al. Bispectral index monitoring of conscious sedation with the combination of meperidine and midazolam during endoscopy. *Clin Gastroenterol Hepatol.* 2008;6(1):102-108. [IIIB]

225. Chisholm CJ, Zurica J, Mironov D, Sciacca RR, Ornstein E, Heyer EJ. Comparison of electrophysiologic monitors with clinical assessment of level of sedation. *Mayo Clin Proc.* 2006;81(1):46-52. [IIA]

226. Yeganeh N, Roshani B, Almasi A, Jamshidi N. Correlation between Bispectral Index and predicted effect-site concentration of propofol in different levels of target-controlled, propofol induced sedation in healthy volunteers. *Arch Iranian Med.* 2010;13(2):126-134. [IIB]

227. *ACR-SIR Practice Parameter for Sedation/Analgesia.* 2014. American College of Radiology/Society of Interventional Radiology. http://www.acr.org/~/media/F194CBB800AB43048B997A75938AB482.pdf. Accessed October 22, 2015. [IVB]

228. American Academy of Pediatrics; American Academy of Pediatric Dentistry; Cote CJ, Wilson S; Work Group on Sedation. Guidelines for monitoring and management of pediatric patients during and after sedation for diagnostic and therapeutic procedures: an update. *Paediatr Anaesth.* 2008;18(1):9-10. [IVB]

229. Qureshi WA, Zuckerman MJ, Adler DG, et al. ASGE guideline: modifications in endoscopic practice for the elderly. *Gastrointest Endosc.* 2006;63(4):566-569. [IVC]

230. Akhtar Abbasi J, Padda Manmeet S. Safety and efficacy of colonoscopy in the elderly: experience in an innercity community hospital serving African American and Hispanic patients. *Ethnicity Dis.* 2011;21(4):412-414. [IIIB]

231. Parlak M, Parlak I, Erdur B, Ergin A, Sagiroglu E. Age effect on efficacy and side effects of two sedation and analgesia protocols on patients going through cardioversion: a randomized clinical trial. *Acad Emerg Med.* 2006;13(5):493-499. [IB]

232. Martinez JF, Aparicio JR, Company L, et al. Safety of continuous propofol sedation for endoscopic procedures in elderly patients. *Rev Esp Enferm Dig.* 2011;103(2):76-82. [IIIB]

233. Travis AC, Pievsky D, Saltzman JR. Endoscopy in the elderly. *Am J Gastroenterol.* 2012;107(10):1495-1501. [VA]

234. *Guidance for Directors of Anesthesia Service for Computer-Assisted Personalized Sedation (CAPS) Devices.* 2014. American Society of Anesthesiologists. https://www.asahq.org/~/media/sites/asahq/files/public/resources/asa%20committees/2014-1-21-final-sedasys-guidance.pdf?la=en. Accessed October 22, 2015. [IVB]

235. Pambianco DJ, Vargo JJ, Pruitt RE, Hardi R, Martin JF. Computer-assisted personalized sedation for upper endoscopy and colonoscopy: a comparative, multicenter randomized study. *Gastrointest Endosc.* 2011;73(4):765-772. [IB]

236. Pambianco DJ, Whitten CJ, Moerman A, Struys MM, Martin JF. An assessment of computer-assisted personalized sedation: a sedation delivery system to administer propofol for gastrointestinal endoscopy. *Gastrointest Endosc.* 2008;68(3):542-547. [IIIC]

237. ASGE Technology Committee; Banerjee S, Desilets D, et al. Computer-assisted personalized sedation. *Gastrointest Endosc.* 2011;73(3):423-427. [IVB]

238. Goudra BG, Singh PM, Chandrasekhara V. SEDASYS® airway, oxygenation, and ventilation: anticipating and managing the challenges. *Dig Dis Sci.* 2014;59(5):920-927. [VA]

239. Pambianco DJ. Future directions in endoscopic sedation. *Gastrointest Endosc Clin North Am.* 2008;18(4):789-799. [VA]

240. US Food and Drug Administration. P080009: Premarket approval letter for SEDASYS Computer-Assisted Personalized Sedation System. May 3, 2013. http://

www.accessdata.fda.gov/cdrh_docs/pdf8/p080009a.pdf. Accessed October 22, 2015.

241. Hosseini Jahromi SA, Hosseini Valami SM, Adeli N, Yazdi Z. Comparison of the effects of intranasal midazolam versus different doses of intranasal ketamine on reducing preoperative pediatric anxiety: a prospective randomized clinical trial. *J Anesth.* 2012;26(6):878-882. [IA]

242. Fallah R, Nakhaei MH, Behdad S, Moghaddam RN, Shamszadeh A. Oral chloral hydrate vs. intranasal midazolam for sedation during computerized tomography. *Indian Pediatr.* 2013;50(2):233-235. [IB]

243. Li BL, Yuen VM, Song XR, et al. Intranasal dexmedetomidine following failed chloral hydrate sedation in children. *Anaesthesia.* 2014;69(3):240-244. [IB]

244. Zhang X, Bai X, Zhang Q, Wang X, Lu L. The safety and efficacy of intranasal dexmedetomidine during electrochemotherapy for facial vascular malformation: a double-blind, randomized clinical trial. *J Oral Maxillofac Surg.* 2013;71(11):1835-1842. [IB]

245. Almenrader N, Passariello M, Coccetti B, Haiberger R, Pietropaoli P. Premedication in children: a comparison of oral midazolam and oral clonidine. *Paediatr Anaesth.* 2007;17(12):1143-1149. [IB]

246. West SK, Griffiths B, Shariff Y, Stephens D, Mireskandari K. Utilisation of an outpatient sedation unit in paediatric ophthalmology: safety and effectiveness of chloral hydrate in 1509 sedation episodes. *Br J Ophthalmol.* 2013;97(11):1437-1442. [IIIA]

247. Finnemore A, Toulmin H, Merchant N, et al. Chloral hydrate sedation for magnetic resonance imaging in newborn infants. *Paediatr Anaesth.* 2014;24(2):190-195. [IIIB]

248. ASGE Ensuring Safety in the Gastrointestinal Endoscopy Unit Task Force; Calderwood AH, Chapman FJ, et al. Guidelines for safety in the gastrointestinal endoscopy unit. *Gastrointest Endosc.* 2014;79(3):363-372.

249. Rozario L, Sloper D, Sheridan MJ. Supplemental oxygen during moderate sedation and the occurrence of clinically significant desaturation during endoscopic procedures. *Gastroenterol Nurs.* 2008;31(4):281-285. [IB]

250. Tae CH, Kang KJ, Min BH, et al. Paradoxical reaction to midazolam in patients undergoing endoscopy under sedation: incidence, risk factors and the effect of flumazenil. *Dig Liver Dis.* 2014;46(8):710-715. [IIIB]

251. Moon YE. Paradoxical reaction to midazolam in children. *Korean J Anesthesiol.* 2013;65(1):2-3. [VB]

252. McKenzie WS, Rosenberg M. Paradoxical reaction following administration of a benzodiazepine. *J Oral Maxillofac Surg.* 2010;68(12):3034-3036. [VB]

253. Ip HY, Chung F. Escort accompanying discharge after ambulatory surgery: a necessity or a luxury? *Curr Opin Anaesthesiol.* 2009;22(6):748-754. [VA]

254. Chung F, Assmann N. Car accidents after ambulatory surgery in patients without an escort. *Anesth Analg.* 2008;106(3):817-820, table of contents. [VA]

255. Horiuchi A, Nakayama Y, Fujii H, Katsuyama Y, Ohmori S, Tanaka N. Psychomotor recovery and blood propofol level in colonoscopy when using propofol sedation. *Gastrointest Endosc.* 2012;75(3):506-512. [IIIB]

256. Cote CJ, Notterman DA, Karl HW, Weinberg JA, McCloskey C. Adverse sedation events in pediatrics: a critical incident analysis of contributing factors. *Pediatrics.* 2000;105(4 Pt 1):805-814. [IIIB]

257. Newman DH, Azer MM, Pitetti RD, Singh S. When is a patient safe for discharge after procedural sedation? The timing of adverse effect events in 1367 pediatric procedural sedations. *Ann Emerg Med.* 2003;42(5):627-635. [IIIB]

258. Trevisani L, Cifala V, Gilli G, Matarese V, Zelante A, Sartori S. Post-Anaesthetic Discharge Scoring System to assess patient recovery and discharge after colonoscopy. *World J Gastrointest Endosc.* 2013;5(10):502-507. [IIA]

259. Wong J, Tong D, De Silva Y, Abrishami A, Chung F. Development of the functional recovery index for ambulatory surgery and anesthesia. *Anesthesiology.* 2009;110(3):596-602. [IIIB]

260. Flumazenil injection solution [package insert]. Rockford, IL: Mylan Institutional LLC; November 2013. [VA]

261. Mathus-Vliegen EM, de Jong L, Kos-Foekema HA. Significant and safe shortening of the recovery time after flumazenil-reversed midazolam sedation. *Dig Dis Sci.* 2014;59(8):1717-1725. [IIA]

262. Basu NN, Kald B, Heath D. Morphine delays discharge following ambulatory surgery: a prospective institutional study. *J Perioper Pract.* 2009;19(8):254-256. [IIIB]

263. Makary L, Vornik V, Finn R, et al. Prolonged recovery associated with dexmedetomidine when used as a sole sedative agent in office-based oral and maxillofacial surgery procedures. *J Oral Maxillofac Surg.* 2010;68(2):386-391. [IIIC]

264. Cruthirds D, Sims PJ, Louis PJ. Review and recommendations for the prevention, management, and treatment of postoperative and postdischarge nausea and vomiting. *Oral Surg Oral Med Oral Pathol Oral Radiol.* 2013;115(5):601-611. [VA]

265. Neville A, Coe K, Thompson J. How long is too long? Recovery time of outpatients with sleep apnea after procedural sedation. *Gastroenterol Nurs.* 2013;36(4):260-264. [IIIB]

266. Centers for Medicare & Medicaid Services. 42 CFR 416: Ambulatory surgical services. 2011. https://www.cms.gov/Regulations-and-Guidance/Legislation/CFCsAndCoPs/ASC.html. Accessed October 22, 2015.

267. Centers for Medicare & Medicaid Services. 42 CFR 482. Conditions of participation for hospitals. 2015. http://www.ecfr.gov/cgi-bin/text-idx?tpl=/ecfrbrowse/Title42/42cfr482_main_02.tpl. Accessed October 22, 2015.

268. Veselis RA, Pryor KO, Reinsel RA, Li Y, Mehta M, Johnson RJ. Propofol and midazolam inhibit conscious memory processes very soon after encoding: an event-related potential study of familiarity and recollection in volunteers. *Anesthesiology.* 2009;110(2):295-312. [IA]

269. Watkins TJ, Bonds RL, Hodges K, Goettle BB, Dobson DA, Maye JP. Evaluation of postprocedure cognitive function using 3 distinct standard sedation regimens for endoscopic procedures. *AANA J.* 2014;82(2):133-139. [IB]

270. Padmanabhan U, Leslie K, Eer AS, Maruff P, Silbert BS. Early cognitive impairment after sedation for colonoscopy: the effect of adding midazolam and/or fentanyl to propofol. *Anesth Analg.* 2009;109(5):1448-1455. [IC]

271. Multisociety sedation curriculum for gastrointestinal endoscopy. *Hepatology.* 2012;56(1):E1-E25. [IVA]

272. Ehrhardt BS, Staubach KC. A program for education, competency, and quality in procedural sedation. *Int Anesthesiol Clin.* 2013;51(2):33-42. [VA]

273. Doig AK. Improving moderate sedation practice with interactive online nursing education. *Commun Nurs Res.* 2009;42:212-212. [IC]

274. DeMaria SJ, Levine A, Cohen LB. Human patient simulation and its role in endoscopic sedation training. *Gastrointest Endosc Clin North Am.* 2008;18(4):801-813. [VB]

275. Tobin CD, Clark CA, McEvoy MD, et al. An approach to moderate sedation simulation training. *Simul Healthc.* 2013;8(2):114-123. [IIC]

276. Keidan I, Gravenstein D, Berkenstadt H, Ziv A, Shavit I, Sidi A. Supplemental oxygen compromises the use of pulse oximetry for detection of apnea and hypoventilation during sedation in simulated pediatric patients. *Pediatrics.* 2008;122(2):293-298. [IB]

277. Hollman GA, Banks DM, Berkenbosch JW, et al. Development, implementation, and initial participant feedback of a pediatric sedation provider course. *Teach Learn Med.* 2013;25(3):249-257. [IIIC]

278. Black SA, Nestel DF, Horrocks EJ, et al. Evaluation of a framework for case development and simulated patient training for complex procedures. *Simul Healthc.* 2006;1(2):66-71. [IIIC]

279. Jensen JT, Konge L, Moller A, Hornslet P, Vilmann P. Endoscopy nurse-administered propofol sedation performance. Development of an assessment tool and a reliability testing model. *Scand J Gastroenterol.* 2014;49(8):1014-1019. [IIIB]

280. Lightdale JR, Weinstock P. Simulation and training of procedural sedation. *Tech Gastrointest Endosc.* 2011;13(3):167-173. [VB]

281. Collins AS, Strother D. Synergy and competence: tools of the trade. *J Nurses Staff Dev.* 2008;24(4):E1-E8. [VB]

282. Jest AD, Tonge A. Using a learning needs assessment to identify knowledge deficits regarding procedural sedation for pediatric patients. *AORN J.* 2011;94(6):567-577. [VB]

283. Shavit I, Keidan I, Hoffmann Y, et al. Enhancing patient safety during pediatric sedation: the impact of simulation-based training of nonanesthesiologists. *Arch Pediatr Adolesc Med.* 2007;161(8):740-743. [IIIB]

284. Jordan C, Thomas MB, Evans ML, Green A. Public policy on competency: how will nursing address this complex issue? *J Contin Educ Nurs.* 2008;39(2):86-91. [VA]

285. Brady M, Kinn S, Stuart P. Preoperative fasting for adults to prevent perioperative complications. *Cochrane Database Syst Rev.* 2003;(4):CD004423. [IA]

286. Bernard PA, Makin CE, Hongying D, Ballard HO. Variability of ASA physical status class assignment among pediatric sedation practitioners. Anesthesiologists Physical Status. *Int J Adolesc Med Health.* 2009;21(2):213-220. [IIIB]

287. *Patient Safety: Rights of Registered Nurses When Considering a Patient Assignment* [Position Statement]. 2009. American Nurses Association. http://www.nursingworld.org/MainMenuCategories/Policy-Advocacy/Positions-and-Resolutions/ANAPositionStatements/Position-Statements-Alphabetically/Patient-Safety-Rights-of-Registered-Nurses-When-Considering-a-Patient-Assignment.html. Accessed October 22, 2015. [IVB]

288. Wiebe ER, Byczko B, Kaczorowski J, McLane AL. Can we safely avoid fasting before abortions with low-dose procedural sedation? A retrospective cohort chart review of anesthesia-related complications in 47,748 abortions. *Contraception.* 2013;87(1):51-54. [IIIA]

289. Manchikanti L, Malla Y, Wargo BW, Fellows B. Preoperative fasting before interventional techniques: is it necessary or evidence-based? *Pain Physician.* 2011;14(5):459-467. [IIIB]

290. Wehrmann T, Riphaus A. Sedation with propofol for interventional endoscopic procedures: a risk factor analysis. *Scand J Gastroenterol.* 2008;43(3):368-374. [IIIB]

291. Mason KP, Green SM, Piacevoli Q. Adverse event reporting tool to standardize the reporting and tracking of adverse events during procedural sedation: a consensus document from the World SIVA International Sedation Task Force. *Br J Anaesth.* 2012;108(1):13-20. [IVB]

292. Lightdale JR, Mahoney LB, Fredette ME, Valim C, Wong S, DiNardo JA. Nurse reports of adverse events during sedation procedures at a pediatric hospital. *J Perianesth Nurs.* 2009;24(5):300-306. [IIIB]

293. Hoerl KH. Accuracy of nurse reported adverse sedation events. *J Radiol Nurs.* 2010;29(3):85-86. [VB]

294. Shin JG, Hwang JH, Lee BS, et al. A case of midazolam anaphylaxis. *Clin Endosc.* 2014;47(3):262-265. [VA]

295. Coruh B, Tonelli MR, Park DR. Fentanyl-induced chest wall rigidity. *Chest.* 2013;143(4):1145-1146. [VA]

296. Patel VJ, Ahmed SS, Nitu ME, Rigby MR. Vasovagal syncope and severe bradycardia following intranasal dexmedetomidine for pediatric procedural sedation. *Paediatr Anaesth.* 2014;24(4):446-448. [VB]

297. Cabrera LS, Santana AS, Robaina PE, Palacios MS. Paradoxical reaction to midazolam reversed with flumazenil. *J Emerg Trauma Shock.* 2010;3(3):307. [VB]

298. Holdcroft A. UK drug analysis prints and anaesthetic adverse drug reactions. *Pharmacoepidemiol Drug Saf.* 2007;16(3):316-328. [IIIB]

299. Rueb GR, Brady WJ, Gilliland CA, et al. Characterizing cardiopulmonary arrest during interventional radiology procedures. *J Vasc Interv Radiol.* 2013;24(12):1774-1778. [IIIB]

300. Sharma VK, Nguyen CC, Crowell MD, Lieberman DA, de Garmo P, Fleischer DE. A national study of cardiopulmonary unplanned events after GI endoscopy. *Gastrointest Endosc.* 2007;66(1):27-34. [IIIA]

301. Cravero JP, Blike GT, Beach M, et al. Incidence and nature of adverse events during pediatric sedation/anesthesia for procedures outside the operating room: report from the Pediatric Sedation Research Consortium. *Pediatrics.* 2006;118(3):1087-1096. [IIIA]

302. Khalid-de Bakker CA, Jonkers DM, Hameeteman W, de Ridder RJ, Masclee AA, Stockbrugger RW. Cardiopulmonary events during primary colonoscopy screening in an average risk population. *Neth J Med.* 2011;69(4):186-191. [IIIB]

303. Karamnov S, Sarkisian N, Grammer R, Gross WL, Urman RD. Analysis of adverse events associated with adult moderate procedural sedation outside the operating room. *J Patient Saf.* September 8, 2014. Epub ahead of print. [IIIA]

304. Jensen JT, Vilmann P, Horsted T, et al. Nurse-administered propofol sedation for endoscopy: a risk analysis during an implementation phase. *Endoscopy.* 2011;43(8):716-722. [IIIB]

305. Vargo JJ. Minimizing complications: sedation and monitoring. *Gastrointest Endosc Clin North Am.* 2007;17(1):11-28. [VA]

306. Becker DE, Haas DA. Recognition and management of complications during moderate and deep sedation. Part 2: cardiovascular considerations. *Anesth Prog.* 2011;58(3):126-138. [VA]

307. Ko CW, Dominitz JA. Complications of colonoscopy: magnitude and management. *Gastrointest Endosc Clin North Am.* 2010;20(4):659-671. [VA]

308. Ginzburg L, Greenwald D, Cohen J. Complications of endoscopy. *Gastrointest Endosc Clin North Am.* 2007;17(2):405-432. [VB]

309. Becker DE, Haas DA. Recognition and management of complications during moderate and deep sedation part 1: respiratory considerations. *Anesth Prog.* 2011;58(2):82-92. [VA]

310. Lourenco-Matharu L, Raval P. An unusual response to intravenous sedation: a case report. *SAAD Dig.* 2014;30:12-15. [VA]

311. Galway UA. An anesthesiologist's focus on sedation and complications of GI endoscopy cases—a case of bilateral pneumothoraces and pneumomediatinum after routine ERCP. *Internet J Anesthesiol.* 2010;23(2):14p-14p. [VB]

312. Malhotra N, Singhal S, Malhotra P. Conscious sedation: a safe approach for management of nonagenarian cataract surgery. *Internet J Anesthesiol.* 2007;13(1):4p-4p. [VB]

313. Garg R, Dehran M. Convulsions with propofol: a rare adverse event. *J Postgrad Med.* 2009;55(1):69-71. [VB]

Acknowledgements

Lead Author
Mary J. Ogg, MSN, RN, CNOR
Perioperative Nursing Specialist
AORN Nursing Department
Denver, Colorado

The author and AORN thank Lisa Spruce, DNP, RN, ACNS, ACNP, ANP, CNOR, Director of Evidence-based Perioperative Practice, AORN, Inc, Denver, Colorado; Elayne Kornblatt Phillips, PhD-BSN, MPH, RN, Clinical Associate Professor, University of Virginia, Charlottesville; Melanie F. Sandoval, PhD, RN, Research Nurse Scientist, Perioperative Services, University of Colorado, Aurora; Deborah S. Hickman, MS, RN, CNOR, CRNFA, Director, Renue Plastic Surgery, Brunswick, Georgia; Kerrie Chambers, MSN, RN, CNOR, CNS-CP, Perioperative Nursing Specialist, AORN Nursing Department, Denver, Colorado; Amy L. Halverson, MD, Associate Professor of Surgery, Northwestern University, Feinberg School of Medicine, Chicago, Illinois; Armin Schubert, MD, MBA, Vice President for Medical Affairs, Ochsner Health System, New Orleans, Louisiana; Brian Cammarata, Partner and Director of Risk Management, Old Pueblo Anesthesia, Tucson, Arizona; Leslie Jeter, MSNA, RN, CRNA, Ambulatory Anesthesia of Atlanta, Georgia; and Ramona L. Conner, MSN, RN, CNOR, Editor-in-Chief, Guidelines for Perioperative Practice, AORN Nursing Department, Denver, Colorado, for their assistance in developing this guideline.

Publication History

Originally published April 1993, *AORN Journal*, as "Recommended practices for monitoring the patient receiving intravenous conscious sedation."

Revised; published in January 1997, *AORN Journal*, as "Recommended practices for managing the patient receiving conscious sedation/analgesia." Reformatted July 2000.

Revised November 2001; published March 2002, *AORN Journal*, as "Recommended practices for managing the patient receiving moderate sedation/analgesia."

Revised 2007; published in *Perioperative Standards and Recommended Practices*, 2008 edition.

Minor editing revisions made to omit PNDS codes; reformatted September 2012 for publication in *Perioperative Standards and Recommended Practices*, 2013 edition.

Minor editing revisions made in November 2014 for publication as "Guideline for managing the patient receiving moderate sedation/analgesia" in *Guidelines for Perioperative Practice*, 2015 edition.

Revised December 2015 for publication in *Guidelines for Perioperative Practice* online.

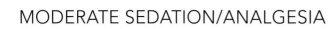

GUIDELINE FOR POSITIONING THE PATIENT

The Guideline for Positioning the Patient has been approved by the AORN Guidelines Advisory Board. It was presented as a proposed guideline for comments by members and others. The guideline is effective May 1, 2017. The recommendations in the guideline are intended to be achievable and represent what is believed to be an optimal level of practice. Policies and procedures will reflect variations in practice settings and/or clinical situations that determine the degree to which the guideline can be implemented. AORN recognizes the many diverse settings in which perioperative nurses practice; therefore, this guideline is adaptable to all areas where operative or other invasive procedures may be performed.

Purpose

This document provides guidance to perioperative team members for positioning patients undergoing operative and other invasive procedures in the perioperative practice setting. Guidance is provided for

- demonstrating respect and privacy during patient positioning;
- conducting preoperative and postoperative nursing assessments specific to patient positioning;
- identifying, selecting, maintaining, and using positioning equipment and devices;
- selecting and using pressure-redistributing support surfaces and prophylactic dressings to prevent pressure injury;
- using neurophysiological monitoring to identify and prevent potential positioning injuries;
- implementing safe practices for positioning patients in the supine, Trendelenburg, reverse Trendelenburg, lithotomy, sitting and semi-sitting, lateral, and prone positions and modifications of these positions;
- implementing safe practices for positioning patients who are pregnant or obese;
- documenting patient positioning and positioning-related activities;
- planning education and verifying competency of personnel responsible for patient positioning;
- developing policies and procedures related to patient positioning; and
- implementing quality improvement programs related to patient positioning.

A discussion of positions or devices used for anesthesia administration, positions for cardiopulmonary resuscitation (CPR), and positions that are preferred or modified for specific procedures are outside the scope of this document. Recommendations for patient moving and handling, transport, transfer, and fall prevention are also outside of the scope of this document. Guidance for preventing deep vein thrombosis (DVT) is outside the scope of this document;

however, because some mechanical methods of DVT prophylaxis are inherently associated with patient positioning, guidance is provided relative to the use of mechanical DVT prophylaxis in combination with specific positions. Guidance related to positioning for robotic procedures is included with the relevant recommendation. There are a vast variety of surgical positions and of positioning equipment and devices, and it would not be possible to address them all in this document; therefore, the information in this guideline is limited to the most commonly used positions and positioning equipment and devices.

Positioning patients is one of the most important tasks performed by perioperative personnel[1,2] and is the responsibility of all members of the surgical team.[2-5] The goals of patient positioning include

- providing exposure of the surgical site[6];
- maintaining the patient's comfort and privacy;
- providing access to intravenous (IV) lines and monitoring equipment;
- allowing for optimal ventilation by maintaining a patent airway and avoiding constriction or pressure on the chest or abdomen;
- maintaining circulation and protecting muscles, nerves, bony prominences, joints, skin, and vital organs from injury;
- observing and protecting fingers, toes, and genitals; and
- stabilizing the patient to prevent unintended shifting or movement.

Positioning the patient is a team effort that includes the perioperative registered nurse (RN), the anesthesia professional, the surgeon, and other perioperative personnel (eg, first assistants, assistive personnel).[1,5,7-9] As patient advocates, perioperative team members are responsible for maintaining the patient's autonomy, dignity, and privacy and for representing the patient's interests throughout the procedure.[10] Some elements of patient positioning are core to anesthesia practice; therefore, the ability of the perioperative team to support the activities of the anesthesia professional is essential. All perioperative team members involved in positioning activities are responsible for

- understanding the physiologic changes that occur during operative and other invasive procedures[9,11-14];
- evaluating the patient's risk for injury based on an assessment of identified needs and the planned operative or invasive procedure[9,13];
- anticipating the surgeon's requirements for surgical access;
- gathering positioning equipment and devices;
- using positioning equipment and devices correctly;
- monitoring the patient during the procedure[1];

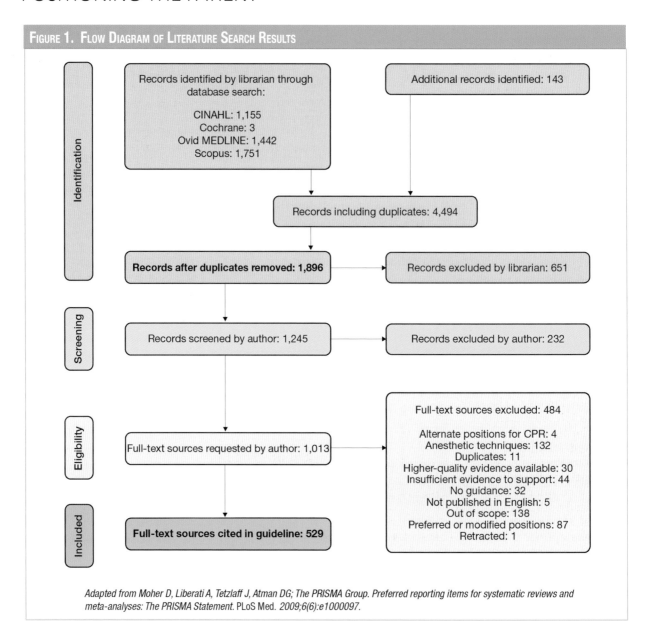

FIGURE 1. FLOW DIAGRAM OF LITERATURE SEARCH RESULTS

Records identified by librarian through database search:

CINAHL: 1,155
Cochrane: 3
Ovid MEDLINE: 1,442
Scopus: 1,751

Additional records identified: 143

Records including duplicates: 4,494

Records after duplicates removed: 1,896

Records excluded by librarian: 651

Records screened by author: 1,245

Records excluded by author: 232

Full-text sources requested by author: 1,013

Full-text sources excluded: 484

Alternate positions for CPR: 4
Anesthetic techniques: 132
Duplicates: 11
Higher-quality evidence available: 30
Insufficient evidence to support: 44
No guidance: 32
Not published in English: 5
Out of scope: 138
Preferred or modified positions: 87
Retracted: 1

Full-text sources cited in guideline: 529

Identification · Screening · Eligibility · Included

Adapted from Moher D, Liberati A, Tetzlaff J, Atman DG; The PRISMA Group. Preferred reporting items for systematic reviews and meta-analyses: The PRISMA Statement. PLoS Med. 2009;6(6):e1000097.

- applying principles of body mechanics and ergonomics during patient positioning;
- respecting the patient's individual positioning limitations; and
- implementing interventions to provide for the patient's comfort and safety and to protect the patient's circulatory, respiratory, musculoskeletal, neurological, and integumentary structures.[2,3,5,13,15]

Incorrectly positioning a surgical patient can result in serious injury to both personnel and the patient.[1,4] Performing patient positioning requires the application of lifting, pushing, or pulling forces and therefore presents a high risk for musculoskeletal injury to the lower back and shoulders of the team members performing these tasks.[16] Because of the effects of sedation, regional anesthesia, or general anesthesia, patients lack normal perception and protective reflexes and are thus at increased risk for positioning injury.[4,17]

Most positioning injuries are caused by mechanisms involving compression or stretching.[13] Stretching leads to nerve compression and ischemic changes from reduced blood flow.[13] Some surgical positions increase the risk for a stretching injury (eg, lateral neck rotation).[13] Compression reduces blood flow and disrupts cellular integrity, resulting in tissue edema, ischemia, and necrosis.[13] Positioning injuries can affect the skin and soft tissues, joints, ligaments and bones, eyes, nerves, and blood and lymph vessels.[4] A positioning injury can be temporary or permanent, and the effects of the injury can range from minor inconvenience to long-term functional restriction, secondary morbidity, or even death.[4,14]

Many positioning injuries are associated with prolonged procedures. The definition of a prolonged procedure is subjective, and the literature does not conclusively define a time parameter for prolonged surgery. The American Society of Anesthesiologists

(ASA) Task Force on Perioperative Visual Loss[18] considers procedures to be prolonged when they exceed an average of 6.5 hours duration (range 2 hours to 12 hours).

Failing to provide appropriate positioning interventions for individuals undergoing operative or other invasive procedures may be deemed negligence or a failure to meet the duty of care owed to the patient.[19] When there is a positioning injury, the doctrine of *res ipsa loquitur* (ie, the thing speaks for itself) may be applicable.[11] Under this doctrine, there is an assumption that the event that caused the injury was under the control of the defendant (eg, surgeon, anesthesia professional, perioperative RN) and would not have occurred if proper care had been provided to the plaintiff (ie, patient).[11] The potential for a patient injury and for litigation underscores the importance of implementing positioning interventions to prevent nerve and tissue damage and thoroughly and accurately documenting the care provided.[11,12]

Evidence Review

A medical librarian conducted a systematic literature search of the databases Ovid MEDLINE®, EBSCO CINAHL®, Scopus®, and the Ovid Cochrane Database of Systematic Reviews. The search was limited to literature published in English from 2008 through February 2016. At the time of the initial search, weekly alerts were created for the topics included in that search. Results from these alerts were provided to the lead author until September 2016. The lead author requested a supplementary search on eye protection and requested additional articles that either did not fit the original search criteria or were discovered during the evidence appraisal process. The lead author and the medical librarian also identified relevant guidelines from government agencies, professional organizations, and standards-setting bodies.

Search terms included *positioning, positioning injury, compression injury, shear, friction, pressure, interface pressure, pressure ulcers, pressure reducing, pressure relieving, positioning surfaces, support surfaces, positioning equipment, positioning devices, safety straps, OR table, OR bed, OR mattress, alternating pressure mattresses, procedure table, padding, foam, gel, viscoelastic, supine, Fowler/Semi-Fowler/ beach chair, lithotomy, lateral, prone, Trendelenburg/ reverse Trendelenburg, jack-knife/Kraske,* and *robotic.* Other subject headings and keywords were included to address specific positioning devices, alternative terms for positions, patient-monitoring indicators, and risk assessment.

Excluded were non-peer-reviewed publications and low-quality evidence when higher-quality evidence was available. In total, 1,013 research and non-research sources of evidence were identified for possible inclusion, and of these, 529 are cited in the guideline (Figure 1).

Included articles were independently evaluated and critically appraised according to the strength and quality of the evidence. Articles identified in the search were provided to the project team for evaluation. The team consisted of the lead author and one evidence appraiser. The articles were reviewed and critically appraised using the AORN Research or Non-Research Evidence Appraisal Tools as appropriate. Each article was then assigned an appraisal score. The appraisal score is noted in brackets after each reference as applicable.

The collective evidence supporting each intervention within a specific recommendation was summarized, and the AORN Evidence Rating Model was used to rate the strength of the evidence. Factors considered in review of the collective evidence were the quality of the evidence, the quantity of similar evidence on a given topic, and the consistency of the evidence supporting a recommendation. The evidence rating is noted in brackets after each intervention.

Note: *The evidence summary table is available at http://www.aorn.org/evidencetables/.*

Editor's note: *Ovid MEDLINE is a registered trademark of the US National Library of Medicine's Medical Literature Analysis and Retrieval System, Bethesda, MD. CINAHL, Cumulative Index to Nursing and Allied Health Literature, is a registered trademark of EBSCO Industries, Birmingham, AL. Scopus is a registered trademark of Elsevier B.V., Amsterdam, The Netherlands.*

Recommendation I

Perioperative team members should provide care that respects the dignity and privacy of each patient[10] during patient positioning.

Perioperative team members are responsible for ensuring equitable, compassionate, and optimal care for all perioperative patients without bias or intolerance.[6,10] Some patients (eg, patients who are obese, patients with disabilities) present additional challenges during patient positioning, and a greater level of advocacy may be required to create an environment of respect and sensitivity.[6]

I.a.   Perioperative team members should implement measures to provide privacy during patient positioning. *[3: Moderate Evidence]*

Maintaining the patient's privacy is essential to preserving the trust developed in the caregiver-patient relationship.[10] Perioperative team members have an obligation to protect patients from undue exposure or unwarranted invasions of privacy.[6,10]

I.a.1.   Perioperative team members should provide privacy during patient positioning by
- keeping windows covered and doors closed in patient care areas,
- restricting access to perioperative patient care areas to authorized personnel only,
- limiting traffic in procedure rooms, and
- exposing only the areas of the patient's body necessary to provide care or access. *[4: Limited Evidence]*

Maintaining the patient's privacy is reflected by implementing processes to protect the patient's auditory and physical privacy.[10] Keeping the patient covered, unless specific exposure of an area of the body is required, will help to keep the patient warm as well as to maintain the patient's dignity during a vulnerable time.[20]

Recommendation II

The perioperative RN should conduct a preoperative patient assessment to identify patients at risk for positioning injury, develop a plan of care, and implement interventions to prevent injury.

Patient assessment is a critical responsibility performed by the perioperative RN to help prevent injury related to patient positioning.[9,21-24] Identifying patients at risk for positioning injury and developing a plan of care is necessary for implementing preventive interventions.[19,23,25-27]

II.a. The perioperative RN should perform a preoperative assessment of factors related to the procedure. Procedural factors should include the

  ○ type of procedure[21,28-30]; *[1: Strong Evidence]*
  ○ estimated length of the procedure[21,25,28-34]; *[1: Strong Evidence]*
  ○ ability of the patient to tolerate the anticipated position[35]; *[1: Strong Evidence]*
  ○ amount of surgical exposure required[5]; *[2: High Evidence]*
  ○ ability of the anesthesia professional to access the patient[21,28]; *[2: High Evidence]* and
  ○ desired procedural position, potential change of position, and positioning devices required.[5,26,29,30,32,34] *[3: Moderate Evidence]*

The type and estimated duration of the surgical procedure are significant factors in estimating the patient's risk for tissue damage.[12,15,30,32,36,37] Lumbley[29] et al found that the types of procedures with the most pressure injuries were abdominal, noncardiac thoracic, and orthopedic. Shaw et al[26] found that orthopedic procedures were a significant predictor of pressure injury. In a systematic review of 23 studies that examined sensory changes or nerve injury after abdominoplasty procedures, Ducic et al[14] found that most patient injuries occurred during surgeries that included more than one procedure type. The researchers noted that combining procedures increased operative time and the risk for positioning injury.[14]

There are variances in the literature as to the specific length of time after which a positioning injury would be expected to occur.[29,33,34,36,38,39] The risk for pressure injury is multifactorial and increases with the length of surgery.[32] In an analysis of 44 claims from the American Association of Nurse Anesthetists (AANA) Foundation Closed Malpractice Claims Database, Fritzlen et al[38] found that 57% (n = 25) of the injuries reported occurred during procedures that lasted longer than 2 hours. O'Connell[36] proposed that procedures lasting longer than 4 hours presented an increased risk for tissue damage in even the healthiest patients. Mills et al[39] conducted a review of records of adult urological robotic procedures and found the median time for procedures during which positioning injuries occurred was 5.5 hours.

The ASA Task Force on Prevention of Perioperative Peripheral Neuropathies[35] suggested that ascertaining whether the patient can tolerate the anticipated surgical position may be helpful to reduce the risk for nerve injury.

Providing sufficient surgical exposure may reduce surgical complications by improving visibility of the surgical site, easing access to the operative area and anatomic structures, and reducing operative time.[2,4,5]

Safe surgical positioning requires that the anesthesia professional assess the patient's range of motion, assess nerve and vascular impairment, participate in the positioning of the patient, have sufficient access to the patient to provide adequate depth of anesthesia, assess the position of the patient intraoperatively, maintain hemodynamic stability and oxygenation, and protect the patient through the use of noninvasive and invasive monitors.[4,5,15,40,41]

Some surgical positions and positioning devices increase the patient's risk for injury.[34] A key causative factor for pressure injury is external pressure on bony prominences for prolonged periods.[42] Pressure points vary based on the surgical position and placement of positioning devices. Straps or adhesive tape used to secure a patient in the desired position during a surgical procedure can be a source of pressure that results in injury.[43]

II.b. Perioperative RNs should participate in the health care organization's pressure injury prevention program by conducting a preoperative assessment of the patient's risk for pressure injury.[44] *[1: Strong Evidence]*

Prevention of pressure injury is an important aspect of perioperative patient care.[45] Surgical positioning presents a risk for skin breakdown and pressure injury.[22,34,46] Risk assessment provides a method for identifying individuals who are susceptible to pressure injuries and for implementing interventions to prevent pressure injury.[19,25,47,48] Use of the same processes and tools for pressure injury risk assessment throughout the health care organization promotes consistency in reporting and enhances communication among caregivers working in different areas or on different shifts.[49] The Centers for Medicare & Medicaid Services no longer pays for health services provided for care related to Stage 3 and Stage 4 pressure injuries that develop during a hospital admission.[50] This regulation provides strong impetus for perioperative RNs to be cognizant of risk factors that can contribute to pressure injury.[27]

II.b.1. Perioperative RNs should use a structured risk assessment tool for preoperative assessment of the patient's risk for pressure injury. [1: Strong Evidence]

Evidence supports the use of a risk assessment tool.[3,19,51] Risk assessment tools provide

- practical frameworks for assessment,
- operational definitions of risk factors that have clinical relevance and can be reliably measured,
- clinical reminders of risks, and
- an auditable standard.[3,19,51]

Risk assessment tools do not necessarily include assessment of all key factors that may increase the patient's risk for pressure injury, and they are limited in their ability to determine the importance of one risk factor compared with another or to determine the cumulative effects of multiple risk factors.[19] The use of a risk assessment tool does not replace the need for a comprehensive patient assessment conducted by a qualified perioperative RN using sound clinical judgment.[19]

There is a lack of agreement as to which risk assessment tool is most effective for predicting the risk for pressure injury in perioperative patients.[19] Pressure injury risk assessment tools identified in the literature include the Braden Scale,[52] Munro Scale,[53,54] and Scott Triggers tool[55] (Table 1).

The Braden Scale is widely used for pressure injury risk assessment, but it does not address risk factors specific to surgical patients.[56,57] In a meta-analysis of three pooled studies, He et al[57] found that the Braden Scale had a low predictive validity for assessing pressure injury risk in surgical patients. The Braden Scale has been used as a preoperative tool to assess older adult frailty,[23] which may be a predictor of postoperative complications because the older adult's frailty level is an indicator of vulnerability to stressors resulting from diminished physiologic reserves associated with the aging process.[23] The Munro Scale and the Scott Triggers tool were developed to help perioperative RNs identify surgical patients at risk for pressure injury.[53-55]

II.b.2. The pressure injury risk assessment should include evaluation and documentation of the patient's

- age,[17,21,25,27,30,31,51,56] [1: Strong Evidence]
- nutritional status,[19,21,23,25,30,37,44,51,58] [1: Strong Evidence]
- laboratory test values,[17,19,21,25,37,59] [1: Strong Evidence]

POSITIONING THE PATIENT

- comorbidities affecting tissue perfusion (eg, diabetes, peripheral vascular disease),[4,19,21,23,25,27,30,31,37,51,56,60,61] [1: Strong Evidence]
- skin condition (eg, color, turgor, integrity, temperature, moisture, pre-existing pressure injury),[6,19,21,27,30,31,37,43,44,51,56,61-64] [1: Strong Evidence]
- ASA physical status classification,[64,65] [2: High Evidence]
- body mass index (BMI),[12,17,21,25,27,30-32,64] [2: High Evidence] and
- peripheral pulses (ie, rate, rhythm, symmetry, amplitude).[37] [3: Moderate Evidence]

The risk for skin and pressure injury is high in both older and very young patients.[2] Patients 65 years and older are particularly vulnerable to positioning injury.[1,31,37,43] Older adults may also have conditions such as osteoporosis, osteoarthritis, or coronary artery disease that can increase their risk for positioning injury.[1,22,31]

Both inadequate nutritional intake and poor nutritional status can increase the risk for pressure injury.[19,38] Patients who are malnourished are at increased risk for pressure injury because they do not have the stored reserves that help the body promote effective healing and protect itself from injury.[19,43,49,66-68] Inadequate nutrition increases the risk for tissue damage, delayed wound healing, sepsis, and wound infection.[23] Undernourished and malnourished states may be more prevalent in the older adult population.[23] Despite the appearance of having a nutritional reserve, patients who are obese may be at risk for nutritional deficits.[58,69] Patients who have undergone previous weight loss surgery are also vulnerable to nutritional deficits that may increase their risk for pressure injury.[69]

Evidence related to the relevance of laboratory test values as indicators of malnutrition and pressure injury is limited.[19] Data have not clearly demonstrated specific laboratory markers of nutritional status that best predict pressure injury in perioperative patients.[42] Patients with low hematocrit (ie, < 38%) and hemoglobin levels (ie, < 14.1 g/dL) are at greater risk for positioning injury than patients with normal hematocrit (ie, men 40% to 54%; women 36% to 48%) and hemoglobin levels (ie, men 13.5 g/dL to 17.5 g/dL; women 12.0 g/dL to 15.5 g/dL).[2,15,19,42,49] Serum albumin and prealbumin levels are not considered reliable indicators of nutritional status[19]; however, low albumin levels (ie, 40 g/L ± 7.1 g/L) may interfere with healing, placing the patient at increased risk for pressure injury.[42] Reduced albumin levels may also be indicators of an

TABLE 1. PRESSURE INJURY RISK ASSESSMENT TOOLS: ADULT

Tool	Braden Scale	Munro Scale	Scott Triggers Tool
Indicators	• Sensory perception • Moisture • Activity • Mobility • Nutrition • Friction and shear[1]	Preoperative • Mobility • Nutritional status • Body mass index • Weight loss within the past 30 to 180 days • Age • Comorbidities[3] Intraoperative • American Society of Anesthesiologists physical status classification • Type of anesthesia • Temperature • Hypotension • Moisture • Surface/motion • Position[3] Postoperative • Length of perioperative duration • Blood loss[3]	• Age older than 62 years • Serum albumin level < 3.5 g/L or body mass index < 19 kg/m^2 or > 40 kg/m^2 • American Society of Anesthesiologists physical status classification of III or higher • Estimated surgery time longer than 180 minutes[5]
Scoring	Each indicator is assessed and scored from 1 to 4 for a total score of 6 to 23.[1] Lower scores are indicative of a greater risk for pressure injury.[1]	Preoperative, intraoperative, and postoperative indicators are scored as low, medium, and high risk for each phase of care.[4] The level of risk may change throughout the perioperative period.[4] The cumulative score reflects the patient's risk for pressure injury.[4]	Each indicator is considered a trigger. Patients with 2 or more triggers are considered to be at high risk for pressure injury.[5]
Patient Population	Validated tool for assessing the patient's risk for pressure injury.[1] Does not assess risk factors specific to surgical patients.[2]	Developed specifically for the perioperative patient.[3,4]	Developed specifically for the perioperative patient.[5]

REFERENCES

1. Bergstrom N, Braden BJ, Laguzza A, Holman V. The Braden Scale for Predicting Pressure Sore Risk. Nurs Res. 1987;36(4):205-210.

2. He W, Liu P, Chen HL. The Braden Scale cannot be used alone for assessing pressure ulcer risk in surgical patients: a meta-analysis. Ostomy Wound Manage. 2012;58(2):34-40.

3. Munro Pressure Ulcer Risk Assessment Scale for Perioperative Patients—Adults. AORN, Inc. https://www.aorn.org/-/media/aorn/guidelines/tool-kits/pressure-ulcer/munro-pressure-ulcer-risk-assessment-scale.xlsx?la=en. Accessed March 10, 2017.

4. Cardinal Health/AORN Pressure Ulcer Prevention Project. Instructions for the Munro Pressure Ulcer Risk Assessment Scale for Perioperative Patients for Adults. AORN, Inc. https://www.aorn.org/-/media/aorn/guidelines/tool-kits/pressure-ulcer/instructions-for-munro-risk-assessment-scale.pdf?la=en. Accessed March 10, 2017.

5. Scott SM. Progress and challenges in perioperative pressure ulcer prevention. J Wound Ostomy Continence Nurs. 2015;42(5):480-485.

inflammatory response that increases metabolism and secondarily increases the risk for malnutrition.[19]

Comorbidities that affect tissue perfusion and oxygenation may increase the potential for pressure injury.[15,19,35,38,42,49,67,70] General anesthetics administered to surgical patients result in some degree of vasodilation that subsequently leads to hypotension and reduced tissue perfusion.[15,27,33,34,36,49,64,71,72] Hypoperfusion of tissue under pressure in an immobile patient can be a significant fac-

tor related to the development of pressure injury in a perioperative patient.[29] Patients with diabetes, respiratory disease, and vascular disease are at increased risk for injury as a result of reduced tissue perfusion and oxygenation.[42]

Patients with preexisting peripheral vascular disease have baseline limb ischemia and may not tolerate positions (eg, lithotomy position) that lead to additional reductions in perfusion.[73] In a retrospective review of 222 patients who developed pressure injuries after undergoing surgery lasting at least 2 hours, Lumbley et al[29] found that patient comorbidities affecting tissue perfusion in combination with malnutrition and cachexia resulted in a predisposition toward intraoperative pressure injuries. In an analysis of 44 cases from the AANA Foundation Closed Malpractice Claims Database, Fritzlen et al[38] found that 55% (n = 24) of the patients who were injured had preexisting pathological conditions that placed them at increased risk for injury. When abnormal body habitus (ie, BMI ≤ 21kg/m² or BMI > 28 kg/m²) was included as a preexisting condition, the percentage of patients who were injured increased to 70% (n = 31).

A skin risk assessment evaluates the condition of the patient's skin and factors that may put the patient at risk for pressure injury (eg, decreased turgor, cool temperature).[43] Preoperative visual assessment of the patient's skin, bony prominences, and body surfaces that will be subjected to pressure, friction, or shear force during the procedure may help direct interventions to prevent pressure injuries. A preoperative skin assessment establishes a baseline for comparison with a postoperative skin assessment.[31] Alterations in skin color, moisture, temperature, texture, mobility, and turgor may lead to the development of a pressure injury or the progression of an existing pressure injury.[19,22] Breaks in skin integrity increase a patient's risk for infection or pressure injury and can lead to psychological distress and challenges in pain management.[47]

The skin of older adults (ie, ≥ 65 years) is fragile and prone to shear injuries.[37] The skin of older adults is less elastic; the dermis is thin and has less collagen, muscle, and adipose tissue than the skin of younger adults.[22,31,36,41-43,56] These changes leave the older adult's skin more susceptible to pressure, bruising, skin tears, infection, impaired thermoregulation, and slow healing.[23,36,41,42,56,66] Skin assessments may be more difficult in patients who are obese because of the patient's size, lack of landmarks, and chronic conditions.[6,74]

The presence of excess moisture on the skin disrupts the skin's natural protective barrier and weakens the elasticity of the skin.[61] Moisture increases the potential for skin damage caused by skin maceration that intensifies the negative effects of pressure, shear, and friction.[19,31,56,61,75]

All surgical patients are at risk for pressure injury, but the presence of certain factors puts some patients at higher risk.[8,22,25,30,31,49,51,56,76] Mills et al[39] conducted a review of records of 334 adult urological robotic surgeries to identify risk factors associated with positioning injuries. The researchers found that ASA physical status classification was significantly associated with pressure injury. In a nonexperimental study to evaluate the number of injuries caused by surgical positioning and to identify risk factors predictive of pressure injury, Menezes et al[65] prospectively evaluated 172 patients undergoing elective surgery in the supine, lateral, and lithotomy positions for development of a pressure injury. The results of the study showed a significant association between pressure injury and patients with an ASA classification of II or III (n = 19; 90.5%) compared to patients with an ASA classification of I (n = 2; 9.5%).

In a case series with retrospective chart analysis and review of intraoperative neurophysiological monitoring data from 398 patients, Silverstein et al[77] found that BMI was a significant predictor of generalized upper extremity neural compromise. Patients who are obese may be at increased risk for positioning injury because they may not tolerate traditional surgical positions as well as patients of normal weight.[1,24,32,49] In the prospective study conducted by Menezes et al,[65] the results also showed a significant association between pressure injury and patients with a BMI ≥ 30 kg/m² (n = 15; 71.4%) compared to patients with a BMI < 30 kg/m² (n = 6; 28.6%). Patients who are thin or underweight and have decreased body mass are more susceptible to skin and pressure injury than patients of normal weight because they have less adipose tissue to protect nerves and bony prominences.[2,12,32,42,68]

Preoperative assessment of the rate, rhythm, symmetry, and amplitude of peripheral pulses provides a baseline for comparison after patient positioning and placement of positioning devices.

II.b.3. A structured pediatric risk assessment tool may be used for preoperative assessment of the risk for pressure injury in pediatric patients.[44] *[1: Strong Evidence]*

Using a risk assessment tool that is appropriate to the population may increase the accuracy of risk prediction.[19,44,47,78] Because of differences in anatomic structure, the sites most susceptible to pressure injury in the pediatric population differ from those in the adult population.[19,43,78] For example, the occipital region is at increased risk for skin breakdown in infants and toddlers in the supine position because they have a disproportionately large head size.[19,48]

Neonates are vulnerable to skin and pressure injuries because of an immature and underdeveloped epidermis and dermis.[15,19,78] The skin of children may be more resilient to normal and shear pressures than the skin of older adults because it is supported with sufficient collagen and elastin.[45] Neonates and children are at higher risk for nutritional deficiencies because of smaller appetites and dietary intake in combination with an increased nutritional requirement necessary to meet normal growth needs.[19]

Pediatric and neonatal pressure injury risk assessment tools identified in the literature include the Braden Q Scale,[45,47,48,79] the Braden Q + P Scale,[47] the Glamorgan Scale,[47,79,80] and the Neonatal Skin Risk Assessment Scale[81] (Table 2).

II.c.   The perioperative RN should perform a preoperative assessment of patient-specific factors that may increase the patient's risk for positioning injury. Patients should be assessed for the presence of

- critical devices (eg, catheters, drains)[21,28]; [1: Strong Evidence]
- jewelry or body piercings[28]; [3: Moderate Evidence]
- braided hair, hair accessories, or hair extensions; [3: Moderate Evidence]
- superficial implants (eg, dermal, iris) or implanted critical devices (eg, pacemaker, implantable chemotherapy port)[4,21,31]; [3: Moderate Evidence] and
- prosthetics (eg, prosthetic limb) or corrective devices (eg, orthopedic immobilizer).[28] [4: Limited Evidence]

Critical devices are those for which there is a risk of significant clinical impact to the patient if the device is dislodged or does not perform as expected.[82] Examples of critical devices include vascular access devices, endotracheal tubes, nasogastric feeding tubes, and indwelling urinary catheters.[82] Pressure injuries can occur as a result of pressure on the skin from critical devices.[19] Critical devices may have tubes or other attachments that can become entrapped in skin folds, resulting in skin damage, especially in patients who are obese.[19] Critical devices may have been placed in locations that limit the ability for pressure to be redistributed.[83] Notably, children are particularly vulnerable to pressure injury from iatrogenic sources such as tubing, cardiac leads, probes, identification bands, and security tags.[15,43]

The presence of jewelry or body piercings may lead to surgical site infection, electrical burns, airway obstruction, or pressure injury.[63,84,85]

Braided hair or hair that has been secured in an accessory (eg, barrette, bobby pin, ponytail holder) create an area of sufficient pressure to compress and injure the skin and soft tissue

between the skull and the surface on which the patient's head is resting.[63,86] Hair accessories may have plastic or metal components, and hair extensions may be attached to the scalp with metal clips, tapes, or adhesives that could lead to pressure injuries.[86]

The presence of a superficial implant or implanted critical device can increase the patient's risk for injury from pressure on the implant or device.[87] Dermal implants are decorative shapes implanted under the skin to create a silhouette of the molded shape on the surface of the skin.[85,88,89] The implant can be made of silicone, Teflon®, or metal.[85,88,89] Subdermal implants have components that are completely embedded under intact skin and cannot be removed.[85,88,89] Transdermal and microdermal implants have anchors that lie under the skin with metal pieces that penetrate through the skin[85] to which jewelry can be attached.[88,89] In some cases, the attached jewelry can be removed.[88,89] Patients with dermal implants may be at increased risk for skin breakdown or pressure injury resulting from pressure at the implant site.[88,89] The damage from pressure at the implant site may not be immediately visible because the pressure injury may initially manifest in the deeper tissue.[89]

Patients with iris implants or eye jewelry who are positioned in the prone position may be at increased risk for ocular injury. Consultation with an ophthalmologist regarding methods for reducing direct pressure on the eye or preventing corneal abrasion may be necessary to prevent a position-related injury.[88]

Prosthetics or corrective devices may create pressure on the skin and soft tissue if left in place during the procedure.

II.c.1.   A patient's jewelry, body piercings, hair accessories, or other items that may pose a risk for positioning injury should be removed before the patient is transferred to or positioned on the operating room (OR) bed.[21,28] [3: Moderate Evidence]

Some jewelry or piercings may interfere with the surgical site or become entangled in bedding or caught on equipment while the patient is being moved and can cause injuries as a result of accidental removal. Patients positioned on jewelry, body piercings, hair accessories, hair extensions, or braids may be subject to pressure injuries.[84-86,90]

II.c.2.   Patients should not be positioned directly on critical or superficial implanted devices.[19] When positioning the patient on a critical or implanted device cannot be prevented,

- the patient and critical devices that are able to be repositioned should be repositioned during the procedure[15,19,63] and

TABLE 2. PRESSURE INJURY RISK ASSESSMENT TOOLS: PEDIATRIC AND NEONATAL

Tool	Braden Q Scale	Braden Q + P Scale	Glamorgan Scale	Neonatal Skin Risk Assessment Scale
Indicators	• Mobility • Activity • Sensory perception • Moisture • Friction and shear • Nutritional status • Tissue perfusion[1]	• Height and weight • American Society of Anesthesiologists physical status classification • Surgical position • Length of procedure • Devices • Underlying condition • Sensory perception • Moisture • Mobility • Nutrition • Friction and shear • Tissue perfusion (ie, capillary refill > 2 seconds or oxygen saturation < 95%)[2]	• Mobility • Hard surfaces • Peripheral perfusion • Nutritional status • Anemia (ie, hemoglobin levels < 9.0 g/dL) • Pyrexia (ie, temperature > 100.4° F [38° C] more than 4 hours) • Low serum albumin levels (ie, < 3.5 g/L) • Weight (< 10th percentile) • Incontinence (inappropriate for age)[3]	• General skin condition • Mental state • Mobility • Activity • Nutritional status • Moisture[4]
Scoring	Each indicator is assessed and scored from 1 to 4 for a total score of 7 to 28.[1] Lower scores are indicative of a greater risk for pressure injury.[1]	Each indicator is assessed using a weighted yes/no scoring system.[2] Higher scores are indicative of a greater risk for pressure injury.[2]	Each indicator is assigned a weighted score.[3] Higher scores are indicative of a greater risk for pressure injury.[3]	Each indicator is assessed and scored from 1 to 4 for a total score of 6 to 24.[4] Lower scores are indicative of a greater risk for pressure injury.[4]
Patient Population	Validated tool for assessing the pediatric patient's risk for pressure injury.[1]	Developed specifically for the perioperative pediatric patient.[2]	Validated tool for assessing the pediatric patient's risk for pressure injury.[3]	Validated tool for assessing the neonatal patient's risk for pressure injury.[4]

REFERENCES

1. Quigley SM, Curley MA. Skin integrity in the pediatric population: preventing and managing pressure ulcers. J Soc Pediatr Nurs. 1996;1(1):7-18.

2. Galvin PA, Curley MA. The Braden Q+P: a pediatric perioperative pressure ulcer risk assessment and intervention tool. AORN J. 2012;96(3):261-270.

3. Willock J, Anthony D, Richardson J. Inter-rater reliability of the Glamorgan Paediatric Pressure Ulcer Risk Assessment Scale. Paediatr Nurs. 2008;20(7):4-19.

4. Huffines B, Logsdon MC. The Neonatal Skin Risk Assessment Scale for predicting skin breakdown in neonates. Issues Compr Pediatr Nurs. 1997;20(2):103-114.

• repositioning interventions and repositioning intervals should be based on the individual patient and the device(s).[19]
[1: Strong Evidence]

Pressure injuries can occur as a result of prolonged pressure on the skin from critical or implanted devices.[19,91] Repositioning the patient and critical device redistributes pressure from pressure points and from the device.[15,19,42,91] Simple position changes (eg, changing degree of lateral rotation, elevating the head of the bed) may be sufficient to redistribute pressure and prevent injury.[19]

II.c.3. Critical devices should be supported and secured in a manner that decreases pressure and tension and does not damage skin.[19,83]
[1: Strong Evidence]

Securing critical devices is paramount to patient safety.[82] Supporting critical devices may help to decrease pressure and prevent

pressure injury.[19] Effectively supporting critical devices may require the use of adhesive tape or medical adhesives. Although the tape or adhesive may successfully secure the device, the application process can cause tension to the surrounding tissue, increasing shear and causing pressure from the device onto the adjacent skin.[83] The use of adhesive tape or medical adhesives for securing and supporting critical devices can be especially damaging in very young and older patients who have fragile skin.[15]

II.c.4. Prophylactic dressings may be used to prevent pressure injury from critical devices.[19]
[1: Strong Evidence]

The evidence review did not reveal any studies specific to the use of prophylactic dressings for prevention of pressure injury from critical devices in perioperative patients; however, there is evidence to support the use of dressings as a prophylactic intervention to prevent pressure injury related to compression from critical devices (ie, tracheostomy tubes and ties, ventilation and nasal continuous positive airway pressure [CPAP] masks, nasotracheal tubes).[92-95] In a study to determine the efficacy of prophylactic dressings for preventing pressure injury in patients undergoing noninvasive ventilation applied through a face mask, Weng[92] concluded that the use of prophylactic dressings increased patient comfort and reduced the incidence of pressure injury.

Kuo et al[93] conducted a retrospective review of the records of 134 pediatric tracheostomy patients and concluded that the use of a silver-impregnated polyurethane foam dressing placed under the tracheostomy tube and ties reduced the occurrence of postoperative pressure injury from the tracheostomy tube and ties.

In a quasi-experimental study, Huang et al[94] found that the application of a dressing and cushioning material significantly reduced the size and severity of nasal ala pressure injuries attributable to nasotracheal intubation during oral and maxillofacial surgery.

Günlemez et al[95] investigated the efficacy of silicone gel sheeting applied to the nares of preterm infants ventilated with nasal CPAP. They concluded that the use of the silicone gel sheeting reduced the incidence and severity of nasal injury (ie, bleeding, crusting, excoriation, columella necrosis) associated with nasal CPAP.

II.d. The perioperative RN should communicate with surgical team members regarding the patient's risk for positioning injury. *[3: Moderate Evidence]*

Communication of the preoperative assessment findings to surgical team members is necessary for providing safe patient care.[88]

II.d.1. Perioperative team members should collaborate to determine interventions to be implemented to mitigate the patient's risk for injury.[28,29,62] *[3: Moderate Evidence]*

Applying appropriate interventions (eg, changing the surgical approach or position, providing extra padding to redistribute pressure, collaborating with personnel from other departments [eg, radiology, ophthalmology] to determine contraindications or revisions to the plan of care) may help prevent patient injury.[88]

Ulm et al[96] retrospectively reviewed the records of 831 patients who underwent robotic gynecological surgery to determine the incidence of position-related injury. The researchers found that only seven patients

(0.8%) experienced a position-related injury. They concluded that the reason for the infrequent occurrence of position-related injury was the use of a collaborative team approach for preventing patient injury.

II.d.2. Interventions that will be implemented to prevent positioning injury should be discussed during the preoperative briefing[28] and reviewed during the postoperative debriefing. *[3: Moderate Evidence]*

Collaborative preprocedure assessment and planning and postprocedure review may improve efficiency and communication among team members and may help to reduce or eliminate potential injuries associated with patient positioning.[3,6,97,98]

Recommendation III

Perioperative team members should identify and provide the positioning equipment and devices required for the operative or invasive procedure.[21,23,24]

Perioperative team members determine the equipment and devices to be used based on the planned procedure, surgeon's preferences, and risk factors identified during the preoperative patient assessment. Safe patient care requires that the patient's position
- provide optimal exposure for the surgical team[2,4,41];
- allow for the placement of positioning equipment and devices[21,41];
- incorporate modifications necessary to accommodate the patient's physical needs[21,41]; and
- provide sufficient access for the anesthesia professional to administer the necessary depth of anesthesia, maintain hemodynamic stability and oxygenation, and preserve and protect invasive infusion sites and monitoring devices.[4,5,15,40]

III.a. Before the patient's arrival in the procedure room, the perioperative RN should identify and resolve potential conflicts in the availability of positioning equipment. *[3: Moderate Evidence]*

Procedures may be delayed and the patient's safety may be compromised when the equipment necessary to correctly and safely position the patient is not available.[6]

III.a.1. Perioperative personnel should confirm the availability of required positioning equipment when the procedure is scheduled. *[5: Benefits Balanced with Harms]*

Verifying the availability of positioning equipment at the time of scheduling may help prevent delays in patient care.

III.b. The perioperative RN should confirm that the OR is set up correctly for the planned procedure before the patient arrives in the procedure room.[24] *[2: High Evidence]*

Patient safety may be compromised when the room arrangement is not specific to the planned procedure and its laterality.[99]

III.c.   The correct patient position and positioning equipment should be verified during the time out.[100] *[2: High Evidence]*

The World Health Organization[100] recommends including a discussion of issues and concerns related to positioning equipment as part of the time out. Using effective methods to improve communication and involve all members of the perioperative team may help to reduce errors and improve patient safety.[99,101,102]

Recommendation IV

Perioperative team members should select, clean, inspect, and maintain positioning equipment, devices, and support surfaces and should ensure they are repaired or replaced when damaged, defective, or obsolete.[9,28]

Clean and functional equipment and devices contribute to patient and personnel safety. Failures in surface integrity can contribute to bacterial growth and patient skin breakdown. Equipment, devices, and support surfaces may have a finite life span.[19] Use of damaged, defective, or obsolete equipment and devices poses a risk for injury to patients and personnel.

IV.a.   Processes and procedures for evaluating, selecting, and purchasing positioning equipment and devices should be developed and implemented.[103] *[2: High Evidence]*

Patient and health care worker safety, quality, and cost containment are primary concerns of perioperative personnel as they participate in evaluating and selecting equipment and devices for use in the perioperative setting.[103] The technology used to design and create positioning equipment, devices, and support surfaces continues to evolve; therefore, it is important for perioperative team members to be informed by current evidence regarding the use of these products.

IV.a.1.   Personnel performing positioning activities should actively participate in the process of identifying and selecting positioning equipment and devices.[6] *[3: Moderate Evidence]*

Personnel performing positioning activities are a reliable source of feedback regarding desired features, functionality, and safety design of positioning equipment and devices.

IV.a.2.   An inventory of positioning equipment, devices, and support surfaces sufficient to meet the anticipated demand should be maintained.[4] *[2: High Evidence]*

Positioning needs vary with each patient. Without the necessary equipment, optimal positioning may not be possible. Working without the necessary equipment, substituting equipment of a lesser quality, or using equipment designed for other purposes increases the risk for injuries to patients and personnel. Having an adequate inventory of devices and equipment improves efficiency, lessens the potential for patient care to be delayed, and decreases the possibility of conflict that may arise when the needed equipment is not available.

In a nonexperimental study to examine problems associated with surgical patient positioning, Sørensen et al[8] sent an electronic questionnaire to 833 perioperative RNs employed at four public university hospitals in Denmark. There were 481 responses (57.7%) to the survey. The results showed there was an overall lack of OR beds, positioning equipment, and devices available for patient arm and leg support. The lack of available equipment unduly complicated the positioning process. At times, it was necessary for personnel to spend time and effort searching for equipment, particularly equipment and devices required for the prone and lateral positions. The inadequate supply of equipment and devices also required personnel to either compete for or share the equipment. The researchers concluded that the lack of sufficient quantities of positioning equipment and devices presented a risk to patient and personnel safety.

IV.b.   A multidisciplinary team should determine the type of support surfaces that will be used for perioperative patients. Multidisciplinary team members may include wound, ostomy, and continence care RNs; perioperative RNs; infection preventionists; supply chain managers; and other involved personnel. *[1: Strong Evidence]*

Evidence regarding the most effective pressure-redistributing support surface is inconclusive, and further research is warranted to determine the effectiveness of support surfaces in the perioperative setting.[30,31,51,104-109]

In an effort to provide clinical guidance for selecting a support surface based on individual patient needs, the Wound, Ostomy and Continence Nurses Society has developed an evidence- and consensus-based algorithm for support surface selection that uses the Braden Scale mobility and moisture subscale scores to drive selection of support surfaces.[109] The algorithm can be adapted to include specific products used by the health care organization.[109]

King and Bridges[105] conducted a quasi-experimental study to determine peak skin interface pressures when using three support surfaces—an OR bed mattress, a polyurethane convoluted foam overlay on an OR bed mattress, and a viscoelastic dry polymer gel overlay on an OR bed mattress—with participants in the supine and lateral positions. The researchers found that in the supine position, participants' sacral pressures were significantly higher on the OR bed mattress with the foam overlay than on the OR bed mattress alone or with the gel overlay. Heel pressures were significantly lower on the OR bed mattress with the foam overlay than on the OR bed mattress alone or with the gel overlay. In the lateral position, participants' trochanter pressures were significantly higher on the OR bed mattress with the foam overlay than on the OR bed mattress with the gel overlay. Most of the participants reported that the foam overlay was the most comfortable surface and the gel overlay was the least comfortable surface. The researchers concluded that adding a foam or gel overlay to an OR bed mattress did not reduce skin interface pressures.

Hoshowsky and Schramm[104] conducted a randomized controlled trial (RCT) to examine the effects of two OR bed mattresses—a vinyl-covered 2-inch (5.1-cm) foam mattress and a nylon fabric-covered 2-inch (5.1-cm) foam-and-gel mattress—and one viscoelastic dry polymer gel overlay on intraoperative pressure injury formation. The researchers found that both the foam-and-gel mattress and the viscoelastic gel overlay were significantly more effective than the foam mattress in preventing skin changes and pressure injury, but the viscoelastic gel overlay was the most effective surface for preventing pressure injury.

Scott[55] evaluated the efficacy of a 4-inch (10.2 cm) multi-layer pressure-redistributing surface compared with a 2-inch (5.1-cm) foam OR bed mattress. The author found that patients were eight times more likely to develop a pressure injury when positioned on the foam surface compared with the multi-layer pressure-redistributing surface.

Deane et al[110] conducted a quasi-experimental study to determine whether changes in skin interface pressures could be related to the OR bed surface material. The researchers measured the interface pressure between the participants' skin and an OR bed mattress, an OR bed mattress covered with a convoluted foam overlay, and an OR bed mattress covered with a viscoelastic gel overlay. They found the interface pressures for the OR bed mattress with the convoluted foam overlay were not statistically lower than for the OR bed mattress alone. The interface pressures for the OR bed mattress with the viscoelastic gel overlay were significantly higher than for the OR bed mattress with the convoluted foam overlay.

Wu et al[107] conducted a quasi-experimental study to evaluate the efficacy of high-density foam pads compared with viscoelastic polymer pads in the prevention of pressure injury. The researchers found that the average and peak pressures measured at the points padded with the viscoelastic polymer were significantly lower than at the points padded with high-density foam; however, there was not a significant difference in the number of pressure injuries.

Reddy[106] conducted a systematic review of 64 RCTs, systematic reviews, and observational studies to determine the effects of surfaces used to prevent pressure injuries. Based on evidence of a moderate quality, the researcher concluded that viscoelastic foam mattresses reduced the incidence of pressure injuries in people at risk compared with foam mattresses; however, the most effective mattress was undetermined. The researcher also concluded that using pressure-redistributing overlays on OR beds was more effective than no overlay for preventing pressure injuries, but this conclusion was supported by only very low-quality evidence.

In a Cochrane systematic review of support surfaces for pressure injury prevention, McInnes et al[108] analyzed 59 RCTs and quasi-randomized trials, published or unpublished, that assessed the effects of any support surface for prevention of pressure injury in any patient group or setting. The researchers found that foam alternatives (eg, viscoelastic foam) reduced the incidence of pressure injury in patients at risk for pressure injury. The researchers also found that pressure-redistributing overlays on the OR bed reduced the incidence of postoperative pressure injury.

In a nonexperimental study conducted in a university medical center in Canada, Pham et al[76] calculated the cost of using the existing OR bed mattress and supplemental padding compared with the cost of using a viscoelastic dry polymer gel overlay on top of the OR bed mattress. The researchers found that the use of the viscoelastic gel overlay during procedures lasting 90 minutes or longer decreased the incidence of postoperative pressure injury by 0.51% and resulted in an overall cost savings of $46 per patient ($38.23 in 2017 US dollars).

IV.c. Perioperative team members should verify cleanliness, surface integrity, and correct function of positioning equipment, devices, and support surfaces before use.[5,21,28,41] *[1: Strong Evidence]*

Positioning equipment and devices are exposed to direct patient contact and frequent hand contact and have the potential for surface contamination with microorganisms and body substances.[111,112] Application of rigorous environmental cleaning practices will assist in providing a clean environment for perioperative patients and minimize the risk for exposure of health care personnel and patients to potentially infectious microorganisms.[113]

Loss of surface integrity can create a reservoir for the collection of dirt and debris that may be difficult or impossible to remove during cleaning and can lead to bacterial growth. Surfaces that are irregular, wrinkled, or damaged can contribute to skin breakdown. Some support surfaces (eg, convoluted foam) can lose resilience, hold moisture, prevent air circulation, and harbor microorganisms if not replaced when soiled.[43] Inspection and evaluation provide an opportunity to identify and remove from service soiled or defective items that might put patients at risk for infection or injury.

IV.c.1. Soiled, damaged, or defective surfaces, devices, and equipment should be removed from service and cleaned, repaired, or replaced. *[5: Benefits Balanced with Harms]*

Removal from service, followed by cleaning, repair, and replacement of soiled, damaged, or defective equipment and devices helps prevent further damage from use and reduces the risk for patient infection or injury to patients or personnel.

IV.d. Preventive maintenance and repair should be performed at established intervals on all equipment and devices used for patient positioning.[28] *[3: Moderate Evidence]*

Regular preventive maintenance promotes optimal functioning of equipment and devices and decreases the risk for injury to patients and personnel.

IV.d.1. The schedule for preventive maintenance and repair should align with the manufacturer's instructions for use (IFU). *[5: Benefits Balanced with Harms]*

The manufacturer is the most reliable source for determining preventive maintenance schedules. Between January 2009 and January 2016, the US Food and Drug Administration (FDA)[114] received more than 1,000 medical device reports associated with slippage or movement of neurosurgical head holders that resulted in more than 700 injuries. The FDA determined that slippage of the neurosurgical head holders was multifactorial and not specific to any manufacturer or brand of device; however, one cause of the slippage was found to be a lack of preventive maintenance. The FDA suggested the risk for injury could be mitigated by following the manufacturer's instructions for cleaning, maintaining, and replacing the neurosurgical head holder based on the manufacturer's suggested life expectancy of the device (ie, number of uses or length of time the device has been in use). The FDA also recommended inspecting the neurosurgical head holder system before and after each use, removing any parts of the system that appear to be damaged, and returning defective items to the manufacturer for repair or replacement.

IV.d.2. Preventive maintenance and repair should be performed by qualified individuals. *[5: Benefits Balanced with Harms]*

Preventive maintenance requires special skills and knowledge that includes systematic inspection, testing, measurement, adjustment, parts replacement, and detection and correction of device or equipment malfunction either before it occurs or before it develops into a major failure. Having qualified personnel perform preventive maintenance and repair increases the probability that repair and service will be performed correctly.

Recommendation V

Perioperative team members should use OR beds, positioning equipment and devices, and support surfaces correctly.[28]

Patients and health care workers are at risk for injury if OR beds, positioning equipment and devices, and support surfaces are not used correctly.

V.a. Operating room beds and attachments should be used in accordance with the manufacturer's IFU.[5,24] *[3: Moderate Evidence]*

Patient injuries resulting from failure to follow the positioning equipment manufacturer's IFU have been reported.[115,116] Dauber and Roth[115] reported the case of an obese patient undergoing spinal fusion surgery in the prone position on a spinal table. When a slight axial rotational adjustment was made to the patient's position, the table rapidly tilted vertically, causing the patient to fall to the floor. The patient's vital signs remained stable, and neither the endotracheal tube nor the indwelling IV catheter became dislodged; however, the patient immediately developed a large subgaleal hematoma. During a root cause analysis of the event, it was determined that the incident was caused by a failure to correctly activate the table-locking mechanism.

Ahmad et al[116] reported two incidents of muscle necrosis and anterior thigh compartment syndrome caused by incorrect placement of Jackson table attachments. Both patients were injured as a result of a failure to follow the manufacturer's IFU. The Jackson table has adjustable pads designed to support the iliac crest and thighs. The iliac crest pads are designed by the manufacturer to be higher than the thigh pads. When the thigh and iliac crest pads are reversed (either in error or deliberately to achieve a greater degree of lumbar lordosis, as was the reason in these cases), the higher iliac crest pad creates a greater degree of focal pressure on the thighs that can lead to patient injury.

V.a.1. The perineal post on the fracture table should be padded and placed in accordance with the manufacturer's IFU.[117] *[3: Moderate Evidence]*

Incorrect placement of the perineal post of the fracture table can lead to perineal pressure injury, pudendal neuropathy, or erectile dysfunction.[36,117-119] Accurate post placement and sufficient padding around the perineal post can help to prevent these injuries.[36,117-120]

V.b.   Positioning equipment and devices and support surfaces should be used in accordance with the manufacturer's IFU. *[3: Moderate Evidence]*

In an expert opinion article, Chitlik[9] described an incident that illustrates the importance of following the manufacturer's IFU when using vacuum-packed positioning devices. Rather than disconnecting the suction and closing the valve on the device per the manufacturer's IFU, personnel were leaving the suction attached to the device during the procedure. This resulted in the device deflating during the procedure, losing its capacity to keep the patient in the desired position. When the device deflated, there was a tendency for the patient to slide toward the head of the bed, which necessitated repositioning interventions.

V.b.1.   Positioning equipment and devices should be designed and intended for use in positioning surgical patients.[63] *[4: Limited Evidence]*

Using equipment and devices intended for use in positioning surgical patients decreases the risk for injury to patients and personnel.

V.b.2.   Perioperative personnel should verify compatibility between positioning devices and support surfaces before use. *[5: Benefits Balanced with Harms]*

Manufacturers may permit or preclude the use of certain devices or surfaces with their products. Using products or surfaces that are not compatible with each other increases the risk for injury to patients or personnel.

V.b.3.   Neurosurgical head holder systems and their accessories should be used in accordance with the manufacturer's IFU.[114] *[3: Moderate Evidence]*

Between January 2009 and January 2016, the FDA received more than 1,000 medical device reports associated with slippage or movement of neurosurgical head holders that resulted in more than 700 injuries.[114] These reports described injuries that included skull fractures, hematomas, and facial bruises and lacerations, as well as surgical procedures that were delayed, prolonged, or terminated. The FDA determined that slippage of the neurosurgical head holders was multifactorial and not specific to any manufacturer or brand of device; however, the FDA recommended that health care providers

- follow the manufacturer's IFU,
- use the manufacturer-recommended accessories with the neurosurgical head holder system, and
- report adverse events associated with the neurosurgical head holder system to the manufacturer and to the FDA through MedWatch: The FDA Safety Information and Adverse Event Reporting Program.[114,121]

The risk for adverse events associated with neurosurgical head holder systems may be greater in the pediatric population because of the varying thickness of the developing cranium.[122] In a survey of 164 neurosurgeons who treated pediatric patients, 158 (96%) of whom reported using cranial fixation pins in their practice, 89 (54%) of the neurosurgeons reported having experienced complications directly related to the use of cranial fixation pins, including cranial fracture, epidural or subdural hematoma, scalp laceration, or cerebrospinal fluid leak.[123]

Poli et al[122] reported the case of a 7-year-old boy who underwent a left suboccipital craniectomy in the prone position. The patient's head was fixed in a Mayfield neurosurgical head holder system. At the end of the procedure, a computerized axial tomography scan revealed a left hemispheric epidural hematoma with a small depressed skull fracture at the site of one of the pins. The patient underwent immediate surgical evacuation of the hematoma and was discharged 13 days later.

V.c.   Operating room beds and positioning equipment and devices should have the weight and size capacity and the articulation abilities necessary for safe movement and care of the patient. *[3: Moderate Evidence]*

Accommodating the unique needs of individual patients is necessary to prevent injury to patients and personnel.[6,74] Operating room bed and positioning device requirements may vary based on the patient's height and weight.

In a qualitative analysis of 863 perioperative incident reports from six institutions in the Midwest, Chappy[124] identified specific events that affected perioperative patient safety during a 3-year period. Sixteen incidents involved patient positioning (2%), and of these, 10 reports (63%) involved patients who were too heavy for the OR bed or bed attachment specifications. In all 10 of these procedures, the OR bed or attachment was used in spite of the weight restrictions because alternative OR beds or equipment were not available. Notably, in all procedures, there was a note in the perioperative record that the surgeon was informed of the weight restriction before the start of the procedure.

V.c.1.   Designated facility personnel should ensure that positioning equipment and devices with a weight limit are clearly labeled. *[5: Benefits Balanced with Harms]*

Recommendation VI

Perioperative personnel should identify potential hazards associated with positioning activities and should establish safe practices.

Positioning patients and using positioning equipment and devices during perioperative care can result in injury to both patients and personnel.[6,16,125] Identifying potential hazards and establishing safe practices may reduce the risk for patient and personnel injury.

VI.a. An adequate number of personnel, devices, and equipment should be available during patient positioning activities to ensure patient and personnel safety.[4-6,41,58,125] *[2: High Evidence]*

Having a sufficient number of personnel to position the patient helps maintain the patient's physiologic body alignment and provide support for the patient's extremities[28] and also reduces the physical demands placed on the personnel performing the task.[16,41,58,125,126] In a qualitative study to capture the perceptions of perioperative team members related to patient and personnel safety during prone positioning, Asiedu et al[127] analyzed open-ended questionnaires and conducted interviews with members of the spine positioning team from a large midwestern teaching and research hospital. The participants reported that limited numbers of available personnel was one of the major challenges faced during prone positioning. The availability of personnel was affected by daily staffing patterns. When the number of personnel was limited (as sometimes occurred during lunch or dinner breaks or during emergency procedures performed outside of normal operating hours), perioperative team members were required to move patients without the number of personnel needed to move the patient safely.

The participants also reported that the difficulty of positioning very large patients could be a source of anxiety and stress to the positioning team and that the receiver role (ie, the person catching the patient during the flip from the supine position on the transport gurney to the prone position on the OR bed) was more challenging than the sender role (ie, the person flipping the patient away from himself or herself). The difficulty of the receiver role was increased with larger patients because it took longer, required more energy, and increased the risk for injury.[127]

VI.b. When on the OR bed, the patient should be attended at all times by at least one surgical team member.[28] *[3: Moderate Evidence]*

A lack of clear communication about who is responsible for watching the patient after the safety straps are removed or before the patient is transferred to the OR bed has been reported as a contributing factor for patient falls in the perioperative setting.[128]

In an incident reported by Redman and McNatt,[129] an 8-month-old infant had been extubated and was lying quietly on the OR bed after an inguinal hernia repair. The anesthesia professional was standing at the head of the bed with her right hand on the child's head. Her body was turned to the left side as she manipulated the anesthesia machine with her left hand. The RN circulator had turned to observe the anesthesia professional when the child suddenly moved from a supine position and fell head-first off the left side of the bed. The RN circulator reacted quickly and was able to cushion the child's fall with her left hand. The child's body came to rest on the top of the RN's shoes. The child was immediately returned to the OR bed alert and awake with no evidence of injury.

Noting that gurneys and patient beds have side rails but OR beds do not, the authors developed a set of portable, cushioned side rails that could be attached to the OR bed to prevent pediatric patient falls. The authors proposed that using the side rails increased the margin of safety, but cautioned that the use of the side rails was not a substitute for constant attendance, vigilant observation, and other safety measures (eg, safety straps) commonly used to prevent patient falls.[129]

VI.c. Positioning of the patient should be coordinated among team members. Methods to achieve coordinated positioning may include
○ verifying that all team members are ready for positioning to occur or
○ implementing a countdown to begin positioning.
[3: Moderate Evidence]

Failure to coordinate positioning activities can result in sliding or pulling the patient and shear forces or friction on the patient's skin. Shearing occurs when the patient's skin remains stationary and the underlying tissues shift or move, as might occur when the patient is pulled or dragged without support to the skeletal system.[43,75] Shearing leads to blood vessel constriction that can increase the risk for ischemia and tissue necrosis.[75,130] Friction occurs when skin surfaces rub against a rough stationary surface,[43] leading to increased shedding of layers of epidermis and an increased susceptibility to pressure injury.[75,130]

Asiedu et al[127] analyzed open-ended questionnaires and conducted interviews with members of the spine positioning team from a large midwestern teaching and research hospital. The participants suggested implementing an audible and visual "pause" before any patient movement to ensure that equipment is set up correctly (eg, wheels locked) and that all positioning personnel are ready for the transfer or positioning to occur, as a method to prevent patient and personnel injury.

VI.c.1.   Team members should
- communicate about the presence of critical devices (eg, catheters, drainage tubes),
- take measures to secure them during positioning, and
- confirm correct placement and patency after positioning.

[3: Moderate Evidence]

Positioning activities can dislodge critical devices.[131]

Recommendation VII

Perioperative team members should position patients on surfaces that reduce the potential for pressure injury.

All perioperative patients are at risk for pressure injury because they are immobile during the procedure; placed on a relatively hard surface; unable to feel pain caused by pressure, friction, and shear forces; and unable to change position to relieve the pressure.[19] Before coming to the OR, a patient may have been transported to the emergency department by ambulance and may have waited for many hours on a hard surface.[31] A patient may have undergone a diagnostic procedure that required remaining in one position for a prolonged period. Some surgical procedures require that the patient be positioned on a hard surface (eg, vacuum-packed positioning device) to maintain the patient's position.[34] Patients are also at risk because of the use of vasoactive medications and the effects of anesthesia on hemodynamic status and tissue perfusion.[31]

VII.a.   Patients should be positioned on surfaces that are smooth and wrinkle-free.[4,22,61,118] *[2: High Evidence]*

Wrinkles in the surface beneath the patient can increase the risk for skin breakdown or pressure injury.[4,22,63]

VII.b.   Patients should not be positioned on multiple layers of sheets, blankets, or other materials.[4,19,61-63,71,132] *[1: Strong Evidence]*

Bed linen and other layers of material (eg, disposable incontinence pads) may be needed for patient comfort and to manage moisture or drainage[19]; however, placing blankets or other materials between the support surface and the patient reduces the pressure-redistributing effect of the support surface.[4,34,62,63,71,133]

In an organizational improvement project to establish the most effective method for preparing the surface of the OR bed to decrease pressure, Campbell[132] evaluated the sacral pressure readings of 20 patients undergoing peripheral vascular surgery. The author found that each layer of cloth or material placed between the patient and the OR bed mattress decreased the pressure-redistributing performance of the OR bed mattress and significantly increased sacral pressure readings. Increasing the number of layers of materials under the patient from three layers to nine layers increased pressure readings from an average of 41.2 mmHg to 73.8 mmHg. The author recommended decreasing the number of sheets and blankets beneath the patient.

VII.c.   Patients should not be positioned on warming blankets, if possible.[25,132,134] *[3: Moderate Evidence]*

Warming blankets placed under surgical patients increase tissue metabolism and multiply the body's demand for oxygen, nutrients, and by-product removal. When patients are anesthetized, hypotensive, and immobile, they may not be able to meet this increased demand and are thus more susceptible to tissue damage.[25,132]

Grous et al[134] conducted a nonexperimental descriptive study to identify factors contributing to pressure injury in 33 patients undergoing operative procedures lasting longer than 10 hours. The researchers observed patient positioning and the placement of all positioning and warming devices. The patients were assessed for pressure injury within 48 hours after surgery. The researchers found that of the 15 patients (46%) who developed pressure injures, 12 (80%) had been placed on warming blankets during the procedure. The researchers recommended that warming blankets not be placed under patients undergoing surgical procedures.

Notably, in some patient populations (eg, neonates) there are limited options for placement of warming blankets, and positioning the patient on a warming blanket may be an effective method for preventing hypothermia. In these cases, it is necessary to evaluate the benefit of reducing the potential for pressure injury compared with the risk for hypothermia.

VII.d.   Perioperative patients should be positioned on surfaces that redistribute pressure. *[1: Strong Evidence]*

Positioning perioperative patients on surfaces that redistribute pressure may reduce the risk for pressure injury.[15,31,51,118] Pressure redistribution is the ability of a supportive material to distribute the load over a broader surface or contact area.[75,109] Pressure redistribution is accomplished by envelopment and immersion.[75] Envelopment is the ability of the support surface to conform and shape itself to the patient's body.[19,75,109] An enveloping support surface increases contact area and reduces pressure.[19,75] Immersion is the depth that a patient's body descends into the support surface.[19,75,109] The greater the level of immersion, the greater the amount of body surface area that is contacted.[19,75] The greater the surface area, the lower the overall pressure.[19,75] Notably, the patient's body can be immersed too deeply into the surface, leading to a "bottoming out" effect.[75] Bottoming out occurs when the support surface becomes fully compressed under the weight of the patient's body, resulting in the patient lying directly on a hard surface.[75] To prevent bottoming out, it is important that support surfaces provide at least 1 inch (2.5 cm) of supportive material between the bed and the patient's body.[104,135]

Using surfaces that reduce tissue interface pressures may be effective in redistributing pressure and lowering the patient's risk for a pressure injury.[75,105] Interface pressures greater than 32 mmHg may occlude capillary blood flow and lead to diminished tissue perfusion and ischemic injury that later manifests as a pressure injury.[36,104,136] However, devices used to measure interface pressure may underestimate pressures at the point where deep tissue injury occurs.[137] In addition, because of variability in individual patients, interface pressure alone may not be sufficient to evaluate the effectiveness of a particular surface in redistributing pressure and preventing pressure injury.[43,75] The duration of pressure may be more of a contributing factor than the intensity of the pressure.[19,105] Pressure injuries may be caused by high pressures applied for short periods or low pressures applied for long periods.[138]

Support surfaces that are designed to redistribute pressure may be constructed of various materials or combinations of materials that include foam, gel, air, or fluid.[19,31,104] Support surfaces may also be designed with structures such as bladders or modules arranged in layers or zones.[19] Support surfaces may be static (ie, lacking in movement) or dynamic.[31,43,104] Dynamic support surfaces are powered to provide movement that alters the immersion and envelopment characteristics of the surface, controls the temperature and humidity between the support surface and the patient, and redistributes pressure.[19] Controlling the temperature and humidity slows metabolic activity, decreases circulatory demand, inhibits sweating, and reduces skin hydration to decrease the risk for pressure injury.[75]

Static surfaces such as viscoelastic polymer (ie, gel) overlays are designed to reduce shearing and to support the patient's weight without becoming fully compressed under the weight of the patient's body.[30,31,61] Gel overlays are radiolucent, latex-free, and reusable.[30]

Foam overlays come in various depths and densities.[30] Foam density (ie, kg/m³) affects the lifespan of the foam padding and its ability to support the weight that is placed on it during a specified period of time.[139] Indentation load deflection indicates how much weight is required to compress the foam padding to 25% of its original size.[139] No evidence exists regarding the optimal foam density and indentation

load deflection for preventing pressure injury in perioperative patients. Using a 3-inch (7.6-cm) low-density foam may not be as effective as using a 2-inch (5.1-cm) high-density foam. Some foam products may be ineffective when used with a patient who is obese because of compression resulting from the patient's weight.[74] Most foam products have a weight limit of approximately 253.5 lb (115 kg); however, some viscoelastic foam mattresses can support up to 694.5 lb (315 kg).[62]

Static air overlays have multiple chambers that allow air exchange between compartments when the patient lies on the surface. Dynamic air overlays or powered devices include air overlays and mattress replacements that can be customized to fit the articulation of various OR bed sections. Alternating air overlays are designed to alternate inflation and deflation of chambers so that pressure points are constantly changing.[30,31]

Simulated fluid immersion technology maintains the patient in a simulated fluid environment designed to redistribute pressure and eliminate pressure points by displacing the patient's weight throughout a simulated fluid medium.[140,141] The system allows the immersion properties of the mattress to be adjusted to the individual patient.[141] Worsley et al[141] found the simulated fluid immersion mattress provided a high level of pressure redistribution with low peak pressures over the body in supine, sitting, and lateral positions. Kirkland-Walsh et al[142] measured full-body interface pressures in four different support surfaces and found the simulated fluid immersion surface produced the lowest average sacral pressure (22.1 mmHg). Further research is needed to determine whether simulated surfaces reduce the risk for pressure injury in perioperative patients.[140-142]

There are a vast variety of pressure-redistributing surfaces available for use with perioperative patients. It is essential that perioperative patients be positioned on surfaces that redistribute pressure; however, selection of appropriate support surfaces for the perioperative practice setting is a complex process that warrants evaluation and review by a multidisciplinary team (See Recommendation IV.b).

VII.d.1. Towels, sheets, and blankets should not be used as positioning devices.[61-63] *[3: Moderate Evidence]*

Using rolled or folded towels, sheets, or blankets as positioning devices increases pressure, contributes to friction injuries, and decreases the pressure-redistributing properties of the support surface.[6,25,61-63]

VII.d.2. Pillows may be used for patient positioning. *[3: Moderate Evidence]*

Notably, pillows provide only a minimal amount of pressure redistribution.[62,63]

VII.d.3. A vacuum-packed positioning device may be used.[143] *[3: Moderate Evidence]*

Using a vacuum-packed positioning device provides stability and helps maintain the patient in the desired position.[143] Vacuum-packed positioning devices are designed to reduce pressure injury by providing a surface on which the patient's weight is evenly distributed and supported.[144] However, after decompression, these devices can increase pressure on nerves and over bony prominences.[34,145] When a vacuum-packed positioning device is used to support a patient in the lateral position, the patient's circulatory system may be compromised not only by the tight restraint provided by the device, but also by the overall effects of gravity on the patient's body and the horizontal body posture.[34]

Stephenson et al[145] described the case of a 14-year-old boy who underwent thoracoscopic resection of a right-sided mediastinal mass in the left lateral position on a vacuum-packed positioning device. The procedure lasted 3 hours. During his follow up visit 6 days after surgery, the patient complained of a 2-day history of shooting and burning left-leg pain and an area of numbness on the lateral aspect of the thigh. He was limping because of the pain, but had no motor deficit. The patient was diagnosed with a lateral femoral cutaneous neuropathy. Six weeks after surgery the patient's pain and numbness had decreased but was still present.

VII.d.4. Positioning devices (eg, shoulder supports) should be placed beneath the patient and not beneath the OR bed mattress or the overlay placed on top of the OR bed mattress. *[3: Moderate Evidence]*

Placing positioning devices beneath the OR bed mattress or overlay decreases the pressure-redistributing properties of the mattress or overlay.[31,63]

VII.d.5. Repositioning activities intended to prevent pressure injury should continue in patients who are placed on pressure-redistributing surfaces.[19,109] *[1: Strong Evidence]*

Repositioning is helpful for providing pressure relief and comfort even when a pressure-redistributing surface is used.[19] The damaging effects of pressure are related to both magnitude and duration.[109] Repositioning activities reduce the duration of pressure.[109]

VII.e. Perioperative patients identified as being at high risk for pressure injury should be positioned on high-specification reactive foam surfaces, if possible. *[1: Strong Evidence]*

The National Pressure Ulcer Advisory Panel (NPUAP), European Pressure Ulcer Advisory Panel (EPUPA), and Pan Pacific Pressure Injury Alliance (PPPIA)[19] recommend the use of high-specification reactive foam surfaces for perioperative patients at high risk for pressure injury. High-specification surfaces are pressure-redistributing pads or mattresses composed of high-density or viscoelastic foam that conforms to the body contours.[146] These surfaces may include multiple layers of foams of various grades and types.[19,62] Properties of a high-specification foam mattress include

- a density of 35 kg/m³,
- an indentation force deflection of 35 to 130,
- hardness (ie, the ability to push back and carry weight) of 130 Newtons,
- a support factor of 1.75 to 2.4,
- a depth of 5.9 inches (150 mm), and
- a mattress cover with a moisture vapor transmission rate of 33 g/m²/24 hours.[19]

A reactive support surface is designed to reduce the risk for pressure injury by changing its load distribution in response to an applied load (ie, the patient's weight).[19] Reactive support surfaces provide deep immersion and a high degree of envelopment to reduce high pressure concentrations over bony prominences.[19] Using high-specification reactive foam surfaces may be an effective strategy to reduce the incidence of pressure injury in perioperative patients.[62,63]

In a Cochrane systematic review of support surfaces for pressure injury prevention, McInnes et al[108] analyzed 59 RCTs and quasi-randomized trials, published and unpublished, that assessed the effects of any support surface for prevention of pressure injury in any patient group or setting. The researchers concluded that the use of high-specification foam mattresses was indicated for patients at high risk for pressure injury.

VII.e.1. Perioperative patients should be placed on high-specification reactive or alternating pressure support surfaces before and after surgery,[19] if possible. *[1: Strong Evidence]*

The NPUAP, EPUPA, and PPPIA[19] recommend the use of high-specification reactive alternating pressure support surfaces for perioperative patients before and after surgery. Positioning a patient on a high-specification surface reduces the risk for pressure injury when the patient is immobile or sedated.

VII.f. Perioperative personnel should use additional pressure-redistributing padding to support the patient and redistribute pressure from bony prominences and other pressure points.[6,19,23,28,51,58,147] *[1: Strong Evidence]*

Placing padding between the patient and hard surfaces and using additional padding on bony prominences and other pressure points increases patient comfort, helps redistribute pressure, and decreases the potential for nerve or pressure injury.[5,23,36,41,62,68,118,147] Patients who are obese may require additional padding because the excess weight of the patient puts additional pressure on areas that contact the OR bed or positioning devices used.[24] Older adults may have musculoskeletal diseases or deformities (eg, arthritis, kyphotic spines) that necessitate additional padding.[23,60]

Notably, the use of excessive padding that creates misalignment or additional pressure or is applied too tightly does not redistribute pressure and can cause pressure injury.[35,143]

VII.g. Prophylactic dressings may be applied to bony prominences (eg, heels, sacrum) or other areas subjected to pressure, friction, and shear. *[2: High Evidence]*

There is evidence to support the use of prophylactic dressings for prevention of pressure injury[148-154]; however, further research is warranted regarding the use of prophylactic dressings in perioperative patients.

The use of prophylactic dressings may reduce the effects of pressure, shear, and friction on healthy skin at increased risk for pressure injury.[150] In a nonexperimental study to identify the modes of action by which prophylactic dressings prevented pressure injury, Call et al[151] tested nine commercially available dressings and found that the use of prophylactic dressings reduced the forces of shear, pressure, and friction placed on patients at risk for pressure injury. The researchers found that the dressings were able to effectively redirect these forces to wider areas and minimize the mechanical loads placed on skeletal structures. The use of prophylactic dressings significantly reduced the amount of shear delivered to the skin by several mechanisms, including
- displacing the shear force outside of the dressing area;
- using silicone adhesives to absorb shear;
- providing bulk to absorb shear;
- having multiple layers of foam to create a displacement plane for absorbing shear; and
- stretching, molding, and conforming to the skin surface to absorb pressure.

The researchers noted that adhesion was an important element of the effectiveness of the dressing because insufficient adhesion allowed the dressing to easily release from the skin, whereas excessive adhesion led to cell stripping or disruption of granulation when used over a healing wound. The researchers concluded that prophylactic dressings were useful to enhance but not replace pressure injury prevention programs.

In an RCT to investigate the effectiveness of multi-layered soft silicone border foam dressings in preventing pressure injury, Santamaria et al[148] randomly allocated 440 critically ill patients to either a control group (n = 221) that received the usual care for pressure injury prevention or an experimental group (n = 219) that received the usual care plus a silicone border foam dressing applied to the sacrum and a silicone border foam dressing applied to each of their heels. The researchers found there were significantly fewer patients with pressure injuries in the experimental group (n = 5; 3.1%) compared with the control group (n = 20; 13.1%). The researchers concluded that the multilayered soft silicone border foam dressings were effective in preventing pressure injuries in critically ill patients.

Moore and Webster[150] conducted a Cochrane systematic review of four RCTs to evaluate the efficacy of dressings in preventing pressure injury in people of any age without pre-existing pressure injury but considered to be at risk for pressure injury in any health care setting. The researchers concluded that although prophylactic dressings reduced the incidence of pressure injury, the results were compromised by the low quality of the trials included.

VII.g.1. A multidisciplinary team should determine the type of prophylactic dressings that will be used in the perioperative setting as part of the health care organization's pressure injury prevention program. Multidisciplinary team members may include wound specialists; wound, ostomy, and continence care RNs; infection preventionists; perioperative RNs; supply chain managers; and other involved personnel. *[2: High Evidence]*

There are numerous types of prophylactic dressings, including
- semipermeable film dressings (ie, a thin polyurethane membrane coated with a layer of acrylic adhesive),
- hydrocolloid dressings (ie, a dressing containing a dispersion of gelatin, pectin, and carboxymethylcellulose together with other polymers and adhesives that form a flexible wafer), and
- foam dressings (ie, open cell, hydrophobic, polyurethane foam sheet).[150]

The use of a prophylactic dressing alters the temperature and humidity of the skin surface.[155] The amount of moisture trapped next to the skin, the amount of moisture that escapes from the dressing, and the amount of heat that is trapped by the dressing can affect the suitability of the dressing for use in preventing pressure injury.[155]

Each dressing is unique and its effectiveness in preventing pressure injury is based on the materials from which it is constructed, the number of layers in the dressing, the presence of perforations or micropores in the films used, the concentration of thermally dense polymers, the amount of air entrapment in the foam, and the amount of moisture accumulated under the dressing.[155]

VII.g.2. Prophylactic dressings used for prevention of pressure injury should be sized according to the manufacturer's IFU. *[3: Moderate Evidence]*

Correct sizing of the prophylactic dressing helps ensure effective redistribution of pressure, shear, and friction forces from areas of risk.[151]

VII.g.3. Multiple layers of prophylactic dressings should not be used.[83] *[3: Moderate Evidence]*

Using multiple layers of prophylactic dressings can increase the amount of pressure, shear, and friction applied to the skin.[83,151]

VII.g.4. Prophylactic dressings should be replaced if damaged, displaced, loosened, or moist.[19] *[1: Strong Evidence]*

The effectiveness of the dressing may be compromised if damaged, displaced, loosened, or moist.

VII.g.5. Safe positioning practices intended to prevent pressure injury should continue in patients receiving prophylactic dressings.[19,153] *[1: Strong Evidence]*

The use of prophylactic dressings does not negate the need for positioning interventions to prevent pressure injury.[19,151]

Recommendation VIII

Perioperative team members should implement safe positioning practices.

Patients undergoing surgical procedures are at increased risk for injury caused by compression or stretching of tissues during positioning.[2,3,7] The patient who is sedated or has received a regional or general anesthetic may not be able to communicate or sense numbness, tingling, tissue temperature changes, or limitation of mobility; therefore, a proactive approach by the perioperative team is necessary to prevent positioning injury.[41]

VIII.a. The patient's head and neck should be maintained in a neutral position without extreme lateral rotation.[28,118] *[3: Moderate Evidence]*

Extreme lateral rotation of the patient's head and neck can result in a brachial plexus stretching injury.[5,7,11,41,68,118,143,156-161] Extreme lateral rotation of the neck can also compress and twist muscles and vessels.[160,162] Direct compression on the neck muscles can lead to compartment syndrome.[162] Reperfusion of the muscles after repositioning of the head to its neutral physiologic position can lead to facial and neck swelling, angioedema, upper airway edema, and muscular edema that further increases compartment pressures and worsens muscle ischemia.[162] Extreme neck rotation can also precipitate paraplegia in patients with preexisting spinal cord pathology.[163]

There have been reports of postoperative infection of the salivary glands (ie, sialadenitis), also known as "anesthesia mumps" associated with extreme lateral rotation and extension of the head.[164-168] Compression of the patient's tongue from the airway maintenance device in combination with lateral rotation and flexion of the head can occlude the Stensen duct, which drains the parotid gland, or the Wharton duct, which drains the submandibular gland, leading to salivary stasis and secondary bacterial infection.[164-168] Compression or kinking of the arterial or venous vasculature can obstruct venous return to the head and neck or decrease blood supply to the salivary glands, resulting in an ischemic sialadenitis.[160,165]

In some cases, the degree of lateral neck rotation required for visualization may be reduced by tilting the table away from the surgeon. Morrison et al[169] suggested that tilting the operating bed 15 degrees improved visibility and reduced pain and the risk for brachial plexus injury associated with lateral rotation of the neck for prolonged periods during rhytidectomy procedures.

VIII.b. The patient's head should be repositioned or other actions (eg, removing the head strap) should be taken to reduce scalp pressure during the procedure, if possible. *[3: Moderate Evidence]*

Alopecia, resulting from ischemic changes in the scalp may occur after exposure to prolonged pressure during surgical procedures.[170,171] Repositioning the patient's head may help prevent pressure alopecia and occipital neuropathy; however, changing the patient's head position during the procedure may be difficult and could potentially dislodge or change the position of the airway maintenance device.

Multiple cases of alopecia have been reported that occurred following surgical procedures lasting longer than 4 hours.[170-177] In all cases, the authors suggested that the alopecia could have been prevented by repositioning of the patient's head during the procedure.

VIII.b.1. The patient's scalp may be massaged during the procedure. *[3: Moderate Evidence]*

Some authors have suggested that massaging the patient's scalp during the procedure may be an effective method of preventing alopecia that occurs after prolonged surgery.[175-177] There are some benefits associated with massage (eg, encourages hyperemia, increases tissue suppleness, reduces edema); however, massage may also damage underlying tissue.[178] Further research is warranted.

VIII.c. The patient's eyes should be protected when the patient is under general anesthesia. *[3: Moderate Evidence]*

Corneal abrasions or other ocular injuries can occur in anesthetized patients as a result of direct trauma to the unprotected eye or a failure of the eye to fully close.[179-181] General anesthesia reduces tear production and can lead to corneal drying.[179-181] Corneal abrasion can result from increased intraocular pressure and edema, as might occur when the patient is in the Trendelenburg position.[179-182]

In a literature review to determine the etiology of perioperative corneal abrasions and compare ocular protection strategies, Grixti et al[181] examined eight RCTs and one historical controlled study. The authors found that passive closure of the eyelids did not provide sufficient protection of the eyes. They noted that an unprotected, closed eye requires constant vigilance by the anesthesia professional to prevent reopening, thus posing a distraction from other duties. Passive closure may also be impractical during certain types of surgical procedures because of the placement of surgical drapes or the position of the patient.

The evidence shows that none of the available methods of corneal protection for patients undergoing general anesthesia are completely effective, and all may be associated with adverse effects.[181,183] Kocatürk et al[183] assessed the efficacy of hypoallergenic adhesive tape, antibiotic ointment, artificial liquid tear gel, and ocular lubricant for perioperative protection of patients' eyes in 184 patients undergoing spinal surgery in the prone position. The researchers found that all of the methods were suitable for protecting against corneal injuries, but all methods resulted in temporary symptoms during the postoperative period (ie, adhesive lids, foreign body sensation, burning, stinging, photophobia, blurred vision, dryness, conjunctival congestion, chemosis).

VIII.c.1. The patient's eyelids may be taped closed. *[3: Moderate Evidence]*

Grixti et al[181] found that taping the eyelids with adhesive or cellophane provided ocular protection. They recommended horizontal taping rather than vertical taping because the patient's eyelids may open under vertical taping, whereas horizontal taping achieves complete closure of the eyes by apposition of the upper and lower eyelids. The authors also recommended taping the patient's eyelids immediately after induction (as soon as the eyelid reflex disappears) and before tracheal intubation to reduce the risk for mechanical trauma to the cornea (unless rapid-sequence induction is being performed).

Taping the eyelids provides protection but impedes the anesthesia professional's ability to perform direct observation of the eyes and assess pupillary reactions. There are also potential hazards associated with eyelid taping. If the tape is placed incorrectly, mechanical trauma or exposure keratopathy can occur. Ocular surface contact with the adhesive substance or the edge of the tape can denude the exposed cornea. Periodic monitoring of the tape is necessary to verify that it has not become displaced. Other undesirable reactions to eyelid taping may include allergy to the tape material, breakdown of eyelid skin, or trauma to the eyelashes. The authors suggested that the tape be removed from upper to lower eyelid before the patient's emergence from anesthesia to help prevent corneal abrasion and ocular injury that might occur if the patient opens his or her eyes prematurely under the tape.

VIII.c.2. Transparent dressings may be used for eyelid closure. *[3: Moderate Evidence]*

The application of bio-occlusive transparent dressings provides complete and uniform lid closure and reduces tear film evaporation, thus creating a moist environment and preventing corneal desiccation.[181] The conformity of the transparent dressing also allows sealing at the periphery, reducing the risk of displacement.[181]

VIII.c.3. The patient's eyes may be lubricated. *[3: Moderate Evidence]*

Ocular lubricants may not be necessary for the majority of patients because the decreased tear production associated with general anesthesia is not detrimental to the ocular surface, provided the eyelids are taped closed.[181] A patient with pre-existing dry eye syndrome or other ocular surface disorders may require ocular lubrication.[181] The use of ocular lubrication may also be necessary for a patient with facial burns or other facial injuries that preclude taping of the eyelids.[181] When deemed necessary, preservative-free, water-based formulations are indicated, as these have a low complication rate.[181] Repeated applications of lubricant at regular intervals during the procedure may compensate for diminished tear production, but may also present an increased risk for corneal abrasion.[181]

VIII.c.4. Goggles may be used for ocular protection. Goggles should not be used when the patient is in the prone position and a face positioner is used.[184] *[3: Moderate Evidence]*

Goggles provide mechanical protection against ocular surface trauma, but they are ineffective in preventing corneal desiccation.[181] When the patient is in the prone position and goggles are used in combination with a face positioner, the goggles can become displaced and cause pressure on the globe.[181,184]

POSITIONING THE PATIENT

VIII.d. The anesthesia professional should check the patient's airway maintenance device after patient positioning and should implement corrective actions as indicated. *[3: Moderate Evidence]*

Changes in patient position during positioning could lead to changes in airway maintenance device position or intracuff pressure. An increase in intracuff pressure may cause damage to the tracheal mucosa.[185] A decrease in intracuff pressure may cause an air leak, resulting in inadequate ventilation and increased risk for aspiration.[185]

In a nonexperimental study to determine whether changes in head and neck position could lead to changes in endotracheal tube intracuff pressure, Olsen et al[185] measured intracuff pressures in 84 patients ages 0.9 years to 17 years undergoing adenotonsillectomy procedures. The researchers found the intracuff pressure increased in 46 patients (54.8%), decreased in 28 patients (33.3%), and remained constant in 10 patients (11.9%). The researchers concluded that regular monitoring of the endotracheal tube intracuff pressure and rechecking of intracuff pressure after positioning activities is indicated.

VIII.e. The patient's neck should not be hyperextended for prolonged periods. *[3: Moderate Evidence]*

Hyperextension of the neck can stretch the brachial plexus,[186] lead to cardiovascular complications associated with compression or mechanical manipulation of the carotid sinus,[187] or injure the spinal cord.[188]

VIII.f. Perioperative team members should verify the patient's body is in physiologic alignment when the patient is positioned. *[4: Limited Evidence]*

Maintaining the patient's physiologic body alignment and supporting extremities and joints reduces the potential for injury.[28,189]

VIII.g. The patient's body should be prevented from contact with metal portions of the OR bed and other hard surfaces.[37] *[3: Moderate Evidence]*

Ulnar or radial nerve injury can occur if the patient's arm is allowed to rest against the metal surface of the OR bed.[41,68,156]

VIII.h. The patient's extremities should be prevented from unintentionally dropping or hanging below level of the OR bed. *[3: Moderate Evidence]*

Allowing the patient's arm to fall or hang off the OR bed can cause radial (if supinated) or median (if pronated) nerve injury.[11,12,143] Allowing the patient's leg to fall or hang off the OR bed can injure the lateral femoral cutaneous nerve.[157]

In a qualitative analysis of 863 perioperative incident reports from six institutions in the Midwest, Chappy[124] identified specific events that affected perioperative patient safety during a 3-year period. Sixteen of the reported incidents involved patient positioning (2%). Three of these incidents (19%) involved patients' legs not being effectively secured to the OR bed and falling off the bed during the procedure. Notably, this was only discovered at the end of the procedure when the surgical drapes were removed.

VIII.i. The location of patient's hands, fingers, feet, toes, and genitals should be monitored during positioning activities, including changes in the configuration of the OR bed. *[3: Moderate Evidence]*

Monitoring the location of the patient's hands, fingers, feet, toes, and genitals ensures they are in a position that is clear of OR bed breaks, sources of compression, or other potential hazards.[36,37]

VIII.j. Safety restraints and monitoring devices (eg, blood pressure cuffs, pulse oximetry sensors) should be applied in a manner that safely secures the patient and allows the accessory device to function effectively without nerve, tissue, or circulatory compression.[6,58] *[3: Moderate Evidence]*

Applying safety restraints reduces the patient's risk of falling off the OR bed. Any device, secured too tightly can result in patient injury.[190] Securing restraints or monitoring accessories too tightly or placing them over superficial nerves or bony prominences can occlude blood vessels or cause nerve or pressure injury.[38,41,143,191-195] Blood pressure cuffs applied too tightly can cause ulnar or radial nerve trauma.[28,143,156] The radial nerve is vulnerable to injury when the arms are secured too tightly to the arm boards.[28,156] The skin of older adults is fragile and may be prone to injury from tape, tight restraints, and monitoring accessories.[37]

VIII.j.1. The perioperative RN should verify placement, tightness, and security of safety restraints after positioning or repositioning activities, including changes in OR bed configuration, and should take corrective actions as indicated. *[4: Limited Evidence]*

Verifying placement, tightness, and security of safety restraints reduces the risk for patient injury from restraints that may have come undone or shifted during patient positioning.[196]

VIII.j.2. The perioperative RN should assess the patient's relevant pulses after securing safety straps and implement corrective actions as indicated. *[3: Moderate Evidence]*

Checking the relevant pulses after securing safety straps verifies adequate perfusion and allows the perioperative RN to assess color, capillary refill time, and pulses and compare them to baseline levels.[191]

VIII.k. Patients with spinal cord lesions should be positioned in a manner that prevents direct pressure on the lesion.[197] *[3: Moderate Evidence]*

Preventing direct pressure on spinal cord lesions prevents injury to neural elements within the lesion and violation of the cerebrospinal fluid space.[197] Drummond et al[197] reported the case of a 32-year-old man with a history of spina bifida who underwent revision of an artificial urinary sphincter. The patient had a meningomyelocele that had been repaired when he was an infant. He had been diagnosed with a pseudomeningocele within the previous 3 years. The patient was positioned in the lithotomy position with additional padding placed under his left hip to minimize pressure on the pseudomeningocele. The procedure lasted 1.25 hours. When he arrived in the postanesthesia care unit, the patient was confused, and during the next 5 hours he was oriented only to person and spoke in monosyllables.

Magnetic resonance imaging performed 2.5 months after the surgery revealed cerebral atrophy. The patient had persistent cognitive impairment, short-term memory impairment, and word-finding difficulty. The pseudomeningocele was predominantly to the left of the midline; therefore, the lithotomy position and the positioning devices used to reduce pressure on the pseudomeningocele had actually applied rather than relieved pressure. The pressure on the pseudomeningocele resulted in inadequate cerebral perfusion and a permanent injury to the patient. The authors concluded that preventing direct pressure on meningoceles or meningomyeloceles is essential for preventing patient injury.

VIII.l. Neurophysiological monitoring may be used intraoperatively to identify potential positioning injuries. *[2: High Evidence]*

Neurophysiological monitoring (eg, somatosensory evoked potential [SSEP], transcranial electrical motor evoked potential [TCeMEP]) is used during surgical procedures to detect changes in the electrophysiological conduction of peripheral nerves and central nervous system pathways that may signal nervous system damage.[77,198-203] The field has evolved from monitoring the function of the spinal cord to monitoring for neural compromise that can occur outside an operative field during a surgical procedure (eg, a positioning injury).[77] Peripheral nerves in the upper extremities or the brachial plexus can become entrapped, compressed, stretched, or ischemic from pressure (eg, arms on arm boards), stretching (eg, taping of shoulders in cervical spine surgeries), dislocation or subluxation of the shoulder, or compression (eg, arm tucking, use of blood pressure cuffs).[200] With the advent of electrophysiology in the OR, neural function can be monitored, and compromise can be detected before a potential injury becomes irreversible.[77,198,200,202,203] Implementing repositioning interventions to reverse neurological conduction changes identified by SSEP monitoring may prevent peripheral nerve injury.[161,198,200-203]

In a prospective cohort observational study to evaluate the use of SSEP monitoring to detect position-related brachial plexus injury during cranial surgery, Jellish et al[204] conducted a focused preoperative and postoperative neurological examination of the brachial plexus on 65 patients undergoing cranial surgery. The patients were positioned in the supine position with the head turned to the contralateral side and secured with a neurosurgical head holder system. The researchers found that six patients (9.2%) developed significantly decreased SSEP amplitude changes after positioning. All of the SSEP changes occurred within the first hour after positioning. The patients' arms were repositioned when the SSEP changes were noted, preventing a positioning injury. The researchers concluded that upper extremity nerve stress can be detected in real time using SSEP monitoring and that neurophysiological monitoring can be an effective method of protecting patients from position-related nerve injury.

In a nonexperimental study of 485 consecutive patients who underwent microvascular decompression surgery, Ying et al[205] evaluated the effectiveness of SSEP monitoring for detecting peripheral nerve and brachial plexus injuries caused by incorrect positioning. The researchers found that 14 patients (2.89%) experienced a significant change of SSEP (n = 6 ulnar nerve, n = 8 median nerve). All of the changes occurred within 10 minutes after positioning. The researchers concluded that continuous intraoperative SSEP monitoring was a useful and valid technique to minimize intraoperative neurological injuries.

Using TCeMEP monitoring in addition to SSEP monitoring may help to validate the SSEP findings and provide additional coverage for emerging motor nerve injury that is not detectable using SSEP monitoring alone.[199,206,207]

Schwartz et al[206] conducted a retrospective review of 3,806 patients who underwent anterior cervical spine surgery with neurophysiological monitoring consisting of SSEP, TCeMEP, and electromyography. The researchers found that 69 patients (1.8%) showed intraoperative evidence of potential neurological injury, prompting repositioning interventions that included releasing shoulder countertraction; repositioning the patient's arms; loosening the sheet used to tuck the patient's arms; reducing shoulder abduction; adding padding to support the shoulders, forearms, or wrists; or flexing the neck. The brachial plexus was the site of potential injury in 45 of these cases (65.2%). The events most often signaling impending neurologic injury were shoulder taping and the application of countertraction (n = 39; 56.5%), hyperextension of the neck (n = 19; 27.5%), and tucking the patient's arms (n = 11; 15.9%). In all but four cases, there was complete resolution of the monitoring signals within 5 minutes of the intervention. None of the patients sustained any postoperative neurological deficit associated with a positioning injury. The researchers concluded that the results of the study demonstrated the important role of SSEP and TCeMEP monitoring in identifying altered neural function secondary to surgical positioning and allowing for prompt intervention to avoid untoward neurological sequelae.

Eager et al[208] conducted a retrospective review of 2,069 patients who underwent spine surgery with neurophysiological monitoring consisting of SSEP, TCeMEP, and electromyography. The researchers found 32 cases (1.5%) with possible intraoperative neurological events, and in 17 cases (53.1%), intraoperative neurophysiological monitoring changes affected the course of the surgery and potentially prevented postoperative neurological deficits. In four of the 17 cases (23.5%), the potential neurological injury was resolved by a change in patient positioning methods. The researchers noted the importance of multimodality intraoperative neurophysiological monitoring for spinal surgery.

VIII.m. Perioperative team members should monitor the patient's position after positioning activities and during the procedure and implement corrective actions as indicated. *[3: Moderate Evidence]*

Proactively monitoring the patient's position helps identify potential positioning problems and reduces the risk for injury.[191] Monitoring the patient's position after positioning activities verifies physiologic alignment; padding of pressure points; and clearance of fingers, toes, and genitals, and allows for necessary adjustments in the patient's position.[209] Even when correctly positioned, a patient may shift, especially during a prolonged procedure; therefore, regular intraoperative monitoring of the patient's position is necessary to detect or prevent positioning injury.[118,196]

Song et al[196] proposed conducting a second time out 3 to 4 hours after the procedure has started during robotic surgeries with extended operating times. They recommended leaving the robot arms docked and the patient draped, but turning on the room lights and examining the patient under the drapes to verify extremity placement and padding and to examine pressure points and check the tightness of safety restraints. The authors also recommended evaluating the patient's position for slippage, confirming the patient's head position and eye protection, and assessing for any changes in skin color. The authors theorized that conducting a second time out could enhance patient safety and improve the quality of care provided.

VIII.m.1. After positioning or repositioning the patient, perioperative team members should verify there are no areas where devices or equipment are resting against the patient.[63,210] *[3: Moderate Evidence]*

Changing the patient's position may expose or damage otherwise protected body tissue. The patient may be injured when positioning equipment is added or removed, the OR bed is adjusted, or the patient is moved on the OR bed.[210] Devices or equipment resting against the patient increase the risk for tissue or nerve damage in surgical patients.[62,210-212]

VIII.m.2. Scrubbed personnel should not lean against the patient.[6] *[3: Moderate Evidence]*

Scrubbed personnel leaning against the patient increases the risk for tissue or nerve damage in the surgical patient.[62]

VIII.n. Repositioning interventions may be implemented during the procedure. *[1: Strong Evidence]*

Repositioning involves changing the patient's position for the purpose of redistributing pressure.[19] Repositioning the patient redistributes pressure from pressure points and positioning devices.[15,19,42] Simple position changes (eg, changing the degree of lateral rotation, elevating the head of the bed, moving the limbs) may be sufficient to redistribute pressure and prevent injury.[19,67]

VIII.n.1. Repositioning interventions and repositioning intervals should be based on the individual patient and the specific situation.[19] *[1: Strong Evidence]*

Repositioning options may be limited or impossible for some perioperative patients.

VIII.n.2. Patients undergoing robotic procedures should be undocked from the robotic system before repositioning is initiated. *[3: Moderate Evidence]*

Adjusting the OR bed or the patient's position is not possible without undocking the robot.[20,179]

Recommendation IX

Perioperative team members should implement safe practices when positioning the patient in the supine or modifications of the supine position.

The supine position is the most frequently used position for surgical procedures because it provides access to a number of body areas.[5,7,28,191] The supine position causes extra pressure on the skin over the occiput, scapulae, olecranon processes, sacrum, coccyx, and calcaneum.[5,36,28]

IX.a. When positioning the patient in the supine position, the patient should be positioned as described in Recommendations VIII. and IX.

Guidance for safe positioning practices is provided in Recommendation VIII.

Guidance for safe practices in positioning the patient in the supine position is provided in this section (Recommendation IX).

IX.b. The patient's arms should be
- tucked at the sides with a draw sheet,
- secured at the sides with arm guards,
- flexed and secured across the body, or
- extended on arm boards.[5,143] *[3: Moderate Evidence]*

The position of the arms is determined by the needs of the surgical team and the physical limitations of the patient.

IX.b.1. When the patient's arms are tucked at the sides and secured with a draw sheet,
- the patient's arms should be in a neutral position[35,38,159] with the palms facing the body and without hyperextension of the elbows[6,36,159]; *[1: Strong Evidence]*
- the patient's elbows and hands may be protected with extra padding[36]; *[1: Strong Evidence]*
- the draw sheet should be pulled up between the patient's body and arm, placed over the patient's arm, and tucked between the patient and the OR bed mattress[36] (Figure 2); *[3: Moderate Evidence]*
- the draw sheet should be tucked snugly enough to secure the patient's arm, but not so tightly as to become a pressure source[74]; *[3: Moderate Evidence]* and
- the draw sheet should extend from the mid-upper arm (ie, above the elbows) to the fingertips. *[5: Benefits Balanced with Harms]*

Neutral position is a position during which the body part distal to the joint (eg, hand is distal to wrist, forearm is distal to elbow) is not inverted or everted, adducted or abducted, flexed or extended.[213] Hyperextension of the elbow can stretch the median nerve.[7,35,156]

Padding at the elbow and hand helps redistribute pressure from the ulnar nerve and may decrease the risk for upper extremity neuropathy.[7,35,214]

Using a draw sheet that extends from the mid-upper arm to the fingertips, placing the sheet over the arm, and tucking the draw sheet between the patient's body and the OR bed mattress prevents the patient's arms from falling outside of the mattress and coming to rest on the metal portion of the OR bed.[36]

If the draw sheet is tucked too tightly, it can create a pressure or nerve injury or a compartment syndrome.[7,36,38,74,143,215]

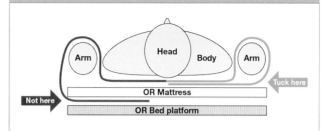

FIGURE 2. TUCKING THE ARMS WITH A DRAW SHEET

The draw sheet is pulled up between the patient's body and arm, placed over the patient's arm, and tucked between the patient and the OR bed mattress.
Illustration by Kurt Jones.

Tucking the patient's arms may interfere with physiological monitoring (eg, blood pressure, arterial catheter) and could result in an unrecognized infiltrated IV in the tucked arm.

IX.b.2. When the patient's arms are extended on arm boards,
- the arms should be supinated (ie, palms facing up),[7,28,36,118,143] *[1: Strong Evidence]*
- the arm boards should be padded,[7,36,118] *[3: Moderate Evidence]*
- the arm boards should be level with the OR bed mattress,[156] *[3: Moderate Evidence]*
- the arms should be abducted less than 90 degrees,[2,5-7,28,118,143] *[3: Moderate Evidence]*
- the arms should not be positioned above the head,[11,36] *[3: Moderate Evidence]*
- the arms and wrists should be maintained in neutral alignment[7,36,118,191] and should not be hyperextended,[6,12,195] *[3: Moderate Evidence]* and
- the arms should be secured to the arm boards.[28,36] *[3: Moderate Evidence]*

Placing the patient's palms up decreases pressure on the ulnar nerve.[35,118] When the patient's arms are pronated (ie, palms down), the ulnar nerve is more vulnerable to compression injury.[214]

The use of padded arm boards may decrease the risk for upper extremity neuropathy.[35,156]

Placement of the patient's abducted arm onto an arm board at a lower level than the OR bed mattress stretches the brachial plexus.[156]

The risk for brachial plexus injury and occlusion of the subclavian or axillary arteries is increased when the patient's arm is abducted more than 90 degrees.[11,12,36,38,68,143,156-158,191,214,216-218] The risk is further increased in patients who are thin and when both arms are extended and abducted.[68] Turning the patient's head to the side while the arms are extended on arm boards also increases stretch on the brachial plexus.[158] When the patient's arms are extended on arm boards and the patient slides caudally, excessive abduction of the arms can occur and cause a brachial neuropathy.[216] Notably, it may be difficult to ascertain the full degree of arm abduction in patients with large arms.[217]

Extreme abduction of the arm so that the hand rests above the head places considerable stretch on the brachial plexus.[11,219]

Maintaining the patient's arms and wrists in neutral alignment reduces the risk for a positioning injury.[36,220] Patients with a large muscle mass or a large amount of adipose tissue in the upper arm may be at increased risk for hyperextension when the arm is extended on an arm board.[195]

In a quasi-experimental study to evaluate the effect of wrist hyperextension (as used for insertion and stabilization of intraarterial catheters) on median nerve function, Chowet et al[221] analyzed median nerve conduction in 12 volunteer research participants. The participants were placed in the supine position with their right wrists hyperextended to 65 degrees and 85 degrees. The researchers recorded compound action potentials every 10 minutes for 2 hours. Subsequently, they released the participants' hands from hyperextension and recorded the potentials. The participants' left wrists served as the controls. The researchers concluded that wrist hyperextension for arterial line placement and stabilization was likely to result in profound impairment of median nerve function. They recommended that the patient's wrists be returned to the neutral position after arterial line placement.

Securing the arms to the arm boards reduces the risk of the patient's arms falling off the arm board.

IX.c.   A pillow or pad may be placed under the patient's lumbosacral area. *[3: Moderate Evidence]*

The effects of general anesthesia may reduce or eliminate paraspinal muscle tone, leading to loss of the patient's normal lordotic curve (ie, inward curvature of the lumbar and cervical regions of the spine).[5,144] Use of a lumbosacral pad may help prevent postoperative back pain by supporting the patient's physiologic lordotic curvature.[7,41]

IX.d.   The patient's knees should be flexed approximately 5 degrees to 10 degrees.[222] *[1: Strong Evidence]*

Positioning the knees in slight flexion prevents popliteal vein compression and reduces the patient's risk for DVT.[19,223] Extending the patient's legs and elevating the heels may increase pressure at the sacrum and allow the knee to hyperextend, compressing the popliteal vein and increasing the risk for DVT.[137,223-226]

Huber and Huber[224] conducted an observational study to determine the incidence of popliteal vein compression in 50 patients undergoing surgery in the supine position. The researchers used duplex ultrasonography to determine the amount of popliteal vein compression when the patient's knees were flexed and extended. The researchers found that of the 90 popliteal veins studied, 39 (43%) were completely occluded and an additional 19 (21%) decreased in diameter when the patient's heels were elevated. The researchers also found that BMI was a significant factor in popliteal vein compression. Patients with a BMI > 25 kg/m^2 were 1.33 times more likely to have popliteal vein compression than patients with a BMI < 25 kg/m^2. Patients with a BMI > 30 kg/m^2 were 1.67 times more likely to have popliteal compression than patients with a BMI < 25 kg/m^2.

In a subsequent pilot study to clarify the association between popliteal vein compression and DVT, Huber et al[223] scanned the popliteal veins of 54 patients who presented to a vascular laboratory for ultrasonic scanning to determine the presence of a DVT. The researchers found that five of 18 patients with popliteal vein compression had a DVT (27.7%), and five of 36 patients without popliteal vein compression had a DVT (16.7%). This difference was statistically significant. The researchers concluded there was an association between popliteal vein compression and an increased likelihood of developing a DVT. They recommended that patients undergoing surgery in the supine position have their heels elevated and their knees slightly flexed to prevent popliteal vein compression. The researchers emphasized caution when placing anything behind the popliteal fossa, as the weight of the patient's leg could be sufficient to compress the popliteal vein. They recommended using a supportive device that redistributes the weight of the leg over a larger area.

IX.d.1.   A soft pillow may be placed under the patient's knees. *[3: Moderate Evidence]*

The effects of general anesthesia relax and lengthen the hamstring, allowing the patient's knees to hyperextend.[5] Placing a pillow under the patient's knees may prevent hyperextension of the knees and help relieve pressure on the patient's lower back.[5,36,191] Using a soft pillow reduces the risk for popliteal compression[222] and provides protection for the common peroneal and tibial nerves[191] but may not be sufficient to prevent popliteal vein compression in some patients.[223]

IX.e. The safety strap should be placed approximately 2 inches (5 cm) above the patient's knees.[191] *[3: Moderate Evidence]*

Placing the safety strap on the patient's upper thighs or below the patient's knees does not effectively restrain the patient's legs to the OR bed. Placing the safety strap directly over the patient's knees increases the risk for nerve injury from compression of the common peroneal nerve against the head of the fibula.[191]

IX.f. The patient's legs should be parallel and the ankles uncrossed.[2,28] *[3: Moderate Evidence]*

Keeping the patient's legs parallel with ankles uncrossed reduces pressure to the occiput, scapulae, thoracic vertebrae, olecranon processes, ischial tuberosities, sacrum, coccyx, and calcaneum.[17,105]

IX.g. The patient's heels should be elevated off the underlying surface.[19,105,191] *[1: Strong Evidence]*

Offloading the supine patient's heels (ie, suspending the heels above the OR bed surface) increases perfusion and helps prevent pressure injury.[224] In a quasi-experimental study to examine heel skin temperatures in 18 adult patients during the first 3 days after hip surgery, Wong et al[227] placed temperature sensors on the plantar surfaces of each foot, close to the patient's heels. Temperature measurements were taken when the patients' heels were

○ suspended above the bed surface for 20 minutes,
○ on the bed surface for 15 minutes, and
○ suspended again above the bed surface for 15 minutes.

The researchers found there was a trend for heel skin temperature to increase after the patients' heels were placed on the bed surface for 15 minutes, and this increase in temperature continued after the patients' heels were removed from the bed surface. The researchers recommended keeping the patients' heels off the bed surface at all times to prevent heel skin temperature changes, enhance heat dissipation, and prevent deep tissue damage.

King and Bridges[105] conducted a quasi-experimental study to determine the peak skin interface pressures of three support surfaces (ie, an OR bed mattress, a polyurethane convoluted foam overlay on the OR bed mattress, and a viscoelastic dry polymer gel pad overlay on the OR bed mattress) with participants in the supine and lateral positions. The researchers found that heel pressures were increased on all three surfaces, suggesting that elevating the patient's heels off the surface is indicated whenever possible.

In an RCT to determine the effectiveness of offloading the heels in preventing pressure injury, Donnelly et al[228] inspected the heels of [239] older patients with fractured hips each day during their admission period. The patients were randomly allocated to either the control group positioned on pressure-redistributing surfaces (n = 119) or the experimental group positioned on pressure-redistributing surfaces plus heel elevation using a commercially available heel-suspension boot (n = 120). The researchers found that 31 patients (26%) in the control group developed pressure injuries compared with eight patients (7%) in the experimental group. The researchers concluded that offloading the heels reduced the incidence of pressure injuries.

Notably, heel elevation may increase the risk for sacral pressure injury. In a prospective cohort study to identify risk factors associated with pressure injury in patients undergoing surgical procedures lasting longer than 3 hours, Primiano et al[229] collected and analyzed data on 258 patients. The researchers found that 21 patients (8.1%) developed a pressure injury, and five of those patients (23.8%) had their heels elevated during surgery. The findings of the study indicated that although heel elevation may have prevented pressure injury to the patients' heels, it may have contributed to the development of sacral pressure injury. The researchers recommended further research to investigate whether prolonged heel elevation is consistently linked to increased risk for sacral pressure injury.

IX.g.1. Pressure on the heels should be redistributed by
  • using a heel-suspension device designed to elevate the heel and distribute the weight of the patient's leg along the calf[19] (Figure 3) *[1: Strong Evidence]* or
  • elevating and supporting the patient's calves with a pressure-redistributing surface that is wide enough to accommodate the externally rotated malleolus.[222] *[3: Moderate Evidence]*

Elevating the heels in a manner that distributes the weight of the patient's leg along the calf without putting pressure on the Achilles tendon and without hyperextending the knee is the most effective way to prevent pressure injuries to the heel and sacrum.[137] Positioning devices used to reduce pressure injury to the heels are designed to work in one of three ways:
  • by cradling the heel in a gel or foam surface,
  • by offloading the heel by supporting the Achilles tendon, or
  • by providing a surface that distributes the weight of the patient's leg along the calf.[137]

Devices designed to offload the heels by cradling the heel in a gel or foam surface or by supporting the Achilles tendon may increase pressure at the sacrum and/or Achilles tendon and allow the knee to

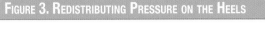

FIGURE 3. REDISTRIBUTING PRESSURE ON THE HEELS

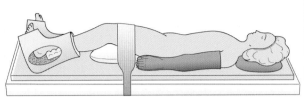

Heel-suspension devices are designed to elevate the heel and distribute the weight of the patient's leg along the calf without placing pressure on the Achilles tendon.

Illustration by Kurt Jones.

hyperextend, compressing the popliteal vein and increasing the risk for DVT.[137,226] Offloading the heels by supporting the Achilles tendon may also increase intra-compartmental pressure and lead to a compartment syndrome.[230]

Redistributing the weight of the patient's leg along the calf reduces the risk for pressure injury to the skin over the sacrum and the Achilles tendon.[222] Malkoun et al[137] investigated interface pressures at the calf, heel, Achilles tendon, and lateral malleolus using three commercially available heel positioning devices, a prototype heel-suspension device that provided heel elevation through distribution of the weight along the calf, and a standard OR bed mattress. The researchers found the interface pressures were significantly lower when devices that elevated the heel were used compared with devices designed to redistribute heel pressure. They also found that use of the prototype device resulted in significantly lower interface pressures at the Achilles tendon and the lateral malleolus than the other heel positioning devices.

Using a wide support surface helps prevent localized pressure on the lateral malleolus if the leg rotates externally.[222]

IX.h. Perioperative team members should protect the patient's feet from hyperflexion and hyperextension.[2] *[3: Moderate Evidence]*

The patient's feet may become hyperflexed or hyperextended from the weight of blankets, drapes, or equipment (eg, the Mayo stand) resting on the patient's foot.

IX.i. When using a hyperlordotic position (ie, supine with arched spine), the patient should not be hyperextended beyond a physiologic degree.[143] *[3: Moderate Evidence]*

Excessive arching of the lumbar spine (ie, beyond what is characteristic of normal functioning[231]) can stress the joints and ligaments, leading to postoperative back pain and femoral

neuropathy.[144,232] Arching the spine lengthens and flattens the major vessels and can impede blood flow, leading to changes in intraspinal perfusion and causing either congestion or ischemia of the spinal canal.[144]

Recommendation X

Perioperative team members should implement safe practices when positioning the patient in the Trendelenburg or modifications of the Trendelenburg position.

In the Trendelenburg position, the patient's feet are higher than the patient's head by 15 degrees to 30 degrees.[5] This position moves the abdominal viscera cephalad to improve surgical access to the pelvic organs.[5,233] Trendelenburg position causes a redistribution of the blood supply from the lower extremities into the central and pulmonary circulation.[69,179,234] Limb perfusion decreases.[235] Trendelenburg position also decreases venous return from the head, leading to venous pooling and increased intraocular pressure.[69,143,179,180,236-241] Swelling of the eyes, lips, tongue, and larynx can occur as a result of venous stasis.[7,179,182,242,243] Laryngeal swelling can lead to respiratory distress and the need to reintubate or delay extubation.[179,243]

Evidence related to the potential for cerebral desaturation in the Trendelenburg position indicates that the Trendelenburg position does not negatively affect cerebral oxygenation or autoregulation (ie, the mechanisms that maintain blood flow at physiologic levels during changes in blood pressure).[244-248] However, the Trendelenburg position does cause an elevation in cerebral blood volume and cerebrospinal fluid volume that raises intracranial pressure and may cause cerebral edema.[5,7,249] Researchers have also found that the increase in intracranial pressure associated with the Trendelenburg position may be predicted by a corresponding increase in optic nerve sheath diameter, which can be measured noninvasively using ocular sonography, allowing patients to be screened intraoperatively for increasing intracranial pressure.[250-253]

Patients who are positioned in the Trendelenburg position for prolonged periods may be at risk for postoperative vision loss.[254,255] Postoperative vision loss can be caused by an ischemic process that occurs as a result of decreased blood supply from the arteries of the optic nerve or by venous stasis that occurs as a result of decreased venous outflow.[180,242,254] Some researchers have found the increased intraocular pressure associated with the Trendelenburg position poses a risk for postoperative vision loss, particularly in patients with pre-existing ocular disease.[238-241,256,257] Grosso et al[255] found that pneumoperitoneum led to mild and reversible intraocular pressure increases; however, pneumoperitoneum in combination with the Trendelenburg position led to a greater increase in intraocular pressure. Older patients who have elevated baseline intraocular pressure are at greater risk for ischemic optic neuropathy, and ophthalmology consultation may be warranted before surgery to reduce the risk for injury in these patients.[179,180,182,238,239,241,255]

PATIENT CARE

The Trendelenburg position causes an increase in lower esophageal sphincter pressure.[258] To ventilate the lungs in this position, the patient's diaphragm pushes against the displaced abdominal contents, which increases the risk for the alveoli to collapse, resulting in atelectasis and hypoxemia.[7,69,143,234,258,259] Choi et al[259] found that the Trendelenburg position, in combination with pneumoperitoneum, enhanced atelectasis formation and decreased lung volume and lung compliance, leading to increased end-tidal carbon dioxide ($ETCO_2$) pressures. These pressures were significantly greater in older patients (ie, > 65 years) compared with middle-aged patients (ie, 45 years to 65 years).

Pulmonary functional residual capacity may be additionally impaired during laparoscopic or robotic surgery because of pneumoperitoneum.[58,179] According to Kilic et al,[260] prolonged use (ie, > 2 hours) of the steep (ie, 40-degree to 45-degree) Trendelenburg position can cause upper airway edema and reduced lung compliance. These effects may be more pronounced in patients who are obese.[260] In a retrospective review of 1,032 obese patients who underwent robotic gynecological surgery at two academic institutions, Wysham et al[261] found that only 33 patients (3%) had pulmonary complications. However, the researchers stipulated that older patients may be at increased risk for pulmonary complications when positioned in the Trendelenburg position.[261]

Evidence regarding the hemodynamic effects of the Trendelenburg position is inconclusive. Stretching of the peritoneum, either by pressure from an abdominal mass or pneumoperitoneum in combination with the Trendelenburg position, can cause bradycardia.[262] Some researchers have found that the Trendelenburg position produces negative hemodynamic effects (eg, reduced stroke volume, reduced cardiac output).[263-266] Lowenstein et al[264] suggested that women with cardiovascular disease, particularly those with arrhythmias or peripheral vascular disease, may not tolerate the hemodynamic changes associated with the steep Trendelenburg position. Other researchers have found the Trendelenburg position produces no negative hemodynamic effects[267-269] and may even improve hemodynamic function.[270,271] Further research is warranted to evaluate the hemodynamic effects of the Trendelenburg position.

Wen et al[272] conducted a retrospective review of 175,699 patients who underwent radical prostatectomy procedures during 2008 and 2009 using data extracted from the Nationwide Inpatient Sample database. The researchers found that positioning complications occurred in 0.4% of cases (n = 703). The steep (ie, 25-degree to 45-degree) Trendelenburg position was not associated with positioning complications in this sample.

X.a. When positioning the supine patient in the Trendelenburg position, the patient should be positioned as described in Recommendations VIII, IX, and X.

Guidance for safe practices in positioning the supine patient is provided in Recommendations VIII and IX.

Guidance for safe practices in positioning the patient in Trendelenburg position is provided in this section (Recommendation X).

X.b. When positioning the lithotomy patient in Trendelenburg position, the patient should be positioned as described in Recommendation VIII, X, and XII.

Guidance for safe practices in positioning the patient in the lithotomy position is provided in Recommendations VIII and XII.

Guidance for safe practices in positioning the patient in Trendelenburg position is provided in this section (Recommendation X).

X.c. The degree of Trendelenburg position should be minimized as much as possible.[4] *[2: High Evidence]*

There is no agreement in the literature as to the degree of Trendelenburg that constitutes "steep" or "maximum"[233,273]; however, a 30-degree to 45-degree OR bed tilt is generally considered a steep angle.[20,179,233,274] Using a more pronounced degree of Trendelenburg position places a greater physiologic strain on the patient's body and increases the potential for complications (eg, intracranial hypertension, respiratory deterioration).[233,273] The combination of pneumoperitoneum and steep degrees of Trendelenburg can lead to moderate to severe adverse hemodynamic changes (eg, reduced stroke volume, cardiac output, left ventricular end-diastolic volume[266]) and facial, ocular, and upper airway edema.[233,273,275] Retinal detachment and blindness may also result from prolonged use of the steep Trendelenburg position.[233,273]

In a study to investigate the influence of the angle of Trendelenburg position on cardiovascular and respiratory homeostasis, Kadono et al[275] found that cardiovascular and respiratory parameters were negatively affected and tended to worsen with steeper Trendelenburg. The researchers recommended completing the procedure efficiently and using the smallest degree of Trendelenburg possible.

Ghomi et al[233] conducted a descriptive study to explore the necessity of using steep (ie, 30-degree to 40-degree) Trendelenburg position in robotic gynecological surgery and to evaluate whether a lesser degree of Trendelenburg position could be used effectively. When adequate pneumoperitoneum had been achieved, the patients were placed in the degree of Trendelenburg that obtained sufficient exposure of the surgical field as determined by the primary surgeon. When the robotic portion of the procedure was completed, the degree of Trendelenburg position was measured. The surgeon and surgical team were blinded to the recorded degree of Trendelenburg. The researchers found that the median degree of Trendelenburg used was 16.4 degrees. The researchers concluded that robotic-assisted gynecological surgery could be performed using a modest degree of Trendelenburg without increasing complications or operating time.

In a quasi-experimental study to estimate the Trendelenburg angle required to perform robotic gynecological surgical procedures, Gould et al[273] measured the angle of Trendelenburg determined by the surgeons to be sufficient to perform the procedure (ie, the small bowel and sigmoid colon were displaced out of the surgical field). The researchers found the mean angle most commonly selected by the surgeons was 28.1 degrees. This difference was statistically significant when compared with the 40-degree angle the surgeons commonly used at the researchers' facility.

Raz et al[276] conducted an RCT to evaluate whether modifying the Trendelenburg position so that the patient's head and shoulders remained in a horizontal position would reduce the increase in intraocular pressure associated with the Trendelenburg position. The researchers compared intraocular pressures in 50 patients undergoing robotic-assisted laparoscopic radical prostatectomy. They found that modifying the Trendelenburg position had a significantly positive effect on patient safety by lowering intraocular pressure and accelerating its recovery to the normal range without affecting the surgery.

X.d. **The patient should be in the Trendelenburg position for the shortest time possible.**[4,9,274,277-279] *[2: High Evidence]*

Reducing the length of time the patient is placed in Trendelenburg position decreases the potential for complications or patient injury.

The Trendelenburg position increases cephalic and intracranial pressures and can lead to otological complications,[278] cerebral edema,[249] and neurological complications (eg, stupor).[279] In a prospective cohort study, Schramm et al[274] found that steep (ie, 40-degree to 45-degree) Trendelenburg position in combination with pneumoperitoneum slowly impaired cerebrovascular autoregulation during the course of robotic-assisted prostate surgeries. The researchers recommended minimizing the length of time the patient is in the Trendelenburg position.

Patients who are positioned in the Trendelenburg position for long periods are at risk for postoperative vision loss associated with increased intraocular pressure.[180,237,242,280-282] The increase in intraocular pressure is directly correlated with the amount of time in Trendelenburg position.[242,283]

In a systematic review of the literature to identify the number and type of peripheral nerve injuries associated with laparoscopic colorectal surgery involving the Trendelenburg position, Codd et al[284] suggested that reducing procedural times or returning the OR bed to a horizontal position at specified times during the procedure could help to reduce pressure on the brachial plexus and reduce the patient's risk for nerve injury associated with the Trendelenburg position.

Patients positioned in Trendelenburg position during prolonged procedures are also at risk for developing rhabdomyolysis.[285] Mattei et al[285] conducted a prospective study of 60 consecutive patients undergoing robotic-assisted radical prostatectomy with extended pelvic lymph node dissection and found that prolonged periods (ie, 2.8 hours to 7.8 hours) in steep (ie, 30-degree) Trendelenburg position increased the patient's risk for developing rhabdomyolysis. The researchers recommended reducing the time the patient is in the Trendelenburg position.

X.e. Patients in the Trendelenburg position should be repositioned into the supine or reverse Trendelenburg position at established intervals during the procedure, if possible. *[3: Moderate Evidence]*

Returning the patient to the supine position, or a position in which the ocular level is above the heart, will help to reduce intraocular pressure and facilitate return to baseline levels.[182,238] Reducing intraocular pressure may reduce the risk for postoperative vision loss.[182]

In a systematic review of eight papers reporting data on ocular complications in robotic surgery on 142 patients, Gkegkes et al[254] found that the most frequent complication was increased intraocular pressure. The researchers also found that elevated intraocular pressure and ischemic damage to the optic nerve could possibly be prevented by the introduction of intervals of reverse Trendelenburg positioning.

X.e.1. Repositioning interventions and repositioning intervals should be
- based on the individual patient and the specific situation[19] *[1: Strong Evidence]* and
- established by the perioperative team before the beginning of the procedure, if possible.[182] *[3: Moderate Evidence]*

The evidence does not determine a time limit for the use of the Trendelenburg position or for repositioning intervals. Barr et al[249] suggested repositioning every 3 hours. Freshcoln and Diehl[182] suggested attempting a supine intervention for 5 minutes after 4 hours of steep Trendelenburg. There are numerous physiologic patient variables (eg, age, comorbidities, medications) that can affect the length of time a patient can tolerate the Trendelenburg position without injury.[255]

Current evidence also does not identify how long the patient needs to be supine or in the reverse Trendelenburg position before being repositioned back into Trendelenburg position.

X.f. Perioperative team members should implement measures to prevent the patient from sliding on the OR bed.[4,20,58] *[1: Strong Evidence]*

The Trendelenburg position places the patient at risk for sliding cephalad.[9,286] Patient sliding increases the risk for skin breakdown as a result of friction and gravitational forces that pull the patient toward the head of the bed.[9,139,179] Preventing the patient from sliding on the OR bed decreases shear and reduces the potential for pressure on the brachial plexus.[4,20,179] A shift in the patient's position could place undue strain on the abdominal wall and also increase the risk for trauma to intra-abdominal structures.[179,286]

Shifting of the patient's trunk may also lead to suboptimal positioning of the extremities, increasing the risk for nerve injury from stretching or compression.[9,179,286] Preventing the patient from sliding on the OR bed is important for preventing patient injury that may occur in robotic-assisted procedures if the patient's position shifts after the device is docked.[9,32,139] If the patient slips while the robotic system is engaged, incisional tears could occur at the port sites that could cause hernias.[20] These effects may be increased in patients who are obese because they are more susceptible to downward shifting.[179]

X.f.1. Measures to prevent patients from sliding may include using
- convoluted foam or viscoelastic gel overlays,[139,179,286,287] *[1: Strong Evidence]*
- vacuum-packed positioning devices,[139,288] *[3: Moderate Evidence]* or
- other positioning devices designed for this purpose.[289,290] *[4: Limited Evidence]*

Evidence regarding the most effective methods and surfaces to prevent patients from sliding on the OR bed is inconclusive. Further research is warranted.

X.g. After positioning in the Trendelenburg position, the anesthesia professional should check the patient's airway maintenance device and take corrective actions as indicated.[5,144] *[3: Moderate Evidence]*

When the patient is placed into the Trendelenburg position, cephalad migration of the carina causes a shortening of the trachea, allowing the airway maintenance device to migrate distally, toward the right main bronchus.[69,144,291]

An increase in airway maintenance device cuff pressure may also occur during surgery in the Trendelenburg position.[292] Wu et al[292] evaluated endotracheal cuff pressure changes before and after supine and Trendelenburg position in 70 patients undergoing laparoscopic surgery. The researchers found there was a significant increase in endotracheal tube cuff pressure after

insufflation and after position changes, especially when patients were in the Trendelenburg position.

X.h. The patient's arms should be
- tucked at the sides with a draw sheet (See Recommendation IX.b.1) or
- secured at the sides with arm guards.

[3: Moderate Evidence]

Tucking or securing the patient's arms at the sides reduces the potential for patient injury. Extending the patient's arms on arm boards can lead to excessive abduction of the arms and cause a brachial neuropathy when the patient slides caudally.[216]

X.i. Shoulder braces should not be used,[9,159,277,293] if possible. *[2: High Evidence]*

Compression over the acromion by shoulder braces can injure the brachial plexus.[4,12,32,69,159,293] This injury is exacerbated by the muscle-relaxing, joint-mobilizing effects of general anesthesia.[4,214,293]

In a quasi-experimental study to investigate surgical positions that place the patient at risk for stretch-induced neuropathies, Coppieters et al[293] analyzed the effect of arm and neck positions in three different shoulder positions in 25 male volunteers. The tests were performed with and without fixation of the shoulder girdle to simulate the presence and absence of a shoulder brace. The researchers found that shoulder fixation resulted in a significantly reduced range of motion, even when the fixation was applied over the acromioclavicular joint. The researchers discouraged the use of shoulder braces and suggested that if they were used, it would be important to position the patient on a nonsliding surface, to monitor the pressure of the shoulder braces regularly during the procedure, and to consider the effect of the absence of protective reflexes in an anesthetized patient.

The pressure exerted on the brachial plexus by the shoulder braces increases as the angle of Trendelenburg increases.[4,294] In a prospective descriptive study to measure the pressure placed on the shoulders and to compare the pressures during varying degrees of Trendelenburg position, Suozzi et al[294] studied three different patient positioning systems (ie, two shoulder support systems and a vacuum-packed positioning device with shoulder supports). A total of 23 volunteer participants were placed in the lithotomy position with arms tucked and tilted to 5-degree, 10-degree, 15-degree, 20-degree, 25-degree, and 30-degree Trendelenburg position. The researchers measured the pressure on the shoulders at each angle of Trendelenburg for each device.

The researchers found that as the degree of Trendelenburg increased, the shoulder pressure increased for all of the positioning systems tested. The results showed that in the 30-degree Trendelenburg position, the vacuum-packed positioning device transmitted the least amount of pressure to the shoulders and the shoulder support systems transmitted the most pressure to the shoulders. The researchers theorized this may have been caused by the larger surface area of the vacuum-packed positioning device compared with the other positioning systems. When questioned as to which positioning system was the most comfortable, 74% (n = 17) of the participants stated that they preferred the vacuum-packed positioning device.[294]

X.i.1.　If shoulder braces are used,
- the point of contact should be at the level of the acromioclavicular joints,[4,12] *[1: Strong Evidence]*
- the braces should be padded,[4,12] *[2: High Evidence]* and
- the patient's arms should be tucked at his or her sides. *[2: High Evidence]*

If the shoulder brace is placed proximal to the neck, excessive pressure to the clavicle can compress the brachial plexus as it exits the thorax between the clavicle and the first rib.[35,68,143,156,214] If the shoulder brace is placed lateral to the neck, it can place an upward force on the shoulder while the patient's head and neck are experiencing downward gravitational forces.[12,67,214] The opposing upward and downward forces can result in a stretching and compression injury to the brachial plexus.[12,67,156,214,293]

Providing sufficient padding and placing the shoulder braces at the level of the acromioclavicular joint may help to prevent brachial plexus injury.[12]

The combination of arm abduction and shoulder braces may increase the risk for brachial plexus injury.[4,295,296]

X.j.　Circumferential wrist restraints should not be used.[277] *[3: Moderate Evidence]*

Using circumferential wrist restraints to prevent patient sliding can pull the humeral head downward and cause a brachial plexus injury.[277] Shveiky et al[277] conducted a literature review to explore the anatomy, pathophysiology, diagnosis, and treatment of position-related brachial plexus injuries associated with laparoscopic- and robotic-assisted surgery. The authors reviewed 24 reported cases of brachial plexus injury and found the Trendelenburg position was used in all 24 cases, with shoulder braces used in nine cases (37.5%). Most patients recovered during the course of 1 week to 9 months; however, in one case, there was a permanent disability.

The authors found that in the Trendelenburg position, whether the patient's arms were tucked at the sides or extended on arm boards, the patient was more likely to slide down the OR bed toward the head. Circumferential wrist restraints pulled the humeral head and shoulder girdle downward, increasing the risk for brachial plexus injury. The authors recommended using the smallest degree of Trendelenburg position necessary; reducing operative times to the extent possible; avoiding lateral rotation of the patient's neck; avoiding abduction, external rotation, and extension of the upper extremities; not using shoulder braces or circumferential wrist restraints; and regularly assessing the patient's position during surgery.

X.k.　Trendelenburg position should not be used for patients who are extremely obese (ie, BMI > 40 kg/m²), if possible.[234] *[3: Moderate Evidence]*

Vaughan and Wise[297] enrolled 64 extremely obese patients (ie, 313.0 lb ± 69.2 lb [142.0 kg ± 31.4 kg]) undergoing jejunoileal bypass procedures in a quasi-experimental study to investigate the intraoperative arterial oxygenation pattern in obese patients undergoing abdominal surgeries in the Trendelenburg position. The patients were divided into two groups. Group 1 patients (n = 25) were maintained in the supine position. Group 2 patients (n = 39) were maintained in a 15-degree Trendelenburg position. The researchers found that a change from supine to 15-degree Trendelenburg position resulted in a significant reduction in mean partial pressure of oxygen in arterial blood (PaO_2).

The researchers suggested not using the Trendelenburg position for patients who are extremely obese; however, if using this position is absolutely necessary, they recommended careful monitoring of the patient's arterial blood gases. The researchers also noted that although obese, the study participants were otherwise healthy, young individuals (ie, 22.9 years to 43.7 years). Obese individuals with heart, lung, liver, or kidney disease are at increased risk for ineffective oxygenation when positioned in the Trendelenburg position.[297]

Notably, in some cases the benefits of using minimally invasive surgical approaches may exceed the potential harms of using the Trendelenburg position in extremely obese patients.

Recommendation XI

Perioperative team members should implement safe practices when positioning the patient in the reverse Trendelenburg or modifications of the reverse Trendelenburg position.

In the reverse Trendelenburg position, the patient's head is positioned 15 degrees to 30 degrees higher than the feet. The surgical site is elevated above the level of the heart to improve drainage of body fluids away from the surgical site, reducing intracranial pressure and decreasing bleeding in the surgical field.[7,144] Pulmonary function and hemoglobin saturation are improved.[6] Venous pooling in the lower body can result in hypotension. Venous air embolism (VAE) is a potentially lethal complication of this position.[7]

XI.a. When positioning the supine patient in reverse Trendelenburg position, the patient should be positioned as described in Recommendations VIII, IX, and XI.

Guidance for safe practices in positioning the supine patient is provided in Recommendations VIII and IX.

Guidance for safe practices in positioning the patient in the reverse Trendelenburg position is provided in this section (Recommendation XI).

XI.b. A padded foot board should be used.[21] *[3: Moderate Evidence]*

Using a padded foot board helps prevent the patient from sliding downward on the OR bed and reduces the potential for injury to the peroneal and tibial nerves from foot and ankle flexion.[6,21]

XI.b.1. The perioperative RN should assess and monitor the patient's feet during the procedure and implement corrective actions as indicated. *[3: Moderate Evidence]*

Assessing and monitoring the patient's feet during the procedure confirms physiologic alignment and placement against the foot board, prevents rotation and increased pressure on the ankle, and may help to prevent circulatory or nerve damage.[6]

XI.c. Patients undergoing abdominal myomectomy procedures may be positioned in the 10-degree reverse Trendelenburg position. *[1: Strong Evidence]*

Positioning patients undergoing myomectomy procedures in the reverse Trendelenburg position may reduce the risk for VAE. An et al[298] conducted an RCT to determine the incidence and grade of VAE during abdominal myomectomy in the supine position compared with the reverse Trendelenburg position. The researchers enrolled 84 women, ASA classification I or II, who were scheduled for myomectomy under general anesthesia into the study and randomly allocated them into the supine group (n = 40) or the 10-degree Trendelenburg group (n = 44). The incidence and grade of VAE was significantly lower in the reverse Trendelenburg group than in the supine group, and the researchers recommended using the 10-degree reverse Trendelenburg position for abdominal myomectomy procedures.

Recommendation XII

Perioperative team members should implement safe practices when positioning the patient in the lithotomy or modifications of the lithotomy position.

The lithotomy position provides surgical exposure for vaginal, rectal, and urological procedures.[209] Modifications of the lithotomy position include low, standard, high, hemi, and exaggerated, depending on how high the legs and pelvis are elevated for the procedure.[36,144]

- Low: The patient's hips are flexed until the angle between the posterior surface of the patient's thighs and the OR bed surface is 40 degrees to 60 degrees. The patient's lower legs are parallel with the OR bed.[144]
- Standard: The patient's hips are flexed until the angle between the posterior surface of the patient's thighs and the OR bed surface is 80 degrees to 100 degrees. The patient's lower legs are parallel with the OR bed.[144]
- Hemi: The patient's nonoperative leg is positioned in standard lithotomy. The patient's operative leg may be placed in traction.[144]
- High: The patient's hips are flexed until the angle between the posterior surface of the patient's thighs and the OR bed surface is 110 degrees to 120 degrees. The patient's lower legs are flexed.[144]
- Exaggerated: The patient's hips are flexed until the angle between the posterior surface of the patient's thighs and the OR bed surface is 130 degrees to 150 degrees. The patient's lower legs are almost vertical.[144]

Raising the patient's legs shifts the blood from the legs into the central circulation and decreases perfusion of the legs.[36,299] This results in an increase in cardiac output and venous return.[36,299] Respiratory complications can occur in the lithotomy position because the patient's abdominal organs shift when the legs are placed in leg holders.[36,209] This increases pressure on the diaphragm and can cause respiratory compromise.[7,36,69,209] In patients who are obese, there is additional chest weight and abdominal pressure, leading to an increased respiratory workload and an increased risk for aspiration.[69,209,234]

XII.a. When positioning the patient in lithotomy position, the patient should be positioned as described in Recommendations VIII, IX.b, and XII.

Guidance for safe practices in positioning the patient is provided in Recommendations VIII and IX.b.

Guidance for safe practices in positioning the patient in the lithotomy position is provided in this section (Recommendation XII).

XII.a.1. The patient's hands and fingers should be protected from injury when the foot of the OR bed is raised, lowered, or reattached.[5,21,36,37,143] *[3: Moderate Evidence]*

If tucked at his or her sides, the patient's hands and fingers are in danger of injury when the bottom of the OR bed is raised, lowered, or reattached.[5,209]

XII.b. The patient should be in the lithotomy position for the shortest time possible.[12,21,68,209,300-315] *[2: High Evidence]*

The length of time a patient may remain in the lithotomy position without risk for injury is unknown.[73,300,316] Case reports in the literature describe complications associated with prolonged time in the lithotomy position, including

- unilateral lower-leg muscle contusion after 6 hours[317];
- unilateral lower-leg compartment syndrome after 4.5 hours,[318] 5 hours,[319] 6 hours,[314,320] 10 hours,[310] and 12 hours[310];
- unilateral lower-leg compartment syndrome and thrombosis of the common iliac artery after 6 hours[321];
- bilateral lower-leg compartment syndrome after 90 minutes,[315] 4.25 hours,[313] 5 hours,[319] and 7 hours[308];
- bilateral lower-leg and left forearm compartment syndrome after 11 hours[309];
- bilateral thigh compartment syndrome, rhabdomyolysis, and acute renal failure after 6 hours[322];
- bilateral gluteal compartment syndrome after 6 hours[311]; and
- rhabdomyolysis and acute renal failure after 5.5 hours.[323]

Notably, Sadeghian et al[324] reported a bilateral femoral neuropathy in a 20-year-old man after only 30 minutes in the lithotomy position. The risk for injury is multifactorial and may be related to the patient's condition as well as the position.[73,300,302,306-308,320,323,325] The reason some patients develop an injury and others do not remains unknown.[302] The longer the patient's legs are maintained in the lithotomy position, the greater the potential for developing a neuropathy, neurovascular complication, or compartment syndrome.[32,68,73,313,320-323] The addition of Trendelenburg position to the lithotomy position increases the potential for injury because the vertical distance between the heart and the lower limbs is increased.[301,302,305,307,308,313,314]

In a review of the literature on compartment syndrome, Bauer et al[302] found that 70.6% of compartment syndrome cases (n = 10) were identified after surgery lasting longer than 5 hours. The authors concluded that time spent in the lithotomy position was the most important and potentially avoidable risk factor for development of compartment syndrome.

In a retrospective observational study to investigate the incidence and circumstances of lower extremity compartment syndrome occurring after gynecological surgery, Bauer et al[307] found that reported cases of postoperative compartment syndrome occurred after surgeries longer than 2 hours in all cases and longer than 4 hours in 76.2% of cases (n = 16).

XII.b.1. Patients in the lithotomy position should be repositioned at established intervals during the procedure, if possible. *[3: Moderate Evidence]*

Evidence indicates that repositioning the patient at established intervals during the procedure may reduce the risk for compartment syndrome or other injuries associated with prolonged lithotomy position.[302,303,310,311,314,318,326]

XII.b.2. Repositioning interventions and repositioning intervals should be
- based on the individual patient and the specific situation[19] *[1: Strong Evidence]* and
- established by the perioperative team before the beginning of the procedure, if possible.[182] *[4: Limited Evidence]*

Evidence regarding the most effective repositioning strategies (ie, whether it is sufficient to lower the patient's legs or whether the legs need to be completely removed from the leg holders) or repositioning intervals for the lithotomy position is inconclusive. Taking the patient's limbs out of lithotomy position at predetermined intervals may help to prevent position-related patient injury[73,300]; however, lowering the patient's legs while in the leg holders may be sufficient to prevent injury.

The length of time after which the patient's legs need to be repositioned is unknown and may be affected by physiologic patient variables (eg, age, comorbidities, medications).[255] The literature suggests implementing repositioning interventions at intervals ranging from 2 to 4 hours.[249,302,303,305,306,315,327-329]

Sharma and Doble[330] suggested having perioperative team members provide regular updates (ie, hourly) of the time the patient's legs have been elevated in the lithotomy position.

Current evidence does not identify how long the patient needs to be repositioned before being returned to the lithotomy position.

XII.c. The safety restraint should not be placed over the patient's chest or abdomen. *[5: Benefits Balanced with Harms]*

Correct placement of the safety restraint is difficult in the lithotomy position. The literature does not discuss best practices for placement of the safety restraint when the patient is in the lithotomy position. The perioperative RN may not be able to place the restraint low across the patient's pelvis without restricting access to the surgical site. Use of a safety restraint that is placed high or too tight across the abdomen increases the risk for pressure injury or restricting respiration. The patient's legs may seem to be secure in the leg holders with his or her arms tucked at the sides; however, there is still a risk that the patient will shift on the procedure bed, especially when being moved in and out of Trendelenburg position, which is often used in conjunction with the lithotomy position. Safe positioning practices require the patient be attended at all times by at least one surgical team member when on the OR bed[28] (See Recommendation VI.b).

XII.d. The patient's buttocks should be even with the lower break of the procedure bed and positioned in a manner that securely supports the sacrum on the bed surface.[143] *[3: Moderate Evidence]*

Supporting the patient's sacrum reduces the potential for injury.[143]

XII.d.1. When the patient is in the exaggerated lithotomy position, the patient's sacrum should be supported.[144] *[5: Benefits Balanced with Harms]*

Placing a positioning support beneath the sacrum when the patient is in the exaggerated lithotomy position helps to support the patient's hips.

XII.e. The patient's hips should be positioned in a manner that prevents excessive flexion, rotation, or abduction.[209,304,310,331] *[3: Moderate Evidence]*

Excessive flexion (ie, more than 80 degrees to 90 degrees) or abduction (ie, more than 30 degrees to 45 degrees) puts stress on the patient's hip joints and can cause a femoral, sciatic, obturator, or common peroneal neuropathy.[5,11,12,68,209,214,331-333] The longer the patient is in an extreme lithotomy position, the more likely an injury is to occur.[331]

When candy cane–shaped leg holders are used, the patient's hips are particularly vulnerable to excessive rotation and hyperabduction.[209,334]

Patients who are obese are at increased risk for injury to joints, muscles, nerves, and soft tissue because the difficulty in identifying anatomic landmarks can make safe levels of knee and hip flexion hard to determine.[209] Overabduction can occur because of the size and weight of the patient's thighs and the need to create sufficient space for the surgical team.[209]

Notably, in a nonexperimental study, Pannucci et al[335] found that intraoperative positioning of the lower extremities represented a modifiable risk factor for prevention of DVT. The researchers used duplex ultrasound to measure common and proximal femoral vein diameter, peak systolic velocity, and volume flow in 12 healthy patients positioned supine with knee flexion at zero degrees, 30 degrees, 60 degrees, and 90 degrees. They found that in the common femoral vein, hip flexion at 90 degrees was associated with a significant increase in mean volume flow compared with hip flexion at zero degrees. The researchers concluded that when leg holders were used, hip flexion of 90 degrees maximized venous drainage from the legs.

XII.f. Leg holders should be placed at an even height.[12] *[3: Moderate Evidence]*

Placing the leg holders at an even height reduces the potential for injury that might occur if one leg is positioned higher than the other.[12]

XII.g. The patient's legs should be supported over the largest surface area of the leg possible.[36,159,300] *[3: Moderate Evidence]*

Supporting the leg over the largest surface area possible redistributes pressure and helps to prevent pressure injury.[159,300]

Boot-type leg holders support the entire leg, reducing the potential for nerve and pressure injury because pressure is evenly distributed over the leg and the foot.[159,209] Navarro-Vicente et al[336] conducted a prospective analysis of patients who underwent major colorectal abdominal surgery in a university hospital in Spain. The researchers found that eight (0.3%) of 2,304 patients developed a peripheral nerve injury. There was no association between nerve injury and patient age, sex, BMI, ASA classification, or urgent surgery; however, the use of a vacuum-packed positioning device and boot-type leg holders seemed to be protective for nerve injury in both the upper and lower limbs.

Knee-crutch leg holders support the weight of the patient's leg at the knee and may not redistribute pressure, increasing pressure on the popliteal space, which can injure the posterior and common peroneal nerves and the popliteal artery.[209,332] Increased pressure associated with knee-crutch leg holders can obstruct or slow venous and lymphatic return, increase the risk for hypoperfusion to the lower extremities, and increase intracompartmental pressures.[325] Mizuno and Takahashi[325] investigated external pressure applied to the calf region when using knee-crutch leg holders and found that external pressure measurements were higher in men than in women, and pressure levels significantly increased with increases in height, weight, and BMI for all participants.

Patients who are placed in lithotomy with Trendelenburg position and patients with a high BMI may be at increased risk for pressure injury even when boot-type leg holders are used. Yamada et al[337] measured contact pressures of the lower extremities in 138 patients undergoing robotic-assisted radical prostatectomy procedures in the lithotomy position with 25-degree Trendelenburg. The researchers found that 33 patients (23.9%) required adjustments in leg position because of high contact pressures (ie, > 32 mmHg). Contact pressures were significantly higher when the lithotomy with 25-degree Trendelenburg position was used than when a horizontal lithotomy position was used. The researchers also found a significant correlation between increased contact pressures and higher BMI levels.

XII.g.1. When using candy cane–shaped leg holders, additional padding should be placed around the patient's foot and ankle.[209] *[3: Moderate Evidence]*

When candy cane–shaped leg holders are used, the weight of the patient's leg is supported by the foot straps.[209] Placing additional padding around the foot and ankle may help to redistribute pressure over a larger area and decrease the potential for injury to the distal sural and plantar nerves.[209]

XII.h. The patient's heels should be placed in the lowest position possible.[300,306] *[3: Moderate Evidence]*

Evidence supports using the lowest possible lithotomy position and when possible, positioning the legs at or below the level of the heart.[301,302,304,306,307,312,318,329,338] In the high and exaggerated lithotomy positions, the calf is in a more vertical position and the legs are supported at the heel, placing the heel at risk for pressure injury.[300] The risk for compartment syndrome, rhabdomyolysis, and acute renal failure may also increase as the legs are elevated.[329,338] There is a reduction in lower limb arterial pressure and an increase in venous pressure in the high and exaggerated lithotomy positions that results in an increase in compartmental pressure, reducing blood flow and leading to local ischemia.[329,338]

In a prospective study, Liu et al[339] assigned 99 patients undergoing hysterectomy procedures into three groups. Group 1 patients underwent laparoscopic-assisted hysterectomy in the low lithotomy position (n = 36), Group 2 patients underwent vaginal hysterectomy in the standard lithotomy position (n = 32), and Group 3 patients underwent abdominal hysterectomy in the supine position (n = 31). The researchers measured lower extremity venous pressures at the start of the surgery and at 5, 10, and 45 minutes. The researchers found that Group 1 patients had the highest venous pressures and Group 3 patients had the lowest. The researchers concluded that both low lithotomy position with pneumoperitoneum and standard lithotomy position without pneumoperitoneum increased lower extremity venous pressures; therefore, placing the patient's heels in a lower position represented a modifiable risk factor for prevention of DVT.

XII.i. The patient's legs should not rest against the leg holder posts.[209,331] *[3: Moderate Evidence]*

The common peroneal nerve is vulnerable to injury from the fibular neck resting against the vertical post of the leg holder when the patient is in the lithotomy position.[11,12,214,331] An injury to the common peroneal nerve can cause a paresthesia of the lateral lower leg and dorsum of the foot and result in foot drop.[209,214,331] Pressure from the lower extremities resting against leg holder posts raises compartment pressures and also increases the risk for inadequate lower-extremity perfusion.[314]

XII.i.1. Scrubbed personnel should not lean against the patient's thighs.[214,301,331,334] *[3: Moderate Evidence]*

Leaning against the patient's inner thigh increases abduction and external rotation of the thighs and can cause a femoral neuropathy.[214,331,334]

XII.j. The patient's legs should be slowly and simultaneously placed into the leg holders by a minimum of two people (ie, a minimum of one person per leg).[21,36,41] *[2: High Evidence]*

Slowly and simultaneously raising and lowering the patient's legs allows the patient to adjust to the sudden shift in circulatory volume.[36,209,299] Patients with pre-existing depressed cardiac function may not tolerate sudden hemodynamic changes.[299] Having a minimum of two people move the patient's legs simultaneously into the leg holders helps avoid torsional stresses at the hip joint and pelvis and prevent injury to patients and personnel.[21,41,340] In some cases, additional personnel (eg, two people per leg) may be needed to safely place the patient's legs into the leg holders.[340]

XII.k. The patient's legs should be removed from the leg holders in a two-step process:
  1. A minimum of two people (ie, a minimum of one person per leg) should remove the legs slowly and simultaneously from the leg holders and bring them together before the legs are lowered to the OR bed.[209] *[3: Moderate Evidence]*
  2. The patient's legs should be simultaneously lowered to the OR bed. *[5: Benefits Balanced with Harms]*

Raising or lowering the patient's legs too rapidly can result in fluid volume shifts that affect blood pressure.[209] Having a minimum of two people move the patient's legs simultaneously out of the leg holders helps avoid torsional stresses at the hip joint and pelvis and prevent patient and personnel injury.[41] In some cases, additional personnel (eg, two people per leg) may be needed to safely remove the patient's legs from the leg holders.[340]

At the end of the procedure, the patient's overall circulating blood volume may be depleted when the patient's legs are lowered to the OR bed because of the blood returning quickly into the patient's peripheral circulation.[36] Simultaneously lowering the patient's legs to the OR bed may help to prevent rapid or unexpected circulatory changes.

Notably, the practice of slowly and simultaneously removing the legs from the leg holders, bringing the legs together before the legs are lowered to the OR bed, and then lowering one leg at a time to the OR bed is not incorrect and may further help to prevent rapid circulatory changes; however, there is no evidence to show this is necessary.

XII.l. Graduated compression stockings and/or intermittent pneumatic compression devices may be used on patients in the lithotomy position. *[3: Moderate Evidence]*

Evidence related to best practices for use of graduated compression stockings and intermittent pneumatic compression devices on patients in the lithotomy position is inconclusive. Extrinsic compression applied to the legs by graduated compression stockings or intermittent pneumatic compression devices may increase intracompartmental pressures, and this may be compounded by a prolonged lithotomy position.[309,312,314,315] It has been suggested that the combination of the lithotomy position and intermittent pneumatic compression devices impairs perfusion to muscles, which, because of the elevation of the legs in lithotomy position, are already subject to reduced perfusion.[314,341] The reperfusion of muscles caused by the cycling of the compression devices may exacerbate the potential for compartment syndrome by increasing compartmental pressures and extravasation through damaged endothelium.[315,341] For this reason it may be preferable to use other methods of venous thromboembolic prophylaxis.[312]

Rao and Jayne[304] recommended avoiding the combined use of graduated compression stockings and intermittent pneumatic compression devices, but also advised exercising the utmost of caution before omitting their combined use because the risk for DVT and pulmonary embolism is much greater than the risk for compartment syndrome. Raza et al[306] suggested that if both graduated compression stockings and pneumatic intermittent compression devices were used, it would be important to monitor the patient for potential signs of compartment syndrome, especially after a prolonged procedure.

Pfeffer et al[342] conducted a nonexperimental study to assess the effects of a pneumatic compression device on compartmental pressures in the lower leg with the leg positioned in lithotomy position. The researchers measured pressures in the tibialis anterior muscle compartment of 25 healthy volunteers with the leg supine and in the lithotomy position with and without intermittent compression. Three different leg holders were used for the lithotomy position that provided support behind the knee (knee-crutch), under the calf (boot-type), and at the ankle (candy cane–shaped).

The lithotomy position with support behind the knee or calf increased intracompartmental pressure. The addition of intermittent compression significantly decreased pressure during lithotomy and in the supine position. The researchers found that the lithotomy position with support at the ankle significantly decreased compartmental pressures. The researchers concluded that the changes in com-

partmental pressures in the lithotomy position were dependent on the type of leg holder used. The results of the study also showed that the use of intermittent compression significantly reduced compartmental pressures in the lower leg. The researchers cautioned that these results may not be applicable if the intermittent pneumatic compression devices are used with graduated compression stockings because of the constant pressure provided by the stockings.

Thromboembolic events are a serious and sometimes fatal event, and the risk for these events may be greater than the risk for compartment syndrome.[305,318,327] The patient's individual risk factors as well as the benefits and potential harms of not providing adequate DVT prophylaxis require careful evaluation.[303,305,318] It may be reasonable to continue the use of graduated compression stockings and intermittent pneumatic compression devices for thromboprophylaxis in patients undergoing surgical procedures in the lithotomy position.[327]

XII.m. The hemi-lithotomy position should not be used, if possible.[12] *[3: Moderate Evidence]*

Placing the patient's nonoperative leg in a hemi-lithotomy position predisposes it to the development of well-leg compartment syndrome.[12,328,343,344] In patients with an increased muscle mass, the hemi-lithotomy position can be sufficient to induce a compartment syndrome.[328] In a prospective study of 10 patients undergoing intramedullary nailing of a fractured femur in the hemi-lithotomy position, Tan et al[345] found that placement of the uninjured leg in the hemi-lithotomy position immediately increased the calf compartment pressure by more than 18 mmHg, and this pressure remained elevated until the leg was taken down. The researchers proposed that the immediate increase in compartment pressure was the direct result of mechanical compression from the leg holder. When the leg is elevated in the holder, the weight of it causes a decrease in the volume of the calf compartments pressing against the leg holder, causing the pressure within the compartments to rise. The researchers recommended avoiding the use of the hemi-lithotomy position.

Using a leg holder that allows the calf to remain free from pressure, rather than using a standard leg holder, may decrease the risk for compartment syndrome associated with the hemi-lithotomy position.[344]

Recommendation XIII

Perioperative team members should implement safe practices when positioning the patient in the sitting or semi-sitting or modifications of the sitting or semi-sitting position.

The sitting position is also known as the Fowler position. The semi-sitting position is also known as the semi-Fowler or beach chair position. These positions are used for access to the shoulder, posterior cervical spine, or posterior or lateral head.[144]

The sitting and semi-sitting positions are variants of the supine position with the head, neck, and torso elevated 20 degrees to 90 degrees, the hips flexed 45 degrees to 60 degrees, and the knees flexed 30 degrees.[118,346-348] These positions may be accompanied by 10 degrees to 15 degrees of Trendelenburg position.[118,346]

Advantages of the sitting or semi-sitting positions include improved surgical exposure and visual alignment with critical anatomy, access to the patient's airway, ease of mechanical ventilation, reduced intracranial pressure, reduced facial swelling, improved lung excursion and diaphragmatic activity, and reduced blood pooling in the surgical field.[7,144,191,347-353]

Complications that may arise from the use of the sitting or semi-sitting positions include VAE, hemodynamic instability, pneumocephalus, quadriplegia, and compressive peripheral neuropathy.[191,348,351,352,354] A known patent foramen ovale may be a contraindication to the sitting or semi-sitting position because of the potential for a VAE to pass into the systemic arterial circulation.[348,349] There is a risk for cerebrovascular insult with these positions, and this risk is magnified when the patient is hypotensive.[353,354] There is a risk for poor venous return from the lower extremities and pooling of blood in the patient's pelvis in the sitting or semi-sitting position.[350]

The sitting or semi-sitting position may also affect bispectral index values, which are used to evaluate depth of anesthesia and prevent patient awareness during surgery.[355] Lee et al[355] found there was a significant decrease in bispectral index values associated with a change from the supine to the semi-sitting position, and this could potentially affect interpretation of the depth of anesthesia.

XIII.a.   When positioning the patient in sitting or semi-sitting position, the patient should be positioned as described in Recommendations VIII and XIII.

      Guidance for safe practices in positioning the patient is provided in Recommendation VIII.

      Guidance for safe practices in positioning the patient in the sitting or semi-sitting position is provided in this section (Recommendation XIII).

XIII.b.   In the sitting or semi-sitting position, the degree of patient head elevation should be minimized as much as possible. *[2: High Evidence]*

      A lesser degree of patient head elevation may reduce the incidence of hypotension and the potential for subsequent cerebral desaturation.[356,357] The sitting and semi-sitting positions may cause hypotensive, bradycardic events leading to cerebral desaturation.[356,358,359] There is evidence to suggest a strong positive correlation between the degree of head elevation in the sitting or semi-sitting position and cerebral desaturation events.[356,358,360-365] Cerebral desaturation puts the brain at risk for ischemic injury, and

the anesthetized patient is unable to express that cerebral blood flow has been reduced.[363] The consequences of cerebral desaturation include cognitive decline, organ morbidity, stroke, and death.[354,359] In the sitting and semi-sitting positions, there is a reduction in mean arterial pressure[366] and a significant decrease in cerebral artery blood flow velocity and autoregulatory response[366-368] that could lead to ischemia[368] or cognitive decline.[366]

Salazar et al[362] reviewed the literature to determine the incidence of postoperative neurocognitive deficits, number of reported complications, and incidence of postoperative cerebral desaturation events in patients who underwent arthroscopic surgery in the sitting or semi-sitting position. The authors analyzed 10 studies with a composite enrollment of 24,701 patients undergoing shoulder surgery in the sitting or semi-sitting position and found only one case of postoperative neurocognitive deficit (0.004%). The authors also identified four case reports of six patients with catastrophic neurocognitive complications after shoulder surgery in the sitting or semi-sitting position. In addition, the authors analyzed seven studies where a total of 287 patients were monitored for cerebral desaturation events. The authors found that the mean incidence of cerebral desaturation events was 41.1%.

There is also evidence to suggest that despite hypotension occurring in the sitting or semi-sitting position, its correlation with decreased cerebral desaturation or autoregulation has yet to be determined.[353,364,369-371] The role of hypoperfusion in cerebral infarction is unclear.[353] As well, there is a lack of evidence to define the degree and duration of cerebral desaturation required to produce a definitive and measurable neurocognitive decline.[356,372] In a blinded prospective study, Yadeau et al[369] measured cerebral oximetry levels in 99 patients undergoing ambulatory shoulder arthroscopy in the sitting position with a mean head to heart distance of 12.6 inches (32 cm). The researchers found that hypotension occurred 76% of the time with a mean duration of 71 minutes, but cerebral desaturation occurred only 0.77% of the time with a mean duration of 7 minutes. The researchers suggested that despite the presence of hypotension, adequate cerebral perfusion was maintained.

Tange et al[370] evaluated tissue oxygen index values in 30 patients undergoing shoulder surgery in the 60-degree semi-sitting position. They found that as long as the patient's blood pressure was maintained above 60 mmHg, the semi-sitting position did not alter cerebral oxygenation. To evaluate changes in cerebral tissue oxygen index values associated with the 60-degree semi-sitting position and the 90-degree sitting position, Mori et al[373] enrolled

28 healthy patients, 33 patients with one cardiovascular risk factor, and 30 patients with more than one cardiovascular risk factor (N = 91) in a prospective study. Cardiovascular risk factors included cardiac diseases, diabetes mellitus, hypertension, hypercholesterolemia, and smoking. The researchers found that the tissue oxygen index values were in the normal range of 70% before and during anesthesia in all groups.

Pin-on et al[371] conducted a comprehensive retrospective review of the records of 5,177 patients who underwent surgery in the sitting or semi-sitting position and found there were no ischemic brain injuries.

XIII.c. The patient's head should be maintained in a neutral position without excessive flexion, extension, or rotation.[349,374] *[3: Moderate Evidence]*

Maintaining the patient's head in a neutral position when the patient is in a sitting or semi-sitting position can be challenging; however, extremes of neck flexion, extension, or rotation can result in patient injury.[346,375] Flexion of the head against the chest can lead to venous and lymphatic congestion, resulting in macroglossia.[376] Amukoa et al[374] recommended maintaining a minimum space of 1 inch (2.5 cm) between the patient's chin and chest to preserve airway patency and allow venous drainage from the face and tongue. Lindroos et al[348] also suggested that a 2-fingerbreadth distance between the patient's chin and sternum is mandatory. Hyperextension of the patient's neck could result in a spinal cord injury.[349,375] Rotation of the patient's neck while in a sitting or semi-sitting position could result in a neuropathy caused by compression and stretching of the glossopharyngeal, vagus, and hypoglossal nerves.[350]

XIII.c.1. Perioperative team members should assess and monitor the patient's head position after positioning activities and during the procedure and implement corrective actions as indicated.[374,375] *[3: Moderate Evidence]*

Assessing and monitoring the patient's head position may help prevent patient injury. Rhee and Cho[377] described two cases of hypoglossal nerve palsy after shoulder surgery. Both patients (ie, a 41-year-old man and a 71-year-old man) were positioned in a 70-degree semi-sitting position for the diagnostic shoulder arthroscopy and a 30-degree semi-sitting position for the open Bankhart repair. In both cases, the procedure lasted approximately 90 minutes. In addition, in both cases, the patients' heads were immobilized by an adhesive plaster strip from the headrest across the forehead and a second adhesive plaster strip across the chin. After surgery, both patients reported difficulty pronouncing words, and they were diagnosed with a unilateral hypoglossal neurop-

athy that resolved within 6 weeks. The authors concluded that the most likely cause of both injuries was the change from the 70-degree to 30-degree semi-sitting position. They speculated that the change in position affected the position of the head and neck and led to unintended compression on the hypoglossal nerve.

Liang[378] opined on the duty of the perioperative team members to monitor the patient's head position during surgical procedures in describing the case of an obese woman who underwent cervical spinal surgery in the sitting position with her head flexed toward her chest. The surgeon and perioperative RN taped the patient's head to a horseshoe-shaped head positioner to prevent it from moving during the procedure but did not provide any additional padding to the patient's head or neck. When the procedure was completed, the patient was transferred to the postanesthesia care unit, where she lapsed into a coma after 20 minutes. When she emerged from the coma, the patient was only able to move one finger and to slightly move one foot. The physicians concluded that she had suffered bilateral strokes from carotid artery obstruction resulting in permanent paraplegia.

The patient sued the surgeon, anesthesiologist, and RN anesthetist. Expert physicians testifying at the trial agreed that the carotid artery obstruction resulted from the patient's chin resting on her sternum, either during the positioning process or sometime during the surgery. On cross examination, both anesthesia professionals acknowledged an obligation to inspect the patient during the procedure and ensure the patient's head is not in a position that might lead to clinical problems. If their inspections reveal a need to reposition the patient, their obligation is to inform the surgeon so that the issue can be addressed. The appeals court also observed that the only way to be assured that the patient's head remains in the correct position is through visual inspection and monitoring. Although they had attached monitors to the patient, neither of the anesthesia professionals had lifted the drapes to check the position of the patient's head. This failure to verify the patient's position was determined to be the cause of the injury to the patient.[378]

XIII.c.2. A horseshoe-shaped head positioner should not be used,[349] if possible. *[3: Moderate Evidence]*

Using a horseshoe-shaped head positioner may cause pressure on the lesser occipital or the greater auricular nerve, resulting in a neuropathy.[349,379] The greater auricular nerve is vulnerable to injury because of its superficial location.[379,380]

XIII.d. In the sitting or semi-sitting position, the patient's arms or nonoperative arm should be flexed across the body and secured.[21,118,144,346] *[3: Moderate Evidence]*

Flexing the patient's arm(s) across the body provides surgical access and a physiologic position.

XIII.d.1. The patient's operative arm may be
- held by the surgeon or surgical assistant or
- supported by an arm-positioning device designed for this purpose.[118,347]
[3: Moderate Evidence]

Using an arm-positioning device during shoulder surgery may improve visibility within the joint and provide tension on the tissues being repaired.[347] If an arm holder is not used, an assistant may be required to apply traction or joint distraction.[347]

XIII.d.2. Extension and external rotation of the patient's operative arm should be minimized as much as possible.[158] *[3: Moderate Evidence]*

Minimizing extension and external rotation of the patient's operative arm may help to prevent injury. Evidence does not define the safe limit of extension or external rotation.[158]

XIII.e. The patient's buttocks should be padded.[21] *[3: Moderate Evidence]*

Padding the patient's buttocks helps prevent excessive pressure on the sciatic nerve and coccyx.[191] Prolonged pressure on the buttocks during surgery in the sitting position can lead to muscle trauma and spasm of the piriformis muscle and resultant compression of the sciatic nerve.[381,382]

XIII.f. The patient's knees should be flexed 30 degrees.[118,346-349] *[3: Moderate Evidence]*

Flexing the patient's knees reduces stretching of the sciatic nerve and may help to prevent a postoperative neuropathy.[383]

Notably, there is no evidence to specify the necessary degree of flexion required to prevent neuropathy; however, several authors have recommended 30 degrees of knee flexion in the sitting or semi-sitting position.[118,346-348]

XIII.g. After the patient is moved into a sitting or semi-sitting position, the perioperative RN should
- prevent the patient's abdominal pannus from resting on the thighs, if possible, and
- verify placement and security of the safety restraint across the patient's thighs. *[3: Moderate Evidence]*

Satin et al[384] described occurrences of lateral femoral cutaneous nerve palsy in four obese patients undergoing shoulder surgery in the semi-sitting position with a safety restraint applied across the thighs. The procedure times ranged from 95 minutes to 220 minutes. All patients reported severe pain and numbness in the anterolateral thighs after surgery, and in all cases, the pain and numbness resolved within 3 to 6 months. The authors noted that in patients who are obese, abdominal distention, increased visceral weight, or abundance of adipose tissue may cause the abdominal wall to bend over itself, pushing on the inguinal ligament and forcing the iliac fascia surrounding the lateral femoral cutaneous nerve to compress the underlying nerve. The authors concluded that the injuries in the reported cases were likely caused by external compression from the abdominal pannus resting on the patient's thighs. They recommended preventing the patient's abdominal pannus from resting on the thighs and reassessing the tightness of the restraint after the patient is moved into the semi-sitting position.

Notably, some methods of securing the abdominal pannus away from the thighs (eg, taping the abdomen) could lead to patient injury (eg, skin breakdown, abdominal compression); therefore, when attempting to prevent the patient's abdominal pannus from resting on the thighs, it is necessary to implement safe positioning practices and to evaluate the benefits compared with potential harms of the methods used.

A correctly placed safety restraint across the patient's thighs can tighten when the patient is moved into a sitting or semi-sitting position.[384]

XIII.h. Sequential compression devices may be used when the patient is in the sitting or semi-sitting position.[349] *[1: Strong Evidence]*

Using sequential compression devices limits venous pooling and enhances venous return from the legs.[349,374,385,386]

Kwak et al[385] conducted an RCT to investigate the effect of intermittent pneumatic sequential compression devices on the incidence of hypotension and other hemodynamic variables in the semi-sitting position. The researchers randomly assigned 50 healthy patients undergoing elective shoulder arthroscopy under general anesthesia to either the control group (n = 25) or the sequential compression devices group (n = 25). They measured hemodynamic variables before induction and at 5 minutes after the induction of anesthesia in the supine position and again at 1, 3, and 5 minutes after the patient was raised to a 70-degree semi-sitting position. The researchers found that the incidence of hypotension was significantly higher in the control group (n = 16; 64%) than in the sequential compression devices group (n = 7; 28%). The mean arterial pressure, cardiac index, and stroke volume index were also significantly higher in the sequential compression devices group than in the control group. The researchers concluded that the use of intermittent pneumatic sequential compression devices reduced the incidence of hypotension and supported venous return from the legs when patients were in the semi-sitting position.

XIII.i. The sitting position should not be used for patients with ventriculoperitoneal shunts, if possible. *[3: Moderate Evidence]*

Prabhakar et al[387] reported the case of a 4-year-old girl with a ventriculoperitoneal shunt who underwent an elective midline suboccipital craniectomy in the sitting position for removal of a pineal tumor. The surgery lasted 4 hours. During a postoperative position change, the authors noted a large pneumocephalus and a right parietal hematoma. The surgeons performed a burr hole evacuation of the hematoma, and the pneumocephalus resolved without intervention. The authors concluded that the ventriculoperitoneal shunt tube led to excessive drainage of cerebrospinal fluid that resulted in intracranial hypotension and rupture of bridging veins, leading to the pneumocephalus and hematoma. They recommended not using the sitting position for patients with ventriculoperitoneal shunts.

XIII.j. The perioperative team should be prepared to detect and implement interventions to manage VAE events.[388-390] *[3: Moderate Evidence]*

Venous air embolism can occur when air or gas is drawn into the circulation by the veins above the level of the heart and is most likely to occur during neurosurgery or open shoulder surgery in the sitting or semi-sitting position.[347-349,351,352,389-392] Rushatamukayanunt et al[391] found that the incidence of VAE was significantly higher in the sitting position (41.3%) than the horizontal positions (ie, prone and lateral; 11.0%). Venous air embolism can occur in any position in which the operative site is higher than the right atrium[388] and may also occur in the supine, reverse Trendelenburg, lateral, or prone positions.[191,388-391]

Venous air embolism can pass into the systemic arterial circulation and lead to ischemia of vital organs.[348] It can lead to cardiovascular collapse caused by obstruction of outflow from the heart with pulmonary hypertension and paradoxical air embolism.[351] The incidence of VAE is not well tolerated in patients with chronic obstructive pulmonary disease, and thus, chronic obstructive pulmonary disease may be a contraindication to using the sitting position.[352]

Successful treatment of VAE requires prompt recognition and rapid and simultaneous implementation of multiple interventions by the perioperative team.[351,388-391] If not diagnosed and treated immediately, VAE can be fatal.[388,391]

Notably, in addition to air, there are other potential embolic sources (eg, atherosclerotic plaque, thromboemboli, fat, bone).[349] Perelló et al[393] reported the case of a 49-year-old woman who developed a bone embolism during a craniectomy performed in the sitting position. At the end of the procedure, the patient had an episode of atrial bigeminy accompanied by an abrupt decrease in ETCO$_2$. The patient was diagnosed with a VAE, and the surgeons attempted to aspirate the air through her central venous catheter; however, rather than air, they recovered bone fragments.

XIII.j.1. Venous air embolism should be managed by
- ventilating the patient with 100% oxygen[351,374,389,390,394];
- controlling bone, dural sinus, and muscle bleeding[340,351,394];
- filling the surgical wound with irrigation fluid or packing it with saline-soaked sponges[348,351,374,389,394];
- placing the patient in left lateral and Trendelenburg position[351,374,390,394];
- attempting to aspirate entrained air from a right atrial catheter[351,374,389,390];
- initiating cardiac compressions with the patient in supine and Trendelenburg position[374,389,390];
- administering IV fluids and vasopressors[351,374,389,390];
- implementing transesophageal echocardiography[394]; and
- using ETCO$_2$.[394] *[3: Moderate Evidence]*

The goal of air embolism management is to prevent further air entry, reduce the volume of entrained air, and provide hemodynamic support.[388-390]

Ventilating the patient with 100% oxygen maximizes patient oxygenation, aids elimination of nitrogen, and reduces embolus volume.[389,390]

Controlling bone, dural sinus, and muscle bleeding and filling the surgical wound with irrigation fluid or packing it with saline-soaked sponges helps prevent further entrainment of air.[389]

Changing the patient's position may help prevent air from traveling through the right side of the heart into the pulmonary arteries.[388,390]

Aspiration of entrained air from a central venous catheter in the right atrium may be effective; however, there are no data to support emergent catheter insertion for air aspiration during an acute VAE event.[389,390]

Initiating cardiac compressions may help to break large bubbles into smaller ones and force air out of the right ventricle into the pulmonary vessels, thus improving cardiac output.[390]

Infusion of IV fluids optimizes myocardial perfusion and may help to push the blocked airlock into the lungs where it can be absorbed.[389,390] Volume expansion increases intravascular volume and central venous pressure and may reduce further gas entry.[351,388] Administration of vasopressors increases the force and speed of ventricular contractions.[389,390]

Implementing transesophageal echocardiography may help to confirm the diagnosis of VAE.[394]

Using ETCO$_2$ can assist in assessing cardiac output and monitoring the progression and resolution of VAE.[394]

XIII.j.2. Bilateral jugular compression may be used when managing VAE.[348,374,389]

Applying jugular compression may be effective in limiting the entry of air into the chest and right atrium from sources in the face and head by increasing venous pressure; however, increased intracranial pressure and subsequent decreased cerebral perfusion may be a direct consequence of this technique.[389,390] Additional concerns include the potential for direct carotid artery compression resulting in possible dislodgement of atheromatous plaque, venous engorgement leading to cerebral edema, and carotid sinus stimulation resulting in severe bradycardia.[389,390]

Recommendation XIV

Perioperative team members should implement safe practices when positioning the patient in the lateral or modifications of the lateral position.

In the lateral position, the patient is positioned on the nonoperative side.[5,144] In a right lateral position, the patient is lying on his or her right side.[144] This position provides exposure for a left-sided procedure.[144] In a left lateral position, the patient is lying on his or her left side. This position provides exposure for a right-sided procedure. The dependent side is the reference point for documentation.

The lateral position is used for orthopedic procedures involving the hip and, with some modification, for kidney and thoracic procedures.[5,21,36,191] The lateral position may be preferred to the prone position for patients who are obese, as the bulk of the patient's panniculus can be displaced off the abdomen.[74]

A patient in the lateral position is at risk for injury from pressure on vulnerable points on the dependent side (ie, ear, acromion process, olecranon, iliac crest, greater trochanter, lateral knee, malleolus).[21] In a retrospective review of position-related complications in 71 patients undergoing surgery in the lateral position, Furuno et al[395] found that one patient developed rhabdomyolysis and one patient developed a transient peroneal nerve palsy, but 22 patients developed Stage 1 pressure injuries (31%), and 12 patients developed Stage 2 pressure injuries (17%).

During prolonged surgery in the lateral position, the patient can experience local muscle compression with ischemia and subsequent reperfusion injury leading to compartment syndrome or rhabdomyolysis.[396] Woernle et al[396] examined serum creatinine kinase (CK) levels as

markers of muscle injury in 150 patients undergoing neurosurgical procedures in the supine or prone (n = 100) or lateral (n = 50) positions. The researchers found that postoperative CK levels were significantly elevated after procedures in the lateral position. Elevated CK levels may lead to acute renal, hepatic, and respiratory complications. The researchers concluded that the elevated CK levels resulted from increased pressure associated with the lateral position.

The weight of the abdomen is shifted away from the diaphragm; however, prolonged lateral positioning can lead to vascular congestion and relative hypoventilation in the dependent lung.[7,69,234] In the lateral position, the dependent lung receives a larger blood flow and the upper lung is easier to ventilate (ie, ventilation-perfusion mismatch).[7,36] Patients with pre-existing cardiac or pulmonary disease may not be able to tolerate these physiologic changes.[36,397]

Patients with osteoporosis or other degenerative orthopedic diseases may be at risk for fracture or spinal misalignment when placed in the lateral position.[21,37,398]

In a prospective observational study of 29 consecutive patients undergoing thoracic surgery in the lateral position, Hemmerling et al[399] measured cerebral saturation to detect differences between the upper and lower hemispheres. The researchers found significantly higher saturation levels in the upper hemisphere compared with the lower hemisphere. Notably, there may be no clinical impact associated with this finding.

XIV.a. The patient should be in the lateral position for the shortest time possible.[110,400,401] *[3: Moderate Evidence]*

Reducing the length of time the patient is placed in lateral position decreases the potential for rhabdomyolysis.[400,401] Dakwar et al[402] performed a retrospective review of 315 patients who underwent minimally invasive spinal surgery in the lateral position. The authors found that five patients (1.6%) developed rhabdomyolysis and acute renal failure. They concluded that the etiology of the rhabdomyolysis was likely multifactorial; however, all patients had been secured in the lateral position with safety straps and adhesive tape for the entire procedure, and all patients had operative times longer than 4 hours.

XIV.a.1. Patients in the lateral position may be repositioned at established intervals during the procedure. *[3: Moderate Evidence]*

Evidence indicates that repositioning the patient at established intervals during the procedure may reduce the risk for compartment syndrome or other injury associated with prolonged lateral position.[110,400]

XIV.a.2. Repositioning interventions and repositioning intervals should be
- based on the individual patient and the specific situation[19] *[1: Strong Evidence]* and

- established by the perioperative team before the beginning of the procedure, if possible.[182] *[4: Limited Evidence]*

XIV.b. A head positioner or pillow should be placed under the patient's head.[21] *[3: Moderate Evidence]*

Supporting the patient's head helps maintain cervical and thoracic alignment and prevent lateral flexion of the neck that could stretch the brachial plexus.[5,11,36,144] Using a head positioner may help to reduce pressure on the dependent ear.[5]

XIV.b.1. The patient's dependent ear should be assessed and monitored after positioning and during the procedure and corrective actions implemented as indicated.[36] *[3: Moderate Evidence]*

Assessing and monitoring the patient's dependent ear verifies it is not folded.

XIV.b.2. A horseshoe-shaped head positioner should not be used, if possible. *[3: Moderate Evidence]*

Mechanical compression from a horseshoe-shaped head positioner has been reported as a cause of postoperative facial edema and acute unilateral parotid enlargement in the lateral position.[403]

XIV.c. The patient's arms may be supported and secured on two level and parallel arm boards, with one arm on each arm board, the upper arm above the lower arm, and both arms abducted less than 90 degrees.[36,144]

- The lower arm should be positioned on the same plane as the OR bed mattress, with the forearm and wrist in a neutral position and the palm up.[36]
- The upper arm should be positioned on the same plane as the shoulder, with the forearm and wrist in a neutral position and the palm down.[36]

[3: Moderate Evidence]

Incorrect placement of the patient's arms could cause a stretching or compression injury.[143,156]

XIV.c.1. The patient's operative arm may be
- held by the surgeon or surgical assistant or
- suspended by a positioning device designed for this purpose.

If the patient's arm is suspended, it should not be abducted more than 90 degrees.[11,118] *[3: Moderate Evidence]*

The risk for brachial plexus injury and occlusion of the subclavian or axillary arteries is increased when the patient's arm is abducted more than 90 degrees.[11,12,36,38,68,143,156-158,191,214]

XIV.d. An axillary roll should be placed under the patient's dependent thorax, distal to the axil-lary fold, at the level of the seventh to ninth rib.[21,36,41,118,143,144,191,404] *[3: Moderate Evidence]*

Using an axillary roll improves compliance of the patient's dependent hemithorax and improves cardiac output.[118,144,191] Placing the axillary roll below the axilla provides support for the rib cage, reduces pressure on the head of the dependent humerus, and avoids compression of the axillary neurovascular bundle.[5,7,11,36,118,144,191]

Notably, the term *axillary roll* is a misnomer. The word axillary implies an incorrect and potentially dangerous location for the positioning support.[144] Placing the axillary roll in the axilla can injure the long thoracic nerve,[404] cause vascular obstruction, or compromise IV infusions or intra-arterial monitors if present in the dependent arm.[144] The word roll may imply that the positioning support is composed of a rolled sheet or towel. Rolled sheets and towels do not redistribute pressure.

XIV.d.1. A device designed for use as an axillary support should be used. *[5: Benefits Balanced with Harms]*

Using devices designed for use as axillary supports reduces the potential for patient injury that might occur when a device is used that is not designed for this purpose (eg, an IV bag).

XIV.d.2. The axillary support should be wide enough to spread its lifting ability over the area of several contiguous ribs.[144] *[5: Benefits Balanced with Harms]*

XIV.d.3. The patient's bilateral radial pulses should be verified after positioning in the lateral position and placement of the axillary roll, and corrective actions should be taken as indicated.[143,191] *[3: Moderate Evidence]*

Verifying bilateral peripheral pulses confirms adequate blood flow in the dependent arm.[36,191,405]

XIV.e. The patient's physiologic spinal alignment should be maintained.[5,11,36,41,144,191] *[3: Moderate Evidence]*

Maintaining the patient's physiologic spinal alignment reduces the potential for injury.[11]

XIV.f. The patient's breasts and abdomen should not be compressed or hang over the edge of the OR bed.[6,191] *[3: Moderate Evidence]*

XIV.g. A safety restraint should be placed across the patient's hips.[144] *[5: Benefits Balanced with Harms]*

Placing a safety restraint across the patient's hips provides stability.[144]

XIV.h. The patient's dependent leg should be flexed at the hip and knee.[21,143,144,191] The patient's upper leg should be straight and supported with pillows between the legs.[21,144,191] *[3: Moderate Evidence]*

715

Flexing the patient's dependent leg provides a wide base of support that helps to stabilize the pelvis.[143,144] Maintaining the patient's upper leg in a straight position provides stability and also ensures that the bony prominences of the upper leg do not rest against the bony prominences of the dependent leg.[144] Placing pillows between the patient's legs facilitates venous drainage and helps to prevent pressure injury.[7,144]

XIV.h.1. The patient's dependent knee, ankle, and foot should be padded.[5,21,118,143] *[3: Moderate Evidence]*

The lateral position increases the risk for injury to the common peroneal nerve.[11] Using padding helps to protect the peroneal nerve on the dependent leg from being compressed between the fibula and the OR bed.[5,11,41]

XIV.i. The degree of bed flexion and the duration of kidney rest elevation used to provide additional exposure (eg, renal procedures, thoracic procedures) should be minimized as much as possible.[110] *[3: Moderate Evidence]*

Flexing the OR bed widens the intercostal spaces.[36,110] Raising the kidney rest increases the amount of flexion and improves exposure.[36,110] However, flexing the OR bed and/or raising the kidney rest increases interface pressures, which may increase the patient's risk for pressure injury.[110]

Deane et al[110] conducted a quasi-experimental study to determine whether changes in interface pressures could be related to BMI, sex, position, or the table surface material. The researchers recruited 20 healthy volunteers (ie, 10 men, 10 women) and grouped them according to BMI (< 25 kg/m^2 = 5 men, 5 women; ≥ 25 kg/m^2 = 5 men, 5 women). The researchers placed the participants in left lateral position with the OR bed flat, half-flexed (ie, 25 degrees), fully-flexed (ie, 50 degrees), half-flexed with the kidney brace elevated, and fully-flexed with the kidney brace elevated. They recorded interface pressures for 5-minute periods in each position. The researchers found that full-bed flexion produced significantly higher pressures than both flat and half-flexed positions. Positions with the kidney rest elevated were also associated with significantly higher pressures than without the kidney rest. The researchers recommended decreasing the amount of bed flexion and limiting the duration of the elevation of the kidney rest.

XIV.i.1. When kidney braces are used,
- the longer brace should be placed anteriorly, against the iliac crest and
- the shorter brace should be placed posteriorly, against the lumbar back.[406]

[3: Moderate Evidence]

If the kidney brace is aligned under the patient's flank rather than the iliac crest,

ventilation of the dependent lung is restricted.[36]

The lateral position requires supports that do not press against the abdomen to avoid impairing venous drainage from the lower limbs.[406]

Recommendation XV

Perioperative team members should implement safe practices when positioning the patient in the prone or modifications of the prone position.

The prone position provides surgical access to the dorsal aspects of the patient's body.[36] The jack-knife, or Kraske, position is a variation of the prone position that provides additional exposure for sacral, rectal, or perineal areas. The knee-chest position is a modification of the prone position that provides exposure for spinal procedures and offers the advantage of reduced abdominal pressure.[191]

The prone position produces an increase in functional residual capacity and alterations in the distribution of both ventilation and perfusion throughout the lungs.[407] These changes improve ventilation/perfusion matching and consequently improve oxygenation.[407]

In a systematic review of the literature, Kwee et al[408] identified 13 potential complications associated with the prone position that included
- increased intra-abdominal pressure,
- increased bleeding,
- abdominal compartment syndrome,
- limb compartment syndrome,
- nerve injuries,
- pressure injuries,
- cardiovascular compromise,
- thrombosis and stroke,
- hepatic dysfunction,
- ocular injuries,
- oropharyngeal swelling,
- airway maintenance device dislodgement, and
- VAE.

Intra-abdominal, intrathoracic, and intraocular pressures are increased in the prone position.[407-411] Changes in intra-abdominal pressure and resultant epidural venous congestion can influence airway pressures and cause increased intraoperative blood loss.[407,409,410,412] The prone position can also cause sudden changes in inferior vena cava pressure.[407,413] These changes can be a contributing factor in the migration of an inferior vena cava filter, especially flexible retrievable filters.[413]

Patients who are obese may have increased intra-abdominal and central venous pressures in the prone position related to increased abdominal girth.[411] These physiologic changes reduce systemic venous return and cardiac output and can lead to reduced end-organ blood flow.[411] Han et al[414] studied the effect of BMI on intra-abdominal pressure and found that intra-abdominal pressures were significantly higher in obese individuals (ie, BMI 25.0 kg/m^2 to 29.9 kg/m^2) than in normal-weight individuals (ie, BMI 18.5 kg/m^2 to 22.9 kg/m^2) when in the prone position. This higher intra-abdominal pressure resulted in significantly increased intraoperative blood loss in obese individuals (495 mL ± 88 mL) compared with normal-weight individuals (435 mL ± 65 mL).

Elevated intra-abdominal pressure significantly increases the risk for abdominal compartment syndrome.[408] Patients who are obese or who have had previous abdominal surgeries are at increased risk for abdominal compartment syndrome when in the prone position.[408]

Elevated intracompartmental pressures associated with the prone position can lead to reduced limb perfusion.[408] Inadequate blood supply to the limbs can result in ischemia, which in turn leads to edema that further increases intracompartmental pressures.[408] Ischemia leads to tissue necrosis, rhabdomyolysis, and renal failure.[408] Factors such as obesity, large muscle mass, peripheral vascular disease, and prolonged procedures augment the patient's risk for limb compartment syndrome.[408]

Surgery in the prone position increases the risk for neuropathic injury to the cervical spine and brachial plexus because of excessive pressure or stretch by flexion, extension, or lateral rotation.[408]

Patients who undergo procedures in the prone position are vulnerable to pressure injury on the face, breasts, lower costal margins, iliac crests, genitalia, knees, and toes.[21,36] Patients with breast implants have a theoretical risk for rupture of the implants if they are placed under direct pressure while the patient is in the prone position.[408] Respiratory function may be decreased as a result of compression on the rib cage and diaphragm.[21,36,69,144]

Hemodynamic changes associated with the prone or jack-knife position (ie, reduced cardiac output and cardiac index, increased systemic vascular resistance[407]) could increase the risk for cardiovascular compromise or collapse in patients with limited cardiovascular reserve.[408,415,416] Hemodynamic changes may be more pronounced in patients with increased thoracic and intra-abdominal pressure or with truncal obesity or when prone positioning is modified to improve surgical access (eg, exaggerated lumbar flexion).[416]

The prone position increases the patient's risk for thrombosis and stroke caused by position-related occlusion of blood flow that may lead to stasis and clotting.[408] Kinking of blood vessels related to lateral rotation of the patient's head increases the potential for intimal injury and thrombosis formation.[408]

Hepatic dysfunction can be a consequence of the increased central venous pressure associated with the prone position.[408,410] Increased central venous pressure in combination with anesthetic-induced hypotension could lead to hypoperfusion and ischemic hepatitis.[408]

General anesthesia decreases tear production and the potential for ocular injuries that include desiccation, irritation, abrasion, laceration, and subsequent inflammation or infection is increased in the prone position.[408] Ocular complications associated with the prone position include increased intraocular pressure, decreased tissue perfusion, conjunctival edema, hemorrhage, chemosis, and postoperative vision loss.[408] Patients who are predisposed to acute angle-closure glaucoma are at high risk for ocular injury even during short procedures because the prone position can shift the lens-iris diaphragm forward so it obstructs aqueous humor outflow and increases intraocular pressure.[408] Several risk factors are associated with postoperative vision loss including prolonged procedural time, high-volume infusion, intraoperative anemia, and hypotension.[417] When these risk factors are combined with a head-down position or extreme rotation of the head to one side, they may result in a loss of vision because of compromised blood flow to the optic nerve.[417]

In the prone position, gravity causes an accumulation of extravascular fluid in any dependent body part, including the hands, feet, face, and conjunctiva.[36] The longer the procedure, the more dramatic the edema.[36] This transient edema can also affect the nose, oropharynx, salivary glands, and tongue. For this reason, it may be necessary to keep the patient intubated during the immediate postoperative period.[36,408]

Both the prone and the lateral position cause dilation of the airway as a result of gravitational effects on anatomic structures. There is an increased risk for airway maintenance device displacement or dislodgement.[408]

The risk for air entrainment through the surgical wound into the venous system and the potential for VAE is greater when the surgical site is elevated above the heart or the patient is hypotensive, as may occur when the patient is in the prone position.[408]

Venous congestion associated with the prone position can lead to a rise in middle ear pressure, although the mechanism and effects of these pressure changes warrant further research.[418]

The prone position may result in impaired cerebral venous drainage with a subsequent reduction in cerebral perfusion[419]; however, the effects of the prone position on cerebral oxygenation and perfusion are inconclusive. Closhen et al[419] found a small increase in cerebral oxygen saturation of less than 5% in patients undergoing orthopedic surgery in the prone position and in awake volunteers. Babakhani et al[420] found that cerebral oxygenation could be maintained in the prone position as long as hypotension and bradycardia were prevented. Deiner et al[421] found that older patients in the prone position were more than twice as likely to experience mild cerebral desaturation as older patients in the supine position.

In a prospective observational study of 30 children ages 13 to 18 years positioned prone for scoliosis correction surgery, Brown et al[422] found there was a reduction in cardiac index and mean arterial pressure, but these changes were not significant. Further research is warranted to determine whether the effects of the prone position on cerebral oxygenation and perfusion are associated with postoperative neurological deficit.

XV.a.   Patients in the prone position should be positioned in 5-degree to 10-degree reverse Trendelenburg, if possible.[18,69,184,283,423-426] *[1: Strong Evidence]*

Positioning surgical patients with the head above the heart helps reduce venous congestion in the eye and orbit and decrease intraocular and intraorbital pressure.[118,236,425,427,428] Positioning the

717

patient in 5-degree to 10-degree reverse Trendelenburg also decreases facial edema.[118] Emery et al[429] conducted an RCT to evaluate intraocular pressures in 63 patients undergoing lumbar spine surgery in the prone position. In 27 patients, the head was maintained in a horizontal position during the surgery. In 25 patients, the head of the OR bed was elevated to 10-degree reverse Trendelenburg position during the surgery. The researchers found that the mean intraocular pressure for the head-elevated group was significantly lower than the mean intraocular pressure for the horizontal group. The researchers concluded that this intervention could mitigate the risk for postoperative blindness associated with increased intraocular pressure.

XV.a.1. The Wilson frame should not be used,[411] if possible. *[2: High Evidence]*

The Wilson frame is sometimes used during lumbar spine surgeries to reduce lumbar lordosis and induce lumbar kyphosis; however, in doing so, the Wilson frame positions the patient's head lower than the heart, which increases orbital venous pressure and exacerbates venous congestion in the head over time.[411,424] In a case-controlled study of 80 patients with ischemic optic neuropathy compared with 315 matched control patients, the ASA Postoperative Visual Loss Study Group[411] found that Wilson frame use was an independent risk factor for postoperative vision loss. The researchers recommended reducing anesthetic time, minimizing blood loss, and not using the Wilson frame as methods for preventing postoperative vision loss associated with ischemic optic neuropathy.

XV.b. The patient should be in the prone position for the shortest time possible.[283,424,430] *[1: Strong Evidence]*

There have been reports of subconjunctival hemorrhage,[431] subperiosteal orbital hemorrhage,[432] Horner syndrome,[433] and postoperative vision loss[423,434-437] after prolonged surgery in the prone position. Intraocular pressure increases in the anesthetized patient in the prone position, and the magnitude of this increase is related to the amount of time spent in the prone position.[236,280,438-442] Intraocular pressure can increase significantly after only a few minutes in the prone position.[283] The most dramatic increases in intraocular pressure occur when the patient is in the prone position with his or her head down (eg, jack-knife).[280,283,438]

Yoshimura et al[441] suggested that measuring intraocular pressures 1 hour after surgery in the prone position could provide an opportunity for implementing interventions to prevent additional increases in intraocular pressure (eg, head-up positioning, reducing operating time).

Eddama[442] also suggested that regular measurement of intraocular pressures during prolonged surgeries provides an opportunity for implementing a change in the patient's position when critical thresholds are reached.

The length of time a patient may remain in the prone position without risk for pressure injury is unknown. Nazerali et al[443] conducted a retrospective review of the records of 10 patients who developed facial pressure injuries after neurosurgery, orthopedic surgery, or plastic surgery in the prone position. The authors found that the mean intraoperative prone time for a surgery complicated by a facial pressure injury was 8.6 hours compared with 3.2 hours for a surgery not complicated by a facial pressure injury. The authors recommended minimizing the patient's time in the prone position.

Sherman et al[444] prospectively identified position-related injuries in 17 patients undergoing 19 prone sacral procedures. The researchers found that five (29%) of the patients developed position-related injuries. One patient developed a transient ulnar nerve palsy attributed to an unrecognized shift in the arm board during the procedure. Three patients, two of whom were extremely obese, developed Stage 1 pressure injuries, and one patient developed a Stage 2 pressure injury. The researchers concluded that extreme obesity and procedural times in excess of 10 hours were risk factors for position-related complications.

Case reports describe compartment syndrome associated with prolonged time in the prone or knee-chest positions, including

○ right anterior thigh compartment syndrome after 5 hours[445] and

○ right lower-leg compartment syndrome with acute renal failure after 6 hours.[446]

The ASA Task Force on Perioperative Visual Loss encourages staging prone procedures that are anticipated to be lengthy.[18] Using a series of staged procedures rather than one prolonged procedure may help minimize the patient's time in the prone position; however, the risks associated with multiple surgeries (eg, infection, unstable spine) may outweigh the benefits of staged procedures.[184,423]

XV.c. The patient's head should be positioned in a neutral position, without excessive flexion, extension, or rotation.[18,36,184,349,374,423,430,447-452] *[1: Strong Evidence]*

Extremes of neck flexion or extension can result in patient injury.[346,375,416]

Positioning the patient's head in the midline, or neutral, position may reduce the risk for cerebral ischemia.[448,453] Maintaining a neutral head position maintains optimal cerebral blood flow and perfusion[449] and minimizes the risk of occluding the carotid or vertebral arteries.[407] Andersen et al[453] conducted a prospective controlled study of 48 patients undergoing spinal surgery in the prone position to determine whether head rotation more than 45 degrees would affect cerebral blood oxygen saturation levels. The researchers measured cerebral blood oxygen saturation levels during anesthesia with the patients' heads in neutral, rotated-left, and rotated-right positions; with the patients' heads in a face positioner; and with the patients' heads resting on a horseshoe-shaped head positioner. The researchers found that when the patients' heads were resting on the horseshoe-shaped head positioner, there was no significant decrease in cerebral blood oxygen saturation levels in the neutral, rotated-left, or rotated-right positions. When the patients' heads were in the face positioner, there was a significant decrease in cerebral oxygen saturation levels when the patients' heads were turned to the right or to the left compared with the midline or neutral position. The researchers recommended using a neutral head position for patients in the prone position.

Using a midline, or neutral position for the head during prone positioning is also preferred because it decreases intraocular pressure, which increases perfusion of the optic nerve and reduces the potential for postoperative vision loss.[450,451,454] Using a midline position also decreases the potential for ocular compression that might occur when the patient's head is turned to the side.[450,452]

XV.c.1. When the patient's head is positioned in the midline, a face positioner designed for this purpose should be used.[5,36,143,184,191] *[3: Moderate Evidence]*

Face positioners provide protection for the patient's forehead, eyes, and chin. They allow the patient's head to remain in the midline while keeping external pressure off the eyes, providing a clear path for the airway maintenance device and allowing a clear view of the patient's face and eyes.[21,36,118,191,455,456]

Evidence related to the safest and most effective face positioner is inconclusive.[455,457,458] Further research is warranted. Nazerali et al[443] conducted a retrospective review of the records of 10 patients who developed facial pressure injuries after neurosurgery, orthopedic surgery, or plastic surgery in the prone position. The authors found the type of face positioner used contributed to facial pressure injury. After changing from a non-face-contoured positioner to a face-contoured positioner, there was a significant decrease in the occurrence of facial pressure injuries. The authors recommended using face-contoured positioners when the patient is in the prone position.

XV.c.2. The position of the patient's face should be assessed and monitored after positioning activities and during the procedure, and corrective actions should be implemented as indicated.[416] *[3: Moderate Evidence]*

Assessing and monitoring the position of the patient's face can help to prevent pressure injury to the eyes, nose, mouth, forehead, and chin.[416] Grover and Jangra[456] suggested positioning a mirror beneath the face positioner to allow the patient's face position to be monitored. Levan et al[459] described the case of a 66-year-old man who underwent spinal surgery in the prone position with his face positioned in a face positioner. The authors took a photograph of the patient's face in the face positioner at the beginning of the procedure and every 30 minutes during the procedure. The authors examined the pictures to assess patient positioning. They found that after 2 hours in the prone position the patient's face had progressively migrated from its initial position, and by 2.5 hours, the patient's nose was contacting the bottom of the face positioner. Perioperative team members repositioned the patient and added padding to maintain the patient's face in the face positioner. No further change in position was required during the 7-hour procedure.

XV.c.3. A horseshoe-shaped head positioner should not be used, if possible. *[3: Moderate Evidence]*

Direct compression from a horseshoe-shaped head positioner has been reported as a cause of postoperative vision loss when the patient is in the prone position.[460,461]

XV.d. Perioperative team members should implement interventions to prevent direct pressure on the patient's eyes.[118,404] *[3: Moderate Evidence]*

There is an increased risk for direct compression on the orbit when the patient is in the prone position.[118,462] Direct pressure on the eye may increase the risk for corneal abrasion or other ocular injuries, including postoperative vision loss.[463,464]

XV.d.1. The patient's eyes should be assessed and monitored after positioning activities and during the procedure, and corrective actions should be implemented as indicated.[184,416,423,456] *[3: Moderate Evidence]*

Assessing and monitoring the patient's eyes verifies there is no direct pressure on the eyes and confirms the patient's position has not changed.[425,465]

In a study to explore the incidence and related risk factors for perioperative eye injuries, Yu et al[466] found that the prone and lateral positions were precipitating factors for eye injury. The researchers recommended careful positioning and intermittent assessment of the patient's eyes during the procedure.

XV.e. The anesthesia professional should assess the patient's airway maintenance device after positioning in the prone position, during the procedure, and after the patient is returned to the supine position and should implement corrective actions as indicated.[407,467] *[3: Moderate Evidence]*

Changes in the patient's position could lead to changes in airway maintenance device position or intracuff pressure.[416] Assessing the patient's airway maintenance device after positioning and during the procedure may prevent patient injury.[468] In a prospective study to determine whether the supine-to-prone position change displaced the endotracheal tube, Minonishi et al[469] measured the insertion depth of the endotracheal tube in 132 patients undergoing spinal surgery in the prone position. The researchers found that moving the patient from supine to prone position displaced the endotracheal tube in 91.7% of patients (n = 121). The endotracheal tubes had moved 0.4 inch (10 mm) or more in 47.9% of the patients (n = 58), and 86.3% of the patients (n = 104) had changes in endotracheal tube cuff pressure.

XV.f. When positioned in the prone position, the patient's arms should be
- tucked at the sides with a draw sheet,[11,36,118,191]
- secured at the sides with arm guards,
- placed on an arm board positioned parallel to the OR bed,[11,36,118,191] or
- placed on an arm rest with adjustment joints designed for this purpose.[36] *[3: Moderate Evidence]*

Placement of the arms is determined by the needs of the surgical team and the physical limitations of the patient.

XV.f.1. When the patient's arms are tucked at the sides and secured with a draw sheet,
- the patient's arms should be in a neutral position,[35,38,159] with the palms facing the body and without hyperextension of the elbows[6,36,159,191]; *[1: Strong Evidence]*
- the draw sheet should be pulled up between the patient's body and arm, placed over the patient's arm, and tucked between the patient and the OR bed mattress[36,191]; *[3: Moderate Evidence]*
- the draw sheet should be tucked snugly enough to secure the patient's arm, but not so tightly as to create a pressure source[74]; *[3: Moderate Evidence]* and
- the draw sheet should extend from the mid upper arm (ie, above the elbows) to the fingertips. *[5: Benefits Balanced with Harms]*

Neutral position is a position during which the body part distal to the joint (eg, hand is distal to wrist, forearm is distal to

elbow) is not inverted or everted, adducted or abducted, flexed or extended.[213] Hyperextension of the elbow can stretch the median nerve.[7,35,156]

Using a draw sheet that extends from the mid upper arm to the fingertips, placing the sheet over the arm, and tucking the draw sheet between the patient's body and the OR bed mattress prevents the patient's arms from falling outside of the mattress and coming to rest on the metal portion of the OR bed.[36]

When the draw sheet is tucked too tightly, it can create a pressure or nerve injury or a compartment syndrome.[7,36,38,74,143,215]

Notably, tucking the patient's arms may interfere with physiological monitoring (eg, blood pressure, arterial catheter) and could result in an unrecognized infiltrated IV in the tucked arm.

XV.f.2. When the patient's arms are placed on arm boards or an arm rest with adjustment joints,
- the arm boards or arm rest should be padded[159,191]; *[1: Strong Evidence]*
- the arm boards or arm rest should be at a level lower than the chest[118,191]; *[3: Moderate Evidence]*
- the arms should be abducted less than 90 degrees, with elbows flexed[5,11,67,143,161]; *[3: Moderate Evidence]*
- the arms should not be positioned above the patient's head[11,21,36,118,191]; *[3: Moderate Evidence]*
- the arms should be pronated (ie, palms facing downward)[5,11,67,143,161]; *[3: Moderate Evidence]*
- the arms and wrists should be maintained in neutral alignment[36,191]; *[3 Moderate Evidence]* and
- the arms should be secured to the arm boards.[28,36] *[3: Moderate Evidence]*

The use of padded arm boards may decrease the risk for upper extremity neuropathy.[35,159]

Positioning the patient's arms at a level lower than the chest provides physiologic alignment.

The risk for brachial plexus injury and occlusion of the subclavian or axillary arteries is increased when the patient's arm is abducted more than 90 degrees.[11,12,36,38,68,143,157-159,161,191,214]

Positioning the patient's arms above the head can cause a stretch injury to the lower trunk and brachial plexus.[11,67,191]

Pronating the patient's arms and maintaining the patient's arms and wrists in neutral alignment reduces the risk for positioning injury.[36]

Securing the arms to the arm boards reduces the risk of the patient's arms falling off the arm board.

XV.g. The patient should be positioned on two chest supports that extend from the clavicle to the iliac crest.[5,21,118,143,191,470,471] *[3: Moderate Evidence]*

Chest supports allow chest and abdominal expansion and decrease intra-abdominal pressure.[5,21,143,191]

Incorrect placement or movement of chest supports can lead to patient injury.[470] The use of the prone position with chest supports placed at the chest or pelvis can result in an acute but reversible change in hepatic blood flow and cardiac output.[472] Placing the chest supports inferior and medial to the iliac crest can result in a neuropathy associated with compression of the lateral femoral cutaneous nerve.[471]

XV.g.1. Chest supports should positioned to permit full lung and abdominal expansion.[5,21,118,143,191,473] *[3: Moderate Evidence]*

Chest supports that do not permit full lung and abdominal expansion may increase intra-abdominal pressure. Increased intra-abdominal pressure impairs vena caval flow and can result in venous engorgement, decreased venous return to the heart, and reduced cardiac output.[7,36,234,423] Engorged epidural veins can increase bleeding at the surgical site during spinal procedures.[7,409] If the abdomen is compressed, there is a risk for mesenteric artery thrombosis and necrotic bowel.[74]

Positioning chest supports in a manner that prevents pressure on the abdomen may be difficult in a patient who is obese or pregnant and requires chest supports that are capable of supporting the patient's weight.[74]

XV.h. The patient's breasts, abdomen, and genitals should be positioned in a manner that frees them from torsion or pressure.[191] *[3: Moderate Evidence]*

Evidence related to best practices for positioning the patient's breasts in the prone position is inconclusive. Some experts recommend diverting the breasts medially because lateral displacement can place traction on the vasculature and can be painful.[5,143] Another expert recommended placing a viscoelastic gel pad above the breast to support the chest and prevent neck compression from breast tissue if the patient's breasts are large and placing a viscoelastic gel pad below the patient's breasts if they are small.[191]

XV.i. The patient's knees should be padded.[5,36,143,191] *[3: Moderate Evidence]*

Providing additional pressure-redistributing padding at the patient's knees helps prevent pressure injury.[5]

XV.j. The patient's toes should be elevated off the bed by placing padding under the patient's shins so the shins are high enough to prevent pressure on the tips of the toes.[5,21,143,191] *[3: Moderate Evidence]*

Placing padding under the patient's shins provides greater pressure redistribution than placing padding under the dorsum of the patient's foot. Preventing pressure on the tips of the patient's toes reduces the incidence of pressure injuries and foot drop.[191]

XV.k. The perioperative RN should assess the patient's pedal pulses after positioning in the knee-chest position and during the procedure and should take corrective actions as indicated.[191] *[3: Moderate Evidence]*

A significant danger of the knee-chest position is the potential for impaired perfusion distal to the knees as a result of vascular kinking in the popliteal space.[191] Checking the patient's pedal pulses verifies adequate perfusion and allows the perioperative RN to assess color, capillary refill time, and pulses and compare them to baseline levels.[191]

XV.l. When the patient is in the prone position, a gurney should be readily accessible. *[1: Strong Evidence]*

A gurney is a height-adjustable patient transport vehicle with wheels that can be locked. A gurney may be necessary to rapidly reposition the patient from prone to supine position for CPR. Turning the patient to supine position for CPR provides superior access to the airway and chest.[407] However, turning the patient from prone to supine position causes a temporary interruption and potential disconnection of patient monitors.[416] The decision to reposition the patient may be determined by the effectiveness of cardiac compressions and defibrillation attempts in the prone position.[416] Additional considerations include the expected duration of interrupted resuscitation for repositioning, the need for access for other resuscitation procedures (eg, chest tube insertion, central venous cannulation), and the condition of the surgical wound (eg, multiple surgical instruments in place).[407,408,416]

Recommendation XVI

Perioperative team members should implement measures to reduce the risk for injuries when positioning patients who are pregnant.

In patients who are pregnant, venous return may be impeded because of compression from the gravid uterus on the maternal aorta and inferior vena cava.[69,474,475] Compression of the aorta reduces uterine and placental perfusion.[476] Compression of the inferior vena cava impedes venous return and decreases cardiac output.[476] At term gestation, the inferior vena cava is nearly completely compressed against the vertebral bodies by the gravid uterus.[7,477,478] Venous return occurs primarily through the collateral veins.[477]

XVI.a. Pregnant women undergoing obstetric surgery should be positioned in a left lateral tilt by

- placing a 4.7-inch (12-cm) wedge-shaped positioning device under the right lumbar region above the iliac crest and below the lower costal region to achieve a 12-degree to 15-degree lateral tilt,[479] [1: Strong Evidence]
- placing a wedge-shaped positioning device under the right pelvis to achieve a 12-degree to 15-degree lateral tilt,[479] [1: Strong Evidence] or
- tilting the OR bed 15 degrees to 45 degrees to the left.[474,476,480] [2: High Evidence]

Implementing patient positions that displace the uterus to the left may help prevent supine hypotensive syndrome caused by the gravid uterus compressing the aorta and inferior vena cava.[7,474,478]

The Association of Women's Health, Obstetric and Neonatal Nurses (AWHONN)[479] recommends maintaining uterine displacement by using a wedge-shaped positioning device under the right lumbar region or under the right pelvis to achieve a 12-degree to 15-degree left lateral tilt.

A lumbar wedge may be more effective in preventing hypotension than a pelvic wedge.[478] When a pelvic wedge is used, the amount of left lateral tilt required to displace the uterus may be affected by the patient's BMI. In an observational study, Harvey et al[481] recommended tilting the OR bed or using an inflatable pelvic wedge designed for this purpose for positioning obese pregnant women rather than using a pelvic wedge to displace the uterus.

Evidence regarding whether to use a pelvic wedge or an OR bed tilt as well as the recommended degree of OR bed tilt is inconclusive. Kinsella and Harvey[482] concluded that a right pelvic wedge and an OR bed tilt were equally effective in producing left lateral tilt sufficient to displace the uterus. Lee et al[476] concluded that aortocaval compression in pregnant patients could be effectively reduced by tilting the OR bed 15 degrees or greater. Higuchi et al[480] concluded that a 30-degree to 45-degree OR bed tilt was necessary to effectively reduce inferior vena cava compression in pregnant women. Archer et al[474] found that an OR bed tilt of 45 degrees was superior to any position with the right side down.

Saravanakumar et al[475] hypothesized that the addition of a reverse Trendelenburg tilt to a left lateral position could effectively relieve aortocaval compression. The researchers obtained magnetic resonance images of six pregnant women (32 weeks to 36 weeks pregnant; BMI 30 kg/m² to 35 kg/m²) in six different positions: right lateral, left lateral, supine with a pelvic polyurethane wedge (7.9 inch; 20 cm), and 5-degree, 10-degree, and 15-degree reverse Trendelenburg. They found inferior vena cava compression was present in all participants in all positions; however, inferior vena cava dimensions were increased in the left lateral position compared to supine with a pelvic wedge. The addition of 15-degree reverse Trendelenburg position to the supine position with a pelvic wedge produced an increase in inferior vena cava diameter, but the increase was not statistically significant.

Notably, tilting the OR bed could make the surgery more difficult for the surgeon and increase the risk for injury to the mother.[483]

In a Cochrane systematic review to determine the most effective maternal position during cesarean section, Cluver et al[483] analyzed 11 RCTs representing a total of 857 women and found there was no change in hypotensive episodes with a right lumbar wedge, left OR bed tilt, right OR bed tilt, or Trendelenburg tilt compared with horizontal supine position. The researchers concluded that a left OR bed tilt might be better than a right OR bed tilt, and a lumbar wedge might be better than a left OR bed tilt. Larger studies with more robust data are needed to confirm these findings.

XVI.b. Women undergoing nonobstetric surgery who are more than 18 weeks pregnant should be positioned in a left lateral tilt during the operative procedure, if possible.[479] [1: Strong Evidence]

The AWHONN[479] recommends using a left lateral tilt whenever possible for women who are more than 18 weeks pregnant.

Recommendation XVII

Perioperative team members should implement measures to reduce the risk for injuries when positioning patients who are obese.

According to the Centers for Disease Control and Prevention, people with a BMI of 30 kg/m² to < 35 kg/m² are classified as Class I obese, people with a BMI of 35 kg/m² to < 40 kg/m² are classified as Class 2 obese, and people with a BMI of 40 kg/m² or higher are classified as Class 3 extremely obese.[484] Obesity is associated with significant physiologic cardiovascular and pulmonary changes, and the surgical position in which the obese patient is placed can further alter cardiovascular and pulmonary function.[69,234] Airway and breathing mechanisms are compromised in obese patients because of

- excess adipose tissue leading to an increased workload for the supportive muscles[74,473,485];
- increased oxygen consumption and carbon dioxide production[74,473,485];

- decreased myocardial compliance (ie, 35% of normal)[74,473,485];
- increased breathing effort and decreased efficiency of air exchange[74,473];
- decreased resting functional residual lung capacity[74,473]; and
- increased incidence of gastroesophageal reflux, hiatal hernia, and abdominal pressure that adds to the risk for aspiration.[74,485]

In a nonexperimental study to demonstrate the relationship between BMI and regional hypoxemia in the lung, Yamane et al[486] measured the PaO_2 and the partial pressure of carbon dioxide from the pulmonary veins of 40 patients. The patients had normal cardiopulmonary function and were undergoing a catheter ablation for atrial fibrillation. The researchers found that the PaO_2 value in the inferior pulmonary veins was significantly lower than in the superior pulmonary veins in supine patients, and the extent of the hypoxemia was proportional to the patient's BMI. These findings demonstrated that even moderate obesity was associated with appreciable regional hypoxemia.

Cardiac output, pulmonary blood flow, and arterial pressure are also increased in obese patients in the supine position.[234] Excess body weight compromises the cardiovascular system by
- increasing metabolic demand and cardiac output,[74,485]
- increasing blood volume,[58,74,485]
- increasing venous return and preload,[69,157]
- increasing the work of the heart and the volume of blood pumped by the heart with each contraction (leading to left ventricular dilation and thickening of the heart muscle),[74,485] and
- causing hypoxia and hypercapnia (leading to pulmonary vasoconstriction and right-sided heart failure).[74]

Patients who are obese may be at increased risk for postoperative rhabdomyolysis caused by traumatic compression of muscle tissue during extended procedures.[487]

XVII.a. The patient's head may be elevated 25 degrees. *[1: Strong Evidence]*

Use of the supine position in patients who are obese can lead to significant reductions in lung volume, increased work of breathing, and hypoxemia.[69,157,234] Patients who are obese may have difficulty breathing in a recumbent position.[24,74,485] The AWHONN[479] suggests that a head-elevated position may be indicated during positioning of women who are obese.

Airway management, ventilation, and intubation may be more difficult in patients who are obese.[69,485] Airway management may be difficult because of the patient's increased neck circumference.[58] A short, thick neck inhibits mobility and makes visualization of the larynx difficult.[24] Ventilating an obese patient is difficult because of the need for high pressure to overcome the weight of the chest and the abdomen when the patient is supine.[74,485] Intubation may be difficult because of the lack of landmarks and the presence of redundant tissue.[74] Large breasts may get in the way of the laryngoscope handle.[24] The weight of the patient's head may make it difficult to lift in order to visualize the larynx.[24]

Elevating the obese patient's head and neck helps establish a patent airway, ease intubation, decrease ventilator pressure, and prevent aspiration.[24,69,74,157] The 25-degree head-elevated position may improve visualization of anatomic structures and provide ergonomic advantages for the anesthesia professional performing the intubation.[488,489]

XVII.a.1. To place the patient in a head-elevated position,
- the back of the OR bed may be elevated[157,490] *[1: Strong Evidence]* or
- a wedge-shaped positioning device that supports the patient's head and shoulders may be used.[157,491] *[3: Moderate Evidence]*

Wedge-shaped positioners are designed to redistribute pressure and reduce the patient's risk for pressure injury.[157] Using a wedge-shaped positioning device that supports the head and shoulders helps prevent strain on the patient's arms and brachial plexus.[69] Although potentially achieving similar results in terms of head elevation, using a stack of towels or blankets does not redistribute pressure, and may not sufficiently support the patient's arms and shoulders, increasing the risk for brachial plexus injury.[157] Using a wedge-shaped positioning device may prevent insufficient or excessive elevation of the patient's head and neck that may occur when too few or too many linens are used.[157] Excessive elevation can inhibit face mask ventilation and make the intubation process and application of cricoid pressure more difficult.[157] Likewise, using irrigation fluid bags to support the patient's head and shoulders is not recommended as these are not designed as positioning devices and may not provide the necessary stability or withstand the weight of an obese patient.[157] Electronically elevating and lowering the back of the OR bed is easier than manually adjusting or removing a stack of linens or a wedge-shaped positioning device and decreases the risk for personnel injury.[157,490]

XVII.b. A wedge-shaped positioning device may be placed under the obese patient's right lumbar region, or a left OR bed tilt of at least 15 degrees may be used. *[3: Moderate Evidence]*

Some obese patients cannot tolerate recumbent positions.[234] In patients with central obesity, venous return may be impeded due to aortocaval compression similar to the effect of a gravid uterus.[69] Compression of the inferior vena cava against the vertebral bodies can lead to severe hypotension in patients who are obese.[7,234] The use of a wedge-shaped positioning device or a 15-degree left lateral OR bed tilt may offset aortocaval compression in obese patients in recumbent positions[69,234]; however, tilting the OR bed laterally for prolonged periods may result in sciatic nerve palsy.[157]

XVII.c. Padded arm guards may be used to contain the obese patient's arms at the sides of the body, if necessary. *[5: Benefits Balanced with Harms]*

Using padded arm guards provides additional width and support and allows the obese patient's arms to be positioned at his or her sides.

Recommendation XVIII

The perioperative RN should collaborate with the perianesthesia RN to identify patient injury caused by intraoperative positioning.[21]

Identifying patients at risk for positioning injury allows for the implementation of preventive interventions.[26] Injuries related to the patient's surgical position may be averted by effective postoperative monitoring and management.[46,492]

XVIII.a. The RN circulator should conduct a postoperative patient assessment to identify patient injury caused by intraoperative positioning.[41,191] *[3: Moderate Evidence]*

The RN circulator has knowledge of pressure points associated with the intraoperative position and of the locations where safety restraints, adhesives, monitoring devices, positioning equipment or devices, and other items that may present a risk for patient injury were placed during the procedure.[60]

The RN circulator also has knowledge of intraoperative factors that may increase the likelihood of a positioning injury (eg, intraoperative blood administration[493]). In a retrospective observational study of 2,695 surgical patients, O'Brien et al[493] found that intraoperative administration of blood products was significantly associated with postoperative pressure injury.

XVIII.a.1. The RN circulator should use a standardized communication tool to provide information from the postoperative assessment to the perianesthesia RN, regarding
- areas of the patient's body that should be assessed and monitored for potential injury,[9] *[3: Moderate Evidence]*
- events during the intraoperative period that may have contributed to a position-related injury,[9,49,61,63] *[3: Moderate Evidence]* and
- the position of the patient during the procedure. *[5: Benefits Balanced with Harms]*

Communicating areas of concern may improve postoperative monitoring and management of potential position-related injuries. Using standardized communication tools helps ensure that necessary patient care information is communicated.

XVIII.b. The perianesthesia RN should
- place the patient in a position other than the surgical position, if possible, and
- monitor areas that are at high risk for positioning injuries.[56,63]
[4: Limited Evidence]

Changing the patient's position after surgery reduces pressure on high-risk areas. Monitoring areas that are at high risk for positioning injuries assists with early recognition and treatment and allows for identification and review of positioning methods that may have contributed to or caused the injury.

XVIII.c. The perianesthesia RN should assess the patient for signs and symptoms of pressure injury.[24,28,494] *[2: High Evidence]*

Early detection and treatment of pressure injury may help prevent skin alteration from progressing to skin loss.[26] Blanchable erythema, especially over a bony prominence, may be a normal, reactive, hyperemic response or the first clinical sign of pressure injury development after surgery.[24,26] Other early signs of pressure injury include changes in skin temperature or texture or pain sensation.[15] Pressure injuries may not appear for 1 to 4 days after surgery.[15,28,56,64] Pressure injuries that occur intraoperatively have a unique purple appearance that originates at the muscle over a bony prominence and progresses outward.[28,56,64]

Minnich et al[495] developed a postoperative skin assessment tool designed to be completed postoperatively by the RN circulator and the perianesthesia RN. Specific skin assessment processes were implemented to allow for rapid discovery and treatment. After using the assessment protocol for more than 3,000 patients over 2 years, the authors found the incidence of pressure injuries dropped from 7.1% to 3.3%.

XVIII.d. The perianesthesia RN should assess the patient for signs and symptoms of extremity nerve dysfunction.[35,416,494] *[1: Strong Evidence]*

Assessment of nerve dysfunction may lead to early recognition and treatment of peripheral neuropathies.[35,65] Signs of nerve injury include a decreased range of motion, impaired limb muscle strength, numbness or tingling, or pain in the limbs or joints not associated with the procedure.[28] Symptoms of nerve damage may appear days or even weeks after the procedure because the symptoms may be confused with pain or immobility caused by the procedure.[28]

Gezginci et al[496] evaluated postoperative pain and neuromuscular complications (ie, paresthesia, numbness, weakness) associated with positioning after robotic-assisted laparoscopic radical prostatectomy in 534 patients. The researchers found that patients who had previous surgeries, comorbidities, and ASA classifications of II and III were at increased risk for neuromuscular complications.

XVIII.e. The perianesthesia RN should assess the patient for signs and symptoms of compartment syndrome. *[3: Moderate Evidence]*

Compartment syndrome presents as swelling; restricted movement; lack of sensation; tightness; severe pain; and, in extreme cases, no extremity pulse.[28] It is associated with significant morbidity and loss of limb function resulting from necrosis of ischemic muscle in the affected compartment as well as potential mortality from the reperfusion that occurs after surgical decompression.[492,497] Compartment syndrome is an acute medical emergency that most often requires urgent surgical treatment.[492,497] A rapid response is necessary to minimize the risk for long-term morbidity or potential mortality.[193]

Patients with compartment syndrome often present with reports of pain that are out of proportion with clinical findings and unrelieved by analgesics.[193,497] Notably, the use of a postoperative epidural can mask the initial pain associated with compartment syndrome.[497]

XVIII.f. The perianesthesia RN should evaluate the patient for signs and symptoms of ocular injury.[18,498] *[1: Strong Evidence]*

Differences in pupillary reactivity, light sensitivity, visual field defects and patient reports of blurred, distorted, or painful vision may be indicative of ocular injury or impending postoperative vision loss.[283,498]

Patient-related risk factors for postoperative vision loss include male sex, preoperative anemia, hypertension, peripheral vascular disease, coronary artery disease, diabetes, use of tobacco, and obesity.[451] Procedure-related risk factors include spinal surgery, cardiac surgery, head-neck surgery, hip and femur surgeries, procedures longer than 6 hours, prone or Trendelenburg position, significant blood loss, and use of the Wilson frame.[451] Anesthetic-related risk factors include limited intravascular fluid administration or excessive crystalloid administration.[451] Patients who are anemic before surgery or have experienced substantial blood loss during the procedure may be at increased risk for ocular injury.[451,499,500]

Recommendation XIX

The health care organization should maintain records of patient care related to patient positioning and organizational processes related to positioning equipment and devices.

Documentation in the patient's medical record provides a description of the perioperative care administered, status of patient outcomes upon transfer, and information to support continuity of care.[10] Documentation provides data for identifying trends and demonstrating compliance with regulatory requirements and accreditation standards. Effective management and collection of health care information that accurately reflects the patient's care, treatment, and services is a regulatory requirement[501-504] and an accreditation standard for both hospitals[505,506] and ambulatory settings.[506-510]

XIX.a. The perioperative RN should document patient care and use of positioning equipment and devices on the intraoperative record. *[1: Strong Evidence]*

Accurate documentation facilitates comprehensive patient care, provides information for retrospective review and research data, and establishes a legal record.[38] Documentation provides a baseline record of the patient's condition.[9] Documentation of specific positioning actions may result in improved positioning processes by helping practitioners focus attention on relevant aspects of patient positioning and by providing information on positioning strategies that improve the quality of patient care.[28,35]

Comprehensive documentation related to patient positioning is necessary for demonstrating that the standard of care was met when defending claims that allege substandard care.[9,11,28,67,416] In an analysis of 44 cases from the AANA Foundation Closed Malpractice Claims Database, Fritzlen et al[38] found that documentation of patient positioning on the anesthesia record was judged as "adequate" in 12 (27%) of the claims studied, and documentation of padding was judged as adequate in eight claims (18%). There was a complete absence of documentation of patient positioning in 24 (55%) of the claims, and a complete absence of documentation of padding in 25 (57%) of the claims in this data set.

Rowen et al[6] suggested achieving consensus after positioning and documenting that all team members agreed that the patient was correctly and safely positioned.

XIX.a.1. Documentation related to positioning the patient should include the
- preoperative assessment[21]; *[4: Limited Evidence]*
- identification and titles of individuals participating in positioning the patient6; *[3: Moderate Evidence]*
- patient's position, including the position of the patient's arms and legs, and any repositioning activities[11,28]; *[3: Moderate Evidence]*
- type and location of positioning equipment or devices[6,43]; *[3: Moderate Evidence]*
- type and location of safety restraints6; *[3: Moderate Evidence]*
- type and location of any additional padding provided[21,28]; *[4: Limited Evidence]*
- specific actions taken to prevent patient injury, especially any actions taken in

response to findings from the preoperative assessment[28,416]; *[3: Moderate Evidence]* and

- postoperative assessment.[24,88] *[3: Moderate Evidence]*

XIX.a.2. The perioperative RN should initiate the health care organization's policies and procedures for establishing and documenting a chain of custody for jewelry or other items that are removed from the patient. The perioperative RN should document

- the type and location of critical devices, superficial implants, jewelry, or other items that cannot be removed and
- any actions taken (eg, use of additional padding) to prevent patient injury from the item that cannot be removed.[21]

[1: Strong Evidence]

Establishing and documenting a chain of custody helps prevent loss or theft of jewelry and other items removed from patients. Some jewelry is easily removed; however, removal of some types of piercing jewelry requires the use of special tools.[85] The goals for nursing interventions are to prevent potential patient injuries or complications and treat actual patient problems.[511] Documenting nursing interventions promotes continuity of patient care and improves the exchange of patient care information among health care team members.[511]

XIX.a.3. Photography used to document injuries related to positioning should be consistent with the health care organization's policies regarding medical photography and video images.[43] *[4: Limited Evidence]*

XIX.b. The health care organization should maintain records related to processes for preventive maintenance and repair of positioning equipment and devices. *[5: Benefits Balanced with Harms]*

Records of preventive maintenance and repair of positioning equipment and devices provide a source of evidence for review during investigation of clinical issues (eg, patient injury). Records of preventive maintenance also provide evidence of maintenance, compliance with manufacturers' IFU, and information that may be useful in determining the need for repair or replacement. Records of repairs may help to identify trends in equipment and device damage and help to define practices that may reduce damage.

Recommendation XX

Personnel with responsibility for positioning patients should receive initial and ongoing education and complete competency verification activities related to patient positioning.

Initial and ongoing education of perioperative personnel facilitates the development of knowledge, skills, and attitudes that affect safe patient care. It is the responsibility of the health care organization to provide initial and ongoing education and to verify the competency of its personnel[10]; however, the primary responsibility for maintaining ongoing competency remains with the individual.[512]

Competency verification activities provide a mechanism for competency documentation and help verify that personnel understand the principles and processes necessary for safe patient positioning.

Ongoing development of knowledge and skills and documentation of personnel participation is a regulatory requirement[501-504] and an accreditation standard for both hospitals[513,514] and ambulatory settings.[514-517]

XX.a. The health care organization should establish education and competency verification activities for its personnel and determine intervals for education and competency verification related to patient positioning. *[3: Moderate Evidence]*

Providing education and verifying competency assists in developing knowledge and skills that may reduce the risk for errors and enhance perioperative team members' appreciation of the potential mechanisms of patient and personnel injury associated with patient positioning.[3,20,51,66,156] Education and competency verification needs and intervals are unique to the facility and to its personnel and processes.

XX.a.1. Education and competency verification activities related to positioning patients should include

- processes for patient assessment,[21,44,133] *[1: Strong Evidence]*
- identification of factors that increase the risk for positioning injury in patients and personnel,[28,44,56,236] *[1: Strong Evidence]*
- identification and effective use of pressure-redistributing support surfaces,[43,44,133] *[1: Strong Evidence]*
- a description of the relevant anatomy and physiology,[28,156,214,331] *[3: Moderate Evidence]*
- a description of the characteristics of special populations served by the health care organization (eg, pregnant patients, obese patients, older patients, pediatric patients),[23,51] *[3: Moderate Evidence]*
- procedures for safe use of positioning equipment and devices,[28,416] *[3: Moderate Evidence]*
- implementation of safe practices for patient positioning,[21,28,236,416] *[3: Moderate Evidence]*
- documentation of positioning activities,[43] *[4: Limited Evidence]* and
- procedures for identifying and reporting patient or personnel injury caused by patient positioning. *[5: Benefits Balanced with Harms]*

XX.b. Personnel should receive education and complete competency verification activities before new support surfaces or positioning equipment or devices are introduced.[28] *[4: Limited Evidence]*

Receiving education and completing competency verification activities before new support surfaces or equipment is introduced helps ensure correct use and promote safe positioning practices.

Recommendation XXI

The health care organization should develop policies and procedures for positioning the patient, revise them as necessary, and make them readily available in the practice setting in which they are used.

Policies and procedures assist in the development of patient safety, quality assessment, and performance improvement activities. Policies and procedures also serve as operational guidelines used to minimize patients' risk for injury or complications, standardize practice, and direct personnel. Policies and procedures establish authority, responsibility, and accountability within the practice setting.

Having policies and procedures that guide and support patient care, treatment, and services is a regulatory requirement[501-504] and an accreditation standard for both hospitals[518,519] and ambulatory settings.[516,519-521]

XXI.a. A multidisciplinary team should develop perioperative policies related to positioning that are consistent with the health care organization's pressure injury prevention program.[51,133] Multidisciplinary team members may include wound specialists; wound, ostomy, and continence care RNs; infection preventionists; perioperative RNs; supply chain managers; and other involved personnel. *[1: Strong Evidence]*

The potential economic impact of pressure injury (eg, expense of treatment, lack of reimbursement) underscores the need for a multidisciplinary approach to prevention.[51]

XXI.b. Policies and procedures related to positioning patients should address
○ processes for patient assessment;
○ procedures for selection, care, and maintenance of positioning equipment and devices;
○ procedures for safe use of positioning equipment and devices for patients and personnel;
○ identification and use of pressure-redistributing support surfaces;
○ procedures for safe patient positioning;
○ processes for identification and reporting of patient or personnel injury caused by patient positioning; and
○ documentation of positioning activities.
[5: Benefits Balanced with Harms]

XXI.c. The manufacturers' IFU for support surfaces and positioning equipment and devices should be readily available and adhered to by personnel responsible for positioning activities. *[5: Benefits Balanced with Harms]*

Instructions for use identify the validated procedures necessary for safe and effective use of support surfaces and positioning equipment and devices.

XXI.c.1. The manufacturer's IFU should be reviewed periodically, and positioning procedures should comply with the most current IFU. *[5: Benefits Balanced with Harms]*

Manufacturers may make modifications to their IFU when new technology becomes available, when regulatory requirements change, or when modifications are made to a device.

Recommendation XXII

The health care organization's quality management program should evaluate patient positioning.

Quality assurance and performance improvement programs can facilitate the identification of problem areas and assist personnel in evaluating and improving the quality of patient care and formulating plans for corrective action. These programs provide data that may be used to determine whether an individual organization is within benchmark goals, and if not, to identify areas that may require corrective action. A quality management program provides a mechanism to evaluate effectiveness of processes, compliance with positioning policies and procedures, and function of positioning equipment and devices.

Collecting data to monitor and improve patient care, treatment, and services is a regulatory requirement[501-504] and an accreditation standard for both hospitals[522,523] and ambulatory settings.[523-527]

XXII.a. The quality assurance and performance improvement program for patient positioning should include
○ periodically reviewing and evaluating positioning activities to verify compliance or to identify the need for improvement,
○ identifying corrective actions directed toward improvement priorities, and
○ taking additional actions when improvement is not achieved or sustained.
[4: Limited Evidence]

Reviewing and evaluating quality assurance and performance improvement activities may identify failure points that contribute to errors in patient positioning and help define actions for improvement and increased competency.[21,56] Taking corrective actions may improve patient safety by enhancing understanding of the principles of and compliance with best practices for patient positioning.

XXII.b. Personnel who participate in patient positioning should participate in ongoing quality assurance and performance improvement activities related to positioning patients by identifying processes that are important for

- monitoring quality,
- developing strategies for compliance,
- establishing benchmarks to evaluate quality indicators,
- collecting data related to the levels of performance and quality indicators,
- evaluating practice based on the cumulative data collected,
- taking action to improve compliance, and
- assessing the effectiveness of the actions taken.

[3: Moderate Evidence]

Participating in ongoing quality assurance and performance improvement activities is a primary responsibility of perioperative personnel engaged in practice.[10]

XXII.c. Checklists may be used as part of the health care organization's quality improvement program for patient positioning. *[3: Moderate Evidence]*

Checklists are designed to prevent adverse events by promoting a team culture, standardizing practice, allowing the detection of potential errors, and improving patient safety.[192] Checklists serve as cognitive aids to improve performance.[40,528] The systematic use of checklists may help guide perioperative team members and reduce the rate of position-related injuries by improving positioning skills without dependence on long-term memory.[40,416,528] Using a checklist may direct additional attention to safe positioning requirements that might otherwise not be implemented.[67] The use of a checklist does not replace vigilant assessment, monitoring, and implementation of established safe practices when positioning patients.[528]

XXII.d. Near misses and adverse events should be reported and documented according to the health care organization's policy and procedure and should be reviewed for potential opportunities for improvement. *[5: Benefits Balanced with Harms]*

Near misses are unplanned events that do not result in injury. Adverse events are events that result in patient injury. Reports of near misses and adverse events can be used to identify actions that may prevent similar occurrences and reveal opportunities for improvement.

XXII.d.1. Reports regarding device malfunction that led to serious injury or death should be submitted to MedWatch: The FDA Safety Information and Adverse Event Reporting Program.[121] *[5: Benefits Balanced with Harms]*

The FDA uses medical device reports to monitor device performance, detect potential device-related safety issues, and contribute to risk-benefit assessments of suspected device-associated deaths, serious injuries, or malfunction.[121] The Manufac-

turer and User Facility Device Experience (MAUDE) database houses reports submitted to the FDA by mandatory reporters (ie, manufacturers, importers, device user facilities) and voluntary reporters (ie, health care professionals, patients, consumers).[529]

Mandatory reporters are required to submit reports when they become aware of information that reasonably suggests that one of their marketed devices may have caused or contributed to a death or serious injury or has malfunctioned and that the malfunction of the device would be likely to cause or contribute to a death or serious injury if the malfunction were to recur.[529] Voluntary reporters are required to submit reports when they become aware of information that reasonably suggests a device may have caused or contributed to a death or serious injury of a patient.[529]

XXII.d.2. Data on patient and health care personnel injuries related to patient positioning should be collected, analyzed, and used for performance improvement. *[5: Benefits Balanced with Harms]*

Editor's note: Teflon is a registered trademark of the Chemours Co, Wilmington, DE.

REFERENCES

1. Dybec RB. Keeping up-to-date on patient positioning. *OR Nurse.* 2013;7(2):16-17. [VC]

2. Lopes CM, Galvão CM. Surgical positioning: evidence for nursing care. *Rev Lat Am Enfermagem.* 2010;18(2):287-294. [VB]

3. Bouyer-Ferullo S. Preventing perioperative peripheral nerve injuries. *AORN J.* 2013;97(1):110-124. [VA]

4. Fleisch MC, Bremerich D, Schulte-Mattler W, et al. The prevention of positioning injuries during gynecologic operations. Guideline of DGGG (S1-Level, AWMF Registry No. 015/077, February 2015). *Geburtshilfe Frauenheilkd.* 2015;75(8):792-807. [IVB]

5. MacDonald JJ, Washington SJ. Positioning the surgical patient. *Anaesth Intensive Care Med.* 2012;13(11):528-532. [VB]

6. Rowen L, Hunt D, Johnson KL. Managing obese patients in the OR. *OR Nurse.* 2012;6(2):26-36. [VB]

7. Washington SJ, Smurthwaite GJ. Positioning the surgical patient. *Anaesth Intensive Care Med.* 2009;10(10):476-479. [VB]

8. Sørensen EE, Kusk KH, Grønkjaer M. Operating room nurses' positioning of anesthetized surgical patients. *J Clin Nurs.* 2016;25(5-6):690-698. [IIIB]

9. Chitlik A. Safe positioning for robotic-assisted laparoscopic prostatectomy. *AORN J.* 2011;94(1):37-45. [VA]

10. Standards of perioperative nursing. In: *Guidelines for Perioperative Practice.* Denver, CO: AORN, Inc; 2015:693-732. https://www.aorn.org/aorn-org/guidelines/clinical-resources/aorn-standards. Accessed March 16, 2017. [IVC]

11. Sawyer RJ, Richmond MN, Hickey JD, Jarratt JA. Peripheral nerve injuries associated with anaesthesia. *Anaesthesia.* 2000;55(10):980-991. [VB]

12. Kuponiyi O, Alleemudder DI, Latunde-Dada A, Eedarapalli P. Nerve injuries associated with gynaecological surgery. *Obstet Gynaecol.* 2014;16(1):29-36. [VA]

13. Johnson RL, Warner ME, Staff NP, Warner MA. Neuropathies after surgery: anatomical considerations of pathologic mechanisms. *Clin Anat.* 2015;28(5):678-682. [VA]

14. Ducic I, Zakaria HM, Felder JM 3rd, Arnspiger S. Abdominoplasty-related nerve injuries: systematic review and treatment options. *Aesthet Surg J.* 2014;34(2):284-297. [IA]

15. Nilsson UG. Intraoperative positioning of patients under general anesthesia and the risk of post-operative pain and pressure ulcers. *J Perianesth Nurs.* 2013;28(3):137-143. [IIIB]

16. Waters T, Short M, Lloyd J, et al. AORN ergonomic tool 2: positioning and repositioning the supine patient on the OR bed. *AORN J.* 2011;93(4):445-449. [VA]

17. Lindgren M, Unosson M, Krantz AM, Ek AC. Pressure ulcer risk factors in patients undergoing surgery. *J Adv Nurs.* 2005;50(6):605-612. [IIIB]

18. Practice advisory for perioperative visual loss associated with spine surgery: an updated report by the American Society of Anesthesiologists Task Force on Perioperative Visual Loss. *Anesthesiology.* 2012;116(2):274-285. [IVA]

19. The National Pressure Ulcer Advisory Panel, European Pressure Ulcer Advisory Panel, Pan Pacific Pressure Injury Alliance. *Prevention and Treatment of Pressure Ulcers: Clinical Practice Guideline.* East Washington, DC: National Pressure Ulcer Advisory Panel; 2014. [IVA]

20. Mangham M. Positioning of the anaesthetised patient during robotically assisted laparoscopic surgery: perioperative staff experiences. *J Perioper Pract.* 2016;26(3):50-52. [VC]

21. Fletcher HC. Preventing skin injury in the OR. *OR Nurse.* 2014;8(3):29-34. [VC]

22. Jacobs A, Rose S. Assessment is more than skin deep in older adults. *OR Nurse.* 2011;5(4):29. [VC]

23. Penprase B, Johnson C. Optimizing the perioperative nursing role for the older adult surgical patient. *OR Nurse.* 2014;8(4):26-34. [VB]

24. Dybec RB. Intraoperative positioning and care of the obese patient. *Plast Surg Nurs.* 2004;24(3):118-122. [VB]

25. Schultz A. Predicting and preventing pressure ulcers in surgical patients. *AORN J.* 2005;81(5):986-1006. [IIIB]

26. Shaw LF, Chang PC, Lee JF, Kung HY, Tung TH. Incidence and predicted risk factors of pressure ulcers in surgical patients: experience at a medical center in Taipei, Taiwan. *Biomed Res Int.* 2014;2014:416896. [IIIB]

27. Tschannen D, Bates O, Talsma A, Guo Y. Patient-specific and surgical characteristics in the development of pressure ulcers. *Am J Crit Care.* 2012;21(2):116-125. [IIIB]

28. ECRI. Patient positioning. *Operating Room Risk Management.* August 2011:2. [VC]

29. Lumbley JL, Ali SA, Tchokouani LS. Retrospective review of predisposing factors for intraoperative pressure ulcer development. *J Clin Anesth.* 2014;26(5):368-374. [IIIB]

30. Armstrong D, Bortz P. An integrative review of pressure relief in surgical patients. *AORN J.* 2001;73(3):645-653. [VB]

31. Walton-Geer PS. Prevention of pressure ulcers in the surgical patient. *AORN J.* 2009;89(3):538-552. [VB]

32. Sukhu T, Krupski TL. Patient positioning and prevention of injuries in patients undergoing laparoscopic and robot-assisted urologic procedures. *Curr Urol Rep.* 2014;15(2):398. [VA]

33. Hayes RM, Spear ME, Lee SI, et al. Relationship between time in the operating room and incident pressure ulcers: a matched case-control study. *Am J Med Qual.* 2015;30(6):591-597. [IIIB]

34. Aronovitch SA. Intraoperatively acquired pressure ulcers: are there common risk factors? *Ostomy Wound Manage.* 2007;53(2):57-69. [IIIB]

35. American Society of Anesthesiologists Task Force on Prevention of Perioperative Peripheral Neuropathies. Practice advisory for the prevention of perioperative peripheral neuropathies: an updated report by the American Society of Anesthesiologists Task Force on Prevention of Perioperative Peripheral Neuropathies. *Anesthesiology.* 2011;114(4):741-754. [IVA]

36. O'Connell MP. Positioning impact on the surgical patient. *Nurs Clin North Am.* 2006;41(2):173-192. [VB]

37. Clayton JL. Special needs of older adults undergoing surgery. *AORN J.* 2008;87(3):557-574. [VB]

38. Fritzlen T, Kremer M, Biddle C. The AANA Foundation Closed Malpractice Claims Study on nerve injuries during anesthesia care. *AANA J.* 2003;71(5):347-352. [IIIB]

39. Mills JT, Burris MB, Warburton DJ, Conaway MR, Schenkman NS, Krupski TL. Positioning injuries associated with robotic assisted urological surgery. *J Urol.* 2013;190(2):580-584. [IIIB]

40. Enchev Y. Checklists in neurosurgery to decrease preventable medical errors: a review. *Balkan Med J.* 2015;32(4):337-346. [VA]

41. Adedeji R, Oragui E, Khan W, Maruthainar N. The importance of correct patient positioning in theatres and implications of mal-positioning. *J Perioper Pract.* 2010;20(4):143-147. [VB]

42. Price MC, Whitney JD, King CA, Doughty D. Wound care. Development of a risk assessment tool for intraoperative pressure ulcers. *J Wound Ostomy Continence Nurs.* 2005;32(1):19-32. [VB]

43. ECRI. Pressure ulcers. *Operating Room Risk Management.* November 2011:2. [VC]

44. Stansby G, Avital L, Jones K, Marsden G; Guideline Development Group. Prevention and management of pressure ulcers in primary and secondary care: summary of NICE guidance. *BMJ.* 2014;348:g2592. [IVA]

45. Curley MA, Razmus IS, Roberts KE, Wypij D. Predicting pressure ulcer risk in pediatric patients: the Braden Q Scale. *Nurs Res.* 2003;52(1):22-33. [IIIB]

46. Sewchuk D, Padula C, Osborne E. Prevention and early detection of pressure ulcers in patients undergoing cardiac surgery. *AORN J.* 2006;84(1):75-96. [IIIB]

47. Galvin PA, Curley MA. The Braden Q+P: a pediatric perioperative pressure ulcer risk assessment and intervention tool. *AORN J.* 2012;96(3):261-270. [VB]

48. Quigley SM, Curley MA. Skin integrity in the pediatric population: preventing and managing pressure ulcers. *J Soc Pediatr Nurs.* 1996;1(1):7-18. [VB]

49. Cherry C, Moss J. Best practices for preventing hospital-acquired pressure injuries in surgical patients. *Can Oper Room Nurs J.* 2011;29(1):6-8. [VB]

50. Centers for Medicare and Medicaid Services (CMS) HHS. Medicaid program; payment adjustment for provider-preventable conditions including health care-acquired conditions. Final rule. *Fed Regist.* 2011;76(108):32816-32838.

51. Stechmiller JK, Cowan L, Whitney JD, et al. Guidelines for the prevention of pressure ulcers. *Wound Repair Regen.* 2008;16(2):151-168. [IVA]

52. Bergstrom N, Braden BJ, Laguzza A, Holman V. The Braden Scale for Predicting Pressure Sore Risk. *Nurs Res.* 1987;36(4):205-210. [VA]

53. Cardinal Health/AORN Pressure Ulcer Prevention Project. Instructions for the Munro Pressure Ulcer Risk Assessment Scale for Perioperative Patients for Adults. AORN, Inc. https://www.aorn.org/-/media/aorn/guidelines/tool-kits/pressure-ulcer/instructions-for-munro-risk-assessment-scale.pdf?la=en. Accessed March 10, 2017.

54. Munro Pressure Ulcer Risk Assessment Scale for Perioperative Patients—Adults. AORN, Inc. https://www.aorn.org/-/media/aorn/guidelines/tool-kits/pressure-ulcer/munro-pressure-ulcer-risk-assessment-scale.xlsx?la=en. Accessed March 10, 2017.

55. Scott SM. Progress and challenges in perioperative pressure ulcer prevention. *J Wound Ostomy Continence Nurs.* 2015;42(5):480-485. [VB]

56. Giachetta-Ryan D. Perioperative pressure ulcers: how can they be prevented? *OR Nurse.* 2015;9(4):22-28. [VC]

57. He W, Liu P, Chen HL. The Braden Scale cannot be used alone for assessing pressure ulcer risk in surgical patients: a meta-analysis. *Ostomy Wound Manage.* 2012;58(2):34-40. [IIIB]

58. Owers CE, Abbas Y, Ackroyd R, Barron N, Khan M. Perioperative optimization of patients undergoing bariatric surgery. *J Obes.* 2012;2012:781546. [VB]

59. Bulfone G, Marzolil I, Wuattrin R, Fabbro C, Palese A. A longitudinal study of the incidence of pressure sores and the associated risks and strategies adopted in Italian operating theatres [Published erratum in: *J Perioper Pract.* 2012;22(5):149]. *J Perioper Pract.* 2012;22(2):50-56. [IIIB]

60. Doerflinger DMC. Older adult surgical patients: presentation and challenges. *AORN J.* 2009;90(2):223-244. [VA]

61. Engels D, Austin M, McNichol L, Fencl J, Gupta S, Kazi H. Pressure ulcers: factors contributing to their development in the OR. *AORN J.* 2016;103(3):271-281. [VA]

62. Black J, Fawcett D, Scott S. Ten top tips: preventing pressure ulcers in the surgical patient. *Wounds Int.* 2014;54(4):14-18. [VB]

63. Pressure Ulcer Prevention in the OR: Recommendations and Guidance. St Paul, MN: Minnesota Hospital Association; 2013. https://www.mnhospitals.org/Portals/0/Documents/ptsafety/skin/OR-pressure-ulcer-recommendations.pdf. Accessed March 10, 2017. [IVC]

64. Fred C, Ford S, Wagner D, Vanbrackle L. Intraoperatively acquired pressure ulcers and perioperative normothermia: a look at relationships. *AORN J.* 2012;96(3):251-260. [IIIA]

65. Menezes S, Rodrigues R, Tranquada R, Müller S, Gama K, Manso T. Injuries resulting from positioning for surgery: incidence and risk factors. *Acta Med Port.* 2013;26(1):12-16. [IIIC]

66. Strasser LA. Improving skin integrity in the perioperative environment using an evidence-based protocol. *J Dermatol Nurses Assoc.* 2012;4(6):351-362. [VA]

67. Winfree CJ, Kline DG. Intraoperative positioning nerve injuries. *Surg Neurol.* 2005;63(1):5-18. [VB]

68. Agostini J, Goasguen N, Mosnier H. Patient positioning in laparoscopic surgery: tricks and tips. *J Visc Surg.* 2010;147(4):e227-e232. [VB]

69. Cullen A, Ferguson A. Perioperative management of the severely obese patient: a selective pathophysiological review. *Can J Anesth.* 2012;59(10):974-996. [VA]

70. Sezer SD, Küçük M, Yüksel H, Odabaşi AR, Şen S, Ogurlu M. Drop foot, an unexpected complication of vaginal hysterectomy. *Turk Jinekoloji ve Obstetrik Dernegi Dergisi.* 2012;9(1):73-76. [VC]

71. Connor T, Sledge JA, Bryant-Wiersema L, Stamm L, Potter P. Identification of pre-operative and intra-operative variables predictive of pressure ulcer development in patients undergoing urologic surgical procedures. *Urol Nurs.* 2010;30(5):289-305. [IIB]

72. Thomas DR. Does pressure cause pressure ulcers? An inquiry into the etiology of pressure ulcers. *J Am Med Dir Assoc.* 2010;11(6):397-405. [VA]

73. Anusionwu IM, Wright EJ. Compartment syndrome after positioning in lithotomy: what a urologist needs to know. *BJU Int.* 2011;108(4):477-478. [VB]

74. Bushard S. Trauma in patients who are morbidly obese. *AORN J.* 2002;76(4):585-589. [VB]

75. Mackey D. Support surfaces: beds, mattresses, overlays—oh my! *Nurs Clin North Am.* 2005;40(2):251-265. [VB]

76. Pham B, Teague L, Mahoney J, et al. Support surfaces for intraoperative prevention of pressure ulcers in patients undergoing surgery: a cost-effectiveness analysis. *Surgery.* 2011;150(1):122-132. [IIIB]

77. Silverstein JW, Matthews E, Mermelstein LE, DeWal H. Causal factors for position-related SSEP changes in spinal surgery. *Eur Spine J.* 2016;25(10):3208-3213. [IIIB]

78. Parnham A. Pressure ulcer risk assessment and prevention in children. *Nurs Child Young People.* 2012;24(2):24-29. [VA]

79. Anthony D, Willock J, Baharestani M. A comparison of Braden Q, Garvin and Glamorgan risk assessment scales in paediatrics. *J Tissue Viability.* 2010;19(3):98-105. [IIIB]

80. Willock J, Anthony D, Richardson J. Inter-rater reliability of Glamorgan Paediatric Pressure Ulcer Risk Assessment Scale. *Paediatr Nurs.* 2008;20(7):14-19. [IIIB]

81. Huffines B, Logsdon MC. The Neonatal Skin Risk Assessment Scale for predicting skin breakdown in neonates. *Issues Compr Pediatr Nurs.* 1997;20(2):103-114. [IIIB]

82. McNichol L, Lund C, Rosen T, Gray M. Medical adhesives and patient safety: state of the science: consensus statements for the assessment, prevention, and treatment of adhesive-related skin injuries. *J Wound Ostomy Continence Nurs.* 2013;40(4):365-380. [IVB]

83. Dyer A. Ten top tips: Preventing device-related pressure ulcers. *Wounds Int.* 2015;6(1):9-13. [VB]

84. Larkin BG. The ins and outs of body piercing. *AORN J.* 2004;79(2):333-342. [VA]

85. Smith FD. Caring for surgical patients with piercings. *AORN J.* 2016;103(6):583-596. [VB]

86. Ogg MJ. Preventing alternate site burns from hair accessories during electrosurgery [Clinical Issues]. *AORN J.* 2012;95(4):545-547. [VB]

87. Cho JK, Han JH, Park SW, Kim KS. Deep vein thrombosis after spine operation in prone position with subclavian venous catheterization: a case report. *Korean J Anesthesiol.* 2014;67(1):61-65. [VA]

88. Denholm B. Caring for surgical patients who have subdermal implants [Clinical Issues]. *AORN J.* 2013;97(3):372-375. [VA]

89. Wanzer LJ, Hick RW. Identifying and minimizing risks for surgical patients with dermal implants. *AORN J.* 2012;96(4):C5-C6. [VB]

90. Guideline for safe use of energy-generating devices. In: *Guidelines for Perioperative Practice.* Denver, CO: AORN, Inc; 2017:129-156. [IVA]

91. Haldar R, Kaushal A, Srivastava S, Singh PK. Paediatric intravenous splint: a cause of pressure injury during neurosurgery in prone position. *Pediatr Neurosurg.* 2016;51(1):55-56. [VB]

92. Weng MH. The effect of protective treatment in reducing pressure ulcers for non-invasive ventilation patients. *Intensive Crit Care Nurs.* 2008;24(5):295-299. [IIB]

93. Kuo CY, Wootten CT, Tylor DA, Werkhaven JA, Huffman KF, Goudy SL. Prevention of pressure ulcers after pediatric tracheotomy using a Mepilex Ag dressing. *Laryngoscope.* 2013;123(12):3201-3205. [IIIB]

94. Huang TT, Tseng CE, Lee TM, Yeh JY, Lai YY. Preventing pressure sores of the nasal ala after nasotracheal tube intubation: from animal model to clinical application. *J Oral Maxillofac Surg.* 2009;67(3):543-551. [IIC]

95. Günlemez A, Isken T, Gokalp AS, Turker G, Arisoy EA. Effect of silicon gel sheeting in nasal injury associated with nasal CPAP in preterm infants. *Indian Pediatr.* 2010;47(3):265-267. [IB]

96. Ulm MA, Fleming ND, Rallapali V, et al. Position-related injury is uncommon in robotic gynecologic surgery. *Gynecol Oncol.* 2014;135(3):534-538. [IIIB]

97. Makary MA, Holzmueller CG, Thompson D, et al. Operating room briefings: working on the same page. *Jt Comm J Qual Patient Saf.* 2006;32(6):351-355. [VB]

98. Makary MA, Holzmueller CG, Sexton JB, et al. Operating room debriefings. *Jt Comm J Qual Patient Saf.* 2006;32(7):407-410, 357. [VB]

99. *AORN Position Statement: Preventing Wrong-Patient, Wrong-Site, Wrong-Procedure Events.* AORN, Inc. http://www.aorn.org/guidelines/clinical-resources/position-statements. Accessed March 10, 2017. [IVB]

100. WHO Surgical Safety Checklist. World Health Organization. http://www.who.int/patientsafety/safesurgery/tools_resources/SSSL_Checklist_finalJun08.pdf?ua=1. Accessed March 10, 2017.

101. UP.01.03.01: A time-out is performed before the procedure. In: *Comprehensive Accreditation and Certification Manual: Critical Access Hospitals.* July 2016 ed. Oakbrook Terrace, IL: Joint Commission Resources; 2016.

102. UP.01.03.01: A time-out is performed before the procedure. In: *Comprehensive Accreditation and Certification Manual: Ambulatory.* July 2016 ed. Oakbrook Terrace, IL: Joint Commission Resources; 2016.

103. Guideline for product selection. In: *Guidelines for Perioperative Practice.* Denver, CO: AORN, Inc; 2017:183-190. [IVB]

104. Hoshowsky VM, Schramm CA. Intraoperative pressure sore prevention: an analysis of bedding materials. *Res Nurs Health.* 1994;17(5):333-339. [IB]

105. King CA, Bridges E. Comparison of pressure relief properties of operating room surfaces. *Perioper Nurs Clin.* 2006;1(3):261-265. [IIB]

106. Reddy M. Pressure ulcers. *BMJ Clin Evid.* 2011;2011:1901. [IIIA]

107. Wu T, Wang ST, Lin PC, Liu CL, Chao YF. Effects of using a high-density foam pad versus a viscoelastic polymer pad on the incidence of pressure ulcer development during spinal surgery. *Biol Res Nurs.* 2011;13(4):419-424. [IIA]

108. McInnes E, Jammali-Blasi A, Bell-Syer SEM, Dumville JC, Middleton V, Cullum N. Support surfaces for pressure ulcer prevention. *Cochrane Database Syst Rev.* 2015;(9):CD001735. [IIB]

109. McNichol L, Watts C, Mackey D, Beitz JM, Gray M. Identifying the right surface for the right patient at the right time: generation and content validation of an algorithm for support surface selection. *J Wound Ostomy Continence Nurs.* 2015;42(1):19-37. [IVA]

110. Deane LA, Lee HJ, Box GN, et al. Third place: flank position is associated with higher skin-to-surface interface pressures in men versus women: implications for laparoscopic renal surgery and the risk of rhabdomyolysis. *J Endourol.* 2008;22(6):1147-1151. [IIB]

111. *Guidelines for Environmental Infection Control in Health-Care Facilities: Recommendations of CDC and the Healthcare Infection Control Practices Advisory Committee (HICPAC).* Atlanta, GA: Centers for Disease Control and Prevention; 2003. https://www.cdc.gov/hicpac/pdf/guidelines/eic_in_HCF_03.pdf. Accessed March 10, 2017. [IVA]

112. Ahmad R, Tham J, Naqvi SG, Butt U, Dixon J. Supports used for positioning of patients in hip arthroplasty: is there an infection risk? *Ann R Coll Surg Engl.* 2011;93(2):130-132. [IIIC]

113. Guideline for environmental cleaning. In: *Guidelines for Perioperative Practice.* Denver, CO: AORN, Inc; 2017:7-28. [IVA]

114. Neurosurgical head holders (skull clamps) and device slippage: FDA safety communication. February 25, 2016. US Food and Drug Administration. https://www.fda.gov/MedicalDevices/Safety/AlertsandNotices/ucm487665.htm. Accessed March 10, 2017. [VA]

115. Dauber MH, Roth S. Operating table failure: another hazard of spine surgery. *Anesth Analg.* 2009;108(3):904-905. [VB]

116. Ahmad FU, Madhavan K, Trombly R, Levi AD. Anterior thigh compartment syndrome and local myonecrosis after posterior spine surgery on a Jackson table. *World Neurosurg.* 2012;78(5):553.e5-553.e8. [VB]

117. Flierl MA, Stahel PF, Hak DJ, Morgan SJ, Smith WR. Traction table-related complications in orthopaedic surgery. *J Am Acad Orthop Surg.* 2010;18(11):668-675. [VA]

118. Bonnaig N, Dailey S, Archdeacon M. Proper patient positioning and complication prevention in orthopaedic surgery. *J Bone Joint Surg Am.* 2014;96(13):1135-1140. [VB]

119. Mallet R, Tricoire JL, Rischmann P, Sarramon JP, Puget J, Malavaud B. High prevalence of erectile dysfunction in young male patients after intramedullary femoral nailing. *Urology.* 2005;65(3):559-563. [IIIB]

120. Toolan BC, Koval KJ, Kummer FJ, Goldsmith ME, Zuckerman JD. Effects of supine positioning and fracture post placement on the perineal countertraction force in awake volunteers. *J Orthop Trauma.* 1995;9(2):164-170. [IIIC]

121. MedWatch: The FDA Safety Information and Adverse Event Reporting Program. US Food and Drug Administration. https://www.fda.gov/Safety/MedWatch/. Accessed March 10, 2017.

122. Poli JC, Zoia C, Lattanzi D, Balbi S. Epidural haematoma by Mayfield head-holder: case report and review of literature. *J Pediatr Sci.* 2013;5:e195. [VA]

123. Berry C, Sandberg DI, Hoh DJ, Krieger MD, McComb JG. Use of cranial fixation pins in pediatric neurosurgery. *Neurosurgery.* 2008;62(4):913-918; discussion 918-919. [IIIB]

124. Chappy S. Perioperative patient safety: a multisite qualitative analysis. *AORN J.* 2006;83(4):871-877. [IIIB]

125. Waters T, Baptiste A, Short M, Plante-Mallon L, Nelson A. AORN ergonomic tool 1: lateral transfer of a patient from a stretcher to an OR bed. *AORN J.* 2011;93(3):334-339. [VA]

126. Waters T, Lloyd JD, Hernandez E, Nelson A. AORN ergonomic tool 7: pushing, pulling, and moving equipment on wheels. *AORN J.* 2011;94(3):254-260. [VA]

127. Asiedu GB, Lowndes BR, Huddleston PM, Hallbeck S. "The Jackson Table is a pain in the...": a qualitative study of providers' perception toward a spinal surgery table. *J Patient Saf.* January 7, 2016. Epub ahead of print. [IIIB]

128. Beyea SC. Preventing patient falls in perioperative settings. *AORN J.* 2005;81(2):393-395. [VB]

129. Redman JF, McNatt SJ. Portable cushioned operating table siderails: an adjunct to pediatric surgery. *South Med J*. 2000;93(11):1081-1082. [VC]

130. Chen HL, Chen XY, Wu J. The incidence of pressure ulcers in surgical patients of the last 5 years: a systematic review. *Wounds*. 2012;24(9):234-241. [IIIB]

131. Shon YJ, Bae SK, Park JW, Kim IN, Huh J. Partial displacement of epidural catheter after patient position change: a case report. *J Clin Anesth*. 2017;37:17-20. [VB]

132. Campbell K. Pressure point measures in the operating room. *J Enterostomal Ther*. 1989;16(3):119-124. [VB]

133. Lupe L, Zambrana D, Cooper L. Prevention of hospital-acquired pressure ulcers in the operating room and beyond: a successful monitoring and intervention strategy program. *Int Anesthesiol Clin*. 2013;51(1):128-146. [VB]

134. Grous CA, Reilly NJ, Gift AG. Skin integrity in patients undergoing prolonged operations. *J Wound Ostomy Continence Nurs*. 1997;24(2):86-91. [IIIB]

135. Whitney J, Phillips L, Aslam R, et al. Guidelines for the treatment of pressure ulcers. *Wound Repair Regen*. 2006;14(6):663-679. [IVB]

136. Landis EM. Micro-injection studies of capillary blood pressure in human skin. *Heart*. 1930;15:209-228. [IIIA]

137. Malkoun M, Huber J, Huber D. A comparative assessment of interface pressures generated by four surgical theatre heel pressure ulcer prophylactics. *Int Wound J*. 2012;9(3):259-263. [IIIB]

138. Kosiak M. Etiology and pathology of ischemic ulcers. *Arch Phys Med Rehabil*. 1959;40(2):62-69. [IIIB]

139. Sutton S, Link T, Makic MB. A quality improvement project for safe and effective patient positioning during robot-assisted surgery. *AORN J*. 2013;97(4):448-456. [VB]

140. Fletcher J, Harris C, Mahoney K. A small-scale evaluation of the Dolphin Fluid Immersion Simulation® Mattress. *Wounds UK*. 2014;10(1):97-100. [VC]

141. Worsley PR, Parsons B, Bader DL. An evaluation of fluid immersion therapy for the prevention of pressure ulcers. *Clin Biomech* (Bristol Avon). 2016;40:27-32. [IIIB]

142. Kirkland-Walsh H, Teleten O, Wilson M, Raingruber B. Pressure mapping comparison of four OR surfaces. *AORN J*. 2015;102(1):61.e1-61.e9. [IIIB]

143. Akhavan A, Gainsburg DM, Stock JA. Complications associated with patient positioning in urologic surgery. *Urology*. 2010;76(6):1309-1316. [VB]

144. Martin JT, Warner MA. *Positioning in Anesthesia and Surgery*. 3rd ed. Philadelphia, PA: Saunders; 1997.

145. Stephenson LL, Webb NA, Smithers CJ, Sager SL, Seefelder C. Lateral femoral cutaneous neuropathy following lateral positioning on a bean bag. *J Clin Anesth*. 2009;21(5):383-384. [VB]

146. National Institute for Health and Care Excellence. *The Prevention and Management of Pressure Ulcers in Primary and Secondary Care. Clinical Guideline No. 179. Methods, Evidence, and Recommendations*. London, UK: National Clinical Guideline Centre; 2014:1-416. [IVA]

147. American College of Surgeons National Surgical Quality Improvement Program, American Geriatrics Society. Optimal Perioperative Management of the Geriatric Patient. American College of Surgeons. https://www.facs.org/~/media/files/quality%20programs/geriatric/acs%20nsqip%20geriatric%202016%20guidelines.ashx. Accessed March 10, 2017. [IVB]

148. Santamaria N, Gerdtz M, Sage S, et al. A randomised controlled trial of the effectiveness of soft silicone multi-layered foam dressings in the prevention of sacral and heel pressure ulcers in trauma and critically ill patients: the border trial. *Int Wound J*. 2015;12(3):302-308. [IB]

149. Brindle CT, Wegelin JA. Prophylactic dressing application to reduce pressure ulcer formation in cardiac surgery patients. *J Wound Ostomy Continence Nurs*. 2012;39(2):133-142. [IIB]

150. Moore ZE, Webster J. Dressings and topical agents for preventing pressure ulcers. *Cochrane Database Syst Rev*. 2013;(8):CD009362. [IB]

151. Call E, Pedersen J, Bill B, et al. Enhancing pressure ulcer prevention using wound dressings: what are the modes of action? *Int Wound J*. 2015;12(4):408-413. [IIIB]

152. Walsh NS, Blanck AW, Smith L, Cross M, Andersson L, Polito C. Use of a sacral silicone border foam dressing as one component of a pressure ulcer prevention program in an intensive care unit setting. *J Wound Ostomy Continence Nurs*. 2012;39(2):146-149. [VB]

153. Chaiken N. Reduction of sacral pressure ulcers in the intensive care unit using a silicone border foam dressing. *J Wound Ostomy Continence Nurs*. 2012;39(2):143-145. [VB]

154. Forni C, Loro L, Tremosini M, et al. Use of polyurethane foam inside plaster casts to prevent the onset of heel sores in the population at risk. A controlled clinical study. *J Clin Nurs*. 2011;20(5-6):675-680. [IIB]

155. Call E, Pedersen J, Bill B, Oberg C, Ferguson-Pell M. Microclimate impact of prophylactic dressings using in vitro body analog method. *Wounds*. 2013;25(4):94-103. [IIIB]

156. Zhang J, Moore AE, Stringer MD. Iatrogenic upper limb nerve injuries: a systematic review. *ANZ J Surg*. 2011;81(4):227-236. [VB]

157. Bale E, Berrecloth R. The obese patient. Anaesthetic issues: airway and positioning. *J Perioper Pract*. 2010;20(8):294-299. [VB]

158. Kam AW, Lam PH, Murrell GAC. Brachial plexus injuries during shoulder arthroplasty: what causes them and how to prevent them. *Tech Shoulder Elbow Surg*. 2015;15(4):109-114. [VA]

159. Colsa Gutierrez P, Viadero Cervera R, Morales-Garcia D, Ingelmo Setien A. Intraoperative peripheral nerve injury in colorectal surgery. An update. *Cir Esp*. 2016;94(3):125-136. [VA]

160. Shimizu S, Sato K, Mabuchi I, et al. Brachial plexopathy due to massive swelling of the neck associated with craniotomy in the park bench position. *Surg Neurol*. 2009;71(4):504-508. [VB]

161. Uribe JS, Kolla J, Omar H, et al. Brachial plexus injury following spinal surgery. *J Neurosurg Spine*. 2010;13(4):552-558. [VB]

162. Lin SP, Sung CS, Chan KH. Compartment syndrome and rhabdomyolysis as a positioning complication following retrosigmoid craniotomy. *Acta Anaesthesiol Taiwan*. 2013;51(4):184-186. [VB]

163. Ortega R, Suzuki S, Sekhar P, Stram JR, Rengasamy SK. Paraplegia after mastoidectomy under general anesthesia. *Am J Otolaryngol*. 2009;30(5):340-342. [VB]

164. Singha SK, Chatterjee N. Postoperative sialadenitis following retromastoid suboccipital craniectomy for posterior fossa tumor. *J Anesth*. 2009;23(4):591-593. [VB]

165. Postaci A, Aytac I, Dikmen B, Oztekin CV. Acute unilateral parotid gland swelling after lateral decubitus position under general anesthesia. *Saudi J Anaesth*. 2012;6(3):295-297. [VB]

166. Hsieh CT, Liu MY, Chen YH, Chang CF. Postoperative acute sialadenitis following posterior fossa surgery. *Neurosciences*. 2011;16(4):378-380. [VB]

167. Kim LJ, Klopfenstein JD, Feiz-Erfan I, Zubay GP, Spetzler RF. Postoperative acute sialadenitis after skull base surgery. *Skull Base*. 2008;18(2):129-133. [VB]

168. Asghar A, Karam K, Rashid S. A case of anesthesia mumps after sacral laminectomy under general anesthesia. *Saudi J Anaesth.* 2015;9(3):332-333. [VC]

169. Morrison CM, Dobryansky M, Warren RJ, Zins JE. The table tilt: preventing traction on the brachial plexus during facelift surgery. *Aesthet Surg J.* 2012;32(4):524. [VC]

170. Khokhar RS, Baaj J, Alhazmi HH, Dammas FA, Aldalati AM. Pressure-induced alopecia in pediatric patients following prolonged urological surgeries: the case reports and a review of literature. *Anesth Essays Res.* 2015;9(3):430-432. [VB]

171. Davies KE, Yesudian P. Pressure alopecia. *Int J Trichology.* 2012;4(2):64-68. [VB]

172. Gollapalli L, Papapetrou P, Gupta D, Fuleihan SF. Post-operative alopecia after robotic surgery in steep Trendelenburg position: a restated observation of pressure alopecia. *Middle East J Anesthesiol.* 2013;22(3):343-345. [VC]

173. Keidan I, Ben-Menchem E. Postoperative occipital nerve injury in a child. *Anaesth Intensive Care.* 2012;40(2):355-356. [VB]

174. Lee C, Choi PD, Scott G, Arkader A. Postoperative alopecia in children after orthopaedic surgery. *J Pediatr Orthop.* 2012;32(7):e53-e55. [VA]

175. Goodenough J, Highgate J, Shaaban H. Under pressure? Alopecia related to surgical duration. *Br J Anaesth.* 2014;113(2):306-307. [VC]

176. Matsushita K, Inoue N, Ooi K, Totsuka Y. Postoperative pressure-induced alopecia after segmental osteotomy at the upper and lower frontal edentulous areas for distraction osteogenesis. *Oral Maxillofac Surg.* 2011;15(3):161-163. [VB]

177. Bagaria M, Luck AM. Postoperative (pressure) alopecia following sacrocolpopexy. *J Robot Surg.* 2015;9(2):149-151. [VB]

178. Duimel-Peeters I, Halfens R, Berger M, Snoeckx L. The effects of massage as a method to prevent pressure ulcers. A review of the literature. *Ostomy Wound Manage.* 2005;51(4):70-80. [VB]

179. Ghomi A. Robotics in practice: new angles on safer positioning. Contemporary OB/GYN. http://contemporaryobgyn.modernmedicine.com/contemporary-obgyn/news/modernmedicine/modern-medicine-feature-articles/robotics-practice-new-angles?page=full. Published October 1, 2012. Accessed March 10, 2017. [VB]

180. Kan KM, Brown SE, Gainsburg DM. Ocular complications in robotic-assisted prostatectomy: a review of pathophysiology and prevention. *Minerva Anestesiol.* 2015;81(5):557-566. [VA]

181. Grixti A, Sadri M, Watts MT. Corneal protection during general anesthesia for nonocular surgery. *Ocul Surf.* 2013;11(2):109-118. [VB]

182. Freshcoln M, Diehl MR. Repositioning during robotic procedures to prevent postoperative visual loss. *OR Nurse.* 2014;8(4):36-41. [VC]

183. Kocatürk O, Kocatürk T, Kaan N, Dayanir V. The comparison of four different methods of perioperative eye protection under general anesthesia in prone position. *J Clin Anal Med.* 2012;3(2):163-165. [IIB]

184. Roth S. Perioperative visual loss: what do we know, what can we do? *Br J Anaesth.* 2009;103(Suppl 1):31-40. [VA]

185. Olsen GH, Krishna SG, Jatana KR, et al. Changes in intracuff pressure of cuffed endotracheal tubes while positioning for adenotonsillectomy in children. *Paediatr Anaesth.* 2016;26(5):500-503. [IIIB]

186. Anghelescu DL, Burgoyne LL, Khan RB. Multiple mechanisms of perioperative brachial plexus injury. *Anaesth Intensive Care.* 2008;36(2):276-278. [VB]

187. Truong AT, Sturgis EM, Rozner MA, Truong DT. Recurrent episodes of asystole from carotid sinus hypersensitivity triggered by positioning for head and neck surgery. *Head Neck.* 2013;35(1):E28-E30. [VB]

188. Li CC, Yie JC, Lai CH, Hung MH. Quadriplegia after off-pump coronary artery bypass surgery: look before you place the neck in an extended position. *J Cardiothorac Vasc Anesth.* 2013;27(2):e16-e17. [VB]

189. Reddy MKR, Arivazhagan A, Chandramouli BA. Intractable hypotension and bradycardia during surgical positioning in atlantoaxial dislocation. *J Neurosurg Anesthesiol.* 2008;20(1):71. [VC]

190. Addas BM. An uncommon cause of brachial plexus injury. *Neurosciences.* 2012;17(1):64-65. [VB]

191. St-Arnaud D, Paquin MJ. Safe positioning for neurosurgical patients. *AORN J.* 2008;87(6):1156-1168. [VA]

192. Ahmed K, Khan N, Khan MS, Dasgupta P. Development and content validation of a surgical safety checklist for operating theatres that use robotic technology. *BJU Int.* 2013;111(7):1161-1174. [VA]

193. Teeples TJ, Rallis DJ, Rieck KL, Viozzi CF. Lower extremity compartment syndrome associated with hypotensive general anesthesia for orthognathic surgery: a case report and review of the disease. *J Oral Maxillofac Surg.* 2010;68(5):1166-1170. [VB]

194. Judge A, Fecho K. Lateral antebrachial cutaneous neuropathy as a result of positioning while under general anesthesia. *Anesth Analg.* 2010;110(1):122-124. [VB]

195. Moore C. Intraoperative median nerve injury. *Int Student J Nurse Anesth.* 2011;10(2):11-14. [VB]

196. Song JB, Vemana G, Mobley JM, Bhayani SB. The second "time-out": a surgical safety checklist for lengthy robotic surgeries. *Patient Saf Surg.* 2013;7(1):19. [VC]

197. Drummond JC, Ciacci JD, Lee RR. Direct pressure on a pseudomeningocele resulting in intraoperative cerebral ischemia. *Can J Anaesth.* 2014;61(7):656-659. [VB]

198. Anastasian ZH, Ramnath B, Komotar RJ, et al. Evoked potential monitoring identifies possible neurological injury during positioning for craniotomy. *Anesth Analg.* 2009;109(3):817-821. [VB]

199. Jahangiri FR, Holmberg A, Vega-Bermudez F, Arlet V. Preventing position-related brachial plexus injury with intraoperative somatosensory evoked potentials and transcranial electrical motor evoked potentials during anterior cervical spine surgery. *Am J Electroneurodiagnostic Technol.* 2011;51(3):198-205. [VB]

200. Silverstein JW, Madhok R, Frendo CD, DeWal H, Lee GR. Contemporaneous evaluation of intraoperative ulnar and median nerve somatosensory evoked potentials for patient positioning: a review of four cases. *Neurodiagn J.* 2016;56(2):67-82. [VB]

201. Chung I, Glow JA, Dimopoulos V, et al. Upper-limb somatosensory evoked potential monitoring in lumbosacral spine surgery: a prognostic marker for position-related ulnar nerve injury. *Spine J.* 2009;9(4):287-295. [IIB]

202. La Neve JE, Zitney GP. Use of somatosensory evoked potentials to detect and prevent impending brachial plexus injury during surgical positioning for the treatment of supratentorial pathologies. *Neurodiagn J.* 2014;54(3):260-273. [VA]

203. Davis SF, Khalek Mohamed Abdel, Giles J, Fox C, Lirette L, Kandil E. Detection and prevention of impending brachial plexus injury secondary to arm positioning using ulnar nerve somatosensory evoked potentials during transaxillary approach for thyroid lobectomy. *Am J Electroneurodiagnostic Technol.* 2011;51(4):274-279. [VB]

204. Jellish WS, Sherazee G, Patel J, et al. Somatosensory evoked potentials help prevent positioning-related

brachial plexus injury during skull base surgery. *Otolaryngol Head Neck Surg.* 2013;149(1):168-173. [IIIA]

205. Ying T, Wang X, Sun H, Tang Y, Yuan Y, Li S. Clinical usefulness of somatosensory evoked potentials for detection of peripheral nerve and brachial plexus injury secondary to malpositioning in microvascular decompression. *J Clin Neurophysiol.* 2015;32(6):512-515. [IIIA]

206. Schwartz DM, Sestokas AK, Hilibrand AS, et al. Neurophysiological identification of position-induced neurologic injury during anterior cervical spine surgery. *J Clin Monit Comput.* 2006;20(6):437-444. [IIIB]

207. Bhalodia VM, Sestokas AK, Tomak PR, Schwartz DM. Transcranial electric motor evoked potential detection of compressional peroneal nerve injury in the lateral decubitus position. *J Clin Monit Comput.* 2008;22(4):319-326. [VB]

208. Eager M, Shimer A, Jahangiri FR, Shen F, Arlet V. Intraoperative neurophysiological monitoring (IONM): lessons learned from 32 case events in 2069 spine cases. *Neurodiagn J.* 2011;51(4):247-263. [IIIA]

209. Bennicoff G. Perioperative care of the morbidly obese patient in the lithotomy position. *AORN J.* 2010;92(3):297-309. [VB]

210. Rosevear HM, Lightfoot AJ, Zahs M, Waxman SW, Winfield HN. Lessons learned from a case of calf compartment syndrome after robot-assisted laparoscopic prostatectomy. *J Endourol.* 2010;24(10):1597-1601. [VA]

211. Pandey R, Elakkumanan LB, Garg R, et al. Brachial plexus injury after robotic-assisted thoracoscopic thymectomy. *J Cardiothorac Vasc Anesth.* 2009;23(4):584-586. [VB]

212. Hobaika AB, Horiguchi CH. Radial nerve lesion after malposition and sedation by continuous target controlled infusion of propofol for extracorporeal shock wave lithotripsy. *Middle East J Anesthesiol.* 2013;22(2):235-236. [VC]

213. Neutral position of a joint. The Free Dictionary. http://medical-dictionary.thefreedictionary.com/neutral+position+of+joint. Accessed March 10, 2017.

214. Bradshaw AD, Advincula AP. Optimizing patient positioning and understanding radiofrequency energy in gynecologic surgery. *Clin Obstet Gynecol.* 2010;53(3):511-520. [VB]

215. Clark JM, Friedell ML, Gupta BR, Davenport WC, Amponsah K. Perioperative compartment syndrome of the hand. *Am Surg.* 2011;77(1):116-118. [VA]

216. Hida A, Arai T, Nakanishi K, Nagaro T. Bilateral brachial plexus injury after liver transplantation. *J Anesth.* 2008;22(3):308-311. [VB]

217. Akinbingol G, Borman H, Maral T. Bilateral brachial plexus palsy after a prolonged surgical procedure of reduction mammaplasty, abdominoplasty, and liposuction. *Ann Plast Surg.* 2002;49(2):219-220. [VC]

218. Tekin L, Akarsu S, Carli A, et al. Brachial plexus lesion due to malpositioning during thyroid surgery: a case report. *J Phys Med Rehabil Sci.* 2011;14(3-4):80-84. [VB]

219. Sabiniewicz R, Ereciński J, Zipser M. Brachial plexus injury as an unusual complication after aortic stent implantation. *Cardiol Young.* 2011;21(2):227-228. [VB]

220. Cristian DA, Grama FA, Burcos T, Poalelungi A. Brachial plexus injury after a left-side modified radical mastectomy associated with patient positioning in the operating room. *Gineco.eu.* 2013;9(3):136-137. [VB]

221. Chowet AL, Lopez JR, Brock-Utne JG, Jaffe RA. Wrist hyperextension leads to median nerve conduction block: implications for intra-arterial catheter placement. *Anesthesiology.* 2004;100(2):287-291. [IIB]

222. Huber D. Preventing deep tissue injury of the foot and ankle in the operating theatre. *Wounds UK.* 2013;9(2):34-38. [VB]

223. Huber D, Huber J, DeYoung E. The association between popliteal vein compression and deep venous thrombosis: results of a pilot study. *Phlebology.* 2013;28(6):305-307. [IIIB]

224. Huber DE, Huber JP. Popliteal vein compression under general anaesthesia. *Eur J Vasc Endovasc Surg.* 2009;37(4):464-469. [IIIB]

225. Levine A, Huber J, Huber D. Changes in popliteal vein diameter and flow velocity with knee flexion and hyperextension. *Phlebology.* 2011;26(7):307-310. [IIIB]

226. O'Connor D, Breslin D, Barry M. Well-leg compartment syndrome following supine position surgery. *Anaesth Intensive Care.* 2010;38(3):595. [VB]

227. Wong VK, Stotts NA, Hopf HW, Dowling GA, Froelicher ES. Changes in heel skin temperature under pressure in hip surgery patients. *Adv Skin Wound Care.* 2011;24(12):562-570. [IIC]

228. Donnelly J, Winder J, Kernohan WG, Stevenson M. An RCT to determine the effect of a heel elevation device in pressure ulcer prevention post-hip fracture. *J Wound Care.* 2011;20(7):309-318. [IA]

229. Primiano M, Friend M, McClure C, et al. Pressure ulcer prevalence and risk factors during prolonged surgical procedures. *AORN J.* 2011;94(6):555-566. [IIIA]

230. O'Shea E, Power K. Well leg compartment syndrome following prolonged surgery in the supine position. *Can J Anaesth.* 2008;55(11):794-795. [VB]

231. Physiologic. The Free Dictionary. http://medical-dictionary.thefreedictionary.com/physiologic. Accessed March 10, 2017.

232. Albrecht P, Grosse J, Neukaeter W. Femoral neuropathy caused by hyperlordotic positioning. *J Anesth.* 2014;28(5):800. [VC]

233. Ghomi A, Kramer C, Askari R, Chavan NR, Einarsson JI. Trendelenburg position in gynecologic robotic-assisted surgery. *J Minim Invasive Gynecol.* 2012;19(4):485-489. [IIIC]

234. Brodsky JB. Positioning the morbidly obese patient for anesthesia. *Obes Surg.* 2002;12(6):751-758. [VB]

235. Ideno S, Miyazawa N, Yamamoto S. Muscle injury following laparoscopic appendectomy. *J Anesth.* 2014;28(5):801. [VB]

236. Kamel I, Barnette R. Positioning patients for spine surgery: avoiding uncommon position-related complications. *World J Orthop.* 2014;5(4):425-443. [VA]

237. Awad H, Santilli S, Ohr M, et al. The effects of steep Trendelenburg positioning on intraocular pressure during robotic radical prostatectomy. *Anesth Analg.* 2009;109(2):473-478. [IIB]

238. Borahay MA, Patel PR, Walsh TM, et al. Intraocular pressure and steep Trendelenburg during minimally invasive gynecologic surgery: is there a risk? *J Minim Invasive Gynecol.* 2013;20(6):819-824. [IIB]

239. Taketani Y, Mayama C, Suzuki N, et al. Transient but significant visual field defects after robot-assisted laparoscopic radical prostatectomy in deep Trendelenburg position. *PLoS One.* 2015;10(4):e0123361. [IIIB]

240. Astuto M, Minardi C, Uva MG, Gullo A. Intraocular pressure during laparoscopic surgery in paediatric patients. *Br J Ophthalmol.* 2011;95(2):294-295. [IIC]

241. Mondzelewski TJ, Schmitz JW, Christman MS, et al. Intraocular pressure during robotic-assisted laparoscopic procedures utilizing steep Trendelenburg positioning. *J Glaucoma.* 2015;24(6):399-404. [IIIB]

242. Molloy BL. Implications for postoperative visual loss: steep Trendelenburg position and effects on intraocular pressure. *AANA J.* 2011;79(2):115-121. [IIIB]

243. Rewari V, Ramachandran R. Prolonged steep Trendelenburg position: risk of postoperative upper airway obstruction. *J Robot Surg.* 2013;7(4):405-406. [VB]

244. Kalmar AF, Dewaele F, Foubert L, et al. Cerebral haemodynamic physiology during steep Trendelenburg position and CO_2 pneumoperitoneum. *Br J Anaesth.* 2012;108(3):478-484. [IIIB]

245. Choi SH, Lee SJ, Rha KH, Shin SK, Oh YJ. The effect of pneumoperitoneum and Trendelenburg position on acute cerebral blood flow-carbon dioxide reactivity under sevoflurane anaesthesia. *Anaesthesia.* 2008;63(12):1314-1318. [IIA]

246. Closhen D, Treiber AH, Berres M, et al. Robotic assisted prostatic surgery in the Trendelenburg position does not impair cerebral oxygenation measured using two different monitors: a clinical observational study. *Eur J Anaesthesiol.* 2014;31(2):104-109. [IIA]

247. Park EY, Koo BN, Min KT, Nam SH. The effect of pneumoperitoneum in the steep Trendelenburg position on cerebral oxygenation. *Acta Anaesthesiol Scand.* 2009;53(7):895-899. [IIIB]

248. Lahaye L, Grasso M, Green J, Biddle CJ. Cerebral tissue O_2 saturation during prolonged robotic surgery in the steep Trendelenburg position: an observational case series in a diverse surgical population. *J Robot Surg.* 2015;9(1):19-25. [IIB]

249. Barr C, Madhuri TK, Prabhu P, Butler-Manuel S, Tailor A. Cerebral oedema following robotic surgery: a rare complication. *Arch Gynecol Obstet.* 2014;290(5):1041-1044. [VB]

250. Chin JH, Seo H, Lee EH, et al. Sonographic optic nerve sheath diameter as a surrogate measure for intracranial pressure in anesthetized patients in the Trendelenburg position. *BMC Anesthesiol.* 2015;15:43. [IIB]

251. Shah SB, Bhargava AK, Choudhury I. Noninvasive intracranial pressure monitoring via optic nerve sheath diameter for robotic surgery in steep Trendelenburg position. *Saudi J Anaesth.* 2015;9(3):239-246. [IA]

252. Kim MS, Bai SJ, Lee JR, Choi YD, Kim YJ, Choi SH. Increase in intracranial pressure during carbon dioxide pneumoperitoneum with steep Trendelenburg positioning proven by ultrasonographic measurement of optic nerve sheath diameter. *J Endourol.* 2014;28(7):801-806. [IIIB]

253. Kim SH, Kim HJ, Jung KT. Position does not affect the optic nerve sheath diameter during laparoscopy. *Korean J Anesthesiol.* 2015;68(4):358-363. [IIIC]

254. Gkegkes ID, Karydis A, Tyritzis SI, Iavazzo C. Ocular complications in robotic surgery. *Int J Med Robot.* 2015;11(3):269-274. [IIIB]

255. Grosso A, Scozzari G, Bert F, Mabilia MA, Siliquini R, Morino M. Intraocular pressure variation during colorectal laparoscopic surgery: standard pneumoperitoneum leads to reversible elevation in intraocular pressure. *Surg Endosc.* 2013;27(9):3370-3376. [IIB]

256. Grosso A, Ceruti P, Morino M, Marchini G, Amisano M, Fioretto M. Comment on the paper by Mondzelewski and colleagues: "Intraocular pressure during robotic-assisted laparoscopic procedures utilizing steep Trendelenburg positioning." *J Glaucoma.* 2015;24(6):399-404. *J Glaucoma.* August 22, 2016. Epub ahead of print. [VB]

257. Hoshikawa Y, Tsutsumi N, Ohkoshi K, et al. The effect of steep Trendelenburg positioning on intraocular pressure and visual function during robotic-assisted radical prostatectomy. *Br J Ophthalmol.* 2014;98(3):305-308. [IIB]

258. De Leon A, Thörn S-E, Ottosson J, Wattwil M. Body positions and esophageal sphincter pressures in obese patients during anesthesia. *Acta Anaesthesiol Scand.* 2010;54(4):458-463. [IIB]

259. Choi DK, Lee IG, Hwang JH. Arterial to end-tidal carbon dioxide pressure gradient increases with age in the steep Trendelenburg position with pneumoperitoneum. *Korean J Anesthesiol.* 2012;63(3):209-215. [IIA]

260. Kilic OF, Borgers A, Kohne W, Musch M, Kropfl D, Groeben H. Effects of steep Trendelenburg position for robotic-assisted prostatectomies on intra- and extrathoracic airways in patients with or without chronic obstructive pulmonary disease. *Br J Anaesth.* 2015;114(1):70-76. [IIB]

261. Wysham WZ, Kim KH, Roberts JM, et al. Obesity and perioperative pulmonary complications in robotic gynecologic surgery. *Am J Obstet Gynecol.* 2015;213(1):33.e1-33.e7. [IIIB]

262. Chin YS. Bradycardia caused by position change. *J Anesth.* 2012;26(3):475-476. [VB]

263. Darlong V, Kunhabdulla NP, Pandey R, et al. Hemodynamic changes during robotic radical prostatectomy. *Saudi J Anaesth.* 2012;6(3):213-218. [IIB]

264. Lowenstein L, Mustafa M, Burke YZ, Mustafa S, Segal D, Weissman A. Steep Trendelenburg position during robotic sacrocolpopexy and heart rate variability. *Eur J Obstet Gynecol Reprod Biol.* 2014;178:66-69. [IIIB]

265. Zorko N, Mekis D, Kamenik M. The influence of the Trendelenburg position on haemodynamics: comparison of anaesthetized patients with ischaemic heart disease and healthy volunteers. *J Int Med Res.* 2011;39(3):1084-1089. [IIC]

266. Russo A, Marana E, Viviani D, et al. Diastolic function: the influence of pneumoperitoneum and Trendelenburg positioning during laparoscopic hysterectomy. *Eur J Anaesthesiol.* 2009;26(11):923-927. [IIIB]

267. Meininger D, Westphal K, Bremerich DH, et al. Effects of posture and prolonged pneumoperitoneum on hemodynamic parameters during laparoscopy. *World J Surg.* 2008;32(7):1400-1405. [IIIB]

268. Kalmar AF, Foubert L, Hendrickx JF, et al. Influence of steep Trendelenburg position and CO(2) pneumoperitoneum on cardiovascular, cerebrovascular, and respiratory homeostasis during robotic prostatectomy. *Br J Anaesth.* 2010;104(4):433-439. [IIIB]

269. Lestar M, Gunnarsson L, Lagerstrand L, Wiklund P, Odeberg-Wernerman S. Hemodynamic perturbations during robot-assisted laparoscopic radical prostatectomy in 45-degree Trendelenburg position. *Anesth Analg.* 2011;113(5):1069-1075. [IIIC]

270. Haas S, Haese A, Goetz AE, Kubitz JC. Haemodynamics and cardiac function during robotic-assisted laparoscopic prostatectomy in steep Trendelenburg position. *Int J Med Robot.* 2011;7(4):408-413. [IIB]

271. Mekiš D, Kamenik M. Influence of body position on hemodynamics in patients with ischemic heart disease undergoing cardiac surgery. *Wien Klin Wochenschr.* 2010;122(Suppl 2):59-62. [IIIB]

272. Wen T, Deibert CM, Siringo FS, Spencer BA. Positioning-related complications of minimally invasive radical prostatectomies. *J Endourol.* 2014;28(6):660-667. [IIIB]

273. Gould C, Cull T, Wu YX, Osmundsen B. Blinded measure of Trendelenburg angle in pelvic robotic surgery. *J Minim Invasive Gynecol.* 2012;19(4):465-468. [IIB]

274. Schramm P, Treiber AH, Berres M, et al. Time course of cerebrovascular autoregulation during extreme Trendelenburg position for robotic-assisted prostatic surgery. *Anaesthesia.* 2014;69(1):58-63. [IIIB]

275. Kadono Y, Yaegashi H, Machioka K, et al. Cardiovascular and respiratory effects of the degree of head-down angle during robot-assisted laparoscopic radical prostatectomy. *Int J Med Robot*. 2013;9(1):17-22. [IB]

276. Raz O, Boesel TW, Arianayagam M, et al. The effect of the modified Z Trendelenburg position on intraocular pressure during robotic assisted laparoscopic radical prostatectomy: a randomized, controlled study. *J Urol*. 2015;193(4):1213-1219. [IB]

277. Shveiky D, Aseff JN, Iglesia CB. Brachial plexus injury after laparoscopic and robotic surgery. *J Minim Invasive Gynecol*. 2010;17(4):414-420. [VB]

278. Addison AB, Inarra E, Watts S. Bilateral otorrhagia: a rare complication of laparoscopic abdominopelvic surgery. *BMJ Case Rep*. December 19, 2014;2014. [VB]

279. Pandey R, Garg R, Darlong V, Punj J, Chandralekha KA. Unpredicted neurological complications after robotic laparoscopic radical cystectomy and ileal conduit formation in steep Trendelenburg position: two case reports. *Acta Anaesthesiol Belg*. 2010;61(3):163-166. [VB]

280. Pinkney TD, King AJ, Walter C, Wilson TR, Maxwell-Armstrong C, Acheson AG. Raised intraocular pressure (IOP) and perioperative visual loss in laparoscopic colorectal surgery: a catastrophe waiting to happen? A systematic review of evidence from other surgical specialities. *Tech Coloproctol*. 2012;16(5):331-335. [IIIB]

281. Mizrahi H, Hugkulstone CE, Vyakarnam P, Parker MC. Bilateral ischaemic optic neuropathy following laparoscopic proctocolectomy: a case report. *Ann R Coll Surg Engl*. 2011;93(5):e53-e54. [VB]

282. Kumar G, Vyakarnam P. Postoperative vision loss after colorectal laparoscopic surgery. *Surg Laparosc Endosc Percutan Tech*. 2013;23(2):e87-88. [VB]

283. Nuzzi R, Tridico F. Ocular complications in laparoscopic surgery: review of existing literature and possible prevention and treatment. *Semin Ophthalmol*. 2016;31(6):584-592. [VB]

284. Codd RJ, Evans MD, Sagar PM, Williams GL. A systematic review of peripheral nerve injury following laparoscopic colorectal surgery. *Colorectal Dis*. 2013;15(3):278-282. [IIIB]

285. Mattei A, Di Pierro GB, Rafeld V, Konrad C, Beutler J, Danuser H. Positioning injury, rhabdomyolysis, and serum creatine kinase-concentration course in patients undergoing robot-assisted radical prostatectomy and extended pelvic lymph node dissection. *J Endourol*. 2013;27(1):45-51. [IIIB]

286. Klauschie J, Wechter ME, Jacob K, et al. Use of anti-skid material and patient-positioning to prevent patient shifting during robotic-assisted gynecologic procedures. *J Minim Invasive Gynecol*. 2010;17(4):504-507. [IIIC]

287. Wechter ME, Kho RM, Chen AH, Magrina JF, Pettit PD. Preventing slide in Trendelenburg position: Randomized trial comparing foam and gel pads. *J Robot Surg*. 2013;7(3):267-271. [IA]

288. Nakayama JM, Gerling GJ, Horst KE, Fitz VW, Cantrell LA, Modesitt SC. A simulation study of the factors influencing the risk of intraoperative slipping. *Clin Ovarian Other Gynecol Cancer*. 2014;7(1-2):24-28. [IIIB]

289. Talab SS, Elmi A, Sarma J, Barrisford GW, Tabatabaei S. Safety and effectiveness of SAF-R, a novel patient positioning device for robot-assisted pelvic surgery in Trendelenburg position. *J Endourol*. 2016;30(3):286-292. [IIIC]

290. Hewer CL. The physiology and complications of the Trendelenburg position. *Can Med Assoc J*. 1956;74(4):285-288. [VB]

291. Kalmar AF, De Wolf AM, Hendrickx JFA. Anesthetic considerations for robotic surgery in the steep Trendelenburg position. *Adv Anesth*. 2012;30(1):75-96. [VA]

292. Wu CY, Yeh YC, Wang MC, Lai CH, Fan SZ. Changes in endotracheal tube cuff pressure during laparoscopic surgery in head-up or head-down position. *BMC Anesthesiol*. 2014;14:75. [IIB]

293. Coppieters MW, Van de Velde M, Stappaerts KH. Positioning in anesthesiology: toward a better understanding of stretch-induced perioperative neuropathies. *Anesthesiology*. 2002;97(1):75-81. [IIB]

294. Suozzi BA, Brazell HD, O'Sullivan DM, Tulikangas PK. A comparison of shoulder pressure among different patient stabilization techniques. *Am J Obstet Gynecol*. 2013;209(5):478.e1-478.e5. [IIIB]

295. Devarajan J, Byrd JB, Gong MC, et al. Upper and middle trunk brachial plexopathy after robotic prostatectomy. *Anesth Analg*. 2012;115(4):867-870. [VA]

296. Eteuati J, Hiscock R, Hastie I, Hayes I, Jones I. Brachial plexopathy in laparoscopic-assisted rectal surgery: a case series. *Tech Coloproctol*. 2013;17(3):293-297. [VB]

297. Vaughan RW, Wise L. Intraoperative arterial oxygenation in obese patients. *Ann Surg*. 1976;184(1):35-42. [IIB]

298. An J, Shin SK, Kwon J-Y, Kim KJ. Incidence of venous air embolism during myomectomy: the effect of patient position. *Yonsei Med J*. 2013;54(1):209-214. [IA]

299. Ghai A, Saini S, Kiran S, Kamal K, Kad N, Bhawna. Influence of lithotomy position on the haemodynamic changes in patients with coronary artery disease. *J Anaesthesiol Clin Pharmacol*. 2008;24(3):359-360. [VB]

300. Roeder RA, Geddes LA, Corson N, Pell C, Otlewski M, Kemeny A. Heel and calf capillary-support: pressure in lithotomy positions. *AORN J*. 2005;81(4):821-830. [IIIB]

301. Wilde S. Compartment syndrome. The silent danger related to patient positioning and surgery. *Br J Perioper Nurs*. 2004;14(12):546-550. [VC]

302. Bauer EC, Koch N, Janni W, Bender HG, Fleisch MC. Compartment syndrome after gynecologic operations: evidence from case reports and reviews. *Eur J Obstet Gynecol Reprod Biol*. 2014;173:7-12. [VA]

303. Karmaniolou I, Staikou C. Compartment syndrome as a complication of the lithotomy position. *West Indian Med J*. 2010;59(6):698-701. [VA]

304. Rao MM, Jayne D. Lower limb compartment syndrome following laparoscopic colorectal surgery: a review. *Colorectal Dis*. 2011;13(5):494-499. [VB]

305. Pridgeon S, Bishop CV, Adshead J. Lower limb compartment syndrome as a complication of robot-assisted radical prostatectomy: the UK experience. *BJU Int*. 2013;112(4):485-488. [IIIB]

306. Raza A, Byrne D, Townell N. Lower limb (well leg) compartment syndrome after urological pelvic surgery. *J Urol*. 2004;171(1):5-11. [VB]

307. Bauer EC, Koch N, Erichsen CJ, et al. Survey of compartment syndrome of the lower extremity after gynecological operations. *Langenbecks Arch Surg*. 2014;399(3):343-348. [IIIB]

308. Chin KY, Hemington-Gorse SJ, Darcy CM. Bilateral well leg compartment syndrome associated with lithotomy (Lloyd Davies) position during gastrointestinal surgery: a case report and review of literature. *Eplasty*. 2009;9:e48. [VB]

309. Galyon SW, Richards KA, Pettus JA, Bodin SG. Three-limb compartment syndrome and rhabdomyolysis after robotic cystoprostatectomy. *J Clin Anesth*. 2011;23(1):75-78. [VB]

310. Awab A, El Mansoury D, Benkabbou A, et al. Acute compartment syndrome following laparoscopic colorectal surgery. *Colorectal Dis*. 2012;14(2):e76. [VC]

311. Keene R, Froelich JM, Milbrandt JC, Idusuyi OB. Bilateral gluteal compartment syndrome

PATIENT CARE

following robotic-assisted prostatectomy. *Orthopedics.* 2010;33(11):852. [VA]

312. Raman SR, Jamil Z. Well leg compartment syndrome after robotic prostatectomy: a word of caution. *J Robot Surg.* 2009;3(2):105-107. [VB]

313. Enomoto T, Ohara Y, Yamamoto M, Oda T, Ohkohchi N. Well leg compartment syndrome after surgery for ulcerative colitis in the lithotomy position: a case report. *Int J Surg Case Rep.* 2016;23:25-28. [VA]

314. Oman SA, Schwarz D, Muntz HG. Lower limb compartment syndrome as a complication of radical hysterectomy. *Gynecol Oncol Rep.* 2016;16:39-41. [VA]

315. Stornelli N, Wydra FB, Mitchell JJ, Stahel PF, Fabbri S. The dangers of lithotomy positioning in the operating room: case report of bilateral lower extremity compartment syndrome after a 90-minutes surgical procedure. *Patient Saf Surg.* 2016;10:18. [VA]

316. Koç G, Tazeh NN, Joudi FN, Winfield HN, Tracy CR, Brown JA. Lower extremity neuropathies after robot-assisted laparoscopic prostatectomy on a split-leg table. *J Endourol.* 2012;26(8):1026-1029. [IIIA]

317. Chikazawa K, Netsu S, Akashi K, Suzuki Y, Konno R, Motomatsu S. Delayed diagnosis of single compartment muscle contusion after radical hysterectomy in the lithotomy position: a case report. *Int J Surg Case Rep.* 2016;26:199-201. [VB]

318. Lawrenz B, Kraemer B, Wallwiener D, Witte M, Fehm T, Becker S. Lower extremity compartment syndrome after laparoscopic radical hysterectomy: brief report of an unusual complication of laparoscopic positioning requirements. *J Minim Invasive Gynecol.* 2011;18(4):531-533. [VB]

319. Boesgaard-Kjer DH, Boesgaard-Kjer D, Kjer JJ. Well-leg compartment syndrome after gynecological laparoscopic surgery. *Acta Obstet Gynecol Scand.* 2013;92(5):598-600. [VB]

320. Ulrich D, Bader AA, Zotter M, Koch H, Pristauz G, Tamussino K. Well-leg compartment syndrome after surgery for gynecologic cancer. *J Gynecol Surg.* 2010;26(4):261-262. [VC]

321. Nakamura K, Aoki H, Hirakawa T, Murata T, Kanuma T, Minegishi T. Compartment syndrome with thrombosis of common iliac artery after gynecologic surgery. *Obstet Gynecol.* 2008;112(2 Pt 2):486-488. [VB]

322. Yang RH, Chu YK, Huang CW. Compartment syndrome following robotic-assisted prostatectomy: rhabdomyolysis in bone scintigraphy. *Clin Nucl Med.* 2013;38(5):365-366. [VC]

323. Guella A, Al Oraifi I. Rhabdomyolysis and acute renal failure following prolonged surgery in the lithotomy position. *Saudi J Kidney Dis Transpl.* 2013;24(2):330-332. [VB]

324. Sadeghian H, Arasteh H, Motiei-Langroudi R. Bilateral femoral neuropathy after transurethral lithotomy in the lithotomy position: report of a case. *J Clin Neuromuscul Dis.* 2016;17(4):225-226. [VB]

325. Mizuno J, Takahashi T. Male sex, height, weight, and body mass index can increase external pressure to calf region using knee-crutch-type leg holder system in lithotomy position. *Ther Clin Risk Manag.* 2016;12:305-312. [IIIB]

326. Hsu KL, Chang CW, Lin CJ, Chang CH, Su WR, Chen SM. The dangers of hemilithotomy positioning on traction tables: case report of a well-leg drop foot after contralateral femoral nailing. *Patient Saf Surg.* 2015;9:18. [VB]

327. Sajid MS, Shakir AJ, Khatri K, Baig MK. Lithotomy-related neurovascular complications in the lower limbs after colorectal surgery. *Colorectal Dis.* 2011;13(11):1203-1213. [VB]

328. Noordin S, Allana S, Wajid. Well leg compartment syndrome: the debit side of hemilithotomy position. *J Ayub Med Coll Abbottabad.* 2009;21(1):166-168. [VA]

329. Sharma N, Doble A. A case of compartment syndrome of the thighs following urethroplasty. *Br J Med Surg Urol.* 2009;2(2):82-84. [VB]

330. Sharma N, Doble A. Response to the letter to the editor "Well leg compartment syndrome following radical cystectomy and urinary diversion in the supine position." *Br J Med Surg Urol.* 2009;2(6):260. [VB]

331. Bradshaw AD, Advincula AP. Postoperative neuropathy in gynecologic surgery. *Obstet Gynecol Clin North Am.* 2010;37(3):451-459. [VB]

332. Mizuno J, Takahashi T. Factors that increase external pressure to the fibular head region, but not medial region, during use of a knee-crutch/leg-holder system in the lithotomy position. *Ther Clin Risk Manag.* 2015;11:255-261. [IIIB]

333. Wilson M, Ramage L, Yoong W, Swinhoe J. Femoral neuropathy after vaginal surgery: a complication of the lithotomy position. *J Obstet Gynaecol.* 2011;31(1):90-91. [VB]

334. Tondare AS, Nadkarni AV, Sathe CH, Dave VB. Femoral neuropathy: a complication of lithotomy position under spinal anesthesia. *Can Anaesth Soc J.* 1983;30(1):84-86. [VB]

335. Pannucci CJ, Henke PK, Cederna PS, et al. The effect of increased hip flexion using stirrups on lower-extremity venous flow: a prospective observational study. *Am J Surg.* 2011;202(4):427-432. [IIIB]

336. Navarro-Vicente F, Garcia-Granero A, Frasson M, et al. Prospective evaluation of intraoperative peripheral nerve injury in colorectal surgery. *Colorectal Dis.* 2012;14(3):382-385. [IIIB]

337. Yamada Y, Fujimura T, Fukuhara H, et al. Measuring contact pressure of lower extremities in patients undergoing robot-assisted radical prostatectomy. *Urol Int.* 2016;96(3):268-273. [IIIB]

338. Vijay MK, Vijay P, Kundu AK. Rhabdomyolysis and myogloginuric acute renal failure in the lithotomy/exaggerated lithotomy position of urogenital surgeries. *Urol Ann.* 2011;3(3):147-150. [VC]

339. Liu X, Wang X, Meng X, Wang H, An Z. Effects of patient position on lower extremity venous pressure during different types of hysterectomy. *J Obstet Gynaecol Res.* 2015;41(1):114-119. [IIIB]

340. Guidance statement: safe patient handling and movement in the perioperative setting. In: *Guidelines for Perioperative Practice.* Denver, CO: AORN, Inc; 2015:733-752. [IVB]

341. Pearce A. Bilateral lower limb compartment syndrome following radical cystectomy and urinary diversion in the supine position. *Br J Med Surg Urol.* 2009;2(6):258-259. [VB]

342. Pfeffer SD, Halliwill JR, Warner MA. Effects of lithotomy position and external compression on lower leg muscle compartment pressure. *Anesthesiology.* 2001;95(3):632-636. [IIIB]

343. Chung JH, Ahn KR, Park JH, et al. Lower leg compartment syndrome following prolonged orthopedic surgery in the lithotomy position—a case report. *Korean J Anesthesiol.* 2010;59(Suppl):S49-S52. [VA]

344. Meyer RS, White KK, Smith JM, Groppo ER, Mubarak SJ, Hargens AR. Intramuscular and blood pressures in legs positioned in the hemilithotomy position: clarification of risk factors for well-leg acute compartment syndrome. *J Bone Joint Surg Am.* 2002;84-A(10):1829-1835. [IIIB]

345. Tan V, Pepe MD, Glaser DL, Seldes RM, Heppenstall RB, Esterhai JL Jr. Well-leg compartment pressures during hemilithotomy position for fracture fixation. *J Orthop Trauma.* 2000;14(3):157-161. [IIIB]

346. Peruto CM, Ciccotti MG, Cohen SB. Shoulder arthroscopy positioning: lateral decubitus versus beach chair. *Arthroscopy.* 2009;25(8):891-896. [VA]

347. Li X, Eichinger JK, Hartshorn T, Zhou H, Matzkin EG, Warner JP. A comparison of the lateral decubitus and beach-chair positions for shoulder surgery: advantages and complications. *J Am Acad Orthop Surg.* 2015;23(1):18-28. [VA]

348. Lindroos AC, Niiya T, Randell T, Romani R, Hernesniemi J, Niemi T. Sitting position for removal of pineal region lesions: the Helsinki experience. *World Neurosurg.* 2010;74(4-5):505-513. [IIIB]

349. Gardner BM. The beach chair position. *S Afr Fam Pract.* 2015;57(2):S6-S9. [VA]

350. Cogan A, Boyer P, Soubeyrand M, Hamida FB, Vannier JL, Massin P. Cranial nerves neuropraxia after shoulder arthroscopy in beach chair position. *Orthop Traumatol Surg Res.* 2011;97(3):345-348. [VB]

351. Basaldella L, Ortolani V, Corbanese U, Sorbara C, Longatti P. Massive venous air embolism in the semi-sitting position during surgery for a cervical spinal cord tumor: anatomic and surgical pitfalls. *J Clin Neurosci.* 2009;16(7):972-975. [VC]

352. Dilmen OK, Akcil EF, Tureci E, et al. Neurosurgery in the sitting position: retrospective analysis of 692 adult and pediatric cases. *Turk Neurosurg.* 2011;21(4):634-640. [IIIB]

353. Friedman DJ, Parnes NZ, Zimmer Z, Higgins LD, Warner JJ. Prevalence of cerebrovascular events during shoulder surgery and association with patient position. *Orthopedics.* 2009;32(4). [IIIC]

354. Meex I, Genbrugge C, De Deyne C, Jans F. Cerebral tissue oxygen saturation during arthroscopic shoulder surgery in the beach chair and lateral decubitus position. *Acta Anaesthesiol Belg.* 2015;66(1):11-17. [VA]

355. Lee SW, Choi SE, Han JH, Park SW, Kang WJ, Choi YK. Effect of beach chair position on bispectral index values during arthroscopic shoulder surgery. *Korean J Anesthesiol.* 2014;67(4):235-239. [IIIB]

356. Pant S, Bokor DJ, Low AK. Cerebral oxygenation using near-infrared spectroscopy in the beach-chair position during shoulder arthroscopy under general anesthesia. *Arthroscopy.* 2014;30(11):1520-1527. [IIIB]

357. Mazzon D, Danelli G, Poole D, Marchini C, Bianchin C. Beach chair position, general anesthesia and deliberated hypotension during shoulder surgery: a dangerous combination! *Minerva Anestesiol.* 2009;75(5):281-282. [VB]

358. Moerman AT, De Hert SG, Jacobs TF, De Wilde LF, Wouters PF. Cerebral oxygen desaturation during beach chair position. *Eur J Anaesthesiol.* 2012;29(2):82-87. [IIIB]

359. Triplet JJ, Lonetta CM, Levy JC, Everding NG, Moor MA. Cerebral desaturation events in the beach chair position: correlation of noninvasive blood pressure and estimated temporal mean arterial pressure. *J Shoulder Elbow Surg.* 2015;24(1):133-137. [IIIB]

360. Murphy GS, Szokol JW, Marymont JH, et al. Cerebral oxygen desaturation events assessed by near-infrared spectroscopy during shoulder arthroscopy in the beach chair and lateral decubitus positions. *Anesth Analg.* 2010;111(2):496-505. [IIIB]

361. Meex I, Vundelinckx J, Buyse K, et al. Cerebral tissue oxygen saturation values in volunteers and patients in the lateral decubitus and beach chair positions: a prospective observational study. *Can J Anaesth.* 2016;63(5):537-543. [IIIB]

362. Salazar D, Hazel A, Tauchen A J, Sears BW, Marra G. Neurocognitive deficits and cerebral desaturation during shoulder arthroscopy with patient in beach-chair position: a review of the current literature. *Am J Orthop (Belle Mead NJ).* 2016;45(3):E63-E68. [IIIB]

363. Dippmann C, Winge S, Nielsen HB. Severe cerebral desaturation during shoulder arthroscopy in the beach-chair position. *Arthroscopy.* 2010;26(9 Suppl):S148-S150. [VB]

364. Salazar D, Sears B, Acosta A, et al. Effect of head and neck positioning on cerebral perfusion during shoulder arthroscopy in beach chair position. *J Surg Orthop Adv.* 2014;23(2):83-89. [IIIB]

365. Laflam A, Joshi B, Brady K, et al. Shoulder surgery in the beach chair position is associated with diminished cerebral autoregulation but no differences in postoperative cognition or brain injury biomarker levels compared with supine positioning: the anesthesia patient safety foundation beach chair study. *Anesth Analg.* 2015;120(1):176-185. [IIIB]

366. Hanouz JL, Fiant AL, Gérard JL. Middle cerebral artery blood flow velocity during beach chair position for shoulder surgery under general anesthesia. *J Clin Anesth.* 2016;33:31-36. [IIIB]

367. Buget MI, Atalar AC, Edipoglu IS, et al. Patient state index and cerebral blood flow changes during shoulder arthroscopy in beach chair position. *Braz J Anesthesiol.* 2016;66(5):470-474. [IIIB]

368. McCulloch TJ, Liyanagama K, Petchell J. Relative hypotension in the beach-chair position: effects on middle cerebral artery blood velocity. *Anaesth Intensive Care.* 2010;38(3):486-491. [IIIB]

369. Yadeau JT, Liu SS, Bang H, et al. Cerebral oximetry desaturation during shoulder surgery performed in a sitting position under regional anesthesia. *Can J Anaesth.* 2011;58(11):986-992. [IIIB]

370. Tange K, Kinoshita H, Minonishi T, et al. Cerebral oxygenation in the beach chair position before and during general anesthesia. *Minerva Anestesiol.* 2010;76(7):485-490. [IIIB]

371. Pin-on P, Schroeder D, Munis J. The hemodynamic management of 5177 neurosurgical and orthopedic patients who underwent surgery in the sitting or "beach chair" position without incidence of adverse neurologic events. *Anesth Analg.* 2013;116(6):1317-1324. [IIIA]

372. Lee JH, Min KT, Chun YM, Kim EJ, Choi SH. Effects of beach-chair position and induced hypotension on cerebral oxygen saturation in patients undergoing arthroscopic shoulder surgery. *Arthroscopy.* 2011;27(7):889-894. [IIIB]

373. Mori Y, Yamada M, Akahori T, et al. Cerebral oxygenation in the beach chair position before and during general anesthesia in patients with and without cardiovascular risk factors. *J Clin Anesth.* 2015;27(6):457-462. [IIIB]

374. Amukoa P, Reed A, Thomas JM. Use of the sitting position for pineal tumour surgery in a five-year-old child. *S Afr J Anaesth Analg.* 2011;17(6):388-392. [VB]

375. Rains DD, Rooke GA, Wahl CJ. Pathomechanisms and complications related to patient positioning and anesthesia during shoulder arthroscopy. *Arthroscopy.* 2011;27(4):532-541. [VB]

376. Vermeersch G, Menovsky T, De Ridder D, De Bodt M, Saldien V, Van de Heyning P. Life-threatening macroglossia after posterior fossa surgery: a surgical positioning problem? *B-ENT.* 2014;10(4):309-313. [VB]

377. Rhee YG, Cho NS. Isolated unilateral hypoglossal nerve palsy after shoulder surgery in beach-chair position. *J Shoulder Elbow Surg.* 2008;17(4):e28-e30. [VB]

378. Liang BA. Judgment notwithstanding the verdict: the anesthesiologist's duty to monitor head position in the perioperative period. *J Clin Anesth.* 2009;21(5):369-370. [VA]

379. Ng AK, Page RS. Greater auricular nerve neuropraxia with beach chair positioning during shoulder surgery. *Int J Shoulder Surg.* 2010;4(2):48-50. [VB]

380. LaPrade CM, Foad A. Greater auricular nerve palsy after arthroscopic anterior-inferior and posterior-inferior labral tear repair using beach-chair positioning and a standard universal headrest. *Am J Orthop (Belle Mead NJ).* 2015;44(4):188-191. [VB]

381. Wang JC, Wong TT, Chen HH, Chang PY, Yang TF. Bilateral sciatic neuropathy as a complication of craniotomy performed in the sitting position: localization of nerve injury by using magnetic resonance imaging. *Childs Nerv Syst.* 2012;28(1):159-163. [VB]

382. Kiermeir D, Banic A, Rosler K, Erni D. Sciatic neuropathy after body contouring surgery in massive weight loss patients. *J Plast Reconstr Aesthet Surg.* 2010;63(5):e454-e457. [VB]

383. Rawlani V, Lee MJ, Dumanian GA. Bilateral sciatic neurapraxia following combined abdominoplasty and mastopexy. *Plast Reconstr Surg.* 2010;125(1):31e-32e. [VC]

384. Satin AM, DePalma AA, Cuellar J, Gruson KI. Lateral femoral cutaneous nerve palsy following shoulder surgery in the beach chair position: a report of 4 cases. *Am J Orthop (Belle Mead NJ).* 2014;43(9):E206-E209. [VA]

385. Kwak HJ, Lee JS, Lee DC, Kim HS, Kim JY. The effect of a sequential compression device on hemodynamics in arthroscopic shoulder surgery using beach-chair position. *Arthroscopy.* 2010;26(6):729-733. [IA]

386. Woo KY, Kim EJ, Lee JH, Lee SG, Ban JS. Recurrent paroxysmal supraventricular tachycardia in the beach chair position for shoulder surgery under general anesthesia. *Korean J Anesthesiol.* 2014;65(6 Suppl):S75-S76. [VB]

387. Prabhakar H, Singh GP, Ali Z, Bindra A. Surgery in sitting position in patient with ventriculoperitoneal shunt in situ may be hazardous! *Childs Nerv Syst.* 2009;25(12):1531-1532. [VB]

388. Pandey V, Varghese E, Rao M, et al. Nonfatal air embolism during shoulder arthroscopy. *Am J Orthop (Belle Mead NJ).* 2013;42(6):272-274. [VB]

389. Mirski MA, Lele AV, Fitzsimmons L, Toung TJ. Diagnosis and treatment of vascular air embolism. *Anesthesiology.* 2007;106(1):164-177. [VB]

390. Natal BL. Venous air embolism treatment & management. Medscape. http://emedicine.medscape.com/article/761367-treatment. Accessed March 10, 2017. [VB]

391. Rushatamukayanunt P, Seanho P, Muangman S, Raksakietisak M. Severe venous air embolism related to positioning in posterior cranial fossa surgery in Siriraj Hospital. *J Med Assoc Thai.* 2016;99(5):511-516. [IIIB]

392. Sandwell S, Kimmell KT, Silberstein HJ, et al. 349 safety of the sitting cervical position for elective spine surgery. *Neurosurgery.* 2016;63(Suppl 1):203. [IIIC]

393. Perelló L, Gracia I, Fabregas N. Bone embolism during neurosurgery in sitting position. *J Neurosurg Anesthesiol.* 2013;25(1):93. [VC]

394. Ariadne Labs, Brigham and Women's Hospital, Harvard School of Public Health. *Operating Room Crisis Checklists: Crisis Checklist Package.* 2013. Project Check. http://www.projectcheck.org/uploads/1/0/9/0/1090835/or_crisis_checklists_package_10-11-13.pdf. Accessed March 10, 2017.

395. Furuno Y, Sasajima H, Goto Y, et al. Strategies to prevent positioning-related complications associated with the lateral suboccipital approach. *J Neurol Surg B Skull Base.* 2014;75(1):35-40. [IIIB]

396. Woernle CM, Sarnthein J, Foit NA, Krayenbuhl N. Enhanced serum creatine kinase after neurosurgery in lateral position and intraoperative neurophysiological monitoring. *Clin Neurol Neurosurg.* 2013;115(3):266-269. [IIB]

397. Achar SK, Paul C, Varghese E. Unilateral pulmonary edema after laparoscopic nephrectomy. *J Anaesthesiol Clin Pharmacol.* 2011;27(4):556-558. [VB]

398. Danish SF, Wilden JA, Schuster J. Iatrogenic paraplegia in 2 morbidly obese patients with ankylosing spondylitis undergoing total hip arthroplasty. *J Neurosurg Spine.* 2008;8(1):80-83. [VB]

399. Hemmerling TM, Kazan R, Bracco D. Inter-hemispheric cerebral oxygen saturation differences during thoracic surgery in lateral head positioning. *Br J Anaesth.* 2009;102(1):141-142. [IIC]

400. Kim TK, Yoon JR, Lee MH. Rhabdomyolysis after laparoscopic radical nephrectomy—a case report. *Korean J Anesthesiol.* 2010;59(Suppl):S41-S44. [VB]

401. De Tommasi C, Cusimano MD. Rhabdomyolysis after neurosurgery: a review and a framework for prevention. *Neurosurg Rev.* 2013;36(2):195-202. [VA]

402. Dakwar E, Rifkin SI, Volcan IJ, Goodrich JA, Uribe JS. Rhabdomyolysis and acute renal failure following minimally invasive spine surgery: report of 5 cases. *J Neurosurg Spine.* 2011;14(6):785-788. [VB]

403. Rowell J, Lynn AM, Filardi TZ, Celix J, Ojemann JG. Acute unilateral enlargement of the parotid gland immediately post craniotomy in a pediatric patient: a case report. *Childs Nerv Syst.* 2010;26(9):1239-1242. [VA]

404. Ameri E, Behtash H, Omidi-Kashani F. Isolated long thoracic nerve paralysis—a rare complication of anterior spinal surgery: a case report. *J Med Case Rep.* 2009;3:7366. [VB]

405. Jain V, Davies M. Axillary artery compression in park bench position during a microvascular decompression. *J Neurosurg Anesthesiol.* 2011;23(3):264. [VC]

406. Newton G, White E. Femoral artery occlusion in obese patients in the lateral position. *Anaesthesia.* 2010;65(8):863. [VC]

407. Edgcombe H, Carter K, Yarrow S. Anaesthesia in the prone position. *Br J Anaesth.* 2008;100(2):165-183. [VA]

408. Kwee MM, Ho YH, Rozen WM. The prone position during surgery and its complications: a systematic review and evidence-based guidelines. *Int Surg.* 2015;100(2):292-303. [IVA]

409. Koh JC, Lee JS, Han DW, Choi S, Chang CH. Increase in airway pressure resulting from prone position patient placing may predict intraoperative surgical blood loss. *Spine.* 2013;38(11):E678-E682. [IIIB]

410. DePasse JM, Palumbo MA, Haque M, Eberson CP, Daniels AH. Complications associated with prone positioning in elective spinal surgery. *World J Orthop.* 2015;6(3):351-359. [VA]

411. Postoperative Visual Loss Study Group. Risk factors associated with ischemic optic neuropathy after spinal fusion surgery. *Anesthesiology.* 2012;116(1):15-24. [IIIA]

412. Akinci IO, Tunali U, Kyzy AA, et al. Effects of prone and jackknife positioning on lumbar disc herniation surgery. *J Neurosurg Anesthesiol.* 2011;23(4):318-322. [IC]

413. Chalhoub V, Tohmé J, Richa F, Dagher C, Yazbeck P. Inferior vena cava filter migration during the prone position for spinal surgery: a case report. *Can J Anesth.* 2015;62(10):1114-1118. [VB]

414. Han IH, Son DW, Nam KH, Choi BK, Song GS. The effect of body mass index on intra-abdominal pressure

and blood loss in lumbar spine surgery. *J Korean Neurosurg Soc.* 2012;51(2):81-85. [IIB]

415. Borodiciene J, Gudaityte J, Macas A. Lithotomy versus jack-knife position on haemodynamic parameters assessed by impedance cardiography during anorectal surgery under low dose spinal anaesthesia: a randomized controlled trial. *BMC Anesthesiol.* 2015;15(1):1-9. [IA]

416. Chui J, Craen RA. An update on the prone position: continuing professional development. *Can J Anaesth.* 2016;63(6):737-767. [VA]

417. Shriver MF, Zeer V, Alentado VJ, Mroz TE, Benzel EC, Steinmetz MP. Lumbar spine surgery positioning complications: a systematic review. *Neurosurg Focus.* 2015;39(4):E16. [IIIB]

418. Degerli S, Acar B, Sahap M, Polat A, Horasanli E. Investigation of middle ear pressure changes during prone position under general anesthesia without using nitrous oxide. *J Craniofac Surg.* 2013;24(6):1950-1952. [IIB]

419. Closhen D, Engelhard K, Dette F, Werner C, Schramm P. Changes in cerebral oxygen saturation following prone positioning for orthopaedic surgery under general anaesthesia: a prospective observational study. *Eur J Anaesthesiol.* 2015;32(6):381-386. [IIA]

420. Babakhani B, Heroabadi A, Hosseinitabatabaei N, et al. Cerebral oxygenation under general anesthesia can be safely preserved in patients in prone position: a prospective observational study. *J Neurosurg Anesthesiol.* June 2, 2016. Epub ahead of print. [IIIB]

421. Deiner S, Chu I, Mahanian M, Lin HM, Hecht AC, Silverstein JH. Prone position is associated with mild cerebral oxygen desaturation in elderly surgical patients. *PLoS One.* 2014;9(9):e106387. [IIB]

422. Brown ZE, Gorges M, Cooke E, Malherbe S, Dumont GA, Ansermino JM. Changes in cardiac index and blood pressure on positioning children prone for scoliosis surgery. *Anaesthesia.* 2013;68(7):742-746. [IIB]

423. Shifa J, Abebe W, Bekele N, Habte D. A case of bilateral visual loss after spinal cord surgery. *Pan Afr Med J.* 2016;23:119. [VA]

424. Li A, Swinney C, Veeravagu A, Bhatti I, Ratliff J. Postoperative visual loss following lumbar spine surgery: a review of risk factors by diagnosis. *World Neurosurg.* 2015;84(6):2010-2021. [VA]

425. Nickels TJ, Manlapaz MR, Farag E. Perioperative visual loss after spine surgery. *World J Orthop.* 2014;5(2):100-106. [VA]

426. Dereine T, van Pesch V, Van Boven M, Hantson P. Transient perioperative visual loss after an elective neurosurgical procedure. *Acta Anaesthesiol Belg.* 2013;64(3):109-113. [VB]

427. Grant GP, Szirth BC, Bennett HL, et al. Effects of prone and reverse Trendelenburg positioning on ocular parameters. *Anesthesiology.* 2010;112(1):57-65. [IIB]

428. Carey TW, Shaw KA, Weber ML, DeVine JG. Effect of the degree of reverse Trendelenburg position on intraocular pressure during prone spine surgery: a randomized controlled trial. *Spine J.* 2014;14(9):2118-2126. [IC]

429. Emery SE, Daffner SD, France JC, et al. Effect of head position on intraocular pressure during lumbar spine fusion: a randomized, prospective study. *J Bone Joint Surg (Am).* 2015;97(22):1817-1823. [IB]

430. Lee LA, Newman NJ, Wagner TA, Dettori JR, Dettori NJ. Postoperative ischemic optic neuropathy. *Spine.* 2010;35(9 Suppl):S105-S116. [VA]

431. Akhaddar A, Boucetta M. Subconjunctival hemorrhage as a complication of intraoperative positioning for lumbar spinal surgery. *Spine J.* 2012;12(3):274. [VC]

432. Russell DJ, Dutton JJ. Bilateral spontaneous subperiosteal orbital hemorrhages following endoscopic retrograde cholangiopancreatography. *Ophthal Plast Reconstr Surg.* 2011;27(3):e49-e50. [VC]

433. Guillaume JE, Gowreesunker P. Horner's syndrome in the prone position—a case report. *Acta Anaesthesiol Belg.* 2013;64(3):119-121. [VC]

434. Stang-Veldhouse KN, Yeu E, Rothenberg DM, Mizen TR. Unusual presentation of perioperative ischemic optic neuropathy following major spine surgery. *J Clin Anesth.* 2010;22(1):52-55. [VB]

435. Quraishi NA, Wolinsky JP, Gokaslan ZL. Transient bilateral post-operative visual loss in spinal surgery. *Eur Spine J.* 2012;21(Suppl 4):S495-S498. [VB]

436. Goni V, Tripathy SK, Goyal T, Tamuk T, Panda BB, Shashidhar BK. Cortical blindness following spinal surgery: very rare cause of perioperative vision loss. *Asian Spine J.* 2012;6(4):287-290. [VB]

437. Reddy A, Foroozan R, Edmond JC, Hinckley LK. Dilated superior ophthalmic veins and posterior ischemic optic neuropathy after prolonged spine surgery. *J Neuroophthalmol.* 2008;28(4):327-328. [VB]

438. Kendrick H. Post-operative vision loss (POVL) following surgical procedures. *J Anesth Clin Res.* 2012;3(1). [VB]

439. Agah M, Ghasemi M, Roodneshin F, Radpay B, Moradian S. Prone position in percutaneous nephrolithotomy and postoperative visual loss. *Urol J.* 2011;8(3):191-196. [IIIB]

440. Szmuk P, Steiner JW, Pop RB, et al. Intraocular pressure in pediatric patients during prone surgery. *Anesth Analg.* 2013;116(6):1309-1313. [IIIB]

441. Yoshimura K, Hayashi H, Tanaka Y, Nomura Y, Kawaguchi M. Evaluation of predictive factors associated with increased intraocular pressure during prone position spine surgery. *J Anesth.* 2015;29(2):170-174. [IIIB]

442. Eddama M. Re: Raised intraocular pressure and perioperative visual loss in laparoscopic colorectal surgery: a catastrophe waiting to happen? A systematic review of evidence from other surgical specialties. *Tech Coloproctol.* 2013;17(2):247. [VA]

443. Nazerali RS, Song KR, Wong MS. Facial pressure ulcer following prone positioning. *J Plast Reconstr Aesthet Surg.* 2010;63(4):e413-e414. [VB]

444. Sherman CE, Rose PS, Pierce LL, Yaszemski MJ, Sim FH. Prospective assessment of patient morbidity from prone sacral positioning. *J Neurosurg Spine.* 2012;16(1):51-56. [VB]

445. Dahab R, Barrett C, Pillay R, De Matas M. Anterior thigh compartment syndrome after prone positioning for lumbosacral fixation. *Eur Spine J.* 2012;21(Suppl 4):S554-S556. [VB]

446. Gupta R, Batra S, Chandra R, Sharma VK. Compartment syndrome with acute renal failure: a rare complication of spinal surgery in knee-chest position. *Spine.* 2008;33(8):E272-E273. [VB]

447. Minami K, Iida M, Iida H. Case report: central venous catheterization via internal jugular vein with associated formation of perioperative venous thrombosis during surgery in the prone position. *J Anesth.* 2012;26(3):464-466. [VB]

448. Harman F, Yayci F, Deren S, et al. Acute cerebellar ischemia after lumbar spinal surgery: a rare clinical entity. *J Anesth.* 2012;26(6):947-948. [VC]

449. Hojlund J, Sandmand M, Sonne M, et al. Effect of head rotation on cerebral blood velocity in the prone position. *Anesthesiol Res Pract.* 2012;2012:647258. [IIB]

450. Ooi EI, Ahem A, Zahidin AZ, Bastion ML. Unilateral visual loss after spine surgery in the prone position for extradural haematoma in a healthy young man. *BMJ Case Rep.* December 13, 2013;2013. [VC]

451. Pin-On P, Boonsri S. Postoperative visual loss in orthopedic spine surgery in the prone position: a case report. *J Med Assoc Thai.* 2015;98(3):320-324. [VB]

452. Yu YH, Chen WJ, Chen LH, Chen WC. Ischemic orbital compartment syndrome after posterior spinal surgery. *Spine.* 2008;33(16):E569-E572. [VB]

453. Andersen JD, Baake G, Wiis JT, Olsen KS. Effect of head rotation during surgery in the prone position on regional cerebral oxygen saturation: a prospective controlled study. *Eur J Anaesthesiol.* 2014;31(2):98-103. [IIB]

454. Nuri Deniz M, Erakgun A, Sertoz N, Guven Yilmaz S, Ates H, Erhan E. The effect of head rotation on intraocular pressure in prone position: a randomized trial. *Rev Bras Anestesiol.* 2013;63(2):209-212. [IB]

455. Uribe AA, Baig MN, Puente EG, Viloria A, Mendel E, Bergese SD. Current intraoperative devices to reduce visual loss after spine surgery. *Neurosurgical Focus.* 2012;33(2):E14. [VB]

456. Grover VK, Jangra K. Perioperative vision loss: a complication to watch out. *J Anaesthesiol Clin Pharmacol.* 2012;28(1):11-16. [VA]

457. Grisell M, Place HM. Face tissue pressure in prone positioning: a comparison of three face pillows while in the prone position for spinal surgery. *Spine.* 2008;33(26):2938-2941. [IIB]

458. McMichael JC, Place HM. Face tissue pressures in prone positioning: a comparison of 3 pillows. *J Spinal Disord Tech.* 2008;21(7):508-513. [IIIC]

459. Levan P, O'Rourke M, Presta M, Bryam S. The use of mobile smartphone technology to enhance positioning of a prone patient for thoracic spine surgery. *Internet J Anesthesiol.* 2012;30(3):1. [VB]

460. Asok T, Aziz S, Faisal HA, Tan AK, Mallika PS. Central retinal artery occlusion and ophthalmoplegia following spinal surgery in the prone position. *Med J Malaysia.* 2009;64(4):323-324. [VB]

461. Song JS, Yim JH, Lee KB. Unilateral blindness after posterior cervical spinal surgery: a case report. *Neurosurg Q.* 2015;25(1):78-81. [VC]

462. Epstein NE. Perioperative visual loss following prone spinal surgery: a review. *Surg Neurol Int.* 2016;7(Suppl 13):S347-S360. [VB]

463. Kitthaweesin K, Moontawee K, Thanathanee O. Sudden visual loss and total ophthalmoplegia after brain surgery. *Neuroophthalmology.* 2009;33(1-2):59-61. [VB]

464. Takahashi Y, Kakizaki H, Selva D, Leibovitch I. Bilateral orbital compartment syndrome and blindness after cerebral aneurysm repair surgery. *Ophthal Plast Reconstr Surg.* 2010;26(4):299-301. [VC]

465. Woodruff C, English M, Zaouter C, Hemmerling TM. Postoperative visual loss after plastic surgery: case report and a novel continuous real-time video monitoring system for the eyes during prone surgery. *Br J Anaesth.* 2011;106(1):149-151. [VC]

466. Yu HD, Chou AH, Yang MW, Chang CJ. An analysis of perioperative eye injuries after nonocular surgery. *Acta Anaesthesiol Taiwan.* 2010;48(3):122-129. [IIIB]

467. Walker BJ, Rampersad SE. Iatrogenic endotracheal tube obstruction with foam face padding. *Paediatr Anaesth.* 2009;19(5):544-545. [VB]

468. Chae YJ, Kim JY, Yoo JY, Choi YH, Park KS. Tongue bite in a patient with tracheostomy after prone position—a case report. *Korean J Anesthesiol.* 2011;60(5):365-368. [VB]

469. Minonishi T, Kinoshita H, Hirayama M, et al. The supine-to-prone position change induces modification of endotracheal tube cuff pressure accompanied by tube displacement. *J Clin Anesth.* 2013;25(1):28-31. [IIIB]

470. Lee JA, Jeon YS, Jung HS, Kim HG, Kim YS. Acute compartment syndrome of the forearm and hand in a patient of spine surgery—a case report. *Korean J Anesthesiol.* 2010;59(1):53-55. [VB]

471. Cho KT, Lee HJ. Prone position-related meralgia paresthetica after lumbar spinal surgery: a case report and review of the literature. *J Korean Neurosurg Soc.* 2008;44(6):392-395. [VA]

472. Chikhani M, Evans DL, Blatcher AW, et al. The effect of prone positioning with surgical bolsters on liver blood flow in healthy volunteers. *Anaesthesia.* 2016;71(5):550-555. [IIIB]

473. Debbarma S, Garg S, Kumar K, Anuradha S, Dewan R. Obesity and respiratory complications. *J Int Med Sci Acad.* 2008;21(3):151-153. [VB]

474. Archer TL, Suresh P, Shapiro AE. Cardiac output measurement, by means of electrical velocimetry, may be able to determine optimum maternal position during gestation, labour and caesarean delivery, by preventing vena caval compression and maximising cardiac output and placental perfusion pressure. *Anaesth Intensive Care.* 2011;39(2):308-311. [VB]

475. Saravanakumar K, Hendrie M, Smith F, Danielian P. Influence of reverse Trendelenburg position on aortocaval compression in obese pregnant women. *Int J Obstet Anesth.* 2016;26:15-18. [IIIC]

476. Lee SW, Khaw KS, Ngan Kee WD, Leung TY, Critchley LA. Haemodynamic effects from aortocaval compression at different angles of lateral tilt in non-labouring term pregnant women. *Br J Anaesth.* 2012;109(6):950-956. [IIIB]

477. Baird EJ, Arkoosh VA. Hemodynamic effects of aortocaval compression and uterine contractions in a parturient with left ventricular outflow tract obstruction. *Anesthesiology.* 2012;117(4):879. [VC]

478. Zhou ZQ, Shao Q, Zeng Q, Song J, Yang JJ. Lumbar wedge versus pelvic wedge in preventing hypotension following combined spinal epidural anaesthesia for caesarean delivery. *Anaesth Intensive Care.* 2008;36(6):835-839. [IB]

479. Association of Women's Health, Obstetric and Neonatal Nurses. *Perioperative Care of the Pregnant Woman. Evidence-based Clinical Practice Guideline.* Washington, DC: AWHONN; 2011. [IVA]

480. Higuchi H, Takagi S, Zhang K, Furui I, Ozaki M. Effect of lateral tilt angle on the volume of the abdominal aorta and inferior vena cava in pregnant and nonpregnant women determined by magnetic resonance imaging. *Anesthesiology.* 2015;122(2):286-293. [IIIA]

481. Harvey NL, Hodgson RL, Kinsella SM. Does body mass index influence the degree of pelvic tilt produced by a Crawford wedge? *Int J Obstet Anesth.* 2013;22(2):129-132. [IIIB]

482. Kinsella SM, Harvey NL. A comparison of the pelvic angle applied using lateral table tilt or a pelvic wedge at elective caesarean section. *Anaesthesia.* 2012;67(12):1327-1331. [IIIB]

483. Cluver C, Novikova N, Hofmeyr GJ, Hall DR. Maternal position during caesarean section for preventing maternal and neonatal complications. *Cochrane Database Syst Rev.* 2013;3:007623. [IA]

484. Defining adult overweight and obesity. Centers for Disease Control and Prevention. https://www.cdc.gov/obesity/adult/defining.html. Accessed March 10, 2017.

485. Donohoe CL, Feeney C, Carey MF, Reynolds JV. Perioperative evaluation of the obese patient. *J Clin Anesth.* 2011;23(7):575-586. [VA]

486. Yamane T, Date T, Tokuda M, et al. Hypoxemia in inferior pulmonary veins in supine position is dependent on obesity. *Am J Respir Crit Care Med.* 2008;178(3):295-299. [IIIB]

487. Cheema UY, Vogler CN, Thompson J, Sattovia SL, Vallurupalli S. Protracted hypocalcemia following post-thyroidectomy lumbar rhabdomyolysis secondary to evolving hypoparathyroidism. *Ear Nose Throat J.* 2015;94(3):113-116. [VB]

488. Lee BJ, Kang JM, Kim DO. Laryngeal exposure during laryngoscopy is better in the 25 degrees back-up position than in the supine position. *Br J Anaesth.* 2007;99(4):581-586. [IIIB]

489. Collins JS, Lemmens HJ, Brodsky JB, Brock-Utne JG, Levitan RM. Laryngoscopy and morbid obesity: a comparison of the "sniff" and "ramped" positions. *Obes Surg.* 2004;14(9):1171-1175. [IB]

490. Rao SL, Kunselman AR, Schuler HG, DesHarnais S. Laryngoscopy and tracheal intubation in the head-elevated position in obese patients: a randomized, controlled, equivalence trial. *Anesth Analg.* 2008;107(6):1912-1918. [IA]

491. Cattano D, Melnikov V, Khalil Y, Sridhar S, Hagberg CA. An evaluation of the rapid airway management positioner in obese patients undergoing gastric bypass or laparoscopic gastric banding surgery. *Obes Surg.* 2010;20(10):1436-1441. [IIB]

492. Banicek J, McGarvey D. The effect of patient positioning during lengthy surgery on postoperative health. *Nurs Times.* 2010;106(3):15. [VC]

493. O'Brien DD, Shanks AM, Talsma A, Brenner PS, Ramachandran SK. Intraoperative risk factors associated with postoperative pressure ulcers in critically ill patients: a retrospective observational study. *Crit Care Med.* 2014;42(1):40-47. [IIIB]

494. American Society of PeriAnesthesia Nurses. *2017-2018 Perianesthesia Nursing Standards Practice Recommendations and Interpretive Statements.* Cherry Hill, NJ: ASPAN; 2017. [IVB]

495. Minnich L, Bennett J, Mercer J. Partnering for perioperative skin assessment: a time to change a practice culture. *J Perianesth Nurs.* 2014;29(5):361-366. [VA]

496. Gezginci E, Ozkaptan O, Yalcin S, Akin Y, Rassweiler J, Gozen AS. Postoperative pain and neuromuscular complications associated with patient positioning after robotic assisted laparoscopic radical prostatectomy: a retrospective non-placebo and non-randomized study. *Int Urol Nephrol.* 2015;47(10):1635-1641. [IIIB]

497. Kalin A, Harihran V, Tudor F. Unicompartment compartment syndrome following laparascopic colonic resection. *BMJ Case Rep.* July 9, 2013;2013. [VB]

498. Hoff JM, Varhaug P, Midelfart A, Lund-Johansen M. Acute visual loss after spinal surgery. *Acta Opthalmol.* 2010;88(4):490-492. [VB]

499. Price TP, Ivashchenko A, Schurr MJ. Perioperative visual loss after excision and autografting of a thermal burn to the back. *Burns.* 2014;40(4):e31-e34. [VB]

500. Yilmaz M, Kalemci O. Visual loss after lumbar discectomy due to cortical infarction: case report. *J Neurol Sci.* 2013;30(2):422-426. [VC]

501. *State Operations Manual Appendix A—Survey Protocol, Regulations and Interpretive Guidelines for Hospitals.* Rev 151. November 20, 2015. Centers for Medicare & Medicaid Services. https://www.cms.gov/Regulations-and-Guidance/Guidance/Manuals/downloads/som107ap_a_hospitals.pdf. Accessed March 10, 2017.

502. *State Operations Manual Appendix L—Guidance for Surveyors: Ambulatory Surgical Centers.* Rev 137. April 1, 2015. Centers for Medicare & Medicaid Services. https://www.cms.gov/Regulations-and-Guidance/Guidance/Manuals/downloads/som107ap_l_ambulatory.pdf. Accessed March 10, 2017.

503. 42 CFR 482. Conditions of participation for hospitals. US Government Publishing Office. https://www.gpo.gov/fdsys/granule/CFR-2011-title42-vol5/CFR-2011-title42-vol5-part482. Accessed March 10, 2017.

504. 42 CFR 416. Ambulatory surgical services. US Government Publishing Office. https://www.gpo.gov/fdsys/granule/CFR-2011-title42-vol3/CFR-2011-title42-vol3-part416. Accessed March 10, 2017.

505. RC.01.01.01: The hospital maintains complete and accurate medical records for each individual patient. In: *Hospital Accreditation Standards.* 2016 ed. Oakbrook Terrace, IL: Joint Commission Resources; 2016.

506. MS.16: Medical record maintenance. In: *NIAHO Interpretive Guidelines and Surveyor Guidance.* Version 11 ed. Milford, OH: DNV GL - Healthcare; 2014: 37.

507. RC.01.01.01: The organization maintains complete and accurate clinical records. In: *Standards for Ambulatory Care.* Oakbrook Terrace, IL: Joint Commission Resources; 2016.

508. Clinical records and health information. In: *Accreditation Handbook for Ambulatory Health Care.* Skokie, IL: Accreditation Association for Ambulatory Health Care, Inc; 2016:51-53.

509. Medical records: operating room records. In: *Regular Standards and Checklist for Accreditation of Ambulatory Surgery Facilities.* Version 14.4 ed. Gurnee, IL: American Association for Accreditation of Ambulatory Surgery Facilities, Inc; 2016:60-63.

510. Medical records: procedure room records. In: *Procedural Standards and Checklist for Accreditation of Ambulatory Surgery Facilities.* Version 3 ed. Gurnee, IL: American Association for Accreditation of Ambulatory Surgery Facilities; 2011:64-66.

511. Guideline for patient information management. In: *Guidelines for Perioperative Practice.* Denver, CO: AORN, Inc; 2017:591-616. [IVA]

512. Jordan C, Thomas MB, Evans ML, Green A. Public policy on competency: how will nursing address this complex issue? *J Contin Educ Nurs.* 2008;39(2):86-91. [VB]

513. HR.01.05.03: Staff participate in ongoing education and training. In: *Comprehensive Accreditation Manual: CAMH for Hospitals.* 2016 ed. Oakbrook Terrace, IL: Joint Commission Resources; 2016.

514. MS.10: Continuing education. In: *NIAHO Interpretive Guidelines and Surveyor Guidance.* Version 11 ed. Milford, OH: DNV GL - Healthcare; 2014:30.

515. HR.01.05.03: Staff participate in ongoing education and training. In: *Comprehensive Accreditation Manual: CAMAC for Ambulatory Care.* 2016 ed. Oakbrook Terrace, IL: Joint Commission Resources; 2016.

516. Governance. In: *Accreditation Handbook for Ambulatory Health Care.* 2016 ed. Skokie, IL: Accreditation Handbook for Ambulatory Health Care, Inc; 2016:33-40.

517. Personnel: personnel records; individual personnel files. In: *Regular Standards and Checklist for Accreditation of Ambulatory Surgery Facilities.* 2016 ed. Gurnee, IL: American Association for Accreditation of Ambulatory Surgery Facilities, Inc; 2016:74-75.

518. LD.04.01.07: The hospital has policies and procedures that guide and support patient care, treatment, and services. In: *Hospital Accreditation Standards.* 2016 ed. Oakbrook Terrace, IL: Joint Commission Resources; 2016.

519. SS.1:Organization. In: *NIAHO Interpretive Guidelines and Surveyor Guidance.* Version 11 ed. Milford, OH: DNV GL - Healthcare; 2014:80-82.

520. LD.04.01.07: The organization has policies and procedures that guide and support patient care, treatment, or services. In: *Standards for Ambulatory Care.* 2016 ed. Oakbrook Terrace, IL: Joint Commission Resources; 2016.

521. Personnel: personnel records. In: *Procedural Standards and Checklist for Accreditation of Ambulatory Surgery Facilities.* Version 3 ed. Gurnee, IL: American Association for Accreditation of Ambulatory Surgery Facilities, Inc; 2011:77-79.

522. PI.03.01.01: The hospital improves performance on an ongoing basis. In: *Hospital Accreditation Standards*. 2016 ed. Oakbrook Terrace, IL: Joint Commission Resources; 2016.

523. QM.1: Quality management system. In: *NIAHO Interpretive Guidelines and Surveyor Guidance*. Version 11 ed. Milford, OH: DNV GL - Healthcare; 2014:10-17.

524. PI.03.01.01: The organization improves performance. In: *Standards for Ambulatory Care*. 2016 ed. Oakbrook Terrace, IL: Joint Commission Resources; 2016.

525. Quality management and improvement. In: *Accreditation Handbook for Ambulatory Health Care*. 2016 ed. Skokie, IL: Accreditation Association for Ambulatory Health Care, Inc; 2016:46-50.

526. Quality assessment/quality improvement: quality improvement. In: *Regular Standards and Checklist for Accreditation of Ambulatory Surgery Facilities*. Version 14.4 ed. Gurnee, IL: American Association for Accreditation of Ambulatory Surgery Facilities; 2016:64.

527. Quality assessment/quality improvement: unanticipated operative sequelae. In: *Regular Standards and Checklist for Accreditation of Ambulatory Surgery Facilities*. Version 14.4 ed. Gurnee: IL, American Association for Accreditation of Ambulatory Surgery Facilities, Inc; 2016:66-69.

528. Salkind EM. A novel approach to improving the safety of patients undergoing lumbar laminectomy. *AANA J*. 2013;81(5):389-393. [VC]

529. MAUDE—Manufacturer and User Facility Device Experience. US Food and Drug Administration. https://www.accessdata.fda.gov/scripts/cdrh/cfdocs/cfmaude/search.cfm. Accessed March 10, 2017.

Acknowledgements

LEAD AUTHOR
Sharon A. Van Wicklin, MSN, RN, CNOR, CRNFA(E), CPSN-R, PLNC
Senior Perioperative Practice Specialist
AORN Nursing Department
Denver, Colorado

The author and AORN thank Marie A. Bashaw, DNP, RN, NEA-BC, CNOR, Assistant Professor, Wright State University College of Nursing and Health, Dayton, Ohio; Rodney W. Hicks, PhD, RN, FNP-BC, FAANP, FAAN, Professor, College of Graduate Nursing, Western University of Health Sciences, Pomona, California; Lynn J. Reede, DNP, MBA, CRNA, FNAP, Senior Director, Professional Practice, American Association of Nurse Anesthetists, Park Ridge, Illinois; Jay Bowers, BSN, RN, CNOR, TNCC, Clinical Educator, West Virginia University Healthcare, Morgantown; Diana L. Wadlund, MSN, ACNP-C, CRNFA, Nurse Practitioner, Paoli Hospital, Paoli, Pennsylvania; and Donna Ford, MSN, RN-BC, CNOR, CRCST, Staff Registered Nurse, Mayo Clinic, Rochester, Minnesota, for their assistance in developing this guideline.

PUBLICATION HISTORY
Originally published November 1990, *AORN Journal*.

Revised November 1995; published August 1996, *AORN Journal*.

Revised and reformatted; published January 2001, *AORN Journal*.

Revised 2007; published in *Perioperative Standards and Recommended Practices*, 2008 edition.

Minor editing revisions made to omit PNDS codes; reformatted September 2012 for publication in *Perioperative Standards and Recommended Practices*, 2013 edition.

Minor editing revisions made in November 2014 for publication as "Guideline for positioning the patient" in *Guidelines for Perioperative Practice*, 2015 edition.

Revised April 2017 for publication in *Guidelines for Perioperative Practice* online.

PATIENT CARE

GUIDELINE FOR TEAM COMMUNICATION

The Guideline for Team Communication has been approved by the AORN Guidelines Advisory Board. It was presented as a proposed guideline for comments by members and others. The guideline is effective January 15, 2018. The recommendations in the guideline are intended to be achievable and represent what is believed to be an optimal level of practice. Policies and procedures will reflect variations in practice settings and/or clinical situations that determine the degree to which the guideline can be implemented. AORN recognizes the many diverse settings in which perioperative nurses practice; therefore, this guideline is adaptable to all areas where operative or other invasive procedures may be performed.

Purpose

This document provides guidance for improving perioperative team communication through a culture of safety that incorporates team training, simulation training, standardized transfer of patient information (commonly referred to as hand overs or hand offs), briefings, time outs, surgical safety checklists, and debriefings. In 1999, the Institute of Medicine report *To Err Is Human: Building a Safer Health System* stated that between 44,000 and 98,000 hospital patients die annually as a result of medical errors in the United States.[1] Subsequent studies have estimated the incidence to be as high as 180,000 to 400,000 deaths annually.[2] Since this landmark report, the health care industry has embraced the need for change. Numerous organizations have written position statements on the importance of team communication and the use of a safe surgery checklist to reduce the incidence of medical errors.[3-9]

The collective evidence[10-13] demonstrates that communication breakdowns in the perioperative setting are a factor in events that adversely affect patients. Seventy percent of adverse events in the surgical environment are caused by breakdowns in communication among health care providers.[14,15] The perioperative environment is stressful, and perioperative team members are under increasing pressure from numerous demands and complex functions that lend themselves to error. Despite these pressures, patient safety is a top priority for perioperative RNs and cannot be sacrificed for efficiency. Communication tools and team training programs provide a foundation to improve the chances that communication is conveyed effectively and received accurately. The surgical safety checklist is one tool that the literature supports as improving communication in the perioperative environment.[16-62] The use of checklists in hand overs, briefings, and debriefings provides a defense against adverse events.[46,63,64]

Successful perioperative team communication requires a high-reliability team with a shared goal. According to Wahr et al,[50] high-reliability teams have six elements in common: communication, coordination, cooperation, cognition, conflict resolution, and coaching. An understanding by each team member of his or her role and responsibilities is necessary to achieve a successful surgical outcome for the patient. Beginning with the patient's decision to consent to the procedure, valuable information is collected and handed over to multiple personnel during the patient's surgical encounter. Effective communication among team members is important for understanding the surgical plan for each individual patient. A shared mental model increases the effectiveness of communication between team members because each team member is knowledgeable about his or her own role, other team members' roles, and how these roles interrelate. As the surgery progresses, a shared mental model facilitates timely communication and response by each team member to changes in the surgical plan.[50]

Communication is a process that consists of sending and receiving messages; however, a variety of distractions can impede the ability to send or receive the message accurately. Distractions can be internal or external. Internal distractions are related to the individual's nontechnical skills and individual resilience to human factors (eg, hunger, thirst, anxiety, anger, fatigue) when communicating within the team.[65] External or environmental distractions can be divided into two types: essential and nonessential. Essential distractions come from components necessary for patient care, such as equipment alarms, telephones, pagers, and equipment noise. Nonessential distractions occur in the environment but are not necessary for patient care, such as irrelevant conversations, music, and interruptions from personnel not essential to the procedure. Hierarchical and personal relationships among the individuals on the team can be barriers to effective communication. Other individual barriers include educational background, language preference, culture, race, and gender.[63]

Interprofessional team members send and receive multiple messages throughout a patient's surgical experience. Mohorek[66] described the Linear Model of Communication as a conceptual framework for hand overs between physicians and described different reasons for errors during the hand-over process. Viewing the flow of communication in a linear model may be beneficial for mapping out the critical messages that are covered in each team conversation and for preventing repetition of information that is not critical.

Nontechnical skills, including situational awareness, decision making, leadership, communication,

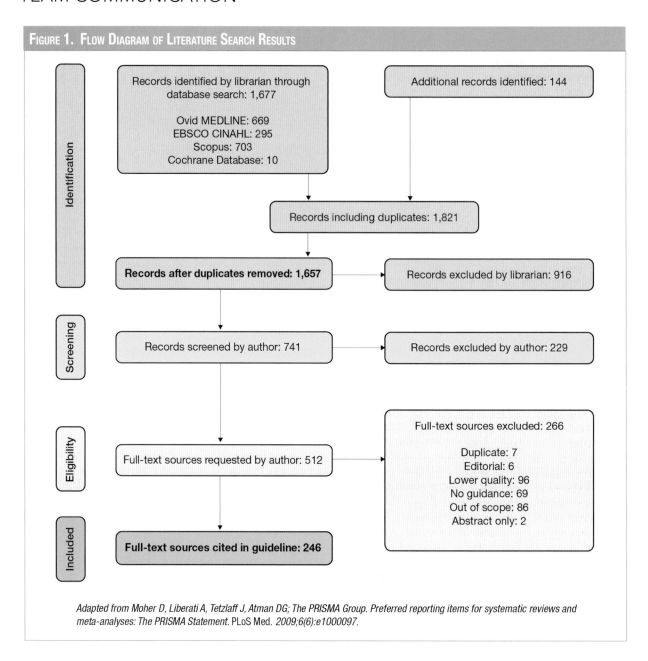

FIGURE 1. FLOW DIAGRAM OF LITERATURE SEARCH RESULTS

Adapted from Moher D, Liberati A, Tetzlaff J, Atman DG; The PRISMA Group. Preferred reporting items for systematic reviews and meta-analyses: The PRISMA Statement. PLoS Med. *2009;6(6):e1000097.*

and teamwork, may affect team communications. Nontechnical skills have been extensively studied in aviation and have been added to training programs for pilots. Although tools for observing nontechnical skills have been validated for other professional roles in the perioperative setting, a standardized tool has not been developed for observing nontechnical skills in the perioperative registered nurse (RN) role. Validated tools for observing nontechnical skills in the perioperative environment include Observational Teamwork Assessment for Surgery (OATS),[67,68] Anesthetist Non-Technical Skills (ANTS),[69] Nontechnical Skills for Surgeons (NOTSS),[14,70-72] and Scrub Practitioners' List of Intraoperative Nontechnical Skills (SPLINTS).[69]

The following topics are outside the scope of this document: workplace violence, bullying, incivility, and workplace safety. Although disruptive behavior is mentioned in the description of the literature, guidance for addressing disruptive behavior is also outside the scope of this document.

Evidence Review

A medical librarian conducted a systematic search of the databases Ovid MEDLINE®, EBSCO CINAHL®, Scopus®, and the Cochrane Database of Systematic Reviews. The search was limited to literature published in English from 2011 through April 2017. At the time of the initial search, weekly alerts were created on the topics included in that search. Results from these alerts were provided to the lead author until July 2017. The lead author requested additional articles that either did not fit the original search criteria or were discovered during the evidence appraisal process. The lead author and the medical librarian also identified relevant guidelines from government agencies, professional organizations, and standards-setting bodies.

Search terms included subject headings such as *operating rooms, communication, patient handoff, clinical protocols, intraoperative complications, interdisciplinary communication, hand off (patient safety),* and *Universal Protocol.* Additional keywords and phrases included *time-out, briefings, debriefings, passive, assertive, sentinel event, never event, TeamSTEPPS, system reliability, misinformation, miscommunication,* and *process improvement.*

Included were research and non-research literature in English, complete publications, and publications with dates within the time restriction. Excluded were non-peer-reviewed publications and older evidence within the time restriction when more recent evidence was available. Editorials, news items, and brief items were excluded. Low-quality evidence was excluded when higher-quality evidence was available (Figure 1).

Articles identified in the search were provided to the project team for evaluation. The team consisted of the lead author, a coauthor, and one evidence appraiser. The lead author divided the search results into topics and assigned the members of the team to review and critically appraise each article using the AORN Research or Non-Research Evidence Appraisal Tools as appropriate. The literature was independently evaluated and appraised according to the strength and quality of the evidence. Each article was then assigned an appraisal score. The appraisal score is noted in brackets after each reference, as applicable.

The collective evidence supporting each intervention within a specific recommendation was summarized, and the AORN Evidence Rating Model was used to rate the strength of the evidence. Factors considered in the review of the collective evidence were the quality of the evidence, the quantity of similar evidence on a given topic, and the consistency of evidence supporting a recommendation. The evidence rating is noted in brackets after each intervention.

Note: *The evidence summary table is available at http://www.aorn.org/evidencetables/.*

Editor's note: *MEDLINE is a registered trademark of the US National Library of Medicine's Medical Literature Analysis and Retrieval System, Bethesda, MD. CINAHL, Cumulative Index to Nursing and Allied Health Literature, is a registered trademark of EBSCO Industries, Birmingham, AL. Scopus is a registered trademark of Elsevier B.V., Amsterdam, The Netherlands.*

Recommendation I

The health care organization should establish administrative processes to create a patient safety culture and encourage individual team members to actively engage in and support the culture.

Commitment to a patient safety culture in the perioperative setting improves patient care, teamwork, and communication, which reduces the patient's risk for adverse events.[73,74] In a patient safety culture, perioperative team members reduce risk by communicating safety concerns. Team members adapt and modify their

behavior by learning from mistakes or by receiving rewards for use of safety behaviors.[75] The pillars of a patient safety culture—trust, report, and improve—provide a foundation for health care organizations to achieve high levels of patient safety.[76]

Establishing a patient safety culture is a system-level intervention to improve patient safety. Investigations in the aviation, nuclear power, and oil and gas industries have found that major factors in accidents were system failures.[75,77]

I.a. The health care organization should promote respect among team members by
- encouraging honesty;
- fostering learning;
- encouraging collaborative practice;
- encouraging team members to speak up;
- holding team members accountable for their behavior;
- maintaining adequate staffing systems;
- providing expert, credible, and visible leadership;
- providing opportunities for shared decision making at all levels; and
- recognizing the value of each team member's contributions.[1,76,78]

[3: Moderate Evidence]

Promoting respectful behaviors among team members facilitates effective communication and teamwork and encourages individuals to speak up when a variance may lead to an unsafe outcome. Effective teamwork, a systems approach, and blameless communication are the best strategies for building a patient safety culture.[79-82] A nonexperimental study conducted by Kolbe et al[82] provides evidence that team communication is improved when there is a positive relationship between speaking-up behavior and technical team performance. The researchers defined speaking up as "explicitly communicating task-relevant observations, requesting clarification, or explicitly challenging or correcting a task-relevant decision or a procedure."[82(p1100)] They found that speaking up during the briefing was associated with speaking up later when a situation became more critical.

In the Silence Kills study, a nonexperimental study conducted by VitalSmarts, AORN, and the American Association of Critical-Care Nurses, the researchers surveyed RNs (N = 4,235) about three concerns identified in an earlier study: dangerous shortcuts, incompetence, and disrespect.[83] The survey responses indicated that 82% (n = 3,472) of the respondents worked with people who demonstrated disrespectful behaviors such as condescending responses, insults, rude comments, yelling, shouting, swearing, or name calling. Forty-six percent of the RN respondents (n = 1,948) identified that disrespect prevented them from communicating effectively and undermined their professional credibility. Forty-nine percent (n = 2,075) stated that they spoke to their managers about the person who was being disrespectful, and 16% (n = 678) spoke to the person who was demonstrating disrespectful behaviors. The researchers concluded that health care organizations that created an environment where RNs were personally, socially, and structurally supported to speak up increased the incidence of respectful behavior.

Adequate staffing systems in a healthy perioperative practice environment respects the needs of perioperative team members.[78]

I.b.   The health care organization should hold the executives and managers at all levels accountable for promoting a patient safety culture. [3: Moderate Evidence]

The collective evidence[22,80,82,84-97] supports the need for leaders to promote factors that shape the sense of safety for the perioperative team. An expert panel convened by the National Patient Safety Foundation advised that leaders should consistently prioritize safety and the well-being and safety of the health care workforce through the use of standardized definitions of safety terms and measurement of safety outcomes.[98]

A nonexperimental study conducted by Vital-Smarts, AORN, and the American Association of Critical-Care Nurses[83] found that only 41% (n = 341) of perioperative RN managers (N = 832) followed up on reported deviations from safety protocols that could have caused patient harm.

I.b.1.   Health care organization leaders should encourage the reporting of errors, unsafe conditions, and intimidating behaviors.[50,81,99,100] [2: High Evidence]

Health care organization leaders provide the foundation for building a patient safety culture. A patient safety culture reflects actions that provide safe care in the health care organization.[84] Disruptive behavior has an adverse effect on staff relationships, communication flow, and patient care. The collective evidence[50,81,99-103] identifies that disruptive behavior can cause increased workplace stress, contribute to dysfunctional teams, reduce the quality of care for patients and their family members, and increase the risk of litigation. Leaders of high-reliability teams foster a patient safety culture by discouraging disruptive team member behaviors and encouraging behaviors that promote reporting of safety concerns.

I.c.   The health care organization should use human factor analysis in the development of processes for establishing a patient safety culture. [2: High Evidence]

A patient safety culture incorporates human factor analysis to decrease adverse events or errors. The collective evidence[82,83,104-108] demonstrates that the use of standardization, checklists, and protocols mitigates the human factor risk. The perioperative team should be constantly adapting to mitigate human factor risk and promote resilience in the environment. Maxfield et al[83] reported that 85% (n = 2,020) of RN survey respondents had used tools that minimize human factor errors, such as checklists, hand-over tools, and drug interaction warning systems. These tools identify problems that may have been missed, to assist in prevention of unintentional slips and errors.

I.d.   The health care organization should establish an environment that promotes resilience in individual team members. [3: Moderate Evidence]

The collective evidence[50,90,109] supports the relationship between human error and personal factors, such as fatigue, nutritional state, emotional states including anger and stress, multitasking, and loss of awareness of what is happening. Brennan et al[90] describes using the mnemonic HALT (Hungry, Anxious or angry, Late or lonely, and Tired) to assess team members' abilities to perform their roles. The researchers concluded that a team member can use the mnemonic to stop himself or herself from potentially creating an error or to inform and help if they observe any of these factors in another team member.

I.e.   The health care organization should establish patient safety goals. [5: Benefits Balanced with Harms]

Establishing patient safety goals guides the team in working toward a patient safety culture.

I.f.   The health care organization should implement clear, just, and transparent processes for recognizing human and system errors and distinguishing these from unsafe, blameworthy actions. [3: Moderate Evidence]

Errors are frequently the consequence of system failures.[110-112] Reason defined errors as "all those occasions in which a planned sequence of mental or physical activities fails to achieve its intended outcome, and when these failures cannot be attributed to the intervention of some chance agency."[111(p9)] These errors can be slips, lapses, or mistakes in memory or actions when executing the action or plan.

In a just culture, determination of individual and system errors is balanced with personal accountability and system improvement. People are encouraged to provide essential safety-related information but are also clear about where the line must be drawn between acceptable and unacceptable behavior. Blaming an individual for an error may be more immediate than taking the time to investigate and correct the system issue that was the root cause. However, blaming does not help personnel or the health care organization understand how mistakes occur, fix a broken system, or help an individual improve his or her performance, and it will not stop unsafe acts from occurring.[110-112]

I.f.1. When an error is caused by a system failure, the health care organization should take steps to improve the system.[28,111,113] *[3: Moderate Evidence]*

I.f.2. When an error is caused by the action of an individual, the health care organization should provide the individual with counseling, coaching, or other corrective action.[95,114-116] *[3: Moderate Evidence]*

I.g. The health care organization should establish a process for conflict resolution. *[3: Moderate Evidence]*

The collective evidence[101-103,117-119] indicates that conflicts are inevitable in the high-volume, complex, and constantly changing perioperative environment. Providing a process to resolve conflict in a constructive manner may decrease frustration and stress in the workplace. In a quasi-experimental study, Saxton[118] conducted a survey of 17 perioperative nurses before and after they attended a two-day Crucial Conversations® workshop. In the post-workshop survey, 71% of the participants (n = 12) reported having more confidence in their ability to address disruptive physician behavior.

I.h. The health care organization should establish an interdisciplinary team with authority and responsibility to provide oversight for the patient safety culture. *[1: Strong Evidence]*

Establishing an interdisciplinary team of key stakeholders who oversee the implementation of team training and system design provides a forum for discussion of barriers to the patient safety culture.[50,53,120] The National Surgical Patient Safety Summit[3] recommends having a centralized and coordinated oversight committee to monitor the patient safety culture.

I.h.1. The interdisciplinary team should include
- nurses,
- support personnel,
- surgeons,
- anesthesia professionals,
- perioperative services executives,
- quality management personnel, and
- risk management personnel.[50,53,120]
[3: Moderate Evidence]

I.h.2. The interdisciplinary team should
- oversee the implementation of the culture of safety and team training;
- develop and implement the communication tools that will be used for briefing, time out, debriefing, and hand overs;
- review the safety measures and identify actions to be taken to sustain safety measures; and

- report safety data to the perioperative executive team.[50,53,120]
[1: Strong Evidence]

I.i. Perioperative team leaders should be identified and should provide leadership by
- organizing the team,
- identifying and articulating clear goals,
- assigning tasks and responsibilities,
- monitoring and modifying the plan,
- reviewing the team's performance,
- managing and allocating resources,
- facilitating information sharing,
- encouraging team members to assist one another,
- facilitating conflict resolution in the learning environment, and
- modeling effective teamwork.
[3: Moderate Evidence]

The collective evidence[50,96,113,121-123] supports the need for strong leadership in teams. Henrickson Parker et al[96] conducted a literature review on surgeon leadership skills. The review revealed two common categories for leadership: task focus and team focus. A team supported by a leader who can focus on both the task and the team can work well together and accomplish goals. Although the authors found many studies on leadership theory and leadership in the workplace, only one study was conducted in the perioperative setting. The authors found that the perception of teamwork differed among surgeons and nursing personnel. Nurses viewed good leadership as good collaboration where their input is respected, whereas surgeons defined collaboration as having a team that can anticipate needs and follow instructions.

Further research is needed to determine ideal intraoperative leadership behaviors for safe surgical practice and whether the surgeon should lead the team or maintain focus on the task of performing surgery.

I.j. The health care organization should reduce barriers to effective communication, including
- facility design barriers,[124-127] *[2: High Evidence]*
- irrelevant conversations,[127,128] *[2: High Evidence]*
- noise levels,[126,129,130] *[2: High Evidence]*
- social setting barriers (eg, status, hierarchy),[101] *[3: Moderate Evidence]*
- distractions,[124,131] *[3: Moderate Evidence]* and
- interruptions.[126,127,131,132] *[3: Moderate Evidence]*

The collective evidence[124-127,130-132] supports that distractions lead to miscommunication and adverse events.

Jothiraj et al[131] conducted a qualitative study in which they observed anesthesiologists in 32 separate procedures during which distractions were recorded by two trained medical student observers. Distractions caused by another anesthesiologist were frequent, and in one-third of those events, the distraction had an observable effect on the anesthesiologist caring for the patient. The authors suggested that the anesthesiologists needed to address themselves as causes of distractions and the potential impact on patient safety.

In an observational study, Keller et al[129] compared peak noise levels on the influence of communication in the surgical setting. The results showed that high noise peaks reduced the frequency of patient-related communication, and communication was impaired because the noise was distracting. The researcher recommended interventions to reduce the noise level in the OR.

Weigl et al[132] conducted an observational study that compared the effect of intraoperative interruptions on surgeons' perceived workload in orthopedic surgery. The researchers observed 56 elective procedures and determined that intraoperative interruptions occurred an average of 9.78 times per hour. The interruptions that occurred most often included people entering or exiting the OR (30.6%) and telephone- or pager-related disruptions (23.6%). The researchers determined that interruptions contributed to the deterioration of the surgeon's mental focus.

I.j.1.   Personnel should refrain from nonessential activities to minimize distractions during important tasks (ie, the sterile cockpit rule) or during critical communication phases of the procedure (eg, briefing, time out, debriefing, induction of or emergence from anesthesia, count process, specimen handling).[113,131-134] *[3: Moderate Evidence]*

The collective evidence[113,131-133] supports that mental fatigue and stress can be reduced when a hand over is performed in a private, quiet setting with minimal interruptions and distractions where the participants can focus their attention on the information being provided.

I.j.2.   Strategies should be implemented to decrease distractions or interruptions. Strategies may include
- identifying sources of noise that can be reduced,[113,134]
- leaving cell phones and pagers outside of the OR or procedure room,[134]
- prioritizing conversations during critical phases of care,
- muting cell phones,[134,135]
- limiting nonessential conversation,[135]
- controlling voice level and tone,[134]
- setting equipment alarms and alerts to the lowest audible level,[135]
- limiting the number of people in the OR,[134]
- limiting overhead paging,[134]

- displaying "quiet please" posters,[113,134] and
- providing education on the importance of minimizing interruptions.[113]
[3: Moderate Evidence]

I.j.3.   When a distraction or interruption occurs that could affect patient safety, a safety pause should be implemented by any perioperative team member. A safety pause may consist of
- identifying a safety event,
- calling for a safety pause and communicating the concern,
- resolving the event with a team response to the concern, and
- discussing the event during the debriefing process and identifying ways to improve patient care.[108,132]
[3: Moderate Evidence]

A safety pause provides an opportunity for any perioperative team member to pause patient care when he or she perceives that a distraction or interruption is causing potentially unsafe conditions.[108,134]

In an organizational experience described by Meginniss et al,[108] personnel used a standardized communication technique called "Time-out for patient safety." This technique provided a critical language for safety situations and empowered the team members to speak up when they had a safety concern.

I.k.   The perioperative team members should collaborate and support each other by
- crosschecking and monitoring;
- asking a question, making a request, or voicing a concern;
- using the chain of command;
- giving timely and specific feedback for peer coaching;
- questioning attitudes; and
- reading back and verifying the receipt of critical patient information.[95,114-116]
[3: Moderate Evidence]

The collective evidence[95,114-116] supports collaboration among team members that improves accurate communication. When individuals ask for more information at the hand over, the hand over is perceived as more accurate. Boyd et al[116] found that reading back techniques increased the transfer of critical patient information between team members.

I.l.   Perioperative team members should speak up and address behavior they have observed that may lead to patient harm by
- collecting the facts;
- assuming the best intent of each team member;
- helping the team member as well as the patient;

○ making the conversation safe to prevent defensiveness;

○ using facts and data as much as possible;

○ avoiding telling negative stories or making accusations; and

○ diffusing or deflecting the person's anger and emotion.[83]

[2: High Evidence]

A perioperative team member's willingness to speak up is dependent on whether he or she perceives it is safe to do so, that there is opportunity to do so, that doing so will be effective, and that he or she has credibility with other members of the team.[105] Nembhard et al[105] conducted a qualitative study in which they interviewed 99 surgeons, anesthesia professionals, and nursing personnel at 12 randomly selected hospitals in the United States about their willingness to speak up. They found that factors such as tenure, work configuration, culture, benchmarking, and external environment influenced the health professionals' sense of safety, efficacy, opportunity, or legitimacy, all of which affected their belief about the risk and benefit of speaking up and willingness to speak up. They also found the team members would speak up for three purposes: to learn for themselves, to inform others, and to protect patients. The researchers concluded that leaders can influence or elicit a willingness to voice concerns by attending to these factors.

Raemer et al[107] conducted a randomized controlled trial in which they concluded that an educational intervention alone was ineffective in improving the speaking-up behaviors of practicing nontrainee anesthesiologists. The anesthesiologists (N = 337) completed a survey after participating in a simulation course designed to observe speaking-up behavior in different simulated scenarios. The five most frequently mentioned hurdles to speaking up were uncertainty about the issue, stereotypes about others on the team, unfamiliarity with the individual they were speaking to, respect for other's experience, and the repercussion expected. The five most frequently mentioned strategies to increase speaking up were realizing the speaking-up problem, having a speaking-up rubric, certainty about the consequences of speaking up, familiarity with the individual they were speaking to, and getting a second opinion or getting help.[107]

Recommendation II

The health care organization should establish and implement a standardized hand-over process for the transfer of patient information between individuals and teams.

The collective evidence[136-150] suggests that communication failure and incomplete or missing patient information are the most common causes of sentinel events and pose a significant threat to patient safety. Communication failures during transfer of information are common in the perioperative setting and can compromise patient safety and contribute to inefficiency.[138] A standardized hand-over process may improve patient safety by promoting optimal communication by all perioperative team members during the transfer of patient information, which is a critical phase in a patient's perioperative experience.

II.a. The health care organization should establish an interdisciplinary team at the facility level to develop a standardized hand-over process. *[2: High Evidence]*

A standardized hand-over process helps to identify risks during the perioperative phases so the team can take action to minimize threats to patient safety. In a systematic review of nonexperimental studies, Moller et al[151] recognized that patient hand over is an ever-changing and complex process designed to analyze and address the challenges in the local setting. The author recommended that the hand-over process be designed to fit the context in which it will take place.

II.a.1. The interdisciplinary team should include
• perioperative RNs,
• perianesthesia RNs,
• RNs from receiving patient care units,
• surgeons,
• anesthesia professionals,
• licensed independent practitioners
• allied health care providers, and
• support personnel
[5: Benefits Balanced with Harms]

II.b. The hand-over process should include
○ assigning the roles and responsibilities of team members,
○ individualizing the hand over for the specific patient population (eg, child, adult) and level of acuity (eg, severity of symptoms, complexity of surgery, comorbid conditions),
○ notifying the receiving team member that the patient is being transferred and of the potential equipment needs before the patient's arrival,
○ completing urgent tasks before starting the hand-over communication,
○ limiting the hand-over conversation to only patient-specific discussions,
○ allowing only one person to speak at a time,
○ keeping distractions and interruptions (eg, personal conversations) to a minimum with only urgent clinical interruptions allowed,
○ using supporting documentation (eg, lab test results), and
○ providing an opportunity for participants to voice concerns and ask questions.[151]
[2: High Evidence]

A structured hand-over process that includes strategies for safe patient care helps to identify and mitigate risks to patient safety.[151]

In a systematic review of quasi-experimental and nonexperimental studies, Segall et al[152]

identified recommendations for hand-over structure and information transfer. The researchers found an association between poor quality hand-over processes and adverse patient safety events.

II.b.1.   The interdisciplinary team should assign team member roles and responsibilities for the hand-over process.[153,154] *[3: Moderate Evidence]*

Ambiguous roles and responsibilities can cause confusion during the hand-over process and can contribute to potential patient harm. In a nonexperimental study, McElroy et al[153] identified that team member participation was important to the development of a high-quality hand-over process. The physical presence of all team members was clearly identified as key to conveying all of the patient care issues that need to be addressed between transferring and receiving team members.

In a qualitative study, McElroy et al[154] found that clarifying team member roles and expectations decreased ambiguity and the risk of patient harm. The researchers determined that there were varying degrees of team member participation in the hand-over process, and roles within a team determined the team members' perspectives of the hand-over process.

II.c.   Perioperative team members should use the read-back method when communicating patient information to other team members. *[3: Moderate Evidence]*

The read-back method improves communication during hand overs. In a nonexperimental study conducted by Boyd et al,[116] postanesthesia care unit nurses and anesthesia assistants participated in 88 simulated scenarios involving a clinical crisis. Participants used either a read-back method, verbal acknowledgement without read-back, or no verbal reply to respond to patient information. Participants who used the read-back method were 8.27 times more likely to correctly recall information and those that responded verbally were 3.16 times more likely to correctly recall information compared to participants who gave no verbal response.

II.d.   The perioperative team should use standardized hand-over tools, checklists, or protocols. *[2: High Evidence]*

The collective evidence[46,64,143,155-163] demonstrates that the use of standardized tools, protocols, and checklists improves the quality of information transfer and decreases communication breakdowns during hand overs.

In a systematic review of quasi-experimental and nonexperimental studies, Pucher et al[46] found that using a checklist or standardized process may improve transfers of patient information.

In a randomized controlled trial, Salzwedel et al[64] implemented use of a written checklist in a university hospital. The researchers observed 40 hand overs before the checklist implementation and 80 hand overs after implementation. They determined that the percentage of overall items included in the hand over were significantly increased with use of the checklist. The researchers concluded that the quality of patient hand overs was improved because of the additional patient information relayed with the use of a written checklist.

In a quality improvement (QI) project, Petrovic et al[164] implemented use of a perioperative hand-over tool to improve postprocedural patient transfers. The tool established a mandate that all members of the hand-over team be present at the bedside and provided a series of structured steps that guided the hand over. The authors found that implementation of the tool resulted in improved information sharing, increased team satisfaction, and decreased distractions during the hand over.

II.d.1.   The perioperative team may use evidence-based tools during the hand over, such as
- SBAR: situation, background, assessment, recommendation[157,160]; *[2: High Evidence]*
- I PASS the BATON: introduction, patient, assessment, situation, safety concerns, (the) background, actions, timing, ownership, next[165]; *[3: Moderate Evidence]*
- SWITCH: surgical procedure, wet, instruments, tissue, counts, have you any questions[158]; *[3: Moderate Evidence]* and
- SURgical PAtient Safety System (SURPASS)[56]. *[2: High Evidence]*

In a prospective intervention study, Randmaa et al[160] implemented the SBAR communication tool in anesthetic clinics in two hospitals. The researchers used preassessment and postassessment data to determine the number of incident reports generated because of communication errors. In the intervention group using the SBAR tool, there was a significant improvement in communication accuracy, and the number of incident reports resulting from communication errors decreased from 31% of all incident reports in the year before the tool implementation to 11% of all incident reports in the year after the implementation.

Eberhardt[157] reported on an organizational experience in which a team comprised of medical/surgical and perioperative RNs implemented the SBAR hand-over tool to standardize the hand-over process between the medical-surgical unit and the OR. The team implemented a pilot test and refined the tool based on the feedback from the perioperative and medical-surgical RNs. The team then implemented the process throughout the facility and received positive responses from all the RNs who used it in the hand-over process.

As part of TeamSTEPPS®, the mnemonic I PASS THE BATON was created to structure the critical communication elements that need to be conveyed during a hand over or patient care transition.[165]

Johnson et al[158] developed the SWITCH intraoperative tool in response to identified inconsistencies in communication of essential information during the transfer of patient care from one perioperative care provider to another. The tool enabled the perioperative team to have a standardized reporting process, address communication barriers, and maintain focus on patient care during critical moments, such as shift changes, thereby improving patient safety.

The SURPASS checklist was developed as a multidisciplinary checklist designed to follow the patient from admission to discharge, and it can be used for the hand-over process. In a quasi-experimental study, deVries et al[56] compared rates of complication in patients before (n = 3,760) and after (n = 3,820) implementation of the SURPASS checklist. The researchers found that the total number of complications per 100 patients decreased from 27.3 to 16.7.

II.e. The interdisciplinary team should include all phases and locations of patient care in a standardized hand-over process design. Phases of care should include

- scheduling,
- preadmission,
- preoperative,
- intraoperative, and
- postoperative.

Locations of care may include the

- primary care provider's office,
- surgeon's office,
- scheduling department,
- preanesthesia testing unit,
- presurgical testing unit,
- preoperative holding area,
- OR or procedure room,
- postanesthesia care unit, and
- other areas where postoperative care is provided (eg, medical/surgical ward, intensive care unit).

[2: High Evidence]

The collective evidence[143,146,152] indicates that poor standardization, incomplete transfer of information, incomplete team involvement, and absence of clinical task execution are barriers to effective postoperative hand overs. Hand overs can be inconsistent, and items deemed important may vary by team member, patient population, patient acuity, and facility.

II.e.1. The hand-over process for the scheduling to the preoperative phase should include verification of

- the correct patient and procedure including site and side;
- completion of the history and physical;
- completion of required consultations;
- informed consent;
- preoperative orders;
- an anesthesia consult as needed;
- implant, instrumentation, and equipment needs; and
- the identification of the patient's caregiver who will be present at the preoperative visit.[56,166]

[3: Moderate Evidence]

In a nonexperimental study, Wu and Aufses[167] reviewed scheduling errors reported in one institution's adverse event reporting system and identified that in 17,606 surgeries, there were 151 errors in scheduling. The most common scheduling errors were wrong-side booking (eg, left, right), incomplete booking (eg, additional procedures added after booking, bilateral cases scheduled for one side), and wrong approach (eg, laparoscopic versus open). The incomplete booking and wrong approach scheduling errors resulted in delays and increased cost to the health care organization. The researchers concluded that scheduling errors were infrequent but caused disruptions in OR team dynamics, delays, and substantial costs.

In a literature review, Zahiri et al[166] found that the first encounter with the patient is crucial for ensuring that the correct and compete medical record is available to prevent wrong site surgery. The authors recommended that the surgeon perform a thorough history and physical and that this information be entered meticulously into the patient's medical record; that the consent be completed with the patient and immediately placed in the patient's medical record; and that a standardized, efficient scheduling process be instituted in the surgeon's office to decrease risk to the patient as a result of scheduling errors.

II.e.2. The hand-over process for the preoperative to the intraoperative phase may include information on

- the correct patient and procedure;
- the correct operative side/site;
- the history and physical;
- the patient's allergies;
- the patient's current medications and adjustments if needed (eg, anticoagulants, antibiotics);
- significant diagnostic test results;
- medications given or prescribed;
- anticoagulation prophylaxis, if applicable;

- patient mobility issues;
- blood products available, if ordered; and
- a plan for communicating with the patient's significant other.[56]

[2: High Evidence]

II.e.3. The hand-over process during the intraoperative phase for personnel change may include information on

- the correct patient and procedure,
- the correct operative side/site,
- special considerations or precautions,
- intraoperative imaging,
- the type of incision and dressing needed,
- the postoperative plan of care,
- medications or other solutions on the sterile field,
- blood products given or available,
- current blood loss,
- urine output,
- the presence of drains,
- implants needed,
- instruments needed and the location of the instruments,
- specimen management,
- grafts (eg, type, location),
- the status of counts (eg, sponges, needles, instruments) and the location of counted items (eg, body cavities, off the sterile field),
- the status of documentation, and
- a plan for communicating with the patient's significant other.[146,158]

[3: Moderate Evidence]

II.e.4. The hand-over process for the intraoperative to postoperative phase may include information on

- the patient's circulation, airway, and breathing[133,143];
- the patient's name, age, weight, vital signs[143,152];
- the patient's allergies[143,146,152];
- the patient's diagnosis and pertinent medical history[146,152];
- the procedure performed[143,146,152];
- surgical complications and corrective interventions[146,152];
- time in the OR[146];
- the patient's current condition (eg, hemodynamic status)[143,152];
- the patient's skin condition[143];
- the pressure injury risk assessment;
- the patient's hypothermia status[146];
- the type of anesthesia[146,152];
- complications from the anesthesia[152];
- intraoperative medications administered, including dose and time[146,152];
- IV fluids and lines present[146,152];
- drains and tubes present[143];
- wound packing (eg, type, location)[143];
- blood products used, including type and amount[152];
- estimated blood loss[146,152];
- any intraoperative testing performed (eg, radiograph, echocardiogram)[152];
- surgical site information (eg, dressings, tubes, drains, packing)[152];
- the postoperative management plan and orders,[152] including
  - anticipated recovery concerns[152];
  - the monitoring plan and the acceptable range of physiological variables[152];
  - the plan for pain management[152];
  - the plan for IV fluids, medications, antibiotics, and venous thromboembolism prophylaxis[146,152];
  - the plan for feeding and oral hydration[143,146,152];
  - disposition of the patient (eg, discharge or admission)[143]; and
  - the receiving patient care unit, if applicable[143];
- special considerations or precautions; and
- a plan for communicating with the patient's significant other.

[3: Moderate Evidence]

II.e.5. The hand-over process for patients being transferred directly from the OR to an intensive care unit (ICU) should include activities before and upon arrival.

The perioperative RN should prepare for the hand over before arrival at the ICU, by

- notifying the ICU before leaving the OR or at predetermined notification time frames established by the interdisciplinary team[145,168,169];
- notifying the ICU of ventilator settings, if applicable[145,168,169];
- verifying that all transport equipment is available and functioning correctly[168];
- creating a written or digital OR summary data sheet for the ICU team[168];
- notifying the ICU if the patient will need isolation precautions and what type[143];
- notifying the ICU to prepare monitors, drains, IV fluids, and medications before the patient's arrival[133,169]; and
- disentangling patient device tubing and lines before leaving the OR.[143,169]

[3: Moderate Evidence]

On arrival at the ICU, the hand-over process should include completion of patient care tasks and communication of patient information, including

- a call for a safety pause at the start of the hand over[169];
- a review of hand-over elements from the intraoperative to postoperative phases (See Recommendation II.e.4.);
- connection of the breathing circuit to the ICU ventilator[143];

- a check of oxygenation and ventilation status (eg, breath sounds, chest expansion, oxygen saturation)[148,169];
- connection of the patient to monitoring equipment[169];
- connection of chest tubes to suction[169];
- communication of the anesthesia details by the anesthesia professional (eg, type of induction, central line, arterial lines placed, complications)[144,145,148,169];
- communication of the surgery details by the surgeon (eg, surgery performed, cardiopulmonary bypass time, cross clamp time, transesophageal echocardiogram results)[144,145,148,169];
- discussion by the team of postoperative details (eg, blood loss, blood products administered, blood products currently available, pacemaker, vital signs, intracardiac pressures, medications administered, fluid volume, sedatives, laboratory test results, tubes, drains)[144,145,148,169];
- confirmation that medications and IV drips are correctly labeled[144,145,148,169];
- discussion of the expected postoperative course, potential complications or risks, and anticipatory guidance[145,168,169]; and
- discussion of specific concerns for the patient.[144,145,147,148,168,169]

[3: Moderate Evidence]

The collective evidence[133,143-145,147,148,153,168,169] suggests that hand overs to an intensive care setting can be difficult because of the acuity of the patient; the numerous drains, lines, and tubes present; distractions and noise; and the lack of all team members being present during the hand-over process, all of which can increase a patient's risk for harm.

Developing protocols and checklists for use in hand overs between the OR and the ICU increases team-member involvement, reduces errors, and may improve efficiencies during the hand-over process.[133,143-145,147,148,153,168,169]

In a qualitative study, McElroy et al[168] assessed systems and processes involved in the hand over between the OR and the ICU. Using a failure modes, effects, and criticality analysis, the researchers identified 37 individual steps in the hand-over process. The researchers found 81 process failures, 22 of which were in critical processes. The processes with the greatest risk to cause harm were lack of preliminary OR to ICU communication, team members being absent during the hand over, and equipment malfunctioning during transport.

Chen et al[133] conducted an observational, cross-sectional study of hand-over communications between the OR and the pediatric cardiac ICU in one facility. The team used a protocol that included the "sterile cockpit"

environment where all hand-over team participants refrained from nonessential activities to decrease distractions during the hand-over process. The researchers concluded that the hand-over process in a sterile cockpit environment decreased distraction and improved discussion about the anticipated patient course.

Recommendation III

The health care organization should establish and implement a standardized briefing process before the surgical procedure.

The collective evidence[114,120,170-178] supports the use of briefings to improve teamwork and team communication and improve the quality of patient care by increasing efficiency, decreasing interruptions and delays, and improving patient outcomes. Briefing improves team communication by allowing teams to develop a shared mental model.[179]

Thanapongsathorn et al[172] reported on an organizational experience in which a project team implemented a preoperative briefing that included the entire perioperative team. The perioperative team met before each procedure, and the briefing lasted no longer than 10 minutes. The project team collected team satisfaction data and found that the briefings increased the level of satisfaction for teamwork and decreased operative time because preventable delays were identified before the start of the surgery.

Although evidence supports the performance of the time out just before the incision, further research is needed to determine the ideal timing for the briefing.[50,63,66,180]

III.a. The interdisciplinary team should create a standardized briefing process with input from perioperative team members representing individual service lines (eg, cardiac, orthopedic, neurosurgical, obstetric). *[3: Moderate Evidence]*

Johnston et al[171] reported on an organizational experience in which they developed an auditing tool to determine how preoperative briefings were conducted at an academic medical center. They found a high degree of variability in participation among team members and across service lines and highlighted the need for service-specific customization of the briefing process.

III.a.1. The briefing process should include
- introduction of the team members[175,181];
- the patient's name and identifiers (the patient may participate)[171,173,175];
- the consent signed[171];
- the planned procedure and side[171,173];
- the goals of the procedure[175];
- the estimated length of the procedure[173];
- a review of laboratory results and radiographs[171,172,175];
- the planned intraoperative patient position[171,173,175];
- the pressure injury risk assessment;

- the planned patient skin antisepsis[171];
- that the needed equipment is available,[175];
- that the needed instruments are available[172];
- the patient's known allergies or sensitivities[171];
- special considerations or precautions[173,175];
- a fire risk assessment[182]; and
- questions, safety concerns, and equipment concerns.[173,175]

[3: Moderate Evidence]

III.a.2. The briefing process may include information about
- venous thromboembolism prophylaxis[171,175];
- difficult airway or risk of aspiration[171];
- antibiotic administration[170,171,175];
- anticipated antibiotic redosing[171,175];
- the need for glucose management[171,175];
- the plan for regional, neuraxial, or local anesthesia[173];
- anticipated blood loss[171,173,175];
- planned pneumatic tourniquet use[173];
- availability of blood and blood products[171,172,175];
- availability of implants[175];
- intraoperative imaging needed[171]; and
- the postoperative plan of care.[173]

[3: Moderate Evidence]

III.b. The briefing may be guided by the use of a checklist.[170] *[3: Moderate Evidence]*

In a quasi-experimental study, Lingard et al[170] assessed the effect of a checklist-driven preoperative team briefing on the timing of the administration of prophylactic antibiotics. The percentage of patients who received on-time administration of antibiotics improved from 77.6% in the pre-intervention phase to 87.6% in the post-intervention phase.

III.c. All unnecessary activities and conversations should come to a stop when the briefing is initiated.[120,134,183,184] *[1: Strong Evidence]*

Distractions and interruptions during critical conversations and phases of perioperative care can contribute to surgical errors.

Recommendation IV

The patient's identity, procedure, and procedural site including laterality must be verified and the site marked.[185]

Identifying the correct site on the patient's body where the procedure or surgery is to be performed helps to decrease the risk for wrong site surgery.[120,185,186] Site marking is required by the Centers for Medicare & Medicaid Services (CMS).[185] All accrediting agencies with CMS deemed status require site marking.

The Universal Protocol was developed by The Joint Commission to provide guidance for prevention of wrong site, wrong procedure, and wrong person surgery.[186] The protocol consists of three steps: preprocedure verification, patient site marking, and a time out. The World Health Organization also recommends site marking for cases involving laterality or multiple structures or levels.[120]

IV.a. The site marking process must be consistent throughout the health care organization and not open to interpretation.[185,186] *[1: Regulatory Requirement]*

Consistent site marking processes applied throughout the health care organization decrease confusion and risk for wrong site surgery.

IV.a.1. The health care organization should identify procedures that will require site marking.[120,186] *[1: Strong Evidence]*

IV.a.2. At a minimum, site marking should be performed when there is more than one possible location for the surgery to occur.[186] *[5: Benefits Balanced with Harms]*

IV.b. The procedure site must be marked before the procedure begins.[120,185,186] *[1: Regulatory Requirement]*

Marking the site before the procedure helps to promote patient involvement and minimize the risk for wrong site surgery.

IV.b.1. The patient or the patient's representative should be involved in the marking of the site if possible.[186] *[5: Benefits Balanced with Harms]*

IV.b.2. The procedure site must be marked by a licensed independent practitioner who is accountable and will be present when the procedure is performed.[185,186] *[1: Regulatory Requirement]*

IV.b.3. Site marking may be delegated to another individual as defined in health care organization policy, which may include
- a postgraduate medical student who is being supervised by the licensed independent practitioner performing the procedure, is familiar with the patient, and will be present when the surgery or procedure is performed or
- a person who has a collaborative or supervisory agreement with the licensed independent practitioner performing the procedure, is familiar with the patient, and will be present when the procedure or surgery is performed (an advanced practice RN or physician assistant).[186]

[5: Benefits Balanced with Harms]

IV.b.4. The mark should be made at or near the procedure site and be visible after surgical skin antisepsis and draping.[186] *[5: Benefits Balanced with Harms]*

IV.b.5. For patients who refuse site marking or for cases when it is anatomically or technically impossible (eg, mucosal surfaces, the perineum, teeth) or impractical (eg, minimal access procedures that involve a lateralized internal organ, whether through a natural orifice or percutaneous access; procedures on premature infants for whom marking may cause a permanent tattoo), the facility should create an alternative marking process.[186] *[5: Benefits Balanced with Harms]*

IV.b.6. For spinal procedures, in addition to skin marking, intraoperative imaging techniques should be used to determine the exact vertebral level.[120,186,187] *[3: Moderate Evidence]*

Recommendation V

The perioperative team must perform a time out before an operative or invasive procedure begins.[185]

The collective evidence[26,50,120,166,183-185,188,189] supports the time out as a tool to prevent wrong site surgeries. The purpose of the time out is to conduct a final check that the correct patient, correct site, and correct procedure are identified. During a time out, all activities are stopped so that the perioperative team can focus on the factors that contribute to a wrong person, wrong site, and wrong procedure surgery and other risks to patient safety.[120,184,189] A time out provides an opportunity for all perioperative team members to speak up and address any concerns or problems that would affect the safety of the patient.

V.a. The time out should be a standardized process as defined by the facility. *[5: Benefits Balanced with Harms]*

A standardized process is most effective when it is conducted consistently throughout the facility.

V.a.1. A designated perioperative team member should call for the time out to begin.[183] *[3: Moderate Evidence]*

V.a.2. The time out should involve all members of the perioperative team. The participating team members must include the individual performing the procedure, the anesthesia professional, the RN circulator, the scrub person, and any other team members who will be participating in the procedure from the beginning.[120,189] *[2: Strong Evidence]*

V.a.3. If two or more procedures are being performed on the same patient and the person performing the procedure is different, a time out should be conducted before each procedure.[120,189] *[1: Strong Evidence]*

V.a.4. During the time-out process, the team must confirm, at a minimum, the correct patient, site, and procedure to be performed.[120,185,189] *[1: Regulatory Requirement]*

V.a.5. All unnecessary activities and conversations in the OR should come to a stop when the time out is called.[120,183,184] *[1: Strong Evidence]*

V.a.6. If perioperative team members have not introduced themselves, each person should state his or her name and role on the team.[188] *[3: Moderate Evidence]*

V.a.7. Any patient safety concerns or concerns about the procedure should be discussed during the time out.[120,188] *[1: Strong Evidence]*

V.a.8. The time out should be documented as completed in accordance with facility policy (amount and type of documentation).[189] *[5: Benefits Balanced with Harms]*

V.b. A time out should be performed before regional anesthesia procedures.[21] *[3: Moderate Evidence]*

Barrington et al[21] conducted a literature review to describe the phenomenon of wrong site regional anesthetic blocks and to identify preventive strategies. The authors found that the incidence of wrong regional block procedures may be as frequent as 7.5 per 10,000 procedures. They identified factors that contribute to wrong regional blocks, including scheduling changes, poor communication, incomplete documentation, patient position change, physician distraction, lack of surgical consent, inadequate supervision of residents, lack of situational awareness, fatigue, site marking not visible, cognitive overload, and failure to perform a time out. The authors recommended performing a time out immediately before all regional anesthesia procedures and repeating the time out with any patient position change or procedures performed by a different team.

V.c. The health care organization should identify when a subsequent or second time out may be performed for a lengthy procedure. *[3: Moderate Evidence]*

Patients who are undergoing lengthy surgical procedures are at increased risk for positioning and nerve injuries and other complications. In an organizational experience, Song et al[190] implemented a second time out in their facility that was aimed at reducing patient complications and addressing problems encountered during lengthy robotic surgeries. The authors developed a standardized surgical checklist to address potential problems and improve patient safety. The second time out provided an opportunity for members of the perioperative team to discuss concerns for patient safety and address issues unique to robotic surgery. The implementation of the second time out received positive feedback from the perioperative team, and there was minimal intrusion into the surgical procedure time.

V.d. The perioperative team should use a standardized surgical safety checklist during the time-out process. *[2: High Evidence]*

The collective evidence[16-62] supports the use of a standardized safe surgery checklist during the time-out process to improve communication, reduce the potential for error, reduce patient complications, improve adherence to critical processes and safety measures, and decrease surgical mortality. A surgical safety checklist is designed to enhance communication and teamwork and helps create an environment in which perioperative team members' input is solicited and welcomed and information sharing is encouraged.[53]

In a systematic review of quasi-experimental and nonexperimental studies, Treadwell et al[16] found that the use of a safe surgery checklist, such as the World Health Organization (WHO) Surgical Safety Checklist or the SURPASS checklist, could potentially decrease patient morbidity and mortality in surgery. Safe surgery checklists were associated with fewer complications, improved communication, improvements in facility safety culture, and increased detection of potential safety issues.

Thomassen et al[17] also conducted a systematic review of quasi-experimental and nonexperimental studies and found that safe surgery checklists could be used in all clinical settings to increase compliance with national guidelines, reduce the number of safety events, decrease morbidity and mortality, and mitigate errors attributable to human factors. The researchers did not find evidence that the safe surgery checklists had negative effects on patient safety or quality of care.

In another systematic review, Russ et al[18] found that patient outcomes could be improved when perioperative teams used a safe surgery checklist because the use of the checklist improved teamwork and communication.

Lyons and Popejoy[19] conducted a systematic review with meta-analysis on the effects of the use of a safe surgery checklist on teamwork, communication, morbidity, mortality, and safety. The researchers found that using a checklist improved team communication and teamwork, reduced morbidity and mortality, and improved compliance with safety measures.

Bock et al[25] conducted a quasi-experimental retrospective comparative analysis of administrative outcome data before and after implementation of a surgical safety checklist in one large hospital in Italy. The researchers collected data 3 months before and 3 months after checklist implementation (N = 10,741 procedures). Thirty- and 90-day all-cause mortality were the outcomes for this study. The introduction of the surgical safety checklist was associated with a significant reduction in 90-day all-cause mortality (2.4% [n = 129] compared with 2.2% [n = 118] after the surgical safety checklist implementation). The implementation of the safe surgery checklist was not associated with a reduction of 30-day all-cause mortality.

The evidence conflicts about the actual rate of improved surgical mortality with checklist use. Urbach et al[191] surveyed 101 hospitals in Canada in a nonexperimental study to determine operative mortality, rates of surgical complications, lengths of hospital stay, and rates of hospital readmission and emergency department visits within 30 days after discharge among patients undergoing a variety of surgical procedures before and after adoption of a safe surgery checklist. The researchers found no significant reduction in operative mortality after checklist implementation. In addition, there were no reductions in risk of surgical complications, hospital readmissions, or emergency department visits after the safe surgery checklist implementation. The researchers noted that a greater effect from the use of the safe surgery checklist may occur with intensive team training or increased monitoring for compliance. The researchers also acknowledged that the safe surgery checklist may be beneficial in improving teamwork and communication.

In a prospective study, Sewell et al[192] evaluated the outcomes of mortality, early complications, and personnel perceptions of the WHO Surgical Safety Checklist after an educational program was instituted to increase use of a safe surgery checklist in one facility. The researchers reviewed 480 patient procedures before the educational program and 485 after the educational program. They determined that the use of the checklist for emergency and elective orthopedic patients at their facility was not associated with a significant reduction in early major complications or mortality. The educational program significantly increased the accurate use of the checklist and improved personnel perceptions of the WHO Surgical Safety Checklist.

Standardized checklist formats include the WHO Surgical Safety Checklist,[120] the SURPASS Checklist,[93] and AORN's Comprehensive Surgical Checklist.

V.e. The interdisciplinary team should adapt the safe surgery checklist to the patient population served. *[2: High Evidence]*

The collective evidence[20,27,32,35,36,47,52-55,59,193-196] supports the customization of checklists based on specialized surgical procedures and unique characteristics of patients, with input from all members of the perioperative team.

V.e.1. The checklist should be developed with input from perioperative team members representing individual service lines. *[2: High Evidence]*

Input from individual team members helps to identify care relevant to specific patient populations, provide meaning to the safe surgery checklist, and decrease variability.

Fargen et al[32] reported on the experience of one organization that implemented a three-part, 20-item checklist specific to the neurointerventional service line. Nurses, physicians, and radiology technologists were surveyed after each neurointerventional procedure 4 weeks before and 4 weeks after checklist implementation. Seventy-one procedures were performed before checklist implementation and 60 after implementation. Post-checklist surveys indicated that communication improved and the number of adverse events was significantly lower after checklist use (ie, decreased from 25 to six adverse events).

V.f.   The perioperative team should use memory aid tools such as whiteboards, electronic whiteboards, or other tools to guide safe surgery checklist use. *[2: High Evidence]*

Using tools as a memory aid helps to increase compliance with the safe surgery checklist. In a quasi-experimental study, Mainthia et al[39] implemented an electronic checklist system in all ORs in one institution. They performed direct observations of 80 cases 1 month before and 1 month and 9 months after implementation of the electronic tool (N = 240). The researchers found that the core elements of the time out were performed approximately 50% of the time before implementation and approximately 80% at both 1 month and 9 months postintervention. The researchers concluded that implementing an electronic whiteboard for checklist use dramatically increased compliance with performing preprocedural time outs.

Recommendation VI

The health care organization should establish and implement a standardized debriefing process.

The collective evidence[23,50,53,59,114,174-176,179,192] supports the use of debriefings to improve teamwork and team communication, foster continuous team learning, and improve the quality of patient care by identifying defects or system barriers in care and allowing teams to learn from those defects.

The debriefing process is an active process with engagement from all members of the perioperative team focusing on specific events and applying what they learned to their practice. Debriefings allow the perioperative team to identify opportunities to improve efficiency and patient safety, identify any defects in care, and discuss the plan for the transition of patient care from the OR to another team.[50,53,175]

In an organizational experience report, Van Herzeele et al[179] identified that the debriefing process fosters team learning because members of the perioperative team can discuss what went well and what needs improvement in individual patient cases, allowing them to improve team performance.

Although evidence supports the performance of the time out just before the incision, further research is needed to determine the ideal timing for the debriefing.[50,63,66,180]

VI.a.   An interdisciplinary team should create a standardized debriefing process with input from perioperative team members representing individual service lines. *[3: Moderate Evidence]*

Input from individual team members helps to identify care relevant to specific patient populations, which provides meaning to the debriefing process. Hicks et al[175] implemented a standardized debriefing process for patients undergoing colorectal surgery and structured the process to include focused questions relevant to colorectal surgery. They recognized that although it can be labor intensive to engage frontline providers, a debriefing process relevant to individual service lines may prove to be more sustainable and acceptable than one created with a top-down approach.

VI.a.1.   The debriefing process may include a discussion of
- counts performed and confirmed[175];
- the procedure performed[176];
- labeling and disposition of specimen containers[175];
- equipment and instrumentation issues[175];
- missing supplies[176];
- blood loss[175];
- glycemic control[175];
- pain management[175];
- venous thromboembolism prophylaxis[175];
- the wound classification[176];
- team members' concerns regarding the recovery and management of the patient[192]; and
- safety concerns and questions.[176]
[3: Moderate Evidence]

VI.b.   All unnecessary activities and conversations in the OR or procedure room should come to a stop when the debriefing is called.[120,183,184] *[1: Strong Evidence]*

VI.c.   The debriefing may be guided by the use of a checklist. *[5: Benefits Balanced with Harms]*

Recommendation VII

The health care organization's quality management program should evaluate and monitor team communication and the culture of safety.

Quality assurance and performance improvement programs can facilitate the identification of problem areas and assist personnel in evaluating and improving the quality of patient care and formulating plans for corrective action. These programs provide data that may be used to determine whether an individual organization is within benchmark goals, and if not, to identify areas that may require corrective action. A quality management program provides a mechanism to evaluate effectiveness of processes and compliance with team communication policies and procedures.

Collecting data to monitor and improve patient care, treatment, and services is a regulatory requirement[197-200] and an accreditation standard for both hospitals[201,202] and ambulatory settings.[203,204]

Sustaining a change in culture requires an organization to commit to high reliability and monitoring of quality initiatives. Health care organizations can be distracted by new initiatives and lose track of improvements that were gained in QI initiatives, like team training, effective communication, and a culture of safety.[205] A white paper published by the Institute for Healthcare Improvement (IHI)[206] described systems for sustaining improvement developed by 10 outstanding health care systems. The IHI framework outlines key factors for implementing a high-performing medical system. This framework defines primary drivers of high-performing systems as quality control, QI, and establishing a culture of high-performance management. Creating positive trust relationships encourages and sustains frontline personnel engagement in quality control and QI. The IHI framework further defined 13 secondary drivers: standardization, accountability, visual management, problem solving, escalation, integration, prioritization, assimilation, implementation, policy, feedback, transparency, and trust.

VII.a. The health care organization should review patterns of error causality to develop QI projects. *[3: Moderate Evidence]*

The collective evidence[92,97,110,188,207-212] supports increased error reporting to assist with improving health care systems. The use of reporting to analyze system failures and develop QI initiatives helps decrease the potential for human error.

In a nonexperimental study, Rogers et al[213] reviewed alleged surgical errors that resulted in patient injury in 258 of the 444 (58%) malpractice claims reported from four malpractice liability insurers. Surgeon reviewers looked at each case to determine the factors that led to a surgical error. The reviewers found that most of the 258 cases involved more than one clinician and one-third involved chains of events contributing to patient harm, such as communication breakdowns, lack of supervision, technology failures, and patient-related factors. The researchers concluded that malpractice claims can be a source for surgical error analysis.

Reason[111] developed the Swiss Cheese Model, which illustrates how a chain of errors can "slip through the holes" as a result of failures in system defenses, barriers, and safeguards. High-reliability organizations develop strong systems and provide individual support to keep the "holes" from aligning and leading to an adverse event. Failure in the defense developed to decrease error can be attributed to two reasons: active failure and latent failure. Reason described resilient high-reliability systems with error management programs that use a system approach by reviewing all factors such as the person, the team, the task, the workplace, and the institution as a whole.

VII.b. The health care organization may implement a huddle to discuss safety concerns. *[3: Moderate Evidence]*

The collective evidence[214-216] supports the use of Healthcare Utilizing Deliberate Discussion Linking Events (HUDDLE) as a QI tool for managers to check in on safety issues on a daily basis and escalate concerns quickly to resolve potential safety concerns in the system.

Morrison and Sanders[216] reported on an organizational experience in which huddles were used to improve communication and teamwork on a unit. The huddle was performed 15 minutes after change-of-shift reports. All personnel were expected to attend, and a huddle champion (ie, charge nurse) summarized key points at the end of the huddle to refocus on the safety issues identified. Each member was given an opportunity to speak and share ideas.

VII.c. The health care organization should develop patient safety indicators that measure the patient safety culture. *[2: High Evidence]*

The collective evidence[16-33,35-38,40,42-45,48,49,51,53] supports the reporting of morbidity, mortality, and adverse event data to measure patient safety. Adverse event reporting has been reported to increase when a just culture is established. Providing information on improvements in patient safety keeps the team members engaged in high-reliability teams. Two expert opinions challenge this reporting mechanism because there are so many factors involved in morbidity and mortality of patients.[191,192]

VII.c.1. Dashboards of patient safety indicators should be developed and available for the perioperative team. *[4: Limited Evidence]*

Dashboards provide personnel with visual information on progress in improving safety and sustaining safety measures.[217]

VII.c.2. Patient safety indicators should be reviewed with perioperative team members. *[5: Benefits Balanced with Harms]*

Recommendation VIII

Personnel should receive initial and ongoing education and complete competency verification activities related to team communication and a patient safety culture.

Initial and ongoing education of perioperative personnel facilitates the development of knowledge, skills, and attitudes that affect safe patient care. It is the responsibility of the health care organization to provide initial and ongoing education and to verify the competency of its personnel[53,218]; however, the primary responsibility for maintaining ongoing competency remains with the individual.

Competency verification activities provide a mechanism for competency documentation and help verify that personnel understand the principles and processes necessary for safe patient care.

Ongoing development of knowledge and skills and documentation of personnel participation is a regulatory requirement[198-200] and an accreditation standard for both hospitals and ambulatory settings.

VIII.a. The health care organization should establish education and competency verification activities for its personnel and determine intervals for education and competency verification related to a patient safety culture and team communication. *[3: Moderate Evidence]*

Education and competency verification needs and intervals are unique to the facility and to its personnel and processes. Formal didactic instruction and competency verification is implemented to relay the importance of team communication for patient safety, strategies for safe and effective team communication, and expectations regarding team communication processes.[218]

VIII.b. The health care organization should provide perioperative team training. *[2: High Evidence]*

The collective evidence and guidance from professional organizations[3,5,6,50,179,219,220] support team training as an effective intervention for improving communication and teamwork in the perioperative setting. Team training may reduce the risk for human error (eg, safety omissions) while improving team communication and attitudes.

The collective evidence[14,69-72,96,221-225] indicates that approximately half of all adverse events could have been prevented and that the underlying causes are often attributable to human factors and nontechnical skills of personnel rather than to a lack of technical training or expertise. Generic nontechnical skills such as communication, teamwork, leadership, situational awareness, and decision making have been found to be critical for safety in most high-risk occupations.

Teamwork is dependent on individual performance and the performance of the team collectively through communication, cooperation, coordination, cognition, conflict resolution, and leadership. Improving communication in the perioperative environment requires an environment in which open communication is encouraged and the removal of hierarchical barriers.[50,63]

VIII.b.1. Perioperative team training should incorporate principles of human factor analysis. *[3: Moderate Evidence]*

Human factors, including repetition, stress, and fatigue, can impede team performance.[75,84,90]

In an organizational experience report, Hu et al[84] investigated the etiology and reso-

lution of unanticipated events in the OR during 10 high-acuity surgical procedures. The researchers developed a tool to track deviations caused by human factors and classified the deviations as either delays or safety compromises. Delays were defined as complete halts in forward progress for the entire team lasting more than 2 minutes. Safety compromises were defined as episodes of increased risk of harm to the patient. The researchers found there were multiple deviations per procedure (ie, one every 79.5 minutes). The researchers developed a conceptual model that illustrates the occurrence of the safety compromises in the OR. Communication and organizational structure was frequently identified as the root causes in both types of deviations. Strategies to resolve deviations were categorized as vigilance, communication, coordination, cooperation, and leadership.[84]

VIII.b.2. Perioperative team training should incorporate the safe surgery checklist. *[2: High Evidence]*

Providing team training on checklist use fosters team communication and team building, which are necessary components to have in place before checklist implementation.[53] The collective evidence[16,22-24,29,31,34,38,42,44,45,49,54,57,59,61-63,192,226-231] supports team training with the implementation of a safe surgery checklist to foster mutual understanding among team members, improve communication, flatten the surgical hierarchy, promote team responsibility and accountability, and build toward high reliability in perioperative teams. Using a safe surgery checklist without training is little more than a tick-box exercise that has no real meaning to perioperative teams. Training and input from all perioperative team members is essential to achieving a significant commitment to a patient safety culture.

Rydenfalt[226] conducted an observational study to examine the actual usage of each component of safe surgery checklists in 24 surgical procedures. Overall, the safe surgery checklist was used 96% of the time; however, all of the individual items on the checklist were only completed 54% of the time. The researchers determined that the time-out process could be improved by educating and training perioperative team members on how the safe surgery checklist affects patient safety and by designing safe surgery checklists with input from the perioperative teams that will use them.

Puget et al[62] conducted a literature review to examine how the safe surgery checklist could be used as a communication tool with a focus on team attitudes and behaviors in the OR. The authors determined that implementation strategy is important, and perioperative leaders need to assess the patient safety climate at the facility to make the surgical safety checklist relevant to those who will be using it rather than a challenge to team use. In addition, customizing the safe surgery checklist allows teams to have a feeling of ownership and increases compliance with use of the safe surgery checklist.

Ariadne labs created a safe surgery checklist implementation guide for hospitals and ambulatory surgery centers that can be used as a resource for team leaders to design their own safe surgery checklist, support implementation efforts, avoid common problems, and improve team buy in.[53]

VIII.c. Perioperative team training should include all team members. *[3: Moderate Evidence]*

Team training reduces professional silos during perioperative team interactions. Paige et al[223] reported on an organizational experience of implementing interprofessional simulation-based training. The authors defined interprofessional education as bringing together two or more students from different health care professions to learn with, from, and about each other. Core interprofessional competencies were categorized into four major domains: values and ethics for interprofessional practice, roles and responsibilities, interprofessional communication, and teamwork.[223] The authors noted the value of interprofessional education in the OR where team dynamics continue to be less than ideal. The OR environment has been described as a silo where the interaction among team members is more multiprofessional than interprofessional. Communication between team members with differing roles (eg, physician to nurse, nurse to technician) is a challenge because of educational level, cultural background, and hierarchical barriers. The silo mentality is perpetuated and fosters a less than ideal OR culture. The authors list several problems caused by silos of professional practice, such as lack of communication, role confusion, heightened tension, and ineffective teamwork.

VIII.c.1. Perioperative team members should actively participate in team training. *[2: High Evidence]*

The collective evidence[16-62] indicates that team training is effective for improving team communication and reducing patient morbidity. A statement from the American Heart Association[50] reported that poor teamwork contributes to errors and that team training reduces the incidence of errors. Therefore, the American Heart Association recommends that all cardiac OR team members participate in team training to improve

communication, leadership, and situational awareness.

Crew Resource Management is a team training program widely used in health care. In a quasi-experimental study that took place in five hospitals in the United Kingdom, McCulloch et al[232] compared the effectiveness of Crew Resource Management team training, standard operating procedures (SOPs), and Lean thinking for promoting compliance with completion of the WHO Surgical Safety Checklist. Using the Oxford Nontechnical Skills Assessment (NOTECHS) II, the researchers compared the effectiveness of each intervention independently, a combination of team training with SOPs, and a combination of team training with Lean thinking. The researchers found that the group using team training combined with SOPs improved compliance with nontechnical skills and technical team performance when completing the WHO checklist. The researchers asserted that the use of SOPs and Lean thinking empowered the team to make changes to the process for completing the WHO checklist and improve their work environment.

The evidence[121,233,234] indicates that implementing TeamSTEPPS® in the perioperative setting may improve teamwork as part of QI processes. Tibbs and Moss[233] conducted a QI program implementing Team-STEPPS and recommended that perioperative team members participate in team training to improve communication and team relationships.

Medical Team Training is a program developed by the Veterans Health Administration that emphasizes communication and teamwork with the use of checklist-driven operative briefings and debriefings.[235] One difference in the Medical Team Training Program compared to other Crew Resource Management-based programs is that the training faculty members work with an implementation team, including surgical personnel, for a two-month planning and preparation phase before implementation.[235] In a retrospective cohort study of 119,383 procedures in Veterans Health Administration facilities, Young-Xu et al[235] found that facilities participating in the Medical Team Training program (n = 42) had a significantly lower surgical morbidity rate than facilities that were not participating in the program (n = 32). This study demonstrated an important link between improvement of teamwork in the OR and improvement of a measurable patient outcome, surgical morbidity.

VIII.d. Perioperative team training should include simulation scenarios that incorporate the health care organization's standardized communication tools for briefing, time out, debriefing, and hand overs *[2: High Evidence]*

The collective evidence[16,22-24,29,31,34,38,42,44,45,49,54,57,59,61-63,192,226-231,235,236] supports the use of simulation with interprofessional groups for improving communication and decreasing adverse outcomes from lack of communication in critical patient care moments, such as time out and hand overs.

In addition, the evidence[93,123,237-240] suggests that interprofessional training with simulation-based scenarios is effective in improving nontechnical skills and teamwork. The evidence also supports using either video recordings or observational scenarios to assess team skills and improve communication.[93,237,239,241-245]

VIII.d.1. Perioperative team training should include simulation training with all perioperative team members.[150,163,246] *[3: Moderate Evidence]*

Simulation training for the hand-over process helps to improve interprofessional communication. In an organizational experience report, Weinger et al[246] used formal education and simulation training to train perioperative team members in the hand-over process. They concluded that this education and training process significantly improved interprofessional communication.

Pukenas et al[163] evaluated the percentage of hand-over omissions plus errors by surgical residents before and after simulation training using a hand-over checklist in a qualitative study. The researchers found that the communication failure rate (incorrect and omitted items) decreased from 29.7% to 16.8% after initial training and additionally decreased to 13.2% 1 year after the simulation training was completed.

VIII.d.2. Perioperative team training observers should provide feedback to participants on nontechnical skills. *[3: Moderate Evidence]*

The collective evidence[68-72,222,244] supports the use of observational tools to assess nontechnical skills, such as situational awareness, decision making, leadership, communication, and teamwork. Further research is needed to validate a tool for observation of nontechnical skills in the perioperative RN.

In a quasi-experimental study, Dedy et al[72] trained 11 surgical residents on nontechnical skills and used the NOTSS rating system to score observed behaviors in four categories: situational awareness, decision making, communication and teamwork, and leadership. The residents were observed and given baseline scores and individual feedback based on the observations. Then, each resident and the educator developed a plan to change target behaviors identified

for improvement or to maintain performance. Scores on nontechnical skills improved significantly after the training. Participants reported that the intervention was useful and they believed it was important to incorporate debriefing and feedback on nontechnical skills into surgical training.

Editor's note: Crucial Conversations is a registered trademark of VitalSmarts, Provo, UT. TeamSTEPPS is a registered trademark of the US Department of Health and Human Services, Washington, DC, and the US Department of Defense, Washington, DC.

Glossary

Active failure: An error that is the result of an individual's failure and occurs at the point of contact between a human and an aspect of a larger system.

Briefing: A short dialogue for planning before the start of an operative or invasive procedure to discuss team formation, assign essential team roles, establish expectations and climate, and anticipate outcomes.

Debriefing: A short dialogue conducted after the procedure has concluded that is designed to improve team performance and effectiveness.

Distraction: An event that causes a diversion of attention or concentration during performance of a task.

Error: An act of commission (doing something wrong) or omission (failing to do what is right) that leads to an undesirable outcome or significant potential for such an outcome. These can be slips, lapses, or mistakes in memory or actions when executing the action or plan.

Hand over: The transfer of patient information from one person to another during transitions of care.

High-reliability team: A team that is organized to anticipate and detect defects, maintain stable operations, and respond to abnormalities.

Interruption: An unplanned or unexpected event causing discontinuation of a task.

Just culture: A culture that balances personal accountability and system improvement.

Latent failure: An error that is a result of organizational system or design failure that allows active errors to occur and cause harm.

Licensed independent practitioner: A physician, dentist, nurse practitioner, nurse midwife, or any other individual permitted by law and the organization to provide care and services without direction or supervision, within the scope of the individual's license and consistent with individually granted clinical privileges.

Noise: Any sound that interferes with normal hearing and is undesired.

Patient safety culture: A culture in which every perioperative team member places value on safety and commits to personal responsibility for patient safety.

Read-back method: A dialogue in which the listener verbally repeats patient information so that the sender can confirm the correctness of the message.

Resilience: Human adaptation to an imperfect system.

Root cause analysis: A retrospective process for identifying basic or causal factor(s) underlying variation in performance, including the occurrence or possible occurrence of a sentinel event.

Shared mental model: The perception of, understanding of, or knowledge of a situation or process that is shared among team members through communication.

Site marking: The act of identifying the correct site on the patient's body where the operative or invasive procedure is to be performed.

Sterile cockpit: An environment in which personnel refrain from nonessential activities to minimize distractions during important tasks.

Time out: The pause in patient care activity taken by the surgical team immediately before the start of the procedure to conduct a final assessment that the correct patient, site, positioning, and procedure are identified and that, as applicable, all relevant documents, related information, and necessary equipment are available.

REFERENCES

1. Institute of Medicine. Kohn LT, Corrigan JM, Donaldson MS, eds. *To Err Is Human: Building a Safer Health System.* Washington, DC: National Academy Press; 2000.

2. Makary MA, Daniel M. Medical error—the third leading cause of death in the US. *BMJ.* 2016;353:i2139. [VB]

3. *Information Statement: Surgical Patient Safety.* American Academy of Orthopaedic Surgeons. https://www.aaos.org/uploadedFiles/PreProduction/About/Opinion_Statements/advistmt/1049%20Surgical%20Patient%20Safety.pdf. Published 2016. Accessed September 28, 2017. [VA]

4. *Information Statement: Surgical Site and Procedure Confirmation.* American Academy of Orthopaedic Surgeons. https://www.aaos.org/uploadedFiles/PreProduction/About/Opinion_Statements/advistmt/1043%20Surgical%20Site%20and%20Procedure%20Confirmation.pdf. Published March 2015. Accessed September 28, 2017. [VA]

5. *Information Statement: Consistency for Safety in Orthopaedic Surgery.* American Academy of Orthopaedic Surgeons. https://www.aaos.org/uploadedFiles/PreProduction/About/Opinion_Statements/advistmt/1042%20Consistency%20for%20Safety%20in%20Orthopaedic%20Surgery.pdf. Published March 2015. Accessed September 28, 2017. [VA]

6. *Information Statement: Surgeon and Surgical Team Concentration.* American Academy of Orthopaedic Surgeons. https://www.aaos.org/uploadedFiles/PreProduction/About/Opinion_Statements/advistmt/1041%20Surgeon%20and%20Surgical%20Team%20Concentation.pdf. Published December 2014. Accessed September 28, 2017. [VA]

7. American College of Surgeons (ACS) Committee on Perioperative Care. Revised statement on safe surgery checklists, and ensuring correct patient, correct site, and correct procedure surgery. *Bull Am Coll Surg.* 2016;101(10):52. [VA]

8. American College of Surgeons (ACS) Committee on Perioperative Care. Statement on distractions in the operating room. *Bull Am Coll Surg.* 2016;101(10):42-44. [VA]

9. American College of Surgeons (ACS); American Society of Anesthesiologists. Statement on physician-led team-based surgical care. *Bull Am Coll Surg.* 2016;101(8):50. [VA]

10. Ajlan AM, Harsh GR 4th. The human factor and safety attitudes in neurosurgical operating rooms. *World Neurosurg.* 2015;83(1):46-48. [VA]

11. Arriaga AF, Elbardissi AW, Regenbogen SE, et al. A policy-based intervention for the reduction of communication breakdowns in inpatient surgical care: results from a Harvard surgical safety collaborative. *Ann Surg.* 2011;253(5):849-854. [IIA]

12. Barzallo Salazar MJ, Minkoff H, Bayya J, et al. Influence of surgeon behavior on trainee willingness to speak up: a randomized controlled trial. *J Am Coll Surg.* 2014;219(5):1001-1007. [IA]

13. Braaf S, Manias E, Finch S, Riley R, Munro F. Healthcare service provider perceptions of organisational communication across the perioperative pathway: a questionnaire survey. *J Clin Nurs.* 2013;22(1-2):180-191. [IIIA]

14. Michinov E, Jamet E, Dodeler V, Haegelen C, Jannin P. Assessing neurosurgical non-technical skills: an exploratory study of a new behavioural marker system. *J Eval Clin Pract.* 2014;20(5):582-588. [IIIB]

15. Update: sentinel event statistics. *Jt Comm Perspect.* 2006;26(10):14-15.

16. Treadwell JR, Lucas S, Tsou AY. Surgical checklists: a systematic review of impacts and implementation. *BMJ Qual Saf.* 2014;23(4):299-318. [IIIA]

17. Thomassen Ø, Storesund A, Søfteland E, Brattebø G. The effects of safety checklists in medicine: a systematic review. *Acta Anaesthesiol Scand.* 2014;58(1):5-18. [IIIA]

18. Russ S, Rout S, Sevdalis N, Moorthy K, Darzi A, Vincent C. Do safety checklists improve teamwork and communication in the operating room? A systematic review. *Ann Surg.* 2013;258(6):856-871. [IIIA]

19. Lyons VE, Popejoy LL. Meta-analysis of surgical safety checklist effects on teamwork, communication, morbidity, mortality, and safety. *West J Nurs Res.* 2014;36(2):245-261. [IA]

20. Arriaga AF, Bader AM, Wong JM, et al. Simulation-based trial of surgical-crisis checklists. *N Engl J Med.* 2013;368(3):246-253. [IIA]

21. Barrington MJ, Uda Y, Pattullo SJ, Sites BD. Wrong-site regional anesthesia: review and recommendations for prevention? *Curr Opin Anaesthesiol.* 2015;28(6):670-684. [VA]

22. Bergs J, Lambrechts F, Simons P, et al. Barriers and facilitators related to the implementation of surgical safety checklists: a systematic review of the qualitative evidence. *BMJ Qual Saf.* 2015;24(12):776-786. [IB]

23. Berrisford RG, Wilson IH, Davidge M, Sanders D. Surgical time out checklist with debriefing and multidisciplinary feedback improves venous thromboembolism prophylaxis in thoracic surgery: a prospective audit. *Eur J Cardiothorac Surg.* 2012;41(6):1326-1329. [IIIB]

24. Bliss LA, Ross-Richardson CB, Sanzari LJ, et al. Thirty-day outcomes support implementation of a surgical safety checklist. *J Am Coll Surg.* 2012;215(6):766-776. [IIA]

25. Bock M, Fanolla A, Segur-Cabanac I, et al. A comparative effectiveness analysis of the implementation of surgical safety checklists in a tertiary care hospital. *JAMA Surg.* 2016;151(7):639-646. [IIA]

26. Starling J 3rd, Coldiron BM. Outcome of 6 years of protocol use for preventing wrong site office surgery. *J Am Acad Dermatol.* 2011;65(4):807-810. [VB]

27. Calland JF, Turrentine FE, Guerlain S, et al. The surgical safety checklist: lessons learned during implementation. *Am Surg.* 2011;77(9):1131-1137. [IB]

28. Collins SJ, Newhouse R, Porter J, Talsma A. Effectiveness of the surgical safety checklist in correcting errors: a literature review applying Reason's Swiss Cheese Model. *AORN J.* 2014;100(1):65-79. [VA]

29. Conley DM, Singer SJ, Edmondson L, Berry WR, Gawande AA. Effective surgical safety checklist implementation. *J Am Coll Surg.* 2011;212(5):873-879. [VB]

30. Cullati S, Le Du S, Rae AC, et al. Is the surgical safety checklist successfully conducted? An observational study of social interactions in the operating rooms of a tertiary hospital. *BMJ Qual Saf.* 2013;22(8):639-646. [IIIB]

31. Cullati S, Licker M, Francis P, et al. Implementation of the surgical safety checklist in Switzerland and perceptions of its benefits: cross-sectional survey. *PLoS One.* 2014;9(7):e101915. [IIIB]

32. Fargen KM, Velat GJ, Lawson MF, Firment CS, Mocco J, Hoh BL. Enhanced staff communication and reduced near-miss errors with a neurointerventional procedural checklist. *J Neurointerv Surg.* 2013;5(5):497-500. [VB]

33. Gordon BM, Lam TS, Bahjri K, Hashmi A, Kuhn MA. Utility of preprocedure checklists in the congenital cardiac catheterization laboratory. *Congenit Heart Dis.* 2014;9(2):131-137. [IIB]

34. Graling PR. Designing an applied model of perioperative patient safety. *Clin Scholars Rev.* 2011;4(2):104-114. [VA]

35. Hawranek M, Gasior PM, Buchta P, et al. Periprocedural checklist in the catheterisation laboratory is associated with decreased rate of treatment complications. *Kardiol Pol.* 2015;73(7):511-519. [IIB]

36. Helmiö P, Blomgren K, Takala A, Pauniaho SL, Takala RS, Ikonen TS. Towards better patient safety: WHO Surgical Safety Checklist in otorhinolaryngology. *Clin Otolaryngol.* 2011;36(3):242-247. [IIB]

37. Hullfish KL, Miller T, Pastore LM, et al. A checklist for timeout on labor and delivery: a pilot study to improve communication and safety. *J Reprod Med.* 2014;59(11-12):579-584. [VA]

38. Jones S. Your life in WHO's hands: The World Health Organization Surgical Safety Checklist: a critical review of the literature. *J Perioper Pract.* 2011;21(8):271-274. [VA]

39. Mainthia R, Lockney T, Zotov A, et al. Novel use of electronic whiteboard in the operating room increases surgical team compliance with pre-incision safety practices. *Surgery.* 2012;151(5):660-666. [IIA]

40. Nissan J, Campos V, Delgado H, Matadial C, Spector S. The automated operating room: a team approach to patient safety and communication. *JAMA Surg.* 2014;149(11):1209-1210. [IIIC]

41. Norton EK, Singer SJ, Sparks W, Ozonoff AI, Baxter J, Rangel S. Operating room clinicians' attitudes and perceptions of a pediatric surgical safety checklist at 1 institution. *J Patient Saf.* 2016;12(1):44-50. [IIIA]

42. Nugent E, Hseino H, Ryan K, Traynor O, Neary P, Keane FBV. The surgical safety checklist survey: a national perspective on patient safety. *Ir J Med Sci.* 2013;182(2):171-176. [IIIA]

43. Oak SN, Dave NM, Garasia MB, Parelkar SV. Surgical checklist application and its impact on patient safety in pediatric surgery. *J Postgrad Med.* 2015;61(2):92-94. [IIC]

44. Papaconstantinou HT, Jo CH, Reznik SI, Smythe WR, Wehbe-Janek H. Implementation of a surgical safety checklist: impact on surgical team perspectives. *Ochsner J.* 2013;13(3):299-309. [IIA]

45. Porter AJ, Narimasu JY, Mulroy MF, Koehler RP. Sustainable, effective implementation of a surgical preprocedural checklist: an "attestation" format for all operating team members. *Jt Comm J Qual Patient Saf.* 2014;40(1):3-9. [IIIC]

46. Pucher PH, Johnston MJ, Aggarwal R, Arora S, Darzi A. Effectiveness of interventions to improve patient handover in surgery: a systematic review. *Surgery.* 2015;158(1):85-95. [IIIA]

47. Raman J, Leveson N, Samost AL, et al. When a checklist is not enough: how to improve them and what else is needed. *J Thorac Cardiovasc Surg.* 2016;152(2):585-592. [VA]

48. Silva Araújo MP, de Oliveira AC. "Safe surgery saves lives" program contributions in surgical patient care: integrative review. *Rev Enferm UFPE.* 2015;9(4):7448-7457. [VA]

49. Takala RS, Pauniaho SL, Kotkansalo A, et al. A pilot study of the implementation of WHO surgical checklist in Finland: improvements in activities and communication. *Acta Anaesthesiol Scand.* 2011;55(10):1206-1214. [IIIB]

50. Wahr JA, Prager RL, Abernathy JH, et al. Patient safety in the cardiac operating room: human factors and teamwork: a scientific statement from the American Heart Association. *Circulation.* 2013;128(10):1139-1169. [IVA]

51. Walker IA, Reshamwalla S, Wilson IH. Surgical safety checklists: do they improve outcomes? *Br J Anaesth.* 2012;109(1):47-54. [VB]

52. Zeeni C, Carabini L, Gould RW, et al. The implementation and efficacy of the Northwestern High Risk Spine Protocol. *World Neurosurg.* 2014;82(6):e815-e823. [VA]

53. *Safe Surgery Checklist Implementation Guide.* Boston MA: Ariadne Labs; 2015. Safe Surgery 2015. http://www.safesurgery2015.org/uploads/1/0/9/0/1090835/safe_surgery_implementation_guide__092515.012216_.pdf. Accessed September 28, 2017. [VA]

54. Berlinger N, Dietz E. Time-out: the professional and organizational ethics of speaking up in the OR. *AMA J Ethics.* 2016;18(9):925-932. [VB]

55. Dagey D. Using simulation to implement an OR cardiac arrest crisis checklist. *AORN J.* 2017;105(1):67-72. [VA]

56. de Vries EN, Prins HA, Crolla RM, et al. Effect of a comprehensive surgical safety system on patient outcomes. *N Engl J Med.* 2010;363(20):1928-1937. [IIA]

57. Haynes AB, Weiser TG, Berry WR, et al. Changes in safety attitude and relationship to decreased postoperative morbidity and mortality following implementation of a checklist-based surgical safety intervention. *BMJ Qual Saf.* 2011;20(1):102-107. [IIA]

58. Safe surgery saves lives: surgical safety checklist. In: *The ORNAC Standards for Perioperative Registered Nursing Practice.* 12th ed. Kingston, Ontario: Operating Room Nurses Association of Canada (ORNAC); 2015:34-35. [IVB]

59. Russ S, Rout S, Caris J, et al. Measuring variation in use of the WHO Surgical Safety Checklist in the operating room: a multicenter prospective cross-sectional study. *J Am Coll Surg.* 2015;220(1):1-11.e4. [IIIA]

60. Position statement: surgical safety. In: *2014-2015 ACORN Standards for Perioperative Nursing.* Adelaide, South Australia: The Australian College of Operating Room Nurses; 2014:154-156. [IVB]

61. Michael R, Della P, Zhou H. The effectiveness of the Surgical Safety Checklist as a means of communication in the operating room. *ACORN.* 2013;26(2):48-52. [IIIA]

62. Pugel AE, Simianu VV, Flum DR, Dellinger EP. Use of the surgical safety checklist to improve communication and reduce complications. *J Infect Public Health.* 2015;8(3):219-225. [VB]

63. Gillespie BM, Withers TK, Lavin J, Gardiner T, Marshall AP. Factors that drive team participation in surgical safety checks: a prospective study. *Patient Saf Surg.* 2016;10(1):3. [IIIA]

64. Salzwedel C, Bartz HJ, Kühnelt I, et al. The effect of a checklist on the quality of post-anaesthesia patient handover: a randomized controlled trial. *Int J Qual Health Care.* 2013;25(2):176-81. [IA]

65. Sexton JB, Schwartz SP, Chadwick WA, et al. The associations between work-life balance behaviours, teamwork climate and safety climate: cross-sectional survey introducing the work-life climate scale, psychometric properties, benchmarking data and future directions. *BMJ Qual Saf.* 2017;26(8):632-640. [IIIA]

66. Mohorek M, Webb TP. Establishing a conceptual framework for handoffs using communication theory. *J Surg Educ.* 2015;72(3):402-409. [VB]

67. Hull L, Arora S, Kassab E, Kneebone R, Sevdalis N. Observational teamwork assessment for surgery: content validation and tool refinement. *J Am Coll Surg.* 2011;212(2):234-243.e1-e5. [IIIB]

68. Sharma B, Mishra A, Aggarwal R, Grantcharov TP. Non-technical skills assessment in surgery. *Surg Oncol.* 2011;20(3):169-177. [IIIB]

69. Mitchell L, Mitchell J. "Pass the buzzy thing, please." Recognising and understanding information: an essential non-technical skill element for the efficient scrub practitioner. *J Perioper Pract.* 2011;21(6):203-205. [IIC]

70. Spanager L, Beier-Holgersen R, Dieckmann P, Konge L, Rosenberg J, Oestergaard D. Reliable assessment of general surgeons' non-technical skills based on video-recordings of patient simulated scenarios. *Am J Surg.* 2013;206(5):810-817. [IIB]

71. Geraghty AM, McIlhenny C. Human factor skills in the surgical environment. *Br J Hosp Med (Lond).* 2016;77(1):14-16. [VC]

72. Dedy NJ, Fecso AB, Szasz P, Bonrath EM, Grantcharov TP. Implementation of an effective strategy for teaching nontechnical skills in the operating room: a single-blinded nonrandomized trial. *Ann Surg.* 2016;263(5):937-941. [IIA]

73. Han SJ, Rolston JD, Lau CY, Berger MS. Improving patient safety in neurologic surgery. *Neurosurg Clin North Am.* 2015;26(2):143-147. [VB]

74. Hemingway MW, O'Malley C, Silvestri S. Safety culture and care: a program to prevent surgical errors. *AORN J.* 2015;101(4):404-415. [VA]

75. El Bardissi AW, Sundt TM. Human factors and operating room safety. *Surg Clin North Am.* 2012;92(1):21-35. [VA]

76. *Leading a Culture of Safety: A Blueprint for Success.* Boston, MA: National Patient Safety Foundation; 2017.

77. Espin S, Lingard L, Baker GR, Regehr G. Persistence of unsafe practice in everyday work: an exploration of organizational and psychological factors constraining safety in the operating room. *Qual Saf Health Care.* 2006;15(3):165-170. [IIIB]

78. *AORN Position Statement on a Healthy Perioperative Practice Environment.* AORN, Inc. https://www.aorn.org/guidelines/clinical-resources/position-statements. Updated 2015. Accessed September 29, 2017. [IVB]

79. Lipira LE, Gallagher TH. Disclosure of adverse events and errors in surgical care: challenges and strategies for improvement. *World J Surg.* 2014;38(7):1614-1621. [VB]

80. Merry AF, Weller J, Mitchell SJ. Improving the quality and safety of patient care in cardiac anesthesia. *J Cardiothorac Vasc Anesth.* 2014;28(5):1341-1351. [VA]

81. Tsao K, Browne M. Culture of safety: a foundation for patient care. *Semin Pediatr Surg.* 2015;24(6):283-287. [VA]

82. Kolbe M, Burtscher MJ, Wacker J, et al. Speaking up is related to better team performance in simulated anesthesia inductions: an observational study. *Anesth Analg.* 2012;115(5):1099-1108. [IIIB]

83. Maxfield D, Grenny J, Lavandero R, Groah L. *The Silent Treatment: Why Safety Tools and Checklists Aren't Enough to Save Lives.* Provo, UT: VitalSmarts; 2011. [IIIA]

84. Hu YY, Arriaga AF, Roth EM, et al. Protecting patients from an unsafe system: the etiology and recovery of intraoperative deviations in care. *Ann Surg.* 2012;256(2):203-210. [VA]

85. Hickson GB, Pichert JW, Webb LE, Gabbe SG. A complementary approach to promoting professionalism: identifying, measuring, and addressing unprofessional behaviors. *Acad Med.* 2007;82(11):1040-1048. [VA]

86. Reiter CE, Pichert JW, Hickson GB. Addressing behavior and performance issues that threaten quality and patient safety: what your attorneys want you to know. *Prog Pediatr Cardiol.* 2012;33(1):37-45. [VA]

87. Lane-Fall MB, Brooks AK, Wilkins SA, Davis JJ, Riesenberg LA. Addressing the mandate for hand-off education: a focused review and recommendations for anesthesia resident curriculum development and evaluation. *Anesthesiology.* 2014;120(1):218-229. [VA]

88. Prati G, Pietrantoni L. Attitudes to teamwork and safety among Italian surgeons and operating room nurses. *Work.* 2014;49(4):669-677. [IIIA]

89. Vannucci A, Kras JF. Decision making, situation awareness, and communication skills in the operating room. *Int Anesthesiol Clin.* 2013;51(1):105-127. [VA]

90. Brennan PA, Mitchell DA, Holmes S, Plint S, Parry D. Good people who try their best can have problems: recognition of human factors and how to minimise error. *Br J Oral Maxillofac Surg.* 2016;54(1):3-7. [VA]

91. Kirschbaum KA, Rask JP, Brennan M, Phelan S, Fortner SA. Improved climate, culture, and communication through multidisciplinary training and instruction. *Am J Obstet Gynecol.* 2012;207(3):200.e1-200.e7. [VB]

92. Singer SJ, Rivard PE, Hayes JE, Shokeen P, Gaba D, Rosen A. Improving patient care through leadership engagement with frontline staff: a Department of Veterans Affairs case study. *Jt Comm J Qual Patient Saf.* 2013;39(8):349-360. [VA]

93. Bearman M, O'Brien R, Anthony A, et al. Learning surgical communication, leadership and teamwork through simulation. *J Surg Educ.* 2012;69(2):201-207. [IIIB]

94. The Joint Commission. The essential role of leadership in developing a safety culture. *Sentinel Event Alert.* 2017;57. https://www.jointcommission.org/assets/1/18/SEA_57_Safety_Culture_Leadership_0317.pdf. Accessed September 29, 2017. [VA]

95. Huang LC, Conley D, Lipsitz S, et al. The surgical safety checklist and teamwork coaching tools: a study of inter-rater reliability. *BMJ Qual Saf.* 2014;23(8):639-650. [IIIA]

96. Henrickson Parker S, Yule S, Flin R, McKinley A. Towards a model of surgeons' leadership in the operating room. *BMJ Qual Saf.* 2011;20(7):570-579. [VA]

97. Taylor AM, Chuo J, Figueroa-Altmann A, Di Taranto S, Shaw KN. Using four-phased unit-based patient safety

walkrounds to uncover correctable system flaws. *Jt Comm J Qual Patient Saf.* 2013;39(9):396-403. [VA]

98. *Free from Harm: Accelerating Patient Safety Improvement Fifteen Years After* To Err is Human. Boston, MA: National Patient Safety Foundation; 2015. http://c.ymcdn.com/sites/www.npsf.org/resource/resmgr/PDF/Free_from_Harm.pdf. Accessed September 29, 2017.

99. Figueroa MI, Sepanski R, Goldberg SP, Shah S. Improving teamwork, confidence, and collaboration among members of a pediatric cardiovascular intensive care unit multidisciplinary team using simulation-based team training. *Pediatr Cardiol.* 2013;34(3):612-619. [VB]

100. Gillespie BM, Gwinner K, Chaboyer W, Fairweather N. Team communications in surgery—creating a culture of safety. *J Interprof Care.* 2013;27(5):387-393. [IIIA]

101. Rosenstein A. Managing disruptive behaviors in the health care setting: focus on obstetrics services. *Am J Obstet Gynecol.* 2011;204(3):187-182. [VB]

102. Walrath JM, Dang D, Nyberg D. An organizational assessment of disruptive clinician behavior: findings and implications. *J Nurs Care Qual.* 2013;28(2):110-121. [VA]

103. Swiggart WH, Dewey CM, Hickson GB, Finlayson AJ, Spickard WA Jr. A plan for identification, treatment, and remediation of disruptive behaviors in physicians. *Front Health Serv Manage.* 2009;25(4):3-11. [VA]

104. Hu YY, Arriaga AF, Peyre SE, Corso KA, Roth EM, Greenberg CC. Deconstructing intraoperative communication failures. *J Surg Res.* 2012;177(1):37-42. [VB]

105. Nembhard IM, Labao I, Savage S. Breaking the silence: determinants of voice for quality improvement in hospitals. *Health Care Manage Rev.* 2015;40(3):225-236. [IIIA]

106. Reid J, Bromiley M. Clinical human factors: the need to speak up to improve patient safety. *Nurs Stand.* 2012;26(35):35-40. [VA]

107. Raemer DB, Kolbe M, Minehart RD, Rudolph JW, Pian-Smith MC. Improving anesthesiologists' ability to speak up in the operating room: a randomized controlled experiment of a simulation-based intervention and a qualitative analysis of hurdles and enablers. *Acad Med.* 2016;91(4):530-539. [IA]

108. Meginniss A, Damian F, Falvo F. Time out for patient safety. *J Emerg Nurs.* 2012;38(1):51-53. [VB]

109. Sexton JB, Thomas EJ, Helmreich RL. Error, stress, and teamwork in medicine and aviation: cross sectional surveys. *BMJ.* 2000;320(7237):745-749. [IIIA]

110. Stein JE, Heiss K. The Swiss Cheese Model of adverse event occurrence—closing the holes. *Semin Pediatr Surg.* 2015;24(6):278-282. [VA]

111. Reason J. *Human Error.* New York, NY: Cambridge University Press; 1990:302. [VA]

112. Herzer KR, Mirrer M, Xie Y, et al. Patient safety reporting systems: sustained quality improvement using a multidisciplinary team and "good catch" awards. *Jt Comm J Qual Patient Saf.* 2012;38(8):399-347. [VA]

113. Pape TM. The role of distractions and interruptions in operating room safety. *Perioper Nurs Clin.* 2011;6(2):101-111. [VA]

114. Kleiner C, Link T, Maynard MT, Halverson Carpenter K. Coaching to improve the quality of communication during briefings and debriefings. *AORN J.* 2014;100(4):358-368. [VA]

115. McCulloch P, Mishra A, Handa A, Dale T, Hirst G, Catchpole K. The effects of aviation-style non-technical skills training on technical performance and outcome in the operating theatre. *Qual Saf Health Care.* 2009;18(2):109-115. [VB]

116. Boyd M, Cumin D, Lombard B, Torrie J, Civil N, Weller J. Read-back improves information transfer in simulated clinical crises. *BMJ Qual Saf.* 2014;23(12):989-993. [IIIB]

117. Patel B, Johnston M, Cookson N, King D, Arora S, Darzi A. Interprofessional communication of clinicians using a mobile phone app: a randomized crossover trial using simulated patients. *J Med Internet Res.* 2016;18(4):e79. [IB]

118. Saxton R. Communication skills training to address disruptive physician behavior. *AORN J.* 2012;95(5):602-611. [IIA]

119. Simmons A. "Territorial games" aim to help curb disruptive behavior in the OR. *OR Manager.* 2014;30(1):24-26. [VC]

120. *Implementation Manual WHO Surgical Safety Checklist 2009: Safe Surgery Saves Lives.* Geneva, Switzerland: World Health Organization; 2009. http://apps.who.int/iris/bitstream/10665/44186/1/9789241598590_eng.pdf. Accessed September 29, 2017. [IVA]

121. Plonien C, Williams M. Stepping up teamwork via TeamSTEPPS. *AORN J.* 2015;101(4):465-470. [VB]

122. Sentinel events (SE). In: *Comprehensive Accreditation Manual.* E-edition. Oakbrook Terrace, IL: The Joint Commission; 2017:SE-1–SE-20.

123. Klipfel JM, Carolan BJ, Brytowski N, Mitchell CA, Gettman MT, Jacobson TM. Patient safety improvement through in situ simulation interdisciplinary team training. *Urol Nurs.* 2014;34(1):39-46. [VA]

124. Al-Hakim LG, Xiao Y. On the day of surgery: how long does preventable disruption prolong the patient journey? *Int J Health Care Qual Assur.* 2012;25(4):322-342. [IIIB]

125. Steeples LR, Hingorani M, Flanagan D, Kelly SP. Wrong intraocular lens events—what lessons have we learned? A review of incidents reported to the national reporting and learning system: 2010-2014 versus 2003-2010. *Eye.* 2016;30(8):1049-1055. [IIIA]

126. Campbell G, Arfanis K, Smith AF. Distraction and interruption in anaesthetic practice. *Br J Anaesth.* 2012;109(5):707-715. [IIIA]

127. Stewart DE, Tlusty SM, Taylor KH, et al. Trends and patterns in reporting of patient safety situations in transplantation. *Am J Transplant.* 2015;15(12):3123-3133. [IIIA]

128. Wheelock A, Suliman A, Wharton R, et al. The impact of operating room distractions on stress, workload, and teamwork. *Ann Surg.* 2015;261(6):1079-1084. [IIIA]

129. Keller S, Tschan F, Beldi G, Kurmann A, Candinas D, Semmer NK. Noise peaks influence communication in the operating room. an observational study. *Ergonomics.* 2016;59(12):1541-1552. [IIIB]

130. Way TJ, Long A, Weihing J, et al. Effect of noise on auditory processing in the operating room. *J Am Coll Surg.* 2013;216(5):933-938. [IIA]

131. Jothiraj H, Howland-Harris J, Evley R, Moppett IK. Distractions and the anaesthetist: a qualitative study of context and direction of distraction. *Br J Anaesth.* 2013;111(3):477-482. [IIIB]

132. Weigl M, Antoniadis S, Chiapponi C, Bruns C, Sevdalis N. The impact of intra-operative interruptions on surgeons' perceived workload: an observational study in elective general and orthopedic surgery. *Surg Endosc.* 2015;29(1):145-153. [IIIB]

133. Chen JG, Wright MC, Smith PB, Jaggers J, Mistry KP. Adaptation of a postoperative handoff communication process for children with heart disease: a quantitative study. *Am J Med Qual.* 2011;26(5):380-386. [VB]

134. *AORN Position Statement on Managing Distractions and Noise During Perioperative Patient Care.* https://www.aorn.org/guidelines/clinical-resources/

position-statements. Updated 2014. Accessed September 29, 2017. [IVB]

135. Wright MI. Implementing no interruption zones in the perioperative environment. *AORN J*. 2016;104(6):536-540. [VA]

136. Saleem AM, Paulus JK, Vassiliou MC, Parsons SK. Initial assessment of patient handoff in accredited general surgery residency programs in the United States and Canada: a cross-sectional survey. *Can J Surg*. 2015;58(4):269-277. [IIIA]

137. Nagpal K, Abboudi M, Manchanda C, et al. Improving postoperative handover: a prospective observational study. *Am J Surg*. 2013;206(4):494-501. [IIA]

138. Nagpal K, Arora S, Vats A, et al. Failures in communication and information transfer across the surgical care pathway: interview study. *BMJ Qual Saf*. 2012;21(10):843-849. [IIIB]

139. Manser T, Foster S. Effective handover communication: an overview of research and improvement efforts. *Best Pract Res Clin Anaesthesiol*. 2011;25(2):181-191. [VA]

140. Grover A, Duggan E. Chinese whispers in the post anaesthesia care unit (PACU). *Ir Med J*. 2013;106(8):241-243. [VB]

141. Evanina EY, Monceaux NL. Anesthesia handoff: a root cause analysis based on a near-miss scenario. *Clin Scholars Rev*. 2012;5(2):132-136. [VB]

142. Chard R, Makary MA. Transfer-of-care communication: nursing best practices. *AORN J*. 2015;102(4):329-342. [VA]

143. Petrovic MA, Aboumatar H, Scholl AT, et al. The perioperative handoff protocol: evaluating impacts on handoff defects and provider satisfaction in adult perianesthesia care units. *J Clin Anesth*. 2015;27(2):111-119. [IIA]

144. Agarwal HS, Saville BR, Slayton JM, et al. Standardized postoperative handover process improves outcomes in the intensive care unit: a model for operational sustainability and improved team performance. *Crit Care Med*. 2012;40(7):2109-2115. [VA]

145. Breuer RK, Taicher B, Turner DA, Cheifetz IM, Rehder KJ. Standardizing postoperative PICU handovers improves handover metrics and patient outcomes. *Pediatr Crit Care Med*. 2015;16(3):256-263. [IIA]

146. Siddiqui N, Arzola C, Iqbal M, et al. Deficits in information transfer between anaesthesiologist and post-anaesthesia care unit staff: an analysis of patient handover. *Eur J Anaesthesiol*. 2012;29(9):438-445. [IIIB]

147. Craig R, Moxey L, Young D, Spenceley NS, Davidson MG. Strengthening handover communication in pediatric cardiac intensive care. *Paediatr Anaesth*. 2012;22(4):393-399. [IIA]

148. Joy BF, Elliott E, Hardy C, Sullivan C, Backer CL, Kane JM. Standardized multidisciplinary protocol improves handover of cardiac surgery patients to the intensive care unit. *Pediatr Crit Care Med*. 2011;12(3):304-308. [IIB]

149. Raiten JM, Lane-Fall M, Gutsche JT, et al. Transition of care in the cardiothoracic intensive care unit: a review of handoffs in perioperative cardiothoracic and vascular practice. *J Cardiothorac Vasc Anesth*. 2015;29(4):1089-1095. [VB]

150. Johner AM, Merchant S, Aslani N, et al. Acute general surgery in Canada: a survey of current handover practices. *Can J Surg*. 2013;56(3):E24-E28. [IIIB]

151. Møller TP, Madsen MD, Fuhrmann L, Østergaard D. Postoperative handover: characteristics and considerations on improvement: a systematic review. *Eur J Anaesthesiol*. 2013;30(5):229-242. [IIIA]

152. Segall N, Bonifacio AS, Schroeder RA, et al; Durham VA Patient Safety Center of Inquiry. Can we make postoperative patient handovers safer? A systematic review of the literature. *Anesth Analg*. 2012;115(1):102-115. [IIIA]

153. McElroy LM, Daud A, Lapin B, et al. Detection of medical errors in kidney transplantation: a pilot study comparing proactive clinician debriefings to a hospital-wide incident reporting system. *Surgery*. 2014;156(5):1106-1115. [IIIA]

154. McElroy LM, Macapagal KR, Collins KM et al. Clinician perceptions of operating room to intensive care unit handoffs and implications for patient safety: a qualitative study. *Am J Surg*. 2015;210(4):629-635. [IIIB]

155. Agarwala AV, Firth PG, Albrecht MA, Warren L, Musch G. An electronic checklist improves transfer and retention of critical information at intraoperative handoff of care. *Anesth Analg*. 2015;120(1):96-104. [VA]

156. Schuster KM, Jenq GY, Thung SF, et al. Electronic handoff instruments: a truly multidisciplinary tool? *J Am Med Inform Assoc*. 2014;21(e2):e352-e357. [VB]

157. Eberhardt S. Improve handoff communication with SBAR. *Nursing*. 2014;44(11):17-20. [VC]

158. Johnson F, Logsdon P, Fournier K, Fisher S. SWITCH for safety: perioperative hand-off tools. *AORN J*. 2013;98(5):494-507. [VA]

159. Morris AM, Hoke N. Communication is key in the continuum of care. *OR Nurse*. 2015;9(5):14-19. [VC]

160. Randmaa M, Mårtensson G, Swenne CL, Engström M. SBAR improves communication and safety climate and decreases incident reports due to communication errors in an anaesthetic clinic: a prospective intervention study. *BMJ Open*. 2014;4(1):e004268. [IIA]

161. Ryan S, O'Riordan JM, Tierney S, Conlon KC, Ridgway PF. Impact of a new electronic handover system in surgery. *Int J Surg*. 2011;9(3):217-220. [IIIB]

162. Weiss MJ, Bhanji F, Fontela PS, Razack SI. A preliminary study of the impact of a handover cognitive aid on clinical reasoning and information transfer. *Med Educ*. 2013;47(8):832-41. [VA]

163. Pukenas EW, Dodson G, Deal ER, Gratz I, Allen E, Burden AR. Simulation-based education with deliberate practice may improve intraoperative handoff skills: a pilot study. *J Clin Anesth*. 2014;26(7):530-538. [IIIA]

164. Petrovic MA, Martinez EA, Aboumatar H. Implementing a perioperative handoff tool to improve post-procedural patient transfers. *Jt Comm J Qual Patient Saf*. 2012;38(3):135-142. [VA]

165. Department of Defense Patient Safety Program. *Healthcare Communications Toolkit to Improve Transitions in Care*. Falls Church, VA: TRICARE Management Activity; 2005. https://www.oumedicine.com/docs/ad-obgyn-workfiles/handofftoolkit.pdf?sfvrsn=2. Accessed September 29, 2017. [IVA]

166. Zahiri HR, Stromberg J, Skupsky H, et al. Prevention of 3 "never events" in the operating room: fires, gossypiboma, and wrong-site surgery. *Surg Innov*. 2011;18(1):55-60. [IVB]

167. Wu RL, Aufses A Jr. Characteristics and costs of surgical scheduling errors. *Am J Surg*. 2012;204(4):468-473. [IIIA]

168. McElroy LM, Collins KM, Koller FL, et al. Operating room to intensive care unit handoffs and the risks of patient harm. *Surgery*. 2015;158(3):588-594. [IIB]

169. Fabila TS, Hee HI, Sultana R, Assam PN, Kiew A, Chan YH. Improving postoperative handover from anaesthetists to non-anaesthetists in a children's intensive care unit: the receiver's perception. *Singapore Med J*. 2016;57(5):242-253. [VA]

PATIENT CARE

170. Lingard L, Regehr G, Cartmill C, et al. Evaluation of a preoperative team briefing: a new communication routine results in improved clinical practice. *BMJ Qual Saf.* 2011;20(6):475-482. [IIB]

171. Johnston FM, Tergas AI, Bennett JL, et al. Measuring briefing and checklist compliance in surgery: a tool for quality improvement. *Am J Med Qual.* 2014;29(6):491-498. [VA]

172. Thanapongsathorn W, Jitsopa J, Wongviriyakorn O. Interprofessional preoperative briefing enhances surgical teamwork satisfaction and decrease operative time: a comparative study in abdominal operation. *J Med Assoc Thai.* 2012;95(Suppl 12):S8-S14. [VA]

173. Jain AL, Jones KC, Simon J, Patterson MD. The impact of a daily pre-operative surgical huddle on interruptions, delays, and surgeon satisfaction in an orthopedic operating room: a prospective study. *Patient Saf Surg.* 2015;9(1):8. [VA]

174. Bethune R, Sasirekha G, Sahu A, Cawthorn S, Pullyblank A. Use of briefings and debriefings as a tool in improving team work, efficiency, and communication in the operating theatre. *Postgrad Med J.* 2011;87(1027):331-334. [VA]

175. Hicks CW, Rosen M, Hobson DB, Ko C, Wick EC. Improving safety and quality of care with enhanced teamwork through operating room briefings. *JAMA Surg.* 2014;149(8):863-868. [VA]

176. Bandari J, Schumacher K, Simon M, et al. Surfacing safety hazards using standardized operating room briefings and debriefings at a large regional medical center. *Jt Comm J Qual Patient Saf.* 2012;38(4):154-160. [VA]

177. Symons NRA, Wong HWL, Manser T, Sevdalis N, Vincent CA, Moorthy K. An observational study of teamwork skills in shift handover. *Int J Surg.* 2012;10(7):355-359. [VA]

178. Einav Y, Gopher D, Kara I, et al. Preoperative briefing in the operating room: shared cognition, teamwork, and patient safety. *Chest.* 2010;137(2):443-449. [IIIA]

179. Van Herzeele I, Sevdalis N, Lachat M, Desender L, Rudarakanchana N, Rancic Z. Team training in ruptured EVAR. *J Cardiovasc Surg.* 2014;55(2):193-206. [VA]

180. Gillespie BM, Gwinner K, Fairweather N, Chaboyer W. Building shared situational awareness in surgery through distributed dialog. *J Multidiscip Healthc.* 2013;6:109-118. [IIIA]

181. Birnbach DJ, Rosen LF, Fitzpatrick M, Paige JT, Arheart KL. Introductions during time-outs: do surgical team members know one another's names? *Jt Comm J Qual Patient Saf.* 2017;43(6):284-288. [IIIB]

182. Guideline for a safe environment of care, part 1. In: *Guidelines for Perioperative Practice.* Denver, CO: AORN, Inc; 2017:243-268. [IVA]

183. Clarke JR, Waddell L, Wolff DD Jr. Quarterly update on wrong-site surgery: how to do an effective time-out in the dark. *Penn Patient Saf Advis.* 2014;11(2):88-92. [VA]

184. Weiser TG, Berry WR. Review article: perioperative checklist methodologies. *Can J Anesth.* 2013;60(2):136-142. [VB]

185. Revised guidance related to new & revised regulations for hospitals, ambulatory surgical centers (ASCs), rural health clinics (RHCs) and federally qualified health centers (FQHCs). 2015. Centers for Medicare & Medicaid Services. https://www.cms.gov/Medicare/Provider-Enrollment-and-Certification/SurveyCertificationGenInfo/Downloads/Survey-and-Cert-Letter-15-22.pdf. Accessed September 29, 2017.

186. UP.01.02.01: Mark the procedure site. In: *Comprehensive Accreditation Manual.* E-dition. Oakbrook Terrace, IL: The Joint Commission; 2017.

187. Mayer JE, Dang RP, Duarte Prieto GF, Cho SK, Qureshi SA, Hecht AC. Analysis of the techniques for thoracic- and lumbar-level localization during posterior spine surgery and the occurrence of wrong-level surgery: results from a national survey. *Spine J.* 2014;14(5):741-748. [IIIB]

188. Yoon RS, Alaia MJ, Hutzler LH, Bosco JA 3rd. Using "near misses" analysis to prevent wrong-site surgery. *J Healthc Qual.* 2015;37(2):126-132. [VA]

189. A time-out is performed before the procedure. In: *Comprehensive Accreditation Manual.* E-dition. Oakbrook Terrace, IL: The Joint Commission; 2017.

190. Song JB, Vemana G, Mobley JM, Bhayani SB. The second "time-out": a surgical safety checklist for lengthy robotic surgeries. *Patient Saf Surg.* 2013;7(1):19. [VA]

191. Urbach DR, Govindarajan A, Saskin R, Wilton AS, Baxter NN. Introduction of surgical safety checklists in Ontario, Canada. *N Engl J Med.* 2014;370(11):1029-1038. [IIIA]

192. Sewell M, Adebibe M, Jayakumar P, et al. Use of the WHO Surgical Safety Checklist in trauma and orthopaedic patients. *Int Orthop.* 2011;35(6):897-901. [VA]

193. Fourcade A, Blache JL, Grenier C, Bourgain JL, Minvielle E. Barriers to staff adoption of a surgical safety checklist. *BMJ Qual Saf.* 2012;21(3):191-197. [IIB]

194. Lyons VE, Popejoy LL. Time-out and checklists: a survey of rural and urban operating room personnel. *J Nurs Care Qual.* 2017;32(1):E3-E10. [IIIB]

195. Cima R, Dankbar E, Lovely J, et al. Colorectal surgery surgical site infection reduction program: a National Surgical Quality Improvement Program-driven multidisciplinary single-institution experience. *J Am Coll Surg.* 2013;216(1):23-33. [VB]

196. Maniar RL, Sytnik P, Wirtzfeld DA, et al. Synoptic operative reports enhance documentation of best practices for rectal cancer. *J Surg Oncol.* 2015;112(5):555-560. [IIIA]

197. *State Operations Manual Appendix A—Survey Protocol, Regulations and Interpretive Guidelines for Hospitals.* Rev 151; 2015. Centers for Medicare & Medicaid Services. https://www.cms.gov/Regulations-and-Guidance/Guidance/Manuals/downloads/som107ap_a_hospitals.pdf. Accessed September 29, 2017.

198. *State Operations Manual Appendix L—Guidance for Surveyors: Ambulatory Surgical Centers.* Rev. 137; 2015. Centers for Medicare & Medicaid Services. https://www.cms.gov/Regulations-and-Guidance/Guidance/Manuals/downloads/som107ap_l_ambulatory.pdf. Accessed September 29, 2017.

199. 42 CFR 482. Conditions of participation for hospitals. 2011. Government Publishing Office. https://www.gpo.gov/fdsys/granule/CFR-2011-title42-vol5/CFR-2011-title42-vol5-part482. Accessed September 29, 2017.

200. 42 CFR 416. Ambulatory surgical services. 2011. Government Publishing Office. https://www.gpo.gov/fdsys/granule/CFR-2011-title42-vol3/CFR-2011-title42-vol3-part416. Accessed September 29, 2017.

201. Patient safety systems for hospitals. In: *Comprehensive Accreditation Manual for Hospitals.* Oakbrook Terrace, IL: The Joint Commission; 2017:PS-1–PS-50. https://www.jointcommission.org/assets/1/18/CAMH_04a_PS.pdf. Accessed September 29, 2017. [VA]

202. NIAHO: National Integrated Accreditation for Healthcare Organizations. Surgical services (SS). In: *Interpretive Guidelines and Surveyor Guidance.* Version 11. Milford, OH: DNV GL Healthcare USA, Inc; 2014:80-91.

203. Quality assessment/quality improvement: quality improvement. In: *Regular Standards and Checklist for Accreditation of Ambulatory Surgery Facilities.* Version 14.5. Gurnee, IL: American Association for Accreditation of Ambulatory Surgery Facilities, Inc; 2017:64.

204. Quality assessment/quality improvement: unanticipated operative sequelae. In: *Regular Standards and Checklist for Accreditation of Ambulatory Surgery Facilities*. Version 14.5. American Association for Accreditation of Ambulatory Surgery Facilities, Inc; 2017:66-69.

205. Cassin BR, Barach PR. Making sense of root cause analysis investigations of surgery-related adverse events. *Surg Clin North Am*. 2012;92(1):101-115. [VA]

206. Scoville R, Little K, Rakover J, Luther K, Mate K. *Sustaining Improvement*. IHI White Paper. Cambridge, MA: Institute for Healthcare Improvement; 2016. http://www.ihi.org/resources/Pages/IHIWhitePapers/Sustaining-Improvement.aspx. Accessed September 29, 2017. [VA]

207. Blackmore CC, Bishop R, Luker S, Williams BL. Applying lean methods to improve quality and safety in surgical sterile instrument processing. *Jt Comm J Qual Patient Saf*. 2013;39(3):99-105. [VB]

208. Wakeam E, Hyder JA, Ashley SW, Weissman JS. Barriers and strategies for effective patient rescue: a qualitative study of outliers. *Jt Comm J Qual Patient Saf*. 2014;40(11):503-513. [IIIB]

209. Johnson M, Sanchez P, Suominen H, et al. Comparing nursing handover and documentation: forming one set of patient information. *Int Nurs Rev*. 2014;61(1):73-81. [IIIB]

210. Pronovost PJ, Armstrong CM, Demski R, et al. Creating a high-reliability health care system: improving performance on core processes of care at Johns Hopkins Medicine. *Acad Med*. 2015;90(2):165-172. [VA]

211. Chassin MR, Loeb JM. High-reliability health care: getting there from here. *Milbank Q*. 2013;91(3):459-490. [VA]

212. Lin M, Heisler S, Fahey L, McGinnis J, Whiffen TL. Nurse knowledge exchange plus: human-centered implementation for spread and sustainability. *Jt Comm J Qual Patient Saf*. 2015;41(7):303-312. [VA]

213. Rogers SO Jr, Gawande AA, Kwaan M, et al. Analysis of surgical errors in closed malpractice claims at 4 liability insurers. *Surgery*. 2006;140(1):25-33. [IIIA]

214. Glymph DC, Olenick M, Barbera S, Brown EL, Prestianni L, Miller C. Healthcare utilizing deliberate discussion linking events (HUDDLE): a systematic review. *AANA J*. 2015;83(3):183-188. [VA]

215. Krenzischek DA, Xie Y, Petrovic M, et al. The perioperative handoff protocol: application of a multidisciplinary model to promote teamwork and reduce perioperative miscommunication. *J Perianesth Nurs*. 2011;26(3):188-189. [VC]

216. Morrison D, Sanders C. Huddling for optimal care outcomes. *Nursing*. 2011;41(12):22-24. [VB]

217. Park KW, Smaltz D, McFadden D, Souba W. The operating room dashboard. *J Surg Res*. 2010;164(2):294-300. [VB]

218. Johnson JK, Arora VM, Bacha EA, Barach PR. Improving communication and reliability of patient handovers in pediatric cardiac care. *Prog Pediatr Cardiol*. 2011;32(2):135-139. [VB]

219. HR.01.05.03: Staff participate in ongoing education and training. In: *Comprehensive Accreditation and Certification Manual*. E-dition. Oakbrook Terrace, IL: The Joint Commission; 2016.

220. Committee on Development of High Performance Teamwork; American College of Surgeons. Statement on high-performance teams. *Bull Am Coll Surg*. 2010;95(2):23-24. [IVC]

221. Larsson J, Holmström IK. How excellent anaesthetists perform in the operating theatre: a qualitative study on non-technical skills. *Br J Anaesth*. 2013;110(1):115-121. [IIIB]

222. McClelland G. Assessing scrub practitioner non-technical skills: a literature review. *J Perioper Pract*. 2015;25(1-2):12-18. [VA]

223. Paige JT, Garbee DD, Brown KM, Rojas JD. Using simulation in interprofessional education. *Surg Clin North Am*. 2015;95(4):751-766. [VA]

224. Rudarakanchana N, Van Herzeele I, Desender L, Cheshire NJW. Virtual reality simulation for the optimization of endovascular procedures: current perspectives. *Vasc Health Risk Manag*. 2015;11:195-202. [VB]

225. Willems A, Waxman B, Bacon AK, Smith J, Peller J, Kitto S. Interprofessional non-technical skills for surgeons in disaster response: a qualitative study of the Australian perspective. *J Interprof Care*. 2013;27(2):177-183. [IIIA]

226. Rydenfalt C, Johansson G, Odenrick P, Akerman K, Larsson PA. Compliance with the WHO Surgical Safety Checklist: deviations and possible improvements. *Int J Qual Health Care*. 2013;25(2):182-187. [VB]

227. Nurok M, Sundt TM 3rd, Frankel A. Teamwork and communication in the operating room: relationship to discrete outcomes and research challenges. *Anesthesiol Clin*. 2011;29(1):1-11. [IIIB]

228. Marshall MB, Emerson D. Patient safety in the surgical setting. *Thorac Surg Clin*. 2012;22(4):545-550. [VA]

229. Bohmer AB, Kindermann P, Schwanke U, et al. Long-term effects of a perioperative safety checklist from the viewpoint of personnel. *Acta Anaesthesiol Scand*. 2013;57(2):150-157. [IIIA]

230. Braaf S, Manias E, Riley R. The "time-out" procedure: an institutional ethnography of how it is conducted in actual clinical practice. *BMJ Qual Saf*. 2013;22(8):647-655. [IIIB]

231. Weiser TG, Porter MP, Maier RV. Safety in the operating theatre—a transition to systems-based care. *Nat Rev Urol*. 2013;10(3):161-173. [VA]

232. McCulloch P, Morgan L, New S, et al. Combining systems and teamwork approaches to enhance the effectiveness of safety improvement interventions in surgery: the safer delivery of surgical services (S3) program. *Ann Surg*. 2017;265(1):90-96. [IIA]

233. Tibbs SM, Moss J. Promoting teamwork and surgical optimization: combining TeamSTEPPS with a specialty team protocol. *AORN J*. 2014;100(5):477-488. [VA]

234. Li Y. Evidence summary. TeamSTEPPS. The Joanna Briggs Institute EBP Database, JBI@Ovid. 2017;JBI5271. [IVA]

235. Young-Xu Y, Neily J, Mills PD, et al. Association between implementation of a medical team training program and surgical morbidity. *Arch Surg*. 2011;146(12):1368-1373. [IIA]

236. Nurok M, Evans LA, Lipsitz S, Satwicz P, Kelly A, Frankel A. The relationship of the emotional climate of work and threat to patient outcome in a high-volume thoracic surgery operating room team. *BMJ Qual Saf*. 2011;20(3):237-242. [IIB]

237. Brown LL, Overly FL. Simulation-based interprofessional team training. *Clin Pediatr Emerg Med*. 2016;17(3):179-184. [VB]

238. Burke C, Grobman W, Miller D. Interdisciplinary collaboration to maintain a culture of safety in a labor and delivery setting. *J Perinat Neonatal Nurs*. 2013;27(2):113-123. [IIIB]

239. Cumin D, Boyd MJ, Webster CS, Weller JM. A systematic review of simulation for multidisciplinary team training in operating rooms. *Simul Healthc*. 2013;8(3):171-179. [IIIA]

240. Gardner AK, Scott DJ. Concepts for developing expert surgical teams using simulation. *Surg Clin North Am*. 2015;95(4):717-728. [VB]

241. Andrew B, Plachta S, Salud L, Pugh CM. Development and evaluation of a decision-based simulation for assessment of team skills. *Surgery.* 2012;152(2):152-157. [IIIB]

242. Arain NA, Hogg DC, Gala RB, et al. Construct and face validity of the American College of Surgeons/Association of Program Directors in Surgery laparoscopic troubleshooting team training exercise. *Am J Surg.* 2012;203(1):54-62. [IIIA]

243. Bilotta FF, Werner SM, Bergese SD, Rosa G. Impact and implementation of simulation-based training for safety. *Sci World J.* 2013;2013:652956. [VA]

244. Pena G, Altree M, Field J, et al. Nontechnical skills training for the operating room: a prospective study using simulation and didactic workshop. *Surgery.* 2015;158(1):300-309. [IIIB]

245. Nicksa GA, Anderson C, Fidler R, Stewart L. Innovative approach using interprofessional simulation to educate surgical residents in technical and nontechnical skills in high-risk clinical scenarios. *JAMA Surg.* 2015;150(3):201-207. [IIIB]

246. Weinger MB, Slagle JM, Kuntz AH, et al. A multimodal intervention improves postanesthesia care unit handovers. *Anesth Analg.* 2015;121(4):957-971. [VA]

Acknowledgments

LEAD AUTHOR
Mary C. Fearon, MSN, RN, CNOR
Perioperative Practice Specialist
AORN Nursing Department
Denver, Colorado

CO-AUTHOR
Lisa Spruce, DNP, RN, CNS-CP, CNOR, ACNS, ACNP, FAAN
Director, Evidence-Based Perioperative Practice
AORN Nursing Department
Denver, Colorado

CONTRIBUTING AUTHORS
Ramona L. Conner, MSN, RN, CNOR, FAAN
Editor-in-Chief, Guidelines for Perioperative Practice
AORN Nursing Department
Denver, Colorado

Amber Wood, MSN, RN, CNOR, CIC, FAPIC
Senior Perioperative Practice Specialist
AORN Nursing Department
Denver, Colorado

The authors and AORN thank Janice Neil, PhD, CNE, RN, Associate Professor, East Carolina College of Nursing, Greenville, North Carolina; Barbara L. Nalley, MSN, CRNP, CNOR, Manager, Jackson Surgical Assistants, Crofton, Maryland; David R. Urbach, MD, Clinical Epidemiology MSc, University Health Network, Toronto, Canada; Marie A. Bashaw, DNP, RN, NEA-BC, CNOR, Assistant Professor, Wright State University College of Nursing and Health, Dayton, Ohio; Jennifer Butterfield, MBA, RN, CNOR, CASC, Administrator/CEO, Lakes Surgery Center, Northville, Michigan; Susan Ruwe, MSN, RN, CPHQ, CIC, Senior Infection Preventionist, Carle Foundation Hospital, Argenta, Illinois; Donna Prichard, MA, BSN, RN, NE-BC, CNOR, Director of Perioperative Services, Interfaith Medical Center, Brooklyn, New York; Juan A. Sanchez, MD, MPA, Associate Professor of Surgery, Johns Hopkins University School of Medicine, Chair of Surgery, Saint Agnes Hospital, Baltimore, MD; Marisa Merlino, MHA, RN-BC, CNOR, CSSM, Staff Nurse II, Scott & White Memorial Hospital, Temple, Texas; and Vangie Dennis, BSN, RN, CNOR, CMLSO, Director of Patient Care Practice, Emory Clinic Ambulatory Surgery Center, Duluth, Georgia, for their assistance in developing this guideline.

PUBLICATION HISTORY
Originally published January 2018 in *Guidelines for Perioperative Practice.* Supersedes the "Guideline for transfer of patient care information."

GUIDELINE FOR PREVENTION OF VENOUS THROMBOEMBOLISM

The Guideline for Prevention of Venous Thromboembolism has been approved by the AORN Guidelines Advisory Board. It was presented as a proposed guideline for comments by members and others. The guideline is effective November 1, 2017. The recommendations in the guideline are intended to be achievable and represent what is believed to be an optimal level of practice. Policies and procedures will reflect variations in practice settings and/or clinical situations that determine the degree to which the guideline can be implemented. AORN recognizes the many diverse settings in which perioperative nurses practice; therefore, this guideline is adaptable to all areas where operative or other invasive procedures may be performed.

Purpose

This document provides guidance to perioperative team members for developing and implementing a protocol for prevention of venous thromboembolism (VTE), including prevention of deep vein thrombosis (DVT) by mechanical and pharmacologic prophylaxis and prevention of pulmonary embolism (PE) as a complication of DVT.

According to the Centers for Disease Control and Prevention,[1] approximately 900,000 people in the United States experience VTE each year. Approximately 33% of patient deaths related to VTE in the United States occur following a surgical procedure.[2] Among people who develop VTE,

- 50% have long-term complications (eg, swelling, pain, discoloration, scaling in the affected limb) as part of a condition called post-thrombotic syndrome,[1]
- 33% have a recurrence within 10 years,[1,3]
- 10% to 30% die within 1 month of diagnosis,[1]
- 25% with PE experience sudden death as the first symptom,[1,3] and
- 4% who survive PE develop chronic thromboembolic pulmonary hypertension.[4]

Treatment for VTE involves therapeutic anticoagulation, often for a minimum of 3 months; this treatment is associated with minor bruising and hematoma as well as major bleeding events that can be fatal.[4] Patients who have survived VTE have experienced anxiety, adverse effects from anticoagulant treatment, financial burden, loss of function, and fear of recurrence.[4]

Hospital-associated VTE, including DVT and PE, has been identified as a major public health concern.[1,4] Although as many as 70% of hospital-associated VTE cases could be prevented, fewer than half of hospitalized patients receive preventive measures according to the standard of care.[1] The gap between evidence-based practice and actual clinical practice for VTE prevention is concerning and presents a major opportunity for improvement in patient care.[4]

Prevention of VTE is also important for reducing economic burden,[5,6] as costs attributed to VTE in surgical patients have been found to be 1.5 times greater than costs for care of patients without VTE, and the expenses may persist for up to 5 years.[3,7] Although the prevention of VTE should be a priority for the entire health care organization, the particular risks facing surgical patients makes it critical that perioperative RNs take an active role in VTE prevention.[8-12]

All perioperative patients, including children, may be at risk for VTE because of immobility, vessel injury, compression of tissue caused by retraction, and patient positioning requirements. As such, recommendations for prevention of VTE are applicable to all perioperative patients, including children. The patient may have one or more of the three primary causative factors of venous thrombus formation, which is commonly referred to as Virchow's triad (ie, venous stasis, vessel wall injury, hypercoagulability). Although DVT usually occurs in the lower extremities, it also may occur in the upper extremities.[13-20]

Pulmonary embolism may result as a complication of DVT, although PE may occur independently from DVT.[21] Further research is needed to determine the ideal means to prevent PE and whether a reduction in DVT will lead to a reduction in the incidence of PE.[21]

The selection of VTE prophylaxis, including inferior vena cava filter use, is a medical decision and is outside the scope of this document. The following topics are also outside the scope of this document:
- diagnosis of VTE,
- treatment of VTE and complications (eg, post-thrombotic syndrome, venous stasis ulcers, chronic thromboembolic pulmonary hypertension),
- arterial thrombosis,
- superficial vein thrombosis,
- thrombosis at the surgical site (eg, flap, brain, portal vein thrombosis),
- use of regional anesthesia with DVT prophylaxis,
- laboratory testing of D-dimer levels to assess VTE risk,
- conditions that were studied as potential risk factors and found not to be associated with VTE (eg, use of cement, preoperative travel, Asian ethnicity, hemophilia, arthroscopy, laparoscopic cholecystectomy, shoulder procedures, non-oncologic otorhinolaryngology procedures),
- thromboprophylaxis for a patient with an implanted stent,
- anticoagulation for cardiac bypass,
- medication administration, and
- recommendations for bridging anticoagulant therapy.

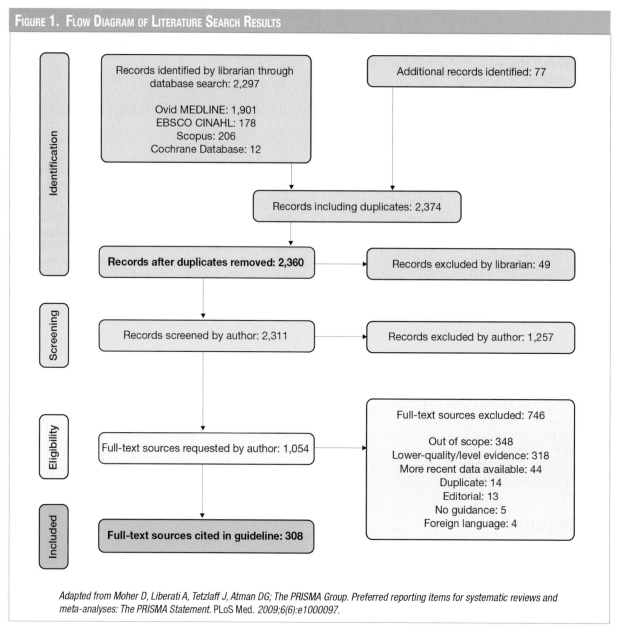

FIGURE 1. FLOW DIAGRAM OF LITERATURE SEARCH RESULTS

Records identified by librarian through database search: 2,297

Ovid MEDLINE: 1,901
EBSCO CINAHL: 178
Scopus: 206
Cochrane Database: 12

Additional records identified: 77

Records including duplicates: 2,374

Records after duplicates removed: 2,360

Records excluded by librarian: 49

Records screened by author: 2,311

Records excluded by author: 1,257

Full-text sources requested by author: 1,054

Full-text sources excluded: 746

Out of scope: 348
Lower-quality/level evidence: 318
More recent data available: 44
Duplicate: 14
Editorial: 13
No guidance: 5
Foreign language: 4

Full-text sources cited in guideline: 308

Identification

Screening

Eligibility

Included

Adapted from Moher D, Liberati A, Tetzlaff J, Atman DG; The PRISMA Group. Preferred reporting items for systematic reviews and meta-analyses: The PRISMA Statement. PLoS Med. 2009;6(6):e1000097.

Evidence Review

A medical librarian conducted a systematic search of the databases Ovid MEDLINE®, EBSCO CINAHL®, Scopus®, and the Cochrane Database of Systematic Reviews. The search was limited to literature published in English from 2011 through April 2016. A second search of the same databases was performed using the same topics as in the initial search for literature published from 2016 to March 2017. The lead author requested additional articles that either did not fit the original search criteria or were discovered during the evidence appraisal process. The lead author and the medical librarian also identified relevant guidelines from government agencies, professional organizations, and standards-setting bodies.

Search terms included subject headings such as *operating rooms, venous thrombosis, thromboembolism, compression garments, intermittent pneumatic compression, risk factors, Caprini, prophylaxis, foot inflation device,* and *thromboprophylaxis*. Additional keywords and phrases included the names of relevant pharmaceuticals.

Inclusion criteria were research and non-research literature in English, complete publications, and publication dates within the time restriction when available. Excluded were non-peer-reviewed publications, older evidence within the time restriction when more recent evidence was available, research conducted in nonsurgical patient populations (eg, stroke, critical care), and research on mechanical prophylaxis for indications other than prevention of VTE (eg, pain control, lymphedema, ischemia). Editorials, news items, and brief items were excluded. Lower-level and lower-quality evidence was excluded when higher-quality evidence was available, and literature outside the time restriction was excluded when literature within the time restriction was available. In total, 1,054 research and non-research sources of evidence were identified for possible inclusion, and of these, 308 are cited in the guideline (Figure 1).

Articles identified in the search were provided to the project team for evaluation. The team consisted of the lead author and two evidence appraisers. The lead author divided the search results into topics and assigned members of the team to review and critically appraise each article using the AORN Research or Non-Research Evidence Appraisal Tools as appropriate. The literature was independently evaluated and appraised according to the strength and quality of the evidence. Each article was then assigned an appraisal score. The appraisal score is noted in brackets after each reference, as applicable.

The collective evidence supporting each intervention within a specific recommendation was summarized, and the AORN Evidence Rating Model was used to rate the strength of the evidence. Factors considered in the review of the collective evidence were the quality of the evidence, the quantity of similar evidence on a given topic, and the consistency of evidence supporting a recommendation. The evidence rating is noted in brackets after each intervention.

Note: *The evidence summary table is available at http://www.aorn.org/evidencetables/.*

Editor's note: *MEDLINE is a registered trademark of the US National Library of Medicine's Medical Literature Analysis and Retrieval System, Bethesda, MD. CINAHL, Cumulative Index to Nursing and Allied Health Literature, is a registered trademark of EBSCO Industries, Birmingham, AL. Scopus is a registered trademark of Elsevier B.V., Amsterdam, The Netherlands.*

Recommendation I

The health care organization should establish and implement a protocol for the prevention of VTE.

Using an organization-wide protocol that is developed using evidence-based, professional guidelines and that includes clinical decision support for prophylactic choices prompts health care providers to give consistent and effective care for the prevention of VTE.[4]

I.a.   The VTE protocol should be developed by an interdisciplinary team, including
  ○ a clinical team leader;
  ○ a quality improvement facilitator;
  ○ process owners, including frontline personnel from each discipline (eg, pharmacists, RNs, surgeons, anesthesia professionals);
  ○ information technology and health information system experts; and
  ○ patient representatives.[4]
  [3: Moderate Evidence]
  The Agency for Healthcare Research and Quality recommends assembling an effective, interdisciplinary team that is empowered and supported by the health care organization's leaders to facilitate achieving meaningful improvement in VTE prevention.[4]

I.b.   The VTE protocol should
  ○ be evidence-based;
  ○ standardize assessment of VTE and bleeding risk;
  ○ provide clinical decision support for evidence-based prophylaxis based on level of risk for VTE and bleeding at critical phases of care (eg, admission, transfer of care, post surgery); and
  ○ be easy to use in clinical practice.[4]
  [3: Moderate Evidence]
  Protocols for VTE prevention establish best practice at the local level.[4]

I.b.1.   The VTE protocol should include a standardized VTE risk assessment model.[4]
  [3: Moderate Evidence]
  The Agency for Healthcare Research and Quality recommends using a standardized VTE risk assessment model to improve the reliability of the VTE protocol.[4] Qualitative and quantitative VTE risk assessment models have been validated in various perioperative patient populations.[4,22-44] A limitation of the evidence is that there is no consensus regarding a preferred VTE risk assessment tool.[4]

I.b.2.   The VTE protocol should include a standardized bleeding risk assessment model.[4]
  [3: Moderate Evidence]
  The Agency for Healthcare Research and Quality recommends using a standardized bleeding risk assessment model to improve the reliability of the VTE protocol.[4] Bleeding risk is evaluated concurrently with the VTE risk assessment and may be influenced by patient- or procedure-specific factors.[4]

I.b.3.   The VTE protocol should include a start time (eg, upon admission, before surgery, after surgery) for all types of prophylaxis based on the clinical condition of the patient. *[5: Benefits Balanced with Harms]*
  The risk for VTE formation begins with preoperative immobility and administration of anesthesia and continues throughout the postoperative phase of care until the patient regains mobility.[45] Some prophylactic measures, such as pharmacologic methods, may be contraindicated because of the increased risk for bleeding and may need to be started postoperatively when the risk for bleeding decreases.[2]

I.b.4.   The VTE protocol may include specialty- or procedure-specific (eg, orthopedic, cardiac) clinical decision support for prophylaxis. *[5: Benefits Balanced with Harms]*

I.c.   The health care organization should use a clinical decision support system with alerts to notify clinicians of a potential lapse in prophylaxis according to the VTE protocol. *[3: Moderate Evidence]*

The collective evidence[4,46,47] indicates that clinical decision support systems and alerts can improve compliance with the VTE protocol and reduce the patient's risk for VTE. Borab et al[46] conducted a systematic review with meta-analysis of 11 nonexperimental studies in which computerized clinical decision support systems were implemented for VTE prevention in surgical patients. The researchers found that these systems significantly increased compliance with recommended prophylaxis and significantly reduced the risk for VTE events.

In a systematic review with meta-analysis of 54 randomized controlled trials (RCTs) and quasi-experimental studies, Kahn et al[47] found that use of alerts significantly improved prescription of prophylaxis, especially as part of a multifaceted intervention to improve compliance. However, this systematic review did not find a significant benefit for reduction of VTE.

When alerts are used as a strategy to improve compliance with the VTE protocol, notifying the clinician of only critical events indicating a lapse in care, rather than all screening events, may reduce the risk of alert fatigue from unnecessary alerts.[4]

Recommendation II

The perioperative RN should complete a preoperative patient assessment to determine VTE risk factors.

The preoperative assessment provides information necessary to determine the individual patient's risk for VTE and identify prophylaxis measures recommended by the health care organization's VTE protocol.

II.a.   The preoperative patient assessment should include VTE risk factors that contribute to venous stasis, vessel wall injury, and hypercoagulability, including
  ○ age greater than 40 years[2,48]; *[1: Strong Evidence]*
  ○ cancer (ie, active or occult) or cancer treatment[48-50]; *[1: Strong Evidence]*
  ○ obesity[33,48,51-66]; *[1: Strong Evidence]*
  ○ previous history of VTE or stroke[2,48,67-70]; *[1: Strong Evidence]*
  ○ prolonged bed rest (> 3 days) or immobilization[2,48]; *[1: Strong Evidence]*
  ○ varicose veins[48,71-74]; *[1: Strong Evidence]*
  ○ presence of a central venous catheter[2,75-77]; *[1: Strong Evidence]*
  ○ trauma[2,48,78-80]; *[1: Strong Evidence]*
  ○ spinal cord injury[2,48,81,82]; *[1: Strong Evidence]*
  ○ inherited or acquired thrombophilia[48,67,83,84]; *[1: Strong Evidence]*
  ○ estrogen therapy (ie, oral contraceptive, hormone replacement therapy)[48,67,85-89]; *[1: Strong Evidence]*
  ○ critical care admission[48]; *[1: Strong Evidence]*
  ○ dehydration[48]; *[1: Strong Evidence]*

  ○ comorbidities, including
    • heart disease[90-92] (eg, congestive heart failure,[93-96] hypertension,[71,97] pacemaker[98]),
    • metabolic or endocrine disease (eg, Cushing's disease[99,100]),
    • respiratory disease[95,101] (eg, chronic obstructive pulmonary disease[33,94]),
    • acute infectious disease[33,102-104] (eg, sepsis[2,27,105,106]), and
    • inflammatory conditions[107] (eg, inflammatory bowel disease,[54,108-112] rheumatoid arthritis,[113] psoriasis[114])[48];
    [1: Strong Evidence]
  ○ pregnancy and the postpartum period[67,115-117]; *[2: High Evidence]*
  ○ smoking[54,58,118-120]; *[2: High Evidence]*
  ○ steroid therapy[121-124]; *[2: High Evidence]*
  ○ American Society of Anesthesiologists physical status classification of 3 or higher[27,30,64,90,92,111,125,126]; *[2: High Evidence]*
  ○ recent surgery (ie, within 30 days)[27,58,122]; *[2: High Evidence]*
  ○ preoperative hospitalization[122]; *[2: High Evidence]*
  ○ blood transfusion[127-131]; *[3: Moderate Evidence]*
  ○ known non-O blood type[128,132]; *[3: Moderate Evidence]*
  ○ obstructive sleep apnea[120]; *[3: Moderate Evidence]* and
  ○ asplenia.[133] *[3: Moderate Evidence]*

  The collective evidence indicates that patients with any of these risk factors exhibit a greater potential for developing VTE.

II.a.1.   The preoperative patient assessment should include procedure-related VTE risk factors, including
  • duration of surgery (ie, surgery and general anesthesia time longer than 90 minutes or longer than 60 minutes for procedures involving the lower limb or pelvis[48])[27,48,55,58,64,65,71,131,134-140]; *[1: Strong Evidence]*
  • the intraoperative patient position (eg, excessive hip flexion, hyperextension of the knee, reverse Trendelenburg)[141]; *[1: Strong Evidence]*
  • use of a pneumatic tourniquet, especially during prolonged periods of inflation[142]; *[1: Strong Evidence]*
  • major orthopedic surgery (eg, hip arthroplasty, knee arthroplasty, hip fracture surgery)[48,143-147]; *[1: Strong Evidence]*
  • bariatric surgery[48,51,53,55,56,60-63,138,148]; *[1: Strong Evidence]*
  • cardiothoracic surgery[2,48,149,150]; *[1: Strong Evidence]*
  • vascular surgery[48,151-153]; *[1: Strong Evidence]*
  • general surgery involving the abdomen or pelvis (eg, hepatic resection[131,154-156])[2,27,48,157,158]; *[1: Strong Evidence]*

- urologic surgery involving the abdomen or pelvis (eg, nephrectomy)[2,48,159-161]; *[1: Strong Evidence]*
- neurosurgery[2,48,124,162-165]; *[1: Strong Evidence]*
- spine surgery[2,35,48,64,96,166-172]; *[1: Strong Evidence]*
- immobilizing cast of a lower limb[48]; *[1: Strong Evidence]*
- open procedure[60,61,95,111,173-178]; *[2: High Evidence]*
- emergency procedure[125,157]; *[2: High Evidence]*
- concurrent procedures[27,101,125,179-181]; *[2: High Evidence]*
- transplant surgery[182-192]; *[2: High Evidence]*
- cesarean delivery[115-117]; *[2: High Evidence]*
- major foot and ankle surgery (eg, Achilles tendon rupture, total ankle arthroplasty, ankle fracture)[193-200]; *[2: High Evidence]*
- major hand, wrist, or elbow surgery (eg, elbow arthroplasty)[201]; *[3: Moderate Evidence]*
- procedures involving hardware placement[202]; *[3: Moderate Evidence]* and
- major plastic surgery (eg, body contouring, abdominoplasty, breast reconstruction).[31,66,181,203] *[3: Moderate Evidence]*

II.b.   The perioperative RN should consult and collaborate with perioperative team members regarding the need for and selection of prophylaxis based on the organizational protocol and the individual patient's VTE risk factor assessment. *[5: Benefits Balanced with Harms]*

The perioperative RN has a professional responsibility to advocate for the patient regarding the need for and selection of VTE prophylaxis by consulting and collaborating with other professional colleagues regarding patient care.

Recommendation III

The perioperative RN should implement mechanical VTE prophylaxis in a safe and effective manner as prescribed.

Mechanical prophylaxis is used for prevention of VTE in patients undergoing operative and invasive procedures. Nursing interventions are necessary to decrease the potential for complications associated with mechanical VTE prophylaxis. Mechanical prophylaxis includes the use of intermittent pneumatic compression devices, use of graduated compression stockings, early ambulation, and foot and ankle exercises.

The benefit of using mechanical prophylaxis modalities is reduction of VTE risk without increasing the risk for bleeding.[45] Mechanical prophylaxis is often used in combination with pharmacologic prophylaxis. Unless a patient is at low risk for VTE or is at high risk for bleeding complications, mechanical

prophylaxis alone is not recommended for effective VTE prevention.[49,50,204]

The American College of Chest Physicians (ACCP)[2] recommends mechanical prophylaxis for all surgical patients, including early ambulation for patients at very low risk for VTE and intermittent pneumatic compression devices for patients at low, moderate, or high risk for VTE. The American Society for Metabolic and Bariatric Surgery (ASMBS)[51] recommends mechanical prophylaxis and early ambulation for all patients who undergo bariatric surgery. The American College of Foot and Ankle Surgeons (ACFAS)[193] recommends a multimodal approach for preventing VTE in high-risk patients undergoing foot and ankle surgery, which includes early mobilization and use of intermittent pneumatic compression devices and graduated compression stockings. The ERAS® (Enhanced Recovery After Surgery) guidelines[205-207] also recommend mechanical prophylaxis (ie, intermittent pneumatic compression devices and graduated compression stockings) as part of a multimodal approach.

III.a.   When prescribed, intermittent pneumatic compression devices should be functioning and graduated compression stockings should be applied before the administration of regional or general anesthesia.[48] *[1: Strong Evidence]*

Regional or general anesthesia dilates the calf veins due to the loss of leg muscle tone. According to Caprini,[45] the best theoretical approach to prophylaxis is to minimize venous stasis and dilation, starting before the anticipated confinement of surgery and continuing throughout the entire period of risk. The National Institute for Clinical Excellence (NICE)[48] guidelines recommend starting mechanical prophylaxis for surgical patients at admission.

III.b.   The perioperative RN should perform interventions for safe and effective use of intermittent pneumatic compression devices. *[5: Benefits Balanced with Harms]*

Evidence indicates that patients may be harmed by wearing intermittent pneumatic compression devices for prevention of VTE.[208,209] The harms caused by intermittent pneumatic compression devices may include pressure injury[208] and hypothermia.[209] Another potential harm associated with intermittent pneumatic compression devices may be a fall when the patient ambulates. However, Boelig et al[210] found that patient falls were rarely associated with sequential compression device use in one health care organization database (0.45% of total patient falls). The harms may be mitigated by interventions implemented by the perioperative RN to facilitate the patient's wearing of intermittent pneumatic compression devices in accordance with the manufacturer's instructions for use, prevent pressure injury, and prevent unplanned hypothermia.

The benefits of intermittent pneumatic compression include a reduction in VTE rates similar to those for pharmacologic prophylaxis methods while also reducing the risk for major bleeding in surgical patients.[211-214] Research has demonstrated that the addition of intermittent pneumatic compression to pharmacologic prophylaxis significantly reduces the risk for VTE compared to either modality alone.[212,215-219] Although the exact mechanism of VTE prevention by intermittent pneumatic compression devices is unknown, evidence suggests that intermittent pneumatic compression devices reduce venous stasis, improve venous return from the lower extremities, and cause flow-induced endothelial reactions that increase fibrinolytic activity.[45,213,220,221] Foot inflation devices reduce venous stasis by simulating natural walking and providing compression to the plantar venous plexus.

For mechanical prophylaxis, the ACCP[2,143] recommends the use of intermittent pneumatic compression devices in preference to graduated compression stockings because of the risk for skin complications associated with the stockings. The American Congress of Obstetricians and Gynecologists (ACOG)[115,222,223] also preferentially recommends intermittent pneumatic compression for all patients undergoing gynecologic surgical procedures or cesarean delivery. In an RCT involving 108 high-risk patients undergoing gynecological pelvic surgery, Gao et al[224] found that a combination of intermittent pneumatic compression and graduated compression stockings significantly reduced VTE rates compared with use of graduated compression stockings alone. Further research is needed to determine whether graduated compression stockings limit the hemodynamic performance of intermittent pneumatic compression devices by preventing filling of veins.[225]

Morris and Woodcock[225] conducted a systematic review to compare intermittent pneumatic compression and graduated compression stockings and found weak and potentially biased nonexperimental evidence indicating that intermittent pneumatic compression was superior in effectiveness to graduated compression stockings for VTE prevention. The researchers urged caution in interpreting the results, and warned that insufficient evidence that one is more effective does not imply strong evidence of equivalency.

The limitations of the evidence are that optimal compression techniques (eg, sequential, simultaneous, cycle method), area of compression (eg, foot, calf, entire leg), and time of inflation are unknown. Several intermittent pneumatic compression devices have been cleared by the US Food and Drug Administration with a wide variety of design features that provide inflation on the foot, calf, or entire leg. In subgroup analysis of a systematic review, Pavon et al[212] did not find any significant differences in effectiveness based on intermittent pneumatic compression device mode of inflation or device location. Only one study in the systematic review compared various lengths of pneumatic compression devices; this study found that calf-length pneumatic compression was more effective than plantar compression for reduction of thigh swelling, although no cases of DVT or PE were reported.[226] Several studies have found that venous foot pump devices are safe and effective for prevention of VTE,[227-229] although one study did not find a difference in VTE rates with foot pump use.[230]

III.b.1. The perioperative RN should assess the patient for potential contraindications related to use of the intermittent pneumatic compression device, including
- any leg condition (eg, dermatitis, recent skin graft, gangrene) that pneumatic compression may exacerbate,[2,48] *[1: Strong Evidence]*
- known allergy or sensitivity to the sleeve or tubing material,[48] *[1: Strong Evidence]*
- cardiac failure or pulmonary edema from congestive heart failure,[48,220] *[1: Strong Evidence]*
- any factor that prevents correct fitting of sleeves (eg, exceeding the size limit, severe leg edema, deformity),[48,231] *[1: Strong Evidence]*
- pre-existing DVT, *[5: Benefits Balanced with Harms]* and
- severe arteriosclerosis or other ischemic vascular disease. *[5: Benefits Balanced with Harms]*

In a nonexperimental study, Hou et al[232] found that application of intermittent pneumatic compression in patients with pre-existing DVT was safe. The International Compression Club[220] has stated that further research is needed in this area.

III.b.2. The perioperative RN should notify the prescriber and anesthesia professional of any identified contraindications related to use of the intermittent pneumatic compression device. *[5: Benefits Balanced with Harms]*

III.b.3. Sleeves for intermittent pneumatic compression devices should be applied according to the manufacturer's instructions for use. *[5: Benefits Balanced with Harms]*

III.b.4. When the manufacturer's instructions for use require the use of stockinet, graduated compression stockings, or other material under the sleeves, the material should be wrinkle-free when applied to the skin. *[5: Benefits Balanced with Harms]*

Some manufacturers may recommended stockinet, graduated compression stockings, or other materials for skin protection under the sleeves. Smooth, wrinkle-free under-sleeve material may reduce the risk of skin injury.

III.b.5. During application of the sleeve, the tubing on the external surface of the sleeve should be placed facing away from the patient's skin and away from locations that may create a pressure injury. *[5: Benefits Balanced with Harms]*

Placement of the tubing between the patient's skin and the sleeve may lead to a pressure injury. Tubing may also cause pressure injury depending on the patient's position.

III.b.6. The perioperative RN should verify that the sleeves for intermittent pneumatic compression devices are applied correctly, connected to the device pump, and operating and that the tubing is away from locations that may create a pressure injury after the patient is transferred to the OR bed or repositioned. *[5: Benefits Balanced with Harms]*

III.b.7. When intermittent pneumatic compression is used, interventions should be implemented to prevent unplanned hypothermia as recommended in the AORN Guideline for Prevention of Unplanned Patient Hypothermia.[209,233] *[1: Strong Evidence]*

Use of intermittent pneumatic compression may increase the patient's risk for hypothermia. In an RCT, Huh et al[209] found that temperatures dropped significantly for patients wearing calf- or thigh-length sequential compression devices compared with patients not wearing the devices. The researchers recommended temperature monitoring and active warming methods because of the core temperature drop noted in the group wearing the sequential compression devices.

III.b.8. Sleeves for intermittent pneumatic compression devices used on the sterile field should be sterile (See the AORN Guideline for Sterile Technique).[234] *[1: Strong Evidence]*

Failure to adhere to aseptic practices during invasive procedures has been associated with surgical site infections.[234]

Intermittent pneumatic compression devices are used on the sterile field. Research has shown that patients undergoing bilateral total knee arthroplasty are twice as likely to develop VTE as patients undergoing unilateral arthroplasty.[235] In a retrospective study of a single clinician's experience,[236] sterile intermittent pneumatic compression devices were applied to 157 patients undergoing bilateral total knee arthroplasty when the tourniquet was not

inflated, as part of a multimodal approach for VTE prevention.

III.b.9. Intermittent pneumatic compression devices used during procedures with intra-operative magnetic resonance imaging (MRI) should be MRI safe (ie, nonferromagnetic).[237] *[3: Moderate Evidence]*

Intermittent pneumatic compression devices that are not MRI safe can become lethal projectiles, causing harm to personnel and patients or damage to the scanner.[237] Two nonexperimental studies showed that use of intermittent pneumatic compression devices during intraoperative MRI significantly reduced the risk of DVT.[238,239] Maybody et al[239] found that the sleeves and tubing of an intermittent compression device were MRI safe, although the control unit was not MRI safe. To comply with MRI safety requirements, the control unit was placed in the MRI control room and connected to the sleeves using extended tubing. Use of the extended tubing did not cause device failure or interfere with the procedure.

III.b.10. The intermittent pneumatic compression device should remain on for a minimum of 18 hours daily during the intraoperative and immediate postoperative period unless removal is necessitated by patient care needs.[2,48,143] *[1: Strong Evidence]*

The ACCP and NICE guidelines[2,48,143] recommend that patients wear intermittent pneumatic compression devices for as much time as possible to obtain the optimal benefit for VTE prevention. In a nonexperimental study of patients undergoing urologic surgery (N = 100), Ritsema et al[240] found that noncompliance with wearing sequential compression devices was more likely to be caused by hospital factors, such as availability of equipment and timely restarting of the devices by nursing personnel, than by patient factors.

III.b.11. The intermittent pneumatic compression device should be portable. *[1: Strong Evidence]*

The collective evidence[2,143,235,241-246] supports that mobile compression devices are safe and effective for prevention of VTE in surgical patients. In an RCT, Obi et al[241] investigated patient compliance (N = 67) with intermittent pneumatic compression device use for battery-powered devices (n = 35) compared to stationary devices that must remain plugged into the electrical outlet (n = 32). The researchers found that use of portable, battery-operated intermittent pneumatic compression devices significantly increased patient compliance compared to use of stationary devices.

III.b.12. The intermittent pneumatic compression device should be capable of recording wear time. *[1: Strong Evidence]*

The collective evidence[2,143,235,241-246] supports use of intermittent pneumatic compression devices that record wear time as a mechanism to monitor patient adherence. In a systematic review with meta-analysis of eight nonexperimental studies, Craigie et al[247] found that as many as 25% of hospitalized surgical patients were not compliant with wearing mechanical prophylaxis.

III.c. The perioperative RN should perform interventions for safe and effective use of graduated compression stockings. *[5: Benefits Balanced with Harms]*

The collective evidence[2,48,248-252] indicates that patients may be harmed by wearing graduated compression stockings for prevention of VTE when graduated compression stockings are incorrectly worn or sized. The harms may include skin injury[2,48]; nerve injury[248,249]; compartment syndrome[250]; and tourniquet effect, which increases the risk for VTE.[251,252] The harms may be mitigated by interventions implemented by the perioperative RN to facilitate the patient's wearing of graduated compression stockings in accordance with the manufacturer's instructions for use.

Although the exact mechanism of graduated compression stockings function is unknown, evidence suggests that exerting graded pressure distally to proximally in combination with muscular contraction displaces blood from the superficial to deep venous system of the leg. This displacement of blood increases the velocity and volume of blood flow in the deep system, thereby potentially preventing VTE.[253] Sachdeva et al[253] conducted a systematic review with meta-analysis and found that graduated compression stockings were effective in reducing the risk for VTE in hospitalized surgical patients, although the included research was conducted primarily with patients undergoing general and orthopedic surgery. In another systematic review, Mandavia et al[254] did not find a clear benefit of graduated compression stockings in addition to pharmaceutical prophylaxis in surgical inpatients when compared to patients receiving only pharmaceutical prophylaxis.

A limitation of the evidence is that the effect of graduated compression stockings alone for prevention of VTE is not clear because stockings are often used in combination with other interventions, including intermittent pneumatic compression devices and pharmaceutical prophylaxis.

III.c.1. The perioperative RN should assess the patient for potential contraindications related to the use of graduated compression stockings, including
- any skin conditions (eg, dermatitis, recent skin graft, leg ulcer) that stockings may exacerbate,[2,48]
- any vascular conditions (eg, peripheral vascular disease, peripheral arterial bypass grafting, severe arteriosclerosis) that stockings may exacerbate,[2,48,231]
- severe peripheral neuropathy or other sensory impairment,[48]
- gangrene,[48]
- known allergy or sensitivity to stocking material,[48]
- cardiac failure or pulmonary edema from congestive heart failure,[48] and
- any factor that prevents correct fitting of stockings (eg, exceeding the size limit, severe leg edema, deformity).[48,231]

[1: Strong Evidence]

III.c.2. The perioperative RN should notify the prescriber and anesthesia professional of any identified contraindications related to the use of the graduated compression stockings. *[5: Benefits Balanced with Harms]*

III.c.3. The perioperative RN should assess the patient's ability to wear thigh-length graduated compression stockings in accordance with the manufacturer's instructions for use and the patient's preference for length (ie, thigh or knee length). When thigh-length graduated compression stockings are contraindicated based on the patient assessment, the perioperative RN should collaborate with the prescriber to determine whether knee-length graduated compression stockings may be substituted for thigh-length stockings. *[5: Benefits Balanced with Harms]*

The evidence regarding the ideal length for graduated compression stockings conflicts. The ACCP[2] recommends that surgical patients wear thigh-length graduated compression stockings instead of knee length, citing evidence showing greater benefit for prevention of VTE in stroke patients who wore thigh-length stockings. For hospitalized surgical patients, three systematic reviews with meta-analysis[255-258] found insufficient high-quality evidence to determine a statistical difference in effectiveness between thigh- and knee-length graduated compression stockings. Because of this conflicting evidence and the theory that prevention of VTE with graduated compression stockings is unlikely to be effective when patient compliance is low,[259] the authors of one systematic review[256] suggested a pragmatic approach of providing thigh-length graduated compression stockings only to patients who can consistently use the stockings according to the manufacturer's instructions.

An RCT conducted with Turkish patients undergoing abdominal-pelvic surgeries (N = 219) directly compared patient satisfaction with thigh- and knee-length graduated compression stockings. Ayhan et al[260] found that patients who wore low-pressure (ie, 15 mmHg to 18 mmHg), knee-length stockings (n = 73) were more satisfied and had fewer problems than those who wore low-pressure, thigh-length stockings (n = 73) or moderate-pressure (20 mmHg to 30 mmHg), knee-length stockings (n = 73). The researchers monitored the patients 5 to 7 days after surgery using duplex ultrasonography and found no patients in the study had experienced DVT.

Another study recommended considering patient preference based on evidence showing similar hemodynamic performance between thigh- and knee-length graduated compression stockings. In this quasi-experimental study, Lattimer et al[261] found that graduated compression stockings significantly improved all hemodynamic performance tests, including venous filling index, venous volume, and time to fill 90% of venous volume, regardless of length (ie, thigh- or knee-length) or compression class (18 mmHg to 21 mmHg versus 23 mmHg to 32 mmHg). The majority of patients in the study (62%, n = 21) preferred knee-length graduated compression stockings. The authors recommended basing stocking selection on patient preference because of a lack of significance in hemodynamic performance by length or compression class.

Further research is needed to determine the most effective graduated compression stocking length for prevention of VTE in surgical patients, patient adherence,[259] and cost.

III.c.4. Graduated compression stockings should be fitted to the individual patient. The patient's legs should be measured separately and according to the manufacturer's instructions.[2,48] [1: Strong Evidence]

Incorrect sizing of graduated compression stockings may cause injury to the patient or reduce the effectiveness for VTE prevention. The ACCP[2] recommends that the stockings be fitted to ensure efficacy, with pressure at the ankle between 18 mmHg and 23 mmHg. Measuring each of the patient's legs is necessary because there may be enough variability in length and circumference to require a different stocking size for each leg.

An insufficient range of stocking sizes may contribute to the use of an incorrectly sized stocking. In a nonexperimental study,

Bowling et al[252] found that one facility had only three of six sizes of stockings available. Only 14% of stockings showed gradation in accordance with the manufacturers' intended compression, and 23% of stockings exerted more pressure at the calf than the ankle, thereby creating a tourniquet effect, which increases the risk for VTE. The authors discussed that a wide variety of sizes was necessary to achieve individual patient fit, although available products in larger sizes increased in length but not girth at the calf. In addition to the lack of all available sizes of stockings, patients were not universally remeasured for size 24 hours after surgery in accordance with facility policy, which may have contributed to the poor fit.

In a nonexperimental study, Thompson et al[251] implemented a protocol for sizing knee-length stockings in patients undergoing total hip and knee replacements (N = 57). The standardized protocol significantly improved correct sizing of stockings, reduced the proportion of patients with proximal indentation from stockings, reduced the number of patients with reverse gradients, and improved patient compliance with wearing stockings.

Compartment syndrome has been reported as a result of incorrect stocking size. Hinderland et al[250] reported a case of lateral leg compartment syndrome after ankle surgery in a patient's nonoperative extremity. The authors attributed the compartment syndrome to a graduated compression stocking that was a size too small. The patient complained of severe pain when he awoke from surgery. Removal of the stocking and intermittent pneumatic compression device provided minimal relief of the patient's pain. No defect was found with the pneumatic compression device. The patient was assessed for compartment syndrome; however, the compartment pressures were initially normal. The patient returned 2 days later with severe, increasing pain and underwent surgical decompression fasciotomy of the lateral leg compartment, split-thickness skin graft, and 3 weeks of non-weight bearing of bilateral extremities. The patient was able to return to full activity 4 months after surgery with no muscle deficits, although he was treated for mild neuropraxia of the foot.

III.c.5. Graduated compression stockings should be applied according to the manufacturer's written instructions. After application, the perioperative RN should verify that the
- stockings are not rolled up the foot or down the leg,
- stockings are smooth when fitted,

- toe holes lie underneath the toes,
- heel patches are in the correct position, and
- thigh gussets are positioned on the patient's inner thighs.
[5: Benefits Balanced with Harms]

III.c.6.   The perioperative RN should verify that the graduated compression stockings have not rolled up the foot or down the leg during transfer to and from the OR bed or during procedural positioning. [5: Benefits Balanced with Harms]

III.c.7.   Patients who develop postoperative leg edema should have their stockings removed, legs remeasured, and stockings refitted.[48,252] [1: Strong Evidence]

Postoperative leg edema may alter the fit of the graduated compression stockings, which may reduce the pressure exerted at the ankle and reduce the effectiveness of the stockings.[252] The NICE[48] guidelines recommend remeasurement and refitting of graduated compression stockings for patients with postoperative leg edema or swelling.

At a single facility that required stocking remeasurement at 24 hours after surgery, Bowling et al[252] found that the remeasurement was not taking place according to recommendations from NICE. Only 14% of stockings worn by patients had gradation in accordance with the manufacturers' intended compression, and 23% of stockings exerted more pressure at the calf than the ankle, which increases the risk for VTE.

In a nonexperimental study, Thompson et al[251] implemented a protocol for refitting knee-length graduated compression stockings 48 hours after surgery for patients undergoing total hip and knee replacements. The standardized protocol significantly improved correct sizing of stockings, reduced the proportion of patients with proximal indentation from stockings, reduced the number of patients with reverse gradients, and improved patient compliance with wearing the stockings.

III.c.8.   Elastic bandages should not be used as a replacement for graduated compression stockings. [5: Benefits Balanced with Harms]

Potential harms of using elastic bandages include risk for skin, pressure, and nerve injury. Elastic bandages may not provide a protective effect for VTE due to variability in pressure exerted and inability to control for tourniquet effect. Inconsistent bandaging technique may be associated with poor patient outcomes.[220] Further research is needed to determine the safety and efficacy of using elastic bandages for VTE prevention.

III.d.   Graduated compression stockings and intermittent pneumatic compression devices may be used on patients in the lithotomy position (See the AORN Guideline for Positioning the Patient).[141] [1: Strong Evidence]

The risk for VTE may be greater than the risk for compartment syndrome when mechanical prophylaxis is used for a patient in the lithotomy position, and it may be reasonable to continue the use of graduated compression stockings and intermittent pneumatic compression devices for thromboprophylaxis in patients undergoing surgical procedures in the lithotomy position.[141]

III.e.   The perioperative RN should assess the patient for adverse effects related to the use of mechanical VTE prophylaxis, including
- skin injury[2,48,208]; [1: Strong Evidence]
- hypothermia from the use of intermittent pneumatic compression devices[209]; [1: Strong Evidence]
- numbness, tingling, discomfort, or pain[248-250]; [3: Moderate Evidence]
- proximal indentation from knee-length graduated compression stockings[251]; [3: Moderate Evidence] and
- ischemia. [5: Benefits Balanced with Harms]

Skin injury,[2,48,208] nerve injury,[248,249] compartment syndrome,[250] and vascular compromise (eg, ischemia) are potential complications related to use of mechanical VTE prophylaxis.

In a nonexperimental study, Thompson et al[251] identified proximal indentation on the calves of patients wearing knee-length graduated compression stockings and found that patients with proximal indentation were significantly more likely to have reverse gradients (41%) than patients without proximal indentation (8%). The researchers implemented a protocol for refitting knee-length stockings 48 hours after surgery and found that the standardized protocol significantly reduced the proportion of patients with proximal indentation from stockings (53% to 19%).

III.e.1.   The VTE protocol should specify when mechanical VTE prophylaxis (ie, intermittent pneumatic compression device, graduated compression stockings) should be removed for patient assessment and patient care activities (eg, ambulation, before discharge, transfer of care). [5: Benefits Balanced with Harms]

III.e.2.   When evidence of complications related to the use of mechanical VTE prophylaxis is present, the perioperative RN should
- remove the stocking and compression device,[48] [1: Strong Evidence]
- notify the physician and anesthesia professional, [5: Benefits Balanced with Harms] and
- document actions taken. [5: Benefits Balanced with Harms]

III.e.3. When patient injury or equipment failure occur during the use of intermittent pneumatic compression devices,

- the intermittent pneumatic compression device should be removed from service;
- all sleeve and tubing accessories should be retained if possible; and
- the adverse event details, including device identification and maintenance and service information, should be reported according to the health care organization's policy and procedures.

[5: Benefits Balanced with Harms]

Retaining the intermittent pneumatic compression device, sleeves, and tubing accessories facilitates the incident investigation.

III.f. The patient should ambulate as soon as possible after surgery. [1: Strong Evidence]

Ambulation decreases venous stasis by creating natural compression of the venous system through muscle contraction and compression of the venous foot pump. Several guidelines[2,48,51,85,144,193] recommend early ambulation or mobilization as a postoperative intervention to prevent VTE. The NICE[48] guidelines recommend encouraging mobilization as soon as possible after surgery for all surgical patients. Other guidelines recommend early ambulation for a specific surgical procedure, VTE risk level, or patient population. For example, the ACCP[2] recommends early ambulation as the only method of VTE prophylaxis for patients undergoing general and abdominal-pelvic surgery who are at very low risk for VTE. Similarly, the ACOG[85] recommends early ambulation for low-risk patients undergoing gynecologic surgery who do not require other mechanical or pharmaceutical prophylaxis. The American Academy of Orthopaedic Surgeons[144] recommends early mobilization after elective hip and knee arthroplasty, in addition to mechanical and pharmaceutical prophylaxis. The ACFAS[193] recommends a multimodal approach that includes early mobilization and weight bearing for preventing VTE in high-risk patients undergoing foot and ankle surgery. The ASMBS[51] recommends early ambulation for all patients who have undergone bariatric surgery in addition to mechanical and pharmaceutical prophylaxis based on the patient's risk assessment.

Early mobilization is also included in multimodal protocols for improving recovery of surgical patients, including ERAS[205-207,262] and fast-track[263-267] protocols. The ERAS guidelines for elective rectal/pelvic surgery recommend a care plan that supports patient independence and mobilization, with patients out of bed for 2 hours on the day of surgery and 6 hours on postoperative days thereafter.[207] The ERAS guidelines for gynecologic/oncology surgery recommend encouraging the patient to mobilize within 24 hours after surgery.[206] Fast-track protocols for patients undergoing hip and knee arthroplasty include mobilization as soon as 2 to 4 hours[263,264] or 3 to 5 hours[267] after surgery.

Further research is needed to compare multimodal protocols with early mobilization to a protocol without early mobilization to determine the specific benefits of early mobilization.[264]

The benefits of early postoperative ambulation outweigh the harms. Benefits of ambulation include reduced VTE complications, reduced pulmonary complications, reduced muscle atrophy, reduced hospital length of stay, and counteracting insulin resistance from immobilization.[205,206] Postoperative ambulation is a low-cost intervention for VTE prevention.[144] Benefits of early mobilization may include a reduced need for prolonged pharmaceutical prophylaxis, although further research is needed.[263-265] The harms may include patient falls.

III.f.1. The perioperative RN should assess the patient's risk for falls and implement measures to prevent falls during postoperative ambulation. [5: Benefits Balanced with Harms]

III.f.2. The perioperative RN should collaborate with the perioperative team to minimize barriers to postoperative ambulation, including

- inadequate pain control,[205,206,264]
- pain management techniques that reduce patient mobility (eg, regional anesthesia),
- an indwelling urinary catheter,[205,206]
- IV infusion,[205,206] and
- lack of patient motivation (eg, sedation).[205]

[1: Strong Evidence]

The evidence supports that barriers to early postoperative ambulation include inadequate pain control,[264] IV fluid infusion, an indwelling urinary catheter, lack of patient motivation, and pre-existing comorbidities.[205,206] Compliance with a multimodal ERAS protocol may minimize these barriers.[206] Pain management techniques that limit the patient's mobility, such as regional anesthesia, may also be a barrier to postoperative ambulation.

III.g. The perioperative RN should instruct the patient to perform postoperative foot and ankle exercises. [2: High Evidence]

Foot and ankle exercises decrease venous stasis by creating natural compression of the venous system through muscle contraction. The ACFAS[193] recommends early rehabilitation and mobilization of the operative limb, including ankle exercises, to reengage the calf muscle pump as part of a multimodal approach for VTE prevention in high-risk patients. Wang et al[268] found that patients in an RCT who were selected to perform active ankle movements postoperatively for 7 days (n = 96) had fewer occurrences of thrombosis and DVT, less swelling of the thigh and calf, and improved maximum venous outflow and capacity, which may prevent formation of DVT, than patients who did not perform ankle movements (n = 78). The active ankle movements included a range of movement to 20-degree dorsal flexion, 30-degree varus and valgus, and 40-degree plantar flexion at a frequency of 30 times per minute, 20 times per day.

Shimizu et al[269] found that a novel leg apparatus to facilitate active ankle movement improved venous flow in the femoral veins of eight healthy volunteers after 1 minute of exercise compared to application of intermittent pneumatic compression for 10 minutes. The novel leg apparatus enabled movement from the supine position to 30-degree dorsiflexion, 60-degree plantar flexion, combined flexion and rotation of the ankle, flexion and extension of the knee and hip, and combined leg motion.

The limitations of the evidence are that research has not confirmed the effect of foot and ankle exercises on VTE development. Further research is needed to determine the optimal method, sequence, and frequency of foot and ankle exercises.

The benefits of the patient performing foot and ankle exercises outweigh the harms. Benefits include improvement of blood flow in the lower extremities, which may prevent VTE.[268,269] The effect of benefits may be limited by the patient's ability to perform foot and ankle exercises in the full range of motion (eg, because of a rigid cast[193] or contractures) or to contract muscles in the lower extremities (eg, because of paralysis).

Recommendation IV

The perioperative RN should implement pharmacologic VTE prophylaxis in a safe and effective manner as prescribed.

Nursing interventions are necessary to decrease the risk of potential complications from pharmacologic prophylaxis that may be used throughout the perioperative period. Pharmacologic prophylaxis consists of administering anticoagulant medications that inhibit blood clotting. The pharmacologic regimen may include medications such as low molecular weight heparin, low-dose unfractionated heparin, warfarin, factor Xa inhibitors (ie, fondaparinux, rivaroxaban, apixaban), dabigatran, vitamin K antagonists, or aspirin.

IV.a. The perioperative RN should assess the patient for potential contraindications related to use of pharmacologic VTE prophylaxis, including
- active bleeding[2,48,270]; *[1: Strong Evidence]*
- previous major bleeding[2,143,270,271]; *[1: Strong Evidence]*
- known, untreated bleeding disorder[2,48,270]; *[1: Strong Evidence]*
- severe renal or hepatic failure[2,48,143,270,271]; *[1: Strong Evidence]*
- thrombocytopenia[2,48,270,271]; *[1: Strong Evidence]*
- acute stroke[2,48]; *[1: Strong Evidence]*
- uncontrolled systemic hypertension[2,48,270,271]; *[1: Strong Evidence]*
- lumbar puncture or epidural or spinal anesthesia within the previous 4 hours or planned within the next 12 hours[2,48,270-272]; *[1: Strong Evidence]*
- concomitant use of anticoagulants, antiplatelet therapy, or thrombolytic drugs[2,48,143,270,271]; *[1: Strong Evidence]*
- procedures in which bleeding complications may have especially severe consequences (eg, craniotomy, spinal surgery, spinal trauma, reconstructive procedures involving a free flap)[2,270]; *[1: Strong Evidence]*
- bacterial endocarditis[270,271]; *[2: High Evidence]*
- allergy to medication[271]; *[2: High Evidence]*
- pregnancy[270]; *[5: Benefits Balanced with Harms]*
- ophthalmic surgery[270]; *[5: Benefits Balanced with Harms]* and
- prosthetic heart valve.[270] *[5: Benefits Balanced with Harms]*

IV.a.1. The perioperative RN should notify the prescriber of any identified contraindications. *[5: Benefits Balanced with Harms]*

IV.b. The perioperative RN should assess the patient for adverse effects related to the use of pharmacologic VTE prophylaxis, including
- bleeding[2,270,271]; *[1: Strong Evidence]*
- hematoma formation[2,270]; *[1: Strong Evidence]*
- thrombocytopenia[2,270,271]; *[1: Strong Evidence]*
- osteoporosis and osteopenia[271]; *[2: High Evidence]*
- skin necrosis[270,273]; *[3: Moderate Evidence]*
- calciphylaxis[270]; *[5: Benefits Balanced with Harms]*
- atheroembolism[270]; *[5: Benefits Balanced with Harms]* and
- injection site irritation, pain, bruising, bleeding, or itching.[270] *[5: Benefits Balanced with Harms]*

IV.b.1. The perioperative RN should notify the prescriber and anesthesia professional of any identified adverse effects. *[5: Benefits Balanced with Harms]*

Recommendation V

The perioperative RN should provide the patient and the patient's designated caregiver(s) with instructions regarding prevention of VTE and prescribed prophylactic measures.

Education related to VTE prevention may reduce the patient's risk for developing VTE by increasing the patient's awareness and, potentially, compliance with prophylaxis.[274]

V.a. The perioperative RN should provide the patient and the patient's designated caregiver(s) with verbal and written instructions on the prevention of VTE,[48,274,275] including

- common signs and symptoms of DVT or PE (eg, leg pain, swelling, unexplained shortness of breath, wheezing, chest pain, palpitations, anxiety, sweating, coughing up blood)[48]; *[1: Strong Evidence]*

- the importance of seeking medical help and who to contact if the patient suspects DVT, PE, or an adverse effect[48]; *[1: Strong Evidence]*

- the importance of adhering to the entire duration of prescribed VTE prophylaxis[48]; *[1: Strong Evidence]*

- who to contact if the patient has any problems using the prescribed VTE prophylaxis[48]; *[1: Strong Evidence]*

- the importance of mobilization, including ambulation and foot and ankle exercises[48]; *[1: Strong Evidence]*

- maintaining adequate hydration[48,276]; *[1: Strong Evidence]*

- preventive measures to use when travelling long distances after surgery, including frequent ambulation, calf muscle exercise, and wearing fitted, knee-length graduated compression stockings[277]; *[1: Strong Evidence]*

- elevating the legs[276]; *[3: Moderate Evidence]*

- avoiding clothing that constricts the lower extremities; *[5: Benefits Balanced with Harms]*

- avoiding sitting with knees bent or legs crossed for long periods of time; *[5: Benefits Balanced with Harms]* and

- avoiding sitting or standing for long periods of time. *[5: Benefits Balanced with Harms]*

Venous thromboembolism frequently develops or becomes evident after the patient is discharged. One analysis of the National Surgical Quality Improvement Program database found that 30% of patients with VTE were diagnosed after hospital discharge.[111] Education provides the patient with the signs and symptoms of VTE, an awareness of VTE prevention measures, and information about when to seek medical help. Three audits of patients' preoperative knowledge found that patients lacked of awareness of risk for VTE and methods of prevention.[274,275,278] One quasi-experimental study found that implementation of targeted patient education on VTE risk and prevention significantly improved patient awareness.[274]

V.b. The perioperative RN should provide the patient receiving mechanical prophylaxis and the patient's designated caregiver(s) with preoperative and postoperative instructions, including

- the benefits of mechanical prophylaxis[48];

- the importance of compliance[2,48,143,247,259];

- the importance of wearing sized, graduated compression stockings in accordance with the manufacturer's instructions for use[2,48];

- instructions for removal, laundering, and reapplication of graduated compression stockings[48,249];

- instructions for removal and reapplication of the intermittent compression device immediately after ambulation[2,143];

- the importance of postoperative ambulation[48];

- potential complications, including
  - skin injury (eg, marking, blistering),[2,48,208]
  - ischemia (eg, discoloration), and
  - numbness, tingling, discomfort, or pain[248-250]; and

- who to contact if the patient has any problems using the prescribed mechanical prophylaxis.[48]

[1: Strong Evidence]

Education helps the patient understand the potential complications of mechanical prophylaxis as well as the importance of compliance with its correct use.

V.b.1. The perioperative RN should assess the patient's ability to remove and replace intermittent pneumatic compression devices and graduated compression stockings or the availability of someone to help the patient.[48] *[1: Strong Evidence]*

V.b.2. The perioperative RN should monitor the patient's use of intermittent pneumatic compression devices and graduated compression stockings and compliance with the manufacturer's instructions for use. If these are not being used correctly, the RN should assist the patient and provide reeducation.[48] *[1: Strong Evidence]*

V.b.3. The perioperative RN should provide the patient prescribed an alternative mechanical prophylaxis device (ie, continuous passive motion,[279] electrical calf muscle stimulation[280]) and the patient's designated caregiver(s) with preoperative and postoperative instructions for use of the device. *[5: Benefits Balanced with Harms]*

V.c. The perioperative RN should provide the patient receiving pharmacologic VTE prophylaxis and the patient's designated caregiver(s) with preoperative and postoperative instructions, including

- the importance of following through with medication-related laboratory tests[270];

- the importance of continuing medication post discharge as prescribed[270];

- who to contact if the patient has any problems self-administering the prescribed pharmacologic prophylaxis[48];

- the importance of not stopping medication or of not starting a new medication, including over-the-counter medications (eg, aspirin, ibu-profen), without consulting the physician[270];

○ potential adverse effects and when to seek medical attention[281];

○ interactions with herbal and other over-the-counter preparations (eg, ginger, ginkgo biloba, ginseng, garlic, chamomile)[270,282];

○ reporting signs of bleeding, including
  • unusual bruising,
  • pink or brown urine,
  • red or black tarry stools,
  • coughing up blood,
  • vomiting blood or vomit that looks like coffee grounds,
  • pain, swelling, or discomfort in a joint,
  • recurring nose bleeds,
  • unusual bleeding from gums, or
  • cuts that do not stop bleeding[270,282];

○ reporting signs of epidural hematoma if the patient underwent any spine procedures, including
  • back pain,
  • tingling or numbness,
  • muscle weakness, or
  • incontinence[270];

○ avoiding eating large amounts of food high in vitamin K such as green, leafy vegetables;

○ avoiding certain activities (eg, contact sports)[282];

○ using an electric razor when shaving[282];

○ using a soft toothbrush and waxed dental floss gently[282];

○ informing health care workers about pharmacologic prophylaxis before undergoing any procedures (eg, dental work, laboratory tests)[270,282];

○ carrying or wearing medical identification to let health care providers know that the patient takes anticoagulation therapy[282]; and

○ informing the physician if the patient is breastfeeding.[270]

[5: Benefits Balanced with Harms]

Education assists the patient in understanding the potential complications of pharmacologic prophylaxis, as well as the importance of compliance as prescribed.

Recommendation VI

Documentation should reflect activities for prevention of VTE.

Documentation in the patient's medical record provides a description of the perioperative care administered, status of patient outcomes upon transfer, and information to support continuity of care.[283] Documentation provides data for identifying trends and demonstrating compliance with regulatory requirements and accreditation standards. Effective management and collection of health care information that accurately reflects the patient's care, treatment, and services is a regulatory requirement[284-287] and an accreditation standard for both hospitals[288,289] and ambulatory settings.[289-293]

VI.a. Documentation should be recorded in a manner consistent with the health care organization's policies and procedures and should include

○ pharmacologic prophylaxis administration (eg, medication, dose, time, route),[281] *[2: High Evidence]*

○ presence of VTE risk factors,[294] *[3: Moderate Evidence]*

○ contraindications to mechanical or pharmacologic prophylaxis and actions taken,[294] *[3: Moderate Evidence]*

○ adverse effects from mechanical or pharmacologic prophylaxis and actions taken,[294] *[3: Moderate Evidence]*

○ patient education provided,[221,294] *[3: Moderate Evidence]*

○ the reason for any variance from the VTE protocol,[4] *[3: Moderate Evidence]*

○ the type and size of the intermittent pneumatic compression sleeve and graduated compression stockings applied,[294] *[3: Moderate Evidence]*

○ results of a fall risk assessment and measures taken to prevent patient falls during postoperative ambulation, *[5: Benefits Balanced with Harms]*

○ application and removal times for all mechanical prophylactic measures, *[5: Benefits Balanced with Harms]*

○ intermittent pneumatic compression device identification (eg, serial or biomedical number) and settings, *[5: Benefits Balanced with Harms]* and

○ results of a patient skin assessment for mechanical prophylactic measures. *[5: Benefits Balanced with Harms]*

Miller[294] conducted an audit of graduated compression use in surgical patients (N = 80) at a teaching hospital in Australia. Limb measurement, stocking size, and patient education were not documented for any patient. Assessment for DVT risk factors was documented for 17.5% of patients and daily skin assessment was recorded for 29% of patients. The author recommended using a documentation tool to ensure consistency of VTE risk assessment, assessment for contraindications to graduated compression stockings, patient education, and monitoring of patients wearing stockings for complications and compliance.

Recommendation VII

Personnel should receive initial and ongoing education and complete competency verification activities related to VTE prevention.

Initial and ongoing education of perioperative personnel facilitates the development of knowledge, skills, and attitudes that affect safe patient care. It is the responsibility of the health care organization to provide initial and ongoing education and to verify the competency of its personnel[283]; however, the primary responsibility for maintaining ongoing competency remains with the individual.[295]

Competency verification activities provide a mechanism for competency documentation and help verify that personnel understand the principles and processes necessary for safe patient care.

Ongoing development of knowledge and skills and documentation of personnel participation is a regulatory requirement[284-287] and an accreditation standard for both hospitals[296,297] and ambulatory settings.[297-300]

VII.a. The health care organization should establish education and competency verification activities for its personnel and determine intervals for education and competency verification related to VTE prevention.[47] *[2: High Evidence]*

Providing education and verifying competency assists in developing knowledge and skills that may improve compliance with the VTE protocol and thus may reduce the patient's risk for VTE. In a systematic review with meta-analysis, Kahn et al[47] found that educational interventions to improve use of VTE prophylaxis significantly improved the quality of prophylaxis, especially when combined with other interventions as part of a multifaceted systems approach.

Education and competency verification needs and intervals are unique to the facility or health care organization and to its personnel and processes.

VII.a.1. Education and competency verification activities related to VTE prevention should include
- the pathophysiology of VTE formation;
- VTE protocol and updates;
- assessment for VTE risk factors, including patient- and procedure-specific risk factors;
- manufacturers' instructions for use and sizing of graduated compression stockings;
- manufacturers' instructions for use and sizing of intermittent pneumatic compression devices;
- contraindications and adverse effects of mechanical prophylaxis;
- the importance of compliance with mechanical prophylaxis;
- contraindications and adverse effects of pharmacologic prophylaxis; and
- the importance of patient education on prevention of VTE and prescribed prophylactic measures.

[5: Benefits Balanced with Harms]

Recommendation VIII

The health care organization's quality management program should evaluate the outcomes of VTE prophylaxis and protocol compliance.

Quality assurance and performance improvement programs can facilitate the identification of problem areas and assist personnel in evaluating and improving the quality of patient care and formulating plans for corrective action. These programs provide data that may be used to determine whether an individual organization is within benchmark goals, and if not, to identify areas that may require corrective action. A quality management program provides a mechanism to evaluate effectiveness of processes, including processes in the VTE prevention protocol.

Collecting data to monitor and improve patient care, treatment, and services is a regulatory requirement[284-287] and an accreditation standard for both hospitals[301,302] and ambulatory settings.[302-306]

VIII.a. The quality assurance and performance improvement program for VTE prevention should include
- monitoring the rate of perioperative venous thromboembolism, including DVT and PE[4,307,308];
- assessing compliance with prophylaxis according to the health care organization's VTE prevention protocol[4];
- addressing barriers to compliance with prophylaxis, including complications from prophylaxis use[4];
- identifying common failure modes in VTE prevention processes[4]; and
- providing ongoing evaluation, feedback to perioperative team members, and refinement of the VTE protocol as needed.[4]

[3: Moderate Evidence]

Editor's note: *ERAS (Enhanced Recovery After Surgery) is a registered trademark of the ERAS Society, Stockholm, Sweden.*

Glossary

Atheroembolism: A cholesterol embolism, with or without calcified matter, originating from an atheroma of the aorta or other diseased artery.

Calciphylaxis: A condition of induced systemic hypersensitivity in which tissues respond to challenging agents with local calcification.

Proximal indentation: An indentation of the proximal calf from graduated compression stockings, creating a reverse gradient.

Reverse gradient: A condition in which proximal pressures from graduated compression stockings are higher than distal pressures, causing the advantageous pressure gradient for venous thromboembolism to reverse, which compromises venous return and increases the risk for venous thromboembolism. Synonym: tourniquet effect.

Thrombophilia: A condition in which the blood coagulates faster than normal.

REFERENCES

1. Venous thromboembolism (blood clots). Centers for Disease Control and Prevention. https://www.cdc.gov/ncbddd/dvt/index.html. Accessed August 24, 2017. [VA]

2. Gould MK, Garcia DA, Wren SM, et al. Prevention of VTE in nonorthopedic surgical patients: Antithrombotic Therapy and Prevention of Thrombosis, 9th ed: American College of Chest Physicians Evidence-Based Clinical Practice Guidelines. *Chest*. 2012;141(2 Suppl):e227S-e277S. [IVA]

3. Heit JA. Epidemiology of venous thromboembolism. *Nat Rev Cardiol*. 2015;12(8):464-474. [VB]

4. Maynard G. *Preventing Hospital-Associated Venous Thromboembolism: A Guide for Effective Quality Improvement*. 2nd ed. [AHRQ Publication No. 16-0001-EF]. Rockville, MD: Agency for Healthcare Research and Quality; 2016. https://www.ahrq.gov/sites/default/files/publications/files/vteguide.pdf. Accessed August 24, 2017. [VA]

5. Vekeman F, LaMori JC, Laliberté F, et al. Risks and cost burden of venous thromboembolism and bleeding for patients undergoing total hip or knee replacement in a managed-care population. *J Med Econ*. 2011;14(3):324-334. [IIIA]

6. Baser O, Supina D, Sengupta N, Wang L, Kwong L. Clinical and cost outcomes of venous thromboembolism in Medicare patients undergoing total hip replacement or total knee replacement surgery. *Curr Med Res Opin*. 2011;27(2):423-429. [IIIA]

7. Cohoon KP, Leibson CL, Ransom JE, et al. Direct medical costs attributable to venous thromboembolism among persons hospitalized for major operation: a population-based longitudinal study. *Surgery*. 2015;157(3):423-431. [IIIA]

8. Adams A. Proactivity in VTE prevention: a concept analysis. *Br J Nurs*. 2015;24(1):20-25. [VA]

9. Findlay J, Keogh M, Cooper L. Venous thromboembolism prophylaxis: the role of the nurse. *Br J Nurs*. 2010;19(16):1028-1032. [VB]

10. Frostick S. Pharmacological thromboprophylaxis and total hip or knee replacement. *Br J Nurs*. 2016;25(1):45-53. [VB]

11. McNamara SA. Prevention of venous thromboembolism. *AORN J*. 2014;99(5):642-647. [VB]

12. Collins R, MacLellan L, Gibbs H, MacLellan D, Fletcher J. Venous thromboembolism prophylaxis: the role of the nurse in changing practice and saving lives. *Aust J Adv Nurs*. 2010;27(3):83-89. [VA]

13. Smith T, Daniell H, Hing C. Upper extremity deep vein thrombosis in orthopaedic and trauma surgery: a systematic review. *Eur J Orthop Surg Traumatol*. 2011;21(2):79-85. [IIIB]

14. Desai K, Dinh TP, Chung S, Pierpont YN, Naidu DK, Payne WG. Upper extremity deep vein thrombosis with tourniquet use. *Int J Surg Case Rep*. 2015;6C:55-57. [VB]

15. Durant TJS, Swanson BT, Cote MP, Allen DA, Arciero RA, Mazzocca AD. Upper extremity deep venous thromboembolism following arthroscopic labral repair of the shoulder and biceps tenodesis: a case report. *Int J Sports Phys Ther*. 2014;9(3):377-382. [VB]

16. Garofalo R, Notarnicola A, Moretti L, Moretti B, Marini S, Castagna A. Deep vein thromboembolism after arthroscopy of the shoulder: two case reports and a review of the literature. *BMC Musculoskelet Disord*. 2010;11:65. [VB]

17. Oofuvong M, Oearsakul T, Chittithavorn V, Viboonjuntra P. Upper extremity deep vein thrombosis related to fatal massive pulmonary embolism after spinal surgery. *J Med Assoc Thai*. 2012;95(2):279-281. [VB]

18. Saleh H, Pennings A, Elmaraghy A. Venous thromboembolism after shoulder arthroplasty: a report of three cases. *Acta Orthop Traumatol Turc*. 2015;49(2):220-223. [VB]

19. Wood J, Halen JV, Samant S. Upper extremity deep vein thrombosis and pulmonary embolus after radial forearm free flap: a case report and literature review. *J Reconstr Microsurg*. 2014;30(4):275-278. [VB]

20. Yamamoto T, Tamai K, Akutsu M, Tomizawa K, Sukegawa T, Nohara Y. Pulmonary embolism after arthroscopic rotator cuff repair: a case report. *Case Rep Orthop*. 2013;2013:801752. [VB]

21. Parvizi J, Parmar R, Raphael IJ, Restrepo C, Rothman RH. Proximal deep venous thrombosis and pulmonary embolus following total joint arthroplasty. *J Arthroplasty*. 2014;29(9):1846-1848. [IIIA]

22. Bikdeli B, Sharif-Kashani B, Shahabi P, et al. Comparison of three risk assessment methods for venous thromboembolism prophylaxis. *Blood Coagul Fibrinolysis*. 2013;24(2):157-163. [IIIB]

23. Hewes PD, Hachey KJ, Zhang XW, et al. Evaluation of the Caprini model for venothromboembolism in esophagectomy patients. *Ann Thorac Surg*. 2015;100(6):2072-2078. [IIIB]

24. Lobastov K, Barinov V, Schastlivtsev I, Laberko L, Rodoman G, Boyarintsev V. Validation of the Caprini risk assessment model for venous thromboembolism in high-risk surgical patients in the background of standard prophylaxis. *J Vasc Surg*. 2016;4(2):153-160. [IIIB]

25. Pannucci CJ, Bailey SH, Dreszer G, et al. Validation of the Caprini risk assessment model in plastic and reconstructive surgery patients. *J Am Coll Surg*. 2011;212(1):105-112. [IIIB]

26. Pannucci CJ, Barta RJ, Portschy PR, et al. Assessment of postoperative venous thromboembolism risk in plastic surgery patients using the 2005 and 2010 Caprini risk score. *Plast Reconstr Surg*. 2012;130(2):343-353. [IIIB]

27. Pannucci CJ, Basta MN, Fischer JP, Kovach SJ. Creation and validation of a condition-specific venous thromboembolism risk assessment tool for ventral hernia repair. *Surgery*. 2015;158(5):1304-1313. [IIIA]

28. Pannucci CJ, Laird S, Dimick JB, Campbell DA, Henke PK. A validated risk model to predict 90-day VTE events in postsurgical patients. *Chest*. 2014;145(3):567-573. [IIIA]

29. Nam D, Nunley RM, Johnson SR, Keeney JA, Clohisy JC, Barrack RL. The effectiveness of a risk stratification protocol for thromboembolism prophylaxis after hip and knee arthroplasty. *J Arthroplasty*. 2016;31(6):1299-1306. [IIIA]

30. Shaikh M, Jeong HS, Mastro A, Davis K, Lysikowski J, Kenkel JM. Analysis of the American Society of Anesthesiologists physical status classification system and Caprini risk assessment model in predicting venous thromboembolic outcomes in plastic surgery patients. *Aesthet Surg J*. 2016;36(4):497-505. [IIIB]

31. Iorio ML, Venturi ML, Davison SP. Practical guidelines for venous thromboembolism chemoprophylaxis in elective plastic surgery. *Plast Reconstr Surg*. 2015;135(2):413-423. [IVC]

32. Cassidy MR, Rosenkranz P, McAneny D. Reducing postoperative venous thromboembolism complications with a standardized risk-stratified prophylaxis protocol and mobilization program. *J Am Coll Surg*. 2014;218(6):1095-1104. [VA]

33. Shah DR, Wang H, Bold RJ, et al. Nomograms to predict risk of in-hospital and post-discharge venous thromboembolism after abdominal and thoracic surgery: an American College of Surgeons National Surgical Quality Improvement Program analysis. *J Surg Res*. 2013;183(1):462-471. [IIIA]

34. Stroud W, Whitworth JM, Miklic M, et al. Validation of a venous thromboembolism risk assessment model in

gynecologic oncology. *Gynecol Oncol.* 2014;134(1):160-163. [IIIB]

35. Goz V, McCarthy I, Weinreb JH, et al. Venous thromboembolic events after spinal fusion: which patients are at high risk? *J Bone Joint Surg Am.* 2014;96(11):936-942. [IIIA]

36. Cavazza S, Rainaldi MP, Adduci A, Palareti G. Thromboprophylaxis following cesarean delivery: one site prospective pilot study to evaluate the application of a risk score model. *Thromb Res.* 2012;129(1):28-31. [IIB]

37. Shuman AG, Hu HM, Pannucci CJ, Jackson CR, Bradford CR, Bahl V. Stratifying the risk of venous thromboembolism in otolaryngology. *Otolaryngol Head Neck Surg.* 2012;146(5):719-724. [IIIB]

38. Janus E, Bassi Λ, Jackson D, Nandurkar H, Yates M. Thromboprophylaxis use in medical and surgical inpatients and the impact of an electronic risk assessment tool as part of a multi-factorial intervention. A report on behalf of the elVis study investigators. *J Thromb Thrombolysis.* 2011;32(3):279-287. [IIIA]

39. Novis SJ, Havelka GE, Ostrowski D, et al. Prevention of thromboembolic events in surgical patients through the creation and implementation of a computerized risk assessment program. *J Vasc Surg.* 2010;51(3):648-654. [IIA]

40. Bahl V, Hu HM, Henke PK, Wakefield TW, Campbell DAJ, Caprini JA. A validation study of a retrospective venous thromboembolism risk scoring method. *Ann Surg.* 2010;251(2):344-350. [IIIA]

41. Connelly CR, Laird A, Barton JS, et al. A clinical tool for the prediction of venous thromboembolism in pediatric trauma patients. *JAMA Surg.* 2016;151(1):50-57. [IIIA]

42. Atchison CM, Arlikar S, Amankwah E, et al. Development of a new risk score for hospital-associated venous thromboembolism in noncritically ill children: findings from a large single-institutional case-control study. *J Pediatr.* 2014;165(4):793-798. [IIIA]

43. Prentiss AS. Early recognition of pediatric venous thromboembolism: a risk-assessment tool. *Am J Crit Care.* 2012;21(3):178-183. [IIIC]

44. Caprini JA. Identification of patient venous thromboembolism risk across the continuum of care. *Clin Appl Thromb Hemost.* 2011;17(6):590-599. [VA]

45. Caprini JA. Mechanical methods for thrombosis prophylaxis. *Clin Appl Thromb Hemost.* 2010;16(6):668-673. [VA]

46. Borab ZM, Lanni MA, Tecce MG, Pannucci CJ, Fischer JP. Use of computerized clinical decision support systems to prevent venous thromboembolism in surgical patients: a systematic review and meta-analysis. *JAMA Surg.* 2017;152(7):638-645. [IIIC]

47. Kahn SR, Morrison DR, Cohen JM, et al. Interventions for implementation of thromboprophylaxis in hospitalized medical and surgical patients at risk for venous thromboembolism. *Cochrane Database Syst Rev.* 2013;(7):CD008201. [IIA]

48. Venous thromboembolism: reducing the risk for patients in hospital. Clinical guideline. NICE: National Institute for Health and Care Excellence. http://www.nice.org.uk/guidance/cg92. Published January 2010. Updated June 2015. Accessed August 24, 2017. [IVA]

49. Farge D, Debourdeau P, Beckers M, et al. International clinical practice guidelines for the treatment and prophylaxis of venous thromboembolism in patients with cancer. *J Thromb Haemost.* 2013;11(1):56-70. [IVA]

50. Lyman GH, Bohlke K, Khorana AA, et al. Venous thromboembolism prophylaxis and treatment in patients with cancer: American Society of Clinical Oncology clinical practice guideline update 2014. *J Clin Oncol.* 2015;33(6):654-656. [IVA]

51. American Society for Metabolic and Bariatric Surgery Clinical Issues Committee. ASMBS updated position statement on prophylactic measures to reduce the risk of venous thromboembolism in bariatric surgery patients. *Surg Obes Relat Dis.* 2013;9(4):493-497. [IVC]

52. Hoefnagel D, Kwee LE, van Putten EHP, Kros JM, Dirven CMF, Dammers R. The incidence of postoperative thromboembolic complications following surgical resection of intracranial meningioma. A retrospective study of a large single center patient cohort. *Clin Neurol Neurosurg.* 2014;123:150-154. [IIIB]

53. Agarwal R, Hecht TEH, Lazo MC, Umscheid CA. Venous thromboembolism prophylaxis for patients undergoing bariatric surgery: a systematic review. *Surg Obes Relat Dis.* 2010;6(2):213-220. [IIIB]

54. Pellino G, Sciaudone G, Candilio G, De Fatico GS, Canonico S, Selvaggi F. Predictors of venous thromboembolism after colorectal surgery in a single unit. *Acta Chir Belg.* 2015;115(4):288-292. [IIIB]

55. Finks JF, English WJ, Carlin AM, et al. Predicting risk for venous thromboembolism with bariatric surgery: results from the Michigan Bariatric Surgery Collaborative. *Ann Surg.* 2012;255(6):1100-1104. [IIIA]

56. Stein PD, Matta F. Pulmonary embolism and deep venous thrombosis following bariatric surgery. *Obes Surg.* 2013;23(5):663-668. [IIIA]

57. Wang L, Pryor AD, Altieri MS, et al. Perioperative rates of deep vein thrombosis and pulmonary embolism in normal weight vs obese and morbidly obese surgical patients in the era post venous thromboembolism prophylaxis guidelines. *Am J Surg.* 2015;210(5):859-863. [IIIA]

58. Nwaogu I, Yan Y, Margenthaler JA, Myckatyn TM. Venous thromboembolism after breast reconstruction in patients undergoing breast surgery: an American College of Surgeons NSQIP analysis. *J Am Coll Surg.* 2015;220(5):886-893. [IIIA]

59. Parkin L, Sweetland S, Balkwill A, et al. Body mass index, surgery, and risk of venous thromboembolism in middle-aged women: a cohort study. *Circulation.* 2012;125(15):1897-1904. [IIIA]

60. Jamal MH, Corcelles R, Shimizu H, et al. Thromboembolic events in bariatric surgery: a large multi-institutional referral center experience. *Surg Endosc.* 2015;29(2):376-380. [IIIA]

61. Winegar DA, Sherif B, Pate V, DeMaria EJ. Venous thromboembolism after bariatric surgery performed by bariatric surgery center of excellence participants: analysis of the bariatric outcomes longitudinal database. *Surg Obes Relat Dis.* 2011;7(2):181-188. [IIIA]

62. Becattini C, Agnelli G, Manina G, Noya G, Rondelli F. Venous thromboembolism after laparoscopic bariatric surgery for morbid obesity: clinical burden and prevention. *Surg Obes Relat Dis.* 2012;8(1):108-115. [IIIA]

63. Bartlett MA, Mauck KF, Daniels PR. Prevention of venous thromboembolism in patients undergoing bariatric surgery. *Vasc Health Risk Manag.* 2015;11:461-477. [IIIA]

64. Schoenfeld AJ, Herzog JP, Dunn JC, Bader JO, Belmont PJ Jr. Patient-based and surgical characteristics associated with the acute development of deep venous thrombosis and pulmonary embolism after spine surgery. *Spine.* 2013;38(21):1892-1898. [IIIA]

65. Swenson CW, Berger MB, Kamdar NS, Campbell DAJ, Morgan DM. Risk factors for venous thromboembolism after hysterectomy. *Obstet Gynecol.* 2015;125(5):1139-1144. [IIIA]

66. Wes AM, Wink JD, Kovach SJ, Fischer JP. Venous thromboembolism in body contouring: an analysis of

17,774 patients from the National Surgical Quality Improvement databases. *Plast Reconstr Surg.* 2015;135(6):972e-980e. [IIIA]

67. Anderson JAM, Weitz JI. Hypercoagulable states. *Crit Care Clin.* 2011;27(4):933-952. [VA]

68. Allen D, Sale G. Lower limb joint replacement in patients with a history of venous thromboembolism. *Bone Joint J.* 2014;96-B(11):1515-1519. [IIIB]

69. Liem TK, Huynh TM, Moseley SE, et al. Symptomatic perioperative venous thromboembolism is a frequent complication in patients with a history of deep vein thrombosis. *J Vasc Surg.* 2010;52(3):651-657. [IIIB]

70. Pedersen AB, Sorensen HT, Mehnert F, Overgaard S, Johnsen SP. Risk factors for venous thromboembolism in patients undergoing total hip replacement and receiving routine thromboprophylaxis. *J Bone Joint Surg Am.* 2010;92(12):2156-2164. [IIIA]

71. Qu H, Li Z, Zhai Z, et al. Predicting of venous thromboembolism for patients undergoing gynecological surgery. *Medicine.* 2015;94(39):e1653. [IIIB]

72. Testroote MJG, Wittens CHA. Prevention of venous thromboembolism in patients undergoing surgical treatment of varicose veins. *Phlebology.* 2013;28(Suppl 1):86-90. [IIIB]

73. Sutton PA, El-Dhuwaib Y, El-Duhwaib Y, Dyer J, Guy AJ. The incidence of post operative venous thromboembolism in patients undergoing varicose vein surgery recorded in hospital episode statistics. *Ann R Coll Surg Engl.* 2012;94(7):481-483. [IIIB]

74. Chen K, Yu GF, Huang JY, et al. Incidence and risk factors of early deep venous thrombosis after varicose vein surgery with routine use of a tourniquet. *Thromb Res.* 2015;135(6):1052-1056. [IIIA]

75. Minami K, Iida M, Iida H. Case report: central venous catheterization via internal jugular vein with associated formation of perioperative venous thrombosis during surgery in the prone position. *J Anesth.* 2012;26(3):464-466. [VB]

76. Smith BR, Diniz S, Stamos M, Nguyen NT. Deep venous thrombosis after general surgical operations at a university hospital: two-year data from the ACS NSQIP. *Arch Surg.* 2011;146(12):1424-1427. [IIIB]

77. Wang TF, Wong CA, Milligan PE, Thoelke MS, Woeltje KF, Gage BF. Risk factors for inpatient venous thromboembolism despite thromboprophylaxis. *Thromb Res.* 2014;133(1):25-29. [IIIB]

78. Holley AB, Petteys S, Mitchell JD, et al. Venous thromboembolism prophylaxis for patients receiving regional anesthesia following injury in Iraq and Afghanistan. *J Trauma Acute Care Surg.* 2014;76(1):152-159. [IIIB]

79. Dahl OE, Harenberg J, Wexels F, Preissner KT. Arterial and venous thrombosis following trauma and major orthopedic surgery: molecular mechanisms and strategies for intervention. *Semin Thromb Hemost.* 2015;41(2):141-145. [VA]

80. Allen CJ, Murray CR, Meizoso JP, et al. Risk factors for venous thromboembolism after pediatric trauma. *J Pediatr Surg.* 2016;51(1):168-171. [IIIA]

81. Matsumoto S, Suda K, Iimoto S, et al. Prospective study of deep vein thrombosis in patients with spinal cord injury not receiving anticoagulant therapy. *Spinal Cord.* 2015;53(4):306-309. [IIIB]

82. Giorgi Pierfranceschi M, Donadini MP, Dentali F, et al. The short- and long-term risk of venous thromboembolism in patients with acute spinal cord injury: a prospective cohort study. *Thromb Haemost.* 2013;109(1):34-38. [IIB]

83. Hunt BJ. Venous thromboembolism and thrombophilia testing. *Medicine (United Kingdom).* 2013;41(4):234-237. [VB]

84. Banks-Gonzales V, Ruppert SD. Thrombophilia and hypercoagulation: risk assessment and screening. *J Nurse Pract.* 2012;8(8):649-655. [VA]

85. Committee on Practice Bulletins—Gynecology, American College of Obstetricians and Gynecologists. ACOG Practice Bulletin No. 84: Prevention of deep vein thrombosis and pulmonary embolism. *Obstet Gynecol.* 2007;110(2 Pt 1):429-440. [IVC]

86. Amar S, Van Boven M, Rooijakkers H, Momeni M. Massive postoperative pulmonary embolism in a young woman using oral contraceptives: the value of a preoperative anesthetic consult. *Acta Anaesthesiol Belg.* 2014;65(2):73-75. [VA]

87. Barsoum MK, Heit JA, Ashrani AA, Leibson CL, Petterson TM, Bailey KR. Is progestin an independent risk factor for incident venous thromboembolism? A population-based case-control study. *Thromb Res.* 2010;126(5):373-378. [IIIA]

88. Paresi RJ Jr, Myers RS, Matarasso A. Contraceptive vaginal rings: do they pose an increased risk of venous thromboembolism in aesthetic surgery? *Aesthet Surg J.* 2015;35(6):721-727. [VB]

89. Alaia MJ, Zuskov A, Davidovitch RI. Contralateral deep venous thrombosis after hip arthroscopy. *Orthopedics.* 2011;34(10):e674-e677. [VB]

90. Zeng Y, Shen B, Yang J, Zhou Z, Kang P, Pei F. Preoperative comorbidities as potential risk factors for venous thromboembolism after joint arthroplasty: a systematic review and meta-analysis of cohort and case-control studies. *J Arthroplasty.* 2014;29(12):2430-2438. [IIIA]

91. Markovic-Denic L, Zivkovic K, Lesic A, Bumbasirevic V, Dubljanin-Raspopovic E, Bumbasirevic M. Risk factors and distribution of symptomatic venous thromboembolism in total hip and knee replacements: prospective study. *Int Orthop.* 2012;36(6):1299-1305. [IIIB]

92. Singh JA, Jensen MR, Harmsen WS, Gabriel SE, Lewallen DG. Cardiac and thromboembolic complications and mortality in patients undergoing total hip and total knee arthroplasty. *Ann Rheum Dis.* 2011;70(12):2082-2088. [IIIB]

93. Haskins IN, Amdur R, Sarani B, Vaziri K. Congestive heart failure is a risk factor for venous thromboembolism in bariatric surgery. *Surg Obes Relat Dis.* 2015;11(5):1140-1145. [IIIA]

94. Kapoor A, Labonte AJ, Winter MR, et al. Risk of venous thromboembolism after total hip and knee replacement in older adults with comorbidity and co-occurring comorbidities in the Nationwide Inpatient Sample (2003-2006). *BMC Geriatrics.* 2010;10:63. [IIIB]

95. Masoomi H, Buchberg B, Reavis KM, Mills SD, Stamos M, Nguyen NT. Factors predictive of venous thromboembolism in bariatric surgery. *Am Surg.* 2011;77(10):1403-1406. [IIIB]

96. Gephart MGH, Zygourakis CC, Arrigo RT, Kalanithi PSA, Lad SP, Boakye M. Venous thromboembolism after thoracic/thoracolumbar spinal fusion. *World Neurosurg.* 2012;78(5):545-552. [IIIA]

97. Huang L, Li J, Jiang Y. Association between hypertension and deep vein thrombosis after orthopedic surgery: a meta-analysis. *Eur J Med Res.* 2016;21(1):13. [IIIC]

98. Delos D, Rodeo SA. Venous thrombosis after arthroscopic shoulder surgery: pacemaker leads as a possible cause: pacemaker leads as a possible cause. *HSS J.* 2011;7(3):282-285. [VB]

99. Barbot M, Daidone V, Zilio M, et al. Perioperative thromboprophylaxis in Cushing's disease: what we did

and what we are doing? *Pituitary*. 2015;18(4):487-493. [IIIA]

100. Manetti L, Bogazzi F, Giovannetti C, et al. Changes in coagulation indexes and occurrence of venous thromboembolism in patients with Cushing's syndrome: results from a prospective study before and after surgery. *Eur J Endocrinol*. 2010;163(5):783-791. [IIIB]

101. Masoomi H, Paydar KZ, Wirth GA, Aly A, Kobayashi MR, Evans GRD. Predictive risk factors of venous thromboembolism in autologous breast reconstruction surgery. *Ann Plast Surg*. 2014;72(1):30-33. [IIIA]

102. Monn MF, Hui X, Lau BD, et al. Infection and venous thromboembolism in patients undergoing colorectal surgery: what is the relationship? *Dis Colon Rectum*. 2014;57(4):497-505. [IIIA]

103. Baker D, Sherrod B, McGwin GJ, Ponce B, Gilbert S. Complications and 30-day outcomes associated with venous thromboembolism in the pediatric orthopaedic surgical population. *J Am Acad Orthop Surg*. 2016;24(3):196-206. [IIIA]

104. Barmparas G, Fierro N, Lamb AW, et al. Clostridium difficile increases the risk for venous thromboembolism. *Am J Surg*. 2014;208(5):703-709. [IIIA]

105. Donze JD, Ridker PM, Finlayson SRG, Bates DW. Impact of sepsis on risk of postoperative arterial and venous thromboses: large prospective cohort study. *BMJ*. 2014;349:g5334. [IIIA]

106. Hatch Q, Nelson D, Martin M, et al. Can sepsis predict deep venous thrombosis in colorectal surgery? *Am J Surg*. 2016;211(1):53-58. [IIIA]

107. Albayati MA, Grover SP, Saha P, Lwaleed BA, Modarai B, Smith A. Postsurgical inflammation as a causative mechanism of venous thromboembolism. *Semin Thromb Hemostas*. 2015;41(6):615-620. [VA]

108. Wilson MZ, Connelly TM, Tinsley A, Hollenbeak CS, Koltun WA, Messaris E. Ulcerative colitis is associated with an increased risk of venous thromboembolism in the postoperative period: the results of a matched cohort analysis. *Ann Surg*. 2015;261(6):1160-1166. [IIIA]

109. Kaplan GG, Lim A, Seow CH, et al. Colectomy is a risk factor for venous thromboembolism in ulcerative colitis. *World J Gastroenterol*. 2015;21(4):1251-1260. [IIIB]

110. Merrill A, Millham F. Increased risk of postoperative deep vein thrombosis and pulmonary embolism in patients with inflammatory bowel disease: a study of National Surgical Quality Improvement Program patients. *Arch Surg*. 2012;147(2):120-124. [IIIA]

111. Moghadamyeghaneh Z, Hanna MH, Carmichael JC, Nguyen NT, Stamos MJ. A nationwide analysis of postoperative deep vein thrombosis and pulmonary embolism in colon and rectal surgery. *J Gastrointest Surg*. 2014;18(12):2169-2177. [IIIA]

112. Colorectal Writing Group for Surgical Care and Outcomes Assessment Program-Comparative Effectiveness Research Translation Network (SCOAP-CERTAIN) Collaborative; Nelson DW, Simianu VV, et al. Thromboembolic complications and prophylaxis patterns in colorectal surgery. *JAMA Surg*. 2015;150(8):712-720. [IIIA]

113. Mameli A, Marongiu F. Thromboembolic disease in patients with rheumatoid arthritis undergoing joint arthroplasty: update on prophylaxes. *World J Orthop*. 2014;5(5):645-652. [IIIB]

114. Ahlehoff O, Gislason GH, Lindhardsen J, et al. Psoriasis carries an increased risk of venous thromboembolism: a Danish nationwide cohort study. *PLoS One*. 2011;6(3):e18125. [IIIA]

115. James A; Committee on Practice Bulletins—Obstetrics. Practice Bulletin No. 123: Thromboembolism in pregnancy. *Obstet Gynecol*. 2011;118(3):718-729. [IVB]

116. D'Alton ME, Friedman AM, Smiley RM, et al. National partnership for maternal safety: consensus bundle on venous thromboembolism. *Obstet Gynecol*. 2016;128(4):688-698. [IVB]

117. Tepper NK, Boulet SL, Whiteman MK, et al. Postpartum venous thromboembolism: incidence and risk factors. *Obstet Gynecol*. 2014;123(5):987-996. [IIIA]

118. Musallam KM, Rosendaal FR, Zaatari G, et al. Smoking and the risk of mortality and vascular and respiratory events in patients undergoing major surgery. *JAMA Surg*. 2013;148(8):755-762. [IIIA]

119. Sweetland S, Parkin L, Balkwill A, et al. Smoking, surgery, and venous thromboembolism risk in women: United Kingdom cohort study. *Circulation*. 2013;127(12):1276-1282. [IIIA]

120. Deflandre E, Degey S, Opsomer N, Brichant J, Joris J. Obstructive sleep apnea and smoking as a risk factor for venous thromboembolism events: review of the literature on the common pathophysiological mechanisms. *Obes Surg*. 2016;26(3):640-648. [VB]

121. Kantar RS, Haddad AG, Tamim H, Jamali F, Taher AT. Venous thromboembolism and preoperative steroid use: analysis of the NSQIP database to evaluate risk in surgical patients. *Eur J Intern Med*. 2015;26(7):528-533. [IIIA]

122. Greaves SW, Holubar SD. Preoperative hospitalization is independently associated with increased risk for venous thromboembolism in patients undergoing colorectal surgery: a National Surgical Quality Improvement Program database study. *Dis Colon Rectum*. 2015;58(8):782-791. [IIIA]

123. Lieber BA, Han J, Appelboom G, et al. Association of steroid use with deep venous thrombosis and pulmonary embolism in neurosurgical patients: a national database analysis. *World Neurosurg*. 2016;89:126-132. [IIIA]

124. Rolston JD, Han SJ, Bloch O, Parsa AT. What clinical factors predict the incidence of deep venous thrombosis and pulmonary embolism in neurosurgical patients? *J Neurosurg*. 2014;121(4):908-918. [IIIA]

125. Mueller MG, Pilecki MA, Catanzarite T, Jain U, Kim JYS, Kenton K. Venous thromboembolism in reconstructive pelvic surgery. *Am J Obstet Gynecol*. 2014;211(5):552. e1-552.e6. [IIIA]

126. Miller TJ, Jeong HS, Davis K, et al. Evaluation of the American Society of Anesthesiologists physical status classification system in risk assessment for plastic and reconstructive surgery patients. *Aesthet Surg J*. 2014;34(3):448-456. [IIIB]

127. Ghazi L, Schwann TA, Engoren MC, Habib RH. Role of blood transfusion product type and amount in deep vein thrombosis after cardiac surgery. *Thromb Res*. 2015;136(6):1204-1210. [IIIB]

128. Tollefson MK, Karnes RJ, Rangel L, Carlson R, Boorjian SA. Blood type, lymphadenectomy and blood transfusion predict venous thromboembolic events following radical prostatectomy with pelvic lymphadenectomy. *J Urol*. 2014;191(3):646-651. [IIIA]

129. Xenos ES, Vargas HD, Davenport DL. Association of blood transfusion and venous thromboembolism after colorectal cancer resection. *Thromb Res*. 2012;129(5):568-572. [IIIA]

130. Yang S, Ding W, Yang D, et al. Prevalence and risk factors of deep vein thrombosis in patients undergoing lumbar interbody fusion surgery: a single-center cross-sectional study. *Medicine*. 2015;94(48):e2205. [IIIB]

131. Turley RS, Reddy SK, Shortell CK, Clary BM, Scarborough JE. Venous thromboembolism after hepatic resection: analysis of 5,706 patients. *J Gastrointest Surg*. 2012;16(9):1705-1714. [IIIA]

132. Wang JK, Boorjian SA, Frank I, et al. Non-O blood type is associated with an increased risk of venous thromboembolism after radical cystectomy. *Urology.* 2014;83(1):140-145. [IIIB]

133. Ha LP, Arrendondo M. Fatal venous thromboembolism after splenectomy: pathogenesis and management. *J Am Osteopath Assoc.* 2012;112(5):291-300. [VB]

134. Abel EJ, Wong K, Sado M, et al. Surgical operative time increases the risk of deep venous thrombosis and pulmonary embolism in robotic prostatectomy. *JSLS.* 2014;18(2):282-287. [IIIA]

135. Kim JYS, Khavanin N, Rambachan A, et al. Surgical duration and risk of venous thromboembolism. *JAMA Surg.* 2015;150(2):110-117. [IIIA]

136. Kimmell KT, Walter KA. Risk factors for venous thromboembolism in patients undergoing craniotomy for neoplastic disease. *J Neurooncol.* 2014;120(3):567-573. [IIIA]

137. Kim BD, Hsu WK, De Oliveira GSJ, Saha S, Kim JYS. Operative duration as an independent risk factor for postoperative complications in single-level lumbar fusion: an analysis of 4588 surgical cases. *Spine.* 2014;39(6):510-520. [IIIA]

138. Chan MM, Hamza N, Ammori BJ. Duration of surgery independently influences risk of venous thromboembolism after laparoscopic bariatric surgery. *Surg Obes Relat Dis.* 2013;9(1):88-93. [IIIA]

139. Montoya TI, Leclaire EL, Oakley SH, et al. Venous thromboembolism in women undergoing pelvic reconstructive surgery with mechanical prophylaxis alone. *Int Urogynecol J.* 2014;25(7):921-926. [IIIA]

140. Leung ASM, Fok MWM, Fung BKK. Fatal bilateral lower-limb deep vein thrombosis and pulmonary embolism following single digit replantation. *Hong Kong Med J.* 2015;21(3):283-285. [VB]

141. Guideline for positioning the patient. In: *Guidelines for Perioperative Practice.* Denver, CO: AORN, Inc; 2017: e1-e72. [IVA]

142. Guideline for care of patients undergoing pneumatic tourniquet-assisted procedures. In: *Guidelines for Perioperative Practice.* Denver, CO: AORN, Inc; 2017:157-182. [IVA]

143. Falck-Ytter Y, Francis CW, Johanson NA, et al. Prevention of VTE in orthopedic surgery patients: antithrombotic therapy and prevention of thrombosis, 9th ed: American College of Chest Physicians Evidence-Based Clinical Practice Guidelines. *Chest.* 2012;141(2 Suppl):e278S-e325S. [IVA]

144. Mont MA, Jacobs JJ, Boggio LN, et al. Preventing venous thromboembolic disease in patients undergoing elective hip and knee arthroplasty. *J Am Acad Orthop Surg.* 2011;19(12):768-776. [IVA]

145. Januel J, Chen G, Ruffieux C, et al. Symptomatic in-hospital deep vein thrombosis and pulmonary embolism following hip and knee arthroplasty among patients receiving recommended prophylaxis: a systematic review. *JAMA.* 2012;307(3):294-303. [IIIA]

146. Zhang J, Chen Z, Zheng J, Breusch SJ, Tian J. Risk factors for venous thromboembolism after total hip and total knee arthroplasty: a meta-analysis. *Arch Orthop Trauma Surg.* 2015;135(6):759-772. [IIIA]

147. Lewis CG, Inneh IA, Schutzer SF, Grady-Benson J. Evaluation of the first-generation AAOS clinical guidelines on the prophylaxis of venous thromboembolic events in patients undergoing total joint arthroplasty: experience with 3289 patients from a single institution. *J Bone Joint Surg Am.* 2014;96(16):1327-1332. [IIB]

148. Steele KE, Schweitzer MA, Prokopowicz G, et al. The long-term risk of venous thromboembolism following bariatric surgery. *Obes Surg.* 2011;21(9):1371-1376. [IIIA]

149. Di Nisio M, Peinemann F, Porreca E, Rutjes AWS. Primary prophylaxis for venous thromboembolism in patients undergoing cardiac or thoracic surgery. *Cochrane Database Syst Rev.* 2015;(6):CD009658. [IB]

150. Ho KM, Bham E, Pavey W. Incidence of venous thromboembolism and benefits and risks of thromboprophylaxis after cardiac surgery: a systematic review and meta-analysis. *J Am Heart Assoc.* 2015;4(10):e002652. [IIIA]

151. Aziz F, Patel M, Ortenzi G, Reed AB. Incidence of postoperative deep venous thrombosis is higher among cardiac and vascular surgery patients as compared with general surgery patients. *Ann Vasc Surg.* 2015;29(4):661-669. [IIIA]

152. Ramanan B, Gupta PK, Sundaram A, et al. In-hospital and postdischarge venous thromboembolism after vascular surgery. *J Vasc Surg.* 2013;57(6):1589-1596. [IIIA]

153. Scarborough JE, Cox MW, Mureebe L, Pappas TN, Shortell CK. A novel scoring system for predicting postoperative venous thromboembolic complications in patients after open aortic surgery. *J Am Coll Surg.* 2012;214(4):620-626. [IIIA]

154. Aloia TA, Geerts WH, Clary BM, et al. Venous thromboembolism prophylaxis in liver surgery. *J Gastrointest Surg.* 2016;20(1):221-229. [IVC]

155. Ejaz A, Spolverato G, Kim Y, et al. Defining incidence and risk factors of venous thromboembolism after hepatectomy. *J Gastrointest Surg.* 2014;18(6):1116-1124. [IIIA]

156. Newhook TE, Lapar DJ, Walters DM, et al. Impact of postoperative venous thromboembolism on postoperative morbidity, mortality, and resource utilization after hepatectomy. *Am Surg.* 2015;81(12):1216-1223. [IIIB]

157. Bouras G, Burns EM, Howell A, Bottle A, Athanasiou T, Darzi A. Risk of post-discharge venous thromboembolism and associated mortality in general surgery: a population-based cohort study using linked hospital and primary care data in england. *PLoS One.* 2015;10(12):e0145759. [IIIA]

158. Humes DJ, Walker AJ, Hunt BJ, Sultan AA, Ludvigsson JF, West J. Risk of symptomatic venous thromboembolism following emergency appendicectomy in adults. *Br J Surg.* 2016;103(4):443-450. [IIIA]

159. Violette PD, Cartwright R, Briel M, Tikkinen KAO, Guyatt GH. Guideline of guidelines: thromboprophylaxis for urological surgery. *BJU Int.* 2016;118(3):351-358. [VA]

160. Tikkinen KAO, Agarwal A, Craigie S, et al. Systematic reviews of observational studies of risk of thrombosis and bleeding in urological surgery (ROTBUS): introduction and methodology. *Syst Rev.* 2014;3:150. [IIIB]

161. Tyson MD, Castle EP, Humphreys MR, Andrews PE. Venous thromboembolism after urological surgery. *J Urol.* 2014;192(3):793-797. [IIIA]

162. Salmaggi A, Simonetti G, Trevisan E, et al. Perioperative thromboprophylaxis in patients with craniotomy for brain tumours: a systematic review. *J Neurooncol.* 2013;113(2):293-303. [IB]

163. Harris DA, Lam S. Venous thromboembolism in the setting of pediatric traumatic brain injury. *J Neurosurg Pediatr.* 2014;13(4):448-455. [IIIA]

164. Algattas H, Kimmell KT, Vates GE, Jahromi BS. Analysis of venous thromboembolism risk in patients undergoing craniotomy. *World Neurosurg.* 2015;84(5):1372-1379. [IIIA]

165. Kimmell KT, Jahromi BS. Clinical factors associated with venous thromboembolism risk in patients

undergoing craniotomy. *J Neurosurg.* 2015;122(5):1004-1011. [IIIA]

166. Sansone JM, del Rio AM, Anderson PA. The prevalence of and specific risk factors for venous thromboembolic disease following elective spine surgery. *J Bone Joint Surg Am.* 2010;92(2):304-313. [IIIA]

167. Oglesby M, Fineberg SJ, Patel AA, Pelton MA, Singh K. The incidence and mortality of thromboembolic events in cervical spine surgery. *Spine.* 2013;38(9):E521-E527. [IIIA]

168. Fineberg SJ, Oglesby M, Patel AA, Pelton MA, Singh K. The incidence and mortality of thromboembolic events in lumbar spine surgery. *Spine.* 2013;38(13):1154-1159. [IIIA]

169. Schairer WW, Pedtke AC, Hu SS. Venous thromboembolism after spine surgery. *Spine.* 2014;39(11):911-918. [IIIA]

170. Hohl JB, Lee JY, Rayappa SP, et al. Prevalence of venous thromboembolic events after elective major thoracolumbar degenerative spine surgery. *J Spinal Disord Tech.* 2015;28(5):E310-E315. [IIIA]

171. Cox JB, Weaver KJ, Neal DW, Jacob RP, Hoh DJ. Decreased incidence of venous thromboembolism after spine surgery with early multimodal prophylaxis: clinical article. *J Neurosurg Spine.* 2014;21(4):677-684. [IIIA]

172. Jain A, Karas DJ, Skolasky RL, Sponseller PD. Thromboembolic complications in children after spinal fusion surgery. *Spine.* 2014;39(16):1325-1329. [IIIA]

173. Barber EL, Neubauer NL, Gossett DR. Risk of venous thromboembolism in abdominal versus minimally invasive hysterectomy for benign conditions. *Am J Obstet Gynecol.* 2015;212(5):609.e1-609.e7. [IIIA]

174. Buchberg B, Masoomi H, Lusby K, et al. Incidence and risk factors of venous thromboembolism in colorectal surgery: does laparoscopy impart an advantage? *Arch Surg.* 2011;146(6):739-743. [IIIA]

175. Shapiro R, Vogel JD, Kiran RP. Risk of postoperative venous thromboembolism after laparoscopic and open colorectal surgery: an additional benefit of the minimally invasive approach? *Dis Colon Rectum.* 2011;54(12):1496-1502. [IIIA]

176. Cui G, Wang X, Yao W, Li H. Incidence of postoperative venous thromboembolism after laparoscopic versus open colorectal cancer surgery: a meta-analysis. *Surg Laparosc Endosc Percutan Tech.* 2013;23(2):128-134. [IA]

177. Xie YZ, Fang K, Ma WL, Shi ZH, Ren XQ. Risk of postoperative deep venous thrombosis in patients with colorectal cancer treated with open or laparoscopic colorectal surgery: a meta-analysis. *Indian J Cancer.* 2015;51(Suppl 2):e42-e44. [IB]

178. Autorino R, Zargar H, Butler S, Laydner H, Kaouk JH. Incidence and risk factors for 30-day readmission in patients undergoing nephrectomy procedures: a contemporary analysis of 5276 cases from the national surgical quality improvement program database. *Urology.* 2015;85(4):843-849. [IIIA]

179. Saad AN, Parina R, Chang D, Gosman AA. Risk of adverse outcomes when plastic surgery procedures are combined. *Plast Reconstr Surg.* 2014;134(6):1415-1422. [IIIA]

180. Fischer JP, Wes AM, Tuggle CT, Wu LC. Venous thromboembolism risk in mastectomy and immediate breast reconstruction: analysis of the 2005 to 2011 American College of Surgeons National Surgical Quality Improvement Program data sets. *Plast Reconstr Surg.* 2014;133(3):263e-273e. [IIIA]

181. Tran BH, Nguyen TJ, Hwang BH, et al. Risk factors associated with venous thromboembolism in 49,028 mastectomy patients. *Breast.* 2013;22(4):444-448. [IIIA]

182. Elboudwarej O, Patel JK, Liou F, et al. Risk of deep vein thrombosis and pulmonary embolism after heart transplantation: clinical outcomes comparing upper extremity deep vein thrombosis and lower extremity deep vein thrombosis. *Clin Transplant.* 2015;29(7):629-635. [IIIA]

183. Annamalai A, Kim I, Sundaram V, Klein A. Incidence and risk factors of deep vein thrombosis after liver transplantation. *Transplant Proc.* 2014;46(10):3564-3569. [IIIA]

184. Cherian TP, Chiu K, Gunson B, et al. Pulmonary thromboembolism in liver transplantation: a retrospective review of the first 25 years. *Transplant Int.* 2010;23(11):1113-1119. [IIIA]

185. Emuakhagbon V, Philips P, Agopian V, Kaldas FM, Jones CM. Incidence and risk factors for deep venous thrombosis and pulmonary embolus after liver transplantation. *Am J Surg.* 2016;211(4):768-771. [IIIA]

186. Alvarez-Alvarez RJ, Barge-Caballero E, Chavez-Leal SA, et al. Venous thromboembolism in heart transplant recipients: incidence, recurrence and predisposing factors. *J Heart Lung Transplant.* 2015;34(2):167-174. [IIIA]

187. Abualhassan N, Aljiffry M, Thalib L, Coussa R, Metrakos P, Hassanain M. Post-transplant venous thromboembolic events and their effect on graft survival. *Saudi J Kidney Dis Transpl.* 2015;26(1):1-5. [IIIB]

188. Salami A, Qureshi W, Kuriakose P, Moonka D, Yoshida A, Abouljoud M. Frequency and predictors of venous thromboembolism in orthotopic liver transplant recipients: a single-center retrospective review. *Transplant Proc.* 2013;45(1):315-319. [IIIB]

189. Verhave JC, Tagalakis V, Suissa S, Madore F, Hebert M, Cardinal H. The risk of thromboembolic events in kidney transplant patients. *Kidney Int.* 2014;85(6):1454-1460. [IIIB]

190. Ooi CY, Brandao LR, Zolpys L, et al. Thrombotic events after pediatric liver transplantation. *Pediatr Transplant.* 2010;14(4):476-482. [IIIB]

191. Saez-Gimenez B, Berastegui C, Loor K, et al. Deep vein thrombosis and pulmonary embolism after solid organ transplantation: an unresolved problem. *Transplant Rev.* 2015;29(2):85-92. [VB]

192. Arshad F, Lisman T, Porte RJ. Hypercoagulability as a contributor to thrombotic complications in the liver transplant recipient. *Liver Int.* 2013;33(6):820-827. [VB]

193. Fleischer AE, Abicht BP, Baker JR, Boffeli TJ, Jupiter DC, Schade VL. American College of Foot and Ankle Surgeons' clinical consensus statement: risk, prevention, and diagnosis of venous thromboembolism disease in foot and ankle surgery and injuries requiring immobilization. *J Foot Ankle Surg.* 2015;54(3):497-507. [IVB]

194. Calder JDF, Freeman R, Domeij-Arverud E, van Dijk CN, Ackermann PW. Meta-analysis and suggested guidelines for prevention of venous thromboembolism (VTE) in foot and ankle surgery. *Knee Surg Sports Traumatol Arthrosc.* 2016;24(4):1409-1420. [IIIA]

195. Mangwani J, Sheikh N, Cichero M, Williamson D. What is the evidence for chemical thromboprophylaxis in foot and ankle surgery? Systematic review of the English literature. *Foot.* 2015;25(3):173-178. [IIIB]

196. Barg A, Henninger HB, Hintermann B. Risk factors for symptomatic deep-vein thrombosis in patients after total ankle replacement who received routine chemical thromboprophylaxis. *J Bone Joint Surg Br.* 2011;93(7):921-927. [IIIA]

197. Basques BA, Miller CP, Golinvaux NS, Bohl DD, Grauer JN. Risk factors for thromboembolic events after surgery for ankle fractures. *Am J Orthop (Belle Mead NJ).* 2015;44(7):E220-E224. [IIIA]

198. Altintas F, Ozler T, Guven M, Ozkut AT, Ulucay C. Deep venous thrombosis and pulmonary embolism as rare complications after hallux valgus surgery: case report and literature review. *J Am Podiatr Med Assoc*. 2013;103(2):145-148. [VB]

199. Kadous A, Abdelgawad AA, Kanlic E. Deep venous thrombosis and pulmonary embolism after surgical treatment of ankle fractures: a case report and review of literature. *J Foot Ankle Surg*. 2012;51(4):457-463. [VB]

200. Makhdom AM, Garceau S, Dimentberg R. Fatal pulmonary embolism following Achilles tendon repair: a case report and a review of the literature. *Case Rep Orthop*. 2013;2013:401968. [VB]

201. Roberts DC, Warwick DJ. Venous thromboembolism following elbow, wrist and hand surgery: a review of the literature and prophylaxis guidelines. *J Hand Surg Br*. 2014;39(3):306-312. [VA]

202. Mathur M, Shafi I, Alkhouli M, Bashir R. Surgical hardware-related iatrogenic venous compression syndrome. *Vasc Med*. 2015;20(2):162-167. [VA]

203. Pannucci CJ, MacDonald JK, Ariyan S, et al. Benefits and risks of prophylaxis for deep venous thrombosis and pulmonary embolus in plastic surgery: a systematic review and meta-analysis of controlled trials and consensus conference. *Plast Reconstr Surg*. 2016;137(2):709-730. [IIIA]

204. Zareba P, Wu C, Agzarian J, Rodriguez D, Kearon C. Meta-analysis of randomized trials comparing combined compression and anticoagulation with either modality alone for prevention of venous thromboembolism after surgery. *Br J Surg*. 2014;101(9):1053-1062. [IA]

205. Gustafsson UO, Scott MJ, Schwenk W, et al. Guidelines for perioperative care in elective colonic surgery: Enhanced Recovery After Surgery (ERAS®) Society recommendations. *Clin Nutr*. 2012;31(6):783-800 18p. [IVA]

206. Nelson G, Altman AD, Nick A, et al. Guidelines for postoperative care in gynecologic/oncology surgery: Enhanced Recovery After Surgery (ERAS®) Society recommendations—part II. *Gynecol Oncol*. 2016;140(2):323-332. [IVA]

207. Nygren J, Thacker J, Carli F, et al. Guidelines for perioperative care in elective rectal/pelvic surgery: Enhanced Recovery After Surgery (ERAS®) Society recommendations. *Clin Nutr*. 2012;31(6):801-816. [IVA]

208. Skillman J, Thomas S. An audit of pressure sores caused by intermittent compression devices used to prevent venous thromboembolism. *J Perioper Pract*. 2011;21(12):418-420. [VB]

209. Huh J, Cho YB, Yang MK, Yoo YK, Kim DK. What influence does intermittent pneumatic compression of the lower limbs intraoperatively have on core hypothermia? *Surg Endosc*. 2013;27(6):2087-2093. [IC]

210. Boelig MM, Streiff MB, Hobson DB, Kraus PS, Pronovost PJ, Haut ER. Are sequential compression devices commonly associated with in-hospital falls? A myth-busters review using the patient safety net database. *J Patient Saf*. 2011;7(2):77-79. [IIIA]

211. Eppsteiner RW, Shin JJ, Johnson J, van Dam RM. Mechanical compression versus subcutaneous heparin therapy in postoperative and posttrauma patients: a systematic review and meta-analysis. *World J Surg*. 2010;34(1):10-19. [IB]

212. Pavon JM, Adam SS, Razouki ZA, et al. Effectiveness of intermittent pneumatic compression devices for venous thromboembolism prophylaxis in high-risk surgical patients: a systematic review. *J Arthroplasty*. 2016;31(2):524-532. [IIIA]

213. Arverud E, Azevedo J, Labruto F, Ackermann PW. Adjuvant compression therapy in orthopaedic surgery-an evidence-based review. *Eur Orthop Traumatol*. 2013;4(1):49-57. [VB]

214. Feng JP, Xiong YT, Fan ZQ, Yan LJ, Wang JY, Gu ZJ. Efficacy of intermittent pneumatic compression for venous thromboembolism prophylaxis in patients undergoing gynecologic surgery: a systematic review and meta-analysis. *Oncotarget*. 2017;8(12):20371-20379. [IIIB]

215. O'Connell S, Bashar K, Broderick BJ, et al. The use of intermittent pneumatic compression in orthopedic and neurosurgical postoperative patients. A systematic review and meta-analysis. *Ann Surg*. 2016;263(5):888-899. [IIIA]

216. Sadaghianloo N, Dardik A. The efficacy of intermittent pneumatic compression in the prevention of lower extremity deep venous thrombosis. *J Vasc Surg*. 2016;4(2):248-256. [IIIB]

217. Kakkos SK, Warwick D, Nicolaides AN, Stansby GP, Tsolakis IA. Combined (mechanical and pharmacological) modalities for the prevention of venous thromboembolism in joint replacement surgery. *J Bone Joint Surg Br*. 2012;94(6):729-734. [IIB]

218. Sobieraj DM, Coleman CI, Tongbram V, et al. Comparative effectiveness of combined pharmacologic and mechanical thromboprophylaxis versus either method alone in major orthopedic surgery: a systematic review and meta-analysis. *Pharmacotherapy*. 2013;33(3):275-283. [IIB]

219. Parry K, Sadeghi A, van der Horst S, Westerink J, Ruurda JP, van Hillegersberg R. Intermittent pneumatic compression in combination with low-molecular weight heparin in the prevention of venous thromboembolic events in esophageal cancer surgery. *J Surg Oncol*. 2017;115(2):181-185. [IIIB]

220. Delos Reyes AP, Partsch H, Mosti G, Obi A, Lurie F. Report from the 2013 meeting of the international compression club on advances and challenges of compression therapy. *J Vasc Surg Venous Lymphat Disord*. 2014;2(4):469-476. [VA]

221. Larkin BG, Mitchell KM, Petrie K. Translating evidence to practice for mechanical venous thromboembolism prophylaxis. *AORN J*. 2012;96(5):513-527. [VB]

222. Committee opinion no 610: chronic antithrombotic therapy and gynecologic surgery. *Obstet Gynecol*. 2014;124(4):856-862. [IVC]

223. Rahn DD, Mamik MM, Sanses TVD, et al. Venous thromboembolism prophylaxis in gynecologic surgery: a systematic review. *Obstet Gynecol*. 2011;118(5):1111-1125. [IIIA]

224. Gao J, Zhang Z, Li Z, et al. Two mechanical methods for thromboembolism prophylaxis after gynaecological pelvic surgery: a prospective, randomised study. *Chin Med J (Engl)*. 2012;125(23):4259-4263. [IB]

225. Morris RJ, Woodcock JP. Intermittent pneumatic compression or graduated compression stockings for deep vein thrombosis prophylaxis? A systematic review of direct clinical comparisons. *Ann Surg*. 2010;251(3):393-396. [IIIB]

226. Zhao JM, He ML, Xiao ZM, Li TS, Wu H, Jiang H. Different types of intermittent pneumatic compression devices for preventing venous thromboembolism in patients after total hip replacement. *Cochrane Database Syst Rev*. 2012;11:CD009543. [IIC]

227. Pour AE, Keshavarzi NR, Purtill JJ, Sharkey PF, Parvizi J. Is venous foot pump effective in prevention of thromboembolic disease after joint arthroplasty: a meta-analysis. *J Arthroplasty*. 2013;28(3):410-417. [IIA]

228. Dohm M, Williams KM, Novotny T. Micro-mobile foot compression device compared with pneumatic compression device. *Clin Orthop Relat Res*. 2011;469(6):1692-1700. [IB]

229. Pitto RP, Koh CK. Flowtron foot-pumps for prevention of venous thromboembolism in total hip and knee replacement. *J Orthop.* 2015;12(1):35-38. [IIIA]

230. Sakai T, Izumi M, Kumagai K, et al. Effects of a foot pump on the incidence of deep vein thrombosis after total knee arthroplasty in patients given edoxaban: a randomized controlled study. *Medicine.* 2016;95(1):e2247. [IB]

231. Wickham N, Gallus AS, Walters BNJ, Wilson A; NHMRC VTE Prevention Guideline Adaptation Committee. Prevention of venous thromboembolism in patients admitted to Australian hospitals: summary of National Health and Medical Research Council clinical practice guideline. *Intern Med J.* 2012;42(6):698-708. [IVA]

232. Hou H, Yao Y, Zheng K, et al. Does intermittent pneumatic compression increase the risk of pulmonary embolism in deep venous thrombosis after joint surgery? *Blood Coagul Fibrinolysis.* 2016;27(3):246-251. [IIIB]

233. Guideline for prevention of unplanned patient hypothermia. In: *Guidelines for Perioperative Practice.* Denver, CO: AORN, Inc; 2017:567-590. [IVA]

234. Guideline for sterile technique. In: *Guidelines for Perioperative Practice.* Denver, CO: AORN, Inc; 2017:75-104. [IVA]

235. Levy YD, Hardwick ME, Copp SN, Rosen AS, Colwell CWJ. Thrombosis incidence in unilateral vs simultaneous bilateral total knee arthroplasty with compression device prophylaxis. *J Arthroplasty.* 2013;28(3):474-478. [IIIB]

236. Morris JK, Fincham BM. Intermittent pneumatic compression for venous thromboembolism prophylaxis in total knee arthroplasty. *Orthopedics.* 2012;35(12):e1716-e1721. [IIB]

237. Guideline for minimally invasive surgery. In: *Guidelines for Perioperative Practice.* Denver, CO: AORN, Inc; 2017:629-658. [IVA]

238. Frisius J, Ebeling M, Karst M, et al. Prevention of venous thromboembolic complications with and without intermittent pneumatic compression in neurosurgical cranial procedures using intraoperative magnetic resonance imaging. A retrospective analysis. *Clin Neurol Neurosurg.* 2015;133:46-54. [IIIB]

239. Maybody M, Taslakian B, Durack JC, et al. Feasibility of intermittent pneumatic compression for venous thromboembolism prophylaxis during magnetic resonance imaging-guided interventions. *Eur J Radiol.* 2015;84(4):668-670. [IIIB]

240. Ritsema DF, Watson JM, Stiteler AP, Nguyen MM. Sequential compression devices in postoperative urologic patients: an observational trial and survey study on the influence of patient and hospital factors on compliance. *BMC Urol.* 2013;13:20. [IIIB]

241. Obi AT, Alvarez R, Reames BN, et al. A prospective evaluation of standard versus battery-powered sequential compression devices in postsurgical patients. *Am J Surg.* 2015;209(4):675-681. [IB]

242. Sobieraj-Teague M, Hirsh J, Yip G, et al. Randomized controlled trial of a new portable calf compression device (Venowave) for prevention of venous thrombosis in high-risk neurosurgical patients. *J Thromb Haemost.* 2012;10(2):229-235. [IB]

243. Colwell CWJ, Froimson MI, Anseth SD, et al. A mobile compression device for thrombosis prevention in hip and knee arthroplasty. *J Bone Joint Surg Am.* 2014;96(3):177-183. [IIA]

244. Haynes J, Barrack RL, Nam D. Mobile pump deep vein thrombosis prophylaxis: just say no to drugs. *Bone Joint J.* 2017;99-B(1 Suppl A):8-13. [IIIB]

245. Nam D, Nunley RM, Johnson SR, Keeney JA, Barrack RL. Mobile compression devices and aspirin for VTE prophylaxis following simultaneous bilateral total knee arthroplasty. *J Arthroplasty.* 2015;30(3):447-450. [IIIB]

246. Hardwick ME, Pulido PA, Colwell CWJ. A mobile compression device compared with low-molecular-weight heparin for prevention of venous thromboembolism in total hip arthroplasty. *Orthop Nurs.* 2011;30(5):312-316. [IA]

247. Craigie S, Tsui JF, Agarwal A, Sandset PM, Guyatt GH, Tikkinen KAO. Adherence to mechanical thromboprophylaxis after surgery: a systematic review and meta-analysis. *Thromb Res.* 2015;136(4):723-726. [IIIA]

248. Kim JH, Kim WI, Kim JY, Choe WJ. Peroneal nerve palsy after compression stockings application. *Saudi J Anaesth.* 2016;10(4):462-464. [VB]

249. Guzelkucuk U, Skempes D, Kumnerddee W. Common peroneal nerve palsy caused by compression stockings after surgery. *Am J Phys Med Rehabil.* 2014;93(7):609-611. [VB]

250. Hinderland MD, Ng A, Paden MH, Stone PA. Lateral leg compartment syndrome caused by ill-fitting compression stocking placed for deep vein thrombosis prophylaxis during surgery: a case report. *J Foot Ankle Surg.* 2011;50(5):616-619. [VB]

251. Thompson A, Walter S, Brunton LR, et al. Anti-embolism stockings and proximal indentation. *Br J Nurs.* 2011;20(22):1426-1430. [IIIB]

252. Bowling K, Ratcliffe C, Townsend J, Kirkpatrick U. Clinical thromboembolic detterrent stockings application: Are thromboembolic detterrent stockings in practice matching manufacturers application guidelines. *Phlebology.* 2015;30(3):200-203. [IIIB]

253. Sachdeva A, Dalton M, Amaragiri SV, Lees T. Graduated compression stockings for prevention of deep vein thrombosis. *Cochrane Database Syst Rev.* 2014;(12):CD001484. [IA]

254. Mandavia R, Shalhoub J, Head K, Davies AH. The additional benefit of graduated compression stockings to pharmacologic thromboprophylaxis in the prevention of venous thromboembolism in surgical inpatients. *J Vasc Surg Venous Lymphat Disord.* 2015;3(4):447-455.e1. [IB]

255. Sajid MS, Desai M, Morris RW, Hamilton G. Knee length versus thigh length graduated compression stockings for prevention of deep vein thrombosis in postoperative surgical patients. *Cochrane Database Syst Rev.* 2012;(5):CD007162. [IB]

256. Wade R, Paton F, Rice S, et al. Thigh length versus knee length antiembolism stockings for the prevention of deep vein thrombosis in postoperative surgical patients; a systematic review and network meta-analysis. *BMJ Open.* 2016;6(2):e009456. [IA]

257. Wade R, Sideris E, Paton F, et al. Graduated compression stockings for the prevention of deep-vein thrombosis in postoperative surgical patients: a systematic review and economic model with a value of information analysis. *Health Technol Assess.* 2015;19(98):1-220. [IA]

258. Loomba RS, Arora RR, Chandrasekar S, Shah PH. Thigh-length versus knee-length compression stockings for deep vein thrombosis prophylaxis in the inpatient setting. *Blood Coagul Fibrinolysis.* 2012;23(2):168-171. [IIB]

259. Feist WR, Andrade D, Nass L. Problems with measuring compression device performance in preventing deep vein thrombosis. *Thromb Res.* 2011;128(3):207-209. [VB]

260. Ayhan H, Iyigun E, Ince S, Can MF, Hatipoglu S, Saglam M. A randomised clinical trial comparing the patient comfort and efficacy of three different graduated compression stockings in the prevention of postoperative deep vein thrombosis. *J Clin Nurs.* 2015;24(15-16):2247-2257. [IB]

261. Lattimer CR, Azzam M, Kalodiki E, Makris GC, Geroulakos G. Compression stockings significantly improve hemodynamic performance in post-thrombotic syndrome irrespective of class or length. *J Vasc Surg.* 2013;58(1):158-165. [IIB]

262. Bell BR, Bastien PE, Douketis JD; Thrombosis Canada. Prevention of venous thromboembolism in the Enhanced Recovery After Surgery (ERAS) setting: an evidence-based review. *Can J Anaesth.* 2015;62(2):194-202. [VB]

263. Glassou EN, Pedersen AB, Hansen TB. Risk of re-admission, reoperation, and mortality within 90 days of total hip and knee arthroplasty in fast-track departments in Denmark from 2005 to 2011. *Acta Orthop.* 2014;85(5):493-500. [IIIA]

264. Husted H, Otte KS, Kristensen BB, Orsnes T, Wong C, Kehlet H. Low risk of thromboembolic complications after fast-track hip and knee arthroplasty. *Acta Orthop.* 2010;81(5):599-605. [IIIB]

265. Jorgensen CC, Jacobsen MK, Soeballe K, et al. Thromboprophylaxis only during hospitalisation in fast-track hip and knee arthroplasty, a prospective cohort study. *BMJ Open.* 2013;3(12):e003965. [IIIA]

266. Jorgensen CC, Kehlet H; Lundbeck Foundation Centre for Fast-track Hip and Knee Replacement Collaborative Group. Early thromboembolic events. *Thromb Res.* 2016;138:37-42. [IIIB]

267. Khan SK, Malviya A, Muller SD, et al. Reduced short-term complications and mortality following enhanced recovery primary hip and knee arthroplasty: results from 6,000 consecutive procedures. *Acta Orthop.* 2014;85(1):26-31. [IIIB]

268. Wang Z, Chen Q, Ye M, Shi G, Zhang B. Active ankle movement may prevent deep vein thrombosis in patients undergoing lower limb surgery. *Ann Vasc Surg.* 2016;32:65-72. [IB]

269. Shimizu Y, Kamada H, Sakane M, et al. A novel apparatus for active leg exercise improves venous flow in the lower extremity. *J Sports Med Phys Fitness.* 2016;56(12):1592-1597. [IIC]

270. DailyMed. US National Library of Medicine. https://dailymed.nlm.nih.gov/dailymed/. Accessed August 28, 2017.

271. Mahan CE, Spyropoulos AC. ASHP therapeutic position statement on the role of pharmacotherapy in preventing venous thromboembolism in hospitalized patients. *Am J Health Syst Pharm.* 2012;69(24):2174-2190. [IVB]

272. Horlocker TT, Wedel DJ, Rowlingson JC, et al. Regional anesthesia in the patient receiving antithrombotic or thrombolytic therapy: American Society of Regional Anesthesia and Pain Medicine Evidence-Based Guidelines (Third Edition). *Reg Anesth Pain Med.* 2010;35(1):64-101. [IVA]

273. Karuppiah SV, Johnstone AJ. Skin necrosis associated with thromboprophylaxis after total knee replacement. *Case Rep Orthop.* 2014;2014:139218. [VB]

274. Sadideen H, O'Callaghan JM, Navidi M, Sayegh M. Educating surgical patients to reduce the risk of venous thromboembolism: an audit of an effective strategy. *JRSM Short Rep.* 2011;2(12):97. [IIB]

275. Haymes A. Venous thromboembolism: patient awareness and education in the pre-operative assessment clinic. *J Thromb Thrombolysis.* 2016;41(3):459-463. [IIIB]

276. Keiter JE, Johns D, Rockwell WB. Importance of postoperative hydration and lower extremity elevation in preventing deep venous thrombosis in full abdomino-plasty: a report on 450 consecutive cases over a 37-year period. *Aesthet Surg J.* 2015;35(7):839-841. [IIIB]

277. Guyatt GH, Akl EA, Crowther M, Gutterman DD, Schünemann HJ. Executive summary: Antithrombotic Therapy and Prevention of Thrombosis, 9th ed: American College of Chest Physicians Evidence-Based Clinical Practice Guidelines. *Chest.* 2012;141(2 Suppl):7S-47S. [IVA]

278. Alzoubi KH, Khassawneh BY, Obeidat B, Asfoor SS, Al-azzam SI. Awareness of patients who undergo cesarean section about venous thromboembolism prophylaxis. *J Vasc Nurs.* 2013;31(1):15-20. [IIIA]

279. He ML, Xiao ZM, Lei M, Li TS, Wu H, Liao J. Continuous passive motion for preventing venous thromboembolism after total knee arthroplasty. *Cochrane Database Syst Rev.* 2012;1:CD008207. [IA]

280. Lobastov K, Barinov V, Laberko L, Obolensky V, Boyarintsev V, Rodoman G. Electrical calf muscle stimulation with Veinoplus device in postoperative venous thromboembolism prevention. *Int Angiol.* 2014;33(1):42-49. [IIB]

281. Guideline for Medication Safety. In: *Guidelines for Perioperative Practice.* Denver, CO: AORN, Inc; 2017:295-333. [IVB]

282. Eisenstein DH. Anticoagulation management in the ambulatory surgical setting. *AORN J.* 2012;95(4):510-521. [VB]

283. Standards of perioperative nursing. In: *Guidelines for Perioperative Practice.* Denver, CO: AORN, Inc; 2015:693-732. https://www.aorn.org/aorn-org/guidelines/clinical-resources/aorn-standards. Accessed August 24, 2017. [IVC]

284. *State Operations Manual Appendix A—Survey Protocol, Regulations and Interpretive Guidelines for Hospitals.* Rev 151; 2015 Centers for Medicare & Medicaid Services. https://www.cms.gov/Regulations-and-Guidance/Guidance/Manuals/downloads/som107ap_a_hospitals.pdf. Accessed August 24, 2017.

285. *State Operations Manual Appendix L—Guidance for Surveyors: Ambulatory Surgical Centers.* Rev. 137; 2015. Centers for Medicare & Medicaid Services. https://www.cms.gov/Regulations-and-Guidance/Guidance/Manuals/downloads/som107ap_l_ambulatory.pdf. Accessed August 24, 2017.

286. 42 CFR 482. Conditions of participation for hospitals. 2011. Government Publishing Office. https://www.gpo.gov/fdsys/granule/CFR-2011-title42-vol5/CFR-2011-title42-vol5-part482. Accessed August 24, 2017.

287. 42 CFR 416. Ambulatory surgical services. 2011. Government Publishing Office. https://www.gpo.gov/fdsys/granule/CFR-2011-title42-vol3/CFR-2011-title42-vol3-part416. Accessed August 24, 2017.

288. RC.01.01.01: The hospital maintains complete and accurate medical records for each individual patient. In: *The Joint Commission Comprehensive Accreditation and Certification Manual.* E-dition. Oakbrook Terrace, IL: The Joint Commission; 2016.

289. MS.16: Medical record maintenance. In: *National Integrated Accreditation for Healthcare Organizations (NIAHO): Interpretive Guidelines and Surveyor Guidance.* Version 11. Milford, OH: DNV-GL Healthcare; 2014:37. http://cms.ipressroom.com.s3.amazonaws.com/107/files/20146/DNVGL+Healthcare+-+NIAHO+Acc

reditation+Requirements+and+Interpretive+Guidelines+-+Rev+11.pdf. Accessed August 24, 2017.

290. RC.01.01.01: The organization maintains complete and accurate clinical records. In: *The Joint Commission Comprehensive Accreditation and Certification Manual.* E-dition. Oakbrook Terrace, IL: The Joint Commission; 2016.

291. Clinical records and health information. In: *Accreditation Handbook for Ambulatory Health Care.* Skokie, IL: Accreditation Association for Ambulatory Health Care, Inc; 2016:51-53. https://www.aaahc.org/Global/Handbooks/2016/HB16_FNL-interactive_v2.pdf. Accessed August 24, 2017.

292. Medical records: operating room records. In: *Regular Standards and Checklist for Accreditation of Ambulatory Surgery Facilities.* Version 14.4. Gurnee, IL: American Association for Accreditation of Ambulatory Surgery Facilities, Inc; 2016:60-63.

293. Medical records: procedure room records. In: *Regular Standards and Checklist for Accreditation of Ambulatory Surgery Facilities.* 3rd ed. Gurnee, IL: American Association for Accreditation of Ambulatory Surgery Facilities, Inc; 2011:64-66. https://www.aaaasf.org/docs/default-source/accreditation/standards/standards-manual-and-checklist-v3-(obp).pdf?sfvrsn=5. Accessed August 24, 2017.

294. Miller JA. Use and wear of anti-embolism stockings: a clinical audit of surgical patients. *Int Wound J.* 2011;8(1):74-83. [IIIB]

295. Jordan C, Thomas MB, Evans ML, Green A. Public policy on competency: how will nursing address this complex issue? *J Contin Educ Nurs.* 2008;39(2):86-91. [VB]

296. HR.01.05.03: Staff participate in ongoing education and training. In: *The Joint Commission Comprehensive Accreditation and Certification Manual.* E-dition. Oakbrook Terrace, IL: The Joint Commission; 2016.

297. MS.10: Continuing education. In: *National Integrated Accreditation for Healthcare Organizations (NIAHO): Interpretive Guidelines and Surveyor Guidance.* Version 11. Milford, OH: DNV-GL Healthcare; 2014:30. http://cms.ipressroom.com.s3.amazonaws.com/107/files/20146/DNVGL+Healthcare+-+NIAHO+Accreditation+Requirements+and+Interpretive+Guidelines+-+Rev+11.pdf. Accessed August 24, 2017.

298. HR.01.05.03: Staff participate in ongoing education and training. In: *The Joint Commission Comprehensive Accreditation and Certification Manual.* E-dition. Oakbrook Terrace, IL: The Joint Commission; 2016.

299. Governance. In: *Accreditation Handbook for Ambulatory Health Care.* Skokie, IL: Accreditation Association for Ambulatory Health Care, Inc; 2016:33-40. https://www.aaahc.org/Global/Handbooks/2016/HB16_FNL-interactive_v2.pdf. Accessed August 24, 2017.

300. Personnel: Personnel records; individual personnel files. In: *Regular Standards and Checklist for Accreditation of Ambulatory Surgery Facilities.* Version 14.4. Gurnee, IL: American Association for Accreditation of Ambulatory Surgery Facilities, Inc; 2016:74-75.

301. PI.03.01.01: The hospital improves performance on an ongoing basis. In: *The Joint Commission Comprehensive Accreditation and Certification Manual.* E-dition. Oakbrook Terrace, IL: The Joint Commission; 2016.

302. QM.1: Quality management system. In: *National Integrated Accreditation for Healthcare Organizations (NIAHO): Interpretive Guidelines and Surveyor Guidance.* Version 11. Milford, OH: DNV-GL Healthcare; 2014:10-17. http://cms.ipressroom.com.s3.amazonaws.com/107/files/20146/DNVGL+Healthcare+-+NIAHO+Accreditation+Requirements+and+Interpretive+Guidelines+-+Rev+11.pdf. Accessed August 24, 2017.

303. PI.03.01.01: The organization improves performance. In: *The Joint Commission Comprehensive Accreditation and Certification Manual.* E-dition. Oakbrook Terrace, IL: The Joint Commission; 2016.

304. Quality management and improvement. In: *Accreditation Handbook for Ambulatory Health Care.* Skokie, IL: Accreditation Association for Ambulatory Health Care, Inc; 2016:46-50. https://www.aaahc.org/Global/Handbooks/2016/HB16_FNL-interactive_v2.pdf. Accessed August 24, 2017.

305. Quality assessment/quality improvement: Quality improvement. In: *Regular Standards and Checklist for Accreditation of Ambulatory Surgery Facilities.* Version 14.4. Gurnee, IL: American Association for Accreditation of Ambulatory Surgery Facilities, Inc; 2016:64.

306. Quality assessment/quality improvement: unanticipated operative sequelae In: *Regular Standards and Checklist for Accreditation of Ambulatory Surgery Facilities.* Version 14.4. Gurnee, IL: American Association for Accreditation of Ambulatory Surgery Facilities, Inc; 2016:66-69.

307. *PSI 90: Patient Safety for Selected Indicators.* Technical Specifications. Rockville, MD: Agency for Healthcare Research and Quality; 2015.

308. Venous thromboembolism national hospital inpatient quality measures. In: *Specifications Manual for National Hospital Inpatient Quality Measures.* Version 5.2a. Oakbrook Terrace, IL: The Joint Commission; 2016:VTE-1. https://www.jointcommission.org/assets/1/6/HIQR_SpecsManual_v52a.zip. Accessed August 24, 2017.

Acknowledgements

LEAD AUTHOR
Amber Wood, MSN, RN, CNOR, CIC, FAPIC
Senior Perioperative Practice Specialist
AORN Nursing Department
Denver, Colorado

CONTRIBUTING AUTHOR
Ramona L. Conner, MSN, RN, CNOR, FAAN
Editor-in-Chief, Guidelines for Perioperative Practice
AORN Nursing Department
Denver, Colorado

The authors and AORN thank Heather A. Hohenberger, MSN, RN, CIC, CNOR, CPHQ, FAPIC, System Perioperative Quality Improvement Consultant, Indiana University Health, Indianapolis; Jocelyn M. Chalquist, BSN, RN, CNOR, Surgical Services Educator, Aurora Medical Center-Kenosha, Kenosha, Wisconsin; Barbara L. Nalley, MSN, CRNP, CNOR, Manager, Anne Arundel Medical Group, Annapolis, Maryland; Marie A. Bashaw, DNP, RN, NEA-BC, CNOR, Assistant Professor, Wright State University College of Nursing and Health, Dayton, Ohio; Janice Neil, PhD, RN, CNE, Associate Professor, College of Nursing, East Carolina University, Greenville, North Carolina; Diana L. Wadlund, MSN, ACNP-C, CRNFA, Nurse Practitioner, Paoli Hospital, Paoli, Pennsylvania; Lynn Reed, DNP, MBA, CRNA, FNAP, Senior Director, Professional Practice, American Association of Nurse Anesthetists, Des Plaines, Illinois;

VENOUS THROMBOEMBOLISM

David Urbach, MD, MSc, Clinical Epidemiology, University Health Network, Toronto, Ontario, Canada; Dawn Yost, MSN, RN, CNOR, CSSM, Manager of Training & Development, Surgical Services, West Virginia University Medicine-Ruby Memorial Hospital, Morgantown; Carrie Simpson, BSN, BA, RN-BC, CNOR, Owner & Principal Consultant, CS Perioperative Education Solution, New Orleans, Louisiana; Vangie Dennis, BSN, RN, CNOR, CMLSO, Director of Patient Care Practice, Emory Healthcare and Ambulatory Surgery Centers, Atlanta, Georgia; Jay Bowers, BSN, RN, CNOR, TNCC, Clinical Educator, West Virginia University Healthcare, Morgantown; and Esther Johnstone, DNP, RN, CNOR, Perioperative Practice Specialist, AORN Nursing Department, Denver, Colorado, for their assistance in developing this guideline.

PUBLICATION HISTORY

Originally published March 2011 as "Recommended practices for prevention of deep vein thrombosis" in *Perioperative Standards and Recommended Practices* online.

Reformatted September 2012 for publication in *Perioperative Standards and Recommended Practices*, 2013 edition.

Minor editing revisions made in November 2014 for publication as "Guideline for prevention of deep vein thrombosis" in *Guidelines for Perioperative Practice*, 2015 edition.

Revised November 2017 for publication in *Guidelines for Perioperative Practice* online.

PATIENT CARE

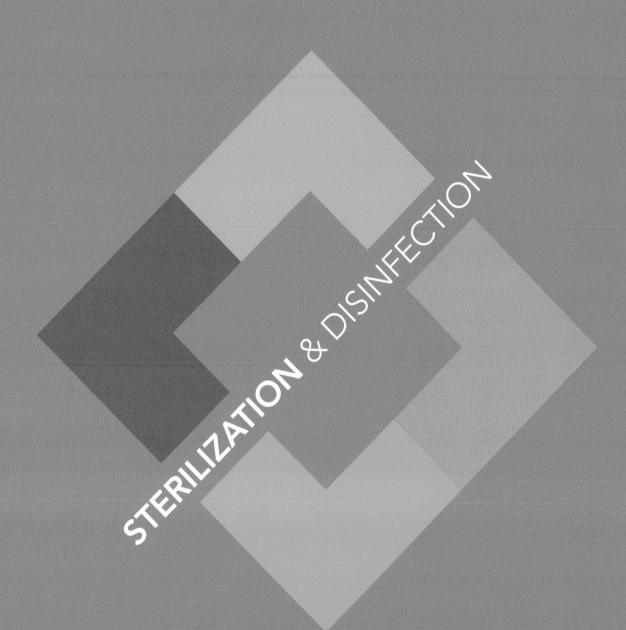

STERILIZATION & DISINFECTION

GUIDELINE FOR PROCESSING FLEXIBLE ENDOSCOPES

The Guideline for Processing Flexible Endoscopes has been approved by the AORN Guidelines Advisory Board. It was presented as a proposed guideline for comments by members and others. The guideline is effective February 1, 2016. The recommendations in the guideline are intended to be achievable and represent what is believed to be an optimal level of practice. Policies and procedures will reflect variations in practice settings and/or clinical situations that determine the degree to which the guideline can be implemented. AORN recognizes the many diverse settings in which perioperative nurses practice; therefore, this guideline is adaptable to all areas where operative or other invasive procedures may be performed.

Purpose

This document provides guidance to perioperative, endoscopy, and sterile processing personnel for processing all types of reusable flexible endoscopes and accessories. Recommendations are provided for design and construction of the endoscopy suite as well as for controlling and maintaining the environment to support processing activities. Guidance is provided for maintaining records of processing for traceability and for quality assurance measures related to processing flexible endoscopes and accessories.

Patients have a right to undergo endoscopic procedures in a safe, clean environment where personnel adhere to consistent, evidence-based practices for processing every flexible endoscope every time care is provided. It is essential that the risk of patient-to-patient transmission of infection via flexible endoscopes be minimized as much as is reasonably possible.

Infections related to endoscopy procedures may be caused by endogenous microorganisms that colonize the mucosal surfaces of the gastrointestinal or respiratory tract and gain access to the bloodstream or other sterile tissues as a consequence of the procedure.[1] Endogenous infections include infections such as cholangitis that may occur after endoscopic procedures of the biliary tract or pneumonia that may occur after endoscopic procedures of the respiratory tract.[1]

Infections related to endoscopy procedures may also be caused by exogenous microorganisms that are transmitted from previous patients or from the inanimate environment by contaminated endoscopes or accessories.[1] The US Food and Drug Administration (FDA) has identified two recurrent themes as contributing to persistent bronchoscope contamination and transmission of exogenous infection:

- a failure to meticulously follow the manufacturer's written instructions for processing and
- the continued use of bronchoscopes despite issues with integrity, maintenance, and mechanical problems.[2]

If flexible endoscopes are not correctly processed, exposure to body fluids and tissue remnants from previous patients may result in the transmission of pathogens to large numbers of subsequent patients.[3] In a systematic search of the literature to clarify the epidemiology of *Klebsiella* species in endoscopy-associated outbreaks, Gastmeier and Vonberg[4] found that insufficient processing was the main reason for subsequent pathogen transmission. The authors concluded that strict adherence to guidelines for processing flexible endoscopes in combination with alertness to the potential for pathogen transmission after endoscopy procedures was required, and that additional studies were needed to determine the true risk of pathogen transmission via flexible endoscopes.

Because of the many different types of flexible endoscopes and the differences in flexible endoscope construction, not all steps discussed in this guideline (eg, leak testing) will apply to all endoscopes; however, some steps (eg, manual cleaning) will apply to all flexible endoscopes. The European Society of Gastrointestinal Endoscopy (ESGE) has proposed a classification of endoscope families[5] based on similar characteristics, including the number, construction, and purpose of the different endoscope channels and their clinical applications.

- Group 1 endoscopes are typically intended for use in the gastrointestinal tract. This group includes endoscopes that have air/water channels, have an instrument/suction channel, and may have an additional instrument or waterjet channel. Examples of Group 1 endoscopes are gastroscopes, colonoscopes, and duodenoscopes with an encapsulated elevator channel.
- Group 2 endoscopes are also intended for use in the gastrointestinal tract. This group includes endoscopes that have air/water channels, have an instrument/suction channel, and may have an additional instrument channel. Group 2 endoscopes also may have an elevator channel and up to two control channels for balloon functions. Examples of Group 2 endoscopes are duodenoscopes with an open elevator channel, echoendoscopes used for endoscopic ultrasound, and enteroscopes.
- Group 3 endoscopes are used in bronchoscopy, otorhinolaryngology applications, gynecology, and urology. This group includes endoscopes with only one channel system for biopsy, irrigation, and suction or endoscopes without any channel. Examples of Group 3 endoscopes are bronchoscopes, cystoscopes, laryngoscopes, and nasendoscopes.

In addition to following the guidance provided in this document, it is critically important for individuals who are responsible for processing Group 1, 2, or 3 flexible endoscopes to follow the manufacturer's instructions for use (IFU), and the IFU for all products and equipment used for processing flexible endoscopes. Processing flexible endoscopes is a complex cycle of multiple steps that includes point-of-use precleaning, transporting, leak testing, cleaning, inspecting, high-level disinfection (HLD) or liquid chemical sterilization, packaging and sterilization, storage, and use (Figure 1).

The complex design of flexible endoscopes increases the efficiency and effectiveness of endoscopic procedures; however, it creates enormous challenges for effective processing.[3] Some parts of the endoscope may be difficult or impossible to access, and effective cleaning of all areas of flexible duodenoscopes may not be possible.[6]

Although single-use devices may meet the quality of reusable endoscopic devices and may provide an option for reducing the risk for transmission of infection,[7-10] a discussion of the potential benefits of single-use flexible endoscopes is outside the scope of this guideline. The use of airborne, contact, or droplet precautions, the various chemicals used as high-level disinfectants or liquid chemical sterilants, the methods used for HLD or low-temperature sterilization, the methods for determining water quality used for processing flexible endoscopes and accessories, the protocols for microbiological surveillance of flexible endoscopes, the management of processing failures, sharps and medication safety, and the ergonomic injuries associated with the endoscopy environment are also outside of the scope of this guideline.

A full discussion of the design and construction of endoscopy suites in hospitals and outpatient facilities, the design of ventilation systems for controlling personnel exposure limits to chemicals used in the endoscopy suite, and the performance and use requirements for eyewash and shower equipment are outside of the scope of this document. However, because the design of the endoscopy suite and the procedures performed in the facility affect the processing of flexible endoscopes, some recommendations have been provided relative to procedure rooms and other elements of the endoscopy suite.

Evidence Review

A medical librarian conducted a systematic search of the databases Ovid MEDLINE®, EBSCO CINAHL®, and Scopus® as well as of the Ovid Cochrane Database of Systematic Reviews. Search results were limited to literature published in English from 1994 through 2014. At the time of the initial search, the librarian established weekly alerts on the search topics and until October 2015, presented relevant results to the lead author. The author and the librarian also identified relevant guidelines and guidance from government agencies, professional organizations, and standards-setting bodies. Finally, during the development of this guideline, the author requested supplementary searches for topics not included in the original search as well as articles and other sources that were discovered during the evidence-appraisal process.

Search terms included the subject headings *endoscopes, disinfection, decontamination, sterilization, disinfectants, detergents, biofilms, infection control, cross-infection, equipment contamination, occupational exposure, protective clothing,* and *hypersensitivity.* Subject headings and key words for specific types of endoscopes, bacteria, disinfectants, and protective devices also were included, as were headings and terms related to the concepts of endoscope storage, methods of reprocessing, disinfection monitoring, infection transmission, disposable and reusable equipment, occupational allergies and injuries, and air pollution and ventilation. Complete search strategies are available upon request.

Excluded were non-peer-reviewed or retracted publications and evidence specific to the mechanism of action or health hazards associated with specific high-level disinfectants or liquid chemical sterilants, rigid endoscopic instrumentation, endoscopic medical treatment protocols, techniques, patient management, or functional design of flexible endoscopes.

In total, 1,257 research and non-research sources of evidence were identified for possible inclusion, and of these, 418 were cited in the guidance document (Figure 2).

Articles identified by the search were provided to the lead author and an evidence appraiser. The lead author and evidence appraiser reviewed and critically appraised each article using the AORN Research or Non-Research Evidence Appraisal Tools as appropriate. The literature was independently evaluated and appraised according to the strength and quality of the evidence. Each article was then assigned an appraisal score. The appraisal score is noted in brackets after each reference, as applicable.

The collective evidence supporting each intervention within a specific recommendation was summarized and the AORN Evidence Rating Model was used to rate the strength of the evidence. Factors considered in the review of the collective evidence were the quality of the evidence, the quantity of similar evidence on a given topic, and the consistency of evidence supporting a recommendation. The evidence rating is noted in brackets after each intervention.

FIGURE 1. FLEXIBLE ENDOSCOPE PROCESSING CYCLE

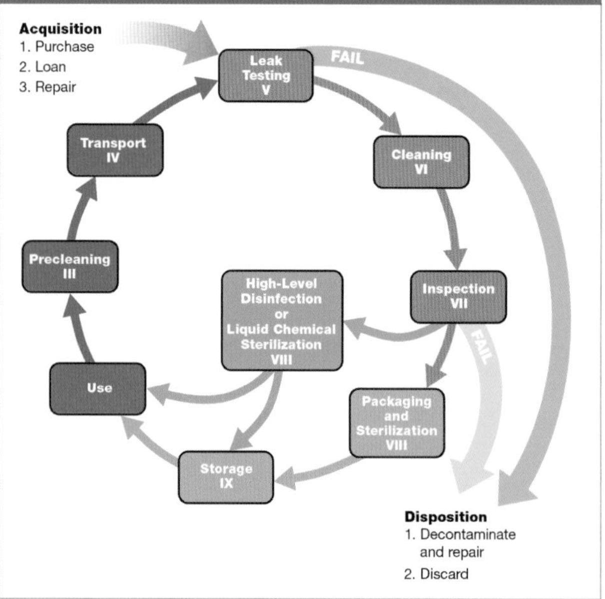

Roman numerals indicate the recommendation number where detailed guidance is provided.

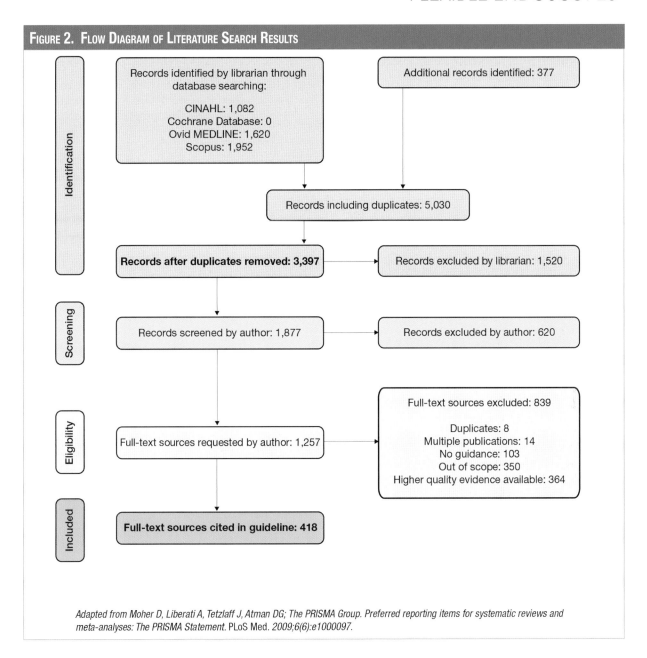

Figure 2. Flow Diagram of Literature Search Results

Adapted from Moher D, Liberati A, Tetzlaff J, Atman DG; The PRISMA Group. Preferred reporting items for systematic reviews and meta-analyses: The PRISMA Statement. PLoS Med. 2009;6(6):e1000097.

Note: *The evidence summary table is available at http://www.aorn.org/evidencetables/.*

Editor's note: *MEDLINE is a registered trademark of the US National Library of Medicine's Medical Literature Analysis and Retrieval System, Bethesda, MD. CINAHL, Cumulative Index to Nursing and Allied Health Literature, is a registered trademark of EBSCO Industries, Birmingham, AL. Scopus is a registered trademark of Elsevier B.V., Amsterdam, The Netherlands.*

Recommendation I

Flexible endoscopes should be processed in an area designed and constructed to support processing activities.[1,11-19]

The endoscopy suite consists of a minimum of three functional areas: procedure room(s), processing room(s),

and patient care area(s).[11] The design of the endoscopy suite, and the procedures performed in the facility affect processing of flexible endoscopes.

The collective evidence supports processing flexible endoscopes in an area designed and constructed for processing activities.[1,11-19]

The benefits are that construction and design to support processing activities may improve efficiency, help to reduce the risk of cross contamination, and provide a safe work environment. The reader should refer to the Facility Guidelines Institute (FGI) *Guidelines for Design and Construction of Hospitals and Outpatient Facilities*[11] for additional guidance.

I.a.   Except for precleaning processes performed at the point of use, endoscope processing should occur in a room where only processing activities are performed and that is physically separated from locations where patient care activities are performed.[12,14,16-18,20-22] *[1: Strong Evidence]*

Limiting endoscope processing activities to designated processing rooms may help prevent contamination of procedure rooms and patient care areas.[22]

I.b.   Endoscope processing may occur in a single endoscopy processing room[14] or in two separate rooms (ie, decontamination room, clean workroom) as shown in Figure 3.[11] *[3: Moderate Evidence]*

The minimum standard for design and construction of hospitals and outpatient care facilities is a single endoscopy processing room containing both decontamination and clean areas.[23]

I.b.1   During the infection control risk assessment, a multidisciplinary team that includes infection preventionists, endoscopy and perioperative RNs, sterile processing personnel, endoscopists, and other involved personnel should determine the potential harms compared with the benefits of performing decontamination and clean activities in separate rooms. *[3: Moderate Evidence]*

Having separate decontamination and clean rooms may avoid the risk of cross contamination from multiple individuals performing both clean and contaminated processing activities in a single area.[23,24]

I.b.2. The endoscopy processing room should include a door[11] that provides access to and from the decontamination area or decontamination room[12] and a separate door that provides access to and from the clean area or clean workroom.[25]

- Automatic sliding doors or foot-operated doors may be used.[21]
- When endoscope processing activities will occur in two separate rooms, either a door or a pass-through window should be provided from the decontamination room to the clean workroom.[12,26]

[2: High Evidence]

Doors to the decontamination area and clean area help contain contaminants within the processing room and help prevent cross contamination.[25] Automatic sliding doors and foot-operated doors facilitate hands-free movement of flexible endoscopes and other items to and from the endoscopy processing room.

I.b.3. An endoscopy processing room with a one-room design should provide

- a minimum of 3 ft (0.9 m) between the decontamination area and the clean work area[11,14] and
- either a separating wall or a barrier that extends a minimum of 4 ft (1.2 m) above the sink rim to separate soiled work areas from clean work areas.[14,23]

[3: Moderate Evidence]

Cross contamination can result when soiled items are placed in close proximity to clean items or are placed on surfaces upon which clean items are later placed. Separation of the decontamination area from the clean area minimizes the potential for contamination of clean and processed flexible endoscopes.[12,13,16,22,23,27]

Hota et al[28] demonstrated that contaminated water droplets had the ability to travel a distance of 39.4 inches (1 m). There is no evidence to indicate that contaminated water droplets from endoscope cleaning activities would be dispersed farther than 39.4 inches (1 m). It is unlikely that microorganisms would be disseminated by air over longer distances because they would be contained within water droplets.[23]

Separating soiled and clean work areas by a distance of at least 3 ft (0.9 m) aligns with current recommendations from the Centers for Disease Control and Prevention (CDC) that patients who require droplet precautions should be placed at least 3 ft from other patients.[29]

FIGURE 3. EXAMPLES OF ENDOSCOPY PROCESSING ROOM DESIGN

Endoscopy Processing Room - One-Room Design

Decontamination Area   Clean Area

Endoscopy Processing Room - Two-Room Design: Decontamination Room and Clean Workroom

Decontamination Room   Clean Workroom

➤ - Soiled receiving
1 - Handwashing station
2 - Eyewash station
3 - Personal protective equipment cabinet
4 - Decontamination sink (3 basins)
5 - Supply cabinet
6 - Work table
7 - Mechanical processor
8 - Steam sterilizer
9 - Low-temperature sterilizer
10 - Pass-through window ➤
11 - Trash
12 - Linen
➤ - Processed endoscopes

Note: These examples are conceptual illustrations of one- and two-room design, equipment placement, and traffic flow. They are not intended to represent complete schematic designs.

TABLE 1. HVAC DESIGN PARAMETERS FOR ENDOSCOPY SUITES

Functional area	Minimum total air changes per hour	Settings for airflow patterns (pressure)	Humidity	Temperature
Endoscopy processing room - One-room design	10	NR	Maximum 60%	60° F to 73° F (16° C to 23° C)
Endoscopy processing room - Two-room design Decontamination room	10	Negative	Maximum 60%	60° F to 73° F (16° C to 23° C)
Clean workroom	10	Positive	Maximum 60%[1]	68° F to 73° F (20° C to 23° C)
Clean/sterile storage room	4	Positive	Maximum 60%	< 75° F (< 24° C)
Endoscopy procedure room	6	NR	Maximum 60%	68° F to 73° F (20° C to 23° C)
Bronchoscopy procedure room	12	Negative	NR	68° F to 73° F (20° C to 23° C)
Sterilizer service access room	10	Negative	NR[2]	NR[2]
Environmental services closet	10	Negative	NR	NR

NR = No Recommendation
[1] Check the manufacturer's instructions for use for storage requirements (eg, reusable linens, chemical indicators, biological indicators)
[2] Check sterilizer manufacturer's specifications

NOTE: The terminology and parameters noted above represent the consensus of a joint heating, ventilation, and air-conditioning (HVAC) task force brought together on April 29, 2015 in Annapolis, Maryland for the purpose of harmonizing the conflicting and sometimes unclear HVAC standards and guidelines established by a variety of professional organizations. The task force included representatives from the American Society of Heating, Refrigerating and Air-Conditioning Engineers (ASHRAE), the American Society for Healthcare Engineering (ASHE), the Association for the Advancement of Medical Instrumentation (AAMI), the Association of periOperative Registered Nurses (AORN), the Facility Guidelines Institute (FGI), and other sterile processing experts and consultants.

Having a wall or physical barrier for separation of the decontamination area provides protection and minimizes the potential for contamination of clean and processed flexible endoscopes.

I.c. The endoscopy processing room should be designed to facilitate a unidirectional workflow from the decontamination area or decontamination room to the clean area or clean workroom and then to clean storage in a separate location.[1,11-15,17,18,20,25,30] *[2: High Evidence]*

A unidirectional flow improves efficiency and helps to contain contaminants within the decontamination area or decontamination room.[11,12,17,18,25,30]

I.d. Heating, ventilation, and air conditioning (HVAC) systems for the endoscopy suite should be designed in compliance with state and local building codes and other guidelines as set forth by the FGI and American Society of Heating, Refrigerating and Air-Conditioning Engineers (ASHRAE).[11,15,31] *[4: Limited Evidence]*

Heating, ventilation, and air conditioning systems control the air quality, temperature, humidity, and air pressure of the room in comparison to the surrounding areas.[32] The HVAC system is intended to reduce the amount of

environmental contaminants (eg, microbial-laden skin squames, dust, lint) in the endoscopy suite.[31,32]

I.d.1. Heating, ventilation, and air conditioning systems in the endoscopy suite should be constructed and designed to meet the parameters shown in Table 1. *[4: Limited Evidence]*

The minimum HVAC values are for new construction or major renovations. They are not intended to be used as values for operating older facilities built when lesser standards were in place.

I.d.2. The minimum number of air changes in the endoscopy suite, including the percentage of outdoor air, should be maintained within the HVAC design parameters at the rate that was applicable at the time of design or of the most recent renovation of the HVAC system.[32] *[4: Limited Evidence]*

Filtered air minimizes the recirculation of indoor contaminants within the area.[32]

I.d.3. The incoming air should be sequentially filtered through two filters. The first filter should be rated as 7 MERV (ie, minimum efficiency reporting value) and the second should be rated as 14 MERV.[11,32] *[4: Limited Evidence]*

The incoming air requires continuous filtration because dust and airborne fungi are present at all times.[32]

Minimum efficiency reporting values measure the effectiveness of the air filters on a scale from 1 to 16.[31] The higher the MERV rating on a filter, the fewer the dust particles and other contaminants that can pass through it.[31]

I.d.4. The airflow direction (ie, pressure relationship of one area to adjacent areas) for the endoscopy suite should be within the HVAC parameters.[32] When endoscope processing activities will occur in two rooms, the pressure relationship should be
- negative in the decontamination room[33] and
- positive in the clean workroom.[33]

[4: Limited Evidence]

There is no recommendation for the pressure relationship when endoscope processing activities will occur in a single room.[33,34]

The direction of the airflow from one room to the adjacent area is engineered to minimize the flow of contaminants from dirty to clean areas.[31] Negative pressure in the decontamination room helps prevent contaminants from flexible endoscopes and other items being processed from reaching surrounding environments.[26] Positive pressure in the clean workroom helps prevent contaminants from surrounding environments from reaching the clean room.[26]

I.d.5. Bronchoscopy procedure rooms should be designed to be under negative pressure to the surrounding areas.[11,32,35,36] For patients who require airborne precautions when a negative pressure room is not available, a portable, industrial grade high-efficiency particulate air (HEPA) filter or portable anteroom system (PAS)-HEPA combination unit may be used to supplement air cleaning.[32,35] *[1: Strong Evidence]*

Use of an airborne infection isolation room; negative pressure room; or portable, industrial grade HEPA filter or PAS-HEPA combination unit helps prevent the spread of airborne pathogens, particularly tuberculosis, rubeola, and varicella zoster, and is recommended during procedures that can generate infectious aerosols (eg, bronchoscopy).[29,36] The reader can refer to the Healthcare Infection Control Practices Advisory Committee "Guideline for isolation precautions: preventing transmission of infectious agents in healthcare settings"[29] and the AORN Guideline for Prevention of Transmissible Infections[35] for additional guidance.

I.d.6. Ventilation within the endoscopy suite must be controlled to meet personnel limits for chemical exposure as required by local, state, and federal Occupational Safety and Health Administration (OSHA) regulations[37,38] and should be accomplished in accordance with industry standards[11,31] and professional guidelines.[18,22,39-46] *[1: Regulatory Requirement]*

I.e. Structural surfaces (eg, doors, floors, walls, ceilings, cabinets, shelves, work surfaces), furniture (eg, tables), and equipment in the endoscopy processing room, procedure rooms, and patient care areas should be smooth and made of materials that are water resistant, stain resistant, and able to withstand frequent cleaning.[11-13,21] *[2: High Evidence]*

Structural surfaces that are smooth and able to withstand frequent cleaning ease the cleaning process. A clean environment will reduce the number of microorganisms present.

I.e.1. Ceiling surfaces in the endoscopy processing room, procedure rooms, and patient care areas should not be composed of perforated, serrated, cut, or highly textured tiles.[11] *[4: Limited Evidence]*

Perforated, serrated, cut, and highly textured ceiling tiles may create a reservoir for the collection of dirt and debris that cannot be removed during cleaning.

I.e.2. Pipes and other fixtures above work areas in the endoscopy suite should be enclosed and tightly sealed.[11,12] *[4: Limited Evidence]*

Providing tight seals and enclosing pipes and other fixtures above work areas helps prevent contamination from dust, condensation, and other potential sources of contamination.[12]

I.e.3. Floor surfaces in endoscopy processing rooms, procedure rooms, and patient care areas should be monolithic.[11] Junctions between floors and walls should have an integral coved wall base that is carried up the wall a minimum of 6 inches (152 mm) and is tightly sealed to the wall.[11,13] *[4: Limited Evidence]*

Seams, joints, or crevices may harbor microorganisms.[12]

I.e.4. The integrity of surfaces within the endoscopy suite should be maintained, and surfaces should be repaired when damaged.[32] *[2: High Evidence]*

Damaged surfaces may shed particles into the environment[12] and may create a reservoir for the collection of dirt and debris that cannot be removed during cleaning.[32] Damage to floor surfaces may create a trip or fall hazard.[32]

I.f. Lighting in the endoscopy suite should be designed in compliance with state and local building codes and other guidelines as set forth by the Illuminating Engineering Society of North America.[47] *[4: Limited Evidence]*

Well-designed lighting facilitates visual inspection of flexible endoscopes and other tasks performed in the endoscopy suite.

I.f.1. Lighting should be designed to provide good visibility for personnel to perform necessary tasks and should be adjustable.[47] *[4: Limited Evidence]*

Although a very high illuminance capability may be required for some tasks, too much light can be uncomfortable. Adjustable lighting improves comfort by allowing personnel to increase or decrease the lighting level as needed to perform the task.[47]

I.g. Hand washing stations in the endoscopy suite must be readily accessible[48] and should be provided in the decontamination room and the clean workroom.[11,21] When endoscope processing activities will occur in a single room, a hand washing station should be provided in the decontamination area.[11] *[1: Regulatory Requirement]*

Providing readily accessible hand washing stations is a regulatory requirement.[48] Hand washing stations that are easy to access facilitate hand washing and may improve hand hygiene compliance.[17] Hand hygiene is required after removal of personal protective equipment (PPE).[35,48]

I.h. A minimum of two decontamination sinks (or one sink with two divisions) should be provided in the endoscopy processing room.[12,13]

○ When two decontamination sinks (or one sink with two divisions) are provided, one sink (or division) should be designated for leak testing and manual cleaning, and the other for rinsing.[12]

○ Three decontamination sinks (or one sink with three divisions) may be provided in the endoscopy processing room.[12] When three decontamination sinks (or one sink with three divisions) are provided, one sink (or division) should be designated for leak testing, the second for manual cleaning, and the third for rinsing.[12,13]

[3: Moderate Evidence]

Sinks are required for functions such as leak testing, cleaning, and rinsing of flexible endoscopes and other items being processed. Separate sinks or divisions facilitate endoscope processing and may help prevent cross contamination.

Silva et al[49] reported a pseudo-outbreak of *Pseudomonas aeruginosa* and *Serratia marcescens* involving 41 patients who underwent bronchoscopy procedures in a 380-bed private hospital in Sao Paulo, Brazil, between December 1994 and October 1996. As part of the investigation, the investigators reviewed and observed endoscopy processing procedures. They found that in addition to other inadequacies in the processing procedures, the same sink was used for both washing and rinsing the bronchoscopes. The pseudo-outbreak resolved with improved processing procedures that included separate sinks for washing and rinsing of the endoscopes.

I.h.1. Decontamination sinks should be deep enough to allow complete submersion of the endoscope and large enough to allow the endoscope to be positioned in the sink without tight coiling.[12,13,15,22,25] *[2: High Evidence]*

Complete submersion of the endoscope minimizes aerosolization during cleaning.[12] Tight coiling of the endoscope may damage the light bundles, internal channels, tubes, or angulation wires.[12]

I.i. Instrument air should be provided in the endoscopy processing room.[50,51] *[4: Limited Evidence]*

Compressed air facilitates flushing and drying of channels and lumens.[12] Clean, filtered air is required for drying lumens and small channels without introducing contaminants into the clean device.

I.j. Eyewash stations, either plumbed or self-contained, must be provided within the endoscopy suite where chemicals that are hazardous to the eyes are located.[52] *[1: Regulatory Requirement]*

It is a regulatory requirement that emergency eyewash stations or showers be immediately accessible in locations where the eyes or body of any person may be exposed to injurious corrosive materials.[52]

Plumbed eyewash stations are connected to a continual source of water that is safe to drink.[53] Self-contained eyewash stations are stand-alone devices that contain flushing fluid.[53]

Many chemicals are eye irritants. Eyewash stations are necessary to provide flushing fluid when the safety data sheet identifies the chemical as a hazard and recommends immediate flushing of the eyes as an emergency first aid measure.

I.j.1. Eyewash stations should be located
- in a well-lit area identified with a highly visible sign positioned within the area served by the eyewash station,[53]
- so that travel time is no greater than 10 seconds from the location of chemical use or storage,[53] and
- on the same level as the hazard, with the path of travel free of obstructions (eg, doors) that may inhibit immediate use of an eyewash station.[53]

[4: Limited Evidence]

I.j.2. Eyewash stations should be positioned with the flushing fluid nozzles not less than 33

FLEXIBLE ENDOSCOPES

inches (83.8 cm) and not more than 45 inches (114.3 cm) from the surface on which the person using the eyewash station stands and a minimum of 6 inches (15.2 cm) from the wall or the nearest obstruction.[53] *[4: Limited Evidence]*

I.j.3. Eyewash stations should not be installed in a location that requires flushing of the eyes in the decontamination sink. *[5: Benefits Balanced with Harms]*

Splashing from the decontamination sink could potentially contaminate the eyes of personnel using the sink.

I.j.4. Once activated, eyewash stations should be capable of delivering tepid (60° F to 100° F [16° C to 38° C]) flushing fluid to both eyes simultaneously at not less than 0.4 gallons (1.5 L) per minute for 15 minutes at a velocity low enough to be noninjurious to the user and without requiring the use of the operator's hands.[53] *[4: Limited Evidence]*

The reader can refer to the current ANSI/International Safety Equipment Association (ISEA) *American National Standard for Emergency Eyewash and Shower Equipment*[53] for additional guidance.

Recommendation II

Flexible endoscopes should be processed in an area controlled and maintained to support processing activities.[1,11-19,24]

The collective evidence supports processing flexible endoscopes in an area where activities such as temperature, humidity, environmental cleaning, surgical attire, traffic patterns, and security are managed in accordance with specific policies and procedures that promote processing activities.[1,11-19,24]

The benefits are that this may improve efficiency, maintain functionality of flexible endoscopes and other medical devices, help to reduce the risk of cross contamination, and provide a safe work environment.

The limitations of the evidence are that no research studies have investigated the link between patient outcomes and flexible endoscopes processed in a controlled area.[30]

II.a. The health care organization should create and implement a systematic process for establishing and monitoring performance of the HVAC system in the endoscopy suite.[27,32] *[4: Limited Evidence]*

Monitoring performance of the HVAC systems helps ensure that the desired HVAC parameters are being achieved and maintained.

II.a.1. Relative humidity should be maintained within the HVAC design parameters for endoscopy suites.[32] *[4: Limited Evidence]*

The effect of relative humidity on bacterial, fungal, and viral growth is inconclusive. Additional research is warranted to determine optimal relative humidity levels for control of environmental contamination.[32]

II.a.2. The room temperature in the endoscopy suite may be intentionally adjusted based on the needs of the patient and the comfort of personnel.[32] *[4: Limited Evidence]*

Maintaining comfort and normothermia of patients in procedure rooms or patient care areas may require that room temperature be adjusted outside of the recommended range. Temperature settings in nonclinical areas may also need to be adjusted to provide comfortable temperatures for personnel based on the activities being performed (eg, a lower temperature may be required in the decontamination area where PPE may be worn for long periods of time).[12]

II.a.3. Personnel who identify an unintentional variance in the predetermined HVAC system parameters in the endoscopy suite should report the variance according to the health care organization's policy and procedure.[32] *[5: Benefits Balanced with Harms]*

Rapid communication between affected and responsible personnel can help facilitate resolution of the variance.[32]

II.a.4. Designated personnel from the health care organization should perform a risk assessment if a variance in the parameters of the HVAC system occurs.[32] *[5: Benefits Balanced with Harms]*

The effect of the HVAC system parameters falling out of range is variable. A small variance for a short period of time may not be of clinical concern, whereas a large variance for a longer period may have clinical significance.[32]

II.a.5. Based on the risk assessment, corrective measures should be taken and may include
- terminal cleaning of surfaces when there is evidence of contamination on surfaces;
- reprocessing or discarding any supplies with packaging that may have been compromised;
- inventorying discarded, damaged supplies to obtain replacements; and
- modifying or updating the HVAC system.[32]
[5: Benefits Balanced with Harms]

II.b. Hand hygiene practices should be implemented in the endoscopy suite in accordance with the AORN Guideline for Hand Hygiene.[54] *[2: High Evidence]*

Hand hygiene has been recognized as a primary method of decreasing health care-associated infections.[54] Health care-associated infections can result in untoward outcomes such as escalated cost of care, increased rates of morbidity and mortality, and longer lengths of stay, as well as the pain and suffering a patient may experience.[54]

STERILIZATION AND DISINFECTION

806

Because of a severe outbreak of *Kelbsiella pneumoniae* producing extended-spectrum beta (ß)-lactamase that occurred in 16 patients undergoing endoscopic retrograde cholangiopancreatography (ERCP) procedures in a hospital in France between December 2008 and August 2009, Aumeran et al[55] observed the duodenoscope processing procedures. They found a lack of personnel compliance with recommended hand hygiene practices, and they concluded that the hands of personnel may have been a source or vehicle for transmission of the outbreak strain.

II.b.1. Hand washing sinks should not be used to clean flexible endoscopes.[12,20,22] *[4: Limited Evidence]*

Cleaning endoscopes in hand washing sinks could contaminate the sink, faucet, and hands of personnel subsequently washed in the same sink.[12]

II.b.2. Decontamination sinks should not be used for hand washing.[12] *[4: Limited Evidence]*

Hand washing in the decontamination sinks could contaminate the endoscope or other items subsequently washed in the same sink.[12]

II.c. Processes and procedures for environmental cleaning in the endoscopy suite should be carried out in accordance with the AORN Guideline for Environmental Cleaning.[56] *[1: Strong Evidence]*

A clean environment will minimize the exposure risk of health care personnel and patients to potentially infectious microorganisms.[56]

II.d. Clean surgical attire and head coverings should be worn in the processing room and procedure rooms of the endoscopy suite. *[5: Benefits Balanced with Harms]*

Surgical attire is worn to provide a high level of cleanliness and hygiene within the endoscopy environment and to promote patient and worker safety.[57] Head coverings contain hair and minimize microbial dispersal.[57]

II.e. Personnel working in the endoscopy suite must wear PPE. *[1: Regulatory Requirement]*

It is a regulatory requirement that PPE be worn whenever splashes, spray, spatter, or droplets of blood, body fluids, or other potentially infectious materials may be generated and eye, nose, or mouth contamination can be reasonably anticipated.[48] Employers are required to ensure that employees are protected when exposed to eye or face hazards from liquid chemicals.[59]

II.e.1. Personal protective equipment should be worn in accordance with the AORN Guideline for Prevention of Transmissible Infections,[35] the AORN Guideline for Surgical Attire,[57] and the AORN Guideline for Cleaning and Care of Surgical Instruments.[58] *[1: Strong Evidence]*

II.e.2. Personnel working in the endoscopy processing room and handling contaminated flexible endoscopes should wear PPE that includes

- surgical masks in combination with eye protection devices, such as goggles, glasses with solid side shields, or chin-length face shields;
- fluid-resistant gowns;
- general purpose utility gloves with cuffs that extend beyond the cuff of the gown; and
- fluid-resistant shoe covers.

[1: Strong Evidence]

Contaminated flexible endoscopes are a potential source of transmissible pathogens.[58] Personal protective equipment helps to protect processing and procedural personnel from exposure to blood, body fluids, and other potentially infectious materials.[58]

Surgical masks in combination with eye protection devices can protect the wearer's face, eyes, nose, and mouth from exposure to hazardous chemicals as well as pathogenic microorganisms, body fluids, and other potentially infectious materials.[57] The mucous membranes of the nose, mouth, and eyes may act as portals of entry to infectious agents.[60] In addition to the risk for injury from a direct splash to the eye, there is also a risk of developing conjunctivitis or a systemic infection.[60] Skin may also act as a portal when its integrity is compromised by trauma or disease.[60]

Kaye[61] reported an unusual complication of inoculation in the eye by effluent from the open biopsy port of a flexible esophagoscope. The patient was diagnosed with herpetic esophagitis. After esophageal brushings and biopsies had been obtained, the endoscopist attempted air inflation and a jet of fluid was directed from the patient's esophagus into the endoscopist's right eye, which was immediately flushed with copious amounts of water. One week later, the endoscopist noted an itchy papule beneath the right eyelid that developed into multiple conjunctival vesicles. Conjunctival cultures were positive for Herpes simplex virus (HSV). The endoscopist subsequently developed a sore throat (also culture-positive for HSV), neck stiffness, lymphadenopathy, and splenomegaly that resolved within a week. The conjunctival HSV reappeared approximately two weeks later and resolved without further recurrence. The author concluded that although this was a rare event, it is conceivable that diseases such as tuberculosis and hepatitis could be transmitted in a similar way. The author recommended that endoscopists keep their faces away from the biopsy port and seal it as soon as the forceps have been withdrawn. In all likelihood, the splashing of fluid into the endoscopist's eye would have been prevented by the use of protective eyewear.

Fluid-resistant gowns can prevent transfer of microorganisms from contaminated items to skin.[58]

General purpose utility gloves can minimize the potential for punctures, nicks, and cuts, and exposure of the hands and forearms to blood, body fluids, and other potentially infectious materials.[58] Wearing utility gloves with cuffs that extend beyond the cuff of the gown helps provide protection from fluids during cleaning of flexible endoscopes and other items in the decontamination sink.[58]

Fluid-resistant shoe covers can protect shoes from splashes, splatters, and spills.[58]

II.e.3. Hand hygiene should be performed after removal of PPE.[29] *[1: Strong Evidence]*

The CDC recommends performing hand hygiene after removal of PPE.[29] Hands may become contaminated when removing PPE. Damage to PPE in the form of tears, punctures, and abrasions may occur and be undetected, exposing the wearer to microbial contamination and bloodborne pathogens.[60]

II.e.4. Reusable PPE must be decontaminated and the integrity of the PPE verified between uses.[48] Reusable PPE must be discarded if there are signs of deterioration or its ability to function as a barrier has been compromised.[48] *[1: Regulatory Requirement]*

Decontaminating reusable PPE and verifying its integrity between uses is a regulatory requirement.[48] Reusable gloves, gowns, aprons, and protective eyewear or face shields may become contaminated and their integrity compromised during use.

II.f. Personnel working in the endoscopy suite should be immunized against vaccine-preventable diseases in accordance with the AORN Guideline for Prevention of Transmissible Infections.[35] *[1: Strong Evidence]*

Personnel may come into contact with patients or infectious material from patients that may put them at risk for exposure and possible transmission of vaccine-preventable diseases.[35]

II.g. Traffic patterns within the endoscopy suite should facilitate movement of patients, personnel, equipment, and supplies into, through, and out of defined areas within the endoscopy suite. *[5: Benefits Balanced with Harms]*

Effective traffic patterns support safe patient care, workplace safety, and security.[32]

II.g.1. Processing room doors should be kept closed except during the entry and exit of personnel. *[5: Benefits Balanced with Harms]*

Keeping the doors closed helps prevent contaminated particles from entering or leaving the room and maintains the pressure differential required for decontamination rooms. Keeping the door closed also assists with venting contaminated room air out of the building, minimizing contamination of adjacent areas.[32]

II.h. Designated personnel from the health care organization, in consultation with security personnel or law enforcement representatives, should develop a security plan for the endoscopy suite.[32] *[5: Benefits Balanced with Harms]*

Including the endoscopy suite in the facility-wide plan takes into consideration the unique security risks created by the presence of high-value equipment, medications, and supplies and the variable hours during which the suite may be unoccupied.[32] Security personnel and law enforcement representatives have expertise in identifying security risks and in prevention and mitigation tactics.[32]

II.h.1. Security measures should be selected based on a risk assessment and may include the use of devices (eg, alarm systems, video surveillance, shatter-proof glass) or controls (eg, locked doors, tracking systems, visitor logs).[32] *[5: Benefits Balanced with Harms]*

Security measures provide for the safety of patients, personnel, and visitors.[32]

II.i. Processes and procedures for purchasing, evaluating, and selecting flexible endoscopes, accessories, equipment, and other items and products related to the use and processing of flexible endoscopes should be carried out in accordance with the AORN Guideline for Product Selection.[62] *[2: High Evidence]*

Patient and worker safety, quality, and cost containment are primary concerns of endoscopy personnel as they participate in evaluating and selecting medical devices and products for use in endoscopy settings.[62]

II.i.1. Endoscopes, accessories, and equipment used in the endoscopy suite should have manufacturer-validated IFU. *[1: Strong Evidence]*

Manufacturers of reusable devices cleared by the FDA provide validated cleaning and processing instructions and guidance on how to process devices between uses. Items cannot be assumed to be correctly processed unless the manufacturer's IFU are derived from validation testing and the instructions have been followed.[58]

Validation by the manufacturer provides objective evidence that the requirements for the specific intended use of the product or device can be consistently fulfilled.[63-65]

II.i.2. Prepurchase evaluation of flexible endo-scopes, accessories, and equipment should include
- ensuring that the facility has the capa-bility to comply with the manufactur-er's IFU,
- confirming that the manufacturer's IFU can be replicated, and
- verifying compatibility with other rele-vant manufacturers' IFU.

[5: Benefits Balanced with Harms]

Manufacturers' IFU vary widely. Some devices or items may have unique require-ments that may not be achievable within the facility.

II.i.3. Endoscope accessories and devices speci-fied by the endoscope or mechanical pro-cessor manufacturer for cleaning and pro-cessing should be obtained at the time of endoscope purchase and used in accor-dance with the IFU.[58] [1: Strong Evidence]

Using accessories and devices that are designed and manufactured to the endo-scope or mechanical processor manufactur-er's specifications helps ensure the endo-scope can be used effectively and facilitates performance of cleaning and processing procedures.[58]

II.j. Processes and procedures for managing new, loaned, and repaired endoscopes, accessories, and equipment in the endoscopy suite should be carried out in accordance with the AORN Guideline for Cleaning and Care of Surgical Instruments.[58] [1: Strong Evidence]

Adhering to the AORN guideline will help ensure successful management of new, loaned, or repaired items.

II.k. Flexible endoscopes and endoscope accessories should be cleaned and processed by individuals who have received education and completed competency verification activities related to endoscope processing.[15,66] [2: High Evidence]

The collective evidence shows that ensuring flexible endoscopes and endoscope accessories are processed by individuals whose primary duties are to clean and process flexible endo-scopes minimizes variability and improves pro-cessing effectiveness.[67,68] Having individuals who have received education and demonstrated competency process flexible endoscopes and accessories helps reduce the risk for errors and cross contamination.[66,69] Individuals whose pri-mary duties are to clean and process flexible endoscopes bring a specialized level of knowl-edge to the processing procedure that may include
- an improved understanding of the health and safety issues that can arise when endoscopes are not correctly processed,[69]
- an in-depth knowledge of the structure and operation of the endoscopes they are respon-sible for processing,[69]
- an in-depth knowledge of the structure and operation of the mechanical processors they are using for processing,[69] and
- a desire for additional education related to processing of flexible endoscopes and acces-sories that may improve the quality and stan-dard of processing.[69]

A dedicated team of individuals responsible for processing flexible endoscopes may also allow endoscopy nurses to focus on clinical responsibilities.[69]

Kolmos et al[70] reported a pseudo-outbreak of P aeruginosa in eight consecutive HIV-infected patients undergoing bronchoscopy in Denmark. None of the patients developed signs of respira-tory tract infection that could be ascribed to the organism. The investigators found the source to be P aeruginosa contamination in the suction channels of two bronchoscopes. Due to the lack of a dedicated processing person, the nurses, who were inexperienced with processing proce-dures for flexible bronchoscopes, were not man-ually cleaning the endoscopes. Further, the mechanical processor was not working cor-rectly, so the bronchoscopes were being manu-ally soaked in glutaraldehyde in a location other than the endoscopy processing room. Interviews with the nurses confirmed that the suction channels had not been cleaned for many weeks before the pseudo-outbreak. When the channels were inspected, there were deposits of organic material in both bronchoscopes. The contami-nated bronchoscopes were effectively cleaned and processed, and this stopped the outbreak. The investigators recommended having dedi-cated personnel process flexible bronchoscopes.

Ensuring flexible endoscopes and endoscope accessories are processed by individuals whose primary duties are to clean and process flexible endoscopes may also reduce repair costs and extend the life of the endoscope.[67,68]

McGill et al[71] conducted a nonexperimental study to ascertain the durability of flexible cysto-scopes in relation to their use in the outpatient setting. The researchers prospectively investi-gated cystoscope processing and repair costs for six new cystoscopes from July 1, 2008, through August 31, 2009, and compared these data with retrospective data from the previous eight months. During the prospective study period, the flexible cystoscopes were only processed by urol-ogy nursing personnel skilled in processes for handling and maintaining flexible cystoscopes. The researchers found there was a 43.9% decrease in repair costs and mechanical failure when the nurses processed the endoscopes.

To investigate the causes and costs of flexible ureteroscope damage and to develop recommen-dations to limit damage, Sooriakumaran et al[72]

analyzed repair costs and damage to 35 ureteroscopes sent for repair during a one-year period. The researchers found that the majority (72%) of the damages occurred during the cleaning and processing phase rather than during procedural use. The researchers suggested that having a skilled, dedicated team clean and process the ureteroscopes could help prevent damage and reduce costs.

In an effort to reduce costs and damage to flexible ureteroscopes, Semins et al[73] studied the effect and analyzed the cost per use of having dedicated urology personnel clean and process all ureteroscopes rather than the facility processing personnel who cleaned and processed all other facility items. Between April 2007 and March 2008, when the urology team processed the ureteroscopes, 11 ureteroscopes were processed 478 times. The average number of uses per ureteroscope before repair was necessary was 28.1. The average repair cost per use was $120.63 ($134.33 in 2015 US dollars). During the previous year, when the processing was performed by facility personnel, the average number of uses per ureteroscope before repair was necessary was only 10.8. The average repair cost per use was $418.19 ($465.69 in 2015 US dollars). The authors concluded that having a skilled and dedicated team process ureteroscopes was an effective measure to reduce repair costs and processing-related damage to flexible ureteroscopes.

McDougall et al[74] conducted a quasi-experimental study to determine whether the technique used to clean flexible ureteroscopes or the number of persons handling the endoscope during the cleaning process influenced function or number of repairs. The researchers used a new, flexible ureteroscope for each of two 30-day study periods. During the first study period, the endoscope was leak tested, cleaned, and processed by the endourology support team. During the second study period, the endoscope was leak tested, cleaned, and processed by the surgeon. The researchers found that the function and durability of the endoscope was not affected by the technique used to clean it or the number of people involved in cleaning and processing the endoscope. The function and durability of the endoscope was found to be affected by the demands of the surgical procedure and the technique of the surgeon.

II.k.1. Processing of flexible endoscopes should be performed in the same manner in all processing locations. *[3: Moderate Evidence]*

Smith[75] reported two cases of septicemia caused by *P aeruginosa* following ERCP procedures. The investigators found that the accessory instruments used through the endoscope were cleaned with chlorhexidine gluconate and soaked in glutaraldehyde for one hour. After soaking, they were rinsed with utility water, and the lumens of the endoscope were flushed using single-use syringes. The accessory instruments were then placed into their original shipping containers while still wet and were stored in a cupboard. The syringes were stored in a wet condition and reused. The investigators sampled the syringes and found them to be culture-positive for the same strain of *P aeruginosa* that was found in the septic patients. The bacteria had been introduced into the patients' biliary tract on endoscopy instruments contaminated after disinfection by the syringes used for flushing the endoscope channels. The endoscopes were being processed at multiple sites, with processing personnel following different processing procedures at different sites.

In a case control study of an outbreak of multidrug-resistant *P aeruginosa*, Machida et al[76] found a relationship between the infections and contaminated bronchoscopes. Between June and August 2007, isolates from five patients in the intensive care unit (ICU) and emergency department (ED) of a 1,076-bed university hospital were culture-positive for multidrug-resistant *P aeruginosa*. All of the patients had undergone bronchoscopy procedures in the ICU or ED. The organism was not found in any of the bronchoscopes in use at the hospital; however, the investigators found that the bronchoscopes used in the ICU and the ED were processed differently from other hospital endoscopes.

The researchers retrospectively reviewed medical records from 2006 and found 11 additional patients with multidrug-resistant *P aeruginosa*. The review showed that these patients also had bronchoscopy procedures in the ICU or ED. Processing procedures were reviewed and showed poor compliance with hospital procedures for processing the endoscopes. The manual cleaning step was often skipped when the endoscopes were processed in the ICU or ED. The outbreak ended when effective cleaning and high-level disinfecting processes were established in all processing areas.[78]

II.k.2. Sufficient time and numbers of personnel should be provided to permit thorough cleaning and processing of flexible endoscopes.[58,77,78] *[3: Moderate Evidence]*

Time constraints and insufficient numbers of endoscope processing team members may create a disincentive for personnel to adhere to recommended cleaning and processing procedures.[58]

II.k.3. Endoscopy procedures should be scheduled to allow sufficient time for cleaning and

STERILIZATION AND DISINFECTION

processing of flexible endoscopes.[78] *[3: Moderate Evidence]*

Time constraints may create a disincentive for personnel to adhere to recommended cleaning and processing procedures.[58]

II.k.4.   An inventory of flexible endoscopes and accessories sufficient to meet the anticipated demand should be maintained.[58,77,78] *[3: Moderate Evidence]*

Having an adequate inventory provides sufficient time for personnel to follow correct cleaning and processing procedures.[58,78]

II.k.5.   A multidisciplinary team that includes endoscopy personnel, RNs from departments where bedside endoscopy procedures are performed, infection preventionists, risk managers, endoscopy processing personnel, endoscopists, and other involved personnel should establish policies and procedures requiring that flexible endoscopes used for procedures performed at the bedside or outside of normal operating hours are processed in the same manner as endoscopes used during normal operating hours. *[3: Moderate Evidence]*

Flexible endoscopes are complex and costly devices that require multiple processing steps. Having skilled, dedicated personnel process flexible endoscopes for emergency procedures performed outside of normal operating hours helps ensure that the endoscopes have been processed correctly and are safe to use.[68]

Bou et al[79] conducted a cohort study to identify risk factors for infection following an outbreak of *P aeruginosa* infections in the 27-bed ICU of a community hospital in Spain during July 2003. The investigators identified 17 case patients with 25 *P aeruginosa* infections that included respiratory tract infections (n = 21), a bloodstream infection (n = 1), a urinary tract infection (n = 1), a pressure ulcer (n = 1), and a surgical site infection (n = 1). Ten of the 17 case patients had undergone bronchoscopy procedures in the ICU during a weekend. A review of the weekend processing procedures showed major deviations from hospital policies. Adequate cleaning and HLD were not performed. The weekend procedure involved rinsing the bronchoscope with povidone-iodine and placing the bronchoscope into its storage case without drying. The bronchoscope was then transported to the endoscopy unit where it was stored in a drawer until its next use. On weekdays, the bronchoscope was either manually or mechanically cleaned and high-level disinfected without a sterile water rinse, alcohol flush, or purging with air. Notably, the manufacturer's IFU were

not being followed in the ICU or the endoscopy unit. The researchers concluded that education of processing personnel was necessary to ensure processing was carried out in accordance with published guidelines in all areas of the hospital and during all hours processing procedures were performed.

Srinivasan et al[80] conducted a survey among 46 practicing bronchoscopists to assess their knowledge of recommended guidelines and processing procedures. The survey was distributed to participants in two bronchoscopy courses attended by pulmonologists from the United States. The results of the survey showed that 65% of the bronchoscopists (n = 30) were not familiar with bronchoscope processing guidelines and 39% (n = 18) did not know what processing procedures were used in their own facilities.

To audit processing of flexible endoscopes used during procedures performed outside of normal operating hours, Radford et al[81] conducted a telephone survey of 104 ear, nose, and throat units in England. On-call clinicians from 72 units (69%) agreed to participate. The researchers found that the on-call clinician processed the flexible endoscope in 60 units (83%); however, the on-call clinician had only received education and hands-on instruction on processing procedures in 27 units (38%). In addition, clinicians in 19 units (26%) followed inadequate processing procedures, and clinicians in 16 units (22%) were unsure of the correct processing method. In one case, the clinician admitted to not cleaning the endoscope between procedures. In 35 units (49%), the endoscope was stored in an unsterile carrying case. In seven units (10%), the on-call clinician did not know how the endoscope was stored. The researchers concluded there was an urgent need for compliance with effective processing procedures for flexible endoscopes used for emergent endoscopy procedures performed outside of normal operating hours.

Recommendation III

Flexible endoscopes and accessories should be precleaned at the point of use.

The collective evidence supports precleaning of flexible endoscopes at the point of use as a mechanism for moistening, diluting, softening, and removing organic soils (eg, blood, feces, respiratory secretions) and reducing the formation of biofilm. If organic soil and biofilm are not removed completely, the subsequent HLD or sterilization process might not be effective.[82] The need for precleaning at the point of use is emphasized in numerous clinical practice guidelines.[12,13,15-22,27,44,45,83-85]

The benefits of precleaning flexible endoscopes at the point of use are that it eases[86] and improves[87] the cleaning process and helps reduce the formation of biofilm, which can interfere with HLD or sterilization.[82]

III.a. Precleaning of flexible endoscopes and accessories at the point of use should occur as soon as possible after the endoscope is removed from the patient (or the procedure is completed) and before organic material has dried on the surface or in the channels of the endoscope.[12,13,18-22,27,44,45,83-85,88] *[1: Strong Evidence]*

The presence of dried organic material makes cleaning difficult.[85,89] When using an enzymatic cleaner, dried organic material has to be rehydrated in order for the enzymes to be effective.[90]

In a quasi-experimental laboratory study, Merritt et al[86] evaluated the effects of 12 different cleaning solutions on four microorganisms known to adhere to polystyrene and medical implant materials (ie, *Staphylococcus epidermidis, Candida albicans, Escherichia coli, P aeruginosa*). The results of the study showed that allowing bioburden to dry on surfaces made cleaning very difficult. The researchers recommended that microorganisms, protein, or other materials not be allowed to dry on flexible endoscopes before cleaning.

Biofilm is difficult to remove and may begin to form within minutes after the procedure is completed.[82,85] In an expert opinion article discussing biofilm development on the surfaces of medical devices and the role of biofilm in device processing, Roberts[82] explained that the formation of biofilm begins when a layer of organic material is deposited on the surface of a medical device (Figure 4). Colonizing microorganisms subsequently become attached to this foundational layer. At this point, the microorganisms are loosely attached and can be removed by cleaning.[91]

Nearly irreversible attachment occurs as the microorganisms begin to multiply and form a mature biofilm.[91,92] A mature biofilm consists of layers of bacterial cell clusters embedded in towers of polysaccharides secreted by the microorganisms into their environment.[91-94] Microorganisms within a mature biofilm are protected by the secreted extracellular substances and may not be easily penetrated or killed by antibiotics, HLD, or sterilization.[82,93-96] This protective mechanism may be related to physical, genetic, or physiological characteristics of the bacteria or their ability to produce neutralizing enzymes.[45] The mature biofilm releases colonizing cells to form new biofilms on other surfaces of the device.[82,94]

Certain conditions are necessary for biofilm formation, including

○ the presence of colonizing microorganisms,
○ sufficient nutrients,
○ acceptable temperature conditions for growth, and
○ time required for the formation of biofilm.[82]

Some microorganisms undergo cell division every 20 to 30 minutes; however, it may take several hours for a mature biofilm to form.[82] The time frame within which the cleaning of flexible endoscopes or other reusable medical devices occurs is therefore a key factor in the prevention of biofilm formation and buildup.[82] Performing precleaning and the remaining processing steps within an hour after a procedure may prevent formation of a mature biofilm even under conditions favorable to rapid biofilm development.[82]

Biofilm can form on the inner surface of endoscope channels and is especially prone to form when these inner channels become scratched or damaged.[93] Herrmann et al[87] performed microscopic examinations of the inner surfaces of the suction and biopsy channels of new flexible endoscopes. They found that the channels were only partially smooth and contained small indentations and irregularities where biofilm could form and be retained even after cleaning. They noted that the formation of biofilm in the small indentations and irregularities was even more likely to occur if the endoscope was not cleaned immediately after use.

Effective precleaning processes may help to prevent patient infection. Naas et al[97] reported an outbreak of carbapenemase-producing *Klebsiella pneumoniae* transmitted via a flexible endoscope. Retrospective analysis showed that 17 patients from five regional hospitals in France had undergone endoscopy with the same gastroscope. Of the 17 patients, six were colonized and two developed infections. A review of the endoscope processing procedures revealed that one potential explanation for the contamination was that the precleaning of the endoscope had been delayed for 24 hours, allowing organic material to dry on the device.

III.b. Precleaning should be performed in accordance with the endoscope manufacturer's IFU. *[5: Benefits Balanced with Harms]*

There are multiple types of flexible endoscopes, and recommended precleaning processes may vary among manufacturers.

Variations from the manufacturer's IFU may result in insufficient cleaning or in processing failure.

III.b.1. Steps for performing precleaning should include
• preparing a fresh solution of a cleaning product with properties recommended by the manufacturer[12,15];
• washing the exterior surfaces of the endoscope with a soft, lint-free cloth or sponge saturated with the cleaning solution[12,13,15,19,21,27,44,83-85,89];
• suctioning the cleaning solution through the suction and biopsy channels[12,13,15,19,21,44,85,89];

STERILIZATION AND DISINFECTION

FIGURE 4. BIOFILM FORMATION[1,2]

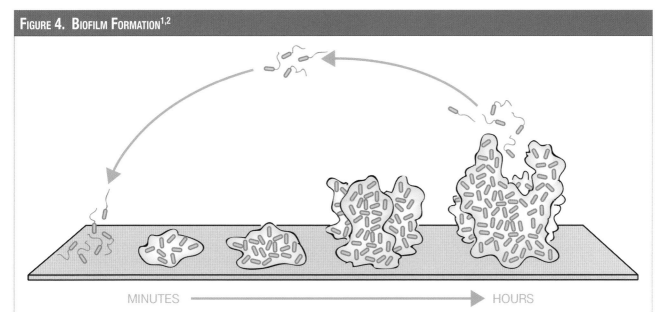

MINUTES ⟶ HOURS

Preconditioning basement layer of organic material is deposited on the surface

Microorganisms proceed with initial attachment to preconditioned surface

Microorganisms multiply and irreversible attachment begins

Mature biofilm forms, consisting of multiple layers of bacterial cell clusters embedded in extracellular polysaccharides

Mature biofilm releases colonizing cells to form new biofilms

REFERENCES
1. Roberts CG. The role of biofilms in reprocessing medical devices. Am J Infect Control. 2013;41(5 Suppl):S77-S80.
2. Pajkos A, Vickery K, Cossart Y. Is biofilm accumulation on endoscope tubing a contributor to the failure of cleaning and decontamination? J Hosp Infect. 2004;58(3):224-229.

- placing the distal end of the endoscope in the cleaning solution and suctioning the solution through the endoscope[12,15,21];
- flushing the air, water, and other channels of the endoscope alternately with the cleaning solution and air,[12,15,16,17,21,83] finishing with air[13,85,89];
- visually inspecting the endoscope for damage[12,19]; and
- discarding the cleaning solution and cleaning cloth or sponge after use.[13,15,83]

[2: High Evidence]

Using a fresh solution for each new cleaning process may help prevent cross contamination of flexible endoscopes.[98] Recommended cleaning solutions vary among endoscope manufacturers. Manufacturers have validated products with specific properties for effective cleaning of their devices.[90]

Washing the external surfaces of the endoscope and flushing the internal channels helps moisten, dilute, soften, and remove organic soils.

Suctioning all channels and cleaning the distal end assists with removing gross soil. Alternating cleaning solution with air may be more effective in loosening and remov-ing organic soils. Finishing with air may help prevent excess fluid from remaining in the channels.[13]

Visually inspecting the endoscope after precleaning helps detect obvious damage to the endoscope.

The cleaning solution and cleaning cloth or sponge may support bacterial growth if stored or reused.[45,99]

III.c. When the precleaning process will be delayed (eg, an endoscope is used for intubation and remains in the procedure room for potential reuse), designated personnel (eg, RN circulator, scrub person) should wipe the external surfaces with a soft, lint-free cloth or sponge saturated with utility or sterile water and suction water through the channels.[85] [3: Moderate Evidence]

Wiping the external surfaces and suctioning water through the channels of the endoscope may help prevent organic soils from drying, reducing bacterial adherence and the risk of biofilm formation until precleaning with a cleaning solution can be accomplished.

Microorganisms readily adhere to surfaces and begin forming biofilm.[82] Biofilm that has formed in lumens is difficult to remove. If not removed, biofilm may reduce the efficacy of subsequent disinfection or sterilization.[45]

Shimono et al[100] reported an outbreak of *P aeruginosa* infections that occurred following thoracic surgery in seven patients. The authors determined that one cause of the outbreak was dried organic material in the bronchoscope that occurred when the bronchoscope was reused several times during the surgeries without any cleaning or flushing between uses.

Recommendation IV

After precleaning at the point of use, contaminated flexible endoscopes and accessories should be transported to the endoscopy processing room.

The collective evidence supports transporting flexible endoscopes from the procedure room to the endoscopy processing room.[12,13,16,17,21,44,84,101]

The benefit of transporting flexible endoscopes to designated decontamination areas is that this may help prevent contamination of procedure rooms and patient care areas and also limits the number of areas where chemicals are used for cleaning and disinfection.[22]

IV.a. Contaminated flexible endoscopes and accessories should be transported to the endoscopy processing room as soon as possible after use. *[3: Moderate Evidence]*

Transporting the contaminated endoscope as soon as possible facilitates the ability to expeditiously initiate the cleaning process and helps prevent organic material from drying on the surface or in the lumens, which facilitates cleaning.[69,86,87]

IV.b. Endoscopes and accessories should be kept wet or damp but not submerged in liquid during transport. *[2: High Evidence]*

Keeping the endoscope and accessories wet helps dilute, soften, and ease removal of organic soils. Allowing organic material to dry on the surface and in the channels of the endoscope makes the cleaning process difficult.[15,24,86]

Submerging the endoscope in liquid during transport may increase the risk of spillage and could lead to fluid invasion if the endoscope has an unknown leak.

IV.c. Contaminated endoscopes and accessories must be transported to the decontamination area in a closed container or closed transport cart.[48] The container or cart must be
○ leak proof,[13,48]
○ puncture resistant,[48] and
○ large enough to contain all contents.[48,84]
[1: Regulatory Requirement]

Transporting items in leak-proof, puncture-resistant containers and in a manner that prevents exposing personnel to blood, body fluids, and other potentially infectious materials is a regulatory requirement.[48]

IV.c.1. The container should be of sufficient size to accommodate the endoscope when the endoscope is coiled in large loops.[12,16] *[3: Moderate Evidence]*

Using containers of sufficient size to fully contain the endoscope and allow loose coiling helps prevent damage to the endoscope.[16,84,102]

In a nonexperimental study to assess the costs of flexible ureterorenoscopy, Collins et al[103] found there was significant damage to a new ureteroscope that produced a crescent-shaped defect in the field of vision after only 12 procedures. The defect was determined to be the result of coiling the ureteroscope too tightly in the cleaning tray.

IV.c.2. The transport cart or container must be labeled with a fluorescent orange or orange-red label containing a biohazard legend (Figure 5).[48] Biohazard labels must be securely affixed so as to prevent separation from the contents.[48] *[1: Regulatory Requirement]*

Labeling containers of biohazardous material is a regulatory requirement[48] and communicates to others that the contents may be biohazardous.

IV.c.3. Flexible endoscopes should be transported in a horizontal position and not suspended.[102] *[3: Moderate Evidence]*

Fluid may leak from the contaminated endoscope if the endoscope is transported vertically. When suspended, the endoscope may become damaged because of compression on dependent components.[102]

IV.c.4. Endoscope accessories should accompany the endoscope[13] but should be contained separately.[12,101,102] *[3: Moderate Evidence]*

Keeping the accessories with the endoscope helps prevent them from being lost or misplaced[13] and supports traceability of the endoscope and accessories as a single unit. Placing the accessories in a separate container helps prevent damage to the endoscope and accessories.[12,101,102]

IV.d. Processing of endoscopes and endoscope accessories should begin as soon as possible after transport to the endoscopy processing room or within the manufacturer's recommended time to processing. *[3: Moderate Evidence]*

Performing processing steps within one hour after a procedure may help prevent formation of biofilm.[15,82]

IV.d.1. When it is not possible to initiate the cleaning process within the endoscope manufacturer's recommended time to cleaning, the manufacturer's IFU for delayed processing should be followed.[12,16] *[3: Moderate Evidence]*

IV.d.2. Flexible endoscopes should not be left soaking in enzymatic cleaning solutions beyond the endoscope manufacturer's designated

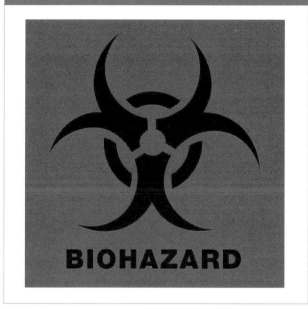

FIGURE 5. BIOHAZARD LEGEND

BIOHAZARD

contact time unless this is recommended in the manufacturer's IFU for delayed processing. *[3: Moderate Evidence]*

Alfa and Howie[104] demonstrated the ability of microorganisms to replicate in enzymatic cleaning solutions when held at room temperature (77° F [25° C]). Soaking endoscopes in enzymatic cleaning solutions beyond the manufacturer's designated contact time may increase the potential for microbial contamination, biofilm formation, ineffective disinfection or sterilization, and moisture damage to the endoscope.[99]

IV.d.3. A procedure should be developed and implemented for recording the times that the procedure is completed and cleaning is initiated. *[5: Benefits Balanced with Harms]*

A process for recording the times that the procedure ended and cleaning was initiated enables processing personnel to ascertain how long the endoscope has been awaiting processing, to establish priority order, and to determine whether routine processing within the manufacturer's recommended time to cleaning is achievable, and if not, to implement the manufacturer's procedures for delayed processing.

IV.e. Transport carts or containers used for flexible endoscopes should be mechanically cleaned and thermally disinfected or manually cleaned and chemically disinfected with a compatible Environmental Protection Agency (EPA)-registered hospital-grade disinfectant after each use.[69] *[2: High Evidence]*

Cleaning and disinfecting transport carts and containers after each use helps prevent cross contamination that could occur if clean items were placed on contaminated transport carts.[69] Disinfectants that are incompatible with the cart or container surface may cause damage to the cart or container and may be ineffective when applied to the incompatible surface.

Recommendation V

Flexible endoscopes designed to be leak tested, should be leak tested after each use, after any event that may have damaged the endoscope, and before use of a newly purchased, repaired, or loaned endoscope.

Not every endoscope requires leak testing.

The collective evidence supports leak testing as a method to help ensure the endoscope has not been compromised and is safe to use.[1,12,13,15-17,19,21,44,83-85,89,93,105,106]

Leak testing detects openings in the external surfaces and internal channels of the endoscope that could permit water, chemicals, or organic material to enter portions of the endoscope not intended for fluids.[106] These materials may accumulate from the time the integrity of the endoscope is breached until the time the leak is identified. Leak testing may be accomplished by manual or mechanical methods and may be performed using a wet (ie, under water) or dry process.[65]

The benefits of leak testing are that it reduces damage and repair costs and decreases the potential for patient infection or injury that might result from use of an endoscope that is not completely sealed.[85,89,107]

Khan et al[108] conducted a prospective quasi-experimental study to determine whether leak testing flexible ureteroscopes after ureterorenoscopy and laser fragmentation of renal calculi procedures reduced damage and repair costs. The new ureteroscope used for the Group 1 procedures (n = 95) was not leak tested after each procedure. The new ureteroscope used for the Group 2 procedures (n = 98) was leak tested after each procedure. Both groups were comparable for surgeon's years of experience, stone location, size and number of stones, access sheath usage, and duration of lasering. During the study period, October 2010 to March 2011, there were seven repairs costing $46,264.40 in Group 1 ($49,322.39 in 2015 US dollars) and three repairs costing $9,952.80 in Group 2 ($10,610.66 in 2015 US dollars). The researchers concluded that leak testing of flexible ureteroscopes significantly reduced the costs of maintenance and repair by promoting early recognition of damage, allowing for earlier repair, and preventing further use of a damaged ureteroscope.

In an effort to determine the longevity of flexible ureteroscopes used in the urology department of a London hospital, Bultitude et al[101] analyzed data for the number of procedures and repairs required for each of four new ureteroscopes used during 375 procedures. The results showed that on average, each ureteroscope was used 94 times, required two repairs, and was used for 36 procedures between each repair. To extend the life of the ureteroscope and help prevent unnecessary repairs, the authors recommended having dedicated personnel process the endoscopes, transporting endoscopes separately from the rest of the supplies and equipment, and performing a leak test after every procedure in order to detect and repair minor problems before they become major problems.

Leak testing may decrease the risk for an infection transmitted by a flexible endoscope. Ramsey et al[109] reported an outbreak of *Mycobacterium tuberculosis* transmitted from a patient with active tuberculosis to at least two patients via a contaminated bronchoscope. Examination of the bronchoscope revealed a small leak in the external sheath of the bronchoscope tip. The hole had not been discovered previously because leak testing was not routinely performed after bronchoscope use. The hole allowed the *M tuberculosis* from the index case to be delivered directly to the distal airways of subsequent patients.

Côtre et al[110] identified 117 bronchoalveolar lavage samples contaminated with *Enterobacteraceae* during three consecutive outbreaks among 418 patients between March 2001 and October 2001 in a 700-bed hospital in France. The source of the contamination was found to be a loose port of the biopsy channel of two of the seven bronchoscopes used in the endoscopy suite. The bronchoscopes were subsequently recalled by the manufacturer due to a potential design flaw. The researchers speculated that leak testing performed after each procedure might have allowed for much earlier detection of the problem.

In a report that illustrates the importance of leak testing in preventing patient injury, Krishna et al[111] described two cases of caustic mucosal injury of the larynx from exposure to glutaraldehyde retained in a damaged endoscope channel. The same laryngoscope was used for both patients. After examination, the laryngoscope was found to have retained glutaraldehyde because of an undetected perforation in the lining of the working channel. Both patients required inpatient admission with airway monitoring, and one patient required admission to the ICU. After treatment with antibiotics and steroids, the patients recovered with no further problems. The authors did not state whether leak testing was included in the processing of the laryngoscope in question; however, they concluded that leak testing was an important and necessary aspect of processing to determine whether the instrument channel had been damaged and to confirm the integrity of the laryngoscope.

V.a.   Leak testing should be performed before manual cleaning and before the endoscope is placed into cleaning solutions.[1,12,13,16,84,89] *[2: High Evidence]*

Performing leak testing before cleaning verifies the integrity of the endoscope and helps prevent damage that might occur during the cleaning process if the endoscope has been compromised.

The addition of cleaning solution to the water used for leak testing may discolor the water or introduce bubbles, limiting the ability of the person performing the leak test to see the entire endoscope or bubbles from the endoscope that indicate leaks.[16,107] Leaks may also go undetected because bubbles from leaks may be assumed to be bubbles from the cleaning solution.[107]

V.b.   Leak testing should be performed in accordance with the endoscope and leak-testing equipment manufacturers' IFU.[12,13,15-17,44,85] *[2: High Evidence]*

There are multiple types of endoscopes and leak-testing equipment. Steps to complete leak testing may vary among manufacturers.

V.b.1.   Steps to perform leak testing should include
- removing all port covers and function valves;
- pressurizing the endoscope to the recommended pressure[12,13,16,21,83,84,107];
- placing the endoscope in a loose configuration[12,13,16,21,83,107];
- manipulating all moving parts, including the elevator and angulating the bending section of the distal end[12,13,16,84,107];
- actuating video switches; and
- maintaining pressure and inspection for a minimum of 30 seconds.[12]

[2: High Evidence]

Underpressurizing may allow a leak to go undiscovered; overpressurizing may stress seals and cause damage to the endoscope.[107]

Tight coiling of the endoscope may hide leaks;[12] loose coiling helps remove structural impediments and improves visibility.[107]

Angulating the bending section of the distal end exposes the surfaces to maximum extension and helps reveal leaks.[12,107]

Maintaining pressure and inspection for a minimum of 30 seconds may help reveal small leaks. Evidence for leak testing time is based on expert opinion. The AAMI[12] recommends 30 seconds. Thomas[107] recommended 90 seconds in order to help detect leaks that may not be detected immediately.

V.c.   When an endoscope fails a leak test, it should be removed from service and repaired or replaced (see Recommendation VII.d.1.).[12,13,83-85] *[3: Moderate Evidence]*

Removing the endoscope from service will prevent further damage to the endoscope[84] and will prevent the damaged endoscope from being used.

Recommendation VI

After leak testing and before high-level disinfection or sterilization, flexible endoscopes should be manually cleaned.

The collective evidence indicates that cleaning is the most important step in the processing of flexible endoscopes.[18,22,85,93,112-114] Because of the body cavities they enter, some flexible endoscopes acquire high levels of microbial contamination.[45,112,113] Some flexible endoscopes contain multiple channels and ports that can easily collect organic material.[45,93] The environment in which flexible endoscopes are used provides optimal conditions for contamination and growth of biofilm.[93] When inadequately cleaned, contaminated endoscopes may be vectors of normal bacterial flora as well as pathogenic bacteria.[115,116] When endoscopes

STERILIZATION AND DISINFECTION

are effectively cleaned, bioburden is reduced to a level that does not present a challenge to subsequent disinfection or sterilization.[46,112,114,117]

In a landmark study, Chu et al[113] investigated and compared the bioburden levels on the exterior surfaces of the insertion tube and in the suction channels of colonoscopes immediately after use and after manual cleaning. The colonoscopes were collected from a free-standing endoscopy center and a hospital. Ten colonoscopes were sampled immediately after use, and 10 colonoscopes were sampled immediately after manual cleaning. The results of this randomized controlled trial showed that immediately after use, the level of bioburden on the exterior surfaces of the insertion tubes ranged from 1.2×10^4 to 1.5×10^6 colony forming units (CFU)/device. The level of bioburden in the suction channels ranged from 1.3×10^7 to 2.0×10^{10} CFU/device. After manual cleaning, the level of bioburden on the exterior surfaces of the insertion tube decreased to a range of 8.2×10^2 to 9.5×10^4 CFU/device, establishing that manual cleaning achieved a mean reduction of greater than 1 log. The level of bioburden in the suction channels decreased to a range of 1.3×10^3 to 4.3×10^5 CFU/device, establishing that manual cleaning achieved a mean reduction of 5.5 logs. The 4-log difference can be attributed to the fact that the suction channel is the working channel of the device through which suction occurs and accessories are inserted into the intended locations, so this lumen is exposed to a greater volume of intestinal material.

If endoscopes are not adequately cleaned, the disinfection or sterilization process can fail and increase the possibility for transmission of infectious microorganisms from one patient to another.[112,114,116,117] Some disinfectants are inactivated in the presence of organic material.[1,16]

In a quasi-experimental laboratory study to demonstrate the effectiveness of a high-level disinfectant (ie, orthophalaldehyde), Alfa and Sitter[115] sampled 10 bronchoscopes, 10 gastroscopes, and 10 colonoscopes immediately after use. They found the level of bioburden for the bronchoscopes was 6.4×10^5 CFU/mL^{-1}, the level of bioburden for the gastroscopes was 1.7×10^5 CFU/mL^{-1}, and the level of bioburden for the colonoscopes was 5.2×10^5 CFU/mL^{-1}. The researchers noted that the average load of microorganisms was higher for the gastroscopes than for the bronchoscopes, reflecting the higher number of bacteria in the gastrointestinal tract compared with the respiratory tract, and was likewise higher for the colonoscopes than for the gastroscopes due to the higher concentration of microorganisms in the colon compared with the upper gastrointestinal tract or the bronchi. The endoscopes were cleaned and disinfected, and the residual microbial load was monitored by sampling the suction channels. The researchers found that the cleaning process alone removed up to 10^3 organisms, leaving fewer organisms for the disinfectant to kill. The cleaning and disinfection procedure achieved more than a 5-$\log_{10}$ reduction in bacterial load. The researchers emphasized the need to combine effective cleaning with the high-level disinfectant to ensure maximum efficacy of the disinfectant.

Cleaning is a process that uses friction, cleaning solution, and water to remove organic and inorganic debris to the extent necessary for further processing or for the intended use.[12,58,89,93,112,117] Cleaning removes rather than kills microorganisms. The effectiveness of the cleaning process can vary based on a number of factors including the type of device being cleaned, the design of the device being cleaned, the person performing the cleaning, the amount of time spent cleaning, and the site where the device is cleaned.[112] Routine cleaning procedures may not effectively remove biofilm from endoscope channels. Biofilm remaining in the lumen of an endoscope may prevent effective HLD or sterilization.[92,115]

In a quasi-experimental laboratory study, Pajkos et al[92] assessed 13 biopsy channels and 12 air channels removed from 13 endoscopes that had been sent to an endoscope processing center in Sydney, Australia. The endoscopes were of various ages from 13 different hospitals, and no information was provided to the researchers as to the reason for servicing or how frequently the endoscopes had been used. The researchers used scanning electron microscopy (SEM) to examine the endoscope channels for the presence of biofilm. The SEM showed that biofilm was present on five of the 13 biopsy channels and on all 12 of the air channel samples. In addition, the researchers found surface defects that included cracks, grooves, and pits in many of the channels. The researchers concluded that cleaning had not removed all biofilm from any of the channels, and they noted that the presence of biofilm could lead to failure of the HLD process by inactivating or preventing penetration of the disinfectant.

Alfa and Howie[104] investigated whether the repeated exposure to high levels of microorganisms and the wet and dry conditions that occur during the use and processing of flexible endoscopes could lead to an accumulation of organic material in endoscope channels, and whether this biofilm buildup presented a greater challenge to remove than traditional biofilm that forms when a surface is exposed to microorganisms and continually bathed in fluid. The results of the study showed that the biofilm buildup facilitated high levels of organism survival and reduced the efficacy of the two high-level disinfectants evaluated during the study (ie, glutaraldehyde, accelerated hydrogen peroxide). The researchers theorized that these results provided an explanation for the persistence of residual levels of biofilm remaining in endoscope channels even when the endoscopes were correctly processed. As flexible endoscopes are repeatedly used and processed, the load of bioburden increases, reducing the efficacy of the high-level disinfectant and increasing the risk for pathogen transmission.

The benefits of manual cleaning are that it removes visible soil and reduces the amount of microbial contamination and biofilm formation on and in the endoscope.[16,83,84] If microbial contamination and biofilm are not removed completely, the surface under the bioburden may not be disinfected or sterilized.[16,22,83,84,104,112,114,116] Manual cleaning helps ensure effective HLD or sterilization and may protect the patient from exposure to contaminated endoscopes that could result in transmissible infections.[114,118]

VI.a. Manual cleaning should occur as soon as possible after leak testing. *[3: Moderate Evidence]*

Initiating the cleaning process as soon as possible after leak testing helps prevent the formation of biofilm.[82,83] Biofilm is difficult to remove

FLEXIBLE ENDOSCOPES

and may begin to form within minutes after the procedure is completed.[82] If biofilm is present on or in the endoscope, the subsequent HLD or sterilization process may not be effective.[82,95,96]

VI.b. Manual cleaning should be performed in accordance with the endoscope manufacturer's IFU. *[3: Moderate Evidence]*

There are multiple types of endoscopes. Steps to complete cleaning may vary among manufacturers. Adherence to the manufacturer's IFU may minimize the risk for infection.[6]

VI.c. Manual cleaning should be performed using the type of water recommended by the endoscope manufacturer. *[4: Limited Evidence]*

Recommendations for the type of water to be used for manual cleaning may vary among endoscope manufacturers. Utility water is often adequate for precleaning, manual cleaning, and rinsing; however, water quality is affected by the presence of dissolved minerals, solids, chlorides, and other impurities and by its acidity and alkalinity.[119] The pH level of the water affects the performance of cleaning solutions.[119] Untreated water quality fluctuates over time, varies with geographic location and season, and can affect the outcome of cleaning actions.[119]

VI.d. Manual cleaning should be performed using a cleaning solution recommended by the endoscope manufacturer. *[2: High Evidence]*

There are multiple types of endoscopes. Recommended cleaning solutions may vary among manufacturers. Following the endoscope manufacturer's IFU decreases the possibility of selecting and using cleaning solutions that may damage the endoscope.

The chemical actions of cleaning solutions vary and are intended for different applications. The pH and rinsability of cleaning products also vary. Some cleaning solutions target specific types of bioburden (eg, protein, lipids); others are intended for general purpose cleaning.[90] General purpose cleaners function primarily as surfactants.[65,120]

Enzymatic cleaners contain one or a combination of enzymes to help break down organic material and facilitate its removal.[65,90,120,121] Enzymes are specific in terms of the soils they remove. Protease enzymes target proteins.[120,121] Amylase enzymes target carbohydrates, starches, and sugars.[90,120-122] Lipase enzymes break down fats and oils.[90,120-122] Cellulase enzymes break down cellulose.[90] Enzymatic cleaners attempt to remove biofilm by decomposing the extracellular polysaccharides surrounding and protecting the embedded microorganism.[95] Because the diversity of extracellular polysaccharides in the biofilm is unique to the microorganism, a mixture of enzymes may be needed for sufficient degradation of bacterial biofilm.[91]

Enzymatic cleaners are effective at room temperature (ie, 68° F to 72° F [20° C to 22° C]) but

function more effectively at warmer temperatures.[19,69,89,120] A temperature that is too hot (ie, ≥ 140° F [≥ 60° C]) denatures proteins and may negate the desired enzymatic activity.[69,120]

Enzymatic cleaners are often recommended for cleaning flexible endoscopes and other medical devices because they help remove proteins, lipids, and carbohydrates by breaking down large molecules into smaller, water-soluble molecules that are easily rinsed away after cleaning[83,122]; however, the collective evidence conflicts regarding the benefits of using enzymatic cleaning solutions compared with nonenzymatic cleaners that may contain disinfectants or other chemicals to enhance cleaning and reduce viable bioburden.[91,95,123] Decontamination is a physical or chemical process that removes or reduces the number of microorganisms or infectious agents and renders reusable medical devices safe for use, handling, or disposal.[12,45,58] Decontamination requires a microbicidal process after cleaning.[12,58] Microbicidal cleaning solutions do not eliminate the need for HLD or sterilization, but they may reduce the risk of exposure to biohazardous substances for processing personnel.[22,120]

In a quasi-experimental laboratory study, Merritt et al[86] evaluated the effects of 12 different cleaning products, including enzymatic and nonenzymatic cleaning solutions, on organisms known to adhere to polystyrene and medical implant materials (ie, *S epidermidis, C albicans, E coli, P aeruginosa*). The results of the study showed that the enzymatic cleaners were effective at cleaning contaminated surfaces and removed all of the microorganisms while the solutions without enzymes were no more effective than utility water.

In a quasi-experimental laboratory study conducted to determine the effectiveness of five enzymatic and nine nonenzymatic cleaners on *E coli* biofilm, Henoun Loukili et al[123] found that of the six products with the highest effectiveness scores (ie, mean percent activity of detergent > 70%), three were enzymatic cleaners and three were nonenzymatic cleaners. The three enzymatic cleaners had the highest scores (ie, 92%, 90%, 89%). The researchers concluded that enzymatic cleaners were not more effective than nonenzymatic cleaners. A major limitation of the study was that the enzymatic solutions were used at room temperature (ie, 68° F to 77° F [20° C to 25° C]), which may not have been in accordance with the manufacturers' recommendations and may have affected overall performance. Another limitation was that the biofilm was prepared on a glass surface that is not representative of the materials used in many medical devices, including flexible endoscopes.

In a study to compare the effectiveness of enzymatic and nonenzymatic cleaners on *E coli* biofilm on the inner surface of gastroscopes,

STERILIZATION AND DISINFECTION

818

Fang et al[124] randomly and equally assigned 15 Teflon® tubes coated with biofilm to one of three groups:

○ Group 1 tubes were treated with a one-minute wash with water, followed by a three-minute wash with enzymatic cleaner, followed by a one-minute wash with water.
○ Group 2 tubes were treated with a one-minute wash with water, followed by a three-minute wash with nonenzymatic cleaner, followed by a one-minute wash with water.
○ Group 3 tubes were treated with a one-minute wash with water, followed by a three-minute wash with sterile distilled water, followed by a one-minute wash with water.

The researchers found that although none of the cleaning solutions completely eliminated the biofilm, there was a 2.39-$\log_{10}$ CFU/tube reduction of bacterial burden in the nonenzymatic group compared with a 0.23-$\log_{10}$ CFU/tube reduction of bacterial burden in the enzymatic group. The researchers concluded that the nonenzymatic cleaners were more effective than the enzymatic cleaners. A limitation of this study was the use of only one bacterial biofilm. Another limitation was that the enzymatic cleaner was noted to be most effective at a temperature higher than room temperature (ie, 68° F [20° C]), but was used at 59° F (15° C). The researchers believed this temperature was more representative of the temperature at which enzymatic cleaning solutions are often used in actual practice.

In a study to evaluate the effects of various cleaning products and contact times on the removal of biofilm from flexible endoscopes, Ren et al[95] randomly and equally assigned 60 Teflon tubes coated with *E coli* biofilm to one of four groups:

○ Group 1 tubes were treated with enzymatic cleaner 1.
○ Group 2 tubes were treated with enzymatic cleaner 2.
○ Group 3 tubes were treated with a nonenzymatic cleaner.
○ Group 4 tubes were treated with sterile water for injection.

The researchers found a statistically significant difference between the amount of residual biofilm in the enzymatic groups (Group 1 = 4.61 ± 0.52 CFU/cm²; Group 2 = 4.67 ± 0.59 CFU/cm²) compared with the nonenzymatic group (1.29 ± 0.13 CFU/cm²). Both enzymatic and nonenzymatic cleaners demonstrated the ability to remove biofilm; however, the amount of biofilm removal was greater with the nonenzymatic cleaner. A limitation of this study was the use of only one bacterial biofilm, although the researchers noted that *E coli* is a major component of normal intestinal flora and source of bacterial contamination of gastrointestinal endoscopes.[95]

In a quasi-experimental laboratory study, Vickery et al[125] tested the efficacy of four enzymatic cleaning solutions and one nonenzymatic cleaning product on Teflon and polyvinyl chloride tubes coated with *E coli* biofilm. The researchers found that the nonenzymatic cleaner resulted in a 4.7-$\log_{10}$ CFU/cm² reduction in biofilm bacteria, while the most effective enzymatic cleaner resulted in only a 1.57-$\log_{10}$ CFU/cm² reduction. Notably, the nonenzymatic cleaner used in the study was a quaternary ammonium disinfectant and for this reason would be expected to have a greater bacterial log reduction compared with cleaning solutions that are not microbicidal.[126]

Alfa and Jackson[121] conducted a quasi-experimental laboratory study to evaluate the cleaning and bactericidal effectiveness of a hydrogen peroxide-based nonenzymatic cleaner compared with two enzymatic cleaners. Test organisms (*Enterococcus faecalis, Salmonella choleraesuis, Staphylococcus aureus, P aeruginosa*) were suspended in artificial test soil on polyvinyl chloride carriers and then exposed to the cleaning solutions. The nonenzymatic cleaner demonstrated a 5-$\log_{10}$ CFU/carrier reduction in microbial load, even in the presence of a dried organic challenge of *E faecalis* and *S aureus*. The researchers found that none of the enzymatic cleaners achieved this level of log reduction.

Marion et al[127] recommended an approach for removing biofilm that involved the use of detachment-promoting cleaners in endoscope channels and automated washer-disinfectors. The researchers contaminated the operating channel of three new endoscopes with biofilm developed from human serum inoculated with a bacterial culture of *P aeruginosa, S epidermidis, Enterobacter cloacae*, and *K pneumoniae*. One endoscope was left untreated; two endoscopes were treated with different detachment-promoting cleaners. The treated endoscopes underwent a static brushing procedure that involved immersing the endoscope in the selected cleaner and brushing the contaminated operating channel for one minute using the manufacturer's recommended cleaning brush, simulating a manual cleaning process. The treated endoscopes also underwent a dynamic flushing procedure that involved the use of a peristaltic pump to circulate the cleaner through the operating channel, simulating a mechanical cleaning process. The researchers examined the internal surfaces of the operating channel using SEM and found that the biofilm was completely removed by the detachment-promoting cleaners.

Perret-Vivancos et al[128] reported the case of a highly contaminated colonoscope that was effectively treated with a combination of biofilm detachment-promoting agents. The treatment included application of a multienzymatic solution designed to digest the foundation where the biofilm was anchored, followed by an enriched detergent solution designed to detach the biofilm as a single unit. After the first treatment, the authors found there was a decrease in the contamination level but the biofilm was not completely eliminated. A second identical treatment was applied and showed a significant reduction in the amount of biofilm. After a third treatment, the biofilm was almost totally removed.

The authors speculated that using these detachment-promoting cleaners could represent an approach to biofilm control that might improve the efficacy of cleaning and reduce the risk of transmitting infections. In addition, these cleaners have the potential to reduce costs by allowing for salvage of endoscopes contaminated with biofilm or as a preventive mechanism to avoid accumulation of biofilm in endoscope channels.[128] Further research is warranted.

VI.d.1.   If the manufacturer's recommended cleaning solution is not available, processing personnel should contact the endoscope manufacturer for recommendations for other cleaning solutions that may be used. *[5: Benefits Balanced with Harms]*

VI.d.2.   Manual cleaning should be performed using a freshly prepared cleaning solution.[12,13,15,16,27,69,83,84,89,98] Cleaning solutions should be changed before they become cloudy or discolored, and before there are visible particulates in the solution. *[2: High Evidence]*

Using a freshly prepared solution for each new cleaning process helps prevent cross contamination.[12,13,15,16,27,69,83,84,89,98] Cleaning solutions are not microbicidal and may support bacterial growth if stored or reused beyond their expiration date.[45,65,84,99,129] Repeated use of cleaning solutions decreases the amount of active ingredients in the solution and reduces cleaning efficacy. Residual contaminants in cleaning solutions could increase the potential for cross contamination.[96] Bioburden is deposited in the cleaning solution during the cleaning process. Changing the cleaning solution minimizes bioburden.

In a nonexperimental study to investigate biofilm on endoscope channels, Ren-Pei et al[96] collected 66 endoscope suction and biopsy channels and 13 water and air channels from 66 endoscopy centers in hospitals throughout China. They used SEM to examine biofilm on the inner surface of the channels. A total of 36 suction and biopsy channels (54.5%) and 10 water and air channels (76.9%) were found to have biofilm.

After examining the endoscope channels, the researchers sent a questionnaire to each of the 66 endoscopy centers to explore the correlation between endoscope processing procedures and the amount of biofilm in the endoscope channels. They divided the responses (N = 66) into hospitals without biofilm on endoscopes (Group A; n = 30), and hospitals with biofilm on endoscopes (Group B; n = 36). The researchers found that the proportion of reuse of enzymatic cleaning solutions in Group A was 60% (18 of 30), whereas in Group B the proportion was 91.6% (33 of 36) and in some cases, the cleaning solution was reused more than four times. The researchers concluded that the formation of biofilm on the endoscope channels could be related to reuse of cleaning solutions.[96]

VI.d.3.   Additional products should not be added to the cleaning solution unless this is recommended by the manufacturer. *[4: Limited Evidence]*

Adding products that are not recommended by the manufacturer could cause a chemical reaction that could damage the endoscope or render the cleaning solution ineffective.[83]

VI.d.4.   The cleaning solution manufacturer's IFU should be followed for
- water quality, hardness, and pH[58,119];
- concentration and dilution[19,20,58,65,83,98];
- water temperature[20,58,83,120];
- contact time[16,58,65,83,84,98,120];
- conditions of storage[58]; and
- use life and shelf life.[58,69,98]

[2: High Evidence]
Deviations from the manufacturer's IFU may render the cleaning product ineffective.[129]

Water quality, including hardness, and pH can alter the effectiveness of cleaning solutions.[25,90,119] The enzymes used in enzymatic cleaners may be most effective at a neutral pH and may be inactivated by a high or low pH.[98]

Using the product in the concentration recommended by the manufacturer helps ensure consistent and accurate cleaning chemistry.[77] A weak solution may not effectively break down proteins and other organic material; a strong solution may produce an increased number of bubbles, creating air pockets that prohibit surface contact of the cleaning chemical with the endoscope.[122,129] Undiluted or under-diluted enzymatic cleaning solutions are difficult to remove and may lead to residual cleaning solutions and proteinaceous material in the endoscope that provide a foundation for biofilm formation and lead to processing failures.

If the water temperature is not warm enough, the cleaning product may not mix with the water as intended,[122,129] and the enzymes may not be able to effectively dissolve and remove organic soil.[25] If the temperature is too hot, it may cause coagulation of proteins and fix proteinaceous soil to the endoscope.[25]

Contact of the cleaning solution with all surfaces of the endoscope for the minimum contact time is necessary for effective cleaning.[16,120,121]

Enzymes used in enzymatic cleaners can lose their effectiveness over time.[83,90,98] The cleaning solution may be ineffective if used beyond the defined period of useful life or the expiration date.

Hutchisson and LeBlanc[98] conducted a quasi-experimental study to demonstrate the need to follow the manufacturer's IFU when using enzymatic cleaning solutions. The researchers tested five colonoscopes used during procedures at a Texas hospital after precleaning at the point of use, and then manually cleaned them using a low-sudsing enzymatic cleaner in the following formulations:

- Endoscope 1: 1 oz of low-sudsing enzymatic cleaner in 1 gallon of water followed by a water rinse.
- Endoscope 2: 2 oz of low-sudsing enzymatic cleaner in 1 gallon of water followed by a water rinse.
- Endoscope 3: 4 oz of low-sudsing enzymatic cleaner in 1 gallon of water followed by a water rinse.
- Endoscope 4: 1 oz of low-sudsing enzymatic cleaner in 1 gallon of water with no rinse.
- Endoscope 5: undiluted low-sudsing enzymatic cleaner followed by a water rinse.

The manufacturer's IFU called for 1 oz of enzymatic cleaner in 1 gallon of water.

After manual cleaning, the colonoscopes were mechanically processed, rinsed, and disinfected with orthophalaldehyde. They were hung vertically to dry without an alcohol flush. An absorbent white cloth was placed on the floor of the endoscope cabinet to catch effluent dripping from the distal tips of the endoscopes. Orthophalaldehyde reacts with residual bioburden to form dark stains. The researchers observed no staining of proteinaceous material with Endoscope 1 that had been cleaned with correctly diluted cleaning solution followed by a water rinse. The researchers observed some staining with Endoscope 4 that had been cleaned with correctly diluted cleaning solution but not rinsed. They observed significant staining with Endoscopes 2, 3, and 5 that were cleaned with underdiluted and nondiluted cleaning solution and then rinsed.[98]

The results of the study demonstrated that when endoscopes were cleaned using incorrect dilutions of cleaning solutions, small amounts of residual proteinaceous material was left on the interior and exterior surfaces of the endoscope. There could be a buildup of this residual material over time, which raises concerns about cleaning effectiveness as well as the potential negative effect of residual buildup on the optimal functioning and life of the endoscope.[98]

VI.d.5.   An automated titration unit may be used to concentrate cleaning products at a consistent ratio.[58] *[5: Benefits Balanced with Harms]*

The concentration of the solution can vary when it is mixed manually. Using a titration unit can aid in accurate measurement of the chemical during preparation of the cleaning solution and help personnel to consistently obtain the recommended concentration of the cleaning product.[58]

VI.d.6.   Cleaning solutions should be changed when the temperature of the solution does not meet the temperature specified in the manufacturer's IFU.[77] A digital temperature measuring device may be used to monitor the temperature of the cleaning solution. *[4: Limited Evidence]*

Cleaning solutions may not be effective when used at temperatures outside of the manufacturer-specified parameters.

VI.e.   The endoscope should be completely submerged in the cleaning solution during the cleaning process.[12,13,16,20,22,65,84,85,89] Removable parts (eg, valves, buttons, caps) should be detached from the endoscope and submerged if recommended by the endoscope manufacturer's IFU.[85] *[2: High Evidence]*

Cleaning the endoscope under the surface of the solution helps prevent splashing of the contaminated solution and reduces the potential for aerosolization and exposure to biohazardous substances.[16] Detaching removable parts and completely submerging the endoscope and removable parts helps ensure contact between the cleaning solution and all surfaces of the endoscope.[65]

VI.f.   All exterior surfaces of the endoscope (Figure 6) should be cleaned with a soft, lint-free cloth or sponge saturated with the cleaning solution.[1,12,13,15,16,18,19,22,27,65,83,84,89,105] *[2: High Evidence]*

Washing the external surfaces of the endoscope helps remove organic material that remains after precleaning.

VI.g.   All accessible channels and the distal end of the endoscope should be cleaned with a cleaning

FLEXIBLE ENDOSCOPES

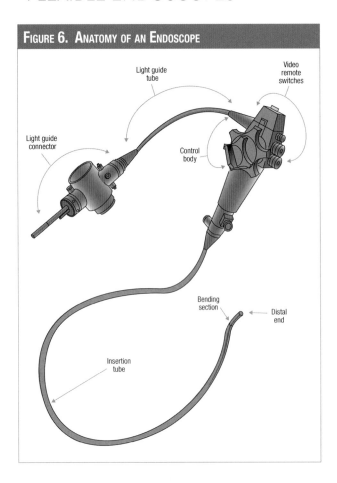

FIGURE 6. ANATOMY OF AN ENDOSCOPE

brush of the length, width, and material recommended by the endoscope manufacturer.[1,13,15,18,19,22,45,65,83,85,89,105,129] The endoscope valves should be manually actuated while cleaning.[12,19,22] *[2: High Evidence]*

The collective evidence supports thorough and careful brushing of the accessible endoscope channels (Figure 7) with a correctly-sized brush as a method of dislodging and removing organic material and biofilm.[1,18,45] Cleaning the distal end helps ensure there is no debris or tissue lodged in or around the water nozzle and suction biopsy channel.[85] The presence and buildup of organic material in the lumens of endoscopes can have significant implications, including toxic reactions, device damage, inadequate disinfection or sterilization, increased risk of biofilm development, and the potential transmission of infection.[130,131]

Using the correct-size brush increases contact between the brush and the walls of the endoscope channels and maximizes the amount of soil removed.[19,129] If the brush is too small, it will not make contact with the organic material or channel walls.[129] If the brush is too large, it may get lodged in the channel and cause damage to the internal channels, or the bristles may be deflected upward, only swiping the sides of the channel and not effectively removing organic material or contacting the channel walls.[129] Some

endoscopes will require the use of two different brush sizes for effective cleaning.[129]

Manually actuating the valves during cleaning helps ensure brushing of all internal parts.[12,19]

Pineau and De Philippe[132] assessed 206 samples from flexible endoscopes (ie, 87 colonoscopes, 93 gastroscopes, 26 bronchoscopes) from four different hospitals in France for levels of bioburden. In this nonexperimental study, the researchers compared samples that had been collected

- after point-of-use precleaning (n = 30);
- after point-of-use precleaning and manual brushing of channels (n = 34);
- after point-of-use precleaning, manual brushing of channels, and double washing and rinsing in a mechanical processor (n = 111); and
- after point-of-use precleaning, manual brushing of channels, double washing and rinsing in a mechanical processor, and HLD in a mechanical processor (n = 31).

The researchers found that brushing significantly reduced the contamination present in the endoscope channels after point-of-use precleaning. Brushing endoscope channels reduced the number of viable bacteria by at least 2.5-$\log_{10}$/cm^2. The researchers concluded that brushing was important for reducing contamination remaining in endoscopes after point-of-use precleaning.

In a quasi-experimental laboratory study, Dietze et al[133] investigated the influence of design on the efficacy of manual cleaning of endoscope channels. The researchers tested two duodenoscopes and two gastroscopes. The air channels of one duodenoscope (A) and one gastroscope (B) were freely accessible and able to be flushed and brushed. The air channels of the other duodenoscope (C) and the other gastroscope (D) were only able to be flushed. The researchers contaminated the air channels of all four endoscopes with blood containing *Enterococcus faecium* as a test organism. They implemented manual cleaning by flushing and brushing for endoscopes A and B and flushing only for endoscopes C and D and then calculated the recovery rates.

The researchers found that the rate of microorganisms recovered after flushing alone was between 4.8 x 10^5 CFU/180 mL and 5.8 x 10^5 CFU/180 mL. The rate of microorganisms recovered after flushing and brushing was between 1.6 x 10^7 CFU/180 mL and 2.3 x 10^7 CFU/180 mL. This indicated that the cleaning rate for flushing alone was only 2.6% of the cleaning rate obtained by flushing and brushing.[133]

In a quasi-experimental study, Ishino et al[134] alternately assigned endoscopes used for upper gastrointestinal examinations into Group A (n = 20), where the air and water channels were brushed three times with a sterile, correctly

STERILIZATION AND DISINFECTION

822

sized brush, and Group B (n = 22), where the air and water channels were not brushed. The researchers examined the endoscope channels using a protein-staining dye and found no residual protein in the air channels of either Group A or Group B endoscopes. The water channels of the Group A endoscopes also had no residual protein; however, one water channel from the Group B endoscopes did have residual protein. The researchers concluded that the proteinaceous material remaining in the water channel of the non-brushed endoscope was likely organic debris, and unless removed by brushing, this material could become fixed on the inner surface of the endoscope channels and become a potential source of infection.

Bajolet et al[118] reported transmission of an extended-spectrum ß-lactamase-producing *P aeruginosa* in four patients who underwent esophagogastroduodenoscopy (EGD) procedures with the same gastroscope between May 2011 and August 2011. The gastroscope had been purchased in January 2011. Microbiological sampling before its first use showed negative results. Observation of the endoscope processing procedures during the investigation identified cleaning failures that included inadequate brushing and flushing of the channels and the use of a single-diameter cleaning brush for all gastrointestinal endoscopes. The investigators concluded that the lack of sufficient cleaning and the use of an incorrectly sized brush may have supported the development of a persistent biofilm that contributed to patient-to-patient transmission of a serious infection.

Agerton et al[135] reported a case of transmission of multidrug-resistant *M tuberculosis* (MDR-TB) caused by a contaminated bronchoscope. Five patients from a South Carolina community who were family members or close friends were diagnosed with tuberculosis. Three additional patients were hospitalized in the same facility as one of the five patients diagnosed with tuberculosis. These three patients had bronchoscopy procedures performed with the same bronchoscope in the same hospital within 17 days of the tuberculosis patient. As a result of the contaminated bronchoscope, two patients had false-positive MDR-TB cultures from specimens obtained during their bronchoscopy procedures, and one patient developed and died from MDR-TB. A review of the processing procedures for bronchoscopes revealed that leak-testing equipment was available but never used, manual cleaning time averaged less than three minutes, and a cleaning brush was passed through the endoscope only one time.

VI.g.1. The elevator mechanism and the recesses surrounding it should be cleaned and brushed with a cleaning brush of the length, width, and material recommended by the endoscope manufacturer.[1,6,13,15,22,45,65,83,85,89,129]

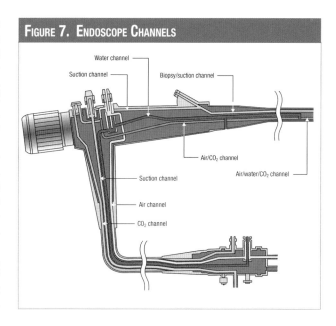

FIGURE 7. ENDOSCOPE CHANNELS

Water channel
Suction channel
Biopsy/suction channel
Air/CO₂ channel
Air/water/CO₂ channel
Suction channel
Air channel
CO₂ channel

The elevator should be raised and lowered throughout the manual cleaning process.[6,85] *[2: High Evidence]*

Some duodenoscopes have a movable elevator channel at the distal end (Figure 8) that allows the accessory instrument to access the pancreatic and biliary ducts.[6] The collective evidence shows that the complex design of the duodenoscope improves the efficiency and effectiveness of ERCP procedures; however, some parts of the endoscope may be extremely difficult to access, and this creates challenges for cleaning.[6] In fact, effective cleaning of all areas of the duodenoscope may not be possible.[6] The moving parts of the elevator mechanisms contain microscopic crevices that may not be reachable with a brush.[6] Residual body fluids and organic material may remain in these crevices after cleaning and disinfection.[6] If this fluid or material contains microbial contamination, subsequent patients may be exposed to serious infections.[6,136,137] Although the risk of infection transmission associated with these complex devices cannot be completely eliminated, the benefits of treatment outweigh the risks in appropriately selected patients.[138]

Raising and lowering the elevator during the cleaning process helps ensure that no organic material is lodged in the moveable mechanism and allows for more effective brushing of all surfaces, including the base of the elevator apparatus.[6,85,139]

Alrabaa et al[136] reported seven cases of carbapenemase-producing *K pneumoniae* in patients from two tertiary hospitals in South Florida between June 2008 and January 2009. All seven patients had ERCP procedures at the same outpatient endoscopy center within 60 days before the outbreak.

STERILIZATION AND DISINFECTION

Six patients had undergone procedures with a common endoscope.[140] The endoscope was examined and found to have residual organic material under the elevator that cultured positive for carbapenemase-producing *E coli, Pseudomonas*, and *Serratia* species.[140] The investigators observed processing procedures at the endoscopy center and found the cleaning procedure for the duodenoscopes was inadequate. The manufacturer's IFU that required cleaning with a brush the complex terminal part of the endoscope that contains the elevator was not followed, and bioburden remained under the elevator of the endoscope after the cleaning process was completed. The investigators concluded that processing duodenoscopes was more complex than processing traditional endoscopes, and additional steps were required to ensure effective decontamination.[140]

The CDC[141] reported an outbreak of New Delhi metallo-ß-lactamase-1 (NDM-1)-producing *E coli* involving 28 colonized and 10 infected patients. All 38 patients were exposed while undergoing ERCP in a Chicago hospital between January 2013 and September 2013. After manual cleaning and mechanical processing, the terminal section of a side-viewing duodenoscope used for five of the case patients remained culture-positive for NDM-1-producing *E coli* and carbapenemase-producing *K pneumoniae*, despite no obvious lapses in protocol. Although cultured from the same endoscope, no colonization or infections were identified from this second strain of carbapenem-resistant *Enterobacteriaceae*. The CDC observed that the design of ERCP endoscopes makes them particularly challenging to clean and disinfect. In an independent inspection of the hospital's procedures, the Centers for Medicare & Medicaid Services reported that the hospital was using unapproved cleaning solutions and brushes and failed to process the endoscopes as recommended by the manufacturer.[142,143]

Wendorf et al[137] described an outbreak of AmpC-producing *E coli* at a medical center in Seattle between November 2012 and August 2013. Thirty-two patients who had undergone ERCP procedures were found to harbor one of two genetically similar strains of the organism.[144,145] The investigators found no violations of the recommended processing procedures. During the investigation, the endoscope manufacturer observed personnel manually cleaning and inspecting the endoscopes and concluded that the cleaning process was not only consistent with manufacturer guidelines, it was above the industry standard. Even after implementing procedures that included enhanced manual cleaning, the investigators found that gastrointestinal bacteria continued to be recovered from the endoscope elevator channels.[137]

Nine endoscopes, which included the eight endoscopes in use during the outbreak plus an additional endoscope, were evaluated by the manufacturer. The manufacturer found that all of the endoscopes (whether in need of repair or not) harbored pathogenic bacteria in the elevator channel and continued to have positive cultures even after repair. Notably, three of the endoscopes had passed leak tests at the hospital but failed the manufacturer's leak test, and seven endoscopes were determined to have at least one critical defect. The investigators concluded that obscure mechanical defects in combination with the difficulty of cleaning the elevator channel facilitated the transmission of the infection.

Kola et al[146] reported an outbreak of carbapenemase-resistant *K pneumoniae* (CRKP) associated with a contaminated duodenoscope in a German university hospital. Between December 2012 and January 2013, CRKP was cultured from 12 patients staying on four different wards. Molecular typing confirmed the close relation between all 12 isolates. Six of the patients were from the same ward; they were immediately transferred to separate rooms and placed on contact precautions. The remaining six patients had all undergone ERCP procedures with the same duodenoscope. Culturing the duodenoscope did not recover CRKP.

The investigators reviewed processing procedures for the duodenoscope and could find not deviations from the manufacturer's IFU; however, they did obtain positive cultures for *Enterococci*, which they suggested was indicative of insufficient cleaning. The duodenoscope was sent to the manufacturer who found a defective distal cap. The outbreak ended when the duodenoscope was removed from service. The investigators concluded that the processing procedures may not have been sufficient in every case because of the complex physical design of the distal end of the duodenoscope.[146]

Verfaillie et al[147] reported a large outbreak of Verona integron-encoded metallo-ß-lactamase (VIM)-2-producing *P aeruginosa* linked to the use of a duodenoscope with a sealed elevator channel intended to obviate the need for special cleaning measures. Between January 2012 and April 2012, 30 patients were identified with a VIM-2-positive *P aeruginosa*; 22 of these patients had undergone ERCP with the same duodenoscope. The investigators confirmed that the strain in all 22 cases was identical to the strain that was cultured from the recess under the forceps elevator of the duodenoscope. Dismantling the distal end of the duodenoscope revealed that the sealed elevator channel design may have hampered effective cleaning. The outbreak resolved when the endoscope was withdrawn from clinical use.

VI.g.2. A clean brush should be used for each endoscope cleaning. Brushes and other items used to clean endoscope channels should be visually inspected before use and should not be used if the integrity of the brush or other cleaning item is in question.[89] *[3: Moderate Evidence]*

Using a clean brush for each cleaning of the endoscope helps prevent cross contamination. Verifying the brush is intact and safe to use (ie, the protective tip is present, the coiling is braided, all bristles are present, the delivery tube is not kinked) assists with effective cleaning and helps prevent damage to the endoscope.[129]

Behnia et al[148] reported a pseudo-outbreak of *Stenotrophomonas maltophilia* and *Acinetobacter baumannii* in six patients in a community hospital in Augusta, Georgia. The source was traced to a contaminated bronchoscope that had been used in two ICUs at the same hospital. The investigators reviewed the processing procedures for the bronchoscope and found that brushes intended for single-use were being shared between several different bronchoscopes and were not discarded after each use.

VI.g.3. The accessible channels of the endoscope should be brushed multiple times until no debris appears on the brush.[12,13,15,16,20,21,27,45,65,83,85,89] Debris should be removed from the brush before the brush is retracted back through the channel and after each pass by swirling the brush in the cleaning solution and rinsing it.[13,15,16,,65,83,85,89] *[2: High Evidence]*

Cleaning and rinsing the cleaning brush after each pass removes visible debris and helps prevent it from being redeposited in the endoscope channel.[12,13]

VI.g.4. New technologies for brush design and lumen cleaning may be used when compatible with the endoscope. *[3: Moderate Evidence]*

There is discussion in the literature regarding the need for enhanced brush design to improve cleaning efficacy, decrease brushing time and effort, and reduce the potential for exposure of processing personnel to biohazardous material.

In a quasi-experimental laboratory study to evaluate protein deposits and removal in the channels of flexible endoscopes, Hervé

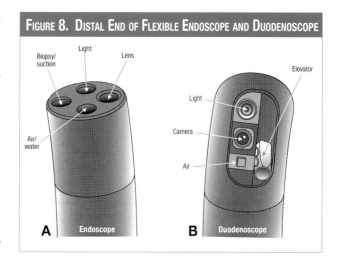

FIGURE 8. DISTAL END OF FLEXIBLE ENDOSCOPE AND DUODENOSCOPE

and Keevil[130] took 8-inch (20-cm) sections of new endoscope biopsy and air and water channels and contaminated them with artificial test soil. An enzymatic cleaner and single-use endoscope brushes were used to clean the soiled channel sections by inserting the brush head at one end of the channel section and pushing it out the other end. This brushing maneuver was repeated several times. The channel sections were then flushed with deionized water and purged with air. After cleaning, dye was injected into the lumen, which was then rinsed with deionized water and purged with air. The channel sections were examined with an episcopic differential contrast/epifluorescence microscope.

The researchers found that brushing the channels did not remove proteinaceous residues because endoscope channels adsorb proteins as a thin film on the internal surfaces. Brushing did have some beneficial effect; however, brushing also appeared to increase microcontamination. The researchers suggested that because prions represent the proteinaceous contamination most resistant to decontamination, this inability to completely remove proteinaceous contamination could be problematic in countries with a population at risk for variant Creutzfeldt-Jakob disease (vCJD); however, the risk of transmission was unclear. They posited that the cleaning outcome could be improved with better brush design.[130]

New technologies for brush design and lumen cleaning may be more effective and less damaging to the internal lumens of flexible endoscopes. Charlton[149] compared the cleaning efficacy of a lumen-cleaning device to three lumen-cleaning brushes (ie, triple-headed brush, single-use brush, reusable brush). The lumen-cleaning device had elastomer discs designed to make contact with the internal walls of the endoscope channels and wipe soil from the surface as it is pulled through the channel. In this nonexperimental laboratory study, the researchers applied simulated blood soil to the lumens of two different-sized endoscope channels (ie, 2.8 mm, 5.0 mm) that had been removed from used endoscopes during servicing. The lumen-cleaning device was passed through the soiled lumens one time. The lumen-cleaning brushes were pushed down and then pulled up through the lumen three times. The researchers found there was very little residual soil in the lumen cleaned with the lumen-cleaning device and substantial quantities of soil in the lumens cleaned with the lumen-cleaning brushes. The lumen-cleaning device removed significantly more soil (92%) compared with the lumen-cleaning brushes (52% to 65%).

The researchers noted that multiple passes with a brush was more time-consuming than a single pass with the lumen-cleaning device. They suggested that the lumen-cleaning device was safer to use than a brush because the lumen-cleaning device emerged only once from the contaminated channel compared with the cleaning motion for brushing that requires the brush to emerge multiple times from the contaminated channel. As the tip of the brush emerges from the lumen, the bristles have the potential to flick soil into the environment, onto other parts of the endoscope, or onto other instruments, increasing the risk for cross contamination and the potential for biohazardous spray and splatter. Brushes may also increase the formation of biofilm by causing surface abrasion or grooves in the channel wall. Notably, this study was funded by the manufacturer of the lumen-cleaning device.[149]

Charlton[150] conducted a second nonexperimental study in a clinical setting to compare the lumen-cleaning device used in the previous laboratory study to reusable lumen-cleaning brushes. The study was completed during a four-day period in an endoscopy clinic of a major hospital in Sydney, Australia. Immediately after the endoscope was removed from the patient, a sterile saline solution was flushed down the biopsy channel of the endoscope and submitted for microbiological sampling. The endoscope was cleaned using either one pass of the lumen-cleaning device (n = 26), or three passes (ie, pushed down and then pulled up through the lumen) of the reusable cleaning brush (n = 27), and a second microbiological sample was submitted.

The researchers found no significant difference between the effectiveness of the lumen-cleaning device compared with the

reusable lumen-cleaning brushes. The lumen-cleaning devices reduced CFU by 3.302-$\log_{10}$/cm². The reusable lumen-cleaning brushes reduced CFU by 3.003-$\log_{10}$/cm². The researchers concluded that one pass of the lumen-cleaning device was as effective as three passes of the reusable lumen-cleaning brushes. Notably, this study was funded by the manufacturer of the lumen-cleaning device.[150]

A report of a study prepared by Highpower Validation Testing & Lab Services[151] detailed the methods used to evaluate and compare the cleaning efficacy of a unique microfiber endoscopic channel brush and the endoscope manufacturer's recommended cleaning brush. The researchers extracted the endoscope cleaning channels, inoculated them with artificial test soil containing blood and protein, allowed the soil to dry for 24 hours, and compared the effectiveness of the brushes in removing the soil. The results showed that the microfiber channel brush removed 99.98% of the soil (ie, a 4-log reduction). The manufacturer's recommended cleaning brush removed 93.35% of the soil (ie, a 1.2-log reduction). Notably, this study was funded by the manufacturer of the microfiber endoscopic channel brush. Further research is warranted.

VI.h. The channels of the endoscope should be flushed with cleaning solution.[12,15-17,19-21,27,89] A cleaning adapter or automatic flushing system may be used when compatible with the endoscope.[12] [2: High Evidence]

Flushing all internal channels helps dislodge and remove organic material and biofilm and exposes these surfaces to the cleaning solution.[27] Cleaning adapters and automatic flushing systems facilitates opening of the ports and cleaning of the channels.[1]

VI.i. The exterior surfaces and internal channels of the endoscope should be flushed and rinsed with utility water until all cleaning solution and residual debris is removed.[12,13,15-17,20,27,83-85,89] [2: High Evidence]

Thorough flushing of the channels and rinsing of the endoscope with utility water helps remove residual debris and cleaning solutions and prevents dilution of the high-level disinfectant or liquid chemical sterilant.[13,16,65,89,90] If not adequately rinsed, enzymatic cleaning solutions may contribute to protein buildup within the endoscope channels.[131]

VI.j. The exterior surfaces of the endoscope should be dried with a soft, lint-free cloth or sponge and all channels purged with instrument air.[12,13,15,16,84,89] [2: High Evidence]

Moisture remaining on the surface or in the endoscope lumens may dilute the high-level disinfectant or interfere with the sterilization process, potentially reducing its effectiveness.[13,16,84] Hydrogen peroxide vapor and hydrogen peroxide gas plasma sterilization cycles may abort in the presence of excess moisture.[40] Ethylene oxide combines with water to form ethylene glycol (ie, antifreeze), which is toxic and not removed during aeration.[41]

VI.k. Reusable parts (eg, valves, buttons, port covers, tubing, water bottles), accessories (eg, forceps), and cleaning implements (eg, brushes, channel cleaning adapters) should be cleaned, brushed, rinsed, and high-level disinfected or sterilized.[1,12,13,17-21,27,44,83,89,152,153] *[1: Strong Evidence]*

Effective processing of reusable endoscope parts and accessories is necessary for safe and successful treatment of patients.[120,152,154] Reusable brushes that are not decontaminated can cause contaminants to be transferred from one device to another.[58]

The FDA[155] has received reports that, in the absence of a valve to prevent backflow, patient fluids such as blood and stool can travel through the auxiliary water channel and into the water inlet and irrigation system; however, there have been no reports of infection directly attributed to backflow. The FDA recommends that the following be processed or replaced after each patient use:

○ any device directly connected to the auxiliary water inlet (up to and including the distal valve in the fluid pathway),[155]

○ the one-way valve in the auxiliary water channel of an endoscope with an internal one-way valve,[155] and

○ any device directly connected to the biopsy channel (up to and including the distal one-way valve in the fluid path).[155]

The Department of Veterans Affairs[156] reported an incident involving a patient who underwent a colonoscopy procedure. During the procedure, the endoscopy team noticed blood in the tubing of the auxiliary water system used for irrigation during procedures. The equipment was taken out of service and an investigation was initiated. The investigators found that a required one-way valve had not been used during the procedure, the tubings had been incorrectly connected, and the tubings were not being disinfected or discarded according to the manufacturer's IFU. Notably, both connectors were the same color and roughly the same size and shape. The investigators were unable to determine when or why the switch occurred. Likewise, they were unable to determine how long the required one-way valve had not been in use.

VI.k.1. Water and irrigation bottles should be high-level disinfected or sterilized at least daily.[22,44,45,93,153] There should be no residual water or moisture remaining in the water-bottle assembly.[153,157] *[1: Strong Evidence]*

Water bottles consist of the water container, cap, and tubing used for insufflation of air and lens washing.[153] Irrigation bottles consist of the water container, tubing, and accessories used to flush water through the endoscope.[153]

Water and irrigation bottles can be a source of endoscope contamination[22]; however, the optimal frequency for replacing, disinfecting, or sterilizing them has not been established and warrants further research.[44] Residual water remaining in the water-bottle assembly may support bacterial growth.

VI.k.2. Sterile water should be used to fill water and irrigation bottles.[1,22,44,45,93,153] *[1: Strong Evidence]*

The collective evidence conflicts regarding the need for sterile water in the water and irrigation bottles, and further research is warranted. The American Society for Gastrointestinal Endoscopy (ASGE) recommends using utility water in irrigation bottles because the rates of bacterial contamination are similar with the use of utility water and sterile water and neither has been associated with clinical infections.[30] This conflicts with the recommendation for using sterile water provided in the "Multisociety guideline on processing flexible gastrointestinal endoscopes."[44] Using sterile water is also recommended by some professional organizations to help prevent contamination from organisms in utility water[1,22,44,45,153]; however, there is a small amount of evidence that indicates this may not be necessary.[158-160]

In a two-phase quasi-experimental study to determine whether the endoscope water source holds potential for transmission of infection, Puterbaugh et al[158] compared utility water in clean water bottles (Phase 1; n = 303) with sterile water in sterile water bottles (Phase 2; n = 106). The researchers took cultures of the water in the bottles before starting and after completing the day's procedures. The researchers found that 29 (9.6%) of the samples from Phase 1 were positive for normal flora found in city water. Four of the samples from Phase 2 (3.8%) were positive for similar bacteria. They concluded that the use of utility water in clean water bottles carried no greater risk than using sterile water in sterile water bottles.

Wilcox et al[159] conducted a quasi-experimental study in a university teaching hospital to determine whether there was a need for sterile water in the water bottles used during endoscopy procedures. During a 12-week period, the water bottles were sterilized weekly and then filled with either sterile or utility water. At the end of each week, the remaining water in the bottles was cultured. During the study period, 437 procedures were performed and 36 cultures were submitted. Nine of the cultures were positive, including three cultures from bottles where sterile water had been used. The bacterial isolates included *Flavobacterium* species (n = 5), *Acinetobacter* species (n = 4), *Pseudomonas* species (n = 2), and *Stenotrophomonas maltophilia* (n = 1). Colony counts ranged from 900/mL to more than 10,000/mL. No patient developed infections from any of the organisms recovered. The researchers concluded that the use of utility water compared with sterile water may be reasonable and may also reduce costs.

In response to this study, Patton et al[161] countered that utility water contains minerals that can leave deposits on flexible endoscopes and in the channels of the endoscope. The mineral deposits could lead to a costly repair or a need to replace the endoscope. The author estimated repair costs at $1,000 to $5,500 ($1,470.59 to $8,088.24 in 2015 US dollars) and noted that the cost of a 1,000 mL bottle of sterile water was $2.38 ($3.50 in 2015 US dollars); therefore, several cases of sterile water were less expensive than a single repair. The author concluded that using sterile water would not only decrease the risk of transmission of pathogenic organisms, it would also decrease the need for repair or replacement of the endoscope.

In an expert opinion piece, Rockey[160] debated the need for sterile water in water bottles, stating there was no evidence to support the concern that using utility water could damage the endoscope and contending that it would take years for mineral deposits to form. If mineral deposits were to form on the internal channels of the endoscope, they would likely be washed away by the force of the fluid flushed through the channels during mechanical processing. The author further stated that using sterile water is necessary when entering sterile body cavities, but should not be necessary when entering portions of the gastrointestinal tract that are not sterile since utility water is acceptable for drinking. Likewise, utility water is used in other body systems without complication (eg, oxygen humidification).

VI.k.3. Insulated electrosurgical devices used during endoscopic procedures should be processed in accordance with the AORN Guideline for Cleaning and Care of Surgical Instruments[58] and handled in accordance with the AORN Guideline for Electrosurgery.[162] *[1: Strong Evidence]*

VI.l. Single-use parts, accessories, and cleaning implements may be used when compatible with the endoscope. *[1: Strong Evidence]*

The intricate design and configuration of certain components and accessories used with flexible endoscopes represent a significant challenge to cleaning.[154] Using single-use products may be helpful in reducing the risk of cross contamination from reusable products.[18,27,120] Using single-use brushes may help ensure that a clean brush is used each time.[58]

Parente[154] conducted a nonexperimental study to evaluate the difficulty with manual cleaning and disinfection of endoscopic biopsy port valves. The researchers collected 15 reusable biopsy port valves from three endoscopy centers across the United States. The valves had been reprocessed and were deemed to be clean, disinfected, and ready for use. The biopsy port valves were examined using brightfield microscopy and then further studied to identify potential sources of contamination using Fourier transform infrared spectroscopy. The researchers found that eight of the 15 valves (53.3%) exhibited some form of debris or potential contamination. Testing confirmed the debris to be proteinaceous material. The researchers also found that many of the valves were damaged, increasing the potential for leakage and providing reservoirs for bacterial colonization. At least one valve came from each of the three facilities. The researchers concluded that single-use biopsy port valves provided a higher degree of patient safety.

VI.l.1. Single-use parts, accessories, and cleaning implements should be discarded after use and should not be reprocessed.[1,13,15,22,27,45,83] *[2: High Evidence]*

Wilson et al[163] reported a pseudo-outbreak of *Aureobasidium* species found in 10 broncheoalveolar lavage fluid cultures taken from nine patients between June 1998 and August 1998. Based on the clinical and laboratory data, there did not appear to be a true infection in any of the patients; however, all of the patients had their bronchoscopy procedures performed in the same outpatient bronchoscopy suite. The investigators observed the processing procedures and found that single-use plastic stopcocks were routinely being reused. The stopcocks were attached to sterile syringes containing sterile water used for the broncheoalveolar lavage. After each use, the stopcocks were manually washed and placed into a mechanical processor. Notably, the manufacturer of the mechanical processor did not recommend disinfecting the stopcocks in this manner.

STERILIZATION AND DISINFECTION

After HLD, the stopcocks were stored in a sterile, plastic container with a screw top. At the time of the investigation, the container held approximately 20 stopcocks. There was no record of how many times each stopcock was being reused. Culture of the stopcocks yielded heavy growth of *Aurebasidium* species. The practice of reusing the single-use stopcocks was discontinued.[163]

Recommendation VII

Flexible endoscopes, accessories, and associated equipment should be visually inspected for cleanliness, integrity, and function before use, during the procedure, after the procedure, after cleaning, and before disinfection or sterilization.

The collective evidence supports visual inspection of endoscopes, accessories, and equipment after cleaning and throughout use and processing as a method to help identify residual organic material and defective items in need of repair.[1,12,13,21,58,65,90]

The benefits are that visual inspection and evaluation provide an opportunity to identify and remove from service soiled or defective items that might put patients at risk for infection or injury until these items are cleaned or repaired.[24,58]

VII.a. Before use, all new, repaired, refurbished, and loaned endoscopes, accessories, or other equipment should be visually inspected and processed according to the manufacturer's IFU. *[5: Benefits Balanced with Harms]*

It is not possible to verify how all new, repaired, refurbished, or loaned equipment and devices have been handled, cleaned, inspected, or processed before receipt in the facility. Failure to correctly clean, inspect, or process an item may lead to transmission of pathogenic microorganisms from a contaminated device and create a risk for patient injury or infection.

Visually inspecting endoscopes, accessories, and equipment upon receipt and before processing can help verify there are no obvious defects and may prevent damaged or malfunctioning endoscopes from being used on patients.

VII.b. Endoscopes, accessories, and equipment should be visually inspected and evaluated for
  o cleanliness,[12,13,21,58,65]
  o missing parts,[1,58]
  o clarity of lenses,[58,106]
  o integrity of seals and gaskets,[58,106]
  o moisture,[58]
  o physical or chemical damage,[106] and
  o function.[12,13,21,58,65,106]
[2: High Evidence]
Visual inspection and evaluation helps detect the presence of residual soil and identify items in need of repair.

VII.c. Lighted magnification should be used to inspect endoscopes and accessories for cleanliness and damage.[12,13,65] *[2: High Evidence]*

An endoscope that appears clean may harbor debris that cannot be seen without magnification. Lighted magnification may increase the ability to identify residual soil or damage.

VII.c.1. Internal channels of flexible endoscopes may be inspected using an endoscopic camera or borescope. *[2: High Evidence]*

Endoscopic cameras and borescopes penetrate the lumen and allow for improved visual inspection.[12,58]

VII.d. Defective endoscopes, accessories, and equipment should be removed from service and repaired or replaced.[1,13,58] *[2: High Evidence]*

Identification of defective endoscopes, accessories, and equipment and removal from service reduces the risk of a defective item being used and helps prevent further damage from use.[84]

VII.d.1. Medical equipment being sent for repair must be decontaminated to the fullest extent possible and a biohazard label attached before transportation.[48] *[1: Regulatory Requirement]*

Decontaminating and labeling medical equipment before transport is a regulatory requirement and communicates to others which portions of the device being transported are contaminated.[48]

Incorrectly preparing the item being sent for repair may further damage the item and expose personnel handling the item to contaminants.

The manufacturer or service representative may provide recommendations that align with regulatory requirements for safe processes to follow for return or repair of the endoscope.[85]

Recommendation VIII

After manual cleaning and inspection, flexible endoscopes and endoscope accessories should be high-level disinfected or sterilized.[45]

The Spaulding classification system, developed by Earl Spaulding in 1968, classifies items as critical, semicritical, or noncritical.[117] The level of processing required (ie, sterilization, HLD, intermediate-level disinfection [ILD], low-level disinfection) is based on the nature of the item that requires processing and the manner in which the item is to be used.[117] The classification system has been used by infection preventionists and others for more than 47 years.[164]

According to the Spaulding classification, devices that enter sterile tissue or the vascular system are considered critical items.[117] When critical items, such as biopsy forceps, are contaminated with microorganisms, the risk of infection transmission is substantial.[117] Therefore, Spaulding et al[117] recommended that critical items be processed by sterilization. Sterilization eliminates all microbial life, including pathogenic and nonpathogenic microorganisms and bacterial spores.[117] Notably, sterilization is a validated process used to render a product free from all forms of viable microorganisms.[155] Liquid chemical sterilization may not convey the same sterility assurance as sterilization using thermal or other low-temperature sterilization methods.[155]

Items such as flexible endoscopes that come in contact with nonintact skin or mucous membranes, are considered to be semicritical.[117] Mucous membranes provide a barrier to common bacterial spores, but not to organisms such as tubercle bacilli and viruses.[117] Therefore, Spaulding et al[117] recommended that semicritical items be processed by sterilization, or at a minimum, by HLD. High-level disinfection eliminates all pathogenic microorganisms except for small numbers of bacterial spores.[46,117]

VIII.a. A multidisciplinary team that includes infection preventionists, endoscopy and perioperative RNs, sterile processing personnel, endoscopists, and other involved personnel should conduct a risk assessment to determine whether items that secondarily enter sterile tissue or the vascular system (ie, via a mucous membrane) should be sterile. *[3: Moderate Evidence]*

At a meeting of the Gastroenterology-Urology Devices Panel convened by the FDA in May 2015 to seek expert scientific and clinical opinion related to reprocessing of duodenoscopes and other flexible endoscopes, Rutala proposed a modification of the Spaulding system wherein items that secondarily enter sterile tissue or the vascular system are considered to be critical items (Table 2).[165] Devices secondarily entering sterile tissue would include devices that enter sterile tissue by way of a mucous membrane, such as a bronchoscope, a cystoscope, or a duodenoscope.[165] For example, a bronchoscope enters the bronchi through the mouth or nose, a cystoscope enters the bladder through the urethra, and a duodenoscope enters the bile or pancreatic ducts through the mouth. Requiring sterilization of items that secondarily enter sterile tissue or the vascular system may help prevent patient infection.

The collective evidence shows there are challenges to implementing the current Spaulding classification system when processing complex, heat-sensitive devices such as flexible endoscopes.[120] Because of the heavy microbial load that may be present on some flexible endoscopes and the difficulty in cleaning and disinfecting long, narrow channels, current HLD processes may not be adequate to ensure flexible endoscopes are safe for use on patients.[166]

The Spaulding classification does not address how to process semicritical items used in conjunction with critical items.[120] Although flexible endoscopes are categorized as semicritical, the accessory devices used in combination with flexible endoscopes may be critical items

because they enter sterile tissue or the vascular system.[120] These critical items are passed through an endoscope categorized as semicritical, which requires a minimum of HLD rather than sterilization.[120] Endoscopic accessories may emerge from the distal end of the endoscope and contact the mucosal surface of the bowel, bladder, or esophagus before they are used for the procedure. In addition, the Spaulding classification does not address the need for inactivating certain types of infectious agents, such as prions.[120] Thus, there are concerns about whether semicritical items should be sterilized rather than high-level disinfected.[165,167]

Incidents of reduced susceptibility to aldehyde disinfectants and high-level disinfectant failure also have been reported.[164,168,169] Tschudin-Sutter et al[168] detected *P aeruginosa* in 23 of 73 routine samples (32%) obtained from endoscopes during November 2009, and in 29 of 99 investigational samples (29%) obtained between November 4, and December 7, 2009. The investigators observed endoscope processing procedures and found no lapses; however, they noted that the drying time on the mechanical processor had been reduced from 10 minutes to 5 minutes to expedite turnaround time.

Environmental samples were obtained, and *P aeruginosa* was detected in the rinsing water and in the drain of one of the mechanical processors. The pathogen could not be detected in the water pipes or in any of the cleaning solutions or disinfectants used for processing the endoscopes. Infectious disease specialists reviewed medical records and detected six patients with lower respiratory tract and bloodstream infections possibly caused by the pseudo-outbreak strain. The investigators found that the glutaraldehyde-based disinfectant demonstrated no activity against the microorganism when used in the recommended concentration and at the recommended temperature. They concluded the *P aeruginosa* was resistant to the glutaraldehyde disinfectant.[168]

In a quasi-experimental study to investigate the potential for bacterial resistance in mechanical processors using aldehyde disinfectants, Fisher et al[169] randomly sampled three mechanical processors in the United States using aldehydes for HLD of flexible endoscopes. The researchers found bacterial contamination after disinfection in all of the mechanical processors and found that some mycobacteria isolates demonstrated significant resistance to glutaraldehyde and orthophalaldehyde disinfectants. The researchers concluded that bacteria can survive aldehyde-based HLD and may pose a cross contamination risk to patients.

In some outbreaks and pseudo-outbreaks, resolution was only achieved when the endoscope was sterilized by ethylene oxide.[166,170-172] Epstein et al[170] conducted a case control study

TABLE 2. SPAULDING CLASSIFICATION MODIFICATION FOR CRITICAL ITEMS[1-3]

Classification	Disinfection Level	Effectiveness
Critical Items that directly **or secondarily (ie, via a mucous membrane)** enter sterile tissue or the vascular system **(eg, bronchoscope, cystoscope, duodenoscope)**. Sterile tissue and the vascular system are at a high risk of infection if contaminated with microorganisms.	**Sterilization** Use saturated steam if possible. Use ethylene oxide, dry heat, ozone, low-temperature hydrogen peroxide gas, or liquid chemical sterilization for heat-sensitive items.	Sterilization eliminates all microbial life, including pathogenic and nonpathogenic microorganisms and bacterial spores.

REFERENCES

1. Spaulding EH, Lawrence CA, Block SS, Reddish GF. Chemical disinfection of medical and surgical materials. In: Lawrence CA, Block SS, Reddish GF, eds. Disinfection, Sterilization, and Preservation. Philadelphia, PA: Lea & Febiger; 1968:517-531.
2. Rutala WA. Weber DJ; the Healthcare Infection Control Practices Advisory Committee (HICPAC). Guideline for Disinfection and Sterilization in Healthcare Facilities, 2008. Atlanta, GA: Centers for Disease Control and Prevention; 2008.
3. Rutala WA. ERCP Scopes: A Need to Shift from Disinfection to Sterilization? Meeting of the FDA Gastroenterology and Urology Devices Panel of the Medical Devices Advisory Committee [transcript]. Annapolis, MD: Free State Reporting, Inc; May 14, 2015.

to identify the source and interrupt transmission of NDM-producing carbapenem-resistant *E coli* in a tertiary care hospital in northeastern Illinois. The investigators identified 39 case patients from January 2013 through December 2013, of whom 35 had undergone ERCP procedures in the same hospital. No lapses in duodenoscope processing were identified; however, NDM-producing *E coli* that shared a 92% genetic similarity to all case patients was recovered from a processed duodenoscope. After the investigators changed from using from HLD with orthophalaldehyde to sterilization with ethylene oxide, the duodenoscopes were culture-negative and no additional case patients were identified.

Between October and December 2010, Chang et al[173] identified ertapenem-resistant *E cloacae* in the urine cultures of 15 patients who had undergone ureteroscopy with the same ureteroscope. The investigators did not find any breaches in the processing procedures. The endoscope was culture-positive for the ertapenem-resistant *E cloacae*. The ureteroscope was meticulously cleaned and high-level disinfected for an additional five minutes beyond the manufacturer's recommended HLD time. The ureteroscope was sampled, and the results were again culture-positive. The ureteroscope was sterilized with ethylene oxide, sampled, and found to be culture-negative.

Smith et al[174] questioned current processing guidelines for duodenoscopes in a report describing transmission of carbapenem-resistant *Enterobacteriaceae*. Between May and November 2013, three patients at a Wisconsin medical center were identified as having NDM-1 carbapenem-resistant *E coli* after undergoing ERCP procedures with the same duodenoscope. The investigators observed the processing procedures and found no lapses. They sampled the duodenoscope and found it was culture-negative; however, the evidence was sufficiently strong to implicate the duodenoscope as the mode of

transmission. The duodenoscope was sterilized with ethylene oxide and no additional infections were diagnosed. The researchers noted that for procedures in which duodenoscopes were used, there may be a risk of transmission of infection despite HLD.

Müller et al[175] described infections of multi-drug-resistant *P aeruginosa* in two patients who had undergone ERCP procedures with the same duodenoscope for which sterilization by ethylene oxide did not eliminate the organism. The endoscope was quarantined and sampled and found to be culture-positive for the same strain of *P aeruginosa* as the infected patients. The endoscope was manually cleaned, soaked in 2% glutaraldehyde for 10 hours, sampled, and again found to be culture-positive. The duodenoscope was then sterilized with ethylene oxide, sampled, and once again found to be culture-positive. The endoscope was returned to the manufacturer for replacement of all internal channels. The investigators concluded that constant vigilance related to processes for cleaning and HLD was needed to ensure safe and effective processing of endoscopes.

Notably, many facilities do not have the capability of performing ethylene oxide sterilization. Sterilization and aeration using ethylene oxide may take 12 to 15 hours or more.[166] Penetration of ethylene oxide into long, narrow lumens is a concern, and flexible endoscopes may not have been validated by the manufacturer for sterilization with ethylene oxide.[120]

In a quasi-experimental laboratory study, Alfa et al[176] assessed the effect of serum and salt on the performance of two 100% ethylene oxide sterilizers, two ion plasma sterilizers, a vaporized hydrogen peroxide sterilizer, and a 12/88 ethylene oxide sterilizer. The researchers inoculated test carriers with *E coli*, *E faecalis*, *P aeruginosa*, *Mycobacterium chelonae*, *Bacillus stearothermophilus* spores, *Bacillus subtilis* spores, and *Bacillus circulans* spores; subjected them to sterilization; and calculated the residual bacterial load. The inoculum was prepared with and without 10% serum and 0.65% salt. The researchers found that all of the sterilizers effected a 6-log reduction of the bacterial inoculum; however, none of the sterilizers could effect a 6-log reduction in the presence of 10% serum and 0.65% salt. The researchers commented that the inability of sterilizers to reliably eliminate microorganisms in narrow channels in the presence of serum and salt raises concerns about the practice of using ethylene oxide sterilization as a mechanism for controlling outbreaks related to contaminated flexible endoscopes. Bile salts are the major organic component in bile whose function is to emulsify fats and facilitate intestinal absorption.[177]

In a second, similar study, Alfa et al[178] compared the ability of a liquid chemical sterilant and ethylene oxide to sterilize long, narrow lumens. The researchers found that the liquid chemical sterilant achieved a 6-log reduction in bacterial load compared with a 2.5- to 6-log reduction for ethylene oxide. The researchers noted that residual salt appeared to be a major problem for ethylene oxide sterilization, and this raised questions about the practice of using ethylene oxide to sterilize flexible endoscopes used in procedures where there might be residual protein, serum, blood, or salt remaining in the lumen. These data support the need to ensure effective cleaning of narrow lumens before initiating any HLD or sterilization method.

In a quasi-experimental study to assess cleaning and sterilization efficacy in narrow-lumened devices using artificial test soil and to assess the use of artificial test soil as a worst-case organic challenge to the microbial killing efficacy of various sterilization methods, Alfa et al[179] inoculated the biopsy channel of a flexible endoscope with artificial test soil containing 10^8 CFU/mL of *Geobacillus stearothermophilus, M chelonae*, and *E faecalis.* Suboptimal cleaning (ie, no brushing, no immersion, only flushing) was compared to optimal manual cleaning (ie, brushing, flushing, immersion) for organic soil removal. The sterilization efficacy of pre-vacuum steam, 100% ethylene oxide, and peracetic acid was evaluated in the presence of this organic challenge. The researchers found that suboptimal cleaning resulted in less than 99% removal of hemoglobin, carbohydrate, and endotoxin, whereas optimal cleaning resulted in greater than 99% removal. The survival of *G stearothermophilus* and *E faecalis* in lumens after sterilization suggested that high residual soil loads affect the efficacy of the sterilization process.

VIII.b. After manual cleaning and inspection and when compatible with the endoscope manufacturer's IFU, flexible endoscopes and accessories should be either mechanically cleaned and mechanically processed by exposure to a high-level disinfectant or a liquid chemical sterilant or should be mechanically cleaned and sterilized. *[1: Strong Evidence]*

Mechanical processing includes mechanical cleaning, mechanical HLD or sterilization, and mechanical rinsing. The collective evidence shows that mechanical processing improves cleaning effectiveness, increases efficiency, minimizes personnel exposure to biohazardous materials, and can be more successfully monitored for quality and consistency.[1,12,15,16,18,22,45,83,85,93,114,122,180-183]

Although mechanical processing is more effective than manual processing, recommendations from professional organizations supporting mechanical processing are inconsistent. Some experts[93,105,120,182] and clinical practice guidelines[13,17-22,122] recommend using only mechanical processing, while other experts[89] and clinical practice guidelines[15,16,27,44,83,84] support the use of manual methods.

Unless the manufacturer of the mechanical processor has validated the processor to exclude manual cleaning, mechanical processing does not eliminate the need for manual cleaning.[122] The sequence of manual cleaning followed by mechanical cleaning most effectively removes bioburden and helps prevent the buildup of dead microorganisms that may occur when incompletely cleaned devices are subjected to HLD or sterilization.[120] The physical force of the water pressure used by mechanical processors to flush endoscope channels allows the bioburden to be physically lifted and removed by the flow of fluid.[120,182,184]

In a quasi-experimental study to evaluate the effectiveness of five methods of HLD for removal of biofilm in endoscopes, Balsamo et al[185] used Teflon tubes to simulate the channels of flexible endoscopes. The researchers contaminated the tubes with *P aeruginosa* biofilm and subjected them to one of five processing methods:

- manual processing using 2% glutaraldehyde,
- mechanical processing using 2% glutaraldehyde,
- manual processing using 0.09% to 0.15% active peracetic acid,
- mechanical processing using 35% peracetic acid, or
- mechanical processing using acidic electrolytic water.

The researchers found that none of the processing methods completely removed the biofilm. Mechanical processing using 2% glutaraldehyde or 35% peracetic acid were the most effective in removing the biofilm. The biofilm remained attached to 35.7% of the sample segments (15 of 42) and was completely removed in 26% of the sample segments (11 of 42). There

STERILIZATION AND DISINFECTION

was a statistically significant difference between manual and mechanical processing methods.

Ubhayawardana et al[182] conducted a nonexperimental study to evaluate the effectiveness of manual processing for removal of bioburden from side-view endoscopes used for ERCP procedures in a tertiary referral endotherapy unit in Sri Lanka. The researchers obtained samples from 102 different flexible side-view endoscopes before and after processing and then tested them for microbial growth. The researchers found that despite strict adherence to recommended processing protocols, the average culture-positive rates from the endoscope tips was 90% (92 of 102) before processing and 21% (21 of 102) after processing. The culture-positive rate from the working channel after processing was 10% (10 of 102). Notably, manual processing was completed in the procedure room, and this may have contributed to the high culture-positive rate. *Klebsiella* and *Candida* species were the most common microorganisms found. The results of this study suggest that processing of the endoscope tip was less effective than processing of the working channels. The researchers concluded that there was a high culture-positive rate after manual processing of side-view endoscopes.

Some mechanical processors also provide a thermal or chemical decontamination process that removes or reduces the number of microorganisms or infectious agents and renders reusable medical devices safe for use, handling, or disposal.[12,45,58,90]

In addition to improved cleaning and decontamination, mechanical processors may also provide improved rinsing of disinfectants and reduce the potential for patient injury associated with residual disinfectants remaining in the endoscope. In a nonexperimental laboratory study, Farina et al[186] determined residual levels of glutaraldehyde in two gastroscopes and two colonoscopes following manual and automatic disinfection procedures. The researchers found that residual glutaraldehyde levels were much higher after manual disinfection (< 0.2 to 159.5 mg/L) than after mechanical disinfection (< 0.2 to 6.3 mg/L).

Mechanical processors may reduce the risk of cross contamination from one load to another by allowing for single-use cleaning and disinfecting solutions.[122]

Using mechanical processors reduces the potential for breaches in recommended processing protocols associated with human error and noncompliance.[67,122,139,182] Audits have shown that personnel do not consistently adhere to guidelines for processing, and this has led to outbreaks of infection.[15,45] Procedures for manual processing of flexible endoscopes may be inadequate or inconsistent and may vary signifi-cantly from one health care facility to another, as well as within the same facility.[89,180]

Studies from the United States[80,181,187-189] and other countries[131,190-207] have demonstrated varying degrees of compliance with recommended processing procedures.

Ofstead et al[181] conducted a prospective multisite observational study to evaluate procedures, employee perceptions, and occupational health issues related to processing flexible endoscopes. The researchers collected data from two gastroenterology specialty centers, two multispecialty hospitals, and one outpatient surgery center from five geographically diverse regions in the United States. The researchers found that when performing manual processing, personnel performed all required steps for only one of 69 endoscopes processed (1.4%). When performing mechanical processing, personnel performed all required steps for 86 of 114 endoscopes processed (75.4%). Steps commonly omitted during manual processing included brushing, forced-air drying, and flushing with 70% isopropyl alcohol. The only step routinely omitted during mechanical processing was the final external drying of the endoscope after removal from the processor.

In an examination of the peer-reviewed and non-peer-reviewed literature to identify lapses in processing flexible endoscopes reported in North America from 2005 to 2012, Dirlam Langlay et al[187] found that lapses occurred in various types of facilities and in all major steps of processing. Lapses included failing to

○ comply with established guidelines,
○ preclean endoscopes before processing,
○ correctly contain contaminated endoscopes,
○ adequately brush endoscope channels,
○ adequately clean the elevator channel of duodenoscopes,
○ perform adequate HLD,
○ correctly program mechanical processors,
○ report malfunctioning mechanical processors, and
○ document processing personnel competency.

These lapses may have resulted in patient exposure to potentially contaminated gastrointestinal endoscopes.

In a study to determine common practices for endoscope processing at regional endoscopy centers, Moses and Lee[188] sent anonymous questionnaires to 367 members of the Society of Gastroenterology Nurses and Associates (SGNA) in Pennsylvania, Delaware, Virginia, Maryland, and the District of Columbia. The survey was completed by 230 members (63%), the majority of whom (59%; n = 136) practiced in hospital-based endoscopy units performing more than 3,000 procedures a year. The results of the study showed wide variation in the manual cleaning process. Only 70% (n = 161) suctioned cleaning solution through the endoscope channels and also brushed channels and valves. There was variation in the number of times the channels were brushed, with the majority (37%; n = 85) brushing three to five times. In 6% of the units (n = 14), manual cleaning was the only processing step, and 18% (n = 42) reported omitting manual cleaning before mechanical processing.

Surveyors from the Centers for Medicare & Medicaid Services[189] assessed adherence to infection control practices in 68 ambulatory surgery centers in three states (ie, 32 in Maryland, 16 in North Carolina, 20 in Oklahoma). The surveyors assessed compliance with hand hygiene, injection safety and medication handling, equipment processing, environmental cleaning, and handling of blood glucose monitoring equipment. They found that overall, 46 (67.6%) of the surgery centers had at least one lapse in infection control, and 12 (17.6%) had identified lapses in three or more infection control categories. Errors in processing included failing to adequately clean instruments before sterilization or HLD (four of 60; 6.7%); failing to use chemical or biologic indicators in sterilizer loads (two of 55; 3.6%); failing to prepare, test, or replace high-level disinfectants (eight of 48; 16.7%); failing to document HLD or sterilization (two of 66; 3%); failing to store sterilized or disinfected equipment in a clean area (one of 65; 1.5%); and reprocessing single-use devices (four of 10; 40%).

Although mechanical processors provide many advantages compared with manual processing, there are some disadvantages. Mechanical processors require preventive maintenance to ensure safe and effective operation.[122,180] The use of contaminated or defective mechanical processors for cleaning, disinfecting, or rinsing can result in inadequate processing[22,122,183] that has been associated with outbreaks of endoscopy-related infections and pseudo-infections[100,208-219] and patient injury.[220,221] In addition, the presence of biofilm has been detected in mechanical processors.[208,209]

An Endoscope Task Force was established to review endoscope processing incidents in England from 2003 to 2004 and to make recommendations to prevent recurrences. The task force found there were a total of 18 incidents. Eight of the incidents (44%) involved failures to adequately clean endoscope channels. Seven incidents (39%) involved problems with mechanical processors. In one incident, a pump had failed, and due to the lack of a functional alarm system, the failure to irrigate endoscopes with cleaning solution and disinfectant was not being signaled. Another incident involved a malfunction in which the cleaning solution was frothing excessively. The cause was identified as a faulty valve; however, processing personnel had removed the pressure sensors and alarm systems from the machine to stop the signal when it was incorrectly deemed that there was nothing wrong. An additional incident involved an incorrect adaptor. Three incidents involved the incorrect use of cleaning solutions.[222]

Vanhems et al[223,224] described the possible transmission of pathogens to 236 persons exposed to an endoscope processed in a defective mechanical processor in a gastrointestinal endoscopy unit. In March 2002, a nurse from the digestive diseases unit questioned the "tactile sensation" of the gastrointestinal endoscopes after they had been mechanically processed. The manufacturer was contacted and determined that the pump for injecting disinfectants into the biopsy channels was malfunctioning and the alarm system designed to detect such a flaw was also malfunctioning. The endoscopes had not been disinfected, and patients had potentially been exposed to contaminants. Notably, the endoscopes had been manually cleaned before being placed into the mechanical processor. A total of 197 (83.5%) patients found to be at risk for infection completed follow-up. No acute infection was observed. The investigators noted that the problem was identified because of the subjective perception of an experienced nurse.

The time required for mechanical processing may be longer[180] or shorter[225] than the time required for manual processing, and costs may be increased[180] or offset by financial gains as a result of increased productivity.[226] The consistency of mechanical processing also may minimize the potential for damage and the need for repairs.[67]

Alfa et al[225] compared the efficacy of the cleaning phase of a mechanical processor with optimal manual cleaning in a quasi-experimental laboratory study. A bronchoscope, gastroscope, and colonoscope were each inoculated with artificial test soil containing *P aeruginosa* and *E faecalis* and then allowed to dry for one hour. The endoscopes were either manually cleaned following the endoscope manufacturer's IFU or mechanically processed following the IFU for the processor. The results showed a greater than 90% reduction in soil levels for both manual and mechanical cleaning. Manual cleaning was slightly better for exterior surfaces, and mechanical cleaning was slightly better for removal of microorganisms from the channels. The researchers noted that manual cleaning time varied between 15 to 25 minutes per endoscope, depending on the type of endoscope being cleaned. This was substantially longer than the six to seven minutes of cleaning time required for mechanical cleaning of endoscopes.

Forte and Shum[227] used a time and motion study to compare the costs of personnel resources and consumable supplies associated with mechanical processors that do and do not require manual cleaning before processing. For three days, the researchers timed and observed two technicians who performed all endoscope processing activities. The researchers found that the total time to process endoscopes was significantly shorter when the technicians used the processor that did not require manual cleaning. The difference in median time to process was 12.6 minutes per colonoscope, 6.31 minutes per gastroscope, and 5.66 minutes per bronchoscope. The amount of time saved per day was 6.2 hours. The researchers determined that the cost of consumable supplies was slightly higher per processing with use of the processor that did not require manual cleaning ($8.91 [$9.50 in 2015 US dollars]) compared with use of the processor that did require manual cleaning ($8.31 [$8.86 in 2015 US dollars]).

Funk and Reaven[226] used data from peer-reviewed published literature and country-specific market research to compare manual processing to mechanical processing relative to productivity, need for endoscope repair, and infection transmission in India, China, and Russia. The researchers found that conversion to mechanical processing had a positive effect on financial performance, paying back the capital investment within 14 months in China and within seven months in Russia. In India, the additional revenue generated by the change to mechanical processing offset nearly all of the operating costs.

VIII.b.1. After precleaning and leak testing, and when directed by the mechanical processor manufacturer's IFU, mechanical processing may be accomplished without manual cleaning. *[2: High Evidence]*

The mechanical processor manufacturer has validated the processes required for effective processing without manual cleaning.[90]

In a quasi-experimental laboratory study to assess the efficacy of a mechanical processor that did not require manual cleaning before use, Alfa et al[228] evaluated patient-used duodenoscopes (n = 15), bronchoscopes (n = 10), colonoscopes (n = 15), and gastroscopes (n = 15). The endoscopes had been precleaned at the point of use and mechanically processed without additional manual cleaning before processing. All endoscope channels and two external surface sites were sampled to determine residual organic and microbial load. The results of the study showed that 99.7% of lumens and 98.8% of surfaces met or surpassed the predetermined cleaning endpoints for protein (< 6.4 µg/cm^2) and bioburden (< 4-$\log_{10}$ viable bacteria/cm^2) residuals.

The researchers also conducted simulated use testing by inoculating the channels and two surface sites of bronchoscopes (n = 3), colonoscopes (n = 3), and duodeno-

scopes (n = 3) with artificial test soil containing 10^8 CFU/mL of *E faecalis, P aeruginosa,* and *C albicans.* The endoscopes were allowed to dry for one hour before sampling. The results showed that 100% of both lumens and surface sites met or surpassed the cleaning end points for protein and bioburden residuals.[228]

VIII.c. Mechanical processing should be performed in accordance with the endoscope manufacturer's IFU and the mechanical processor manufacturer's IFU.[17] *[3: Moderate Evidence]*

There are multiple types of flexible endoscopes and mechanical processors. Instructions for use may vary among manufacturers. Even slight deviations from the recommended protocols can lead to the survival of microorganisms and an increased risk for infection.[225] Kressel and Kidd[208] reported a pseudo-outbreak of *M chelonae* and *Methylobacterium mesophilicum* caused by a contaminated mechanical processor in an academic medical center between July 1998 and October 1998. An unusual number of fungal cultures obtained during bronchoscopy procedures (26 of 131; 20%) grew *M chelonae.* The 26 cultures came from 22 patients; however, none of the patients had clinical evidence of pulmonary mycobacterial infection.

The investigators sampled the bronchoscopes, the mechanical processors, and the glutaraldehyde from the mechanical processors, and obtained positive results for *M chelonae.* They discovered that because of time constraints, employees had modified the connections required for the alcohol flush, rendering it inadequate. As a result, the mechanical processors became contaminated with biofilm that could not be removed. The processors then contaminated the bronchoscopes. The outbreak ended when the facility purchased a new mechanical processor.[208]

VIII.c.1. Processing personnel should verify compatibility between the endoscope and the mechanical processor before processing.[1,16,18,27,44] *[1: Strong Evidence]*

Compatibility between the endoscope and the mechanical processor is necessary to ensure effective processing of the endoscope and to prevent patient infection.[180]

Larson et al[219] investigated a potential outbreak of tuberculosis in a community hospital in New York in October 2000. Three patients had bronchoscopy specimen cultures that were positive for *M tuberculosis*; however, only one patient had clinical signs and symptoms consistent with tuberculosis. The three culture-positive specimens of *M tuberculosis* were obtained within nine days of each other from the same bronchoscope. A review of the processing procedures showed that the mechanical processor was not approved for use with the bronchoscope by the bronchoscope manufacturer.

VIII.c.2. Flexible endoscopes and accessories should be positioned within the mechanical processor in a manner that ensures contact of the processing solutions with all surfaces of the endoscope. *[4: Limited Evidence]*

Contact of all surfaces of the endoscope with processing solutions is necessary to achieve effective processing.

The complexity of flexible endoscopes and the variety of processing equipment available make it essential to follow the manufacturers' IFU to achieve optimal processing.

In a nonexperimental study to determine whether the noncritical portions of a flexible laryngoscope could harbor microorganisms, Bhatt et al[229] randomly sampled six flexible laryngoscopes from the eyepiece and handle immediately before use and after subsequent HLD wherein only the shaft of the endoscope was immersed in the high-level disinfectant. The researchers found there was bacterial growth in 41% (seven of 17) of samples. The results of the study demonstrate that despite HLD of the endoscope shaft, the noncritical portions of the endoscope can harbor microorganisms, and complete submersion of the endoscope is necessary to achieve complete processing.

VIII.c.3. Processing personnel should ensure all connectors between the endoscope and the mechanical processor are connected correctly.[13,20,44,69] *[1: Strong Evidence]*

Correct connections are necessary to ensure exposure of all surfaces of the endoscope to the processing solutions.[20,44]

Mechanical processors may require that endoscope channels be fitted with flow restrictors or tubing connectors to regulate fluid outflow.[225] The restrictors and tubing direct fluids into specific channels, thereby ensuring perfusion of the channels with necessary fluid flow dynamics.[225] Because of the complexity of the channels and their internal connections, it is critical that the correct connection tubing and flow restrictors be used to achieve adequate flow dynamics.[225] Flow restrictors and tubing connectors are often specific to the make and model of the flexible endoscope.[225]

The CDC[212] reported three clusters of culture-positive bronchoscopy specimens obtained from patients at local health care facilities in New York between 1996 and 1998. The first cluster involved five patients at a health care facility whose bronchial specimens yielded *M tuberculosis* with the same genetic pattern, suggestive of a com-

mon source. Samples taken from the bronchoscopes used during the procedures were negative. The investigators identified an inconsistency between the processing procedures recommended in the manufacturer's IFU and those followed by processing personnel. The biopsy port cap was not replaced before the bronchoscope was placed into the mechanical processor, and this led to a 50% reduction in flow and a 25% reduction in pressure, resulting in processing failure.

The second cluster involved bronchial specimens that were culture-positive for *Mycobacterium avium-intracellulare* from seven patients who had all undergone bronchoscopy with the same bronchoscope. The investigators found that the bronchoscope was being processed in a mechanical processor using the connectors provided by the bronchoscope manufacturer rather than the connectors recommended by the mechanical processor manufacturer.[212]

The third cluster involved 18 patients at a health care facility who had bronchial specimens that grew imipenem-resistant *P aeruginosa* (IRPA). None of the patients had IRPA isolated from sputum samples obtained before bronchoscopy, and all but one isolate had identical genetic patterns. The investigators found that the bronchoscopes were not being connected to the mechanical processor in accordance with the mechanical processor manufacturer's IFU.[212] The investigators concluded that there was a need for processing personnel to review and adhere to manufacturer's IFU and ensure correct connections between the endoscope and the mechanical processor.

Sorin et al[230] reported 18 isolates of IRPA from 18 patients who underwent bronchoscopy procedures during a three-month period immediately after implementation of a new mechanical processor. Three patients demonstrated clinical signs and symptoms of infection and were treated with antibiotics. A representative of the mechanical processor manufacturer noted several incorrect connections from the bronchoscope to the processor. The investigators concluded that the incorrect connections led to an insufficient flow of the chemical sterilant through the bronchoscope lumen, resulting in incomplete processing of the bronchoscope.

VIII.c.4. Processing personnel should monitor mechanical processing cycles to verify they are completed as programmed. If a mechanical processing cycle is interrupted, the entire cycle should be repeated.[16,17,20,21,44,83] *[1: Strong Evidence]*

Monitoring mechanical processing cycles helps ensure processing parameters have been achieved. Effective processing cannot be assured when the cycle has been interrupted.[16,44,83]

VIII.d. Mechanical processing of flexible endoscopes should be performed using critical water.[119]
[4: Limited Evidence]

Critical water meets the following parameters:

○ hardness: < 1 mg/L calcium carbonate,[119]
○ pH: 5 to 7,[119]
○ chloride: < 1 mg/L,[119]
○ bacteria: < 10 CFU/mL,[119] and
○ endotoxin: < 10 endotoxin units (EU)/mL.[119]

Water quality is affected by the presence of dissolved minerals, solids, chlorides, and other impurities and by its acidity and alkalinity.[119] Untreated water quality fluctuates over time, varies with geographic location and season, and can affect the outcome of cleaning actions.[119]

Hard water can decrease the effectiveness of cleaning solutions and disinfectants, and can also adversely affect the performance of mechanical processors.[119] Deposits can form on medical devices that may prevent microorganisms and organic material from being removed during cleaning.[119] Hard water may be incompatible with some high-level disinfectants and liquid chemical sterilants.[119]

Water with pH levels that are acidic or alkaline may affect the performance of cleaning solutions (especially enzymatic cleaning solutions), disinfectants, or sterilants.[119]

Controlling bacterial and endotoxin levels in water used for processing flexible endoscopes helps reduce the risk for patient infection.[119]

VIII.e. Mechanical processing should be performed using cleaning, disinfectant, and sterilant solutions and chemicals recommended by the endoscope manufacturer and the mechanical processor manufacturer.[13,18,20,22,44,45,46,83,84] *[1: Strong Evidence]*

There are multiple types of endoscopes and mechanical processors. Recommended cleaning and disinfectant or sterilant solutions may vary among manufacturers.

The chemical actions of cleaning, disinfectant, and sterilant solutions vary and are intended for different applications. Following the manufacturers' IFU decreases the possibility of selecting and using solutions that may damage the endoscope or mechanical processor.[44,45]

VIII.e.1. Chemicals and solutions used in the mechanical processor should be used at the concentration, volume, temperature, and contact time recommended by the mechanical processor manufacturer.[13,18-20,40,43,44,69]

• If recommended by the mechanical processor manufacturer, a test strip or other FDA-cleared testing device specific for the disinfectant and minimum effective concentration of the active ingredient should be used for monitoring solution potency.[1,40,43]

• If a solution falls below its minimum effective concentration, it should be discarded, even if the designated expiration date has not been reached.[40,43]
[1: Strong Evidence]

Some mechanical processors may require the use of a test strip or device to verify efficacy of the high-level disinfectant or liquid chemical sterilant used for processing.[40] The concentration of a high-level disinfectant or liquid chemical sterilant will decrease with dilution by water, the presence of organic material, evaporation of the solution, and exposure of the solution to light.[40] Checking the concentration of the high-level disinfectant or liquid chemical sterilant before use reduces the risk of inadequate processing.[40] High-level disinfection solution potency cannot be guaranteed when the solution falls below the minimum effective concentration. Incorrect dilution, volume, temperature, or contact time may result in a processing failure.[40,69,93,131]

VIII.e.2. Chemicals and solutions used for cleaning and processing flexible endoscopes and endoscope accessories must be handled in accordance with local, state, and federal regulations and the manufacturer's IFU.[38]

• The safety data sheets must be readily accessible to employees within the workplace.[38]
• Chemical spill kits must be stored in close proximity to areas where chemicals or other hazardous materials are stored.[38]
[1: Regulatory Requirement]

Cleaning products, high-level disinfectants, and liquid chemical sterilants can be hazardous to the individuals who are using them. It is a regulatory requirement that employers have a program to ensure that information about the identification, hazards, composition, safe handling practices, and emergency control measures of a chemical is readily available to employees.[38] When employees have information about the chemicals being used, they can take steps to reduce exposure, establish safe work practices, and implement first aid measures when necessary. Chemical spill kits enable prompt response by providing items that may be required in the cleanup of spills, leaks, or other discharges of hazardous materials.

VIII.e.3. The following products should not be used for processing flexible endoscopes:
• skin antiseptics,[1]
• hypochlorites,[1,45]
• phenolics,[1,45] and
• quaternary ammonium compounds.[1,45]
[1: Strong Evidence]

Skin antiseptics (eg, povidone-iodine, chlorhexidine gluconate) are not formulated as disinfectants.[1] Hypochlorites (eg, bleach) are corrosive and may be inactivated by organic material.[1,45] Phenolics (eg, ortho-benzyl-para-chlorophenol) may cause tissue irritation and injury to mucous membranes.[1,45] Quaternary ammonium compounds (eg, benzalkonium chloride) do not provide adequate disinfection of flexible endoscopes.[1,45]

Esteban et al[231] reported a pseudo-outbreak of 15 *Aeromonas hydrophila* isolates from colon biopsies between January 1998 and May 1998. The investigators found that the endoscopes had been manually cleaned with an enzymatic cleaning solution and rinsed with utility water and then placed into a quaternary ammonium solution for 20 minutes. The pseudo-outbreak ended when the quaternary ammonium solution was replaced with 2% glutaraldehyde for HLD.

VIII.f. Following disinfection, the endoscope and endoscope channels should be mechanically rinsed and flushed with critical or sterile water.[1,15,19,20,22,44,83,89,93] Endoscope accessories and removable parts should be rinsed with critical or sterile water. *[1: Strong Evidence]*

Thorough rinsing and flushing with critical water helps prevent patient injury associated with disinfectant or sterilant retained in the endoscope.[1,45,186,232-240] Utility water may contain microorganisms and endotoxins that can be deposited on the endoscope during the final rinse.[1,119] Tissue contaminated with endotoxins can cause severe inflammation.[119] Outbreaks of endoscopy-related infections and pseudo-infections have been linked to rinsing flexible endoscopes with utility water.[49,93,241] Using critical or sterile water reduces the potential for introducing microbes into the endoscope.[65]

Farina et al[186] conducted a nonexperimental study to determine residual levels of 2% glutaraldehyde in flexible endoscopes after manual and mechanical HLD. In a total of 92 measurements taken after manual HLD (n = 24) and mechanical HLD (n = 68) for two gastroscopes and two colonoscopes, the researchers found that residual levels of glutaraldehyde were higher and more variable after manual HLD (< 0.2 mg/mL to 159.5 mg/mL) than after mechanical HLD (< 0.2 mg/mL to 6.3 mg/mL). The researchers concluded that residual 2% glutaraldehyde levels (especially after manual disinfection) could be high enough to be toxic and a cause of colitis or proctitis following endoscopy.

In an attempt to reduce processing time, Kim and Baek[233] changed from using 2% glutaraldehyde to process flexible endoscopes in their endoscopy unit to using a peracetic acid compound. After the change, the researchers observed a series of 12 patients who experienced colonic mucosal pseudolipomatosis. The protocol for mechanical disinfection included a 60-second rinse cycle. The researchers reviewed the processing records and found that the colonic pseudolipomatosis occurred only when one of six nurses was on duty. The nurse sometimes rinsed the endoscopes for only 10 seconds and at other times omitted the mechanical rinsing cycle, opting to manually rinse the endoscopes under running water. No more cases occurred after the 60-second rinse cycle was reinstated. The researchers noted that this case highlighted the importance of completing all processing steps and following the manufacturer's IFU when using mechanical processors.

Wendleboe et al[242] investigated an outbreak of seven *P aeruginosa* infections associated with outpatient cystoscopy performed by a urologist in New Mexico from January to April 2007. The investigators found multiple breaches in processing procedures including rinsing of the cystoscope in unsterile water after processing. Specifically, sterile water was placed in a container and replaced every two weeks or when it began to smell. The outbreak resolved when improved procedures for processing flexible cystoscopes were implemented.

VIII.g. A multidisciplinary team that includes infection preventionists, endoscopy and perioperative RNs, endoscopy processing personnel, endoscopists, and other involved personnel should conduct a risk assessment to determine whether endoscope lumens should be flushed with 70% to 90% ethyl or isopropyl alcohol. *[1: Strong Evidence]*

Flushing endoscope lumens with alcohol may not be necessary if the endoscope is effectively dried.[243] Because of the fixative properties of alcohol, this practice is not recommended in some countries.[18-20,22,69,93]

Alfa and Sitter[243] conducted a prospective, quantitative assessment of the effect of drying on the bacterial load in duodenoscopes used for ERCP procedures. The researchers sampled 42 duodenoscopes that had been manually cleaned and then mechanically processed at two, 24, and 48 hours after disinfection. They found that 21 duodenoscopes (50%) were contaminated. There was visible moisture remaining in the suction channel even though processing personnel had followed the mechanical processor manufacturer's IFU. The bacterial counts ranged from 1×10^1 CFU/mL^{-1} to 1×10^7 CFU/mL^{-1}. The researchers added 10 minutes of drying time to 19 of the 21 contaminated duodenoscopes, either by purging the lumens of the endoscopes with instrument air or by adding 10 minutes of drying time in the mechanical processor. The results showed that there were no microorganisms detected after the additional drying time. The researchers concluded that the additional 10 minutes of drying time prevented bacterial growth in the endoscopes and eliminated the need for an alcohol flush.

Many clinical practice guidelines[1,15,16,19,44-46,83] and experts in the field[89,93,244] recommend manual or mechanical flushing of endoscope lumens with alcohol because it facilitates drying of the endoscope lumens by binding with residual water and enhancing evaporation.[1,16,65] Alcohol prevents colonization and transmission of waterborne bacteria.[46,65,89] Some mechanical processors automatically flush the endoscope with 70% isopropyl alcohol, others do not.

Wang et al[245] reported a pseudo-infection of *M chelonae* involving 25 patients with 25 positive isolates (ie, 18 bronchial, one soft tissue, one plural, five corneal) between September 1992 and December 1992. The investigators found the suction channels of four different bronchoscopes to be the sources of contamination and noted that the processing procedure did not include flushing the suction channels with 70% isopropyl alcohol. The bronchoscope processing procedures were modified to include flushing the endoscope lumens with 70% isopropyl alcohol after mechanical processing, and no further episodes of cross contamination or infection occurred.

In a quasi-experimental study to analyze whether flushing endoscope lumens with 70% ethyl alcohol after processing reduced the risk of microbiological contamination, Gavalda et al[246] sampled 18 different bronchoscopes after processing. The samples were collected on a monthly basis during a four-year period. Nine of the bronchoscopes were processed manually, and nine were processed mechanically. A total of 620 samples was obtained. The researchers found that 564 samples (91%) tested negative, and 56 samples (9%) tested positive, of which two (3.3%) contained pathogenic microorganisms. Only one positive sample (0.6%) was detected among the 167 samples from endoscopes flushed with alcohol after disinfection. The researchers recommended flushing bronchoscope channels with 70% ethyl alcohol after each disinfection cycle.

VIII.h. After mechanical processing, the exterior surfaces of the endoscope should be dried with a soft, lint-free cloth or sponge.[15,16,22,83,89]

- The endoscope channels should be dried by purging with instrument air or mechanically dried with a mechanical processor drying system.[1,15,16,19,22,44-46,83,89,131,244]
- Removable parts and endoscope accessories should be dried.[16]

[1: Strong Evidence]

Some mechanical processors have drying systems, others do not.

The collective evidence shows that effectively drying the internal and external surfaces of the endoscope is as important as effective cleaning and disinfection or sterilization.[244] The

long, narrow channels of the endoscope make it difficult to verify thorough drying.[157] Any moisture remaining on the exterior and interior surfaces of the endoscope can facilitate microbial growth and biofilm formation during storage.[19,46,65,93,131] Because bacteria can double in population every 20 to 30 minutes, an inadequately dried endoscope contaminated with only one or two viable bacteria can, after eight hours of storage, be contaminated with tens of thousands of bacteria.[247] These multiplying bacteria could pose a risk for infection.[247]

In a nonexperimental study to mimic disinfection and drying of biofilm in contaminated endoscopes, Kovaleva et al[248] prepared single species biofilm (ie, *C albicans, Candida parapsilosis, P aeruginosa,* or *S maltophilia*) and dual species biofilm (ie, *C parapsilosis* with *P aeruginosa* or *C parapsilosis* with *S maltophilia*) in sterile tissue culture plates and treated the single and dual strains with 1% peracetic acid. The culture plates were incubated at 122° F (50° C) for two hours to mimic the drying process, and then sealed and incubated at room temperature (ie, 68° F to 72° F [20° C to 22° C]), for one, three, and five days to mimic the storage process. The researchers found that there was no biofilm regrowth when the drying process was applied, but regrowth of all biofilms occurred when the drying process was not implemented. The researchers concluded that thorough drying was an important factor in the maintenance of bacteria-free endoscopes.

In a nonexperimental study, Ren-Pei et al[96] investigated biofilm on endoscope channels. The researchers collected 66 endoscope suction and biopsy channels and 13 water and air channels from 66 endoscopy centers in hospitals throughout China and used SEM to examine biofilm on the inner surface of the channels. A total of 36 suction and biopsy channels (54.5%) and 10 water and air channels (76.9%) were found to have biofilm.

After examining the endoscope channels, the researchers sent a questionnaire to each of the 66 endoscopy centers to explore the correlation between endoscope processing procedures and the amount of biofilm found in the endoscope channels. They divided the responses (N = 66) into hospitals without biofilm on endoscopes (Group A; n = 30), and hospitals with biofilm on endoscopes (Group B; n = 36). The researchers found that the proportion of endoscopy centers using an alcohol flush and compressed air drying in Group A was 76.6% (23 of 30) compared with 38.9% (14 of 36) in Group B. The researchers concluded that the formation of biofilm on the endoscope channels could be related to inadequate drying.[96]

Purging the endoscope channels with instrument air or using a mechanical drying system facilitates drying without introducing

STERILIZATION AND DISINFECTION

contaminants into the clean device, removes residual alcohol, and reduces the likelihood of contamination of the endoscope by waterborne pathogens and the transmission of pathogens that may result in patient infection.[1,22,44,45,89,99,157]

Bajolet et al[118] reported transmission of an extended-spectrum ß-lactamase-producing *P aeruginosa* in four patients who underwent an EGD procedure with the same gastroscope between May and August 2011. The gastroscope had been purchased in January 2011. Microbiological sampling before its first use showed negative results. The investigators observed processing procedures and found the endoscopes were still wet at the end of the cleaning process and were not adequately dried before storage. They concluded that the moist environment in the channels of the endoscope had supported development of a persistent biofilm that contributed to transmission of a serious infection.

Hagan et al[249] reported a pseudo-infection of *Rhodotorula rubra* related to a contaminated bronchoscope in a Kansas City medical center. Between October and November 1992, bronchoscopy specimens from 11 patients yielded growth of *R rubra*. The outbreak ended when investigators initiated changes to the processing procedures that included adding an alcohol flush and purging the lumens of the bronchoscope with air for three minutes.

Carbonne et al[250] reported an outbreak of *K pneumoniae* carbapenemase-producing *K pneumoniae* type 2 that was detected in two hospitals in France during September 2009. Of the 13 patients, seven had been examined with the same duodenoscope that had been used to examine the source patient. The investigators found that the cleaning and disinfection processes were consistent with French national guidelines; however, the drying process was not optimal. The procedures were revised to include a systematic drying step after each disinfection cycle, and no additional cases were identified.

Because of a severe outbreak of *K pneumoniae* producing extended-spectrum ß-lactamase that occurred in 16 patients undergoing ERCP procedures in a hospital in France between December 2008 and August 2009, Aumeran et al[55] observed the duodenoscope processing procedures. They found that the duodenoscopes were not fully dried before they were stored. The investigators hypothesized that bacteria were introduced into the channels of the duodenoscope during the procedures, and despite repeated cleaning and disinfection, the contamination persisted because the moisture remaining in the endoscope channels created conditions favorable to the persistence and growth of the involved organism. The infection was transmitted to 12 patients. Implementing adequate drying of the endoscopes and ensuring that the

elevator channel was dry before storage led to an abrupt termination of the outbreak.

VIII.i. A multidisciplinary team that includes infection preventionists, endoscopy and perioperative RNs, endoscopy processing personnel, endoscopists, and other involved personnel should conduct a risk assessment to determine the potential harms compared with the benefits of initiating one or more enhanced methods for processing duodenoscopes.[138] *[3: Moderate Evidence]*

Initiating enhanced processing methods for duodenoscopes may decrease the potential for pathogenic microorganisms to remain on the endoscope after processing.[138,165,251] Before processing, gastrointestinal endoscopes carry a microbial load of approximately 10^7 to 10^{10} (ie, 10,000,000 to 10,000,000,000) organisms.[112,113,115,252] Cleaning results in a 2-log to 6-log reduction.[253,254] High-level disinfection results in a 4-log to 6-log reduction.[254]

Theoretically, if a flexible endoscope carried a microbial load of 10^{10}, and cleaning reduced the microbial load by 2-log (10^{-2}), and this was followed by HLD that resulted in a 4-log reduction (10^{-4}), the device would still have a 4-log (10^4) microbial load after processing (ie, 10,000 microorganisms). Repeat HLD or sterilization would increase the margin of safety and further decrease the number of pathogenic microorganisms remaining on the endoscope.[165,251]

The sterility assurance level for sterile items is 10^{-6}.[77] A 6-log reduction theoretically reduces a population of 1 million microorganisms to zero.[77]

VIII.i.1. Enhanced methods for processing flexible duodenoscopes may include implementing HLD followed by
- endoscope quarantine until the duodenoscope is culture-negative,[138,165,251]
- a liquid chemical sterilant processing system,[138,165,251]
- a second HLD,[138,165,251]
- ethylene oxide sterilization,[138,165,251] or
- FDA-cleared low-temperature sterilization.[165,251]

[3: Moderate Evidence]

Culturing duodenoscopes after every processing cycle and quarantining the endoscope until culture results are known may be an effective method for assessing processing effectiveness.

Ross et al[144] implemented a process for quarantining flexible duodenoscopes following an outbreak of multidrug-resistant *E coli* that occurred in a Seattle medical center between November 2012 and August 2013. Thirty-two patients were found to harbor one of two genetically similar strains of the organism. All of the patients had undergone ERCP procedures. The investigators were unable to find any lapses in HLD or infection control procedures. The genetic strain of *E coli* was identified by culture on four of eight duodenoscopes, three of which required critical repairs despite a lack of noticeable malfunction. Twenty new duodenoscopes were purchased to implement the quarantine process.

After mechanical processing performed in accordance with the manufacturer's IFU, cultures were taken of the duodenoscope, mechanical processing was repeated after culturing, and the duodenoscope was hung vertically in a storage cabinet with passive airflow for 48 hours. If the culture report was negative, the endoscope was released for use. If bacterial pathogens were identified, the duodenoscope was reprocessed, cultured, and quarantined for an additional 48 hours and only released if the cultures were negative. During a one-year period, a total of 1,524 cultures were collected from the duodenoscopes, of which 200 (13.1%) were positive for bacterial growth. The majority, 171 (85.5%) grew common skin flora and nonpathogenic organisms. The remaining 29 (14.5%) were positive for pathogenic bacterial growth. In two cases, the duodenoscopes required more than one repeat cycle of HLD in order to be culture-negative. The two endoscopes were returned to the manufacturer for inspection, and one had to be taken out of service. The investigators concluded that the quarantine process was successful in ending the outbreak of duodenoscope-related infections.

Because some duodenoscopes may have persistent microbial contamination despite HLD, repeat HLD or sterilization may provide a greater margin of safety.[138] Using a liquid chemical sterilant system after HLD may provide a greater margin of safety and may be effective for heat-sensitive devices such as flexible endoscopes; however, because this process may require rinsing with unsterile water after sterilization, the endoscope may not remain completely free of all viable microorganisms.[138]

Ethylene oxide sterilization following HLD may also provide a greater margin of safety, and may be effective for heat-sensitive devices such as flexible endoscopes; however, it can fail in the presence of organic material, it is costly and not accessible to all health care facilities, and it may affect the material and mechanical properties of the duodenoscope.[138]

Performing HLD followed by HLD, liquid chemical sterilization, low-temperature sterilization, or ethylene oxide sterilization has not been validated by the endoscope, mechanical processor, or sterilizer manufacturers, and further research is warranted.

VIII.j.   Processes and procedures for packaging and sterilizing flexible endoscopes and endoscope accessories should be carried out in accordance with the AORN Guideline for Selection and Use of Packaging Systems for Sterilization[255] and the AORN Guideline for Sterilization.[256] *[1: Strong Evidence]*

Sterilization provides the highest level of assurance that processed items are free of viable microbes.[15]

Packaging systems permit sterilization of the contents within the package, protect the integrity of the sterilized contents, prevent contamination of the contents until the package is opened for use, and permit the aseptic delivery of the contents.[255]

VIII.j.1.   Endoscopic accessories (eg, biopsy forceps) that enter sterile tissue or the vascular system should be packaged and sterilized.[27,44,256] *[1: Strong Evidence]*

Devices that enter sterile tissue or the vascular system are considered critical items.[117]

VIII.k.   Precautions to minimize the risk for transmission of prion diseases from flexible endoscopes and endoscope accessories should be carried out in accordance with the AORN Guideline for Cleaning and Care of Surgical Instruments.[58] *[1: Strong Evidence]*

Prions are a unique class of infectious proteins that cause fatal neurological diseases.[257] Examples of prion diseases are Gertsmann-Straüssler-Schienker syndrome, fatal familial insomnia syndrome, and Creutzfeldt-Jakob disease (CJD).[257] Creutzfeldt-Jakob disease is a rare and ultimately fatal degenerative disease that belongs to a group of neurological disorders known as transmissible spongiform encephalopathies (TSEs).[20] Variant Creutzfeldt-Jakob disease is acquired from cattle with bovine spongiform encephalopathy, or "mad cow disease."[46,167,257,258]

The collective evidence shows there are concerns about the potential for endoscopic transmission of prions and other TSEs, including CJD, and vCJD.[46,122] For an endoscope to act as a vehicle for transmission of prions, contact with infective tissue is required.[46,257]

In CJD, the prions accumulate in the central nervous system and are transmitted by exposure to infectious brain, pituitary, or eye tissue. Because flexible endoscopes do not come in contact with brain, pituitary, or eye tissue, endoscopic transmission of CJD or other TSEs is unlikely.[46,257]

In vCJD, the prions accumulate in both central nervous system and lymphoid tissue.[167,258] Patients with vCJD have infectivity detectable

FLEXIBLE ENDOSCOPES

TABLE 3. RECOMMENDATIONS FOR PROCESSING FLEXIBLE ENDOSCOPES USED WITH HIGH-RISK PATIENTS		
Type of patient	**Type of tissue**	**Method of processing**
High-risk: • Patients with known prion disease • Patients with familial history of CJD, Gerstmann-Sträussler-Scheinker syndrome, or familial insomnia syndrome • Patients with a known mutation in the PrP (prion protein) gene (involved in familial transmissible spongiform encephalopathies [TSEs]) • Patients with a history of dura mater transplantation • Patients with electroencephalograph findings or laboratory evidence suggesting of TSE (eg, markers of neuronal injury such as 14-3-3 protein) • Patients with a known history of cadaver-derived pituitary hormone injection	High-risk: • brain (including dura mater) • spinal cord • posterior eye (including retina or optic nerve) • pituitary gland	Discard
	Low-risk: • cerebrospinal fluid • kidney • liver • spleen • lung • placenta • olfactory epithelium • lymph nodes	No recommendation (Unresolved issue) • Conduct a risk assessment with a multidisciplinary team to determine whether to process or discard • Discard neurosurgical endoscopes with central nervous system contact
	No-risk: • peripheral nerve • intestine • bone marrow • blood • leukocytes • serum • thyroid gland • adrenal gland • heart • skeletal muscle • adipose tissue • gingiva • prostate • testis • tears • saliva • sputum • urine • feces • semen • vaginal secretions • milk • sweat	Process in accordance with the AORN Guideline for Cleaning and Care of Surgical Instruments

REFERENCES

1. *Rutala WA, Weber DJ; Society for Healthcare Epidemiology of America. Guideline for disinfection and sterilization of prion-contaminated medical instruments.* Infect Control Hosp Epidemiol. *2010;31(2):107-117.*
2. *Guideline for cleaning and care of surgical instruments. In:* Guidelines for Perioperative Practice. *Denver, CO: AORN, Inc; 2015:615-650.*

in the appendix, spleen, tonsils, thymus, and lymph nodes.[20,46,93,167,257,258] The prions responsible for vCJD are found in abundance in the Peyer patches located in the terminal ileum.[20,167] Aggregates of lymphoid prions are also found in the large intestine and the stomach.[167] Transmission of vCJD via a flexible gastrointestinal endoscope is therefore theoretically possible because of the lymphatic distribution of prions. The risk for transmission is greater during invasive interventional procedures (eg, biopsy, polypectomy, mucosal resection, sphincterotomy) than during noninterventional procedures[20,258]; however, there have been no reports of such transmission described in the literature.[93,167,258]

VIII.k.1. Flexible endoscopes and accessories used during endoscopy procedures on high-risk patients should be processed as shown in Table 3. *[1: Strong Evidence]*

Prions are highly resistant to conventional physical and chemical disinfection and sterilization and can remain infectious for years.[46,167,257,258]

Methods for processing instruments contaminated with prions are unsuitable for semicritical, heat-labile devices such as flexible endoscopes.[20,257] Current recommendations for processing instruments exposed to prions include decontamination with concentrated sodium hydroxide (ie, lye) or sodium hypochlorite (ie, bleach), which are corrosive to flexible endoscopes, followed

STERILIZATION AND DISINFECTION

by prolonged steam sterilization, which most flexible endoscopes cannot tolerate.[93,257] Dry heat, glutaraldehyde, and ethylene oxide are not effective disinfection or sterilization methods for flexible endoscopes contaminated with prions.[20,93,258] Aldehyde disinfectants (eg, glutaraldehyde, orthophalaldehyde) may anchor prion proteins within endoscope channels and also render them more difficult to remove. For this reason, aldehyde disinfectants are not recommended for HLD in some countries.[20,167,258] Further research is warranted relative to the use of cleaning chemistries and low-temperature sterilization technologies for inactivating prions.[257]

Discarding the endoscope and accessories after use on high-risk tissue from high-risk patients ensures the endoscope and accessories will not be used on subsequent patients and eliminates the risk of inadequate prion inactivation or patient-to-patient transmission of prion disease.

There is no recommendation for processing critical or semicritical devices contaminated with low-risk tissue from high-risk patients. Although low-risk tissue has been found to transmit CJD, this has been demonstrated only when low-risk tissue has been inoculated into the brain of a susceptible animal.[257]

Flexible endoscopes contaminated with no-risk tissue do not present a risk for prion transmission.

VIII.l. A multidisciplinary team that includes infection preventionists, endoscopy and perioperative RNs, endoscopy processing personnel, endoscopists, and other involved personnel should conduct a risk assessment to determine whether single-use endoscope sheaths will be used with compatible flexible endoscopes, and if used, whether, and under what circumstances the endoscope will be disinfected using ILD or HLD. *[3: Moderate Evidence]*

Flexible endoscopes contact mucous membranes and are considered semicritical items requiring a minimum of HLD[117,259]; however, the collective evidence shows that when compatible with the sheath, and used in accordance with the sheath manufacturer's IFU, flexible endoscopes may be effectively processed using 70% isopropyl alcohol (an ILD)[45] rather than HLD, and processing time is reduced.[83,89,260-264]

In a quasi-experimental study to compare the efficacy of various high-level disinfectants against mycobacteria when used in combination with manual cleaning, Foliente et al[253] found that 70% isopropyl alcohol was as effective against mycobacteria as two high-level disinfectants. The researchers inoculated five colonoscopes and five duodenoscopes with *M chelonae*. Each endoscope was manually cleaned,

and then exposed to one of two high-level disinfectants (ie, 2% glutaraldehyde, 7.5% hydrogen peroxide), 70% isopropyl alcohol, a liquid chemical sterilant (ie, 0.2% peracetic acid), or ethylene oxide sterilization. The researchers sampled the endoscopes after inoculation, manual cleaning, and disinfection or sterilization. The results showed the average number of microorganisms recovered after inoculation was 9.4×10^6 CFU. After manual cleaning, the average number of microorganisms was 9.9×10^3 CFU, reflecting a 3-log reduction. The researchers found no mycobacteria after exposure to ethylene oxide or 0.2% peracetic acid. The average number of microorganisms after exposure to 70% alcohol was 19 CFU/endoscope and after exposure to the high-level disinfectants was 13 CFU/endoscope for 2% glutaraldehyde and 40 CFU/endoscope for 7.5% hydrogen peroxide.

Sheaths reduce but do not eliminate the risk of contamination and do not eliminate the need for manual cleaning of the endoscope after use.[89] The endoscope may also be contaminated by the soiled hands or gloves of personnel during application or removal of the sheath.[89] The sheath may be breached or may break or tear during use,[89] potentially exposing the patient to a flexible endoscope processed by ILD rather than HLD. Sheath failure may not be obvious.[259]

Lawrentschuk and Chamberlain[260] described their experience of using a flexible cystoscope with a single-use endoscope sheath designed to function as a microbial barrier on 200 consecutive patients. The authors found that using the single-use sheath eliminated the need for HLD or sterilization, thus saving time and minimizing personnel exposure to hazardous chemicals. Notably, the sheath failed in 5% of procedures. The authors noted that using the sheath reduced contact of the cystoscope with body fluids and chemicals, and this reduced contact could theoretically prolong the life of the endoscope.

In a nonexperimental study to evaluate the use of endoscope sheaths as barriers to viruses on flexible ear, nose, and throat endoscopes, Baker et al[261] challenged the sheaths by applying laser-drilled holes (2 μg to 30 μg) and inoculating the sheaths with suspensions of bacteriophage (1.0×10^8 plaque-forming units (PFU)/mL). The sheath and the endoscope were sampled to recover any virus particles that had penetrated through the holes in the sheath. The researchers found that up to 500 virus particles could pass through the 30 μg holes, indicating a very low viral passage. The researchers concluded that meticulous cleaning of the endoscope followed by ILD provided an instrument that was safe to use on patients.

Elackattu et al[262] conducted a quasi-experimental study to evaluate the number of microorganisms on patient-used flexible nasopharyngolaryngoscopes with and without endoscope sheaths. The researchers took samples from multiple sites on 100 flexible nasopharyngolaryngoscopes. The endoscopes were assigned to either the sheath group (n = 50) or the HLD group (n = 50). Samples were taken from the handle of the endoscopes and the lower third of the insertion shaft of the endoscopes before and after use. The results showed that one in 50 endoscope insertion shafts was culture-positive in both groups. There were no positive cultures of handles in the HLD group; however, there were four positive cultures of handles in the sheath group. The sheath method averaged 89 seconds to process, whereas the HLD method averaged 14 minutes. The researchers concluded that using the endoscope sheath reduced processing time and was a safe method for preventing transmission of infection from one patient to the next. Notably, this study was funded by a grant from the sheath manufacturer.

In a randomized controlled trial to investigate the function and processing of flexible gastroscopes, Mayinger et al[263] compared the performance of 50 sheathed with 50 unsheathed gastroscopes using a 10-point analog rating scale. The researchers recorded processing times, took samples before and after use and processing, and examined the endoscope sheaths for leaks or tears. The researchers found no leaks or tears in any of the endoscope sheaths. Microbial contamination was found in 10% (five of 50) of the unsheathed endoscopes processed by HLD and in 16% (eight of 50) of the sheathed endoscopes. The processing time for the sheathed system was significantly shorter at 8.9 minutes compared with 48.4 minutes for processing by HLD. Based on the results of the analog rating scale, the endoscopists preferred the unsheathed endoscope, while the processing personnel preferred the sheathed endoscope for its ease of processing.

Alvarado et al[264] conducted a randomized controlled trial to determine whether sheathed nasopharyngoscopes could provide reliable protection against bacterial contamination and obviate the need for HLD. The researchers obtained baseline samples at three time periods from the control heads and insertion shafts of three nasopharyngoscopes used in 100 clinical examinations. The samples were obtained

○ before application of the sheath and the procedure,
○ immediately after the procedure and removal of the sheath, and
○ after point-of-use precleaning, disinfection with 70% isopropyl alcohol, and drying.

The researchers found no bacteria on any of the endoscopes after processing. No sheath showed loss of barrier integrity during leak testing. The researchers concluded that after following point-of-use precleaning, disinfection with 70% isopropyl alcohol, and drying pro-

cesses, the endoscopes were safe to use. This study was funded by a grant from the sheath manufacturer.[264]

In an evaluation to measure image clarity, ease of use, and handling performance of a flexible bronchoscope and single-use sheath, Colt et al[265] measured the performance using a linear rating scale of 1 (poor) to 5 (excellent) after use on 24 patients at three tertiary care centers. The mean performance ratings were > 4.0 for image clarity, illumination, lack of fogging, distal tip angulation, and ease of transnasal passage. All other ratings were > 3.0, with the lowest for handling comfort. The authors concluded that the single-use sheath had the potential to reduce bronchoscope downtime by eliminating the need for HLD between procedures. This study was supported in part by the sheath manufacturer.

Using endoscope sheaths may potentially extend the life of the endoscope[83,89,260,266]; however, sheaths increase the diameter of the endoscope and this may lead to patient discomfort.[266,267] Securely fitted sheaths may also cause damage to the delicate tip of the endoscope when the sheath is removed.[266]

In a nonexperimental study to evaluate bacterial contamination of flexible cystoscopes protected by single-use sheaths, Jorgensen et al[267] leak tested 100 cystoscopes and then sampled the cystoscopes after removal of the sheath and after ILD. The researchers found that all samples had less than 5 CFU/sample. The researchers concluded that processing flexible cystoscopes using ILD was an acceptable alternative to HLD, provided there was a low risk for pathogen transmission. Using the sheath reduced processing time between four and 31 minutes per procedure. The researchers noted that using the sheaths resulted in some reduced visualization for the urologist and increased discomfort for the patient.

Street et al[266] audited the costs of disinfection practices in a UK hospital between July 2003 and January 2004 and found that endoscope sheaths had damaged two flexible laryngoscopes with repair costs totaling $15,551.77 (£10,252 [$19,735.77 and £13,029.32 in 2015]). The cause of the damage in one instance was determined to be the sheath being incorrectly fitted, and in the other, the sheath being left on the endoscope overnight. The lining of each flexible endoscope was torn about 2 cm from the tip. Sheaths tightly grip the tip of the flexible endoscope and can shear off the lining of the tip when removed. The authors also opined that the use of sheaths increased patient discomfort and the likelihood of trauma to the nasal mucosa because of the increased diameter of the endoscope, which they calculated to be a 12% increase.

STERILIZATION AND DISINFECTION

VIII.l.1.   Single-use endoscope sheaths should be discarded after each use. *[3: Moderate Evidence]*

Discarding the endoscope sheath after use helps ensure it is not used on subsequent patients. Brake et al[207] conducted a survey of 171 otolaryngologists to compare practices in Canada for disinfection of flexible nasopharyngoscopes. The researchers found that 36.4% of otolaryngologists who used endoscope sheaths were unsure whether the sheaths were to be discarded after use, and 18.2% believed that sheaths were intended to be used multiple times. Only 63.6% always cleaned the nasopharyngoscopes between sheath uses, and 9.1% did not know how often the endoscopes were cleaned between uses. The researchers did not disclose how many of the otolaryngologists who responded to the survey used endoscope sheaths.

VIII.l.2.   If approved for ILD by the multidisciplinary team, the endoscope and single-use endoscope sheath should be visually inspected after each use.[83] *[4: Limited Evidence]*

Inspection of the endoscope sheath confirms the integrity of the sheath and may determine the subsequent level of processing (ie, HLD or ILD).[83]

VIII.l.3.   If the sheath is intact, the endoscope may be disinfected by
- washing all external surfaces with a soft, lint-free cloth or sponge saturated with the endoscope manufacturer's recommended cleaning solution[1,12,13,15,16,18,19,22,27,65,83,84,89,105];
- rinsing the exterior surfaces of the endoscope with utility water until all cleaning solution and residual debris is removed[12,13,15-17,20,27,83-85,89];
- wiping the external surfaces of the endoscope with 70% isopropyl alcohol[83]; and
- drying the external surfaces of the endoscope with a soft, lint-free cloth or sponge.[83]

[2: High Evidence]

The manufacturer has validated the sheath to be impermeable to penetration by microorganisms and has validated that sheath application and removal can be accomplished without contamination of the endoscope. The barrier properties of the sheath have been validated, and a minimum of ILD is required before application of a new sheath.[268]

VIII.l.4.   If the endoscope sheath is torn or any portion of the endoscope appears soiled or wet, the endoscope should be cleaned and processed by HLD or sterilization.[83] *[4: Limited Evidence]*

If the endoscope has been contaminated due to a torn sheath, processing by ILD may not be sufficient to prevent patient-to-patient transmission of pathogenic microorganisms, and HLD is required.[89]

VIII.l.5.   If an endoscope is to be used without the sheath for a subsequent patient, it should be processed by HLD or sterilization, even though the sheath appears intact and the endoscope was processed by ILD.[12] *[5: Benefits Balanced with Harms]*

VIII.l.6.   If the endoscope is only used with a single-use sheath, the multidisciplinary team, should conduct a risk assessment to establish intervals for leak testing, inspection, and HLD or sterilization. *[5: Benefits Balanced with Harms]*

VIII.m.   A multidisciplinary team that includes infection preventionists, endoscopy and perioperative RNs, endoscopy processing personnel, endoscopists, and other involved personnel should conduct a risk assessment to determine whether chlorine dioxide wipes may be used for disinfection of non-channeled flexible endoscopes when compatible with the endoscope and used in accordance with the disinfectant manufacturer's IFU. *[3: Moderate Evidence]*

Chlorine dioxide wipes incorporate a three-step process for cleaning and disinfecting non-channeled flexible endoscopes that includes cleaning, disinfection, and rinsing; however, chlorine dioxide has not been cleared by the FDA as a high-level disinfectant for processing reusable medical equipment.[269]

Non-channeled flexible endoscopes can become contaminated with mucous, debris, microorganisms, and blood during use.[270] Non-channeled flexible endoscopes contact mucous membranes and are considered semicritical items requiring a minimum of HLD.[117]

Bhattacharyya and Kepnes[271] conducted a quasi-experimental study to determine whether HLD rendered non-channeled flexible laryngoscopes free of nonviral infectious microorganisms. The researchers sampled six laryngoscopes after HLD at the beginning, middle, and end of two clinical workdays (n = 36), and after contamination with saliva on two additional days (n = 12). The researchers recovered only one positive culture (2.1%) for mold species. No cultures were positive for bacteria. The researchers concluded that HLD was effective and provided a flexible laryngoscope that was safe for patient use.

Protocols for processing non-channeled flexible endoscopes are derived from protocols for processing channeled flexible endoscopes, which carry a much higher bioload after use and have different design properties than non-channeled endoscopes.[272,273] Other technologies may be effective for processing non-channeled endoscopes.

In a quasi-experimental study to compare various methods for processing non-channeled flexible laryngoscopes, Liming et al[274] applied eight different processes to patient-used endoscopes, sampled the endoscopes after processing, and compared the results. The methods applied included a

- 30-second wash with utility water,
- 30-second scrub with antimicrobial soap,
- 30-second wipe with 70% isopropyl alcohol,
- 30-second scrub with antimicrobial soap followed by a 30-second wipe with 70% isopropyl alcohol,
- 30-second wipe with a germicidal cloth,
- 12-minute soak in orthophyalaldehyde,
- 15-minute soak in orthophyalaldehyde, and
- 20-minute soak in orthophyalaldehyde.

The researchers found that each of the methods used was statistically efficacious in removing bacterial contamination and equally as effective as HLD. The researchers concluded that fast, cost-effective practices were acceptable for processing non-channeled flexible endoscopes.

In a quasi-experimental study to determine the efficacy of various cleaning and disinfecting methods in reducing bacterial and fungal loads on flexible fiberoptic laryngoscopes, Chang et al[272] contaminated clean endoscopes with *S aureus* and *C albicans*. The researchers exposed the contaminated endoscopes to

- 20-, 15-, 10-, and five-minute soaks in orthophalaldehyde after precleaning in an enzymatic cleaning solution;
- 20-, 15-, 10-, and five-minute soaks in orthophalaldehyde without precleaning in an enzymatic cleaning solution;
- a five-minute soak in enzymatic cleaning solution;
- a 30-second wipe with antibacterial soap and water;
- a 30-second wipe with 70% isopropyl alcohol;
- a 30-second wipe with antibacterial soap followed by a 30-second wipe with 70% isopropyl alcohol; and
- a 30-second wipe with a germicidal cloth.

All exposures were followed by a 30-second rinse with utility water. The results showed that all exposures except the five-minute soak in enzymatic cleaning solution were successful in completely eliminating the *S aureus* and *C albicans* from the contaminated endoscopes. The researchers concluded that short and simple cleaning and disinfecting protocols for non-channeled endoscopes were acceptable without sacrificing efficacy and patient safety.

In a nonexperimental study to evaluate the efficacy of chlorine dioxide wipes for disinfection of flexible nasendoscopes, Tzanidakis et al[273] randomly sampled the handles and distal tips of 31 endoscopes from a number of otolaryngology outpatient clinics. The samples were taken immediately before and after use on patients and immediately after cleaning. The researchers found that none of the samples were culture-positive after disinfection with the chlorine dioxide wipes. Three of the samples from the handles of the nasendoscope were positive for *S aureus* before use on the patient, demonstrating the potential for contamination of the area of the nasendoscope that is handled during transport that occurs after cleaning and before use. The researchers concluded that the chlorine dioxide wipes provided a safe and effective alternative to mechanical processing but recommended that personnel perform hand hygiene and don gloves before handling flexible endoscopes.

Javed et al[270] conducted a survey of 200 ear, nose, and throat outpatient departments in the United Kingdom to investigate practices for disinfection of flexible nasal endoscopes. The response to the survey was 61% (n = 121). The researchers found that the preferred method for disinfection of nasal endoscopes was chlorine dioxide wipes (58%; n = 70); however, mechanical processors were also used (34%; n = 41), as were flexible sheaths (7%; n = 8). Precleaning at the point of use using an enzymatic cleaning solution was performed by the vast majority of respondents (65%; n = 79). Notably, the researchers found the use of 2% glutaraldehyde as a high-level disinfectant was rare (0.8%; n = 1).

The use of chlorine dioxide wipes may be more costly than mechanical processing[270] but less costly than use of single-use endoscope sheaths.[266] Phua et al[275] evaluated the efficacy and cost-effectiveness of chlorine dioxide wipes compared with mechanical processing for processing flexible nasendoscopes. The researchers contaminated clean nasendoscopes with *S epidermidis*, exposed them to disinfection using either chlorine dioxide wipes (n = 50) or mechanical processing (n = 50), and then sampled the endoscopes. The researchers used *S epidermidis* as the test organism because it is representative of the normal flora found in the nasopharynx and larynx. The samples showed *S epidermidis* in 2% of samples (one of 50) from the chlorine dioxide group and 28% of samples (14 of 50) from the mechanical processor group. The researchers estimated costs over a 10-year period and determined that even with the expense of installation and maintenance, the mechanical processor would be less costly than the chlorine dioxide wipes and would provide an annual cost savings of approximately $25,355.82 (£16,715 [$26,467.45 in 2015 US dollars and £17,473.49 in 2015 British pounds]).

Street et al[266] audited the costs of disinfection practices in a UK hospital between July 2003 and January 2004. After determining that the cost of single-use sheaths averaged $6079.94 (£4008 [$7715.66 in 2015 US dollars and £5093.79 in 2015 British pounds]) per month, the authors introduced the use of chlorine dioxide wipes and achieved a monthly cost savings of $4770.81 (£3145 [$6054.33 in 2015 US dollars and £3997 in 2015 British pounds]).

Recommendation IX

Flexible endoscopes and endoscope accessories should be stored in a manner that minimizes contamination and protects the device or item from damage.[1,12,13,16,44,45,65,83]

The collective evidence supports effective storage of flexible endoscopes and endoscope accessories as a means of helping to ensure devices are safe for patient use.[1,12,13,16,44,45,83] The benefits of effective storage are that it helps protect the endoscopes and endoscope accessories from damage and reduces contamination.[1,12,13,16,44,45,83] Some evidence is limited due to inconsistency in outcome measures, small sample sizes,[276-282] and lack of a control.[283-287] There is no consensus regarding maximum safe storage times.[1,12,13,15,16,18-22,27,44,83]

IX.a. Cabinets used for storage of flexible endoscopes should be situated in a secure location in the clean workroom of the endoscopy processing room in a two-room design or in a separate clean area close to, but not within, the endoscopy procedure room.[65,288] *[3: Moderate Evidence]*

Situating the storage cabinet in a secure location helps protect inventories of flexible endoscopes and supplies that are vulnerable to misappropriation.[69,288] Locating the storage cabinet in the clean workroom or in a clean area outside of the procedure room helps prevent contamination of processed endoscopes.[69]

IX.a.1. Storage cabinets should have doors,[23] and be located at least 3 ft (0.9 m) from any sink.[23] *[3: Moderate Evidence]*

Ensuring storage cabinets have doors and are separated from sinks by at least 3 ft (0.9 m) provides protection and reduces the potential for processed flexible endoscopes to be contaminated by water droplets.[12,13,16,22,23,27]

IX.b. Flexible endoscopes should be stored in accordance with the endoscope and storage cabinet manufacturers' IFU. *[5: Benefits Balanced with Harms]*

Following the manufacturers' IFU helps ensure safe and effective storage of endoscopes.

IX.b.1. Flexible endoscopes should be stored in a drying cabinet.[15,18,27,69] *[2: High Evidence]*

The collective evidence shows that optimal storage of flexible endoscopes facilitates drying, decreases the potential for contamination, and provides protection from environmental contaminants.[69,85,288]

A wide variety of storage cabinets are available.[20] Drying cabinets include a drying system that circulates HEPA-filtered air through the cabinet while filtered air under pressure is forced through the endoscope channels.[69,276,278] The internal and external surfaces of the endoscope are continuously dried, suppressing bacterial growth.[12,20,69,276,277] Studies related to the efficacy of drying cabinets compared with other methods of storage showed that drying cabinets effectively limited bacterial proliferation during storage.[276-278,283]

In a quasi-experimental study to determine whether bacterial growth occurred in flexible endoscopes during a 72-hour storage period in a drying cabinet, Foxcroft et al[276] processed 55 endoscopes, sampled the endoscopes, stored 40 of the endoscopes in a drying cabinet designed for horizontal storage of the endoscopes, and placed 15 of the endoscopes in an open storage cabinet in the endoscopy unit designed for vertical storage of the endoscopes. Each endoscope in the drying cabinet was connected individually to the HEPA-filtered air source. The cabinet was opened eight times daily to simulate normal use. At the end of the 72-hour storage period, the endoscopes were removed and sampled.

The researchers found that of a total of 64 samples collected from the endoscopes stored in the drying cabinet, only one sample (taken immediately after processing) showed bacterial growth (1 CFU coagulase-negative *Staphylococcus*). The researchers theorized this was likely the result of laboratory contamination since no other cultures from the endoscope were positive. Of the 44 samples collected from the endoscopes stored in the open cabinet, only one sample (taken immediately after processing) showed bacterial growth (1 CFU *Streptococcus*, 1 CFU *Propionbacterium*). The researchers also placed culture plates in the storage cabinets to evaluate and compare environmental contaminants within the cabinets. They found that the culture plates from the drying cabinet had significantly fewer organisms detected than the culture plates placed in the open cabinet. The researchers concluded that a 72-hour storage time did not result in increased bacterial counts in any of the stored endoscopes.[276]

Grandval et al[283] evaluated the microbial levels of endoscopes after clinical use and processing, followed by 72 hours of storage in

- a drying cabinet designed for horizontal storage of the endoscopes (Group 1; n = 41 [colonoscopes = 13; gastroscopes = 21; duodenoscopes = 7]),
- a dedicated storage cabinet designed for vertical storage of the endoscopes without daily disinfection (Group 2; n = 41

[colonoscopes = 17; gastroscopes = 17; duodenoscopes = 7]), and

- a dedicated storage cabinet designed for vertical storage of the endoscopes with daily disinfection (Group 3; n = 41 [colonoscopes = 20; gastroscopes = 15; duodenoscopes = 6]).

The researchers found that 100% of the Group 1 endoscopes had a contamination level consistent with the preset target level (< 5 CFU/endoscope), and 56% of these (n = 23) were completely free of contamination. Of the Group 2 and 3 endoscopes, 88% (n = 36) had a contamination level consistent with the preset target level. Of the Group 2 endoscopes, 41% (n = 17) were completely free of contamination, and of the Group 3 endoscopes, 61% (n = 25) were completely free of contamination. The researchers concluded that the use of a drying cabinet was the most effective method for maintaining microbial loads within the preset target level.[283]

In a quasi-experimental study of the efficacy of a drying cabinet, Pineau et al[277] artificially contaminated one colonoscope, one gastroscope, and one enteroscope with *P aeruginosa*; stored them first inside and then outside of a drying cabinet designed for vertical storage of the endoscopes; and then sampled the endoscopes at 12, 24, 28, and 72 hours. The results showed that when the endoscopes were stored in the drying cabinet, microbial contamination levels were lower than the number of bacteria initially introduced. The researchers theorized that the level would continue to decrease considerably thereafter. For endoscopes stored outside of the drying cabinet, microbial levels were stable or increased. These data demonstrated the advantages of drying cabinets in limiting bacterial proliferation in the internal channels of endoscopes during storage.

Wardle[278] conducted a quasi-experimental study to determine whether gastroscopes and colonoscopes stored in a drying cabinet designed for vertical storage of the endoscopes grew microorganisms in the channels within 72 hours. The researcher evaluated the microbial levels of two gastroscopes and six colonoscopes after clinical use and processing followed by 72 hours of storage in a drying cabinet. The results showed there was no microbial growth in any of the endoscopes. The researcher concluded that flexible endoscopes could be stored in the drying cabinet and used without reprocessing for up to 72 hours but speculated that because of the effectiveness of the cabinet, the endoscopes could be safely used after storage for up to one week.

IX.b.2. If a drying cabinet is not available, flexible endoscopes may be stored in a closed cabinet with HEPA-filtered air that provides positive pressure and allows air circulation around the flexible endoscopes.[1,13,19,27,65,85] *[3: Moderate Evidence]*

Ventilation promotes continued drying of the endoscope. Using HEPA-filtered air may help prevent bacterial growth in the endoscope. Positive pressure may help prevent contamination of stored endoscopes.

IX.b.3. Flexible endoscopes should not be stored in the original shipment cases.[12,15,27,45,65,83,84] *[1: Strong Evidence]*

The cases are difficult to clean, may be contaminated,[45] and are designed for shipping only.[65]

IX.c. Flexible endoscopes that have been mechanically processed should be stored in a cabinet that is either

- designed and intended by the cabinet manufacturer for horizontal storage of flexible endoscopes or
- of sufficient height, width, and depth to allow flexible endoscopes to hang vertically, without coiling and without touching the bottom of the cabinet.[1,12,13,15-20,27,44,45,65,85,93]

[1: Strong Evidence]

Some drying cabinets are designed by the manufacturer for horizontal storage of flexible endoscopes. Using a cabinet of sufficient height, depth, and width helps prevent damage that might occur from one endoscope hitting another.[16] Hanging flexible endoscopes vertically helps prevent coiling or kinking of the endoscope.[12,17,65]

IX.d. Flexible endoscopes should be stored with all valves open[22] and removable parts detached but stored with the endoscope.[1,13,15,16,18-20,22,27,44,83,85] *[1: Strong Evidence]*

Leaving valves open and removable parts detached facilitates drying of the endoscope.[85] Insufficient drying creates an environment conducive to microbial growth and promotes the formation of biofilm.[82] Storing removable parts with the endoscope helps prevent loss and facilitates traceability.[13,22]

Alfa et al[131] surveyed 37 hospitals across Canada and collected samples from the biopsy channel of duodenoscopes to assess processing practices and evaluate levels of bioburden in patient-ready duodenoscopes. The researchers found that 43% of centers (n = 16) were compliant with national processing guidelines. All of the samples with low levels of organisms (< 200 CFU/mL) had gram-positive organisms, whereas the samples with more than 200 CFU/mL had predominantly gram-negative organisms. *S maltophilia* was the most common organism (ie, in six of eight samples). The researchers suggested that this was likely caused by growth of

STERILIZATION AND DISINFECTION

water-related organisms resulting from removable parts being left on the endoscope during storage.

IX.e. Flexible endoscopes should be clearly identifiable with a distinct visual cue as processed and ready for use.[12,17,19,45,65,83] *[1: Strong Evidence]*

Identifying endoscopes that are ready for use and distinguishing them from unprocessed endoscopes may help prevent use of a contaminated endoscope.[12,65]

After identifying two incidents in which used, contaminated flexible endoscopes were returned to the clean storage area without HLD, Nomides et al[289] created a visual cue that would readily identify endoscopes that had been processed and were ready for patient use. Infection prevention and sterile processing team members worked with a manufacturer to develop a green locking tie that was applied to the endoscopes after processing. The tie prevented the endoscope from being used until removal by the user.[289]

Personnel who processed flexible endoscopes were educated about the new system and the use of locking ties was implemented in all areas where endoscopes were processed. Endoscopes with the locking tie were readily identified as processed and ready for patient use. If there was no tie on the endoscope, it was processed and a tie was applied before storage. After implementation of this system, 94% of the endoscopy suites were compliant, and no additional incidents of using contaminated endoscopes were identified. The authors concluded that the use of a distinct, visual cue was an effective way to identify processed endoscopes and improve patient safety.

IX.f. Flexible endoscopes and storage cabinets should be visually inspected for cleanliness before endoscopes are placed into or removed from storage.[13]
- If there is any evidence of contamination of the endoscope (eg, soil, moisture), the endoscope should be reprocessed before use.[13]
- If there is any evidence of contamination of the cabinet (eg, wet spots, soil, fecal odor), all endoscopes in the cabinet should be removed and reprocessed and the cabinet should be cleaned.

[2: High Evidence]

Reprocessing endoscopes that could be contaminated helps ensure they are safe for use. Visible soil in the storage cabinet may indicate that one or more of the stored endoscopes is contaminated. Soil in the cabinet may contaminate endoscopes stored in the cabinet.[13]

IX.g. Personnel should wear clean, low-protein, powder-free, natural rubber latex gloves or latex-free gloves when handling processed flexible endoscopes and when transporting them to and from the storage cabinet. *[2: High Evidence]*

Sterile gloves are not required for handling processed flexible endoscopes unless the endoscope is intended to be placed on a sterile field.

Wearing clean gloves may lessen contamination of processed flexible endoscopes by the hands of personnel.[69] Using low-protein, powder-free natural rubber latex gloves or latex-free gloves can minimize latex exposure and the risk of reactions in both health care workers and patients.[42] Studies related to storage of flexible endoscopes have confirmed endoscope contamination from the hands of personnel and environmental surfaces.[279-282,284,286,287]

Muscarella[290] described the case of a processed endoscope randomly selected from an endoscope storage cabinet for surveillance purposes that yielded positive growth for both patient-borne and environmental bacteria. To investigate the potential for disease transmission, a second colonoscope was sampled immediately after use (ie, the positive control), and a third colonoscope that had been sterilized with ethylene oxide was also sampled (ie, the negative control). Environmental surfaces were sampled, as were the hands and fingernails of personnel who handled the endoscopes. The investigator found that the bacteria from the insertion tube of the negative control and contaminated colonoscope yielded *S aureus* identical to the strain cultured from the fingernails of a newly hired team member. These results suggested that the team member's hands and fingernails were the source of the bacteria and contamination of the colonoscope after processing. The investigator recommended that personnel wear clean gloves when handling processed endoscopes to prevent contamination of endoscopes before they are used on patients.

IX.h. A multidisciplinary team that includes infection preventionists, endoscopy and perioperative RNs, endoscopy processing personnel, endoscopists, and other involved personnel should establish a policy to determine the maximum storage time that processed flexible endoscopes are considered safe to use without reprocessing. *[3: Moderate Evidence]*

The collective evidence regarding the maximum safe storage time for processed endoscopes is inconclusive. Recommendations from professional organizations for maximum storage times for flexible endoscopes are not in agreement; recommended storage times range from three hours to one month (Table 4).

There is limited evidence to definitively establish the length of time that processed flexible endoscopes remain safe for use during storage. Studies have shown that when correctly processed, flexible endoscopes may be safe to use for 48 hours to 56 days after processing.[279,280,282,284-287] There are benefits to reducing unnecessary processing that include reduced processing costs (eg, personnel, processing supplies), reduced

849

FLEXIBLE ENDOSCOPES

TABLE 4. RECOMMENDATIONS FROM PROFESSIONAL ORGANIZATIONS FOR FLEXIBLE ENDOSCOPE STORAGE TIME	
Professional organization	**Storage time**
American College of Chest Physicians[27] American Associates for Bronchology	No recommendation
American Urological Association[83] Society of Urologic Nurses and Associates	7 to 10 days
American Society for Gastrointestinal Endoscopy[44]	10 to 14 days
Association for the Advancement of Medical Instrumentation[12]	Based on risk assessment
Association for Professionals in Infection Control[1]	No recommendation
Association of periOperative Registered Nurses	Based on risk assessment
British Society of Gastroenterology[20]	Up to 1 month per cabinet manufacturer
British Thoracic Society[18]	Per manufacturer
Department of Health: United Kingdom[51]	3 hours unless stored in a way validated to extend usable storage life or in a sterile package
Dutch Nurses Association: Division Gastroenterology and Hepatology[21] Sterilization Association of the Netherlands Dutch Society of Experts on Sterile Medical Devices Dutch Society for Infection Prevention and Control in the Health Care Setting	Up to 1 month in a drying or dust-free storage cabinet
European Society of Gastrointestinal Endoscopy[22] European Society of Gastroenterology and Endoscopy Nurses and Associates	Based on risk assessment
Gastroenterological Society of Australia[15] Gastroenterological Nurses College of Australia	72 hours • bronchoscopes (intubating) • colonoscopes • endoscopic ultrasound (radial) • enteroscopes (stored with continuous airflow) • gastroscopes 12 hours • bronchoscopes • duodenoscopes • endoscopic ultrasound (linear) • enteroscopes (stored hanging vertically)
Health Service Executive United Kingdom[13]	72 hours
Society of Gastroenterology Nurses and Associates[16]	7 days when processed and stored according to professional guidelines and manufacturer's instructions
World Gastroenterology Organisation[19] World Endoscopy Organization	No recommendation

wear and tear on the endoscope and processing equipment, and lower replacement and repair costs.[280,286] Safe storage times may be affected by factors unique to the facility including the type of endoscopes processed and stored, processing effectiveness (eg, level of residual contamination), storage conditions (eg, restricted access, drying cabinet, HEPA-filtered air), compliance with manufacturers' IFU (ie, endoscope, mechanical processor, storage cabinet), frequency of use, and patient population.[22]

In a nonexperimental study to evaluate the survival of aerobic bacteria and fungi in gastrointestinal endoscopes that were processed after routine procedures and stored in an endoscope cabinet over the weekends, Alfa et al[285] tested all channels from 20 flexible gastrointestinal endoscopes (ie, five gastroscopes, nine colonoscopes, six duodenoscopes) used at an endoscopy clinic. The endoscopes were sampled for the presence of bacteria and fungi every Monday morning during a seven-month period. Bacteria and fungi were detected in 50.1% (n = 192) of the 383 channels tested. Of the 141 endoscopes tested, 14.1% (n = 20) had detectable microbial growth in at least one channel. The researchers concluded that with correct processing and drying, flexible endoscopes were safe to use for 48 to 72 hours after processing.

STERILIZATION AND DISINFECTION

Osborne et al[284] conducted a prospective, observational study to determine a safe shelf life for flexible endoscopes in a four-suite gastroenterology unit. All flexible endoscopes in active clinical use (ie, 23 endoscopes) during a three-week period were sampled before storage and when removed from storage (N = 194). The median shelf life ranged from 5.27 hours to 165.35 hours. The researchers found that 15.5% of samples were culture-positive (n = 30); however, only 0.5% were positive for pathogenic microorganisms (n = 1). The researchers concluded that when processed and stored correctly, the endoscopes were safe to use for at least 120 hours.

Rejchrt et al[279] evaluated the bacterial load of gastroscopes, duodenoscopes, and colonoscopes stored in a dust-proof cabinet for five days. After clinical use, the endoscopes were cleaned at the point of use, manually cleaned, mechanically processed without an alcohol flush, sampled, and then stored hanging vertically in the cabinet. The researchers sampled the endoscopes for aerobic and anaerobic bacteria, including bacterial spores, and for *Candida* species after five days of storage. The results showed that all endoscopes were culture-negative after processing. A total of 135 samples were obtained after storage, four of which were positive for normal skin flora (*Corynebacterium pseudodiphteriae, S epidermidis*). Notably, these samples were taken from the external surface of the endoscopes. All of the samples from the internal channels of the endoscopes were negative.

In a second phase of the study, 10 endoscopes were mechanically processed and stored in a dust-proof cabinet for five days and then sampled. All 10 samples were culture-negative. The researchers concluded that when correctly processed and stored, flexible endoscopes were safe to use for up to five days without reprocessing.[279]

Riley et al[287] conducted a nonexperimental, simulated study to establish an acceptable duration of storage before reprocessing for flexible colonoscopes processed with a liquid chemical sterilant. The researchers artificially contaminated all channels of a colonoscope with *S aureus, P aeruginosa*, and *B subtilis*. The endoscope was manually cleaned, sampled, processed, and stored by hanging vertically in a ventilated endoscope storage cabinet. The endoscope was sampled five times after 24 hours of storage and five times after 168 hours of storage. The results showed no growth at 24 hours. At 168 hours, there was no bacterial growth on four of five occasions (80%) and sparse growth (< 5 CFU/mL) of two non-test organisms (ie, coagulase-negative *Staphylococcus* [skin flora], *Micrococcus* species [skin and environmental flora]). The researchers theorized that the presence of the organisms was not a result of inadequate processing but of contamination during testing procedures or storage. The researchers concluded that when correctly processed and stored, flexible endoscopes were safe to use for a period of seven days before reprocessing.

In a multiphase study to assess the microbiological load of endoscopes after HLD, Vergis et al[280] evaluated four duodenoscopes and three colonoscopes. In Phase 1, the endoscopes were sampled daily after HLD for a period of two weeks. This process was repeated in Phase 2. In Phase 3, the endoscopes were sampled daily after HLD for a period of seven days. The researchers found that in Phase 1, six of 70 samples (8.6%) were culture-positive. No cultures were positive in Phase 2. In Phase 3, one endoscope had a positive culture for *S epidermidis*, a low-virulence skin organism. The researchers concluded that with correct processing and storage, flexible endoscopes were safe to use for a period of at least seven days and possibly up to 14 days before reprocessing.

Brock et al[286] conducted a prospective, observational study to demonstrate whether flexible endoscopes were safe to use after storage for as long as 21 days before reprocessing. The researchers tested four duodenoscopes, two gastroscopes, and four colonoscopes. Immediately after use, the endoscopes were precleaned at the point of use, leak tested, manually cleaned, mechanically processed, flushed with alcohol, dried, sampled, and stored in a dust-free endoscope storage cabinet until removed for sampling at seven, 14, and 21 days. Notably, the cabinet was also used for storing endoscopes in active clinical use and was left open during the day but closed at night for security.

The results showed there were 33 positive cultures from 28 of the 96 sites tested, resulting in a 29.2% overall contamination rate. Of the culture-positive samples, 29 were typical skin or environmental contaminants, and thus clinically insignificant. Four potential pathogens were sampled that included *Enterococcus, C parapsilosis*, alpha-hemolytic *Streptococcus*, and *Aureobasidium pullulans*; however, the researchers theorized they were likely clinically insignificant as each was only recovered at one time point at one site and all grew in low concentrations. There were no true pathogenic isolates. The researchers concluded that correctly processed and stored flexible endoscopes were safe to use for a period of 21 days before reprocessing.[286]

Saliou and Baron[291] responded that the level of bacterial colonization in the study might have been underestimated by the researchers' use of sterile water for culture sampling. Brock et al[291] responded that the sampling methods they used were acceptable and were recommended by professional organizations such as ESGE, the CDC, and the Gastroenterological Society of Australia.

In a quasi-experimental study to examine bacterial growth in colonoscopes after various storage times, Ingram et al[282] sampled four new colonoscopes for anaerobic and aerobic bacteria after processing and after storage for three, five, seven, 14, 21, 28, 42, and 56 days. The colonoscopes were stored vertically in an open-air storage area. The results showed that none of the endoscopes were culture-positive after three, five, or seven days of storage. After 14 days of storage, one of the endoscopes had fewer than 2 CFU of *S epidermidis* and *Staphylococcus hominis*, both common skin flora. The only other microbial growth was ≤ 1 CFU of *S epidermidis* noted in one of the endoscopes after 42 days of storage. None of the endoscopes had bacterial growth at 56 days. The researchers concluded that when correctly processed and stored, the period of time for which flexible endoscopes were considered safe to use before reprocessing could be extended to 56 days; however, further research examining viral and fungal growth on stored endoscopes was warranted.

Schmelzer et al[292] conducted a systematic review to evaluate the evidence related to endoscope storage time and included 10 studies that measured the length of endoscope storage time and microbial growth. They concluded that flexible endoscopes were safe to use for a period of seven days before reprocessing; however, the acceptable length of storage was dependent on effective processing, thorough drying, controlled storage, and microbiological surveillance.

IX.h.1. The multidisciplinary team should establish a policy for removing and reprocessing the endoscope before use if the maximum storage time has been exceeded. *[5: Benefits Balanced with Harms]*

IX.i. Storage cabinets used for flexible endoscopes should be cleaned and disinfected with an EPA-registered hospital-grade disinfectant when visibly soiled and on a regular (eg, daily, weekly) basis.[13,15,16,65] *[2: High Evidence]*

Visible soil in the storage cabinet may contaminate endoscopes stored in the cabinet.[13] Areas and equipment that are not cleaned according to a schedule may be missed during routine cleaning procedures and become environmental reservoirs for dust, debris, and microorganisms.

IX.i.1. A multidisciplinary team that includes infection preventionists, endoscopy and perioperative RNs, endoscopy processing personnel, endoscopists, and other involved personnel should should establish a policy to determine the cleaning frequency of the storage cabinet. *[5: Benefits Balanced with Harms]*

Facilities with high volumes of endoscopy procedures will require more frequent cleaning of the storage cabinet.

IX.j. Sterilized items (eg, biopsy forceps) should be stored in a sterile storage area and in accordance with the AORN Guideline for Sterilization.[256] *[4: Limited Evidence]*

Limiting exposure to moisture, dust, or excessive handling decreases potential contamination of sterilized items.[77,256]

Recommendation X

The health care organization should maintain records of flexible endoscope processing and procedures.

Records provide data for the identification of trends and demonstration of compliance with regulatory requirements and accreditation agency standards.

Highly reliable data collection is necessary to demonstrate the health care organization's progress toward quality care outcomes.[293] Effective management and collection of health care information that accurately reflects the patient's care, treatment, and services is a regulatory requirement[294-297] and an accreditation agency standard for both hospitals[298,299] and ambulatory settings.[299-306]

X.a. Records related to flexible endoscope processing should include the
  ○ date[12,13,15,83] and time,[12,13,83]
  ○ identity of the endoscope and endoscope accessories,[12,13,15,20,83,84]
  ○ method and verification of cleaning and results of cleaning verification testing,[13,15,83,84]
  ○ number or identifier of the mechanical processor or sterilizer and results of process efficacy testing,[3,12,13,15,20,83,84]
  ○ identity of the person(s) performing the processing,[3,12,13,83]
  ○ lot numbers of processing solutions,[12,15]
  ○ disposition of defective items or equipment,[3] and
  ○ maintenance of water systems, endoscopes and endoscope accessories, and processing equipment.[3,12,15,83]
  [2: High Evidence]

Records of flexible endoscope processing enable traceability in the event of a processing failure.[13,20,69,77,84] Records of endoscopes, mechanical processors or sterilizers, and processing solutions provide a source of evidence for review during investigation of clinical issues, including infections and pseudo-infections.[44] Records of water systems, endoscopes and accessories, and processing equipment maintenance provide evidence of maintenance,[69] compliance with manufacturers' IFU, and information that may be useful in determining the need for repair or replacement. Records of repairs may help to identify trends in endoscopes and processing equipment damage and help to define practices that may reduce damage.

X.b. Records related to flexible endoscope procedures should include the
- date[3,12,15,84] and time,[3,12,84]
- identity of the patient,[3,12,13,15,20,44,84]
- procedure,[3,12,44,84]
- identity of the licensed independent practitioner performing the procedure,[12,84] and
- identity of the endoscope and endoscope accessories used during the procedure.[3,12,13,15,18,20,44,69,84]

[2: High Evidence]

Records of endoscopy procedures enable traceability in the event of a processing failure.[13,18,20,69,77,84]

X.c. Records should be maintained for a time period specified by the health care organization.[77]
[4: Limited Evidence]

Recommendation XI

Personnel with responsibility for processing flexible endoscopes should receive initial and ongoing education and complete competency verification activities related to processing flexible endoscopes.

Initial and ongoing education of endoscopy personnel facilitates the development of knowledge, skills, and attitudes that affect safe patient care. It is the responsibility of the health care organization to provide initial and ongoing education and to verify the competency of its personnel[307]; however, the primary responsibility for maintaining ongoing competency remains with the individual.[308]

Competency verification activities provide a mechanism for competency documentation and help verify that personnel processing flexible endoscopes and accessories understand the principles and processes necessary for effective processing and reducing the risk of infection from flexible endoscopes and mechanical processors.

Ongoing development of knowledge and skills and documentation of personnel participation is a regulatory requirement[294-297] and an accreditation agency standard for both hospitals[309,310] and ambulatory settings.[310-316]

XI.a. The health care organization should establish education and competency verification activities for its personnel and determine intervals for education and competency verification related to processing flexible endoscopes and accessories. *[4: Limited Evidence]*

Education and competency verification needs and intervals are unique to the facility and to its personnel and processes.

To determine whether deficiencies existed in the processing of contaminated flexible sigmoidoscopes in family practice and internal medicine offices and whether education of office personnel resulted in a correction of identified deficiencies, Jackson and Ball[317] conducted a prospective review of processing before and after an educational course. A total of 25 persons from 19 offices (ie, 14 family

practice, five internal medicine) attended one of three separate educational sessions. The course included both didactic and hands-on instruction. The instructor was a certified gastroenterology RN with infection prevention experience.

The researchers reviewed standards published by the SGNA, the Association for Professionals in Infection Control and Epidemiology (APIC), the ASGE, and the CDC, and selected 17 common standards as those most critical to effective endoscope processing. All of the participants completed a questionnaire based on the 17 standards before the course and again two months after the course. The researchers found that before the educational course, the 19 offices had between four and 11 deficiencies per office, with an average of 6.8 deficiencies per office. After the educational course, deficiencies ranged from zero to eight, with an average of 0.9 deficiencies per office. The researchers concluded that before the educational course, personnel from the family practice and internal medicine offices were insufficiently educated to perform flexible endoscope processing and that endoscopes were not being processed in accordance with standards. However, after the educational course, personnel processed the endoscopes according to the standards.

Lunn et al[318] reported their experience with endoscope repairs before and after implementing an educational program designed to improve handling of flexible endoscopes and equipment. The authors retrospectively reviewed the cost of endoscope repair in the three years preceding and in the five years following an educational program that included both didactic and hands-on components. The authors found that the cost of repairs during the three years before the educational program averaged $42 per procedure ($62.18 in 2015 US dollars). After the educational program, the repair costs dropped dramatically to $8 per procedure ($10.63 in 2015 US dollars). These reduced costs were realized despite an average 10% increase in the number of procedures being performed each year. The authors concluded that an educational program was effective in decreasing the costs of endoscope and equipment repairs.

XI.b. Education and competency verification activities related to processing flexible endoscopes and accessories should include
- controlling and maintaining an environment that supports processing actions[1,12,19,44];
- precleaning at the point of use[3,12,17,19,44,69,84,85];
- transporting[3,12,17,19,44,69,84,85];
- leak testing[3,12,17,19,44,69,84,85];
- manual cleaning[3,12,17,19,44,69,84,85];
- inspecting[3,12,17,19,44,69,84,85];
- HLD, liquid chemical sterilization, packaging and sterilization[3,12,17,19,44,69,84,85];
- storage[12];

- ○ maintaining records of processing and procedures for traceability[12]; and
- ○ quality assurance measures.[2,3]

[2: High Evidence]

Providing education and verifying competency helps reduce the risk of processing errors.[66]

XI.c.   Personnel should receive education and complete competency verification activities before new flexible endoscopes, accessories, cleaning and processing solutions, equipment, or procedures are introduced. *[5: Benefits Balanced with Harms]*

Receiving education and completing competency verification activities before new endoscopes, accessories, cleaning and processing solutions, equipment, or procedures are introduced helps ensure safe practices in the endoscopy suite.

Recommendation XII

Policies and procedures for processing flexible endoscopes should be developed, reviewed periodically, revised as necessary, and readily available in the practice setting in which they are used.

Policies and procedures assist in the development of patient safety, quality assessment, and performance improvement activities. Policies and procedures also serve as operational guidelines used to minimize patients' risk for injury or complications, standardize practice, direct personnel, and establish continuous performance improvement programs. Policies and procedures establish authority, responsibility, and accountability within the practice setting.

Having policies and procedures that guide and support patient care, treatment, and services is a regulatory requirement[294-297] and an accreditation agency standard for both hospitals[319,320] and ambulatory settings.[312,320-326]

XII.a.   Policies and procedures related to processing flexible endoscopes should address
- ○ controlling and maintaining an environment that supports processing actions[30];
- ○ precleaning at the point of use[12];
- ○ transporting[12];
- ○ leak testing[12];
- ○ manual cleaning[12];
- ○ inspecting[12];
- ○ HLD, liquid chemical sterilization, packaging, and sterilization[12];
- ○ storage[12];
- ○ maintaining records of processing and procedures for traceability[12]; and
- ○ quality assurance measures.[2,3]

[3: Moderate Evidence]

Effective processing of flexible endoscopes and accessories begins with clear and detailed policies and procedures.

XII.b.   The manufacturers' IFU should be readily available to and followed by the personnel responsible for processing flexible endoscopes. The manufacturer's IFU should be reviewed periodically, and processing practices should comply with the most current IFU. *[4: Limited Evidence]*

Instructions for use identify the validated processes necessary to achieve effective processing.[77] Manufacturers may make modifications to their IFU when new technology becomes available, when regulatory requirements change, or when modifications are made to a device.

XII.c.   Policies and procedures for managing loaned endoscopes, accessories, and equipment should be developed in accordance with the AORN Guideline for Cleaning and Care of Surgical Instruments.[58] *[4: Limited Evidence]*

The systematic management of loaned instrumentation reduces loss and helps ensure effective processing through increased collaboration, communication, and accountability.[58]

Recommendation XIII

The health care organization's quality management program should evaluate processing of flexible endoscopes.

Quality assurance and performance improvement programs can facilitate the identification of problem areas and assist personnel in evaluating and improving the quality of patient care and formulating plans for corrective action. These programs provide data that may be used to determine whether an individual organization is within benchmark goals, and if not, to identify areas that may require corrective action. A quality management program provides a mechanism to evaluate effectiveness of processes, compliance with manufacturer's IFU, endoscopy processing policies and procedures, and function of equipment.

Collecting data to monitor and improve patient care, treatment, and services is a regulatory requirement[294-297] and an accreditation agency standard for both hospitals[327-334] and ambulatory settings.[332-345]

XIII.a.   The quality assurance and performance improvement program for processing flexible endoscopes should include
- ○ periodically reviewing and evaluating processing activities to verify compliance or to identify the need for improvement,
- ○ identifying corrective actions directed toward improvement priorities, and
- ○ taking additional actions when improvement is not achieved or sustained.

[3: Moderate Evidence]

Reviewing and evaluating quality assurance and performance improvement activities may identify failure points that contribute to errors in processing flexible endoscopes and help define actions for improvement and increased competency.[85] Taking corrective actions may improve patient safety by enhancing understanding of the principles of and compliance with best practices for processing flexible endoscopes.

Evans[346] described a quality improvement initiative undertaken to improve processing of flexible cystoscopes following anecdotal reports of an increased incidence of urinary tract infections after cystoscopy procedures. The author first conducted a literature search to determine best practices for processing flexible cystoscopes. She reviewed the manufacturer's IFU to ensure cystoscopes were being processed in a manner consistent with the IFU, conducted a gap analysis to identify problematic areas, and developed a plan to address them. She then shadowed clinical personnel for two days and conducted interviews to ensure that personnel understood and adhered to best practices for effective processing. The author developed a process improvement tool to audit compliance, and provided remediation on an ongoing basis as needed. The quality improvement process was successful in improving processing of flexible cystoscopes and enhancing patient safety.

XIII.b. Personnel participating in endoscopy procedures or responsible for processing flexible endoscopes and accessories should participate in ongoing quality assurance and performance improvement activities related to processing flexible endoscopes by identifying processes that are important for
- monitoring quality,
- developing strategies for compliance,
- establishing benchmarks to evaluate quality indicators,
- collecting data related to the levels of performance and quality indicators,
- evaluating practice based on the cumulative data collected,
- taking action to improve compliance, and
- assessing the effectiveness of the actions taken.
[2: High Evidence]

Participating in ongoing quality assurance and performance improvement activities is a primary responsibility of endoscopy personnel engaged in practice.[307]

XIII.c. The health care organization should monitor compliance with the use of PPE in the endoscopy suite. *[3: Moderate Evidence]*

The collective evidence shows there are lapses in compliance with the use of PPE.[190,347,348]

In a survey commissioned by the Disinfection Management Committee of the Korean Society of Gastrointestinal Endoscopy, Park et al[190] assessed compliance of 100 nurses and nursing assistants from the endoscopy units of eight secondary or tertiary Korean hospitals with Korean national guidelines for processing flexible endoscopes. The researchers found that the activity with the lowest compliance was wearing protective eyewear, with only 32% of respondents

complying; 72% complied with wearing surgical masks, and 80% complied with wearing gloves. The researchers concluded that education combined with periodic surveillance could improve compliance.

Angtuaco et al[347] conducted a survey of 250 gastroenterologists and gastrointestinal endoscopy nurses from the American Board of Internal Medicine and the SGNA to determine and compare compliance with standard precautions and the use of PPE. A total of 77 gastroenterologists and 157 gastrointestinal endoscopy nurses responded to the survey. The results of the survey showed that
- 32% of the gastroenterologists (n = 25) and 50% of the nurses (n = 79) washed their hands before and after contact with patients.
- 5% of the gastroenterologists (n = 4) and 30% of the nurses (n = 47) wore gloves during patient contact.
- 14% of the gastroenterologists (n = 11) and 21% of the nurses (n = 33) wore face shields during procedures.
- 29% of the gastroenterologists (n = 22) and 46% of the nurses (n = 72) wore protective gowns during procedures.

When asked to provide an assessment of their own compliance with standard precautions and use of PPE, 45% of gastroenterologists (n = 35) and 60% of nurses (n = 94) reported that they always complied. The researchers concluded that compliance with standard precautions for both groups was low, but was greater for the nurses than for the gastroenterologists.[347]

In a survey of 300 randomly selected gastrointestinal endoscopy units in Spain to assess compliance with occupational risk prevention measures, Baudet et al[348] received responses from 196 units (65%). The researchers found that personnel in
- 19% of the units (n = 38) wore protective eyewear,
- 99% of the units (n = 195) wore gloves,
- 46% of the units (n = 90) wore masks, and
- 21% of the units (n = 42) wore protective gowns.

The researchers concluded that compliance with occupational risk prevention measures in Spain was lacking and improvement was needed.

XIII.d. A multidisciplinary team that includes facility engineers, endoscopy processing personnel, infection preventionists, and other involved personnel should establish a policy to determine processes for monitoring and auditing facility water quality to ensure compliance with requirements for endoscope processing as specified in the endoscope, processing equipment, and processing products manufacturers' IFU. Water quality and water filtration systems should be assessed at established intervals[119,213,214,216,247,349-358]

and after major maintenance to the water supply system.[359] *[1: Strong Evidence]*

Water quality varies seasonably and after water-source maintenance. Periodic testing can indicate whether the chemical combination used to condition the water used for endoscope processing requires adjusting.[119] Water-quality checks measure objective performance criteria (eg, pH, hardness) that have a direct effect on the outcomes.[119] The quality of the water is a consideration when determining the necessary level of filtration.[119,215,353,354,357,359-362] The need for repairs or modifications to the water treatment system can be identified from a water-quality check.[119] Monitoring water quality also assists in determining the performance of the filters and whether replacement is necessary.[353,356,358] Failing to regularly replace filters may result in bacterial growth on the filter and contamination of the water supply.[354,356] Contamination of the water supply may increase the patient's risk for infection. Monitoring water quality provides an opportunity for controlling exposure of the endoscope to waterborne contamination and subsequent exposure of patients to potential pathogens.[214,358,361,363]

Quality processes can be enhanced by audits that are conducted on a regular basis.[119,358,362] Regular monitoring and auditing of water quality may help prevent incidents related to contaminated water,[247,349,350,352,353,362,364] including infection[365] and pseudo-infection.[213-216,356,357,359,360]

Rossetti et al[357] reported 16 isolates of *Mycobacterium gordonae* from 267 patients undergoing bronchoscopy procedures. This finding was significant because in the previous seven years only one isolate of *M gordonae* was found among 1,368 patients. The investigators found there had been a failure in water filter replacement and water system maintenance. Replacement of the water filters and restoration of periodic assessment of water quality ended the pseudo-infections.

Rosengarten et al[215] reported a cluster of *Burkholderia cepacia* pseudo-infections associated with a contaminated mechanical processor in a bronchoscopy unit. Bronchoalveolar lavage samples obtained from three patients on three consecutive days grew organisms identified as *B cepacia* on culture; however, there were no clinical manifestations of infection in any of the patients. All of the patients had been examined with the same bronchoscope. Examination of the mechanical processor revealed that the 0.2-micrometer bacteria-retentive filter on the water supply line was missing, and this missing filter was the probable cause of the cluster of pseudo-infections. The mechanical processor was thoroughly cleaned and disinfected, and the missing filter was replaced. Subsequent samples were negative for *B cepacia*. The investigators concluded that a failure to follow the manufacturer's IFU by not installing the 0.2-micrometer filter had enabled bacteria to enter the mechanical processor and contaminate it and the bronchoscopes.

Chroneou et al[213] described a pseudo-outbreak of *M chelonae* in bronchoalveolar lavage fluid that was traced to a contaminated mechanical processor. The investigators obtained environmental samples from 17 different components of the processor, from the brushes used to clean the bronchoscopes, and from the utility water used to rinse the bronchoscopes. The investigators found the source of the outbreak was a filtration system malfunction that occurred because of a failure to change the water filters on schedule. It was not clear who had the responsibility for changing the filters at the scheduled time. Developing a process to ensure the water filters were changed on a monthly basis and assigning this responsibility to biomedical personnel eliminated the pseudo-outbreak strain.

XIII.e. A multidisciplinary team that includes facility engineers, endoscopy processing personnel, infection preventionists, and other involved personnel should collaborate with manufacturer service personnel to determine schedules for preventive maintenance of flexible endoscopes, mechanical processors, and other equipment (eg, the drying cabinet) used for processing flexible endoscopes. *[2: High Evidence]*

A regular program of preventative maintenance helps identify and mitigate potential risks.[22] Mechanical processors that are not maintained or functioning correctly may cause processing failures of flexible endoscopes and increase the risk for transmission of infection.[209,218,367] Schlenz and French[209] reported an outbreak of multidrug-resistant *P aeruginosa* infection involving 11 patients, eight of whom had undergone bronchoscopy procedures with two of three facility bronchoscopes that had been processed in a malfunctioning mechanical processor. There were no maintenance records, and no maintenance had been performed on the processor since its purchase one year previously. The tubing, filter, and pump system had to be replaced before the processor was free of *Pseudomonas* species. The bronchoscopes had likewise not been maintained and required replacement parts. The investigators concluded that regular, controlled, professional maintenance of mechanical processors and bronchoscopes was necessary for safe, effective processing of flexible endoscopes.

In a study to monitor the quality of gastrointestinal endoscope processing, Chiu et al[367] randomly sampled flexible endoscopes immediately after completion of mechanical processing. During the study, the researchers found that the endoscopes processed in one particular mechanical processor were culture-positive in spite of manual cleaning and mechanical processing. The service representative discovered that a relief valve from the mechanical processor was damaged and loose. After the valve was replaced, subsequent cultures were negative. The researchers recommended that mechanical processors undergo preventive maintenance at least every three to six months.

Méan et al[218] reported an incident involving 72 patients who underwent endoscopy procedures. The endoscopes used during the procedures were mechanically processed in a malfunctioning mechanical processor. The malfunction was reported by a nurse who became alarmed when the processor printed a validation ticket even though there was no cleaning solution in the mechanical processor. The processing failure was caused by a malfunction of the sensor whose function was to control the level of cleaning solution in the processor. An undetermined number of cleaning cycles had been skipped; however, the manual cleaning and HLD cycles were completed correctly. The investigators concluded that this incident highlighted the importance of regular preventive maintenance for mechanical processors.

Regular maintenance and replacement of endoscope lumens contaminated with biofilm may help to prevent transmission of infection.[368] In some cases, outbreaks of infection[136,217,365,369,370] and pseudo-infection[368] transmitted via flexible endoscopes were only stopped when the scope was sent to the manufacturer for repair and replacement of the lumen.[368]

DiazGranados et al[371] reported a cluster of 12 patients with respiratory cultures positive for P aeruginosa, 11 of whom had undergone bronchoscopy with the same bronchoscope. Processing procedures were reviewed by the infection prevention team and found to be acceptable. Despite appropriate processing, P aeruginosa was recovered from the bronchoscope. The investigators found that the bronchoscope had been in use for 16 months, and during that time, regular visual inspections and leak testing had been performed. The bronchoscope had been submitted to the manufacturer for repair three times but not for preventive maintenance, and the last repair was performed eight months before the pseudo-outbreak. The bronchoscope was sent to the manufacturer who found multiple defects including kinking of the forceps channel tube, damage to the bending section sheath cover, pinching of the insertion tube, and peeling of the light-guide tube coating. The investigators concluded that regular preventive maintenance inspections were necessary to prevent similar occurrences.

Corne et al[368] investigated an outbreak of P aeruginosa infections (n = 9) and pseudo-infections (n = 7). Inspection of the internal channels of the involved bronchoscopes revealed large surface defects in the internal channels. The researchers theorized the defects were caused by biopsy forceps. The breaches in the internal channels prevented effective cleaning and processing of the endoscopes even though processing personnel adhered to the manufacturer's IFU. The outbreaks were controlled when the manufacturer replaced the inner channels of the bronchoscopes and the facility began using single-use biopsy forceps. The investigators concluded that the outbreaks emphasized the need to establish maintenance procedures for detecting damage to the internal channels of flexible bronchoscopes.

Qiu et al[369] investigated a duodenoscope that was manually cleaned and mechanically processed multiple times but continued to be culture-positive for P aeruginosa. The duodenoscope was sent to the manufacturer, who replaced the internal lumens of the device. Thereafter, the duodenoscope was culture-negative.

Zweigner et al[217] reported an outbreak of carbapenem-resistant K pneumoniae involving eight patients. A review of the processing procedures did not identify any deviations from the manufacturer's IFU. The outbreak ended when the bronchoscopes associated with the infections (n = 2) were submitted to the manufacturer who found defects in the internal channels of both endoscopes. The investigators concluded that the outbreak underlined the importance of regular preventive maintenance for flexible endoscopes.

In a CDC Epidemic Intelligence Service[370] investigation to review a duodenoscope-associated cluster of carbapenem-resistant Bacteriaceae infections in which no breaches in processing or device defects were identified to explain transmission, the investigators returned all duodenoscopes with positive cultures (n = 8) to the manufacturer for assessment. Only one duodenoscope was returned because it was not functioning correctly. The remaining seven duodenoscopes were returned as part of the investigation and had no obvious defects or functional issues. They had undergone and passed leak tests after each use and were functioning without any noticeable problems.

The manufacturer identified critical repair issues in all eight duodenoscopes that included cracks, leak test failures, frayed bending sections, and other issues related to biopsy forceps passage (eg, breaches in the biopsy channel). Notably, there was no preventive maintenance schedule recommended by the manufacturer. The investigators concluded that the lack of preventive maintenance was concerning. A process for the manufacturer to regularly inspect and service duodenoscopes was established that included random selection of duodenoscopes that were then sent to the manufacturer at predetermined intervals.[370]

Damage may occur with repetitive use of endoscopes that suggests a need for limiting the duration a reusable device is used.[372] Lee et al[372] conducted a quasi-experimental study to compare differences in surface alterations between not-aged and simulated-aged samples of endoscope materials. The researchers inoculated the samples with *E coli, P aeruginosa,* and *Mycobacterium terrae* artificial test soil, and then exposed the endoscope materials to identical processing conditions. The researchers found significantly more abrasions, cracks, and holes in the aged samples. They concluded that surface alterations on the samples of the endoscope material increased during repetitive use and processing. The possibility of accumulation of microorganisms and organic substances increased accordingly, and this also increased the risk of infection transmission.

XIII.e.1. The schedule for preventive maintenance should align with the manufacturer's IFU.[13,21,58,366] *[2: High Evidence]*

XIII.e.2. The frequency of preventive maintenance should be based on variables that are unique to the facility.[366] *[2: High Evidence]*

Variables unique to the facility, such as the type of endoscopes that are used, the amount of use of the endoscopes, the type of damage that occurs to the endoscope, the thoroughness of the cleaning processes, the implements that are used to clean the endoscopes, the type of water used in the facility, and other factors may affect the need to increase or decrease the frequency of preventative maintenance.

XIII.e.3. Mechanical processors should be tested for performance on installation; at regular, established intervals (eg, daily, weekly); after major repairs; and after changes in programmed parameters (eg, temperature, cycle time).[21,58] *[2: High Evidence]*

Testing the function of mechanical processors confirms the equipment is operating correctly. Effective processing is dependent on correctly functioning equipment.

XIII.e.4. Preventive maintenance should be performed by qualified individuals.[21,22,85] *[4: Limited Evidence]*

Preventive maintenance requires special skills and knowledge that includes systematic inspection, testing, measurement, adjustment, detection, parts replacement, and correction of device or equipment malfunction either before it occurs or before it develops into major failure. Having qualified personnel perform preventive maintenance increases the probability that repair and service will be performed correctly.[58]

XIII.f. Manual cleaning of flexible endoscopes should be verified using cleaning verification tests when new endoscopes are purchased and at established intervals (eg, after each use, daily). *[3: Moderate Evidence]*

The collective evidence shows that manual cleaning is a learned skill subject to human error.[373] Cleaning verification tests are used to verify the ability of the cleaning process to remove, or reduce to an acceptable level, the organic soil and microbial contamination that occurs during use of a reusable device.[77,374] Cleaning verification tests include adenosine triphosphate (ATP) and chemical reagent tests for detecting clinically relevant soils (eg, protein, carbohydrate). Periodic verification of cleaning effectiveness may help reduce errors in manual cleaning and improve effectiveness.[90,183,373] No single method of cleaning verification has been established as a standard for assessing the outcome of endoscope processing.[45]

Efficacy of cleaning has traditionally been evaluated visually; however, visual inspection alone, even with magnification, is not sufficient to determine cleanliness of complex devices such as flexible endoscopes.[12,90,374,375] Visual inspection is subjective. Infectious microorganisms are not visible to the naked eye. It is also not possible to visually inspect the lumens of flexible endoscopes.[12,90,374] Residual soil may remain and prevent effective subsequent HLD or sterilization.[375]

There is a need for rapid testing methods to detect residual soil and verify the adequacy of manual cleaning.[376] Although no studies have been conducted linking clinical outcomes with using monitors for cleaning verification,[377] auditing the manual cleaning of flexible endoscopes provides an objective method for verifying cleanliness and helps ensure that insufficiently cleaned flexible endoscopes are recleaned before HLD or sterilization.[90,183,377,378]

Alfa et al[252] conducted a quasi-experimental study to determine the type and amount of soil found in various types of flexible endoscopes before and after cleaning. The researchers' intent was that the determination of expected soil levels would help establish parameters for worst-case soil cleaning efficacy benchmarks. The researchers assessed suction channels from 10 bronchoscopes, 10 duodenoscopes, and 10 colonoscopes immediately after use for levels of bilirubin, hemoglobin, protein, sodium ion, carbohydrate, endotoxin, and viable bacteria. An additional set of endoscope suction channels (ie, 10 bronchoscopes, 10 duodenoscopes, 10 colonoscopes) were evaluated for the same components after manual cleaning but before mechanical processing for subsequent clinical use. The researchers found the worst-case soil levels in the suction channels were

○ protein: 115 µg/cm^2,

- sodium ion: 7.4 micromole/cm²,
- hemoglobin: 85 µg/cm²,
- bilirubin: 299 nanomole/cm²,
- carbohydrate: 29.1 µg/cm²,
- endotoxin: 9852 EU/cm², and
- bacteria: 7.1-log10 CFU/cm².

After cleaning, the levels of protein, endotoxin, and sodium ion were reduced five- to tenfold. Carbohydrate and bilirubin were reduced to undetectable levels. The average load of viable bacteria was reduced from between 3-log$_{10}$ to 5-log$_{10}$ CFU/cm². Residual hemoglobin was only detectable in bronchoscopes. The researchers concluded the data demonstrated that cleaning reduced or eliminated many components of organic soil, but a substantial amount of viable bacteria and protein may still remain on the endoscope.[252]

In a study to evaluate contamination of patient-used endoscopes using visual inspection and rapid cleaning verification tests and to determine which testing instruments and methods could be used for quality improvement initiatives related to flexible endoscope processing, Visrodia et al[375] sampled endoscopes used for gastrointestinal procedures after precleaning at the point of use and after manual cleaning. During 37 examinations of 12 endoscopes, the researchers visually inspected 121 endoscope components and conducted 249 rapid cleaning verification tests. The researchers found that regardless of whether there was visible soil on the endoscope after precleaning at the point of use, all endoscopes had high levels of ATP and detectable blood or protein. Although there was no visible soil on any of the endoscopes after manual cleaning, 82% had at least one positive cleaning verification test. The researchers concluded that relying solely on visual inspection after manual cleaning and before HLD was insufficient to ensure processing effectiveness. The researchers theorized that using more than one cleaning verification testing method may be necessary to ensure contamination is consistently detected before endoscopes are processed and used on patients.

In a quasi-experimental study to determine whether colonoscope and gastroscope contamination that occurred during clinical use persisted despite processing in accordance with US guidelines, Ofstead et al[379] performed microbiological cultures and rapid cleaning verification tests for ATP, protein, hemoglobin, and carbohydrate residue during 60 examinations of 15 endoscopes (ie, two new and 13 patient-used [ie, seven colonoscopes, six esophagogastroduodenoscopes without elevator channels]). Benchmarks were set at ATP < 200 relative light units (RLU), protein 120 µg/ml, carbohydrate 210 µg/ml, and hemoglobin 0.25 µg/ml. The researchers assessed endoscope contamination immediately after point-of-use precleaning, manual cleaning, HLD, and overnight storage. The researchers found that

- after point-of-use precleaning, 13 of 13 endoscopes (100%) had detectable protein, hemoglobin, and ATP, and 12 of 13 (92%) harbored viable microorganisms.
- after manual cleaning, 12 of 13 endoscopes (92%) had protein or ATP exceeding the benchmarks and six endoscopes (46%) had at least one positive culture.
- after HLD, eight of 11 endoscopes (73%) were positive for contamination exceeding benchmarks, and viable microorganisms were found on seven endoscopes (64%).
- after overnight storage, nine of 11 endoscopes (82%) were positive, and one of 11 (9%) harbored microorganisms.

Viable microorganisms were recovered from patient-ready endoscopes after all processing steps including HLD. The researchers concluded that despite processing in accordance with US guidelines, viable microorganisms persisted on patient-used flexible endoscopes, and this suggested that current guidelines might not be sufficient to ensure successful processing. The results of the study also suggested that rapid cleaning verification tests were valid and reliable and that it might be beneficial to test for both protein and ATP because one was often present without the other. Assessing the efficacy of manual cleaning using rapid cleaning verification tests allowed processing personnel to be immediately informed when test results exceeded established benchmarks. Endoscopes could then be recleaned before HLD or sterilization.[379]

Hansen et al[380] compared ATP testing with microbiological culturing by examining 108 flexible endoscopes (ie, 40 gastroscopes, eight duodenoscopes, 42 bronchoscopes, 18 colonoscopes) after processing. Benchmarks for positive ATP were set at < 30 RLU and < 100 RLU based on the manufacturer's IFU. The researchers considered all microbiological growth to be positive, regardless of the species or number of CFU. The researchers found that 26% of the endoscopes had bacterial growth (n = 28 [ie, nine gastroscopes, one duodenoscope, 13 bronchoscopes, five colonoscopes]). Using < 30 RLU as the benchmark, 62% of the endoscopes were positive for ATP (n = 67 [ie, 25 gastroscopes, six duodenoscopes, 24 bronchoscopes, 12 colonoscopes]). Using < 100 RLU as the benchmark, 19% were positive for ATP (n = 21; [ie, seven gastroscopes, one duodenoscope, eight bronchoscopes, five colonoscopes]). The researchers concluded that it was beneficial to implement ATP testing as a method to identify ineffective cleaning of flexible endoscopes and the need for recleaning before HLD or sterilization.

XIII.f.1. A multidisciplinary team that includes infection preventionists, endoscopists, endoscopy processing personnel, and other involved individuals should establish the type of cleaning verification test to be performed. *[2: High Evidence]*

There are a number of tests that can be used to assess cleaning efficacy.[90,373,378,381] Chemical tests involve the use of a reagent and observing for a color change that indicates the presence of organic markers such as protein or blood.[90,373,381]

In a dual phase (ie, simulated-use, in-use) study to validate the use of an audit tool composed of reagent test strips in 43 endoscopy clinics across Canada, Alfa et al[381] collected samples from 30 patient-used endoscopes (ie, 10 colonoscopes, 10 duodenoscopes, 10 gastroscopes) and tested them for residual protein, carbohydrate, and hemoglobin using the audit tool test strips. The test strips had three reagent pads designed to rapidly detect organic residuals of protein, carbohydrate, and hemoglobin after manual cleaning. The researchers confirmed that the audit tool flagged endoscopes with residual protein, hemoglobin, or carbohydrate.[373] In the second phase of the study, the researchers sent prototype testing kits to 44 endoscopy clinics in 23 health care facilities across Canada and conducted a survey to obtain feedback from processing personnel using a 5-point analog rating scale. The results of the survey showed that processing personnel valued the audit tool and thought it was important for confirming the adequacy of manual cleaning. Respondents also thought the test was easy to use, that it should be used on some endoscopes daily, and that it should be part of the quality assurance program for the endoscopy unit.[381]

Quantitative tests provide a measurement against which cleaning results can be compared.[90] Adenosine triphosphate bioluminescence is an example of a quantitative test.[378] The item to be tested is swabbed to collect ATP, the swab is inserted into a reaction tube, and the ATP on the swab reacts with the chemicals in the reaction tube.[58] The reaction tube is then inserted into a hand-held luminometer that converts the ATP released from microorganisms or human cells into a light signal, which is measured in RLU.[58]

Obee et al[374] conducted a nonexperimental study to compare the efficacy of endoscope processing using microbiological surveillance and ATP bioluminescence. Following visual observation of manual cleaning, the researchers sampled eight different areas on 63 gastrointestinal endoscopes (N = 504) before, during, and after processing. The benchmarks for positive results were set at ATP > 500 RLU and microbiological culture ≥ 3 CFU/sample. The researchers found that a total of 32 cultures (6.3%) and 95 ATP tests (18.8%) were positive; however, after processing, only three cultures (0.6%) and one ATP test (0.2%) were positive. The researchers concluded that ATP provided a rapid means of assessing the efficacy of manual cleaning before HLD.

In a prospective study carried out in a gastrohepatology unit to evaluate using ATP bioluminescence to verify manual cleaning of flexible endoscopes, Fernando et al[382] obtained samples from the lumens of endoscopes and tested the endoscopes using ATP in 120 endoscopic procedures. The samples were obtained before the procedure, after the procedure, after manual cleaning, and after mechanical processing. The ATP benchmark was set at < 100 RLU. If the after-processing benchmark was exceeded, the endoscope was reprocessed and retested. The researchers found the average RLU reading before the procedure was 48 RLU. After the procedure, the average reading was 124,052 RLU. After manual cleaning the average reading was 1,423 RLU, and after mechanical processing, the average reading was 144 RLU. The corresponding culture results before the procedure were all negative. After the procedure, only four cultures were negative. After manual cleaning, 26 cultures were negative, and after mechanical processing, all cultures were negative. Twenty-one (18%) of the post-mechanical processing cultures were initially positive; however, after reprocessing, the cultures were negative. The researchers concluded that ATP testing had the potential to play an important role in verifying that flexible endoscopes had been effectively processed and were safe to use. They posited that because the results were available so rapidly, the test could be easily performed before every procedure.

In a nonexperimental study to evaluate ATP, microbial load, and protein as potential indicators of gastrointestinal endoscope cleanliness, Fushimi et al[383] sampled exterior surfaces and interior suction/accessory channels of 12 endoscopes used in 41 patients. The researchers found that before cleaning, the ATP levels were 10,417 RLU from the exterior surfaces and 30,281 RLU from the channels. After cleaning, these values decreased to 82 RLU and 104 RLU, respectively. Before cleaning, the microbial load was 5,143 CFU/sample exterior and 95,827 CFU/sample channels. After cleaning, the microbial load was 1 CFU/sample exterior and 104 CFU/sample channels. Before cleaning, the protein level was 36 μg/sample channels; after cleaning, the level was 20 µg/sample. There was a significant change in ATP and microbial load; however, the decrease in protein levels was not significant. The researchers concluded that ATP measurement provided a reliable, rapid, and practical assessment of endoscope cleanliness for routine monitoring in the clinical setting.

In a quasi-experimental, three-phase study, Sciortino et al[384] investigated and evaluated the use of a portable luminometer system for detecting contamination after cleaning and HLD of flexible endoscopes. In Phase 1, the researchers conducted a microbiological analysis of 15 endoscopes (ie, five processed, one cleaned, nine contaminated). The researchers found that the five processed endoscopes were culture-negative. The other 10 endoscopes were culture-positive. Notably, the internal channel of one of the culture-positive endoscopes was visibly contaminated with feces, yet had been cleaned but not disinfected for patient use.

In Phase 2, the researchers examined 31 endoscopes and tested them before cleaning, after cleaning, after HLD, and after storage at one- to two-week intervals. The researchers found that of the 31 endoscopes tested, eight (25.8%) were sterile (0 RLU; < 1 CFU), 12 (38.7%) were clean (< 5,000 RLU; < 50 CFU), and 11 (35.5%) were contaminated (> 5,000 RLU; > 50 CFU).[384]

In Phase 3, the researchers tested 63 endoscopes that had been processed and stored for reuse. The results showed that none of the endoscopes were sterile, 10 (15.9%) were clean, and 53 (84.1%) were contaminated.[384]

The researchers found that the storage room was moist and humid, and there was an open window 16 ft from the storage cabinet. The researchers observed there were disadvantages of ATP testing that included a lack of specificity for certain pathogenic microorganisms. In addition, the swab did not reach into crevices and could not be used deep inside internal channels without potential damage to the endoscope. Regardless, the researchers concluded that application of the ATP test was beneficial because it enabled monitoring of processing problems that could be addressed and immediately corrected.[384]

In response to a study by Visrodia et al[375] that supported the use of rapid cleaning verification tests, Whiteley et al[385] criticized ATP systems because of the lack of correlation between ATP and specific pathogens of concern and because of the measurement variability between commercially branded devices. In reply, Visrodia et al[386] countered

that their research[375] had shown that flexible endoscopes with and without visually apparent organic soil had high levels of blood, protein, and ATP. The intent of their study was to identify methods for rapidly evaluating the effectiveness of manual cleaning in the clinical setting. The ATP testing system provided a numerical result reflecting the amount of ATP present, and these data can assist in quality monitoring of flexible endoscope processing and help ensure the adequacy of manual cleaning before mechanical processing.

There are quantitative tests that can be used for cleaning verification testing of other residual soils, including

- protein,
- carbohydrate,
- hemoglobin,
- endotoxin,
- lipid,
- sodium ion,
- bioburden, and
- total organic carbon.[90]

Quantitative testing can be used as part of a quality monitoring program to observe for trends and to monitor performance of a manual or a mechanical process.[58] Readings that trend lower indicate effective cleaning, whereas readings that trend higher may indicate a need for improved manual cleaning processes.[58] Further research is warranted.

XIII.f.2. The multidisciplinary team should establish the benchmarks for the cleaning verification tests to be performed. *[2: High Evidence]*

Standards for clinically significant levels of residual soil remaining after cleaning are lacking,[90] and this lack of widely accepted residual soil benchmarks has limited the implementation of rapid cleaning verification testing.[373,377,378,387]

Manufacturers may establish quantitative benchmarks for cleaning verification tests to measure manual cleaning of flexible endoscopes.[58] Endoscopes not meeting this reference point after manual cleaning require recleaning before HLD or sterilization.[58] However, variability has been identified as a concern in the use of hand-held ATP monitors, and this variability is greatest at the boundary between acceptable and unacceptable cleanliness verification.[388] Variability may also lead to poor repeatability.[388] The RLU reading scale has not been quantified against a known standard and therefore cannot be calibrated, diminishing interbrand compatibility.[388] An additional concern is the risk for random error, which may be undetectable in single monitoring samples.[388]

FLEXIBLE ENDOSCOPES

Whiteley et al[388] investigated the reliability of ATP bioluminometers and documented precision and variability measurements using known and quantitative standard methods. The researchers subjected four commercially branded ATP bioluminometers to known quantities of various bacteria in suspension cultures. The researchers found that the variability of commercial ATP bioluminometers was unacceptably high. They concluded that the advantages of the ATP rapid response test were undermined by the imprecision of the instrument.

However, studies have demonstrated the adequacy of an ATP benchmark of < 200 RLU for ATP[252,378,387] for both manual[387] and pump-assisted manual cleaning.[389] In a simulated-use, quasi-experimental study to validate the use of ATP for monitoring manual cleaning of flexible endoscopes, Alfa et al[387] contaminated all channels of a duodenoscope with artificial test soil containing 106 CFU of *P aeruginosa* and *E faecalis*. Residual levels of ATP, protein, hemoglogin, and bioburden were calculated from an uncleaned, partially cleaned, and fully cleaned duodenoscope. The benchmarks for clean were set at ATP < 200 RLU, protein < 6.4mg/cm², hemoglobin < 2.2 mg/cm², and bioburden < 4-$\log_{10}$ CFU/cm². The researchers found that the benchmarks for protein, hemoglobin, and bioburden were met if ATP < 200 RLU was achieved. The researchers concluded that effectively cleaned flexible endoscopes would have < 200 RLU of ATP.

In a quasi-experimental study to determine whether the published benchmarks[252,378,387] for protein (< 6.4 µg/cm²), bioburden (< 4-$\log_{10}$ CFU/cm²), and ATP (< 200 RLU) were relevant for pump-assisted manual cleaning, Alfa et al[389] sampled the suction biopsy channel of patient-used endoscopes after precleaning at the point of use (ie, 10 colonoscopes, 10 duodenoscopes, 10 gastroscopes) and after pump-assisted manual cleaning (ie, 20 colonoscopes, 20 duodenoscopes, 20 gastroscopes) and then tested them for protein, bioburden, and ATP levels. The researchers found that after pump-assisted manual cleaning, 25% of gastroscopes (n = 5) exceeded the ATP benchmark, whereas all duodenoscopes (n = 20) and colonoscopes (n = 20) were below the benchmark level. The protein and bioburden residuals were also consistently lower than existing benchmarks after pump-assisted cleaning. The researchers concluded that the benchmark for protein could be lowered to < 2 µg/cm², and the benchmark for bioburden could be lowered to < 2-$\log_{10}$ CFU/cm², for pump-assisted

manual cleaning; however, the ATP benchmark of < 200 RLU was still adequate.

XIII.f.3. The multidisciplinary team should evaluate the need to implement protocols for cleaning verification testing of flexible duodenoscopes with elevator channels. *[2: High Evidence]*

Duodenoscopes with elevator channels pose a particular challenge for cleaning because of the design of the intricate distal end that provides access to the pancreatic and bile ducts. Even in cases where processing personnel performed all required processing steps, multidrug-resistant microorganisms have been transmitted to patients via flexible endoscopes, resulting in colonization, infection, or death.[137,170,171]

Alfa et al[378] conducted a quasi-experimental study to verify that the ATP benchmark of < 200 RLU was achievable in a busy endoscopy clinic. The researchers sampled all channels from patient-used colonoscopes (n = 20) and duodenoscopes (n = 20) after manual cleaning and tested them for residual ATP. Benchmarks for achieving adequate cleaning were set at ATP < 200 RLU, protein < 6.4 µg/cm², and bioburden < 4-$\log_{10}$ CFU/cm². The researchers found that 96% (115 of 120) of manually cleaned endoscopes met the ATP benchmark of < 200 RLU. All 120 endoscopes tested had protein and bioburden levels lower than the benchmark levels. The researchers recommended the use of ATP testing after manual cleaning as an audit tool to confirm adequacy of cleaning. Notably, the five endoscopes that exceeded benchmark levels were duodenoscopes with elevator channels. The researchers suggested these data indicated that the elevator channel required additional monitoring to verify cleaning adequacy.

Bommarito et al[390] tested three types of flexible endoscopes (ie, 30 duodenoscopes, 116 gastroscopes, 129 colonoscopes) with ATP at five different hospitals, and determined the number of cleaning failures using < 200 RLU as the benchmark. The researchers observed that the failure rates in the manual cleaning step was highest for duodenoscopes (33%; n = 10) and gastroscopes (24%; n = 28), and lowest for colonoscopes (3%; n = 4). The researchers suggested that a more rigorous protocol was needed for manual cleaning of upper gastrointestinal endoscopes, and cleaning verification testing helped ensure cleaning effectiveness.

XIII.g. A multidisciplinary team that includes infection preventionists, endoscopists, endoscopy processing personnel, microbiologists, laboratory personnel, risk managers, and other involved individuals should evaluate the need to implement a

STERILIZATION AND DISINFECTION

862

program for regular microbiologic surveillance cultures of flexible endoscopes and mechanical processors. *[2: High Evidence]*

The collective evidence regarding the need for routine microbiological surveillance cultures is inconclusive. Routine microbiological surveillance culturing of flexible endoscopes after processing, during storage, or before use has not been advised in current US guidelines. The CDC,[45] APIC,[1] and the "Multisociety guideline on reprocessing flexible endoscopes"[44] representing ASGE, the Society for Healthcare Epidemiology of America (SHEA), AORN, and APIC do not recommend routine microbiologic sampling of flexible endoscopes except when focused microbiologic testing is indicated as a result of clinical or epidemiologic findings that suggest endoscopy-related transmission of infection.

A program of regular microbiological surveillance culturing of flexible endoscopes and mechanical processors is advised in the processing guidelines of several international organizations, including the combined Gastroenterological Society of Australia (GESA), Gastroenterological Nurses College of Australia (GENCA), and Australian Gastrointestinal Endoscopy Association (AGEA)[15] the combined ESGE and European Society of Gastroenterology and Endoscopy Nurses and Associates (ESGENA) committee,[391] and the Steering Group for Flexible Endoscope Cleaning and Disinfection (SFERD).[21] However, there are variances among the recommendations.

Routine surveillance microbiological culturing is supported in the literature as an effective method for monitoring the effectiveness and quality of processing, reinforcing best practices, evaluating the effectiveness of corrective interventions, and detecting endoscopes requiring service.[93,183,281,367,392-400]

Chiu et al[401] assessed the effectiveness of mechanical processing of double-balloon enteroscopes by collecting and analyzing samples before and after processing of oral and anal route enteroscopes. Before processing, the positive culture rate was 83.9% (26 of 31) for the oral route enteroscopes, and 100% (26 of 26) for the anal route enteroscopes. After processing, the positive culture rate was 12.9% (four of 31) for the oral route enteroscopes, and 19.2% (five of 26) for the anal route enteroscopes. The researchers concluded that surveillance culture monitoring was an effective method for assessing the effectiveness of HLD of double-balloon enteroscopes.

In a nonexperimental study to evaluate the quality of gastrointestinal endoscope processing and the advantages of microbiological culture surveillance of flexible endoscopes, Saviuc et al[393] conducted a retrospective analysis of the results of endoscope sampling performed from

October 1, 2006, to December, 31, 2014, in a gastrointestinal unit of a French teaching hospital equipped with 89 flexible endoscopes and three mechanical processors. The compliance rate was defined as the proportion of results that met target (< 5 CFU and absence of indicator microorganisms) and alert (≤ 5 to ≤ 25 CFU and absence of indicator microorganisms). Indicator microorganisms included *Enterobacteriaceae, Pseudomonas, S maltophilia, S aureus, Acinetobacter,* and *Candida.* A total of 846 samples were taken, and the researchers found the overall compliance rate was 86% (n = 728). A total of 14% (n = 118) samples carried indicator microorganisms. The researchers concluded that microbiological surveillance was indispensable for monitoring processing, reinforcing good practices, and detecting endoscopes in need of service.

Bisset et al[402] monitored patient-ready endoscopes during an 80-week period to determine the efficacy of decontamination procedures in a busy endoscopy center. The researchers sampled the internal surface of the endoscopes from 1,376 upper gastrointestinal procedures and 987 lower gastrointestinal procedures after mechanical processing. The researchers found that both gastroscopes (1.8%; n = 25) and colonoscopes (1.9%; n = 19) were equally likely to grow bacteria, with all numbers of bacteria < 10 organisms/mL. A change in procedure to processing endoscopes with the buttons attached to the endoscope resulted in a cluster of culture-positive results. No clinically untoward consequences were observed, but the researchers concluded that cultures after changes in protocols were necessary to confirm that the change in protocol did not alter processing effectiveness.

Routine microbiological surveillance may also help to identify the source of contamination and rectify processing methods to prevent transmission of infection.[367,394,398,400] Tunuguntla and Sullivan[394] performed 300 cultures at three- to six-month intervals on 12 flexible endoscopes between 1994 and 2003. In 1995, they found that all but two endoscopes were culture-positive for *Pseudomonas* species ranging from 1,000 CFU/mL to 7,000 CFU/mL. The culture-positive endoscopes were reprocessed and recultured, but again were culture-positive for *Pseudomonas* with CFU ranging from 20,000 CFU/mL to 75,000 CFU/mL. The authors then investigated the water source and mechanical processors and found that one of the processors was culture-positive for 50,000 CFU/mL of *Pseudomonas* due to a contaminated water source. The contaminated mechanical processor was replaced and the water source was changed, resulting in negative cultures. The authors theorized that these deficiencies in processing might have led to patient infection and would not have been detected except for routine culture surveillance.

Microbiological sampling of rinse water used during mechanical processing may reduce the risk of patient infection or pseudo-infection from waterborne bacteria.[247]

In a literature review to determine the need for microbiological culturing of rinse water used in mechanical processors, Muscarella[247] discussed the regulatory requirement[403,404] and recommendations[45,77,256] for validating the sterilization process using biological indicators to ensure that conditions for sterilization have been achieved and the similar need for verifying that utility water passed through water filtration systems, such as those connected to mechanical processors used for flexible endoscopes, is cultured. The filtered water used to rinse the endoscope may be labeled "sterile" or "bacteria free"; however, there is no way to know whether the rinse water actually meets this claim if it is not routinely sampled. Routine sampling of the rinse water may also provide information about the effectiveness of the water filtration system.

Endoscopes are complex devices. There may be debris and bacterial growth in inaccessible portions of the endoscope. Viruses such as hepatitis B and C and HIV cannot be cultured using standard methods.[138] Commonly used disinfectants may inhibit cultures. There may be false-positive results from contaminated equipment or skin. A negative culture does not guarantee that the scope has been adequately processed. Surveillance cultures of processed endoscopes have not been validated by correlating viable counts on an endoscope with infection after an endoscopic procedure.[44,45] Notably, the false-positive rate, the false-negative rate, and the limits of detection also have not been established.[138] The sensitivity of routine cultures may be unreliable for detecting the organisms associated with outbreaks.

Between May and November 2013, three patients at a Wisconsin medical center were identified as having NDM-1 carbapenem-resistant E coli after undergoing ERCP procedures with the same duodenoscope. Smith et al[174] observed the endoscope processing procedures and found no lapses. The investigators obtained three cultures from the duodenoscope: one sonication culture, one brush culture with the elevator channel open, and one brush culture with the elevator channel closed. Despite these measures, the duodenoscope was culture-negative; however, the evidence was sufficiently strong to implicate the duodenoscope as the mode of transmission. The investigators concluded that it was questionable whether routine surveillance cultures would have led to an earlier identification of endoscope colonization since the NDM-1-producing E coli was not able to be isolated from the implicated duodenoscope.

Kola et al[146] reported an outbreak of CRKP in a German university hospital associated with a contaminated duodenoscope. Between December 2012 and January 2013, CRKP was cultured from 12 patients staying on four different wards. Molecular typing confirmed the close relation between all 12 isolates. Six of the patients were from the same ward; they were immediately transferred to separate rooms and placed on contact precautions. The remaining six patients had all undergone ERCP procedures using the same duodenoscope. Culturing of the duodenoscope did not recover CRKP. The investigators reviewed processing procedures for the duodenoscope and could find no deviations from the manufacturer's IFU; however, they did obtain positive cultures for Enterococci, which they suggested was indicative of insufficient cleaning. The investigators concluded that although culturing of the duodenoscope did not recover CRKP, it did not exclude it as the vehicle of transmission. They theorized that flushing the channels with normal saline may not have been sensitive enough to reveal the contamination, particularly after the endoscope had been processed several times before sampling, as it was in this case.

Fraser et al[405] conducted a case-control study following an outbreak of multidrug-resistant P aeruginosa sepsis in five patients who underwent ERCP procedures with the same duodenoscope. The endoscope, which was on loan from the manufacturer, had been processed and cultured with negative results one month earlier before being put into clinical use. The investigators concluded that the organism that caused the outbreak had most likely been transmitted from patient to patient by the loaned endoscope. In an attempt to prevent such an outbreak, endoscopes at the facility had been cultured quarterly before the outbreak; however, the outbreak occurred despite a negative surveillance culture of the implicated endoscope. The investigators suggested that routine cultures were not helpful in preventing the outbreak and were therefore of no benefit. They theorized that the endoscopist's awareness of the potential for opportunistic infection following ERCP procedures was more valuable than routine endoscope surveillance cultures.

The use of surveillance cultures is confounded by the delay in feedback and the frequent isolation of nonpathogenic organisms resulting from environmental contamination.[44,93] The need to quarantine flexible endoscopes until the culture results have been obtained may not allow for rapid reuse of the tested endoscope and could also lead to delays in patient care.[138]

Microbiological culturing is resource-intensive, and requires additional expenditures for microbiological testing and time for personnel to collect and process samples.[138,367,406] Culturing for bacterial load is impractical for many endoscopy centers that may not have access to microbiology laboratories.[138] Implementing a recommendation for routine surveillance cultures may require that some facilities outsource culture testing to qualified microbiologists. This could be quite costly, and it might also be difficult for facilities to find a laboratory that is willing to perform the necessary culture testing. Outsourcing surveillance culturing to environmental or contract laboratories may also lead to uncertainty in interpretation of results.[138]

Gillespie et al[407] conducted a review of microbiological testing conducted between January 1, 2002, and December 31, 2006, at two health campuses in Southern Australia in which, together, more than 3,500 endoscopic procedures were performed annually. Bronchoscopes, duodenoscopes, and mechanical processors were microbiologically sampled every four weeks. Gastroscopes and colonoscopes were cultured every three months. Positive cultures were investigated and followed up by the endoscopy and infection prevention teams. Costs for processing team members to sample the endoscopes were calculated at weekend pay rates because the samples were obtained outside of normal operating hours. Time to sample was calculated at 22 minutes per sample and $10.54 ($AUD 15) per hour. During the five-year period, 2,374 microbiological tests were undertaken. The annual cost of microbiological testing was $14,109.55 ($AUD 20,080). The total cost of testing over five years was $70,547.75 ($AUD 100,400). In 2015, this would equate to a sampling cost of $12.53 ($AUD 17.83) per hour, an annual cost of $83,885.55 ($AUD 119,369.14), and a five-year cost of $419,427.75 ($AUD 596,845.70).

XIII.g.1. The multidisciplinary team should establish the methods and frequencies for microbiological surveillance culturing of flexible endoscopes and mechanical processors. *[2: High Evidence]*

Standards for performing microbiological cultures, including the frequency of testing and the interpretation of results have not been determined.[44,45,93,183,367,399] A protocol for culturing and a sampling method has not yet been validated.[93,399] Different techniques may be required for different portions of the endoscope. For example, a swab-rinse technique may be recommended for sampling exterior surfaces and the distal opening of the suction/biopsy channel port.[93] A flush/brush/flush technique with rinsing through the channels using a sterile fluid and sterile cleaning brush to obtain samples through the biopsy port may be recommended for sampling the interior surface of the endoscope channels.[93] A flush technique may be recommended when brushing the channel lumens is not possible.[93]

Anterograde sampling, where the last-rinse water from the endoscope is collected inside the mechanical processor at the distal end of the endoscope, or retrograde sampling, where the suction/biopsy channel and the air/water channel are each manually flushed with sterile fluid from the distal to the proximal end, may be recommended.[93] Collection of microbiological samples requires the use of sterile technique and this may be difficult when culturing a long, flexible instrument.[407] It may be necessary to have more than one person perform the collection to prevent contamination. Developing effective standardized procedures for obtaining the cultures, as well as the actions to be implemented based on the results of the cultures, is challenging.

In a five-year (ie, February 2006 to January 2011) prospective quasi-experimental study to assess the effectiveness of HLD by comparing cultured samples from biopsy channels of gastrointestinal endoscopes and the internal surfaces of mechanical processors, Chiu et al[392] collected rinse samples from 420 biopsy channels (ie, 300 gastroscopes, 120 colonoscopes) and swab samples from mechanical processors and examined them for the presence of aerobic and anaerobic bacteria and mycobacteria. The researchers found the number of culture-positive samples obtained from the biopsy channels (13.6%; 57 of 420) was significantly higher than that obtained from the mechanical processors (1.7%; seven of 420). In addition, the number of culture-positive samples obtained from the biopsy channels of gastroscopes (10.7%; 32 of 300) and colonoscopes (20.8%; 25 of 120) was significantly higher than those obtained from the mechanical processors used for HLD of gastroscopes (2.0%; six of 300) and the mechanical processors used for HLD of colonoscopes (0.8%; one of 120).

The researchers concluded that culturing rinse samples from biopsy channels provided a better indication of the effectiveness of HLD of gastrointestinal endoscopes than culturing swab samples from the inner surfaces of mechanical processors. They recommended using rinse samples for performing regular surveillance monitoring of flexible endoscopes. Lu et al[408] described the same study but concluded that swab culturing was also a useful method for monitoring the contamination level of the mechanical processor and the effectiveness of the HLD process.[392]

Because of a severe outbreak of *K pneumoniae* producing extended-spectrum ß-lactamase that occurred in 16 patients undergoing ERCP procedures in a hospital in France between December 2008 and August 2009, Aumeran et al[55] observed duodenoscope processing procedures. They found that the duodenoscopes were not fully dried before they were stored. The investigators hypothesized that bacteria was introduced into the channels of the duodenoscope during the procedures, and despite repeated cleaning and disinfection, the contamination persisted because the moisture remaining in the endoscope channels created conditions favorable to the persistence and growth of the involved organism. The infection was transmitted to 12 patients. Surveillance cultures of the endoscopes were repeatedly negative during the outbreak, but the epidemic strain was finally isolated by flushing and brushing the duodenoscope channels.

In an expert opinion piece, Muscarella[409] discussed the limitations of surveillance culturing demonstrated by the Aumeran report[55] and the false-negative result that erroneously confirmed the endoscope was safe for patient use. Only when the sampling technique was modified to include brushing of the endoscope's suction channel in addition to flushing it was the effectiveness of sampling sufficient to culture the outbreak strain. Recovery of bacteria from a sampled channel confirms that the sampling technique effectively recovered microorganisms from the endoscope (ie, a true positive result), whereas non-recovery does not necessarily confirm effective processing.

Recommendations regarding the frequency of surveillance conflict. The ESGE-ESGENA[391] recommends periodic microbiological surveillance of endoscopes, mechanical processors, and the water used in endoscopy concurrently, at intervals no greater than three months.[44] The GESA and the GENCA[15] recommend sampling of mechanical processors, duodenoscopes, bronchoscopes, and ultrasound instruments at four-week intervals, and sampling of all other gastrointestinal endoscopes at three-month intervals. The SFERD[21] recommends microbial testing of water following installation of mechanical processors or water treatment systems, and additionally recommends quarterly testing and testing following incidents or after process-altering repairs. The SFERD recommends annual microbiological culturing of endoscopes and mechanical processors as well as supplemental culturing of loaned endoscopes and culturing of endoscopes and mechanical processors following repair, outbreak, or

when deemed necessary by supervisory personnel.

XIII.g.2. The multidisciplinary team should establish benchmarks for microbial levels in flexible endoscope channels and mechanical processors. *[3: Moderate Evidence]*

Correlations with patients' clinical outcomes is preferred for validation of benchmarks for microbial levels in flexible endoscope channels; however, this type of validation is difficult to perform. The introduction of low-virulence microorganisms to the gastrointestinal tract does not necessarily mean that the patient will have clinical symptoms or develop an infection. In a non-experimental study to define a realistic benchmark for residual microbial levels that could be achieved 99% of the time in a routine clinical setting, Alfa et al[285] tested all channels of 20 flexible gastrointestinal endoscopes (ie, five gastroscopes, nine colonoscopes, six duodenoscopes) used at an endoscopy clinic. The endoscopes were sampled for the presence of bacteria and fungi every Monday morning during a seven-month period. Bacteria and fungi were detected in 5.7% (n = 22) of the 383 channels tested. Of the 141 endoscopes tested, 14.1% (n = 20) had detectable microbial growth in at least one channel. The samples from only two channels grew > 100 CFU/mL of bacteria. The researchers recommended that < 100 CFU/mL be used as a clinically relevant benchmark for the number of bacteria detected from processed endoscopes.

XIII.g.3. The multidisciplinary team should evaluate the need to implement a program for regular microbiological culturing of duodenoscopes.[138] *[3: Moderate Evidence]*

Routine or periodic surveillance culturing may help to assess the adequacy of duodenoscope processing and identify duodenoscopes with persistent contamination despite processing in accordance with the manufacturer's IFU.[138,410]

The ECRI recommends performing baseline cultures on all duodenoscope channels and elevator mechanisms using a media specific for carbapenem-resistant *Enterobacteriaceae* followed by regular surveillance culturing for carbapenem-resistant *Enterobacteriaceae* as well as quarantining cultured duodenoscopes until negative results are received. The ECRI further recommends that if current resources will not allow for culturing each duodenoscope after each use, weekly culturing may be considered. If cultures are positive, the ECRI recommends reprocessing and repeat culturing, and if the repeat culture is positive, permanently removing the endoscope from service or sending it back to the manufacturer for additional assessment.[411]

The CDC has provided interim guidance for performing culture surveillance for bacterial contamination of duodenoscopes or other endoscopes that have an elevator mechanism (eg, endoscopic ultrasound) after processing.[410,412,413] The CDC guidance is intended to supplement and not replace or modify manufacturer recommended processing procedures.[410] The interim protocol provided by the CDC may change as new information becomes available.[410]

XIII.g.4. Duodenoscopes with positive cultures of ≤ 10 CFU of low-concern organisms should be considered in the context of typical culture results at the facility.[410] *[3: Moderate Evidence]*

Small numbers (< 10 CFU) of low-concern organisms (ie, organisms less often associated with disease and potentially a result of contamination of cultures during collection), such as coagulase-negative staphylococci (excluding *Staphylococcus lugdunensis, Bacillus* species, and diptheroids) might occasionally be detected. Levels of low-concern organisms can vary depending on the processing procedures in the facility.[410]

XIII.g.5. Duodenoscopes with positive cultures of any quantity of high-concern organisms should be taken out of service and corrective actions initiated that may include
- quarantining the duodenoscope, reprocessing it, and repeating post-processing cultures until it is culture-negative[410];
- reviewing the manufacturer's IFU to ensure compliance with processing procedures[410];
- notifying infection prevention and other relevant personnel to initiate corrective actions, as necessary[410];
- following the manufacturer's IFU for having the duodenoscope evaluated for defects[410]; or
- reviewing positive cultures among affected patients to determine whether other clusters of pathogens could have been transmitted.[410]

[3: Moderate Evidence]

Positive cultures of organisms of high concern (ie, organisms more often associated with disease), such as gram-negative bacteria (eg, *E coli, K pneumoniae, Enterobacteriaceae, P aeruginosa*), *S aureus*, and *Enterococcus* necessitate corrective actions.[410]

XIII.g.6. If a cluster of suspected or confirmed endoscopy-related infections is identified, the infection preventionist should initiate an investigation in consultation with a health care epidemiologist and the multidisciplinary team.[3,12,17] *[3: Moderate Evidence]*

Initiating an investigation helps determine possible routes of infection and end further transmission.

Weber and Rutala[416] proposed a 15-step sequential approach to assist health care facilities in evaluating and managing potential failures of processing semicritical and critical items that includes
1. confirming failure of processing;
2. immediately removing from service any potentially incorrectly processed semicritical or critical item;
3. not using a questionable mechanical processor until correct functioning has been restored;
4. informing key stakeholders;
5. conducting a thorough evaluation to determine the cause of the processing failure;
6. preparing a list of potentially exposed patients;
7. assessing whether the processing failure increased the patients' risk for infection;
8. informing an expanded list of stakeholders of the processing failure;
9. developing a hypothesis for the processing failure and initiating corrective action;
10. developing a method to assess potential adverse patient events;
11. considering notifying appropriate state and federal authorities;
12. considering patient notification;
13. if patients are notified, considering whether they require medical evaluation for possible postexposure therapy with anti-infectives or additional follow-up to detect infection and offering it, if warranted;
14. developing a detailed plan to prevent similar failures in the future; and
15. performing an after-action report.

The reader can refer to the ASGE guideline for reprocessing failure[414] and other relevant documents[66,223,224,415-417] for additional guidance.

XIII.g.7. If a breach in protocol for endoscope processing is recognized, the infection preventionist, epidemiologist, and multidisciplinary team should perform an assessment and investigation to determine whether patient notification is required, and if so, how patients will be notified and followed.[17,78] *[3: Moderate Evidence]*

Health care facilities have an ethical obligation to inform affected patients in a timely manner when a significant breach in processing occurs.[414] Prompt notification allows patients to take precautions to minimize the risk of transmitting the infection to others and allows for early serologic testing.[414] Where a breach in processing has been determined to pose a negligible patient risk, health care providers have to consider the ethical issue of a patient's right to know compared with the potential for causing unnecessary patient distress in a situation where the risk for infection may be very small.[414-416] Reporting a processing-related outbreak may also cause patients to avoid potential life-saving endoscopic procedures because of an unwarranted fear of infection.[414]

XIII.h. Adverse events should be reported and documented according to the health care organization's policy and procedure and should be reviewed for potential opportunities for improvement. [5: Benefits Balanced with Harms]

Reports of adverse events and near misses can be used to identify actions that may prevent similar occurrences and reveal opportunities for improvement.

XIII.h.1. Near misses (ie, unplanned events that do not result in injury) should be investigated and corrective action taken to prevent serious adverse events. [5: Benefits Balanced with Harms]

XIII.h.2. Reports regarding device malfunction leading to serious injury or death should be submitted to MedWatch: The FDA Safety Information and Adverse Event Reporting Program.[418] [5: Benefits Balanced with Harms]

The FDA uses medical device reports to monitor device performance, detect potential device-related safety issues, and contribute to risk-benefit assessments of suspected device-associated deaths, serious injuries, or malfunction. The MAUDE (ie, Manufacturer and User Facility Device Experience) database houses reports submitted to the FDA by mandatory reporters (ie, manufacturers, importers, device user facilities) and voluntary reporters (ie, health care professionals, patients, consumers).[418]

Mandatory reporters are required to submit reports when they become aware of information that reasonably suggests that one of their marketed devices may have caused or contributed to a death or serious injury or has malfunctioned and that the malfunction of the device would be likely to cause or contribute to a death or serious injury if the malfunction were to recur.[418] Voluntary reporters are required to submit reports when they become aware of information that reasonably suggests a device may have caused or contributed to a death or serious injury of a patient.[418]

Editor's note: *Teflon is a registered trademark of the Chemours Co, Wilmington, DE.*

Glossary

Adenosine triphosphate (ATP): A substance present in all living cells that provides energy for many metabolic processes and is involved in making ribonucleic acid.

Adsorb: The adhesion by gases, solutes, or liquids in an extremely thin layer of molecules to the surfaces of solid bodies or liquids with which they come in contact.

Analog rating scale: An instrument for measuring subjective phenomena in which a subject selects from a gradient of alternatives arranged in linear fashion.

Bacteriophage: A virus that lives within a bacterium, replicating itself and eventually destroying the bacterial cell.

Benchmark: A standard or point of reference against which things may be compared or measured.

Bioburden: The degree of microbial load; the number of viable organisms contaminating an object.

Biofilm: A thin layer of microorganisms adhering to the surface of a structure, which may be organic or inorganic, together with the polysaccharides that they secrete.

Biohazard: A biological or chemical substance that is dangerous to human beings and the environment.

Borescope: A device used to inspect the inside of an instrument through a small opening or lumen of the instrument.

Colonic mucosal pseudolipomatosis: A rare, benign complication of a colonoscopy involving a characteristic white, slightly elevated lesion usually preceded by an effervescent release of molecular oxygen.

Colony-forming unit: A measure of the number of viable bacterial cells in a sample.

Coved wall base: Molding or trim used to create a curved transition from the wall to the floor.

Critical water: Water that is extensively treated to remove microorganisms and other materials.

Decontamination: The process of removing pathogenic microorganisms from objects so they are safe to handle, use, or discard.

Decontamination sink: A sink located in the decontamination room or endoscopy processing room that is used for endoscope processing tasks, such as leak testing, cleaning, and rinsing of flexible endoscopes and other reusable items.

Drying cabinet: A medical device designed for storage of flexible endoscopes that circulates continuous filtered air through each endoscope channel and within the cabinet.

Endoscopy suite: A facility or unit within a facility designed for care of the patient undergoing procedures requiring the use of an endoscope. The suite includes waiting rooms, offices, lounges, endoscopy procedure rooms, other patient care areas, and endoscopy processing rooms.

Endotoxin: A toxic substance present in the outer membrane of gram-negative bacteria that is released from the cell when it disintegrates.

Enzymes: Proteins that act as catalysts to bring about specific biochemical reactions.

Hand washing station: An area that includes a sink, a hands-free faucet, cleansing solutions, and a means for drying the hands.

High-concern organisms: Organisms often associated with disease, such as gram-negative bacteria (eg, *Escherichia coli, Klebsiella pneumoniae, Enterobacteriaceae, Pseudomonas aeruginosa*), *Staphylococcus aureus,* and *Enterococcus.* Positive cultures of organisms of high concern require corrective action.

High-level disinfectant: A germicide that inactivates all microbial pathogens, except bacterial endospores.

High-level disinfection: Processes that kill all microbial pathogens, but not necessarily all bacterial spores.

Hypochlorites: Oxidizing agents composed of chlorine and oxygen.

Infection control risk assessment: A documented process to proactively identify and plan safe design elements, including consideration of long-range infection prevention; identify and plan for internal and external building areas and sites that will be affected during construction/renovation; identify potential risk for transmission of airborne and waterborne biological contaminants during construction and/or renovation and commissioning; and develop infection control risk mitigation recommendations to be considered.

Instrument air: A medical gas that falls under the general requirements for medical gases as defined by the *NFPA 99: Health Care Facilities Code,* is not respired, is compliant with the *ANSI/ISA S-7.0.01: Quality Standard for Instrument Air,* and is filtered to 0.01 micron, free of liquids and hydrocarbon vapors, and dry to a dew point of -40° F (-40° C).

Intermediate-level disinfection: A process that destroys all vegetative bacteria, including tubercle bacilli, lipid and some nonlipid viruses, and fungi, but not bacterial spores.

Liquid chemical sterilant: A chemical that has been validated to provide microbial kill adequate to obtain clearance by the US Food and Drug Administration for a sterilization label claim.

Log reduction: A 10-fold reduction in the number of live bacteria. A 1-log reduction would reduce 100 bacteria to 10.

Low-concern organisms: Organisms less often associated with disease and potentially a result of contamination of cultures during collection, such as coagulase-negative staphylococci. Levels of low-concern organisms can vary depending on the processing procedures in the facility.

Mechanical processor: A device that mechanically cleans, rinses, and exposes flexible endoscopes and accessories to a high-level disinfectant or liquid chemical sterilant.

Minimum efficiency reporting value (MERV): A measure of the effectiveness of air filters on a rating scale of 1 to 16. The higher the MERV rating, the more effective the filter.

Monolithic: A single-piece surface with no seams or joints unless the surface joints are chemically or heat welded.

Patient care area: An area used for the provision of patient care (eg, monitoring, evaluation, treatments).

pH: A numeric scale used to specify the acidity or alkalinity of an aqueous solution. Solutions with a pH lower than 7 (ie, the pH of water) are acidic and solutions with a pH higher than 7 are alkaline or basic.

Phenolics: Germicides derived from carbolic acid.

Plaque-forming unit: A measure of the number of particles capable of forming plaques per unit volume, such as virus particles.

Polysaccharide: A carbohydrate consisting of bonded sugar molecules.

Prions: A unique class of infectious proteins that cause fatal neurological diseases and are resistant to disinfection and sterilization.

Procedure room: A room designated for the performance of procedures that do not require a restricted environment but may require the use of sterile instruments or supplies.

Processing room: A room dedicated to cleaning, decontaminating, inspecting, and preparing surgical instruments and other medical devices (eg, flexible endoscopes) for high-level disinfection or sterilization.

Pseudo-infection: Laboratory evidence of the presence of pathogenic microorganisms in the absence of infection.

Pseudo-outbreak: An episode of false increased disease incidence due to enhanced surveillance (eg, microbiological culturing) or other factors (eg, laboratory contamination, false positive test).

Quaternary ammonium compounds: Disinfectants derived from ammonium in which the nitrogen atom is attached to four organic groups.

Reagent: A substance that is used to test for the presence of another substance by causing a chemical reaction.

Shelf life: The period of time during which a stored product remains effective, useful, or suitable for use.

Skin antiseptics: Products with antimicrobial activity that are applied to the skin to reduce the number of microbial flora.

Sterility assurance level (SAL): The probability of a single viable microorganism remaining on an item after sterilization. An SAL of 10-6 means there is less than or equal to one chance in 1 million that a single viable microorganism is present on a sterilized item.

Sterilization: Processes by which all microbial life, including pathogenic and nonpathogenic microorganisms and spores, are killed.

Surfactant: A substance that reduces the surface tension of a liquid in which it is dissolved.

Surgical attire: Nonsterile apparel designated for the perioperative practice setting that includes two-piece pantsuits, scrub dresses, cover jackets, head coverings, shoes, masks, and protective eyewear.

Transmissible spongiform encephalopathies (TSEs): Fatal prion diseases that affect the brain and nervous system. The development of tiny holes in the brain causes it to appear like a sponge, hence the term *spongiform.*

Use life: The defined period for safe use of a product after the container is opened.

Utility water: Water obtained directly from a faucet that has not been purified, distilled, or otherwise treated. Synonym: tap water

STERILIZATION AND DISINFECTION

869

FLEXIBLE ENDOSCOPES

Validation: Confirmation by examination and provision of objective evidence, performed by the manufacturer, that the particular requirements for a specific intended use can be consistently fulfilled.

Variant Creutzfeldt-Jakob Disease (vCJD): A fatal degenerative neurological disease caused by a prion. The human form of bovine spongiform encephalopathy (ie, mad cow disease).

REFERENCES

1. Alvarado CJ, Reichelderfer M. APIC guideline for infection prevention and control in flexible endoscopy. Association for Professionals in Infection Control. *Am J Infect Control.* 2000;28(2):138-155. [IVB]

2. Infections associated with reprocessed flexible bronchoscopes: FDA safety communication. US Food and Drug Administration. http://www.fda.gov/MedicalDevices/Safety/AlertsandNotices/ucm462949.htm. Accessed December 9, 2015. [VA]

3. Preventing cross-contamination in endoscope processing: FDA safety communication. US Food and Drug Administration. http://www.fda.gov/MedicalDevices/Safety/AlertsandNotices/ucm190273.htm. Accessed December 9, 2015. [VB]

4. Gastmeier P, Vonberg RP. *Klebsiella* spp. in endoscopy-associated infections: we may only be seeing the tip of the iceberg. *Infection.* 2014;42(1):15-21. [VA]

5. Kampf B, Makowski T, Weiss H, et al. ESGE newsletter. Definition of "endoscope families" as used in EN ISO 15883-4. *Endoscopy.* 2013;45(2):156-157. [VB]

6. Design of endoscopic retrograde cholangiopancreatography (ERCP) duodenoscopes may impede effective cleaning: FDA safety communication. US Food and Drug Administration. http://www.fda.gov/MedicalDevices/Safety/AlertsandNotices/ucm434871.htm. Accessed December 9, 2015. [VA]

7. Boylu U, Oommen M, Thomas R, Lee BR. In vitro comparison of a disposable flexible ureteroscope and conventional flexible ureteroscopes. *J Urol.* 2009;182(5):2347-2351. [IIIB]

8. Piepho T, Werner C, Noppens RR. Evaluation of the novel, single-use, flexible aScope for tracheal intubation in the simulated difficult airway and first clinical experiences. *Anaesthesia.* 2010;65(8):820-825. [VB]

9. Pujol E, Lopez AM, Valero R. Use of the Ambu® aScope in 10 patients with predicted difficult intubation. *Anaesthesia.* 2010;65(10):1037-1040. [VB]

10. Tvede MF, Kristensen MS, Nyhus-Andreasen M. A cost analysis of reusable and disposable flexible optical scopes for intubation. *Acta Anaesthesiol Scand.* 2012;56(5):577-584. [VB]

11. *Guidelines for Design and Construction of Hospitals and Outpatient Facilities.* Chicago, IL: Facility Guidelines Institute; 2014. [IVC]

12. *ANSI/AAMI ST91:2015 Flexible and Semi-rigid Endoscope Processing in Health Care Facilities.* Arlington, VA: Association for the Advancement of Medical Instrumentation; 2015. [IVC]

13. Health Service Executive Advisory Group. *HSE Standards and Recommended Practices for Endoscope Reprocessing Units.* Tipperary, Ireland: HSE; 2012. [IVB]

14. CLARIFICATION: requirements for an endoscopy equipment processing room. *Jt Comm Perspect.* 2012;32(3):13-14. [VA]

15. *Infection Control in Endoscopy.* 3rd ed. Victoria, Australia: Gastroenterological Society of Australia and the Gastroenterological Nurses College of Australia; 2010. [IVB]

16. *Standards of Infection Prevention in Reprocessing Flexible Gastrointestinal Endoscopes.* Chicago, IL: Society of Gastroenterology Nurses and Associates, Inc; 2016. https://www.sgna.org/Portals/0/Standards%20for%20reprocessing%20endoscopes_FINAL.pdf. Accessed October, 27, 2016. [IVB]

17. Hookey L, Armstrong D, Enns R, Matlow A, Singh H, Love J. Summary of guidelines for infection prevention and control for flexible gastrointestinal endoscopy. *Can J Gastroenterol.* 2013;27(6):347-350. [VA]

18. Du Rand IA, Blaikley J, Booton R, et al. British Thoracic Society guideline for diagnostic flexible bronchoscopy in adults. *Thorax.* 2013;68(Suppl 1):i1-i44. [IVA]

19. World Gastroenterology Organisation/World Endoscopy Organization. *Endoscope Disinfection—A Resource-Sensitive Approach.* World Endoscopy Organisation. http://www.worldendo.org/assets/downloads/pdf/guidelines/wgo_weo_endoscope_disinfection.pdf. Accessed December 9, 2015. [IVC]

20. Guidance on decontamination of equipment for gastrointestinal endoscopy. 2014. British Society of Gastroenterology. http://www.bsg.org.uk/clinical-guidance/general/guidelines-for-decontamination-of-equipment-for-gastrointestinal-endoscopy.html. Accessed December 9, 2015. [IVA]

21. *Professional Standard Handbook Cleaning and Disinfection Flexible Endoscopes.* Version 3.1 ed. The Netherlands: Steering Group for Flexible Endoscope Cleaning and Disinfection; 2014. [IVB]

22. Beilenhoff U, Neumann CS, Rey JF, et al. ESGE-ESGENA Guideline: cleaning and disinfection in gastrointestinal endoscopy. *Endoscopy.* 2008;40(11):939-957. [IVC]

23. Formal Interpretations: *Guidelines for Design and Construction of Hospitals and Outpatient Facilities,* 2014. Facility Guidelines Institute. http://fgiguidelines.org/pdfs/FGI-interps_2014Guidelines_141222.pdf. Accessed December 9, 2015. [VA]

24. Choice Framework for local Policy and Procedures 01-06—Decontamination of flexible endoscopes: Policy and management. 2013. UK Department of Health. https://www.gov.uk/government/uploads/system/uploads/attachment_data/file/192522/Decontamination_of_flexible_endoscopes.pdf. Accessed December 9, 2015. [IVB]

25. Choice Framework for local Policy and Procedures 01-06—Decontamination of flexible endoscopes: Design and installation. 2013. UK Department of Health. https://www.gov.uk/government/uploads/system/uploads/attachment_data/file/148560/CFPP_01-06_Design_and_installation_Final.pdf. Accessed December 9, 2015. [IVB]

26. Burlingame BL. Airflow in endoscope cleaning rooms [Clinical Issues]. *AORN J.* 2013;98(5):541-542. [VA]

27. Mehta AC, Prakash UBS, Garland R, et al. American College of Chest Physicians and American Association for Bronchoscopy Concensus Statement: Prevention of flexible bronchoscopy-associated infection. *Chest.* 2005;128(3):1742-1755. [IVC]

28. Hota S, Hirji Z, Stockton K, et al. Outbreak of multidrug-resistant *Pseudomonas aeruginosa* colonization and infection secondary to imperfect intensive care unit room design. *Infect Control Hosp Epidemiol.* 2009;30(1):25-33. [VB]

29. Siegel JD, Rhinehart E, Jackson M, Chiarello L; Healthcare Infection Control Practices Advisory Committee. 2007 Guideline for Isolation Precautions: Preventing Transmission of Infectious Agents in Healthcare Settings. *Am J Infect Control.* 2007;35(10 Suppl 2):S65-S164. [IVA]

STERILIZATION AND DISINFECTION

30. ASGE Ensuring Safety in the Gastrointestinal Endoscopy Unit Task Force; Calderwood AH, Chapman FJ, et al. Guidelines for safety in the gastrointestinal endoscopy unit. *Gastrointest Endosc.* 2014;79(3):363-372. [IVB]

31. Overview of health care HVAC systems. In: *HVAC Design Manual for Hospitals and Clinics.* 2nd ed. Atlanta, GA: American Society of Heating, Refrigerating and Air-Conditioning Engineers; 2013. [IVC]

32. Guideline for a safe environment of care, part 2. In: *Guidelines for Perioperative Practice.* Denver, CO: AORN, Inc; 2015:265-290. [IVA] 33. Table 7.1: Design parameters. In: *ANSI/ASHRAE/ASHE 170-2013: Ventilation of Health Care Facilities.* Atlanta, GA: American Society of Heating, Refrigerating and Air-Conditioning Engineers; 2013. [IVC]

34. *Interpretation IC 170-2013-4 of ANSI/ASHRAE/ASHE Standard 170-2013 Ventilation of Health Care Facilities.* Atlanta, GA: American Society of Heating, Refrigerating and Air-Conditioning Engineers; January 27, 2015. [IVC]

35. Guideline for prevention of transmissible infections. In: *Guidelines for Perioperative Practice.* Denver, CO: AORN, Inc; 2015:419-454. [IVA]

36. Tan HL, Lo PLC, Eng CTP. Bronchoscopy during SARS: perspectives from a non-SARS designated hospital. *J Bronchol.* 2006;13(4):223-225. [VB]

37. Occupational Safety and Health Act of 1970 (Public Law 91-596, December 29, 1970, as amended through January 1, 2004). Occupational Safety and Health Administration. https://www.osha.gov/pls/oshaweb/owadisp.show_document?p_table=OSHACT&p_id=2743. Accessed December 9, 2015.

38. 29 CFR 1910.1200: Hazard Communication. 2011. Occupational Safety and Health Administration. https://www.osha.gov/pls/oshaweb/owadisp.show_document?p_table=standards&p_id=10099. Accessed December 9, 2015.

39. *Industrial Ventilation: A Manual of Recommended Practice for Design.* Cincinnati, OH: ACGIH; 2013. [IVC]

40. *ANSI/AAMI ST58: Chemical Sterilization and High-level Disinfection in Health Care Facilities.* Arlington, VA: Association for the Advancement of Medical Instrumentation; 2013. [IVC]

41. *ANSI/AAMI ST41: Ethylene Oxide Sterilization in Health Care Facilities: Safety and Effectiveness.* Arlington, VA: Association for the Advancement of Medical Instrumentation; 2012. [IVC]

42. Guideline for a safe environment of care, part 1. In: *Guidelines for Perioperative Practice.* Denver, CO: AORN, Inc; 2015:239-264. [IVA]

43. Guideline for high-level disinfection. In: *Guidelines for Perioperative Practice.* Denver, CO: AORN, Inc; 2015:601-614. [IVB]

44. ASGE Quality Assurance In Endoscopy Committee; Petersen BT, Chennat J, et al. Multisociety guideline on reprocessing flexible gastrointestinal endoscopes: 2011. *Gastrointest Endosc.* 2011;73(6):1075-1084. [IVA]

45. Rutala WA. Weber DJ; the Healthcare Infection Control Practices Advisory Committee (HICPAC). *Guideline for Disinfection and Sterilization in Healthcare Facilities, 2008.* Atlanta, GA: Centers for Disease Control and Prevention; 2008. [IVA]

46. SGNA Practice Committee 2013-14. Guideline for use of high-level disinfectants and sterilants for reprocessing flexible gastrointestinal endoscopes. *Gastroenterol Nurs.* 2015;38(1):70-80. [IVB]

47. *ANSI/IESNA RP-29-06: Lighting for Hospitals and Health Care Facilities.* RP-29-06 ed. New York, NY: Illuminating Engineering Society of North America; 2006. [IVC]

48. 29 CFR §1910.1030: Bloodborne Pathogens. Occupational Safety and Health Administration. http://www.osha.gov/pls/oshaweb/owadisp.show_document?p_table=STANDARDS&p_id=10051. Accessed December 9, 2015.

49. Silva CV, Magalhaes VD, Pereira CR, Kawagoe JY, Ikura C, Ganc AJ. Pseudo-outbreak of *Pseudomonas aeruginosa* and *Serratia marcescens* related to bronchoscopes. *Infect Control Hosp Epidemiol.* 2003;24(3):195-197. [VC]

50. *NFPA 99: Health Care Facilities Code Handbook.* Quincy, MA: National Fire Protection Association; 2015. [IVC]

51. *ANSI/ISA S7.0.01-1996 Quality Standard Instrument Air.* Research Triangle Park, NC: Instrument Society of America; 1996. [IVC]

52. 29 CFR 1910.151: Medical and First Aid. Occupational Safety and Health Administration. https://www.osha.gov/pls/oshaweb/owadisp.show_document?p_table=STANDARDS&p_id=9806. Accessed December 9, 2015.

53. American National Standards Institute/International Safety Equipment Association. *American National Standard for Emergency Eyewash and Shower Equipment.* Arlington, VA: International Safety Equipment Association; 2009. [IVC]

54. Guideline for hand hygiene. In: *Guidelines for Perioperative Practice.* Denver, CO: AORN, Inc; 2015:31-42. [IVB]

55. Aumeran C, Poincloux L, Souweine B, et al. Multidrug-resistant *Klebsiella pneumoniae* outbreak after endoscopic retrograde cholangiopancreatography. *Endoscopy.* 2010;42(11):895-899. [VA]

56. Guideline for environmental cleaning. In: *Guidelines for Perioperative Practice.* Denver, CO: AORN, Inc; 2015:9-30. [IVA]

57. Guideline for surgical attire. In: *Guidelines for Perioperative Practice.* Denver, CO: AORN, Inc; 2015:97-120. [IVA]

58. Guideline for cleaning and care of surgical instruments. In: *Guidelines for Perioperative Practice.* Denver, CO: AORN, Inc; 2015:615-650. [IVA]

59. 29 CFR 1910.133: Eye and Face Protection. Occupational Safety and Health Administration. https://www.osha.gov/pls/oshaweb/owadisp.show_document?p_table=STANDARDS&p_id=9778. Accessed December 9, 2015.

60. ASGE Technology Committee; Pedrosa MC, Farraye FA, et al. Minimizing occupational hazards in endoscopy: personal protective equipment, radiation safety, and ergonomics. *Gastrointest Endosc.* 2010;72(2):227-235. [VB]

61. Kaye MD. Herpetic conjunctivitis as an unusual occupational hazard (endoscopists' eye). *Gastrointest Endosc.* 1974;21(2):69-70. [VB]

62. Guideline for product selection. In: *Guidelines for Perioperative Practice.* Denver, CO: AORN, Inc; 2015:179-186. [IVB]

63. 21 CFR Chapter 1. Subchapter H: Medical Devices. 2015. US Food and Drug Administration. https://www.accessdata.fda.gov/scripts/cdrh/cfdocs/cfCFR/CFRSearch.cfm?CFRPart=820. Accessed December 9, 2015.

64. *Reprocessing Medical Devices in Health Care Settings: Validation Methods and Labeling Guidance for Industry and Food and Drug Administration Staff.* Silver Spring, MD: US Food and Drug Administration; 2015.

65. Rudy SF, Adams J, Waddington C. Implementing the SOHN-endorsed AORN guidelines for reprocessing reusable upper airway endoscopes. *ORL Head Neck Nurs.* 2012;30(1):6-15. [VB]

66. Weber DJ. Managing and preventing exposure events from inappropriately reprocessed endoscopes. *Infect Control Hosp Epidemiol.* 2012;33(7):657-660. [VA]

67. Statham MM, Willging JP. Automated high-level disinfection of nonchanneled flexible endoscopes: duty cycles and endoscope repair. *Laryngoscope.* 2010;120(10):1946-1949. [IIIB]

68. Hutson P. Staffing the endoscopy department: what is the appropriate skill mix? *Gastrointest Nurs.* 2011;9(1):28-33. [VB]

69. Choice Framework for local Policy and Procedures 01-06—Decontamination of flexible endoscopes: Operational management. 2013. UK Department of Health. https://www.gov.uk/government/uploads/system/uploads/attachment_data/file/148559/CFPP_01-06_Operational_mgmt_Final.pdf. Accessed December 9, 2015. [IVB]

70. Kolmos HJ, Lerche A, Kristoffersen K, Rosdahl VT. Pseudo-outbreak of *Pseudomonas aeruginosa* in HIV-infected patients undergoing fiberoptic bronchoscopy. *Scand J Infect Dis.* 1994;26(6):653-657. [VC]

71. McGill JJ, Schaeffer AJ, Gonzalez CM. Durability of flexible cystoscopes in the outpatient setting. *Urology.* 2013;81(5):932-937. [IIIB]

72. Sooriakumaran P, Kaba R, Andrews HO, Buchholz NP. Evaluation of the mechanisms of damage to flexible ureteroscopes and suggestions for ureteroscope preservation. *Asian J Androl.* 2005;7(4):433-438. [IIIB]

73. Semins MJ, George S, Allaf ME, Matlaga BR. Ureteroscope cleaning and sterilization by the urology operating room team: the effect on repair costs. *J Endourol.* 2009;23(6):903-905. [VB]

74. McDougall EM, Alberts G, Deal KJ, Nagy JM 3rd. Does the cleaning technique influence the durability of the <9F flexible ureteroscope? *J Endourol.* 2001;15(6):615-618. [IIC]

75. Smith F. *Pseudomonas* infection. *Nurs Times.* 1994;90(46):55-56. [VB]

76. Machida H, Seki M, Yoshioka N, et al. Correlation between outbreaks of multidrug-resistant *Pseudomonas aeruginosa* infection and use of bronchoscopes suggested by epidemiological analysis. *Biol Pharm Bull.* 2014;37(1):26-30. [IIIB]

77. *ANSI/AAMI ST79: Comprehensive Guide to Steam Sterilization and Sterility Assurance in Health Care Facilities.* Arlington, VA: Association for the Advancement of Medical Instrumentation; 2013. [IVC]

78. Centers for Disease Control and Prevention. *Immediate Need for Healthcare Facilities to Review Procedures for Cleaning, Disinfecting, and Sterilizing Reusable Medical Devices.* Health Alert Network. September 11, 2015. http://stacks.cdc.gov/view/cdc/34153. Accessed December 9, 2015. [VB]

79. Bou R, Aguilar A, Perpinan J, et al. Nosocomial outbreak of *Pseudomonas aeruginosa* infections related to a flexible bronchoscope. *J Hosp Infect.* 2006;64(2):129-135. [IIIB]

80. Srinivasan A, Wolfenden LL, Song X, Perl TM, Haponik EF. Bronchoscope reprocessing and infection prevention and control: bronchoscopy-specific guidelines are needed. *Chest.* 2004;125(1):307-314. [IIIB]

81. Radford PD, Unadkat SN, Rollin M, Tolley NS. Disinfection of flexible fibre-optic endoscopes out-of-hours: confidential telephone survey of ENT units in England—10 years on. *J Laryngol Otol.* 2013;127(5):489-493. [IIIC]

82. Roberts CG. The role of biofilms in reprocessing medical devices. *Am J Infect Control.* 2013;41(5 Suppl):S77-S80. [VA]

83. Joint AUA/SUNA white paper on reprocessing of flexible cystoscopes. *J Urol.* 2010;184(6):2241-2245. [VC]

84. Cavaliere M, Iemma M. Guidelines for reprocessing nonlumened heat-sensitive ear/nose/throat endoscopes. *Laryngoscope.* 2012;122(8):1708-1718. [VB]

85. Lind N, Ninemeier JD, Bird BT; International Association of Healthcare Central Service Materiel Management. *Central Service Technical Manual.* Chicago, IL: International Association of Healthcare Central Service Materiel Management; 2007. [IVC]

86. Merritt K, Hitchins VM, Brown SA. Safety and cleaning of medical materials and devices. *J Biomed Mater Res.* 2000;53(2):131-136. [IIB]

87. Herrmann IF, Heeg P, Matteja B, et al. Silent risks and hidden dangers in endoscopy: what to do? *Acta Endoscopica.* 2008;38(5):493-502. [IIIC]

88. Alfa MJ. Medical-device reprocessing. *Infect Control Hosp Epidemiol.* 2000;21(8):496-498. [VA]

89. Muscarella LF. Prevention of disease transmission during flexible laryngoscopy. *Am J Infect Control.* 2007;35(8):536-544. [VA]

90. *TIR 30: A Compendium of Processes, Materials, Test Methods, and Acceptance Criteria for Cleaning Reusable Medical Devices.* Arlington, VA: Association for the Advancement of Medical Instrumentation; 2011. [IVC]

91. Johansen C, Falholt P, Gram L. Enzymatic removal and disinfection of bacterial biofilms. *Appl Environ Microbiol.* 1997;63(9):3724-3728. [IIIC]

92. Pajkos A, Vickery K, Cossart Y. Is biofilm accumulation on endoscope tubing a contributor to the failure of cleaning and decontamination? *J Hosp Infect.* 2004;58(3):224-229. [IIC]

93. Kovaleva J, Peters FT, van der Mei HC, Degener JE. Transmission of infection by flexible gastrointestinal endoscopy and bronchoscopy. *Clin Microbiol Rev.* 2013;26(2):231-254. [VA]

94. Costerton JW, Stewart PS, Greenberg EP. Bacterial biofilms: a common cause of persistent infections. *Science.* 1999;284(5418):1318-1322. [VB]

95. Ren W, Sheng X, Huang X, Zhi F, Cai W. Evaluation of detergents and contact time on biofilm removal from flexible endoscopes. *Am J Infect Control.* 2013;41(9):e89-e92. [IB]

96. Ren-Pei W, Hui-Jun X, Ke Q, Dong W, Xing N, Zhao-Shen L. Correlation between the growth of bacterial biofilm in flexible endoscopes and endoscope reprocessing methods. *Am J Infect Control.* 2014;42(11):1203-1206. [IIIB]

97. Naas T, Cuzon G, Babics A, et al. Endoscopy-associated transmission of carbapenem-resistant *Klebsiella pneumoniae* producing KPC-2 beta-lactamase. *J Antimicrob Chemother.* 2010;65(6):1305-1306. [VB]

98. Hutchisson B, LeBlanc C. The truth and consequences of enzymatic detergents. *Gastroenterol Nurs.* 2005;28(5):372-376. [IIB]

99. Alfa MJ. Can biofilm prevent high level disinfection? *J GENCA.* 2006;16(1):23-24. [VA]

100. Shimono N, Takuma T, Tsuchimochi N, et al. An outbreak of *Pseudomonas aeruginosa* infections following thoracic surgeries occurring via the contamination of bronchoscopes and an automatic endoscope reprocessor. *J Infect Chemother.* 2008;14(6):418-423. [VB]

101. Bultitude MF, Dasgupta P, Tiptaft RC, Glass JM. Prolonging the life of the flexible ureterorenoscope. *Int J Clin Pract.* 2004;58(8):756-757. [VB]

102. Thomas LA. Transporting the endoscope. *Gastroenterol Nurs.* 2005;28(2):145-146. [VB]

STERILIZATION AND DISINFECTION

103. Collins JW, Keeley FX Jr, Timoney A. Cost analysis of flexible ureterorenoscopy. *BJU Int.* 2004;93(7):1023-1026. [IIIC]

104. Alfa MJ, Howie R. Modeling microbial survival in buildup biofilm for complex medical devices. *BMC Infect Dis.* 2009;9:56. [IIB]

105. Yanaihara H, Hamasuna R, Takahashi S, et al. Current controversial issues in the decontamination process for urological endoscopes. *Int J Urol.* 2012;19(1):5-6. [VB]

106. Endoscope inspections fraught with challenges. *Healthc Purchasing News.* 2013;37(11):16-18. [VB]

107. Thomas LA. Essentials for endoscopic equipment. Leak testing. *Gastroenterol Nurs.* 2005;28(5):430-432. [VB]

108. Khan F, Mukhtar S, Marsh H, et al. Evaluation of the pressure leak test in increasing the lifespan of flexible ureteroscopes. *Int J Clin Pract.* 2013;67(10):1040-1043. [IIB]

109. Ramsey AH, Oemig TV, Davis JP, Massey JP, Torok TJ. An outbreak of bronchoscopy-related *Mycobacterium tuberculosis* infections due to lack of bronchoscope leak testing. *Chest.* 2002;121(3):976-981. [VC]

110. Cetre JC, Nicolle MC, Salord H, et al. Outbreaks of contaminated broncho-alveolar lavage related to intrinsically defective bronchoscopes. *J Hosp Infect.* 2005;61(1):39-45. [IIIB]

111. Krishna PD, Statham MM, Rosen CA. Acute glutaraldehyde mucosal injury of the upper aerodigestive tract due to damage to the working channel of an endoscope. *Ann Otol Rhinol Laryngol.* 2010;119(3):150-154. [VB]

112. Chu NS, Favero M. The microbial flora of the gastrointestinal tract and the cleaning of flexible endoscopes. *Gastrointest Endosc Clin N Am.* 2000;10(2):233-244. [VA]

113. Chu NS, McAlister D, Antonoplos PA. Natural bioburden levels detected on flexible gastrointestinal endoscopes after clinical use and manual cleaning. *Gastrointest Endosc.* 1998;48(2):137-142. [IC]

114. Kampf G, Fliss PM, Martiny H. Is peracetic acid suitable for the cleaning step of reprocessing flexible endoscopes? *World J Gastrointest Endosc.* 2014;6(9):390-406. [VA]

115. Alfa MJ, Sitter DL. In-hospital evaluation of orthophthalaldehyde as a high level disinfectant for flexible endoscopes. *J Hosp Infect.* 1994;26(1):15-26. [IIB]

116. Weber DJ, Rutala WA. Lessons from outbreaks associated with bronchoscopy. *Infect Control Hosp Epidemiol.* 2001;22(7):403-408. [VA]

117. Spaulding EH, Lawrence CA, Block SS, Reddish GF. Chemical disinfection of medical and surgical materials. In: Lawrence CA, Block SS, Reddish GF, eds. *Disinfection, Sterilization, and Preservation.* Philadelphia, PA: Lea & Febiger; 1968:517-531. [VA]

118. Bajolet O, Ciocan D, Vallet C, et al. Gastroscopy-associated transmission of extended-spectrum beta-lactamase-producing *Pseudomonas aeruginosa. J Hosp Infect.* 2013;83(4):341-343. [VA]

119. *Technical Information Report 34: Water for the Reprocessing of Medical Devices.* Atlanta, GA: Association for the Advancement of Medical Instrumentation; 2014. [IVC]

120. Alfa MJ. Methodology of reprocessing reusable accessories. *Gastrointest Endosc Clin N Am.* 2000;10(2):361-378. [VA]

121. Alfa MJ, Jackson M. A new hydrogen peroxide-based medical-device detergent with germicidal properties: comparison with enzymatic cleaners. *Am J Infect Control.* 2001;29(3):168-177. [IIB]

122. Rey JF, Kruse A, Neumann C; ESGE (European Society of Gastrointestinal Endoscopy); ESGENA (European Society of Gastrointestinal Endoscopy Nurses and Associates). ESGE/ESGENA technical note on cleaning and disinfection. *Endoscopy.* 2003;35(10):869-877. [VB]

123. Henoun Loukili N, Zink E, Grandadam S, Bientz M, Meunier O. Effectiveness of detergent-disinfecting agents on *Escherichia coli* 54127 biofilm. *J Hosp Infect.* 2004;57(2):175-178. [IIC]

124. Fang Y, Shen Z, Li L, et al. A study of the efficacy of bacterial biofilm cleanout for gastrointestinal endoscopes. *World J Gastroenterol.* 2010;16(8):1019-1024. [IB]

125. Vickery K, Pajkos A, Cossart Y. Removal of biofilm from endoscopes: evaluation of detergent efficiency. *Am J Infect Control.* 2004;32(3):170-176. [IIB]

126. Sava A. Biofilm digestion: more confusion than answers. *Am J Infect Control.* 2005;33(10):614. [VB]

127. Marion K, Freney J, James G, Bergeron E, Renaud FN, Costerton JW. Using an efficient biofilm detaching agent: an essential step for the improvement of endoscope reprocessing protocols. *J Hosp Infect.* 2006;64(2):136-142. [IIB]

128. Perret-Vivancos C, Marion K, Renaud FN, Freney J. Efficient removal of attached biofilm in a naturally contaminated colonoscope using detachment-promoting agents. *J Hosp Infect.* 2008;68(3):277-278. [VB]

129. Thomas LA. Essentials for endoscopic equipment. Manual cleaning. *Gastroenterol Nurs.* 2005;28(6):512-513. [VB]

130. Herve R, Keevil CW. Current limitations about the cleaning of luminal endoscopes. *J Hosp Infect.* 2013;83(1):22-29. [IIC]

131. Alfa MJ, Olson N, Degagne P, Jackson M. A survey of reprocessing methods, residual viable bioburden, and soil levels in patient-ready endoscopic retrograde cholangiopancreatography duodenoscopes used in Canadian centers. *Infect Control Hosp Epidemiol.* 2002;23(4):198-206. [IIIA]

132. Pineau L, De Philippe E. Evaluation of endoscope cleanliness after reprocessing: a clinical-use study. *Zentralsterilisation.* 2013;21(1):15-27. [IIIB]

133. Dietze B, Kircheis U, Schwarz I, Martiny H. Freely accessible endoscope channels improve efficacy of cleaning. *Endoscopy.* 2001;33(6):523-528. [IIB]

134. Ishino Y, Ido K, Koiwai H, Sugano K. Pitfalls in endoscope reprocessing: brushing of air and water channels is mandatory for high-level disinfection. *Gastrointest Endosc.* 2001;53(2):165-168. [IIB]

135. Agerton T, Valway S, Gore B, et al. Transmission of a highly drug-resistant strain (strain W1) of *Mycobacterium tuberculosis.* Community outbreak and nosocomial transmission via a contaminated bronchoscope. *JAMA.* 1997;278(13):1073-1077. [VA]

136. Alrabaa SF, Nguyen P, Sanderson R, et al. Early identification and control of carbapenemase-producing *Klebsiella pneumoniae*, originating from contaminated endoscopic equipment. *Am J Infect Control.* 2013;41(6):562-564. [VA]

137. Wendorf KA, Kay M, Baliga C, et al. Endoscopic retrograde cholangiopancreatography-associated AmpC *Escherichia coli* outbreak. *Infect Control Hosp Epidemiol.* 2015;36(6):634-642. [IIIA]

138. Supplemental measures to enhance duodenoscope reprocessing: FDA safety communication. US Food and Drug Administration. http://www.fda.gov/MedicalDevices/Safety/AlertsandNotices/ucm454766.htm. Accessed December 9, 2015. [VA]

139. Edmiston CE Jr, Spencer M. Endoscope reprocessing in 2014: why is the margin of safety so small? *AORN J.* 2014;100(6):609-615. [VA]

140. An outbreak of carbapenem-resistant *Klebsiella pneumoniae* infections associated with endoscopic

STERILIZATION AND DISINFECTION

retrograde cholangiopancreatography (ERCP) procedures at a hospital. *Am J Infect Control.* 2010;38(5):e141. [VB]

141. Notes from the field: New Delhi metallo-ß-lactamase–producing *Escherichia coli* associated with endoscopic retrograde cholangiopancreatography—Illinois, 2013. *Morb Mortal Weekly Rep.* 2014;62(51):1051. [VA]

142. Advocate Lutheran General Hospital. Report No. 8196. January 16, 2014. Association of Health Care Journalists. http://www.hospitalinspections.org/report/8196. Accessed December 9, 2015.

143. Muscarella LF. Risk of transmission of carbapenem-resistant Enterobacteriaceae and related "superbugs" during gastrointestinal endoscopy. *World J Gastrointest Endosc.* 2014;6(10):457-474. [VA]

144. Ross AS, Baliga C, Verma P, Duchin J, Gluck M. A quarantine process for the resolution of duodenoscope-associated transmission of multidrug-resistant *Escherichia coli. Gastrointest Endosc.* 2015;82(3):477-483. [VA]

145. *Meeting of the FDA Gastroenterology and Urology Devices Panel of the Medical Devices Advisory Committee* [transcript]. Annapolis, MD: Free State Reporting, Inc; May 14, 2015. [VA]

146. Kola A, Piening B, Pape UF, et al. An outbreak of carbapenem-resistant OXA-48-producing *Klebsiella pneumonia* associated to duodenoscopy. *Antimicrob Resist Infect Control.* 2015;4:8-015-0049-4. eCollection 2015. [VA]

147. Verfaillie CJ, Bruno MJ, F Voor In 't Holt A, et al. Withdrawal of a novel-design duodenoscope ends outbreak of a VIM-2-producing *Pseudomonas aeruginosa. Endoscopy.* 2015;47(6):493-502. [VA]

148. Behnia MM, Amurao K, Clemons V, Lantz G. Pseudo-outbreak of *Stenotrophomonas maltophilia* and *Acinetobacter baumannii* by a contaminated bronchoscope in an intensive care unit. *Tanaffos.* 2010;9(3):44-49. [VB]

149. Charlton TS. A comparison of the efficacy of lumen-cleaning devices for flexible gastrointestinal endoscopes. *Aust Infect Control.* 2007;12(3):81. [IIIC]

150. Charlton TS. A comparison of two devices for the manual cleaning of flexible gastrointestinal endoscopes in a clinical setting. *Aust Infect Control.* 2007;12(4):130-130, 132, 134, passim. [IIIB]

151. *Final report: Comparative Brush Study of the Cygnus Medical Dragon Tail Cleaning Brush and the Olympus Single Use Combination Cleaning Brush Protein Analysis.* Study No. 1504-244. Rochester, NY: Highpower Validation Testing & Lab Services; 2015. [IIB]

152. Society of Gastroenterology Nurses and Associates. Reprocessing of endoscopic accessories and valves. *Gastroenterol Nurs.* 2013;36(4):291-292. [IVB]

153. Society of Gastroenterology Nurses and Associates. *Position Statement on Reprocessing of Water Bottles Used During Endoscopy.* Updated 2011. http://www.ascquality.org/Library/endoscopereprocessingtoolkit/SGNA%20Water%20Bottle%20Reprocessing.pdf. Accessed December 9, 2015. [IVB]

154. Parente DM. Could biopsy port valves be a source for potential flexible endoscope contamination? *Infect Control Today.* 2007;11(5). [IIIC]

155. Liquid chemical sterilization. US Food and Drug Administration. http://www.fda.gov/MedicalDevices/ProductsandMedicalProcedures/GeneralHospitalDevicesandSupplies/ucm208018.htm. Accessed December 9, 2015.

156. Veterans Affairs Office of Inspector General. *Use and Reprocessing of Flexible Fiberoptic Endoscopes at VA Medical Facilities.* Report No. 09-01784-146. Washington, DC: Department of Veterans Affairs; 2009. [VA]

157. Muscarella LF. Disinfecting endoscopes immediately before the first patient of the day. *AORN J.* 2001;73(6):1159-1163. [VA]

158. Puterbaugh M, Barde C, Van Enk R. Endoscopy water source: tap or sterile water? *Gastroenterol Nurs.* 1997;20(6):203-206. [IIC]

159. Wilcox CM, Waites K, Brookings ES. Use of sterile compared with tap water in gastrointestinal endoscopic procedures. *Am J Infect Control.* 1996;24(5):407-410. [IIC]

160. Rockey DC. Endoscopy: dollars and sense. *Gastroenterology.* 1995;108(6):1957. [VB]

161. Patton RF, Wilcox CM, Blakely J. Benefits of sterile water use in an endoscopic laboratory [4] (multiple letters). *Am J Infect Control.* 1998;26(3):366-367. [VC]

162. Guideline for electrosurgery. In: *Guidelines for Perioperative Practice.* Denver, CO: AORN, Inc; 2015:121-138. [IVB]

163. Wilson SJ, Everts RJ, Kirkland KB, Sexton DJ. A pseudo-outbreak of *Aureobasidium* species lower respiratory tract infections caused by reuse of single-use stopcocks during bronchoscopy. *Infect Control Hosp Epidemiol.* 2000;21(7):470-472. [VB]

164. Rutala WA, Weber DJ. New developments in reprocessing semicritical items. *Am J Infect Control.* 2013;41(5 Suppl):S60-S66. [VA]

165. *Meeting of the FDA Gastroenterology and Urology Devices Panel of the Medical Devices Advisory Committee* [transcript]. Annapolis, MD: Free State Reporting, Inc; May 15, 2015. [VA]

166. Rutala WA, Weber DJ. Gastrointestinal endoscopes: a need to shift from disinfection to sterilization? *JAMA.* 2014;312(14):1405-1406. [VA]

167. Puzey A. Managing the risks of prion disease transmission through flexible endoscopy. *Gastrointest Nurs.* 2010;8(2):18-25. [VA]

168. Tschudin-Sutter S, Frei R, Kampf G, et al. Emergence of glutaraldehyde-resistant *Pseudomonas aeruginosa. Infect Control Hosp Epidemiol.* 2011;32(12):1173-1178. [VA]

169. Fisher CW, Fiorello A, Shaffer D, Jackson M, McDonnell GE. Aldehyde-resistant mycobacteria bacteria associated with the use of endoscope reprocessing systems. *Am J Infect Control.* 2012;40(9):880-882. [IIC]

170. Epstein L, Hunter JC, Arwady MA, et al. New Delhi metallo-beta-lactamase-producing carbapenem-resistant *Escherichia coli* associated with exposure to duodenoscopes. *JAMA.* 2014;312(14):1447-1455. [IIIA]

171. McCool S, Clarke L, Querry A, et al. Carbapenem-resistant Enterobacteriaceae (CRE) *Klebsiella pneumonia* (KP) Cluster Analysis Associated with GI Scopes with Elevator Channel [poster]. 2013. Infectious Diseases Society of America. https://idsa.confex.com/idsa/2013/webprogram/Handout/id1798/POSTER188_1619.pdf. Accessed December 9, 2015. [VA]

172. Campagnaro RL, Teichtahl H, Dwyer B. A pseudo-epidemic of *Mycobacterium chelonae*: contamination of a bronchoscope and autocleaner. *Aust New Zealand J Med.* 1994;24(6):693-695. [VB]

173. Chang CL, Su LH, Lu CM, Tai FT, Huang YC, Chang KK. Outbreak of ertapenem-resistant *Enterobacter cloacae* urinary tract infections due to a contaminated ureteroscope. *J Hosp Infect.* 2013;85(2):118-124. [IIIB]

174. Smith ZL, Oh YS, Saeian K, et al. Transmission of carbapenem-resistant Enterobacteriaceae during ERCP: time to revisit the current reprocessing guidelines. *Gastrointest Endosc.* 2015;81(4):1041-1045. [VA]

175. Müller S, Maguilnilk I, Konkewicz LR, Barth AL, Kuchenbecker RS. Biofilm in duodenoscope: hospital infection by pan-resistant aeruginosa pseudomonas

related to endoscopic retrograde cholangiopancreatography (ERCP). *J GENCA*. 2010;20(1):13-14. [VC]

176. Alfa MJ, DeGagne P, Olson N, Puchalski T. Comparison of ion plasma, vaporized hydrogen peroxide, and 100% ethylene oxide sterilizers to the 12/88 ethylene oxide gas sterilizer. *Infect Control Hosp Epidemiol*. 1996;17(2):92-100. [IIB]

177. Boyer JL. Bile formation and secretion. *Compr Physiol*. 2013;3(3):1035-1078. [VA]

178. Alfa MJ, DeGagne P, Olson N, Hizon R. Comparison of liquid chemical sterilization with peracetic acid and ethylene oxide sterilization for long narrow lumens. *Am J Infect Control*. 1998;26(5):469-477. [IIB]

179. Alfa MJ, DeGagne P, Olson N. Validation of ATS as an appropriate test soil to assess cleaning and sterilization efficacy in narrow lumened medical devices such as flexible endoscopes. *Zentralsterilisation*. 2005;13(6):387-402. [IIB]

180. Muscarella LF. Automatic flexible endoscope reprocessors. *Gastrointest Endosc Clin N Am*. 2000;10(2):245-257. [VA]

181. Ofstead CL, Wetzler HP, Snyder AK, Horton RA. Endoscope reprocessing methods: a prospective study on the impact of human factors and automation. *Gastroenterol Nurs*. 2010;33(4):304-311. [IIIA]

182. Ubhayawardana DL, Kottahachchi J, Weerasekera MM, Wanigasooriya IW, Fernando SS, De Silva M. Residual bioburden in reprocessed side-view endoscopes used for endoscopic retrograde cholangiopancreatography (ERCP). *Endosc Int Open*. 2013;1(1):12-16. [IIIB]

183. Kenters N, Huijskens EG, Meier C, Voss A. Infectious diseases linked to cross-contamination of flexible endoscopes. *Endosc Int Open*. 2015;3(4):E259-E265. [VA]

184. Vickery K, Ngo QD, Zou J, Cossart YE. The effect of multiple cycles of contamination, detergent washing, and disinfection on the development of biofilm in endoscope tubing. *Am J Infect Control*. 2009;37(6):470-475. [IIB]

185. Balsamo AC, Graziano KU, Schneider RP, Antunes Junior M, Lacerda RA. Removing biofilm from an endoscopic: evaluation of disinfection methods currently used. *Rev Esc Enferm USP*. 2012;46(Spec): 91-98. [IIB]

186. Farina A, Fievet MH, Plassart F, Menet MC, Thuillier A. Residual glutaraldehyde levels in fiberoptic endoscopes: measurement and implications for patient toxicity. *J Hosp Infect*. 1999;43(4):293-297. [IIIC]

187. Dirlam Langlay AM, Ofstead CL, Mueller NJ, Tosh PK, Baron TH, Wetzler HP. Reported gastrointestinal endoscope reprocessing lapses: the tip of the iceberg. *Am J Infect Control*. 2013;41(12):1188-1194. [VA]

188. Moses FM, Lee JS. Current GI endoscope disinfection and QA practices. *Dig Dis Sci*. 2004;49(11-12):1791-1797. [IIIB]

189. Schaefer MK, Jhung M, Dahl M, et al. Infection control assessment of ambulatory surgical centers. *JAMA*. 2010;303(22):2273-2279. [IIIA]

190. Park JB, Yang JN, Lim YJ, et al. Survey of endoscope reprocessing in Korea. *Clin Endosc*. 2015;48(1):39-47. [IIIB]

191. Przytulski K, Reguła J. Disinfection of endoscopes and sterilization of accessories for gastrointestinal endoscopy in Polish units—analysis of the questionnaire. *Gastroenterol Pol*. 2004;11(3):241-243. [IIIC]

192. Yamada G, Takahashi H, Abe S. A survey of bronchoscope reprocessing procedure in Japan [2]. *J Bronchol*. 2005;12(3):184-185. [IIIC]

193. Zhang X, Kong J, Tang P, et al. Current status of cleaning and disinfection for gastrointestinal endoscopy in China: a survey of 122 endoscopy units. *Dig Liver Dis*. 2011;43(4):305-308. [IIIB]

194. Akamatsu T, Tabata K, Hironga M, Kawakami H, Uyeda M. Transmission of *Helicobacter pylori* infection via flexible fiberoptic endoscopy. *Am J Infect Control*. 1996;24(5):396-401. [IIIB]

195. Ahuja V, Tandon RK. Survey of gastrointestinal endoscope disinfection and accessory reprocessing practices in the Asia-Pacific region. *J Gastroenterol Hepatol*. 2000;15(Suppl):G78-G81. [IIIB]

196. Barbosa JM, Souza AC, Tipple AF, Pimenta FC, Leao LS, Silva SR. Endoscope reprocessing using glutaraldehyde in endoscopy services of Goiania, Brazil: a realidade em servicos de endoscopia de Goiania, GO. *Arq Gastroenterol*. 2010;47(3):219-224. [IIIB]

197. Fratila O, Tantau M. Cleaning and disinfection in gastrointestinal endoscopy: current status in Romania. *J Gastrointest Liver Dis*. 2006;15(1):89-93. [IIIC]

198. Heudorf U, Exner M. German guidelines for reprocessing endoscopes and endoscopic accessories: guideline compliance in Frankfurt/Main, Germany. *J Hosp Infect*. 2006;64(1):69-75. [IIIC]

199. Honeybourne D, Neumann CS. An audit of bronchoscopy practice in the United Kingdom: a survey of adherence to national guidelines. *Thorax*. 1997;52(8):709-713. [IIIC]

200. Lubbe DE, Fagan JJ. South African survey on disinfection techniques for the flexible nasopharyngoscope. *J Laryngol Otol*. 2003;117(10):811-814. [IIIC]

201. Orsi GB, Filocamo A, Di Stefano L, Tittobello A. Italian National Survey of Digestive Endoscopy Disinfection Procedures. *Endoscopy*. 1997;29(8):732-738. [IIIC]

202. Soares JB, Goncalves R, Banhudo A, Pedrosa J. Reprocessing practice in digestive endoscopy units of district hospitals: results of a Portuguese National Survey. *Eur J Gastroenterol Hepatol*. 2011;23(11):1064-1068. [IIIB]

203. Spinzi G, Fasoli R, Centenaro R, Minoli G; SIED Lombardia Working Group. Reprocessing in digestive endoscopy units in Lombardy: results of a regional survey. *Dig Liver Dis*. 2008;40(11):890-896. [IIIB]

204. Ribeiro MM, de Oliveira AC, Ribeiro SM, Watanabe E, de Resende Stoianoff MA, Ferreira JA. Effectiveness of flexible gastrointestinal endoscope reprocessing. *Infect Control Hosp Epidemiol*. 2013;34(3):309-312. [IIIB]

205. Lakhani R, Smithard A, Bleach N. How clean is your scope? A completed audit cycle of the disinfection of nasendoscopes. *Ann R Coll Surg Engl*. 2010;92(7):587-590. [IIB]

206. Banfield GK, Hinton AE. A national survey of disinfection techniques for flexible nasendoscopes in UK ENT out-patient departments. *J Laryngol Otol*. 2000;114(3):202-204. [IIIC]

207. Brake MK, Lee BS, Savoury L, et al. Survey of nasopharyngoscope decontamination methods in Canada. *J Otolaryngol Head Neck Surg*. 2010;39(6):714-722. [IIIB]

208. Kressel AB, Kidd F. Pseudo-outbreak of *Mycobacterium chelonae* and *Methylobacterium mesophilicum* caused by contamination of an automated endoscopy washer. *Infect Control Hosp Epidemiol*. 2001;22(7):414-418. [VB]

209. Schelenz S, French G. An outbreak of multidrug-resistant *Pseudomonas aeruginosa* infection associated with contamination of bronchoscopes and an endoscope washer-disinfector. *J Hosp Infect*. 2000;46(1):23-30. [VB]

210. Blanc DS, Parret T, Janin B, Raselli P, Francioli P. Nosocomial infections and pseudoinfections from contaminated bronchoscopes: two-year follow up using molecular markers. *Infect Control Hosp Epidemiol*. 1997;18(2):134-136. [IIIB]

211. Maloney S, Welbel S, Daves B, et al. *Mycobacterium abscessus* pseudoinfection traced to an automated

endoscope washer: utility of epidemiologic and laboratory investigation. *J Infect Dis.* 1994;169(5):1166-1169. [IIIB]

212. Centers for Disease Control and Prevention (CDC). Bronchoscopy-related infections and pseudoinfections—New York, 1996 and 1998. *MMWR Morb Mortal Wkly Rep.* 1999;48(26):557-560. [VA]

213. Chroneou A, Zimmerman SK, Cook S, et al. Molecular typing of *Mycobacterium chelonae* isolates from a pseudo-outbreak involving an automated bronchoscope washer. *Infect Control Hosp Epidemiol.* 2008;29(11):1088-1090. [VC]

214. Gillespie TG, Hogg L, Budge E, Duncan A, Coia JE. *Mycobacterium chelonae* isolated from rinse water within an endoscope washer-disinfector. *J Hosp Infect.* 2000;45(4):332-334. [VC]

215. Rosengarten D, Block C, Hidalgo-Grass C, et al. Cluster of pseudoinfections with *Burkholderia cepacia* associated with a contaminated washer-disinfector in a bronchoscopy unit. *Infect Control Hosp Epidemiol.* 2010;31(7):769-771. [VA]

216. Ramirez J, Ahmed Z, Gutierrez CN, Byrd RP Jr, Roy TM, Sarubbi FA. Impact of atypical mycobacterial contamination of bronchoscopy on patient care: report of an outbreak and review of the literature. *Infect Dis Clin Pract (Baltim Md).* 1998;7(6):281-285. [VC]

217. Zweigner J, Gastmeier P, Kola A, Klefisch F-R, Schweizer C, Hummel M. A carbapenem-resistant *Klebsiella pneumoniae* outbreak following bronchoscopy. *Am J Infect Control.* 2014;42(8):936-937. [VB]

218. Mean M, Mallaret MR, Bichard P, Shum J, Zarski JP. Gastrointestinal endoscopes cleaned without detergent substance following an automated endoscope washer/disinfector dysfunction. *Gastroenterol Clin Biol.* 2006;30(5):665-668. [VC]

219. Larson JL, Lambert L, Stricof RL, Driscoll J, McGarry MA, Ridzon R. Potential nosocomial exposure to *Mycobacterium tuberculosis* from a bronchoscope. *Infect Control Hosp Epidemiol.* 2003;24(11):825-830. [VA]

220. Kara M, Turan I, Polat Z, Dogru T, Bagci S. Chemical colitis caused by peracetic acid or hydrogen peroxide: a challenging dilemma. *Endoscopy.* 2010;42(Suppl 2):E3-E4. [VC]

221. Cammarota G, Cesaro P, Cazzato A, et al. Hydrogen peroxide-related colitis (previously known as "pseudolipomatosis"): a series of cases occurring in an epidemic pattern. *Endoscopy.* 2007;39(10):916-919. [VC]

222. Gamble HP, Duckworth GJ, Ridgway GL. Endoscope decontamination incidents in England 2003-2004. *J Hosp Infect.* 2007;67(4):350-354. [VB]

223. Vanhems P, Gayet-Ageron A, Ponchon T, et al. Follow-up and management of patients exposed to a flawed automated endoscope washer-disinfector in a digestive diseases unit. *Infect Control Hosp Epidemiol.* 2006;27(1):89-92. [VB]

224. Vanhems P, Gayet-Ageron A, Ponchon T, et al. Erratum: Follow-up and management of patients exposed to a flawed automated endoscope washer-disinfector in a digestive diseases unit (Infection Control and Hospital Epidemiology [January 2006] 27 [89-91]). *Infect Control Hosp Epidemiol.* 2006;27(4):431.

225. Alfa MJ, Olson N, DeGagne P. Automated washing with the Reliance Endoscope Processing System and its equivalence to optimal manual cleaning. *Am J Infect Control.* 2006;34(9):561-570. [IIB]

226. Funk SE, Reaven NL. High-level endoscope disinfection processes in emerging economies: financial impact of manual process versus automated endoscope reprocessing. *J Hosp Infect.* 2014;86(4):250-254. [IIIC]

227. Forte L, Shum C. Comparative cost-efficiency of the EVOTECH endoscope cleaner and reprocessor versus manual cleaning plus automated endoscope reprocessing in a real-world Canadian hospital endoscopy setting. *BMC Gastroenterology.* 2011;11:105. [IIIB]

228. Alfa MJ, DeGagne P, Olson N, Fatima I. EVOTECH endoscope cleaner and reprocessor (ECR) simulated-use and clinical-use evaluation of cleaning efficacy. *BMC Infect Dis.* 2010;10:200. [IIA]

229. Bhatt JM, Peterson EM, Verma SP. Microbiological sampling of the forgotten components of a flexible fiberoptic laryngoscope: what lessons can we learn? *Otolaryngol Head Neck Surg.* 2014;150(2):235-236. [IIIC]

230. Sorin M, Segal-Maurer S, Mariano N, Urban C, Combest A, Rahal JJ. Nosocomial transmission of imipenem-resistant *Pseudomonas aeruginosa* following bronchoscopy associated with improper connection to the Steris System 1 processor. *Infect Control Hosp Epidemiol.* 2001;22(7):409-413. [IIIB]

231. Esteban J, Gadea I, Fernandez-Roblas R, et al. Pseudo-outbreak of *Aeromonas hydrophila* isolates related to endoscopy. *J Hosp Infect.* 1999;41(4):313-316. [VC]

232. West AB, Kuan SF, Bennick M, Lagarde S. Glutaraldehyde colitis following endoscopy: clinical and pathological features and investigation of an outbreak. *Gastroenterology.* 1995;108(4):1250-1255. [VC]

233. Kim SJ, Baek IH. Colonic mucosal pseudolipomatosis: disinfectant colitis? *Gastroenterol Nurs.* 2012;35(3):208-213. [IIIB]

234. Rozen P, Somjen GJ, Baratz M, Kimel R, Arber N, Gilat T. Endoscope-induced colitis: description, probable cause by glutaraldehyde, and prevention. *Gastrointest Endosc.* 1994;40(5):547-553. [VC]

235. Tsai MS, Chiu HH, Li JH. Education and imaging. Gastrointestinal: glutaraldehyde proctocolitis. *J Gastroenterol Hepatol.* 2008;23(9):1460. [VC]

236. Yen HH, Chen YY. Glutaraldehyde colitis. *Endoscopy.* 2006;38(Suppl 2):E98. [VB]

237. Mohamad MZ, Koh KS, Chong VH. Gluteraldehyde-induced colitis: a rare cause of lower gastrointestinal bleeding. *Am J Emerg Med.* 2014;32(6):685.e1-685.e2. [VC]

238. Mee AS, Bower M. Risk factors for pancreatitis [2]. *Gut.* 1997;40(2):289. [VC]

239. Stein BL, Lamoureux E, Miller M, Vasilevsky CA, Julien L, Gordon PH. Glutaraldehyde-induced colitis. *Can J Surg.* 2001;44(2):113-116. [VC]

240. Caprilli R, Viscido A, Frieri G, Latella G. Acute colitis following colonoscopy. *Endoscopy.* 1998;30(4):428-431. [VC]

241. Bennett SN, Peterson DE, Johnson DR, Hall WN, Robinson-Dunn B, Dietrich S. Bronchoscopy-associated *Mycobacterium xenopi* pseudoinfections. *Am J Respir Crit Care Med.* 1994;150(1):245-250. [IIIA]

242. Wendelboe AM, Baumbach J, Blossom DB, Frank P, Srinivasan A, Sewell CM. Outbreak of cystoscopy related infections with *Pseudomonas aeruginosa*: New Mexico, 2007. *J Urol.* 2008;180(2):588-592. [IIIB]

243. Alfa MJ, Sitter DL. In-hospital evaluation of contamination of duodenoscopes: a quantitative assessment of the effect of drying. *J Hosp Infect.* 1991;19(2):89-98. [IIIA]

244. Muscarella LF. Inconsistencies in endoscope-reprocessing and infection-control guidelines: the importance of endoscope drying. *Am J Gastroenterol.* 2006;101(9):2147-2154. [VA]

245. Wang HC, Liaw YS, Yang PC, Kuo SH, Luh KT. A pseudoepidemic of *Mycobacterium chelonae* infection caused by contamination of a fibreoptic bronchoscope suction channel. *Eur Respir J.* 1995;8(8):1259-1262. [IIIC]

246. Gavalda L, Olmo AR, Hernandez R, et al. Microbiological monitoring of flexible bronchoscopes after high-level disinfection and flushing channels with alcohol: results and costs. *Respir Med.* 2015;109(8):1079-1085. [IIB]

247. Muscarella LF. Application of environmental sampling to flexible endoscope reprocessing: the importance of monitoring the rinse water. *Infect Control Hosp Epidemiol.* 2002;23(5):285-289. [VA]

248. Kovaleva J, Degener JE, van der Mei HC. Mimicking disinfection and drying of biofilms in contaminated endoscopes. *J Hosp Infect.* 2010;76(4):345-350. [IIIB]

249. Hagan ME, Klotz SA, Bartholomew W, Potter L, Nelson M. A pseudoepidemic of *Rhodotorula rubra*: a marker for microbial contamination of the bronchoscope. *Infect Control Hosp Epidemiol.* 1995;16(12):727-728. [VC]

250. Carbonne A, Thiolet JM, Fournier S, et al. Control of a multi-hospital outbreak of KPC-producing *Klebsiella pneumoniae* type 2 in France, September to October 2009. *Euro Surveill.* 2010;15(48):pii:19734. [VA]

251. Rutala WA, Weber DJ. ERCP scopes: what can we do to prevent infections? *Infect Control Hosp Epidemiol.* 2015;36(6):643-648. [VA]

252. Alfa MJ, Degagne P, Olson N. Worst-case soiling levels for patient-used flexible endoscopes before and after cleaning. *Am J Infect Control.* 1999;27(5):392-401. [IIA]

253. Foliente RL, Kovacs BJ, Aprecio RM, Bains HJ, Kettering JD, Chen YK. Efficacy of high-level disinfectants for reprocessing GI endoscopes in simulated-use testing. *Gastrointest Endosc.* 2001;53(4):456-462. [IIC]

254. Rutala WA, Weber DJ. FDA labeling requirements for disinfection of endoscopes: a counterpoint. *Infect Control Hosp Epidemiol.* 1995;16(4):231-235. [VB]

255. Guideline for selection and use of packaging systems for sterilization. In: *Guidelines for Perioperative Practice.* Denver, CO: AORN, Inc; 2015:651-664. [IVA]

256. Guideline for sterilization. In: *Guidelines for Perioperative Practice.* Denver, Co: AORN, Inc; 2015:665-692. [IVA]

257. Rutala WA, Weber DJ; Society for Healthcare Epidemiology of America. Guideline for disinfection and sterilization of prion-contaminated medical instruments. *Infect Control Hosp Epidemiol.* 2010;31(2):107-117. [IVA]

258. Widmer A. Prions and endoscopy: an unresolved problem. *Zentralsterilisation.* 2004;12(Suppl 1):70-77. [VB]

259. Cooke RP, Goddard SV. Endoscopes and protective sheaths. *J Hosp Infect.* 2002;52(2):153-154. [VC]

260. Lawrentschuk N, Chamberlain M. Sterile disposable sheath system for flexible cystoscopes. *Urology.* 2005;66(6):1310-1313. [VC]

261. Baker KH, Chaput MP, Clavet CR, Varney GW, To TM, Lytle CD. Evaluation of endoscope sheaths as viral barriers. *Laryngoscope.* 1999;109(4):636-639. [IIIC]

262. Elackattu A, Zoccoli M, Spiegel JH, Grundfast KM. A comparison of two methods for preventing cross-contamination when using flexible fiberoptic endoscopes in an otolaryngology clinic: disposable sterile sheaths versus immersion in germicidal liquid. *Laryngoscope.* 2010;120(12):2410-2416. [IIB]

263. Mayinger B, Strenkert M, Hochberger J, Martus P, Kunz B, Hahn EG. Disposable-sheath, flexible gastroscope system versus standard gastroscopes: a prospective, randomized trial. *Gastrointest Endosc.* 1999;50(4):461-467. [IB]

264. Alvarado CJ, Anderson AG, Maki DG. Microbiologic assessment of disposable sterile endoscopic sheaths to replace high-level disinfection in reprocessing: a

265. Colt HG, Beamis JJ, Harrell JH, Mathur PM. Novel flexible bronchoscope and single-use disposable-sheath endoscope system. A preliminary technology evaluation. *Chest.* 2000;118(1):183-187. [VB]

266. Street I, Hamann J, Harries M. Audit of nasendoscope disinfection practice. *Surgeon.* 2006;4(1):11-13. [VC]

267. Jorgensen PH, Slotsbjerg T, Westh H, Buitenhuis V, Hermann GG. A microbiological evaluation of level of disinfection for flexible cystoscopes protected by disposable endosheaths. *BMC Urol.* 2013;13:46. [IIIB]

268. Guidance for manufacturers seeking marketing clearance of ear, nose, and throat endoscope sheaths used as protective barriers: guidance for industry. US Food and Drug Administration. http://www.fda.gov/RegulatoryInformation/Guidances/ucm073746.htm. Accessed December 9, 2015.

269. FDA-cleared sterilants and high level disinfectants with general claims for processing reusable medical and dental devices—March 2015. http://www.fda.gov/MedicalDevices/DeviceRegulationandGuidance/ReprocessingofReusableMedicalDevices/ucm437347.htm. Accessed December 9, 2015.

270. Javed F, Sood S, Banfield G. Decontamination methods for flexible nasal endoscopes. *Br J Nurs.* 2014;23(15):850-852. [IIIB]

271. Bhattacharyya N, Kepnes LJ. The effectiveness of immersion disinfection for flexible fiberoptic laryngoscopes. *Otolaryngol Head Neck Surg.* 2004;130(6):681-685. [IIB]

272. Chang D, Florea A, Rowe M, Seiberling KA. Disinfection of flexible fiberoptic laryngoscopes after in vitro contamination with *Staphylococcus aureus* and *Candida albicans. Arch Otolaryngol Head Neck Surg.* 2012;138(2):119-121. [IIB]

273. Tzanidakis K, Choudhury N, Bhat S, Weerasinghe A, Marais J. Evaluation of disinfection of flexible nasendoscopes using Tristel wipes: a prospective single blind study. *Ann R Coll Surg Engl.* 2012;94(3):185-188. [IIIB]

274. Liming B, Funnell I, Jones A, Demons S, Marshall K, Harsha W. An evaluation of varying protocols for high-level disinfection of flexible fiberoptic laryngoscopes. *Laryngoscope.* 2014;124(11):2498-2501. [IIB]

275. Phua CQ, Mahalingappa Y, Karagama Y. Sequential cohort study comparing chlorine dioxide wipes with automated washing for decontamination of flexible nasendoscopes. *J Laryngol Otol.* 2012;126(8):809-814. [IIB]

276. Foxcroft L, Monaghan W, Faoagali J. Controlled study of the Lancer FD8 drying/storage cabinet for endoscopes. *J GENCA.* 2008;18(2):5-11. [IIB]

277. Pineau L, Villard E, Duc DL, Marchetti B. Endoscope drying/storage cabinet: interest and efficacy. *J Hosp Infect.* 2008;68(1):59-65. [IIC]

278. Wardle B. Endoscope storage cabinets. *J GENCA.* 2007;17(3):5. [IIC]

279. Rejchrt S, Cermak P, Pavlatova L, McKova E, Bures J. Bacteriologic testing of endoscopes after high-level disinfection. *Gastrointest Endosc.* 2004;60(1):76-78. [IIC]

280. Vergis AS, Thomson D, Pieroni P, Dhalla S. Reprocessing flexible gastrointestinal endoscopes after a period of disuse: is it necessary? *Endoscopy.* 2007;39(8):737-739. [IIB]

281. Marino M, Grieco G, Moscato U, et al. Is reprocessing after disuse a safety procedure for bronchoscopy?: a cross-sectional study in a teaching hospital in Rome. *Gastroenterol Nurs.* 2012;35(5):324-330. [IIB]

282. Ingram J, Gaines P, Kite R, Morgan M, Spurling S, Winsett RP. Evaluation of medically significant bacteria in colonoscopes after 8 weeks of shelf life in open air storage. *Gastroenterol Nurs.* 2013;36(2):106-111. [IIB]

283. Grandval P, Hautefeuille G, Marchetti B, Pineau L, Laugier R. Evaluation of a storage cabinet for heat-sensitive endoscopes in a clinical setting. *J Hosp Infect.* 2013;84(1):71-76. [IIIB]

284. Osborne S, Reynolds S, George N, Lindemayer F, Gill A, Chalmers M. Challenging endoscopy reprocessing guidelines: a prospective study investigating the safe shelf life of flexible endoscopes in a tertiary gastroenterology unit. *Endoscopy.* 2007;39(9):825-830. [IIIB]

285. Alfa MJ, Sepehri S, Olson N, Wald A. Establishing a clinically relevant bioburden benchmark: a quality indicator for adequate reprocessing and storage of flexible gastrointestinal endoscopes. *Am J Infect Control.* 2012;40(3):233-236. [IIIB]

286. Brock AS, Steed LL, Freeman J, Garry B, Malpas P, Cotton P. Endoscope storage time: assessment of microbial colonization up to 21 days after reprocessing. *Gastrointest Endosc.* 2015;81(5):1150-1154. [IIIB]

287. Riley R, Beanland C, Bos H. Establishing the shelf life of flexible colonoscopes. *Gastroenterol Nurs.* 2002;25(3):114-119. [IIIB]

288. Thomas LA. Essentials for endoscopic equipment. Recommended care and handling of flexible endoscopes: endoscope storage. *Gastroenterol Nurs.* 2005;28(1):45-46. [VB]

289. Nomides N, Sweeney J, Sturm L, et al. Ready for patient use? Implementing a visual cue for high level disinfected endoscopes. *Am J Infect Control.* 2014;42:S40-S41. [VA]

290. Muscarella LF. The study of a contaminated colonoscope. *Clin Gastroenterol Hepatol.* 2010;8(7):577-580.e1. [VA]

291. Saliou P, Baron R. Method for assessing the microbial contamination of GI endoscopes. *Gastrointest Endosc.* 2015;82(3):582. [VA]

292. Schmelzer M, Daniels G, Hough H. Safe storage time for reprocessed flexible endoscopes: a systematic review. *JBI Database System Rev Implement Rep.* 2015;13(9):187-243. [IIIC]

293. Guideline for health care information management. In: *Guidelines for Perioperative Practice.* Denver, CO: AORN, Inc; 2015:491-512. [IVB]

294. *State Operations Manual Appendix A—Survey Protocol, Regulations and Interpretive Guidelines for Hospitals.* Rev. 105. Washington, DC: Department of Health and Human Services, Centers for Medicare & Medicaid Services. 2014.

295. *State Operations Manual Appendix L—Guidance for Surveyors: Ambulatory Surgical Centers.* Rev. 99. Washington, DC: Department of Health and Human Services, Centers for Medicare & Medicaid Services. 2014.

296. 42 CFR 482. Conditions of participation for hospitals. 2013. US Government Publishing Office. https://www.gpo.gov/fdsys/granule/CFR-2011-title42-vol5/CFR-2011-title42-vol5-part482/content-detail.html. Accessed December 10, 2015.

297. 42 CFR 416: Ambulatory surgical services. 2013. US Government Publishing Office. https://www.gpo.gov/fdsys/granule/CFR-2011-title42-vol3/CFR-2011-title42-vol3-part416. Accessed December 10, 2015.

298. RC.01.01.01: The hospital maintains complete and accurate medical records for each individual patient. In: *Hospital Accreditation Standards.* 2014 ed. Oakbrook Terrace, IL: Joint Commission Resources; 2014.

299. MS.16 Medical record maintenance. In: *NIAHO Interpretive Guidelines and Surveyor Guidance.* 10.1 ed. Milford, OH: DNV Healthcare Inc; 2012:29.

300. RC.01.01.01: The organization maintains complete and accurate clinical records. In: *Standards for Ambulatory Care 2014: Standards, Elements of Performance, Scoring, Accreditation Policies.* Oakbrook Terrace, IL: Joint Commission Resources; 2014.

301. Clinical records and health information. In: *2014 Accreditation Handbook for Ambulatory Health Care.* Skokie, IL: Accreditation Association for Ambulatory Health Care; 2014:37-39.

302. Medical records: pre-operative medical record. In: *Regular Standards and Checklist for Accreditation of Ambulatory Surgery Facilities.* Version 14 ed. Gurnee, IL: American Association for Accreditation of Ambulatory Surgery Facilities; 2014:59-60.

303. Medical records: operating room records. In: *Regular Standards and Checklist for Accreditation of Ambulatory Surgery Facilities.* Version 14 ed. Gurnee, IL: American Association for Accreditation of Ambulatory Surgery Facilities; 2014:62-64.

304. Medical records: general. In: *Regular Standards and Checklist for Accreditation of Ambulatory Surgery Facilities.* Version 14 ed. Gurnee, IL: American Association for Accreditation of Ambulatory Surgery Facilities; 2014:58-59.

305. Medical records: general. In: *Procedural Standards and Checklist for Accreditation of Ambulatory Surgery Facilities.* Version 3 ed. Gurnee, IL: American Association for Accreditation of Ambulatory Surgery Facilities; 2011:60-61.

306. Medical records: procedure room records. In: *Procedural Standards and Checklist for Accreditation of Ambulatory Surgery Facilities.* Version 3 ed. Gurnee, IL: American Association for Accreditation of Ambulatory Surgery Facilities; 2011:64-66.

307. Standards of perioperative nursing practice. In: *Guidelines for Perioperative Practice.* Denver, CO: AORN, Inc; 2015:693-708. [IVB]

308. Jordan C, Thomas MB, Evans ML, Green A. Public policy on competency: how will nursing address this complex issue? *J Contin Educ Nurs.* 2008;39(2):86-91. [VA]

309. HR.01.05.03: Staff participate in ongoing education and training. In: *Comprehensive Accreditation Manual: CAMH for Hospitals.* 2014 ed. Oakbrook Terrace, IL: Joint Commission Resources; 2014.

310. MS.10 Continuing education. In: *NIAHO Interpretive Guidelines and Surveyor Guidance.* 10.1 ed. Milford, OH: DNV Healthcare Inc; 2012:24.

311. HR.01.05.03: Staff participate in ongoing education and training. In: *Comprehensive Accreditation Manual: CAMAC for Ambulatory Care.* 2014 ed. Oakbrook Terrace, IL: Joint Commission Resources; 2014.

312. Governance. In: *2014 Accreditation Handbook for Ambulatory Health Care.* Skokie, IL: Accreditation Association for Ambulatory Health Care; 2014:19-26.

313. Personnel: personnel records; individual personnel files. In: *Regular Standards and Checklist for Accreditation of Ambulatory Surgery Facilities.* Version 14 ed. Gurnee, IL: American Association for Accreditation of Ambulatory Surgery Facilities; 2014:75-76.

314. Personnel: knowledge, skill & CME training. In: *Regular Standards and Checklist for Accreditation of Ambulatory Surgery Facilities.* Version 14 ed. Gurnee, IL: American Association for Accreditation of Ambulatory Surgery Facilities; 2014:77-78.

STERILIZATION AND DISINFECTION

315. Personnel: personnel safety. In: *Procedural Standards and Checklist for Accreditation of Ambulatory Surgery Facilities.* Version 3 ed. Gurnee, IL: American Association for Accreditation of Ambulatory Surgery Facilities; 2011:79-80.

316. Personnel: knowledge, skill & CME training. In: *Procedural Standards and Checklist for Accreditation of Ambulatory Surgery Facilities.* Version 3 ed. Gurnee, IL: American Association for Accreditation of Ambulatory Surgery Facilities; 2011:79.

317. Jackson FW, Ball MD. Correction of deficiencies in flexible fiberoptic sigmoidoscope cleaning and disinfection technique in family practice and internal medicine offices. *Arch Fam Med.* 1997;6(6):578-582. [IIC]

318. Lunn W, Garland R, Gryniuk L, Smith L, Feller-Kopman D, Ernst A. Reducing maintenance and repair costs in an interventional pulmonology program. *Chest.* 2005;127(4):1382-1387. [VB]

319. LD.04.01.07: The hospital has policies and procedures that guide and support patient care, treatment, and services. In: *Hospital Accreditation Standards.* 2014 ed. Oakbrook Terrace, IL: Joint Commission Resources; 2014.

320. SS.1: Organization. In: *NIAHO Interpretive Guidelines and Surveyor Guidance.* 10.1 ed. Milford, OH: DNV Healthcare Inc; 2012:70-71.

321. LD.04.01.07: The organization has policies and procedures that guide and support patient care, treatment, or services. In: *Standards for Ambulatory Care 2014: Standards, Elements of performance, Scoring, Accreditation policies.* Oakbrook Terrace, IL: Joint Commission Resources; 2014.

322. Personnel: personnel safety. In: *Regular Standards and Checklist for Accreditation of Ambulatory Surgery Facilities.* Version 14 ed. Gurnee, IL: American Association for Accreditation of Ambulatory Surgery Facilities; 2014:79.

323. Personnel: personnel records. In: *Procedural Standards and Checklist for Accreditation of Ambulatory Surgery Facilities.* Version 3 ed. Gurnee, IL: American Association for Accreditation of Ambulatory Surgery Facilities; 2011:77-79.

324. 200.35: High Level Disinfection of Endoscopes. In: *Regular Standards and Checklist for Accreditation of Ambulatory Surgery Facilities.* Gurnee, IL: American Association for Accreditation of Ambulatory Surgery Facilities; 2014:28.

325. 200.40: Instrument Processing. In: *Regular Standards and Checklist for Accreditation of Ambulatory Surgery Facilities.* Gurnee, IL: American Association for Accreditation of Ambulatory Surgery Facilities; 2014:28.

326. 200.30: Procedures—Sterilization. In: *Procedural Standards and Checklist for Accreditation of Ambulatory Surgery Facilities.* Gurnee, IL: American Association for Accreditation of Ambulatory Surgery Facilities; 2011:34-36.

327. PI.03.01.01: The hospital improves performance on an ongoing basis. In: *Hospital Accreditation Standards.* 2014 ed. Oakbrook Terrace, IL: Joint Commission Resources; 2014.

328. IC.02.01.01: The hospital implements its infection prevention and control plan. In: *Comprehensive Accreditation Manual for Hospitals e-dition.* Washington, DC: The Joint Commission; August 2014.

329. IC.02.02.01: The hospital reduces the risk of infections associated with medical equipment, devices, and supplies. In: *Comprehensive Accreditation Manual for Hospitals e-dition.* Washington, DC: The Joint Commission; August 2014.

330. IC.03.01.01: The hospital evaluates the effectiveness of its infection prevention and control plan. In: *Comprehensive Accreditation Manual for Hospitals e-dition.* Washington, DC: The Joint Commission; August 2014.

331. EC.02.04.03: The hospital inspects, tests, and maintains medical equipment. In: *Hospital Accreditation Standards.* 2015 ed. Oakbrook Terrace, IL: Joint Commission Resources; 2015.

332. Quality management system. In: *NIAHO Interpretive Guidelines and Surveyor Guidance.* 10.1 ed. Milford, OH: DNV Healthcare Inc; 2012:10-16.

333. Infection prevention and control. In: *NIAHO Accreditation Requirements Interpretive Guidelines & Surveyor Guidance.* 10.1 ed. Milford, OH: DNV Healthcare; 2012.

334. Physical environment. PE.1 Facility. In: *NIAHO Accreditation Requirements Interpretive Guidelines & Surveyor Guidance Revision.* 10.1 ed. Milford, OH: DNV Healthcare; 2012.

335. PI.03.01.01: The organization improves performance. In: *Standards for Ambulatory Care 2014: Standards, Elements of Performance, Scoring, Accreditation Policies.* Oakbrook Terrace, IL: Joint Commission Resources; 2014.

336. IC.02.01.01: The organization implements infection prevention and control activities. In: *Comprehensive Accreditation Manual for Ambulatory Care e-dition.* Washington, DC: The Joint Commission; August 2014.

337. IC.02.02.01: The organization reduces the risk of infections associated with medical equipment, devices, and supplies. In: *Comprehensive Accreditation Manual for Ambulatory Care e-dition.* Washington, DC: The Joint Commission; August 2014.

338. IC.03.01.01: The organization evaluates the effectiveness of its infection prevention and control activities. In: *Comprehensive Accreditation Manual for Ambulatory Care e-dition.* Washington, DC: The Joint Commission; August 2014.

339. EC.02.04.03: The organization inspects, tests, and maintains medical equipment. In: *Ambulatory Accreditation Standards.* 2015 ed. Oakbrook Terrace, IL: Joint Commission Resources; 2015.

340. Quality managment and improvement. In: *Accreditation Handbook for Ambulatory Health Care.* Skokie, IL: Accreditation Association for Ambulatory Health Care; 2014:32-36.

341. Infection prevention and control and safety. In: *Accreditation Handbook for Ambulatory Health Care.* Skokie, IL: Accreditation Association for Ambulatory Health Care; 2014:40-43.

342. Faciliites and environment. In: *Accreditation Handbook for Ambulatory Health Care.* Skokie, IL: Accreditation Association for Ambulatory Health Care; 2014:44-45.

343. Quality assessment/quality improvement: quality improvement. In: *Regular Standards and Checklist for Accreditation of Ambulatory Surgery Facilities.* Version 14 ed. Gurnee, IL: American Association for Accreditation of Ambulatory Surgery Facilities; 2014:65.

344. Quality assessment/quality improvement: unanticipated operative sequelae. In: *Regular Standards and Checklist for Accreditation of Ambulatory Surgery Facilities.* Version 14 ed. Gurnee, IL: American Association for Accreditation of Ambulatory Surgery Facilities; 2014:68-70.

345. Operating room policy, environment, and procedures: equipment. In: *Regular Standards and Checklist for Accreditation of Ambulatory Surgery Facilities.* Version 14 ed. Gurnee, IL: American Association for Accreditation of Ambulatory Surgery Facilities; 2014:45.

STERILIZATION AND DISINFECTION

346. Evans P. Cystoscope reprocessing safety: one practice's experience. *AAACN Viewpoint.* 2014;36(2):10-11. [VB]

347. Angtuaco TL, Oprescu FG, Lal SK, et al. Universal precautions guideline: self-reported compliance by gastroenterologists and gastrointestinal endoscopy nurses—a decade's lack of progress. *Am J Gastroenterol.* 2003;98(11):2420-2423. [IIIC]

348. Baudet JS, Martín JM, Sánchez del Rio A, Aguirre-Jaime A. Occupational risk prevention in endoscopy units: a pending issue. *Rev Esp Enferm Dig.* 2011;103(2):83-88. [IIIB]

349. Joint Working Group of the Hospital Infection Society (HIS) and the Public Health Laboratory Service (PHLS). Rinse water for heat labile endoscopy equipment. *J Hosp Infect.* 2002;51(1):7-16. [IVA]

350. Kovaleva J, Degener JE, van der Mei HC. Methylobacterium and its role in health care-associated infection. *J Clin Microbiol.* 2014;52(5):1317-1321. [VA]

351. Phillips G, McEwan H, Butler J. Quality of water in washer-disinfectors. *J Hosp Infect.* 1995;31(2):152-154. [VC]

352. Marek A, Smith A, Peat M, et al. Endoscopy supply water and final rinse testing: five years of experience. *J Hosp Infect.* 2014;88(4):207-212. [VA]

353. Cooke RP. Hazards of water. *J Hosp Infect.* 2004;57(4):290-293. [VB]

354. Cooke RP, Whymant-Morris A, Umasankar RS, Goddard SV. Bacteria-free water for automatic washer-disinfectors: an impossible dream? *J Hosp Infect.* 1998;39(1):63-65. [IIIC]

355. Curtis B, Cooke RPD, Whymant-Morris A, Umasankar RS, Goddard SV. Testing water quality for automatic washer-disinfectors (multiple letters) [5]. *J Hosp Infect.* 1999;42(1):74-76. [VB]

356. Falkinham JO 3rd. Hospital water filters as a source of *Mycobacterium avium* complex. *J Med Microbiol.* 2010;59(Pt 10):1198-1202. [VC]

357. Rossetti R, Lencioni P, Innocenti F, Tortoli E. Pseudoepidemic from *Mycobacterium gordonae* due to a contaminated automatic bronchoscope washing machine. *Am J Infect Control.* 2002;30(3):196-197. [VB]

358. Khalsa K, Smith A, Morrison P, et al. Contamination of a purified water system by *Aspergillus fumigatus* in a new endoscopy reprocessing unit. *Am J Infect Control.* 2014;42(12):1337-1339. [VB]

359. Mitchell DH, Hicks LJ, Chiew R, Montanaro JC, Chen SC. Pseudoepidemic of *Legionella pneumophila* serogroup 6 associated with contaminated bronchoscopes. *J Hosp Infect.* 1997;37(1):19-23. [VB]

360. Kiely JL, Sheehan S, Cryan B, Bredin CP. Isolation of *Mycobacterium chelonae* in a bronchoscopy unit and its subsequent eradication. *Tuber Lung Dis.* 1995;76(2):163-167. [VC]

361. Phillips L. Identification and resolution of contamination causes found in flexible endoscopes. *Gastroenterol Nurs.* 1997;20(1):9-11. [VC]

362. Hubner NO, Assadian O, Poldrack R, et al. Endowashers: an overlooked risk for possible post-endoscopic infections. GMS *Krankenhhyg Interdiszip.* 2011;6(1):o13. [IIB]

363. Robertson P, Smith A, Mead A, et al. Risk-assessment-based approach to patients exposed to endoscopes contaminated with *Pseudomonas spp. J Hosp Infect.* 2015;90(1):66-69. [VB]

364. Phillips G, McEwan H, McKay I, Crowe G, McBeath J. Black pigmented fungi in the water pipe-work supplying endoscope washer disinfectors. *J Hosp Infect.* 1998;40(3):250-251. [VC]

365. Imbert G, Seccia Y, La Scola B. *Methylobacterium sp.* bacteraemia due to a contaminated endoscope. *J Hosp Infect.* 2005;61(3):268-270. [VC]

366. Choice Framework for local Policy and Procedures 01-06—Decontamination of flexible endoscopes: Validation and verification. 2013. UK Department of Health. https://www.gov.uk/government/uploads/system/uploads/attachment_data/file/148562/CFPP_01-06_Validation_Final.pdf. Accessed December 10, 2015. [IVB]

367. Chiu KW, Fong TV, Wu KL, et al. Surveillance culture of endoscope to monitor the quality of high-level disinfection of gastrointestinal reprocessing. *Hepatogastroenterology.* 2010;57(99-100):531-534. [IIC]

368. Corne P, Godreuil S, Jean-Pierre H, et al. Unusual implication of biopsy forceps in outbreaks of *Pseudomonas aeruginosa* infections and pseudo-infections related to bronchoscopy. *J Hosp Infect.* 2005;61(1):20-26. [VB]

369. Qiu L, Zhou Z, Liu Q, Ni Y, Zhao F, Cheng H. Investigating the failure of repeated standard cleaning and disinfection of a *Pseudomonas aeruginosa*-infected pancreatic and biliary endoscope. *Am J Infect Control.* 2015;43(8):e43-e46. [VB]

370. Hunter J, Epstein L. *Epi-Aid trip report: cluster of plasmid-mediated AmpC-producing carbapenem-resistant Enterobacteriaceae (CRE)—Washington, 2014.* Atlanta, GA: Department of Health and Human Services, Centers for Disease Control and Prevention; 2014. [VA]

371. DiazGranados CA, Jones MY, Kongphet-Tran T, et al. Outbreak of *Pseudomonas aeruginosa* infection associated with contamination of a flexible bronchoscope. *Infect Control Hosp Epidemiol.* 2009;30(6):550-555. [IIIA]

372. Lee DH, Kim DB, Kim HY, et al. Increasing potential risks of contamination from repetitive use of endoscope. *Am J Infect Control.* 2015;43(5):e13-e17. [IIB]

373. ASGE Technology Committee; Komanduri S, Abu Dayyeh BK, et al. Technologies for monitoring the quality of endoscope reprocessing. *Gastrointest Endosc.* 2014;80(3):369-373. [VB]

374. Obee PC, Griffith CJ, Cooper RA, Cooke RP, Bennion NE, Lewis M. Real-time monitoring in managing the decontamination of flexible gastrointestinal endoscopes. *Am J Infect Control.* 2005;33(4):202-206. [IIIB]

375. Visrodia KH, Ofstead CL, Yellin HL, Wetzler HP, Tosh PK, Baron TH. The use of rapid indicators for the detection of organic residues on clinically used gastrointestinal endoscopes with and without visually apparent debris. *Infect Control Hosp Epidemiol.* 2014;35(8):987-994. [IIB]

376. Petersen BT. Monitoring of endoscope reprocessing: accumulating data but best practices remain undefined. *Infect Control Hosp Epidemiol.* 2014;35(8):995-997. [VA]

377. Alfa MJ. Monitoring and improving the effectiveness of cleaning medical and surgical devices. *Am J Infect Control.* 2013;41(5 Suppl):S56-S59. [VA]

378. Alfa MJ, Fatima I, Olson N. The adenosine triphosphate test is a rapid and reliable audit tool to assess manual cleaning adequacy of flexible endoscope channels. *Am J Infect Control.* 2013;41(3):249-253. [IIA]

379. Ofstead CL, Wetzler HP, Doyle EM, et al. Persistent contamination on colonoscopes and gastroscopes detected by biologic cultures and rapid indicators despite reprocessing performed in accordance with guidelines. *Am J Infect Control.* 2015;43(8):794-801. [IIB]

380. Hansen D, Benner D, Hilgenhoner M, Leisebein T, Brauksiepe A, Popp W. ATP measurement as method to monitor the quality of reprocessing flexible endoscopes. *Ger Med Sci.* 2004;2:o04. [IIIB]

381. Alfa MJ, Olson N, Degagne P, Simner PJ. Development and validation of rapid use scope test strips to determine the efficacy of manual cleaning for flexible endoscope channels. *Am J Infect Control.* 2012;40(9):860-865. [IIIA]

382. Fernando G, Collignon P, Beckingham W. ATP bioluminescence to validate the decontamination process of gastrointestinal endoscopes. *Healthc Infect.* 2014;19(2):59-64. [IIA]

383. Fushimi R, Takashina M, Yoshikawa H, et al. Comparison of adenosine triphosphate, microbiological load, and residual protein as indicators for assessing the cleanliness of flexible gastrointestinal endoscopes. *Am J Infect Control.* 2013;41(2):161-164. [IIIB]

384. Sciortino CV Jr, Xia EL, Mozee A. Assessment of a novel approach to evaluate the outcome of endoscope reprocessing. *Infect Control Hosp Epidemiol.* 2004;25(4):284-290. [IIC]

385. Whiteley GS, Derry C, Glasbey T. Sampling plans for use of rapid adenosine triphosphate (ATP) monitoring must overcome variability or suffer statistical invalidity. *Infect Control Hosp Epidemiol.* 2015;36(2):236-237. [VA]

386. Visrodia KH, Ofstead CL, Wetzler HP, Tosh PK, Baron TH. Reply to Whiteley et al. *Infect Control Hosp Epidemiol.* 2015;36(2):237-238. [VA]

387. Alfa MJ, Fatima I, Olson N. Validation of adenosine triphosphate to audit manual cleaning of flexible endoscope channels. *Am J Infect Control.* 2013;41(3):245-248. [IIB]

388. Whiteley GS, Derry C, Glasbey T, Fahey P. The perennial problem of variability in adenosine triphosphate (ATP) tests for hygiene monitoring within healthcare settings. *Infect Control Hosp Epidemiol.* 2015;36(6):658-663. [IIIA]

389. Alfa MJ, Olson N, Murray BL. Comparison of clinically relevant benchmarks and channel sampling methods used to assess manual cleaning compliance for flexible gastrointestinal endoscopes. *Am J Infect Control.* 2014;42(1):e1-e5. [IIA]

390. Bommarito M, Thornhill GA, Morse DJ. A multi-site field study evaluating the effectiveness of manual cleaning of flexible endoscopes with an ATP detection system. *Am J Infect Control.* 2013;41(6 Suppl):S24. [IIIC]

391. Beilenhoff U, Neumann CS, Rey JF, et al. ESGE-ESGENA guideline for quality assurance in reprocessing: microbiological surveillance testing in endoscopy. *Endoscopy.* 2007;39(2):175-181. [IVC]

392. Chiu KW, Tsai MC, Wu KL, Chiu YC, Lin MT, Hu TH. Surveillance cultures of samples obtained from biopsy channels and automated endoscope reprocessors after high-level disinfection of gastrointestinal endoscopes. *BMC Gastroenterol.* 2012;12:120. [IIA]

393. Saviuc P, Picot-Gueraud R, Shum Cheong Sing J, et al. Evaluation of the quality of reprocessing of gastrointestinal endoscopes. *Infect Control Hosp Epidemiol.* 2015;36(9):1017-1023. [IIIA]

394. Tunuguntla A, Sullivan MJ. Monitoring quality of flexible endoscope disinfection by microbiologic surveillance cultures. *Tenn Med.* 2004;97(10):453-456. [VB]

395. Merighi A, Contato E, Scagliarini R, et al. Quality improvement in gastrointestinal endoscopy: microbiologic surveillance of disinfection. *Gastrointest Endosc.* 1996;43(5):457-462. [VC]

396. Moses FM, Lee J. Surveillance cultures to monitor quality of gastrointestinal endoscope reprocessing. *Am J Gastroenterol.* 2003;98(1):77-81. [VA]

397. Bretthauer M, Jorgensen A, Kristiansen BE, Hofstad B, Hoff G. Quality control in colorectal cancer screening: systematic microbiological investigation of endoscopes used in the NORCCAP (Norwegian Colorectal Cancer Prevention) trial. *BMC Gastroenterol.* 2003;3:15. [IIIA]

398. Buss AJ, Been MH, Borgers RP, et al. Endoscope disinfection and its pitfalls—requirement for retrograde surveillance cultures. *Endoscopy.* 2008;40(4):327-332. [VA]

399. Hong KH, Lim YJ. Recent update of gastrointestinal endoscope reprocessing. *Clin Endosc.* 2013;46(3):267-273. [VA]

400. Kovaleva J, Meessen NE, Peters FT, et al. Is bacteriologic surveillance in endoscope reprocessing stringent enough? *Endoscopy.* 2009;41(10):913-916. [VA]

401. Chiu KW, Lu LS, Wu KL, et al. Surveillance culture monitoring of double-balloon enteroscopy reprocessing with high-level disinfection. *Eur J Clin Invest.* 2012;42(4):427-431. [IIIC]

402. Bisset L, Cossart YE, Selby W, et al. A prospective study of the efficacy of routine decontamination for gastrointestinal endoscopes and the risk factors for failure. *Am J Infect Control.* 2006;34(5):274-280. [IIIA]

403. Infection Control Devices Branch Division of General and Restorative Devices Office of Device Evaluation Center for Devices and Radiological Health Food and Drug Administration. Guidance on Premarket Notification [510(k)] Submissions for Sterilizers Intended for Use in Health Care Facilities. March 1993. US Food and Drug Administration. http://www.fda.gov/downloads/medicaldevices/deviceregulationandguidance/guidancedocuments/ucm081341.pdf. Accessed December 10, 2015.

404. Addendum to: Guidance on Premarket Notification [510(k)] Submissions for Sterilizers Intended for Use in Health Care Facilities. September 19, 1995. US Food and Drug Administration. http://www.fda.gov/RegulatoryInformation/Guidances/ucm080300.htm. Accessed December 10, 2015.

405. Fraser TG, Reiner S, Malczynski M, Yarnold PR, Warren J, Noskin GA. Multidrug-resistant *Pseudomonas aeruginosa* cholangitis after endoscopic retrograde cholangiopancreatography: failure of routine endoscope cultures to prevent an outbreak. *Infect Control Hosp Epidemiol.* 2004;25(10):856-859. [IIIC]

406. Nelson DB. Recent advances in epidemiology and prevention of gastrointestinal endoscopy related infections. *Curr Opin Infect Dis.* 2005;18(4):326-330. [VB]

407. Gillespie EE, Kotsanas D, Stuart RL. Microbiological monitoring of endoscopes: 5-year review. *J Gastroenterol Hepatol.* 2008;23(7 Pt 1):1069-1074. [IIIB]

408. Lu LS, Wu KL, Chiu YC, Lin MT, Hu TH, Chiu KW. Swab culture monitoring of automated endoscope reprocessors after high-level disinfection. *World J Gastroenterol.* 2012;18(14):1660-1663. [IIIA]

409. Muscarella LF. Investigation and prevention of infectious outbreaks during endoscopic retrograde cholangiopancreatography. *Endoscopy.* 2010;42(11):957-959. [VA]

410. Interim duodenoscope surveillance protocol. Centers for Disease Control and Prevention. http://www.cdc.gov/hai/organisms/cre/cre-duodenoscope-surveillance-protocol.html. Accessed December 10, 2015. [VA]

411. H0245 01: *ECRI institute Recommends Culturing Duodenoscopes as a Key Step to Reducing CRE Infections* [Hazard Report]. Plymouth Meeting, PA: ECRI Institute. March 3, 2015. [VA]

412. Interim duodenoscope sampling method. Centers for Disease Control and Prevention. http://www.cdc.gov/hai/settings/lab/lab-duodenoscope-sampling.html. Accessed December 10, 2015. [VB]

413. Interim duodenoscope culture method. Centers for Disease Control and Prevention. http://www.cdc.gov/

STERILIZATION AND DISINFECTION

hai/settings/lab/lab-duodenoscope-culture-method.html. Accessed December 10, 2015. [VB]

414. Banerjee S, Nelson DB, Dominitz JA, et al. Reprocessing failure. *Gastrointest Endosc.* 2007;66(5):869-871. [IVA]

415. Patel PR, Srinivasan A, Perz JF. Developing a broader approach to management of infection control breaches in health care settings. *Am J Infect Control.* 2008;36(10):685-690. [VA]

416. Weber DJ, Rutala WA. Assessing the risk of disease transmission to patients when there is a failure to follow recommended disinfection and sterilization guidelines. *Am J Infect Control.* 2013;41(5):S67-S71. [VA]

417. Holodniy M, Oda G, Schirmer PL, et al. Results from a large-scale epidemiologic look-back investigation of improperly reprocessed endoscopy equipment. *Infect Control Hosp Epidemiol.* 2012;33(7):649-656. [IIIA]

418. MAUDE—Manufacturer and User Facility Device Experience. https://www.accessdata.fda.gov/scripts/cdrh/cfdocs/cfmaude/search.cfm. Accessed December 9, 2015.

Acknowledgements

LEAD AUTHOR
Sharon A. Van Wicklin, MSN, RN, CNOR, CRNFA(E), CPSN-R, PLNC
Senior Perioperative Practice Specialist
AORN Nursing Department
Denver, Colorado

CONTRIBUTING AUTHORS
Ramona Conner, MSN, RN, CNOR
Editor-in-Chief, Guidelines for Perioperative Practice
AORN Nursing Department
Denver, Colorado

Cynthia Spry, MA, MS, RN, CNOR(E), CSPDT
Independent Consultant
New York, New York

The authors and AORN thank Marie A. Bashaw, DNP, RN, NEA-BC, CNOR, Assistant Professor, Wright State University College of Nursing and Health, Dayton, Ohio; Cori L. Ofstead, MSPH, President and CEO, Ofstead & Associates, Inc, St Paul, Minnesota; John E. Eiland, RN, MS, Senior Research Associate, Ofstead & Associates, Inc, St Paul, Minnesota; Judith Goldberg, DBA, MSN, RN, CNOR, CSSM, CHL, CRCST, Director, Patient Care Services, Perioperative and Procedural Services, Lawrence + Memorial Hospital, New London, Connecticut; Sheryl P. Eder, MSN, RN, CNOR, CRCST, Director, Sterile Processing Department, LeeSar Regional Service Center, Fort Myers, Florida; Angela Hewitt, MD, MS, Associate Professor, Division of Infectious Diseases, Associate Medical Director, Department of Infection Control and Epidemiology, Associate Medical Director, Nebraska Biocontainment Unit, Director, Infectious Diseases Outpatient Clinics, University of Nebraska Medical Center, Omaha; Heather A. Hohenberger, BSN, RN, CIC, CNOR, CPHQ, Quality Improvement Consultant, Perioperative Services, Indiana University Health, Indianapolis; and Donna Ford, MSN, RN-BC, CNOR, CRCST, Nursing Education Specialist, Mayo Clinic, Rochester, Minnesota, for their assistance in developing this guideline.

PUBLICATION HISTORY
Originally published February 1993, *AORN Journal.*
Revised November 1997; published January 1998. Reformatted July 2000.
Revised November 2002; published in *Standards, Recommended Practices, and Guidelines,* 2003 edition.
Reprinted February 2003, *AORN Journal.*
Revised November 2008; published in *Perioperative Standards and Recommended Practices,* 2009 edition.
Reformatted September 2012 for publication in *Perioperative Standards and Recommended Practices,* 2013 edition.
Minor editing revisions made in November 2014 for publication as Guideline for Cleaning and Processing Flexible Endoscopes and Endoscope Accessories in *Guidelines for Perioperative Practice,* 2015 edition.
Revised February 2016 for publication in *Guidelines for Perioperative Practice,* 2016 edition.
Minor editing revisions made in October 2016 for publication in *Guidelines for Perioperative Practice,* 2017 edition.

STERILIZATION AND DISINFECTION

GUIDELINE FOR MANUAL CHEMICAL HIGH-LEVEL DISINFECTION

The Guideline for Manual Chemical High-Level Disinfection has been approved by the AORN Guidelines Advisory Board. It was presented as a proposed guideline for comments by members and others. The guideline is effective January 15, 2018. The recommendations in the guideline are intended to be achievable and represent what is believed to be an optimal level of practice. Policies and procedures will reflect variations in practice settings and/or clinical situations that determine the degree to which the guideline can be implemented. AORN recognizes the many diverse settings in which perioperative nurses practice; therefore, this guideline is adaptable to all areas where operative or other invasive procedures may be performed.

Purpose

High-level disinfection is a process that deactivates all types of microorganisms with the exception of bacterial spores and prions.[1] The purpose of this document is to provide guidance to health care personnel for

- performing safe and effective manual chemical high-level disinfection of reusable semicritical items and
- preventing patient and health care worker injury associated with the handling and use of liquid chemical high-level disinfectants (HLDs).

The Spaulding classification system defines reusable medical items as critical, semicritical, or noncritical.[2] The level of processing required (ie, sterilization; high-, intermediate-, or low-level disinfection) is based on the manner in which the item is to be used.[2] Items that contact mucous membranes (eg, endocavity ultrasound probes) or nonintact skin are considered to be semicritical.[2] Spaulding[2] recommended that semicritical items be processed by sterilization or, at a minimum, by high-level disinfection.

Failure to correctly perform high-level disinfection can lead to transmission of pathogens via contaminated medical or surgical devices.[3,4] The vast majority of patient infections and exposures related to processing medical or surgical devices have involved high-level disinfection of reusable semicritical items.[3] In a recent safety report, The Joint Commission[5] noted that processes for high-level disinfection of equipment and devices are frequently found to be inadequate, especially in ambulatory care centers and decentralized locations in hospitals. Breaches in the performance of high-level disinfection can result in outbreaks of viral or bacterial organisms.[5]

High-level disinfectants are harmful to human tissue and the environment.[6] Health hazards associated with the use of HLDs vary from minor irritation of mucous membranes to more serious injury (eg, chemical burns).[1] Health care organizations are responsible for informing health care workers about chemical hazards in the workplace and for implementing measures to reduce personnel exposure and mitigate identified hazards.[7] Implementing safe processes for handling and using chemical HLDs is essential for preventing injury to both patients and personnel.[6]

Guidance for the following topics is outside of the scope of this document:

- processing critical items for sterilization;
- processing semicritical items using thermal high-level disinfection (ie, pasteurization);
- processing flexible endoscopes and accessories and other semicritical items using mechanical (ie, automated) processes for high-level disinfection or liquid chemical sterilization (See the AORN Guideline for Processing Flexible Endoscopes[8]);
- processing endocavity ultrasound probes and other semitcritical items using nebulized hydrogen peroxide mist;
- processing semicritical items potentially contaminated with prions;
- processing noncritical items for intermediate- or low-level disinfection;
- assessing risk and notifying patients regarding high-level disinfection failures; and
- using specific HLDs.

Evidence Review

A medical librarian conducted a systematic literature search of the Ovid MEDLINE®, CINAHL®, and Scopus® databases and the Cochrane Database of Systematic Reviews for meta-analyses, randomized and nonrandomized trials and studies, and systematic and nonsystematic reviews. The initial search was conducted in August 2014, and an additional search was performed in December 2016. In each search, the results were limited to literature published in English in the 5 years prior to the search date. The medical librarian established continuing alerts on the topics covered in this guideline and provided relevant results to the lead author. During the development of this guideline, the author requested supplementary searches for topics not included in the original search as well as articles and other sources that were discovered during the evidence-appraisal process. The lead author and the medical librarian also identified and obtained relevant guidelines from government agencies, standards-setting bodies, and other professional organizations.

Search terms included *high-level disinfection, semi-critical item or device, automated endoscope reprocessor, Spaulding schema or criteria, peracetic acid, hydrogen peroxide, glutaraldehyde, ortho-phthalaldehyde, thermal or heat disinfection, pasteurization, medical device washer, equipment contamination or reuse, anesthesia equipment, disease*

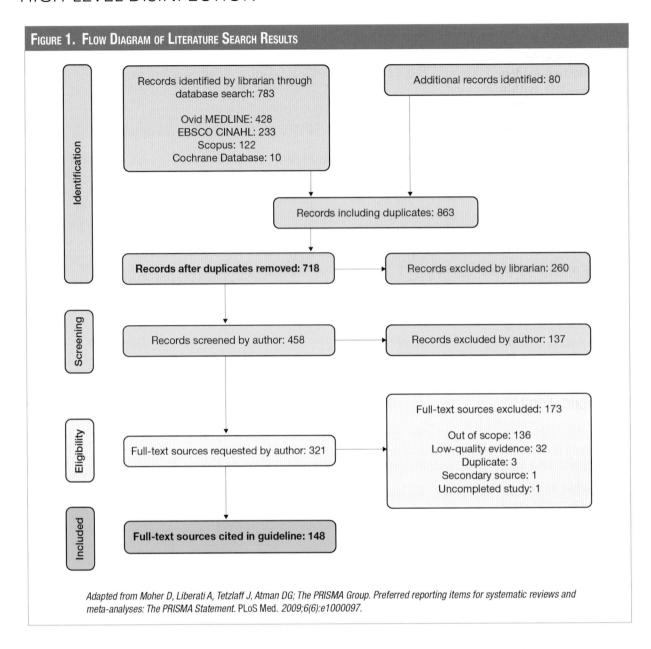

FIGURE 1. FLOW DIAGRAM OF LITERATURE SEARCH RESULTS

Records identified by librarian through database search: 783

Ovid MEDLINE: 428
EBSCO CINAHL: 233
Scopus: 122
Cochrane Database: 10

Additional records identified: 80

Records including duplicates: 863

Records after duplicates removed: 718

Records excluded by librarian: 260

Records screened by author: 458

Records excluded by author: 137

Full-text sources requested by author: 321

Full-text sources excluded: 173

Out of scope: 136
Low-quality evidence: 32
Duplicate: 3
Secondary source: 1
Uncompleted study: 1

Full-text sources cited in guideline: 148

Identification

Screening

Eligibility

Included

Adapted from Moher D, Liberati A, Tetzlaff J, Atman DG; The PRISMA Group. Preferred reporting items for systematic reviews and meta-analyses: The PRISMA Statement. PLoS Med. 2009;6(6):e1000097.

transmission, cross-infection, biofilm, bacteria, micro-bial, spores, fungus, prion, Creutzfeldt-Jacob syndrome, Klebsiella, Pseudomonas aeruginosa, carbapenemase-producing Enterobacteriaceae, Staphylococcus aureus, Pseudomonas putida, Mycobacterium massiliense, storage, shelf life, cabinet, transport, protective clothing, eye protective devices, occupational disease or exposure, hypersensitivity, health personnel, medical waste disposal, waste management, and documentation. Subject headings and key words for specific types of endoscopes also were included.

Included were research and non-research literature in English, complete publications, and publication dates within the time restriction when available. Excluded were non-peer-reviewed publications, older evidence within the time restriction when more recent evidence was available, and research and non-research evidence related to thermal high-level disinfection, specific disinfectants, workplace safety and occupational illness not

related to high-level disinfection, sterile processing activities not associated with high-level disinfection, environmental and surface disinfection, and high-level disinfection of single-use devices. Editorials, news items, and brief items were excluded. Low-quality evidence was excluded when higher-quality evidence was available, and literature outside the time restriction was excluded when literature within the time restriction was available. In total, 321 research and non-research sources of evidence were identified for possible inclusion, and of these, 148 are cited in the guideline (Figure 1).

Articles identified in the search were provided to the project team for evaluation. The team consisted of the lead author and one evidence appraiser. The lead author and the evidence appraiser critically appraised each reference using the AORN Research or Non-Research Evidence Appraisal Tools as appropriate. The literature was independently evaluated and appraised according to the strength and quality of the evidence.

Each reference was then assigned an appraisal score. The appraisal score is noted in brackets after each reference, as applicable.

The collective evidence supporting each intervention and activity within a specific recommendation was summarized and the AORN Evidence Rating Model was used to rate the strength of the evidence. Factors considered in the review of the collective evidence were the quality of the evidence, the quantity of similar evidence on a given topic, and the consistency of evidence supporting a recommendation. The evidence rating is noted in brackets after each intervention and activity statement.

Note: *The evidence summary table is available at http://www.aorn.org/evidencetables/.*

Editor's note: *MEDLINE is a registered trademark of the US National Library of Medicine's Medical Literature Analysis and Retrieval System, Bethesda, MD. CINAHL, Cumulative Index to Nursing and Allied Health Literature, is a registered trademark of EBSCO Industries, Birmingham, AL. Scopus is a registered trademark of Elsevier B.V., Amsterdam, The Netherlands.*

Recommendation I

Reusable semicritical items may be processed using manual methods when manual chemical high-level disinfection is the only processing method recommended by the manufacturer.

Some reusable semicritical items cannot be sterilized or mechanically processed.

I.a.   The health care organization should appoint an interdisciplinary team of key stakeholders to conduct a risk assessment to identify reusable semicritical items used within the facility that may be processed by manual chemical high-level disinfection when recommended by the device manufacturer. *[5: Benefits Balanced with Harms]*

Having an interdisciplinary team conduct a risk assessment allows for a comprehensive, holistic review of the organization's needs by individuals with a range of relevant knowledge and skills and a variety of perspectives.

I.b.   Reusable semicritical items that are manufacturer-validated for sterilization should be sterilized, if possible. *[3: Moderate Evidence]*

Reusable semicritical items processed by high-level disinfection present a greater risk of disease transmission than items processed by sterilization.[3] Sterilization eliminates all microbial life, including pathogenic and nonpathogenic microorganisms and bacterial spores.[2] Correctly sterilized and handled items are rarely associated with patient infection[9]; however, some sterilization methods can affect the material and mechanical properties of the item. Sterilization may not be possible for all reusable semicritical devices in all health care facilities.

I.c.   The interdisciplinary team should conduct a risk assessment to determine whether each semicritical item that secondarily enters sterile tissue or the vascular system (ie, via a mucous membrane) should be sterile. *[3: Moderate Evidence]*

Sterilization provides the greatest margin of safety and assurance that the item is safe for use.[3,10] Because of the heavy microbial load that may be present on some semicritical items (eg, flexible gastrointestinal endoscopes) and the difficulty of cleaning and disinfecting items with lumens and long, narrow channels, current high-level disinfection processes may not be adequate to ensure all items that enter sterile tissue via a mucous membrane are safe for use on patients.[11]

High-level disinfection may not effectively eliminate some viruses, bacteria, mycobacteria, and protozoa.[12] There have been reports of increased resistance profiles in some bacteria (including mycobacteria) to glutaraldehyde-based HLDs. Lorena et al[13] and Duarte et al[14] reported on an outbreak of postoperative infections due to *Mycobacterium massiliense* BRA100 involving 197 patients. All involved hospitals (N = 63) were using 2% glutaraldehyde for high-level disinfection of endoscopic instruments unable to tolerate steam sterilization. The outbreak resolved when use of the glutaraldehyde-based HLD was discontinued.

Tschudin-Sutter et al[15] detected *Pseudomonas aeruginosa* in 23 of 73 routine samples obtained from endoscopes and in 29 of 99 subsequent samples obtained from the endoscopes. The investigators found that the glutaraldehyde-based HLD used for disinfection of the endoscopes demonstrated no activity against *P aeruginosa* when used at the manufacturer's recommended concentration and temperature. They concluded the *P aeruginosa* was resistant to the glutaraldehyde-based disinfectant.

Some HLDs may not be effective against certain types of viral pathogens.[12] Meyers et al[16] conducted a nonexperimental laboratory study of the susceptibility of infectious human papillomavirus (HPV) type 16 to commonly used clinical disinfectants (N = 11), including glutaraldehyde and ortho-phalaldehyde. The researchers found that both glutaraldehyde and ortho-phalaldehyde did not demonstrate any significant reduction of infectivity of the virus. Because HLDs are commonly used to disinfect vaginal and rectal endocavity ultrasound probes, further research is warranted, and when possible, sterilization may be the preferred method for processing these and other semicritical items.[10]

I.d.   Reusable semicritical items that are manufacturer-validated for high-level disinfection or liquid chemical sterilization using automated methods should be mechanically processed.[8] *[1: Strong Evidence]*

885

The collective evidence shows that using automated methods (ie, mechanical processing) for high-level disinfection or sterilization of reusable semicritical items improves cleaning effectiveness, increases efficiency, and minimizes personnel exposure to hazardous substances (eg, chemical, biological).[1,17,18] Mechanical processors contain the disinfection process, reducing worker exposure to HLDs.[19-24] Mechanical processing methods can also be more successfully monitored for quality and consistency than manual methods of high-level disinfection.[1,17,18]

Ubhayawardana et al[18] conducted a nonexperimental study in the endotherapy unit of a university teaching hospital in Sri Lanka to evaluate the quality of manual processes for high-level disinfection of flexible side-view endoscopes. The researchers collected and analyzed 102 samples obtained from the tip and working channel of the endoscopes after manual chemical high-level disinfection. The results of the study showed that 20% (n = 21) of tips and 9% (n = 10) of channels were culture-positive. The researchers concluded that using mechanical processing methods for high-level disinfection increased processing effectiveness, reduced bioburden, and decreased human variability.

I.e. Endocavity ultrasound probes should be processed by high-level disinfection or sterilization.[1,3,25-34] *[1: Strong Evidence]*

Endocavity ultrasound probes are introduced into a variety of body orifices (eg, vagina, rectum, trachea).[25] These probes contact mucosal tissue and are therefore classified as semicritical devices that require cleaning and a minimum of high-level disinfection.[2,25] The Centers for Disease Control and Prevention (CDC)[1] and the American Institute of Ultrasound Medicine[26] recommend that endocavity probes, used with or without a sheath or cover, be processed with high-level disinfection at a minimum.

The collective evidence shows that endocavity ultrasound probes present a high risk of contamination with pathogenic microorganisms after ultrasound procedures and that disinfection by methods other than high-level disinfection or sterilization may not be sufficient to eliminate the organisms even when a sheath or cover is used.[27-31,35]

Westerway et al[27] conducted a blinded prospective study in the ultrasound unit of a private clinic and public hospital in Australia. They collected and analyzed a total of 129 samples from transvaginal and transabdominal ultrasound probes. The samples from the probes were collected after use (transvaginal: n = 28; transabdominal: n = 32), after low-level disinfection (transvaginal: n = 26; transabdominal: n = 32), and after high-level disinfection (transvaginal: n = 9; transabdominal: n = 2). The researchers found that although a sheath or cover was used with all of the probes, 60% (n = 19) of the transabdominal and 14% (n = 4) of the transvaginal probes showed bacterial contamination after use. Contaminating pathogenic species on the transabdominal probes included *Staphylococcus haemolyticus* and *Staphylococcus warneri*. After low-level disinfection, 3% (n = 1) of the transabdominal probes and 4% (n = 1) of the transvaginal probes remained contaminated. No contaminating bacteria were detected on any of the probes after high-level disinfection.

Inadequately disinfected endocavity probes also increase the risk for transmission of HIV, hepatitis B virus, hepatitis C virus, *Neisseria gonorrhea*, *Chlamydia trachomatis*, *Trichomonas vanginalis*, and HPV.[28] In a random probability distribution computer simulation performed to produce hypothetical cohorts for a population of 4 million annual ultrasound examinations in France, Leroy et al[29] estimated the number of patients infected by HIV, herpes simplex virus, hepatitis B virus, hepatitis C virus, HPV, cytomegalovirus, and *C trachomatis*. The simulation showed that despite the use of a sheathed probe and low-level disinfection, the probability of infection from a contaminated probe ranged from 1% to 6%, depending on the pathogen. For cases of HIV, this would result in approximately 60 infected patients per year. The researchers recommended using high-level disinfection for vaginal and rectal endocavity ultrasound probes.

Casalegno et al[30] conducted a prospective study in two phases in the gynecology department of a university hospital in France. In the first phase, the researchers collected and analyzed 217 samples from endocavity ultrasound probes after these were used for patient examination. In the second phase, the researchers collected and analyzed 200 samples before the probe was used for patient examination. Despite the use of sheathed probes, human DNA was detected in 36 (18%) of the post-examination samples, and 61 (28%) of the pre-examination samples. Seven post-examination samples (3.5%) were HPV positive, and six pre-examination samples (2.8%) were HPV positive, with four samples (2%) positive for high-risk HPV. The researchers recommended replacing the current method of processing (ie, low-level disinfection with quaternary ammonium compound wipes) with a more stringent high-level disinfection process.

In a prospective study conducted in a French radiology center, M'Zali et al[31] collected and analyzed a total of 300 samples from endocavity ultrasound probes for HPV (n = 100), *C trachomatis* (n = 100), and commensal or environmental bacteria (n = 100). The samples were collected after disinfection of the probes with wipes impregnated with a quaternary ammonium compound and chlorhexidine. The researchers found HPV on 13% of the samples (n = 13), *C trachomatis* on 20% of the samples (n = 20), and commensal or environmental bacterial flora on 86% of the samples (n = 86). The researchers concluded that endocavity ultrasound probes remained contaminated after low-level disinfection.

Notably, not all HLDs may be effective against all pathogens that could potentially be found on endocavity ultrasound probes. Ryndock et al[35] conducted a nonexperimental study to compare the efficacy of immersion in a liquid chemical HLD (ie, ortho-phalaldehyde) and exposure to nebulized hydrogen peroxide mist against HPV type 16 and HPV type 18 on endocavity ultrasound probes. The researchers found the liquid chemical HLD had only minimal efficacy against HPV. The HPV type 16 was highly resistant to the ortho-phalaldehyde, demonstrating only a $0.52\ \log_{10}$ reduction in viral infectivity. The HPV type 18 was also highly resistant to the ortho-phalaldehyde, demonstrating only a $0.39\ \log_{10}$ reduction in viral activity. The nebulized hydrogen peroxide mist method showed greater than $5\ \log_{10}$ reductions for both HPV type 16 and HPV type 18.

Recommendation II

The interdisciplinary team should select HLDs that will be used within the health care organization.

It is the responsibility of the health care organization to select HLDs using a systematic evaluation process that includes compliance with federal, state, and local regulations and a review of product safety, effectiveness, materials compatibility, and cost-effectiveness[36] (See the AORN Guideline for Medical Device and Product Evaluation[37]).

II.a.   The interdisciplinary team should select a US Food and Drug Administration (FDA)-cleared HLD for high-level disinfection of reusable semicritical items. *[1: Regulatory Requirement]*

The FDA regulates HLDs used to process medical devices and surgical instruments.[38] Notably, the FDA uses the term *liquid chemical sterilant* in conjunction with the term *high-level disinfectant* based on the position that, given sufficient time, many HLDs are also indicated for use as liquid chemical sterilants.[38,39] The reader can refer to the "FDA-cleared sterilants and high-level disinfectants with general claims for processing reusable medical and dental devices"[38] for additional information.

II.b.   The interdisciplinary team should select the HLD based on a risk assessment of the potential health hazards associated with the disinfectant.[40] *[3: Moderate Evidence]*

Health hazards associated with exposure to HLDs can be serious. Reported reactions have included

○ headache,[20,23]
○ ocular irritation and conjunctivitis,[20,23]
○ nasal membrane irritation and rhinitis,[20]
○ cough,[20]
○ skin staining,[22,41]
○ contact dermatitis,[20,24,42-45]
○ occupational asthma,[20,24,45-51] and
○ allergic reactions including anaphylaxis.[22,52,53]

Input from a variety of stakeholders can assist health care organizations with decisions related to potential health hazards and selection of HLDs for use in the facility.[54]

Rideout et al[54] surveyed personnel from 51 acute care hospitals in Canada to gather information about the decision-making process for selection of HLDs. The researchers found the decision about which HLD to use generally involved more than one person or personnel from more than one department. Members of the team selecting HLDs for use in the facility most frequently included personnel performing high-level disinfection and personnel from occupational health, infection prevention, and regional health departments. The researchers also found the greatest concern of team members selecting HLDs was protecting the health of individuals using the HLDs.

II.c.   The interdisciplinary team should assess compatibility of the HLD and the HLD manufacturer's instructions for use (IFU) with existing semicritical items and current processes, products, and equipment used for high-level disinfection within the facility. *[5: Benefits Balanced with Harms]*

Having an interdisciplinary team evaluate compatibility requirements helps ensure that the new HLD will be compatible with existing products and processes, or if not compatible, helps clarify the need for additional items or equipment necessary for use of the HLD being evaluated.

Recommendation III

The interdisciplinary team should determine the locations where HLDs will be stored within the health care organization.

Confining HLDs to designated storage locations may help to mitigate the risk for spills and exposure of personnel.

III.a.   High-level disinfectants must be stored in accordance with

○ safety data sheet (SDS) information;
○ manufacturer's IFU; and
○ federal, state, and local regulations[7] (eg, requirements for storage of flammable or combustable items, patient and personnel safety requirements).

[1: Regulatory Requirement]

Safe and compliant storage of HLDs reduces the potential for exposure and injury to patients and personnel.

III.b. High-level disinfectants should be stored in a secure location.[36] *[4: Limited Evidence]*

Storing HLDs in secure locations may help prevent accidental damage to the HLD containers and unauthorized removal or use of HLDs.[36]

III.c. High-level disinfectants should be stored within the manufacturer's recommended temperature range.[36] *[4: Limited Evidence]*

Manufacturers' IFU recommend product storage at specified temperatures.

III.d. Activated HLDs should be stored in covered containers[20] with tight-fitting lids.[19,24] *[3: Moderate Evidence]*

Keeping containers tightly closed helps prevent spills; reduces the potential for personnel exposure to vapors; and decreases evaporation of the HLD, which could lead to a change in HLD concentration.[36]

III.d.1. Containers of activated HLDs should be clearly labeled with the contents and reuse-life dates.[36] *[4: Limited Evidence]*

Labeling containers of activated HLDs communicates to others the contents and period of time the HLD solution may be used.

III.d.2. If it is necessary to transport activated HLDs from one designated location to another, they should be transported in closed containers with tight-fitting lids[19,21] that are clearly labeled with the contents.[36] *[3: Moderate Evidence]*

Transporting HLDs in closed containers with tight-fitting lids reduces the potential for spills.[19] Labeling containers communicates the contents to others.

Recommendation IV

Manual chemical high-level disinfection should occur in areas controlled and maintained to support processing activities.

Performing manual chemical high-level disinfection in locations that are controlled and maintained to support high-level disinfection processes minimizes contamination of the environment, reduces the risk for cross contamination, decreases personnel exposure to hazardous chemicals, improves efficiency, and enhances process control and monitoring (See the AORN Guideline for Processing Flexible Endoscopes[8]).

IV.a. The interdisciplinary team should determine the locations where manual chemical high-level disinfection will occur within the health care organization. *[5: Benefits Balanced with Harms]*

Confining manual chemical high-level disinfection to locations determined by an interdisciplinary team may help reduce the risk for patient and personnel exposure.

IV.b. High-level disinfection should occur in an area where access is limited to authorized personnel.[19] *[3: Moderate Evidence]*

Confining high-level disinfection processes reduces the potential for exposure of unauthorized personnel.[19,21,36]

IV.b.1. Warning signs may be posted at the entrance to the disinfection area.[19] *[3: Moderate Evidence]*

Warning signs may reduce the potential for exposure by preventing unauthorized personnel from entering the area.[19,36]

IV.c. Manual chemical high-level disinfection should occur in a designated area that is separate from locations where patient care activities are performed.[1] *[1: Strong Evidence]*

Performing high-level disinfection in designated areas helps prevent contamination of patient care areas and reduces the potential for adverse exposure effects on patients.[36] Local exhaust and ventilation systems used in areas where high-level disinfection is performed might not be recommended for areas where patient care activities are carried out.[36]

IV.d. High-level disinfection should occur in a designated clean area that is separate from the decontamination area. *[4: Limited Evidence]*

Separating the clean area from the area where devices are cleaned and prepared for high-level disinfection reduces the risk of device contamination that might occur when both clean and contaminated processing activities are performed in a single area.[36] Droplets and aerosols created during cleaning of soiled instruments or other items can cause cross contamination of nearby clean items or surfaces.[55]

IV.d.1. If the clean and decontamination areas are located within the same room, the area where high-level disinfection will occur should be separated from the decontamination area by
- a minimum of 3 ft (0.9 m)[56] and
- a separating wall or a barrier that extends a minimum of 4 ft (1.2 m) above the sink rim.[57]

[3: Moderate Evidence]

Hota et al[58] demonstrated that contaminated water droplets had the ability to travel a distance of 1 m (39 inches). Based on the results of this report, the Facility Guidelines Institute determined it is unlikely that microorganisms from a decontamination area would be disseminated by air over distances longer than 1 m because they would be contained within water droplets.[57] Separating decontamination and clean work areas by a distance of at least 3 ft aligns with current recommendations from the CDC that patients who require droplet precautions are separated by at least

3 ft from other patients.[59] Having a wall or physical barrier for separation of the decontamination area provides protection and minimizes the potential for contamination of items that have been processed by high-level disinfection.

IV.e. The workflow for high-level disinfection processes should be designed to facilitate a unidirectional flow that prevents recontamination of the item during or after completion of the disinfection process.[56,60] *[2: High Evidence]*

A unidirectional flow improves efficiency and helps contain contaminants within the decontamination area.[56,60]

IV.f. High-level disinfection should occur in an area with sufficient space to permit freedom of movement of personnel during the disinfection process.[19,61] *[3: Moderate Evidence]*

Crowded work spaces may increase the potential for spills.[19]

IV.g. High-level disinfection should not be performed in areas near potential sources of contamination.[36] *[4: Limited Evidence]*

Performing high-level disinfection in areas near scrub sinks, hoppers, waste or linen containers, or other potential sources of contamination increases the potential for cross contamination.[36]

IV.h. High-level disinfection should not be performed in high-traffic areas.[36] *[4: Limited Evidence]*

Performing high-level disinfection in high-traffic areas increases the potential for spills and cross contamination.[36]

Recommendation V

Personnel should prepare reusable semicritical items to be processed by high-level disinfection according to the device manufacturer's IFU.

The device manufacturer is responsible for ensuring the device can be effectively cleaned and for providing validated cleaning instructions.[36] Preparing the device for high-level disinfection by effective cleaning, rinsing, purging, and drying is a critical step necessary to reduce bioburden and moisture to a level that does not present a challenge to subsequent high-level disinfection.

V.a. If precleaning is recommended by the device manufacturer, personnel should preclean the device in accordance with the device manufacturer's IFU. *[5: Benefits Balanced with Harms]*

Precleaning recommendations and procedures vary among manufacturers. Deviations from the manufacturer's IFU may result in insufficient cleaning of the item or high-level disinfection failure.[8]

V.a.1. Precleaning should occur at the point of use. *[1: Strong Evidence]*

Precleaning at the point of use assists with moistening, diluting, softening, and

removing organic soils and reducing the formation of biofilm that might prevent effective high-level disinfection.[1,8,55,62]

V.b. After precleaning at the point of use or after use, personnel must transport contaminated items to be prepared for high-level disinfection in a closed container or closed transport cart.[63] *[1: Regulatory Requirement]*

Transporting items to the decontamination area in a manner that prevents exposing personnel to blood, body fluids, and other potentially infectious materials is a regulatory requirement.[63]

V.b.1. The container or cart must be leak proof,
- puncture resistant,
- large enough to contain all contents, and
- labeled with a fluorescent orange or orange red label containing a biohazard legend.[63]

[1: Regulatory Requirement]

Securing and labeling containers of biohazardous material is a regulatory requirement and communicates to others that the contents may be biohazardous.[63]

V.b.2. Semicritical items should be kept wet or damp, but not submerged in liquid during transport. *[3: Moderate Evidence]*

Keeping the items wet helps dilute, soften, and ease removal of organic soils.[64] Dried organic materials and debris can make the item more difficult to clean and potentially lead to the formation of biofilm.[64] Submerging the device in liquid during transport may increase the risk of spillage and could lead to fluid invasion if the device has an unknown leak.

V.c. After transport of items to the decontamination area, personnel should leak test items designed to be leak tested in accordance with the device and leak-testing equipment manufacturers' IFU.[8] *[1: Strong Evidence]*

Not every device requires leak testing. Leak testing helps detect breaches in the integrity of the device being tested.[60] Leak testing also helps reduce damage and repair costs and decreases the potential for patient infection or injury that might result from use of a device that is not completely sealed.

V.d. After transport of items to the decontamination area or after leak testing, personnel should clean the items in accordance with the device manufacturers' IFU.[8,55] *[1: Strong Evidence]*

The collective evidence shows that cleaning is essential to successful high-level disinfection because HLDs are inactivated by or less effective in the presence of organic material.[1,4,6,26,33,34,65] There have been reports of endocavity ultrasound probes or portions of endocavity ultrasound probes not being cleaned or being inadequately cleaned before disinfection, leading to residual contamination remaining on the

HIGH-LEVEL DISINFECTION

device.[32,66,67] Reducing the level of microbial contamination on the item is necessary when performing high-level disinfection because there is a lower margin of safety (ie, a reduced ability to inactivate high levels of bacteria) compared with sterilization.[68] Effective cleaning can reduce bioburden to a level that does not inhibit high-level disinfection.[6]

Some HLDs may fix organic soil and blood to the surface of the item being disinfected.[69] Effective cleaning and removal of fixed soils before manual chemical high-level disinfection is necessary for successful high-level disinfection.[69] In a nonexperimental laboratory study, Kampf et al[69] found that exposure to disinfectants and liquid chemical sterilants led to variable amounts of blood fixation on the surface of surgical instruments processed by high-level disinfection. The glutaraldehyde-based disinfectants showed blood fixation between 77% and 100%. The peracetic acid-based disinfectants showed fixation rates between 19% and 78%. The researchers concluded that effective cleaning before disinfection was essential for effective high-level disinfection or liquid chemical sterilization.

V.e. After cleaning, personnel should rinse the item and flush any lumens or channels with utility water in accordance with the device manufacturer's IFU.[8] *[2: High Evidence]*

Thorough rinsing and flushing helps dislodge and remove residual debris and cleaning solutions.[70] If not adequately rinsed, enzymatic cleaning solutions may contribute to protein buildup within device channels.[70] Unless prohibited by the device manufacturer's IFU, using utility water is acceptable during the cleaning process. In some cases, a final rinse with water treated to remove organic and inorganic substances may be recommended by the device manufacturer to prevent staining and help ensure effective high-level disinfection or sterilization.

V.f. After rinsing, personnel should remove visible moisture from the external surfaces of the device using a clean, lint-free cloth.[8,60] *[2: High Evidence]*

Water remaining on the surface of the device can dilute the HLD.[36] If sufficiently diluted, the concentration of the active ingredients in the HLD can be reduced to a level that is too low to effectively eliminate certain microorganisms within the recommended exposure time.[36]

V.f.1. Device lumens should be purged with instrument air in accordance with the device manufacturer's IFU.[8,60] *[2: High Evidence]*

Water remaining in the lumens of devices can dilute the HLD.[36]

V.g. After removing visible moisture and purging, personnel should inspect the item for cleanliness, damage, and function.[8,9,55,60,71-73] *[2: High Evidence]*

Inspection helps identify residual soil or organic material that might put patients at risk for infection and allows soiled items to be removed from service until they are sufficiently cleaned.[9,71,73] Inspection also identifies damaged and defective items and allows them to be removed from service until repaired or replaced.[72]

V.g.1. Items should be inspected using lighted magnification.[8,55,60] *[2: High Evidence]*

An item that appears clean may harbor debris that cannot be seen without magnification.[8,55] Lighted magnification may increase the ability of personnel to identify soiled or damaged items.[8,55]

V.g.2. Internal channels and lumens may be inspected using an endoscopic camera or a borescope.[8,55] *[2: High Evidence]*

Endoscopic cameras and borescopes penetrate the lumen and allow for improved inspection.[8] Retained organic material in lumens can lead to patient injury.[9,73]

V.g.3. Soiled items should be recleaned.[71] *[1: Strong Evidence]*

Residual soil remaining on the item can prevent effective high-level disinfection.[1,4,6,26,33,34,65]

V.g.4. Damaged or defective items should be removed from service and repaired or replaced.[55,60] *[2: High Evidence]*

Using damaged or defective instruments or devices can cause or contribute to patient injury.[72]

Recommendation VI

Personnel must prepare and use HLDs in accordance with the disinfectant and device manufacturers' IFU.[74]

Label claims, contraindications for use, and requirements for effective high-level disinfection are unique to each HLD. Failing to follow the manufacturer's IFU can jeopardize the effectiveness of the disinfection process or the performance of the device.[36] In the United States, HLDs are regulated under the Federal Insecticide, Fungicide, and Rodenticide Act (FIFRA).[74,75] Under FIFRA, any substance or mixture of substances intended to prevent, destroy, repel, or mitigate any pest (including microorganisms, but excluding those in or on living humans or animals) is required to be registered before sale or distribution.[74,75]

The device manufacturer is responsible for registering the device, ensuring the device can be effectively disinfected, and providing validated instructions for high-level disinfection.[36] Users of products registered under FIFRA are required to follow the manufacturer's IFU.[74,75] Failure to follow the manufacturer's IFU is

STERILIZATION AND DISINFECTION

890

considered a misuse of the product and is potentially subject to enforcement action under FIFRA.[74,75]

VI.a.   The interdisciplinary team should monitor processes for manual chemical high-level disinfection and the use of HLDs within the health care organization. *[4: Limited Evidence]*

Oversight of high-level disinfection processes by an interdisciplinary team supports safe use of HLDs and implementation of work practices that will reduce occupational and patient exposure to HLDs.[36] Reducing the risk of patient infection associated with inadequate disinfection or sterilization of medical devices is a regulatory requirement[76-79] and an accreditation agency standard for both hospitals[80,81] and ambulatory settings.[81-84]

VI.b.   Before performing high-level disinfection, personnel should verify compatibility of the HLD with the item to be processed by high-level disinfection.[6,26] *[2: High Evidence]*

Using an HLD that is not compatible with the item may void the device warranty.[6] Not all HLDs are safe for use with all endocavity ultrasound probes.[26] Incompatibility between a device and a disinfectant may result in changes in appearance, integrity, and performance of the device.[3,6] Materials such as metals, alloys, and plastics and their polymers can be adversely affected by exposure to certain chemicals.[36] Some materials might become brittle and crack.[36] Others (eg, polymeric adhesives) might dissolve. Still others might swell or become distorted.[36] Any of these effects could cause the device to malfunction or fail.[36]

VI.c.   Personnel should use activated HLDs at the concentration recommended by the disinfectant manufacturer.[36,85] *[3: Moderate Evidence]*

The minimum recommended concentration (MRC) or minimum effective concentration (MEC) and reuse-life date are established by the manufacturer.[6] Using the HLD at the recommended concentration reduces the potential for inadequate disinfection.[36]

Howie et al[86] conducted a quasi-experimental laboratory study to determine the efficacy of optimal and suboptimal concentrations of two HLDs—glutaraldehyde and activated hydrogen peroxide—for inactivating enveloped and non-enveloped viruses, bacteria, yeast, and mycobacteria. The researchers found that when used at the manufacturer's recommended concentration, 2.6% glutaraldehyde inactivated all test organisms except a specific *Mycobacterium chelonae* strain. When used at the manufacturer's recommended concentration, 7% activated hydrogen peroxide inactivated all test organisms, including *M chelonae*. A substantial number and variety of microorganisms survived exposure when the disinfectants were diluted. The researchers noted that these findings underscore the importance of and need for quality

assurance monitoring of the HLD concentration before each use because HLDs can be used for multiple days. Dilution, evaporation, chemical breakdown, neutralization from accumulated proteins, or other actions that may limit the biocidal activity can occur before the reuse-life date of the HLD has been reached.

VI.c.1.   A test strip or other FDA-cleared testing device specific to the disinfectant and the active ingredient in the disinfectant should be used before each use of the HLD solution.[6,36,85] *[2: High Evidence]*

Solution test strips are used to determine whether the concentration of the active ingredient in the HLD is above or below the MRC or MEC.[36] The concentration of the active ingredient in an HLD solution decreases with dilution by water, the presence of organic or inorganic soil, time, evaporation of the solution, and exposure of the solution to light.[6,36] High-level disinfectant solution potency cannot be guaranteed when the solution concentration falls below the MRC or MEC.[36,87]

VI.c.2.   Test strips or testing devices should be used and stored in accordance with the test strip or testing device manufacturer's IFU.[36,85] *[3: Moderate Evidence]*

VI.c.3.   Efficacy testing of the test strip or testing device should be performed as recommended by the test strip or testing device manufacturer's IFU.[6,36] *[2: High Evidence]*

Test strips can deteriorate and become less accurate over time.[6]

VI.c.4.   If the test strip or testing device indicates the concentration of the active ingredient is inadequate, the solution should be discarded, even if the designated reuse-life date has not been reached.[6,36] *[2: High Evidence]*

VI.d.   Personnel should use activated HLDs at the temperature recommended by the disinfectant manufacturer.[36,85,87] *[3: Moderate Evidence]*

VI.d.1.   The temperature of the HLD solution should be verified before each use with a thermometer calibrated within the applicable range. *[4: Limited Evidence]*

Monitoring the solution temperature helps ensure effectiveness of the HLD and confirms the HLD is being used at the manufacturer's recommended temperature.[36]

VI.d.2.   The accuracy of thermometers used to measure temperature of the HLD solution should be verified at established intervals. *[5: Benefits Balanced with Harms]*

Verifying accuracy of thermometers helps ensure correct temperature measurement.

VI.e. Personnel should use activated HLDs at the volume recommended by the disinfectant manufacturer.[36] *[4: Limited Evidence]*

Using the HLD at the recommended volume helps ensure complete immersion and contact with all surfaces of the device.[36]

VI.e.1. If it is necessary to add activated HLD solution to an existing container of activated HLD solution (eg, the solution has evaporated, there is insufficient volume of solution to immerse the device), personnel should
- consult the HLD manufacturer's IFU to verify adding activated solution is an acceptable practice,
- test the activated HLD solution after the additional solution has been added to verify MRC or MEC, and
- not use the activated HLD solution beyond the original solution container's reuse-life date.

[5: Benefits Balanced with Harms]

VI.f. Personnel should use the type of soaking container recommended by the HLD manufacturer. *[4: Limited Evidence]*

Using the type of container recommended by the manufacturer helps ensure there is no interaction between the container and the active or inert ingredients in the HLD.[36]

VI.f.1. The soaking container should be large enough to contain the volume of solution recommended by the HLD manufacturer while reducing the surface contact area to the smallest amount possible.[19] *[3: Moderate Evidence]*

Using the smallest container possible that holds the HLD manufacturer's recommended volume of solution helps reduce the amount of HLD that is used and decreases the potential for exposure and spills.

VI.g. Personnel should discard activated HLDs on or before the manufacturer's recommended reuse-life date, even if the concentration of the ingredients is at or above the MRC or MEC.[36] *[4: Limited Evidence]*

Following the manufacturer's IFU for the period of time the disinfectant can be used may help prevent use of an ineffective HLD solution.

VI.h. Personnel should inspect the HLD solution before use.[36] The HLD solution should be discarded if precipitates are present or if the solution appears cloudy.[36] *[4: Limited Evidence]*

Inspection before use may help prevent use of a contaminated HLD solution. The presence of precipitates or a cloudy solution may indicate the solution has been contaminated.[36]

VI.i. Personnel should handle the HLD solution in a manner that minimizes agitation of the solution and personnel exposure.[19] *[3: Moderate Evidence]*

Reducing solution agitation helps decrease exposure levels.[19] Solution agitation may be increased during tasks such as
- activating and pouring HLD solutions into or out of soaking containers,
- opening the soaking container,
- immersing items to be disinfected,
- handling soaked items,
- removing items from the soaking container, and
- disposing of HLD solutions into the sanitary sewer.[19]

VI.j. Personnel should disassemble the item to be processed by high-level disinfection according to the manufacturer's IFU.[1,88] *[1: Strong Evidence]*

Disassembling the item helps ensure all surfaces are exposed to the disinfectant. Rutala et al[88] conducted a nonexperimental laboratory study to investigate the effectiveness of high-level disinfection of a probe used in ultrasound-guided prostate biopsy. The researchers inoculated the interior lumen of the biopsy needle guide, the outside surface of the biopsy needle guide, and the interior lumen of the ultrasound probe with 107 colony-forming units (CFU) of *P aeruginosa*. After inoculation, the researchers immersed the probe in an HLD for the manufacturer's recommended contact time and then assessed the probe for microbial contamination. They found that disinfection (defined by the researchers as a reduction in bacterial load greater than 7 $\log_{10}$ CFU) could only be achieved if the needle guide was removed from the probe. When the needle guide was left in the probe during immersion, disinfection was not achieved (ie, the reduction in bacterial load was only 1 $\log_{10}$ CFU). The disinfection failure occurred because the microorganisms that contaminated the surfaces of the probe lumen and outside surfaces of the needle guide were not exposed to the HLD and were able to survive the disinfection process. The researchers recommended disassembling the device before high-level disinfection. However, some items cannot be disassembled or are designed by the device manufacturer to remain assembled during high-level disinfection or sterilization.

VI.k. Personnel should immerse the item to be disinfected in the HLD solution.[1] *[1: Strong Evidence]*

Complete immersion helps ensure all surfaces of the device are in contact with the HLD. It is not possible to ensure that all surfaces of an incompletely immersed item (eg, an item that floats on the surface of the disinfectant solution) will be effectively processed by high-level disinfection.[1]

Some cryosurgical probes are not fully immersible.[1,3] Manufacturers of endocavity ultrasound transducers may advise against submersion of the transducer handle because only the head portion of an ultrasound transducer contacts the patient's mucous membranes[25] and because the handle is not fully sealed.[32] The handle does not directly contact the patient, but it does contact the gloved hands of the technician during positioning of the probe and is therefore in need of high-level disinfection due to potential contamination from mucous membrane secretions.[25]

In a prospective cross-sectional study conducted at an ultrasound clinic and public hospital in Australia, Ngu et al[32] collected samples from 152 transducer handles that were cleaned and dried after routine use. The researchers randomly separated the transducers into two study groups. In the first group (n = 77), the transducer head was processed by high-level disinfection using 2.4% glutaraldehyde, but the handle was not disinfected (per usual practice). In the second group (n = 75), both the transducer head and handle were disinfected using a nebulized hydrogen peroxide mist. The researchers found that residual bacteria, including pathogenic bacteria, persisted on 80.5% (n = 62) of the handles that were not disinfected. Bacterial contamination on the handles that were disinfected was significantly lower at 5.3% (n = 4). The researchers concluded that ultrasound transducer handles could become contaminated with clinically significant organisms if they were not completely immersed or were processed using a method that did not disinfect the handle.

VI.k.1. If a portion of the device cannot be immersed in the HLD,
- the portion of the device that can be immersed should be immersed, and
- the portion of the device that cannot be immersed should be disinfected in accordance with the device manufacturer's IFU.[1,3]

[1: Strong Evidence]

VI.k.2. Items that cannot be immersed in the HLD should be
- replaced with fully immersible items or
- processed by high-level disinfection using the device manufacturer's validated methods that do not involve immersion in a liquid HLD.[1,3] *[1: Strong Evidence]*

High-level disinfection of the entire device reduces the potential for cross contamination and transmission of infection.[25] Methods found to be acceptable for high-level disinfection of both the endocavity probe head and handle include ultraviolet C light[89,90] or nebulized hydrogen peroxide mist.[3,10,33,91-93]

VI.l. Personnel should flush and completely fill lumens and ports with the HLD solution while the item is immersed.[94] *[3: Moderate Evidence]*

Eliminating air bubbles and flushing and filling lumens and ports with the HLD solution helps ensure that all surfaces of the item are exposed to the disinfectant. Rutala et al[94] conducted a nonexperimental laboratory study of channeled cystoscopes to examine the effectiveness of immersion compared with immersion and perfusion of the channel with the HLD. The researchers inoculated the channel of a flexible cystoscope with a suspension of test organisms (ie, vancomycin-resistant *Enterobacteriaceae*, carbapenem-resistant *Enterobacteriaceae*, *Klebsiella pneumoniae*), allowed the cystoscope to dry, and then immersed the cystoscope in an HLD for the manufacturer's recommended contact time. They found that high-level disinfection (defined by the researchers as a reduction in bacterial load greater than 7 $\log_{10}$ CFU) did not occur unless the cystoscope channel was actively perfused with the HLD while the device was completely submerged. Failure to fully perfuse the channel achieved only minimal reduction in bacterial contamination; however, complete inactivation (ie, a reduction equal to 8 $\log_{10}$ CFU) was achieved when the channel was actively perfused.

VI.l.1. Moving parts should be actuated while the item is immersed in the HLD solution. *[5: Benefits Balanced with Harms]*

Actuating moving parts helps ensure that all surfaces of the item are exposed to the disinfectant.

VI.m. Personnel should immerse the item to be disinfected in the HLD solution for the full duration of the disinfectant manufacturer's recommended contact time.[1,26,85] *[1: Strong Evidence]*

Immersion for the full duration of the recommended contact time helps ensure that all surfaces of the item are exposed to the disinfectant and that any microorganisms on the device are completely inactivated.

VI.m.1. If there is a discrepancy between the disinfectant and device manufacturers' recommended contact times, the device should be immersed for the longer of the recommended contact times. *[5: Benefits Balanced with Harms]*

Using the longer recommended contact time may provide a margin of safety and help ensure the device is adequately disinfected.

VI.m.2. A timing device should be used to verify the exposure time. *[5: Benefits Balanced with Harms]*

Using a timing device helps ensure the item was exposed to the HLD for the full duration of the HLD manufacturer's recommended contact time.

VI.n. Rinsing sinks or containers should be located as close as possible to the HLD soaking tray.[19] *[3: Moderate Evidence]*

Locating the rinsing sinks or soaking containers in close proximity to the HLD soaking tray minimizes the potential for dripping HLDs onto other surfaces.[19]

VI.o. After high-level disinfection, personnel should thoroughly rinse and flush the item as described in the device manufacturer's IFU.[6,26] *[2: High Evidence]*

The collective evidence shows that thorough rinsing and flushing helps prevent patient injury associated with HLD remaining on the device.[6,52,53,95,96] High-level disinfectants not completely rinsed from the device can injure mucous membranes.[6] There have been reports of serious patient injury including toxic anterior segment syndrome,[95] anaphylaxis,[52,53] and bowel injury[96,97] associated with inadequate rinsing of medical devices and surgical instruments processed by high-level disinfection. Thorough rinsing reduces the potential for patient exposure to the disinfectant chemical.[6] Thorough rinsing also decreases the potential for HLDs to be absorbed into and subsequently released from the device.[52,53]

VI.o.1. The device should be rinsed with critical or sterile water. *[4: Limited Evidence]*

Using critical or sterile water reduces the potential for introducing microorganisms onto the disinfected device. Some manufacturers recommend rinsing with utility water; however, utility water may contain microorganisms and endotoxins that can be deposited on the item during the rinsing process.[98] Tissue contaminated with endotoxins can experience severe inflammation.[98]

Gillespie et al[99] reported an outbreak of *P aeruginosa* in four patients who underwent transrectal ultrasound-guided prostate biopsy. The authors concluded that rinsing the biopsy needle guide, a device intended for use on the sterile field, with utility water was a cause of the outbreak.

VI.o.2. If not defined in the HLD manufacturer's IFU, the interdisciplinary team should establish the frequency for changing rinse water and rinsing containers. At a minimum, the rinse water and rinsing containers should be changed daily. *[5: Benefits Balanced with Harms]*

Some HLD manufacturer's do not specify how often the rinse water and rinsing containers are to be changed. In that case, the frequency of changing rinse water and rinsing containers is best determined by an interdisciplinary team because the number and type of devices undergoing high-level disinfection is unique to the facility.

Wendelboe et al[100] investigated an outbreak of seven *P aeruginosa* infections associated with outpatient cystoscopy performed by a urologist in New Mexico from January to April 2007. The investigators found multiple breaches in processing procedures, including rinsing of the cystoscope in unsterile water after high-level disinfection. Specifically, sterile water was placed in a rinsing container and replaced every 2 weeks or when it began to smell. The outbreak was resolved when improved procedures for processing flexible cystoscopes were implemented.

VI.p. When removing the device from the HLD and when rinsing the device, personnel should handle it in a controlled manner that prevents the disinfected item from coming into contact with the soaking or rinsing containers. *[5: Benefits Balanced with Harms]*

Handling the device in a controlled manner prevents contamination of the device by unintended contact with surfaces or items.

VI.q. After rinsing, if the device will be stored for future use, personnel should
  ○ dry the external surfaces of the device with a clean, lint-free cloth and
  ○ dry device lumens with instrument air.[1,6]
[1: Strong Evidence]

Moisture remaining on the external or internal surfaces of the device can facilitate microbial growth during storage.[1,6,70] Clean, filtered air is required for drying lumens and small channels without introducing contaminants into the clean device.

VI.r. If the device will be placed on a sterile field, personnel should rinse, dry, contain, transport and place the device on the sterile field using sterile technique.[1,3] *[1: Strong Evidence]*

Using sterile technique is necessary to maintain a sterile field (See the AORN Guideline for Sterile Technique).[101] Notably, a sterile field ceases to be sterile when a device that has not been sterilized is placed upon it.

VI.r.1. The device may be covered with a sterile sheath or drape (eg, camera drape).[1,3] *[1: Strong Evidence]*

Covering the device with a sterile sheath or drape may help to maintain a sterile field and reduce the risk of patient infection.[1,3]

Recommendation VII

Personnel should protect reusable semicritical items that have been processed by high-level disinfection from contamination until the item is delivered to the point of use.[1]

Protecting disinfected items is necessary to prevent contamination.

VII.a. Personnel should transport items that are processed by high-level disinfection immediately before use to the point of use using aseptic technique.[36] *[4: Limited Evidence]*

Using aseptic technique during transport to the point of use helps prevent contamination of the device.

VII.b. Personnel should transport and store items that are processed by high-level disinfection and stored before use in accordance with the device manufacturer's IFU and in a manner that protects the device from damage or contamination. *[5: Benefits Balanced with Harms]*

Correct storage and protection of items that have been processed by high-level disinfection may reduce the potential for contamination of processed devices.

VII.b.1. Devices that have been processed by high-level disinfection and will be stored before use should be clearly identifiable with a distinct visual cue as processed and ready for use.[1] *[1: Strong Evidence]*

Identifying items that have been processed by high-level disinfection and are ready for use may help to prevent use of a contaminated device.[1]

VII.b.2. If the item will be stored in a cabinet or other storage device, the storage cabinet or storage device manufacturer's IFU should be followed. *[3: Moderate Evidence]*

Following the storage cabinet manufacturer's IFU may prevent contamination of the item being stored in the cabinet and reduce the risk of patient infection. Stigt et al[102] reported a pseudo-outbreak of *Stenotrophomonas maltophilia* in the cultures of bronchial aspirations obtained from three patients via two different bronchoscopes. The pseudo-outbreak was caused by inadequate disinfection of ultrasound endoscopes. The contaminated ultrasound endoscopes subsequently contaminated bronchoscopes stored in the same drying cabinet via the connecting tubes in the cabinet. The authors found the humidity of the air being blown through the channels in the drying cabinet was higher than that recommended by the drying cabinet manufacturer. Excessively humidified air led to inadequate drying that promoted the outgrowth of residential microorganisms in the inadequately disinfected ultrasound endoscopes.

VII.b.3. Personnel should visually inspect storage cabinets and disinfected devices for cleanliness before the item is placed into or removed from storage.[60]
- If there is any evidence of contamination of the disinfected device (eg, soil, moisture), the item should be reprocessed before use.[60]
- If there is any evidence of contamination of the storage cabinet (eg, wet spots, soil, odor), all items in the cabinet should be removed and reprocessed and the cabinet should be cleaned.[60] *[2: High Evidence]*

Visible soil in the storage cabinet may indicate that one or more of the stored items is contaminated. Soil in the cabinet could also contaminate other items stored in the cabinet.[60] Reprocessing items that might be contaminated helps ensure they are safe for use.

VII.b.4. Personnel should wear clean, latex-safe gloves when handling items that have been processed by high-level disinfection and when transporting them to and from the storage cabinet. *[1: Strong Evidence]*

Wearing gloves may lessen the risk of contamination of processed items by the hands of personnel. Using latex-safe gloves can minimize latex exposure and the risk of reactions in both health care workers and patients.[103] Sterile gloves are not required for handling processed items unless they are intended to be placed on a sterile field.

Recommendation VIII

The health care organization must provide a safe environment for personnel who handle or use HLDs.[7]

High-level disinfectants are harmful to human tissue and the environment; therefore, implementing safe processes for handling and use is essential for the safety of patients and personnel.[6] It is a regulatory requirement that employers have a program to ensure that information about the identification, hazards, and composition of chemicals and safe handling practices and emergency control measures for chemicals is communicated and readily available to personnel.[7]

VIII.a. The health care organization must develop a written hazard communication program for all chemicals used within the facility.[7] *[1: Regulatory Requirement]*

It is a regulatory requirement that employers provide their employees with information about the hazards of all chemicals used in the workplace.[7]

VIII.a.1. The hazard communication program must include a list of the hazardous chemicals present in the facility and information about
- the specific hazards of each chemical,
- the SDS, and
- how the chemicals will be labeled.[7]
[1: Regulatory Requirement]

VIII.a.2. Safety data sheets for each chemical used in the facility must be readily accessible to personnel within the workplace.[7] *[1: Regulatory Requirement]*

Safety data sheets provide information about the chemical hazards; safety precautions for handling, storing, and transporting the chemical; signs and symptoms of toxic exposure; and first aid treatments after exposure. Providing personnel with information about the chemicals being used in the workplace is a regulatory requirement[7] that allows personnel to implement procedures to reduce exposure, establish safe work practices, and apply first aid measures when necessary.

VIII.b. The health care organization must develop a chemical spill control and cleanup plan.[7] *[1: Regulatory Requirement]*

Developing a chemical spill control and cleanup plan is a regulatory requirement[7] that promotes a rapid, efficient, and effective response to chemical spills.[36]

VIII.b.1. The spill control plan should
- designate the individuals responsible for managing spill cleanup,
- include the HLD manufacturer's recommendations for emergency response and cleanup procedures,
- specify the location of spill control supplies and required personal protective equipment (PPE),
- delineate respiratory protection requirements for HLDs,
- identify methods for preventing the dispersal of HLDs to other areas of the facility through the general ventilation system,
- describe evacuation procedures for non-essential personnel,
- outline medical treatment plans for exposed individuals,
- explain site-specific reporting requirements, and
- define education and competency verification requirements for personnel.[19]

[2: High Evidence]

Effective management of chemical spills reduces the amount of vapor dispersed into the air and the potential for contact with skin, eyes, and mucous membranes.[6]

VIII.b.2. Chemical spill kits should be stored in close proximity to areas where HLDs and other hazardous materials are stored or used.[19] *[3: Moderate Evidence]*

Readily accessible chemical spill kits enable a prompt response by providing items that may be required in the cleanup of spills, leaks, or other discharges of hazardous materials.

VIII.c. The health care organization must provide single-action eyewash stations, either plumbed or self-contained, in areas where HLDs that are hazardous to the eyes are located.[104] *[1: Regulatory Requirement]*

It is a regulatory requirement that emergency eyewash stations or showers be immediately accessible in locations where the eyes or body of any person may be exposed to injurious corrosive materials.[104] Many HLDs are eye irritants. Eyewash stations are necessary to provide flushing fluid when the SDS identifies the chemical as a hazard and recommends immediate flushing of the eyes as an emergency first aid measure.[21] The reader can refer to the *American National Standard for Emergency Eyewash and Shower Equipment*[105] for additional guidance.

VIII.d. The health care organization must control and maintain ventilation in areas where HLDs will be handled or used, to meet limits for chemical exposure of personnel as required by federal, state, and local regulations.[7,106] *[1: Regulatory Requirement]*

Ventilation control and maintenance of ventilation systems should be accomplished in accordance with industry standards[56,107] and professional guidelines.[1,6,36,108-110] *[1: Strong Evidence]*

Controlling ventilation systems to provide adequate ventilation dilutes vapor and reduces personnel exposure to HLD fumes.[20,23,24] Maintaining ventilation systems helps ensure correct and continued functioning.[6]

VIII.d.1. Rooms where manual chemical high-level disinfection is performed should have a minimum of 10 air changes per hour.[19,21,36,56,107] *[3: Moderate Evidence]*

VIII.d.2. Additional ventilation (eg, local exhaust ventilation) necessary to control personnel exposure within the threshold limit values should be installed at the point of release of HLD vapors.[19,36] Local exhaust ventilation systems for high-level disinfection processes may include a
- local exhaust hood (eg, laboratory fume hood) or
- self-contained, freestanding, recirculating exhaust ventilation system (eg, ductless fume hood).[19]

[3: Moderate Evidence]

Local exhaust ventilation captures and removes vapor at the source before it can escape into the general work environment.[19,21,36] Local exhaust hoods capture HLD vapor and conduct it into the exhaust system (via the hood) where it is transported through a duct system and discharged to the outside.[19,36] Ductless fume hoods have ventilated enclosures that draw air out of the hood, pass it through an air-cleaning filter, and discharge the cleaned air back into the work area.[19,36] Local exhaust ventilation is not required for all HLDs.

VIII.d.3. Enclosed work stations may be used. *[3: Moderate Evidence]*

Enclosed work stations help manage air flow and reduce exposure to HLD fumes. Work stations also provide an enclosed area for soaking trays that helps protect personnel from splashes and spills.[19]

VIII.d.4. Doors to areas where high-level disinfection is performed should remain closed.[19] *[3: Moderate Evidence]*

Keeping doors closed helps maintain air pressure differentials to surrounding areas.[19]

VIII.e. The health care organization should monitor exposure levels in areas where HLDs are handled or used if there is a potential for chemical vapors to be dispersed into the air in amounts that may be hazardous to health care personnel.[19,36] *[3: Moderate Evidence]*

Health care organizations have a responsibility to minimize health care worker exposure to chemical vapors.[36] Monitoring exposure levels helps ensure a safe work environment and enables monitoring results to be compared with recommended threshold limit values for HLDs.[19] Monitoring is not required for all HLDs. The reader can refer to the American Conference of Governmental Industrial Hygienists[111] and the Occupational Safety and Health Administration Occupational Chemical Database[112] for information regarding permissible exposure limits and validated sampling methods for HLDs.

VIII.e.1. When exposure monitoring is required, at a minimum, exposure levels should be evaluated
- after initial use of the HLD[19]; *[3: Moderate Evidence]*
- whenever there is a significant change in protocol, work practices, or caseload[19]; *[3: Moderate Evidence]*
- after major heating, ventilation, or air conditioning equipment repairs or disruptions[6,19]; *[2: High Evidence]* and
- when personnel have concerns about or symptoms of overexposure.[19] *[3: Moderate Evidence]*

VIII.f. Personnel should use HLD transfer pumps or safety nozzles whenever possible.[19,21] *[3: Moderate Evidence]*

Transfer pumps reduce personnel exposure by containing the release of HLD vapor within a closed system during transfer of HLDs from one container to another.[19] Safety nozzles reduce the potential for splashing when HLD solutions are poured.[19]

VIII.g. The health care organization must develop and implement a written respiratory protection program for required respirator use.[113] *[1: Regulatory Requirement]*

Respirators are required as part of the respiratory protection program for certain chemicals if the limits for chemical exposure of personnel cannot be achieved by using engineering controls (eg, local exhaust ventilation) or when using engineering controls is not feasible.[113]

VIII.h. The health care organization must ensure that personnel handling HLDs or performing high-level disinfection wear PPE.[63,114-116] *[1: Regulatory Requirement]*

Employers are required to ensure that employees are protected when exposed to eye or face hazards from liquid chemicals, bloodborne pathogens or other potentially infectious material, or mechanical irritants capable of causing injury or impairment through absorption, inhalation, or physical contact.[1,20,63,114-116]

In a retrospective review of health care personnel seen for injuries related to chemical exposures at a University of North Carolina hospital between 2003 and 2012, Weber et al[24] found that splashes to mucous membranes were reported by 30 health care personnel, with 19 splashes to the eye; however, 33 personnel reported exposure events in which no injury occurred because they were wearing PPE.

VIII.h.1. Personal protective equipment worn during manual chemical high-level disinfection should include
- masks,
- protective eyewear (eg, goggles),
- chemical-resistant gloves recommended by the glove and disinfectant manufacturers for use with the HLD,[36] and
- additional PPE as recommended by the SDS (eg, respirators, impervious gowns, aprons).
[1: Strong Evidence]

The specific PPE worn for each task depends on the potential for and the anticipated length of exposure[1] (See the AORN Guideline for Prevention of Transmissible Infections,[117] the AORN Guideline for Surgical Attire,[118] and the AORN Guideline for Cleaning and Care of Surgical Instruments[55]). Personnel handling or using HLDs are vulnerable to injury from a direct chemical splash.[24] Surgical masks in combination with eye protection devices protect the wearer's eyes, nose, face, and mouth from exposure to hazardous chemicals. Goggles or safety glasses are necessary whenever there is a potential for a chemical to contact the eyes.[21,114] Eye glasses or contact lenses do not provide sufficient protection from chemical splashes.[6]

Skin may also act as a portal of entry. Employers are required to ensure workers' hands are protected from exposure to potential skin absorption of substances such as chemical HLDs.[116] Chemical resistance and glove permeability vary among glove manufacturers. Polyvinyl chloride, neoprene, and latex examination gloves may not provide adequate skin protection from HLDs.[19]

Additional PPE may be needed based on the task and the recommendations of the SDS.

VIII.h.2. Gloves should be fitted at the wrist and long enough to provide protection of the forearm or clothing from splashes or seepage.[6,21,36] *[2: High Evidence]*

Wearing close-fitting, elbow-length gloves or protective sleeves provides protection of the hands and forearms.[19]

VIII.h.3. Personnel should inspect gloves for integrity after donning, before contact with the HLD, and throughout use.[101] *[3: Moderate Evidence]*

Careful inspection of glove integrity after donning and before contact with the HLD may reveal holes and defects in the unused product that may have occurred during the manufacturing or donning process and could allow for the passage of the HLD through the glove to the hands of personnel. Careful inspection of glove integrity throughout use may prevent unnoticed glove perforation that may present an increased risk for direct contact with the HLD.

VIII.h.4. Personnel should perform hand hygiene after removal of PPE.[59] *[1: Strong Evidence]*

The CDC recommends performing hand hygiene after removal of PPE.[59] Hands may become contaminated when removing PPE. Damage to PPE in the form of tears, punctures, and abrasions may occur and be undetected, exposing the wearer to chemical hazards.

VIII.h.5. Reusable PPE must be
- verified for integrity before each use,
- decontaminated after each use, and
- discarded if there are signs of deterioration or if its ability to function as a barrier has been compromised.[63]
[1: Regulatory Requirement]

VIII.i. The health care organization must dispose of HLDs in accordance with federal, state, and local regulations.[119-121] *[1: Regulatory Requirement]*

The US Environmental Protection Agency regulates the treatment, storage, and disposal of hazardous chemical wastes under the Resource Conservation and Recovery Act.[119,120] States are permitted to administer their own hazardous waste program providing they enact laws that are at least as stringent as the federal laws.[121] State regulations are often more restrictive than federal regulations.[122] Local governments also have laws and regulations pertaining to the disposal of hazardous materials.[123]

VIII.i.1. If there are no disposal restrictions, activated HLDs may be disposed of, along with copious amounts of cold water, into a drain connected to the sanitary sewer system.[19,21,36] *[3: Moderate Evidence]*

Some local regulations may prohibit disposal of HLDs into the sewer system or may require neutralization before disposal.[19]

VIII.i.2. When recommended by the disinfectant manufacturer, a neutralizer should be added to the activated HLD before disposal. *[5: Benefits Balanced with Harms]*

High-level disinfectant vapors may increase when the solution is poured out of a soaking container. Adding a neutralizer may reduce exposure levels.

VIII.i.3. Activated HLDs, including neutralized HLDs, should not be disposed of into septic systems.[19,36] *[3: Moderate Evidence]*

Disposing of HLDs in a septic system can disrupt the biodegradation process by killing beneficial microorganisms.[19,36]

VIII.i.4. When the activated HLD is discarded into a sink, the sink should be
- close to the area where the HLD is stored and
- large enough to accommodate the volume of HLD being discarded.[36]
[4: Limited Evidence]

Discarding the HLD into a sink that is in close proximity and of sufficient size reduces the potential for spills.

VIII.i.5. When the HLD is discarded from a reusable soaking container, the soaking container should, at a minimum, be cleaned and dried before reuse. *[5: Benefits Balanced with Harms]*

Cleaning and drying soaking containers that have been used to store HLDs reduces the potential for cross contamination and helps ensure that residual HLD has been removed from the container.

VIII.i.6. Empty HLD containers should be disposed of in accordance with the disinfectant manufacturer's IFU.[19,36] *[3: Moderate Evidence]*

Disposing of empty HLD containers in accordance with the disinfectant manufacturer's IFU may prevent accidental chemical exposure or inappropriate use of containers.[36]

Recommendation IX

The health care organization should maintain records of manual chemical high-level disinfection processes.

Records provide data for the identification of trends and demonstration of compliance with regulatory requirements and accreditation agency standards. Highly reliable data collection is necessary to demonstrate the health care organization's progress toward quality care outcomes.[124] Effective management and collection of health care information that accurately reflects the patient's care, treatment, and services is a regulatory requirement[76-79] and an accreditation agency standard for both hospitals[125,126] and ambulatory settings.[126-130]

IX.a.   Records related to manual chemical high-level disinfection should include the
- date and time of high-level disinfection[36];
- HLD solution lot number[36];
- HLD solution shelf-life date[36];
- HLD solution activation date[36];
- HLD solution reuse-life date[36];
- results of solution test strip testing, if applicable[36];
- results of MRC or MEC testing, if applicable[36];
- HLD solution temperature[36];
- HLD solution exposure time[36];
- quantity and description of the device or item[36];
- unique device identification number, if available[36];
- identity of the person performing high-level disinfection[36];
- identity of the patient on whom the device was used, if possible[36]; and
- identity of the physician and procedure where the device was used, if possible.[36]

[4: Limited Evidence]

Maintaining records of manual chemical high-level disinfection helps ensure that parameters for correct high-level disinfection have been met,[85] enables retrieval of HLD solutions in the event of a recall, and establishes traceability and accountability.

IX.b.   Records of manual chemical high-level disinfection should be maintained for a time period specified by the health care organization.
[5: Benefits Balanced with Harms]

Recommendation X

The health care organization should provide initial and ongoing education and competency verification activities related to manual chemical high-level disinfection for personnel who are handling and using chemical HLDs.[5,6,21,36]

Initial and ongoing education of perioperative personnel facilitates the development of knowledge, skills, and attitudes that affect safe patient care. It is the responsibility of the health care organization to provide initial and ongoing education and to verify the competency of its personnel; however, the primary responsibility for maintaining ongoing competency remains with the individual.

Competency verification activities provide a mechanism for competency documentation and help verify that personnel understand the principles and processes necessary for safe and effective manual chemical high-level disinfection. Having competent personnel perform manual chemical high-level disinfection increases the likelihood that personnel will adhere to best practices and reduces the potential for exposure and adverse events to both patients and personnel.[36] Advances and developments in high-level disinfection processes, the emergence of new diseases and micro-

organisms, the increasing complexity of medical devices, and the responsibility for implementing safe and effective processing of reusable semicritical devices underscore the need for health care organizations to ensure that manual chemical high-level disinfection is performed by educated and competent personnel.[36] Ongoing development of knowledge and skills and documentation of personnel participation is a regulatory requirement[76-79] and an accreditation agency standard for both hospitals[131,132] and ambulatory settings.[132-135]

X.a.   The health care organization must provide education about the written hazard communication program for personnel who use, handle, or may be exposed to HLDs.[7,103] *[1: Regulatory Requirement]*

Personnel who have received education and completed competency verification activities related to the plan may have a greater understanding of how to reduce potential adverse effects associated with exposure to hazardous chemicals.

X.a.1.   Education related to the hazard communication program must include
- an explanation of the SDS and chemical labeling system, and how to obtain and use this hazard information;
- methods and observations that may be used to detect the presence or release of all chemicals used in the workplace;
- the physical and health hazards of all chemicals used in the workplace; and
- the measures personnel can take to protect themselves, including specific procedures the organization has implemented to protect personnel from exposure to chemicals used in the workplace (eg, emergency procedures, PPE).[7]

[1: Regulatory Requirement]

Henn et al[136] surveyed 4,657 members of professional practice organizations representing RNs, technologists/technicians, dental professionals, respiratory therapists, and others who reported handling HLDs in the previous 7 days. The results showed that 44% of the respondents did not always wear protective gowns, 42% did not always wear eye and face protection, and 9% did not always wear gloves. The most frequent explanation provided for not wearing PPE was that "exposure was minimal," even though 12% of the respondents reported direct skin contact with an HLD in the previous 7 days. The researchers noted the results of the survey indicated the respondents did not fully recognize the hazards and potential adverse health effects of HLD exposure and the need for PPE.

X.b.   The health care organization should establish education and competency verification activities for its personnel and determine intervals for education and competency verification related to manual chemical high-level disinfection. *[3: Moderate Evidence]*

Manual chemical high-level disinfection is a complex process requiring performance by educated and competent personnel.[85] The Joint Commission has identified sufficient education and competency verification of personnel performing high-level disinfection processes as one of the areas most frequently needing improvement in health care facilities.[85]

Education and competency verification needs and intervals are unique to the facility and to its personnel and processes. Educational and skill mastery needs will vary among personnel and may also vary among organizational processing sites.[137,138] Some personnel will require greater levels of remediation and reinforcement.[139]

X.b.1.   The health care organization should ensure that the personnel responsible for providing education and competency verification to individuals who perform manual chemical disinfection are sufficiently educated and competent to do so.[5,85] *[3: Moderate Evidence]*

X.c.   Education and competency verification activities related to manual chemical high-level disinfection should include
- ○ information about devices and disinfectants approved by the interdisciplinary team for manual chemical high-level disinfection; *[5: Benefits Balanced with Harms]*
- ○ procedures for safe and effective preparation and use of chemical HLDs,[20,21,110] *[2: High Evidence]*
- ○ elements of a safe environment for personnel who are performing manual chemical high-level disinfection, including the location and use of
  - • SDS,
  - • eyewash stations,
  - • chemical spill kits, and
  - • PPE[1,21,110]; *[1: Strong Evidence]*
- ○ requirements for maintaining records of manual chemical high-level disinfection; *[5: Benefits Balanced with Harms]*
- ○ quality assurance measures for manual chemical high-level disinfection; *[5: Benefits Balanced with Harms]* and
- ○ processes for reporting adverse events and occupational exposure incidents related to manual chemical high-level disinfection. *[5: Benefits Balanced with Harms]*

Recommendation XI

The health care organization should develop policies and procedures for manual chemical high-level disinfection that are reviewed periodically, revised as necessary, and readily available in the practice setting in which they are used.

Policies and procedures assist in the development of patient safety, quality assessment, and performance improvement activities. Policies and procedures also serve as operational guidelines used to minimize patients' risk for injury or complications, standardize practice, direct personnel, and support continuous performance improvement programs. Policies and procedures establish authority, responsibility, and accountability within the practice setting. Having policies and procedures that guide and support patient care, treatment, and services is a regulatory requirement[76-79] and an accreditation agency standard for both hospitals[81,140] and ambulatory settings.[81,134,141,142]

XI.a.   Policies and procedures related to manual chemical high-level disinfection should address
- ○ devices and disinfectants approved by the interdisciplinary team for manual chemical high-level disinfection, *[5: Benefits Balanced with Harms]*
- ○ procedures for safe and effective preparation and use of chemical HLDs,[21,143] *[2: High Evidece]*
- ○ elements of a safe environment for personnel who are performing manual chemical high-level disinfection, *[5: Benefits Balanced with Harms]*
- ○ maintaining records of manual chemical high-level disinfection, *[5: Benefits Balanced with Harms]*
- ○ quality assurance measures for manual chemical high-level disinfection, *[5: Benefits Balanced with Harms]* and
- ○ processes for reporting adverse events related to manual chemical high-level disinfection. *[5: Benefits Balanced with Harms]*

XI.b.   The manufacturers' IFU for all components of the high-level disinfection process (eg, device, equipment, supplies, HLD solutions) should be readily available to and followed by personnel responsible for manual chemical high-level disinfection.[5] *[4: Limited Evidence]*

Instructions for use identify the manufacturers' validated processes and procedures necessary to achieve effective manual chemical high-level disinfection.

XI.b.1.   The health care organization should review the device and HLD manufacturers' IFU at established intervals and should verify that manual chemical high-level disinfection practices are in compliance with the most current IFUs.[110] *[2: High Evidence]*

Manufacturers may make modifications to their IFUs when new technology becomes available, when regulatory requirements change, or when modifications are made to their product.

Recommendation XII

The health care organization's quality management program should evaluate manual chemical high-level disinfection processes.[5]

Quality assurance and performance improvement programs can facilitate the identification of problem areas and assist personnel in evaluating and improving the quality of patient care and formulating plans for corrective action. These programs provide data that may be used to determine whether an individual organization is within benchmark goals, and if not, to identify areas that may require corrective action. A quality management program provides a mechanism to evaluate effectiveness of manual chemical high-level disinfection processes, compliance with manufacturer's IFU, and equipment function. Collecting data to monitor and improve patient care, treatment, and services is a regulatory requirement[76-79] and an accreditation agency standard for both hospitals[144,145] and ambulatory settings.[145-148]

XII.a. The quality assurance and performance management program for manual chemical high-level disinfection should include
- ○ periodically reviewing and evaluating manual chemical high-level disinfection to verify compliance with or to identify the need for improvement with established processes for manual chemical high-level disinfection,
- ○ identifying corrective actions directed toward improvement priorities, and
- ○ taking additional actions when improvement is not achieved or sustained.

[3: Moderate Evidence]

Reviewing and evaluating quality assurance and performance improvement activities may identify failure points that contribute to errors in manual chemical high-level disinfection and help define actions for improvement. Monitoring compliance with established safe practices can increase workplace safety and help reduce personnel exposure to HLDs. Taking corrective actions may improve patient safety by verifying that personnel understand the principles of and comply with best practices for manual chemical high-level disinfection.

Nayebzadeh[23] conducted a nonexperimental study to investigate the effects of work practices and work-related symptoms among health care workers handling HLDs. The researcher observed work practices and interviewed 53 health care workers in 19 different locations from five hospitals in Canada about the frequency of HLD spills, use of PPE, and HLD-exposure symptoms. The researcher found that only 15% (n = 8) of the workers used face protection when handling HLDs. Almost 50% (n = 26) reported experiencing at least one chemical spill in the previous 12 months. The researcher concluded that monitoring and verifying compliance with safe work practices could significantly reduce worker exposure and health effects caused by exposure to HLDs.

XII.b. Personnel participating in manual chemical high-level disinfection should take part in ongoing quality assurance and performance improvement activities related to manual chemical high-level disinfection by
- ○ monitoring quality;
- ○ developing strategies for compliance,
- ○ establishing benchmarks to evaluate quality indicators,
- ○ collecting data related to the levels of performance and quality indicators,
- ○ evaluating practice based on the cumulative data collected,
- ○ taking action to improve compliance, and
- ○ assessing the effectiveness of the actions taken.

[5: Benefits Balanced with Harms]

Participating in ongoing quality assurance and performance improvement activities is a primary responsibility of health care personnel engaged in clinical practice.

XII.c. Adverse events and occupational exposure incidents related to manual chemical high-level disinfection should be reported and documented after each event according to the health care organization's policy and procedure and should be reviewed for potential opportunities for improvement.[20,24,110] *[2: High Evidence]*

Reporting and reviewing adverse events and near misses can be useful for identifying actions that may prevent similar occurrences and revealing opportunities for improvement.

Glossary

Activation: The process by which a high-level disinfectant becomes chemically operative after combination with another chemical.

Chemical-resistant gloves: Gloves with varying levels of resistance to challenge chemicals based on the glove manufacturer's test data for breakthrough time, degree of degradation, and permeation rate.

Critical water: Water that is extensively treated to remove microorganisms and other materials.

Endotoxin: A toxic substance that is released when a bacterial cell disintegrates.

High-level disinfection: A process that deactivates all types of microorganisms with the exception of bacterial spores and prions.

Instrument air: A medical gas that falls under the general requirements for medical gases as defined by the *NFPA 99: Health Care Facilities Code,* is not respired, is compliant with the *ANSI/ISA S-7.0.01: Quality Standard for Instrument Air,* and is filtered to 0.01 micrometer, free of liquids and hydrocarbon vapors, and dry to a dew point of -40 F (-40 C).

Minimum effective concentration (MEC): The minimum concentration of a liquid chemical germicide that achieves the claimed microbicidal activity as determined by dose-response testing.

Minimum recommended concentration (MRC): The minimum concentration at which the manufacturer tested the product and validated its performance.

Pseudo-outbreak: An episode of false increased disease incidence due to enhanced surveillance (eg, microbiological culturing) or other factor (eg, laboratory contamination, false positive test).

Purging: The removal of visible moisture from a device after rinsing.

Reuse life: The period of time an activated high-level disinfectant solution can be used, provided the concentration of the active ingredient remains at or above the manufacturers' specified minimum recommended concentration.

Semicritical items: Items that contact mucous membranes or nonintact skin.

Shelf-life: The period of time during which a stored product remains effective, useful, or suitable for use.

Threshold limit value: The airborne concentration of a substance not to be exceeded during any part of the working exposure.

Utility water: Water obtained directly from a faucet that has not been purified, distilled, or otherwise treated. Synonym: tap water.

References

1. Rutala WA, Weber DJ; Healthcare Infection Control Practices Advisory Committee. *Guideline for Disinfection and Sterilization in Healthcare Facilities, 2008.* Washington, DC: Centers for Disease Control and Prevention; 2008. https://www.cdc.gov/infectioncontrol/pdf/guidelines/disinfection-guidelines.pdf. Updated February 2017. Accessed October 5, 2017. [IVA]

2. Spaulding EH, Lawrence CA, Block SS, Reddish GF. Chemical disinfection of medical and surgical materials. In: Lawrence CA, Block SS, Reddish GF, eds. *Disinfection, Sterilization, and Preservation.* Philadelphia, PA: Lea & Febiger; 1968:517-531. [VA]

3. Rutala WA, Weber DJ. Reprocessing semicritical items: current issues and new technologies. *Am J Infect Control.* 2016;44(5):e53-e62. [VA]

4. Rutala WA, Weber DJ. Cleaning, disinfection, and sterilization in healthcare facilities. In: *APIC Text of Infection Control and Epidemiology.* Arlington, VA: Association for Professionals in Infection Control and Epidemiology; 2016. [IVB]

5. Improperly sterilized or HLD equipment—a growing problem. *Quick Safety.* 2017(33):1-5. https://www.jointcommission.org/assets/1/23/qs_33a_2017.pdf. Accessed October 5, 2017. [VC]

6. *Guideline for Use of High-Level Disinfectants & Sterilants in the Gastroenterology Setting.* Chicago, IL: Society of Gastroenterology Nurses and Associates, Inc; 2017:13. [IVB]

7. 29 CFR 1910.1200: Hazard communication: toxic and hazardous substances. Occupational Safety and Health Administration. https://www.osha.gov/pls/oshaweb/owadisp.show_document?p_table=standards&p_id=10099. Accessed October 5, 2017.

8. Guideline for processing flexible endoscopes. In: *Guidelines for Perioperative Practice.* Denver, CO: AORN, Inc; 2017:717-800. [IVA]

9. Tosh PK, Disbot M, Duffy JM, et al. Outbreak of *Pseudomonas aeruginosa* surgical site infections after arthroscopic procedures: Texas, 2009. *Infect Control Hosp Epidemiol.* 2011;32(12):1179-1186. [IIIA]

10. Rutala WA, Weber DJ. Disinfection and sterilization in health care facilities: an overview and current issues. *Infect Dis Clin North Am.* 2016;30(3):609-637. [VA]

11. Rutala WA, Weber DJ. Gastrointestinal endoscopes: a need to shift from disinfection to sterilization? *JAMA.* 2014;312(14):1405-1406. [VA]

12. McDonnell G, Burke P. Disinfection: is it time to reconsider Spaulding? *J Hosp Infect.* 2011;78(3):163-170. [VA]

13. Lorena NS, Pitombo MB, Cortes PB, et al. *Mycobacterium massiliense* BRA100 strain recovered from postsurgical infections: resistance to high concentrations of glutaraldehyde and alternative solutions for high level disinfection. *Acta Cir Bras.* 2010;25(5):455-459. [IIIB]

14. Duarte RS, Lourenco MC, Fonseca Lde S, et al. Epidemic of postsurgical infections caused by *Mycobacterium massiliense. J Clin Microbiol.* 2009;47(7):2149-2155. [IIIB]

15. Tschudin-Sutter S, Frei R, Kampf G, et al. Emergence of glutaraldehyde-resistant *Pseudomonas aeruginosa. Infect Control Hosp Epidemiol.* 2011;32(12):1173-1178. [VA]

16. Meyers J, Ryndock E, Conway MJ, Meyers C, Robison R. Susceptibility of high-risk human papillomavirus type 16 to clinical disinfectants. *J Antimicrob Chemother.* 2014;69(6):1546-1550. [IIIB]

17. Ofstead CL, Wetzler HP, Snyder AK, Horton RA. Endoscope reprocessing methods: a prospective study on the impact of human factors and automation. *Gastroenterol Nurs.* 2010;33(4):304-311. [IIIA]

18. Ubhayawardana DL, Kottahachchi J, Weerasekera MM, Wanigasooriya IW, Fernando SS, De Silva M. Residual bioburden in reprocessed side-view endoscopes used for endoscopic retrograde cholangiopancreatography (ERCP). *Endosc Int Open.* 2013;1(1):12-16. [IIIB]

19. Best practices for the safe use of glutaraldehyde in health care. 2006. Occupational Safety and Health Administration. http://www.osha.gov/Publications/3258-08N-2006-English.html. Accessed October 5, 2017. [VA]

20. Cohen NL, Patton CM. Worker safety and glutaraldehyde in the gastrointestinal lab environment. *Gastroenterol Nurs.* 2006;29(2):100-104. [VB]

21. ECRI. Ethylene oxide, formaldehyde, and glutaraldehyde. *Operating Room Risk Management.* 2012;1A. [VB]

22. Pala G, Moscato G. Allergy to ortho-phthalaldehyde in the healthcare setting: advice for clinicians. *Expert Rev Clin Immunol.* 2013;9(3):227-234. [VA]

23. Nayebzadeh A. The effect of work practices on personal exposure to glutaraldehyde among health care workers. *Ind Health.* 2007;45(2):289-295. [IIIB]

24. Weber DJ, Consoli SA, Rutala WA. Occupational health risks associated with the use of germicides in health care. *Am J Infect Control.* 2016;44(5):e85-e89. [IIIB]

25. Alfa MJ. Intra-cavitary ultrasound probes: cleaning and high-level disinfection are necessary for both the probe head and handle to reduce the risk of infection transmission. *Infect Control Hosp Epidemiol.* 2015;36(5):585-586. [VA]

26. Guidelines for cleaning and preparing external- and internal-use ultrasound probes between patients, safe handling, and use of ultrasound coupling gel. The American Institute of Ultrasound in Medicine. http://www.aium.org/officialStatements/57. Approved May 2017. Accessed October 5, 2017. [IVC]

27. Westerway SC, Basseal JM, Brockway A, Hyett JA, Carter DA. Potential infection control risks associated with ultrasound equipment—a bacterial perspective. *Ultrasound Med Biol.* 2017;43(2):421-426. [IIIB]

28. Shokoohi H, Armstrong P, Tansek R. Emergency department ultrasound probe infection control: challenges and solutions. *Open Access Emerg Med*. 2015;7:1-9. [VB]

29. Leroy S, M'Zali F, Kann M, Weber DJ, Smith DD. Impact of vaginal-rectal ultrasound examinations with covered and low-level disinfected transducers on infectious transmissions in France. *Infect Control Hospital Epidemiol*. 2014;35(12):1497-1504. [IIIB]

30. Casalegno JS, Le Bail Carval K, Eibach D, et al. High risk HPV contamination of endocavity vaginal ultrasound probes: an underestimated route of nosocomial infection? *PLoS One*. 2012;7(10):e48137. [IIIB]

31. M'Zali F, Bounizra C, Leroy S, Mekki Y, Quentin-Noury C, Kann M. Persistence of microbial contamination on transvaginal ultrasound probes despite low-level disinfection procedure. *PLoS One*. 2014;9(4):e93368. [IIIB]

32. Ngu A, McNally G, Patel D, Gorgis V, Leroy S, Burdach J. Reducing transmission risk through high-level disinfection of transvaginal ultrasound transducer handles. *Infect Control Hosp Epidemiol*. 2015;36(5):581-584. [IIIB]

33. Combs CA, Fishman A. A proposal to reduce the risk of transmission of human papilloma virus via transvaginal ultrasound. *Am J Obstet Gynecol*. 2016;215(1):63-67. [VA]

34. Chu K, Obaid H, Babyn P, Blondeau J. Bacterial contamination of ultrasound probes at a tertiary referral university medical center. *AJR Am J Roentgenol*. 2014;203(5):928-932. [VB]

35. Ryndock E, Robison R, Meyers C. Susceptibility of HPV16 and 18 to high level disinfectants indicated for semi-critical ultrasound probes. *J Med Virol*. 2016;88(6):1076-1080. [IIIB]

36. *ANSI/AAMI ST58:2013 Chemical Sterilization and High-Level Disinfection in Health Care Facilities*. Arlington, VA: Association for the Advancement of Medical Instrumentation; 2013. [IVC]

37. Guideline for medical device and product evaluation. In: *Guidelines for Perioperative Practice*. Denver, CO: AORN, Inc; 2017:e135-e142. [IVB]

38. FDA-cleared sterilants and high level disinfectants with general claims for processing reusable medical and dental devices—March 2015. US Food and Drug Administration. http://www.fda.gov/MedicalDevices/DeviceRegulationandGuidance/ReprocessingofReusableMedicalDevices/ucm437347.htm. Accessed October 5, 2017.

39. Wallace CA. New developments in disinfection and sterilization. *Am J Infect Control*. 2016;44:e23-e27. [VB]

40. Hawley B, Casey ML, Cox-Ganser JM, Edwards N, Fedan KB, Cummings KJ. Notes from the field: Respiratory symptoms and skin irritation among hospital workers using a new disinfection product—Pennsylvania, 2015. *MMWR Morb Mortal Wkly Rep*. 2016;65(15):400-401. [VB]

41. Abdulla FR, Adams BB. Ortho-phthalaldehyde causing facial stains after cystoscopy. *Arch Dermatol*. 2007;143(5):670. [VC]

42. Anderson SE, Umbright C, Sellamuthu R, et al. Irritancy and allergic responses induced by topical application of ortho-phthalaldehyde. *Toxicol Sci*. 2010;115(2):435-443. [IIIA]

43. Suneja T, Belsito DV. Occupational dermatoses in health care workers evaluated for suspected allergic contact dermatitis. *Contact Derm*. 2008;58(5):285-290. [IIB]

44. Warshaw EM, Schram SE, Maibach HI, et al. Occupation-related contact dermatitis in North American health care workers referred for patch testing: cross-sectional data, 1998 to 2004. *Dermatitis*. 2008;19(5):261-274. [IIIB]

45. Fujita H, Ogawa M, Endo Y. A case of occupational bronchial asthma and contact dermatitis caused by ortho-phthalaldehyde exposure in a medical worker. *J Occup Health*. 2006;48(6):413-416. [VB]

46. Arif AA, Delclos GL. Association between cleaning-related chemicals and work-related asthma and asthma symptoms among healthcare professionals. *Occup Environ Med*. 2012;69(1):35-40. [IIIB]

47. Robitaille C, Boulet LP. Occupational asthma after exposure to ortho-phthalaldehyde (OPA). *Occup Environ Med*. 2015;72(5):381. [VB]

48. Walters GI, Moore VC, McGrath EE, Burge PS, Henneberger PK. Agents and trends in health care workers' occupational asthma. *Occup Med (Lond)*. 2013;63(7):513-516. [IIIB]

49. Bakerly ND, Moore VC, Vellore AD, Jaakkola MS, Robertson AS, Burge PS. Fifteen-year trends in occupational asthma: data from the shield surveillance scheme. *Occup Med (Lond)*. 2008;58(3):169-174. [IIIB]

50. Copeland S, Nugent K. Persistent and unusual respiratory findings after prolonged glutaraldehyde exposure. *Int J Occup Environ Med*. 2015;6(3):177-183. [VB]

51. Donnay C, Denis MA, Magis R, et al. Under-estimation of self-reported occupational exposure by questionnaire in hospital workers. *Occup Environ Med*. 2011;68(8):611-617. [IIIB]

52. Ryu M, Kobayashi T, Kawamukai E, Quan G, Furuta T. Cytotoxicity assessment of residual high-level disinfectants. *Biocontrol Sci*. 2013;18(4):217-220. [IIIB]

53. Suzukawa M, Yamaguchi M, Komiya A, Kimura M, Nito T, Yamamoto K. Ortho-phthalaldehyde-induced anaphylaxis after laryngoscopy. *J Allergy Clin Immunol*. 2006;117(6):1500-1501. [VB]

54. Rideout K, Teschke K, DimichWard H, Kennedy SM. Considering risks to healthcare workers from glutaraldehyde alternatives in high-level disinfection. *J Hosp Infect*. 2005;59(1):4-11. [IIIB]

55. Guideline for cleaning and care of surgical instruments. In: *Guidelines for Perioperative Practice*. Denver, CO: AORN, Inc.; 2017:815-850. [IVA]

56. American Society for Healthcare Engineering, Facility Guidelines Institute. *Guidelines for Design and Construction of Hospitals and Outpatient Facilities*. Chicago, IL: American Society for Healthcare Engineering; 2014. [IVC]

57. Guidelines interpretations. Facility Guidelines Institute. https://www.fgiguidelines.org/guidelines/interpretations-2/. Accessed October 5, 2017. [VA]

58. Hota S, Hirji Z, Stockton K, et al. Outbreak of multidrug-resistant *Pseudomonas aeruginosa* colonization and infection secondary to imperfect intensive care unit room design. *Infect Control Hosp Epidemiol*. 2009;30(1):25-33. [VB]

59. Siegel JD, Rhinehart E, Jackson M, Chiarello L; the Healthcare Infection Control Practices Advisory Committee. 2007 Guideline for isolation precautions: preventing transmission of infectious agents in healthcare settings. Centers for Disease Control and Prevention. https://www.cdc.gov/infectioncontrol/guidelines/isolation/. Updated 2017. Accessed October 5, 2017. [IVA]

60. HSE National Decontamination of Reusable Invasive Medical Devices Advisory Group, ed. *Health Service Executive Standards and Recommended Practices for Endoscope Reprocessing Units*. Version 2.2. Tipperary, Ireland: Health Service Executive; 2012. [IVB]

61. Bringhurst J. Special problems associated with reprocessing instruments in outpatient care facilities. *Am J Infect Control*. 2016;44:e63-e67. [VA]

62. Roberts CG. The role of biofilms in reprocessing medical devices. *Am J Infect Control*. 2013;41(5 Suppl):S77-S80. [VA]

63. 29 CFR 1910.1030: Bloodborne pathogens. US Government Publishing Office. https://www.ecfr.gov/cgi-bin/

text-idx?SID=a71fad4cc5d7ca4d71154a2c80a4f88f&mc=true&node=se29.6.1910_11030&rgn=div8. Accessed October 5, 2017.

64. Merritt K, Hitchins VM, Brown SA. Safety and cleaning of medical materials and devices. *J Biomed Mater Res.* 2000;53(2):131-136. [IIB]

65. Rutala WA, Weber DJ. Disinfection, sterilization, and antisepsis: an overview. *Am J Infect Control.* 2016;44:e1-e6. [VA]

66. Gray RA, Williams PL, Dubbins PA, Jenks PJ. Decontamination of transvaginal ultrasound probes: review of national practice and need for national guidelines. *Clin Radiol.* 2012;67(11):1069-1077. [IIIB]

67. Sanz GE, Theoret J, Liao MM, Erickson C, Kendall JL. Bacterial contamination and cleanliness of emergency department ultrasound probes. *CJEM.* 2011;13(6):384-389. [IIIB]

68. Alfa MJ. Current issues result in a paradigm shift in reprocessing medical and surgical instruments. *Am J Infect Control.* 2016;44:e41-e45. [VA]

69. Kampf G, Bloss R, Martiny H. Surface fixation of dried blood by glutaraldehyde and peracetic acid. *J Hosp Infect.* 2004;57(2):139-143. [IIIB]

70. Alfa MJ, Olson N, DeGagne P, Jackson M. A survey of reprocessing methods, residual viable bioburden, and soil levels in patient-ready endoscopic retrograde cholangiopancreatography duodenoscopes used in Canadian centers. *Infect Control Hosp Epidemiol.* 2002;23(4):198-206. [IIIA]

71. Alfa MJ. Monitoring and improving the effectiveness of cleaning medical and surgical devices. *Am J Infect Control.* 2013;41(5 Suppl):S56-S59. [VA]

72. Yasuhara H, Fukatsu K, Komatsu T, Obayashi T, Saito Y, Uetera Y. Prevention of medical accidents caused by defective surgical instruments. *Surgery.* 2012;151(2):153-161. [IIIA]

73. Parada SA, Grassbaugh JA, Devine JG, Arrington ED. Instrumentation-specific infection after anterior cruciate ligament reconstruction. *Sports Health.* 2009;1(6):481-485. [IIIB]

74. Federal insecticide, fungicide, and rodenticide act [as amended through P.L. 112–177, effective Sept. 28, 2012]. US Senate Committee on Agriculture, Nutrition, & Forestry. https://www.agriculture.senate.gov/imo/media/doc/FIFRA.pdf. Accessed October 5, 2017.

75. Summary of the federal insecticide, fungicide, and rodenticide act. US Environmental Protection Agency. https://www.epa.gov/laws-regulations/summary-federal-insecticide-fungicide-and-rodenticide-act. Accessed October 5, 2017.

76. *State Operations Manual Appendix A—Survey Protocol, Regulations and Interpretive Guidelines for Hospitals.* Rev 151; 2015 Centers for Medicare & Medicaid Services. https://www.cms.gov/Regulations-and-Guidance/Guidance/Manuals/downloads/som107ap_a_hospitals.pdf. Accessed October 5, 2017.

77. *State Operations Manual Appendix L—Guidance for Surveyors: Ambulatory Surgical Centers.* Rev. 137; 2015. Centers for Medicare & Medicaid Services. https://www.cms.gov/Regulations-and-Guidance/Guidance/Manuals/downloads/som107ap_l_ambulatory.pdf. Accessed October 5, 2017.

78. 42 CFR 482. Conditions of participation for hospitals. 2011. Government Publishing Office. https://www.gpo.gov/fdsys/granule/CFR-2011-title42-vol5/CFR-2011-title42-vol5-part482. Accessed October 5, 2017.

79. 42 CFR 416. Ambulatory surgical services. 2011. Government Publishing Office. https://www.gpo.gov/fdsys/granule/CFR-2011-title42-vol3/CFR-2011-title42-vol3-part416. Accessed October 5, 2017.

80. IC.02.02.01: The hospital reduces the risk of infections associated with medical equipment, devices, and supplies. In: *Hospital Accreditation Standards.* Oakbrook Terrace, IL: Joint Commission Resources; 2017.

81. SS.1: Organization. In: *NIAHO Interpretive Guidelines and Surveyor Guidance.* Version 11. Milford, OH: DNV-GL Healthcare; 2014:80-82.

82. IC.02.02.01: The organization reduces the risk of infections associated with medical equipment, devices, and supplies. In: *Standards for Ambulatory Care.* Oakbrook Terrace, IL: Joint Commission Resources; 2017.

83. Infection prevention and control and safety. In: *Accreditation Handbook for Ambulatory Health Care.* Skokie, IL: Accreditation Association for Ambulatory Health Care, Inc.; 2016:54-57.

84. Operating room policy, environment, and procedures. In: *Regular Standards and Checklist for Accreditation of Ambulatory Surgery Facilities.* Version 14.5. Gurnee, IL: American Association for Accreditation of Ambulatory Surgery Facilities, Inc; 2017:24-36.

85. High-level disinfection and sterilization: know your process. *Jt Comm Perspect.* 2014;34(2):9. [VB]

86. Howie R, Alfa MJ, Coombs K. Survival of enveloped and non-enveloped viruses on surfaces compared with other micro-organisms and impact of suboptimal disinfectant exposure. *J Hosp Infect.* 2008;69(4):368-376. [IIIB]

87. Maillard JY. Innate resistance to sporicides and potential failure to decontaminate. *J Hosp Infect.* 2011;77(3):204-209. [VB]

88. Rutala WA, Gergen MF, Weber DJ. Disinfection of a probe used in ultrasound-guided prostate biopsy. *Infect Control Hosp Epidemiol.* 2007;28(8):916-919. [IIIB]

89. Kac G, Podglajen I, Si-Mohamed A, Rodi A, Grataloup C, Meyer G. Evaluation of ultraviolet C for disinfection of endocavitary ultrasound transducers persistently contaminated despite probe covers. *Infect Control Hosp Epidemiol.* 2010;31(2):165-170. [IIIB]

90. Bloc S, Mercadal L, Garnier T, et al. Evaluation of a new disinfection method for ultrasound probes used for regional anesthesia: ultraviolet C light. *J Ultrasound Med.* 2011;30(6):785-788. [IIIC]

91. Vickery K, Gorgis VZ, Burdach J, Patel D. Evaluation of an automated high-level disinfection technology for ultrasound transducers. *J Infect Public Health.* 2014;7(2):153-160. [IIIB]

92. Rutala WA, Gergen MF, Sickbert-Bennett E. Effectiveness of a hydrogen peroxide mist (trophon) system in inactivating healthcare pathogens on surface and endocavitary probes. *Infect Control Hosp Epidemiol.* 2016;37(5):613-614. [IIIB]

93. Johnson S, Proctor M, Bluth E, et al. Evaluation of a hydrogen peroxide-based system for high-level disinfection of vaginal ultrasound probes. *J Ultrasound Med.* 2013;32(10):1799-1804. [IIIB]

94. Rutala WA, Gergen MF, Bringhurst J, Weber DJ. Effective high-level disinfection of cystoscopes: is perfusion of channels required? *Infect Control Hosp Epidemiol.* 2016;37(2):228-231. [IIB]

95. Unal M, Yucel I, Akar Y, Oner A, Altin M. Outbreak of toxic anterior segment syndrome associated with glutaraldehyde after cataract surgery. *J Cataract Refract Surg.* 2006;32(10):1696-1701. [VA]

96. Karpelowsky JS, Maske CP, Sinclair-Smith C, Rode H. Glutaraldehyde-induced bowel injury after laparoscopy. *J Pediatr Surg.* 2006;41(6):e23-e25. [VB]

97. Nazik H, Bodur S, Api M, Aytan H, Narin R. Glutaraldehyde-induced bowel injury during gynecologic

laparoscopy. *J Minim Invasive Gynecol.* 2012;19(6):756-757. [VB]

98. *AAMI TIR 34: 2014. Water for the Reprocessing of Medical Devices.* Arlington, VA: Association for the Advancement of Medical Instrumentation; 2014. [IVC]

99. Gillespie JL, Arnold KE, Noble-Wang J, et al. Outbreak of *Pseudomonas aeruginosa* infections after transrectal ultrasound-guided prostate biopsy. *Urology.* 2007;69(5):912-914. [VB]

100. Wendelboe AM, Baumbach J, Blossom DB, Frank P, Srinivasan A, Sewell CM. Outbreak of cystoscopy related infections with *Pseudomonas aeruginosa*: New Mexico, 2007. *J Urol.* 2008;180(2):588-592. [IIIB]

101. Guideline for sterile technique. In: *Guidelines for Perioperative Practice.* Denver, CO: AORN, Inc; 2017:75-104. [IVA]

102. Stigt JA, Wolfhagen MJ, Smulders P, Lammers V. The identification of *Stenotrophomonas maltophilia* contamination in ultrasound endoscopes and reproduction of decontamination failure by deliberate soiling tests. *Respiration.* 2015;89(6):565-571. [VB]

103. Guideline for a safe environment of care, part 1. In: *Guidelines for Perioperative Practice.* Denver, CO: AORN, Inc; 2017:243-268. [IVA]

104. 29 CFR 1910.151: Medical services and first aid. Occupational Safety and Health Administration https://www.osha.gov/pls/oshaweb/owadisp.show_document?p_table=STANDARDS&p_id=9806. Accessed October 5, 2017.

105. *ANSI/ISEA Z358.1-2014 American National Standard for Emergency Eyewash and Shower Equipment.* Arlington, VA: International Safety Equipment Association; 2014. [IVC]

106. Occupational safety and health act of 1970 (PL 91-596). Occupational Safety and Health Administration. https://www.osha.gov/pls/oshaweb/owadisp.show_document?p_table=OSHACT&p_id=2743. Accessed October 5, 2017.

107. Overview of health care HVAC systems. *In: HVAC Design Manual for Hospitals and Clinics.* Atlanta, GA: American Society of Heating, Refrigerating and Air-Conditioning Engineers; 2013:1-18. [IVC]

108. *Industrial Ventilation: A Manual of Recommended Practice for Design.* Cincinnati, OH: American Conference of Governmental Industrial Hygienists; 2016. [IVC]

109. Guideline for a safe environment of care, part 2. In: *Guidelines for Perioperative Practice.* Denver, CO: AORN, Inc; 2017:269-294. [IVA]

110. National Institute for Occupational Safety and Health, ed. *Evaluation of Ortho-phthalaldehyde in Eight Healthcare Facilities.* HHE report no. 2006-0238-3239. Cincinnati, OH: US Department of Health and Human Services, Centers for Disease Control and Prevention, National Institute for Occupational Safety and Health; 2015. [IIIA]

111. TLV / BEI introduction. American Conference of Governmental Industrial Hygienists. http://www.acgih.org/tlv-bei-guidelines/tlv-bei-introduction. Accessed October 5, 2017.

112. OSHA occupational chemical database. Occupational Safety and Health Administration. https://www.osha.gov/chemicaldata/. Accessed October 5, 2017.

113. 29 CFR 1910.134: Personal protective equipment: respiratory protection. Occupational Safety and Health Administration. https://www.osha.gov/pls/oshaweb/owadisp.show_document?p_table=STANDARDS&p_id=12716. Accessed October 5, 2017.

114. 29 CFR 1910.133: Personal protective equipment: eye and face protection. US Government Publishing Office. http://www.ecfr.gov/cgi-bin/text-idx?SID=138cf8e943da8b05e30a2d25732e5a51&mc=true&node=se29.5.1910_1133&rgn=div8. Accessed October 5, 2017.

115. 29 CFR 1910.132: Personal protective equipment: general requirements. Occupational Safety and Health Administration. https://www.osha.gov/pls/oshaweb/owadisp.show_document?p_table=STANDARDS&p_id=9777. Accessed October 5, 2017.

116. 29 CFR 1910.138: Personal protective equipment: hand protection. Occupational Safety and Health Administration. https://www.osha.gov/pls/oshaweb/owadisp.show_document?p_table=STANDARDS&p_id=9788. Accessed October 5, 2017.

117. Guideline for prevention of transmissible infections. In: *Guidelines for Perioperative Practice.* Denver, CO: AORN, Inc; 2017:507-542. [IVA]

118. Guideline for surgical attire. In: *Guidelines for Perioperative Practice.* Denver, CO: AORN, Inc; 2017:105-128. [IVA]

119. Resource conservation and recovery act (RCRA) laws and regulations. US Environmental Protection Agency. https://www.epa.gov/rcra. Accessed October 5, 2017.

120. 42 USC 6901: Congressional findings. US Government Publishing Office. https://www.gpo.gov/fdsys/pkg/USCODE-2011-title42/html/USCODE-2011-title42-chap82.htm. Accessed October 5, 2017.

121. 42 USC 6926: Authorized state hazardous waste programs. US Government Publishing Office. https://www.gpo.gov/fdsys/granule/USCODE-2010-title42/USCODE-2010-title42-chap82-subchapIII-sec6926. Accessed October 5, 2017.

122. Introduction to hospital waste management. In: *Healthcare Risk Control.* Vol 3. Plymouth Meeting, PA: ECRI, Inc; 2011:1-13. [VB]

123. Management of hazardous chemicals and waste. In: *Healthcare Risk Control.* Vol 3. Plymouth Meeting, PA: ECRI, Inc; 2017:1-15. [VB]

124. Guideline for patient information management. In: *Guidelines for Perioperative Practice.* Denver, CO: AORN, Inc; 2017:591-616. [IVA]

125. RC.01.01.01: The hospital maintains complete and accurate medical records for each individual patient. In: *Hospital Accreditation Standards.* Oakbrook Terrace, IL: Joint Commission Resources; 2017.

126. MS.16: Medical record maintenance. In: *NIAHO Interpretive Guidelines and Surveyor Guidance.* Version 11. Milford, OH: DNV-GL Healthcare; 2014:37.

127. RC.01.01.01: The organization maintains complete and accurate clinical records. In: *Standards for Ambulatory Care.* Oakbrook Terrace, IL: Joint Commission Resources; 2017.

128. Clinical records and health information. In: *Accreditation Handbook for Ambulatory Health Care.* Skokie, IL: Accreditation Association for Ambulatory Health Care, Inc; 2016:51-53.

129. Medical records: operating room records. In: *Regular Standards and Checklist for Accreditation of Ambulatory Surgery Facilities.* Version 14.5. Gurnee, IL: American Association for Accreditation of Ambulatory Surgery Facilities; 2017:60-63.

130. Medical records: procedure room records. In: *Procedural Standards and Checklist for Accreditation of Ambulatory Surgery Facilities.* Version 3. Gurnee, IL: American Association for Accreditation of Ambulatory Surgery Facilities, Inc; 2011:64-66.

131. HR.01.05.03: Staff participate in ongoing education and training. In: *Comprehensive Accreditation Manual:*

CAMH for Hospitals. Oakbrook Terrace, IL: Joint Commission Resources; 2017.

132. MS.10: Continuing education. In: *NIAHO Interpretive Guidelines and Surveyor Guidance*. Version 11. Milford, OH: DNV-GL Healthcare; 2014:30.

133. HR.01.05.03: Staff participate in ongoing education and training. In: *Comprehensive Accreditation Manual: CAMAC for Ambulatory Care*. Oakbrook Terrace, IL: Joint Commission Resources; 2017.

134. Governance. In: *Accreditation Handbook for Ambulatory Health Care*. Skokie, IL: Accreditation Association for Ambulatory Health Care, Inc; 2016:33-40.

135. Personnel: personnel records; individual personnel files. In: *Regular Standards and Checklist for Accreditation of Ambulatory Surgery Facilities*. Gurnee, IL: American Association for Accreditation of Ambulatory Surgery Facilities, Inc; 2017:74-75.

136. Henn SA, Boiano JM, Steege AL. Precautionary practices of healthcare workers who disinfect medical and dental devices using high-level disinfectants. *Infect Control Hosp Epidemiol*. 2015;36(2):180-185. [IIIB]

137. Taneja N, Gill SS, Biswal M, et al. Working awareness of healthcare workers regarding sterilisation, disinfection, and transmission of bloodborne infections and device-related infections at a tertiary care referral centre in north India. *J Hosp Infect*. 2010;75(3):244-245. [IIIC]

138. Bailey C, Kay R, Starling P, et al. A health system approach to improving high level disinfection practices. *Am J Infect Control*. 2015;43:S14. [VC]

139. Rettig SL, Hoegg CL, Teszner E, Smathers SA, Satchell L, Sammons J. Ensuring competency of high-level disinfection (HLD) practices in non-central processing department (CPD) locations. *Am J Infect Control*. 2015;43:S22. [VB]

140. LD.04.01.07: The hospital has policies and procedures that guide and support patient care, treatment and services. In: *Hospital Accreditation Standards*. Oakbrook Terrace, IL: Joint Commission Resources; 2017.

141. LD.04.01.07: The organization has policies and procedures that guide and support patient care, treatment, or services. In: *Standards for Ambulatory Care*. Oakbrook Terrace, IL: Joint Commission Resources; 2017.

142. Personnel: personnel records. In: *Procedural Standards and Checklist for Accreditation of Ambulatory Surgery Facilities*. Version 3. Gurnee, IL: American Association for Accreditation of Ambulatory Surgery Facilities, Inc; 2011:77-79.

143. Steege AL, Boiano JM, Sweeney MH. NIOSH health and safety practices survey of healthcare workers: training and awareness of employer safety procedures. *Am J Ind Med*. 2014;57(6):640-652. [IIIA]

144. PI.03.01.01: The hospital improves performance on an ongoing basis. In: *Hospital Accreditation Standards*. Oakbrook Terrace, IL: Joint Commission Resources; 2017.

145. QM.1: Quality management system. In: *NIAHO Interpretive Guidelines and Surveyor Guidance*. Version 11. Milford, OH: DNV-GL Healthcare; 2014:10-17.

146. PI.03.01.01: The organization improves performance. In: *Standards for Ambulatory Care*. Oakbrook Terrace, IL: Joint Commission Resources; 2017.

147. Quality management and improvement. In: *Accreditation Handbook for Ambulatory Health Care*. Skokie, IL: Accreditation Association for Ambulatory Health Care, Inc; 2016:46-50.

148. Quality assessment/quality improvement: quality improvement. In: *Regular Standards and Checklist for Accreditation of Ambulatory Surgery Facilities*. Version 14.5. Gurnee, IL: American Association for Accreditation of Ambulatory Surgery Facilities, Inc; 2017:64.

Acknowledgments

LEAD AUTHOR

Sharon A. Van Wicklin, MSN, RN, CNOR, CRNFA(E), CPSN-R, PLNC, FAAN
Senior Perioperative Practice Specialist
AORN Nursing Department
Denver, Colorado

The author and AORN thank Gerald McDonnell, BSc, PhD, Senior Director, Johnson & Johnson Family of Companies, Raritan, New Jersey; Susan G. Klacik, BS, CRCST, ACE, CHL, FCS, President, Klacik Consulting LLC, Canfield, Ohio; Judith L. Goldberg, DBA, MSN, RN, CNOR, CSSM, CHL, Director, Perioperative and Procedural Services, Lawrence & Memorial Hospital, Waterford, Connecticut; Marie A. Bashaw, DNP, RN, NEA-BC, CNOR, Assistant Professor, Wright State University, Dayton, Ohio; Susan Ruwe, MSN, RN, CPHQ, CIC, Senior Infection Preventionist, Carle Foundation Hospital, Urbana, Illinois; Bernard C. Camins, MD, MSc, Associate Professor of Medicine, University of Alabama at Birmingham; Dawn Myers Yost, MSN, RN, CNOR, CSSM, Manager, Training and Development Surgical Services/ Business Manager, West Virginia University Hospitals/ West Virginia University Medicine, Morgantown; and Jane Flowers, MSN, RN, CNOR, NEA-BC, CRCST, Manager, Sterile Processing, University of Maryland Shore Regional Health, Easton, for their assistance in developing this guideline.

PUBLICATION HISTORY

Originally published August 1980, *AORN Journal*, as AORN "Recommended practices for sterilization and disinfection."

Format revision July 1982; revised February 1987.

Revised October 1992 as "Recommended practices for disinfection"; published as proposed recommended practices for September 1994 as "Recommended practices for chemical disinfection."

Revised 1998 as "Recommended practices for high-level disinfection"; published March 1999, *AORN Journal*.

Revised November 2004; published in *Standards, Recommended Practices, and Guidelines*, 2005 edition. Reprinted February 2005, *AORN Journal*.

Revised November 2008; published in *Perioperative Standards and Recommended Practices*, 2009 edition.

Minor edition revisions made in November 2009 for publication in *Perioperative Standards and Recommended Practices*, 2010 edition.

Reformatted September 2012 for publication in *Perioperative Standards and Recommended Practices*, 2013 edition.

Minor editing revisions made in November 2014 as "Guideline for high-level disinfection" in *Guidelines for Perioperative Practice*, 2015 edition.

Revised January 2018 for publication in *Guidelines for Perioperative Practice*, 2018 edition.

GUIDELINE FOR CLEANING AND CARE OF SURGICAL INSTRUMENTS

The Guideline for Cleaning and Care of Surgical Instruments has been approved by the AORN Guidelines Advisory Board. It was presented as a proposed guideline for comments by members and others. The guideline is effective November 15, 2014. The recommendations in the guidelines are intended to be achievable and represent what is believed to be an optimal level of practice. Policies and procedures will reflect variations in practice settings and/or clinical situations that determine the degree to which the guideline can be implemented. AORN recognizes the many diverse settings in which perioperative nurses practice; therefore, this guideline is adaptable to all areas where operative and other invasive procedures may be performed.

Purpose

This document provides guidance for cleaning surgical instruments, including point-of-use cleaning, selecting cleaning chemicals, and determining water quality. Guidance is also provided for decontaminating, transporting, inspecting, and care of surgical instruments. Processing of laryngoscope blades and handles and ophthalmic instruments, special precautions necessary to minimize the risk for transmitting prion diseases from contaminated instruments, and the use of personal protective equipment (PPE) that must be worn during cleaning and care of instruments are also addressed. The recommendations are general recommendations, as it is not possible to make a separate recommendation for every instrument used.

Sterilization, packaging for terminal sterilization, high-level disinfection, and processing of flexible endoscopes are outside the scope of this document. Guidance for these topics is provided in the AORN Guideline for Sterilization,[1] Guideline for High-Level Disinfection,[2] Guideline for Selection and Use of Packaging Systems for Sterilization,[3] and Guideline for Cleaning and Processing Flexible Endoscopes and Endoscope Accessories.[4]

Evidence Review

On August 2, 2013, a medical librarian conducted a systematic search of the databases MEDLINE®, CINAHL®, and the Cochrane Database of Systematic Reviews for meta-analyses, systematic reviews, randomized controlled and non-randomized trials and studies, case reports, letters, reviews, and guidelines. The search was limited to literature published in English from January 2008 through June 2013.

Search terms included *surgical instruments, equipment reuse, surgical procedures, instrument reprocessing, cross infection, infection control, surgical wound infection, surgical site infection, equipment contamination, washing system, washer-disinfector, medical device washer, presoak, soak, disinfection, decontamination, sterilization, detergents, sterile water, water purification, water microbiology enzymatic detergents, non-enzymatic detergents, ultrasonic, impingement, maintenance, storage, transport, case cart, inspection, magnification, staining, corrosion, adenosine triphosphate, photobacterium, luciferases, luminescent measurements, microbial sensitivity tests, ninhydrin, antineoplastic agents, toxic anterior segment syndrome, toxic endothelial cell deconstruction, prion diseases, Creutzfeldt-Jakob syndrome, fatal familial insomnia,* and *Gerstmann-Straussler-Scheinker. Surgical instruments* as a broad search term was augmented by the inclusion of terms related to specific instruments, such as *laryngoscopes, blades, forceps, scalpels, dilators, lumens, drills,* and *retractors.*

At the time of the initial search, the librarian established weekly alerts on the search topics and until June 2014, presented relevant results to the lead author. During the development of this guideline, the author requested supplementary literature searches and additional literature that either did not fit the original search criteria or was discovered during the evidence-appraisal process; this additional literature included book chapters and manufacturers' materials. The librarian and author also identified relevant guidelines from government agencies and standards-setting bodies.

Articles were excluded if they addressed the use of a device or the care of patients rather than the practices associated with instrument processing. Articles related to processing single-use devices were excluded as outside the scope of this document. Articles that were clearly biased or written as product promotion for marketing purposes also were excluded.

Articles identified in the search were provided to the lead author and assigned evidence reviewer for review and critical appraisal using the AORN Research or Non-Research Evidence Appraisal Tools as appropriate. The literature was independently evaluated and appraised by the lead author and evidence reviewer according to the strength and quality of the evidence. Each article was then assigned an appraisal score determined by consensus. The appraisal score is noted in brackets after each reference as applicable.

The evidence supporting each activity and intervention statement within a specific recommendation was summarized, and the AORN Evidence-Rating Model was used to rate the strength of the collective evidence. Factors considered in the review of the collective body of evidence were the quality of similar evidence on a given topic, the consistency of the evidence supporting a recommendation, and the potential benefits and harms. The assigned evidence rating is noted in brackets after each intervention and activity statement.

Editor's note: MEDLINE is a registered trademark of the US National Library of Medicine's Medical Literature Analysis and Retrieval System, Bethesda, MD. CINAHL, Cumulative Index to Nursing and Allied Health Literature, is a registered trademark of EBSCO Industries, Birmingham, AL.

Recommendation I

All instruments and devices used in surgery should be cleared by the US Food and Drug Administration (FDA) for use in surgery and have written, manufacturer-validated cleaning and decontamination instructions for use (IFU).

Manufacturers of reusable instruments and devices cleared by the FDA provide validated cleaning and decontamination instructions and instructions on how to process devices between uses. Items cannot be assumed to be clean, decontaminated, or sterile unless the manufacturer's IFU are derived from validation testing and the user has followed those instructions. Instructions for use provide users with validated techniques for processing instruments.[5,6]

I.a. A multidisciplinary team consisting of sterile processing personnel, perioperative registered nurses (RNs), physicians, infection preventionists, and other stakeholders should develop a mechanism for evaluating and selecting the products that require cleaning and decontamination and the associated cleaning products that will be used at the health care facility.[7] *[2: High Evidence]*

Involvement of a multidisciplinary team in the product selection process allows input from personnel with expertise beyond that of the clinical end users. Facility areas in which personnel are responsible for cleaning, decontamination, and care of instruments may include operating rooms (ORs), sterile processing areas, procedure areas, physician offices, and clinics where processing is performed. Personnel working in these areas have information concerning equipment and resource capabilities that will help determine the facility's ability to follow the manufacturer's written IFU.

A standardized product evaluation and selection process that includes input from key personnel may assist in the selection of functional and reliable products that are safe, cost-effective, and environmentally friendly; promote quality care; and prevent duplication or rapid obsolescence.[7]

I.b. Before the purchase of surgical instruments and other devices used for surgical or other procedures performed in the facility, a designated person responsible for processing surgical instruments should obtain and evaluate

the applicable manufacturer's written IFU, including
- instructions for precleaning at the point of use,
- transport of the soiled device,
- cleaning,
- decontamination,
- inspection,
- functionality testing,
- packaging,
- high-level disinfection, and
- sterilization,

to determine whether the facility has the capability to comply with the manufacturer's instructions. *[2: High Evidence]*

Cleaning, decontamination, and handling instructions recommended by device manufacturers vary widely. Some instruments may require special cleaning, packaging, sterilization, or maintenance procedures that cannot be provided by the facility.[6,8-12]

I.b.1. A designated person responsible for processing surgical instruments should review the instrument manufacturer's written IFU to determine the requirements for replicating the validated cleaning and processing methods. *[5: Benefits Balanced with Harms]*

I.b.2. The manufacturer's written IFU should be reviewed for requirements related to
- utilities (eg, water, compressed air);
- cleaning equipment;
- device disassembly required for cleaning;
- accessories (eg, adaptors for creating a correct connection between the device and equipment, utilities, and cleaning equipment);
- accessories for cleaning lumens, ports, and internal parts;
- cleaning agents;
- lubricants; and
- procedures for handling, cleaning, disinfecting, testing, packaging, and sterilizing.[5,6,13,14]

[4: Limited Evidence]

I.b.3. Prepurchase evaluation of the health care facility's capability to comply with the instrument manufacturer's instructions for care and cleaning should include determining requirements for cleaning and decontaminating equipment (eg, washer/decontaminators, ultrasonic cleaners, forced-air dryers, sinks, detergents, brushes, adaptors, lubricants) and whether
- the instructions are clear and understandable to personnel who will be handling the instrument or device,
- a water supply of the specified quality is available, and
- utilities (eg, electrical, ventilation, steam supply) are in place.

[4: Limited Evidence]

The instrument manufacturers' IFU provide instructions for cleaning and processing that are required to achieve the validated results.[6]

Recommendation II

Before use, all new, repaired, refurbished, and loaned instruments and devices should be cleaned and decontaminated, inspected, and sterilized or high-level disinfected according to the instrument or device manufacturer's written IFU.

It is not possible to verify how all new, repaired, refurbished, and loaned instruments and devices have been handled, cleaned, inspected, or processed before receipt in the facility. Failure to clean, inspect, disinfect, or sterilize an item may lead to transmission of pathogenic microorganisms from a contaminated device and create a risk for patient injury, including surgical site infection (SSI).[15-25]

Inspecting instruments and devices upon receipt and before processing in accordance with the manufacturer's written IFU can help verify that there are no obvious defects and may prevent damaged or incorrectly functioning devices from being used in patient care.[26]

Cleaning and decontamination remove soil that may interfere with subsequent processing and reduce or eliminate viable microorganisms, thereby rendering devices safe to handle.[2,10]

II.a. The manufacturer's written IFU should be readily available to the personnel responsible for processing instruments and devices used for surgical or other procedures performed in the facility.[27] *[1: Strong Evidence]*

Instructions for use identify the processes necessary to achieve effective decontamination and sterility.[10]

II.a.1. Manufacturer's IFU should be reviewed periodically, and processing practices should comply with the most current IFU. *[3: Moderate Evidence]*

Manufacturers may make modifications to their IFU when new technology becomes available, when regulatory requirements change, or when modifications are made to a device.[28]

II.b. Accessories specified by the device manufacturer for cleaning and processing should be obtained at the time of the device purchase and used in accordance with the IFU. *[4: Limited Evidence]*

Using accessories that are designed and manufactured to the device manufacturer's specifications facilitates performance of the required cleaning and processing procedures.[6]

II.c. Instruments and related accessories should be removed from external shipping containers and web-edged or corrugated cardboard boxes before transfer into the decontamination area. *[4: Limited Evidence]*

External shipping containers and web-edged cardboard boxes may collect dust, debris, and insects during transport and may carry contaminants into the facility.[1,10]

II.d. Instruments should be inspected for defects and correct function upon receipt.[29,30] Instrument inspection should include verifying
- tip integrity and alignment,
- security of screws,
- ability of ratchets to hold,
- sharpness of cutting edges,
- integrity of box locks,
- freedom of moveable parts, and
- insulation integrity (for instruments used for electrosurgery).

[3: Moderate Evidence]

Inspection of instruments before processing may minimize the risk of damaged, nonfunctioning, or incorrectly functioning instruments being used in patient care.

II.e. A multidisciplinary team appointed by the health care facility should establish policies and procedures for managing loaned items (eg, instruments). The policies and procedures should include
- a process for requesting and communicating the need for loaned instrument sets;
- time requirements for preprocedure delivery, product testing, and processing (ie, cleaning, decontaminating, inspecting, packaging, sterilizing) and for postprocedure processing and pick-up;
- requirements for education and competency verification of personnel before new or loaned instrumentation is used;
- a process for obtaining and reviewing manufacturers' written IFU;
- delivery requirements (eg, location, documentation);
- a process for returning the item(s) to the lender;
- time requirements for vendor retrieval;
- inventory requirements and a process for taking inventory;
- processes for care, cleaning, decontaminating, inspecting, packaging, and sterilizing before use;
- responsibility for ensuring each instrument set weighs no more than 25 lb (11.3 kg);
- method of transport;
- processes for point-of-use and postprocedure cleaning and decontamination; and
- documentation of processes and transactions related to loaned instruments.[31,32]

[4: Limited Evidence]

A successful loaned instrument management program begins with clear and detailed policies and procedures developed in collaboration with all stakeholders.[29]

II.e.1. Loaned instruments should be cleaned, decontaminated, inspected, and sterilized by the receiving health care organization before use. *[4: Limited Evidence]*

Conditions of transport vary, and an event could occur during transport that could compromise sterility or cause damage to the instruments before they are received at the facility. Inspection verifies that the instruments have no visible defects or damage. Parameters of inhouse sterilization can be verified immediately after a cycle is complete. Even if the instruments have been sterilized in another health care facility, the user will have no record of the sterilization process in the event of a recall.[29,30]

II.e.2. Before processing and preferably before receipt of loaned instruments, a designated person responsible for processing surgical instruments should obtain and review the manufacturers' written IFU for cleaning. *[3: Moderate Evidence]*

When instructions are received in advance, preparations can be made for cleaning and sterilization before the arrival of the instruments. Advance preparation can prevent potential delays in patient care and help ensure correct cleaning and sterilization procedures are followed. Review of processing instructions before receipt of the instruments may improve the efficiency of processing.[33]

II.e.3. The accessories needed to process loaned instruments according to the manufacturer's written IFU should be received before processing.[5] *[4: Limited Evidence]*

Accessories specified in the manufacturer's written IFU are those the manufacturer has determined are needed to perform required cleaning procedures.[6]

II.e.4. Loaned instruments should be requested when the surgery is scheduled and delivered to the health care facility in sufficient time to allow inhouse inventorying, inspection, disassembly, cleaning, packaging, and terminal sterilization in accordance with the manufacturer's written IFU.[29,32] *[4: Limited Evidence]*

When there is insufficient time to process instruments according to the manufacturers' written IFU, patient safety may be at risk.[29,32,34] Management of loaned instruments requires planning. Requesting the instruments well in advance of the surgical procedure allows adequate time for the vendor to deliver the instruments and for facility personnel to perform the required cleaning; decontamination; inspection; sterilization; and if needed, product quality assurance testing procedures.

II.e.5. Loaned instruments and accessories should be removed from external shipping containers and web-edged or corrugated cardboard boxes before transfer into the decontamination area. *[4: Limited Evidence]*

External shipping containers and web-edged cardboard boxes may collect dust, debris, and insects during transport and may carry contaminants into the facility.[1,10]

II.e.6. The recipient should inventory and document the type and quantity of loaned instruments and confirm receipt with the lender upon delivery.[29] *[3: Moderate Evidence]*

Inventory lists of instruments help provide verification that the instrument set is complete upon receipt. Taking inventory is critical to verifying that all required instruments have been received and are available for use during the procedure. When an inventory is not performed, it is not possible to determine whether the instruments that were intended to be delivered were actually received and that all instruments are returned to the lender. If an instrument critical to the procedure is not available when needed, the surgeon may not be able to perform the procedure as planned and patient care may be compromised or delayed.[16,35]

II.e.7. Loaned instruments should be inspected for defects and correct function upon receipt.[29,30] Instrument inspection should include verifying

- tip integrity and alignment,
- security of screws,
- ability of ratchets to hold,
- sharpness of cutting edges,
- integrity of box locks,
- freedom of moveable parts, and
- insulation integrity (for instruments used for electrosurgery).

[3: Moderate Evidence]

Inspection of instruments before processing may minimize the risk of damaged, nonfunctioning, or incorrectly functioning instruments being used in patient care.

II.e.8. Loaned instruments, regardless of whether they were processed in another health care facility, should be considered contaminated and should be delivered directly to a sterile processing area and decontaminated as soon as possible after delivery.[10,29] *[3: Moderate Evidence]*

It is not possible to know under what conditions instruments were processed at another facility or for the receiving facility to monitor or control events that may contaminate items during transport. The receiving facility is responsible for providing the surgical patient with sterile products and is therefore responsible for monitoring the cleaning and sterilization process.[19,29,30]

STERILIZATION AND DISINFECTION

The evidence review for this guideline found only one published article related to the condition of loaned instruments. This limited, single-facility, quality assurance project evaluated the cleanliness of loaned instruments upon receipt. A total of 139 sets were visually inspected and tested for blood residue during a two-month period. Six sets (4.3%) were visibly contaminated. Twenty-three sets (16.5%) tested positive for blood residue. The authors recommended that that all loaned instruments be enclosed in biohazard containers, that some method of documentation of the decontamination and quality assurance processes used by the lending institution be included with each shipment, that designated receiving areas be established, that institutions establish standard procedures for loaned instrumentation, and that the procedure be communicated not only to sterile processing personnel and the hospital infection prevention committee, but also to perioperative personnel.[33]

II.e.9. Loaned instruments should be disassembled, cleaned, decontaminated, and inspected before they are returned to the vendor or lending facility.[1,30] *[3: Moderate Evidence]*

Instruments used in surgery may be contaminated with blood, body fluids, or other potentially infectious materials and may pose a safety risk to health care and other personnel if they are not handled or decontaminated correctly.[10]

II.e.10. Loaned instruments should be inventoried and documentation should be provided to the lender and receiver regarding the processing and disposition of items after decontamination.[29,30] *[3: Moderate Evidence]*

Documentation makes it possible to determine where an instrument may have been lost or damaged and provides a description of the steps taken to help ensure the return of items that are safe to handle.

Recommendation III

Instruments should be cleaned and decontaminated as soon as possible after use.

Cleaning instruments as soon as possible after use can help prevent formation of biofilm and dried blood. When blood or other bioburden is allowed to dry on instruments, it can become more difficult to remove. The effectiveness of disinfection or sterilization can be compromised when thorough cleaning is not accomplished.[6,10,19,28]

III.a. Preparation for decontamination of instruments should begin at the point of use.[10,12,28] *[2: High Evidence]*

Moistening and removing gross soil at the point of use can help prevent organic material and debris from drying on instruments. Organic material and debris are more difficult to remove from surgical instruments when they are allowed to dry. Removal of organic material and debris at the point of use can improve the efficacy and effectiveness of cleaning and decontamination.[2,6,10]

III.b. Instruments should be kept free of gross soil during the procedure. *[2: High Evidence]*

Gross soil left to dry on instruments can affect the efficacy of subsequent disinfection and sterilization processes.[2,10,22,36-38]

III.b.1. During the procedure, the scrub person should remove gross soil from instruments by wiping the surfaces with a sterile surgical sponge moistened with sterile water. Saline should not be used to wipe instrument surfaces. *[3: Moderate Evidence]*

Blood, organic material, debris, and saline are highly corrosive to instrument surfaces and can cause corrosion, rusting, and pitting when allowed to dry on surgical instruments. These materials can be difficult to remove from all surfaces during the cleaning and decontamination process, reducing the efficacy of the subsequent sterilization process.[6,10,12,36]

III.b.2. Periodically during the procedure, the scrub person should use sterile water to irrigate instruments with lumens. *[1: Strong Evidence]*

Irrigating instrument lumens periodically throughout a procedure removes gross soil and may reduce the risk of biofilm formation. Biofilm can form on many surfaces but is particularly problematic when it forms in lumens because it is difficult to see and remove. After a biofilm forms, mechanical action is required to remove it.[38]

In an experimental longitudinal study, Vickery et al[38] grew a mature biofilm of *Pseudomonas aeruginosa* on 20 Teflon® endoscope tubings and subjected them to 20 decontamination and recontamination cycles. Decontamination consisted of a manual wash followed by a 2% glutaraldehyde disinfection in an automated endoscope reprocessor. This process was repeated 20 times. At the 20th cycle, 90% of the tubing was biofilm free. The researchers concluded that washing endoscopes under high flow rates with some detergents removed established biofilms. Although the researchers examined endoscopes, the results of this study may be applicable to decontamination of other lumened instruments.

If not removed, a biofilm can reduce the efficacy of subsequent disinfection or sterilization processes.[2,10,28,38]

911

STERILIZATION AND DISINFECTION

III.c. All instruments opened onto the sterile field in the operating or procedure room should be cleaned and decontaminated whether or not they have been used.[10,28] *[3: Moderate Evidence]*

Scrubbed persons may touch and contaminate instruments without being aware of it. Instruments that were used may come in contact with unused items. Airborne microorganisms may come in contact with instruments that have not been used. Contamination of unused instruments on the sterile field can occur without the occurrence being noticed.[12]

III.d. In preparation for transport to a decontamination area, sharp instruments must be segregated from other instruments and confined in a puncture-resistant container. *[1: Regulatory Requirement]*

Segregation of sharps from other instruments minimizes the risk of injury to personnel handling instruments during cleaning and decontamination. The Occupational Safety and Health Administration (OSHA) prohibits processes that require employees to place their hands into basins of sharp instruments because of the risk for percutaneous exposure to bloodborne pathogens.[39] The reader should refer to the Guideline for Sharps Safety[40] for guidance related to preventing sharps injuries.

III.d.1. Disposable sharps (eg, scalpel blades, suture needles) must be removed and discarded into a closeable, puncture-resistant container that is leak-proof on its sides and bottom and is labeled or color-coded as biohazardous.[39,40] *[1: Regulatory Requirement]*

III.e. When an instrument is composed of more than one piece, it should be opened and disassembled according to the manufacturer's written IFU and arranged in a manner that will permit contact of cleaning solutions with all surfaces of the instruments. *[1: Strong Evidence]*

When surfaces cannot be contacted by cleaning solutions, thorough cleaning cannot be achieved; thus, these surfaces can retain organic material and debris. These retained materials can prevent contact of cleaning solutions and disinfecting or sterilizing agents with instrument surfaces, reduce the effectiveness of subsequent disinfection or sterilization processes,[2,10,12] and cause patient injury if they are not removed before sterilization.[17,21,23,41] Further research is warranted to determine the clinical significance of retained organic material and debris on instruments during disinfection and sterilization processes.

In a case series investigation, Parada et al[23] characterized the relationship between sterilization failure and SSIs. During a 14-week period, the investigators collected laboratory data on five patients who sustained SSIs after anterior cruciate ligament reconstruction and determined the infection rate was 12.2%. Before this

period, the infection rate for anterior cruciate ligament reconstruction was 0.3%. The investigators found gross organic material inside an instrument common to all the surgical procedures. The inadequate removal of debris had occurred because there was no brush available with a diameter small enough to clean the cannula on the device.

III.f. Delicate instruments should be protected from damage during transport to a decontamination area. Delicate and other easily damaged instruments, such as fiberoptic cords, rigid endoscopes, and microsurgical instruments, should be placed on top of heavier instruments or segregated into separate containers.[10,12] *[3: Moderate Evidence]*

Instruments may shift during transport, causing heavy instruments to damage more-delicate instruments.

III.g. Instruments should be kept moist until they are cleaned. A towel moistened with water placed over the instruments may be used. Saline should not be used. *[3: Moderate Evidence]*

Keeping instruments moist helps prevent blood, organic materials, and debris from drying and adhering to the instruments. Dried organic materials and debris can make instruments more difficult to clean and potentially lead to the formation of biofilm. Prolonged exposure of instruments to saline can cause pitting.[10,12]

III.g.1. Instruments that cannot be cleaned immediately should be treated with an instrument cleaner according to the device and the instrument cleaner manufacturers' written IFU.[8,10,12] *[2: High Evidence]*

Treating instruments with an instrument cleaner at the point of use can help prevent rusting and corrosion; prevent blood, organic materials, and debris from drying on the instruments; and inhibit biofilm formation.[8,10]

III.g.2. Liquids used to soak contaminated items at the point of use should be discarded before transport. When disposal of the solution is not feasible, it must be transported in a leak-proof container to the decontamination area for disposal.[39] *[1: Regulatory Requirement]*

Contaminated liquids may be spilled during transport, presenting a risk of contaminating the environment and exposing personnel to blood, body fluids, and other potentially infectious materials.[10,12,39]

Recommendation IV

Contaminated instruments must be contained during transport to a decontamination area.[10,39]

Containment of contaminated instruments decreases the potential for injury to personnel or their exposure to blood, body fluids, or other potentially infectious materials and helps prevent damage to the instruments during transport.

IV.a. Contaminated instruments should be transported to the decontamination area as soon as possible after completion of the procedure. *[1: Strong Evidence]*

Removal of blood, organic materials, and debris from instruments becomes more difficult after they have dried.[2,10,37,42]

IV.b. Soiled instruments must be transported to the decontamination area in a closed container or enclosed transport cart. The container or cart must be
- leak proof,[39]
- puncture resistant,[39]
- large enough to contain all contents, and
- labeled with a fluorescent orange or orange-red label containing a biohazard legend.[39]

[1: Regulatory Requirement]

Transporting soiled instruments in a manner that prevents exposing personnel to bloodborne pathogens and other potentially infectious materials is an OSHA requirement.[39]

Labeling the transport containment device communicates to others that the contents are potentially infectious.

IV.b.1. Biohazard labels should be affixed so as to prevent separation from the contents. When appropriate to the configuration of the contents, a red bag or red container may be used instead of a label to indicate contaminated waste.[39] *[1: Regulatory Requirement]*

IV.b.2. If the instrument containment device has been contaminated, it must be either cleaned at the point of use or placed inside another containment device and labeled as biohazardous.[39,43] *[1: Regulatory Requirement]*

Contact with contaminated surfaces can transmit potentially infectious microorganisms.[39,43] The reader should refer to the AORN Guideline for Prevention of Transmissible Infections[44] for guidance.

IV.b.3. Contaminated instruments and other items should be separated from clean and sterile supplies before transport to the processing area. *[4: Limited Evidence]*

Separation of soiled instruments from clean supplies minimizes the risk of cross-contamination.[10]

Recommendation V

Instruments should be cleaned and decontaminated in an area separate from locations where clean items are handled.[10,45,46]

Physical separation of decontamination areas from areas where clean items are handled minimizes the risk of cross-contamination. Cross-contamination can result when soiled items are placed in close proximity to clean items or are placed on surfaces upon which clean items are later placed. Droplets and aerosols created during cleaning of soiled instruments can cause cross-contamination of any nearby clean items or surfaces.

V.a. The sterile processing area should have
- separate clean and decontamination spaces, which may be rooms or areas;
- decontamination and clean spaces that are separated by one of three methods:
  - a wall with a door or pass-through,
  - a partial wall or partition that is at least 4 ft high and at least the width of the counter, or
  - a distance of 4 ft between the instrument washing sink and the area where the instruments are prepared for sterilization;
- separate sinks for washing instruments and for hand hygiene;
- decontaminating equipment (eg, automated washer, ultrasonic cleaner); and
- storage space for PPE and cleaning supplies in the decontamination area.

[4: Limited Evidence]

The requirements for processing reusable medical devices do not vary by location. Equivalent procedures, supplies, and equipment are needed in all locations where sterile processing is performed.[45,46]

V.b. Instruments should not be cleaned or decontaminated in scrub or hand sinks. *[5: Benefits Balanced with Harms]*

Cleaning soiled instruments in a scrub or hand sink can contaminate the sink and faucet, which are intended to be used for clean activities (eg, hand washing, surgical hand antisepsis).

V.c. The decontamination area must contain
- an eyewash station[10,47,48] and
- a hand-washing sink.[39]

[1: Regulatory Requirement]

The Occupational Safety and Health Administration requires that an eyewash station be provided where chemicals that are hazardous to the eyes are located.[47] Hand hygiene facilities are required by OSHA for use after removal of PPE.[39]

V.c.1. Eyewash stations, either plumbed or self contained, must be provided within the immediate area where chemicals such as instrument cleaning solutions or disinfectants that are hazardous to the eyes are located.[47,49] Eyewash stations should be located so that travel time is no greater than 10 seconds from the location of chemical use or storage, or should be immediately available if the chemical is caustic or is a strong acid.[49] Eyewash stations should be located on the same level as the hazard, with the path of travel free of obstructions (eg, doors) that may inhibit immediate use of the eyewash station.[49] Eyewash stations should

- be identified with a highly visible sign[49];
- deliver warm water (ie, 60° F to 100° F [15.6° C to 37.8° C]) at a rate of 1.5 L/minute for 15 minutes[49];
- be designed to flush both eyes simultaneously using a hands-free, stay-open feature[49];
- be flushed weekly to remove stagnant water, which may contain microbial contamination, from thoe system[49]; and
- be tested regularly and maintained in accordance with the manufacturer's written IFU.[49]

    [1: Regulatory Requirement]

V.d. The decontamination area should contain

- automated equipment consistent with the types of instruments to be cleaned and decontaminated,
- adaptors and accessories to connect instruments with cleaning equipment and utilities,
- a filtered medical-grade compressed air supply,[10] and
- access to water of appropriate quality for rinsing instruments (eg, deionized or reverse-osmosis water).

    [1: Strong Evidence]

Automated cleaning and decontamination provides an effective level of cleaning that is difficult to replicate consistently using manual methods.[50-52] Compressed air is used to clear lumens of detergent and rinse water after cleaning.

V.e. The decontamination area should be stocked with the accessories and supplies needed to clean and decontaminate instruments in accordance with the manufacturers' written IFU.[10] Supplies should include

- brushes or other devices intended to remove organic material and debris from lumens, with a diameter and length appropriate to the lumen to be cleaned;
- enzymatic and nonenzymatic detergent;
- soft, low-linting cleaning cloths;
- testing equipment;
- a source of treated water (eg deionized, reverse osmosis, filtered);
- 70% to 90% alcohol;
- a thermometer; and
- a measuring device.

    [4: Limited Evidence]

Brushes or devices of the correct size used in accordance with the brush or device manufacturer's IFU can facilitate cleaning of lumens. The instrument manufacturer's IFU may recommend either an enzymatic or a nonenzymatic detergent for cleaning. Soft, low-linting cleaning cloths may prevent scratches to the surface of instruments and prevent lint from adhering to the surfaces of the instruments.

Treated water is used for final rinsing. Impurities in untreated water can leave residues on instruments that may lead to corrosion, pitting, or staining.[10,51,53] A thermometer is used to measure that the detergent solution is within the recommended temperature range as specified by the detergent manufacturer's written IFU. Measuring devices are used to mix detergents at the concentration specified by the detergent manufacturer's written IFU.

V.f. The decontamination area heating, ventilation, and air conditioning (HVAC) system should be maintained within the HVAC design parameters at the rate that was applicable according to regulatory and professional guidelines at the time of design or most recent renovation of the HVAC system.[46] *[4: Limited Evidence]*

The HVAC system controls the air quality, temperature, humidity, and pressure of the room in comparison with the surrounding areas. The HVAC system is designed in accordance with the American Society of Heating, Refrigerating and Air-Conditioning Engineers (ASHRAE)[54] and local regulatory requirements to reduce the amount of environmental contaminants and to provide a comfortable environment for occupants in the area.[46]

V.f.1. A multidisciplinary team that includes infection preventionists, perioperative RNs, sterile processing personnel, representatives from facility maintenance, and other stakeholders representing the health care organization should develop and implement a systematic process for monitoring HVAC performance parameters in the decontamination area and a mechanism for resolving variances.[46] *[4: Limited Evidence]*

The HVAC parameters recommended by ASHRAE and the Facilities Guidelines Institute for decontamination areas are

- 2 outdoor air changes per hour,[45,54]
- 6 total air changes per hour,[45,54]
- negative air pressure,[45,54] and
- temperature between 72° F and 78° F (22° C and 26° C).[45,54]

Room temperature may be intentionally adjusted to accommodate the individual comfort needs of the occupants.[45] Negative pressure helps prevent contaminated air from entering into positive-pressure, clean areas. The evidence on the effect of relative humidity on bacterial, fungal, and viral growth is inconclusive. Further research is warranted to determine optimal relative humidity levels to control environmental contamination.

In a descriptive study, Panagopoulou et al[55] examined air and surface fungal levels of two buildings in a Greek tertiary care hospital during a 12-month period. Each room in building A had a separate air-conditioning unit. Building B had a central air-conditioning unit. The researchers determined that, independent of the method of air-conditioning, the fungal levels were higher during the months in which the temperature and humidity levels were higher.

In a literature review on the effects of humidity on bacterial survival, Tang[56] found that various levels of humidity created differing responses in different strains of bacteria. The responses included structural changes and death. The bacterial survival rates were dependent on the species. The author was unable to find a link between humidity and bacterial survival.

In a laboratory setting, Thompson et al[57] found that aerosolized *Staphylococcus epidermidis*, used as a surrogate for *Staphylococcus aureus*, survived at relative humidity levels of < 20%, 40% to 60%, 70% to 80%, and > 90%. The researchers concluded that *S epidermidis* was not affected by the level of relative humidity.

In a literature review of the effect of temperature and humidity on viruses, Memarzadeh[58] reviewed 120 articles and found no conclusive evidence supporting a maximum or minimum relative humidity level to decrease the survival rate of viruses and the ability of viruses to cause diseases.

The ASHRAE guidelines related to room temperature ranges for the decontamination area are the accepted professional guidelines for HVAC systems in the United States.[54] Personnel working in the decontamination area and wearing PPE may become uncomfortable at room temperatures above 72° F (22° C). Lower room temperatures may contribute to the comfort of personnel wearing PPE.

V.f.2.   Designated personnel should perform a risk assessment of the decontamination area if a variance in the parameters of the HVAC system occurs. Based on the risk assessment, measures should be taken to restore the area to full functionality after the HVAC system variance has been corrected.[46] *[5: Benefits Balanced with Harms]*

The evidence review did not reveal any evidence of clinical significance related to the degree of variance in the HVAC system design parameters. The effect of the HVAC system parameters falling out of range is variable. A small variance for a short period of time may not be of clinical concern, whereas a large variance for a longer period may have clinical significance. Further research on this topic is warranted.

V.f.3.   Personnel who identify an unintentional variance (ie, variances other than intentional temperature adjustments) in the pre-

determined HVAC system parameters should report the variance according to the health care organization's policy and procedure.[46] *[5: Benefits Balanced with Harms]*

Rapid communication between affected and responsible personnel may help facilitate resolution of the variance.

Recommendation VI

Personnel working in the decontamination area and handling contaminated instruments must wear PPE.[39]

Contaminated instruments are a potential source of transmissible pathogens. Personnel in the decontamination area are at risk for exposure to blood, body fluids, and other potentially infectious materials. Personal protective equipment helps to protect the individual from exposure to infectious materials.

VI.a.   Personal protective equipment consistent with exposure risks in the decontamination area must be worn,[39] including
- a fluid-resistant gown with sleeves,
- gloves (ie, general purpose utility gloves with a cuff that extends beyond the cuff of the gown),
- a mask and eye protection or a full face shield, and
- shoe covers or boots designed for use as PPE.[39]

[1: Regulatory Requirement]

Splashes, splatters, and skin contact can be reasonably anticipated by personnel handling contaminated instruments. Fluid-resistant gowns can prevent transfer of microorganisms from contaminated items to skin.[10] General purpose utility gloves can minimize the potential for punctures, cuts, and nicks and exposure of the hands to blood, body fluids, and other potentially infectious materials.[10] Utility glove cuffs that extend beyond the cuff of the gown help to provide adequate fluid protection during instrument cleaning in a sink. A mask and eye protection or a full face shield can protect the face and eyes from contact with contaminated aerosols and chemicals used for cleaning purposes.[10] Fluid-resistant shoe covers can protect shoes from contaminants and splashes, splatters, and spills.

VI.a.1.   Personal protective equipment should be placed where it is readily available to personnel entering an area in which there is a risk of exposure to transmissible pathogens.[27] *[1: Regulatory Requirement]*

There is potential for exposure to transmissible pathogens in the decontamination area, and OSHA requires the employer to provide PPE.[39] Placing PPE in an area readily available to decontamination area personnel can facilitate compliance with OSHA requirements for wearing PPE when there is danger of exposure to blood, body fluids, or other potentially infectious materials.

VI.b. Hand hygiene must be performed after PPE is removed.[39] *[1: Regulatory Requirement]*

Perforations can occur in gloves, and hands can become contaminated during removal of PPE; OSHA requires hand hygiene after removal of PPE.[39]

VI.c. Reusable PPE must be cleaned and decontaminated and its integrity confirmed between uses. *[1: Regulatory Requirement]*

Personal protective equipment is appropriate only if it does not permit potentially infectious materials to pass through and contact the individual.[39] Reusable gloves, gowns, aprons, face shields, and eye wear can become contaminated and their integrity compromised during use. Decontamination and confirmation of integrity helps to protect the wearer from exposure.

Recommendation VII

The type of water used for cleaning should be consistent with the manufacturers' written IFU and the intended use of the equipment and cleaning product.[6,10,28,53]

Water quality is affected by the presence of dissolved minerals, solids, chlorides, and other impurities and by its acidity and alkalinity (ie, pH).[53,59] Minerals can cause deposits, scale, or water spots to form on instruments.[53,59] Excessive chlorides can cause pitting.[53,59] The pH level affects the performance of enzymatic and detergent agents.[6,53,59] Untreated water quality fluctuates over time, varies with geographic location and season, and can affect the outcome of cleaning actions.[51,53,60]

VII.a. The final rinse should be performed with treated (eg, distilled, reverse osmosis, filtered) water of a quality that will not stain or cause damage to instruments or contribute to recontamination of the instrument.[10] *[4: Limited Evidence]*

Untreated water can contain contaminants, including endotoxins, which can be deposited on instruments during the final rinse. Rinsing with treated water can prevent deposits of impurities or contaminants on instruments.[10,51]

Endotoxins are heat stable and may not be destroyed by subsequent steam sterilization. Tissue contaminated with endotoxins can cause severe inflammation.[53]

Treated water can prevent spotting, stains, deposits, and corrosion on the surfaces of instruments.[53,59]

VII.b. Device-processing personnel, in collaboration with clinical engineering personnel, should perform a water-quality assessment periodically[53] and after major maintenance to the water supply system to determine water quality relative to the requirements for cleaning as specified in the detergent and cleaning equipment manufacturers' written IFU. *[2: High Evidence]*

Water quality varies seasonally and after water-source maintenance. Periodic testing can indicate whether the chemical combination used to condition the cleaning and decontamination water requires adjusting. Water-quality checks determine the hardness (ie, mineral content) of the water and any impurities present.

Water quality that does not meet the requirements specified in the detergent or the cleaning equipment manufacturers' IFU can adversely affect the efficacy of cleaning chemistries.[6,53] The need for repairs or modifications to the treatment system can be identified from a water-quality check.[53]

A nonexperimental study by Harnroongroj et al[60] compared 32 first-burst water samples with 29 running tap samples of water supplied to an OR and found the bacterial count in first-burst water was three times higher than in running tap water. This research was performed in Thailand and may not be generalizable to the United States.

In a nonexperimental study to determine the effectiveness of a commercially available test for determining the presence of organic soil on instruments after cleaning in automated washers, Alfa et al[51] found that surgical instruments cleaned in automated washers may have visually undetected high post-cleaning residuals of carbohydrate and endotoxin. An objective of the researchers was to determine the level of protein, hemoglobin, carbohydrate, and endotoxin before and after cleaning in an automated washer. The researchers evaluated five types of surgical instruments from plastic surgery trays for residuals both before and after cleaning. Of a total of 25 instruments tested, 21 (84%) had substantially higher carbohydrate levels and 15 (60%) had higher endotoxin levels after cleaning than before cleaning. The results of the study suggest that endotoxins remaining on surgical instruments after cleaning in automated washers may be related to water quality. The researchers recommended monitoring of water quality.

Recommendation VIII

Surgical instrument, cleaning product, and cleaning equipment manufacturers' validated, written IFU should be reviewed for compatibility during selection and followed during use of cleaning products and equipment for cleaning and decontaminating surgical instruments.[10]

The intended use of cleaning products and cleaning equipment varies. Following the manufacturers' written IFU decreases the possibility of selecting and using cleaning products and equipment that may damage instruments.[6]

VIII.a. A multidisciplinary team that includes infection preventionists, perioperative RNs, sterile processing personnel, and other stakeholders representing the health care organization should develop a mechanism for evaluating and selecting products for cleaning surgical instruments. *[4: Limited Evidence]*

The chemical actions of cleaning products vary, and products are intended for different applications. Some cleaning products target specific types of bioburden (eg, protein, lipids, other organic material); others are intended for general purpose cleaning.

Some cleaning products contain one or more enzymes to break up soil and facilitate its removal.[6,61] Enzymes are specific in terms of the soils they remove.[6,61] Some enzymatic detergents contain more than one enzyme and are intended to be used as all-purpose detergents; others are intended for a specific type of soil.[6,61] Protease enzymes target blood and body salts.[6] Amylases target carbohydrates, starches, and sugars.[6,61] Lipases break down fats and oils.[6,61] The pH and the rinsability of cleaning products vary.

Cleaning equipment manufacturers' requirements for selection and use of cleaning products also vary. Some instrument manufacturers' written IFU specifically recommend against using some cleaning agent formulations.

VIII.a.1. Neutral detergents with a pH of 7 that are low foaming and easy to remove during rinsing should be used for manual or mechanical cleaning unless contraindicated by the device or cleaning equipment manufacturer's IFU. *[1: Strong Evidence]*

Detergents help to dislodge solids from the surface of instruments. Neutral pH or slightly alkaline detergents are compatible with most instruments and work well with enzymes that may be added to detergents to help break down and facilitate removal of organic materials.[2] Detergents that are low foaming facilitate observation of the cleaning process.[5]

VIII.a.2. Cleaning products should
- be nonabrasive,
- be low foaming,
- be easy to remove during rinsing,
- be biodegradable,
- provide for soil dispersion,
- be nontoxic in the specific-use dilution,
- be effective for clinically relevant soils under specified conditions,
- have a long shelf life,
- be cost-effective, and
- be able to be tested for effective concentration.[6]

[4: Limited Evidence]

Cleaning products that are nonabrasive can help protect the surface of instruments from damage. Cleaning products that are low foaming are less likely to interfere with the action of mechanical cleaning equipment. Cleaning products that are easy to remove facilitate removal of detergent during rinsing.[6] Cleaning products that are nontoxic contribute to personnel safety. Use of cleaning products that are effective on clinically relevant soils may increase the efficacy of the cleaning process.

VIII.b. Cleaning products must be handled according to the safety data sheets (SDSs) and the manufacturers' written IFU. The SDSs must be readily accessible to employees within the workplace.[62] *[1: Regulatory Requirement]*

Highly acidic or alkaline cleaning agents are corrosive and can cause injury to skin or mucus membranes.[6] Exposure to enzymatic detergents can cause asthma.[2] Access to the cleaning product IFU and SDS provides opportunities for personnel to use the product correctly and obtain information useful for implementing processes that prevent injury.[48]

VIII.c. The cleaning product manufacturer's written IFU should be followed for[2,10]
- water quality, hardness, and pH;
- concentration and dilution;
- water temperature;
- contact time;
- conditions of storage; and
- shelf life and use life.

[1: Strong Evidence]

Water quality, including hardness and pH, can affect the effectiveness of cleaning products.[53] Using the product in the concentration recommended by the manufacturer's written IFU helps to ensure consistent and accurate cleaning chemistry.[10] The manufacturer has determined the correct temperature and contact time to facilitate cleaning with the specific product. Shelf life and use life indicate the time span or use after which the cleaning product's effectiveness cannot be assured. Using the product after expiration or at a temperature other than specified in the IFU can render the product ineffective.[6]

VIII.c.1. An automated titration unit may be used to efficiently concentrate chemicals at a consistent ratio. *[5: Benefits Balanced with Harms]*

The concentration of the solution can vary when it is mixed manually. Use of a titration unit can aid in accurate measurement of the chemical during preparation of the cleaning solution and help personnel to consistently obtain the recommended concentration of the cleaning product.

VIII.d. Abrasive devices and products should not be used to clean instruments unless their use is specified in the device manufacturer's written IFU.[10] *[4: Limited Evidence]*

Abrasive devices and products, such as metal scouring pads, scouring powders, and bleach can cause permanent damage to instrument surfaces and can result in pitting, providing a place that can harbor microorganisms and debris. In some circumstances, the device manufacturer may recommend using a metal brush.[10] In circumstances in which instruments were used on prion-contaminated tissue, the guidelines for processing may recommend use of a corrosive chemical[63,64] (See Recommendation XIII).

VIII.d.1. Brushes or other items used to clean crevices and lumens should have a diameter and length appropriate for the area within or on the instrument or device being cleaned and be made of a material specified as compatible by the instrument or device manufacturer.[10] *[4: Limited Evidence]*

Tissue and debris can become lodged in crevices, box locks, lumens, and other areas of instruments. Use of a brush intended for these difficult-to-clean areas may be required to effectively remove organic material and debris.[10,23]

VIII.d.2. Brushes used to clean lumens should
- meet the requirement for cleaning as specified in the instrument or device manufacturer's written IFU,[10]
- be long enough to clean the entire length of the lumen and exit at the distal end,
- contact the inner surface of the lumen without collapsing,
- have bristles soft enough to prevent damage to the internal lumen surface, and
- be either designed for single use and discarded after each use or be reusable and decontaminated at least daily or more frequently as needed.[10]

[4: Limited Evidence]

Brushes that are too short to exit the distal length of a lumen can push debris to a point in the lumen but fail to remove it. Brushes with bristles that are too small or too large in diameter can prevent thorough cleaning. Bristles that are abrasive can damage instruments.

Reusable brushes that are not decontaminated can cause contaminants to be transferred from one device to another. Use of single-use disposable brushes helps ensure that a clean brush is used each time.

Recommendation IX

Surgical instruments and equipment should be cleaned and decontaminated according to the manufacturer's validated, written IFU.[10]

Cleaning of instruments (ie, removal of organic and inorganic soil) is the first step in decontamination and can be accomplished through manual or mechanical processes. The instrument and equipment manufacturers have determined the manual or mechanical steps and processes necessary to effectively clean a device.[6,10] Decontamination (ie, rendering instruments safe to handle) may require a microbiocidal process after cleaning (eg, wiping with 70% to 90% alcohol). Factors that determine whether a microbiocidal process is required after cleaning include device materials and design (see Recommendation XIII).

IX.a. Manual cleaning as specified in the instrument manufacturer's written IFU should be used for instruments that cannot tolerate mechanical cleaning.[12] *[3: Moderate Evidence]*

Manual cleaning is often recommended for devices that cannot tolerate the action of mechanical cleaning or cannot be immersed (eg, power drills, delicate microsurgical instruments, flexible endoscopes, cameras). Seals on lensed instruments can be damaged when processed through ultrasonic equipment.[10] Mechanical cleaning of devices when the manufacturer's written IFU recommend against it can result in damage to instruments and can limit the associated warranty.

IX.a.1. In preparation for manual cleaning, instruments should be disassembled and ports, valves, stop cocks, ratchets, and joints should be opened.[10,12] *[3: Moderate Evidence]*

Opening and disassembling instruments facilitates contact of the cleaning solution with all surfaces of the instruments.

IX.a.2. Instruments should be rinsed in cool water before washing.[6,10] *[4: Limited Evidence]*

Hot water can denature blood proteins, which makes them more difficult to remove.[10] Cool water can help to prevent coagulation of blood on instruments and can help remove gross soil from lumens, joints, and crevices.[2,6,10] Rinsing with cool water can wash away water-soluble blood proteins and prevent denaturing.[10]

IX.a.3. Unless contraindicated in the device manufacturer's written IFU, the instrument should be submerged for cleaning in a solution of water and detergent intended for cleaning surgical instruments. The detergent should be compatible with the device to be cleaned and used at the concentration and temperature specified in the detergent manufacturer's IFU.[10] *[4: Limited Evidence]*

Full submersion of the instrument in the cleaning solution reduces the risk of splashing potentially contaminated cleaning solution onto personnel and into the environment. The concentration and temperature of the cleaning solution specified in the detergent IFU have been validated by the detergent manufacturer as necessary for the detergent to be effective.[6]

IX.a.4. Lumens should be flushed with cleaning solution and brushed with a brush of the length, diameter, type, and material specified in the device manufacturer's IFU.[6] *[4: Limited Evidence]*

Brushing is necessary to ensure detergent contact of the cleaning solution within lumens. Brushes that are too short cannot contact the entire lumen. Brushes with a diameter that is too small will not contact all surfaces within the lumen.[65]

IX.a.5. Devices with lumens should be immersed in the cleaning solution in a vertical position.[10] *[4: Limited Evidence]*

Air may become trapped within lumens when the device is soaked in a horizontal position. Entrapped air may prevent contact of the cleaning solution with the surfaces within the lumen.

IX.b. Cleaning solutions should be changed before they become heavily soiled, when the temperature of the solution does not meet the temperature specified in the manufacturer's written IFU, and as needed.[10] *[4: Limited Evidence]*

Bioburden is deposited in the cleaning solution during the cleaning process. Frequent changes of the cleaning solution can help to minimize bioburden. Following the manufacturer's written IFU helps facilitate effective cleaning.

IX.c. Instruments that require lubrication should be lubricated with a type of lubricant that is recommended by the instrument manufacturer and is compatible with the subsequent sterilization method. *[3: Moderate Evidence]*

Instruments require different types of lubricant depending on the design of the device or the sterilization method. Oil-based lubricants may be recommended for the internal mechanisms of powered devices. Water-soluble lubricants are compatible with steam sterilization.[12] Following the device manufacturer's instructions for lubrication can facilitate selection and use of the correct lubricant.

IX.d. Mechanical methods (eg, ultrasonic cleaner, washer disinfector/decontaminator) should be used for cleaning surgical instruments unless otherwise specified by the instrument manufacturer.[5,6,50] *[1: Strong Evidence]*

Mechanical cleaning is preferred over manual cleaning because it is reproducible and provides consistent detergent concentration, temperature control, and washing and rinsing processes, whereas manual cleaning is subject to variation among personnel.[5,50-52] Mechanical cleaning reduces the risk to personnel of exposure to blood, body fluids, other potentially infectious materials, and other hazards.[5,6] Mechanical cleaning is more easily monitored for quality than manual cleaning.[6]

IX.d.1. When mechanical equipment incorporates cleaning accessories specifically intended for use with specific types of instruments (eg, robotic or laparoscopic instruments), these accessories should be used according to the equipment and device manufacturers' written IFU.[6] *[4: Limited Evidence]*

IX.e. Ultrasonic cleaners may be used to remove soil from hard-to-access areas of instruments.[10] *[3: Moderate Evidence]*

Ultrasonic cleaners can provide an effective means of removing soil from hard-to-reach areas, such as joints and crevices.[6] Ultrasonic cleaners vary by design, intended use, operation, and maintenance. Some ultrasonic cleaners are designed and intended for use on specific instruments. Instructions for use will vary accordingly.[66]

IX.e.1. Cleaning products compatible with the ultrasonic cleaner should be used.[6] *[3: Moderate Evidence]*

Ultrasonic cleaners remove debris through a process of cavitation. Cleaning chemistries that are not compatible with the ultrasonic cleaner can interfere with the cavitation process and result in inadequate cleaning.[67]

IX.e.2. Ultrasonic cleaning device manufacturers' written IFU should be followed regarding degassing the cleaning solution before instrument processing. *[3: Moderate Evidence]*

Water contains air bubbles that can interfere with the cavitation process if not removed.[67]

IX.e.3. Gross soil should be removed from instruments before they are placed in the ultrasonic cleaner. *[4: Limited Evidence]*

Ultrasonic cleaners are not designed to remove gross soil. They are designed to remove debris from joints, crevices, lumens, and hard-to-reach areas.[10]

IX.e.4. Only instruments made of similar metals should be combined in the ultrasonic cleaner unless otherwise specified in the instrument manufacturer's written IFU.[10] Instruments composed of brass, copper, aluminum, or chrome should not be mixed with instruments made of stainless steel in an ultrasonic cleaner.[6] *[4: Limited Evidence]*

Placing instruments made of dissimilar metals in the ultrasonic cleaner can cause the transfer of ions from one instrument to another (ie, electroplating), which can result in etching and pitting of the instrument. Damage to the finish of the instrument can create surface imperfections that can harbor microorganisms and debris.[6]

IX.e.5. Only instruments compatible with the ultrasonic cleaning process should be subjected to ultrasonic cleaning. *[3: Moderate Evidence]*

Some instruments, such as lensed instruments, air-powered drills, flexible endoscopes, and chrome-plated instruments, will sustain damage if cleaned in an ultrasonic cleaner.[67] Lenses may loosen, internal components of air-powered drills may sustain damage if immersed, and chrome plating can loosen.[68]

IX.e.6. Instruments with lumens should be thoroughly submerged and filled with cleaning solution.[6] If the ultrasonic cleaner includes adaptors or connections for internal lumen flushing, these should be attached to lumens that are intended to be cleaned. *[3: Moderate Evidence]*

The presence of air prevents the cleaning solution from contacting the inner lumen of instruments and affects the cavitation process.[10,67]

IX.e.7. Instruments should be thoroughly rinsed after ultrasonic cleaning.[8] The rinse should be performed with treated (eg, distilled, reverse osmosis, filtered) water of a quality that will not stain or cause damage to the instruments or contribute to recontamination of the instruments.[10] *[2: High Evidence]*

Rinsing removes the cleaning solution. Solution in the cleaner may contain debris that can be deposited on the instruments as they are removed.[8]

IX.e.8. The lid should be closed when the ultrasonic cleaner is in use. *[3: Moderate Evidence]*

A closed lid prevents aerosolization of contaminants.[66]

IX.e.9. The cleaning solution in the ultrasonic cleaner should be changed before it becomes visibly soiled, when the temperature of the solution does not meet the temperature specified in the manufacturer's written IFU, and as needed.[10,67] *[3: Moderate Evidence]*

Organic material and debris that is lifted from instruments during the ultrasonic processing is deposited in the solution and can become a growth medium for bacteria and other microorganisms. The effectiveness of the cleaning can be reduced when the cleaning solution is heavily soiled. Some manufacturer's written IFU specify using a fresh cleaning solution each time an ultrasonic cycle is run. Following the manufacturer's written IFU helps facilitate effective cleaning.

IX.e.10. Ultrasonic cleaners should be emptied, cleaned, disinfected, rinsed, and dried at least daily or, preferably, after each use.[10] If not contraindicated by the ultrasonic cleaner manufacturer's written IFU, the chamber should be wiped with 70% to 90% alcohol and dried with a lint-free cloth.[8,69] *[2: High Evidence]*

Inadequately cleaned ultrasonic cleaners and endotoxins have been associated with toxic anterior segment syndrome (TASS).[70] Fluid in the ultrasonic cleaner can harbor gram-negative bacteria.[8,69,71,72] Growth of these bacteria can result in the production of endotoxins, which are heat resistant, can survive steam sterilization, and can cause serious consequences for patients.[8,71,72] Alcohol promotes drying, inhibits microbial growth, and can prevent biofilm formation.[67,69]

IX.f. Mechanical washer disinfectors/decontaminators should be used according to the manufacturer's written IFU.[10] *[4: Limited Evidence]*

Washer disinfector equipment designs vary among manufacturers and models. Following the manufacturer's written IFU will help ensure that the equipment is used correctly and functions as intended.

IX.f.1. Surgical instruments and their containment devices and accessories should be positioned in the washer disinfector in a manner that ensures contact of the cleaning solution with all surfaces of the items.[10]
- Items composed of more than one part should be disassembled according to the manufacturer's IFU. Small parts should be contained.
- Instruments should be placed in open mesh-bottom pans.
- Ports and stopcocks should be opened.
- Stylets should be removed from lumened instruments.
- Instrument ratchets should be in the open position.
- Items with surfaces that will retain water should be placed on edge.
- Electrical cords and insulated instruments should be segregated from sharp instruments.

[4: Limited Evidence]

Preparing and positioning items as described above helps ensure contact of the cleaning solution with all surfaces of the instrument. Contact with the cleaning solution is critical to effective cleaning and decontamination.[10] Containing small parts helps to prevent loss. Placing on edge the items with surfaces that will retain water helps prevent water retention. Sharp items can damage the softer material of cords and cables and can damage insulation coverings.

IX.f.2. The instrument manufacturer's written IFU should be followed during use of automated washing equipment, including placement of the instrument within mechanical washers, cycle parameters, and any other specific cleaning requirements. *[4: Limited Evidence]*

The variety of equipment available and the complexity of devices make it essential to consult and follow the manufacturer's IFU to achieve optimal cleaning effectiveness.[10]

IX.f.3. The operator of the mechanical washer should consult with the mechanical washer manufacturer's written IFU to determine
- the level of decontamination that is achieved (eg, low-level, intermediate) and
- how to monitor the cycle to determine that the parameters necessary to render the processed items safe to handle are met (see Recommendation XVII).

[5: Benefits Balanced with Harms]

Recommendation X

Surgical instruments should be inspected and evaluated for cleanliness and correct working order after decontamination and if soiled or defective, should be removed from service until they are cleaned or repaired.[10]

Items that are not clean or do not function correctly can put a patient at risk for injury or SSI.[17,20,22,23,69] Inspection and evaluation provide an opportunity to identify soiled or damaged instruments and to remove these items from service until they are cleaned or repaired.

X.a. Items should be inspected and evaluated for
- cleanliness;
- correct alignment;
- corrosion, pitting, burrs, nicks, cracks;
- sharpness of cutting edges;
- wear and chipping of inserts and plated surfaces;
- missing parts;
- integrity of insulation on insulated devices;
- integrity of cords and cables;
- clarity of lenses;
- integrity of seals and gaskets;
- presence of moisture;
- correct functioning; and
- other defects.

[2: High Evidence]

Use of instruments that are not thoroughly cleaned, are damaged, or do not function correctly poses a risk to patient safety.[17,20,23,24,26,73,74]

X.a.1. Powered equipment should be checked before use to verify that power ceases when the device is turned off and that the device is functioning as intended. Instruments that require power to operate should be attached to the power source for testing as specified in the manufacturer's written IFU. *[4: Limited Evidence]*

Power that does not cease when a powered device is turned off can cause harm to personnel or patients.[6] Verifying that instruments requiring a power source are func-

tioning as intended may help to prevent injury to patients and personnel.

X.a.2. Instruments that require assembly or that work with an accessory instrument should be assembled to confirm correct fit and that locking mechanisms work as intended. After inspection, these instruments should be disassembled before packaging for sterilization.[75] *[3: Moderate Evidence]*

Attachments and accessory items not designed to the instrument manufacturer's specifications may not fit or seal correctly and may be ejected with force and pose a risk to patients and personnel. Disassembling items before sterilization helps ensure that the sterilant contacts all surfaces of the item being sterilized.

X.a.3. Lighted magnification should be used to inspect hard-to-clean areas of devices for cleanliness. *[3: Moderate Evidence]*

An instrument that appears clean to the naked eye may harbor debris that cannot be seen without magnification.[76]

Lipscomb et al[77] compared the results of 202 cleaned and decontaminated instruments by first visually examining them and then examining them using microscopic analysis (ie, episcopic differential interference contrast microscopy). Visual inspection by the researchers showed that 37% of the instruments (75 of 202) had a low level of contamination, and 4% (eight of 202) had a high level of contamination. The microscopic assessment showed 66% (133 of 202) were severely contaminated and 27% (55 of 202) were moderately contaminated.

X.a.4. The internal channels of reusable arthroscopic shavers should be inspected using an endoscopic camera or borescope.[78] *[2: High Evidence]*

It is not possible to visually inspect lumens without a device that can penetrate the lumen. Retained organic material or debris in lumens can lead to patient injury.[22,23]

In a 2007 case-control study, Tosh et al[22] reported on an outbreak of *Pseudomonas aeruginosa* SSI in seven patients on whom the same arthroscopic shaver was used. Upon investigation, the researchers found debris in a lumen of the shaver although the shaver had undergone repeated decontamination and sterilization procedures. The researchers concluded that the retained surgical debris allowed the bacteria to survive the sterilization process, and the subsequent use of the shaver was likely related to the SSI outbreak.

The FDA recommends that the inside of the device be inspected and that consideration be given to using a 3-mm videoscope to inspect the channels of the shaver hand piece.[78]

X.a.5. Insulated devices should be visually examined and tested using equipment designed to detect insulation failure. *[2: High Evidence]*

Electrode insulation damage caused during use or processing may create an alternate pathway for the electrical current to leave the active electrode and cause patient injury. Some insulation failures are not visible. Damage to insulation may not be seen during visual inspection.[20]

In a two-part study, Espada et al[26] tested 78 robotic and 298 insulated laparoscopic instruments for insulation failure using a porosity detector. The researchers found that 25 of 78 robotic instruments (32%) had an insulation defect, but only seven of 25 defects (28%) were visible to the naked eye. Thirty-nine of the 298 laparoscopic instruments (13%) had an insulation defect, but only 27 of the 39 defects (69%) were visible to the naked eye.

In a nonexperimental study that examined insulated instruments from four hospitals, Montero et al[20] used a porosity detector to detect insulation failure. The researchers found that 33 of 226 insulated instruments (15%) had an insulation failure. There was no significant difference in insulation failure between hospitals that routinely checked for failure and those that did not.

Serious patient injury, such as thermal bowel injury, can occur when instruments with insulation defects are used.[26]

X.b. Defective instruments should be identified, removed from service, and repaired or discarded.[10] *[4: Limited Evidence]*

Identification of defective instruments and removal from service facilitates segregation of these instruments from instruments to be used when assembling sets. Removing defective instruments from service reduces the risk that defective instruments will be used.[10]

X.c. Instruments should be thoroughly dried before they are assembled in packaging systems in preparation for sterilization.[10] *[4: Limited Evidence]*

Moisture can interfere with sterilization processes.[10] Excess moisture on instrument surfaces can alter the content of steam and can pose a challenge for effective heating of the instrument during steam sterilization.[10] Hydrogen peroxide vapor and hydrogen peroxide gas plasma sterilization cycles may abort in the presence of excess moisture.[79] Ethylene oxide combines with water to form ethylene glycol (ie, antifreeze), which is toxic and is not removed during aeration.[80]

Recommendation XI

Special precautions should be taken during processing of intraocular ophthalmic instruments.[8]

Prevention of toxic anterior segment syndrome (TASS), an acute inflammation of the anterior segment of the eye, requires thorough cleaning and rinsing of intraocular instruments and strict adherence to the manufacturer's written IFU and to professional guidelines.[81-83] Toxic anterior segment syndrome is a complication of anterior segment eye surgery and is most commonly associated with cataract surgery.[84] According to the FDA, hundreds of surgical centers in North America reported outbreaks of TASS between 2000 and 2011.[84]

Most instances of TASS appear to be related to instrument processing.[69,70,81-83,85-90] Factors associated with TASS include

- contaminated instruments,
- contaminated ultrasonic cleaners,
- detergent residues (eg, soaps, enzymatic cleaners) remaining on instruments,
- insufficient rinsing of instruments,
- endotoxin residues on instruments,
- steam impurities during steam sterilization,[91]
- use of glutaraldehyde during processing,[92]
- dried debris and residues of ophthalmic viscoelastic (OV) material remaining on instruments,
- use of reusable cannulated instruments, and
- insufficiently dried lumens.[83]

Further research is warranted to determine the multifactorial risk factors for TASS.[83]

In response to a number of TASS outbreaks, the American Society of Cataract and Refractive Surgery (ASCRS) and the American Society of Ophthalmic Registered Nurses issued recommended practices for processing ophthalmic instruments.[8] The ASCRS formed a task force composed of members of industry and the ASCRS to educate surgeons who perform anterior segment eye surgery on the causes, symptoms, and treatment of TASS, and to help investigate outbreaks of TASS.[69] The task force posted a questionnaire on the ASCRS web site to allow surgeons to self-report cases of TASS and provide information about instrument cleaning and processing practices; surgical protocols; substances and techniques used for cleaning phacoemulsification and irrigation/aspiration hand pieces; and products used during the perioperative period, including medications, irrigation fluids, cannulas, and instrument tips.[69,85] The questionnaire has been maintained on the ASCRS web site since June 2007.[85] In addition, members of the TASS task force made site visits at the request of personnel from the facilities reporting TASS cases.[69]

Cutler Peck et al[69] conducted a retrospective analysis of 77 questionnaires submitted to the ASCRS web site from June 1, 2007, through May 31, 2009, and evaluated the findings from 54 TASS task force site visits conducted between October 1, 2005, and May 31, 2009. The researchers found there were common practices associated with TASS that included

- inadequately flushing phacoemulsification and irrigation/aspiration hand pieces,

- using enzymatic cleaners,
- using detergents at the wrong concentration,
- using contaminated fluids in ultrasonic cleaners,
- adding antibiotics to balanced salt solutions,
- using epinephrine with preservatives,
- using preoperative skin antiseptics incorrectly,
- using powdered gloves,
- reusing single-use products, and
- failing to maintain instruments correctly.

The researchers concluded that changing these practices could help prevent TASS.

Bodnar et al[85] conducted a retrospective analysis of 130 questionnaires submitted to the ASCRS web site from June 1, 2007, through March 1, 2012, and of information from 71 site visits conducted by the TASS task force between October 1, 2005, and December 31, 2011. The researchers noted several trends when comparing their data with the data previously analyzed by Cutler Peck et al.[69] When analyzing data obtained from the questionnaires, the researchers found a 26% reduction in sites reporting inadequate flushing of hand pieces and a 27% increase in sites reporting the use of deionized or distilled water for the final rinse. When analyzing data from the site visits, the researchers found a 36% reduction in the use of epinephrine with preservatives and a 36% reduction in the use of enzymatic detergents; however, they found a 21% increase in the handling of intraocular lenses and instrument tips with gloved hands, a 47% increase in poor instrument maintenance, and a 34% increase in use of contaminated fluids in ultrasonic cleaners. The researchers concluded that education had improved some practices but had not improved others.

The findings from these studies indicate a need to improve education of personnel who use or process ophthalmic instruments regarding best practices for care and processing of ophthalmic instruments to prevent TASS.

XI.a.   Immediately after use during the procedure, ophthalmic instruments should be wiped clean with sterile water and a lint-free sponge and flushed or immersed in sterile water according to the manufacturer's written IFU.[8,10] *[1: Strong Evidence]*

Ophthalmic viscoelastic material can harden and dry within minutes, making subsequent removal difficult.[8,10,82,85,88] Keeping OV or other organic material moist can prevent drying and hardening of such material on ophthalmic devices.[8]

Biofilm adheres to the surfaces of instruments and is very difficult to remove. Keeping the OV and organic material moist helps facilitate removal and prevent biofilm formation.

XI.b.   The instrument manufacturer's written instructions for cleaning should be reviewed and followed.[8,10] *[1: Strong Evidence]*

The method of cleaning and the compatibility of cleaning products may vary among instrument manufacturers. Instructions for cannulated instruments indicate the type and volume of solution to be used for rinsing and cleaning and the number of times and for how long the cannula should be flushed.[8,82]

XI.c.   Adequate time, an adequate number of personnel, and sufficient instrument inventory should be provided to permit thorough instrument cleaning and sterilization.[8,10] *[2: High Evidence]*

Time constraints may create a disincentive for personnel to adhere to recommended cleaning and disinfection procedures.[69]

In a retrospective analysis of 77 questionnaires and 54 site visits to identify risk factors associated with TASS, an ASCRS task force reported that 23 of the sites (43%) were noted to have an insufficient number of instrument sets or of personnel to provide adequate time to process ophthalmic instruments. Personnel at six sites (11%) did not follow the manufacturer's written IFU, and four individuals were observed to perform inadequate flushing of phacoemulsification and irrigation/aspiration hand pieces.[69]

XI.c.1.   An inventory of ophthalmic instruments sufficient to meet the anticipated demand should be maintained.[8,10] *[2: High Evidence]*

An adequate instrument inventory provides sufficient time for personnel to follow correct cleaning, decontamination, and terminal sterilization procedures and helps eliminate or reduce the need for immediate-use steam sterilization (IUSS).[8,10,83]

XI.d.   Intraocular instruments should be cleaned in a designated cleaning area. Intraocular instruments should be cleaned separately from general surgical instruments.[10] *[2: High Evidence]*

Procedures for processing ophthalmic instruments differ from those for general surgery instruments.[85] Cleaning intraocular instruments separately from general surgery instruments can help prevent cross-contamination with bioburden from heavily soiled nonophthalmic surgical instruments.[8,10]

XI.e.   Single-use disposable cannulae should be used whenever possible.[8] *[1: Strong Evidence]*

Thorough cleaning of these devices is difficult because the lumens are exceptionally small.[8] Use of reusable cannulae has been associated with TASS.[82,87]

In a 2006 review of the literature to identify possible causes of TASS, Mamalis et al[86] identified detergent residues and denatured OV material on reusable intraocular instruments as possible causes.

XI.f.   The scrub person should flush the irrigation and aspiration ports of phacoemulsification and irrigation/aspiration hand pieces and accessory reusable tips and tubing with sterile water according to the manufacturer's written IFU before disconnecting the hand piece from the unit.[8] *[2: High Evidence]*

Inadequate flushing of phacoemulsification hand pieces has been associated with TASS.[69] When OV material is allowed to dry on phacoemulsification hand pieces, it is difficult to remove. Flushing immediately after the procedure can help prevent OV material from drying. Flushing the hand piece prevents buildup of OV material inside the hand piece, which is difficult to remove during cleaning.[93]

XI.g. Cleaning products used to clean intraocular instruments should be selected and used in accordance with the instrument manufacturer's written IFU.[8,10] *[2: High Evidence]*

Some IFU for ophthalmic instruments recommend against the use of enzymatic detergents.[69]

In a retrospective analysis of questionnaires and site visits to examine instrument cleaning and processing of extraocular and intraocular products used during cataract surgery, Culter-Peck et al[69] identified common practices associated with TASS. They analyzed 77 questionnaires and 54 site visits; 909 cases of TASS were reported. Use of enzymatic cleaners was reported in 36 questionnaires (47%) and observed at 48 sites (89%). The researchers concluded that the benefit of using enzymatic cleaners to clean ophthalmic instruments had not been established and, in fact, was prohibited in some manufacturers' instructions for specific-use products.

In a randomized controlled trial (RCT) to determine whether enzymatic detergents used to clean ophthalmic instruments could cause TASS, Leder et al[94] randomly assigned rabbits into seven treatment groups to receive intracameral injection of three different doses of enzymatic detergent. Although the enzymatic detergent caused a severe inflammatory response, the response did not include TASS. The researchers concluded that given that patient exposure to an enzymatic detergent would be significantly less than the lowest dose used in the experiment, enzymatic detergent on ophthalmic instruments was not a cause of TASS.

Mamalis and Edelhauser raised concerns about the validity and generalizability of the study conducted by Leder et al[94] in a letter to the editor and stated "there are significant differences in the inflammatory reaction of the rabbit, as well as their response to toxic insults, that make it difficult to extrapolate findings from the rabbit to the human."[93(p651)] They noted that the conclusions of the researchers were inconsistent with the results presented in the study and contended that the results of the study actually provided additional support for the role of enzymatic detergents as a potential cause of TASS.

Following the instrument manufacturer's IFU helps ensure compatibility of the cleaning product with the device. Incorrect selection and incorrect detergent dilution has been associated with TASS.[69]

XI.g.1. After cleaning, ophthalmic instruments should be rinsed with a copious amount of water.[8] *[2: High Evidence]*

Thorough rinsing helps remove residual cleaning product. Detergent residue has been identified as a possible cause of TASS, although studies performed on rabbits have not supported enzymatic detergent residues alone as a cause of TASS.[83,94]

In a review of the literature, Ozcelik et al[83] identified detergent residues/soaps, enzymatic cleaners, inappropriate rinsing, and dried debris and OV material residues as potential causes or risk factors for TASS. However, in an RCT to investigate whether enzymatic detergents used to clean ophthalmic instruments could cause TASS, Leder et al[94] concluded that enzymatic detergent residues alone did not cause TASS. The researchers randomly assigned 35 rabbits into seven treatment groups (ie, low, medium, and high detergent concentration of three detergents, plus a control group of untreated rabbits) and injected their eyes with detergent accordingly. The enzymatic detergents caused a severe but unusual response; however, this response has not been reported in humans.

When the instructions for cleaning are strictly followed, it is possible to remove all detergent.[82,87]

XI.g.2. A final rinse should be performed with sterile distilled or sterile deionized water.[8,69,86] *[2: High Evidence]*

Untreated water may contain endotoxins, which are heat stable and as such will remain biologically active after sterilization and which have been implicated in occurrences of TASS.[70,83,85,86]

Residual enzymes and detergents not rinsed from instruments have been associated with TASS.[8,70,85,86]

XI.g.3. After cleaning, lumens should be rinsed with sterile deionized or distilled water. The rinse fluid should be expelled from the lumen into a drain and not back into the rinse water. Lumens should be dried with medical-grade compressed air.[8,83] *[2: High Evidence]*

Rinsing removes detergent and other residue from the lumens. Expelling the lumen rinse into a drain prevents reuse of the rinse water and prevents recontamination of the lumen with debris that has been rinsed out of the lumen. Compressed air forced through the lumen eliminates moisture that can serve as a medium for microbial growth.

XI.g.4. After manual cleaning, unless contraindicated in the manufacturer's written IFU, instruments should be disinfected by wiping and by rinsing lumens with 70% to 90% alcohol and should be dried before they are packaged for sterilization. *[3: Moderate Evidence]*

Wiping with alcohol disinfects the instruments and renders them safe to handle. Endotoxins are removable with alcohol.[88] Rinsing lumens with alcohol facilitates drying.

XI.h. If an ultrasonic cleaner is used, it should be emptied, cleaned, disinfected, rinsed, and dried at least daily or, preferably, after each use.[10] If not contraindicated by the ultrasonic cleaner manufacturer's written IFU, the chamber should be wiped with 70% to 90% alcohol and dried with a lint-free cloth.[8,69] *[2: High Evidence]*

Inadequately cleaned ultrasonic cleaners and endotoxins have been associated with TASS.[70] Fluid in the ultrasonic cleaner can harbor gram-negative bacteria.[8,69,71,72] Growth of these bacteria can result in the production of endotoxins, which are heat resistant, can survive steam sterilization, and can cause serious consequences for patients.[8,71,72] Alcohol promotes drying, inhibits microbial growth, and can prevent biofilm formation.[67,69]

XI.h.1. Ophthalmic instruments should be thoroughly rinsed after ultrasonic cleaning.[8] A final rinse should be performed with treated water before drying, inspecting, and packaging in preparation for sterilization. *[1: Strong Evidence]*

Adequate rinsing removes the cleaning solution. Residual cleaning products have been implicated in the occurrence of TASS.[69,82]

In an RCT, Tamashiro et al[82] filled 30 reusable 25-gauge injection cannulas with OV material and allowed them to dry for 50 minutes. Cannulas were then presoaked, washed using a high-pressure water jet, backwashed with enzymatic detergent in an ultrasonic cleaner, rinsed with tap water, rinsed with sterile distilled water, dried with compressed filtered air, wrapped in surgical-grade paper, and steam sterilized. After sterilization, the cannulas were tested for cytotoxicity. The results showed that all extracts were noncytotoxic. Six of the cannulas were then immersed in enzymatic detergent and rinsed, and the extracts from these were tested for cytotoxicity. The researchers found that the extracts were not cytotoxic; however, they observed changes in cell morphology and a reduction in cell growth. The researchers concluded that the cleaning protocol had the potential to minimize the occurrence of TASS associated with residues of OV material and enzymatic detergents remaining on ophthalmic instruments.

XI.i. After cleaning and decontamination, instruments that have been in contact with OV material should be inspected for residual OV material under magnification.[8] *[1: Strong Evidence]*

Retained OV material has been associated with TASS.[8,69]

Viscoelastic material is difficult to remove during cleaning, especially if it has been allowed to dry. Inspection under magnification can facilitate detection of residual OV material. Although studies conducted on rabbits showed that OV material alone, even if denatured by steam sterilization, did not cause ocular inflammation, the presence of endotoxin in OV material can cause severe ocular reaction.[95]

Buchen et al[96] conducted an RCT to determine the ocular reactivity of rabbits to bacterial endotoxin contained in an aqueous medium and in a cohesive and dispersive OV material. The researchers found that inflammation occurred after injection of as little as 0.02 endotoxin units in OV material and 0.08 endotoxin units in a phosphate buffered saline.

XI.j. Records should be maintained of all cleaning methods, cleaning solutions, and lot numbers of cleaning solutions used with ophthalmic instruments. *[3: Moderate Evidence]*

Records of cleaning methods and solutions can assist in surveillance efforts[84] and be used to facilitate investigation of any suspected or confirmed cases of TASS.

Recommendation XII

Laryngoscope blades and their handles should be cleaned, decontaminated, dried, and stored in a manner that reduces the risk of exposing patients and personnel to potentially pathogenic microorganisms.

Laryngoscope blades and handles may be a potential source of contamination.[97,98] In a comprehensive integrative review, Negri de Sousa et al[97] identified 77 articles that addressed the laryngoscope blade or handle as a potential source of contamination.[97] Based on the quality of the research, the authors selected 20 articles for further review. In five of the studies, blood was found on the laryngoscope blade. None of the studies that investigated the handles found blood.

In a descriptive study of laryngoscope blades and handles, Phillips and Monaghan[99] found that although none of the blades or handles had visible blood, 13 of 65 blades (20%), and 26 of 65 handles (40%) tested positive for occult blood.

XII.a. After each use, laryngoscope blades should be cleaned and high-level disinfected or sterilized according to the manufacturer's written IFU.[2] *[1: Strong Evidence]*

Cleaning and disinfection minimizes the risk of pathogen transmission.[2] Semicritical items are those that contact mucus membranes or nonintact skin.[2] Laryngoscope blades are considered semicritical items that require a minimum of high-level disinfection.[2,100]

Jones et al[101] conducted an investigation of an outbreak of *Serratia marcescens* that involved two geographically distinct neonatal intensive care units during a nine-week period. They found that 17 infants were colonized and three developed septicemia, two of whom died. The investigators found that during the outbreak, two infants had been transferred between the two units and two employees worked in both units. Because of a shortage of laryngoscope blades, the blades had been shared without being sterilized between uses. At one of the facilities, *S marcescens* was isolated from a laryngoscope blade and a sample of breast milk. The outbreak isolates were of the identical serotype and phage type as those identified in the outbreak. The investigators concluded that infection prevention measures, including disinfection of laryngoscope blades, were insufficient at these facilities.

Foweraker[102] reported four cases of *Pseudomonas aeruginosa* infection in a pediatric cardiac intensive care unit. They infections were believed to have been transmitted by a single laryngoscope blade disinfected between uses by wiping with alcohol. Sampling of the laryngoscope blade in question revealed *P aeruginosa* of the identical type as a blood culture from one child who died from the infection. The author recommended thorough cleaning and disinfection of blades and handles to reduce the potential for infection.

XII.b. Laryngoscope handles should be cleaned and low-level disinfected after each use and may be high-level disinfected or sterilized according to the manufacturer's written IFU. *[1: Strong Evidence]*

Laryngoscope handles are classified as noncritical items according to the Spaulding Classification.[2] Noncritical items are those that contact intact skin.[2] According to the Centers for Disease Control and Prevention (CDC), low-level disinfectants are used for noncritical items.[2] Although the laryngoscope handle by itself is a noncritical device, the laryngoscope consists of two parts that are handled concurrently. In a comprehensive, integrative review, Negri de Sousa et al[97] recommended that both parts of the laryngoscope be classified as semicritical.

Laryngoscope handles have a knurled surface (ie, a series of small ridges cut into the metal) to facilitate grip; the rough surface can accumulate bioburden.[97,103] When the laryngoscope blade is folded closed, the tip of the blade is in contact with the handle. Studies have demonstrated the presence of microorganisms on laryngoscope handles.[97,103-105] To date, no studies have demonstrated patient infection as a result of contaminated laryngoscope handles[97]; however, studies have demonstrated the potential for pathogen transmission from the laryngoscope handle to the patient.[103,104]

In a nonexperimental study to identify the extent and nature of contamination of laryngoscope handles considered to be clean and ready for use in the OR, Williams et al[103] cultured 192 laryngoscope handles. The researchers found 99 positive cultures that yielded a total of 128 different microorganisms on the handles.

In a quasi-experimental study, Call et al[104] sampled 60 laryngoscope handles considered to be clean and ready for use in the OR. Samples from 40 handles were sent to the laboratory for aerobic bacterial culture; samples from 20 handles were examined for viral contamination. The researchers found that 30 of the 40 samples sent for bacterial culture (75%) were positive for bacterial contamination, and all 20 of the other handles were negative for viral contamination. The researchers recommended a minimum of low-level disinfection of laryngoscope handles after each use.

Some manufacturer's IFU recommend low-level surface disinfection while others recommend high-level disinfection or sterilization between uses.[106,107]

Recommendations for processing vary within the published literature;[97] however, the Association of Anaesthetists of Great Britain and Ireland suggests that laryngoscope handles do become contaminated with bacteria and blood during use and as such they should be cleaned, disinfected, and sterilized after every use.[108]

Further research is warranted regarding processing protocols and the risk of infection associated with laryngoscope handles.

XII.c. Cleaned and disinfected laryngoscope blades and handles should be packaged and stored in a manner that prevents contamination.[100,107] *[1: Strong Evidence]*

Packaging assists in preventing recontamination of items that have been high-level disinfected. Packaging of laryngoscope blades to prevent recontamination is a CDC recommendation.[2]

XII.c.1. Laryngoscope blades should be stored in individual packages.[107] *[3: Moderate Evidence]*

Storing blades individually minimizes the potential for contaminating multiple blades, which could occur if a contaminated blade is placed back into a package of uncontaminated blades. Individual storage eliminates the need to process multiple blades.[107]

STERILIZATION AND DISINFECTION

Recommendation XIII

Special precautions should be taken to minimize the risk of transmission of prion diseases from contaminated instruments.

Prions are a unique class of infectious proteins that cause fatal neurological diseases known as transmissible spongiform encephalopathies (TSEs).[63] Examples of prion diseases are Gertsmann-Straussler-Scheinker syndrome, fatal familial insomnia syndrome, and Creutzfeldt-Jakob disease (CJD).[63] Variant Creutzfeldt-Jakob Disease (vCJD) is acquired from cattle with bovine spongiform encephalopathy or "mad cow disease."[63] Transmissible spongiform encephalopathies have been described in a number of animal species.[64] To date, with the exception of cattle, there is no evidence of transmission of TSEs to humans from animals.[63]

Creutzfeldt-Jakob disease has been transmitted iatrogenically through direct inoculation (ie, with contaminated cadaveric human growth hormone), use of contaminated cadaveric dura mater, and use of contaminated medical equipment.[63] Human cadaveric growth hormone has been replaced with growth hormone produced using recombinant DNA technology, and cadaveric dura mater is no longer used in neurosurgeries.[63]

Iatrogenic CJD resulting from use of contaminated medical equipment has been reported in two circumstances: two cases from contaminated electroencephalography electrodes and four suspected cases from contaminated neurosurgical devices[63]; all occurred in Europe during the period from 1952 through 1976.[63] No other cases have been reported of transmission from instruments used in other types of surgeries or since that time.[109]

Prions are resistant to conventional physical and chemical sterilization.[63] Special precautions and protocols are required to inactivate prions.[63,109-112] Instrumentation used for neurosurgery procedures performed on a patient suspected or known to have a prion disease is of particular concern because of the high concentrations of prions in the brain and spinal cord.[110]

XIII.a. A multidisciplinary team that includes infection preventionists, perioperative RNs, sterile processing personnel, surgeons, representatives from the clinical pathology laboratory, and other stakeholders should establish, document, and implement evidence-based policies and procedures to minimize the risk of prion disease transmission.[110] These processes should be based on
  ○ the patient's risk of having a prion disease;
  ○ the level of infectivity of the tissue involved, as defined by the World Health Organization (WHO) *Tables on Infectivity Distribution in Transmissible Spongiform Encephalopathies*[110,113]; and
  ○ the intended use of the medical device.
  [1: Strong Evidence]

A defined protocol based on available evidence provides guidance to protect patients and health care workers from prion transmission. Anesthesia professionals, infection preventionists, perioperative team members, risk management personnel, neurosurgeons, and sterile processing personnel are involved when surgery is performed on a patient known or suspected to have a prion disease. A coordinated effort among disciplines is important and may increase the likelihood of developing effective strategies to protect patients and personnel.[110]

Common laboratory methodologies are ineffective in diagnosing prion disease. Diagnosis can be confirmed through neuropathological examinations of brain tissue, usually performed at autopsy. Research to develop additional laboratory techniques for diagnosis is ongoing.[109,114]

The WHO has published clinical diagnostic criteria for CJD.[112] These criteria are used to identify patients at risk of having or developing CJD. Patients at high risk of having or developing prion disease include those with
  ○ progressive dementia consistent with CJD in whom a diagnosis has not been confirmed or ruled out,
  ○ a familial history of a prion disease,
  ○ a history of dura mater transplants, or
  ○ a history of receiving cadaveric-derived pituitary hormone.[63]

Although all prion diseases are infectious, the risk of infection is not the same for all tissue. Based on successful experimental transmission, the risk of infection from tissue types is categorized as high, low, or no risk.[113]
  ○ Tissue from the posterior eye retina or optic nerve, brain, pituitary gland, and spinal cord are categorized as high risk.[113]
  ○ Liver, lung, spleen, kidney, and lymph nodes are categorized as low risk, as are body fluids, blood, and urine.[113,114]

Prions are found in other tissue, and studies to determine whether they can transmit prion disease are ongoing.[111] The definition of high- and low-risk tissue has continued to change.[111] Infectivity in similar tissue can vary according to the type of prion.[111]

Research directed toward understanding tissue infectivity is ongoing.[111] In particular, blood has been studied to determine whether transfusion is a risk factor.[114-119] Four potential cases of vCJD from blood transfusion have been reported.[110,114] The risks associated with having received blood or blood components from a donor with CJD have been studied.[114-119] Although there is no direct evidence of a causal relationship, the long incubation of CJD, as long as 20 years, is a limitation of these studies.[114-119] The risk associated with receipt of blood or blood products from a donor with vCJD is significantly higher than that associated with receipt of blood or blood components from a donor with CJD.[117-119]

There are no known cases of prion disease transmission attributable to the reuse of devices contaminated with blood.[115] Because of the long incubation period of CJD and the discovery of prion protein in tonsils, gut, and muscle, the risk of prion contamination may extend to surgeries on tissue not currently listed as high risk, and categories of high-risk tissue may continue to change.[110,111]

XIII.b. Patients should be screened for the risk of prion disease before surgery, and information about patients identified to be at risk should be communicated to personnel who are directly or indirectly involved in the patient's care (eg, anesthesia professional, surgeon, nurses, infection preventionist, clinical pathology laboratory representatives, sterile processing personnel, risk manager, surgery scheduler).[63] *[1: Strong Evidence]*

Preoperative screening provides a mechanism to identify patients at high risk of having a prion disease. Early communication provides an opportunity to plan for the provision of instruments that can be discarded or taken out of service (ie, quarantined) until a definitive diagnosis is made or to identify alternatives to the use of complex instruments.

Early communication is crucial as it provides an opportunity for review of policies and procedures related to sterilization, disinfection, and environmental cleaning. Early communication may allow time to track the instruments used in surgery, and prevent them from being discarded or returned to service without undergoing special disinfection and sterilization procedures.

XIII.c. Single-use surgical drapes, gowns, and supplies should be used whenever possible and discarded after use.[63,112] *[1: Strong Evidence]*

The use and disposal of single-use gowns and supplies eliminates the need to institute special protocols for laundering and may reduce the risk of exposing personnel to prion-contaminated materials.

Although there is no known correlation between contact with work surfaces and attire worn in surgery with transmission of prion diseases, use of single-use gowns and drapes eliminates the need to determine protocols for reusable drapes and gowns potentially contaminated with prions.

Use and incineration of single-use gowns and drapes is recommended in the 1999 *WHO Infection Control Guidelines for Transmissible Spongiform Encephalopathies*.[112] The more current 2010 Society for Healthcare Epidemiology of America (SHEA) "Guideline for disinfection and sterilization of prion-contaminated medical instruments"[63] recommends that masks, gowns, and protective eyewear be worn if mucus membrane or skin exposure to blood, body fluids, or other potentially infectious materials is anticipated and that laundry be managed according to the OSHA bloodborne pathogens standard.[39,63]

XIII.c.1. Noncritical work surfaces should be covered with fluid-resistant drapes, and if contaminated with high-risk tissue, the drape should be discarded as nonregulated medical waste. Regulated waste, (eg, bulk blood, pathologic waste, sharp devices) should be managed according to state regulations.[63] *[1: Strong Evidence]*

Minimizing contamination of surfaces reduces the need for special precautions or protocols for environmental cleaning.

There are no known studies that correlate prion disease transmission with the disposal of waste contaminated with high-risk tissue from a patient known or suspected to have a prion disease. Previous WHO guidelines[63] recommended incineration of potentially prion-contaminated medical waste; however, current guidelines[112] recommend disposal as nonregulated waste.

XIII.d. If the need for an implant is anticipated, only the implant essential for the specific patient should be delivered to the sterile field. Implants opened and handled by scrubbed personnel after the surgery has started should be discarded and not processed for subsequent use. *[5: Benefits Balanced with Harms]*

Discarding potentially contaminated implants eliminates the risk of implanting a prion-contaminated implant into a patient. Implants, such as screws, are often supplied in racks that hold multiple implants. When sets containing multiple implants are open, there is a risk of cross-contamination of implants that are not used. Removing implants that will not be needed for the patient before sterilizing the tray decreases the amount of implant inventory that will need to be discarded.

XIII.e. Reusable instruments used on high-risk tissue of patients suspected of having prion disease should be easy to clean and should tolerate exposure to an extended steam sterilization cycle. *[1: Strong Evidence]*

Depending on the cleaning management before sterilization (eg, cleaning process, cleaning product), extended steam sterilization cycles may not be necessary. However, at the time of this publication and on the basis of current knowledge, an extended cycle steam sterilization is still recommended as the option for sterilization that provides the greatest margin of safety.[63,111]

XIII.f. Instruments used on high-risk tissue of patients at high risk for prion disease should be designed for single use.[63] If single-use instruments are not available, reusable instruments should be limited to those that are easy to clean. The number of instruments used should be kept to a minimum. *[1: Strong Evidence]*

Use of single-use instruments eliminates the need to implement special processing protocols and eliminates the risk of instruments contaminated with prions being used on another patient. Use of single-use instruments also eliminates the risk of exposure of personnel who process instruments.

Successful cleaning is a critical step in processing instruments exposed to high-risk tissue. When instruments are difficult to clean thoroughly, the potential for incomplete cleaning is increased. The challenge to cleaning is reduced when easy-to-clean devices are used.

XIII.f.1. Single-use brain biopsy sets should be used on all patients undergoing brain biopsy. *[3: Moderate Evidence]*

Creutzfeldt-Jakob disease is often definitively diagnosed by brain biopsy, and whether the patient has a prion disease may not be known at the time of surgery.

Until the later stages of CJD, most patients developing a prion disease cannot be identified.[120] Patients undergoing surgery for a brain biopsy are considered to be at high risk for prion disease.[109] Commercial single-use brain biopsy sets are available, or sets can be assembled using instruments at the end of their useful life and discarding them after use.

XIII.f.2. Rigid, as opposed to flexible, neuroendoscopes should be used for patients with known or suspected prion disease. *[5: Benefits Balanced with Harms]*

Flexible neuroendoscopes contain narrow lumens. Narrow lumens are difficult to clean. Neuroendoscopes may not be compatible with the cleaning procedures and extended steam sterilization cycles recommended for items contaminated with prions.

XIII.f.3. Power drills and saws should not be used for patients with known or suspected prion disease. *[1: Strong Evidence]*

Power drills and saws create aerosols and may splatter potentially infectious material. Although there are no reported cases of occupational transmission of prion disease through exposure to aerosols, much about prions and their infectivity is unknown.[63,109,121]

Stitz and Aguzzi[122] reviewed the literature related to prion-containing aerosols and concluded that although not identified as a source of prion transmission in humans, the high rate of prion transmission by way of aerosols in mice suggested that it was advisable to avoid inhaling aerosols from prion-containing materials.

In a series of experiments that tested the cellular and molecular characteristics of prion propagation after aerosol intranasal exposure in mice, Haybaeck et al[123] demonstrated that prions could be transmitted to mice through aerosols. They exposed both immunocompetent and immunodeficient mice to prion aerosols that were produced by using a nebulizing device with prion-contaminated brain homogenates of concentrations ranging from 0.1% to 20%. All mice exposed to infectious aerosols developed clinical mouse scrapie (a form of TSE) or displayed brain tissue indicative of subclinical prion infection. The longer the exposure time, the shorter the incubation time; notably, exposure of only one minute resulted in infection. The researchers concluded that although there have been no reports of prion transmission to humans by aerosols under normal conditions, it remains prudent to minimize exposure to aerosols that may contain prions. They recommended that prion-containing aerosols be considered a potential vector for prion infection.

Power drills are difficult to clean, and the cleaning and sterilization methods recommended to eliminate prion infectivity may damage these instruments.

XIII.f.4. Single-use instruments that have come in contact with high-risk tissue from patients known or suspected to have a prion disease should be discarded.[63] *[1: Strong Evidence]*

Prions are highly resistant to conventional disinfection and sterilization processes.[10,63,111] Discarding these devices eliminates the risk of inadequate prion inactivation.

XIII.g. Reusable instruments that have come in contact with high-risk tissue from patients known or suspected to have a prion disease should be treated in accordance with the most current infection prevention guidelines.[63] *[1: Strong Evidence]*

Reducing infectivity is crucial to providing instruments that are safe to use on patients. When a potentially contaminated device can be cleaned and prion tissue removed, the risk of prion disease transmission is minimized. There is currently no consensus on the best method of managing instruments that are likely to be contaminated with prions. Until recently, the most referenced guidelines for managing prevention of TSEs were the WHO *Infection Control Guidelines for Transmissible Spongiform Encephalopathies*.[112] These were published in 1999 and were based on studies that

○ did not incorporate conventional cleaning procedures that reduce protein contamination,

- investigated inactivation using tissue homogenates dried onto carriers, and
- investigated inactivation using various strains and concentrations of prions and a variety of tissue.[10,109]

Although they are effective, the WHO guidelines for managing instruments contaminated with prions[112] are impractical and are corrosive to instruments. The more current SHEA "Guideline for disinfection and sterilization of prion-contaminated medical instruments,"[63] published in 2010, reflect research conducted after the WHO publication. These guidelines identify practices that can eliminate prion infectivity with a wide margin of safety.[63]

XIII.g.1. Instruments that cannot be cleaned or require sterilization using low-temperature technologies should not be used or should be discarded.[63] [1: Strong Evidence]

Steam sterilization for an extended cycle time is the only sterilization method recommended in national guidelines at this time.[63] Low-temperature sterilization technologies have not been incorporated into recognized guidelines for inactivating prions.

Research into the effectiveness of gaseous hydrogen peroxide for inactivating prions is ongoing. Several studies have demonstrated that hydrogen peroxide vapor and some hydrogen peroxide gas plasma technologies in combination with specific cleaning agents are effective in inactivating prions, and researchers have suggested that sterilization with gaseous hydrogen peroxide protocols will be practical and widely used in the future.[63,124]

In a quasi-experimental study designed to test the effectiveness of a gaseous hydrogen peroxide sterilization process to inactivate prions, Fichet et al[124] contaminated stainless steel wires with prion-infected brain homogenates and then exposed them to gaseous hydrogen peroxide sterilization. Sterilization parameters included a vacuum process at 86° F (30° C) for three or six pulses. The researchers concluded that exposure under these conditions demonstrated that gaseous hydrogen peroxide was effective in inactivating prions.

In a quasi-experimental study to test effectiveness of decontamination methods to inactivate prions, Yan et al[125] contaminated stainless steel wires with prion-infected brain homogenate material and subjected them to a variety of decontamination and sterilization procedures including exposure to gaseous hydrogen peroxide, steam sterilization, sodium hydroxide, enzymatic detergent, enzymatic detergent plus gaseous hydrogen peroxide, peracetic acid, alkaline detergent, alkaline detergent plus orthophthalaldehyde, alkaline detergent plus steam sterilization, and alkaline detergent plus gaseous hydrogen peroxide. The researchers injected the wires into the brains of living hamsters. Successful processing was defined as a total group survival time of 18 months after implantation. After 18 months, only those hamsters incubated with wires reprocessed with an alkaline detergent followed by sterilization with a four injection gaseous hydrogen peroxide cycle showed no clinical signs of prion disease.

In a quasi-experimental study to determine the effectiveness of hydrogen peroxide gas plasma for inactivating animal and human prions, Rogez-Kreuz et al[126] decontaminated prion-contaminated steel wires with combinations of enzymatic or alkaline detergents and gaseous hydrogen peroxide. The researchers found that gaseous hydrogen peroxide decreased the infectivity of the prions; however, its efficacy was dependent on the concentration of the hydrogen peroxide and the systems used to deliver it. Only one specific model of a hydrogen peroxide gas plasma sterilizer was 100% effective in inactivating prions.

XIII.g.2. Instruments should be kept moist until they are cleaned and decontaminated.[63] Instruments may be kept moist by immersion in water, a wet cloth draped over the instruments, or use of a transport gel or foam.[63] [1: Strong Evidence]

When prions are allowed to dry on instruments, they become highly resistant to removal.[127-129] Dried films of tissue are more resistant to prion inactivation by steam sterilization than tissue that is kept moist.[63]

Prions are hydrophobic and in the absence of moisture can strongly attach to surfaces, particularly stainless steel.[128] Keeping instruments moist until cleaning and decontamination can help reduce the tenacity of prions to adhere to surfaces.

XIII.g.3. Instruments should be decontaminated in a mechanical washer as soon as possible after use.[63] [1: Strong Evidence]

Mechanical washing is preferred because process consistency is more likely than with manual washing, and the mechanical process is more easily monitored. Automation of cleaning helps ensure reproducibility.[74] Mechanical washers employ a validated cycle that is not possible with manual cleaning.

Stainless steel has a high affinity for prion adsorption. The longer prion-contaminated instruments are permitted to dry, the greater the adsorption and the more difficult the prion removal.[128]

XIII.g.4. Cleaning chemicals that have evidence of prionicidal activity and that are compatible with the instruments to be cleaned should be used.[63] *[1: Strong Evidence]*

It is important that product selection decisions take into consideration the combined effect of precleaning, cleaning, disinfection, and sterilization and effectiveness against other infectious diseases and not just the ability to inactivate prions.

The WHO recommendation to soak instruments in 1 N sodium hydroxide (NaOH)[112] is effective at eliminating prion infectivity but, because of incompatibility with most instruments, is impractical. A number of alkaline and enzymatic cleaning agents in combination with steam sterilization have been shown to be effective as well and are compatible with instruments.[63,111]

Some cleaning formulas have a demonstrated ability to remove and inactivate prions.[111,130] However, it has also been shown that some cleaning agents may increase the resistance of prions to subsequent steam sterilization.[111,130] In an investigative study of the effectiveness of innovative physical and chemical methods of prion inactivation, Fichet et al[130] subjected prion-contaminated stainless steel wires to a variety of cleaning chemistries and sterilization technologies. The researchers found that one phenolic formulation increased the resistance of prions to inactivation.

In a quasi-experimental study, McDonnell et al[111] found that cleaning with certain chemical formulations, alkaline formulations in particular, in combination with steam sterilization was an effective prion-decontamination process. The researchers found that low-temperature gaseous hydrogen peroxide sterilization reduced infectivity in both the presence and absence of cleaning.

In an RCT to determine effectiveness of prion inactivation, Schmitt et al[131] subjected prion-contaminated stainless steel wires to either an automated decontamination procedure developed for prion decontamination, or a routine automated alkaline disinfection process used for sterile processing in Germany. The routine procedure included an alkaline wash and thermal disinfection. The specially designed prion decontamination process included an alkaline wash, thermal disinfection, and an oxidizing process using hydrogen peroxide combined with an alkaline detergent. After processing, the researchers implanted the wires into the brains of eight hamsters. The researchers found that the specially designed process was more effective than conventional alkaline cleaning, was as effective as exposure to a steam sterilization process at 273° F (134° C) for two hours, and left no detectable prion infectivity. The researchers also found that although the alkaline cleaning resulted in significant reduction of prion infectivity, it did not eliminate prion infectivity in six of eight animals in which the stainless steel wires were implanted.

XIII.g.5. After decontamination, one of the following three methods recommended by SHEA should be used to steam sterilize instruments exposed to high-risk tissue:
- prevacuum sterilization at 273° F (134° C) for 18 minutes[63,111];
- gravity displacement sterilization at 270° F (132° C) for 60 minutes[63,111]; or
- immersion in 1 N NaOH for 60 minutes, then removal, rinsing with water, and sterilization using one of the cycles noted above (1 N NaOH is a solution of 40 g NaOH in 1 L water).[63,111]

[1: Strong Evidence]

These measures have demonstrated safety and efficacy.[63,111]

The SHEA guidelines state "it is unclear from the published literature which of these options is best for complete inactivation of prions because some studies have revealed excellent but not complete inactivation of the test prions with autoclaving only . . . and the same result for use of NaOH and autoclaving. . . ."[63(p111)]

A fourth option described in the SHEA guidelines is to immerse the contaminated instruments in 1 N NaOH for 60 minutes and heat them in a gravity displacement sterilizer at 250° F (121° C) for 30 minutes, then clean and subject the instruments to routine sterilization.[63] This option is effective for prion inactivation; however, it can damage many devices, especially anodized aluminum-containing devices (depending on the quality and finish of the materials used) and therefore is not recommended by many device manufacturers.[111]

XIII.h. Instruments exposed to high-risk tissue should not be subjected to IUSS.[10,63] *[1: Strong Evidence]*

Steam sterilization cycles for IUSS of surgical instruments are different from those recommended by SHEA for prion inactivation.[63] The steam sterilization cycles recommended by SHEA for instruments exposed to high-risk tissue are supported by prion investigational studies and have been shown to inactivate prions.[63]

XIII.i. Semicritical and critical devices contaminated with low-risk tissue from high-risk patients should be processed using conventional processing procedures.[63] *[1: Strong Evidence]*

Instruments contaminated with low-risk tissue are unlikely to transmit infection after processing using conventional protocols because those instruments would not be used in the central nervous system.[63]

The SHEA guidelines make no recommendation regarding processing of devices exposed to low-risk tissue.[63] Studies to determine the risk associated with low-risk tissues are ongoing, and until evidence indicates that special processing protocols are required to prevent transmission of infection, SHEA makes no recommendation. Transmission of infection from low-risk tissue has only been demonstrated in animal studies of direct inoculation into the brain.[63]

XIII.j. Instruments that require special prion processing procedures should be identified in a manner that alerts personnel who handle and process instruments that the instruments are contaminated or potentially contaminated with prions.[10] *[4: Limited Evidence]*

Awareness that instruments are contaminated or potentially contaminated with prions reduces the risk of these instruments being ineffectively processed and subsequently used on other patients.

XIII.j.1. An instrument-tracking process should be used that provides for tracking of surgical instruments used on high-risk tissue (eg, spinal and brain tissue). *[5: Benefits Balanced with Harms]*

Instrument tracking systems identify items used during the procedure and also identify the patient for whom the items were used.

XIII.k. Noncritical environmental surfaces contaminated with high-risk tissue from a patient known or suspected to have a prion disease should be cleaned and then spot decontaminated with a 1:5 or 1:10 dilution of hypochlorite for a contact time of 15 minutes or with 1 N NaOH.[63,132] *[1: Strong Evidence]*

Because there is no Environmental Protection Agency-registered antimicrobial product specifically for prion-contaminated environmental surfaces, a solution of diluted hypochloride or 1 N NaOH is recommended.[63]

No transmission of prion diseases from environmental surfaces, other than devices used in surgery, has been reported. However, current evidence on prion diseases suggests the need for continued research to better explain transmission. It remains prudent to eliminate highly infectious material from OR surfaces that patients and personnel will be in contact with during subsequent surgeries.

XIII.l. Noncritical environmental surfaces contaminated with low-risk tissue should be cleaned

using standard disinfection processes.[63] *[1: Strong Evidence]*

Transmission of prion disease from surfaces contaminated with low-risk tissue has not been reported.

XIII.m. When a patient is identified postoperatively as having had a prion disease at the time of surgery, special precautions should be taken. Devices determined to be potentially contaminated with high-risk tissue from the patient should be removed from service and decontaminated according to the most current professional guidelines for prion inactivation.[63] *[1: Strong Evidence]*

Inadequately decontaminated instruments may pose a risk to subsequent patients who have contact with the instruments. The current SHEA Guidelines[63] describe six cases of CJD transmitted by neurosurgical instruments in Europe between 1952 through 1976, demonstrating prion survival of several years. Two of these cases occurred in 1967. These patients developed CJD 15 and 18 months after stereotactic electroencephalographic explorations using electrodes that had been implanted earlier in a patient with CJD and sterilized with 70% alcohol and formaldehyde vapor. Two years later, the electrodes were retrieved and implanted into the brain of a chimpanzee who then developed CJD.[63,64] These classic cases are frequently cited in prion-related articles.[110,116,133,134]

XIII.n. Perioperative personnel who may be exposed to prions should review current research on methods of detecting prion infectivity and decontamination methods and incorporate new evidence into practice.[111] *[2: High Evidence]*

Research related to prion disease, tissue infectivity, potential risks of transmission, and effectiveness of cleaning chemistries and sterilization technologies and cycles is ongoing. Incorporating current, evidence-based knowledge into practice may help minimize risks associated with prions.

Recommendation XIV

Documentation of instrument cleaning and disinfection processes should be maintained.

Documentation provides data for the identification of trends and demonstration of compliance with regulatory requirements and accreditation agency standards.

Effective management and collection of health care information that accurately reflects the patient's care, treatment, and services is a regulatory requirement and accreditation agency standard for both hospitals and ambulatory settings.[135-140]

XIV.a. Cleaning and decontamination documentation should include the
 ○ date,
 ○ time,

○ identification of instruments,
○ method and verification of cleaning and results of cleaning audits,
○ number or identifier of the mechanical instrument washer and results of washer efficacy testing,
○ name of the person performing the cleaning and decontamination,
○ lot numbers of cleaning agents,
○ testing results for insulated instruments,
○ disposition of defective equipment, and
○ maintenance of cleaning equipment.
[4: Limited Evidence]
Documentation enables traceability in the event of a failure.[10] Records of washer testing provide a source of evidence for review during investigation of clinical issues, including SSIs. Documentation of equipment maintenance provides evidence that equipment has been maintained.

XIV.b. Records should be maintained for a time period specified by the health care organization and in compliance with local, state, and federal regulations.[1,10] *[4: Limited Evidence]*

Recommendation XV

Perioperative team members with responsibilities for cleaning and care of instruments used in surgery should receive initial and ongoing education and complete competency verification activities related to cleaning and care of surgical instruments.

It is the responsibility of the health care organization to provide initial and ongoing education and to verify the competency of perioperative team members.[141] Initial and ongoing education of perioperative personnel about cleaning and care of instruments facilitates the development of knowledge, skills, and attitudes that affect safe patient care.

Competency verification activities measure individual performance, provide a mechanism for documentation, and help verify that perioperative personnel have an understanding of the principles and processes related to recommended practices for cleaning and care of surgical instruments.

XV.a. Perioperative team members should receive education and complete competency verification activities that address specific knowledge and skills related to cleaning and care of surgical instruments. *[1: Regulatory Requirement]*
Ongoing development of knowledge and skills and documentation of personnel participation is a regulatory requirement and accreditation agency standard for both hospital and ambulatory settings.[135,136,142-144]

XV.a.1. Education regarding cleaning and care of surgical instruments should include
• adherence to manufacturers' IFU,
• methods of cleaning and verification of cleaning,
• types of contamination of medical devices,

• methods of decontamination,
• selection of cleaning chemistries,
• safe use of cleaning chemistries,
• safe use of cleaning equipment,
• how to verify washer cleaning efficacy,
• use of PPE during instrument processing,
• risks and hazards associated with contaminated instruments,
• prions and risks associated with prion-contaminated instruments,
• procedures for decontaminating instruments that are potentially contaminated or known to be contaminated with prions,
• measures to minimize risks of exposure to transmissible pathogens,
• TASS and measures to prevent its occurrence,
• corrective actions to employ in the event of a cleaning failure,
• corrective actions to employ in the event of an equipment or instrument failure,
• new instruments and equipment, and
• evidence-based information about changes in cleaning chemistries and technologies.
[5: Benefits Balanced with Harms]

Recommendation XVI

Policies and procedures for cleaning and care of instruments used in surgery should be developed, reviewed periodically, revised as necessary, and readily available in the practice setting in which they are used.

Policies and procedures assist in the development of patient safety, quality assessment, and performance improvement activities. Policies and procedures also serve as operational guidelines used to minimize patients' risk for injury or complications, standardize practice, direct perioperative personnel, and establish continuous performance improvement programs. Policies and procedures establish authority, responsibility, and accountability within the practice setting.

XVI.a. Policies and procedures regarding cleaning and care of surgical instruments used in surgery should be developed using professional guidelines and validated, written manufacturers' IFU. *[1: Regulatory Requirement]*
Having policies and procedures that guide and support patient care, treatment, and services is a regulatory requirement and an accreditation agency standard for both hospital and ambulatory settings.[135,136,145-148]

XVI.a.1. Policies and procedures related to cleaning and care of surgical instruments should include
• prepurchase evaluation;
• a review of the manufacturer's IFU before purchase or consignment;
• management of loaned instruments, including advance notification, time frame for delivery and pickup, requirements for

INSTRUMENT CLEANING

and delineation of responsibilities for inventory, and processes for care and handling, cleaning, decontamination, packaging, and sterilization of instruments;

- point-of-use cleaning of instruments;
- transport of contaminated instruments;
- precautions to be taken when handling contaminated instruments;
- precautions to be taken when handling cleaning chemistries;
- processes for cleaning and decontaminating instruments after use in surgery;
- care and handling of accessories and supplies necessary for cleaning and decontaminating contaminated instruments;
- processes for manual and automated cleaning;
- use and care of cleaning equipment and cleaning chemistries;
- requirements for water quality used for cleaning instruments;
- methods for processing ophthalmic instruments;
- design of decontamination areas to accommodate efficient workflow;
- requirements for ventilation, temperature, and humidity of decontamination areas;
- use of PPE in relation to cleaning and decontaminating instruments;
- methods for monitoring cleaning processes and cleaning equipment;
- inspection and testing of instruments to determine cleanliness, integrity, and function;
- preparation of instruments for packaging;
- procedures for managing laryngoscope blades and handles;
- criteria for identification and precautions taken for instruments used on patients with known or suspected prion disease;
- documentation of cleaning;
- education and competency verification;
- maintenance of SDSs;
- procedures for reporting exposure to bloodborne pathogens; and
- procedures for reporting adverse events.

[5: Benefits Balanced with Harms]

Recommendation XVII

The health care organization's quality management program should evaluate the cleaning, decontamination, and care of instruments.

Quality assurance and performance improvement programs can facilitate the identification of problem areas and assist personnel in evaluating and improving the quality of patient care and formulating plans for corrective actions. These programs provide data that may be used to determine whether an individual organization is within benchmark goals and, if not, to identify areas that may require corrective actions. A quality

management program provides a mechanism to evaluate effectiveness of processes, compliance with manufacturers' written IFU, sterile processing policies and procedures, and function of equipment.

Collecting data to monitor and improve patient care, treatment, and services is a regulatory requirement and an accreditation agency standard for both hospital and ambulatory settings.[135,136,149-152]

XVII.a. A quality management program should include monitoring of manual and mechanical cleaning. *[2: High Evidence]*

Cleaning is a critical component of instrument processing and can affect the efficacy of a subsequent sterilization processes. Items that have been sterilized after inadequate cleaning processes have caused patient injury.[21-23,153]

XVII.a.1. Mechanical cleaners (eg, washer disinfectors/decontaminators) should be tested for correct function on installation, at least weekly (preferably daily) during routine use, after major repairs, and after significant changes in cleaning parameters (eg, changing cleaning solutions).[10] *[4: Limited Evidence]*

Monitoring washer function provides information about whether the equipment is functioning correctly. Thorough cleaning is dependent on how the equipment is used, how instruments are placed in the machine, and whether the equipment is functioning correctly.

Adequate cleaning is essential to remove or destroy microorganisms and eliminate endotoxins. Testing washer disinfectors/decontaminators on a regular basis verifies that the equipment is functioning correctly or identifies an opportunity for corrective action. Commercial tests to monitor cleaning efficacy of mechanical washer disinfector/decontaminators are available.

XVII.a.2. Manual cleaning should be evaluated using objective measures (eg, chemical reagent tests for detecting clinically relevant soils [eg, protein]) when new types of instruments requiring manual cleaning are processed and periodically at intervals determined by the health care facility. *[5: Benefits Balanced with Harms]*

Manual cleaning is a learned skill and is subject to human error.

XVII.a.3. When verifying the effectiveness of manual cleaning, the instruments most difficult to clean should be used. *[5: Benefits Balanced with Harms]*

Using the most difficult instruments to clean provides a robust measure of cleaning effectiveness.

XVII.a.4. Testing should be performed to assess efficacy of cleaning of medical devices. *[1: Strong Evidence]*

STERILIZATION AND DISINFECTION

Currently, there is no single standard of clean, nor is there a standard test soil. Agreement as to what level of residual soil is acceptable after cleaning and what level of residual soil is clinically significant is also lacking.[5,51]

Efficacy of cleaning has traditionally been evaluated visually. Several studies comparing visual analysis with microscopic analysis have demonstrated that visual inspection alone is not sufficient to determine levels of cleanliness.[21,51,77,154] Visual inspection is subjective. In addition, infectious microorganisms and residues are not visible to the naked eye. It is also not possible to visually inspect most lumens. Even under ideal cleaning conditions, instruments may retain debris.[42]

There are, however, a number of tests that can be used to assess cleaning efficiency.[155-158] Qualitative tests usually involve swabbing a device, immersing it in a reagent, and observing for a color change that indicates the presence of organic markers, such as protein or blood.[5,10,82,158] Quantitative tests provide a measure or action limit against which test results are measured. Adenosine tri-phosphate (ATP) bioluminescence is an example of a quantitative test.[155-157] The item to be tested is swabbed to collect ATP, the swab is inserted into a reaction tube, and the ATP on the swab is released using chemicals in the reaction tube. The reaction tube is then inserted into a hand-held luminometer that converts the ATP released from microorganisms or human cells into a light signal, which is measured in relative light units (ie, RLUs). Manufacturers may establish "benchmark cutoffs" for manual cleaning of instruments (eg, flexible endoscopes) that users can employ so that any instrument failing this quantitative cutoff after cleaning is re-cleaned before disinfection/sterilization.[158]

Quantitative testing can be used in a quality monitoring program to observe for trends and to monitor performance of a washer disinfector/decontaminator or of manual processes.[37,154,159] Readings that trend lower indicate improved cleaning, whereas readings that trend higher can indicate a need for improvement.

XVII.b. Instruments and equipment should be maintained and serviced in accordance with the device manufacturer's written IFU. *[3: Moderate Evidence]*

Preventive maintenance requirements or recommendations are what the device manufacturer has determined are necessary to keep instruments and equipment in optimal working order. Providing instruments and equipment in optimal working order is critical to patient safety.[23]

XVII.b.1. Cleaning equipment should be maintained and serviced in accordance with the equipment manufacturer's written IFU, and maintenance and service should be documented. *[5: Benefits Balanced with Harms]*

The manufacturer has determined that the maintenance requirements specified in the manufacturer's written IFU are necessary for optimal performance.

Documentation of maintenance provides a record that can be used to determine compliance with the IFU. Documentation of service can provide information useful in determining whether equipment needs to be replaced.

XVII.b.2. Instruments and cleaning equipment should be serviced by personnel who are qualified to repair the instruments and equipment in need of service. Instrument or equipment service should be documented. *[5: Benefits Balanced with Harms]*

Instruments and cleaning equipment used in surgery are complex. Having qualified personnel service instruments and equipment increases the probability that repair and service will be performed correctly.

Documentation of instrument repairs may help to identify trends in instrument and cleaning equipment damage and define practices that may reduce damage.

XVII.c. Insulated equipment should be tested for current leakage before use and after decontamination. *[4: Limited Evidence]*

Testing before use and after decontamination allows a defective device to be replaced before use or sterilization and provides an opportunity for corrective action in advance of the surgical procedure.[25]

XVII.d. Adverse events should be reported and documented according to the health care organization's policy and procedure and should be reviewed for potential opportunities for improvement.
- During investigation of SSIs, the cleaning process and its documentation should be reviewed by infection preventionists, perioperative RNs, and designated sterile processing personnel.
- Near misses (ie, unplanned events that do not result in injury, such as organic or inorganic material discovered in a processed instrument tray) should be investigated and corrective action taken to prevent serious adverse events. *[2: High Evidence]*

Surgical site infection has been documented as a result of inadequate cleaning of surgical instruments.[22,23] Reports of near misses can be used to identify actions that should be taken to

INSTRUMENT CLEANING

prevent actual adverse events and can reveal opportunities for improvement.

Editor's note: Teflon is a registered trademark of DuPont, Wilmington, DE.

Glossary

Adsorption: The adhesion of extremely thin layers of molecules to the solid surfaces they contact.

Aerosol: A suspension of fine solid or liquid particles in air.

Borescope: A device used to inspect the inside of an instrument through a small opening or lumen of the instrument.

Cavitation: A process that uses high-frequency sound waves to form microscopic bubbles that become unstable and implode, creating tiny vacuums capable of removing debris from instrument surfaces and crevices.

Cleaning: A process that uses friction, detergent, and water to remove organic debris; the process by which any type of soil, including organic debris, is removed to the extent necessary for further processing or for the intended use. Cleaning removes rather than kills microorganisms.

Creutzfeldt-Jakob disease: A fatal degenerative neurological disease caused by a prion.

Decontamination: Any physical or chemical process that removes or reduces the number of microorganisms or infectious agents and renders reusable medical products safe for handling or disposal. The process by which contaminants are removed, either by hand cleaning or mechanical means, using specific solutions capable of rendering blood and debris harmless and removing them from the surface of an object or instrument.

Distilled water: Water that has been boiled, vaporized, cooled, and condensed to remove impurities.

Electroplating: A process whereby electrical current reduces dissolved metal cations that then form a coating on an electrode, causing a change in the surface properties of a device.

Gross soil: Organic material (eg, blood, tissue, bone) and debris (eg, bone cement) that accumulates on surgical instruments during operative or other invasive procedures.

Homogenate: A tissue that is or has been made homogenous, as by grinding cells into a creamy consistency for laboratory studies. A homogenate usually lacks cell structure.

Hydrophobic: Absence of affinity to water.

Loaned items: Medical devices used in health care facilities that are not owned by the facility.

Lumen: A channel or path through a tubular structure.

Medical-grade compressed air: Air supplied from cylinders, bulk containers, or medical air compressors or reconstituted from oxygen USP and oil-free dry nitrogen NF.

Porosity detector: A high-voltage device designed to find pinholes and flaws in nonconductive coatings. Porosity detectors can only be used to find flaws in coatings when the layer beneath the coating is made of a conductive material.

Product quality assurance testing: A quality assurance process used to verify that a device manufacturer's instructions for sterile processing can be achieved in the health care setting.

Reverse osmosis: A water purifying process whereby water under pressure is passed through a semi-permeable membrane to eliminate impurities.

Toxic anterior segment syndrome (TASS): A complication of ophthalmic surgery involving a severe, non-infectious inflammation of the anterior segment of the eye, caused by various contaminants in solutions, medications, steam, and residue on surgical instruments and supplies.

Transmissible spongiform encephalopathies (TSEs): A fatal prion disease that effects the brain and nervous system. The development of tiny holes in the brain cause it to appear like a sponge, hence the term "spongiform."

Treated water: Water that has been filtered, deionized, distilled, or subjected to reverse osmosis to reduce impurities.

Ultrasonic cleaner: A processing unit that transmits ultrasonic waves through the cleaning solution in a mechanical process known as cavitation. Ultrasonic cleaning is particularly effective in removing soil deposits from hard-to-reach areas.

Validating: A documented procedure performed by manufacturers for obtaining, recording, and interpreting the results required to establish that a process will consistently yield product that complies with predetermined specifications.

Variant Creutzfeldt-Jakob disease (vCJD): A fatal degenerative neurological disease caused by a prion. The human form of bovine spongiform encephalopathy (ie, mad cow disease).

Viscoelastic: A gel injected into the anterior chamber during ophthalmic surgery to maintain the depth of the chamber, protect the corneal endothelium, and stabilize the vitreous.

Washer/decontaminator: A processing unit that, either by use of single or multiple chambers, automatically decontaminates surgical instruments. It employs a cool water rinse, hot water wash, rinse, and drying. An ultrasonic cleaning feature and lubricant rinse may be added.

References

1. Guideline for sterilization. In: *Guidelines for Perioperative Practice.* Denver, CO: AORN, Inc; 2015:665-692. [IVA]

2. *Guideline for Disinfection and Sterilization in Healthcare Facilities*, 2008. Atlanta, GA: Centers for Disease Control and Prevention; 2008. [IVA]

3. Guideline for selection and use of packaging systems for sterilization. In: *Guidelines for Perioperative Practice.* Denver, CO: AORN, Inc; 2015:651-664. [IVA]

4. Guideline for cleaning and processing flexible endoscopes and endoscope accessories. In: *Guidelines for Perioperative Practice.* Denver, CO: AORN, Inc; 2015:589-600. [IVB]

STERILIZATION AND DISINFECTION

5. *ANSI/AAMI TIR30:2011 A Compendium of Processes, Materials, Test Methods, and Acceptance Criteria for Cleaning Reusable Medical Devices.* Arlington, VA: Association for the Advancement of Medical Instrumentation; 2011. [IVC]

6. *AAMI TIR12: 2010 Designing, Testing, and Labeling Reusable Medical Devices for Reprocessing in Health Care Facilities: a Guide for Medical Device Manufacturers.* Arlington, VA: Association for the Advancement of Medical Instrumentation; 2010. [IVC]

7. Guideline for product selection. In: *Guidelines for Perioperative Practice.* Denver, CO: AORN, Inc; 2015:179-186. [IVB]

8. American Society of Cataract and Refractive Surgery, American Society of Ophthalmic Registered Nurses. Recommended practices for cleaning and sterilizing intraocular surgical instruments. *J Cataract Refract Surg.* 2007;33(6):1095-1100. [IVB]

9. Hensell MG. Instrumentation for robotic surgery. *Periop Nurs Clin.* 2010;5(1):69-81. [VA]

10. *ANSI/AAMI ST79: Comprehensive Guide to Steam Sterilization and Sterility Assurance In Health Care Facilities.* Arlington, VA: Association for the Advancement of Medical Instrumentation; 2013. [IVC]

11. Meredith SJ, Sjorgen G. Decontamination: back to basics. *J Periop Pract.* 2008;18(7):285-288. [VA]

12. Spry CC, Brooks Tighe SM. Care and handling of surgical instruments. In: Brooks Tighe S, ed. *Instrumentation for the Operating Room: a Photographic Manual.* 8th ed. St Louis, MO: Elsevier/Mosby; 2012:1-2. [VB]

13. Howlin RP, Harrison J, Secker T, Keevil CW. Acquisition of proteinaceous contamination through the handling of surgical instruments by hospital staff in sterile service departments [corrected]. 2009;10(3):106-111. [IA]

14. Seavey R. Reprocessing in the ambulatory surgery setting. *Healthc Purch News.* 2012;36(12):38-41. [VA]

15. Rutala WA, Weber DJ. Disinfection and sterilization: an overview. *Am J Infect Control.* 2013;41(5):S2-S5. [VA]

16. Hercules PA. Instrument readiness: a patient safety issue. *Perioper Nurs Clin.* 2010;5(1):15-25. [VA]

17. Dancer SJ, Stewart M, Coulombe C, Gregori A, Virdi M. Surgical site infections linked to contaminated surgical instruments. *J Hosp Infect.* 2012;81(4):231-238. [VB]

18. Cordero I. Sharpening and tightening surgical scissors. *Comm Eye Health J.* 2011;24(76):44-45. [VB]

19. Goldberg JL. What the perioperative nurse needs to know about cleaning, disinfection, and sterilization. *Perioper Nurs Clin.* 2010;5(3):263-272. [VB]

20. Montero PN, Robinson TN, Weaver JS, Stiegmann GV. Insulation failure in laparoscopic instruments. *Surg Endosc.* 2010;24(2):462-465. [IIIA]

21. Shimono N, Takuma T, Tsuchimochi N, et al. An outbreak of Pseudomonas aeruginosa infections following thoracic surgeries occurring via the contamination of bronchoscopes and an automatic endoscope reprocessor. *J Infect Chemother.* 2008;14(6):418-423. [VA]

22. Tosh PK, Disbot M, Duffy JM, et al. Outbreak of Pseudomonas aeruginosa surgical site infections after arthroscopic procedures: Texas, 2009. *Infect Control Hosp Epidemiol.* 2011;32(12):1179-1186. [IIIA]

23. Parada SA, Grassbaugh JA, Devine JG, Arrington ED. Instrumentation-specific infection after anterior cruciate ligament reconstruction. *Sports Health.* 2009;1(6):481-485. [VA]

24. Yasuhara H, Fukatsu K, Komatsu T, Obayashi T, Saito Y, Uetera Y. Prevention of medical accidents caused by defective surgical instruments. *Surgery.* 2012;151(2):153-161. [IIIA]

25. Saito Y, Kobayashi H, Uetera Y, Yasuhara H, Kajiura T, Okubo T. Microbial contamination of surgical instruments used for laparotomy. *Am J Infect Control.* 2014;42(1):43-47. [IIIC]

26. Espada M, Munoz R, Noble BN, Magrina JF. Insulation failure in robotic and laparoscopic instrumentation: a prospective evaluation. *Am J Obstetr Gynecol.* 2011;205(2):121.e1-121.e5. [IIIA]

27. *Guide to Infection Prevention for Outpatient Settings: Minimum Expectations for Safe Care.* Atlanta, GA: Centers for Disease Control and Prevention; 2011. [IVA]

28. Spry CC. Care and handling of basic surgical instruments. *AORN J.* 2007;86(Suppl 1):S77-S81. [VA]

29. Seavey R. Reducing the risks associated with loaner instrumentation and implants. *AORN J.* 2010;92(3):322-334. [VA]

30. Huter-Kunish GG. Processing loaner instruments in an ambulatory surgery center. *AORN J.* 2009;89(5):861-866. [VA]

31. Duro M. New IAHCSMM loaner instrumentation position paper and policy template. *AORN J.* 2011;94(3):287-289. [VA]

32. IAHCSMM Position Paper on the Management of Loaner Instrumentation. IAHCSMM. http://www.iahcsmm.org/137-resources/news/association-news/association-archives/767-iahcsmm-releases-loaner-instrumentation-position-paper,-sample-policy.html?highlight=WyJsb2FuZXIiLCJpbnN0cnVtZW50YXRpb24iLCJsb2FuZXIgaW5zdHJ1bWVudGF0aW9uIl0=. Accessed September 29, 2014. [IVC]

33. Winthrop TG, Sion BA, Gaines C. Loaner instrumentation: processing the unknown. *AORN J.* 2007;85(3):566-573. [VB]

34. Seavey R. High-level disinfection, sterilization, and antisepsis: current issues in reprocessing medical and surgical instruments. *Am J Infect Control.* 2013;41(5):S111-S117. [VA]

35. McNamara SA. Instrument readiness: an important link to patient safety. [Patient Safety First]. *AORN J.* 2011;93(1):160-164. [VA]

36. Root CW, Kaiser N, Antonucci C. What, how and why: enzymatic instrument cleaning products in healthcare environments. *Healthc Purchasing News.* 2008;32(11):50. [VA]

37. Azizi J, Anderson SG, Murphy S, Pryce S. Uphill grime: process improvement in surgical instrument cleaning. *AORN J.* 2012;96(2):152-162. [IIA]

38. Vickery K, Ngo Q, Zou J, Cossart YE. The effect of multiple cycles of contamination, detergent washing, and disinfection on the development of biofilm in endoscope tubing. *Am J Infect Control.* 2009;37(6):470-475. [IA]

39. Toxic and Hazardous Substances: Bloodborne Pathogens, 29 CFR §1910.1030 (2012). Occupational Safety and Health Administration. http://www.osha.gov/pls/oshawewb/owadisp.show_document?p_table=STANDARDS&pid=10051. Accessed September 23, 2014.

40. Guideline for sharps safety. In: *Guidelines for Perioperative Practice.* Denver, CO: AORN, Inc; 2015:365-388. [IVA]

41. Bruins MJ, Wijshake D, de Vries-van Rossum SV, Klein Overmeen RG, Ruijs GJ. Otitis externa following aural irrigation linked to instruments contaminated with *Pseudomonas aeruginosa. J Hosp Infect.* 2013;84(3):222-226. [IIIB]

42. Azizi J, Basile RJ. Doubt and proof: the need to verify the cleaning process. *Biomed Instrum Technol.* 2012;Spring(Suppl):49-54. [IIIA]

43. Weber DJ, Rutala WA, Miller MB, Huslage K, Sickbert-Bennett E. Role of hospital surfaces in the transmission of emerging health care-associated pathogens: norovirus, *Clostridium difficile* and Acinetobacter species. *Am J Infect Control.* 2010;38(Suppl 1):S25-S33. [VA]

44. Guideline for prevention of transmissible infections. In: *Guidelines for Perioperative Practice.* Denver, CO: AORN, Inc; 2015:419-451. [IVA]

45. Facility Guidelines Institute, American Society for Healthcare Engineering. *Guidelines for Design and Construction of Hospitals and Outpatient Facilities.* Chicago, IL: American Society for Healthcare Engineering; 2014. [IVC]

46. Guideline for a safe environment of care, part 2. In: *Guidelines for Perioperative Practice.* Denver, CO: AORN, Inc; 2015:265-290. [IVA]

47. Medical services and first aid, 29 CFR §1910.151. Occupational Safety and Health Administration. http://www.gpo.gov/fdsys/granule/CFR-2013-title29-vol5/CFR-2013-title29-vol5-sec1910-151. Accessed September 23, 2014.

48. Guideline for a safe environment of care, part 1. In: *Guidelines for Perioperative Practice.* Denver, CO: AORN, Inc; 2015:239-263. [IVA]

49. *ANSI/ISEA Z358.1-2009: American National Standard for Emergency Eyewash and Shower Equipment.* New York, NY: American National Standards Institute; 2009. [IVC]

50. Alfa MJ, Nemes R. Manual versus automated methods for cleaning reusable accessory devices used for minimally invasive surgical procedures. *J Hosp Infect.* 2004;58(1):50-58. [IA]

51. Alfa MJ, Olson N, Al-Fadhaly A. Cleaning efficacy of medical device washers in North American healthcare facilities. *J Hosp Infect.* 2010;74(2):168-177. [IIIA]

52. Ofstead CL, Wetzler HP, Snyder AK, Horton RA. Endoscope reprocessing methods: a prospective study on the impact of human factors and automation. *Gastroenterol Nurs.* 2010;33(4):304-311. [IIIA]

53. *AAMI TIR34:2007: Water for the Reprocessing of Medical Devices.* Arlington, VA: Association for the Advancement of Medical Instrumentation; 2007. [IVC]

54. American Society of Heating, Refrigerating and Air-Conditioning Engineers. Room design. In: *HVAC Design Manual for Hospitals and Clinics.* 2nd ed. Atlanta, GA: ASHRAE; 2013:151-202. [IVC]

55. Panagopoulou P, Filioti J, Farmaki E, Maloukou A, Roilides E. Filamentous fungi in a tertiary care hospital: environmental surveillance and susceptibility to antifungal drugs. *Infect Control Hosp Epidemiol.* 2007;28(1):60-67. [IIIB]

56. Tang JW. The effect of environmental parameters on the survival of airborne infectious agents. *J R Soc Interface.* 2009;6(Suppl 6):S737-S746. [VB]

57. Thompson KA, Bennett AM, Walker JT. Aerosol survival of Staphylococcus epidermidis. *J Hosp Infect.* 2011;78(3):216-220. [IIIB]

58. Memarzadeh F. Literature review of the effect of temperature and humidity on viruses. *ASHRAE Transactions.* 2012;18(Part I):1049-1060. [VB]

59. *Proper Maintenance of Instruments.* 8th ed. Morfelden-Walldorf, Germany: Arbeitskreis Instrumenten-Aufbereitung [Instrument Working Group]; 2004. [IVC]

60. Harnroongroj T, Leelaporn A, Limsrivanichayakorn S, Kaewdaeng S, Harnroongroj T. Comparison of bacterial count in tap water between first burst and running tap water. *J Med Assoc Thailand.* 2012;95(5):712-715. [IIIC]

61. Enzymatic detergents and contamination control: a guide for instrument reprocessing. Infection Control Today. http://www.infectioncontroltoday.com/articles/2010/06/enzymatic-detergents-and-contamination-control-a.aspx. Accessed September 23, 2014. [VB]

62. Hazard Communication Standard Final Regulatory Text 2012. Occupational Safety and Health Administration. https://www.osha.gov/dsg/hazcom/ghs-final-rule.html. Accessed September 23, 2014.

63. Rutala WA, Weber DJ. Guideline for disinfection and sterilization of prion-contaminated medical instruments. *Infect Control Hosp Epidemiol.* 2010;31(2):107-117. [IVA]

64. Rutala WA, Weber DJ. Creutzfeldt-Jakob disease: recommendations for disinfection and sterilization. *Clin Infect Dis.* 2001;32(9):1348-1356. [IVA]

65. Williamson JE. Brushing up on brush basics. *Healthc Purchasing News.* 2009;33(5):28. [VB]

66. Czyrko C. Ultrasonic cleaners in dental decontamination. *Dent Nurs.* 2012;8(4):210-213. [VB]

67. Kauffman M, Joseph C. Ultrasonic cleaning in the healthcare setting. *Healthc Purchasing News.* 2011;35(1):30-33. [VA]

68. Kohn Rachel. Ultra-sound reasons to use an ultrasonic cleaner for surgical instruments. *Healthc Purchasing News.* 2011;35(5):54-54. [VB]

69. Cutler Peck CM, Brubaker J, Clouser S, Danford C, Edelhauser HE, Mamalis N. Toxic anterior segment syndrome: common causes. *J Cataract Refract Surg.* 2010;36(7):1073-1080. [IIIA]

70. Mamalis N. Toxic anterior segment syndrome update. *J Cataract Refract Surg.* 2010;36(7):1067-1068. [VA]

71. Richburg FA, Reidy JJ, Apple DJ, Olson RJ. Sterile hypopyon secondary to ultrasonic cleaning solution. *J Cataract Refract Surg.* 1986;12(3):248-251. [VA]

72. Kreisler KR, Martin SS, Young CW, Anderson CW, Mamalis N. Postoperative inflammation following cataract extraction caused by bacterial contamination of the cleaning bath detergent. *J Cataract Refract Surg.* 1992;18(1):106-110. [VA]

73. Gilmour D. Instrument integrity and sterility: the perioperative practitioner's responsibilities. *J Perioper Pract.* 2008;18(7):292-296. [VC]

74. Alfa MJ. Monitoring and improving the effectiveness of cleaning medical and surgical devices. *Am J Infect Control.* 2013;41(5 Suppl):S56-S59. [VA]

75. Instrument inspections lead to detections. *Healthc Purchasing News.* 2012;36(11):38-40. [VB]

76. Alfa MJ. The "Pandora's Box" dilemma: reprocessing of implantable screws and plates in orthopedic tray sets. *Biomed Instrum Technol.* 2012;Spring(Suppl):55-59. [VA]

77. Lipscomb IP, Sihota AK, Keevil CW. Comparison between visual analysis and microscope assessment of surgical instrument cleanliness from sterile service departments. *J Hosp Infect.* 2008;68(1):52-58. [IIIB]

78. Ongoing Safety Review of Arthroscopic Shavers. US Food and Drug Administration. http://www.fda.gov/MedicalDevices/Safety/AlertsandNotices/ucm170639.htm. Accessed on Feb 21, 2014.

79. *ANSI/AAMI ST58:2013: 2010 Chemical Sterilization and High-level Disinfection in Health Care Facilities.* Arlington, VA: Association for the Advancement of Medical Instrumentation; 2013. [IVC]

STERILIZATION AND DISINFECTION

80. *ANSI/AAMI ST41:2008/(R)2012: Ethylene Oxide Sterilization in Health Care Facilities: Safety and Effectiveness.* Arlington, VA: Association for the Advancement of Medical Instrumentation; 2012. [IVC]

81. Shunmugam M, Hugkulstone CE, Wong R, Williamson TH. Consecutive toxic anterior segment syndrome in combined phaco-vitrectomy. *Int Ophthalmol.* 2013;33(3):289-290. [VA]

82. Tamashiro NS, Souza RQ, Goncalves CR, et al. Cytotoxicity of cannulas for ophthalmic surgery after cleaning and sterilization: evaluation of the use of enzymatic detergent to remove residual ophthalmic viscosurgical device material. *J Cataract Refract Surg.* 2013;39(6):937-941. [IA]

83. Ozcelik ND, Eltutar K, Bilgin B. Toxic anterior segment syndrome after uncomplicated cataract surgery. *Eur J Ophthalmol.* 2010;20(1):106-114. [VB]

84. FDA collaboration to monitor rare eye condition associated with cataract surgery [FDA News Release]. US Food and Drug Administration. http://www.fda.gov/NewsEvents/Newsroom/PressAnnouncements/ucm284239.htm. Accessed on September 23, 2014. [VB]

85. Bodnar Z, Clouser S, Mamalis N. Toxic anterior segment syndrome: update on the most common causes. *J Cataract Refract Surg.* 2012;38(11):1902-1910. [IIIA]

86. Mamalis N, Edelhauser HF, Dawson DG, Chew J, LeBoyer RM, Werner L. Toxic anterior segment syndrome. *J Cataract Refract Surg.* 2006;32(2):324-333. [VA]

87. McCormick PJ, Kaiser JJ, Schoene MJ, et al. Ophthalmic viscoelastic devices as a cleaning challenge. *Biomed Instrum Technol.* 2013;47(4):347-355. [IIA]

88. Maier P, Birnbaum F, Bohringer D, Reinhard T. Toxic anterior segment syndrome following penetrating keratoplasty. *Arch Ophthalmol.* 2008;126(12):1677-1681. [VA]

89. Mathys KC, Cohen KL, Bagnell CR. Identification of unknown intraocular material after cataract surgery: evaluation of a potential cause of toxic anterior segment syndrome. *J Cataract Refract Surg.* 2008;34(3):465-469. [VB]

90. Providing safe surgical instruments: factors to consider. Infection Control Today. http://www.infectioncontroltoday.com/articles/2008/04/providing-safe-surgical-instruments-factors-to-co.aspx. Accessed September 23, 2014. [VB]

91. Hellinger WC, Hasan SA, Bacalis LP, et al. Outbreak of toxic anterior segment syndrome following cataract surgery associated with impurities in autoclave steam moisture. *Infect Control Hosp Epidemiol.* 2006;27(3):294-298. [VA]

92. Ayaki M, Shimada K, Yaguchi S, Koide R, Iwasawa A. Corneal and conjunctival toxicity of disinfectants—assessing safety for use with ophthalmic surgical instruments. *Regul Toxicol Pharmacol.* 2007;48(3):292-295. [IB]

93. Mamalis N, Edelhauser HF. Enzymatic detergents and toxic anterior segment syndrome. *Ophthalmology.* 2013;120(3):651-652. [VA]

94. Leder HA, Goodkin M, Buchen SY, et al. An investigation of enzymatic detergents as a potential cause of toxic anterior segment syndrome. *Ophthalmology.* 2012;119(7):e30-e35. [IB]

95. Buchen SY, Calogero D, Tarver ME, Hilmantel G, Tang X, Eydelman MB. Evaluation of intraocular reactivity to organic contaminants of ophthalmic devices in a rabbit model. *Ophthalmology.* 2012;119(7):e24-e29. [IB]

96. Buchen SY, Calogero D, Hilmantel G, Eydelman MB. Rabbit ocular reactivity to bacterial endotoxin contained in aqueous solution and ophthalmic viscosurgical devices. *Ophthalmology.* 2012;119(7):e4-e10. [IA]

97. Negri de Sousa AC, Levy CE, Freitas MI. Laryngoscope blades and handles as sources of cross-infection: an integrative review. *J Hosp Infect.* 2013;83(4):269-275. [VA]

98. Simmons SA. Laryngoscope handles: a potential for infection. *AANA J.* 2000;68(3):233-236. [IIA]

99. Phillips RA, Monaghan WP. Incidence of visible and occult blood on laryngoscope blades and handles. *AANA J.* 1997;65(3):241-246. [IIIC]

100. Tablan OC, Anderson LJ, Besser R, et al. Guidelines for preventing health-care–associated pneumonia, 2003: recommendations of CDC and the Healthcare Infection Control Practices Advisory Committee. *MMWR Recomm Rep.* 2004;53(RR-3):1-36. [IVA]

101. Jones BL, Gorman LJ, Simpson J, et al. An outbreak of Serratia marcescens in two neonatal intensive care units. *J Hosp Infect.* 2000;46(4):314-319. [VB]

102. Foweraker JE. The laryngoscope as a potential source of cross-infection. *J Hosp Infect.* 1995;29(4):315-316. [VC]

103. Williams D, Dingley J, Jones C, Berry N. Contamination of laryngoscope handles. *J Hosp Infect.* 2010;74(2):123-128. [IIIB]

104. Call TR, Auerbach FJ, Riddell SW, et al. Nosocomial contamination of laryngoscope handles: challenging current guidelines. *Anesth Analg.* 2009;109(2):479-483. [IIA]

105. Howell V, Thoppil A, Young H, Sharma S, Blunt M, Young P. Chlorhexidine to maintain cleanliness of laryngoscope handles: an audit and laboratory study. *Eur J Anaesthesiol.* 2013;30(5):216-221. [IIIB]

106. Rosing J. What's needed for reprocessing, storage of laryngoscope blades? *OR Manager.* 2011;27(12):15. [VC]

107. Standards FAQs details: laryngoscopes—blades and handles—how to clean, disinfect and store these devices. The Joint Commission. http://www.jointcommission.org/mobile/standards_information/jcfaqdetails.aspx?StandardsFAQId=508&StandardsFAQChapterId=69. Accessed September 23, 2014. [VB]

108. Association of Anaesthetists of Great Britain and Ireland. Infection control in anaesthesia. *Anaesthesia.* 2008;63(9):1027-1036. [IVA]

109. Thomas JG, Chenoweth CE, Sullivan SE. Iatrogenic Creutzfeldt-Jakob disease via surgical instruments. *J Clin Neurosci.* 2013;20(9):1207-1212. [VA]

110. McDonnell G. Prion disease transmission: can we apply standard precautions to prevent or reduce risks? *J Perioper Pract.* 2008;18(7):98-304. [VA]

111. McDonnell G, Dehen C, Perrin A, et al. Cleaning, disinfection and sterilization of surface prion contamination. *J Hosp Infect.* 2013;85(4):268-273. [IIA]

112. *WHO Infection Control Guidelines for Transmissible Spongiform Encephalopathies.* Report of a WHO consultation, Geneva, Switzerland, 23-26 March 1999. World Health Organization. http://www.who.int/csr/resources/publications/bse/WHO_CDS_CSR_APH_2000_3/en/. Accessed September 23, 2014. [IVB]

113. *WHO Tables on Tissue Infectivity Distribution in Transmissible Spongiform Encephalopathies.* Geneva, Switzerland: WHO Press; 2010. [IVA]

114. Barrenetxea G. Iatrogenic prion diseases in humans: an update. *Eur J Obstetr Gynecol Reproduct Biol.* 2012;165(2):165-169. [VB]

115. Henson M, Ireton M, Mortensen JE. Prions: a brief overview. *Amt Events.* 2013;30(2):72-84. [VA]

116. Blattler T. Implications of prion diseases for neurosurgery. *Neurosurg Rev.* 2002;25(4):195-203. [VA]

117. Dorsey K, Zou S, Schonberger LB, et al. Lack of evidence of transfusion transmission of Creutzfeldt-Jakob disease in a US surveillance study. *Transfusion.* 2009;49(5):977-984. [IIIA]

118. Puopolo M, Ladogana A, Vetrugno V, Pocchiari M. Transmission of sporadic Creutzfeldt-Jakob disease by blood transfusion: risk factor or possible biases. *Transfusion.* 2011;51(7):1556-1566. [IIIC]

119. Molesworth AM, Mackenzie J, Everington D, Knight RS, Will RG. Sporadic Creutzfeldt-Jakob disease and risk of blood transfusion in the United Kingdom. *Transfusion.* 2011;51(8):1872-1873. [IIIC]

120. McDonnell Gerald. Prion diseases and device reprocessing: a time gone or a time bomb? *Br J Neurosci Nurs.* 2013;9(5):229-233. [VA]

121. Alcalde-Cabero E, Almazan-Isla J, Brandel J-P, et al. Health professions and risk of sporadic Creutzfeldt-Jakob disease, 1965 to 2010. *Euro Surveill.* 2012;17(15):pii-20144. http://www.eurosurveillance.org/ViewArticle.aspx?ArticleId=20144. Accessed October 1, 2014. [VA]

122. Stitz L, Aguzzi A. Aerosols: an underestimated vehicle for transmission of prion diseases? *Prion.* 2011;5(3):138-141. [VA]

123. Haybaeck J, Heikenwalder M, Klevenz B, et al. Aerosols transmit prions to immunocompetent and immunodeficient mice. *PLoS Pathog.* 2011;7(1):e1001257. [IIB]

124. Fichet G, Antloga K, Comoy E, Deslys JP, McDonnell G. Prion inactivation using a new gaseous hydrogen peroxide sterilisation process. *J Hosp Infect.* 2007;67(3):278-286. [IIB]

125. Yan ZX, Stitz L, Heeg P, Pfaff E, Roth K. Infectivity of prion protein bound to stainless steel wires: a model for testing decontamination procedures for transmissible spongiform encephalopathies. *Infect Control Hosp Epidemiol.* 2004;25(4):280-283. [IIB]

126. Rogez-Kreuz C, Yousfi R, Soufflet C, et al. Inactivation of animal and human prions by hydrogen peroxide gas plasma sterilization. *Infect Control Hosp Epidemiol.* 2009;30(8):769-777. [IIB]

127. Hesp JR, Poolman TM, Budge C, et al. Thermostable adenylate kinase technology: a new process indicator and its use as a validation tool for the reprocessing of surgical instruments. *J Hosp Infect.* 2010;74(2):137-143. [IA]

128. Secker TJ, Hervé R, Keevil CW. Adsorption of prion and tissue proteins to surgical stainless steel surfaces and the efficacy of decontamination following dry and wet storage conditions. *J Hosp Infect.* 2011;78(4):251-255. [IIB]

129. Lipscomb IP, Pinchin H, Collin R, Keevil CW. Effect of drying time, ambient temperature and pre-soaks on prion-infected tissue contamination levels on surgical stainless steel: concerns over prolonged transportation of instruments from theatre to central sterile service departments. *J Hosp Infect.* 2007;65(1):72-77. [IA]

130. Fichet G, Comoy E, Duval C, et al. Novel methods for disinfection of prion-contaminated medical devices. *Lancet.* 2004;364(9433):521-526. [IIB]

131. Schmitt A, Westner IM, Reznicek L, Michels W, Mitteregger G, Kretzschmar HA. Automated decontamination of surface-adherent prions. *J Hosp Infect.* 2010;76(1):74-79. [IA]

132. Lehmann S, Pastore M, Rogez-Kreuz C, et al. New hospital disinfection processes for both conventional and prion infectious agents compatible with thermosensitive medical equipment. *J Hosp Infect.* 2009;72(4):342-350. [IA]

133. Belay ED, Blase JM, Sehulster LA, Maddox RB, Schonberger L. Management of neurosurgical instruments and patients exposed to Creutzfeldt-Jakob disease. *Infect Control Hosp Epidemiol.* 2013;34(12):1272-1280. [VA]

134. Bernoulli C, Siegfried J, Baumgartner G, et al. Danger of accidental person-to-person transmission of Creutzfeldt-Jakob disease by surgery. *Lancet.* 1977;209(8009):478-479. [VB]

135. *State Operations Manual Appendix A—Survey Protocol, Regulations and Interpretive Guidelines for Hospitals. Rev. 105; 3/21/14.* Washington, DC: Department of Health and Human Services, Centers for Medicare & Medicaid; 2014.

136. *State Operations Manual Appendix L: Guidance for Surveyors: Ambulatory Surgical Centers. Rev. 99; 1/31/14.* Washington, DC: Department of Health and Human Services, Centers for Medicare & Medicaid; 2014.

137. RC.01.01.01: The hospital maintains complete and accurate medical records for each individual patient. In: *Hospital Accreditation Standards 2014.* 2014 ed. Oakbrook Terrace, IL: Joint Commission Resources; 2014.

138. RC.01.01.01: The organization maintains complete and accurate clinical records. In: *Standards for Ambulatory Care 2014: Standards, Elements of Performance, Scoring, Accreditation Polices.* Oakbrook Terrace, IL: Joint Commission Resources; 2014.

139. MS.16: Medical record maintenance. In: *NIAHO Interpretive Guidelines and Surveyor Guidance. 10.1* ed. Milford, OH: DNV Healthcare Inc; 2012: 2029.

140. Clinical records and health information. In: *2014 Accreditation Handbook for Ambulatory Health Care.* Skokie, IL: Accreditation Association for Ambulatory Health Care; 2014:37-39.

141. Standards of perioperative nursing practice. In: *Perioperative Standards and Recommended Practices.* Denver, CO: AORN, Inc; 2014:3-42. [IVB]

142. HR.01.05.03: Staff participate in ongoing education and training. In: *Comprehensive Accreditation Manual: CAMH for Hospitals.* 2014 ed. Oakbrook Terrace, IL: Joint Commission Resources; 2014.

143. HR.01.05.03: Staff participate in ongoing education and training. In: *Comprehensive Accreditation Manual: CAMAC for Ambulatory Care.* 2014 ed. Oakbrook Terrace, IL: Joint Commission Resources; 2014.

144. MS.10: Continuing education. In: *NIAHO Interpretive Guidelines and Surveyor Guidance. 10.1 ed.* Milford, OH: DNV Healthcare Inc; 2012:24.

145. LD.04.01.07: The hospital has policies and procedures that guide and support patient care, treatment, and services. In: *Hospital Accreditation Standards 2014.* 2014 ed. Oakbrook Terrace, IL: Joint Commission Resources; 2014.

146. LD.04.01.07: The organization has policies and procedures that guide and support patient care, treatment, or services. In: *Standards for Ambulatory Care 2014: Standards, Elements of Performance, Scoring, Accreditation Polices.* Oakbrook Terrace, IL: Joint Commission Resources; 2014.

147. SS.1: Organization. In: *NIAHO Interpretive Guidelines and Surveyor Guidance. 10.1 ed.* Milford, OH: DNV Healthcare Inc; 2012:70-71.

148. Governance. In: *2014 Accreditation Handbook for Ambulatory Health Care.* Skokie, IL: Accreditation Association for Ambulatory Health Care; 2014:19-26.

149. PI.03.01.01: The hospital improves performance on an ongoing basis. In: *Hospital Accreditation Standards 2014.* 2014 ed. Oakbrook Terrace, IL: Joint Commission Resources; 2014.

150. PI.03.01.01: The organization improves performance. In: *Standards for Ambulatory Care 2014:*

Standards, Elements of Performance, Scoring, Accreditation Polices. Oakbrook Terrace, IL: Joint Commission Resources; 2014.

151. Quality management and improvement. In: *2014 Accreditation Handbook for Ambulatory Health Care.* Skokie, IL: Accreditation Association for Ambulatory Health Care; 2014:32-36.

152. Quality management system. In: *NIAHO Interpretive Guidelines and Surveyor Guidance. 10.1 ed.* Milford, OH: DNV Healthcare Inc; 2012:10-16.

153. Xia Y, Lu C, Zhao J, et al. A bronchofiberoscopy-associated outbreak of multidrug-resistant *Acinetobacter baumannii* in an intensive care unit in Beijing, China. *BMC Infect Dis.* 2012;Dec12:335. [VB]

154. Heathcote R, Stadelmann B. Measuring of ATP bioluminescence as a means of assessing washer disinfector performance and potentially as a means of validating the decontamination process. *Healthc Infect.* 2009;14(4):147-151. [IIIB]

155. Alfa MJ, Fatima I, Olson N. The adenosine triphosphate test is a rapid and reliable audit tool to assess manual cleaning adequacy of flexible endoscope channels. *Am J Infect Control.* 2013;41(3):249-253. [IIIA]

156. Shama G, Malik DJ. The uses and abuses of rapid bioluminescence-based ATP assays. *Int J Hyg Environ Health.* 2013;216(2):115-125. [VA]

157. Anderson RE, Young V, Stewart M, Robertson C, Dancer SJ. Cleanliness audit of clinical surfaces and equipment: who cleans what? *J Hosp Infect.* 2011;78(3):178-181. [IIIB]

158. Alfa MJ, Olson N, DeGagné P, Simner PJ. Development and validation of rapid use scope test strips to determine the efficacy of manual cleaning for flexible endoscope channels. *Am J Infect Control.* 2012;40(9):860-865. [IA]

159. Jagrosse D, Bommarito M, Stahl JB. Monitoring the cleaning of surgical instruments with an ATP detection system. *Am J Infect Control.* 2012;40(5):e90-e91. [IIIC]

Acknowledgements

LEAD AUTHOR
Cynthia Spry, MA, MS, RN, CNOR(E), CBSPDT
Independent Consultant
New York, New York

CONTRIBUTING AUTHOR
Ramona L. Conner, MSN, RN, CNOR
Manager, Standards and Guidelines
AORN Nursing Department
Denver, Colorado

The authors and AORN thank Michelle Alfa, PhD, FCCM, Winnipeg, MB, Canada; Jane Rothrock, PhD, RN, CNOR, FAAN, Professor and Director, Perioperative Programs, Delaware County Community College, Media, PA; Paula Berrett, BS, CRCST, Intermountain Healthcare Urban South Region CP Manager, Utah Valley Regional Medical Center, Provo, Utah; Antonia Hughes, MA, BSN, RN, CNOR, Perioperative Education Specialist, Baltimore Washington Medical Center, Glen Burnie, MD; George D. Allen, PhD, RN, CNOR, CIC, Director of Infection Control, Downstate Medical Center, Fresh Meadows, NY, for their assistance in developing this guideline.

PUBLICATION HISTORY
Originally published February 1988, *AORN Journal.* Revised March 1992.

Revised November 1996; published January 1997, *AORN Journal.*

Reformatted July 2000.

Revised November 2001; published March 2002, *AORN Journal.*

Revised 2007; published in *Perioperative Standards and Recommended Practices*, 2008 edition.

Minor editing revisions made to omit PNDS codes; reformatted September 2012 for publication in *Perioperative Standards and Recommended Practices*, 2013 edition.

Revised September 2014 for online publication in *Perioperative Standards and Recommended Practices.*

Minor editing revisions made in November 2014 for publication in *Guidelines for Perioperative Practice,* 2015 edition.

Evidence ratings revised in *Guidelines for Perioperative Practice,* 2018 edition, to conform to the current AORN Evidence Rating Model.

GUIDELINE FOR SELECTION AND USE OF PACKAGING SYSTEMS FOR STERILIZATION

The Guideline for Selection and Use of Packaging Systems for Sterilization has been approved by the AORN Recommended Practices Advisory Board. It was presented as proposed recommendations for comments by members and others. The guideline is effective November 15, 2013. The recommendations in the guideline are intended to be achievable and represent what is believed to be an optimal level of practice. Policies and procedures will reflect variations in practice settings and/or clinical situations that determine the degree to which the guideline can be implemented. AORN recognizes the many diverse settings in which perioperative nurses practice; therefore, this guideline is adaptable to all areas where operative and other invasive procedures may be performed.

Purpose

This document provides guidance to perioperative personnel for evaluating, selecting, and using packaging systems and for packaging the items to be sterilized and subsequently used in the perioperative setting. Packaging systems should permit sterilization of the contents within the package, protect the integrity of the sterilized contents, prevent contamination of the contents until the package is opened for use, and permit the aseptic delivery of the contents to the sterile field. Packaging systems include woven fabrics, nonwoven materials, paper-plastic pouches, Tyvek®-plastic pouches, plastic-plastic pouches, and containment devices (eg, sterilization containers, instrument cases, cassettes, organizing trays) composed of a variety of materials. This guideline does not include recommendations for cleaning contaminated instruments, loading a sterilizer, or sterilization. The reader should refer to the AORN Guideline for Cleaning and Care of Surgical Instruments[1] and Guideline for Sterilization.[2]

Evidence Review

A medical librarian conducted a systematic literature search of the databases MEDLINE®, CINAHL®, Scopus®, and Cochrane Database of Systematic Reviews for meta-analyses, randomized and nonrandomized trials and studies, systematic and nonsystematic reviews, and opinion documents and letters. Search terms included *surgical equipment, surgical instruments, dental instruments, organizing tray, instrument set, loaner instrument, medical packaging, product packaging, device packaging, product labeling, packaging material, sterilization container, rigid container, instrument case, instrument cassette, packaging system, reusable pack, pouch, heat sealer, sequential wrapping, plastics, textiles, fabrics, Mylar, Tyvek, Kraft, olefin, paper, polypropylene, polypropene, barrier integrity, barrier system, barrier properties, sterility maintenance cover, sterilization, flash sterilization, immediate use sterilization, infection control, microbial colony count, cross infection, equipment contamination, humidity, steam, condensation, equipment reuse, single-use, event-related, time related, time-dependent, event-dependent, outdating, monitoring, quality control, materials testing, indicators and reagents, package integrity, equipment failure, safety management, hospital central supply, sterile processing,* and *hospital purchasing.*

The lead author and the medical librarian identified and obtained relevant guidelines from government agencies, other professional organizations, and standards-setting bodies. The lead author assessed additional professional literature, including some that was cited in other articles provided to the author. The initial search was confined to the years 2005 to 2012 and limited to English-language articles. The time restriction was not applied in subsequent searches. The librarian also established continuing alerts on the topics included in this guideline and provided relevant results to the lead author. The majority of research regarding packaging was related to shelf life and was conducted more than 10 years ago when facilities were transitioning from time-related shelf life to event-related shelf life. Articles addressing other aspects of packaging were quite limited. It is evident from the literature search that there is a need for additional research on all aspects of packaging for sterilization.

Articles identified by the search were provided to a doctorally prepared evidence appraiser and to the lead author for evaluation. Articles were critically appraised using the Johns Hopkins Evidence-Based Practice Model and the Research or Non-Research Evidence-Appraisal Tools as appropriate. The articles were independently evaluated and appraised according to the strength and quality of the evidence. Each article was then assigned an appraisal score as agreed upon by the researcher and the lead author. The appraisal score is noted in brackets after each reference citation, as applicable.

The collective evidence supporting each intervention within a specific recommendation was summarized and used to rate the strength of the evidence using the AORN Evidence Rating Model. Factors considered in review of the collective evidence were the quality of the research, quantity of similar studies on a given topic, and consistency of results supporting a recommendation. The evidence rating is noted in brackets after each intervention.

Editor's note: *MEDLINE is a registered trademark of the US National Library of Medicine's Medical*

Literature Analysis and Retrieval System, Bethesda, MD. CINAHL, Cumulative Index to Nursing and Allied Health Literature, is a registered trademark of EBSCO Industries, Birmingham, AL. Scopus is a registered trademark of Elsevier B.V., Amsterdam, Netherlands. Tyvek is a registered trademark of DuPont, Wilmington, DE. Mylar is a registered trademark of DuPont Tejin Films, Chester, VA.

Recommendation I

Packaging systems and packaging materials should be evaluated before purchase and use.[3]

When packaging systems are compatible with the sterilization method and equipment, the probability is increased that sterility can be achieved and maintained until use of the packaged items.[4-6]

I.a.   Packaging systems should
   ○ have US Food and Drug Administration (FDA) clearance for performance claims for intended use;
   ○ be suitable for the items being sterilized;
   ○ include a manufacturer's instructions for use (IFU);
   ○ be free of toxic ingredients;
   ○ be odor free;
   ○ be low linting;
   ○ be large enough to permit equal distribution of the contents;
   ○ be easy to use for personnel who prepare, transport, and/or open the package;
   ○ permit secure and complete closure of items;
   ○ permit sealing that is tamper-evident;
   ○ permit identification of the contents before opening;
   ○ allow adequate air removal;
   ○ allow sterilant penetration and direct contact with the item(s) and surfaces;
   ○ allow removal of the sterilant;
   ○ be resistant to tears and punctures;
   ○ protect contents from physical damage;
   ○ maintain sterility of the contents until opened;
   ○ permit aseptic delivery of the contents to the sterile field (eg, minimal wrap memory, easy removal of lids from rigid sterilization containers);
   ○ have a favorable cost-benefit ratio; and
   ○ be free of restrictive waste-disposal regulatory requirements.[3,7,8]
   [4: Limited Evidence]

I.a.1.   Prepurchase evaluation of packaging systems should include consideration of the environmental impact of the product throughout its life cycle.[5,9-12]

   Estimates of the amount of waste generated by health care facilities vary, with some estimates as high as 4 billion pounds annually. Much of that waste is generated in the operating room and consists of packaging and disposable supplies.[13,14] Some experts suggest that use of environmentally responsible packaging results in cost savings.[13,15]

I.b.   Before selecting a packaging system, purchasers should evaluate and verify the performance of the packaging system and materials in the environment in which they will be used to determine whether conditions for sterilization, shelf life, transport, storage, and handling can be met.[3] *[4: Limited Evidence]*

I.b.1.   Prepurchase evaluation of packaging materials should determine
   • FDA clearance for performance claims for intended use;
   • ability to verify the manufacturer's IFU through facility product testing;
   • barrier effectiveness;
   • compatibility with the intended sterilization method(s) and cycles used within the facility;
   • biocompatibility;
   • availability of an external chemical indicator (CI);
   • durability;
   • useful product life (including all components);
   • requirements for tracking use;
   • method for tracking use;
   • method for labeling;
   • ability of the seal to maintain package integrity;
   • requirements for disassembly, laundering, or cleaning requirements;
   • maintenance requirements;
   • storage requirements;
   • ease of use;
   • weight;
   • available sizes;
   • ease of transport;
   • ease of aseptic presentation;
   • environmental impact; and
   • cost-effectiveness.

I.c.   Manufacturers' IFU should be evaluated to verify that the packaging system and packaging material are intended for use with both the method(s) of sterilization and the specific equipment to be used.[3] *[4: Limited Evidence]*

   Packaging manufacturers' IFU provide information that identifies correct use with the intended sterilization method(s) and equipment.

I.c.1.   The manufacturer's validation information should be reviewed and evaluated before purchase.

   Validation information may include items such as sterilant penetration, resistance to tears and punctures, barrier performance, use with extended steam sterilization cycles, sterility maintenance, and shelf life.[3,7,16,17]

I.d.   Prepurchase product testing should be performed if the packaging represents a major change in packaging type (eg, a change from using woven to using nonwoven materials, a change from using nonwoven materials to using rigid sterilization containers).[3] *[4: Limited Evidence]*

Product testing is used to verify that adherence to the device manufacturer's instructions for sterilization is achievable in the health care setting.

I.d.1.   Product testing should include
- evaluation of sterilization efficacy by placing biological indicators (BIs) and CIs inside a variety of sets and packages to be processed (eg, basin sets, instrument sets);
- placement of BIs and CIs within the package in the areas that present the greatest challenge to sterilant contact (medical device and packaging manufacturers may be able to assist in identifying challenging areas);
- moisture assessment;
- documentation of product testing activities to include the date of the test, a description of the package and contents, the location of BIs and CIs within the test package, and test results; and
- reprocessing of the product before use.[3]

Recommendation II

Packaging systems should be compatible with the specific sterilization method for which they will be used.

The interaction among packaging systems, medical devices, and sterilizer technologies is complex. Not all packaging systems are suitable for all methods of sterilization.

II.a.   Packaging systems for steam sterilization should permit steam penetration and adequate drying.[3] *[4: Limited Evidence]*

Attention to steam penetration and drying decreases the possibility that steam sterilization efficacy will be adversely affected by humidity; elevation; packaging material; package contents; load; position of items within the sterilizer; size, weight, and density of the pack or rigid sterilization container; and other parameters of the sterilization cycle.[3]

II.b.   Packaging systems for ethylene oxide (EO) should
- be permeable to EO and moisture;
- permit aeration;
- include recommendations for aeration time and parameters; and
- be specified by the packaging manufacturer as for use in EO sterilization.[18]

[4: Limited Evidence]

Woven, nonwoven, and peel-pouch packages and some rigid sterilization container systems can be permeated by EO and do not impede rapid aeration of the contents. However, some packaging materials can retain EO residuals, making them difficult to aerate. Woven materials may absorb a large amount of relative humidity that is needed for EO sterilization.[18]

Sufficient humidity helps maintain adequate hydration of microorganisms, thereby increasing their susceptibility to destruction by EO.[18]

II.c.   Packaging systems used for low-temperature hydrogen peroxide gas plasma sterilization and low-temperature hydrogen peroxide vapor sterilization systems should
- allow hydrogen peroxide sterilants to penetrate packaging materials,
- be compatible (ie, nondegradable, nonabsorbable) with the designated sterilization process, and
- be constructed of a material recommended by the sterilizer manufacturer.

[4: Limited Evidence]

Sterilization methods that use low-temperature hydrogen peroxide gas plasma or low-temperature hydrogen peroxide vapor are affected by absorbable packaging materials (eg, cellulose-based packaging material, textile wrappers, paper-plastic pouches, porous wrap). Absorption of the sterilant (ie, hydrogen peroxide) by paper-plastic pouches or porous wrap has been shown to adversely affect the sterilization process.[19]

II.c.1.   Written documentation of the acceptability of use of low-temperature hydrogen peroxide gas plasma sterilization or low-temperature hydrogen peroxide vapor sterilization systems with specific containment devices should be obtained from the device and sterilizer manufacturers. Only containment devices validated for use in hydrogen peroxide gas plasma or hydrogen peroxide vapor should be used.

II.c.2.   If a rigid sterilization container that requires a filter is used, the filter should be made of noncellulose material.

Not all rigid sterilization containers and their accessories are compatible with low-temperature hydrogen peroxide gas plasma or low-temperature hydrogen peroxide vapor.

II.d.   Packaging systems for ozone sterilization should
- allow ozone to penetrate packaging materials,
- be compatible (ie, nondegradable, nonabsorbable) with the designated sterilization process, and
- be constructed of a material recommended by the sterilizer manufacturer.[19]

[4: Limited Evidence]

Use of packaging systems that are intended for use in ozone sterilizers facilitates compatibility with the ozone sterilization process.[19]

STERILIZATION AND DISINFECTION

Recommendation III

Packaging materials should be processed and stored in a way that maintains the qualities required for sterilization.

Some manufacturers of packaging materials may specify environmental storage condition requirements for their product. Temperature and humidity equilibrium may be necessary to permit adequate sterilant penetration and to avoid superheating. Wrap material that is too dry and stored in areas of low humidity may lead to superheating and sterilization failure.[3,20]

III.a. Reusable woven textiles should be laundered after every use to maintain hydration. *[4: Limited Evidence]*

Resterilization without relaundering may lead to superheating and could create a deterrent to sterilization. Overdrying, heat pressing (eg, ironing), and storage in areas of low humidity may lead to superheating and sterilization failure. In addition, when woven textiles are not rehydrated after sterilization and/or if repeated sterilization is attempted, the textiles may absorb the available moisture present in the steam, thereby possibly creating a dry or superheated steam effect.[3]

III.b. Packaging materials should be stored at room temperature and at a relative humidity that is in accordance with the packaging manufacturer's IFU.[3] *[4: Limited Evidence]*

III.c. Wrapping materials labeled for single-use should be discarded after one sterilization cycle.[21] *[1: Strong Evidence]*

Products labeled as single-use or disposable are intended for one use and are not intended to be reprocessed.[22]

III.c.1. Single-use packaging materials can be recycled if the product is suitable for recycling.[10-14]

III.d. The shelf life of a packaged sterile item should be considered event-related.[2,3] *[1: Strong Evidence]*

The sterility of an item does not change with the passage of time, but may be affected by particular events (eg, amount of handling) or environmental conditions (eg, humidity).[2,3,21]

In a randomized controlled trial, researchers assessed the sterility of 700 porcelain cylinders sterilized in four different packaging materials (125 each of cotton serge fabric, crepe paper, nonwoven wrap, and peel pouches) and then stored for up to six months. The external package was deliberately contaminated with *Serratia marcescens*. No growth of the test microorganisms was identified inside the packages in any of the storage intervals (ie, seven, 14, 28, 90, and 180 days).[23]

In another randomized controlled trial that examined the effect of time on the sterile integrity of single-sealed peel pouches, double-sealed pouches, linen-wrapped devices, and double-linen wrapped trays, a total of 600 sterile packages were studied. A control group of 60 packages was sent for analysis of microbial contamination immediately after sterilization. The remaining 540 sterilized packages were stored at randomly selected storage sites. Samples were tested for microbial contamination at one, three, six, and 12 months. Results showed a nonstatistically significant effect of time on the odds of a nonsterility event.[24]

Recommendation IV

Items to be sterilized should be packaged in a manner that facilitates sterilization and provides for an aseptic presentation of the package contents. Packaging should be used according to the packaging manufacturer's and sterilizer manufacturer's written IFU.

Incorrect packaging may prevent sterilization from occurring. Inappropriate handling can lead to loss of package integrity. Incorrect packaging can make aseptic delivery of the contents to the sterile field difficult or impossible.

IV.a. Packaging materials, including filters for rigid sterilization container systems, should be inspected for defects and extraneous matter before use.[3] Packaging materials with defects should not be used.[4] *[1: Strong Evidence]*

Defective packaging materials can permit migration of pathogens into the package. In an observational study to determine susceptibility of packaging materials to bacterial transmission, nails ranging in size from 1.1 mm to 10.0 mm that were contaminated with three colonies of skin flora were used to make holes in 90 samples of a polypropylene wrap. Results showed bacterial transmission occurred through the entire range of holes.[25]

IV.b. The size of the wrapping material should be selected to achieve adequate coverage of the item(s) being packaged. The item(s) should be wrapped securely to prevent gapping, billowing, or formation of air pockets.[3] *[4: Limited Evidence]*

Gapping, billowing, or air pockets may prevent sterilant contact with the surface of the device or allow penetration of contaminants into the package.[3]

IV.c. Items to be sterilized should be positioned within packages to allow sterilant contact with all surfaces.[3] *[4: Limited Evidence]*

Sterilant contact is necessary for sterilization to be achieved.

IV.d. The total weight of instrument containment devices, including the contents, should not exceed 25 lb.[3,26,27] *[3: Moderate Evidence]*

Instrument sets weighing more than 25 lb are known to be difficult to dry without lengthy drying times and present an increased risk of ergonomic injury to health care personnel.[3,27]

IV.e. Instruments composed of more than one part that can be disassembled should be disassembled unless the manufacturer's written and validated IFU specifies that disassembly is not required.[3] *[4: Limited Evidence]*

Sterilization of assembled instruments can prevent exposure of some areas of the device to the sterilant.[3]

IV.f. Items to be sterilized that have concave or convex surfaces that create potential for water retention should be positioned within packages in a manner that prevents those surfaces from retaining water.[3,4] *[1: Strong Evidence]*

Preventing water retention can help avoid the occurrence of wet packs and sterilization failure.

IV.g. Towels placed within instrument sets should be lint-free, freshly laundered, and thoroughly rinsed by a health care-accredited laundry facility. *[4: Limited Evidence]*

Adequate rinsing reduces the risk of leaving chemical residues that could be transferred from the towels to instruments.[28] Lint left on sterile instruments may be transferred to the surgical wound and may cause a foreign-body reaction.

IV.h. Items to be sterilized should be placed in the package or tray in an open or unlocked position. *[4: Limited Evidence]*

The open or unlocked position facilitates sterilant contact of all surfaces of the item.[3]

IV.h.1. Racks or stringers designed and intended for sterilization can be used to maintain instruments in their open position.[3]

IV.i. Packaging should be performed in a manner that facilitates maintenance of sterility and aseptic presentation of the contents. Sequential wrapping with two single wraps or single wrapping with a doubled-bonded wrap may be used. *[3: Moderate Evidence]*

Sequential wrapping using two nonwoven, disposable, barrier-type wrappers provides a tortuous pathway to impede microbial migration and permits ease of presentation to the sterile field without compromising sterility.

A fused or double-bonded, disposable, nonwoven single wrapper used according to the manufacturer's IFU provides a bacterial barrier comparable to the sequential double wrap.[7] In one study conducted during a five-month period, 200 packs wrapped in two FDA-cleared and manufacturer-validated barrier-type wrappers were compared with 200 packs wrapped in a single FDA-cleared and manufacturer-validated double-bonded, nonwoven wrapper to determine whether the risk of contamination was greater with either method. Results indi-

cated that use of a single double-bonded wrapper was not associated with a greater risk of contamination. A statistically significant reduction in time required to wrap was identified with use of the single double-bonded, disposable, nonwoven wrapper.[12]

IV.j. The health care organization should weigh the risks and benefits of placing a nonvalidated product (ie, count sheet) in instrument trays against the need for inventory control and instrument count procedures. *[5: Benefits Balanced with Harms]*

Although there are no known reports of adverse events related to sterilized count sheets, there is limited research regarding the safety of toners or various papers subjected to any sterilization method. Chemicals used in the manufacturing of paper and toner inks pose a theoretical risk of reaction in some sensitized individuals.

A literature search related to cytotoxicity of count sheets yielded only one study. This limited controlled study, employing commonly used inks and paper under extremely exaggerated conditions, found that label and toner inks transferred to instruments during sterilization were not cytotoxic.[29] Results from this study are not generalizable and definitive conclusions regarding the safety of all count papers and all inks used in count sheets placed within sterilized instrument sets is not possible.

Recommendation V

Chemical indicators specific to the sterilization method selected should be used with each package.[2]

Chemical indicators are used to verify that one or more of the conditions necessary for sterilization have been achieved within each package. External and internal CIs do not verify sterility of the contents.[3,4]

V.a. A CI should be placed on the outside and inside of every package to be processed unless the internal indicator is readable through the package material.[3,4] *[1: Strong Evidence]*

External CIs are used to verify that the package has been exposed to the sterilization process. External indicators are intended to differentiate processed packages from unprocessed packages.

Internal CIs are used to verify that the sterilant has reached the contents of the package and that critical variables of the sterilization process have been met. The number of critical process variables that are monitored with an internal indicator is dependent on the specific type of internal indicator that is used.

V.a.1. A class I CI (ie, process indicator) should be placed externally. Examples of process indicators are indicator tape and indicator labels.

V.a.2. A class III CI (ie, single-parameter indicator), class IV CI (ie, multiparameter indicator), class V CI (ie, integrating indicator), or class VI CI (ie, emulating indicator) should be placed internally.

V.a.3. More than one CI may be required for multi-layered trays and should be placed according to the tray manufacturer's IFU.

V.a.4. The CI manufacturer's written instructions for storage, use, and expiration date should be followed.[3]

V.b. Chemical indicators should be placed in an area within the package that presents a challenge for air removal and sterilant contact. When there is a question concerning the appropriate number and placement of internal CIs, the CI manufacturer, the device manufacturer, and the containment device manufacturer should be consulted for additional information.[2,3] *[4: Limited Evidence]*

The number and placement of internal CIs may be affected by the contents of the package, the configuration of the items within the set, and the packaging or containment device.

Recommendation VI

Reusable woven packaging materials should be inspected and monitored throughout the life of the product.

Multiple launderings and processings will eventually diminish the protective barrier of the material.

VI.a. Textiles should be inspected on a light table for defects (eg, holes, tears, worn spots). Small defects can be repaired using a vulcanized patch; the number of repairs should be kept to a minimum.[3] *[4: Limited Evidence]*

Vulcanized patches do not permit penetration of most sterilants. Keeping the quantity and concentration of patches to a minimum may decrease the risk of compromised penetration of the sterilant.

A search for published literature on the patching of textiles intended for use as a sterilization wrap did not result in any articles that identified the number or placement of patches that could prevent or compromise sterilization of the package contents.

VI.a.1. All woven reusable textiles should be de-linted after washing and before packaging.

VI.a.2. When there is a question about the suitability of a woven wrap, it should be discarded. Defects should not be sewn.

Sewing increases the number of holes in the textile into which microbes can enter.

VI.b. A method should be established to monitor, control, and determine the useful life of reprocessed woven materials. This should include the number of sterilization processes and washing cycles that may occur while maintaining the acceptable barrier quality of the material.[30] *[4: Limited Evidence]*

The barrier qualities of woven materials are diminished by repeated laundering and sterilization cycles. Processes to evaluate material quality after each use are needed to determine suitability for continued use.

VI.b.1. If a printed area (eg, grid system) for marking the number of uses is available on the woven textile, the printed area should be marked each time the item is used. When the grid is full, the item should be removed from service.[30]

VI.b.2. The manufacturer's IFU should be followed for the suggested number of reprocessings.[30]

Recommendation VII

Peel pouches (ie, paper-plastic, Tyvek, Mylar) should be used according to manufacturers' written IFU.[3]

Manufacturers' IFU provide steps that the manufacturers have determined should be followed to achieve and maintain sterility of the package contents.

VII.a. Peel pouches should be used only for small, lightweight, low-profile items (eg, one or two clamps, scissors). Heavy devices, such as drills and weighted vaginal speculums, should not be packaged in peel pouches.[3] *[4: Limited Evidence]*

Heavy or sharp items may compromise the package seal.

VII.b. Peel pouches should not be used within wrapped sets or containment devices unless the pouch manufacturer can supply documented validation for this practice.[3] *[4: Limited Evidence]*

The impervious plastic side of a peel pouch in contact with devices within sets may prevent sterilant from contacting the devices.[3]

VII.c. Double pouching (ie, placing the item within one pouch and then placing this pouch inside another) should not be performed without written instructions from the pouch manufacturer indicating that this practice has been validated and the pouch in question has been cleared by the FDA for this purpose.[3] *[4: Limited Evidence]*

Sterilization validation studies performed by the manufacturer provide confirmation that the pouch will perform as intended when two pouches are used in a single package.

VII.d. Unless otherwise specified in the manufacturer's IFU, when double pouching is used,
- the inner pouch should fit within the outer pouch without folding,[3] and
- the inner pouch should face in the same direction as the outer pouch (ie, plastic or Mylar faces plastic or Mylar, and paper or Tyvek faces paper or Tyvek).[3]

[4: Limited Evidence]

Folding the inner pouch may entrap air and inhibit sterilant contact.[18]

The plastic side of the pouch is impervious to sterilant penetration. The paper side of the pouch permits sterilant penetration. Facing the inner pouch in the same direction as the outer pouch results in paper-to-paper contact through which the sterilant can penetrate. If the paper side of the inner pouch is in contact with the plastic side of the outer pouch, penetration of the sterilant through the paper side of the inner pouch is prevented.[3]

VII.e. When loading the sterilizer, peel pouches should be placed on edge and spaced to permit sterilant contact and drying.[3] *[4: Limited Evidence]*

Separation of pouch packages facilitates sterilant contact with all surfaces of each package.

VII.e.1. Racks designed and intended for sterilization that separate and hold all the pouches in a vertical position can be used to position peel pouches.

VII.f. Peel pouches should be labeled according to the pouch manufacturer's IFU. Labels should be placed on the plastic side of the pouch.[3] *[4: Limited Evidence]*

Writing or placing a label on the paper side of the pouch may compromise the barrier properties by causing damage to the package.[3]

VII.f.1. A marker with nontoxic ink may be used for writing on the plastic side of the pouch.

Use of a nontoxic ink will prevent toxins from being deposited on the package contents. The force of writing with a ballpoint pen or a pencil may cause perforation of the pouch.[3]

Recommendation VIII

A rigid sterilization container should be used, cleaned, inspected, repaired, and maintained according to the manufacturer's written IFU.

Rigid sterilization container design and materials may affect compatibility with the sterilization process (eg, penetration of the sterilant, release of the sterilant and moisture). Directions related to the method of sterilization may vary by manufacturer.

VIII.a. The recommended sterilization method and cycle exposure times for each rigid sterilization container system should be provided by and obtained from the manufacturer.[3] *[4: Limited Evidence]*

Manufacturers of rigid sterilization containers with FDA clearance have validated that their containers will permit sterilization using specific sterilization methods and cycle exposure times.

VIII.a.1. Sterilization efficacy and drying effectiveness of rigid sterilization containers should be evaluated before initial use as well as periodically, according to the manufacturer's written IFU.[3]

Rigid sterilization container systems vary widely in design, mechanics, and construction. Such variables affect the performance of the containers and their compatibility with sterilization methods.

Health care personnel are responsible for ensuring that rigid sterilization container systems are suitable for proposed sterilization uses and are compatible with existing sterilizers.

VIII.b. Before placing cassettes or organizing trays within rigid sterilization containers, users should refer to the containment device or organizing tray manufacturer's IFU to determine whether this practice is acceptable and/or consult with the rigid sterilization container manufacturer and the device manufacturer to determine whether this practice is acceptable.[3] *[4: Limited Evidence]*

Some device manufacturers provide specifications that should be met to ensure sterilization efficacy when cassettes or organizing trays are used within rigid sterilization containers.

VIII.c. The integrity of the rigid container should be inspected after each use. Inspections should include that
- the mating surfaces and edges of the container and lid are free of dents and chips;
- the lid and container fit together properly and securely;
- the filter retention mechanisms and fasteners are secure and not distorted or burred;
- the latching mechanisms are functioning as they should;
- the handles are in working order;
- the integrity of the filter media is not compromised;
- the gaskets are pliable, securely fastened, and without breaks or cuts; and
- the valves are in working order.

[4: Limited Evidence]

Improperly maintained valves, worn gaskets, dents, or other damage may compromise both the integrity of the container and the ability of the container to maintain sterility.[3]

VIII.c.1. Single-use or reusable filters and valve systems should be secured and in proper working order before sterilization. Filter plates should be examined for integrity before and after the sterilization process. Only intact filters should be used. If the filter is damp, dislodged, or has holes, tears, or punctures, the contents should be considered unsterile.

VIII.c.2. Damaged items should be removed from service and repaired or replaced.

949

VIII.d. Rigid sterilization containers should be cleaned after each use.[3] For proper cleaning, all components (eg, filter retention plates) should be disassembled unless otherwise specified in the manufacturer's IFU. *[4: Limited Evidence]*

Retained debris on container surfaces and components can inhibit sterilant contact.

VIII.e. Additional materials (eg, silicone mats, towels) should not be placed within rigid sterilization containers unless the container manufacturer has provided directions for their use.[3] *[4: Limited Evidence]*

Adding materials to the container in a manner that is not in accordance with the manufacturer's IFU may inhibit sterilization and the performance of the container.

VIII.f. Before devices are placed within rigid sterilization containers, the manufacturer's IFU should be consulted to determine limitations related to density of materials, weight, and distribution of contents.[3] *[4: Limited Evidence]*

Following the manufacturer's requirements for density of materials and weight and distribution of contents will facilitate sterilization and optimize the performance of the container.

Recommendation IX

Packages to be sterilized should be labeled.

Accurate labeling provides identification of the package contents as well as information that enables tracking of the sterilizer, sterilization cycle, personnel involved in the sterilization process, and the patient for whom the items were used.[2]

IX.a. Packages should be labeled before sterilization. Package labels should include
- the sterilizer number or unique identifier if more than one sterilizer is in use;
- the cycle or load number[2,3];
- the date of sterilization[2];
- a description of the package contents (eg, major abdominal set, Kerrison rongeur, Kleppinger bipolar forceps); and
- identification of the assembler.

[3: Moderate Evidence]

Package label information allows items to be identified or retrieved in the event of a sterilization processing error or equipment malfunction.[3]

IX.b. Package labels should be visible and remain securely fixed to the package throughout processing, storage, and distribution to the point of use.[3] *[4: Limited Evidence]*

Visible and secure packaging labels are necessary for verification of package contents and tracking of sterilization cycles and personnel involved in the sterilization process.

IX.c. When a marker is used to enter label information, the ink should be nontoxic, nonbleeding, and indelible.[3] *[4: Limited Evidence]*

Using nontoxic, nonbleeding ink may help to prevent toxic deposits on or in sterile packages. Using indelible ink may help to prevent loss of labeling information.[3]

IX.c.1. Writing should be entered on the indicator tape or affixed label of wrapped packages or on the plastic side of peel pouches, and not on the packaging material.[3]

Writing on the wrapper or on the paper side of peel pouches may damage the package and compromise its barrier function.[3]

Recommendation X

Perioperative team members with responsibilities for selection and/or use of packaging systems should receive initial and ongoing education and competency verification on their understanding of selection and use of packaging systems.

It is the responsibility of the health care organization to provide initial and ongoing education and to verify the competency of perioperative team members.[5]

Initial and ongoing education of perioperative personnel about selection and use of packaging systems facilitates the development of knowledge, skills, and attitudes that affect safe patient care.

Periodic education programs provide the opportunity to reinforce principles of packaging and packaging systems evaluation and may be used to introduce relevant new equipment and practices.

Competency verification measures individual performance, provides a mechanism for documentation, and may verify that perioperative personnel have an understanding of the principles and processes related to selection and use of packaging systems.[31-35]

X.a. Perioperative team members should receive education and complete competency verification activities that address specific knowledge and skills related to selection and use of packaging systems. *[1: Regulatory Requirement]*

Ongoing development of knowledge and skills and documentation of personnel participation are regulatory and accreditation requirements for both hospital and ambulatory settings.[36-46]

X.a.1. Education regarding selection and use of packaging systems should include
- adhering to manufacturers' IFU,
- safe use of packaging systems,
- risks and potential hazards associated with packaging,
- measures to minimize risk,
- product testing,
- corrective actions to employ in the event of a failure of the packaging system, and
- new information about changes in packaging technology and its compatibility

with sterilization equipment and processes.

X.b. Relative to the selection and use of packaging systems, the perioperative registered nurse (RN) should

○ participate in ongoing educational activities[5];

○ identify personal learning needs[5];

○ seek experiences to acquire, maintain, and augment personal knowledge and skills proficiency[5];

○ share knowledge and skills[5];

○ communicate pertinent information to perioperative team members[5];

○ contribute to a healthy work environment by using appropriate and courteous verbal and nonverbal communication techniques[5]; and

○ develop and implement conflict resolution skills to manage difficult behavior, promote positive working relationships, and advocate for patient safety.[5]

[3: Moderate Evidence]

Education, collegiality, and collaboration are standards of perioperative nursing and a primary responsibility of the RN who practices in the perioperative setting.[5,47]

Recommendation XI

Policies and procedures for selection and use of packaging systems should be developed, reviewed periodically, revised as necessary, and readily available in the practice setting in which they are used.

Policies and procedures assist in the development of patient safety, quality assessment, and performance activities. Policies and procedures also serve as operational guidelines used to minimize patient risk of injury or complications, standardize practice, direct perioperative personnel, and establish continuous performance improvement programs. Policies and procedures establish authority, responsibility, and accountability within the practice setting.

XI.a. Policies and procedures regarding the selection and use of packaging systems should be developed. *[1: Regulatory Requirement]*

Having policies and procedures that guide and support patient care, treatment, and services is a regulatory and accrediting agency requirement for both hospital and ambulatory settings.[36,37,41,42,48-50]

XI.a.1. Policies and procedures regarding selection and use of packaging systems should include

• prepurchase evaluation;

• assembly of devices within packaging systems;

• weight limitations;

• product testing;

• labeling;

• placement and positioning of packages within the sterilizer;

• storage requirements pre- and post-sterilization;

• shelf life;

• use of internal and external sterilization monitors;

• wrapping requirements and technique;

• use of peel pouches; and

• maintenance of packaging materials, peel pouches, rigid container systems, and heat sealers.

Recommendation XII

Perioperative personnel should participate in a variety of quality assurance and performance improvement activities that are consistent with the health care organization's plan to improve understanding of and compliance with the principles and processes of selection and use of packaging systems.

Quality assurance and performance improvement programs assist in evaluating and improving the quality of packaging items to be sterilized for operative and other invasive procedures. Quality assurance programs provide information used to determine whether packaging practices are in compliance with recognized standards and to identify areas that may require corrective action.

XII.a. The health care organization should establish quality assurance and performance improvement programs to monitor the workplace environment and practices associated with selection and use of packaging systems.[2,3] *[4: Limited Evidence]*

Monitoring the packaging processes allows results to be compared against a predetermined level of quality. Reviewing the findings provides information for identifying problems and trends that can be used to improve practice.[2]

XII.b. Performance improvement activities for selection and use of packaging systems should include monitoring personnel for understanding of the principles and processes of selection and use of packaging systems. *[1: Regulatory Requirement]*

Collecting data to monitor and improve patient care, treatment, and services is a regulatory and accrediting agency requirement for both hospital and ambulatory settings.[36,37,40,51-55]

XII.b.1. Process monitoring for activities related to selection and use of packaging systems should include monitoring compliance with policies and procedures for the following:

• using packaging systems and their IFU;

• verifying the compatibility of packaging systems with sterilization processes;

• storing packaging materials;

• assembling, handling, and packaging wrapped, pouched, and containerized items;

• labeling packages for sterilization;

• determining event-related sterility;

• product testing; and

• investigating wet packs.

STERILIZATION AND DISINFECTION

XII.b.2. The quality assurance and performance improvement program for selection and use of packaging systems should include
- periodically reviewing and evaluating activities to verify compliance or to identify the need for improvement,
- identifying corrective actions directed toward improvement priorities, and
- taking additional actions when improvement is not achieved or sustained.

Reviewing and evaluating quality assurance and performance improvement activities helps to identify failure points that contribute to errors in the use of packaging systems and helps define actions for improvement and increased competency.

Taking corrective actions may improve patient safety by enhancing understanding of the principles of and compliance with the processes for selection and use of packaging systems.

XII.c. Quality assurance testing of packaging systems and related equipment (eg, heat sealers) should be performed before initial use as well as periodically, according to the manufacturers' written IFU.[3] [4: Limited Evidence]

Packaging systems and related equipment vary in design, mechanics, and construction. These variables affect the performance and compatibility of packaging systems with sterilization methods.[2,3]

XII.c.1. The packaging system manufacturer should be consulted to determine the areas within the package that present the greatest challenge.[2]

XII.c.2. Testing and monitoring of heat seal equipment should be performed in accordance with the manufacturer's IFU.

XII.c.3. During periodic product quality assurance testing of packaging systems, sterilization efficacy and drying effectiveness should be evaluated for each sterilizer and cycle used.[2]

Health care organizations are responsible for obtaining and maintaining manufacturers' documentation of methodology and performance testing for packaging systems.[2]

Health care personnel are responsible for ensuring that packaging systems are suitable for proposed sterilization uses and compatible with existing sterilizers.[2]

XII.d. Product testing should be performed whenever there is a major change in packaging systems, such as a change from using wrapping materials to using rigid sterilization containers, or when there are changes to materials, tray configuration, or content density.[2,3]

Two types of tests should be performed:
○ Biological indicators and CIs/integrators/emulating indicators should be placed inside

a set, tray, or pack being tested. The set should be run in a full load and the indicators evaluated for pass or fail results.[3]
○ After steam sterilization, the package should be inspected for any moisture on the outside and/or on its contents (ie, a wet pack).[3]
[4: Limited Evidence]

Product testing verifies the ability to achieve a sterile, dry package and contents in the health care facility.[3]

XII.e. The occurrence of wet packs should be investigated and resolved. *[4: Limited Evidence]*

Internal or external moisture has the potential to compromise the integrity of the barrier material and the sterility of the contents. Moisture present inside the package after steam sterilization is indicative of problems with the packaging or the sterilization process.[3]

XII.e.1. Measures to resolve wet packs should include an evaluation of the
- package weight, density, and configuration;
- packaging materials and methods used;
- load contents and configuration;
- placement of the package on the sterilizer cart;
- compliance with the manufacturer's recommendations for containers, instruments, and wrappers;
- process of removal of the load from the sterilizer after sterilization;
- conditions (eg, temperature, humidity) in the cooldown area;
- location of air-conditioning vents in the cooldown area; and
- water and steam quality.[3,21,56]

Sterilizer performance, utility supply, and steam quality issues may require evaluation by engineering personnel or the sterilizer manufacturer representative.[56]

XII.f. Perioperative RNs should participate in ongoing quality assurance and performance improvement activities related to selection and use of packaging systems by
○ identifying processes that are important for quality monitoring (eg, weight of containment devices not exceeding 25 lb),
○ developing strategies for compliance,
○ establishing benchmarks to evaluate quality indicators,
○ collecting data related to levels of performance and quality indicators,
○ evaluating practice based on the cumulative data collected,
○ taking action to improve compliance, and
○ assessing the effectiveness of the actions taken.
[3: Moderate Evidence]

Participating in ongoing quality assurance and performance improvement activities is a standard of perioperative nursing and a primary responsibility of the RN who is engaged in practice in the perioperative setting.[5]

Glossary

Chemical indicators: Devices used to monitor exposure to one or more sterilization parameters.

- *Class I:* Process indicator that demonstrates that the package has been exposed to the sterilization process to distinguish between processed and unprocessed packages.
- *Class II:* Process indicator that is used for a specific purpose, such as the dynamic air removal test (Bowie-Dick test).
- *Class III:* A single-parameter indicator that reacts to one of the critical parameters of sterilization.
- *Class IV:* A multi-parameter indicator that reacts to one, two, or more of the critical parameters of sterilization.
- *Class V (integrating indicator):* An indicator that reacts to all critical parameters of sterilization.
- *Class VI (emulating indicator):* An indicator that reacts to all critical parameters of a specified sterilization cycle.

Containment device: Reusable rigid sterilization container, instrument case, cassette, or organizing tray intended for the purpose of containing reusable devices for sterilization.

Hydrogen peroxide gas plasma sterilization: A sterilization process that involves the combined use of hydrogen peroxide and low-temperature gas plasma. Gas plasmas are highly ionized gases composed of ions, electrons, and neutral particles.

Hydrogen peroxide vapor sterilization: A sterilization process in which vaporized hydrogen peroxide acts as a sterilant.

Instrument case/cassette: A container with a lid and a base to sterilize devices that permits air removal and sterilant penetration/removal. The devices require wrapping in packaging material if sterility of the contents is to be maintained.

Nonwoven material: Fabric made by bonding fibers together as opposed to weaving threads.

Organizing tray: A reusable metal or plastic tray that permits organization and protection of the contents. Some organizing trays have diagrams for the representative instruments etched onto the surface of the tray to facilitate their identificaton and location within the tray.

Package integrity: Unimpaired physical condition of a final package.

Paper-plastic pouch (peel pouch): A type of packaging made of Mylar® (a polyester film manufactured by DuPont) and paper that is suitable for packaging items to be sterilized in steam or a type of packaging made of Mylar® and Tyvek® (a polyethelene material manufactured by DuPont) that is suitable for packaging items to be sterilized in EO, low-temperature hydrogen gas plasma, or hydrogen peroxide vapor.

Rigid sterilization container system: Specifically designed heat-resistant, metal, plastic, or anodized aluminum receptacles used to package items, usually sur-

gical instruments, for sterilization. The lids and/or bottom surfaces contain steam- or gas-permeable, high-efficiency microbial filters.

Sequential wrapping: A double-wrapping procedure that creates a package within a package.

Shelf life: When this term is used in conjunction with a sterile device, shelf life is considered to be the length of time a device is safe to use.

Sterility maintenance cover (dust cover): A plastic bag, usually 2 to 3 thousandths of an inch (ie, mils) in thickness, applied to a cooled, sterilized item to provide extra protection from dust, moisture, and other environmental contaminates. These covers can be heat-sealed or self-sealed closed.

Sterilization validation studies: Tests performed by a device manufacturer that demonstrate that a sterilization process will consistently yield sterile product under defined parameters.

Superheating: A condition in which dehydrated textiles are subjected to steam sterilization. The superheated package or product becomes too dry, which causes destructive effects on the strength of the cloth fibers. When woven textiles are not re-hydrated after sterilization, and/or if repeated sterilization is attempted, the textiles could absorb the available moisture present in the steam, thereby creating a dry or superheated steam effect and adversely affecting the steam sterilization process.

Useful life: The length of time, as determined by the manufacturer, for which a product maintains acceptable safety and performance characteristics. The manufacturer should provide data to support the useful life of the product.

Wet packs: Packs are considered wet when there is moisture in the form of dampness, droplets, or puddles of water found on or within a textile pack, instrument, basin set, rigid sterilization container, or other containment device after a completed sterilization cycle and after a cool-down period. Wet packs are associated with steam sterilization; however, they can occur with EO sterilization.

Woven textile: A reusable fabric constructed from yarns made of natural and/or synthetic fibers or filaments that are woven or knitted together to form a web in a repeated interlocking pattern.

REFERENCES

1. Guideline for cleaning and care of surgical instruments. In: *Guidelines for Perioperative Practice.* Denver, CO: AORN, Inc; 2015:615-650.

2. Guideline for sterilization. In: *Guidelines for Perioperative Practice.* Denver, CO: AORN, Inc; 2015:665-692.

3. *ANSI/AAMI ST79:2010 & A1:2010, & A2:2011, & A3:2012: Comprehensive Guide to Steam Sterilization and Sterility Assurance in Health Care Facilities.* Arlington, VA: Association for the Advancement of Medical Instrumentation; 2012. [IVC]

4. *Guideline for Disinfection and Sterilization in Healthcare Facilities, 2008.* Centers for Disease Control and Prevention. http://www.cdc.gov/hicpac/disinfection_sterilization/13_0sterilization.html. Accessed on November 8, 2013. [IVA]

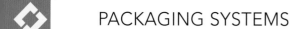

5. Standards of perioperative nursing. In: *Perioperative Standards and Recommended Practices*. Denver, CO: AORN, Inc; 2013:3-20. [IVB]

6. Diab-Elschahawi M, Blacky A, Bachhofner N, Koller W. Challenging the Sterrad 100NX sterilizer with different carrier materials and wrappings under experimental "clean" and "dirty" conditions. *Am J Infect Control*. 2010;38(10):806-810. [IIIB]

7. Rutala WA, Weber DJ. Choosing a sterilization wrap for surgical packs. *Infect Control Today*. May 1, 2000. http://www.infectioncontroltoday.com/articles/2000/05/choosing-a-sterilization-wrap-for-surgicalpacks.aspx. Accessed September 20, 2013. [VC]

8. ANSI/AAMI/ISO 11607-1:2006/(R)2010: Packaging for terminally sterilized medical devices—Part 1: Requirements for materials, sterile barrier systems and packaging. Arlington, VA: Association for the Advancement of Medical Instrumentation; 2010. [IVC]

9. Brusco J, Ogg M. Health care waste management and environmentally preferable purchasing. *AORN J*. 2010;92(6 Suppl):S62-S66. [VB]

10. *EPA's Final Guidance on Environmentally Preferable Purchasing*. August 20, 1999. Environmental Protection Agency. http://www.epa.gov/epp/pubs/guidance/final-guidance.htm. Accessed September 20, 2013. [IVA]

11. *AORN Position Statement: Environmental Responsibility*. http://www.aorn.org/Clinical_Practice/Position_Statements/Position_Statements.aspx. AORN, Inc. Accessed September 20, 2013. [IVB]

12. Laustsen G. Reduce-recycle-reuse: guidelines for promoting perioperative waste management. *AORN J*. 2007;85(4):717-728. [VA]

13. Lee RJ, Mears SC. Greening of orthopedic surgery. *Orthopedics*. 2012;35(6):e940-e944. [VB]

14. Belkin NL. Green nursing: the environment and economics. *AORN J*. 2007;86(1):15-16. [VC]

15. Conrardy J, Hillanbrand M, Myers S, Nussbaum GF. Reducing medical waste. *AORN J*. 2010;91(6):711-721. [IIIB]

16. Herman P, Larsen C. Measuring porous microbial barriers, part 1. Medical Device and Diagnostic Industry. http://www.mddionline.com/article/measuring-porous-microbial-barriers-part-1. Accessed September 20, 2013. [IVA]

17. Herman P, Larsen C. Measuring porous microbial barriers, part 2. Medical Device and Diagnostic Industry. http://www.mddionline.com/article/measuring-porous-microbial-barriers-part-2. Accessed September 20, 2013. [IVA]

18. *ANSI/AAMI ST41:2008: Ethylene Oxide Sterilization in Health Care Facilities: Safety and Effectiveness*. Arlington, VA: Association for the Advancement of Medical Instrumentation; 2008. [IVC]

19. *ANSI/AAMI ST58:2005/(R)2010: Chemical Sterilization and High-level Disinfection in Health Care Facilities*. Arlington, VA: Association for the Advancement of Medical Instrumentation; 2006. [IVC]

20. Kimberly-Clarke. KimGuard Sterilization Wrap. KimGuard One-Step Sterilization Wrap. Directions for use. http://www.njcl.us/images/KIMBERLY_CLARK_WRAP_DIRECTIONS_FOR_USE.PDF. Accessed September 20, 2013.

21. Rutala WA, Weber DJ; Healthcare Infection Control Practices Advisory Committee. *Guideline for Disinfection and Sterilization in Healthcare Facilities, 2008*. Atlanta, GA: Centers for Disease Control and Prevention; 2008. [IVA]

22. *Guidance Documents (Medical Devices and Radiation-Emitting Products) > Labeling Recommendations for Single-Use Devices Reprocessed by Third Parties and Hospitals; Final Guidance for Industry and FDA*. US Food and Drug Administration. http://www.fda.gov/MedicalDevices/DeviceRegulationandGuidance/GuidanceDocuments/ucm071058.htm. Accessed September 20, 2013.

23. Moriya GA, Souza RQ, Pinto FM, Graziano KU. Periodic sterility assessment of materials stored for up to 6 months at continuous microbial contamination risk: laboratory study. *Am J Infect Control*. 2012;40(10):1013-1015. [IA]

24. Joan LSP, Norhashimawati Khor S. Time versus event-related sterility: linen & pouch packaging remain sterile over a year of storage and handling. *Singapore Nurs J*. 2010;37(1):34-42. [IB]

25. Waked WR, Simpson AK, Miller CP, Magit DP, Grauer JN. Sterilization wrap inspections do not adequately evaluate instrument sterility. *Clin Orthop Relat Res*. 2007;462:207-211. [IA]

26. *ANSI/AAMI ST77: Containment Devices for Reusable Medical Device Sterilization*. Arlington, VA: Association for the Advancement of Medical Instrumentation; 2013. [IVC]

27. AORN guidance statement: safe patient handling and movement in the perioperative setting. In: *Perioperative Standards and Recommended Practices*. Denver, CO: AORN; 2013:553-572. [IVB]

28. American Society of Cataract and Refractive Surgery, American Society of Ophthalmic Registered Nurses. Recommended practices for cleaning and sterilizing intraocular surgical instruments. *J Cataract Refract Surg*. 2007;33(6):1095-1100. [IVB]

29. Lucas AD, Chobin N, Conner R, et al. Steam sterilization and internal count sheets: assessing the potential for cytotoxicity. *AORN J*. 2009;89(3):521-531. [IIB]

30. *ANSI/AAMI ST65:2008: Processing of Reusable Surgical Textiles for Use in Health Care Facilities*. Arlington, VA: Association for the Advancement of Medical Instrumentation; 2008. [IVC]

31. Nicholson P, Gillis S, Dunning AM. The use of scoring rubrics to determine clinical performance in the operating suite. *Nurse Educ Today*. 2009;29(1):73-82. [IIIB]

32. Ringerman E, Flint LJ, Hughes DE. An innovative education program: the peer competency validator model. *J Nurses Staff Dev*. 2006;22(3):114-123. [VB]

33. Sportsman S. Competency education and validation in the United States: what should nurses know? *Nurs Forum*. 2010;45(3):140-149. [VA]

34. Stobinski JX. Perioperative nursing competency. *AORN J*. 2008;88(3):417-436. [VB]

35. Whittaker S, Carson W, Smolenski MC. Assuring continued competence—policy questions and approaches: how should the profession respond? *Online J Issues Nurs*. 2000;5(3). http://www.nursingworld.org/MainMenuCategories/ANAMarketplace/ANAPeriodicals/OJIN/TableofContents/Volume52000/No3Sept00/ArticlePreviousTopic/ContinuedCompetence.aspx. Accessed September 20, 2013. [VA]

36. Centers for Medicare & Medicaid Services. *State Operations Manual Appendix A: Survey Protocol, Regulations and Interpretive Guidelines for Hospitals*. Rev.78; 2011.

37. Centers for Medicare & Medicaid Services. *State Operations Manual Appendix L: Guidance for Surveyors: Ambulatory Surgical Centers*. Rev. 76; 2011.

38. HR.01.05.03: Staff participate in ongoing education and training. In: *Comprehensive Accreditation Manual: CAMH for Hospitals*. Oakbrook Terrace, IL: Joint Commission Accreditation; 2013.

STERILIZATION AND DISINFECTION

39. HR.01.05.03: Staff participate in ongoing education and training. In: *Comprehensive Accreditation Manual for Ambulatory Care.* Oakbrook Terrace, IL: The Joint Commission; 2013.

40. Quality management and improvement. In: *2013 Accreditation Handbook for Ambulatory Health Care.* Skokie, IL: Accreditation Association for Ambulatory Health Care; 2013:30-34.

41. Personnel: personnel records. In: *Procedural Standards and Checklist for Accreditation of Ambulatory Surgery Facilities.* Version 3 ed. Gurnee, IL: American Association for Accreditation of Ambulatory Surgery Facilities; 2011:77-79.

42. Personnel: personnel records; resumes. In: *Regular Standards and Checklist for Accreditation of Ambulatory Surgery Facilities.* Version 13 ed. Gurnee, IL: American Association for Accreditation of Ambulatory Surgery Facilities; 2011:77-78.

43. Personnel: knowledge, skill & CME training. In: *Regular Standards and Checklist for Accreditation of Ambulatory Surgery Facilities.* Version 13 ed. Gurnee, IL: American Association for Accreditation of Ambulatory Surgery Facilities; 2011:78-79.

44. Personnel: personnel safety. In: *Regular Standards and Checklist for Accreditation of Ambulatory Surgery Facilities.* Version 13 ed. Gurnee, IL: American Association for Accreditation of Ambulatory Surgery Facilities; 2011:80.

45. Personnel: knowledge, skill & CME training. In: *Procedural Standards and Checklist for Accreditation of Ambulatory Surgery Facilities.* Version 3 ed. Gurnee, IL: American Association for Accreditation of Ambulatory Surgery Facilities; 2011:79.

46. Personnel: personnel safety. In: *Procedural Standards and Checklist for Accreditation of Ambulatory Surgery Facilities.* Version 3 ed. Gurnee, IL: American Association for Accreditation of Ambulatory Surgery Facilities; 2011:79-80.

47. Jordan C, Thomas MB, Evans ML, Green A. Public policy on competency: how will nursing address this complex issue? *J Contin Educ Nurs.* 2008;39(2):86-91. [VA]

48. LD.04.01.07: The hospital has policies and procedures that guide and support patient care, treatment, and services. In: *Hospital Accreditation Standards* 2013. 2013 ed. Oakbrook Terrace, IL: Joint Commission Resources; 2013.

49. LD.04.01.07: The organization has policies and procedures that guide and support patient care, treatment, or services. In: *Standards for Ambulatory Care 2013: Standards, Elements of Performance Scoring Accreditation Polices.* Oakbrook Terrace, IL: The Joint Commission; 2013.

50. Governance. In: *2013 Accreditation Handbook for Ambulatory Health Care.* Skokie, IL: Accreditation Association for Ambulatory Health Care; 2013:17-24.

51. PI.03.01.01: The hospital improves performance on an ongoing basis. In: *Hospital Accreditation Standards 2013.* 2013 ed. Oakbrook Terrace, IL: Joint Commission Resources; 2013.

52. PI.03.01.01: The organization improves performance. In: *Standards for Ambulatory Care 2012: Standards, Elements of Performance Scoring Accreditation Polices.* Oakbrook Terrace, IL: The Joint Commission; 2013.

53. Quality improvement/quality assessment: quality improvement. In: *Procedural Standards and Checklist for Accreditation of Ambulatory Surgery Facilities.* Version 3

ed. Gurnee, IL: American Association for Accreditation of Ambulatory Surgery Facilities; 2011:67.

54. Quality assessment/quality improvement: quality improvement. In: *Regular Standards and Checklist for Accreditation of Ambulatory Surgery Facilities.* Version 13 ed. Gurnee, IL: American Association for Accreditation of Ambulatory Surgery Facilities; 2011:67.

55. Quality assessment/quality improvement: unanticipated operative sequelae. In: *Regular Standards and Checklist for Accreditation of Ambulatory Surgery Facilities.* Version 13 ed. Gurnee, IL: American Association for Accreditation of Ambulatory Surgery Facilities; 2011:69-71.

56. Brown JM, Bliley J. How to solve wet packs, and evaluate water issues. *Mater Manag Health Care.* 2008;17(7):50-52. [VB]

Acknowledgements

LEAD AUTHOR
Cynthia Spry, MA, MS, RN, CNOR, CBSPDT
Independent Consultant
New York, New York

CONTRIBUTING AUTHOR
Ramona Conner, MSN, RN, CNOR
Manager, Standards and Guidelines
AORN Nursing Department
Denver, Colorado

The authors and AORN thank Paula Berrett, BS, CRCST, Intermountain Healthcare Urban South Region CP Manager, Utah Valley Regional Medical Center, Provo, Utah; Paula Morton, MS, RN, CNOR, Director of Perioperative Services, Sherman Health, Elgin, Illinois; Judith Goldberg, DBA, MSN, RN, CNOR, CRCST, Nurse Manager, Pequot Surgical Center, Groton, Connecticut; and Jane Rothrock, PhD, RN, CNOR, FAAN, Professor, Delaware Community College, Media, Pennsylvania, for their assistance in developing this guideline.

PUBLICATION HISTORY
Originally published February 1983, *AORN Journal.*

Revised November 1988, February 1992.

Revised November 1995; published May 1996, *AORN Journal.*

Revised and reformatted; published December 2000, *AORN Journal.*

Revised 2006; published in *Standards, Recommended Practices, and Guidelines,* 2007 edition.

Minor editing revisions made to omit PNDS codes; reformatted September 2012 for publication in *Perioperative Standards and Recommended Practices,* 2013 edition.

Revised September 2013 for online publication in *Perioperative Standards and Recommended Practices.*

Minor editing revisions made in November 2014 for publication in *Guidelines for Perioperative Practice,* 2015 edition.

Evidence ratings revised in *Guidelines for Perioperative Practice,* 2018 edition, to conform to the current AORN Evidence Rating Model.

The Guideline for Sterilization has been approved by the AORN Recommended Practices Advisory Board. It was presented as proposed recommendations for comments by members and others. The guideline is effective June 15, 2012. The recommendations in the guideline are intended to be achievable and represent what is believed to be an optimal level of practice. Policies and procedures will reflect variations in practice settings and/or clinical situations that determine the degree to which the guideline can be implemented. AORN recognizes the various settings in which perioperative nurses practice; therefore, this guideline is adaptable to various practice settings. These practice settings include traditional operating rooms (ORs), ambulatory surgery centers, physicians' offices, cardiac catheterization laboratories, endoscopy suites, radiology departments, and all other areas where operative and other invasive procedures may be performed.

Purpose

This document provides guidance for sterilizing items to be used in the perioperative setting. The creation and maintenance of an aseptic environment has direct influence on patient outcomes. A major responsibility of the perioperative registered nurse (RN) is to minimize patient risk for surgical site infections (SSIs). One of the measures for preventing SSIs is to provide reusable surgical items that are free of contamination at the time of use. This can be accomplished by subjecting them to cleaning and decontamination, followed by a disinfection or sterilization process.

The Spaulding classification system is commonly used to classify patient care items to determine the appropriate level of processing.[1] The Spaulding classification system, developed by Earl Spaulding in 1968, classifies items as noncritical, semicritical, or critical and identifies the appropriate processing method for each category. Infection preventionists and others use this system to determine the correct processing methods for preparing instruments and other items for patient use. According to the Spaulding classification system, the level of processing required is based on the nature of the item that requires processing and the manner in which the item is to be used.

The guideline addresses processing of critical medical devices. Processing of noncritical and semicritical devices is outside the scope of this document. The difference between noncritical and semicritical devices is as follows.

Noncritical devices are devices that contact only intact skin. Noncritical devices require low-level disinfection or cleaning. Examples of noncritical devices include

- tourniquets and blood pressure cuffs,
- stethoscopes, and
- Mayo stands.

Semicritical devices are devices that come in contact with nonintact skin or with mucous membranes and require a minimum of high-level disinfection. Examples of semicritical devices include

- vaginal and rectal probes,
- respiratory therapy equipment,
- bronchoscopes, and
- laryngoscope blades.[2,3]

Sterilization provides the highest level of assurance that surgical items are free of viable microbes.[1] Although these recommendations include several references to cleaning, decontamination, disinfection, and packaging, the major focus is on sterilization.

The guideline includes recommendations for high-temperature sterilization (ie, sterilization by steam), low-temperature sterilization (ie, ethylene oxide, low-temperature hydrogen peroxide gas plasma, low-temperature hydrogen peroxide vapor, dry heat, ozone), and processing using a liquid chemical sterilant system using peracetic acid.

Cleaning, decontamination, disinfection, and packaging of sterile medical devices are outside the scope of this document. The reader should refer to the AORN Guideline for Cleaning and Care of Surgical Instruments[4] and Guideline for High-Level Disinfection[5] for additional guidance.

Evidence Review

A medical librarian conducted a systematic literature search of the databases MEDLINE®, CINAHL®, Scopus®, and Cochrane Database of Systematic Reviews for meta-analyses, randomized and nonrandomized trials and studies, systematic and nonsystematic reviews, and opinion documents and letters. Search terms included *sterilization, ethylene oxide, steam, peracetic acid, dry heat, hydrogen peroxide gas, ozone, hospital equipment and supplies, prostheses and implants, surgical equipment, infusion pumps, disposable equipment, diagnostic equipment, flash sterilization, immediate use, surgical equipment and supplies, equipment contamination, microbial contamination, indicators and reagents, fungi, bacterial contamination, ethylene oxide toxicity*, and *biofilms*, as applicable.

The search was limited to articles published in English between 2005 and 2011. Older articles were included where there were no articles within this time period. Additional articles not identified in the original literature search were obtained by reviewing the reference lists of the original articles. The librarian also established continuing alerts on the sterilization topics. The lead author and medical librarian identified relevant documents from government agencies, standards-setting bodies, and equipment manufacturers, with the lead author requesting other guidelines, professional literature, and book chapters as necessary.

Articles identified by the search were provided to the project team for evaluation. The team consisted of the lead author, two members of the Recommended Practices Advisory Board, two members of the Research Committee, and an ad hoc member of the Evidence Rating Task Force. The lead author divided the search results into topics and assigned members of the team to review and critically appraise each article using the Johns Hopkins Evidence-Based Practice Model and the Research or Non-Research Evidence Appraisal Tools as appropriate. The literature was independently evaluated and appraised according to the strength and quality of the evidence. Each article was then assigned an appraisal score as agreed upon by consensus of the team. The appraisal score is noted in brackets after each reference citation, as applicable.

The collective evidence supporting each intervention within a specific recommendation was summarized and used to rate the strength of the evidence using the AORN Evidence Rating Model. Factors considered in review of the collective evidence were the quality of research, quantity of similar studies on a given topic, and consistency of results supporting a recommendation. The evidence rating is noted in brackets after each intervention.

Editor's note: *MEDLINE is a registered trademark of the US National Library of Medicine's Medical Literature Analysis and Retrieval System, Bethesda, MD. CINAHL, Cumulative Index to Nursing and Allied Health Literature, is a registered trademark of EBSCO Industries, Birmingham, AL. Scopus is a registered trademark of Elsevier B.V., Amsterdam, Netherlands.*

Recommendation I

Patient care items should be processed for reuse based on the intended use of the item.

I.a.   Items that enter sterile tissue or the vascular system are categorized as critical and should be sterile when used.[1,6] Sterilization may be accomplished using a variety of sterilization methods and technologies (eg, steam, ethylene oxide, hydrogen peroxide). *[1: Strong Evidence]*
Examples of critical items include
○ surgical instruments,
○ cutting endoscopic accessories that break the mucosal barrier, and
○ implants.

I.a.1.   If it is determined that in-house reprocessing of single-use devices is feasible, a program for reprocessing of single-use devices that meets US Food and Drug Administration (FDA) requirements and includes policies, procedures, competencies, and educational requirements should be developed. Reprocessing of single-use medical devices is outside the scope of this document.

I.a.2.   If it is determined that in-house reprocessing of single-use items is not feasible and it is still the intention of the facility to target some single-use devices for reprocessing, the facility should investigate the feasibility of using the services of a third-party reprocessing company. Criteria for evaluating the services of a third-party reprocessor and identifying single-use items for reprocessing are outside the scope of this document.

Recommendation II

Devices labeled as single-use should not be reprocessed unless the FDA guidelines for reprocessing of single-use devices can be met.

In 2000 the FDA issued a guidance document for reprocessing of single-use devices.[7] This document details the requirements that a reprocessor must meet. These requirements are the same requirements that the original device manufacturer must meet. They include

• registering as a reprocessing firm and listing all products that are reprocessed;
• submitting reports of associated adverse events to the FDA;
• tracking devices that, in the event of failure, could have serious outcomes;
• correcting or removing from the market unsafe devices; and
• meeting manufacturing and labeling requirements.

An in-depth explanation of these guidelines can be accessed on the FDA web site.[7,8] Meeting these requirements is beyond the capabilities of most health care facilities.

II.a.   Health care facilities considering reprocessing single-use devices should identify devices labeled as single-use that they would like to reprocess, review the FDA guidance document, and, based on the requirements within the document, make a determination as to the feasibility of reprocessing those devices within the facility.[7] *[1: Regulatory Requirement]*

Recommendation III

Items to be sterilized should be cleaned, decontaminated, inspected, packaged, sterilized, and stored in a controlled environment and in accordance with the AORN Guideline for Cleaning and Care of Surgical Instruments[4] and the device manufacturer's validated and written instructions for use.

A controlled environment is intended to facilitate effective decontamination, assembly, sterilization, and storage and to minimize environmental contamination and maintain sterility of sterilized items.

Effective sterilization cannot take place without effective cleaning. The process of sterilization is negatively affected by the amount of bioburden and the number, type, and inherent resistance of microorganisms, including biofilms, on the items to be sterilized.

TABLE 1. ATTIRE AND PERSONAL PROTECTIVE EQUIPMENT REQUIREMENTS[1]

Work area	Scrubs	Head covers	Gloves*	Gowns#	Eye protection+	Masks or face shields±
Decontamination	X	X	X	X	X	X
Preparation and packaging	X	X				
Sterilization processing	X	X				
Sterile storage	X	X				

*Gloves should be waterproof, general-purpose utility, or heavy duty.
#Gowns must be liquid-resistant with sleeves.
+Eye protection includes goggles/eye glasses with side shields or chin-length face shields.
± Masks should be fluid-resistant.
Other protective equipment (such as shoe covers) may be worn as needed. The type and characteristics will depend on the task and degree of anticipated exposure.

REFERENCE

1. Occupational Safety & Health Administration. US Department of Labor. Toxic and hazardous substances. Appendix A: bloodborne pathogens. 29 CFR §1910.1030. Fed Regist. 1991;56(235):64004-64182. Effective December 6, 1991. http://www.osha.gov/pls/oshaweb/owadisp.show_document?p_table=standards&p_id=10051. Accessed April 25, 2012.

Soils, oils, and other materials may shield microorganisms on items from contact with the sterilant or combine with and inactivate the sterilant.[1,6,9]

III.a. Items sterilized outside of the facility in which they will be used, unless they are processed in a commercial FDA-regulated instrument sterilization facility, should be removed from their container or wrapper and cleaned, decontaminated, and sterilized according to the manufacturer's validated and written instructions for use within the organization in which they will be used. [4: Limited Evidence]

Controlled conditions reduce the risk of contamination.[6] It is not possible to know the conditions under which items were cleaned, packaged, and sterilized at another facility or to know the conditions of transport.

III.a.1. Facilities in which instruments are routinely processed at a satellite facility or at a campus site that requires transportation of the sterilized items from one building to another should develop policies and procedures to ensure standardized processing procedures, controlled conditions of transport, and oversight of all aspects of processing and transport. Criteria for such a practice are outside the scope of this document.

III.b. Functional workflow patterns should be established to create and maintain physical separation between the decontamination and sterilization areas.[6,10] [4: Limited Evidence]

Physical separation aids in achieving environmental and microbial control. During manual cleaning of instruments, particulates, aerosolized matter, dust, and microbial counts are elevated. Physical separation and vented airflow to the outside minimizes potential contamination of processed items.[10]

III.b.1. Attire, use of personal protective equipment (PPE), and limitations in personnel access and movement should be based on expected contamination levels (Table 1).

III.b.2. Functional workflow patterns should be established in the following order, from potentially high contamination areas to clean areas:
1. decontamination area,
2. preparation and packaging,
3. sterilization processing,
4. sterile storage, and
5. clean distribution.

A workflow pattern that begins in the decontamination area (ie, dirty) and flows to the clean distribution area can help to prevent clean or sterile items from reentering a contaminated area where they may be recontaminated.

III.b.3. Traffic patterns should be established to protect personnel, equipment, supplies, and instrumentation from sources of potential contamination. Traffic patterns should define access restrictions, movement of personnel, and appropriate attire according to AORN guidelines.[10]

III.c. Room temperature, humidity, and ventilation must be controlled and monitored in accordance with local, state, and federal policy and regulation. Table 2 provides parameters for the controlled environment.[6] [4: Limited Evidence]

Bacteria and fungi thrive at warm temperatures, whereas cooler temperatures may impede bacterial and fungal growth in the decontamination area. Regulated environmental controls in work areas are essential for the comfort of personnel wearing appropriate attire and PPE.[6]

TABLE 2. PARAMETERS FOR CONTROLLED ENVIRONMENTS DURING STERILIZATION[1,2]

Functional area	Airflow	Minimum number of air exchanges per hour	All air exhausted directly to the outdoors	Temperature	Relative humidity
Soiled/ decontaminated	Negative (in)	10 *(6)	Yes	60° F to 65° F (16° C to 18° C)	20% to 60%
Sterilizer equipment access	Negative (in)	10	Yes	75° F to 85° F (24° C to 29° C)	20% to 60%
Sterilizer loading/ unloading	Positive (out)	10	Yes	68° F to 73° F (20° C to 23° C)	20% to 60%
Restrooms/ housekeeping	Negative (in)	10	Yes	68° F to 73° F (20° C to 23° C)	20% to 60%
Preparation and packaging	Positive (out)	10 (downdraft type)	No	68° F to 73° F (20° C to 23° C)	20% to 60%
Textile packaging room	Positive (out)	10 (downdraft type)	No	68° C to 73° F (20° C to 23° C)	20% to 60%
Clean/sterile storage	Positive (out)	4 (downdraft type)	No	≤ 75° F (≤ 24° C)	≤ 70%

* The Facilities Guideline Institute recommends a minimum of 6 air exchanges an hour in decontamination. AAMI recommends 10 exchanges.

Regulatory agencies may enforce the American Society for Healthcare Engineering (ASHE) or AAMI recommendations listed in Table 2. They also may enforce other recommendations, such as the 2000 NFPA 101, which states the relative humidity should be at 35%. As stated in the ASHE document, these parameters are intended to be used for the design of the heating, ventilation, and air conditioning systems and there may be daily fluctuations based on the environmental conditions.

REFERENCES

1. *Association for the Advancement of Medical Instrumentation. ANSI/AAMI ST79:2010, A1:2010 & A2:2011, Comprehensive guide to steam sterilization and sterility assurance in health care facilities. Arlington, VA: Association for the Advancement of Medical Instrumentation; 2010 & 2011. Adapted and reprinted with permission. Further reproduction or distribution prohibited.*
2. *ANSI/ASHRAE/ASHE Addendum D to ANSI/ASHRAE/ASHE Standard 170-2008. Atlanta, GA: American Society of Heating, Refrigerating and Air-Conditioning Engineers; 2010.*

III.d. Monitoring results should be readily retrievable.[6] *[3: Moderate Evidence]*

Monitoring and recording environmental controls in each area will assist in verification that minimum recommended parameters are met and maintained and will identify when corrective action needs to be taken.

A mechanism with memory for history of temperature and humidity can alert personnel if there was a deviation during unmanned times.

III.e. Items to be sterilized should be decontaminated before inspection, packaging, and sterilization.[4,6] *[1: Strong Evidence]*

III.e.1. Health care personnel should use standard precautions when performing decontamination activities.

Standard precautions are designed to protect patients and health care workers from contact with recognized and unrecognized sources of infectious diseases.[11,12]

Recommendation IV

Items to be sterilized should be inspected for cleanliness and proper function in accordance with AORN's Guideline for Cleaning and Care of Surgical Instruments.[4]

Debris remaining on a device may compromise the subsequent sterilization process.[1]

IV.a. Instruments should be inspected for cleanliness and function before packaging and sterilization. *[4: Limited Evidence]*

Although commercially available tests can be used to verify the cleaning process,[1] there is no universally accepted standard for clean. Visual inspection is a subjective assessment that depends on the operator. It has limited efficacy but is commonly used to determine cleanliness. Inspection under magnification and ancillary lighting can assist in viewing residual soil and determining cleanliness.[13]

In one study, investigators rated 91% of cleaned instruments as visually clean. However, upon examination under a microscope, they determined that 84% of the instruments that looked clean contained residual debris.[14]

IV.b. The device manufacturer should be consulted for the appropriate methods for testing function.[6] *[4: Limited Evidence]*

Instruments that malfunction or are not intact when used in surgery have the potential to cause patient harm.

Recommendation V

Items to be sterilized should be packaged in a manner that promotes successful sterilization. Items should be packaged in accordance with AORN's Guideline for Selection and Use of Packaging Systems for Sterilization.[15]

Appropriate packaging increases the probability that sterility can be achieved and maintained to the point of use.[1,16]

V.a. Manufacturers of packaging systems should be consulted for package preparation, configuration, and sterilization. *[4: Limited Evidence]*

V.b. The total weight of an instrument set should not exceed 25 lb.[6,17] *[3: Moderate Evidence]*

   Instrument sets weighing more than 25 lb are known to be difficult to dry without lengthy drying times and present an increased risk of ergonomic injury.[6,15,18,19]

V.c. Combination paper-plastic peel pouches should not be placed in a container or wrapped set unless the pouch or container manufacturer has validated this process.[6] Medical-grade, all-paper pouches or other containment devices validated for use within instrument sets may be used to segregate small items within a set. *[4: Limited Evidence]*

   When placing paper-plastic peel pouches within a wrapped set or rigid sterilization container, it may not be possible to position them in a manner that allows adequate air removal, steam contact, or drying.[6]

Recommendation VI

Saturated steam under pressure should be used to sterilize heat- and moisture-stable items unless otherwise indicated by the device manufacturer.[1]

Saturated steam under pressure is a preferred sterilization method. It has a large margin of safety because of its reliability, consistency, and lethality. It is an effective, inexpensive, and relatively rapid sterilization method for most porous and nonporous materials.[1]

VI.a. Manufacturers' written instructions for operating steam sterilizers should be followed. *[3: Moderate Evidence]*

   Steam sterilizers vary in size, design, and performance characteristics. Steam sterilizers may be large capacity—greater than 2 cubic feet—or small table-top models and may differ in how they generate steam.

   Types of steam sterilizers include gravity-displacement sterilizers that permit only gravity-displacement cycles, dynamic air-removal sterilizers (eg, prevacuum, high vacuum, steam-flush pressure-pulse) that permit only dynamic air-removal cycles, and sterilizers that permit either gravity-displacement or dynamic air-removal cycles.[1]

Health care organizations may use both gravity-displacement cycles and dynamic air-removal cycles. Immediate use steam sterilization (IUSS), formerly referred to as flash sterilization, can be performed in either a gravity-displacement or a dynamic air-removal cycle.[20,21]

Air removal is critical to successful steam sterilization. Medical device manufacturers may validate a specific method of air removal and therefore recommend a specific type of steam sterilization cycle or specify the achievement of certain cycle parameters in their written instructions for use.

Steam sterilizers may be used for both terminal sterilization, which permits storage of items after sterilization, and IUSS.[20]

Cycle parameters vary according to sterilizer and device manufacturers' instructions for use, and whether terminal or IUSS is desired.

Table 3 and Table 4 provide typical minimum sterilization times for gravity-displacement and dynamic air-removal steam sterilization cycles, respectively.

It is critical to refer to the device and container manufacturers' instructions to determine the required cycle. Many devices require extended exposure times and some rigid sterilization containers, such as those intended for IUSS, may require exposure times greater than those identified in the tables (Table 3 and Table 4).

VI.b. Cycle parameters recommended by the device manufacturer should be reconciled with the sterilizer manufacturer's written instructions for the specific sterilization cycle and load configuration.[6,21] *[3: Moderate Evidence]*

   Certain types of devices (eg, some pneumatically powered instruments; specialty orthopedic, neurosurgery, trauma instruments) and implants may require prolonged exposure times or drying times. These cycle times may not have been validated by the sterilizer manufacturer.

VI.b.1. When the sterilizer and the device manufacturers' instructions cannot be reconciled, the device manufacturers' instructions should be followed.[20]

   The device manufacturer has validated the cycle, identified in the instructions for use, that must be used to ensure sterility.

VI.c. A quality monitoring program that includes physical monitors (eg, printouts, digital readings, graphs, gauges), chemical indicators, and biological indicators should be used to verify that conditions necessary for steam sterilization have been met.[6] *[1: Strong Evidence]*

   Attention to sterility monitoring to ensure compliance with recommended guidelines is a critical component of quality assurance. Deviation from recommended practices and recommendations can compromise the quality of sterilization processes.

TABLE 3. TYPICAL MINIMUM CYCLE TIMES FOR GRAVITY-DISPLACEMENT STEAM STERILIZATION[1]

Item	Exposure time at 250° F (121° C)	Exposure time at 270° F (132° C)	Exposure time at 275° F (135° C)	Drying time
Packaged instruments	30 minutes	15 minutes		15 to 30 minutes
Textile packs	30 minutes	25 minutes		15 minutes
			10 minutes	30 minutes
Nonporous items subject to immediate use steam sterilization (IUSS)		See device and container manufacturer instructions for use	See device and container manufacturer instructions for use	See IUSS container manufacturer instructions for use
Nonporous and porous items in mixed load subject to IUSS		See device and container manufacturer instructions for use	See device and container manufacturer instructions for use	See IUSS container manufacturer instructions for use

REFERENCE

1. *Association for the Advancement of Medical Instrumentation. ANSI/AAMI ST79:2010, A1:2010 & A2:2011, Comprehensive guide to steam sterilization and sterility assurance in health care facilities. Arlington, VA: Association for the Advancement of Medical Instrumentation; 2010 & 2011. Adapted and reprinted with permission. Further reproduction or distribution is prohibited.*

VI.c.1. Each sterilization cycle should be monitored to verify that parameters required for sterilization have been met.[1,6]

VI.c.2. The sterilizer operator should review physical monitors to verify cycle parameters for every load.[6]

Physical monitors can provide a rapid means of identification of sterilizer failure. Physical monitors record cycle parameters (eg, time for each phase of the cycle, temperature during each phase of the cycle).

VI.c.3. External and internal chemical indicators should be used with each package.

- A class 1 chemical indicator (ie, process indicator) should be placed on the outside of every package unless the internal indicator is visible through the package material.[6] Examples of process indicators are indicator tape and indicator labels.
- A class 5 chemical indicator (ie, integrating indicator) or class 6 chemical indicator (ie, emulating indicator) should be placed inside every package.[6]
- A class 3 or 4 chemical indicator may be used within a package to meet requirements for internal monitoring.[6]

Chemical indicators are used to verify that one or more of the conditions necessary for sterilization have been achieved within each package.[6]

VI.c.4. Chemical indicators should be placed in an area within the package that presents a challenge for air removal and steam contact. When there is a question concerning the appropriate number and placement of internal chemical indicators, the user should consult with the chemical indicator manufacturer, the device manufacturer,

and the container manufacturer for additional information.

The number and the placement of internal chemical indicators may be affected by the contents of the package, the configuration of the items within the set, and the packaging or container.[6]

VI.c.5. Biological indicators should be used to monitor sterilizer efficacy. Efficacy monitoring should be performed at least weekly and preferably daily.

Frequent sterilizer efficacy monitoring reduces the possibility that items will be processed under suboptimal conditions and for load release.[6] (See Recommendation XX for further recommendations concerning a quality monitoring program and application of monitors.)

VI.c.6. Biological indicators should be used for load release purposes. For example, loads containing an implant should be monitored with a biological indicator and not released for use until the result of the test is available.

VI.d. After steam sterilization, the contents of the sterilizer should be removed from the chamber and left untouched until they are cool enough to handle without concern that retained moisture may act as a wick for bacteria that is on the hands of personnel who touch the package. *[4: Limited Evidence]*

A period of 30 minutes to two hours may be necessary for the cooldown, but there is a lack of scientific evidence to support an exact amount of time needed for cooling. Cooling time will vary according to how hot items are at the end of the cycle, the density and composition of the materials contained within the load, the packaging material, and the temperature and

STERILIZATION AND DISINFECTION

TABLE 4. TYPICAL MINIMUM CYCLE TIMES FOR DYNAMIC AIR-REMOVAL STEAM STERILIZATION[1]

Item	Exposure time at 270° F (132° C)	Exposure time at 275° F (135° C)	Drying times
Packaged instruments	4 minutes		20 to 30 minutes
		3 minutes	16 minutes
Textile packs	4 minutes		5 to 20 minutes
		3 minutes	3 minutes
Nonporous items subject to IUSS	See device and container manufacturer instructions for use	See device and container manufacturer instructions for use	See IUSS container manufacturer instructions for use
Nonporous and porous items in mixed load subject to IUSS	See device and container manufacturer instructions for use	See device and container manufacturer instructions for use	See IUSS container manufacturer instructions for use

REFERENCE

1. Association for the Advancement of Medical Instrumentation. ANSI/AAMI ST79:2010, A1:2010 & A2:2011, Comprehensive guide to steam sterilization and sterility assurance in health care facilities. Arlington, VA: Association for the Advancement of Medical Instrumentation; 2010 & 2011. Adapted and reprinted with permission. Further reproduction or distribution is prohibited.

humidity of the ambient environment.[6] Containers made from plastic may require an extended cooling period to ensure moisture is removed from the container. High-density items retain heat and may require extended cooling times.

At the end of a steam sterilization cycle, packages may contain moisture that migrates out of the package as a gas or water vapor during the drying and cooling period. Depending on the type of packaging, a moist area may be created that can act as a wick and draw bacteria from hands before appropriate cooling and drying.

The potential for the formation of condensation is decreased by allowing the contents of the sterilizer to remain untouched until the equalization of the temperature differential between the chamber and outside environment has occurred.[6]

There is a lack of definitive studies to support cracking the sterilizer door to facilitate drying. However, some sterilizer manufacturers' instructions for use may recommend cracking the sterilizer door.[22]

VI.d.1. Warm or hot items should not be placed on cool or cold surfaces. Items should be allowed to cool on the sterilization rack.

When hot and cold surfaces are brought together, moisture may condense from both inside and outside the package.[6]

VI.d.2. Sterilized packages or containers that have formed condensate should be considered unsterile, and the contents should not be used.[6]

Moisture can compromise the integrity of barrier material and the sterility of the contents. Moisture may indicate problems with the packaging and/or sterilization process.

Recommendation VII

Immediate use steam sterilization (IUSS) should be kept to a minimum and should be used only in selected clinical situations and in a controlled manner.[20,23]

Immediate use steam sterilization may be associated with increased risk of infection to patients.[1] Time constraints may result in pressure on personnel to eliminate or modify one or more steps in the cleaning and sterilization process.

The term *flash sterilization* has historically been used to describe steam sterilization of unwrapped items intended to be used immediately. Flash sterilization cycles have traditionally been either 3 or 10 minutes of exposure, depending on the nature of the device being sterilized or the type of cycle indicated, minimal or no dry time, and no cooldown, thereby making the entire cycle time shorter than the cycle times for wrapped or terminally sterilized items. However, current manufacturers' instructions for use may require a variety of cycle times and the use of single wrappers or flash containers as opposed to sterilizing unwrapped items. The term "flash sterilization" no longer serves to describe the various steam sterilization cycles and processes that are used to process items that are not intended to be stored for later use. For this reason, the more appropriate term is *IUSS*.

Immediate use is considered the shortest time possible between a sterilized item's removal from the sterilizer and its aseptic transfer to the sterile field. The term IUSS has been endorsed by AORN, the Association for Professionals in Infection Control and Epidemiology (APIC), the International Association of Healthcare Central Service Materiel Management (IAHCSMM), the Accreditation Association of Ambulatory Healthcare (AAAHC), and the Association of Surgical Technologists (AST), as well as the ASC Quality Collaboration, which represents the ambulatory surgery center industry.[20]

VII.a. Immediate use steam sterilization should be used only when there is insufficient time to process by the preferred wrapped or container method intended for terminal sterilization. Immediate use steam sterilization should not be used as a substitute for sufficient instrument inventory.[6,23] *[1: Strong Evidence]*

VII.a.1. Items to be steam sterilized for immediate use should be subjected to the same decontamination processes as described in AORN's Guideline for Cleaning and Care of Surgical Instruments.[4] Decontamination should be performed in an area intended, designed, and equipped for decontamination activities.

As with terminal sterilization, proper decontamination is essential for removing bioburden and preparing an item for IUSS. Failures in instrument cleaning have resulted in transmission of infectious agents.[24]

VII.a.2. Immediate use steam sterilization should be performed only if all of the following conditions are met:
- The device manufacturer's written instructions include instructions for IUSS.
- The device manufacturer's written instructions for cleaning, cycle type, exposure times, temperature settings, and drying times (if recommended) are available and followed.
- Items are placed in a containment device that has been validated for IUSS and cleared by the FDA for this purpose and in a manner that allows steam to contact all instrument surfaces.
- The containment device manufacturer's written instructions for use are followed.
- Measures are taken to prevent contamination during transfer to the sterile field.
- Items subjected to IUSS are used immediately and not stored for later use or held from one procedure to another.[6]

VII.b. Packaging and wrapping (eg, textiles, paper-plastic pouches, nonwoven wrappers) should not be used in IUSS cycles unless the sterilizer and the packaging are specifically intended and labeled for this use.[6] *[4: Limited Evidence]*

Cycle parameters vary according to sterilizer design.[21]

VII.b.1. Sterilizer manufacturers' written instructions should be followed and reconciled with packaging and device manufacturers' instructions for sterilization.[6]

VII.c. Each sterilization cycle should be monitored to verify that parameters required for sterilization have been met.[6] *[1: Strong Evidence]*

VII.c.1. The sterilizer operator should use physical monitors to verify cycle parameters for each load.[6]

Physical monitors (eg, printouts, digital reading, graphs, gauges) can indicate immediate sterilizer failure. Physical monitors record cycle parameters (eg, time, temperature) for each cycle.

VII.c.2. Biological and chemical indicators should be used to monitor sterilizer efficacy and to assess whether conditions of sterilization have been achieved.

Although products used to monitor sterilizer efficacy and achievement of required parameters vary according to type of cycle or type of sterilizer, monitoring requirements are the same for all types of steam sterilization. (See Recommendation XX for more detailed recommendations for a quality monitoring program and application of monitors.)

VII.c.3. A class 5 chemical integrating indicator or a class 6 indicator should be used within each sterilization container or tray used for IUSS.[6] Class 6 indicators are cycle-specific and should be used only in the specific cycles for which they are labeled.

VII.d. Devices processed using IUSS should be transported to the point of use in a manner that minimizes the risk of contamination of the item and injury to personnel handling the hot, wet, and possibly heavy trays. *[4: Limited Evidence]*

Immediate use steam sterilized items may be vulnerable to contamination by exposure to the environment and handling by personnel while transporting the sterile device to the point of use. It is important that sterilization processing be carried out in a clean environment and that IUSS devices are transferred to the point of use in a manner that prevents contamination.[20,25]

Because drying time is not usually part of a preprogrammed IUSS cycle, the items processed are assumed to be wet at the conclusion of the cycle and will be hot when removed from the sterilizer chamber immediately after the cycle.

VII.e. Rigid sterilization containers designed and intended for IUSS cycles should be used. *[4: Limited Evidence]*

Rigid IUSS containers protect items so as to reduce the risk of contamination during transport of items to the point of use and facilitate ease of presentation to the sterile field.[6,25]

VII.e.1. After each use, IUSS containers should be cleaned, inspected (eg, for wear of gaskets and other critical components), and maintained according to the manufacturer's written instructions.[6]

VII.e.2. Immediate use steam sterilization containers should be opened and the contents used immediately. Instruments processed in IUSS containers should not be stored for later use or held from one procedure to the next.[20]

VII.e.3. Items processed using IUSS should be differentiated from items processed using terminal sterilization.

VII.f. Immediate use steam sterilization should not be used for implantable devices except in cases of defined emergency when no other option is available.[1,6] *[1: Strong Evidence]*

Implants are foreign bodies and they increase the risk of SSI.[23] Careful planning, appropriate packaging, and inventory management in cooperation with suppliers can minimize the need for IUSS of implantable medical devices.

VII.f.1. When IUSS of an implant is unavoidable, cycle selection should be determined by the manufacturer's written instructions for use, and a biological indicator and a class 5 chemical integrating indicator should be run with the load.[6,21] When an implant is used before the biological indicator results are known and the biological indicator is later determined to have a positive result, the surgeon and infection preventionists should be notified as soon as the results are known. If the implant is not used, it should not be saved as sterile for future use. If, after inspection, it is determined that the implant is suitable for future use, resterilization of the implant is required.[6]

VII.f.2. Every implant should be fully traceable to the patient in whom it was implanted.[6]

VII.g Documentation of cycle information and monitoring results should be maintained in a log (ie, electronic or manual).[6] *[4: Limited Evidence]*

Documentation of cycle information provides a means for tracking items that are processed using IUSS to individual patients and for quality monitoring.

VII.g.1. Immediate use steam sterilization records should include information on each load, including
- the items processed,
- the patient on whom the items were used,
- the type of cycle (eg, gravity-displacement, dynamic air-removal),
- the cycle parameters used (eg, temperature, duration of cycle),
- monitoring results,
- the date and time the cycle was run,
- the operator information (ie, person who initiated the cycle, person who retrieved the item from the sterilizer), and
- the reason for IUSS.[6]

VII.g.2. A record describing what could have been done to prevent IUSS of the implant should be completed and used as part of a quality monitoring system.

A record of IUSS of implants can be helpful in determining problems, trends, or circumstances that can be addressed to prevent IUSS of implants in the future.

Recommendation VIII

Ethylene oxide sterilization is a low-temperature process that may be used for moisture- and heat-sensitive surgical items and when indicated by the device manufacturer.

At sterilizing temperatures, ethylene oxide kills microbes in hard-to-reach areas, and it does so with no damage to devices. Ethylene oxide is an alkylating agent that results in microbial death when used under controlled parameters. Ethylene oxide substitutes for hydrogen atoms on molecules needed to sustain life and, by attaching to these molecules, ethylene oxide stops these molecules' normal life-supporting functions. Some of the key molecules that ethylene oxide disrupts are proteins and DNA. Under low-temperature sterilizing conditions, so much ethylene oxide is used that this disruption proves lethal to microbial life.[26]

VIII.a. Ethylene oxide may be used if alternate methods of sterilization are not available or compatible with the medical devices being processed.[26,27] *[1: Strong Evidence]*

Health care organizations use 100% concentrations of ethylene oxide or ethylene oxide in mixtures with inert diluent gases (eg, carbon dioxide, hydrochlorofluorocarbons [HCFCs]) for ethylene oxide sterilization procedures. Until the 1990s, chlorofluorocarbons (CFCs) were used as diluents for ethylene oxide. Chlorofluorocarbons cause depletion of the ozone layer and are no longer produced in the United States. Hydrochlorofluorocarbons deplete the ozone layer, but to a lesser degree than CFCs.[27]

In 2015 the Environmental Protection Agency (EPA) will begin regulation of HCFCs, and production will terminate.[28] One hundred percent concentrations of ethylene oxide will continue to be available.

VIII.a.1. Users of HCFCs should be aware of and comply with federal, state, and local regulations regarding HCFC use in ethylene oxide sterilizers.

VIII.b. The manufacturer's written instructions should be reviewed to determine whether a heat- or moisture-sensitive item is compatible with ethylene oxide. *[4: Limited Evidence]*

VIII.c. Items, including all lumens, should be clean and dry before being packaged for ethylene oxide sterilization.[26] *[4: Limited Evidence]*

Soil inhibits sterilization, and moisture may produce toxic by-products. The combination of water and ethylene oxide results in the formation of ethylene glycol (a form of antifreeze).

VIII.d. Sterilizer manufacturers' written instructions should be followed for ethylene oxide-sterilization parameters and placement of items within the sterilizer.[26] *[4: Limited Evidence]*

Ethylene oxide sterilizers differ in design and operating characteristics.

VIII.d.1. Items should be placed in ethylene oxide sterilizers in baskets or on loading carts in a manner that allows free circulation and penetration of the ethylene oxide and moisture vapor.[26]

VIII.d.2. Full loads of items with common aeration times should be run unless the sterilizer is equipped with an air pollution control device.[29]

A full load is not the same as a full chamber. What constitutes a full load will vary among facilities.

VIII.e. A quality monitoring program that includes physical, chemical, and biological monitors should be used to verify that conditions necessary for sterilization have been met.[26] *[1: Strong Evidence]*

VIII.e.1. Each sterilization cycle should be monitored to verify that parameters required for sterilization have been met.[26]

VIII.e.2. The sterilizer operator should use physical monitors to verify cycle parameters for every load.

Physical monitors (eg, printouts, digital readings, graphs, gauges) can indicate immediate sterilizer failure. Physical monitors record cycle parameters (eg, time, temperature, humidity, gas concentration).

VIII.e.3. Chemical indicators designed for ethylene oxide monitoring should be used to verify that one or more of the conditions for sterilization have been met. A class 1 chemical indicator should be placed on the outside of every package unless the internal indicator is visible.[6,26] A chemical indicator validated for use in ethylene oxide should be placed inside every package.

VIII.e.4. Biological indicators should be used to monitor sterilizer efficacy and for load release. Every load should be monitored with a biological indicator.[26]

VIII.f. Ethylene oxide penetrates packaging materials. Items sterilized in ethylene oxide sterilizers should be properly aerated in a mechanical aerator to remove ethylene oxide. *[1: Regulatory Requirement]*

Ethylene oxide is a known human carcinogen and a chemical that has the potential to cause adverse reproductive effects in humans. The Occupational Safety and Health Administration (OSHA) has established exposure limits for ethylene oxide in the workplace.[30] If not removed,

ethylene oxide residue absorbed into sterilized items represents a hazard to patients and personnel. Items that are not sufficiently aerated may cause patient or personnel injury (eg, chemical burns). Aeration is the only safe and effective way to remove residual ethylene oxide.[26,31]

Adequate aeration times reduce ethylene oxide vapors and residue to a level safe for exposure of both patients and health care personnel.

Rinsing an inadequately aerated item does not remove ethylene oxide and can create hazardous by-products.

VIII.f.1. Items should be sterilized and properly aerated in a single chamber.[32]

The EPA does not permit transfer of ethylene oxide-sterilized loads to a separate aerator.

VIII.f.2. Health care personnel should wear butyl rubber, nitrile, or neoprene gloves that provide protection to the skin when a situation arises in which it is necessary to handle unaerated ethylene oxide-sterilized items.[26]

Safety measures are necessary to prevent health care personnel from coming in contact with ethylene oxide residues.

VIII.f.3. Required aeration times are validated by the medical device manufacturer and should be established based on
- item composition and size,
- item preparation and packaging,
- density of the load,
- type of ethylene oxide sterilizer/aerator used,
- the device and sterilizer manufacturers' written instructions for use, and
- temperature penetration pattern of the aerator's chamber.[26]

VIII.f.4. All ethylene oxide-sterilized items must be completely aerated before they can be used safely.
- Aeration cycles should not be interrupted to remove items for use.
- Items should remain in aerators until the aeration time has been completed.
- Aeration requirements for the most difficult-to-aerate products may require increased aeration time.

Ethylene oxide vapors and residues diffuse from sterilized items over time. This aeration or degassing process can be expedited by raising the temperature and by increasing the flow of air around the item.

VIII.f.5. Device manufacturers' written instructions should be followed for specific aeration requirements.

VIII.f.6. All aeration cycle parameters should be documented and the correct aeration time and temperature verified.

VIII.f.7. A program for monitoring occupational exposure to ethylene oxide must be established to document that worker exposure to ethylene oxide is below permissible exposure limits established by OSHA.

Compliance with regulations promotes a safe work environment that is within federal and state mandated limits.[30,33]

VIII.g. Personnel who have the potential for exposure should wear ethylene oxide-monitoring badges that meet the National Institute for Occupational Safety and Health standards for accuracy.[26,30,34] *[1: Regulatory Requirement]*

VIII.g.1. The ethylene oxide monitoring program in each organization must comply with OSHA regulations.

General environmental monitoring is not required, although it may provide an indicator of problems with the ventilation or ethylene oxide system. Monitoring of short-term exposures during a 15-minute period also is required while sterilization and aeration activities are being performed.

Permissible limits, as established by OSHA, for exposure to ethylene oxide are 1 part per million (ppm) of airborne ethylene oxide expressed as a time weighted average for an eight-hour work shift in a 40-hour work week, or 5 ppm for short-term exposure.[1,26,30]

VIII.h. Health and safety procedures should be developed for health care personnel who are at risk for exposure to ethylene oxide.[26] *[1: Regulatory Requirement]*

Established procedures help to identify, eliminate, or minimize risk from exposure to hazards as well as facilitate timely responses to accidental exposure and emergencies.

VIII.h.1. Personnel must be informed about the health effects and potential hazards associated with exposure to ethylene oxide.[30]

VIII.h.2. Information on ethylene oxide health effects and potential hazards must be provided at the time of assignment to an area where ethylene oxide is used and at least annually thereafter.[30]

VIII.h.3. Periodic employee and environmental physical assessment and testing should be carried out and documented according to current OSHA regulations.[26,30]

VIII.h.4. Personnel should be familiar with the organization's emergency spill plan.[30]

VIII.h.5. Personnel should be aware of safety procedures that should be implemented following exposure to ethylene oxide. The material safety data sheet (MSDS) for the type of ethylene oxide used should be consulted for specific first-aid measures after exposure. People who have inhaled concentrated ethylene oxide gas

- should seek fresh air immediately,
- may require the administration of oxygen, and
- may require cardiopulmonary resuscitation if respiratory or cardiac collapse occurs.[26,30,31]

VIII.i. Documentation of employee monitoring must be maintained in compliance with federal regulations. *[1: Regulatory Requirement]*

Regulations from OSHA require that documentation of employee breathing zone monitoring must be maintained in employees' health records for the duration of employment plus 30 years after termination of employment.[26,30]

Documentation establishes a continuous history of the work environment.

Recommendation IX

Low-temperature hydrogen peroxide gas plasma sterilization methods should be used to sterilize moisture- and heat-sensitive items and when indicated by the device manufacturer.[35]

Low-temperature hydrogen peroxide gas plasma sterilization uses a combination of hydrogen peroxide vapor and low-temperature hydrogen peroxide gas plasma. In this process, hydrogen peroxide, a strong oxidizing agent, kills microorganisms via the hydroxyl free radical. The hydroxyl free radical, being highly reactive, can attack membrane lipids, DNA, and other essential cell components. The plasma breaks down the hydrogen peroxide into a "cloud" of highly energized species that recombine, converting the hydrogen peroxide into water and oxygen.

Items processed using low-temperature hydrogen peroxide gas plasma do not require aeration because the residuals and by-products are oxygen and water in the form of humidity, and these by-products are nontoxic.[35,36] Items are dry at the end of the cycle. Hydrogen peroxide is an irritant of the eyes, mucous membranes, and skin.[37] It is considered nonmutagenic and noncarcenogenic.[38,39]

IX.a. The sterilizer manufacturer's written instructions for use, monitoring, and maintenance should be followed when using a low-temperature hydrogen peroxide gas plasma sterilization system.[35] *[4: Limited Evidence]*

IX.a.1. Written documentation of the acceptability of low-temperature hydrogen peroxide gas plasma sterilization for specific devices should be obtained from the device and sterilizer manufacturers.

IX.a.2. Devices with lumens should be evaluated to determine whether the lumen diameter and length are within the sterilizer manufacturer's acceptable dimensions as specified in the sterilizer manufacturer's instructions for use.[35,40]

IX.a.3. The placement of items within the chamber should comply with the sterilizer manufacturer's instructions for use.

Correct placement and configuration of items within the chamber facilitates contact of the sterilant with the items to be sterilized. Sterilant contact is essential for sterilization.[6]

IX.b. Items to be sterilized using low-temperature hydrogen peroxide gas plasma sterilization should be clean, thoroughly dry, and packaged in sterilization wraps, pouches, trays, or containers cleared by the FDA for use in hydrogen peroxide gas plasma. *[1: Strong Evidence]*

Liquids and cellulose-based (ie, paper-based) packaging materials or products are not suitable for low-temperature hydrogen peroxide gas plasma sterilization.[1]

IX.b.1. Trays, mats, containers, and other accessories designed and validated for use with low-temperature hydrogen peroxide gas plasma should be used.

IX.c. A quality monitoring program that includes physical monitors (eg, printouts, digital readings, graphs, gauges), chemical indicators, and biological indicators should be used. *[1: Strong Evidence]*

These monitors and indicators verify that conditions necessary for sterilization have been met.[6]

IX.c.1. Each sterilization cycle should be monitored to verify that parameters required for sterilization have been met.[6]

IX.c.2. The sterilizer operator should use physical monitors to verify cycle parameters for every load.

Physical monitors can indicate immediate sterilizer failure. Physical monitors record cycle parameters (eg, pressure, time) for each cycle.

IX.c.3. Chemical and biological indicators should be used to monitor sterilizer efficacy and to assess whether parameters of sterilization have been achieved.[6]

IX.c.4. A class 1 chemical indicator should be placed on the outside of every package unless the internal indicator is visible.[6]

IX.c.5. An FDA-cleared chemical indicator recommended by the manufacturer of the selected sterilization system should be placed within each package to be sterilized.[6,41]

IX.c.6. Biological monitors should be used to assess sterilizer efficacy.[6] Routine sterilizer efficacy monitoring should be performed daily, preferably with every load.[35]

Recommendation X

Low-temperature hydrogen peroxide vapor sterilization methods should be used for moisture- and heat-sensitive items and when indicated by the device manufacturer.

Low-temperature hydrogen peroxide vapor sterilization uses vaporized hydrogen peroxide as the sterilant. For this process, hydrogen peroxide sterilant is introduced into the chamber through a vaporizer under low pressure, creating a vapor that fills the sterilization chamber. As the hydrogen peroxide vapor diffuses and contacts surfaces, an oxidative process inactivates microorganisms. Devices sterilized using this process do not require aeration because the by-products are oxygen and water vapor, which are nontoxic.[1,42]

X.a. The sterilizer manufacturer's written instructions for use, monitoring, and maintenance should be followed when using a low-temperature hydrogen peroxide vapor sterilization system.[35] *[4: Limited Evidence]*

X.a.1. Written documentation of the acceptability of low-temperature hydrogen peroxide vapor should be obtained from the device manufacturer or the sterilizer manufacturer's list of validated devices.

X.a.2. Devices with lumens should be evaluated to determine whether the lumen diameter and length are within the sterilizer manufacturer's acceptable dimensions as specified in the instructions for use.[42]

X.a.3. Items should be placed within the chamber in compliance with the sterilizer manufacturer's instructions for use.

Correct placement and configuration of items within the chamber facilitates contact of the sterilant with the items to be sterilized. Sterilant contact is essential for sterilization.[6]

X.b. Items to be sterilized using low-temperature hydrogen peroxide vapor should be clean, thoroughly dry, and packaged in sterilization wraps, pouches, trays, or containers cleared by the FDA for use in the specific low-temperature hydrogen peroxide vapor system. *[1: Strong Evidence]*

Liquids and cellulose-based (eg, paper-based) packaging materials or products and liquids are not suitable for low-temperature hydrogen peroxide vapor sterilization.[1]

X.b.1. Trays, mats, containers, and other accessories designed and validated for use with low-temperature hydrogen peroxide vapor sterilization should be used.

X.c. A quality monitoring program that includes physical monitors (eg, printouts, digital readings, graphs, gauges), chemical indicators, and biological indicators should be used to verify that conditions necessary for sterilization have been met.[6] *[1: Strong Evidence]*

X.c.1. Each sterilization cycle should be monitored to verify that parameters required for sterilization have been met.[6]

X.c.2. The sterilizer operator should use physical monitors to verify that required sterilization parameters are met for every load.[6]

Physical monitors can indicate immediate sterilizer failure. Physical monitors record cycle parameters (eg, time, pressure) for each cycle.

X.c.3. Chemical and biological indicators should be used to monitor sterilizer efficacy and to assess whether parameters of sterilization have been achieved.[6] Efficacy testing should be performed in accordance with manufacturers' instructions.

X.c.4. A class 1 chemical indicator should be placed on the outside of every package unless the internal indicator is visible.[6]

X.c.5. An FDA-cleared chemical indicator recommended by the manufacturer of the selected sterilization system should be placed within each package to be sterilized.[6,41]

Recommendation XI

Sterilization systems using ozone should be used for moisture- and heat-sensitive items when indicated by the device manufacturer.

Ozone has been cleared by the FDA for use in the sterilization of metal and plastic surgical instruments, including some instruments with lumens.[43] Ozone is a strong oxidizer, which makes ozone sterilization an effective low-temperature sterilization process. Ozone is generated within the sterilizer using only oxygen and water. On completion of the sterilization cycle, ozone is exhausted through a catalytic converter, where it is converted back into the raw materials of oxygen and water. No aeration of sterilized items is necessary because these by-products are nontoxic.[35,36,44]

XI.a. Manufacturers' written instruction for operating, monitoring, and maintaining ozone sterilizers should be followed. *[4: Limited Evidence]*

XI.a.1. Written documentation of the acceptability of ozone sterilization should be obtained from the device manufacturer or the sterilizer manufacturer's list of validated devices.

XI.a.2. Devices with lumens should be evaluated to determine whether lumen diameter and length are within the sterilizer manufacturer's acceptable dimensions as specified in the instructions for use.

XI.b. Items to be sterilized using ozone should be packaged in nonwoven pouches or reusable rigid sterilization containers cleared by the FDA

for use in ozone sterilizers.[35,44] *[3: Moderate Evidence]*

Cellulose-based (eg, paper-based) packaging materials or products are not suitable for ozone sterilization.[43]

XI.c. Items should be placed in the sterilizer chamber in compliance with the sterilizer manufacturer's instructions for use. *[4: Limited Evidence]*

Correct placement and configuration of items in the chamber facilitates contact of the sterilant with the items to be sterilized. Sterilant contact is essential for sterilization.[6]

XI.d. A quality monitoring program that includes physical monitors (eg, printouts, digital readings, graphs, gauges), chemical indicators, and biological indicators should be used to verify that conditions necessary for sterilization have been met.[6] *[1: Strong Evidence]*

XI.d.1. Each sterilization cycle should be monitored to verify that parameters required for sterilization have been met.[6]

XI.d.2. The sterilizer operator should use physical monitors to verify parameters for every load.[6]

Physical monitors can indicate immediate sterilizer failure. Physical monitors record cycle parameters (eg, time, pressure) for each cycle.

XI.d.3. Chemical and biological indicators should be used to monitor sterilizer efficacy and to assess whether parameters of sterilization have been achieved.[6] Efficacy testing should be performed in accordance with manufacturers' instructions.

XI.d.4. A class 1 chemical indicator should be located on the outside of every package unless the internal indicator is visible.[6]

XI.d.5. An FDA-cleared chemical indicator recommended by the manufacturer of the selected sterilization system should be placed within each package to be sterilized.[6,41]

Recommendation XII

Dry-heat sterilization should be used only for materials that are impenetrable to moist heat.[1] Dry heat may be used to sterilize anhydrous (ie, waterless) items that can withstand high temperatures and when indicated by the device manufacturer.

Sharp instruments that would be damaged by the moisture of steam may be sterilized by dry heat.[45] Dental instruments, burrs, reusable needles, glassware, and heat-stable powders and oils are examples of items that can withstand the high temperatures generated by dry-heat sterilization. Dry heat is an oxidation or slow-burning process that coagulates protein in microbial cells. Sterilization is accomplished through the transfer of heat energy to objects on contact. There is no moisture present in a dry-heat process, so microorganisms are destroyed by a very slow process of heat absorption.[46]

Presterilized oils and powders are commercially available and may eliminate the need for a dry heat sterilizer.

XII.a. Dry-heat sterilizers should be used, monitored, and maintained according to the manufacturer's written instructions.[46] *[4: Limited Evidence]*

Dry-heat sterilizers may vary in design and performance characteristics.

XII.b. Only packaging and container materials designed and validated by the packaging manufacturer to withstand the high temperature of dry-heat sterilization should be used.[46] *[4: Limited Evidence]*

If packaging is not formulated for dry-heat sterilization, pouches may char, compromising the package integrity of sterilized items.

XII.b.1. Closed containers or cassettes should be used based on the manufacturer's instructions and biological indicator monitoring results. Closed containers or cassettes may extend the time needed to achieve sterilization.

XII.b.2. Packaging manufacturers should be consulted to confirm the compatibility of the packaging material with sterilizer temperatures before packaging materials are selected for dry-heat sterilization.[46]

Most types of tape are not designed to withstand the high temperatures of dry-heat sterilization. Tape adhesive melts when subjected to dry-heat sterilization and may leave a sticky residue on sterilized packages that degrades, leaving baked-on tape residue on the items, or can result in loss of tape adhesion.[46]

XII.b.3. When possible, small containers should be used for items to be dry-heat sterilized, and package density should be as low as possible.[46]

XII.c. Items should be placed within the sterilizer chamber according to the sterilizer manufacturer's instructions for use. *[4: Limited Evidence]*

Correct placement and configuration of items within the chamber facilitates contact of the sterilant with the items to be sterilized. Sterilant contact is essential for sterilization.[46]

XII.d. The operator should be aware of the hazards associated with dry-heat sterilization and use the appropriate PPE (eg, insulated gloves, transfer handles).[46] *[4: Limited Evidence]*

Burns are the most common safety hazard associated with dry-heat sterilization.[46]

XII.d.1. On completion of a dry-heat sterilization cycle, both the sterilizer chamber and the items in the chamber are very hot and should not be touched.

XII.d.2. Packages should be cooled before being handled or removed from the dry-heat sterilizer.

XII.e. A quality monitoring program that includes physical monitors (eg, printouts, digital readings, graphs, gauges), chemical indicators, and biological indicators should be used to verify that conditions necessary for sterilization have been met.[46] *[1: Strong Evidence]*

XII.e.1. Each sterilization cycle should be monitored to verify that parameters for sterilization have been met.[46]

XII.e.2. The sterilizer operator should use physical monitors to verify parameters for every load.[6]

Physical monitors can indicate immediate sterilizer failure. Physical monitors record cycle parameters (eg, time, pressure) for each cycle.

XII.e.3. A class 1 chemical indicator should be located on the outside of every package unless the internal indicator is visible.[6]

XII.e.4. An FDA-cleared chemical indicator recommended by the manufacturer of the selected sterilization system should be placed within each package to be sterilized.[6,41]

Recommendation XIII

Liquid chemical sterilant instrument processing systems that use peracetic acid as a low-temperature sterilant should be used for devices that are heat-sensitive, can be immersed, are approved for this process by the device manufacturer, and cannot be sterilized using terminal sterilization methods.[47,48]

Peracetic acid is an oxidizing agent that is an effective biocide at low temperatures and is effective in the presence of organic matter.[1] It has a chemical formula of acetic acid plus an extra oxygen atom. This extra oxygen atom is highly reactive, reacts with most cellular components, and causes cellular death. The ability of peracetic acid to inactivate many different critical cell systems is responsible for its broad spectrum antimicrobial activity. As peracetic acid returns to acetic acid (ie, vinegar) and the oxygen decomposes, it is rendered nontoxic and environmentally safe. Following liquid chemical sterilant processing, devices are rinsed with potable tap water that has been passed through pre-filters, subjected to an ultraviolet light treatment, and then passed through two 0.1-micron filter membranes.[47]

XIII.a. Liquid chemical sterilant systems using peracetic acid should be used only to process items validated for processing in liquid peracetic acid.[1,48] *[1: Strong Evidence]*

Items processed in liquid chemical sterilant systems that are not validated for these systems may not be compatible with the sterilant or the process, which could result in damage or an ineffective process.

XIII.a.1. The ability to successfully process devices intended for use with a liquid chemical sterilant system that uses peracetic acid should be validated by the device manufacturer and comply with the liquid chemical sterilant processing system manufacturer's written instructions.[35]

Processing devices that are incompatible with liquid chemical sterilant processing systems can shorten the life of the devices.

XIII.a.2. Documentation of devices that can and cannot be processed in liquid chemical sterilant systems using peracetic acid should be obtained from the device and the liquid chemical sterilant system manufacturers.

XIII.b. Critical items processed in liquid chemical sterilant systems should be used immediately and not stored for later use or held from one procedure to another.[47] [1: Strong Evidence]

Processing trays used in liquid chemical sterilant systems are not intended for storage of processed items.

XIII.c. Systems using liquid peracetic acid should be used, monitored, and maintained according to the manufacturer's written instructions. [4: Limited Evidence]

Peracetic acid is an effective sterilizing agent that does not leave toxic residues on sterilized items when items are rinsed properly. Serious injuries (eg, burns) may result if the chemical is not handled, neutralized, and rinsed properly. Peracetic acid is corrosive to the skin at concentrations of 3.4% or higher and corrosive to the eyes at concentrations of 0.35% or higher.[49]

XIII.d. When using liquid chemical sterilant processing systems, health care personnel should verify proper selection of adapters and connect the device to the appropriate adapters as recommended by the manufacturer of both the device and the liquid chemical sterilant processing system.[50] [3: Moderate Evidence]

Failure to do so may result in failure of the liquid chemical sterilant to contact the lumen of the item.

XIII.e. Items processed in a liquid chemical sterilant system using peracetic acid should be transported to the point of use and used immediately.[1] [1: Strong Evidence]

Items processed with peracetic acid are wet and the cassette or container in which they are processed is not sealed to prevent contamination, thereby increasing the risk of contamination if the items are not used immediately.

XIII.f. A quality monitoring program that includes physical monitors (eg, printouts, digital readings, graphs, gauges) and chemical indicators should be used to verify that conditions necessary for processing have been met.[1,6] [1: Strong Evidence]

XIII.f.1. Each sterilization cycle should be monitored to verify that parameters required for processing have been met.[6]

XIII.f.2. The liquid chemical sterilant processing system operator should use physical monitors to verify that parameters required for processing have been met.[35]

Physical monitors can indicate immediate failure to achieve required parameters.

XIII.f.3. Each cycle should be monitored with a chemical indicator validated for use in the liquid chemical sterilant system according to the manufacturer's instructions for use.[35] Biological indicators have not been cleared by the FDA for use with liquid peracetic acid systems.

Recommendation XIV

A formalized program between the health care organization and health care industry representatives should be established for the receipt and use of loaned instrumentation.[51]

Implementation of tracking and quality controls and procedures is necessary to manage instrumentation and implants that are brought in from outside organizations and companies.[52]

XIV.a. Interdisciplinary collaboration between health care organizations' sterile processing and surgical services personnel and commercial health care industry representatives should be established.[6] [4: Limited Evidence]

The systematic management of loaned instrumentation reduces loss and ensures proper decontamination and sterilization through increased collaboration, communication, and accountability.

XIV.b. The loaned instrumentation program should include processes to
- request loaned instrumentation or implants;
- receive loaned items, including a detailed inventory list;
- obtain manufacturers' written instructions for instrument care, cleaning, assembly, and sterilization;
- determine responsibility for ensuring sets weigh no more than 25 lb;
- clean, decontaminate, and sterilize loaned instrumentation at the receiving facility in accordance with AORN's Guideline for Cleaning and Care of Surgical Instruments[4];
- transport processed loaned instrumentation to the point of use;
- return items to the sterile processing department after the procedure for decontamination, processing, inventory, and return to the health care industry representative; and

○ maintain records of transactions.
[4: Limited Evidence]

XIV.c. The manufacturer's instructions for cleaning, packaging, and sterilizing should be obtained before loaned items are received.[52] *[4: Limited Evidence]*

Advanced delivery of instructions for cleaning, packaging, and sterilizing is useful in determining whether a facility has the required equipment and resources to process loaned instruments according to the device manufacturer's written instructions.

XIV.d. Personnel should coordinate requests for loaned instrumentation in sufficient time for loaned items to be processed by conventional terminal sterilization methods.[52] *[4: Limited Evidence]*

Advanced delivery of loaned items to the receiving health care organization ensures sufficient time to permit inhouse disassembly, cleaning, packaging, quality assurance testing, and sterilization of the instruments before scheduled procedures.

XIV.d.1. Personnel requesting loaned items should specify quantities, estimated time of use and return, and restocking requirements to circumvent the need for IUSS.

XIV.d.2. Late receipt of loaned instruments should not be used to justify IUSS.[23,53]

XIV.e. Sterility assurance related to loaned instruments should begin at the point at which the health care organization assumes responsibility for the items.[6] *[4: Limited Evidence]*

Failures in instrument cleaning have resulted in transmission of infectious agents.[24,53]

XIV.e.1. All loaned instruments, regardless of whether they were processed in another health care facility, should be considered contaminated and delivered directly to the sterile processing department for decontamination.[51] Instruments should be thoroughly cleaned and dried in a manner consistent with AORN's Guideline for Cleaning and Care of Surgical Instruments[4] and the guidelines of the Association for the Advancement of Medical Instrumentation (AAMI)[51] before sterilization.

It is not possible to know under what conditions instruments were processed at another facility. Sterilized instruments may become contaminated during transport.

XIV.e.2. Newly manufactured loaned items should be properly decontaminated before sterilization to remove bioburden and substances (eg, oil, grease) that may remain on the item from the manufacturing process.[6]

XIV.e.3. Loaned instruments should be removed from external shipping containers before transport to the sterile processing area.[6]

External shipping containers may have potentially high microbial contamination because of environmental exposure during transport.

XIV.e.4. Rigid sterilization containers should be thoroughly inspected upon receipt and cleaned and decontaminated according to the container manufacturer's instructions.

XIV.e.5. The type and quantity of loaned items should be inventoried and documented.

XIV.e.6. Implants and instruments should be visually inspected for damage.

XIV.e.7. Manufacturers' instructions for processing and sterilizing loaned items should be followed.

XIV.e.8. Implantable devices should be sterilized with a biological indicator and a class 5 integrating indicator and documented in accordance with regulatory requirements and AORN guidelines.

XIV.e.9. After use, loaned items should be decontaminated and returned to the lender in accordance with the health care organization's policy.

Recommendation XV

Sterilized materials should be labeled and stored in a manner to ensure sterility, and each item should be marked with the sterilization date.[6]

Limiting exposure to moisture, dust, excessive light or handling, and temperature and humidity extremes decreases potential contamination of sterilized items.[6] Factors that contribute to contamination include air movement, humidity, temperature, location of storage, presence of vermin, whether shelving is open or closed, and properties of the packaging material.[1]

XV.a. The shelf life of a packaged sterile item should be considered event-related. *[3: Moderate Evidence]*

Shelf life is dependent on packaging material, storage conditions, transport, and handling. An event must occur to compromise package content sterility. Events that may compromise the sterility of a package include
○ multiple instances of handling that leads to seal breakage or loss of package integrity,
○ moisture penetration, and
○ exposure to airborne contaminants.[6,26,46]
Several studies have resulted in data that support event-related shelf life. One study examined the effect of time on the sterility of peel pouches, paper envelopes, and nylon sleeves and showed no increased rate of contamination over time when packages were placed in covered storage.[54] Another study showed that items covered with 3 mil (3/1,000 inch) polyethylene overwrap were

sterile nine months after sterilization.[1] Another microbiological study examined items after two years of storage and showed no contamination.[55] The prospective study, which was conducted over a two-year period, evaluated the effectiveness of event-related shelf life and included placing 152 items that were terminally sterilized on shelves in various wards. Every three months, several items were tested for microbial contamination and all were found to be sterile.

XV.b. Sterile packages should be stored under environmentally controlled conditions.[6] *[4: Limited Evidence]*

Controlled conditions reduce the risk of contamination of sterile items.

XV.b.1. Room temperature, humidity, and ventilation should be controlled in accordance with local, state, and federal policies and regulations.

Regulatory agencies may enforce American Society for Healthcare Engineering (ASHE)[56] or AAMI[6] recommendations or they may enforce other guidelines. As stated in the ASHE document, these parameters are intended to be used for the design of the heating, ventilation, and air-conditioning (HVAC) systems and there may be daily fluctuations based on the environmental conditions.

Recommendations from AAMI include that temperature in sterile storage areas not exceed 75° F (24° C), that there be a minimum of 4 air exchanges per hour, and that relative humidity is between 20% and 60% and not higher than 70%.[6] The ASHE recommends temperatures in the sterile storage area of between 72° F to 78° F (22° C to 26° C) and that humidity not exceed 60%.[56]

Research on the relationship between temperature, humidity, air exchange, and maintenance of sterility is lacking.

XV.b.2. When selecting a temperature and humidity level or range, the perioperative team should collaborate with infection preventionists and facility engineers and consider the pathogens that pose risk to patients and personnel and the effect of temperature and humidity on those organisms.

Other considerations when determining temperature and humidity levels include personnel comfort and the fact that high temperature and humidity levels may lead to the development of condensate on walls and surfaces, which could serve as a wicking agent for the transmission of microorganisms and result in contamination of sterile items.

XV.b.3. Access to sterile supply areas should be limited to personnel who are trained in handling sterile supplies.

XV.b.4. Sterile storage areas, including racks, shelves, bins, and containers, should be kept clean and dry.[57]

XV.b.5. Supplies should be stored in a manner that allows adequate air circulation and ease of cleaning in compliance with local fire codes and in a manner that reduces the risk of contamination.

Recommendations for supply storage are generally 8 to 10 inches from the floor and 2 inches from outside walls. Fire code regulations specify the minimum clearance between sprinkler heads and stored items, with the typical minimum distance being 18 inches, to allow the sprinkler system to be effective.[58]

XV.b.6. Sterile items should not be stored under sinks or in other locations where they can become wet.[1]

XV.b.7. Sterile items should be stored in closed cabinets or covered carts. Open shelving may be used if it is located in a secure, environmentally controlled, clean area.[1]

XV.b.8. Supplies and equipment should be removed from external shipping containers and web-edged or corrugated cardboard boxes before transfer into the sterile storage area.

External shipping containers and web-edged cardboard boxes may collect dust, debris, and insects during shipment and may carry contaminants into the surgical suite.[6,26,46]

Recommendation XVI

Transportation of sterile items should be controlled.

Sterility is event-related and is dependent on the amount of handling, the conditions during transportation and storage, and the quality of the packaging material.[1]

XVI.a. Sterile items should be transported in covered or enclosed carts with solid-bottom shelves.[6] *[4: Limited Evidence]*

Covered or enclosed carts protect sterile items from exposure to environmental contaminants during transportation.

XVI.b. Carts and reusable covers should be cleaned after each use. *[4: Limited Evidence]*

Contaminants may be picked up from the environment during transport.[6]

STERILIZATION AND DISINFECTION

STERILIZATION

Recommendation XVII

Personnel should receive initial and ongoing education and competency validation for sterilization practices.

Initial and ongoing education of perioperative personnel on sterilization practices facilitates the development of knowledge, skills, and attitudes that affect safe patient care.

Periodic educational programs provide the opportunity to reinforce the principles of sterilization, the compatibility of equipment and accessories, and the potential hazards to patients and personnel; and to introduce new information on technology changes and new applications.

Competency validation measures individual performance and provides a mechanism for documentation. Competency assessment verifies that perioperative personnel have an understanding of sterilization and sterilization practices.

XVII.a. An introduction to and review of policies and procedures should be included in personnel orientation to sterile processing of surgical instruments in the perioperative setting. Continuing education should be provided for employees when new equipment, instruments, and processes are introduced. *[5: Benefits Balanced with Harms]*

Operator and processing errors may be minimized with regularly scheduled education, training, and competency demonstration.

XVII.b. Sterilization-specific education and competency assessment should encompass all sterilization methodologies that are in use in the organization, including
  ○ operation and maintenance of sterilization equipment;
  ○ selection and monitoring of sterilization cycles;
  ○ use of chemical, biological, and physical monitors; and
  ○ documentation requirements.
  [5: Benefits Balanced with Harms]

XVII.c. Education should address topics that include
  ○ orientation to equipment and work areas;
  ○ infection control policies and procedures, including exposure plans;
  ○ potential hazards in the environment and methods of hazard protection;
  ○ safe ergonomic practices;
  ○ use and location of MSDSs; and
  ○ standards, guidelines, recommended practices, and regulations related to instrument processing.
  [5: Benefits Balanced with Harms]

Recommendation XVIII

Documentation should reflect activities related to sterilization.[6]

Documentation demonstrates compliance with regulatory and accrediting agency requirements and identifies trends and quality improvement opportunities.

XVIII.a. Sterilization records should be maintained for the amount of time specified in the health care organization's policies and should be in compliance with professional standards and local, state, and federal regulations.[1,6,26,46] *[3: Moderate Evidence]*

Accurate and complete records are required for process verification and are used in sterilizer function analysis.

XVIII.b. Every sterilization cycle and modality, including steam (eg, gravity-displacement, dynamic air-removal), ethylene oxide, hydrogen peroxide gas plasma, hydrogen peroxide vapor, ozone, and dry heat should be documented. Documentation should include
  ○ contents of each load;
  ○ load identification;
  ○ exposure parameters;
  ○ the operator's name or initials; and
  ○ results of physical, chemical, and biological monitors.[1]
  [1: Strong Evidence]

Recommendation XIX

Policies and procedures for sterilization and sterilization-related processes and practices should be developed, reviewed periodically, revised as necessary, and readily available in the practice setting.

Policies and procedures assist in the development of patient safety, quality assessment, and performance improvement activities. Policies and procedures establish authority, responsibility, and accountability within the facility. They also serve as operational guidelines that are used to minimize patient risk factors for complications, standardize practice, direct perioperative personnel, and establish continual performance improvement programs.

XIX.a. The recommendations for sterilization should be used to guide the development of policies and procedures within individual perioperative practice settings. *[5: Benefits Balanced with Harms]*

XIX.b. Policies and procedures should be developed and implemented for processes including
  ○ routine cleaning of sterilizer chambers, carts, and exterior surfaces;
  ○ transport of contaminated devices and equipment to the decontamination area;
  ○ selection of sterilization modality and cycle;
  ○ evaluation and selection of sterilization equipment and accessories[59];
  ○ release of implants that are not terminally sterilized;
  ○ care and handling of loaned instruments;

STERILIZATION AND DISINFECTION

974

- orientation of and competency review for personnel who are responsible for sterilizing items;
- sterilization of items intended for immediate use;
- documentation of sterilization processes, environmental conditions, load contents, and load numbers;
- sterilization process monitoring;
- sterilization equipment maintenance;
- storage of sterile items;
- transport and distribution of sterile items; and
- product testing.

[5: Benefits Balanced with Harms]

Capital equipment and medical device procurement are collaborative processes that require clinical, business, financial, and legal acumen. Goals of product standardization and value analysis processes are to select functional and reliable products that are safe, cost-effective, and environmentally friendly and that promote quality care and avoid duplication or rapid obsolescence.

XIX.c. The sterilizer manufacturer's written instructions for cleaning, operation, and maintenance should be reviewed and reflected in instrument processing policies and procedures. *[5: Benefits Balanced with Harms]*

XIX.c.1. User manuals for all sterilization equipment should be readily available to the sterilizer operators.

As new sterilization technologies are introduced for use in perioperative practice settings, it is imperative that health care personnel strictly follow manufacturers' written instructions for the operation and maintenance of sterilization equipment and be aware of the occupational hazards that different sterilants may pose to patients, health care personnel, and the environment.

XIX.c.2. Equipment and device manuals that provide instructions for use should be retained for the life of the device and sterilizer.

Recommendation XX

A quality assurance and performance improvement process should be in place to measure patient, process, and system outcome indicators.

Quality assurance and performance improvement programs assist in evaluating the quality of patient care and the formulation of plans for corrective actions. These programs provide data that may be used to determine whether an individual organization is within benchmark goals and, if not, identify areas that may require corrective actions.

XX.a. The health care organization should establish quality control and improvement programs to monitor the workplace environment and practices associated with cleaning, disinfection, and sterilization of surgical instruments.[6] *[4: Limited Evidence]*

Monitoring the sterilization process allows results to be compared to a predetermined level of quality. Reviewing the findings provides information identifying problems and trends, which can be used to improve practice.

XX.a.1. Physical, chemical, and biological monitors should be used to monitor sterilization processes. They should be used for routine load release, routine sterilizer efficacy testing, and sterilizer qualification testing (eg, after installation, relocation, malfunction, major repair, sterilization process failure). Table 5 and Table 6 illustrate recommendations for process monitoring and types of monitors, respectively.

XX.b. All sterilizer failures and corrective actions should be documented and reported to the infection preventionist, quality assurance or risk management committee, and to administrators.[6] *[4: Limited Evidence]*

XX.c. All physical, chemical, and biological monitoring results, including results from controls, should be interpreted by qualified personnel in the time frame specified by the manufacturer of the monitor and should be included in the sterilization records. *[4: Limited Evidence]*

Accurate interpretation and reporting of results promotes safe patient care.[6]

XX.d. Immediate investigation and corrective action should be taken in the event of a physical, chemical, or biological monitor failure.[6] *[4: Limited Evidence]*

XX.d.1. The sterilizer printout should be checked first to determine whether cycle parameters were met. If parameters were not met, the sterilizer should be removed from service, the load should be quarantined, and the cause of the failure should be investigated.[6]

XX.d.2. If the cause of the failure is immediately identified (eg, operator error) or the failure is confined to a single item within the load, the cause should be corrected, the sterilizer returned to service, and the load reprocessed.[6]

XX.d.3. If the cause of the failure is not immediately identified, the load should be quarantined and the sterilizer taken out of service. The cause should be investigated and the sterilizer only returned to service when the cause is identified and rectified.[6]

XX.d.4. If they are retrievable, items that were processed in the suspect sterilizer (ie, back to the last known negative biological indicator test) should be recalled and reprocessed before use.[6] When a tracking system

TABLE 5. STEAM STERILIZATION PROCESS MONITORING RECOMMENDATIONS[1]

Routine load release		Routine sterilizer efficacy monitoring	Sterilizer qualification testing (after installation, relocation, malfunction, major repair, sterilization process failure)	Periodic product quality assurance testing
Nonimplants	Implants			
Physical monitoring of cycle	Physical monitoring of cycle	Physical monitoring of cycle	Physical monitoring of cycle	Physical monitoring of cycle
External and internal chemical indicator (CI) monitoring of packages	External and internal CI monitoring of packages	External and internal CI monitoring of packages	External and internal CI monitoring of packages	Placement of BIs and CIs within product test sample
Optional monitoring of the load with a process challenge device (PCD) containing one of the following: • a biological indicator (BI) • a BI and a class 5 integrating indicator • a class 5 integrating indicator • a class 6 emulating indicator	Monitoring of every load with a PCD containing a BI and a class 5 integrating indicator	Weekly, preferably daily (ie, each day the sterilizer is used), monitoring with a PCD containing a BI; the PCD also may contain a CI For sterilizers larger than 2 cubic feet and for table-top sterilizers, monitoring performed in a fully loaded chamber In immediate use steam sterilization (IUSS) cycles, monitoring performed in an empty chamber For dynamic air-removal sterilizers, daily Bowie-Dick testing in an empty chamber	For sterilizers larger than 2 cubic feet and for IUSS cycles, monitoring of three consecutive cycles in an empty chamber with a PCD containing a BI; the PCD also may contain a CI For table-top sterilizers, monitoring of three consecutive cycles in a fully loaded chamber with a PCD containing a BI; the PCD also may contain a CI For dynamic air-removal sterilizers, monitoring of three consecutive cycles in an empty chamber with a Bowie-Dick test pack	

REFERENCE
1. Association for the Advancement of Medical Instrumentation. ANSI/AAMI ST79:2010, A1:2010 & A2:2011, Comprehensive guide to steam sterilization and sterility assurance in health care facilities. Arlington, VA: Association for the Advancement of Medical Instrumentation; 2010 & 2011. Adapted and reprinted with permission. Further reproduction or distribution prohibited.

is present, it can be used to identify items and the patient or patients on whom the items may have been used before it was known that the items should be retrieved. This information can be used to determine further patient care.

• The positive biological indicator vial should be sent to the laboratory for subculturing for bacilli. The recall should not be delayed during this testing.

• All actions taken in response to a positive biological indicator should be documented.

A positive control should be placed in each incubator each day a test vial is run and incubated. The control and the test vials should be from the same lot.[6]

XX.d.5. Positive biological indicator results should be reported immediately so that appropriate action can be taken.

XX.e. Processed items should be labeled with load control numbers to identify the sterilizer used, the cycle or load number, and the date of sterilization. Where tracking systems exist, documentation should be used to track instruments to the patient on whom they were used. *[4: Limited Evidence]*

Load control numbers allow items to be identified or retrieved in the event of a sterilizer failure or malfunction.[6,26,46]

XX.e.1. Information should be recorded from each sterilization cycle and should include the
• identification of the sterilizer (eg, "sterilizer #1"),
• type of sterilizer and cycle used,
• load control number,
• load contents (eg, major set, Kelly clamps),
• critical parameters for the specific sterilization methodology (eg, exposure time, temperature for steam sterilization),
• operator's name, and

- results of sterilization process monitoring (ie, biological, chemical, physical).[1] Documentation is an important component of a quality control program.

XX.f. Physical monitors should be used to verify that parameters (eg, time, temperature, pressure, humidity, gas concentration) for sterilization have been met. *[4: Limited Evidence]*

Physical monitoring provides real-time assessments of cycle conditions as well as historic records by means of printouts, digital readings, graphs, or gauges. Reviewing data from physical monitoring can readily identify sterilizer malfunctions to expedite corrective actions.[6]

XX.f.1. Recordings of physical data should be used, when available, for all sterilization methods to ascertain that sterilization systems function within manufacturers' specifications.[6,26]

XX.f.2. The printout should be reviewed at the end of each cycle and signed by the sterilizer operator, verifying that all sterilization parameters were met.

XX.g. A sterilization chemical indicator should be used inside and outside of each package that is sterilized.[1,6,26] *[1: Strong Evidence]*

- An external indicator should be used on the outside of each package unless the internal indicator is visible.[6]
- Chemical indicators should be reviewed for a proper end point response (eg, color, migration, other change).
- An FDA-cleared chemical indicator recommended by the manufacturer of the selected sterilization system should be placed within each package to be sterilized.[6]

The purpose of the external chemical indicator is to differentiate between processed and unprocessed items.[41] Chemical indicators do not establish whether the item is sterile, but they do demonstrate that the contents were exposed to the sterilant.[41] Although chemical indicators do not verify sterility, they help detect procedural errors and equipment malfunctions.

XX.g.1. If the interpretation of the external or internal process monitors suggests inadequate processing, the item should not be used.[26,41]

XX.g.2. The internal chemical indicator should be reviewed for a proper end point response (eg, color, migration, other change) before placing the items or tray on the sterile field. If the proper end point is not achieved, items or trays should not be placed on the sterile field.

XX.h. Biological monitors should be used routinely to test for sterilizer efficacy, for sterilizer qualification testing (eg, after installation, relocation, malfunction, major repair, sterilization process failure), for routine load release, for implant load release, and for periodic product quality assurance testing for all sterilization processes.[6] *[4: Limited Evidence]*

XX.h.1. **Steam sterilizers:** *Geobacillus stearothermophilus* biological indicators should be used for routine load release, routine sterilizer efficacy monitoring, sterilizer qualification testing, and periodic product quality assurance testing as follows:

- Routine sterilizer efficacy monitoring should be performed weekly, but preferably daily. A process challenge device (PCD) containing a biological indicator should be used to test sterilizer efficacy.
- If a steam sterilizer is intended to be used for multiple types of cycles (eg, gravity-displacement, dynamic air-removal, IUSS), each sterilization cycle type should be tested.
- If one temperature is used but with different exposure times, only the cycle with the shortest exposure time needs to be tested.[6] The shortest time is the most challenging cycle.
- For table-top sterilizers and for sterilizers larger than 2 cubic feet, efficacy testing should be conducted in a fully loaded chamber.
- Efficacy testing of IUSS cycles should be conducted in an empty chamber unless an IUSS container is used.
- The biological monitor should be placed in the most challenging location within the sterilizer chamber and within the IUSS container as indicated by the sterilizer and container manufacturers.
- Each load containing an implantable device should be monitored with a PCD containing a biological indicator and a class 5 indicator and quarantined until the results of the biological indicator testing are available.
- One biological indicator PCD should be run in three consecutive empty cycles for sterilizer qualification testing.
- Qualification testing for sterilizers larger than 2 cubic feet and for IUSS cycles should be conducted in an empty chamber.
- Qualification testing of table-top sterilizers should be conducted in a fully loaded chamber.

XX.h.2. **Dynamic air-removal steam sterilizers:** A Bowie-Dick air-removal test should be performed daily in an empty chamber as follows:

- A Bowie-Dick air-removal test should be performed each day that the sterilizer is used and should be performed before the first load of the day but after a warm-up cycle is run.

TABLE 6. TYPES AND APPLICATIONS FOR USE OF STEAM STERILIZATION MONITORING DEVICES[1]

Monitor	Frequency of use	Application (release of sterilizer, package, load)
Physical monitors		
Time, temperature, and pressure recorders; displays; digital printouts; and gauges	Should be used in every load of every sterilizer	Part of load release criteria
Chemical indicators (CIs)		
External CIs Class 1 (process indicators)	Should be used on the outside of every package unless the internal CI is visible	Part of routine load and package release criteria
Bowie-Dick-type indicators Class 2 (Bowie-Dick)	For routine sterilizer testing (dynamic air-removal sterilizers only), should be run within a test pack each day in an empty sterilizer before the first processed load	Test of sterilizer for efficacy of air removal and steam penetration; part of release criteria for using the sterilizer for the day
	For sterilizer qualification testing (dynamic air-removal sterilizers only), should be run within a test pack after sterilizer installation, relocation, malfunction, major repair or sterilization process failure; test should be run three times consecutively in an empty chamber after biological indicator (BI) tests	Part of release criteria for placing the sterilizer into service after qualification testing
Internal CIs	Should be used inside each package	Part of routine package release criteria at the use site
	Should be used in periodic product quality assurance testing	Part of release criteria for changes made to routinely sterilized items, load configuration, and/or packaging
		Release criteria should include BI results
Class 3 (single-variable indicator) Class 4 (multi-variable indicator)	May be used to meet internal CI recommendation	Part of routine package release criteria at the use site; not to be used for release of loads
Class 5 (integrating indicator)	May be used to meet internal CI recommendation	Part of routine package release criteria at the use site
	Within a process challenge device (PCD), may be used to monitor non-implant sterilizer loads	Part of load release criteria for nonimplant loads
	Within a PCD, should be used to monitor each sterilizer load containing implants; the PCD also should contain a BI	Part of release criteria for loads containing implants
		Except in emergencies, implants should be quarantined until BI results are known

continued on next page

- A warm-up cycle should be run so that Bowie-Dick testing is performed under the conditions in which the sterilizer will be used.
- The test should be run in accordance with the test manufacturer's instructions before the routine biological indicator testing.
- Whenever a dynamic air-removal sterilizer is installed or relocated, malfunctions, undergoes a major repair, or has a sterilization process failure, three consecutive cycles in an empty chamber should be tested with a biological indicator PCD followed by three consecutive cycles in an empty chamber with a Bowie-Dick air-removal test.[6]
- The air-removal test is designed to detect residual air in the sterilizer chamber.

XX.h.3. **Ethylene oxide sterilizers:** *Bacillus atrophaeus* biological indicators should be used to test sterilizer efficacy. Sterilizer efficacy testing should be performed with every load.[26] Qualification testing should be performed after installation, relocation, malfunction, major repair, or sterilization

Monitor	Frequency of use	Application (release of sterilizer, package, load)
TABLE 6 CONTINUED. TYPES AND APPLICATIONS FOR USE OF STEAM STERILIZATION MONITORING DEVICES[1]		
Class 6 (emulating indicator)	May be used to meet internal CI recommendation	Part of routine package release criteria at the use site
	Within a PCD, may be used to monitor sterilizer loads	Part of load release criteria for non-implant loads
		Part of release criteria for loads containing implants
		Implants should be quarantined until BI results are known, except in emergency situations
BIs	Within a PCD, may be used to monitor nonimplant loads	Part of routine load release criteria
	Within a PCD, should be used in every load containing implants; the PCD also should contain a class 5 integrating indicator	Part of release criteria for loads containing implants
		Implants should be quarantined until BI results are known, except in emergency situations
	Within a PCD, should be used for weekly, but preferably daily (ie, each day the sterilizer is used), routine sterilizer efficacy testing; the PCD also may contain a CI	Except in emergencies, implants should be quarantined until BI results are known
	Should be run in a full load for wrapped items; for table-top sterilization, should be run in a fully loaded chamber; for immediate use steam sterilization, should be run in an empty chamber	Part of sterilizer/load release and recall criteria
		Part of routine release criteria for placing the sterilizer into service after qualification testing
	Within a PCD, should be used for sterilizer qualification testing (after sterilizer installation, relocation, malfunction, major repair, sterilization process failure); the PCD also may contain a CI	Part of release criteria for changes made to routinely sterilized items, load configuration, and/or packaging
	Test should be run three times consecutively in an empty chamber, except for table-top sterilizers, for which the test should be run three times consecutively in a full load	
	Should be used for periodic product quality assurance testing	

REFERENCE
1. *Association for the Advancement of Medical Instrumentation. ANSI/AAMI ST79:2010, A1:2010 & A2:2011, Comprehensive guide to steam sterilization and sterility assurance in health care facilities. Arlington, VA: Association for the Advancement of Medical Instrumentation; 2010 & 2011. Adapted and reprinted with permission. Further reproduction or distribution is prohibited.*

process failure. Qualification testing should be performed in accordance with AAMI guidelines[26] and in consultation with the sterilizer manufacturer.

XX.h.4. **Low-temperature hydrogen peroxide gas plasma sterilizers:** *Geobacillus stearothermophilus* biological indicators should be used for routine load release, routine sterilizer efficacy monitoring, sterilizer qualification testing, and periodic product quality assurance testing.[35] Routine sterilizer efficacy monitoring should be performed at least daily on each cycle type, preferably with each load, as follows:

- The sterilizer manufacturer should be consulted for the specific monitoring product to use and the appropriate placement of the product within the sterilizer.
- For each cycle type enabled on low-temperature hydrogen peroxide gas plasma sterilizers (eg, standard, advanced), one

XX.h.5. **Hydrogen peroxide vapor sterilizer:** *Geobacillus stearothermophilus* biological indicators should be used for routine load release, routine sterilizer efficacy monitoring, sterilizer qualification testing, and periodic product quality assurance testing.[35] Routine sterilizer efficacy monitoring should be performed at least daily on each cycle type, preferably with each load, as follows:

- The sterilizer manufacturer should be consulted for the specific monitoring product to use and the appropriate placement of the product within the sterilizer.
- For each cycle offered (eg, lumen, non-lumen), one biological indicator PCD should be run in three consecutive empty cycles for sterilizer qualification testing.[35]

XX.h.6. **Ozone sterilizers:** *Geobacillus stearothermophilus* biological indicators should be used for routine load release, routine sterilizer efficacy monitoring, sterilizer qualification testing, and periodic product quality assurance testing.[35] Routine sterilizer efficacy monitoring should be performed at least daily, preferably with each load, as follows:

- One biological indicator PCD should be run in three consecutive empty cycles for sterilizer qualification testing.
- The sterilizer manufacturer should be consulted for the specific monitoring product(s) to use and the appropriate placement of the product(s) within the sterilizer.[35]

XX.h.7. **Liquid peracetic acid sterilant systems:** A diagnostic cycle to verify the system is operating according to specification should be run every 24 hours according to the manufacturer's instructions for use.[60] Routine efficacy monitoring considerations include the following:

- Biological indicator monitoring is not required for liquid peracetic acid sterilant systems. A microprocessor monitors use dilution, temperature, and sterilant contact time.[47]
- Chemical indicators may be used according to the equipment manufacturer's instructions for use.

XX.h.8. **Dry-heat sterilizers:** *Bacillus atrophaeus* biological indicators should be used for routine load release, routine sterilizer efficacy monitoring, sterilizer qualification testing, and periodic product quality assurance testing. Routine sterilizer efficacy monitoring

should be performed at least weekly, but preferably daily, as follows:

- Each load containing an implantable device should be monitored with a biological indicator and quarantined until the results of the biological indicator testing are available.
- Sterilizer qualification testing biological indicator PCDs should be run in three consecutive empty cycles.
- Mechanical convection (ie, forced-air) dry-heat sterilizers should be monitored according to the manufacturer's recommendations. Additional monitoring of three consecutive sterilization cycles should be performed after sterilizer installation, relocation, malfunction, major repair, or sterilization process failure.
- Testing should be performed in an empty sterilizer.[46]

XX.i. Preventive maintenance on sterilizers should be performed by qualified personnel on a scheduled basis. *[4: Limited Evidence]*

Periodic inspections, maintenance, and replacement of components that are subject to wear (eg, recording devices, steam traps, filters, valves, drain pipes, gaskets) help maintain proper functioning of sterilizers.[6]

XX.i.1. Inspection and cleaning should be performed as outlined in the manufacturer's written instructions.[46]

Proper inspection and cleaning minimizes sterilizer downtime and helps prevent sterilizer malfunctions.

XX.i.2. Preventive maintenance and repairs should be performed by qualified personnel as specified in the manufacturer's written instructions.

XX.i.3. Maintenance records should be kept for each sterilizer. Information noted in the sterilizer maintenance records should include the

- date of service;
- sterilizer model and serial number;
- sterilizer location;
- description of any malfunction;
- name of the person who is performing the maintenance and the name of his or her company;
- description of the type of service and any parts that are replaced;
- results of biological indicator testing, if performed;
- results of Bowie-Dick testing, if performed;
- name of the person requesting the service, where appropriate; and
- signature and title of the person acknowledging the completed work.

Accurate and complete records are required for sterilization process verification.

XX.j. Quality assurance testing of packaging systems including rigid containers is part of a quality assurance program and should be performed before initial use, as well as periodically, according to the manufacturer's written instructions.[6] *[4: Limited Evidence]*

Rigid sterilization container systems vary widely in design, mechanics, and construction. These variables can affect the performance and compatibility of containers with sterilization methods.

XX.j.1. Sterilization efficacy and drying effectiveness should be evaluated when conducting periodic product quality assurance testing of packaging systems, including sterilization containers for each sterilizer used.

Health care organizations are responsible for obtaining and maintaining manufacturers' documentation of methodology and performance testing for packaging systems.

Health care personnel are responsible for ensuring that container systems are suitable for proposed sterilization uses and are compatible with existing sterilizers.

XX.k. Periodic product testing of routinely processed items representing a product family should be performed on a continual basis.[6] *[4: Limited Evidence]*

Criteria that may be used to identify product families include

o design configuration,
o number of components,
o size or surface area,
o materials of construction,
o surface finish or texture,
o mated surfaces,
o presence of cannulations or lumens,
o the need for disassembly, and
o written processing instructions provided by manufacturers.

Product testing is used to verify that the device manufacturer's instructions for sterilization can be achieved in the health care setting.

Information related to product testing is evolving. Users are advised to review current literature for additional information as it becomes available.

XX.k.1. Product testing should be performed when major changes are made, before first use of loaned instruments, before use of newly purchased sets (eg, new specialty), or when there is no preexisting product family. Examples of major changes include

• significant changes in packaging (eg, changing from wrap to containerized systems),
• weight changes, and
• package configuration changes.

XX.k.2. During product testing of sterilization, conditions such as exposure time should be evaluated with physical, biological, and chemical monitors by strategically placing monitors alongside each other at locations that present the greatest challenge to air evacuation and sterilant penetration and contact.

XX.k.3. The container manufacturer should be consulted to determine the areas within the container that present the greatest challenge.

Glossary

Aeration: Method by which absorbed ethylene oxide (EO) is removed from EO-sterilized items by circulating warm air in an enclosed cabinet specifically designed for this purpose.

Anyhdrous: Items that are free of water.

Bioburden: The degree of microbial load; the number of viable organisms contaminating an object.

Biological indicator: A sterilization process-monitoring device commercially prepared with a known population of highly resistant spores that tests the effectiveness of the method of sterilization being used. The indicator is used to demonstrate that conditions necessary to achieve sterilization were met during the sterilizer cycle being monitored.

Bowie-Dick test (Class 2 chemical indicator): A test designed to detect air leaks, ineffective air removal, and presence of noncondensable gasses in dynamic air-removal steam sterilizers. This test is not a test for sterilization efficacy. It is not used in gravity-displacement sterilizers.

Chemical indicator: A sterilization process-monitoring device used to monitor the attainment of one or more critical parameters required for sterilization. A characteristic color or other visual change indicates a defined level of exposure based on the classification of the chemical indicator used.

• *Class 1:* Process indicator that demonstrates that the package has been exposed to the sterilization process to distinguish between processed and unprocessed packages.

• *Class 2 (Bowie-Dick):* Process indicator that is used to detect air leaks, ineffective air removal, and presence of noncondensable gasses. Used in dynamic air-removal sterilizers.

• *Class 3:* Process indicator that reacts to a single parameter of the sterilization process.

• *Class 4:* Process indicator that reacts to two or more of the critical parameters of sterilization.

• *Class 5 (integrating indicator):* Process indicator designed to react to all critical parameters over a specified range of sterilization cycles; performance has been correlated to the performance of the stated test organism under the labeled conditions of use.

• *Class 6 (emulating indicator):* Process indicator designed to react to all of the critical parameters of a specific cycle.

STERILIZATION

Decontamination area: Area designated for collection, retention, and cleaning of soiled and/or contaminated items.

Downtime: A period of time when an item or device is not operational.

Dynamic air removal: Mechanically assisted air removal from the sterilization chamber. Includes prevacuum and steam-flush pressure-pulse steam sterilizers.

Emergency spill plan: A plan of action for any unanticipated release of ethylene oxide or other hazardous chemicals into the workplace.

Gravity displacement: Type of sterilization cycle in which incoming air displaces residual air through a port or drain near the bottom of the sterilizer chamber.

Immediate use steam sterilization (IUSS): Steam sterilization of patient care items intended for immediate use. Formerly known as "flash sterilization."

Physical monitor: Automated devices (eg, printouts, digital readings, graphs, gauges) that monitor sterilization parameters for the sterilization method in use.

Prevacuum: A steam sterilization cycle in which air is removed from the chamber and load via a series of pressure and vacuum excursions.

Process challenge device (PCD): A device designed to represent a defined challenge or resistance to a sterilization process. A commercially prepared PCD may contain a biological indicator, a chemical indicator, or a biological indicator and a chemical indicator. A PCD is used to test the efficacy of the sterilization process.

Qualification testing: Sterilizer testing performed after installation, relocation, malfunction, major repair, or sterilizer process failure to verify that the sterilizer equipment performs within predetermined limits when used in accordance with the manufacturer's instructions for use.

Short-term exposure limits: Durations of exposure to a potentially toxic or harmful substance lasting for less than 15 minutes that cannot be repeated more than four times per day.

Sterilization: Processes by which all microbial life, including pathogenic and nonpathogenic microorganisms and spores, are killed.

Sterilization process monitoring device: A device used to monitor sterilization processes. Sterilization monitoring devices can be biological, chemical, or mechanical.

Terminal sterilization: A process by which the product is sterilized within a sterile barrier that permits storage for use at a later time.

REFERENCES

1. Rutala WA, Weber DJ; Healthcare Infection Control Practices Advisory Committee. *Guideline for Disinfection and Sterilization in Healthcare Facilities*, 2008. Atlanta, GA: Centers for Disease Control and Prevention; 2008. [IVA]

2. Tablan OC, Anderson LJ, Besser R, et al. Guidelines for preventing health-care–associated pneumonia, 2003: recommendations of CDC and the Healthcare Infection Control Practices Advisory Committee. *MMWR Recomm Rep.* 2004;53(RR-3):1-36. [IVA]

3. Standards FAQ details: how should we process and store laryngoscope blades? The Joint Commission.

October 24, 2011. http://www.jointcommission.org/standards_information/jcfaqdetails.aspx?StandardsFAQ ChapterId=69&StandardsFAQId=386. Accessed April 25, 2012.

4. Guideline for Cleaning and Care of Surgical Instruments. In: *Guidelines for Perioperative Practice.* Denver, CO: AORN, Inc; 2015:615-650.

5. Guideline for high-level disinfection. In: *Guidelines for Perioperative Practice.* Denver, CO: AORN, Inc; 2015:601-614.

6. Association for the Advancement of Medical Instrumentation (AAMI). ANSI/AAMI ST79:2010/A2:2011: Comprehensive guide to steam sterilization and sterility assurance in health care facilities. Arlington, VA: AAMI; 2011. [IVC]

7. Enforcement priorities for single-use devices reprocessed by third parties and hospitals. Food and Drug Administration. Center for Devices and Radiological Health. August 14, 2000. http://www.fda.gov/Medical Devices/DeviceRegulationandGuidance/Guidance Documents/ucm107164.htm. Accessed April 26, 2012.

8. Medical devices; reprocessed single-use devices; termination of exemptions from premarket notification; requirement for submission of validation data. *Fed Regist.* 2005;70(188):56911-56925. https://federalregister.gov/a/05-19510. Accessed April 25, 2012.

9. Diab-Elschahawi M, Blacky A, Bachhofner N, Koller W. Challenging the Sterrad 100NX sterilizer with different carrier materials and wrappings under experimental "clean" and "dirty" conditions. *Am J Infect Control.* 2010;38(10):806-810. doi:10.1016/j.ajic.2010.05.023. [IB]

10. Recommended practices for traffic patterns in the perioperative practice setting. In: *Perioperative Standards and Recommended Practices.* Denver, CO: AORN, Inc; 2011:95-98. [IVB]

11. Occupational Safety & Health Administration. US Department of Labor. Toxic and hazardous substances. Appendix A: bloodborne pathogens. 29 CFR §1910.1030. *Fed Regist.* 1991;56(235):64004-64182. Effective December 6, 1991. http://www.osha.gov/pls/oshaweb/owadisp.show_document?p_table=standards&p_id=10051. Accessed April 25, 2012.

12. Siegel JD, Rhinehart E, Jackson M, Chiarello L; Healthcare Infection Control Practices Advisory Committee. *2007 Guideline for Isolation Precautions: Preventing Transmission of Infectious Agents in Healthcare Settings.* Atlanta, GA: Centers for Disease Control and Prevention; 2007. http://www.cdc.gov/hicpac/pdf/isolation/Isolation2007.pdf. Accessed April 25, 2012. [IVA]

13. Lipscomb IP, Sihota AK, Keevil CW. Comparison between visual analysis and microscope assessment of surgical instrument cleanliness from sterile service departments. *J Hosp Infect.* 2008;68(1):52-58. [IIC]

14. DesCoteaux JG, Poulin EC, Julien M, Guidoin R. Residual organic debris on processed surgical instruments. *AORN J.* 1995;62(1):23-30. [IIIC]

15. Guideline for selection and use of packaging systems for sterilization. In: *Guidelines for Perioperative Practice.* Denver, CO: AORN, Inc; 2015:651-664.

16. Association for the Advancement of Medical Instrumentation. ANSI/AAMI/ISO 11607-1:2006/(R)2010: Packaging for terminally sterilized medical devices—Part 1: Requirements for materials, sterile barrier systems, and packaging systems. Arlington, VA: AAMI; 2010. [IVB]

17. Association for the Advancement of Medical Instrumentation (AAMI). ANSI/AAMI ST77:2006/(R)2010: Containment devices for reusable medical device sterilization. Arlington, VA: AAMI; 2010. [IVC]

18. AORN position statement on ergonomically healthy workplace practices. AORN, Inc. http://www.aorn.org/WorkArea/DownloadAsset.aspx?id=21921. Accessed on April 24, 2012. [IVB]

19. AORN guidance statement: safe patient handling and movement in the perioperative setting. In: *Perioperative Standards and Recommended Practices*. Denver, CO: AORN, Inc; 2011:617-638. [IVB]

20. AAMI, Accreditation Association for Ambulatory Health Care, Inc, AORN, et al. Immediate-use steam sterilization statement. http://www.aami.org/publications/standards/ST79_Immediate_Use_Statement.pdf. Accessed April 25, 2012. [IVC]

21. Association for the Advancement of Medical Instrumentation (AAMI). *ANSI/AAMI ST8: Hospital Steam Sterilizers*. Arlington, VA: AAMI; 2008. [IVC]

22. Clement L, Bliley J. Cracking the steam sterilizer door: dispelling the myth. *Healthc Purchasing News*. 2007:40-42. [VC]

23. Mangram AJ, Horan TC, Pearson ML, Silver LC, Jarvis WR. Guideline for prevention of surgical site infection, 1999. Hospital Infection Control Practices Advisory Committee. *Infect Control Hosp Epidemiol*. 1999;20(4):250-78. doi:10.1086/501620. [IVA]

24. Centers for Disease Control and Prevention (CDC). Bronchoscopy-related infections and pseudoinfections— New York, 1996 and 1998. *MMWR Morb Mortal Wkly Rep*. 1999;48(26):557-560. [IVA]

25. Update: The Joint Commission position on steam sterilization. *Jt Comm Perspect*. 2009;29(7):8, 11.

26. Association for the Advancement of Medical Instrumentation (AAMI). ANSI/AAMI ST41: Ethylene oxide sterilization in health care facilities: safety and effectiveness. Arlington, VA: AAMI; 2008. [IVC]

27. Identification and listing of hazardous waste. 40 CFR §261. *Fed Regist*. 2011;76:74709-74717. Effective December 1, 2011. https://federalregister.gov/a/2011-30152. Accessed April 25, 2012.

28. Ozone layer protection – regulatory programs. Phaseout of HCFCs (class II ozone-depleting substances). US Environmental Protection Agency. http://www.epa.gov/ozone/title6/phaseout/classtwo.html. Accessed April 25, 2012.

29. National emission standards for hospital ethylene oxide sterilizers—EPA. Final rule. *Fed Regist*. 2007;63(248):73611-73625.

30. Ethylene oxide. 29 CFR §1910.1047. July 1, 2010. http://www.osha.gov/pls/oshaweb/owastand.display_standard_group?p_toc_level=1&p_part_number=1910. Accessed April 25, 2012.

31. Steris. Envirosystems ethylene oxide sterilant. [VB]

32. Pesticides: reregistration. Ethylene oxide (ETO): hospitals and healthcare facilities must use a single chamber when sterilizing medical equipment with ETO. US Environmental Protection Agency. http://www.epa.gov/oppsrrd1/reregistration/ethylene_oxide/ethylene_oxide_fs.html. Accessed April 25, 2012.

33. Hazard communication in the 21st century workplace. Occupational Safety & Health Administration. http://www.osha.gov/dsg/hazcom/finalmsdsreport.html. Updated March 2004. Accessed April 25, 2012.

34. Ethylene oxide: Evidence of carcinogenicity. Appendix I: Guidelines for minimizing worker exposure to ethylene oxide. http://www.cdc.gov/niosh/81130_35.html#Appendix I ed. 1981.

35. Association for the Advancement of Medical Instrumentation (AAMI). ANSI/AAMI ST58: Chemical sterilization and high-level disinfection in health care facilities. Arlington, VA: AAMI; 2005. [IVC]

36. Joslyn LJ, Block SS. Gaseous chemical sterilization. In: Block SS, ed. *Disinfection, Sterilization, and Preservation*. 5th ed. Philadelphia, PA: Lippincott Williams & Wilkins; 2001:337-359. [IVA]

37. Occupational safety and health guideline for hydrogen peroxide. Occupational Safety & Health Administration. http://www.osha.gov/SLTC/healthguide lines/hydrogenperoxide/recognition.html. Accessed April 25, 2012.

38. *Material Safety Data Sheet MS 52013: Hydrogen Peroxide Cassette*. Irvine, CA: Advanced Sterilization Products; 2008. [VB]

39. *Material Safety Data Sheet MSDS 09461-0-001: Hydrogen Peroxide Solution*. Irvine, CA: Advanced Sterilization Products; 2008.

40. Rutala WA, Weber DJ, Rutala WA. An overview of disinfection and sterilization in health care facilities. In: Rutala WA, ed. *Disinfection, Sterilization, and Antisepsis: Principles, Practices, Current Issues, and New Research*. Washington, DC: Association for Professionals in Infection Control and Epidemiology; 2007:12-48. [IVA]

41. ANSI/AAMI/ISO 15882: Chemical indicators— guidance for selection, use, and interpretation of results. Arlington, VA: Association for the Advancement of Medical Instrumentation; 2008. [IVC]

42. *510(k) Summary for Amsco V-PROTM 1 Low Temperature Sterilization System*. STERIS Corp. Aug. 4, 2006. http://www.accessdata.fda.gov/cdrh_docs/pdf6/K062297.pdf. Accessed April 24, 2012.

43. TSO3 125L Ozone Sterilizer 510(k) summary. TSO3 Inc. March 15, 2002. http://www.accessdata.fda.gov/cdrh_docs/pdf2/K020875.pdf. Accessed April 24, 2012.

44. Weavers LK, Wickramanayake GB, Block SS. Disinfection and sterilization using ozone. In: Block SS, ed. *Disinfection, Sterilization, and Preservation*. 5th ed. Philadelphia, PA: Lippincott Williams & Wilkins; 2001:205-214. [IVA]

45. Joslyn LJ, Block SS. Sterilization by heat. In: Block SS, ed. *Disinfection, Sterilization, and Preservation*. 5th ed. Philadelphia, PA: Lippincott Williams & Wilkins; 2001:695-728. [IVA]

46. ANSI/AAMI ST40: Table-top dry heat (heated air) sterilization and sterility assurance in health care facilities. Arlington, VA: Association for the Advancement of Medical Instrumentation; 2004. [IVC]

47. *Revised 510(k) Summary for SYSTEM 1E Liquid Chemical Sterilant Processing System*. Mentor, OH: STERIS Corp; 2010. [VB]

48. STERIS System 1E (SS1E) liquid chemical sterilant - K090036. US Food and Drug Administration. http://www.fda.gov/MedicalDevices/ProductsandMedicalProcedures/DeviceApprovalsandClearances/Recently-ApprovedDevices/ucm207489.htm. Updated June 30, 2011. Accessed April 25, 2012.

49. Malchesky PS, Block SS. Medical applications of peracetic acid. In: Block SS, ed. *Disinfection, Sterilization, and Preservation*. 5th ed. Philadelphia, PA: Lippincott Williams & Wilkins; 2001:979-996. [IVA]

50. Petersen BT, Chennat J, Cohen J, et al. Multisociety guideline on reprocessing flexible GI endoscopes: 2011. *Infect Control Hosp Epidemiol*. 2011;32(6):527-537. doi:10.1086/660676. [IVB]

51. Winthrop TG, Sion BA, Gaines C. Loaner instrumentation: processing the unknown. *AORN J*. 2007;85(3):566-573. doi:10.1016/S0001-2092(07)60128-8.

52. ASHCSP/IAHCSMM Position Paper on Loaner Instrumentation. http://www.iahcsmm.org/pdfs/ASHCSP-IAHCSMMLoanerPaper.pdf. [IVC]

53. Villarrubia A, Palacin E, Gomez del Rio M, Martinez P. Description, etiology, and prevention of an outbreak of diffuse lamellar keratitis after LASIK. *J Refract Surg.* 2007;23(5):482-486. [IIIC]

54. Butt WE, Bradley DV Jr, Mayhew RB, Schwartz RS. Evaluation of the shelf life of sterile instrument packs. *Oral Surg Oral Med Oral Pathol.* 1991;72(6):650-654. [IA]

55. Webster J, Lloyd W, Ho P, Burridge C, George N. Rethinking sterilization practices: evidence for event-related outdating. *Infect Control Hosp Epidemiol.* 2003;24(8):622-624. doi:10.1086/502264. [IIB]

56. *ASHRAE/ASHE Standard: Ventilation of Health Care Facilities.* Atlanta, GA: American Society of Heating, Refrigerating, and Air-Conditioning Engineers; 2008. [IVB]

57. Guideline for environmental cleaning. In: *Guidelines for Perioperative Practice.* Denver, CO: AORN, Inc; 2015:9-30.

58. Standard pendent and upright spray sprinklers. In: *NFPA 13: Standard for the Installation of Sprinkler Systems.* 2010 ed. Quincy, MA: National Fire Protection Association; 2010: 51-58. [IVA]

59. Guideline for product selection. In: *Guidelines for Perioperative Practice.* Denver, CO: AORN, Inc; 2015: 179-186.

60. Medical device reporting: manufacturer reporting, importer reporting, user facility reporting, distributor reporting. 65(17) *Fed Regist.* (January 26, 2000) 4112-4121 (codified at 21 CFR §803-804).

Acknowledgments

LEAD AUTHOR
Cynthia Spry, MA, MS, RN, CNOR, CSIT
Independent Consultant
New York, New York

CONTRIBUTING AUTHOR
Ramona Conner, MSN, RN, CNOR
Manager, Standards and Guidelines
AORN Nursing Department
Denver, Colorado

The authors and AORN thank Paula Berrett, BS, CRCST, Intermountain Healthcare Urban South Region CP Manager, Utah Valley Regional Medical Center, Provo, Utah; Patricia A. Graybill-D'Ercole, MSN, RN, CNOR, CRCST, CHL, Consultant, Soyring Consulting, York, Pennsylvania; James X. Stobinski, PhD, RN, CNOR, Director of Education and Credentialing, Competency and Credentialing Institute, Denver, Colorado; and Julia A. Thompson, PhD, RN, APRN, CNOR, Administrative Director, Harris County Hospital District, Houston, Texas, for their assistance in developing this guideline.

PUBLICATION HISTORY
Originally published August 1980, *AORN Journal.* Format revision July 1982.

Revised February 1987, October 1992. Published as proposed recommended practices in July 1994.

Revised; published August 1999, *AORN Journal.* Reformatted July 2000.

Revised November 2005; published March 2006, *AORN Journal.*

Revised 2007; published in *Perioperative Standards and Recommended Practices*, 2008 edition.

Minor editing revisions made in November 2010 for publication in *Perioperative Standards and Recommended Practices*, 2011 edition.

Revised June 2012 for online publication in *Perioperative Standards and Recommended Practices.*

Reformatted September 2012 for publication in *Perioperative Standards and Recommended Practices*, 2013 edition.

Evidence ratings revised 2013 to conform to the AORN Evidence Rating Model.

Minor editing revisions made in November 2014 for publication in *Guidelines for Perioperative Practice*, 2015 edition.

Evidence ratings revised in *Guidelines for Perioperative Practice*, 2018 edition, to conform to the current AORN Evidence Rating Model.

APPENDICES

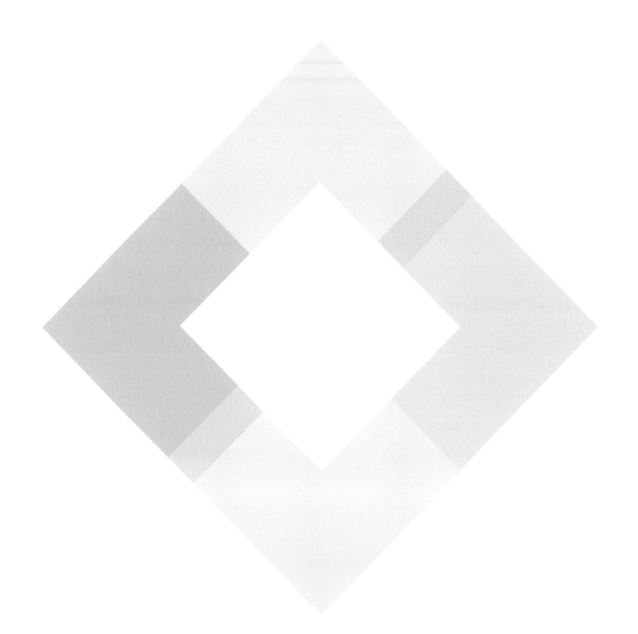

AORN Evidence Rating Model

EVIDENCE RATING	EVIDENCE LEVEL		TYPE OF EVIDENCE	QUALITY LEVEL		
	Research	Non-Research		High	Good	Low
1 REGULATORY	NA	NA	FEDERAL, STATE, OR LOCAL REGULATORY REQUIREMENT	NA	NA	NA
1 STRONG	I		SYSTEMATIC REVIEW-All studies RCTs RANDOMIZED CONTROLLED TRIAL (RCT)	A		
		IV	CLINICAL PRACTICE GUIDELINE CONSENSUS or POSITION STATEMENT	A		
2 HIGH	I		SYSTEMATIC REVIEW-All studies RCTs RCT		B	
	II		SYSTEMATIC REVIEW- All studies Quasi-Experimental or a combination of RCTs and Quasi-Experimental QUASI-EXPERIMENTAL	A		
	III		SYSTEMATIC REVIEW- All studies Non-Experimental or a combination of RCTs, Quasi-Experimental, and Non-Experimental. Any or all studies Qualitative NON-EXPERIMENTAL QUALITATIVE	A		
		IV	CLINICAL PRACTICE GUIDELINE CONSENSUS or POSITION STATEMENT		B	
3 MODERATE	II		SYSTEMATIC REVIEW- All studies Quasi-Experimental or a combination of RCTs and Quasi-Experimental QUASI-EXPERIMENTAL		B	
	III		SYSTEMATIC REVIEW- All studies Non-Experimental or a combination of RCTs, Quasi-Experimental, and Non-Experimental. Any or all studies Qualitative NON-EXPERIMENTAL QUALITATIVE		B	
		V	LITERATURE REVIEW CASE REPORT EXPERT OPINION ORGANIZATIONAL EXPERIENCE	A	B	
4 LIMITED	I		SYSTEMATIC REVIEW-All studies RCTs RCT			C
	II		SYSTEMATIC REVIEW- All studies Quasi-Experimental or a combination of RCTs and Quasi-Experimental QUASI-EXPERIMENTAL			C
	III		SYSTEMATIC REVIEW- All studies Non-Experimental or a combination of RCTs, Quasi-Experimental, and Non-Experimental. Any or all studies Qualitative NON-EXPERIMENTAL QUALITATIVE			C
		IV	CLINICAL PRACTICE GUIDELINE CONSENSUS or POSITION STATEMENT			C
		V	LITERATURE REVIEW CASE REPORT EXPERT OPINION ORGANIZATIONAL EXPERIENCE			C
5 BENEFITS BALANCED WITH HARMS	NA	NA	NO REQUIREMENT-Benefits outweigh potential harms	NA	NA	NA

AORN RESEARCH EVIDENCE APPRAISAL TOOL - STUDY

DATE_____

REVIEWER_____

APPRAISAL SCORE _____

RW#	CITATION

Does this evidence address the perioperative practice question?
☐ Yes ☐ No - Do not proceed with evidence appraisal.

Does this evidence have a major flaw?
☐ No ☐ Yes - Determine level of evidence and score quality as C.
Provide explanation of flaw in comments.

LEVEL OF EVIDENCE

Is this a report of a single research study?
☐ Yes ☐ No (If No, go to the AORN Research Evidence Appraisal Tool - Summary)

INTERVENTION/MANIPULATION The researcher performed an intervention with at least some of the participants (ie, there was some type of treatment being tested).	☐ Yes	☐ No
CONTROL/COMPARISON GROUP The researcher provided standard care or a comparison intervention that was different from the experimental intervention.	☐ Yes	☐ No
RANDOM ASSIGNMENT The researcher assigned participants to a control or treatment group on a random basis (ie, in a manner determined by chance).	☐ Yes	☐ No

YES to Intervention/Manipulation, Control/Comparison Group, and Random Assignment	☐ LEVEL I	Randomized Controlled Trial (RCT)
YES to Intervention/Manipulation or YES to Intervention/Manipulation, and Control/Comparison Group	☐ LEVEL II	Quasi-Experimental (eg, controlled trial, controlled trial without randomization, pre-test/post-test, time series)
NO to Intervention/Manipulation	☐ LEVEL III	Non-Experimental (eg, descriptive, comparative, observational, correlational, case-control, retrospective, cross-sectional)
	☐ LEVEL III	Qualitative (eg, interviews, surveys, focus groups)

ADDITIONAL COMMENTS:

QUALITY OF EVIDENCE	A HIGH	B GOOD	C LOW	NA
PURPOSE/BACKGROUND				
• Was the purpose of the study clearly defined?				■
• Were the research questions clear?				■
• Did the researcher(s) identify what is known and not known about the research questions and how the study would address any gaps in knowledge?				■
• Was the study approved by an institutional review board (IRB)?				
• Were the supporting references the most current available?				■
• Were the supporting references relevant to the research question?				■
RANDOMIZATION				
• Were the subjects randomly assigned to the Intervention and Control groups?				
• Were the subjects and providers blinded to the study group?		■		
CONTROL				
• Was the Control group clearly identified?				
• Was the Control group representative of the sample population?				
• Were the characteristics and/or demographics similar in both the Control and Intervention groups?				
• Were all groups treated equally, except for the Intervention group?				
• Were multiple settings used?				
• If multiple settings were used, were the settings similar?				
INTERVENTION(S)				
• Did the intervention support the research question?				
• Did the intervention(s) for each group contain sufficient details to allow replication?				
SAMPLE SIZE				
• Was an adequate description of sample size determination provided?				
• Was a power analysis performed?		■		
• If no power analysis was performed, did the sample size ensure confidence that the effect of the intervention was demonstrated?	■			
• Was the inclusion/exclusion criteria for the study participants clear?				
• Were all study participants accounted for?				
DATA COLLECTION				
• Was the data collection process clearly described?				■
• Were the methods of statistical analysis clearly described?				
• Was there a discussion of the instrument's validity?				
• Was the precision of each outcome supported with a measurement (eg, confidence interval) to show statistical significance, or lack thereof?				■
• If surveys/questionnaires were used, was the response rate > 25%?				
RESULTS/CONCLUSIONS				
• If tables were presented, was the narrative consistent with the table content?				
• Were the outcomes of the study clearly explained?				■
• Were the conclusions of the researcher(s) consistent with the results of the study?				■
LIMITATIONS/FUTURE RESEARCH				
• Was the discussion of the limitations of the evidence accurate?				■
BIAS				
• Did the researcher(s) implement methods to reduce distortion of the results of the study (eg, blinding)?				■
• Has the effect of the intervention been over- or underestimated by the researcher(s)?				■
VALIDITY				
• Were threats to validity controlled by the study design?				■
GENERALIZABILITY				
• Are the results of the study transferrable or applicable to other settings or populations?				■
FINAL QUALITY SCORE				

AORN RESEARCH EVIDENCE APPRAISAL TOOL - SUMMARY

DATE_____
REVIEWER_____
APPRAISAL SCORE _____

RW#	CITATION

Does this evidence address the perioperative practice question?
☐ Yes ☐ No - Do not proceed with evidence appraisal.

Does this evidence have a major flaw?
☐ No ☐ Yes - Determine level of evidence and score quality as C.
Provide explanation of flaw in comments.

LEVEL OF EVIDENCE

Summary of multiple research studies? ☐ Yes ☐ No (If No, go to the AORN Research Evidence Appraisal Tool - Study)

Comprehensive search strategy and rigorous appraisal?
☐ Yes (Systematic Review) ☐ No (If No, go to the AORN Non-Research Appraisal Tool)

Results from studies combined and analyzed to generate new statistic or effect size (measure of strength of relationship between two variables)	☐ Yes – Systematic Review with Meta-Analysis ☐ No
Concepts from Qualitative studies analyzed and synthesized	☐ Yes – Systematic Review with Meta-Synthesis ☐ No
All studies are randomized controlled trials (RCTs)	☐ LEVEL I
All studies are Quasi-Experimental or a combination of RCTs and Quasi-Experimental	☐ LEVEL II
All studies are Non-Experimental or a combination of RCTs, Quasi-Experimental, and Non-Experimental	☐ LEVEL III
Any or all studies are Qualitative	☐ LEVEL III

ADDITIONAL COMMENTS:

QUALITY OF EVIDENCE	A HIGH	B GOOD	C LOW	NA
PURPOSE/BACKGROUND				
• Was the purpose of the systematic review clearly defined?				▓
• Was the research question clear?				▓
• Did the researcher(s) identify what is known and not known about the research question and how the systematic review would address any gaps in knowledge?				▓
SEARCH				
• Was the search strategy reproducible?				▓
• Were the key search terms stated?				▓
• Were multiple databases searched and identified?				▓
• Was the inclusion/exclusion criteria described?				▓
• Was both published and unpublished literature identified and retrieved where possible?				▓
• Are the types of studies to be included in the review described?				▓
EVIDENCE REVIEW				
• Was there an explanation of the number of studies eliminated at each level of review?				▓
• Were the details of the included studies presented (design, sample, methods, results, outcomes, strengths, limitations)?				▓
• Were methods for appraising the strength of evidence (level and quality) rigorous?				▓
• Was the evidence reviewed and appraised by at least two members of the research team?				▓
• Were the supporting references the most current available?				▓
• Were the supporting references relevant to the research question?				▓
DATA COLLECTION				
• Were methods of statistical analysis described?				
• Were methods of retrieving data from the individual studies described?				
• Was the data extracted by at least two members of the research team?				
RESULTS/CONCLUSIONS				
• Were the conclusions of the researcher(s) consistent with the results of the studies and the overall strength of the evidence?				▓
• Was the strength of the phenomenon being studied quantified in a summary statistic (ie, effect size) that can be compared across the studies?		▓	▓	
LIMITATIONS/FUTURE RESEARCH				
• Were limitations of the review discussed?				▓
FINAL QUALITY SCORE				

| AORN | AORN NON-RESEARCH EVIDENCE APPRAISAL TOOL | DATE_____ REVIEWER_____ APPRAISAL SCORE _____ |

RW#	CITATION

Does this evidence address the perioperative practice question?
☐ Yes ☐ No - Do not proceed with evidence appraisal.

LEVEL OF EVIDENCE

Systematically developed recommendations from recognized experts based on evidence or consensus opinion that guides members of a professional organization in decision-making related to practice or a particular issue of concern	☐ LEVEL IV	Clinical Practice Guideline Consensus or Position Statement
Summary of published literature on a topic of interest without a systematic appraisal of the strength and quality of the evidence	☐ LEVEL V	Literature Review
In-depth analysis of an individual, group, social unit, issue, or event	☐ LEVEL V	Case Report
Advice from an individual(s) with knowledge and expertise on a particular topic or issue	☐ LEVEL V	Expert Opinion
Initiative with a goal to improve the processes or outcome of care being delivered within a particular institution	☐ LEVEL V	Organizational Experience

ADDITIONAL COMMENTS:

QUALITY OF EVIDENCE	A HIGH	B GOOD	C LOW	NA
CLINICAL PRACTICE GUIDELINE/POSITION STATEMENT				
• Was the purpose of the guideline or position statement clearly stated?				
• Was the guideline or position statement developed, reviewed, or revised within the past five years?				
• Were stakeholders involved in the development of the guideline or position statement representative of the specialty?				
• Were the groups to which the recommendations apply and do not apply clearly defined?				
• Was the strategy for developing the guideline or position statement rigorous?				
• Was there a reproducible literature search or other systematic method used to search for evidence?				
• Was a rating scheme or grading method used to determine the quality and strength of the evidence included in the guideline or position statement?				
• Was there an objective description of the type of studies or the consensus process used to support the recommendations?				
• Were the recommendations of the author(s) unbiased and consistent with the literature reviewed?				
• Were the strengths and limitations of the body of evidence clearly described?				
• Were the supporting references the most current available?				
• Were the supporting references relevant to the recommendations?				
• Was the guideline or position statement subjected to a peer review process?				
LITERATURE REVIEW				
• Was the purpose of the literature review clearly stated?				
• Did the author(s) identify what is known and not known about the practice question and how the literature review will address any gaps in knowledge?				
• Were the supporting references the most current available?				
• Were the supporting references relevant to the subject being reviewed?				
• Did the author(s) provide a meaningful analysis and synthesis of the literature reviewed?				
• Were conclusions of the author(s) unbiased and consistent with the literature reviewed?				
• Were the findings of the literature review accurately summarized in tables or figures?				
• Were recommendations made for future practice or study?				
CASE REPORT				
• Was the purpose of the case report clearly stated?				
• Was the case report clearly presented?				
• Were the findings of the case report evidence-based?				
• Was follow-up sufficiently long and complete?				
• Was there a literature review?				
• Did the author(s) provide recommendations for practice?				
• Were the recommendations for practice clearly stated and linked to the findings of the case report?				
EXPERT OPINION				
• Has the individual published or presented on the topic?				
• Was the individual opinion evidence-based?				
• Was the individual opinion clearly stated?				
• Was the individual opinion unbiased and consistent with the evidence?				
ORGANIZATIONAL EXPERIENCE				
• Was the aim of the organizational project clearly stated and focused on assessing and improving current practice?				
• Was the methodology of the project adequately described?				
• Were process or outcome measures for the organizational project identified?				
• Were the results of the organizational project adequately described?				
• Were components of cost/benefit analysis described?				
• Were multiple sites involved?				
FINAL QUALITY SCORE				

GUIDE TO AORN EVIDENCE-RATED GUIDELINES

Evidence rating is a process by which research and non-research evidence is used to support recommendations about clinical decisions. The AORN guidelines provide a rigorous and comprehensive appraisal of the available evidence and link evidence-based recommendations to daily practice.

Recommendation Number:
Each recommendation is identified with a bold font and a Roman numeral.

Recommendation:
Recommendations are broad statements representing what is believed to be optimal and achievable perioperative nursing practice.

Rationale:
Each recommendation statement is followed by a rationale that explains and supports the recommendation.

Activity Number:
Activities are noted by the recommendation Roman numeral and the intervention letter followed by an Arabic numeral.

Activity:
Activity statements describe actions that guide implementation of the intervention.

Recommendation IV

Sterile drapes should be used to establish a sterile field.

Sterile drapes provide a barrier that minimizes the passage of microorganisms from unsterile to sterile areas and reduces the risk of health care-associated infections.[1]

IV.a.   Perioperative team members should place sterile drapes on the patient, furniture, and equipment in the sterile field and should handle them in a manner that prevents contamination.[1] *[1: Strong Evidence]*

In a randomized controlled trial comparing the use of maximal sterile barrier precautions (ie, sterile gown, sterile gloves, surgical cap, full body drape) with the use of only sterile gloves and a small drape during CVC insertion, results showed that maximal sterile barrier precautions led to fewer episodes of catheter colonization and catheter-related bloodstream infections.[61] One program that included using maximal sterile barriers during CVC insertion in 103 intensive care units in Michigan resulted in a 66% decrease in infection rates.[62]

The CDC recommends maximum sterile barrier precautions, including the use of a full body drape, during the placement of CVCs, PICCs, and guidewire exchanges.[8,9]

IV.a.1.   Unsterile equipment (eg, Mayo stands) should be covered on the top, bottom, and sides with sterile barrier materials before being introduced to or brought over a sterile field. Sterile barrier material also should be applied to the portion of the equipment that will be positioned immediately adjacent to the sterile field.

References

1. Mangram AJ, Horan TC, Pearson ML, Silver LC, Jarvis WR; Centers for Disease Control and Prevention (CDC) Hospital Infection Control Practices Advisory Committee. Guideline for prevention of surgical site infection, 1999. *Am J Infect Control.* 1999;27(2):97-132. [IVA]

8. Weber DJ, Rutala WA. Central line-associated bloodstream infections: prevention and management. *Infect Dis Clin North Am.* 2011;25(1):77-102. [IVB]

9. O'Grady NP, Alexander M, Burns LA, et al; Healthcare Infection Control Practices Advisory Committee (HICPAC). *Guidelines for the Prevention of Intravascular Catheter-Related Infections, 2011.* Atlanta, GA: Centers for Disease Control and Prevention; 2011. [IVA]

61. Raad II, Hohn DC, Gilbreath BJ, et al. Prevention of central venous catheter-related infections by using maximal sterile barrier precautions during insertion. *Infect Control Hosp Epidemiol.* 1994;15(4 Pt 1):231-238. [IA]

62. Pronovost P, Needham D, Berenholtz S, et al. An intervention to decrease catheter-related bloodstream infections in the ICU. *N Engl J Med.* 2006;355(26):2725-2732. doi:10.1056/NEJMoa061115. [IIIB]

Intervention Letter:
Interventions are noted by the recommendation Roman numeral followed by a letter.

Intervention:
Interventions are specific practices that guide implementation of the recommendation.

Supporting Evidence:
The intervention statement is followed by a rationale that explains and describes the evidence that supports the intervention.

Evidence Rating:
Using the AORN Evidence Rating Model, the appraisal scores are combined to determine the collective evidence rating for each intervention. The model considers the quality and quantity of the collective evidence. The rating levels are

1: Strong Evidence
1: Regulatory Requirement
2: High Evidence
3: Moderate Evidence
4: Limited Evidence
5: Benefits Balanced with Harms

Evidence Appraisal:
The supporting references are critically appraised and scored according to the strength and quality of the evidence using the AORN Evidence Appraisal Tools. Strength is designated I, II, or III (research) or IV or V (non-research). Quality is designated A (high), B (good), or C (low), for a combined numeral and letter score.

GUIDE TO AMBULATORY SUPPLEMENTS TO THE AORN GUIDELINES

Ambulatory Supplements are provided for five guideline documents.
The Supplements outline additional considerations for perioperative registered nurses practicing in free-standing
ambulatory surgery centers or physician office-based surgery centers.

The *Amb* symbol in the text of a guideline indicates that there is additional information in an Ambulatory Supplement at the end of the document.

TRANSMISSIBLE INFECTIONS

Recommendation XI

Documentation should reflect activities related to infection prevention. *Amb*

Documentation is a professional medicolegal standard.[167] Documentation related to infection prevention is applicable at the systems level and the patient care level. At...
basis fo...
mance, ...
exposur...
mentatio...
clear co...
between ...

XI.a. E...
r...
T...
o...
o...

[1...

XI.b. A...
o...
d...
o...
o...

• an explanation of how the incident occurred.
Some health care employers may be exempt from maintaining a sharps injury log. The requirement to establish and maintain a sharps injury log applies to any employer who is required to maintain a log of occupational injuries and illnesses under

PATIENT AN...

AMBULATORY SUPPLEMENT: TRANSMISSIBLE INFECTIONS

Ambulatory Surgery

Recommendation III

Droplet precautions should be used throughout the perioperative environment (ie, preoperative, intraoperative, postoperative) when providing care to patients who are known or suspected to be infected with microorganisms that can be transmitted by large droplets.[A1]

Amb The facility should screen individuals for infectious agents (eg, influenza, pertussis) transmitted by droplets.[A1] Identification of infected individuals before their admission to the ambulatory surgery center (ASC) may prevent infection transmission.[A1]

Recommendation IV

Airborne precautions should be used when providing care to patients who are known or suspected to be infected with microorganisms that can be transmitted by the airborne route.

IV.h. Elective surgery should be postponed for patients who have suspected or confirmed [tuberculosis] TB until the patient is determined to be noninfectious. If surgery cannot be postponed, perioperative personnel should follow airborne precautions and consult with an infection preventionist.
Amb Personnel in an ASC that provides care to patients with confirmed or suspected TB should follow recommendation IV.
Amb Unless the facility has the capability of establishing a negative pressure room, patients with suspected or confirmed cases of TB should be transferred to or re-scheduled at a facility with a negative pressure room. A negative pressure airborne infection isolation room and a respiratory protection program are needed for airborne infection isolation. Airborne infection isolation is needed for any patient with suspected or confirmed active pulmonary TB.[A1-A3]

Recommendation X

Perioperative personnel should receive initial and ongoing education and competency validation of their understanding of the principles of infection prevention and the performance of standard, contact, droplet, and airborne precautions for prevention of transmissible infections and [multidrug-resistant organisms] MDROs.

PATIENT AND WORKER SAFETY

Amb An ASC that is certified by the Cent... care & Medicaid Services (CMS) mus... staff member trained in infection preven... the facility's infection prevention progra...

Interpretive Guidelines: §416.51(b)(1)
The ASC must designate in writing... fied licensed health care professional... lead the facility's infection control program. The ASC must determine that the individual has had training in the principles and methods of infection control.

Interpretative Guidelines: §416.51(b)(1). In: Centers for Medicare & Medicaid Services. *State Operations Manual Appendix A— Survey Protocol, Regulations and Interpretive Guidelines for Hospitals.* Rev. 89; 2013.

Amb Ambulatory surgery center personnel, including
• medical personnel,
• nursing personnel,
• personnel responsible for on-site sterilization/high-level disinfection processes, and
• environmental services personnel
should receive infection prevention educ...
Amb Infection prevention education... conducted
• upon hire,
• annually, and
• periodically as needed.[A5]

Recommendation XI

Documentation should reflect activities related to infection prevention.

Amb A CMS-certified facility's infection prevention program must document the process of consideration, selection, and implementation of a nationally recognized infection control guideline,[A4] such as the AORN *Perioperative Standards and Re... Practices.*[A6]
Amb Supporting documentation for the... infection tracking and surveillan... should be maintained.[A5]
Amb Infection prevention education record... maintained for all personnel.[A7]

Recommendation XII

Policies and procedures for the prevention and control of transmissible infections and MDROs should be developed, reviewed periodically, revised as necessary, and readily available within the practice setting.

532

Where applicable, the Ambulatory Supplements include text from the Centers for Medicare & Medicaid Services *State Operations Manual.* This text appears within purple brackets.

Relevant text from the guideline is repeated in the Supplement for easy reference and to give context to the ambulatory considerations.

The *Amb* symbol in the Supplement indicates information specific to ambulatory settings.

INDEX

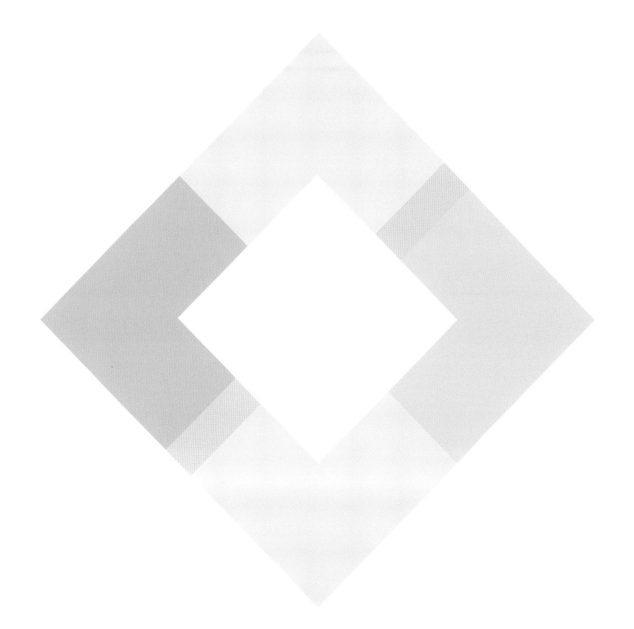

INDEX TO THE 2018 EDITION

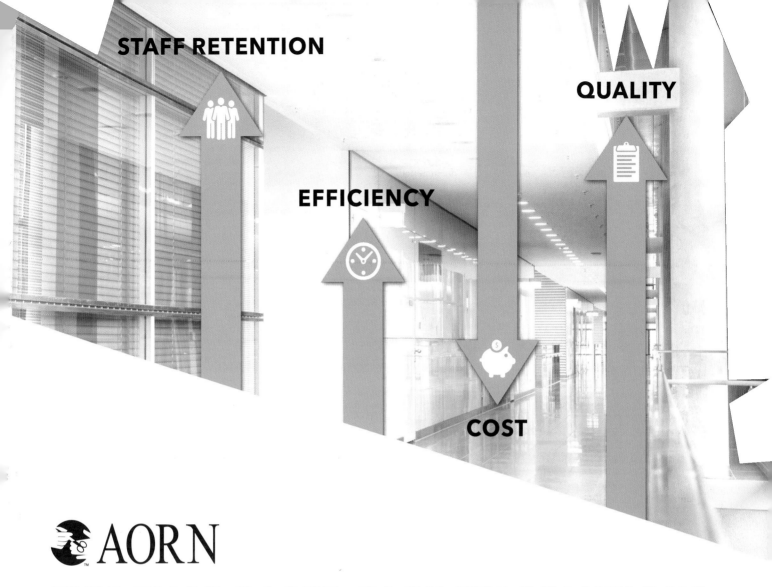

STAFF RETENTION

QUALITY

EFFICIENCY

COST

AORN

EVIDENCE-BASED FACILITY SOLUTIONS

REGULATORY READINESS | SAFE PATIENT OUTCOMES | STANDARDIZED EDUCATION

- *Guidelines for Perioperative Practice*
- Periop 101: A Core Curriculum™
- Periop Mastery Program
- Syntegrity® Perioperative Documentation Solution
- Group Membership
- AORN Career Center

Optimize your business operations. Develop and retain your perioperative team with standardized evidence-based perioperative guidelines.

Learn More at: www.aorn.org/facilitysolutions

MEMBERSHIP BENEFITS YOU WANT
FROM THE PERIOPERATIVE NAME YOU TRUST.

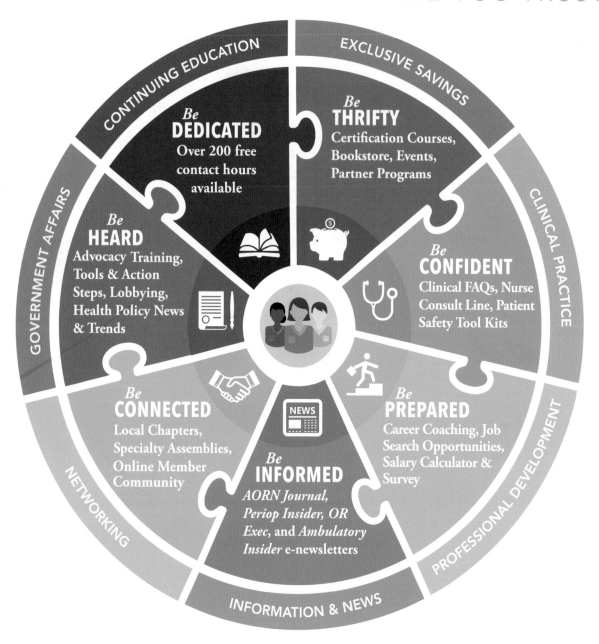

CONTINUING EDUCATION

Be DEDICATED
Over 200 free contact hours available

EXCLUSIVE SAVINGS

Be THRIFTY
Certification Courses, Bookstore, Events, Partner Programs

GOVERNMENT AFFAIRS

Be HEARD
Advocacy Training, Tools & Action Steps, Lobbying, Health Policy News & Trends

CLINICAL PRACTICE

Be CONFIDENT
Clinical FAQs, Nurse Consult Line, Patient Safety Tool Kits

Be CONNECTED
Local Chapters, Specialty Assemblies, Online Member Community

Be INFORMED
AORN Journal, Periop Insider, OR Exec, and *Ambulatory Insider* e-newsletters

Be PREPARED
Career Coaching, Job Search Opportunities, Salary Calculator & Survey

NETWORKING

INFORMATION & NEWS

PROFESSIONAL DEVELOPMENT

PLUS, DON'T MISS OUR NEWEST MEMBER BENEFITS:

Guideline *Essentials*: Implement the Guidelines more effectively with these easy-to-use online resources.

Career coaching: Receive professional guidance and inspiration with a free 90-minute session.

Podcasts: Listen to the *AORN Journal* with monthly summary and full-article podcasts.

Journal *Essentials*: Access on-the-go reading with this digital feature of the *AORN Journal*.

www.aorn.org/renew

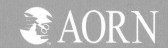